Brief Contents

9th Edition

Clinical Nursing Skills & Techniques

Anne Griffin Perry, RN, MSN, EdD, FAAN
Professor Emerita
School of Nursing
Southern Illinois University—Edwardsville
Edwardsville, Illinois

Patricia A. Potter, RN, MSN, PhD, FAAN
Director of Research
Patient Care Services
Barnes-Jewish Hospital
St. Louis, Missouri

Wendy R. Ostendorf, RN, MS, EdD, CNE
Professor of Nursing
Neumann University
Aston, Pennsylvania

SECTION EDITOR
Nancy Laplante, PhD, RN, AHN-BC
Associate Professor of Nursing
School of Nursing
Widener University
Chester, Pennsylvania

ELSEVIER

ELSEVIER

3251 Riverport Lane
St. Louis, Missouri 63043

Executive Content Strategist: Tamara Myers
Content Development Manager: Jean Sims Fornango/Lisa Newton
Content Development Specialist: Melissa Rawe
Publishing Services Manager: Jeff Patterson
Senior Project Manager: Jodi M. Willard
Design Direction: Brian Salisbury

Printed in the United States of America

Last digit is the print number: 9 8 7 6 5 4 3 2 1

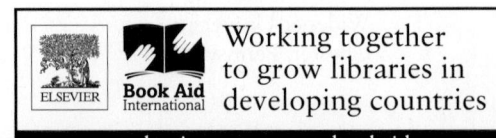

About the Authors

ANNE GRIFFIN PERRY, RN, MSN, EdD, FAAN

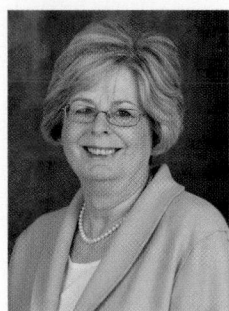

Dr. Anne G. Perry, Professor Emerita at Southern Illinois University—Edwardsville, is a Fellow in the American Academy of Nursing. She received her BSN from the University of Michigan, her MSN from Saint Louis University, and her EdD from Southern Illinois University—Edwardsville. Dr. Perry is a prolific and influential author and speaker. An author for more than 35 years, her work includes four major textbooks (*Essentials for Nursing Practice*, *Fundamentals of Nursing*, *Nursing Interventions & Clinical Skills*, and *Clinical Nursing Skills & Techniques*) and numerous journal articles, abstracts, and nursing research and education grants. She has presented numerous papers at conferences across the United States and internationally. She was one of a few key consultants on *Mosby's Nursing Video Skills* and *Mosby's Nursing Skills Online*.

Dr. Perry is passionate about nursing education and has been involved in education since 1973, first as an instructor and then achieving the rank of Professor and assuming various leadership roles at Saint Louis University School of Nursing. She was a Professor and Associate Dean and Interim Dean at Southern Illinois University—Edwardsville. As a clinician and researcher, Dr. Perry's contributions to pulmonary nursing and nursing language development involve both research and policy making. She has investigated and published findings regarding topics that include weaning from mechanical ventilation, use of the therapeutic intervention scoring system, critical care, and validation of nursing diagnoses.

PATRICIA A. POTTER, RN, MSN, PhD, FAAN

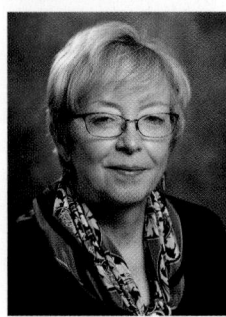

Dr. Patricia Potter received her BSN at the University of Washington in Seattle and her MSN and PhD at Saint Louis University in St. Louis, Missouri. A groundbreaking author for more than 30 years, her work includes four major textbooks (*Essentials for Nursing Practice*, *Fundamentals of Nursing*, *Nursing Interventions & Clinical Skills*, and *Clinical Nursing Skills & Techniques*) and publications in numerous professional journals. She has been an unceasing advocate of evidence-based practice and quality improvement in her roles as administrator, educator and, more recently, director of research.

Dr. Potter has devoted a lifetime to nursing education, practice, and research. She spent a decade teaching at Barnes Hospital School of Nursing and Saint Louis University. She entered into a variety of managerial and administrative roles, ultimately becoming the director of nursing practice at Barnes-Jewish Hospital. In that capacity she sharpened her interest in the development of nursing practice standards and the measurement of patient outcomes in defining nursing practice. Her most recent passion has been in the area of nursing research, specifically cancer family caregiving, the cancer patient symptom experience, fall prevention, and the effects of compassion fatigue on nurses. Recently Dr. Potter has worked with colleagues to develop an inpatient Innovation Unit, which is designed to incorporate current evidence into the selection and development of a unique work team and the creation of a care delivery model and innovative care practices. Dr. Potter is currently a director of research for patient care services at Barnes-Jewish Hospital.

WENDY R. OSTENDORF, RN, MS, EdD, CNE

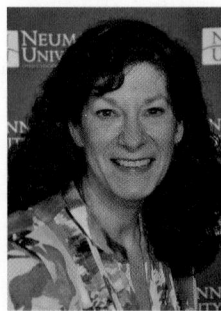

Dr. Wendy R. Ostendorf received her BSN from Villanova University, her MS from the University of Delaware, and her EdD from the University of Sarasota. She currently serves as a professor of nursing in the Division of Nursing and Health Sciences at Neumann University in Aston, Pennsylvania. She has contributed more than 30 chapters to multiple nursing textbooks and has served as author for two major textbooks: *Nursing Interventions & Clinical Skills* and *Clinical Nursing Skills & Techniques*. She has presented more than 25 papers at conferences at the local, national, and international levels.

Professionally, Dr. Ostendorf has a diverse background in pediatric and adult critical care. She has taught at the undergraduate and graduate levels for 35 years. With decades of practice as a clinician, her educational experiences have influenced her teaching philosophy and perceptions of the nursing profession. Dr. Ostendorf's current interests include the history and image of nursing as it has been represented in film. Most recently she was a co-primary research investigator on this topic.

Contributors

Michelle Aebersold, PhD, RN, CHSE, FAAN
Clinical Associate Professor
Director, Simulation and Educational Innovations
University of Michigan School of Nursing
Ann Arbor, Michigan

Marianne Banas, MSN, RN, CCTN, CWCN
Staff Nurse
University of Chicago Hospitals
Chicago, Illinois

Hope V. Bussenius, DNP, APRN, FNP-BC
Assistant Professor
Nell Hodgson Woodruff School of Nursing
Emory University
Atlanta, Georgia

Janice C. Colwell, RN, MS, CWOCN, FAAN
Advanced Practice Nurse, Ostomy and Wound Care
Department of Surgery
The University of Chicago Medicine
Chicago, Illinois

Jane Fellows, MSN, CWOCN
Wound/Ostomy CNS
Advanced Clinical Practice
Duke University Health System
Durham, North Carolina

Susan Jane Fetzer, BA, BSN, MSN, MBA, PhD
Professor
Department of Nursing
College of Health and Human Services
University of New Hampshire
Durham, New Hampshire

Paula Gray, DNP, CRNP, NP-C
Director, Family (Individual Across the Lifespan) CRNP
    Program
Clinical Assistant Professor of Nursing
Widener University School of Nursing
Chester, Pennsylvania

Stephanie Jeffers, PhD, RN
Assistant Professor
Widener University School of Nursing
Chester, Pennsylvania

Alaine Kamm, BSN, MSN
Nurse Practitioner
General Surgery
The University of Chicago Medicine
Chicago, Illinois

Lori Klingman, MSN, RN
Nurse Educator/Faculty Advisor
Ohio Valley Hospital
McKees Rocks, Pennsylvania

Stephen D. Krau, PhD, CNE
Associate Professor
School of Nursing
Vanderbilt University Medical Center
Nashville, Tennessee

Carol Ann Liebold, RN, BSN, CRNI
President/Owner
CarolAnn Liebold, Inc.
Earlton, New York

Nelda K. Martin, RN, ANP-BC, CCNS
Adult Nurse Practitioner/Clinical Nurse Specialist
Heart and Vascular Center
Barnes-Jewish Hospital at Washington University Medical
    Center
St. Louis, Missouri

**Kristen L. Mauk, PhD, DNP, RN, CRRN, GCNS-BC,
    GNP-BC, ACHPN, FAAN**
Professor of Nursing
Director, RN-BSN and MSN programs
Colorado Christian University;
President, International Rehabilitation Consultants/Senior Care
    Central
Ridgway, Colorado

Angela McConachie, FNP, DNP
Assistant Professor
Faculty
Goldfarb School of Nursing at Barnes-Jewish College
St. Louis, Missouri

**Jennifer Painter, MSN, APRN, CNS, RN-BC,
    OCN, AOCNS**
Staff Education Specialist
Nursing School/Faculty Affiliations Coordinator
Student Nurse Extern Program Coordinator
Nursing Development and Education
Institute for Learning, Leadership, & Development (iLead)
John H. Ammon Education Center
Newark, Delaware

**Ann Petlin, RN, MSN, CCNS, CCRN-CSC,
    ACNS-BC, PCCN**
Clinical Nurse Specialist
Cardiothoracic Surgery
Barnes-Jewish Hospital
St. Louis, Missouri

Theresa Pietsch, PhD, RN, CRRN, CNE
Associate Professor
Neumann University
Aston, Pennsylvania

Amy Spencer, MSN, RN-BC
Staff Development Specialist
Christiana Care Health Systems
Newark, Delaware

Diane Rudolphi, MS, RN
Master Instructor
University of Delaware School of Nursing
Newark, Delaware

C.J. Wright-Boon, RN, MSN
Assistant Professor
Saint Francis Medical Center College of Nursing
Peoria, Illinois

Jacqueline Raybuck Saleeby, PhD, RN, BCCS
Associate Professor
Catherine McAuley School of Nursing
Maryville University
St. Louis, Missouri

Rita Wunderlich, RN, PhD, CNE
Associate Professor
Catherine McAuley School of Nursing
Maryville University
St. Louis, Missouri

Felicia Schaps, MSN-Ed, BSN, RN, CRNI, OCN, CNSC, IgCN
Director of Nursing Operations
BioScrip, Inc.
Washington, D.C.

CONTRIBUTORS TO PREVIOUS EDITIONS

We would like to acknowledge the following people who contributed to previous editions of *Clinical Nursing Skills & Techniques*.

Jeannette Adams, PhD, MSN, APRN, CRNI
Della Aridge, RN, MSN
Elizabeth A. Ayello, PhD, MS, BSN, RN, CS, CWOCN
Sylvia K. Baird, BSN, MM
Nicole Bartow, RN, MSN
Margaret Benz, RN, MSN, CSANP
Barbara J. Berger, MSN, RN
Lyndal Guenther Brand, RN, BSN, MSN
Peggy Breckinridge, RN, BSN, MSN, FNP
Victoria M. Brown, RN, BSN, MSN, PhD
Gina Bufe, RN, BSN, MSN(R), PhD, CS
Gale Carli, MSN, MHed, BSN, RN
Ellen Carson, PhD
Maureen Carty, MSN, OCN
Aurelie Chinn, RN, MSN
Mary F. Clarke, MA, RN
Janice C. Colwell, RN, MS, CWOCN
Charlene Compher, PhD, RD, CNSC, LDN, FADA
Kelly Jo Cone, RN, BSN, MS, PhD, CNE
Dorothy McDonnell Cooke, RN, PhD
Eileen Costantinou, RN, BSN, MSN
Sheila A. Cunningham, RN, BSN, MSN
Pamela A. Cupec, RN, MS, ONC, CRRN, ACM
Ruth Curchoe, RN, MSN, CIC
Rick Daniels, RN, BSN, MSN, PhD
Mardell Davis, RN, MSN, CETN
Carolyn Ruppel d'Avis, RN, BSN, MSN
Patricia A. Dettenmeier, RN, BSN, MSN(R), CCRN
Wanda Cleveland Dubuisson, BSN, MN
Sharon J. Edwards, RN, MSN, PhD
Martha E. Elkin, RN, MSN

Deborah Oldenburg Erickson, RN, BSN, MSN
Debra Farrell, BSN, CNOR
Linda Fasciani, RN, BSN, MSN
Jane Fellows, RN, MSN, CWOCN
Susan Jane Fetzer, RN, BA, BSN, MSN, MBA, PhD
Cathy Flasar, MSN, APRN, BC, FNP
Marlene S. Foreman, BSN, MN, RNCS
Carol P. Fray, RN, MA
Leah W. Frederick, RN, MS, CIC
Kathleen Gerhart-Gibson, MSN, RN, CCRN
Paula Goldberg, RN, MS, MSN
Thelma Halberstadt, EdD, MS, BS, RN
Amy Hall, PhD, MS, BSN, RN
Roberta L. Harrison, PhD, RN, CRRN
Linda C. Haynes, PhD, RN
Diane Hildwein, RN, BC, MA
Maureen B. Huhmann, MS, RD
Nancy C. Jackson, RN, BSN, MSN, CCRN
Ruth L. Jilka, RD, CDE
Teresa M. Johnson, RN, MSN, CCRN
Judith Ann Kilpatrick, RN, DNSC
Carl Kirton, RN, BSN, MA, CCRN, ACRN, ANP
Lori Klingman, MSN, RN
Marilee Kuhrik, RN, MSN, PhD
Nancy S. Kuhrik, RN, MSN, PhD
Diane M. Kyle, RN, BSN, MS
Nancy Laplante, PhD, RN, AHN-BC
Louise K. Leitao, RN(c), BSN, MA
Gail B. Lewis, RN, MSN
Ruth Ludwick, PhD, MSN, BSN, RNC, CNS

Mary Kay Macheca, MSN(R), RN, CS, ANP, CDE
Jill Feldman Malen, RN, MS, NS, ANP
Mary K. Mantese, RN, MSN
Elizabeth Mantych, RN, MSN
Tina Marrelli, MSN, MA, RN
Nelda K. Martin, APRN, BC, CCNS, ANP
Kristin L. Mauk, PhD, DNP, RN, CRRN, GCNS-BC, GNP-BC, FAAN
Mary Mercer, RN, MSN
Rita Mertig, MS, BSN, RNC, CNS
Norma Metheny, PhD, MSN, BSN, FAAN
Mary Dee Miller, RN, BSN, MS, CIC
Sharon M.J. Muhs, MSN, RN
Kathleen Mulryan, RN, BSN, MSN
Lynne M. Murphy, RN, MSN
Elaine K. Neel, RN, BSN, MSN
Meghan G. Noble, PhD, RN
Marsha Evans Orr, RN, BS, MS, CS
Pamela L. Ostby, RN, MSN, OCN®
Dula F. Pacquiao, EdD, RN, CTN
Jeanne Marie Papa, MBE, MSN, ACNP-BC, CCRN
Sharon Phelps, RN, BSN, MS
Catherine A. Robinson, BA, RN
Judith Roos, RN, MSN
Mary Jane Ruhland, MSN, RN, BC
Jan Rumfelt, RNC, MSN, EdD
Jacqueline Raybuck Saleeby, PhD, RN, CS
Linette M. Sarti, RN, BSN, CNOR
Phyllis Ann Schiavone, MSN, CRNP
Lois Schick, MN, MBA, CPAN, CAPA
Kelly M. Schwartz, RN, BSN
April Sieh, RN, BSN, MSN

Marlene Smith, RN, BSN, MEd
Julie S. Snyder, MSN, RNC
Laura Sofield, MSN, APRN, BC
Sharon Souter, MSN, BSN
Martha A. Spies, RN, MSN
Paula Ann Stangeland, PhD, RN, CRRN
Patricia A. Stockert, RN, BSN, MS, PhD
E. Bradley Strecker, RN, PhD
Virginia Strootman, RN MS CRNI
Sandra Ann Szekely, RN, BSN
Donna L. Thompson, MSN, CRNP,
  FNP-BC, CCCN

Lynn Tier, RN, MSN, LNC
Nancy Tomaselli, RN, MSN, CS, CRNP,
  CWOCN, CLNC
Riva Touger-Decker, PhD, RD, FADA
Anne Falsone Vaughan, MSN, BSN,
  CCRN
Cynthia Vishy, RN, BSN
Pamela Becker Weilitz, MSN(R), RN, CS,
  ANP
Joan Domigan Wentz, MSN, RN
Laurel Wiersema, RN, MSN

Pamela E. Windle, MS, RN, NE-BC,
  CPAN, CAPA, FAAN
Terry L. Wood, PhD, RN
Patricia H. Worthington, MSN, RN,
  CNSC
Rita Wunderlich, PhD(C), MSN(R),
  CCRN
Rhonda Yancey, BSN, RN
Valerie Yancey, PhD, RN, HNC, CHPN

Reviewers

Michelle Aebersold, PhD, RN, CHSE, FAAN
Clinical Associate Professor
Director, Simulation and Educational Innovations
University of Michigan School of Nursing
Ann Arbor, Michigan

Margaret Barnes, DNP, MSN, RN
Assistant Professor
Indiana Wesleyan University
Marion, Indiana

Karen Benjamin, RN, MSN
RN Educator
University of Wyoming
Laramie, Wyoming

Nakia Best, MSN, RN
PhD Student/Teaching Fellow
University of North Carolina Chapel Hill School of Nursing
Chapel Hill, North Carolina

Anna M. Bruch, RN, MSN
Nursing Professor
Illinois Valley Community College
Oglesby, Illinois

Jennifer A. Brunworth, MSN, RN
Coordinator, Nursing Learning Lab
Clinical Assistant Professor of Nursing
Maryville University
St. Louis, Missouri

Patricia C. Buchsel, RN, MSN, OCN, FAAN
Clinical Instructor
Seattle University of Nursing
Seattle, Washington

Kimberly Clevenger, EdD, MSN, RN, BC
Associate Professor of Nursing
Morehead State University
Morehead, Kentucky

Eileen Costantinou, MSN, RN, BC
Practice Specialist/Senior Coordinator
Barnes-Jewish Hospital
St. Louis, Missouri

Holly Diesel, BA, BSN, MSN, PhD
Associate Professor
Goldfarb School of Nursing at Barnes-Jewish College
St. Louis, Missouri

Julie Eddins, MSN, AG-ACNP-BC, CRNI
Orthopedic Reconstruction Nurse Practitioner
Barnes-Jewish Hospital
St. Louis, Missouri

Yvette Egan, RN, BSN, MS
Clinical Assistant Professor
University of Wisconsin Madison School of Nursing
University of Wisconsin
Madison, Wisconsin

Amber Essman, DNP, MSN, FNP-BC, CNE
Visiting Professor, RN to BSN Online Postlicensure Program
Chamberlain College of Nursing
Grove City, Ohio

Margaret M. Gingrich, RN, MSN, CRNP
Professor of Nursing
Harrisburg Community College
Harrisburg, Pennsylvania

Karen F. Gonzol, BSN, MSN, RN
Retired
Eleanor Wade Custer School of Nursing
Shenandoah University
Winchester, Virginia

Teresa J. Green, MSN, RN, FNP-BC
Associate Professor of Nursing
Morehead State University
Morehead, Kentucky

Jacqueline Guhde, MSN, RN, CNS
Senior Instructor
University of Akron
Akron, Ohio

Kandi Hudson, EdD, RN, CMSRN, CNE
Associate Professor
The Community College of Baltimore County—Essex Campus
Baltimore, Maryland

Vickey Keathley, BSN, MSN, RN
ABSN Clinical Nurse Educator
Duke School of Nursing
Durham, North Carolina

Christina D. Keller, RN, MSN, CHSE
Instructor
Radford University Clinical Simulation Center
Radford University
Radford, Virginia

Lori L. Kelly, BSN, MSN, MBA
Associate Professor of Nursing
Aquinas College School of Nursing
Nashville, Tennessee

Patricia T. Ketchum, MSN
Director of Nursing Laboratories and Lecturer in Nursing
Oakland University School of Nursing
Rochester, Michigan

Vicky J. King, RN, MS, CNE
Nursing Faculty
Cochise College
Sierra Vista, Arizona

Jean LaFollette, RN, BSN, MSN
Instructor, Family Health and Community Health Nursing
Southern Illinois University—Edwardsville
Edwardsville, Illinois

**Diana R. Mager, RN, BSN, MSN, DNP, Board
  Certified Home Health Nursing**
Assistant Professor
Fairfield University School of Nursing
Fairfield, Connecticut

Sheila Matye, DNP, CNE
Web Developer and Manager of Curriculum & Instruction
Chamberlain College of Nursing
Downers Grove, Illinois

Janis Longfield McMillan, RN, MSN, CNE
Assistant Clinical Professor
Northern Arizona University
Flagstaff, Arizona

Sarah Newton, PhD, RN
Director of Undergraduate Programs
School of Nursing
Oakland University
Rochester, Michigan

Rebecca Otten, EdD, MSN, BAHA, RN
Associate Professors, Coordinator Pre-Licensure Programs
California State University, Fullerton
Fullerton, California

Patricia Pence, BSN, MSN, PhD
Nursing Professor
Illinois Valley Community College
Oglesby, Illinois

Jill R. Reed, PhD, APRN-NP
Assistant Professor
UMNC College of Nursing—Kearney Division
Kearney, Nebraska

Diane Rudolphi, MS, RN
Master Instructor
University of Delaware School of Nursing
Newark, Delaware

**Susan Scholtz, RN, PhD, School Nursing
  Certificate**
Associate Professor of Nursing
Moravian College
Bethlehem, Pennsylvania

**Benjamin A. Smallheer, PhD, RN,
  ACNP-BC, CCRN**
Assistant Professor of Nursing
Vanderbilt University School of Nursing
Nashville, Tennessee

Lynette Tanaka, MSN, RN
Assistant Teaching Professor
College of Nursing
University of Missouri—St. Louis
St. Louis, Missouri

Lynne L. Tier, MSN, RN
Assistant Director of Simulation
Adventist University of Health Sciences
Orlando, Florida

Heidi Tymkew, PT, DPT, MHS, CCS
Clinical Specialist
Barnes-Jewish Hospital, Department of Rehabilitation
St. Louis, Missouri

Susan A. Wheaton, RN, BSN, MSN
Lecture/Learning Resource Director
University of Maine
Orono, Maine

Paige D. Wimberley, PhD, APRN, CNS-BC, CNE
Associate Professor of Nursing
Arkansas State University
Jonesboro, Arkansas

Aimee Woda, PhD, RN, MSC
Assistant Professor
Marquette University
Milwaukee, Wisconsin

Lea Wood, DNP, MS(N), BSN-RN
Director of Simulation/Assistant Teaching Professor
University of Missouri
Columbia, Missouri

Jean Yockey, MSN, FNP, CNE
Assistant Professor
University of South Dakota
Vermillion, South Dakota

Melody Ziobro, RN, MS
Assistant Professor of Nursing
Morrisville State College
Morrisville, New York

CLINICAL REVIEWERS

Keith D. Lamb, RRT
Specialist, Surgical Critical Care/Trauma
Christiana Care Health Systems
Newark, Delaware

Manju Maliakal, MSN, CMSRN
Administrative Supervisor
Baylor Scott and White Health
Carrollton, Texas

Marion F. Winkler, PhD, RD, LDN, CNSC
Surgical Nutrition Specialist and Associate Professor of Surgery
Rhode Island Hospital, Department of Surgery
Nutritional Support Service and Alpert Medical School of
  Brown University
Providence, Rhode Island

Preface to the Student

Numerous features are built into this text to help you identify key pieces of information and study more efficiently. Additional study tools and review questions may be found on the companion Evolve site: http://evolve.elsevier.com/Perry/skills

Objectives highlight the primary aims of chapter content.

Evolve media resources are available for every chapter.

22 | Parenteral Medications

SKILLS AND PROCEDURES

Skill 22.1 **Preparing Injections: Ampules and Vials, p. 580**

Procedural Guideline 22.1 **Mixing Parenteral Medications in One Syringe, p. 586**

Skill 22.2 **Administering Intradermal Injections, p. 589**

Skill 22.3 **Administering Subcutaneous Injections, p. 593**

Skill 22.4 **Administering Intramuscular Injections, p. 600**

Skill 22.5 **Administering Medications by Intravenous Bolus, p. 607**

Skill 22.6 **Administering Intravenous Medications by Piggyback, Intermittent Infusion Sets, and Mini-Infusion Pumps, p. 614**

Skill 22.7 **Administering Continuous Subcutaneous Medications, p. 620**

OBJECTIVES

Mastery of content in this chapter will enable the nurse to:
- Correctly prepare injectable medications from a vial and an ampule.
- Identify advantages, disadvantages, and risks of administering medications by each parenteral route.
- Evaluate the effectiveness and outcomes of administering medications by each parenteral route.
- Explain the importance of selecting the proper-size syringe and needle for an injection.
- Discuss factors to consider when selecting injection sites.

- Discuss ways to promote patient comfort while administering an injection.
- Correctly administer intradermal, subcutaneous, and intramuscular injections.
- Compare the risks of three different intravenous routes.
- Correctly administer an intravenous medication by intravenous piggyback, intermittent infusion, or bolus.
- Initiate, maintain, and discontinue a continuous subcutaneous infusion.

MEDIA RESOURCES

evolve http://evolve.elsevier.com/Perry/skills
- Review Questions
- Video Clips

- Audio Glossary
- **NSO** Nursing Skills Online
- Clinical Debrief and Review Questions Answers

SKILL 22.3 ADMINISTERING SUBCUTANEOUS INJECTIONS 599

STEP	RATIONALE

Clinical Decision Point *Aspiration after injecting a subcutaneous medication is not necessary. Piercing a blood vessel in a subcutaneous injection is very rare. Aspiration after injecting heparin and insulin is not recommended (Lilley et al., 2012).*

e. Withdraw needle quickly while placing antiseptic swab or gauze gently over site.

17. Apply gentle pressure to site. *Do not massage site.* (If heparin is given, hold alcohol swab or gauze to site for 30 to 60 seconds.)
18. Help patient to comfortable position.
19. Discard uncapped needle or needle enclosed in safety shield (see illustrations) and attached syringe into puncture- and leak-proof receptacle.

Supporting tissues around injection site minimizes discomfort during needle withdrawal. Dry gauze may minimize patient discomfort associated with alcohol on nonintact skin.
Aids absorption. Massage can damage underlying tissue. Time interval prevents bleeding at site.
Gives patient sense of well-being.
Prevents injury to patients and health care personnel. Recapping needles increases risk for needlestick injury (OSHA, n.d.).

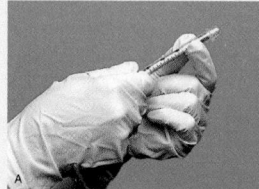

STEP 19 Needle with plastic guard to prevent needlesticks. **A,** Position of guard before injection. **B,** After injection guard locks in place, covering needle.

20. Remove gloves and perform hand hygiene.
21. Stay with patient for several minutes and observe for any allergic reactions.

Reduces transmission of microorganisms.
Dyspnea, wheezing, and circulatory collapse are signs of severe anaphylactic reaction.

EVALUATION

1. Return to room in 15 to 30 minutes and ask if patient feels any acute pain, burning, numbness, or tingling at injection site.
2. Inspect site, noting bruising or induration. Provide warm compress to site.
3. Observe patient's response to medication at times that correlate with onset, peak, and duration of medication. Review laboratory results as appropriate (e.g., blood glucose, partial thromboplastin).
4. **Use Teach-Back:** "I want to be sure I explained to you the reason for this subcutaneous injection. Tell me why you are receiving this injection." Revise your instruction now or develop a plan for revised patient or family caregiver teaching if patient or family caregiver is not able to teach back correctly.

Continued discomfort may indicate injury to underlying bones or nerves.
Bruising or induration indicates complication associated with injection.
Adverse effects of parenteral medications develop rapidly. Evaluate effect of medication on basis of onset, peak, and duration of action.
Determines patient's and family caregiver's level of understanding of instructional topic.

(by the *parenteral* route enter body tissues ... by injection. Injected medications are ... an oral medications. Parenteral routes are ... omiting or cannot swallow, when rapid ... eded, and/or when patients are restricted ... These medication administration proce-... as pose greater risks than those associated ... arenteral medications (see Chapter 21). ... requires a certain set of skills to ensure ... hes the proper location. There are four ... inistration:

... on: Injection into tissues just under the ...

... injection: Injection into the body of a ...

... njection: Injection into the dermis just ...

... ection or infusion: Injection into a vein

STANDARDS OF CARE
- Centers for Medicare & Medicaid Services (CMS), 2015—Preparation and Administration of Drugs
- Infusion Nurses Society, 2016—Infusion Nursing Standards of Practice
- Institute for Safe Medication Practices (ISMP), 2011; 2012; 2015—Safe Medication Preparation
- The Joint Commission, 2016—Patient Identification

PRINCIPLES FOR PRACTICE
- When managing a patient's medications, communicate clearly with the interprofessional team, assess and incorporate the patient's priorities of care and preferences, and use the best evidence when making decisions about patient care.
- Use technology (e.g., bar scanning, electronic medication administration record [MAR]) that is available in your agency when preparing and giving medications.

575

Clinical Decision Points highlight points to consider when performing skills to ensure effective outcomes and promote safety.

Extensive illustrations demonstrate step-by-step procedures for more thorough understanding.

Quick Response codes may be scanned to link to video clips directly from the text page.

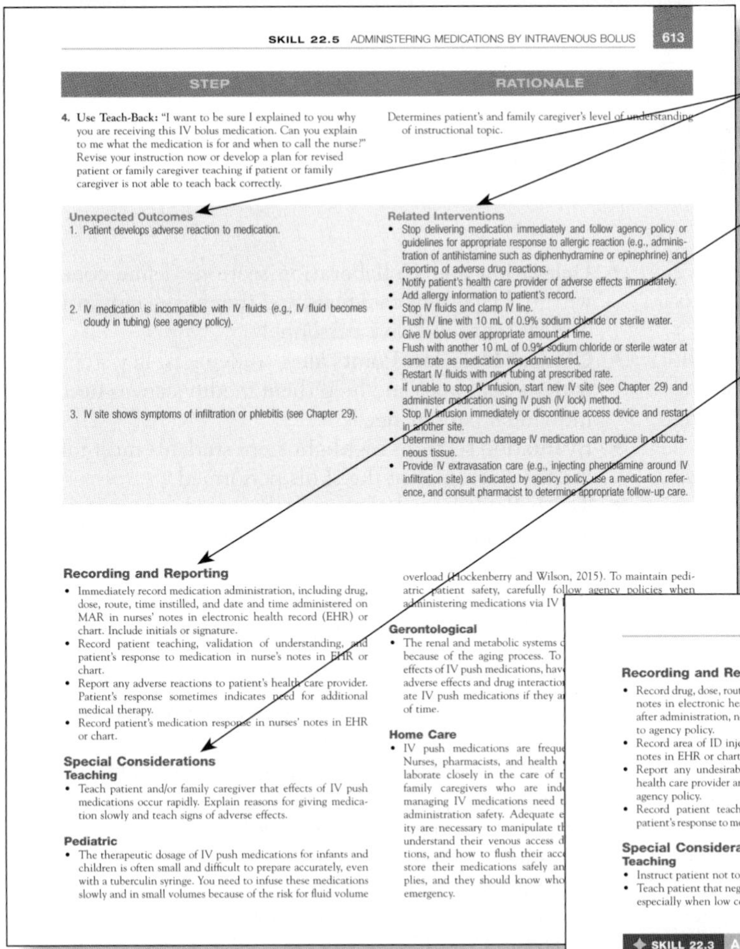

SKILL 22.5 ADMINISTERING MEDICATIONS BY INTRAVENOUS BOLUS 613

STEP	RATIONALE
4. **Use Teach-Back:** "I want to be sure I explained to you why you are receiving this IV bolus medication. Can you explain to me what the medication is for and when to call the nurse?" Revise your instruction now or develop a plan for revised patient or family caregiver teaching if patient or family caregiver is not able to teach back correctly.	Determines patient's and family caregiver's level of understanding of instructional topic.

Unexpected Outcomes	Related Interventions
1. Patient develops adverse reaction to medication.	• Stop delivering medication immediately and follow agency policy or guidelines for appropriate response to allergic reaction (e.g., administration of antihistamine such as diphenhydramine or epinephrine) and reporting of adverse drug reactions. • Notify patient's health care provider of adverse effects immediately. • Add allergy information to patient's record.
2. IV medication is incompatible with IV fluids (e.g., IV fluid becomes cloudy in tubing) (see agency policy).	• Stop IV fluids and clamp IV line. • Flush IV line with 10 mL of 0.9% sodium chloride or sterile water. • Give IV bolus over appropriate amount of time. • Flush with another 10 mL of 0.9% sodium chloride or sterile water at same rate as medication was administered. • Restart IV fluids with new tubing at prescribed rate. • If unable to stop IV infusion, start new IV site (see Chapter 29) and administer medication using IV push (IV lock) method.
3. IV site shows symptoms of infiltration or phlebitis (see Chapter 29).	• Stop IV infusion immediately or discontinue access device and restart in another site. • Determine how much damage IV medication can produce in subcutaneous tissue. • Provide IV extravasation care (e.g., injecting phentolamine around IV infiltration site) as indicated by agency policy, use a medication reference, and consult pharmacist to determine appropriate follow-up care.

Recording and Reporting
- Immediately record medication administration, including drug, dose, route, time instilled, and date and time administered on MAR in nurses' notes in electronic health record (EHR) or chart. Include initials or signature.
- Record patient teaching, validation of understanding, and patient's response to medication in nurse's notes in EHR or chart.
- Report any adverse reactions to patient's health care provider. Patient's response sometimes indicates need for additional medical therapy.
- Record patient's medication response in nurses' notes in EHR or chart.

Special Considerations
Teaching
- Teach patient and/or family caregiver that effects of IV push medications occur rapidly. Explain reasons for giving medication slowly and teach signs of adverse effects.

Pediatric
- The therapeutic dosage of IV push medications for infants and children is often small and difficult to prepare accurately, even with a tuberculin syringe. You need to infuse these medications slowly and in small volumes because of the risk for fluid volume overload (Hockenberry and Wilson, 2015). To maintain pediatric patient safety, carefully follow agency policies when administering medications via IV ...

Gerontological
- The renal and metabolic systems ... because of the aging process. To ... effects of IV push medications, hav... adverse effects and drug interactio... ate IV push medications if they a... of time.

Home Care
- IV push medications are frequ... Nurses, pharmacists, and health ... laborate closely in the care of ... family caregivers who are ind... managing IV medications need ... administration safety. Adequate ... ity are necessary to manipulate ... understand their venous access ... tions, and how to flush their acc... store their medications safely a... plies, and they should know wh... emergency.

Unexpected Outcomes/Related Interventions help you anticipate problems and respond appropriately.

Recording and Reporting guidelines for each skill detail what to document and report.

Special Considerations indicate special teaching considerations, as well as procedure modifications needed for pediatric, gerontological, and home care populations.

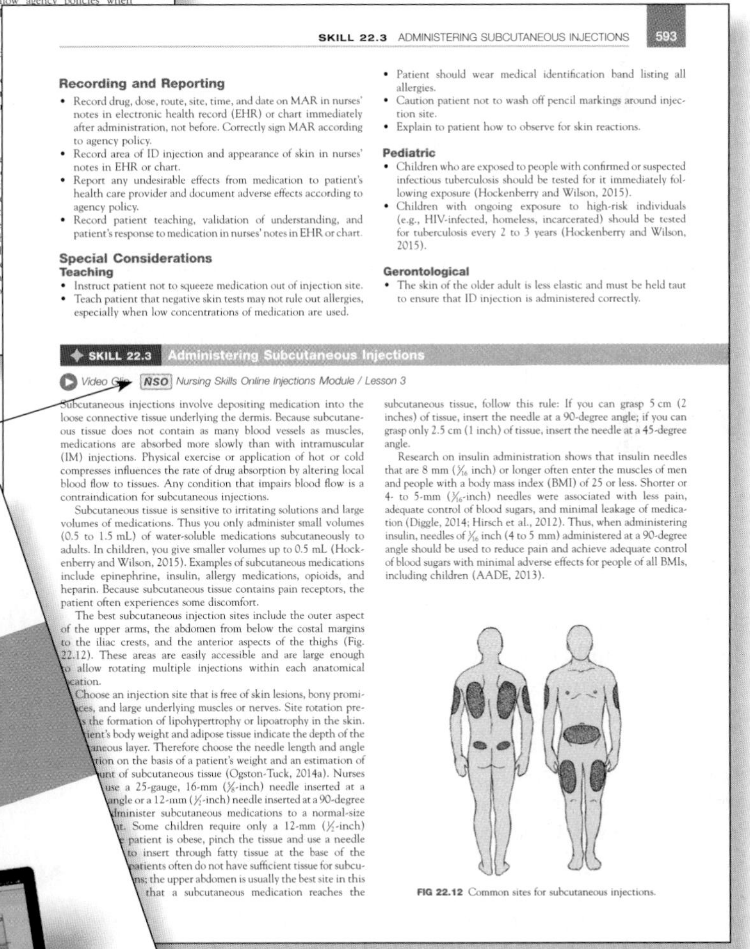

SKILL 22.3 ADMINISTERING SUBCUTANEOUS INJECTIONS 593

Recording and Reporting
- Record drug, dose, route, site, time, and date on MAR in nurses' notes in electronic health record (EHR) or chart immediately after administration, not before. Correctly sign MAR according to agency policy.
- Record area of ID injection and appearance of skin in nurses' notes in EHR or chart.
- Report any undesirable effects from medication to patient's health care provider and document adverse effects according to agency policy.
- Record patient teaching, validation of understanding, and patient's response to medication in nurses' notes in EHR or chart.

Special Considerations
Teaching
- Instruct patient not to squeeze medication out of injection site.
- Teach patient that negative skin tests may not rule out allergies, especially when low concentrations of medication are used.
- Patient should wear medical identification band listing all allergies.
- Caution patient not to wash off pencil markings around injection site.
- Explain to patient how to observe for skin reactions.

Pediatric
- Children who are exposed to people with confirmed or suspected infectious tuberculosis should be tested for it immediately following exposure (Hockenberry and Wilson, 2015).
- Children with ongoing exposure to high-risk individuals (e.g., HIV-infected, homeless, incarcerated) should be tested for tuberculosis every 2 to 3 years (Hockenberry and Wilson, 2015).

Gerontological
- The skin of the older adult is less elastic and must be held taut to ensure that ID injection is administered correctly.

SKILL 22.3 Administering Subcutaneous Injections

Video Clips NSO Nursing Skills Online Injections Module / Lesson 3

Subcutaneous injections involve depositing medication into the loose connective tissue underlying the dermis. Because subcutaneous tissue does not contain as many blood vessels as muscles, medications are absorbed more slowly than with intramuscular (IM) injections. Physical exercise or application of hot or cold compresses influences the rate of drug absorption by altering local blood flow to tissues. Any condition that impairs blood flow is a contraindication for subcutaneous injections.

Subcutaneous tissue is sensitive to irritating solutions and large volumes of medications. Thus you only administer small volumes (0.5 to 1.5 mL) of water-soluble medications subcutaneously to adults. In children, you give smaller volumes up to 0.5 mL (Hockenberry and Wilson, 2015). Examples of subcutaneous medications include epinephrine, insulin, allergy medications, opioids, and heparin. Because subcutaneous tissue contains pain receptors, the patient often experiences some discomfort.

The best subcutaneous injection sites include the outer aspect of the upper arms, the abdomen from below the costal margins to the iliac crests, and the anterior aspects of the thighs (Fig. 22.12). These areas are easily accessible and are large enough to allow rotating multiple injections within each anatomical location.

Choose an injection site that is free of skin lesions, bony prominences, and large underlying muscles or nerves. Site rotation prevents the formation of lipohypertrophy or lipoatrophy in the skin. ...ient's body weight and adipose tissue indicate the depth of the ...aneous layer. Therefore choose the needle length and angle ...tion on the basis of a patient's weight and an estimation of ...unt of subcutaneous tissue (Ogston-Tuck, 2014a). Nurses ...use a 25-gauge, 16-mm (5/8-inch) needle inserted at a ...angle or a 12-mm (1/2-inch) needle inserted at a 90-degree ...dminister subcutaneous medications to a normal-size ...t. Some children require only a 12-mm (1/2-inch) ... patient is obese, pinch the tissue and use a needle ... to insert through fatty tissue at the base of the ...atients often do not have sufficient tissue for subcu...ns; the upper abdomen is usually the best site in this ... that a subcutaneous medication reaches the subcutaneous tissue, follow this rule: If you can grasp 5 cm (2 inches) of tissue, insert the needle at a 90-degree angle; if you can grasp only 2.5 cm (1 inch) of tissue, insert the needle at a 45-degree angle.

Research on insulin administration shows that insulin needles that are 8 mm (5/16 inch) or longer often enter the muscles of men and people with a body mass index (BMI) of 25 or less. Shorter or 4- to 5-mm (3/16-inch) needles were associated with less pain, adequate control of blood sugars, and minimal leakage of medication (Diggle, 2014; Hirsch et al., 2012). Thus, when administering insulin, needles of 3/16 inch (4 to 5 mm) administered at a 90-degree angle should be used to reduce pain and achieve adequate control of blood sugars with minimal adverse effects for people of all BMIs, including children (AADE, 2013).

FIG 22.12 Common sites for subcutaneous injections.

NSO icon links to online course lessons.

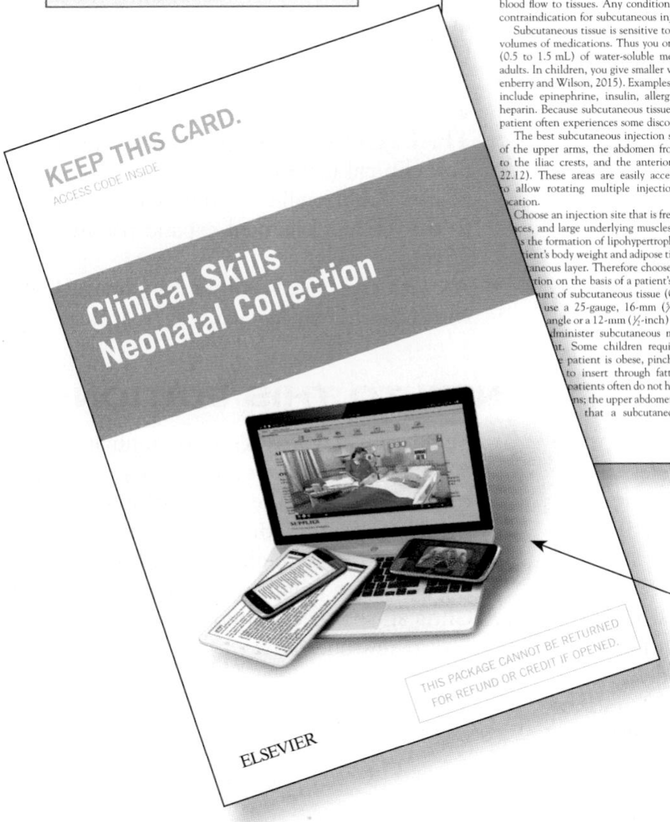
KEEP THIS CARD.
ACCESS CODE INSIDE
Clinical Skills Neonatal Collection
THIS PACKAGE CANNOT BE RETURNED FOR REFUND OR CREDIT IF OPENED.
ELSEVIER

Clinical Skills: Essentials Collection contains 144 entirely new, high-definition video skills.

Preface to the Instructor

The evolution of technology and knowledge influences the way we teach clinical skills to nursing students and improves the quality of care possible for every patient. However, the foundation for success in performing nursing skills remains a competent, well-informed nurse who thinks critically, asks the right questions at the right time, and makes timely decisions. That outcome is the driving factor behind this new edition.

In this ninth edition of *Clinical Nursing Skills & Techniques*, we have created a very different format for our textbook. Each chapter opens by introducing students to key concepts: Standards of Practice, Principles for Practice, Evidence-Based Practice, Patient-Centered Care, and Safety Guidelines. These have been streamlined into a quick, easy-to-read bulleted format. Our new approach emphasizes yet simplifies these important concepts.

In addition, these concepts align with the *Quality and Safety Education for Nurses* (QSEN) initiative. Chapter 1, Using Evidence in Nursing Practice, prepares students to understand and use the evidence-based practice information included in every chapter.

All topics and skills, including sample documentation, have been updated to the most recent standards in nursing practice.

Your students will find that this edition of *Clinical Nursing Skills & Techniques* provides a comprehensive resource that will serve them well through their nursing education and right into their clinical practice careers.

CLASSIC FEATURES

- **Over 200 basic, intermediate, and advanced nursing skills and procedures** are covered.
- **Five-step nursing process format** provides a consistent presentation that helps students apply the process while learning each skill.
- **Skills and Procedures** list and **Objectives** open each chapter.
- **Over 1200 full-color photos and drawings** help students master the material covered.
- **Evidence-Based Practice** sections in each chapter present students with the newest scientific evidence for the procedures presented. Recent research findings are discussed, and their implications for patient care are explored.
- **Patient-Centered Care** sections prepare students to recognize the importance of having patients partner in performing skills in a compassionate and coordinated way based on respect for a patient's cultural preferences, values, and needs (QSEN core competency).
- **Safety Guidelines** sections cover global recommendations on the safe execution of the particular skill set covered in each chapter (QSEN core competency).
- **NSO icon** links text content with the new edition of *Nursing Skills Online*, which has been simultaneously revised with the textbook to provide completely coordinated information.
- **Rationales** are given for steps within skills so students learn the *why* as well as the *how* of each skill. Rationales include citations from the current literature.

- **Delegation and Collaboration** sections define communication within the patient care team and the nurse's responsibility when delegating to assistive personnel.
- **Clinical Decision Points** alert students to key steps that affect patient outcomes and help them modify care as needed to meet individual patient needs.
- **Evaluation** sections highlight steps students must take to evaluate the outcomes of the skills performed.
- **Teach-Back** is included in each evaluation section, where we demonstrate to students how to phrase a Teach-Back question appropriately.
- **Recording and Reporting** sections follow the evaluation discussion and alert students to what information should be documented in each situation.
- **Unexpected Outcomes and Related Interventions** sections inform students to be alert for potential problems and help them determine appropriate nursing interventions.
- **Special Considerations** sections include additional considerations when performing the skill for specific populations of patients or in specific settings and may include:
  - **Teaching Considerations**
  - **Pediatric Considerations**
  - **Gerontological Considerations**
  - **Home Care Considerations**
- **Quick Response codes** (scan with smartphone or tablet with camera to view video clips) on the text pages link video clips to the appropriate skill or procedure, allowing students to view the video immediately after reading the implementation section of the skill.
- **Glossary** (on Evolve) defines all key terms.
- **Additional review questions** (on Evolve) include a brand new set of unique questions for every chapter.
- **TEACH for RN instructor manual** helps you capitalize on the new clinical material in the text, skills video series, and online course. Additional case studies and discussion questions unique to the TEACH manual expand the in-class material available to you.
- As with the eighth edition, an **Image Collection** is available with *Clinical Nursing Skills & Techniques*.

NEW TO THIS EDITION:

- **Standards of Care** sections summarize the most recent evidence-based standards and/or the professional clinical standards recommended for the skills within each chapter.
- **Principles for Practice** sections highlight the key nursing principles that apply to all skills within a chapter.
- **Expanded and improved end-of-chapter exercises** include a Clinical Debrief case study, examples of SBAR communication, and review questions.

Contents

UNIT 13

Care of the Surgical Patient

UNIT 14

Dressings and Wound Care

UNIT 15

Home Care

APPENDIXES

1 | Using Evidence in Nursing Practice

OBJECTIVES

Mastery of content in this chapter will enable the nurse to:

- Discuss how scientific evidence improves the relevance and efficacy of nursing skills.
- Explain the differences between research- and non–research-based evidence.
- Describe the six steps of evidence-based practice.
- Explain the components of a PICO(T) question.

- Discuss the process for critiquing evidence in the literature.
- Identify the elements to review when critiquing a scientific article.
- Discuss ways to apply evidence in nursing practice.
- Explain the importance of identifying outcomes in the evaluation of an evidence-based practice change.

MEDIA RESOURCES

- evolve http://evolve.elsevier.com/Perry/skills
- Review Questions
- Audio Glossary

- Clinical Debrief and Review Questions Answers
- Case Studies

PURPOSE

One of the key messages in the 2010 report of the Institute of Medicine (IOM), The Future of Nursing: Leading Change, Advancing Health, is for nurses to be full partners with physicians and other health care professionals in redesigning health care in the United States (IOM, 2010). To achieve better patient outcomes, new knowledge must be transformed into clinically useful approaches and then successfully implemented across the entire health care team and measured in terms of meaningful impact on performance and health outcomes (Stevens, 2013). Nursing is positioned to lead change and advance health through the use of evidence-based practice (EBP), a process that makes nurses more autonomous in changing health care practices. EBP is a problem-solving approach to clinical practice that combines the best available evidence in combination with a clinician's expertise, patient preferences and values, and available health care resources in making decisions about patient care (Melnyk and Fineout-Overholt, 2014). Through the use of current and relevant scientific evidence, nurses ensure that the skills and procedures performed on patients incorporate best practices for efficiency, patient safety, and clinical effectiveness.

STANDARDS OF CARE

Quality and Safety Education for Nurses (QSEN) Institute: *Pre-Licensure KSA's*, 2014—Evidence-based practice competency

PRINCIPLES FOR PRACTICE

Cathy works on a medical oncology unit where patients undergo chemotherapy and radiation for leukemia, lymphoma, and other forms of cancer. Because of their chemotherapy, many patients experience a drop in their platelet count and clotting factors, increasing their risk for bleeding. Cathy recently cared for a 42-year-old woman who fell while trying to get to the bathroom and hit her head against the bedframe, resulting in a serious intracranial bleed. Cathy discusses the situation with two nurse colleagues and asks, "How can we reduce the number of falls and injuries to our patients on the oncology unit?" The nurse specialist for the unit tells Cathy, "I heard about an approach to fall prevention on one of the surgical floors; it involves hourly rounding. Let's ask this question, "In adult oncology patients, will the use of hourly rounding compared with the current fall prevention protocol affect the incidence of falls during hospitalization?" Feeling frustrated that their existing fall prevention protocol was not effective in reducing falls, the group agrees that the question is the right one to search in the literature.

This clinical case study highlights how professional nurses address problems in their practice.

EBP is a process of making informed decisions about the way nurses care for patients. It all begins with asking clinical questions. Clinical questions lead nurses such as Cathy and her colleagues to find evidence from the research literature, clinical papers, quality improvement data, risk-management trends, and the opinions of nurse experts. Nurses then apply the evidence to make relevant and informed changes in practice such as fall prevention in the case study.

There are elements of all nursing procedures within this textbook that are evidence based. For example, the length of time necessary to wash hands, the technique for determining the position of a feeding tube in the stomach, and the technique for giving an intramuscular injection are based on evidence. Clinical research led to the answers for how these nursing procedures should be performed. The use of such evidence in practice enables clinicians to provide the highest quality of care to their patients and families.

Quality Health Care

The ANA reports that the emphasis in health care today for evidence-based quality improvement and health care transformation underscores the need for redesigning care that is effective, safe, and efficient (Stevens, 2013). The use of EBP is key to achieving quality health care, defined as the degree to which health services for individuals and populations increase the likelihood of desired health outcomes and are consistent with current professional knowledge (IOM, 2013). Implementing health care processes or practices that are known to work (evidence based) in a reliable way is a feature of "quality care." Implementing new knowledge into practice requires a systematic approach that applies evidence to clinical, educational, and administrative practices. EBP is one of the QSEN competencies, with the goal for the QSEN project being to prepare nurses to have the knowledge, skills, and attitudes to continuously improve the quality and safety of the health care systems within which they work (QSEN Institute, 2014). Perhaps what is most important about EBP is that the process encourages all health care providers to question practices and to use evidence in deciding which interventions produce the best outcomes and which do not. Nurses play a key role at the bedside in questioning outdated, illogical, or unsafe practices and then adopting evidence-based interventions that will change patients' health status and achieve desired outcomes.

A Case for Evidence

EBP is a guide for making accurate, timely, and appropriate clinical decisions. It is an interprofessional process for applying the newest knowledge available in health care sciences to the patient's bedside. For example, using a sliding board to transfer a patient from bed to stretcher instead of lifting and using the research-based Braden Scale to routinely assess a patient's risk for skin breakdown are examples of using evidence at the bedside. This textbook demonstrates how to use evidence in nursing procedures or skills and provides the scientific guidelines to perform skills more effectively and improve patient outcomes.

As a professional nurse you need to stay informed and be aware of the most current evidence. Typically new students diligently read their textbooks and assigned scientific articles. A good textbook incorporates current evidence into the practice guidelines and nursing skills at the time it is published. However, because a textbook relies on the scientific literature, some information can become outdated by the time it is published. Articles from nursing and the health care literature are available on almost any topic involving nursing practice. New research is reported every day. Although the scientific basis of nursing practice has grown, there are practices that are still not "research based" (based on findings from well-designed research studies) because findings are inconclusive or researchers have not yet studied the practices. For example, in the past nurses changed intravenous (IV) site dressings daily and applied antibiotic ointment to reduce the incidence of infection at a site. However, there was no evidence at the time to support this practice. IV care was based on tradition. Recent research has shown that topical antibiotics offer no benefit and daily dressing changes are not beneficial unless a dressing becomes soiled or compromised. Today the current standard of care is to cleanse an adult's IV site with chlorhexidine antiseptic solution, not antibiotic ointment, and to change dressings on peripheral catheters if the dressing is damp, loosened, and/or visibly soiled and at least every 5 to 7 days (INS, 2011). The challenge is to obtain the very best, most current information at the right time, when you need it for patient care.

The best evidence comes from well-designed, systematically conducted research studies that are reported in scientific journals. Unfortunately many health care settings do not have a process to help staff adopt new evidence in practice. Nurses in practice settings, unlike educational settings, may not have easy access to databases for scientific literature. Instead they often care for patients on the basis of tradition, preferences, or convenience. Because there are often obstacles to research-based practice in clinical settings, it is important for administrators to provide a supportive environment and adequate facilitation of change. Researchers have found that leadership within health care institutions is vital for the process of implementing EBP in nursing (Sandstrom et al., 2011). Some hospitals have created councils of nurses to lead initiatives to implement and study measures that promote the best standards of care. Hospital-based nursing research centers have also helped sustain a culture of EBP, something that hospitals are focusing on as they move to apply for Magnet designation or redesignation (Ingersoll et al., 2010).

One thing that is unique about EBP is that it includes multiple sources of evidence. When there is no research evidence for a practice question or issue, nurses have a range of non–research-based evidence available (Dearholt et al., 2012). Examples of non–research-based evidence includes consensus or position statements, general literature reviews, quality improvement and risk management data, retrospective or concurrent chart review, and clinicians' expertise. Non–research-based evidence is valuable in informing you about practice issues in your setting (e.g., fall or infection rates). But remember, it is important that you *not* rely on non–research-based evidence alone. Research-based evidence is more likely to be timely, accurate, and relevant. When you face a clinical problem, seek out all sources of evidence to find the best solution in caring for patients.

Even when you use the best evidence available, application and outcomes will differ on the basis of your patients' values, preferences, concerns, and/or expectations. Apply critical thinking competencies to determine whether evidence is relevant and appropriate to your patients and to a clinical situation. For example, some research suggests that spirituality positively affects and enhances patients' physical and psychological health and health promotion behaviors (Conway-Phillips and Janusek, 2014; White, 2013). However, if a patient is reluctant to discuss his or her spirituality and you are unsure of his or her beliefs, an attempt to use spiritual health interventions is inappropriate. Using your clinical expertise and considering patients' cultures, values, and preferences, ensure that you apply new evidence in practice both ethically and appropriately. EBP requires good nursing judgment; it is not finding research evidence and applying it blindly.

Steps of Evidence-Based Practice

There are different models for using EBP. The Johns Hopkins Model includes three phases described as practice question, evidence, and translation (PET) (Dearholt and Dang, 2012). Altogether the PET model includes 18 steps. A simpler model is one described by Melnyk and Fineout-Overholt (2014) that includes six steps:

1. Ask a clinical question.
2. Search for the most relevant and best evidence that applies to the question.
3. Critically appraise the evidence.
4. Apply or integrate evidence along with your clinical expertise, patient preferences, and values in making a practice decision or change.
5. Evaluate the practice decision or change.
6. Communicate and disseminate results.

Ask a Clinical Question

Asking a clinical question is most important because how a problem is posed drives the remaining steps of the EBP process (Dearholt and Dang, 2012). Every day nurses perform interventions (e.g., providing comfort measures, caring for wounds, and offering grief support) that stimulate questions such as, "Why do we use this approach?" and "Is there a better way?" or "This step causes patients distress. What other options are available?" Always think about your practice when caring for patients. Question what does not make sense to you and what you think needs clarification. Include colleagues from other disciplines whose perceptions might help to clarify or examine the clinical problem or issue. As shown in the previous case study, think about a patient care problem or an area of interest that is time consuming, costly, or not logical. Often TJC standards (e.g., the annual patient safety goals) spark questions for you to pose about your patients.

Clinical questions often arise as a result of either a problem- or a knowledge-focused trigger. A problem-focused trigger develops as you care for a patient or notice a trend on a nursing unit. For example, a problem-focused trigger might arise while caring for an unconscious patient: "Which is the best anti-infective solution to use when giving oral care to unconscious patients?" Examples of problem-focused trends include the increase in the number of pressure injuries to patients' skin or tissues or the incidence of urinary tract infections on a nursing unit. A knowledge-focused trigger arises when you ask a question regarding new information about a topic. For example, "What is the current evidence to reduce bloodstream infection in central venous catheters?" Important knowledge sources often include standards and practice guidelines available from national agencies such as the Agency for Healthcare Research and Quality (AHRQ), the INS, the American Association of Critical Care Nurses (AACN), and National Pressure Ulcer Advisory Panel (NPUAP, 2016).

There are two types of clinical questions: background and foreground (Dearholt and Dang, 2012; Straus, 2011). Think of a forest and the trees. A background question gives us a view of a forest. It is broad and general about a condition or idea. For example, "Which interventions reduce falls in oncology patients?" The answer to the question provides general knowledge about the problem, concepts or topic of interest (e.g., falls, fall occurrence among oncology patients, reasons oncology patients fall). In contrast, a foreground question gives us a closer look at the trees in a forest. It is a more specific and focused question that includes specific comparisons (Dearholt and Dang, 2012). A foreground question asks which of two interventions is likely the more effective in addressing a practice issue. For example, "Does hourly rounding compared with a standard fall prevention protocol affect the incidence of falls?" A background question allows you to explore a vast array of options in the literature; whereas a foreground question produces a refined and limited body of evidence specific to your area of interest. In day-to-day clinical

practice it helps to be able to identify foreground questions so the extent of literature to review is limited.

A well-stated foreground question is clearly worded when you use a PICO format. Box 1.1 summarizes the elements of a PICO question. Using key words in a PICO question make it easier to search for evidence in the scientific literature because it restricts a search to only articles pertinent to the PICO terms. The words used in the PICO question are the key terms for your literature search. Examples of PICO questions follow: *In abdominal surgery patients (P), does epidural analgesia (I) compared with patient-controlled analgesia (C) affect pain severity (O)? In medical patients (P) does the use of a case-management model (I) compared with a telephone call-back system (C) improve patient medication adherence (O)?*

An option used in PICO questions involves use of an additional term, "T" for timing. The addition of a Timing factor in a PICOT question allows you to further narrow your question. For example, timing might refer to when an intervention is to be used or a time frame for outcome achievement. Here is an example: *In abdominal surgery patients (P), does epidural analgesia (I) compared with patient-controlled analgesia (C) affect pain severity (O) in the first 48 hours after surgery (T)?*

Well-designed PICO questions do not have to include all four elements. For example, a comparison intervention is not pertinent when a PICO question is about meaning such as, *Do family caregivers (P) of hospice patients feel anxiety (O) when providing hands-on care (I)?* Also, if there is no comparison intervention, only the standard of care, a (C) is not required. The elements of Population, an Intervention or issue of interest, and Outcome are essential for a well-designed PICO question involving an intervention.

A clearly stated PICO question helps to identify knowledge gaps for a specific clinical, educational, or managerial problem or situation. When you form well–thought-out questions, the type of evidence you lack for clinical practice becomes clearer when you

---

BOX 1.1

Developing a PICO Question

P   **Patient, population or problem**
Be succinct. Identify your patients by age, gender, ethnicity, disease, or symptoms.

I   **Intervention or issue of interest**
Which intervention do you think is worthwhile to use in practice? It can be a treatment; a clinical, educational, or administrative intervention; a process of care; an education strategy; or an assessment approach.

C   **Comparison with the intervention**
Does a comparison intervention exist? Which standard of care or current intervention do you usually use now in practice?

O   **Outcome (that is measurable)**
Which result do you wish to achieve or observe as a result of an intervention (e.g., change in patient's behavior, quality of life, physical finding; change in patient's perception, rate of adverse events, costs)?

T   **Time (an optional component for a clinical question)**

Adapted from Dearholt SL, Dang D: *Johns Hopkins nursing evidence-based practice: model and guidelines,* ed 2, Indianapolis, 2012, Sigma Theta Tau International; Purdue Libraries: *Evidence-based practice,* http://guides.lib.purdue.edu/content.php?pid=296535&sid=2435417, 2014. Accessed July 6, 2015; and University of Illinois at Chicago: *Evidence-based medicine,* PICO, 2015, http://researchguides.uic.edu/c.php?g=252338&p=1683349. Accessed July 6, 2015.

search the literature. Examples of different knowledge gaps include the following:

- *Diagnosis:* Questions about the selection and interpretation of diagnostic tests. *Example:* Does the use of a disposable oral thermometer compared with an electronic oral thermometer measure body temperature accurately in a patient with an endotracheal tube?
- *Prognosis:* Questions about a patient's likely clinical outcome. *Example:* Is there a difference in the incidence of deep vein thrombosis in surgical patients wearing sequential compression stockings compared to those who wear elastic stockings?
- *Therapy:* Questions about the selection of the most beneficial treatments. *Example:* Which bowel regimen is most effective in relieving constipation caused by the administration of opioid therapy in oncology patients with chronic pain?
- *Prevention:* Questions about screening and prevention methods to reduce the risk of disease. *Example:* Does the use of social media with education messages compared with informational brochures improve male adolescent's adherence to the human papillomavirus vaccine series?
- *Education:* Questions about best teaching strategies for colleagues, patients, or family members. *Example:* Is the use of motivational interviewing compared with low-literacy teaching booklets more effective to educate low-literacy adults about therapeutic diets?
- *Meaning:* Questions that seek understanding of a phenomenon. *Example:* How do patients with cervical cancer perceive their quality of life?

Search for the Best Evidence

Once you have a clear and concise PICO question, you are ready to search for evidence. Numerous research and non-research resources are available to aid in your search, including government and professional websites, agency procedure manuals, performance improvement reports, and computerized bibliographical databases. Do not hesitate to ask for help to find appropriate evidence. A reference librarian is an excellent resource with whom to collaborate to conduct a literature search. If one is not available, go to your faculty member or an advanced practice nurse within the health care institution.

A reference librarian knows the relevant databases available to you for a literature search about your PICO question (Box 1.2). The databases are repositories of published scientific studies, including peer-reviewed research. A peer-reviewed article is preferable for retrieval because it has been evaluated by a panel of experts familiar with the topic or subject matter of the article. Working with the librarian, you translate the elements of your PICO (T) question into the language or key words that will yield the best articles for your evidence search. For example, consider this PICO question: "Does motivational interviewing (I) compared with media instruction (C) improve oncology patients' (P) adherence to chemotherapy medications (O)?" The key words include oncology patient, motivational interviewing, media instruction, chemotherapy, and adherence. A good librarian will recommend using the indexing language or controlled vocabulary of the database that you are searching. The controlled vocabulary known as Medical Subject Headings (MeSH®) is updated annually from the US National Library of Medicine and contains over 220,000 terms (US National Library of Medicine, 2015). Proper use of MeSH® terms facilitates a more thorough and focused literature search than one you might get from simply trying to search combinations of key words on Google or Yahoo. In the previous example the word

---

BOX 1.2	
Searchable Scientific Literature Databases and Sources	
CINAHL	Cumulative Index of Nursing and Allied Health Literature; database for EBSCO nursing resources; includes studies in nursing, allied health, and biomedicine http://www.cinahl.com
MEDLINE	US National Library of Medicine®; bibliographical database that contains more than 22 million references to journal articles in life sciences with a concentration on biomedicine http://www.nlm.nih.gov/bsd/pmresources.html
EMBASE	Biomedical and pharmaceutical studies and abstracts and articles from biomedical, drug, and medical device conferences http://www.embase.com
PsycINFO	Interprofessional bibliographical resources in psychology and the behavioral and social sciences http://www.apa.org/psycinfo
Cochrane Community— Database of Systematic Reviews	Full text of regularly updated systematic reviews prepared by the Cochrane Collaboration; includes completed reviews and protocols http://community.cochrane.org/cochrane-reviews
National Guidelines Clearinghouse	Public resource for evidence-based clinical practice guidelines. Available through the Agency for Healthcare Research and Quality; contains structured abstracts (summaries) about clinical guidelines and their development; also includes condensed version of guidelines for viewing http://www.guideline.gov/index.aspx
PubMed	Health science library at the US National Library of Medicine; free access to more than 24 million citations for biomedical literature from MEDLINE, life science journals, and online books http://www.nlm.nih.gov

---

oncology might be entered instead as *cancer* to fit the database language; whereas *adherence* might be also entered as *compliance*.

When you work within a database you enter key words to search for articles. Because the vocabulary within published articles is often vague, the words that you select sometimes have one meaning to one author and a very different meaning to another. Each key word generates a set of articles. For example, in the PubMed database *oncology patient* generates over 196,000 articles, *adherence* generates 99,631 articles, and *chemotherapy* generates over 2,600,000 articles. That's a lot of reading! In this example you want to read only articles that address all three of the topics in the same article. There are several ways to reduce those thousands of articles to a more manageable number. One is by using Boolean operators or the function of Search Limits. You narrow a search by combining key terms from your PICO question using the Boolean connector *and*. For example, by entering the combination of "oncology patient *and* chemotherapy *and* adherence" into the literature database, you will only obtain a listing of the articles that contain all three terms; in this case it is 661 articles, which is still quite a few. A librarian can also show you how to use the Search Limits function. Your search can be further narrowed by limiting it by certain categories such as the time frame during which the article was

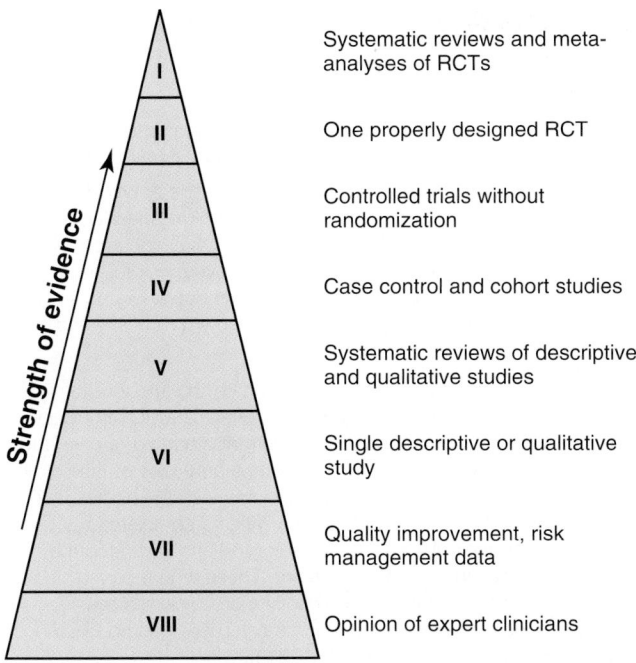

FIG 1.1 The evidence pyramid. *RCT*, Randomized controlled trial.

I — Systematic reviews and meta-analyses of RCTs

II — One properly designed RCT

III — Controlled trials without randomization

IV — Case control and cohort studies

V — Systematic reviews of descriptive and qualitative studies

VI — Single descriptive or qualitative study

VII — Quality improvement, risk management data

VIII — Opinion of expert clinicians

Strength of evidence

written, types of studies, English language publications, or age of patients. In this example, using limits of *humans, 5 years, English,* and *clinical trial,* the search now yields 73 articles. Use of Boolean connectors and Search Limits reduces the number of articles to a manageable number to review for a PICO question.

The pyramid in Fig. 1.1 represents a hierarchy for rating available scientific evidence that you obtain in your search. It is important to learn about the types of studies to help you know which ones have the best scientific evidence and thus which ones you choose to review. The strongest level of evidence is at the top of the pyramid; the weakest is at the bottom. You can use the rating scale of I to VIII when you later critique each article that you obtain in your search of the literature. Table 1.1 describes types of and provides examples of studies in the evidence hierarchy, beginning with the study at the top of the hierarchy, a systematic review.

If your PICO question leads you to an article that is a systematic review, celebrate! A systematic review is the perfect answer to a PICO question. Basically a researcher has asked the same PICO question you have asked and then examined all of the well-designed relevant research studies that ask the same question. The researcher creates a detailed and comprehensive plan and search strategy with the goal of reducing bias in any findings by identifying, appraising, and synthesizing all relevant studies on the topic (Uman, 2011). The researcher sets criteria for the type of studies to review in the search. A systematic review explains if the evidence for which you are searching about a specific question exists and whether it supports a change in practice. A systematic review of well-designed research studies provides the best evidence of the effectiveness of different interventions. A meta-analysis involves using statistical techniques to analyze the data from the studies in the systematic review to determine statistically the strength of the evidence.

A randomized controlled trial (RCT) is a formal experiment for testing therapies and establishing cause and effect. A researcher tests an intervention (e.g., a mobility program or new type of wound covering) against the usual standard of care. Researchers randomly assign subjects in an RCT to either a control or a treatment group. In other words, all of the subjects in the study have an equal chance of being assigned to either group. In that way it is not likely for the two groups to be highly different. The treatment group receives the experimental intervention at the same time the control group receives the usual standard of care. Both groups are measured for the same outcomes to determine if the experimental intervention made a difference. Following completion of an RCT, the researcher knows if the intervention leads to better outcomes than the standard of care. An RCT is an example of a clinical trial, a research study in which one or more human subjects are prospectively assigned to one or more interventions to evaluate the effects of those interventions on health-related biomedical or behavioral outcomes (NIH, 2014).

More often you find articles in the nursing literature that involve controlled trials without randomization (i.e., quasi-experimental studies) or descriptive studies. Even though these types of studies represent a lower level of evidence than RCTs, a study with relevant results helps you decide if your PICO question can be answered. For example if a quasi-experimental study resulted in a positive clinical improvement, even though it was not a statistically significant change, the clinical change might be worth strong consideration for reliable evidence.

The use of clinical experts is at the bottom of the evidence pyramid, but do not consider clinical experts a poor source of evidence. Expert clinicians frequently use evidence as they build their own practice, and they are rich sources of information for clinical problems.

Critique the Evidence

In the case study the nurses on the oncology unit conduct their unit practice committee (UPC) meeting. During the meeting Cathy and her colleagues decide that it is important to include key members of their interprofessional team (pharmacy and physical therapy). The UPC then reviews the articles carefully, using a rapid-appraisal checklist. After the group evaluates the articles for the strength of evidence and synthesizes the findings, they decide that there is evidence for implementing hourly rounding with focused patient assessment to prevent falls. The staff notes that one of the articles recommends hourly rounding during daytime hours and rounding every 2 hours during evening and night hours. Another article summarizes fall risks for patients in an acute care hospital and highlights factors to include in a nursing assessment such as medications (e.g., antihistamines, sedatives, analgesics, and antiemetics).

Critically reviewing and analyzing the available evidence requires a systematic approach. Each source of evidence (e.g., journal article, clinical guideline, expert summary) must be reviewed to determine its value, feasibility, and utility of evidence for making a practice change. Your review should allow you to determine if there is evidence that answers your question. It is important to use an approach that does not bog you down by reviewing every single element of each article. The use of critical appraisal checklists allows you to rapidly review each article from your search and answer four important questions (Centre for Evidence-Based Medicine, 2014):

1. Does this study address a clearly focused question?
2. Did the study use valid methods to address this question?
3. Are the results of the study valid and important?
4. Will these valid, important results help you provide better care for your patients?

Many organizations use appraisal checklists (Fig. 1.2) for recording article reviews. You begin an article review by determining if the question posed by the researcher is clear and concise. Does the article clearly explain the purpose, the research questions addressed, or aims of the study? Is the purpose of the article relevant to your PICO question? Next, is the research study well-designed? This

TABLE 1.1

Types of Studies in the Evidence Hierarchy

Study Type	Description	Example
Systematic review or meta-analysis	An author or panel of experts reviews the evidence from randomized controlled trials (RCTs) (and other defined types of research studies) about a specific clinical question and summarizes the state of the science. In a meta-analysis there is the addition of a statistical analysis that combines data from all studies.	This study aimed to examine the validity of using the Braden Scale in long-term care (LTC) settings. Eleven data sets from nine published studies describing 40,361 residents were analyzed. The appropriateness of the Braden Scale in LTC is questionable given its low specificity and positive predictive value. This means that the scale has high probability that subjects with a positive screening test truly have a risk for a pressure injury; however, if the result on the Braden Scale is positive, the certainty of the person actually having a pressure injury is low (Wilchesky and Lungu, 2015).
RCT	A researcher tests an intervention against the usual standard of care. Participants are randomly assigned to either a control group (receives standard care) or a treatment group (receives the experimental intervention), with both measured on the same outcomes to see if there is a difference.	This study, focusing on patient satisfaction, evaluated the impact of providing clinician photographs on inpatients' recall. The RCT involved three groups. A control group received the current standard of care; the second group received handouts with the names and roles of their clinical care team; and the third group received handouts with the names, roles, and photographs of their clinical care team. Patients completed a survey before discharge on their ability to recall their clinicians and rated the quality of communication with the care team. Those who received photos in the handout correctly identified significantly more clinicians by photograph and identified more clinician names. There was no difference in quality of communication (Appel et al., 2015).
Quasi-experimental study	This research approach tries to show that an intervention causes a particular outcome. This type of study is done when it is not practical, ethical, or possible to randomly assign subjects to experimental and control groups (Dearholt et al., 2012).	Hospitals routinely conduct regular surveillance on the incidence of ventilator-associated pneumonia (VAP) in intensive care units (ICUs). This study asked what would happen to the incidence of VAP if surveillance stopped. Surveillance was interrupted for a year in one ICU (A) and continued in a second (B). The incidence of VAP, mortality, and patient length of stay increased in the A unit. Surveillance provides important data feedback for ongoing performance improvement (Bénet et al., 2012).
Case control or cohort study	Researchers study one group of subjects with a certain condition (e.g., obesity) at the same time as another group of subjects who do not have the condition to determine if there is an association between the condition and predictor variables (e.g., exercise pattern, family history, history of depression).	This study examined nurse practitioner (NP) and physician assistant (PA) participation in direct patient care with ICUs. Patients in ICUs with NPs/PAs had lower mean Acute Physiology Scores and mechanical ventilation rates than ICUs without NPs/PAs). Results support that NPs/PAs are a safe adjunct to the ICU team. The findings support NP/PA management of critically ill patients (Costa et al., 2014).
Descriptive study	Study describes the concepts under study. It sometimes examines the prevalence, magnitude, and/or characteristics of a concept.	This study assessed the risk factors for infection in cancer patients receiving chemotherapy. Data were collected from patient medical records. Risk factors for infection in cancer patients receiving chemotherapy included alkylating agents and underlying diabetes mellitus (Park et al., 2015).
Qualitative study	Study examines individuals' perceptions of experiences with health problems or life events and the contexts in which the experiences occur. A qualitative study provides narrative data from extensive interviews with subjects. A qualitative researcher encourages subjects to tell their story about an event or condition to obtain a full and rich description.	Researchers analyzed interviews from patients and their health care providers following abdominal surgery to develop a conceptual framework for recovery after abdominal surgery. The most important concepts identified were "Energy level," "Sensation of pain," "General physical endurance," and "Carrying out daily routine." Researchers found that no current instruments for measuring recovery include all of these concepts (Lee et al., 2015).
Clinical experts	Accessing clinical experts on a nursing unit is an excellent way to learn about current evidence. Clinical experts often write clinical articles on topics that require application of evidence in the literature.	This article describes how using research and personal experience led to development of an approach to help a preceptor and new nurse make the most of the preceptor experience (Nooe and Kautz, 2015).

question requires knowing the type of study, using the evidence pyramid. For example, if you have an article on an RCT to review, were subjects randomized in the study? Was the sample of subjects large enough to test the intervention effectively? What approach was used in delivering the intervention and measuring the effects? Were all subjects measured for the same outcomes? In contrast, if you read a qualitative study, did the researcher study a sufficient number and representation of subjects, and did the approach allow for a thorough and objective review of findings? Studies that are not designed well cannot provide definitive support for the evidence they aim to produce.

As you read each article, you ask the next question: What are the results and were they important? Do the findings apply to your patients and practice setting? If you have an RCT, you want to know if an intervention worked or not to help decide if it potentially makes sense to use it in your practice. Your analysis of

Example of a Rapid Critical Appraisal Form

- Why was the study done? (Is there a clear explanation of the study purpose?)

- Are the study findings valid?
    How were study participants chosen? How many were chosen?
    Are the study instruments valid and reliable?
    Does the research approach fit the purpose of the study?
    How were accuracy and completeness of data ensured?
    Do the study findings fit the data that were generated?

- What are the results of the study, and are they important?
    Yes
    No
    Unknown

- Is the finding from the study clearly identified?

- Are the results logical, consistent, and easy to follow?

- Are the results plausible and believable?

- How do the results fit with previous research in the area?

- Will the results help me in caring for my patients?

- Do the results apply to my patients?

- How would I use the findings in my practice?

- How would patient and family values be considered in applying these results?

- Do we have the resources to apply this in our practice setting?

FIG 1.2 Example of a rapid critical appraisal form. *(Adapted from Melnyk B, et al: Evidence-based practice in nursing and health care: a guide to best practice, ed 3, Philadelphia, 2014, Wolters Kluwer; and Fineout-Overholt E, et al: Evidence-based practice step by step: critical appraisal of the evidence, Part 1, Am J Nurs 110(7):47, 2010.)*

statistics will help. For example, if an intervention was shown to be "statistically significant," the intervention shows benefit. If instead there was no statistically significant difference, you may reject the value of the intervention. However, if the intervention led to improvement even though not statistically significant, you might still consider it to have clinical value. If you have a descriptive study, you will decide if the information is relevant to your PICO question. For example, were characteristics of the patients in the study similar to those of your own patients?

You might also choose to review a clinical article that explains a clinical practice topic relevant to your PICO question. A clinical article is not rated for its level of evidence; but it can offer useful information, especially if you decide to implement a change related to the practice topic. To learn how to read research and clinical articles, know each of the common elements. This will help you decide if an article is complete and well explained. Articles should include the following elements:

- *Abstract:* A brief summary of the article that tells you if the article is research or clinically based. An abstract summarizes the purpose of the study or clinical topic, the major themes or findings, and the implications for practice.
- *Introduction:* Contains information about the purpose of the article and the importance of the topic for the audience who reads it. There is usually a brief discussion of supporting evidence about why the topic is important from the author's point of view.

After reading the abstract and introduction, decide if you want to continue to read the entire article. You will know if the topic of the article is similar to your PICO question or related closely enough to provide you useful information. Remember that the research question does not need to be the same as yours but close enough to offer useful information. If this is the case, continue to read the next elements of the article:

- *Literature review or background:* A good author offers a detailed background of the level of scientific or clinical information that exists about the topic of the article. The review explains what led the author to conduct a study or report on a clinical topic. Perhaps the article itself does not address your PICO question the way you desire but possibly leads you to other more useful articles. The literature review gives you a good idea of how past research led to the researcher's question.
- *Article narrative:* The "middle section" or narrative of an article differs, depending on whether it is clinical or research based (Melnyk and Fineout-Overholt, 2014). A clinical article describes a clinical topic, which often includes a description of a patient population, the nature of a certain disease or health problem, how it affects patients, and implications for nursing care. Clinical articles often describe how to use a therapy or new technology. A research article describes the conduct of a research study, including its purpose, how the study was designed, and the results. A

narrative of a research article contains several standard subsections:

- *Purpose statement:* Explains the focus or intent of a study. It identifies which concepts will be researched.
- *Methods or design:* Explains how a research study is organized and conducted to answer the research question(s). This is where you learn the type of study (i.e., RCT, case control, or qualitative). You also learn how many subjects or people are in a study. In health care studies subjects sometimes include patients, family members, or health care staff. The language in the methods section is sometimes confusing if it explains details about how the researcher designs the study to minimize bias so as to obtain the most accurate results possible. Use your faculty member as a resource to help interpret this section.
- *Results or Findings:* Clinical and research articles have a summary section. In a clinical article the author explains the clinical implications for the topic. In a research article the author explains the results and how the research question was answered. For example, in a qualitative study there is a thorough summary of subject narratives, which provide a description of themes and ideas that arise from the researcher's analysis of data. There is no statistical analysis of the data collected. A quantitative study includes a full description of the study subjects and a statistical analysis of findings. It is important to learn some of the common statistical terms (Box 1.3). A good author discusses limitations to a study in the results section. The information on limitations helps you decide if you want to use the evidence from the article with your patients.
- *Clinical implications:* A research article includes a section that explains if the findings from the study have clinical implications. The researcher explains how to apply findings in a practice setting for the type of subjects studied.

As you critique each article, complete your critical appraisal checklist. You may choose to rate each article by its level and strength of evidence, using the scale of I to VIII from the evidence pyramid (see Fig. 1.1). It also helps to review multiple articles with a group of colleagues involved in the EBP process. Each person can review a single article; then you can come together as a group to review your total findings. Remember, when reviewing evidence, a recommendation to change practice should not rely solely on a single study or the opinion of a single expert (Poe and White, 2010). Once all evidence has been reviewed, it is time to discuss the third important question: Will the results help you care for your patients?

Use critical thinking to consider the scientific rigor of the evidence and how well it answers your area of interest. Scientific rigor is the extent to which the findings of a study are valid, reliable, and relevant to a patient population of interest. Consider the evidence in light of your patients' concerns and preferences. Your review of articles offers a snapshot conclusion based on combined evidence about one focused topical area. As a clinician, judge whether to use the evidence for a particular patient or group of patients who usually have complex medical histories and patterns of responses (Melnyk and Fineout-Overholt, 2014). Ethically always consider evidence that will benefit patients and do no harm. Decide if the evidence is relevant, is easily applicable in your setting of practice, and has the potential for improving patient outcomes.

There will be times when you find that there is insufficient or no evidence to answer a PICO question. This finding warrants no change in practice because the evidence is weak and inconsistent or absent.

Apply the Evidence—Project Management

If a literature review and critique yield evidence that answers your PICO question and offer evidence that can be applied to practice, the next step is to implement an EBP project. An EBP team must be able to manage an EBP project (such as a new fall prevention protocol) to ensure completion of project tasks and translation of the evidence findings into daily practice (Poe and White, 2010). In other words, a team must introduce practice changes successfully. A successful EBP project involves the following:

1. A sponsor (e.g., an advanced practice nurse, nurse manager, or senior staff nurse) who has the commitment and expertise to make the project succeed.
2. Sufficient resources to accomplish the project, including time (e.g., staff having time to attend meetings, collect data), support of all team members, infrastructure of the unit where change will occur (e.g., how procedures are performed, unit setting), and equipment and supplies (depending on project).
3. Clear identification of outcomes to be measured to determine if the EBP practice change is a success (outcomes are a component of the PICO question, but a team must know how to measure them consistently). **NOTE:** Outcomes should be measured before the pilot to have a baseline to determine if the intervention leads to a change.
4. Time schedule for project. It is recommended you pilot test a practice change a minimum of 3 months and gather outcome measures throughout this time.
5. Communication and orientation plan. It is critical to be sure that all staff involved in any EBP change are informed and educated (if necessary) to be able to perform the practice change.

Common Statistical Terms

Sample Size: Number (n) of individuals in a study.

Significance: A measure that gives the likelihood that a finding or a result of a study is caused by the intervention being tested and not simply by chance. Most researchers set the level of significance at a p value of 0.05 or 0.01. For example, if the effects of an intervention (e.g., hourly rounding) are significant at $p < 0.05$, it means that the likelihood of the effect (fewer falls) occurring by chance is less than 5%; thus it is 95% more likely that the intervention truly had an effect in reducing falls. When a study result has a p value (0.61) greater than that set (e.g., p value 0.05), the researcher has to conclude that the results were possibly by chance and the intervention had no effect.

Confidence interval (CI): The range (e.g., range of a mean score) in which clinicians can expect to get results if they present an intervention in the same way as it was in a study (Fineout-Overholt et al., 2010). The CI tells you the precision of a study. A 95% CI means that clinicians can be 95% confident that their findings will be within the range given in the study.

Effect size: When the effect of an intervention is statistically significant, it does not necessarily mean that it is big, important, or helpful in decision making. It simply means that you can be confident that there is a difference. An effect size greater than 0.05 is considered a large effect.

In the case study, the oncology UPC has completed the literature review. The nurse specialist takes the lead for the team. On the basis of the evidence, the committee members' experiences, a review of the unit fall rate reports, and knowledge of their patients' risk factors, the UPC recommends a new fall prevention program for the unit.

The UPC also recommends piloting the new program for 3 months. The evidence-based program includes several features. The patients on the unit fall during all hours of the day and night; therefore hourly rounding will be implemented around-the-clock. The evidence review revealed information allowing the team to develop a focused fall screening tool and nursing assessments for key fall risk factors. Registered nurses (RNs) will round on patients on all even hours and conduct the focused assessments of fall risk factors for oncology patients identified from the literature such as lower-extremity weakness, impaired gait, general fatigue, and use of antihistamines. The nurses will inform each patient of their personal fall risks.

A project should apply evidence in a manner that integrates well with existing practice for all affected disciplines.

In the case study, if an oncology patient is found to be at high fall risk, the physical therapists will be asked to consult and assess the patient's lower-extremity strength and overall balance and make therapy recommendations. The pharmacy will place alerts on medication administration records so nurses can monitor patients receiving antihistamines before blood transfusions. Nursing assistive personnel (NAP) will round on odd hours and do follow-up observations to be sure that patients have their toileting needs met, are comfortable, and have no further needs. Patients will be told that every hour someone will return to their room for another check.

The nurse specialist has talked with the unit manager, presented the pilot plan, and obtained commitment from the manager to move forward with the project. The UPC works with the manager to create a staff orientation schedule and sets a date for the start of the hourly rounding program pilot. Before the start date the nurse specialist gathers the fall rate data and falls with injuries from the last 3 months for baseline measures. To evaluate the process for program piloting, the team will also collect short surveys from all staff members to determine their reactions to and acceptance of the program.

It is important to have a well-organized EBP project management plan. If the barriers to practice change are excessive, adopting a practice change can be difficult, if not impossible. For example, if the oncology unit's fall program is too difficult for staff to complete, if there is inadequate staffing, or if not all staff are able to attend orientation sessions, the program may not be successful.

Outcome Measurement

During an EBP pilot project, collection of outcome measures is critical. This involves knowing the measures to collect and having a process for consistent reliable data collection.

1. Plan how to collect baseline data on the outcomes that will evaluate the effect of your practice change (e.g., the oncology nurse specialist will be able to use the unit's monthly quality performance report that includes fall rate and fall with injuries. The nurse specialist collects values for 3 months before implementation of the program. The nurse specialist will continue to collect the fall rate and the fall-related injury rate each month, once the new program pilot begins.

   a. Know which outcomes to measure and how to collect the measures consistently (e.g., to measure pain acuity use a self-report pain scale; to measure ambulation determine the distance a patient walks each time).

   b. Be sure that the outcomes are measurable (Box 1.4). Use scales (e.g., pain and Braden Scales), physiological measures (e.g., temperature, blood pressure, pulse oximetry), survey tools, and performance improvement reports.

   c. Choose outcomes that are not costly to collect. Use existing equipment if you can.

   d. Educate team members on the approach to use to collect and record outcomes.

Outcome Measurements

Outcome	Outcome Measure
Fall occurrence	Fall index, falls with injuries
Medication adherence	Pill counts, patient self-report, number of filled prescriptions
Learning discharge instructions (topic specific)	Patient surveys, including questions on topic; nurse observations of patients performing skills (using a rating scale)
Infection occurrence	Monthly infection control reports of laboratory tests on infection incidence

---

e. Limit the number of staff who collect data to ensure better accuracy and consistency in measurement. Be sure that each person collects data the same way, at the same time or frequency, and accurately.

f. Establish a way to record all data.

The goal of any EBP change is to ensure the highest quality of care by using evidence that promotes the best outcomes (Poe and White, 2010). Proper planning is essential before and as you implement your practice change. Once you implement your intervention, monitor the project closely and consider how staff and patients are responding.

Evaluate the Practice Decision or Change

After implementing a practice change, your next step is to evaluate the outcomes. You do this by analyzing the outcome data that you collected before and during the pilot project. Outcome evaluation tells you if your practice change improved conditions, created no change, or worsened conditions. Here are some examples. After using a new, transparent IV dressing, the staff analyzed their audits, which included the incidence of dislodged IVs and the incidence and rating of phlebitis. Their findings showed reduction in the number of catheters that became dislodged and in the onset and severity of phlebitis. The recommendation for this project would continue use of the new dressing. After using a new approach to educating clinic patients about medications and administration schedules, follow-up phone calls to patients found an improved understanding of doses and times to administer. However, patients were not able to explain which side effects to expect. The staff involved with this EBP project created single-page bullet points about common side effects of medications and continued to evaluate the pilot an additional 3 months.

Once an evaluation is complete, you must decide to continue the EBP, make a revision, or discontinue the practice change. Consider not only if the outcomes were met but also whether or not patients, families, or staff were affected in other ways by the change. Analysis of an EBP change may require assistance from statisticians if you or your team members collect extensive data. Be sure to use reliable resources and be thorough in examining all data.

On the oncology unit the UPC made sure that outcome measures were in place before implementing the fall prevention program. The fall rate and falls with injuries were collected from monthly quality performance reports and included each of the 3 months before implementation and then for 3 months after the program began. The UPC designated three staff members to also collect surveys from staff at 1 month and 3 months to see how their colleagues were reacting to the new program. Three months after implementing the program, the oncology unit was cautiously optimistic. The average fall rate for the unit dropped from 5.1 to 3.9; and the injury rate also dropped, from 2 during the first 3 months to only 1 after the pilot began. Although it was not an outcome measure, the nurses observed a decline in patients' use of call lights, which was attributed to their knowing that nurses and assistive personnel would visit frequently. The nursing and physical therapy staff surveys revealed that the majority were enthused and agreed that hourly rounding needed to be a routine part of their unit practice. The nursing staff was able to see that the fall prevention program improved patient outcomes and gave them more time to coordinate care because of fewer distractions from patient calls.

Communicate and Disseminate a Practice Change

Six months after starting the new fall prevention protocol, the fall index of the oncology unit continues to remain low. An added outcome is an improvement in patient satisfaction scores. Cathy submits the protocol for an abstract in the hospital publication, *Nursing Practice*. The outcomes of the oncology UPC project result in the development of hospital-wide hourly rounding protocols. Other units reviewed the literature to customize the nursing assessment to their particular patient needs. The methodical and well-designed EBP project led by the oncology UPC resulted in establishment of an evidence-based standard for other nursing units in the hospital.

After applying evidence, it is important to communicate the change in practice and the results to nursing and other health care colleagues. This is true whether the results are successful or unsuccessful. There are many ways to communicate the outcomes of EBP: talking with a colleague, sharing results in staff meetings, presenting in workshops or seminars, submitting an abstract for a poster presentation, and publishing an article. As a professional you are responsible for communicating important information about nursing practice. Sharing evidence and the effects of any practice change motivates others within a health care setting and makes them excited about potential practice improvements on their work units. When you successfully adopt an EBP way of thinking, it becomes very natural to talk about available evidence and continue seeking solutions for problems in patient care.

SUSTAINING EVIDENCE-BASED PRACTICE CHANGES

Implementing EBP changes in a health care setting takes time and commitment to do it well. What is even more difficult is sustaining the changes over time. Chambers et al. (2013) describe an important process, dynamic sustainability. The process involves continued learning and problem solving and ongoing adaptation of interventions so they continue to fit the practice environments and needs of patients and expectations for ongoing improvement as opposed to diminishing outcomes over time. Competency in EBP requires a commitment to learning new scientific knowledge, working with teams to appropriately apply and later adapt new interventions in practice, and then finding ways to maintain and continue interventions that are consistently effective. Patients expect nursing professionals to be informed and to use the safest and most appropriate interventions. Use of evidence enhances nursing practice and improves patients' outcomes.

◆ CLINICAL DEBRIEF

An orthopedic interprofessional team composed of staff nurses, a physical therapist, and an orthopedic surgeon has been discussing the care of patients undergoing total hip replacements. The surgeon believes that the patients should be reaching a higher level of mobility before being discharged. The physical therapist shares concerns about not being able to see all patients in a timely manner since the number of surgeries performed has increased. The staff nurses have noted that patients' family members always seem interested in their patients' progress. One registered nurse shares a story about a daughter of a patient who spent time coaching her father to walk a bit further, and it seemed to help. The team wonders if the family could be a more involved resource. They want to use an evidence-based approach to improve patient care.

1. Write a PICO question for the orthopedic team's area of clinical interest.
2. The staff nurse who chairs the unit practice committee contacts the hospital librarian to collaborate on a literature search to find articles pertinent to the PICO question. The nurse tells the librarian that the team wants to see if there is evidence for their approach to improving patient mobility. The librarian helps the nurse select indexing language from the database that will be searched. Which alternative MeSH® terms might you give the librarian for the term *mobility*?
3. The staff meets to review the articles obtained from the literature review. Each member selects an article to review. The physical therapist reviews and presents a study involving testing of an educational approach for patients who underwent knee-replacement surgery. Patients were randomly assigned to one of two groups: one group received standard patient education brochures about their surgery, and the other group attended a preoperative teaching class in which

their family caregivers participated. The researcher compared the two groups for the discharge outcomes of length of stay and postoperative ambulation.
   a. Which type of study was reviewed by the physical therapist?
   b. List two reasons why this study might be useful to the interprofessional team in planning their evidence-based practice (EBP) project.
   c. List two reasons why this study might not be useful to the team in planning their EBP project.
4. Identify two ways members of the interprofessional team might decide to measure mobility and how might they reach that decision in the context of who is on the team?

◆ REVIEW QUESTIONS

1. Place the steps of evidence-based practice in the correct order:
   1 _____ Search the literature using MeSH® terms and limits to gather evidence.
   2 _____ Evaluate outcomes of the practice change.
   3 _____ Report the findings in a newsletter to staff.
   4 _____ Apply the evidence by changing a practice protocol.
   5 _____ Identify a problem in practice and ask a PICO question.
   6 _____ Review the articles obtained from the literature review and critique the available evidence.
2. A nurse specialist is reviewing the outcome measures collected during an evidence-based practice (EBP) project on a surgical unit. The EBP

team applied evidence about giving around-the-clock (ATC) analgesics to postoperative patients instead of traditional prn (as needed) medications. The use of ATC analgesics started in September.

a. Review the graph and describe the change in analgesic doses and pain scores.

b. Explain if the changes were to be expected as a result of the EBP change.

	June	July	Aug	Sept	Oct	Nov
Average amount of analgesic doses per patient/day in first 48 h	8.5	9.0	8.1	10.1	11.4	12.0
Average pain scores						
24 h post op	5.4	5.1	4.8	4.1	3.7	3.5
48 h post op	4.9	4.2	4.6	3.9	4.1	3.3

3. An evidence-based practice (EBP) committee on a medicine unit has selected a PICO question and reviewed and critiqued the literature and is now ready to proceed with an EBP project. Which of the following factors are essential for successful EBP project management? (Select all that apply.)

1. A sufficient number of articles providing evidence for the PICO question
2. A sponsor who has the commitment and expertise to make the project succeed
3. Resources to accomplish the project
4. Time schedule for a pilot project
5. Sufficient number of outcomes to be measured to determine that the EBP practice change is a success.

ⓔ *Visit the Evolve site for a complete list of Clinical Debrief and Review Questions answers.*

REFERENCES

Appel L, et al: Put a face to a name: a randomized controlled trial evaluating the impact of providing clinician photographs on inpatients' recall, *Am J Med* 128(1):82, 2015.

Bénet T, et al: Impact of surveillance of hospital-acquired infections on the incidence of ventilator-associated pneumonia in intensive care units: a quasi-experimental study, *Crit Care* 16(4):R161, 2012.

Centre for Evidence-Based Medicine: Critical appraisal tools, 2014, http://www.cebm.net/critical-appraisal/. Accessed July 8, 2015.

Chambers DA, et al: The dynamic sustainability framework: addressing the paradox of sustainment amid ongoing change, *Implement Sci* 8:117, 2013.

Conway-Phillips R, Janusek L: Influence of sense of coherence, spirituality, social support and health perception on breast cancer screening motivation and behaviors in African-American women, *ABNF J* 25(3):72, 2014.

Costa DK, et al: Nurse practitioner/physician assistant staffing and critical care mortality, *Chest* 146(6):1566, 2014.

Dearholt SL, et al: *Johns Hopkins nursing evidence-based practice: model and guidelines*, ed 2, Indianapolis, 2012, Sigma Theta Tau International.

Fineout-Overholt E, et al: Evidence-based practice, step by step: critical appraisal of the evidence, Part II, *Am J Nurs* 110(9):41, 2010.

Infusion Nurses Society (INS): Infusion nursing standards of practice, *J Infus Nurs* 34(1S):2011.

Ingersoll GI, et al: Meeting Magnet research and evidence-based practice expectations through hospital-based research centers, *Nurs Econ* 28(4):226, 2010.

Institute of Medicine (IOM): The future of nursing: leading change, advancing health, Robert Wood Johnson Foundation Initiative on the Future of Nursing at the Institute of Medicine, October 5, 2010, http://www.iom.edu/Reports/2010/The-Future-of-Nursing-Leading-Change-Advancing-Health.aspx. Accessed July 6, 2015.

Institute of Medicine (IOM): Announcement: crossing the quality chasm: the IOM health care quality initiative, 2013, www.iom.edu/Global/News%20Announcements/Crossing-the-Quality-Chasm-The-IOM-Health-Care-Quality-Initiative.aspx. Accessed July 6, 2015.

Lee L, et al: How well are we measuring postoperative "recovery" after abdominal surgery? *Qual Life Res* 24:2583, 2015.

Melnyk BM, Fineout-Overholt E: *Evidence-based practice in nursing and healthcare: a guide to best practice*, ed 3, Philadelphia, 2014, Wolters Kluwer.

National Institute of Health (NIH): *Notice of revised NIH definition of "clinical trial*, 2014. https://grants.nih.gov/grants/guide/notice-files/NOT-OD-15-015.html. Accessed October 24, 2015.

National Pressure Ulcer Advisory Panel: National Pressure Ulcer Advisory Panel (NPUAP) announces a change in terminology form pressure ulcer to pressure injury and updates the stages of pressure injury, Press Release, April 13, 2016, http://www.npuap.org/national-pressure-ulcer-advisory-panel-npuap-announces-a-change-in-terminology-from-pressure-ulcer-to-pressure-injury-and-updates-the-stages-of-pressure-injury/.

Nooe A, Kautz DD: Preceptorship: combining experience with research, *Dimens Crit Care Nurs* 34(2):81, 2015.

Park JH, et al: A retrospective analysis to identify the factors affecting infection in patients undergoing chemotherapy, *Eur J Oncol Nurs* 2015. ii:S1462(15)00052-6. [Epub ahead of print].

Poe SS, White KM: *Johns Hopkins nursing evidence-based practice: implementation and translation*, Indianapolis, 2010, Sigma Theta Tau International.

QSEN Institute: Pre-Licensure KSA's, 2014, http://qsen.org/competencies/pre-licensure-ksas/. Accessed June 20, 2015.

Sandstrom B, et al: Promoting the implementation of evidence-based practice: a literature review focusing on the role of nursing leadership, *Worldviews Evid Based Nurs* 8(4):212, 2011.

Stevens K: The impact of evidence-based practice in nursing and the next big ideas, *Online J Issues Nurs* 18(2):2013.

Straus SE: *Evidence-based medicine: how to practice and teach EBM*, ed 4, Edinburgh, 2011, Elsevier/Churchill Livingstone.

Uman LS: Systematic reviews and meta-analyses, *J Can Acad Child Adolesc Psychiatry* 20(1):57, 2011.

US National Library of Medicine: Fact Sheet: Medical Subject Headings (MeSH®), 2015, http://www.nlm.nih.gov/pubs/factsheets/mesh.html. Accessed July 6, 2015.

White ML: Spirituality self-care effects on quality of life for patients diagnosed with chronic illness, *Self Care Depend Care Nurs* 20(1):23, 2013.

Wilchesky M, Lungu O: Predictive and concurrent validity of the Braden Scale in long-term care: a meta-analysis, *Wound Repair Regen* 23(1):44, 2015.

2 | Admitting, Transfer, and Discharge

OBJECTIVES

Mastery of content in this chapter will enable the nurse to:
- Describe the role communication plays in maintaining continuity of care through a patient's admission, transfer, and discharge from an acute care agency.
- Explain the purpose and importance of discharge planning.
- Identify the ongoing needs of patients in the discharge planning process.
- Explain the role of a patient's family in the admission, transfer, or discharge process.

MEDIA RESOURCES

- evolve http://evolve.elsevier.com/Perry/skills
- Review Questions
- Audio Glossary
- Clinical Debrief and Review Questions Answers

PURPOSE

The coordination of resources and planning a patient's care from admission to discharge or from one level of care to the next is a key role of a nurse. Nurses identify patients' ongoing health care needs and anticipate physical, psychological, and social deficits that have implications for patients to resume normal activities. A nurse involves appropriate family members in a plan of care; provides interventions, including health education; and assists in making health care resources available to patients.

STANDARDS OF CARE

- The Joint Commission (TJC), 2016—Patient identification and medication reconciliation
- The Joint Commission (TJC), 2016—Admission assessment, restraints, and effective communication
- QSEN, 2014—Patient-centered care skills

PRINCIPLES FOR PRACTICE

- Patients and families should be partners in care, sharing in the process of decision making.
- Patient care must be integrated across a variety of settings, services, health care practitioners, and care levels to maintain a continuum of care.
- Transitional care involves nursing actions implemented to ensure coordination and continuity of care for patients who transfer between different settings or levels of care.
- Transitions of care require careful attention to communication to ensure patient safety.
- Discharge planning begins at the time of admission to a hospital, or even earlier when a patient uses an outpatient clinic or testing center to begin his or her care journey.

PATIENT-CENTERED CARE

- In the United States many individuals face greater obstacles to good health on the basis of one or more of the following factors: racial or ethnic group; religion; socioeconomic status; gender; age; mental health; cognitive, sensory, or physical disability; sexual orientation or gender identity; geographical location; or other characteristics historically linked to discrimination or exclusion (USDHHS, 2015). Your admission assessment must incorporate patients' cultural beliefs and practices so you can provide a patient-centered approach to care.
- Be aware of how cultural variables will affect your patient and family assessment, approach to nursing care, and teaching during admission or discharge. It is essential to involve the patient and family caregiver in making decisions about care activities.
- Ask the patient their preferred communication style or language and modify your approach to meet his or her needs as appropriate. Inadequate access to language services compromise patient outcomes (NQF, 2012).

EVIDENCE-BASED PRACTICE

Nurse-to-nurse hand-offs during care transitions (e.g., shift-to-shift or transfer to different service setting) can create important information gaps, omissions, and errors in patient care (Staggers and Blaz, 2013).
- Verbal hand-offs serve important functions beyond information transfer and should be retained in practice. Greater

consideration is needed on analyzing hand-offs from a patient-centered perspective. Hand-off methods should be highly tailored to nurses and their contextual needs in the settings in which they work (Staggers and Blaz, 2013).

- The use of hand-offs performed effectively can result in better communication of patient fall risk or potential for impaired skin integrity and help to prevent patient injury resulting from falls or pressure injuries. In addition, an effective hand-off can improve communication about patients' medications and reduce medication errors (Vandenberg, 2013).
- The use of a standardized hand-off form can reduce hand-off–related errors and help to ensure that critical information is communicated (Zou and Zhang, 2016)

Medication reconciliation involves the process of creating the most accurate list possible of all medications a patient is taking, including drug name, dosage, frequency, and route; and comparing that list against a physician's admission, transfer, and/or discharge orders, with the goal of providing correct medications to the patient at all transition points within a hospital (IHI, 2016).

- Medication reconciliation avoids medication errors such as omissions, duplications, dosing errors, or drug interactions (Kwan et al., 2013; TJC, 2016a).
- Medications need to be reviewed with the patient on admission by either nursing staff or pharmacy. They need to be reviewed once again at discharge and shared with the postdischarge providers to ensure that they understand any changes that were made. This is necessary to reduce adverse drug events and improve patient outcomes (TJC, 2016a).

- A systematic review of the literature demonstrates that medication reconciliation programs targeted at high-risk populations such as the elderly, patients with co-morbidities, and patients on multiple medications can have the greatest impact on reducing adverse drug events (Mueller et al., 2012).
- Successful medication reconciliation interventions include intensive pharmacy staff involvement.

SAFETY GUIDELINES

- Identify whether a patient has a sensory or communication need (e.g., hearing aid, glasses, need for an interpreter).
- Identify if a patient uses any assistive devices and be sure that each is provided and deemed safe to use.
- Screen all patients on admission to a health care setting for possible discharge needs to ensure that appropriate teaching is completed to ensure a safe discharge.
- Include the patient, family caregiver, and relevant health care professionals early in planning care to promote successful transition through the health care system.
- Consider a patient's educational background, health literacy level, and ability to understand instructions.
- Coordinate the health care providers who contribute to a patient's care needs to develop a plan of care for discharge to ensure a safe transition to home or an alternate care facility.
- Help other health care personnel (e.g., dietitian, social worker, pharmacist, physical therapist) assess appropriate resources needed as patients transition through the health care system.

◆ SKILL 2.1   Admitting Patients

Patients enter health care systems in a variety of ways (e.g., hospital, clinic, or physician's or health care provider's offices). The admission process is typically the first experience a patient has with a health care agency. There are common procedures for admitting patients to these settings (Box 2.1). Most patients enter a health care system through a scheduled admission process that often requires an extensive registration. However, some patients require emergency admissions. A patient admitted through the emergency department (ED) is often not able to undergo the same registration process that takes place in a hospital admission office. Level of consciousness, pain, or other symptoms may prevent the patient from being a reliable resource. Family members usually provide

pertinent information for the hospital records while the staff are caring for the patient. In contrast, an older-adult patient with self-care limitations undergoes extensive screening before being accepted as a nursing home resident.

Admission officers, secretaries, and technicians are the personnel involved in the preliminary admission process such as interviewing patients and reviewing information about insurance, demographic data, and agency procedures. Technicians usually collect routine specimens and perform screening procedures such as electrocardiograms (ECGs). A nurse performs the nursing admission assessment (see Chapter 6).

Role of the Admission Personnel

The admission personnel initiate and maintain a courteous and professional relationship with patients while providing information about their safety, legal rights, and privacy. A private interview area gives patients and families a place to reveal important identifying information, including a patient's full legal name, age, birth date, address, next of kin, health care provider, religious preference, occupation, and type of insurance. When a patient has severe hearing impairment, the family or a speech and language pathologist may assist. If a patient does not speak English, a professional interpreter helps during the admission procedure.

The admission personnel secures an identification (ID) band legibly stating a patient's full legal name, hospital or agency number, health care provider, and birth date to the patient's wrist. Health care providers use information from the ID band to identify a patient when performing treatments or procedures. In many

---

BOX 2.1

Common Procedures for Admission to a Health Care System

- Placement of patient in appropriate receiving area
- Explanation of patient's rights (CMS, 2009) and elements of advance directives
- Orientation to relevant health care agency policies and procedures and room environment
- Assessment of patient's health care problems and needs (including risk for falls, pressure injuries, and allergies)
- Preliminary testing and screening (specific for each agency and patient's condition)
- Development of a patient-centered plan of care
- Determination of patient's payment source for health care

agencies an ID band contains a patient's unique bar code that then makes it easy to identify a patient for all ordered procedures. Bar-code wristbands are typically created at the point of admission, and specific patient information is continually updated on the basis of patients' needs (Torres, 2012). If a patient is unconscious, you cannot perform ID until family members arrive or unless you have a bar-code system. Hospital staff provide a patient who has been a victim of crime with an anonymous name on his or her ID band under the agency's "blackout" or "do not publish" procedure.

A patient's legal rights are met by instructing the patient or legal guardian to read the general consent form for treatment. The Centers for Medicare and Medicaid (CMS) (2012a) require all patients to receive information regarding their rights related to health care services at admission; otherwise the hospital will not receive reimbursement for services (Box 2.2). The CMS requires

that information be available in multiple languages and alternate formats (e.g., audio, visual, or written). Other regulatory agencies such as The Joint Commission (TJC) also require agencies to provide for specific patient rights (Box 2.3). Each agency has policies and procedures describing a patient's rights and the role of nurses in ensuring those rights.

The Patient Self-Determination Act, effective December 1, 1991, requires all Medicare- and Medicaid-recipient hospitals to provide patients with information about their right to accept or reject medical treatment. At the time of registration patients receive information about advance directives and are referred to appropriate resources if they want to discuss advance directives or receive help in completing an advance directive document (Box 2.4).

On admission patients must also receive information about the Health Insurance Portability and Accountability Act (HIPAA), a

---

BOX 2.2

Patients' Rights Provided for by CMS

Code of Federal Regulations Title 42, Chapter IV, Part 482, Sec. 482.13 Condition of Participation: Patients' Rights

Standard 1: Notice of Rights
- A hospital must protect and promote each patient's rights.
- A hospital must inform each patient whenever possible or, when appropriate, the patient's representative of the patient's rights in advance of furnishing or discontinuing patient care.
- The hospital must have a process for prompt resolution of patient grievances and must inform each patient whom to contact to file a grievance.

Standard 2: Exercise of Rights
- The patient has the right to participate in the development and implementation of his or her plan of care.
- The patient or his or her representative has the right to make informed decisions regarding his or her care.
- The patient's rights include being informed of his or her health status, involved in care planning and treatment, and able to request or refuse treatment. This right must not be construed as a mechanism to demand the provision of treatment or services deemed medically unnecessary or inappropriate.
- The patient has the right to formulate advance directives and have hospital staff and practitioners who provide care in the hospital comply with these directives.
- The patient has the right to have a family member or representative of his or her choice and his or her own health care provider notified promptly of his or her admission to the hospital.

Standard 3: Privacy and Safety
- The patient has the right to personal privacy.
- The patient has the right to receive care in a safe setting.
- The patient has the right to be free from all forms of abuse or harassment.

Standard 4: Confidentiality of Patient Record
- The patient has the right to the confidentiality of his or her clinical records.
- The patient has the right to access information contained in his or her clinical records within a reasonable time frame.

Standard 5: Restraint or Seclusion
- The patient has the right to be free from physical or mental abuse and corporal punishment.

- The patient has the right to be free from restraints or seclusion of any form that is not medically necessary or is used as a means of coercion, discipline, convenience, or retaliation by staff. A restraint is any manual method, physical or mechanical device, material, or equipment that immobilizes or reduces the ability of a patient to move his or her arms, legs, body, or head freely. A drug used as a restraint is a medication used to manage the patient's behavior or to restrict the patient's freedom of movement and is not a standard treatment or dosage for the patient's medical or psychiatric condition. Seclusion is the involuntary confinement of a patient alone in a room or area from which the patient is physically prevented from leaving.
- A restraint does not include devices such as orthopedically prescribed devices, surgical dressing or bandages, protective helmets, or other methods that involve the physical holding of a patient for the purpose of conducting routine physical examinations or tests, to protect the patient from falling out of bed, or to permit the patient to participate in activities without the risk of physical harm (this does not include a physical escort).
- A restraint or seclusion can only be used if needed to improve the patient's well-being and less restrictive interventions have been determined to be ineffective.
- The use of a restraint or seclusion must be selected only when other less restrictive measures have been found to be ineffective to protect the patient or others from harm and in accordance with the order of a physician or other licensed independent practitioner.
- This order must never be written as a standing order or on an as-needed basis (i.e., prn). The order must be followed by consultation with the patient's treating physician as soon as possible if someone other than the patient's treating physician or health care provider ordered the restraint or seclusion.
- The use of a restraint or seclusion must be:
  - In accordance with a written modification to the patient's plan of care.
  - Implemented in the least restrictive manner possible.
  - In accordance with safe and appropriate restraining techniques.
  - Ended at the earliest possible time.
- The condition of the restrained or secluded patient must be assessed, monitored, and reevaluated continually.
- All staff who have direct patient contact must have ongoing education and training in the proper and safe use of restraints and seclusion.

Modified from Centers for Medicare and Medicaid Services: Medicare and Medicaid programs, hospital conditions of participation: patients' rights; final rule, *Fed Reg* 71(236):71426, 2009.
CMS, Centers for Medicare and Medicaid Services.

federal law finalized in 2003 designed to protect the privacy of patient health information and referred to as *protected health information (PHI)* (US Department of Health and Human Services [USDHHS], 2003). Health information refers to any information (oral or recorded) in any form that is created or received by a health care provider, health plan, public health authority, employer, life insurer, school or university, or health care clearinghouse and relates to the past, present, or future physical or mental health or condition of any individual; the provision of health care to an individual; or the past, present, or future payment for the provision of health care to an individual (HIPAA, 2009). Individually identifiable health information is information that is a subset of health information, including demographic information (e.g., age, social security number, electronic mail address) collected from an individual. Three key concepts of HIPAA are: (1) agencies are required to inform patients of the privacy rights they have and how the

agency will handle their PHI; (2) the agency and the health care providers are to use or disclose a patient's PHI only for the purposes of treatment, payment, or health care operations; and (3) health care providers disclose only the minimum amount of PHI necessary, on a need-to-know basis, to accomplish the purpose of the use. In addition to existing laws, new proposals include allowing patients to know who has accessed their information (USDHHS, 2011). Know your agency-specific policies and procedures related to HIPAA.

Role of the Nurse

On admission to a patient care area, nurses complete a thorough nursing assessment, review any advance directives, and ensure that necessary diagnostic testing is completed. If patients were receiving health care before admission (e.g., home health care, long-term care), a nurse from the sending area provides appropriate information to the receiving nurse for continuity of care. In this situation the nurse from the sending agency should explain to the nurse receiving the hand-off report information about the patient's condition and why he or she is being sent to the acute care setting (Toles et al., 2012).

Admitting personnel collaborate with receiving nursing staff to ensure that a patient's room assignment is based on the patient's condition, health care needs, developmental level, activity level, expected length of stay, and personal preferences. For example, the best room for an older patient who is acutely ill, at risk for falls, and receiving multiple treatments is one close to the nurses' station. The nurse identifies if a patient has any known allergies and, if any exist, places an allergy band on the patient and properly documents the known allergies in the medical record.

When a patient is admitted through the ED, the nurse notifies the nursing division and reports on the patient's admission information, including his or her name; admitting physician or health care provider; chief complaint; and any treatments or testing completed and the outcome, diagnosis, and pertinent information related to the patient's condition (e.g., initial vital signs, allergies, level of consciousness, and intravenous [IV] fluid infusing). An escort takes the patient and family members to the nursing division and introduces them to the nurse assuming the patient's care. The ED nurse shares pertinent observations about the patient's behavior (e.g., anxiety, fear, or level of knowledge regarding need for health care) with the nursing staff to foster continuity of care and help the patient and family cope with a new environment.

Many patients go to a hospital several days in advance for necessary preoperative diagnostic testing. In some cases these patients and their family members also attend preoperative education classes. Other patients have contact with health care providers for the first time when they arrive at a hospital or surgi-center. Patients admitted on the morning of a surgical procedure or treatment are "same-day" admissions. A nurse provides basic instructions about the purpose of the surgery or treatment, preparatory procedures, and postsurgical or posttreatment care. Admission and consent forms, diagnostic tests, preoperative patient teaching (see Chapter 37), and instructions are usually completed before the actual day of surgery. When nurses are able to see patients several days in advance, they use a variety of resources such as classes, videotapes, information booklets, and calls to home for patient teaching.

Nurses actively coordinate the initial admission process for all patients. A patient's condition influences the extent and type of admission activities. Always note the patient's level of fatigue and comfort. For example, when a critically ill patient reaches a hospital nursing division, he or she undergoes extensive examination and treatment procedures immediately. There may be little time

---

BOX 2.3

The Joint Commission Patients' Rights Standards

- Right to an appropriate level of care
- Right to receive safe care
- Respect for cultural values and religious beliefs
- Privacy
- Consent obtained for recording or filming for purposes other than the identification, diagnosis, or treatment of patients
- Confidentiality of information
- Recognition and prevention of potential abuse situation
- Notification of unanticipated outcomes
- Involvement in care decisions
- Information on risks and benefits of investigational studies
- End-of-life care
- Advance directives
- Organ procurement
- Right to have advance directives and to have them followed
- Freedom from unnecessary restraints
- Informed consent for various procedures
- Right to refuse care
- Right to have pain believed and relieved
- Communication with administration
- Education

From The Joint Commission (TJC): *Comprehensive accreditation manual for hospitals,* Chicago, IL, 2016, The Commission.

BOX 2.4

Advance Directives

- An advance directive is a document that gives a patient directions about future medical care or designates another person(s) to make medical decisions if the individual loses decision-making capacity.
- An advance directive conveys the patient's choice in continuing medical care when the patient is unable to speak or make decisions.
- Advance directives may include a living will, power of attorney for health care, or notarized handwritten document.
- A copy of the document should be available in the patient's medical record. If not available, the substance of the advance directive should be documented in the medical record, and a family member should be asked to bring the advance directive to the hospital.
- The attending health care provider is notified of the patient's advance directive.
- Witnesses for an advance directive document should not be medical personnel, nor should they be related to the patient or heirs to the patient's estate. A social worker often fulfills this requirement.

available for you to orient the patient and family to the division or learn of the patient's fears or concerns. When a patient enters a hospital for elective treatment, you have more time to prepare him or her psychologically for hospitalization. Early psychological preparation when a patient is still at home better prepares patients for hospitalization.

Delegation and Collaboration

The skill of completing the nursing assessment during admission to a health care agency cannot be delegated to nursing assistive personnel (NAP). The nurse directs the NAP to:
- Prepare the patient's room with equipment needed before admission.
- Gather and secure the patient's personal care items.
- Escort and orient the patient and family to the nursing unit.
- Collect ordered specimens.

Equipment

- Hospital gown
- Bedpan and urinal (if needed)
- Washbasin, bath towel, and washcloth
- Toiletry items (e.g., soap, toothpaste, hand lotion; *optional* in some hospitals)
- Facial tissues
- Water pitcher and drinking cup
- Kidney or emesis basin
- Disposable thermometer (see agency policy)
- Sphygmomanometer
- Stethoscope
- Clean gloves
- Pulse oximeter (*optional*)
- Documentation forms (see agency policy)

STEP	RATIONALE

ROOM PREPARATION

1. Perform hand hygiene and prepare room equipment and furniture. Prepare bed by adjusting it to the lowest horizontal position if patient is ambulatory. Place bed in high position if patient is arriving by stretcher. Turn down top sheet and bedspread. Arrange room furniture for easy access to bed. Adjust lights, temperature, and ventilation.	Promotes patient's comfort by preventing delays during admission. Proper position of bed lessens likelihood of patient fall during transfer and also reduces risk of back injuries to staff helping patient into bed.
2. Be sure that equipment is in working order. Assemble any special equipment (e.g., suction, oxygen supplies, or IV pole) in patient's room.	Prevents delays in delivering immediate treatment and provides for smooth transition between caregivers.

ASSESSMENT

1. Identify patient using at least two identifiers (e.g., name and birthday or name and medical record number) according to agency policy.	Ensures correct patient. Complies with The Joint Commission standards and improves patient safety (TJC, 2016a).
2. Greet patient and family cordially by name. Introduce yourself by name and job title; explain your responsibilities in patient's care.	Providing personalized care reduces anxiety about admission, clarifies staff roles, and expedites patient requests.
3. If patient does not speak, read, or understand English, arrange for a professional translator to help with the nursing assessment. Use telephone interpreter services as a supplemental system when an interpreter is needed instantly or when services are needed in an unusual or infrequently encountered language (USDHHS, OPHS, 2001).	Translation services are preferable to using family members to promote effective communication.
4. When a patient has a severe hearing impairment, a speech and language pathologist may be of help.	A speech and language pathologist may have augmented hearing devices or resources to facilitate communication of assessment data.
5. Assess patient's general appearance. Note signs or symptoms of physical distress (see Chapter 6).	Provides baseline assessment.

Clinical Decision Point *If patient is having acute physical problems, postpone routine admission procedures and nursing history until his or her needs are met. Complete a focused assessment at this point.*

6. Assess patient's ability to understand and implement health information by asking a health literacy question, such as "How confident are you filling out medical forms by yourself?" (Wallace et al., 2006). The REALM-SF is a reliable and valid tool with a list of seven words you ask a patient to read to determine their level of health literacy on grade scale (e.g., third grade, fourth to sixth grade, seventh and eighth grade and high school) (AHRQ, 2015a).	This helps you determine at what reading level a patient can read, allowing you to select appropriate level of educational material and teaching methods such as Teach-Back (AHRQ, 2015a).

STEP	RATIONALE
7. Assess patient's and family's psychological status by noting verbal and nonverbal behaviors and responses to greetings and explanations.	Anxiety influences how well patient adapts to a health care environment and retains instruction.
8. Assess vital signs (see Chapter 5), height and weight (see Chapter 6), and patient's level of discomfort (using a 0 to 10 scale) (see Chapter 16).	Provides baseline measurement to compare future findings. Determines alterations from normal range.
9. Assess for fall risk using scale with grading criteria agency policy. Ask patient to walk at end of bed and note gait and movement. Consider patient's risk factors (e.g., individual intrinsic factors: co-morbidities (neurological disorders), muscle weakness, unsteady gait, and urinary incontinence (de Jong et al., 2013; Spoelstra et al., 2011); transient factors: postural hypotension, polypharmacy, and use of high-risk medications (e.g., analgesics, antihypertensives) (Chang et al., 2011).	Having a patient walk allows you to more objectively assess his or her gait and level of strength rather than asking the patient if he or she has walking limitations. Provides data to determine patient's risk for injury and whether he or she needs to be placed on fall precautions. For acute care hospital inpatients, the maximum time frame for completing fall risk admission assessments is 24 h (TJC, 2016b).
10. Have family or friends leave room unless patient wishes to have them help with changing into a hospital gown or pajamas. Close door and curtains. Help patient undress and into comfortable position.	Provides for privacy and prepares patient for examination.

11. Obtain nursing history as soon as possible after patient's arrival to nursing division. Apply standards of nursing care adopted by hospital (e.g., functional health patterns). Data include the following:
  a. Patient's perception of illness and health care needs
  b. Past medical history
  c. Presenting signs and symptoms and reason for hospitalization
  d. Completion of a review of health status based on standards such as elimination, respiration, nutrition and metabolism, activity and exercise, self-concept, values and beliefs, cultural factors, social support, and cognitive function
 	
  e. Risk factors for illness
 	
  f. History of allergies, including type of substance and a description of the reaction that patient has previously experienced
	Each patient is to have an admission assessment prepared by a registered nurse (RN) (TJC, 2016a). Each agency sets a time frame for completion of admission assessment (maximum time 24 hours).
	Establishes a baseline of patient's clinical status.
	
	Identifies signs and symptoms in case patient's condition deteriorates.
	Provides a holistic view of patient's health problems and response to those problems.
	
	Allows you to institute preventive care measures and educate patient about health promotion behaviors.
	Patients often have sensitivity to a drug or substance rather than a true allergy; this needs to be clarified. Specify all allergens to prevent accidental exposure.

Clinical Decision Point *Provide patient with allergy arm band listing allergies to foods, drugs, latex, or other substances; document allergies according to agency policy.*

STEP	RATIONALE
g. Detailed medication history, including prescribed, over-the-counter (OTC), and alternative therapies such as herbs and hormones h. Patient's knowledge of health problems and expectations of care	Assesses potential for drug interactions, and information often explains patient's presenting signs and symptoms. Enables you to recognize and meet patient expectations when possible.
12. Apply clean gloves. Conduct physical assessment of appropriate body systems (see Chapter 6). If not obtained in admitting, instruct patient to provide a urine specimen. Inform patient if collecting blood specimens or performing tests. a. A priority is to assess a patient's skin integrity and any current skin breakdown at admission. Use a risk for pressure injury development scale such as the Braden Scale to assess risk for potential skin breakdown. After assessment is complete, remove and dispose of gloves and perform hand hygiene.	Provides objective data for identifying health problems. Unannounced procedures can make patients anxious. Preparation of patient relieves anxiety. Provides baseline data for pressure injury prevention and identifies the presence of any community-acquired pressure injuries when patient is admitted. Existing pressure injuries must be documented within 24 hours of admission (CMS, 2008). Pressure injuries that develop while a patient is hospitalized are considered an adverse event and become the financial responsibility of the agency responsible for their care (CMS, 2008).

STEP	RATIONALE
b. Some hospitals are now requiring assessment of risk for obstructive sleep apnea (OSA) in surgical patients (see Chapter 37). See agency policy. Use the STOP-Bang instrument if available.	STOP-Bang score was validated in obese and morbidly obese surgical patients. For identifying severe OSA, a STOP-Bang score of 4 has high sensitivity of 88%. For confirming severe OSA, a score of 6 is more specific (Chung et al., 2013). Allows you to institute appropriate postoperative observations. OSA is a potentially serious sleep disorder in which breathing repeatedly stops and starts during sleep. Surgical patients with OSA are considered at risk for relaxation of their throat muscles and blockage of the airway during recovery from anesthesia and sedation (D'Arcy, 2013).
13. Check health care providers' orders for treatment measures to initiate immediately.	Delay causes deterioration of patient's condition.
14. Ask patient to identify his or her values regarding health care and needs or expectations of care: "To what extent do you believe being in the hospital will help you? Tell me what you hope will happen during your hospital stay? Tell me what is important to you for your care here to be satisfactory." **NOTE:** Incorporate these questions during the physical examination.	Patient-centered care requires incorporation of patient needs, preferences, and values (QSEN, 2014).
15. Orient patient to patient care unit.	
a. Introduce staff members who enter room. Always introduce patient by last name unless patient indicates otherwise.	Helps patient recognize caregivers. Shows respect for patient.
b. Tell patient and family the name of the nurse manager in charge of the division and explain that person's role in solving problems.	Provides means for patient and family to communicate problems.
c. Explain visiting hours and their purpose (i.e., to provide time to administer needed procedures and give patient time to rest).	Provides knowledge and increases willingness to observe policy for visiting hours.
d. Discuss smoking policy and identify smoking areas for patient and family if available.	A hospital-wide smoking policy that prohibits the use of smoking materials throughout the hospital is required. Some hospitals may have a designated smoking area.
e. Demonstrate use of equipment (e.g., bed, over-bed table, lighting).	Patient's safety depends on patient understanding correct use of equipment.
f. Show patient how to use nurse call light and position it in a convenient place. Have patient demonstrate use of light. Discuss with patient his or her specific fall risks and encourage him or her to ask for help when getting out of bed.	Ensures that patient knows why and how to call for assistance.
g. Escort patient to bathroom (if able to ambulate).	Patient's safety depends in part on understanding how to use toilet facilities.

Clinical Decision Point *Ensure that patient knows how to call for help while in bathroom. (An emergency call light is usually in bathrooms.)*

STEP	RATIONALE
h. Explain hours for mealtime and nourishments to patient and family.	Family often wishes to visit during evening to help with meals.
i. Describe services available (e.g., chaplain, beauty shop, activity therapy).	Offers patient options for making decisions.

NURSING DIAGNOSES

- Anxiety
- Acute pain
- Chronic pain
- Deficient knowledge regarding hospital procedures and planned therapies

- Fear
- Ineffective coping, individual or family
- Powerlessness

- Risk for injury
- Risk for falls

Related factors/Risk factors are individualized based on patient's condition or needs.

STEP	RATIONALE

PLANNING

1. Expected outcomes following completion of procedure:
  - Patient is able to explain purpose and schedule of planned treatments and procedures.

    Understanding treatment plan gives patient a better sense of control and reduces anxiety about the unknown.
  - Patient demonstrates how to call for nurse when help is needed.

    Falls commonly occur when patients attempt to get out of bed without help.
  - Patient is able to ambulate (if condition permits) in room free of obstacles.

    Ensures patient safety and mobility in room.
  - Patient can safely and efficiently use equipment in the room.

    Equipment used in care of patient frequently poses hazards; helps to reduce some anxiety.
  - Patient verbalizes understanding of smoking policy, visiting hours, mealtimes, and services available.

    Knowledge of hospital policies helps patient adapt to the health care environment.
  - Patient self-reports improved comfort.

    Basic pain and comfort measures are effective.

IMPLEMENTATION

1. Perform hand hygiene. Complete patient medication reconciliation by checking home medication list for duplication, omission, or potential drug interactions with newly ordered medications. Update medication list on the basis of health care provider's orders for treatment. Follow agency policy.

Medication reconciliation on admission helps to make sure that patient is taking the correct medications and avoids medication errors (TJC, 2016a).

2. Inform patient about procedures or treatments scheduled for the next shift or day (e.g., visits by health care provider or dietitian). These vary based on nature of patient's condition.

Patient has right to be informed of any scheduled procedures or treatments. Being able to anticipate planned therapies minimizes anxiety.

3. Perform basic comfort measures (positioning, temperature of room) and administer analgesic (if ordered). Remove and dispose of gloves.

Enables patient to participate in planned therapies and education.

4. Complete learning readiness and learning needs assessment for patient and family caregiver.

Identifies patient's and family caregiver's educational needs and learning preferences.

5. Give patient and family caregiver a chance to ask questions about procedures or therapies and to share their personal goals of care. (If patient is unresponsive or unable to understand, review with family.)

Provides opportunity to clarify expectations and misconceptions. Provides for shared decision making.

6. Collect valuables that patient chooses to keep at bedside. Complete clothing and valuables listing sheet (see agency policy); have patient sign. Place valuables in agency safe or send home with family.

Accounts for placement of valuables and prevents loss.

7. Ensure that patient and family have time together alone if desired.

Admission is often stressful and fatiguing. Allows time for decision making.

8. Be sure that call light is within easy reach and bed is in low position.

Provides for patient safety.

9. Perform hand hygiene.

Reduces spread of microorganisms.

EVALUATION

1. Have patient explain own fall risks, hospital policies, tests, and procedures through discussion and questions.

Patient demonstrates learning and understanding through feedback.

2. Ask patient to rate severity of pain on scale of 0 to 10.

Determines if pain severity has decreased.

3. Have patient demonstrate use of call light.

Return demonstration confirms learning.

4. Monitor patient's ability to ambulate independently.

Provides data to judge patient's safety in ambulating without injury.

5. Check patient's room setup regularly.

Determines if care area is free of obstacles.

6. Use Teach-Back: "I want to be sure you understand how to use your call light to contact the nurses if you need assistance getting out of bed. Can you show me how to use it and tell me when you should use it?" Revise your instruction now or develop a plan for revised patient or family caregiver teaching if patient or family caregiver is not able to teach back correctly.

Determines patient's and family caregiver's level of understanding of instructional topic.

STEP	RATIONALE
Unexpected Outcomes 1. Patient is unable to explain hospital policies (e.g., visitation, smoking) or does not know purpose or schedule for tests and procedures. 2. Patient becomes restless, expresses concerns, or displays tension in body movements. 3. Patient falls or is injured.	**Related Interventions** • Schedule follow-up session with patient. • Keep information focused and specific to patient's situation. Include family if helpful. • Give patient time to discuss fears and concerns. • Show caring and compassion so patient becomes willing to communicate openly. • Attend to patient's immediate physical needs. • Inform health care provider of the injury or fall. • Reassess patient's environment, alter care plan as needed, ensure that the environment is free of safety hazards. • Complete incident/adverse event report.

Recording and Reporting

- Record history and assessment findings in appropriate forms/screens of electronic health record (EHR) or chart. Begin to develop nursing plan of care.
- Document your evaluation of patient and family caregiver learning.
- If patient has an advance directive, place copy in the medical record. In the absence of an actual advance directive, document the substance of the directive in the medical record (TJC, 2016a).
- Notify health care provider of patient's arrival; report any unusual findings. Secure admission orders if not previously provided.

Special Considerations
Teaching

- Explain to patient that a different nurse provides care on each shift. Explain time frame for how assignments are made.
- Teaching occurs throughout the admission process. Provide information regarding physical assessment findings, risks for falling, nature of patient's illness, planned diagnostic and treatment procedures, medications, goals of care, and hospital routines.
- In an emergency situation or if patient is unable to perform aspects of his or her care, teach family caregivers about the rationale for any procedures and routines to be used in patient's care.

Pediatric

- Hospitalization is a major crisis for children who feel stress from separation, loss of control, bodily injury, and pain. Separation anxiety is most common from middle infancy throughout the toddler years, especially ages 16 to 30 months. Preschoolers are better able to tolerate brief periods of separation, but their protest behaviors are more subtle than those in younger children (e.g., refusal to eat, difficulty sleeping, withdrawing from others). School-age children are able to cope with separation but have an increased need for parental security and guidance (Hockenberry and Wilson, 2015).
- Explain the rooming-in and visiting policies of the agency. Allow and encourage parental involvement in the child's care. Allow parents to help with routine care activities (e.g., bathing, eating) and, when possible, to remain with the child during procedures.
- Parental input during admission assessment is essential because they can provide input on the child's normal behavior and deviations caused by illness.

Gerontological

- Hospitalized older adults experience functional declines such as new-onset incontinence, malnutrition, deconditioning, pressure injuries, and falls. Interventions that retain functional status (e.g., physical therapy, nutrition consultation) require providing coordinated interdisciplinary care (Touhy and Jett, 2014).
- Patients who typically fall in the hospital are those who have been admitted recently and are unfamiliar with surroundings, have acute illness, take four or more medications, or have been relocated recently. Visual changes that occur with aging often lead to falls in hospitalized older-adult patients (Touhy and Jett, 2014).

◆ SKILL 2.2   Transferring Patients

Patients transfer to different patient care units and agencies to receive alternate forms and levels of therapy and services and to have essential care continued closer to home. When patients transfer, you need to ensure continuity of nursing care by improving transitions across the continuum of care. The goal of a transfer of care is to continue health care to avoid therapeutic interruptions or omissions that may hinder progress toward recovery. Collaborate early with health care providers and members of the interdisciplinary team to ensure efficient patient transfer with optimal patient outcomes. Evidence shows that multiple professionals are necessary to provide more integrated care than individual providers, particularly for patients with complex physiological, psychological, and social needs (Toscan et al., 2012).

When patients move between units or agencies for diagnosis, treatment, and ongoing care, there is a safety risk at each interval. The hand-over (or hand-off) communication that occurs between staff on different units and between and among care teams might not include all the essential information, or information may be misunderstood. Hand-offs serve many functions, from coaching and teaching to team building; but their most important function is information processing: making sure that essential data are transferred for patient safety (Halm, 2013). Substandard or variable hand-offs have contributed to errors, care omissions, treatment delays, inefficiencies from repeated work, inappropriate treatment, adverse events with minor or major harm, increased length of stay, avoidable readmissions, and increased costs (Blouin, 2011; Riesenberg et al., 2010).

When providing a hand-off of a patient to another unit, it is essential to clearly communicate information about the patient's care, treatment, services, and current condition and any recent or anticipated changes in order to meet patient safety goals (TJC, 2016a). Policies and procedures are usually similar throughout an agency. Preventing communication failures begins with structured communication, which is often achieved through the use of standard protocols that identify necessary information for reliable hand-offs. Highly reliable hand-offs incorporate three key elements (Halm, 2013):

1. Face-to-face, two-way communication between health care team members
2. Structured written forms, templates, or checklists that allow clinicians to agree on minimum essential data that create a shared mental model of a patient's situation
3. Content that "captures intention," meaning that clinicians share problems and hypotheses with a predictive diagnosis of the patient's clinical situation (foresight), rather than listing events and completed tasks (hindsight), which has been associated with hand-off errors

Mnemonics such as SBAR (Situation, Background, Assessment, Recommendation) or "I PASS the BATON" (Introduction, Patient, Assessment, Situation, Safety concerns, Background, Actions, Timing, Ownership, Next) are examples of formats to use during communication of transfers that can be tailored for different clinical areas and/or purposes.

In the emergency department (ED), when a patient is transferred from one agency to another, a nurse completes the transfer in compliance with the Emergency Medical Treatment and Labor Act (EMTALA) (CMS, 2012b). EMTALA is a federal law intended to protect patients from being transferred against their wishes and thus defines how an appropriate agency-to-agency transfer is accomplished. An appropriate transfer includes the following steps:

- Informing the patient of the risks and benefits of the transfer
- Obtaining the patient's written consent for transfer
- Having the transferring hospital provide medical treatment within its capacity
- Having available space and qualified personnel for treatment of the patient at the receiving agency and an agreement to accept transfer of the patient and provide treatment
- Making copies of all relevant medical records, including a transfer form, sent by the transferring agency to the receiving agency
- Transporting the patient using qualified personnel and transportation equipment (e.g., ambulance with advanced cardiac life support [ACLS] versus basic life support [BLS]).

Although this law primarily affects the ED, it is important to know EMTALA and the transfer policies for inpatient transfers within the agency itself. Many agencies follow the same policies for all patient transfers.

Delegation and Collaboration

The skill of assessment and decision making conducted during transfers cannot be delegated to nursing assistive personnel (NAP). The nurse directs the NAP to:

- Help the patient with dressing.
- Gather and secure the patient's personal belongings and any equipment that goes with the patient.
- Escort the patient to the nursing unit or transport area.

Equipment

- Transfer forms
- Copies of documents such as medical records, radiology films, laboratory test results (as appropriate)
- Special equipment as needed: wheelchair or stretcher, emesis basin, bedpan and urinal, oxygen tank and tubing, intravenous (IV) pole, cardiac monitor, and emergency medications

STEP	RATIONALE

ASSESSMENT

1. Identify patient using at least two identifiers (e.g., name and birthday or name and medical record number) according to agency policy.

Ensures correct patient. Complies with The Joint Commission standards and improves patient safety (TJC, 2016a).

2. Obtain and review transfer order from sending health care provider. Order includes name of the receiving agency (when applicable), receiving health care provider's name, and statement of patient's stability for transfer.

Health care provider is legally responsible for releasing patient from medical care and arranging for receiving health care provider. Patient has legal right to refuse transfer against medical advice.

3. In collaboration with health care provider and members of the interdisciplinary team, assess reason for patient's transfer (e.g., change in condition, services available at the agency, patient or family preferences regarding patient's location).

Patient needs to have access to agency with best resources to meet health care needs. Health care provider determines patient's physical stability for transfer.

4. Assess individuals at high risk for transitional care problems (e.g., older adults with multiple health issues, depression, non-English speakers, patients with sensory impairments, and low-income patients).

Identifying patients at risk for transitional care problems allows for better continuity of care and improved patient outcomes (Touhy and Jett, 2014). Patients may require consultation with needed resources (e.g., care manager, psychologist) when arriving at destination.

STEP	RATIONALE
5. Explain purpose of transfer thoroughly and provide time to discuss patient's and family's feelings about the change in care setting. As necessary, obtain patient's written consent to transfer. If patient is unable to consent, patient's family provides this consent.	Patients need to be informed of transfer plans in a timely manner (TJC, 2016b). A patient requires adequate psychological preparation. In the event of a clinical emergency in which patient and patient's family are unable to consent, this consent is waived, and patient is transferred to a higher level of care on the basis of the clinical judgment of the health care provider requesting the transfer.
6. Assess patient's current physical condition and determine method for transport. When transferring to a new agency, assess method of transport to transferring vehicle (e.g., wheelchair or stretcher) (consult agency policy).	Determines level of patient stability. Patient's condition often changes quickly and influences stability for transfer and type of support needed during transport.

Clinical Decision Point *Determine if patient's status and safety require life-support equipment. Staff assisting with transfer need training in life-support measures. When transporting to new agency, a vehicle equipped with life-support equipment is necessary.*

STEP	RATIONALE
7. Assess if patient requires pain relief or other medications for symptom management.	Ensures patient's comfort during transfer.
8. Ensure that staff have notified patient's family or significant others of transfer as desired by patient.	Provides adequate communication with family or significant others to help with patient's emotional and psychological adjustment to the transfer (TJC, 2016b).

NURSING DIAGNOSES

- Anxiety
- Deficient knowledge regarding transfer procedure
- Fear
- Powerlessness
- Relocation stress syndrome

Related factors are individualized on the basis of patient's condition or needs.

PLANNING

1. Expected outcomes following completion of procedure:	
• Patient's vital signs and physiological status remain the same following transfer.	Treatments are planned so as not to interrupt physical support of patient during transfer.
• Patient incurs no injury during transport procedures.	Safety measures are successful in transferring patient from wheelchair or stretcher to transport vehicle.
• Patient or family explains purpose of transfer and procedure for transport.	Understanding provides patient with sense of control.
• Receiving nursing staff acquire and confirm written plan of care.	Ensures continuity of care.
2. Arrange for patient's transport to the agency by chosen vehicle (social worker involvement may be necessary).	Transfer needs to occur without delays so patient has access to all needed resources at all times.
3. When transfer is to a new agency, contact the agency and arrange for bed in appropriate setting. Confirm willingness of the agency to accept patient (usually social worker or discharge coordinator completes).	Prevents delays when patient arrives at destination. Receiving hospital ensures that space and qualified personnel are available to treat patients. Hospital also agrees in advance to transfer.

IMPLEMENTATION

1. Make sure that documentation in patient's record is complete, with care plan that has individualized nursing care measures.	Accurate information is necessary for receiving agency to assume patient's care.
2. Complete nursing care transfer form according to agency policy. (When transfer is to a different nursing unit, entire medical record accompanies patient.)	Form summarizes patient's pertinent nursing care needs to ensure continuity of care and prevent unnecessary duplication of services.

STEP	RATIONALE
3. Complete medication reconciliation per agency policy. Check patient's current orders for transfer against the most recent medication administration record and the original home medication list. Communicate updated medication list to next provider of care.	The new medication regimen prescribed at the time of transfer may omit needed medications, unnecessarily duplicate existing therapies, or contain incorrect dosages (AHRQ, 2015b). Ensures that patient receives correct medications at new agency and decreases medication errors (TJC, 2016a).
4. Have NAP gather patient's personal care items, clothing, and valuables. Check the entire room and all storage areas. Secure in suitcase or container.	Prevents loss of articles during transfer.
5. Anticipate problems that patient frequently develops just before or during transfer. Perform necessary nursing therapies such as suctioning or changing a dressing.	Ensures patient's comfort and safety during transport.
6. Help to transfer patient to stretcher or wheelchair using safe patient-handling techniques (see Chapter 11).	It is easier to move patient transported to outside agency by stretcher into transport vehicle.
7. Perform and document final assessment of patient's physical stability.	Minimizes risk of patient developing complications during transfer.

Clinical Decision Point *Priority assessment includes vital signs, clear airway, patency of IV lines and accuracy of infusion rate, and patient's level of consciousness.*

8. When transfer occurs to an outside agency, accompany patient to transport vehicle.	Ensures that medically qualified personnel are in attendance until patient leaves agency/unit.
9. Call receiving agency/unit and notify of impending transfer and patient's status (check agency policy).	Notification of nurse in charge or nurse assuming care of patient ensures better continuity of care at time of patient's arrival.

EVALUATION

1. During the final assessment compare data with the previous findings.	Determines if patient's condition is changing.
2. Inspect patient's alignment and positioning on stretcher/wheelchair.	Proper alignment and positioning reduce risk of an injury occurring during transport.
3. Ensure that equipment needed for transfer is functioning.	Equipment such as oxygen must last through transport for patient safety.
4. Confirm that patient understands transfer and procedures through discussion and questions.	Feedback helps to ensure learning.
5. Determine if receiving agency/nurse has questions about patient's care.	Provides for clear communication during hand-off and continuity of care.
6. **Use Teach-Back:** "I want to be sure you understand why you are being transferred to your new unit. Can you tell me why you are being transferred and what the name of your new unit is?" Revise your instruction now or develop a plan for revised patient or family caregiver teaching if patient or family caregiver is not able to teach back correctly.	Determines patient's and family caregiver's level of understanding of instructional topic.

Unexpected Outcomes

1. Patient's physical status deteriorates during preparation.

2. Patient is confused or uncertain about transfer.
3. Receiving staff misinterpret directions for patient's care.

Related Interventions

- Call health care provider immediately.
- Initiate interventions to stabilize patient's condition.
- Provide clarification or additional explanation.
- Sending agency has nurse or health care provider call to confirm that there are no questions regarding patient's care.

Recording and Reporting

- The nurse sending the patient documents patient's status, including vital signs and other assessment findings regarding patient's condition, nursing plan of care, date and time of transfer, and method of transport on appropriate transfer form.
- Document your evaluation of patient and family caregiver learning.
- Nurse receiving patient documents patient's arrival at agency by recording date and time of arrival, reason for transfer, method

of transport, patient's condition, and care provided at time of arrival.

Special Considerations
Teaching

- A transfer frequently creates anxiety for a patient and family members. Carefully repeat instructions about the transfer when patient and family caregiver are better able to understand your explanation. In this situation be sure to have patient restate any critical information.

Pediatric

- Children need their parents' comfort and security; thus make sure that parents are well informed. Involve older children in any discussion regarding transfers. Allow a parent to accompany the child in the transfer.

Gerontological

- When transferring an older-adult patient to a new agency, relocation is stressful. Ensure that significant support people are still accessible and that patient is thoroughly oriented to new surroundings. Also make sure that patient is able to take important memorabilia and has an opportunity to make decisions about care (Touhy and Jett, 2014).

Long-Term Care

- It is important that patients receive the level of services appropriate to their physical and mental health needs. Participation of social worker or discharge planner in transfer process ensures that transfer to a long-term care facility is appropriate.
- On patient's arrival at long-term care facility, complete a Resident Assessment Instrument (RAI). The RAI consists of the minimum data set (MDS), resident assessment protocols, and utilization guidelines specified in state operations guidelines (Touhy and Jett, 2014).
- Essential components of successful transfer to a long-term care facility are accurate communication of medication lists and advance directives. Possible use of a standardized transfer form can help in accurate communication (Mueller et al., 2012; Toles et al., 2012).

◆ SKILL 2.3   Discharging Patients

Early and comprehensive discharge planning facilitates the transition of a patient or resident from a health care agency to the most independent level of care, whether that is home or another agency. The overall goal of discharge planning is to provide the most appropriate level and quality of care throughout all stages of a patient's illness. The US Department of Health and Human Services (USDHHS) (2014) explains that discharge planning involves:

- Determining the appropriate posthospital/agency discharge destination for a patient.
- Identifying what a patient requires for a smooth and safe transition from the acute care hospital/ post–acute care agency to his or her discharge destination.
- Beginning the process of meeting a patient's identified predischarge and postdischarge needs.

The discharge planning process is comprehensive and interdisciplinary, including all caregivers who are involved in the care of the patient. Every hospitalized patient requires patient-entered discharge planning, and it is equally essential for any patient permanently moving to a different health care agency. The trend toward shorter lengths of stay in acute care settings makes discharge planning increasingly difficult, but all the more essential. The Joint Commission (TJC) identifies the elements of a comprehensive discharge planning model (Box 2.5).

Development of a discharge plan with outcomes mutually accepted by a patient and health care providers is essential (TJC, 2015). Effective discharge planning prepares patients to assume self-care or prepares family caregivers to provide needed support and thus can decrease hospital readmission and promote optimal patient outcomes (Rutherford et al., 2013). The discharge process is simple or complex and occurs in three phases: acute, transitional, and continuing care. In the acute phase medical attention dominates discharge planning efforts. During the transitional phase the need for acute care is still present; but its urgency declines, and patients begin to address and plan for their future health care needs. In the continuing-care phase patients are able to participate in planning and implementing continuing-care activities needed after discharge. In hospitals these phases can occur very quickly, even within hours.

The greatest challenge in effective discharge planning is communication. Patients and families should be full partners in the discharge planning process and thus should be engaged in discussing what will be needed to make the transition in care safe and effective (AHRQ, 2013). When team members communicate during end-of-shift hand-offs, consultations, or huddle sessions, a patient's discharge readiness should be a central topic. Communication is enhanced if an organization has a discharge coordinator or case manager. Staff members in these roles thoroughly assess what each patient's needs will be at discharge, identify available and needed resources, and link patients and families to these resources (e.g., community agencies, Meals on Wheels, rehabilitation sites). The staff also coordinate services (e.g., home health) as appropriate and follow up on patients' progress after discharge.

Discharge from an agency is stressful for a patient and family. Before a patient is discharged, the patient and family need to be prepared with the knowledge and skills to manage care in the home. They also need to know what to expect in regard to any continuing physical problems. Without the necessary equipment and professional resources, a patient risks loss of rehabilitation gains made before discharge. Failure to understand restrictions or

---

BOX 2.5

The Joint Commission Recommendations for Discharge Planning Process

- Address patient communication needs, including patient's preferred language and any sensory or communication impairments.
- Ensure that language services are available for patient and family members.
- Engage patients and families actively in discharge planning and instruction.
- Provide discharge instruction that meets patient needs.
  - Instruction may involve use of pictures, diagrams, or models to illustrate instruction.
  - Use discharge instruction that meets health literacy needs. Materials should be at fifth grade or lower reading level.
- Identify follow-up providers who can meet unique patient needs.
  - Create a list of follow-up providers that offer services and accommodations that meet patient's communication, cultural, religious, mobility, and other needs.
  - Refer patients to appropriate care provider (e.g., community clinic).

Modified from The Joint Commission (TJC): *Advancing effective communication, cultural competence, and patient- and family-centered care: a roadmap for hospitals,* Oakbrook Terrace, IL, 2011, The Joint Commission.

implications of health problems often causes a patient to develop complications. Poor discharge planning ignores a patient's needs within the home and increases the chance of the patient needing to reenter the health care system prematurely.

Delegation and Collaboration

The skills of assessment, care planning, and instruction included in discharging patients cannot be delegated to nursing assistive personnel (NAP). The nurse directs the NAP to:

- Gather and secure personal items and any supplies that patient will take home or to new setting.
- Transport the patient to the discharge transport vehicle.

Equipment

- Wheelchair or stretcher
- Discharge documentation forms (see agency policy)
- Patient instruction sheets
- Plastic bag for personal belongings

STEP	RATIONALE

ASSESSMENT

1. Identify patient using at least two identifiers (e.g., name and birthday or name and medical record number) according to agency policy.

Ensures correct patient. Complies with The Joint Commission standards and improves patient safety (TJC, 2016a).

2. From time of admission, assess patient's discharge needs using nursing history data, including assessments of patient's physical health, functional status, psychosocial support system, financial resources, health values, cultural and ethnic background, level of education, and barriers to care that are needed. Also review ongoing assessment data during your shift of care (e.g., physical examinations and discussions with patient and health care provider). Be sure that the discharge plan is culturally appropriate (e.g., learn the patient's preferences and values about continuing health care after discharge).

Planning for discharge begins at admission and continues throughout patient's stay in an agency to help patient achieve maximum functioning. The discharge planning assessment determines patient's continuing care needs after he or she leaves the acute care hospital/post–acute care agency setting (USDHHS, 2014).

3. Identify risk factors that may increase the chance of patient being readmitted after discharge (TJC, 2013): Diagnoses associated with high readmissions (e.g., heart failure, chronic lung disease); co-morbidities; the need for numerous medications; a history of readmissions, psychosocial and emotional factors such as issues relating to mental health, interpersonal relationships, or family matters; the lack of a family caregiver who could provide support or help with care; older age; financial distress, deficient living environment (e.g., water supply, heating)

Allows you to better prioritize care interventions that manage these risk factors during patient stay in hospital. Conditions affect either patient's ability to become physically or psychologically ready for discharge or ability and readiness of a caregiver to assume patient's care in the home.

4. If patient's destination at discharge will be the home, assess patient's and family caregiver's learning needs as soon as possible (e.g., psychomotor skills, medication management, symptom recognition). Engage patient and family as partners in the discharge teaching plan by having them identify their concerns about discharge.

Improves understanding of health care needs and ability to achieve self-care at home. Inclusion of family caregiver in teaching sessions provides patient with available resource. Engaging patient and family in the assessment supports patient- and family-centered nursing (TJC, 2015).

5. Assess for current barriers to learning (e.g., age, fatigue, pain, lack of motivation). Assess patient's health literacy (see Skill 2.1, Assessment, Step 6).

Determines timing and approach to instruction. Different types of educational materials are effective with different individual learning styles. If printed material is to be used, be sure that material is written at proper reading level.

6. Ask patient and/or family caregiver to describe the home environment and assess for environmental factors that may interfere with self-care (e.g., size of rooms, doorway clearances for wheelchair, steps, lighting, bathroom facilities). (A home care nurse is usually available on referral to help with assessment.)

Environmental factors within patient's home pose safety risks or problems for self-care (see Chapter 43). Early identification of these factors allows you to arrange for home health referral.

7. Collaborate with the interprofessional team to assess patient's anticipated needs after discharge and his or her eligibility for home care reimbursement. Ask these questions: "Does patient have an injury or illness that makes it difficult to leave home (e.g., requires the aid of supportive devices such as a wheelchair or walker; require the use of special transportation; need the assistance of a family caregiver)?" Does the patient have a "skilled need" that requires skills from a specific health care provider?"

These conditions are needed for Medicare reimbursement of home health services. Patient must have a "skilled need" that requires the skills of a licensed nurse, speech therapist, or physical therapist to perform. A health care provider's order is also needed.

STEP	RATIONALE
8. Assess patient's and family's perceptions of continued health care needs outside the hospital. Assess family caregivers' perceived ability to provide care to patient, including their level of social and community support and their ability to manage multiple medications with which the patient is discharged.	Family caregiving is a highly stressful experience. Family members who are not properly prepared for caregiving are frequently overwhelmed by patient's needs, which can lead to unnecessary hospital readmissions.

Clinical Decision Point *It is often necessary to talk with patient and family separately to learn about true concerns or doubts.*

STEP	RATIONALE
9. Assess patient's acceptance of health problems and related restrictions.	Affects willingness to follow therapies and restrictions.

NURSING DIAGNOSES

- Anxiety
- Caregiver role strain
- Deficient knowledge regarding home care restrictions
- Ineffective health management
- Interrupted family processes
- Readiness for enhanced health management
- Relocation stress syndrome
- Self-care deficit: feeding, toileting, dressing/grooming, bathing/hygiene

Related factors are individualized on the basis of patient's condition or needs.

PLANNING

1. Expected outcomes following completion of procedure:	
• Patient or family caregiver explains how health care is to continue in home (or other agency), for which problems to observe and what to do, which treatments or medications patient needs, and when to go to next medical appointment.	Increases likelihood of care not being interrupted in home (or other agency) and reduces chances of unplanned readmission to the hospital.
• Patient is able to demonstrate self-care activities (or family caregiver is able to administer care measures).	Feedback ensures learning.
• Obstacles to patient's mobility and hazards to ambulation in home setting are removed.	Patient is often physically weakened or has physical changes resulting from illness that predispose to injury.

IMPLEMENTATION

1. Preparation before day of discharge:	
a. Partner with patient and family in identifying ways to change physical arrangement of home that will be required to meet patient's needs (see Chapter 43).	Maintains patient's level of independence and ability to retain function within safe environment.
b. Provide patient and family with information about community health care resources (e.g., medical equipment companies, Meals on Wheels, adult day care). Referrals are usually made while patient is in hospital.	Community resources offer services that patient or family cannot provide.
c. Conduct teaching sessions with patient and family as soon as possible during hospitalization. Cover these topics: Description of what life at home will be like; review of medications and dosing schedules; warning signs of possible health problems; explanation of test results; explanation of how to provide therapies or use home medical equipment; review of restrictions resulting from health alterations; and when to make follow-up appointment (AHRQ, 2013). Use appropriate materials such as pamphlets, books, or multimedia resources. Refer patient to reliable and current resources on the Internet.	Gives patient opportunities to practice new skills, ask questions, and obtain necessary feedback to ensure learning. A combination of written and verbal information is effective in improving patient satisfaction and knowledge (TJC, 2015). In some settings electronic programs are available that allow you to tailor patient-specific media instructions.
d. Communicate patient's and family caregiver's response to teaching and proposed discharge plan to other health care team members.	Facilitates continuity and achievement of an individualized discharge plan.

STEP	RATIONALE

2. Procedure on day of discharge:
   a. Encourage patient and family caregiver to ask questions or discuss issues related to home care. A final opportunity to demonstrate learned skills is helpful.

   Allows for final clarification of information previously discussed. Helps relieve anxiety.

   b. Check health care provider's discharge orders for prescriptions, change in treatments, or need for special medical equipment. (Make sure that orders are written as early as possible.) Arrange for delivery and setup of equipment (e.g., hospital bed, oxygen) before patient arrives home.

   Only a health care provider is able to authorize a discharge. Early check of orders permits you to attend to any last-minute treatments or procedures well before discharge.

   c. Determine whether patient or family has arranged for transportation.

   Patient's condition at discharge determines method of transport.

   d. Provide privacy and assistance as patient dresses and packs all personal belongings. Check closets and drawers for belongings. Obtain copy of list of valuables signed by patient and have security or appropriate administrator deliver valuables to patient.

   Prevents loss of personal items. Patient's signature verifies receipt of items and relieves nursing department of liability for losses.

   e. Complete medication reconciliation per agency policy. Check discharge medication orders against the medication administration record and home medication list. Provide patient with prescriptions or pharmacy-dispensed medications ordered by health care provider. Offer a final review of information needed to facilitate safe medication self-administration.

   Decreases risk of medication errors and ensures that patient is receiving correct medication at home (TJC, 2016a). The new medication regimen prescribed at the time of discharge may inadvertently omit needed medications, unnecessarily duplicate existing therapies, or contain incorrect dosages (AHRQ, 2015b). Review provides feedback to determine patient's success in learning about medications

   f. Provide information on follow-up appointments to health care provider's office.

   Provides patient with contact for questions that arise after discharge. Ensures continuity of care to prevent rehospitalization.

   g. Contact agency business office to determine whether patient needs to finalize arrangements for payment of bill. Arrange for patient or family to visit business office.

   Source of concern for many patients is whether agency has accepted insurance or other payment forms.

   h. Acquire utility cart to move patient's belongings. Obtain wheelchair for patient. Transport patients leaving by ambulance on ambulance stretchers.

   Provides for safe transport.

   i. Help patient to wheelchair or stretcher using safe patient handling and transfer techniques (see Chapter 11). Escort patient to entrance of agency where source of transportation is waiting (see agency policy) (see illustrations). Lock wheelchair wheels. Help patient transfer into transport vehicle. Help place personal belongings in vehicle.

   Prevents injury to nurse and patient. Agency policy requires escort to ensure patient's safe exit. Agency's liability ends once patient is safely in vehicle.

   j. Return to division. Notify admitting or appropriate department of time of discharge. Notify housekeeping of need to clean patient's room.

   Allows agency to prepare for admission of next patient.

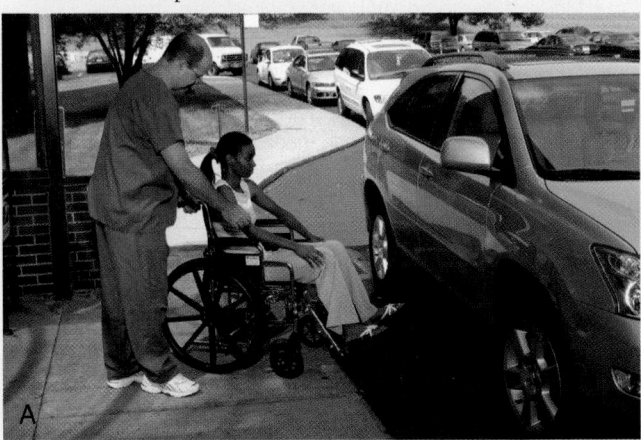
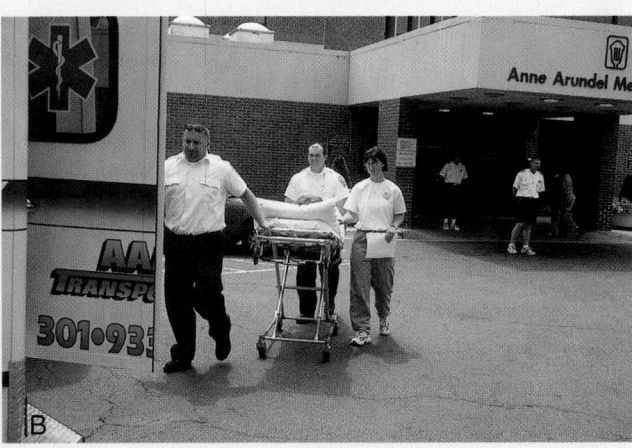

STEP 2i A, Nurse escorts patient to transport vehicle at time of discharge via a wheelchair. **B,** Many patients are discharged via stretcher.

STEP	RATIONALE

EVALUATION

1. Ask patient or family caregiver to describe nature of illness, treatment and medication regimens, and physical signs or symptoms to be reported to a health care provider.

   Measures patient's or family caregiver's learning.

2. Have patient or family caregiver perform any treatments that will continue in the home.

   Return demonstrations allow you to evaluate level of learning.

3. Home care nurse inspects home, identifies obstacles that pose risks for patient, and recommends revisions.

   Provides continuity of care.

4. **Use Teach-Back:** "I want to be sure you understand when your follow-up appointment is. Can you tell me when you are coming back to the clinic?" Revise your instruction now or develop a plan for revised patient or family caregiver teaching if patient or family caregiver is not able to teach back correctly.

   Determines patient's and family caregiver's level of understanding of instructional topic.

Unexpected Outcomes
1. Patient or family caregiver is unable to explain or demonstrate self-care measures.

2. Environmental risks are still present in home.

3. Patient or family caregiver resists discharge plans and refuses assimilation of new roles needed for home care.

Related Interventions
• Provide immediate clarification or additional instruction.
• Plan additional time to demonstrate treatment measures.
• Ask patient to explain which aspect of procedure is difficult to perform and why.
• If patient or family caregiver continues to be unable to correctly demonstrate treatment measures, request referral for home care services.
• Reassess reason for changes not being implemented.
• Home care nurse will problem solve and seek appropriate solution.
• Contact additional resources (e.g., social work, home care, pastoral care).

Recording and Reporting

• Complete documentation of patient's discharge on discharge summary form (Box 2.6). Give patient a signed copy of form.
• Document unresolved problems and description of arrangements made for resolution in nurses' notes in electronic health record (EHR) or chart.
• Document patient's vital signs and status of health problems at time of discharge in nurses' notes in EHR or chart.
• Document your evaluation of patient and family caregiver learning.

Special Considerations
Teaching
• Assess patient's fatigue and pain levels before beginning any instruction. Keep focused on the important teaching topics to cover.

Pediatric
• Once family caregivers have learned how to perform any necessary caregiver skills, have them assume care before child returns home. Many hospitals incorporate a trial period requiring family to manage care before child's discharge home (Hockenberry and Wilson, 2015).
• Complete discharge planning in partnership with children and parents. Over 80% of pediatric discharges are simple and do not require complex teaching or planning (Gibbens, 2010).

Gerontological
• Older adults are interested in more information about community resources and social supports once discharged (Price, 2011).
• Older adults and their families often overestimate their ability to manage care after discharge. They also disagree about what postdischarge care includes. Make referrals to home care to address needs associated with functional decline and help prevent readmission to the hospital.

Home Care

• Assess availability and skill of primary family caregiver (e.g., spouse or friend): assess time availability, ability and willingness to give care, emotional and physical stamina, knowledge of caregiving requirements, and type of relationship held with patient. Assess additional resources, including friends or neighbors who are available to help.
• Inform patient or family caregiver and patient's health care provider about decision to accept or not accept patient for admission to home care agency.

BOX 2.6

Elements of a Written Discharge Summary Form

• Mode of discharge: Ambulatory, wheelchair, stretcher
• Instructions for self-care activities: Activity; diet; medications; special treatments such as wound care, self-catheterization, tracheostomy care
• Reconciled list of discharge medications with dose, frequency, route, reasons for change in medication or for newly prescribed medications
• Signs and symptoms of complications or drug reactions for which to be observant
• Signs and symptoms that patient should consider normal
• Correct settings for any equipment required
• Planned follow-up appointment at health care provider's office, clinic
• Name and contact information of health care provider and/or nursing unit
• Explanation of pertinent emergency procedures
• Patient's signature, showing understanding of instructions

Modified from Louden K: Creating a better discharge summary, *ACP Hospitalist* 3:1, 2009; National Quality Forum (NQF): *National voluntary consensus report, standards for public reporting of patient safety information: a consensus report,* Washington, DC, 2010, NQF.

◆ CLINICAL DEBRIEF

A 69-year-old widow was admitted to the acute care unit with a left-sided stroke. The patient has a history of diabetes mellitus and arthritis. She is able to help with many care activities but requires help with eating. She has a sister who will be her family caregiver. On admission her assessment showed an area of skin breakdown on her left hip, assessed as a stage 1 pressure injury. Her medications on admission were metformin, lisinopril, and St. John's Wort. After 3 days she was transferred to the rehabilitation unit. Her medications on transfer were metformin, lisinopril, and warfarin. She has left-sided weakness from her stroke and will likely require a walker.

1. During the patient's admission assessment, which physical assessment findings are a priority to document and why?
2. During her transfer, which key piece of information, reflecting a potential risk, should be shared during the hand-off with the nurse on the rehabilitation unit?
3. At the time the patient is admitted to rehabilitation, the nurse conducts an assessment in an effort to plan for discharge in 2 weeks. The patient will be going home and staying with her sister for at least a month. During the assessment the nurse learns that the sister is concerned about being able to manage the patient. The sister has heart failure and limited exercise tolerance. Assessment also reveals that her skin has cleared over the left hip. The patient will be trained to use the walker safely in rehabilitation. Write an SBAR to communicate this situation.

◆ REVIEW QUESTIONS

1. The nurse is admitting a patient from the emergency department. Which steps should he or she take to ensure that the patient is safely admitted? (Select all that apply.)
   1. Obtain a list of the patient's medication from the patient
   2. Ask the family to provide interpreter services
   3. Determine patient's level of health literacy
   4. Obtain the patient's history as soon as possible
   5. Wait 24 h before assessing skin integrity
2. The nurse is orienting a student nurse who asks when medication reconciliation is done. The nurse tells her that it is done: (Select all that apply.)
   1. On admission.
   2. On transfer to another level of care.
   3. At the change of every shift.
   4. On discharge.
   5. Once every 24 h.
3. The nurse is preparing the patient on the day of discharge. Which of the following elements are important to address? (Select all that apply.)
   1. Reviewing health care providers' orders
   2. Arranging for transportation
   3. Completing medication reconciliation
   4. Reviewing discharge instructions
   5. Beginning discharge planning

ⓔ *Visit the Evolve site for a complete list of Clinical Debrief and Review Questions answers.*

REFERENCES

Agency for Healthcare Research and Quality (AHRQ): Strategy 4: Care transitions from hospital to home: IDEAL discharge planning, 2013, http://www.ahrq.gov/professionals/systems/hospital/engagingfamilies/strategy4/index.html. Accessed January 17, 2016.

Agency for Healthcare Research and Quality (AHRQ): Healthcare literacy measurement tools, Revised, 2015a, http://www.ahrq.gov/professionals/quality-patient-safety/quality-resources/tools/literacy/index.html. Accessed January 16, 2016.

Agency for Healthcare Research and Quality (AHRQ): Patient safety network: medication reconciliation, 2015b, https://psnet.ahrq.gov/primers/primer/1/medication-reconciliation. Accessed October 26, 2015.

Blouin A: Improving hand-off communications: new solutions for nurse, *J Nurs Care Qual* 26(2):97, 2011.

Centers for Medicare and Medicaid Services (CMS): Hospital-acquired conditions, 2008, https://www.cms.gov/Medicare/Medicare-Fee-for-Service-Payment/HospitalAcqCond/Hospital-Acquired_Conditions.html. Accessed January 10, 2016.

Centers for Medicare and Medicaid Services (CMS): Medicare and Medicaid programs, hospital conditions of participation: patients' rights, final rule, *Fed Regist* 71(236):71426, 2009.

Centers for Medicare and Medicaid Services (CMS): Chapter IV: *Medicare and Medicaid Services, Department of Health and Human Services Centers, Part 482.43, condition of participation, discharge planning,* 2012a, https://www.gpo.gov/fdsys/pkg/CFR-2011-title42-vol5/pdf/CFR-2011-title42-vol5-sec482-43.pdf. Accessed January 16, 2016.

Centers for Medicare and Medicaid Services (CMS): Emergency Medical Treatment & Labor Act (EMTALA), 2012b, https://www.cms.gov/Regulations-and-Guidance/Legislation/EMTALA/. Accessed January 16, 2016.

Chang CM, et al: Medical conditions and medications as risk factors of falls in inpatient older people: a case-control study, *Int J Geriatr Psychiatry* 26(6):602, 2011.

Chung F, et al: Predictive performance of the STOP-Bang score for identifying obstructive sleep apnea in obese patient, *Obes Surg* 23(12):2050, 2013.

D'Arcy Y: Turning the tide on respiratory depression, *Nursing 2014* 43(9):38, 2013.

de Jong MR, et al: Drug-related falls in older patients: implicated drugs, consequences, and possible prevention strategies, *Ther Adv Drug Saf* 4(4):147, 2013.

Gibbens C: Nurse-facilitated discharge for children and their families, *Paediatr Nurs* 22(1):14, 2010.

Halm MA: Nursing handoffs: ensuring safe passage for patients, *Am J Crit Care* 22(2):158, 2013.

HIPAA: HIPAA protected health information: What Does PHI Include? 2009, https://www.hipaa.com/hipaa-protected-health-information-what-does-phi-include/. Accessed January 16, 2016.

Hockenberry MJ, Wilson D: *Wong's nursing care of infants and children*, ed 10, St Louis, 2015, Mosby.

Institute for Healthcare Improvement (IHI): Medication reconciliation to prevent adverse drug events, 2016, http://www.ihi.org/topics/adesmedicationreconciliation/Pages/default.aspx. Accessed January 14, 2016.

Kwan JL, et al: Medication reconciliation during transitions of care as a patient safety strategy: a systematic review, *Ann Intern Med* 158.5(Part_2):397, 2013.

Mueller SK, et al: Hospital-based medication reconciliation practices: a systematic review, *Arch Intern Med* 172(14):1057, 2012.

Price B: How to map a patient's social support network, *Nurs Older People* 23(2):28, 2011.

National Quality Forum (NQF): Healthcare disparities and cultural competence consensus standards: technical report, 2012, http://www.qualityforum.org/Publications/2012/09/Healthcare_Disparities_and_Cultural_Competency_Consensus_Standards_Technical_Report.aspx. Accessed October 25, 2015.

Quality and Safety Education for Nurses (QSEN): Pre-Licensure KSAs, 2014, http://qsen.org/competencies/pre-licensure-ksas/. Accessed January 16, 2016.

Riesenberg L, et al: Nursing handoffs: a systematic review of the literature, *Am J Nurs* 110(4):24, 2010.

Rutherford P, et al: *How-to guide: improving transitions from the hospital to community settings to reduce avoidable rehospitalization*, Cambridge, MA, June 2013, Institute for Healthcare Improvement. http://www.IHI.org.

Spoelstra SL, et al: Fall prevention in hospitals: an integrative review, *Clin Nurs Res*, published online 23 August 2011, https://www.researchgate.net/profile/Sandra_Spoelstra/publication/51591322_Fall_prevention_in_hospitals_an_integrative_review/links/02bfe50e8565723475000000.pdf. Accessed January 16, 2016.

Staggers N, Blaz JW: Research on nursing handoffs for medical and surgical settings: an integrative review, *J Adv Nurs* 69(2):247, 2013.

The Joint Commission (TJC): The need for collaboration across entire care continuum. In *Hot Topics in Healthcare*: Issue number 2, Transitions of care: the need for collaboration, 2013, http://www.jointcommission.org/assets/1/6/toc_hot_topics.pdf. Accessed January 17, 2016.

The Joint Commission (TJC): Transitions of care: engaging patients and families, 2015, http://www.jointcommission.org/assets/1/23/Quick_Safety_Issue_18_November_20151.PDF. Accessed January 14, 2016.

The Joint Commission (TJC): *2016 National Patient Safety Goals*, Oakbrook Terrace, IL, 2016a, The Commission. http://www.jointcommission.org/standards_information/npsgs.aspx. Accessed January 14, 2016.

The Joint Commission (TJC): *The Joint Commission's Electronic Accreditation & Certification Manual*, Oakbrook Terrace, IL, 2016b, The Joint Commission.

Toles MP, et al: Transitions in care among older adults receiving long-term services and supports, *J Gerontol Nurs* 38(11):40, 2012.

Torres A: The role of barcode technology in patient safety and identification, Health Manage Technol, 2012, http://www.healthmgttech.com/the-role-of-barcode-technology-in-patient-safety-and-identification.php. Accessed January 16, 2016.

Toscan J, et al: Integrated transitional care: patient, informal caregiver and health care provider perspectives on care transitions for older persons with hip fracture, *Int J Integr Care* 12(2):2012.

Touhy T, Jett K: *Ebersole and Hess' Gerontological nursing & healthy aging*, ed 4, St Louis, 2014, Mosby.

US Department of Health and Human Services (USDHHS): *Summary of the HIPAA privacy rule*, Washington, DC, 2003, Office for Civil Rights.

US Department of Health and Human Services (USDHHS): HIPAA privacy rule revisions on disclosures accounting, access reporting, *Fed Reg* 76:31426, 2011.

US Department of Health and Human Services (USDHHS): Healthy people 2020, health disparities, 2015, http://www.healthypeople.gov/2020/about/foundation-health-measures/Disparities. Accessed January 14, 2016.

US Department of Health and Human Services (USDHHS) and Centers for Medicare and Medicaid Services (CMS): Discharge planning, 2014, https://www.cms.gov/Outreach-and-Education/Medicare-Learning-Network-MLN/MLNproducts/downloads/Discharge-Planning-Booklet-ICN908184.pdf.

US Department of Health and Human Services (USDHHS), Office of Minority Health (OPHS): National standards for culturally and linguistically appropriate services in health care final report, March 2001, Washington DC, http://minorityhealth.hhs.gov/assets/pdf/checked/finalreport.pdf. Accessed January 16, 2016.

Vandenberg AK: Patient hand offs: facilitating safe and effective transitions of care, Master's Projects. Paper 1. *Scholarworks*, 2013, http://scholarworks.gvsu.edu/cgi/viewcontent.cgi?article=1000&context=kcon_projects. Accessed January 14, 2016.

Wallace LS, et al: BRIEF REPORT: Screening items to identify patients with limited health literacy skills, *J Gen Intern Med* 21(8):874, 2006.

Zou XJ, Zhang YP: Rates of nursing errors and handoff-related errors in a medical unit following implementation of a standardized nursing handoff form, *J Nurs Care Qual* 31(1):61, 2016.

3 | Communication and Collaboration

OBJECTIVES

Mastery of content in this chapter will enable the nurse to:
- Identify guidelines to use in therapeutic communication.
- Explain the communication process.
- Identify the purposes of therapeutic communication and communication in various phases of the nurse-patient relationship.
- Develop skills for therapeutic communication in various phases of the nurse-patient relationship.

- Develop therapeutic communication skills for communicating with patients who have difficulty coping because of feelings such as anxiety, anger, and depression.
- Develop therapeutic communication skills for communication with cognitively impaired patients.
- Develop skills for effective communication with colleagues.

MEDIA RESOURCES

- evolve http://evolve.elsevier.com/Perry/skills
- Review Questions
- Audio Glossary

- Clinical Debrief and Review Questions Answers
- Case Studies

PURPOSE

Communication is the interaction between two or more people. Effective communication positively influences how nursing care is delivered and patient satisfaction with that care. A nurse's responsibility to effectively communicate extends beyond the patient to include family members/significant others and all members of the health care team. The purpose of this chapter is to provide you with a framework to develop effective communication skills that are essential to the delivery of patient-centered care.

STANDARDS OF CARE

- The Joint Commission, 2016—National Patient Safety Goal 1: Improve accuracy of patient identification
- The Joint Commission, 2016—National Patient Safety Goal 2: Improve effectiveness of communication among caregivers
- U.S. Department of Health and Human Services, 2013—National Standards for Culturally and Linguistically Appropriate Services (CLAS) in Health and Health Care

PRINCIPLES FOR PRACTICE

- Nurses must have knowledge of the principles of therapeutic communication, implement the skills of communicating effectively, and possess the attitude of wanting to improve communication skills (Sherwood et al., 2014).
- Communication is an interaction between two or more people that involves the exchange of information between a sender and a receiver, involving the expression of emotions, ideas, and thoughts through verbal (words or written language) and nonverbal (behaviors) exchanges (Fig. 3.1).
- Establish and understand the purpose of a patient interaction. This is an essential quality of effective communication.
- Communication skills provide information and comfort, promote understanding, clarify misinformation, help to develop plans of care, promote interprofessional collaboration, and facilitate wellness through patient teaching.
- Communication includes both spoken and written words. To send an accurate message the sender of verbal communication needs to be aware of the tone, volume, and cadence (pace or rate) of his or her voice.
- Nonverbal communication describes all behaviors that convey messages without the use of words. This type of communication includes body movement, physical appearance, personal space, and touch. Be aware of body language, which includes posture, body position, gestures, eye contact, facial expression, and movement. For clarity make sure that nonverbal communication is consistent with the spoken word.
- Know your attitudes toward a patient or situation. Be aware of your personal feelings to control how you communicate issues.

PATIENT-CENTERED CARE

- Therapeutic communication enables nurses to deliver patient-centered care—care that is respectful of and responsive to individual patient preferences, needs, and values and that ensures

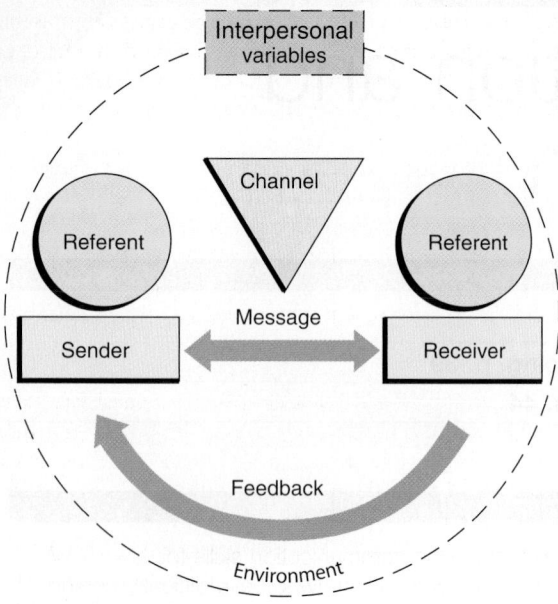

FIG 3.1 Communication is a two-way process.

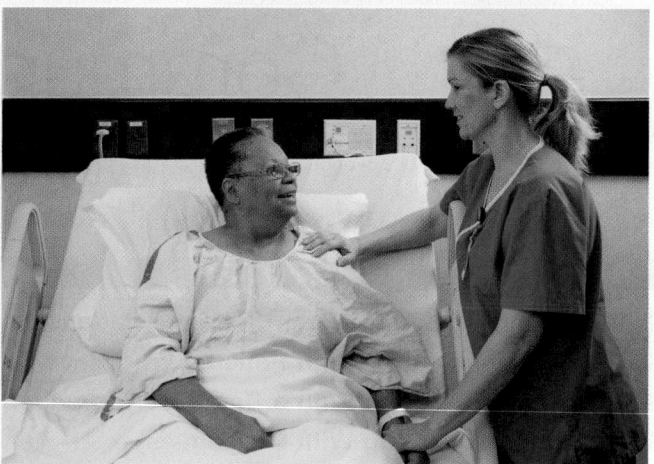

FIG 3.2 An open, relaxed posture conveys interest.

that patient values guide clinical decisions (Institute of Medicine, 2001). It also creates a positive relationship with health care providers and improves patient adherence to treatment regimens.

- Include patients and significant others in collaboration with health care providers to make decisions related to wellness and illness care. Benefits include improved satisfaction with care, self-efficacy, quality of life, and empowerment to manage care (Boykins, 2014; Jahne, 2015; Wittenberg-Lyles et al., 2013).
- Value the importance of assessing patient/family preferences, values, and beliefs when establishing a therapeutic nurse-patient relationship and planning care for a patient (Webster, 2013).
- Understand how culture affects a patient and his or her knowledge and values about health. Nurses need to recognize their own attitudes about working with patients from different backgrounds.
- Be aware of cultural differences such as the use of touch and religious and ethnic practices because these influence methods of communication (Fig. 3.2).
- To avoid misinterpretation of nonverbal cues, be aware of any cultural norms or values (e.g., eye contact) that patients may have (see Skill 3.1).
- Adopt a flexible, respectful attitude that also communicates interest in a patient to bridge any communication barriers that exist because of cultural differences between patient and caregiver.
- When using language assistance:
  - Provide easy-to-understand print and multimedia materials and signage in languages commonly used by populations in the health care agency service area (USDHHS, 2013).
  - Address the patient and family directly when using an interpreter; do not direct questions or comments to the interpreter. Take care to determine if the patient understood (Box 3.1).

EVIDENCE-BASED PRACTICE

Recent studies have examined specific interventions used to effectively communicate with people of varying developmental levels

---

BOX 3.1

Special Approaches for Patients Who Speak Different Languages

- Use a caring tone of voice and facial expressions to help alleviate patients' fears and anxieties.
- Speak slowly and distinctly but not loudly.
- Use gestures, pictures, and role playing to help patients understand.
- Repeat a message in different ways if necessary.
- Be alert to and use words that a patient seems to understand and use them frequently.
- Keep messages simple and repeat them frequently.
- Avoid using medical terms that a patient may not understand.
- Use an appropriate language dictionary or have a medical interpreter or family member make flash cards to communicate key phrases.

From Giger J: *Transcultural nursing: assessment and interventions,* ed 6, St Louis, 2013, Mosby.

and/or people who may have difficulty communicating with others related to a physical or mental illness (Lancioni et al., 2012; Law et al., 2014).

- Speech and language therapy intervention programs have been implemented to help people with brain damage to maximize their communication skills (Blake et al., 2013; Pennington et al., 2004).
- Information and communication technology, including the use of telephones, television, radio, computers, and handheld devices to deliver information promotes treatment compliance among people with severe mental illness. These strategies help those with mental illness who have difficulty remembering to take medication and/or appointment times (Kauppi et al., 2014).
- Effective communication and support from health care providers often reduces psychological distress in patients undergoing cancer treatment. Health care providers may benefit from specific communication skills training to interact more therapeutically with their cancer patients (Moore et al., 2015).
- Health care providers need to consider the needs of older adults for person-centered communication by establishing interpersonal connections with these communication partners.

Specific strategies include use of hearing support, nonverbal communication matching verbal, cultural competence, and communication as tools to prompt resident participation and improved functional independence (Williams, 2013).

- Communicate through the use of printed educational material that focuses on message readability and plain language. Clear communication sends messages that influence a patient's understanding with resulting behavior changes (Genova et al., 2014; USDHHS, 2013).

SAFETY GUIDELINES

- Listen to what and how a patient communicates, including content and verbal and nonverbal messages. Some patients express themselves clearly without difficulty. However, indirect and nonverbal cues communicate a patient's needs (e.g., pain, perceived stress).
- Control external factors in both the environmental setting (temperature of room, privacy issues) and the psychological setting (emotional state of the nurse and patient) that influence or hinder communication. When you are talking with a patient about his or her personal concerns, privacy is important.

- When teaching, try to have a family caregiver present with whom to reinforce the content of the instruction. Use language-appropriate print and multimedia materials. This is necessary for family caregivers to provide needed support when patients return home.
- Controlling noise level and interruptions is also important in an effort to maintain privacy boundaries when communicating with patients (Wittenberg-Lyles et al., 2013).
- Establish and understand the purpose of interaction. This is an essential quality of effective communication
- Guide an interaction depending on the patient's condition and response. Patient needs remain the focus. For example, you establish that the purpose of the interaction is patient teaching; however, the patient just learned about the death of a loved one and expresses the need to talk about the death. You help him or her by grieving first, remaining flexible and creative in the interaction. Or, if the patient complains of increased pain, provide an analgesic.
- When communicating with colleagues, it is important to communicate clearly and to recognize and report errors and nears misses that may compromise patient safety (Sherwood et al., 2014).

♦ **SKILL 3.1** | **Establishing the Nurse-Patient Relationship**

A therapeutic nurse-patient relationship is the foundation of nursing care and involves using a variety of patient-centered therapeutic communication skills (Box 3.2). Communication is essential in nursing since effective communication among patients, families, and health care providers is an essential part of quality care (Bramhall, 2014; Hemsley et al., 2012). The primary goal of therapeutic communication for a nurse is to promote patients' wellness and personal growth. Therapeutic communication empowers patients to make decisions but differs from social communication in that it is patient centered and goal directed with limited disclosure from the professional.

Social communication involves equal opportunity for personal disclosure, and both participants seek to have personal needs met (Keltner et al., 2015). Nurses do not routinely share intimate details of their personal lives with patients. However, they use personal self-disclosure (e.g., outside interests, thoughts about local news, experience as a nurse) cautiously in selected situations. Personal self-disclosure is useful for the following goals: (1) to educate patients, (2) to build therapeutic alliances with patients, and (3) to encourage patients' independence (Halter, 2014). There are times when empathy is essential to establishing and maintaining the nurse-patient relationship. Empathy is being sensitive; it conveys an understanding of a patient's and/or family's feelings and communicating this understanding to them.

Barriers to therapeutic communication include giving an opinion, offering false reassurance, making disingenuous or insincere comments, being defensive, showing approval or disapproval, stereotyping, and asking, "Why?" The use of "why" questions causes increased defensiveness in patients and hinders communication. The therapeutic nurse-patient relationship is goal directed, with a patient moving toward productive modes of interpersonal functioning.

Delegation and Collaboration

All health care providers must practice effective communication. The skill of establishing therapeutic communication cannot be delegated to nursing assistive personnel (NAP). The nurse directs the NAP about:

- The proper way to interact verbally and nonverbally with select patients.
- The need to keep all patient communication confidential.
- Ways to arrange the environment to ensure privacy and confidentiality.
- Special considerations pertaining to communication with patients who are cognitively or sensorially impaired, older, children, and anxious and potentially violent patients.

STEP	RATIONALE

ASSESSMENT

1. Prepare for orientation phase of therapeutic communication. Formulate individualized patient goals, consider time allocation (e.g., patient acuity and medical priorities), formulate initial questions, and mentally prepare to keep one's mind clear of other concerns or distractions. Select the assessment questions most relevant to the clinical situation.

Preparation is part of a planned communication process that facilitates interaction. Planning for the orientation phase helps to identify actual or potential problems, current health status, and experience. Without preparation, a risk exists for casual, non–goal-oriented communication.

BOX 3.2

Therapeutic Communication Techniques

Technique: Listening
Definition: An active process of receiving information and examining one's reaction to messages received
Example: Consider the cultural practices of your patient, maintain appropriate eye contact, and be receptive to nonverbal communications.
Therapeutic Value: Nonverbally communicates your interest and acceptance to a patient
Nontherapeutic Threat: Failure to listen, interrupting patient

Technique: Broad Openings
Definition: Encouraging patient to select topics for discussion
Example: "Can you tell me what you are thinking about?"
Therapeutic Value: Indicates your acceptance valuing of patient's initiative
Nontherapeutic Threat: Domination of interaction by nurse; rejecting responses

Technique: Restating
Definition: Repeating main thought that patient has expressed
Example: "You say that your mother left you when you were 5 years old."
Therapeutic Value: Indicates that you are listening and validates, reinforces, or calls attention to something important that has been said
Nontherapeutic Threat: Lack of validation of your interpretation of message; being judgmental; reassuring; defending

Technique: Clarification
Definition: Attempting to improve your understanding of words, vague ideas, or patient's unclear thoughts or asking patient to explain what he or she means
Example: "I'm not sure what you mean. Could you tell me again?"
Therapeutic Value: Helps to clarify patient's feelings, ideas, and perceptions and provide an explicit correlation between them and patient's actions
Nontherapeutic Threat: Failure to probe; assumed understanding

Technique: Reflection
Definition: Directing back to patient ideas, feelings, questions, or content
Example: "You're feeling tense and anxious, and it's related to a conversation you had with your sister last night?"
Therapeutic Value: Validates your understanding of what patient is saying and signifies empathy, interest, and respect for patient
Nontherapeutic Threat: Stereotyping patient's responses, inappropriate timing of reflections; inappropriate depth of feeling of reflections; inappropriate to the cultural experience and educational level of the patient

Technique: Humor
Definition: Discharging energy through comic enjoyment of the imperfect
Example: "This gives a whole new meaning to 'Just relax.'"
Therapeutic Value: Can promote insight by making conscious any repressed material, resolving paradoxes, tempering aggression, and revealing new options; is a socially acceptable form of sublimation
Nontherapeutic Threat: Indiscriminate use; belittling patient; screen to avoid therapeutic intimacy

Technique: Informing
Definition: Demonstrating skills or giving information
Example: "I think it would be helpful for you to know more about how your medication works."
Therapeutic Value: Helpful in patient education about relevant aspects of patient's well-being and self-care
Nontherapeutic Threat: Giving advice

Technique: Focusing
Definition: Asking questions or making statements that help patient expand on a topic of importance
Example: "I think it would be helpful if we talk more about your relationship with your father."
Therapeutic Value: Allows patient to discuss central issues related to problem and keeps communication process goal directed
Nontherapeutic Threat: Allowing abstractions and generalizations; changing topics

Technique: Sharing Perceptions
Definition: Asking patient to verify your understanding of what patient is thinking or feeling
Example: "You're smiling, but I sense that you're really very angry with me."
Therapeutic Value: Conveys your understanding to patient and has potential for clearing up confusing communication
Nontherapeutic Threat: Challenging patient; accepting literal responses; reassuring; testing; defending

Technique: Theme Identification
Definition: Clarifying underlying issues or problems experienced by patient that emerge repeatedly during nurse-patient relationship
Example: "I've noticed that in all the relationships that you've described you've been hurt or rejected by the man. Do you think this is an underlying issue?"
Therapeutic Value: Allows you to best promote patient's exploration and understanding of important problems
Nontherapeutic Threat: Giving advice; reassuring; disapproving

Technique: Silence
Definition: Using silence or nonverbal communication for a therapeutic reason
Example: Sitting with patient and nonverbally communicating interest and involvement
Therapeutic Value: Allows patient time to think and gain insights, slows the pace of the interaction, and encourages patient to initiate conversation while conveying your support, understanding, and acceptance
Nontherapeutic Threat: Questioning patient: asking for "why" responses; failing to break a nontherapeutic silence

Technique: Suggesting
Definition: Presenting alternative ideas for patient's consideration relative to problem solving
Example: "Have you thought about organizing your medications on a daily schedule? For example, you could use a pill organizer that allows you to sort out medicines to be taken each day or over a week."
Therapeutic Value: Increases patient's perceived options or choices
Nontherapeutic Threat: Giving advice, inappropriate timing; being judgmental

Modified from Keltner N et al: *Psychiatric nursing*, ed 6, St Louis, 2011, Mosby.

STEP	RATIONALE
2. Address patient by name and introduce yourself and role on health care team ("Hello, my name is Jane Smith, and I am the registered nurse assigned to take care of you today. …") Use clear, specific communication, including verbal and nonverbal techniques (e.g., good eye contact, relaxed, comfortable position) to provide information and clarify concerns (see Fig. 3.2). Create a climate of warmth and acceptance.	Congruent verbal and nonverbal communication expresses warmth and respect and helps to establish rapport. The quality of communication in interactions between nurse and patient has important influences on patient outcomes (O'Hagen et al., 2014).
3. Assess the following during initial interaction: patient's needs, coping strategies, defenses, and adaptation styles.	Recurrent themes in patient's responses help to identify problem areas related to health status (e.g., avoidance of questions, request for information, expression of a loss).
4. Determine patient's need to communicate (e.g., constant use of call light, crying, patient who does not understand an illness or who has just been admitted).	Patients in need of support, comfort, knowledge, or encouragement benefit from individualized meaningful communication.
5. Assess reason patient needs health care. Ask patient about health status, lifestyle, support systems, patterns of health and illness, and strengths and limitations.	Nature of illness affects patient's coping ability and effectiveness in communicating needs and concerns. For example, patients who are fearful of a cancer diagnosis and patients who are having joint replacement surgeries probably have differing needs and concerns.
6. Assess for factors about yourself and patient that normally influence communication. Examples of factors include perceptions, values, and beliefs; emotions; sociocultural background; severity of illness; knowledge; age; verbal ability; roles and relationships; environmental setting; physical comfort or discomfort (see illustration).	Communication is a dynamic process influenced by interpersonal and intrapersonal processes. By assessing factors that influence communication, you can more accurately assess a patient's perception of health status (Cronenwett et al., 2007).

STEP 6 Essential and influencing variables of the therapeutic communication environment. *(Modified from Keltner N et al: Psychiatric nursing, ed 6, St Louis, 2011, Mosby.)*

7. Assess personal barriers to communicating with patient (e.g., bias toward patient's condition, anxiety from inexperience).	Barriers prevent you from conveying empathy and caring and obtaining relevant assessment information.
8. Assess patient's language and ability to speak. Does patient have difficulty finding words or associating ideas with accurate word symbols? Does patient have difficulty with expression of language and/or reception of messages? What is patient's primary language?	Assessment determines need for special techniques to address the communication needs of patients with limited English proficiency, hearing impairments, or literacy levels (USDHHS, 2013). Examples include picture boards, computers, sign language, or a medical interpreter (see illustration).

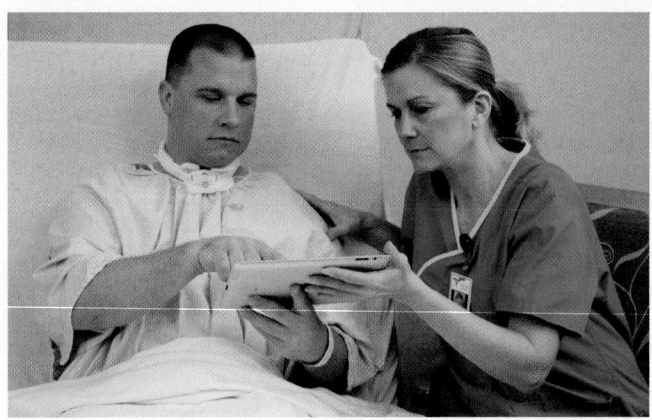

STEP 8 Communication tools for patient who cannot speak.

9. Assess patient's literacy level. Does he or she skip over uncommon or hard words, avoid asking questions, or have difficulty discussing concepts about illness? Assess health literacy by asking these questions: ""How often do you have someone help you read hospital materials?" "How confident are you filling out medical forms by yourself?" and "How often do you have problems learning about your medical condition because of difficulty understanding written information?" (Chew et al., 2004).
   Option: Use a standardized literacy assessment tool available at your institution, such as the Rapid Estimate of Adult Literacy in Medicine (REALM) (Davis et al., 1993) or the Test of Functional Health Literacy in Adults (TOFHLA), also available in Spanish (STOFHLA) (Parker et al., 1995; Smith et al., 2012; Thomason et al., 2015).

Health literacy has a direct effect on health outcomes. Assessing patient's level of health literacy allows you to design more effective communication and patient teaching approaches (Thomason et al., 2015). These three health literacy questions have been found effective screening tests for inadequate health literacy in a general preoperative patient population (Chew et al., 2004).

10. Assess patient's ability to hear. Be sure that hearing aid is functional if worn. Be sure that patient hears and understands words (see Chapter 19).

Patients with hearing deficits require techniques to enhance hearing reception (e.g., speaking in normal tone, speaking so patient can see face).

11. Observe patient's pattern of communication and verbal or nonverbal behavior (e.g., gestures, tone of voice, eye contact).

Observation determines type and manner of communication that you will use.

12. Assess resources available in selecting communication methods:
    a. Review information in medical record and reflect on your past patient communication experiences.

Relying totally on information from patient restricts the quality of interaction. Additional resources provide insight into best methods of communicating.

    b. Consult with family, health care provider, and other health care team members concerning patient's condition, problems, and impressions.

Collaboration with health care team members facilitates your response to patient on the basis of integration of knowledge. Seek information from family after patient approval. Patient privacy must be maintained (Boykins, 2014).

13. Before initiating the working phase of nurse-patient relationship, assess patient's readiness to work toward goal attainment. "We want to work together with you to improve your health. Tell me your goals or what it is that you feel is important for you to recover."

Patient's goals are identified and agreed on by effective communication skills such as restating and clarifying.

14. Consider when patient is due to be discharged or transferred from health care agency. Share that information with patient and family caregiver.

This allows you to anticipate the amount of time available to work with patient and when termination of relationship is to occur.

NURSING DIAGNOSES

- Anxiety
- Deficient knowledge regarding communication skills
- Fear

- Impaired social interaction
- Impaired verbal communication
- Ineffective coping

- Noncompliance
- Readiness for enhanced decision making

Related factors are individualized based on patient's condition or needs.

STEP	RATIONALE

PLANNING

1. Expected outcomes following completion of procedure:
   - Patient expresses ideas, fears, and concerns clearly, asks questions, and openly expresses relief of anxiety.

   Once patients are able to talk directly about emotions, the focus is on coping more effectively with them (Keltner et al., 2015). Asking questions shows an openness to communication.

   - Patient health care goals are identified and achieved.
   - Patient verbalizes understanding of information communicated by nurse.

   Interaction remains patient focused.
   This provides a means to build trust and develop a knowledge base for patient to make decisions.

2. Before engaging in the working phase, prepare patient physically (e.g., deliver pain relief measures, provide for hygiene or elimination), provide a quiet environment, maintain privacy, and reduce distractions or interruptions before beginning discussion.

   Taking care of basic needs promotes an environment for interaction and decreases patient distractions and interruptions.

3. Working phase
   a. Use appropriate communication tools such as iPads or other electronic devices for patients whose initial language is not English.

   Electronic devices such as iPads help with communication and provide translation resources.

   b. Prepare open-ended questions to identify strategies for developing a realistic plan to meet identified health goals of patients (e.g., "Let's talk more about the goals you shared earlier for this hospitalization/visit to the health care agency").

   Open-ended questions promote goal attainment and avoid risk of misinterpretation.

IMPLEMENTATION

1. Working phase: Observe patient's nonverbal behaviors, including body language. If verbal behaviors do not match nonverbal behaviors, seek clarification from patient.

   Congruence between patient's verbal and nonverbal behaviors ensures that you receive the correct message.

2. Explain purpose of interaction when information is to be shared.

   Information and explanation can decrease anxiety about the unknown.

3. Continue to use therapeutic communication skills (see Box 3.2).

   Fosters open, interactive communication with patient as a participant and the focus of the discussion.

4. Identify patient's expectations in seeking health care.

   Identifying expectations conveys a level of interest in patient's needs.

5. Encourage patient to ask for clarification at any time during the communication.

   This gives patient a sense of control and keeps channels of communication open.

6. Set mutual goals.
   a. Use therapeutic communication skills such as restating, reflecting, and paraphrasing to identify and clarify strategies for attainment of mutually agreed-on goals.

   For communication between nurse and patient to be effective, both need to possess the skills and knowledge required for participation within the communicative interaction.

   b. Discuss and prioritize problem areas.

   A patient, nonjudgmental, supportive approach minimizes patient anxiety.

   c. Provide information to patient and help him or her to express needs and feelings.

   Patient is able to respond to help, develop workable solutions based on goals, and fully participate in a realistic plan for his or her well-being.

   d. Use questions carefully and appropriately. Ask one question at a time and allow sufficient time to answer. Use direct questions. Use open-ended statements as much as possible such as, "Tell me about how you're feeling today."

   This helps patient express self and allows you to obtain thorough information about his or her needs and concerns.

Clinical Decision Point *Avoid asking questions about information that may not yet have been disclosed to the patient (e.g., human immunodeficiency virus [HIV] status, diagnostic test results). Avoid asking "why" questions; this causes increased defensiveness in the patient and prevents communication.*

   e. Avoid communication barriers (see Box 3.2).

   Barriers result in a message not being received, being distorted, or not being understood.

STEP	RATIONALE
7. Termination phase: Communicate with the patient.	
a. Prepare by identifying methods of summarizing and synthesizing information pertinent for patient's aftercare (e.g., "What are your plans for follow-up once you return home to maintain your health status?").	Effective communication by summarizing and synthesizing information reinforces behavior change.
b. Use therapeutic communication skills to discuss discharge or termination issues and guide discussion related to specific patient changes in thoughts and behaviors.	Reinforces behaviors/skills learned during working phase of relationship.
c. Summarize with patient what you discussed during interaction, including goal achievement.	Signals the close of interaction and allows you and patient to depart with the same idea. The termination phase consists of evaluation and summary of progress toward prescribed goals. Provides a sense of closure and mutual understanding.

EVALUATION

1. Observe patient's verbal and nonverbal responses to your communication, noting his or her willingness to share information and concerns during orientation phase.	Verbal and nonverbal feedback reveals patient's interest and willingness to communicate and reflects his or her ability to form a therapeutic relationship.
2. Note your response to patient and patient's response to you. Reflect on effectiveness of therapeutic techniques used in establishing rapport with patient.	Sensitivity to one's ability in using therapeutic communication skills helps improve ability to adjust techniques when necessary.
3. During working phase evaluate patient's ability to work toward identified goals. Elicit feedback (verbal and nonverbal) to determine success of goal attainment. Evaluate patient's health status in relation to identified goals. Reevaluate and identify barriers if patient goals are not met.	Feedback is an essential step in evaluating new behaviors. Modifications are necessary if goals cannot be met.
4. During termination phase summarize and restate. Reinforce patient's strengths, outline issues still requiring work, and develop an action plan.	Evaluates patient progress in terms of attainment of mutually agreed-on goals.
5. **Use Teach-Back:** "I want to be sure that you understand the action plan following your discharge. We developed it together, taking into consideration your progress thus far and your strengths and limitations. Describe your action plan." Review the action plan or give patient or family caregiver the plan in a written/other format if he or she is not able to teach back correctly.	Determines patient's and family caregiver's level of understanding of instructional topic.

Unexpected Outcomes	**Related Interventions**
1. Patient continues to verbally and nonverbally express feelings of anxiety, fear, anger, confusion, distrust, and helplessness. Patient often responds to internal and external factors and cues.	• Reassess patient's level of anxiety, fear, and distrust. Attempt to determine the cause of anxiety or fear. • Repeat message to patient at a later time. • Determine influence affecting clear communication (e.g., cultural issues, language issues, literacy issues, physical limitations).
2. Feedback between you and the patient reveals a lack of understanding and ineffective communication.	• Assess for and remove barriers such as literacy level, foreign language issues to communication (USDHHS, 2013). • Repeat message using another approach if possible. • Consider cultural norms associated with eye contact, use of touch, personal space, and nonverbal behaviors (Giger, 2013). • Avoid using medical terms that patient does not understand.
3. You are unable to acquire information about patient's ideas, fears, and concerns. Communication techniques do not promote patient's willingness to communicate openly. Trust is not established. Goals are not identified and therefore cannot be achieved.	• Use alternative communication techniques to promote patient's willingness to communicate openly. • Offer another professional with whom patient can talk to obtain necessary information.
4. Family caregiver answers for patient even when patient is capable of answering.	• Direct question to patient, using his or her name. • Acknowledge answer given by family caregiver; then state that you are interested in patient's response. • Resume interaction after family caregiver has left or encourage family caregiver to take a break for coffee or a meal.

Recording and Reporting

- Record in nurses' notes in electronic health record (EHR) or chart the communication pertinent to patient's health, response to illness or therapies, and responses that demonstrate understanding or lack of understanding (include verbal and nonverbal cues).
- Document teach-back and any changes to teaching plan.
- Report any relevant information obtained through patient's verbal and nonverbal behaviors to members of health care team.

Special Considerations
Teaching Considerations

- Use gestures, pictures, and role playing to help patient understand. Be alert to literacy status; determine if patient is able to access health information adequately. Be alert to words that patient seems to understand and use them frequently.
- Individualize patient teaching to meet patient needs. Always conduct teaching with the purpose of meeting patient's learning needs with consideration for his or her preferred methods for learning.

Pediatric Considerations

- Communicating with children requires an understanding of feelings and thought processes from the child's perspective (Hockenberry and Wilson, 2015).
- Use vocabulary that is familiar to the child, based on his or her level of understanding (age and developmental level). Try to be on same eye level as patient.

- Understand the child's cognitive, developmental, and functional level to select most appropriate communication techniques. Some age-appropriate communication techniques include storytelling and drawing (Hockenberry and Wilson, 2015).

Gerontological Considerations

- Be aware of any cognitive or sensory impairment. Assess each patient individually and avoid stereotyping older adults who have cognitive or sensory impairments (Touhy and Jett, 2014).
- It is important to understand the value of effective communication skills, history, and personality among older adults in terms of providing both human and therapeutic responses. Regression to earlier defenses is normal and adaptive with this population, particularly when facing illness.
- Make sure that older-adult patient with visual or hearing impairment uses assistive devices such as eyeglasses, large-print reading material, or hearing aids to assist in communication (Touhy and Jett, 2014).

Home Care Considerations

- Identify primary family caregiver for patient and adapt techniques to assess level of understanding regarding patient's condition.
- Incorporate communication into patient's daily activities (e.g., bathing and dressing).

◆ **SKILL 3.2** **Communicating With Patients Who Have Difficulty Coping**

Patients in the health care setting sometimes may have difficulty coping for a variety of reasons and thus experience anxiety, anger, and/or depression. You can help the patient decrease or manage his or her ineffective coping symptoms and behaviors through effective communication. Examples of factors that cause anxiety are newly diagnosed illness, separation from loved ones, threat associated with diagnostic tests or surgical procedures, and expectations of life changes. How successfully a patient copes with anxiety depends in part on previous experiences, the presence of other stressors, the significance of the event causing anxiety, and the availability of supportive resources. There are four stages of anxiety with corresponding behavioral manifestations: mild, moderate, severe, and panic (Box 3.3).

Anger is the common underlying factor associated with potential for violence. Patients become angry for a variety of reasons. Anger is often directly related to a patient's experience with illness, or it is associated with previous problems. In the health care setting the nurse has frequent contact with a patient and thus often becomes the target of his or her anger. Understanding how to use de-escalation skills is a useful technique to manage an angry or violent patient and help ensure a safe health care environment for other patients and health care personnel.

Depression is a state of feelings that is more than just sadness. It is a common psychiatric condition that affects a person's ability to function in day-to-day activities. There are many symptoms of depression, the most common being apathy, feelings of sadness, fatigue, guilt, poor concentration, sleep disturbances, and suicidal thoughts. Depression results in both subjective and objective behaviors and patient reports of increased physical complaints (Box 3.4). Some patients report feeling anxious when depressed.

BOX 3.3

Behavioral Manifestations of Anxiety: Stages of Anxiety

Mild Anxiety
- Increased auditory and visual perception
- Increased awareness of relationships
- Increased alertness
- Able to problem solve

Severe Anxiety
- Focus on fragmented details
- Headache, nausea, dizziness
- Unable to see connections between details
- Poor recall

Moderate Anxiety
- Selective inattention
- Decreased perceptual field
- Focus only on relevant information
- Muscle tension; diaphoresis

Panic State of Anxiety
- Does not notice surroundings
- Feeling of terror
- Unable to cope with any problem

BOX 3.4

Symptoms of Depression

Common Symptoms
- Apathy
- Decreased socialization
- Sadness
- Sleep disturbances
- Hopelessness
- Helplessness
- Worthlessness
- Guilt
- Anger

Other Symptoms
- Fatigue
- Decrease in performance of activities of daily living
- Thoughts of death
- Decreased libido
- Feeling inadequate
- Psychomotor agitation
- Verbal berating of self
- Spontaneous crying
- Dependency, passiveness

From Keltner N et al: *Psychiatric nursing*, ed 6, St Louis, 2011, Mosby.

Delegation and Collaboration

The skill of communicating with a patient with difficulty coping cannot be delegated to nursing assistive personnel (NAP). The nurse instructs the NAP about:

- Basic communication skills needed to interact verbally and nonverbally with anxious, angry, or depressed patients.
- Their role as the nurse uses de-escalation techniques.
- Appropriate safety measures for themselves and other patients.

STEP	RATIONALE

ASSESSMENT

STEP	RATIONALE
1. Provide a brief, simple introduction; introduce yourself and explain purpose of interaction.	Ineffective coping behaviors may limit amount of information patient can understand.
2. Assess factors influencing communication with patient (e.g., environment, timing, presence of others, values, experiences, need for personal space because of heightened anxiety).	Identifies effective communication strategies.
3. Assess for possible factors causing patient anxiety (e.g., hospitalization, unknown diagnosis, fatigue).	Understanding the source of anxiety helps in patient support and communication.
4. Discuss possible causes of patient's anxiety, anger, or depression with family members, including past history of the illness, if necessary.	Gathering information about patient from a family perspective is useful because family provides new information or understanding of the situation (Keltner et al., 2015).
5. Observe for physical, behavioral, and verbal cues that indicate that patient is anxious such as dry mouth, sweaty palms, tone of voice, frequent use of call light, difficulty concentrating, wringing of hands, and statements such as, "I'm scared."	Anxiety interferes with usual manner of communication and thus interferes with patient's care and treatment. Extreme anxiety interferes with comprehension, attention, and problem-solving abilities.
6. Assess for physical, behavioral, and verbal cues that indicate that patient is depressed such as feelings of sadness, tearfulness, difficulty concentrating, increase in reports of physical complaints, and statements such as "I'm sad/ depressed."	Depression interferes with usual manner of communication and thus with patient's care and treatment. If depression is severe, it interferes with comprehension, attention, and problem-solving abilities.
7. Assess for possible factors causing patient's depression (e.g., acute or chronic illness, personal vulnerability, recent loss).	Patient's depressive state is sometimes unknown. Understanding the possible cause of depression helps in patient support and communication.
8. Observe for behaviors that indicate that the patient is angry (e.g., pacing, clenched fist, loud voice, throwing objects) and/or expressions that indicate anger (e.g., repeated questioning of nurse, not following requests, aggressive outbursts, threats).	Anger is a normal expression of frustration or response to feeling threatened. However, its expression often interferes with or blocks communication and interactions.
9. Assess factors that influence the angry patient's communication such as refusal to comply with treatment goals, use of sarcasm or hostile behavior, having a low frustration level, or being emotionally immature.	Allows you to accurately evaluate the situation or patient experiences that block or facilitate communication.
10. Assess for resources (e.g., social worker, pastoral care, or family) available to help in communicating with potentially violent patient.	This helps to clarify cause and intervention required to deal with patient's anger.
11. Assess for underlying medical conditions that may potentially lead to violent behavior.	Patients with medical conditions such as traumatic brain injury, dementia, or drug/alcohol withdrawal may exhibit hostile, aggressive behaviors.

Clinical Decision Point *With some violent behaviors (e.g., physical aggression) you may not be able to de-escalate the situation. When this potential exists, know whom to call for assistance (e.g., trained psychology technicians, security staff). Personal safety is paramount.*

NURSING DIAGNOSES

- Anxiety
- Decisional conflict
- Defensive coping
- Hopelessness
- Impaired verbal communication
- Ineffective coping
- Ineffective role performance
- Risk for other-directed violence
- Risk for self-directed violence

Related factors/Risk factors are individualized based on patient's condition or needs.

STEP	RATIONALE

PLANNING

1. Expected outcomes following completion of procedure:
   - Patient discusses factors causing anxiety, anger, or depression

     Reflects success in making patient sense trust and ability to communicate openly.
   - Patient is able to discuss methods to cope with anxiety, anger, or depression

     Gains resources (e.g., use of deep-breathing exercises, guided imagery) to cope with situations that cause anxiety, anger, or depression.
   - Patient states that sensations of anxiety or depression are reduced.

     Communication techniques ease symptoms associated with anxiety and depression and allow patient to focus on problem.

Clinical Decision Point *First acknowledge and take care of anxious patient's physical and emotional discomfort but avoid dwelling on physical complaints. Focus on understanding patient, providing feedback and helping to problem solve, and providing atmosphere of warmth and acceptance.*

   - Patient no longer exhibits verbal and nonverbal expressions of anger.

     De-escalation techniques successfully allow patient to express anger in a constructive way.
2. Prepare for therapeutic intervention by considering patient goals, time allocation, and resources.

   Allows patient to establish rapport, achieve a sense of calm, and begin to analyze source of anxiety.
3. Recognize personal level of anxiety and consciously try to remain calm (breathe slowly and deeply, relax pelvic floor muscles) when communicating with an anxious, angry or depressed patient. Be aware of nonverbal cues that indicate own anxiety (e.g., body language, posture, cadence of speech). Remain nonjudgmental

   Your anxiety increases patient's anxiety. Your personal feelings and values may negatively affect interaction with patient.
4. Prepare a quiet, calm area, allowing ample personal space.

   Decreasing stimuli has a calming effect. Invasion of personal space increases anxiety, anger, or depression.

Clinical Decision Point *First acknowledge and take care of depressed patient's physical and emotional discomfort but avoid dwelling on physical complaints. Focus on understanding patient, providing feedback, and helping to problem solve.*

5. Prepare for de-escalation for an angry patient.
   a. Pause to collect own thoughts, feelings, and reactions.

      Awareness and control of your reaction and responses facilitate more constructive interaction.
   b. Determine what patient is saying.

      Clarification of patient need or concern may help to de-escalate situation.
   c. Prepare the environment to de-escalate a potentially violent patient:

      Potentially violent patient needs to be in an environment with decreased stimuli and have protection from injury to self or against others.

      Encourages patient's expression of anger rather than provokes it.
      (1) Encourage other people, particularly those who provoke anger, to leave room or area.

          Avoids pressuring patient; helps to prevent injury if anger becomes out of control.
      (2) Maintain an adequate distance and open exit. Position yourself closest to door to facilitate escape from a potentially violent situation. Do not block exit so patient feels that escape is unattainable.

          Prevents feeling of being trapped for both you and patient. Feeling trapped may cause a violent outburst. Safety of both parties is paramount.
      (3) When anger begins to disturb others, close door. This is particularly important when patient becomes agitated.

          Agitation and anxiety can spread to others. Some hospital rooms are equipped with security windows and cameras to allow for observation of patients.

Clinical Decision Point *Some patients are disruptive to one another, especially those who are hyperactive, intrusive, or threatening or exhibit bizarre behaviors. For these patients, first try the least-restrictive measures before using more restrictive measures such as seclusion.*

      (4) Reduce disturbing factors in room (e.g., noise, drafts, inadequate lighting).

          Reduces irritants that may heighten anger.

IMPLEMENTATION

1. Use appropriate nonverbal behaviors and active listening skills such as staying with patient at bedside and having a relaxed posture. Focus on understanding the patient's issues.

   Patients experiencing emotionally charged situation may not comprehend a verbally delivered message. Nonverbal messages to patient express interest and help alleviate anxiety.

STEP	RATIONALE
2. Use appropriate verbal techniques that are clear and concise to respond to anxious patient. Use brief statements that acknowledge current state of feelings and provide direction to patient such as, "It seems to me that you're anxious" or "I notice that you seem to want to be alone. Would you like to go to your room to rest?"	Promotes effective communication so patient can explore reasons for anxiety, anger, or depression. Appropriate techniques and statements provide reassurance.
3. Help patient acquire alternative coping strategies such as progressive relaxation, slow deep-breathing exercises, and visual imagery (see Chapter 16).	Coping strategies are nonpharmacological mechanisms to help the patient reduce anxiety and depression and in some cases reduce anger.
4. Provide necessary comfort measures such as analgesics, positioning, or hygiene.	Pain heightens patient's anxiety or depression and can contribute to his or her anger.
5. Use open-ended questions such as, "Tell me about how you're feeling" or "You seem sad. Tell me about your sadness."	Encourages patient to continue talking, facilitating an in-depth discussion of symptoms.
6. Encourage and reward small decisions and independent actions. When necessary, make decisions that patients are not ready to make. Present situations that require no decision making.	Depressed patients are often overly dependent and indecisive.
7. Accept patient as he or she is and focus on his or her positive aspects. Provide positive feedback.	Depressed patients often have low self-esteem. This approach helps to focus on their strengths.
8. Be honest and empathic.	Honesty and empathy facilitate the development of trust.

Clinical Decision Point *If your patient seems depressed, ask him or her about suicidal ideation. Ask "Have you thought about hurting yourself? Tell me how you would do it?" Refer to appropriate mental health professional in agency (if available). Depressed patients are at increased risk for suicide. Other risk factors include general medical conditions, hopelessness, male gender, and increased age. The more developed the plan, the greater the risk of suicide (Keltner et al., 2015).*

9. De-escalation for an angry patient	
a. Maintain personal space. It may be necessary to have someone with you and to keep the room door open. Position yourself between patient and the exit.	Use of personal space may help to de-escalate patient's anger. Positioning promotes health care provider's safety if patient continues to escalate and becomes violent.
b. Maintain nonthreatening verbal and nonverbal approach using a calm, reassuring tone of voice. Use open body language with a concerned, nonthreatening facial expression, open unfolded arms, relaxed posture, and a safe distance. Use gestures that are slow and deliberate rather than sudden and abrupt.	Decreases chance of misinterpretation of message and is less threatening. A relaxed atmosphere prevents further escalation. Creates climate of acceptance for patient.
c. Use therapeutic silence and allow patient to vent feelings. Use active listening for understanding. Do not argue with patient.	Often de-escalates anger. Anger expends emotional and physical energy; patient runs out of momentum and energy to maintain anger at high level. Arguing escalates anger.
d. Respond to anger therapeutically; avoid becoming defensive or angry and encourage verbal expression of anger.	Some depressed patients are angry; understand that anger is a symptom of their depression. Verbal expression often reduces tension.
e. Answer questions calmly and honestly as appropriate. If patient asks power-struggle type of question (challenging or confrontational type) (e.g., "Who said you were in charge?"), redirect and set limits by giving clear, concise expectations. Inform patient of potential consequences without sounding threatening and follow through with consequences if patient does not change behaviors.	A calm, clear communication style helps to set limits on power-struggle types of questions, provides structure for the interaction, and helps diffuse anger (Halter, 2014).
f. If patient is making verbal threats to harm others, remain calm yet professional and continue to set limits on inappropriate behavior.	Angry patient loses ability to process information rationally and therefore may impulsively express anger through intimidation.

Clinical Decision Point *If imminent harm to another is present on discharge, notify proper authorities (e.g., nurse manager, security). A potentially violent patient can be impulsive and explosive; therefore you need to keep personal safety skills in mind. In this case avoid touch.*

g. If patient appears to be calm and anger is defused, explore alternatives to situation or feelings of anger.	Processing with patient can prevent future explosive outbursts and teach patient effective ways of dealing with anger.

STEP	RATIONALE

EVALUATION

1. Observe for continuing presence of physical signs and symptoms or behaviors reflecting anxiety, anger, or depression.
2. Ask patient to describe ways to cope with anxiety, depression, or anger in the future and make decisions about own care.
3. Evaluate patient's ability to discuss factors causing anxiety, depression, or anger.
4. Note patient's ability to answer questions and problem solve.

5. Have patient discuss ways to cope in the future and make decisions about own care.
6. **Use Teach-Back:** "I want to be sure I explained options that will help you manage your anxiety in addition to medication. Describe a few of the exercises we discussed that will help you manage your anxiety." Revise your instruction now or develop a plan for revised patient or family caregiver teaching if patient or family caregiver is not able to teach back correctly.

Observation determines extent to which planned interaction relieved patient's emotions.

This measures patient's ability to assume more health-promoting behavior.

This measures patient's ability to attend or focus on area of concern.

Determines whether anger has lessened so patient is able to focus on alternative coping skills.

Discussion measures patient's ability to assume more health-promoting behavior.

Determines patient's and family caregiver's level of understanding of instructional topic.

Unexpected Outcomes

1. Physical signs and symptoms of anxiety/anger continue. Your interaction has increased patient's anxiety/anger; source of anxiety/anger is not resolved.

2. Patient displays difficulty making decisions by avoiding your efforts at focusing discussion or is unable to discuss real concerns. Anxiety/anger/depression continues to prevent problem solving.
3. Depressive behaviors continue; interaction has been ineffective at relieving depressive symptoms or patient reports suicidal ideation with or without plan.

Related Interventions

• Use refocusing or distraction skills such as relaxation or guided imagery to reduce anxiety (Halter, 2014).
• Reassess factors and remove or alter factors contributing to anxiety/anger.
• Take charge with calm, firm directions. Give as-needed (prn) medications as ordered for anxiety/agitation/escalating behaviors.
• Make sure that fellow staff members are available to help if necessary.
• Be clear and direct when communicating with patient to avoid misunderstanding.
• When used appropriately, touch helps control feelings of panic.
• Continue to use therapeutic communication skills but try different techniques.
• Refer patient to mental health professional for consultation regarding use of pharmacological agents and/or formal psychotherapy to treat depression.
• Refer patient to mental health professional for evaluation and possible admission to an inpatient psychiatric treatment facility.

Recording and Reporting

• Record cause of patient's anxiety/anger/depression and any exhibited signs and symptoms of behaviors on flow sheet or in nurses' notes in electronic health record (EHR) or chart.
• Record de-escalation technique used and patient's response to de-escalation efforts on flow sheet or in nurses' notes in EHR or chart.
• Report methods used to relieve anxiety/anger/depression and patient's response to ensure continuity of care between nurses.
• Report technique used to de-escalate and patient's response to nurse in charge.
• Document your evaluation of patient and family caregiver learning.

Special Considerations
Teaching Considerations
• Teaching patient and family caregiver to identify possible sources of anxiety such as illness, hospitalization, knowledge deficits, or other known stressors gives patient knowledge of anxiety and increases his or her sense of control.

• Patients experiencing emotionally charged situations do not always comprehend instruction. Focus on understanding patient; providing feedback and helping to problem solve; and providing an atmosphere of safety, warmth, and acceptance.
• Teaching patient and family caregiver to identify possible factors that contribute to angry outbursts such as inadequate coping skills, low frustration levels, illness, hospitalization, knowledge deficits, or other known stressors may give patient a sense of control.
• Once anger has been de-escalated, teach patient new adaptive methods of coping with anger.
• Teach patient and family caregiver to identify possible sources of depression. Knowledge of depression increases patient's sense of control over feelings of depression.

Pediatric Considerations
• Children often demonstrate anxiety through physical and behavioral signs but are unable to express anxiety verbally. Some children express anxiety through restless behavior, physical complaints, or behavioral regression. Note any changes in child's behavior that occur during illness or hospitalization (Hockenberry and Wilson, 2015).

- Set limits for inappropriate behaviors exhibited by child such as a time-out. Apply such limits immediately because children tend to have less internal control over their own behaviors (Hockenberry and Wilson, 2015).
- Children often demonstrate symptoms of depression that differ from those of adults. They manifest depression through physical (increased somatic complaints) and behavioral (poor school performance, social isolation) signs and are often unable to express it verbally. Some children express depression through restless behavior or behavioral regression. It is important to note any changes in child's behavior that occur during illness or hospitalization (Hockenberry and Wilson, 2015).

Gerontological Considerations

- Anxiety is one of the most common symptoms seen in older adults. Patients often become ritualistic and intent on performing activities a certain way. Anxiety develops as a result of a specific event or a general pattern of change (e.g., decline in health) (Touhy and Jett, 2014).
- Psychosocial factors such as anxiety and confusion, lack of mobility, and spatial organization of a long-term care facility are factors that decrease social contacts, thus hindering communication with peers and health care providers. This leads to further feelings of isolation, boredom, and increased anxiety.
- Older adults who are socially isolated have multiple medical problems and are more likely to have anxious and/or depressive

symptoms. In addition, they are less likely to seek care for these symptoms.
- Depression among older adults is a major health concern. It is important to differentiate between depression and any underlying medical illness such as cognitive impairment (Touhy and Jett, 2014).
- Suicide risk is increased in older adults because of loss of life partner, health status, independence, and social support system or financial losses (Keltner et al., 2015).

Home Care Considerations

- Anticipation of a home care visit may increase a patient's anxiety and leads to exacerbation of symptoms. Therefore some patients avoid these visits (Halter, 2014).
- Personal safety for nurse against potentially violent patient or family caregiver extends to all health care settings, including patient's home. Assess patient's home and physical surroundings, including possible exits. You may be in a potentially dangerous situation while giving care to patient at home because you are without support from other staff members. Do not enter the home if you feel unsafe; call for help.
- Depression is often present in home care settings. Educate family caregivers about how to identify symptoms. Manage depression on the basis of patient's presenting behaviors with a consideration of any cognitive/physical impairment.

◆ SKILL 3.3   Communicating With a Cognitively Impaired Patient

The act of communicating and expressing oneself is affected by a person's ability. Patients with cognitive impairments pose a challenge for nurses because these patients may have disabilities that negatively affect communication (Carlsson et al., 2014; Lancioni et al., 2012; McGhee, 2011). Acute cognitive impairment or delirium is largely reversible and may be caused by conditions such as infection, polypharmacy, and metabolic changes. Once the cause is identified and treated, the patient's mental status returns to a baseline condition. Chronic types of cognitive impairments are irreversible and progressive. These include dementia (Alzheimer's disease, vascular dementia, frontal-temporal dementia), traumatic brain injury (TBI), and human immunodeficiency virus (HIV)–related cognitive dysfunction.

Cognitive impairments accompanied by communication deficits hinder a patient's ability to initiate conversation and participate in self-care. Since it is time-consuming to interact with these patients, they may be deprived of human contact, which leads to

depression, detachment, and isolation. Patients with cognitive impairments may also be at risk for physical status changes such as infection, falls and injury, and poor nutrition.

There is a potential for a lack of quality nurse-patient interaction and communication, which negatively affects patient outcomes. A patient-centered approach stresses the uniqueness of each patient and his or her individuality when assessing the patient's ability to communicate.

Delegation and Collaboration

The skill of communicating effectively with a cognitively impaired patient cannot be delegated to nursing assistive personnel (NAP). The nurse instructs the NAP about:

- The proper communication skills needed to interact verbally and nonverbally with the cognitively impaired patient.
- The possible causes and signs and symptoms of the patient's cognitive impairment.

STEP	RATIONALE

ASSESSMENT

1. When you first meet a patient, approach from the front. Assess for the physical, behavioral, and verbal cues that indicate that a patient is cognitively impaired. Assess orientation status of patient (person, place, time) and perform a mini-mental examination (see Chapter 6).

2. Assess for possible factors causing patient's cognitive impairment (e.g., acute or chronic illness, fever, medications, fluid and electrolyte imbalance).

You may startle and upset a patient if you touch him or her unexpectedly or approach from behind. If the patient is unable to think, speak, or understand, you need to adjust communication strategies to communicate effectively.

Understanding the possible cause of mental decline helps in conferring with medical team on appropriate therapy and has implications for short-term and long-term communication strategies

STEP	RATIONALE
3. Assess factors influencing communication with patient (e.g., environment, timing, presence of others, values, experiences, prior sensory loss, poor concentration).	Understanding factors that influence communication helps you to identify effective communication strategies (Hemsley et al., 2012).
4. Discuss possible causes of patient's cognitive impairment with family members or caregivers, including current illness, duration, treatment regimen, and past medical history.	Gathering information about patient from a family perspective is useful because family provides new information or understanding of the situation. It is important to establish patient's baseline mental status.
5. Discuss with family how patient typically communicates with them. Consider these questions: Does the patient lose his or her train of thought, struggle to organize words logically, need more time to understand what you're saying, or curse or use offensive language? (Mayo Clinic, 2016).	Allows you to anticipate pattern of patient's communication so you can use effective communication strategies.
6. Ascertain the most effective means of communication with patient (e.g., verbal or written communication, picture board).	Knowing how best to communicate and using alternative communication methods can help identify patient's needs.

NURSING DIAGNOSES

- Acute confusion
- Decisional conflict
- Hopelessness

- Impaired social interaction
- Impaired verbal communication

- Ineffective coping
- Ineffective role performance

Related factors are individualized on the basis of patient's condition or needs.

PLANNING

1. Expected outcomes following completion of procedure: • Patient is able to communicate physical and emotional discomfort needs to nurse.	Use of relevant communication techniques enables patient to express needs (e.g., physical and emotional discomforts) effectively given the limitations related to cognitive impairment.
2. Prepare for communication by considering type of cognitive impairment, communication impairments, time allocation, and resources.	Effective communication allows you to establish rapport with patient and have a quality nurse-patient interaction.
3. Be aware of your nonverbal cues that affect communication with the cognitively impaired patient (e.g., body language, posture, cadence of speech). Remain nonjudgmental.	Frustration in communication with patients with cognitive impairment may negatively affect interaction with patient.
4. Prepare environment physically by providing a quiet, calm area. Reduce distractions such as external noises.	Decreasing stimuli has a calming effect. Ensuring that the environment is quiet and free from distractions enhances the communication experience.

IMPLEMENTATION

1. Approach patient from the front and face him or her when speaking.	This strategy avoids startling the patient and helps to ensure that patient both sees and hears you.
2. Provide brief, simple introduction. Introduce yourself, show respect, and explain purpose of interaction.	Symptoms associated with cognitive impairment limit amount of information that patient can understand.
3. Use appropriate nonverbal behaviors and active listening skills such as staying with patient at bedside or using touch appropriately.	Nonverbal messages to patient express your interest and convey empathy. Use of touch may help with concentration and reassurance.
4. Use clear and concise verbal techniques to respond to patient (Mayo Clinic, 2016). Use simple language and speak slowly; use short and simple sentences. Ask yes-or-no questions.	Appropriate techniques and statements provide reassurance to cognitively impaired patient.
5. Ask one question at a time and allow time for response. Avoid rushing patient. Do not interrupt patient.	This gives patient time to process the information and respond.
6. Repeat sentences using a steady voice and avoid raising your voice or being too quick to guess what patient is trying to express.	Repetition allows time for patient to respond; it can be frustrating for patient if you misinterpret his or her message or pressure him or her to respond.
7. Use augmentative and assistive communication (AAC) devices such as pictogram grid, talking mats, objects, and iPads to facilitate communication.	Talking mats are communication aids that use picture symbols so the patient can place relevant images below a visual scale to indicate feelings (McGhee, 2011).

STEP	RATIONALE
8. Make sure that patient is wearing eyeglasses or hearing aids to help with communication.	Some patients with cognitive impairments forget about eyeglasses or hearing aids and need to be reminded to use these to improve clarity of communication.
9. Do not argue with patient or correct him or her if mistakes are made.	Arguing can lead to increased frustration and agitation.
10. Maintain meaningful interactions with patients and use creative modes of communication on the basis of patient's comfort level and abilities.	Meaningful interactions help patient engage with family or community and surroundings and help reduce a sense of isolation and detachment.
11. Use individualized coping strategies such as progressive relaxation, slow deep-breathing exercises, or visual imagery.	Helps to reduce some anxiety associated with confusion and difficulties in communication.

EVALUATION

1. Observe patient's response for clarity and understanding of messages sent and received.	Observation determines extent to which cognitively impaired patient is able to express self.
2. Observe verbal and nonverbal behaviors.	Observation reveals if patient is comfortable and needs have been met.
3. **Use Teach-Back:** "I want to be sure I explained how this picture board will help you communicate with your family. Tell me how to use the picture board to show your wife that you want to take a shower or take a walk together." Revise your instruction now or develop a plan for revised patient or family caregiver teaching to be implemented at an appropriate time if patient or family caregiver is not able to teach back correctly.	Determines patient's and family caregiver's level of understanding of instructional topic.

Unexpected Outcomes	Related Interventions
1. Messages that are sent and received are not understood.	• Continue to use therapeutic communication skills when interacting with cognitively impaired patient. Be creative in using alternative strategies (e.g., involving family members).
	• Speak to patient as an adult and give time to process information.
2. Patient becomes frustrated, and communication with nurse becomes more challenging.	• Use verbal and nonverbal methods to convey empathy with his or her frustration.
	• Allow for periods of adequate rest; make frequent attempts to interact to minimize social isolation.

Recording and Reporting

- Record both objective and subjective behaviors (associated with cognitive impairment) that patient is displaying and objective behaviors (associated with cognitive impairment) observed on flow sheet or in nurses' notes in electronic health record (EHR) or chart.
- Record and report the methods used to communicate and patient's response.
- Document your evaluation of patient and family caregiver learning.

Special Considerations
Teaching Considerations

- Teach patient and family caregiver how to use various methods to communicate such as pictorial board or communication aids.
- Make teaching modifications with a consideration of impaired concentration and memory related to patient's cognitive status (e.g., present a small amount of material at a time; use simple and short phrases; repeat information as needed).

Pediatric Considerations

- Children may exhibit cognitive impairments because of acute or chronic metabolic or neurological conditions. Communication strategies with children should take into consideration their developmental level. Use pictures and drawings for patients who are unable to read.

Gerontological Considerations

- Many older adults have cognitive impairments that pose serious barriers to the reliability of your assessment; therefore it is important to use effective verbal and nonverbal communication strategies. Poor communication can compromise care, leading to increased anxiety and frustration.
- Patients who have cognitive impairments may exhibit tantrum-like behaviors in response to real or perceived frustration. Use distraction techniques to remove a cognitively impaired older-adult patient from disturbing stimuli or redirect patient to activity that is pleasurable (Touhy and Jett, 2014).

Home Care Considerations

- Manage care on the basis of patient's presenting behaviors with consideration of any cognitive/physical impairment. Include the family caregiver and friends in using effective communication strategies.

✦ SKILL 3.4   Communicating With Colleagues

In health care settings communicating is a key part of everyday practice. You communicate with patients, members of the interprofessional health care team, and external colleagues. This communication occurs face-to-face, over the phone, and in writing. The quality of these interactions is a key component of error prevention; clarity, comprehension, and adherence to treatment plans; and patient outcomes. Nevertheless, communication problems are common in health care settings, and failures in communication pose serious consequences (Judd, 2013; Norgaard et al., 2012). TJC publishes National Patient Safety Goals, one of which is to "improve the effectiveness of communication among caregivers" (TJC, 2016)." Collaboration among physicians, nurses, and other health care professionals increases team members' awareness of one another's type of knowledge and skills, leading to continued improvement in decision making and patient outcomes. Moreover, teamwork and collaboration are essential to quality patient care. Be aware of the differences in communication styles among members of the health care team and adapt your style of communicating to effectively interact with team members (Cronenwett et al., 2007; Happell et al., 2014).

Conflicts among colleagues can indirectly influence the therapeutic nurse-client relationship and negatively affect the delivery of care and patient and health care provider satisfaction (Happell et al., 2014; Moore et al., 2015). Effective communication is necessary to resolve conflict among members of the health care team. Good communication in the form of conflict resolution skills can decrease the risk of conflict and its negative effects.

Standardized communication with the SBAR (Situation-Background-Assessment-Recommendation) is structured to optimize effective communication among members of the health care team. Using SBAR, nurses are better prepared before calling a physician or other professional colleague and when formulating a recommendation based on solid assessment. Nurses are more confident in their judgment, resulting in better patient outcomes (Novak and Fairchild, 2012; DeMeester et al., 2013). Improved communication through the use of structured communication techniques, including bedside reporting with the SBAR framework, streamlines information exchanges and promotes patient safety (e.g., communicating accurate information about test results or medications) (Boykins, 2014). The evidence suggests that bedside reporting gives the oncoming nurse a chance for direct observation of a patient and a chance to ask questions related to the patient's status. This type of interaction promotes accountability between shifts. Bedside reporting and effective communication with the use of SBAR help to decrease adverse events and increase patient and family satisfaction (Cornell et al., 2014; Novak and Fairchild, 2012).

Delegation and Collaboration

The skill of communicating effectively with colleagues can be delegated to nursing assistive personnel (NAP). The nurse instructs the NAP about:

- The proper communication skills needed to effectively interact verbally and nonverbally with colleagues.

STEP	RATIONALE

ASSESSMENT

1. Identify purpose of interaction with colleague.	This sets the stage for the interaction; all members of the communication exchange are aware of purpose of conversation.
2. Assess factors influencing communication with others (e.g., environment, timing, presence of others' cultural beliefs and values, prior experiences).	Assessment allows you to accurately evaluate any barriers to communication or issues that may need to be considered to maintain open, clear channels of communication.
3. Consider level of stress in the situation; do you feel threatened?	Feeling threatened results in a sympathetic stress response that can impair judgment, emotional control, and ability to communicate clearly.

NURSING DIAGNOSES

- Decisional conflict
- Fear
- Ineffective coping

- Deficient knowledge regarding communication skills
- Ineffective role performance

- Impaired social interaction
- Impaired verbal communication

Related factors are individualized based on patient's condition or needs.

PLANNING

1. Prepare for communication with members of the health care team who may have differing needs or concerns. Example: If you feel stressed, try to relax and consciously relax muscles of pelvic floor.	Effective communication allows members of the health care team to establish rapport and have a quality interaction. Adapt own style of communicating (e.g., relaxation) to meet the needs of the health care team.
2. Be aware of your nonverbal cues that affect communication with others. Remain nonjudgmental.	Frustration in communication may negatively affect interaction with others.

STEP	RATIONALE
3. Prepare environment physically; go to a quiet, calm area. Reduce distractions such as external noises.	Factors to consider include privacy, noise control, seating space, and convenience to help to ensure the space needed for effective teamwork.
4. Be aware of hierarchical differences among members of the health care team as a common barrier to effective communication and collaboration.	Intimidating behavior by individuals at the top of a hierarchy can hinder open communication.

IMPLEMENTATION

1. Approach colleague from the front and face him or her when speaking. Maintain appropriate eye contact.	This strategy ensures that colleague both sees and hears you and conveys an attitude of respect.
2. Provide brief, simple introduction; introduce yourself and explain purpose of interaction.	This strategy ensures that colleague understands purpose of interaction.
3. Be aware of your own body language and tone. Assume an open stance; do not fold arms across your chest.	Nonverbal messages convey empathy. Be aware of how your nonverbal communication style may impact others.
4. Acknowledge and respond to a range of views. Allow for equal time for all parties to participate in expressing opinions.	Understand the perspectives of others and support the value of collaboration and teamwork.
5. Use oral communication skills such as: ask open-ended questions; do not assume; do not interrupt; do not blame others. Provide feedback. Use active listening and recognize nonverbal triggers. Ask for clarification when necessary.	Effective communication skills should be used for communicating and resolving conflict.
6. Use a range of workplace written communication methods (e.g., oral, written notes, memos, letters, charts, diagrams).	Standardized communication such as the SBAR method of communication can help streamline information exchanges and promote patient safety.
7. Encourage discussion of both positive and negative feelings to increase the chances of both parties expressing all of their concerns.	Discussion fosters active listening and understanding. All members of the exchange are valued, and their contributions are recognized.
8. Summarize key themes in the discussion and help to develop alternative solutions to the issue.	Conflict resolution involves examining alternative solutions to an issue. It values the influence of system solutions in achieving effective functioning among colleagues (Cronenwett et al., 2007).

EVALUATION

1. Confirm clarity and understanding of messages sent and received.	Determines extent to which members of the exchange understand.
2. Observe verbal and nonverbal behaviors.	Observation reveals if there are any negative emotions or further concerns that contradict a message.

Unexpected Outcomes	Related Interventions
1. Messages that are sent and received are not understood.	• Continue to use therapeutic communication skills when interacting with others. Be creative in using alternative strategies.
2. Frustration among colleagues persists, and communication becomes more challenging.	• Continue to have empathy and use active listening to better understand colleagues.

Recording and Reporting

• As needed, record and report successful communication strategies and pertinent changes to patient's plan of care on flow sheet or in nurses' notes in electronic health record (EHR) or chart.

◆ CLINICAL DEBRIEF

You are assigned to care for Mrs. Jones, an 84-year-old woman who was admitted to the hospital 2 days ago after falling at her son's home. She recently moved in with her son, her only child, following the sudden death of her husband. Her husband had been her primary caregiver since she was diagnosed with Alzheimer's disease 3 years ago. Neither her husband nor her son wanted to put her into a long-term care facility. She had emergency surgery to repair a fractured wrist. During shift report on a medical-surgical unit, the nurse tells you that the patient is withdrawn and confused. In addition, she has difficulty understanding verbal direction from the nursing staff.

When you approach the patient to perform an initial assessment, she is looking out the window and seems disoriented. She appears disheveled, and her lunch tray is untouched. You ask her if she needs help with bathing, dressing, and feeding; but you get a response that you cannot understand. Her impaired communication is causing her increased anxiety, which is further hindering her communication with others and her ability to follow directions.

1. Which steps are necessary to effectively communicate with a cognitively impaired patient?
2. Which strategies would you use to manage/decrease Mrs. Jones' anxiety level? Explain your choice(s).
3. Using the SBAR (Situation-Background-Assessment-Recommendation) format, describe strategies to communicate with the interprofessional team regarding the treatment plan for Mrs. Jones.

◆ REVIEW QUESTIONS

1. Which approach reflects an obstacle to effective nurse-patient communication? (Select all that apply.)
   1. Discussing fears about a patient with members of the health care team
   2. Interrupting patient when he or she does not answer the question posed
   3. Obtaining information about a critically ill patient from his or her family
   4. Admitting a mistake to a patient's family
   5. Giving advice to patient since you are a health care professional
   6. Minimizing concerns/issues of a patient
2. A patient recovering from a bilateral mastectomy for breast cancer tearfully tells the nurse that she is feeling depressed and worthless as a woman. Which communication phrases would not be effective? (Select all that apply.)
   1. "Many women have body image concerns after undergoing this surgery."
   2. "You will feel better soon."
   3. "Tell me more about how you feel."
   4. "Why do you feel depressed and worthless?"
   5. "How long have you been feeling this way?"
   6. "I am sure your husband will still love you no matter what you look like."
3. A patient has a cognitive impairment following a stroke. He lives with his daughter but is in the hospital for pneumonia. The patient is upset because he is unable to describe what he wants to eat. He is loud, and this is annoying to other patients. Which of the following measures would be effective? (Select all that apply.)
   1. Approach the patient from the front and make eye contact.
   2. Explain to the patient that he will benefit by acting calmer and not talking loudly.
   3. Ask patient one question at a time about what he would like to eat.
   4. Use nonverbal communication methods.
   5. Ask family members which communications measures are successful at home.

ⓔ *Visit the Evolve site for a complete list of Clinical Debrief and Review Questions answers.*

REFERENCES

Blake M, et al: An evidence-based systematic review on communication treatments for individuals with right hemisphere brain damage, *Am J Speech Lang Pathol* 22:146, 2013.

Boykins A: Core communication competencies in patient-centered care, *ABNF J* 25(2):40, 2014.

Bramhall E: Effective communication skills in nursing practice, *Nurs Stand* 29(14):53, 2014.

Carlsson E, et al: Communicative strategies used by spouses of individuals with communication disorders related to stroke-induced aphasia and Parkinson's disease, *Int J Lang Commun Disord* 49(6):722, 2014.

Chew LD, et al: Brief questions to identify patients with inadequate health literacy, *Fam Med* 36(8):588, 2004.

Cornell P, et al: Impact of SBAR on nurse shift reports and staff rounding, *Medsurg Nurs* 23(5):334, 2014.

Cronenwett L, et al: Quality and safety education for nurses, *Nurs Outlook* 55:122, 2007.

Davis TC, et al: Rapid estimate of adult literacy in medicine: a shortened screening instrument, *Fam Med* 25(6):391, 1993.

DeMeester K, et al: SBAR improves nurse-physician communication and reduces unexpected death: a pre and post intervention study, *Resuscitation* 84:11926, 2013.

Genova J, et al: The communication assessment checklist in health (CATCH): a tool for assessing quality of printed education materials for clinicians, *J Contin Educ Health Prof* 34(4):232, 2014.

Giger J: *Transcultural nursing: assessment and interventions*, ed 6, St Louis, 2013, Mosby.

Halter MJ: *Varcarolis' Foundations of psychiatric mental health nursing*, ed 7, St Louis, 2014, Mosby.

Happell B, et al: Communication with colleagues: frequency of collaboration regarding physical health of consumers with mental illness, *Perspect Psychiatr Care* 50:33, 2014.

Hemsley B, et al: Nursing the patient with complex communication needs: time as a barrier and a facilitator to successful communication in hospital, *J Adv Nurs* 68(1):116, 2012.

Hockenberry MJ, Wilson D: *Wong's nursing care of infants and children*, ed 10, St Louis, 2015, Mosby.

Institute of Medicine: *Crossing the quality chasm: a new health system for the 21st century*, 2001, National Academy of Sciences. https://www.nationalacademies.org/hmd/~/media/Files/Report%20Files/2001/Crossing-the-Quality-Chasm/Quality%20Chasm%202001%20%20report%20brief.pdf.

Jahne J: Palliative care: patient-centered assessment and communication to improve quality of life, *N M Nurse* 60(4):4, 2015.

Judd M: Broken communication in nursing can kill: teaching communication is vital, *Creat Nurs* 19(2):101, 2013.

Kauppi K, et al: Information and communication technology based prompting for treatment compliance for people with serious mental illness, *Cochrane Database Syst Rev* (6):CD009960, 2014.

Keltner N, et al: *Psychiatric nursing*, ed 7, St Louis, 2015, Mosby.

Lancioni G, et al: Technology-based programs to support forms of leisure engagement and communication for persons with multiple disabilities: two single case studies, *Dev Neurorehabil* 15(3):209, 2012.

Law J, et al: Integrating external evidence of intervention effectiveness with both practice and the parent perspective: development of 'what works' for speech, language, and communication needs, *Dev Med Child Neurol* 57:223, 2014.

Mayo Clinic: Alzheimer's: Tips for effective communication, 2016. http://www.mayoclinic.org/healthy-lifestyle/caregivers/in-depth/alzheimers/art-20047540. Accessed April, 2016.

McGhee J: Effective communication with people who have dementia, *Nurs Stand* 25(25):40, 2011.

Moore PM, et al: Communication skills training for health care professionals working with people who have cancer, *Cochrane Database Syst Rev* (3):CD003751, 2015.

Norgaard B, et al: Communication skills training increases self-efficacy of health care professionals, *J Contin Educ Health Prof* 32(2):90, 2012.

Novak K, Fairchild R: Bedside reporting and SBAR: improving patient communication and satisfaction, *J Pediatr Nurs* 27:760, 2012.

O'Hagen S, et al: What counts as effective communication in nursing? Evidence from nurse educators' and clinicians' feedback on nurse interactions with simulated patients, *J Adv Nurs* 70(6):1344, 2014.

Parker RM, et al: The test of functional health literacy in adults: a new instrument for measuring patients' literacy skills, *J Gen Intern Med* 10(10):537, 1995.

Pennington L, et al: Speech and language therapy to improve the communication skills of children with cerebral palsy, *Cochrane Database Syst Rev* (2):CD003466, 2004.

Sherwood G, et al: A new mindset for quality and safety: the QSEN competencies redefine nurses' roles in practice, *Nephrol Nurs J* 41(1):15, 2014.

Smith P, et al: The relationship between functional health literacy and adherence to emergency department discharge instructions among Spanish-speaking patients, *J Natl Med Assoc* 104(11–12):521, 2012.

The Joint Commission (TJC): *National Patient Safety Goals, 2016,* Oakbrook Terrace, IL, 2016, TJC. http://www.jointcommission.org/standards_information/npsgs.aspx. Accessed April, 2016.

Thomason T, et al: A critique of the Short Test of Functional Health Literacy in Adults, *Clin Nurse Spec* 29(6):308, 2015.

Touhy T, Jett K: *Ebersole & Hess' Gerontological nursing and healthy aging,* ed 4, St Louis, 2014, Mosby.

US Department of Health and Human Services (USDHHS), Office of Minority Health: National standards for culturally and linguistically appropriate services (CLAS) in health and health care, 2013. https://www.thinkculturalhealth.hhs.gov/pdfs/EnhancedNationalCLASStandards.pdf. Accessed April, 2016.

Webster D: Promoting therapeutic communication and patient-centered care using standardized patients, *J Nurs Educ* 52(11):645, 2013.

Williams K: Evidence-based strategies for communicating with older adults in long-term care settings, *J Commun* 20(11):507, 2013.

Wittenberg-Lyles E, et al: Oncology nurse communication barriers to patient-centered care, *Clin J Oncol Nurs* 17(2):152, 2013.

4 | Documentation and Informatics

OBJECTIVES

Mastery of content in this chapter will enable the nurse to:

- List guidelines for effective communication and reporting.
- Describe measures to maintain confidentiality of patient information.
- Identify the purpose of the patient record.
- Describe the elements of a hand-off report and when it would be used.
- Discuss the role of computerization in documentation.
- Write a nurse's progress note using SBAR, SOAP, SOAPIE, PIE, and focus (DAR) charting formats.
- Describe information found in a patient care profile and nursing Kardex.
- Accurately complete a nursing flow sheet.
- Explain guidelines used in documentation of home care and long-term care.
- Describe the role of critical pathways in multidisciplinary documentation.
- Complete an adverse event report accurately.
- Describe the importance of medication reconciliation.

MEDIA RESOURCES

- evolve http://evolve.elsevier.com/Perry/skills
- Review Questions
- Audio Glossary
- Clinical Debrief and Review Questions Answers
- Case Studies

PURPOSE

Documentation is anything entered into a patient's electronic health record (EHR) or written in a patient record. The EHR (Fig. 4.1) is a longitudinal electronic record of patient health information generated by one or more encounters in a care delivery setting (HIMSS, 2015a). Nursing documentation ensures continuity of care, provides legal evidence, and evaluates patient outcomes. The nurse's documentation provides a detailed account of a patient's plan of care, important assessment, and treatment, which must be an accurate and timely evaluation of information. Electronic tools such as computers support documentation and patient care. Informatics focuses on best practices with digital tools (HIMSS, 2015b).

STANDARDS OF CARE

- American Nurses Association (ANA), 2010—Principles for Nursing Documentation Guidance for Registered Nurses
- Centers for Medicare & Medicaid Services (CMS), 2015
- Nursing Informatics, 2014—Scope and Standards of Practice
- Quality and Safety Education for Nurses (QSEN), 2015
- The Joint Commission (TJC), 2015—Accreditation Standards

PRINCIPLES FOR PRACTICE

- All members of the health care team are legally and ethically obligated to keep patient information confidential.
- Documentation occurs within the context of the nursing process, including evidence of patient and family teaching and discharge planning (TJC, 2015a). Agency standards or policies often state the frequency of assessment; thus it is essential to know the standards of your health care agency.
- The North American Nursing Diagnosis Association (NANDA) International (NANDA-I) (2014) has established standardized nursing diagnoses to describe patients' responses to health problems.
- The Nursing Interventions Classification (NIC) provides a label name, definition, and list of activities that a nurse performs to complete an intervention (Center for Nursing and Clinical Effectiveness, 2013a).
- The Nursing Outcomes Classification (NOC) provides an outcome label, a definition, and a list of interventions that can result in the outcome (Center for Nursing and Clinical Effectiveness, 2013b). The use of outcomes is essential when evaluating the achievement of patient care goals and the appropriateness of patient interventions.
- The implementation of NANDA-I, NIC, and NOC promotes consistent nursing language when caring for a patient (Park, 2014).

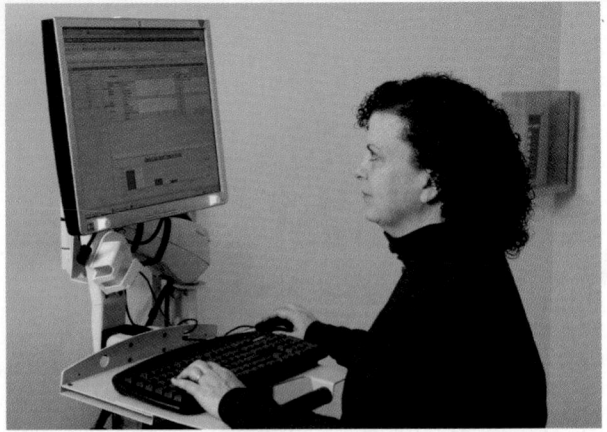

FIG 4.1 Computerized documentation provides many benefits.

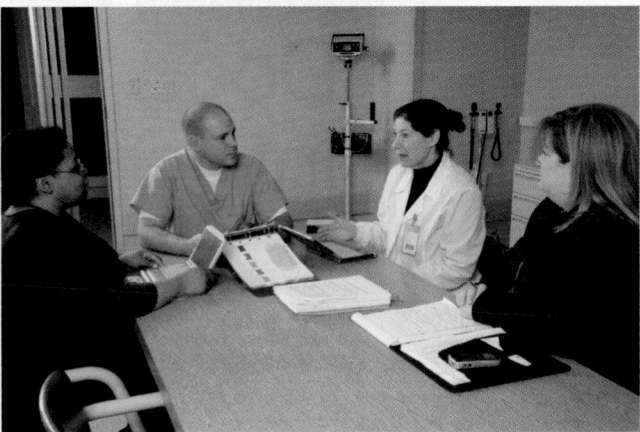

FIG 4.2 Communication among members of the health care team.

- The Health Insurance Portability and Accountability Act of 1996 (HIPAA) protects patients' private health information. HIPAA governs all areas of health information management (e.g., reimbursement, coding, security, and patient records) (USDHHS, 1999).
- The Security Rule of HIPAA (1996) provides standards for the protection of electronic health information. Numerous nursing and medical professional organizations have developed guidelines and strategies for safe computer charting (Box 4.1).
- Although incentives exist to transition from paper health records to EHRs, paper records are still in use in some health care agencies (Perry et al., 2014).
- Comprehensive computer systems in health care delivery have unlimited potential for improving the accuracy, efficiency, and quality of documentation. Meaningful use refers to the use of certified EHRs to improve outcomes, increase patient engagement, and reduce health disparities (see Procedural Guideline 4.4) (HealthIT.gov, 2015).
- Examples of core objectives for meaningful use include clinical-decision support rules; computerized orders; and real-time drug interaction checks. The EHR can support the nurse's decision-making by verifying safety steps in procedures such as medication administration. In addition, clinical data from an EHR can be exchanged more efficiently among the interprofessional team and at transition points in care.
- Accreditation agencies such as TJC specify guidelines for documentation and require health care agencies to monitor and evaluate patient outcomes and appropriateness of care (TJC, 2015a).

PATIENT-CENTERED CARE

- A patient's record or chart is a confidential, permanent legal document containing information relevant to a patient's health care. Nurses and other health care providers record information about a patient's health care after each patient contact. The record is a continuing account of the patient's health status and needs, treatments delivered, results of diagnostic tests, and response to therapy.
- Records and reports communicate specific information about a patient's health status and the interventions that all health care team members contribute toward improving his or her health. Interprofessional communication and documentation are necessary to provide more efficient and effective health care and improve patient outcomes.

BOX 4.1

Use of the Electronic Health Record

- Sign on to the electronic health record (EHR) using only your password.
- Never share passwords and keep your password private.
- Only open EHRs for patients for whom you are caring.
- Review assessment data, problems identified (nursing diagnoses), goals and expected outcomes, and interventions and patient responses during contact with each patient before data entry.
- Follow procedures for entering information in all appropriate program functions.
- Review previously documented entries with those that you enter, noting if there is significant change in patient's status. Report changes to patient's health care provider.
- The copy-and-paste features in EHRs should be used sparingly because of the potential for error (Simpson, 2015).
- Do not leave information about a patient displayed on a monitor where others can see it. Keep a log that accounts for every copy of a computerized file that you have generated from the system.
- Follow agency confidentiality procedures for documenting sensitive material such as diagnosis of human immunodeficiency virus (HIV) infection.
- Know and implement agency protocol to correct documentation errors.
- Never create, change, or delete records unless your agency provides you with this authority.
- Software systems have a system for backup files. If you inadvertently delete part of the permanent record, follow agency policy. It is necessary to type an explanation into the computer file with the date, time, and your initials and submit an explanation in writing to your manager.
- Save information as documentation is completed.
- Protect printouts from computerized records. Shredding printouts and logging in the number of copies generated by each caregiver minimize duplicate records and protect the confidentiality of patient information.
- Workarounds can occur when EHRs are poorly designed; health care providers may fall back on paper charting. Medication errors may increase when nurses are working in a hybrid system. This system uses two formats—a paper and an electronic medical record for the same patient (Gardner and Sparnon, 2014).
- Sign off when you leave the computer.

- Reports are oral or written exchanges of information among caregivers (Fig. 4.2). Reports include information about a patient's clinical status, observations made about his or her behavior, data pertaining to diagnostic tests, and directions for changes in therapy. Common reports given by nurses include telephone reports, transfer reports, and adverse event reports (see Procedural Guideline 4.3).

- When a nurse receives a verbal order or critical test result, the nurse writes down the order or critical test result as it is given and then reads it back to the individual who has given the order. By stating the information back, also called the *read-back*, to the individual giving the order or test result, the nurse verifies that the complete order or test result has been received and understood (Boyd et al., 2014).

- Patient hand-off reports (see Procedural Guideline 4.1), a standardized approach to communication of patient information among caregivers, are being used by many health care agencies.

EVIDENCE-BASED PRACTICE

Computer-based health care records, informatics, and implementation of the electronic patient record all have major implications for patient-centered care, patient engagement, and evidence-based practice (Nursing Informatics, 2014; Rutten et al., 2014). Basic nursing care interventions can be documented to provide meaningful data to the health care team (Englebright et al., 2014).

- Use of EHRs in acute care hospitals demonstrates improvement in patient outcomes for patients diagnosed with acute myocardial infarctions, heart failure, and pneumonia (Appari et al., 2013).

- Quality EHRs allow retrieval of data to improve patient outcomes. For example, data are retrieved from EHRs when patients are identified to their active medication lists. The bar coding of medications can reduce errors because the data retrieved match the right patients to the right medications. (IOM, 2012).

- Recent studies examined benefits and opportunities for further research about EHRs.

  - Nursing outcomes can be measured efficiently with EHRs. Standardized nursing language can be used in EHRs to describe patient problems and interventions. This standardization allows users to extract data for groups of similar populations; analyze outcomes; and, if needed, revise interventions to improve outcomes (Plemmons et al., 2012).

  - Nursing management of chronic diseases such as chronic obstructive pulmonary disease (COPD) can be managed more effectively with EHRs. Evidence suggests that the use of EHRs supporting the implementation of complex interventions is effective to manage exacerbations of COPD. Data can be shared more timely across the health care continuum as patients move among the levels of care. Extraction of data is more efficient because of the standardization of language found in EHRs (Fengping et al., 2015).

  - After 5 years of using an EHR system in an acute care hospital, nurses identified opportunities to improve interprofessional communication and clinical decision making by strengthening the system. Researchers suggest that nurses conduct time-motion studies to evaluate the nursing resources used to maintain and improve EHRs (Harmon et al., 2015).

  - Patients need education, guidance, and support as the health care system transitions to EHRs. The evidence suggests that medical language used in EHRs can be difficult for patients to understand. Some patients are concerned about the security of their health information in cyberspace. Challenges for health care providers include improving access for patients and conveying the value of the EHR to patients (Dontje et al., 2014).

SAFETY GUIDELINES

- Quality documentation and reporting must have the following characteristics: it must be factual, accurate, complete, current, and organized.

  - Factual data contain descriptive, objective information about what a nurse sees, hears, feels, and smells. The only subjective data included in a record are what the patient actually verbalizes. Write subjective information with quotation marks, using the patient's exact words whenever possible. For example, record, "Patients states, 'My stomach hurts.'"

  - The use of exact measurements in documentation establishes accuracy. For example, charting that an abdominal wound is "5 cm (2 inches) in length without redness, edema, or drainage" is more descriptive than "large wound healing well." It is essential to avoid unnecessary words and irrelevant details. For example, the fact that a patient is watching television is only necessary when this activity is significant to the patient's status and plan of care.

  - The information within a recorded entry or a report must be complete, containing appropriate and essential information. Criteria for reporting and recoding information for health problems or nursing activities exist (Table 4.1).

  - TJC standards (2015a) require that "all entries in medical records be dated and a method established to identify the authors of entries." Therefore each entry in a patient's record ends with the caregiver's full name or initials and status. Document interventions performed by another caregiver. For example, "Patient ambulated by Sue Smith, NA." A nursing student enters full name, student nurse abbreviation (e.g., SN, NS), and educational institution such as "David Jones, SN (student nurse), CTCC (Central Texas Community College)." An EHR generates the nurse's name and initials when the entry is submitted.

  - Current documentation includes making timely entries in a patient's record, which avoids omissions and delay in patient care (TJC, 2015a). To increase accuracy and decrease unnecessary duplication, many health care agencies locate medical records near a patient's bedside, which facilitates immediate documentation of care activities. Document the following activities or findings at the time of occurrence:
    - Vital signs
    - Pain assessment and evaluation
    - Administration of medications and treatments
    - Preparation for diagnostic tests or surgery
    - Change in patient's status and who was notified
    - Treatment for a sudden change in patient's status
    - Patient response to intervention
    - Admission, transfer, discharge, or death of a patient

- Military time, a 24-hour system that avoids misinterpretation of AM and PM times, is recommended to record the time of events. The military clock ends with midnight at 2400 and begins 1 minute after midnight at 0001. For example, 1:00 PM is 1300 military time; 10:22 AM is 1022 military time. Fig. 4.3 compares military and civilian times. An EHR generates time of entry when the nurse submits the entry.

- TJC requires health care agencies to standardize abbreviations, symbols, acronyms, and dose designations and establish a list of abbreviations that should never be used (TJC, 2015b). It is essential to know the abbreviation list of the agency in which you work and to use only the accepted abbreviations, symbols, and measures (e.g., metric) so all documentation is accurate and

TABLE 4.1

Examples of Criteria for Reporting and Recording

Topic	Criteria to Report or Record
Assessment	
Subjective data	Description of episode/event in patient's words in quotation marks. Clarify onset, location, description of condition (severity; duration; frequency; precipitating, aggravating, and relieving factors)
Patient behavior (e.g., anxiety, confusion, hostility)	Onset, behaviors exhibited, precipitating factors
Objective data (e.g., rash, tenderness, breath sounds)	Onset, location, description of condition (severity; duration; frequency; precipitating, aggravating, and relieving factors)
Nursing Interventions and Evaluation	
Treatments (e.g., enema, bath, dressing change)	Time administered, equipment used (if appropriate), patient's response (objective and subjective changes) compared to previous treatment (e.g., rated pain 2 on a scale of 0-10 during dressing change or "patient reported no abdominal cramping during enema")
Medication administration	Immediately after administration document: time medication given, dose, route, any preliminary assessment (e.g., pain level, vital signs), patient response or effect of medication (e.g., 1200 "Pain reported at 7 (scale 0-10)." Acetaminophen 6500 mg given PO. 1230: "Patient reports pain level 2 (scale 0-10) at 1330" or "Pruritus and hives developed over lower abdomen 1 hour after penicillin was given")
Patient teaching	Information presented; method of instruction (e.g., discussion, demonstration, videotape, booklet); patient response, including questions and evidence of understanding such as return demonstration or change in behavior
Discharge planning	Measurable patient goals or expected outcomes, progress toward goals, need for referrals

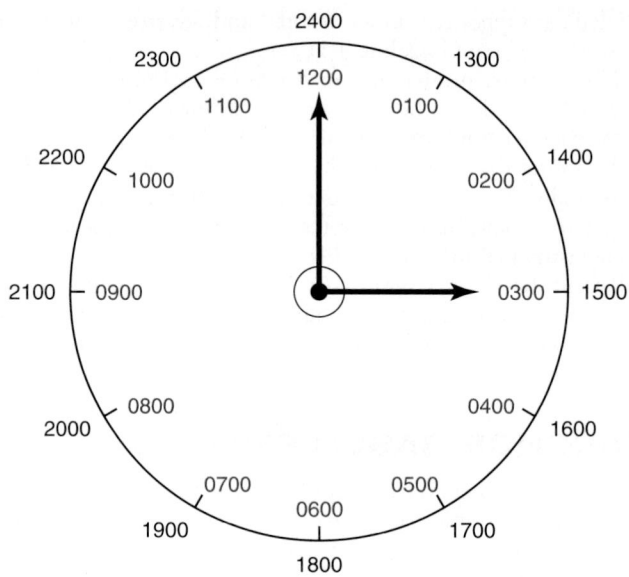

FIG 4.3 Military time clock. Instead of two 12-hour cycles, the military clock is one 24-hour time cycle (e.g., 3 PM is 1500 military time).

BOX 4.2

Official "Do Not Use" Abbreviations

Do Not Use	Potential Problem	Use Instead
U, u (unit)	Mistaken for "0" (zero), the number "4" (four), or "cc"	Write "unit"
IU (International Unit)	Mistaken for IV (intravenous) or the number 10 (ten)	Write "International Unit"
Q.D., QD, q.d., qd (daily)	Mistaken for one another	Write "daily"
Q.O.D., QOD, q.o.d, qod (every other day)	Period after the Q mistaken for "I" and the "O" mistaken for "I"	Write "every other day"
Trailing zero (X.0 mg)	Decimal point is missed	Write X mg
Lack of leading zero (.X mg)		Write 0.X mg
MS	Can mean morphine sulfate or magnesium sulfate	Write "morphine sulfate"
MSO4 and MgSO4	Confused for one another	Write "magnesium sulfate"

The Joint Commission: *Facts about the official "Do Not Use" list,* http://www.jointcommission.org/facts_about_do_not_use_list/. Accessed July 26, 2015.

in compliance with standards. For example, the abbreviation for *every day (qd)* **is no longer used** (Box 4.2; see Chapter 20). If a treatment or medication is needed daily, the written order or care plan should write out the word "*daily*" or "*every day.*" The abbreviation *qd (every day)* can be misinterpreted to mean O.D. *(right eye).*

- Hand-off occurs during shift change or any time the patient changes caregivers. During a hand-off communication process the patient and patient information are transferred to the next caregiver. Hand-off is also used across the health care continuum when patients leave one health system for another. Effective hand-off allows for face-to-face communication when available, which allows the person receiving care of the patient the opportunity to ask questions (Barry, 2014).
  - During hand-off the sender of the patient information initially presents the patient name, room number, age, gender, diagnosis, medical history, discharge planning, and confidential information. This is followed by patient vital signs and

clinical assessments, changes in clinical condition, medication review, fluid balance, and patient safety risk assessment factors. The patient is an active participant in the hand-off process. Once hand-off is completed, the receiver of the information is given an opportunity to ask questions and confirm understanding. Incomplete or comprehensive information can negatively affect a patient's safety. A comprehensive hand-off not only is information sharing but also is the acceptance and effective transfer of all patient authority and responsibility (Joint Commission Center for Transforming Healthcare, nd).

TABLE 4.2

Legal Guidelines for Documentation and Reporting

Guidelines	Rationale	Correct Action
Use only your unique user identification and password to log onto the EHR.	An electronic signature is associated with each user identification and password log-in.	Protect the security of your user identification and password. Once logged on to the computer, do not leave the computer screen unattended.
Do not erase, apply correction fluid, or scratch out errors made while recording in a paper record.	Charting becomes illegible: it appears as if you were attempting to hide information or deface record.	Draw single line through error, write word *error* above it, and sign your name or initials. Then record note correctly. Check agency policy.
Do not write retaliatory or critical comments about patient or care by other health care professionals.	Statements can be used as evidence for nonprofessional behavior or poor quality of care.	Enter only objective descriptions of patient's behavior; use quotations for patient's comments.
Need to add patient information.	New information is acquired.	If additional information is to be added to an existing entry, write the date and time of the new entry on the next available space and mark it as an addendum (date and time of prior note).
	Forgot to chart during a shift.	Write the current date and time in the next available space and mark it as a late entry (date and time/shift missed).
Correct all errors promptly.	Errors in recording can lead to errors in treatment.	Avoid rushing to complete charting; be sure that information is accurate.
Record all facts.	Record must be accurate and reliable.	Be certain that entry is factual; do not speculate or guess.
Record all entries legibly and in black ink for paper records.	Illegible entries can be misinterpreted, causing errors and lawsuits; ink cannot be erased; black ink is more legible when records are photocopied or transferred to microfilm.	Never erase entries or use correction fluid and never use pencil.
If order is questioned, record that you sought clarification.	If you perform an order known to be incorrect, you are just as liable for prosecution as the health care provider.	Do not record "physician made error." Instead, chart that "Dr. Smith was called to clarify order for analgesic."
Chart only for yourself.	You are accountable for information that you enter into chart.	Never chart for someone else. **EXCEPTION:** If caregiver has left unit for day and calls with information that needs to be documented, include the name of the source of information in the entry and that the information was provided via telephone.
Avoid using generalized, empty phrases such as "status unchanged" or "had good day."	Specific information about patient's condition or case can be deleted accidentally if information is too generalized.	Use complete, concise descriptions of care.
Begin each entry with time and end with your signature and title.	This guideline ensures that correct sequence of events is recorded; signature documents who is accountable for care delivered.	Do not wait until end of shift to record important changes that occurred several hours earlier; be sure to sign each entry.

EHR, Electronic health record.

- Five common issues in malpractice caused by inadequate or incorrect documentation include (1) failing to document the correct time of events, (2) failing to record verbal orders or have them signed, (3) charting actions in advance to save time, (4) documenting incorrect data, and (5) failing to give a report or giving an incomplete report to an oncoming shift. You must be aware of the legal guidelines for documentation and reporting (Table 4.2).

COMMON RECORD-KEEPING FORMS OR SCREENS

The patient chart or medical record contains evidence of a patient's health status. The chart includes a variety of forms or screens (as in the case of EHRs) to facilitate quick and comprehensive documentation. Use of these forms helps avoid duplication of information within the record.

Admission Nursing History Forms

A nurse completes a comprehensive nursing history form or screen to gather baseline assessment data when a patient is admitted to a nursing care unit. You use the admission data to form a plan of care and compare it to any changes in a patient's condition. The nursing history guides the admitting nurse through a complete assessment to identify relevant nursing diagnoses or problems for the patient's care plan. Examples of information included in the nursing history are patient allergies, primary spoken/written language, advance directives, disabilities, and mobility/fall risk and medication reconciliation.

Flow Sheets and Graphic Records

Flow sheets and graphic records permit concise documentation of nursing information and patient data over time. They are especially useful for the documentation of routine observations or repeated specific measurements for a patient such as vital signs (see Chapter

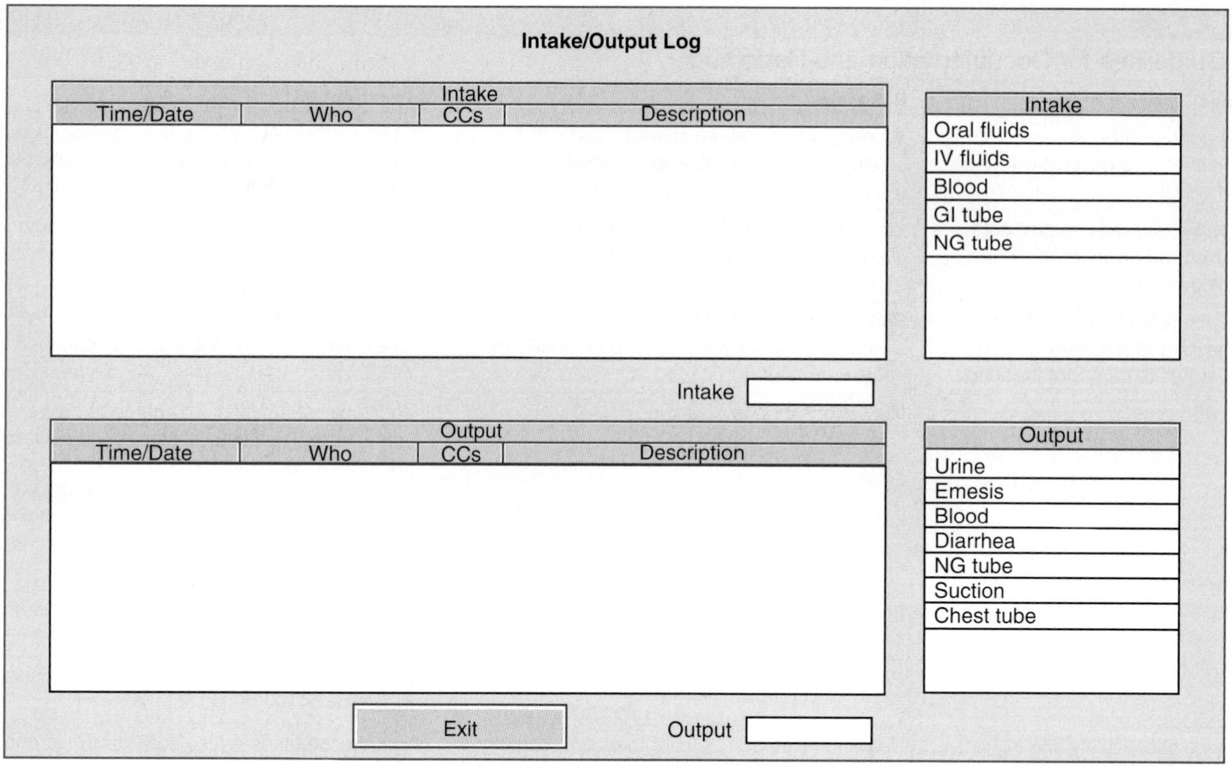

FIG 4.4 Graphic and intake-output record, electronic version. (*Courtesy ER Choice, Irving, TX.*)

5), intake and output, hygiene measures, medication administration (see Chapter 20), and pain assessment. Flow sheets use a format or system for entry of information, usually every 24 hours (Fig. 4.4). When documenting a significant change that you recognize on a flow sheet, describe the change in the progress notes, including the patient's response to nursing interventions. For example, if a patient's blood pressure becomes dangerously low, record in the progress notes the blood pressure, relevant assessment such as pallor or dizziness, and any interventions to raise the blood pressure. Also include an evaluation of the interventions such as repeated blood pressures and relief of dizziness. Other health care providers such as nursing assistants may have the responsibility to document on nursing flow sheets or screens.

Patient Education Record

Many health care agencies have an education record that identifies a patient's knowledge base about his or her diagnosis, treatment, and medications. The goal of patient and family education is to promote health behavior and self-care by involving the patient and/or family in decisions, which improves health outcomes. Standards for patient education include assessment of needs, functional abilities, learning styles, and readiness to learn. Base patient education needs on the assessment and then teach patients about topics such as safe and effective use of medications, nutrition and dietary modifications, safe use of medical equipment, pain control, rehabilitative methods to promote and improve functional abilities, and self-care activities (TJC, 2015a). When documenting on a patient teaching record, be specific about the information and/or skills taught, the patient's learning response, and information given to the patient.

Patient Care Summary or Kardex

Many health care agencies now have computerized systems that provide a concise set of information in the form of a patient care summary. This summary prints out for each patient during each shift. Data are updated automatically as new orders and nursing decisions enter the system.

In some health care settings a Kardex ("cardboard flip-over" file) kept at the nurses' station provides information for daily patient care needs. It has two parts: an activity and treatment section and a nursing care plan section. The updated information in both the patient summary and the Kardex eliminate the need for repeated referral to the chart for routine information throughout the day. The forms do not always become part of the permanent record. Information commonly found on the patient care summary or Kardex includes the following:

- Basic demographic data (e.g., age, religion)
- Primary medical diagnosis
- Current health care provider's orders (e.g., diet, activity, dressing changes)
- Plan of care
- Nursing orders or interventions (e.g., intake and output, comfort measures, teaching)
- Scheduled tests and procedures
- Safety precautions used in the patient's care
- Factors related to activities of daily living
- Nearest relative/guardian or person to contact in an emergency
- Emergency code status
- Allergies

Acuity Records

Many health care agencies use a patient acuity system as a method of determining the intensity of nursing care required for a group of patients. Acuity measurements for patients on a unit serve as a guide for determining staffing needs. An acuity recording system determines the hours of nursing care and number of staff required for a nursing unit.

Typically nurses enter acuity data into a computerized system in the morning. The administrative staff collects the acuity data electronically and uses them to make appropriate staffing decisions. Acuity levels allow the nursing staff to compare patients with one another. For example, an acuity system might rate bathing patients from 1 to 5 (1 is totally dependent, 5 is independent); a patient returning from surgery who requires frequent monitoring and extensive care has an acuity level of 1. On the same continuum another patient awaiting discharge after a successful recovery from surgery has an acuity level of 5. Accurate acuity ratings justify the number and qualifications of staff needed to safely care for patients on a particular unit.

Standardized Care Plans

The trend among many health care agencies is to computerize care plans. These systems provide daily computer-generated care plans, which incorporate several nursing diagnoses or problems in a single nursing or interprofessional plan. These systems improve documentation and facilitate high-quality care that is based on scientific evidence and proven experience (Nunes et al., 2014). Standardized care plans are based on agency standards of clinical practice and are established guidelines used to care for patients with similar health problems. After completing a nursing assessment, identify the patient's nursing diagnosis or health problem and select an appropriate standardized care plan for the patient medical record. Always individualize it for each patient. Most standardized care plans allow for the addition of patient-specific outcomes and target dates for achieving these outcomes.

One advantage of standardized care plans is the establishment of evidence-based standards of care. By using standardized plans nurses learn to recognize the accepted requirements of care for patients. Implementation of digital standardized plans improves continuity of care among professional nurses (Nunes et al., 2014).

One disadvantage of standardized care plans is an increased risk that the unique, individualized therapies needed by patients will go unrecognized. Standardized care plans do not replace professional judgment and decision making. In addition, care plans need to be updated on a regular basis to ensure that content is current and appropriate.

Discharge Summaries

The discharge summary includes essential information for the patient, family caregiver, and health care agency (Box 4.3) and is based on data obtained from the discharge planning process. Discharge planning is a comprehensive process with emphasis placed on preparing a patient for discharge from a health care agency. Nurses enhance discharge planning when they are responsive to changes in a patient's condition and involve the patient and family caregiver in the planning process (An, 2015).

There must be evidence of the involvement of the patient and family caregiver in the discharge planning process so the patient and family have the necessary information and resources to return home (Graham et al., 2013). TJC (2015a) has standards for patient and family education necessary for effective discharge planning. When a patient is discharged from a health care agency, the members of the health care team prepare a discharge summary. It provides important information relating to the patient's ongoing health problems and need for health care after discharge.

Discharge planning achieves specific outcomes that include identifying patients with ongoing health needs, collaborating with other health care professions to determine level of care, matching patients with appropriate referrals and resources, and streamlining the transition to the next level of care (Trossman, 2015). Include

---

BOX 4.3

Discharge Summary Information

- Use clear, concise descriptions in patient's own language.
- Provide step-by-step description of how to perform a procedure (e.g., home medication administration). Reinforce explanation with printed instructions for the patient to take home.
- Provide a detailed list of all prescribed medications.
- Identify precautions to follow when performing self-care or administering medications.
- Review any restrictions that may relate to activities of daily living (e.g., bathing, ambulating, and driving).
- Review signs and symptoms of complications to report to health care provider.
- List names and phone numbers of health care providers and community resources for the patient to contact.
- Identify any unresolved problem, including plans for follow-up and continuous treatment.
- List actual time of discharge, mode of transportation, and who accompanied patient.

---

in the discharge summary the reason for hospitalization; significant findings; current status of the patient; and the teaching plan that is given to the patient or family caregiver, home care, rehabilitation, or long-term care facility (TJC, 2015a). Discharge summaries make the summary concise and instructive. They emphasize previous learning by the patient and family caregiver and care that needs to continue in any restorative care setting.

CHARTING SYSTEMS

A variety of documentation systems (computerized and written) exist for recording patient information and progress (see Box 4.4). The documentation system selected by nursing reflects the philosophy of the health care agency. The same documentation system is used throughout a specific agency, but there are several acceptable methods for recording health care data.

Narrative Documentation

Narrative charting uses a storylike format to document specific information about a patient's conditions and nursing care, usually presented in chronological order. It is useful in emergency situations when the time and order of events are important. Organize a narrative in a clear, concise way (e.g., by using the nursing process to order the data).

Problem-Oriented Medical Records

A problem-oriented medical record (POMR) is a structured method of documenting narratives that emphasizes a patient's problems. This method organizes data using the nursing process, which facilitates communication about patient needs. Data are organized by problem or diagnosis. Ideally all members of the health care team contribute to the list of identified patient problems. This approach helps to coordinate an individualized plan of care with the following sections: database, problem list, care plan, and progress notes.

Patient Database

A database contains all available information pertaining to a patient. This section is the foundation for identifying patient problems and planning care. The database remains active and current for each patient and is revised as new data become available.

PROCEDURAL GUIDELINE 4.1 *Giving a Hand-Off Report*

In addition to written documentation, a nurse provides a change-of-shift report to the next nurse assuming responsibility for patient care. The purpose of the report is to provide continuity of care for the patient. Inaccurate or incomplete shift report can contribute to sentinel events (TJC, 2015d). Nurses give a hand-off report face-to-face, through a written report, with the electronic health record (EHR), or during bedside rounds at each patient's bedside. Bedside reporting can increase patient satisfaction and improve outcomes and is becoming increasingly popular (Spivey, 2014). It is important to have some type of guidelines for reporting to avoid repetitive, irrelevant, and speculative communication (Foster-Hunt et al., 2015). Regardless of the form of the hand-off report, the nurse must maintain confidentiality.

Delegation and Collaboration

The skill of giving a hand-off report cannot be delegated to nursing assistive personnel (NAP). Licensed practical nurses (LPNs) may report on patients for whom they care directly. The nurse directs the NAP to:

- Report to the nurse (e.g., increased pain, changes in vital signs) so there can be assessment, validation, and reporting of any changes in the hand-off report.

Equipment

- Worksheets, patient care summary or nursing Kardex, plan of care, critical pathway, or interprofessional treatment plan
- EHR (if implemented by agency)

Procedural Steps

1. Use an organized format for delivering report that provides a description of patient needs and problems. SBAR (Situation, Background, Assessment, Recommendation) can be used to organize and streamline report (Cornell et al., 2014).
2. Identify the electronic patient record using at least two identifiers (e.g., name and birthday or name and medical record number) according to agency policy (Office of the National Coordination for Health Information Technology, 2014).

3. Gather information from documentation sources, NAP report, or other relevant documents.

Clinical Decision Point *Report only relevant information to next shift to ensure staff's timely responsiveness.*

4. Prioritize information on the basis of patient's needs and problems.
5. For each patient include the following:
   S Situation: Patient's name, gender, age, chief complaint on admission, and current situation
   B Background information: Allergies, emergency code status (i.e., do not resuscitate [DNR]), medical and surgical histories, special needs as related to any physical challenges (e.g., blind, hearing deficit, amputee), and vaccinations
   A Assessment data: Objective observations and measurements made by the nurse during the shift; emphasis on any recent changes.
   Include any relevant information reported by patient, family caregiver, or health care team members such as laboratory data and diagnostic test results. Include therapies or treatments administered during shift and expected outcomes (e.g., medication changes, use of oxygen, referral visits). Describe education given in the teaching plan and patient's/family caregiver's ability to demonstrate learning. Report on evaluation by explaining patient's response and whether outcomes are met.
   Review patient's progress toward discharge during each change-of-shift report.
   R Recommend: Explanation of the priorities to which oncoming nurse must attend, including referrals, nursing orders, and core measures.
   Ask staff from oncoming shift if they have any questions regarding information provided.

Problem List

The problem list includes the patient's physiological, psychological, sociocultural, spiritual, developmental, and environmental needs. Develop a patient's problem list after analyzing the assessment data. Identify and list priority problems in chronological order to serve as an organizing guide for the patient's care. Add new problems as they are identified during the ongoing nursing assessment. When a problem is resolved, record the date and draw a line through the problem and its number. In an electronic system the problem is marked as resolved.

Plan of Care

All disciplines involved in a patient's care contribute to the development of an interprofessional plan of care for a specific problem. For example, for a patient having a nutritional deficit, a nurse recommends feeding approaches, and a registered dietitian recommends types of dietary supplements. Care plan standards require that a plan of care be developed for all patients on admission to a health care agency (TJC, 2015a). Generally these plans include nursing diagnoses, expected outcomes, interventions, and evaluations.

Progress Notes

Health care team members use progress notes to monitor and record the progress of a patient's problem (Box 4.4). Narrative notes, flow sheets, and discharge summaries are formats used to document patient progress (see Procedural Guideline 4.2).

SBAR Documentation. SBAR (Situation, Background, Assessment, Recommendation) is a concrete approach for framing conversations, especially critical ones that require a nurse's immediate attention and action. It allows for an easy and focused way to set expectations for what the team will communicate. SBAR promotes the provision of safe, efficient, timely, and patient-centered communication (Cornell et al., 2014). This method is used for written and verbal communication when a patient's condition changes, for a brief targeted report (e.g., as a preprocedure or postprocedure report) or as a change-of-shift report (Cornell et al., 2014).

SOAP Documentation. One way to structure narrative notes to document patient progress is the SOAP (Subjective data, Objective data, Assessment, and Plan format. Some agencies add an I and E (i.e., SOAPIE). The *I* stands for intervention, and the *E* represents evaluation. The logic for SOAP (IE) notes is similar

---

BOX 4.4

Formats for Recording Progress Notes

Narrative Note
Describes patient data in a narrative paragraph

Example:
Patient states, "I'm dreading this surgery because last time I had a terrible reaction to the anesthesia and such terrible pain when they made me get out of bed." Noted muscle tension and loud, agitated voice. Notified anesthesiologist of patient's prior experience. Discussed alternatives for anesthesia and pain-control options. Stressed importance of activity for circulation/healing. Encouraged to keep nurses informed of pain level/need for medication and that pain may be present but manageable.

SBAR (Acronym for Situation, Background, Assessment, and Recommendation)
System of structured communication used to share information about a patient's condition

Example:
S (Situation): Patient verbalized preoperative fears. Nurse noted muscle tension and loud, agitated voice.
B (Background): Patient fearful of surgery because of past experiences with anesthesia and pain.
A (Assessment): BP: 160/84, T: 98.6°F; P: 86; R: 18. O_2 Saturation: 96%. Skin warm and dry to touch. Respirations even and nonlabored.
R (Recommendation): Encourage patient to discuss preoperative fears. Assess pain level at least every 4 hours after surgery. Provide nonpharmacological pain-management techniques and administer medication as needed.

SOAP (Acronym for Subjective Data, Objective Data, Assessment, and Plan)
Usually based on a numbered list of problems or nursing diagnoses

Example:
S (Subjective data) (the patient's statements regarding the problem): Patient states, "I'm dreading this surgery because last time I had a terrible reaction to the anesthesia and such terrible pain when they made me get out of bed."
O (Objective data) (observations that support or are related to subjective data): Noted muscle tension and loud, agitated voice.
A (Assessment/Analysis) (conclusions reached on basis of data): Fear related to pain/anesthesia.
P (Plan) (plan for dealing with the situation): Notified anesthesiologist, Dr. Martin, of patient's prior experience. Discussed alternatives for anesthesia and pain-control options. Stressed importance of activity for circulation/healing. Encouraged to keep nurses informed of pain level/need for medication and that pain may be present but manageable.

PIE (Acronym for Problem, Intervention, and Evaluation)
Problem-oriented system in which progress notes are written based on a list of identified problems; detailed data may be entered by any member of the health care team

Example:
P (Problem): Patient states, "I'm dreading this surgery because last time I had a terrible reaction to the anesthesia and such terrible pain when they made me get out of bed." Noted muscle tension and loud, agitated voice.
I (Intervention): Notified anesthesiologist, Dr. Martin, of patient's prior experience. Discussed alternatives for anesthesia and pain-control options. Stressed importance of activity for circulation/healing. Encouraged to keep nurses informed of pain level/need for medication and that pain may be present but manageable.
E (Evaluation): Patient stated that she was "very relieved." Stated that she would tell the nurses about pain.

Focus or DAR Charting (Acronym for Data, Action, and Response)
A way to organize progress notes to make them more clear and organized

Example:
D (Data): Patient states, "I'm dreading this surgery because last time I had a terrible reaction to the anesthesia and such terrible pain when they made me get out of bed." Noted muscle tension and loud, agitated voice.
A (Nursing Action): Notified anesthesiologist of patient's prior experience. Discussed alternatives for anesthesia and pain-control options. Stressed importance of activity for circulation/healing. Encouraged to keep nurses informed of pain level/need for medication and that pain may be present but manageable.
R (Patient Response): Patient stated that she was "very relieved." Stated understanding of the importance of informing the nurses about pain.
   NOTE: Some agencies add **P (Plan)** and refer to this as DARP charting.

Example:
P (Plan): Assess pain level at least every 4 hours after surgery. Provide nonpharmacological pain-management techniques and administer medication as needed.

---

to that of the nursing process: collect data about a patient's problems, draw conclusions, and develop a plan of care. Number each SOAP note and title it according to the problem on the list.

PIE Documentation. The PIE (Problem, Intervention, Evaluation) note format of documentation is similar to that of SOAP charting in its problem-oriented nature. However, it differs from the SOAP method in that PIE charting has a nursing origin, whereas SOAP originated from a medical model.

The PIE format simplifies documentation by combining the care plan and progress note into one record. It differs from that of SOAP because there are no assessment data in the narrative note. Assessment data are included in documentation on the flow sheets of each shift. You number or label the PIE notes according to a patient's problems. Resolved problems are dropped from daily documentation after your review. Continuing problems are documented daily.

Focus Charting. Another narrative format is focus charting or DAR (Data, Action, Response). One distinction of focus charting is that it places less importance on patient problems and focuses on patient concerns such as a sign or symptom, condition, nursing diagnosis, behavior, significant event, or change in condition. Each entry includes data (both subjective and objective), actions or nursing interventions, and patient response (e.g., evaluation of effectiveness). Focus charting saves time because it is easy for caregivers to understand, is adaptable to most health care settings, and enables all caregivers to track a patient's condition and progress.

Source Records

In a source record a patient's chart is organized so each discipline (i.e., nursing, medicine, social work, and respiratory therapy) has a separate section in which to record data. The advantage of a source record is that it is easy for caregivers to locate the proper section of the record in which to make entries.

A disadvantage of the source record is that information about a specific problem may be distributed throughout the record. For example, the nurse describes the character of a patient's fractured femur pain and use of repositioning and narcotic analgesia in the nurses' notes and EHR. The health care provider notes in a separate section of the record the patient's bone healing and the plan for casting or surgery. The results of x-ray film examinations that show bone healing are in the radiology results section of the record. The method makes it difficult to find chronological information about patient care or how the team is coordinating care to meet all of the patient's needs.

Charting by Exception

Charting by exception (CBE) is a system of documentation that aims to eliminate redundancy, makes documentation of routine care more concise, emphasizes abnormal findings, and identifies trends in clinical care. CBE is a shorthand method for documenting on the basis of clearly defined standards of practice and predetermined criteria for nursing assessments and interventions. This system involves completing a flow sheet that incorporates standard assessment and intervention criteria by placing a check mark in the appropriate standard box on the flow sheet to indicate normal findings and routine interventions. You write a narrative nurse's note *only* when there is an exception to the established standard or abnormal data are present. Assessments are standardized on

forms so all health care providers evaluate and document findings consistently.

The presumption with CBE is that the nurse assessed the patient and all standards are met unless otherwise documented. Changes in a patient's condition require thorough and precise descriptions of what happened, actions taken, and patient response to treatment. Legal risks in using CBE include difficulty in proving safe care if nurses are not disciplined in documenting exceptions.

Critical Pathways

Critical pathways are a system of documentation that state the goals and important treatment interventions on the basis of best practice and patient expectations by documenting, monitoring, and evaluating variances. Key interventions and expected outcomes are established within an expected time frame for specific diseases (Fig. 4.5). Variances are unexpected occurrences, unmet goals, and interventions not specified within the critical pathway time frame and reflect a positive or negative change. A positive variance occurs when a patient progresses more rapidly than the pathway expected (e.g., use of a Foley catheter is discontinued a day early). A negative variance occurs when the activities on the critical pathway do not happen as predicted or outcomes are unmet (e.g., oxygen therapy is necessary for a new-onset breathing problem). Document the variance and include causative factors, actions taken, patient response, and outcomes. Over time the recurrence of similar variances leads the health care team to revise a critical pathway, particularly if it affects quality of care or length of stay.

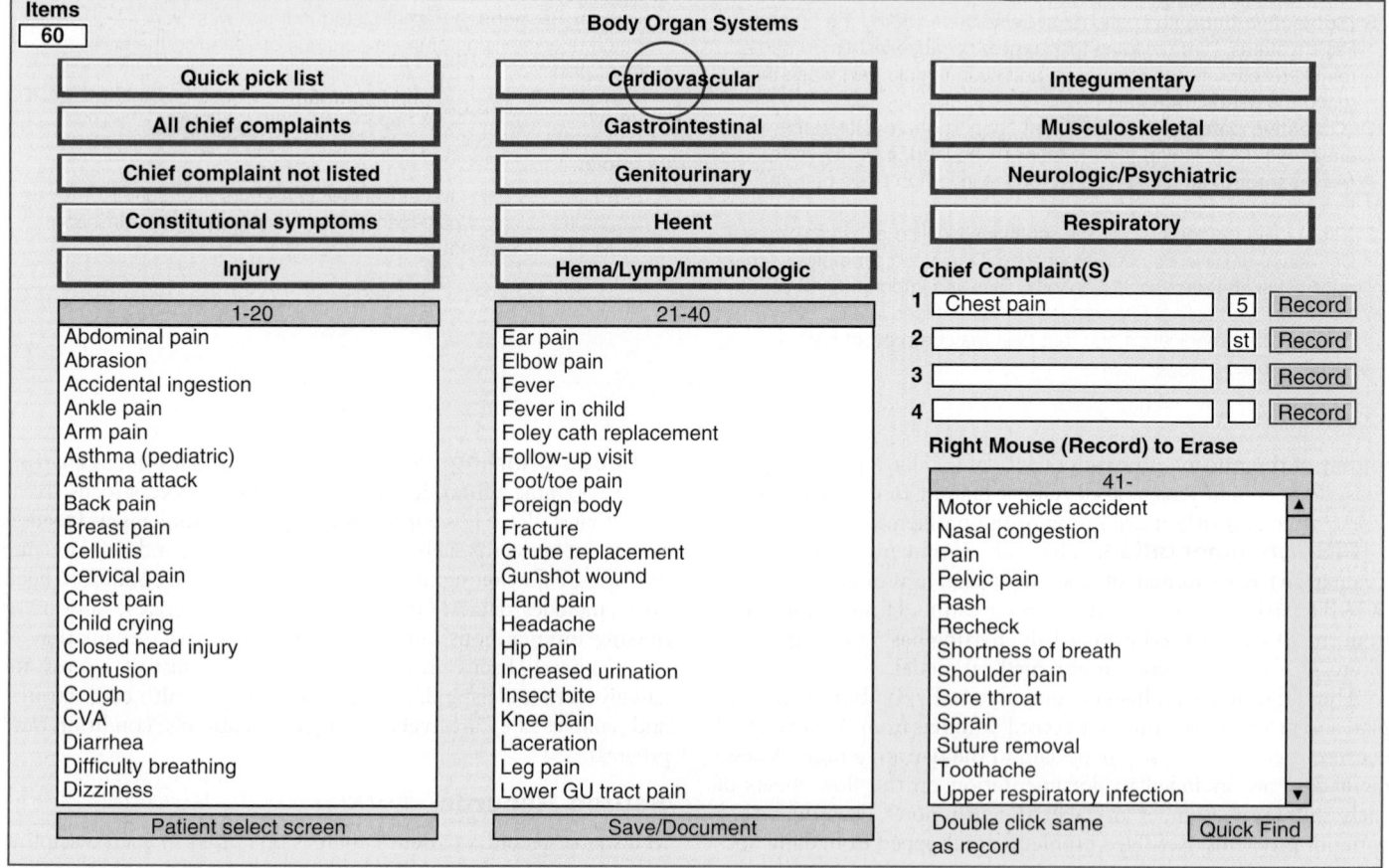

FIG 4.5 Electronic documentation, nursing record. (*Courtesy ER Choice, Irving, TX.*)

PROCEDURAL GUIDELINE 4.2 *Documenting Nurses' Progress Notes*

Accurate documentation reflects the quality of care and provides evidence of each health care team member's accountability in giving care. The purpose of a patient's record is to provide information for communication, education, assessment, research, financial billing, auditing, and legal documentation (Table 4.3).

Because the nursing process directs a nurse's approach to patient care, documentation needs to reflect this process. Nurses record assessment data, changes in a patient's condition, nursing interventions, and an evaluation of the patient's progress toward established outcomes. Prompt documentation of these data increases accuracy and promotes effective communication to all members of the health care team. The nurse caring for the patient is responsible for writing and signing each progress note, which includes full name and title. All caregivers need to be able to read the progress note and have a clear picture of the problem, level of care required, and results of interventions.

Delegation and Collaboration
The skill of documenting nurse progress notes cannot be delegated to nursing assistive personnel (NAP). The nurse instructs the NAP about:
- Which repetitive care activities to document on flow sheets (e.g., vital signs, intake and output [I&O], routine care).
- What to report to the nurse (e.g., increased pain, changes in vital signs) so he or she can reassess, validate, and document any changes in the progress note.

Equipment
- Progress note form (written or electronic)
- Black pen or electronic health record (EHR)

Procedural Steps
1. Identify the electronic patient record using at least two identifiers (e.g., name and birthday or name and medical record number) according to agency policy (Office of the National Coordination for Health Information Technology, 2014).

2. Review assessment data, problems identified, goals and expected outcomes, nursing interventions, and patient response during contact with each patient and before documentation.
3. Document patient information in the narrative format chosen by the health care agency. Follow guidelines for charting to ensure quality documentation.
4. After each patient contact, identify information that needs to be documented. Consider:
   a. Abnormal findings.
   b. Changes in status.
   c. New problems identified.
5. Document in a timely fashion without leaving open spaces between notes and include date and time. In an EHR the date and time are entered automatically by the system.
6. Using agency format, document in chronological order the following:
   a. Pertinent, factual, objective data
   b. Selected subjective data that validates or clarifies
   c. Nursing actions taken
   d. Patient responses to actions taken
   e. Additional plans needing to be implemented
   f. To whom information has been reported, including name and status
7. Sign progress note with full name or first initial and last name and status according to agency policy. Do not leave any open space between this note and the previously written note. Students are usually required to indicate their level of education and school affiliation. In an EHR an electronic signature will be generated when the note is submitted electronically.
8. Review previously documented entries with those that you enter, noting if there is significant change in the patient's status. Report any changes to the patient's health care provider.

TABLE 4.3	
Purposes of Records	
Purpose	**Description**
Communication	The record is a means for health care team members to communicate a patient's *needs* (e.g., individual therapies, patient education, discharge planning) and *progress* (e.g., response to therapies). Anyone reading the record should have a clear understanding of the plan of care.
Education	The record contains a variety of information, including medical and nursing diagnoses, signs and symptoms of disease, successful and unsuccessful therapies, diagnostic findings, and patient behaviors. Students of nursing, medicine, and other health-related disciplines use records as educational resources.
Assessment	Records provide data that nurses use to identify and support nursing diagnoses and plan proper interventions for care. Information from records adds to the nurse's own observations and assessment. Information in medical progress notes allows a nurse to anticipate the status of a patient and conduct an assessment that augments, validates, or confirms health care provider findings.
Research	Statistical data relating to the frequency of clinical disorders, complications, use of specific medical and nursing therapies, recovery from illness, and death can be gathered from patient records. Records describe characteristics of patient populations in a health care agency.
Financial billing	The record is a document that shows the extent to which hospitals should be reimbursed for services. For the agency to obtain full reimbursement, the record needs to show that all health care providers' orders were completed adequately and correctly, and it must reflect results of those orders.

Continued

TABLE 4.3	
Purposes of Records—cont'd	
Purpose	**Description**
Auditing and monitoring	A regular review of information in patient records gives a basis for evaluation of the quality and appropriateness of care provided in an agency. The Joint Commission (2015a) requires health care agencies to establish quality improvement programs to conduct objective, ongoing reviews of patient care. Review of records reveals information about the processes and outcomes of care.
Legal documentation	A medical record must be accurate because it is a legal document. In case of a lawsuit, the medical record, not the nursing care, is on trial. Nursing care may have been excellent; however, care not documented is care not done as far as a court of law is concerned.

PROCEDURAL GUIDELINE 4.3 *Adverse Event Reporting*

An adverse event is any event not consistent with the routine operation of a health care unit or routine care of a patient. Examples include patient falls, needlestick injuries, medication errors, or a visitor becoming ill. The National Quality Forum (2015) identified a standardized list of preventable, serious adverse events that facilitate reporting of such events (Box 4.5). Completion of an occurrence report happens when there is actual or potential patient injury (near miss) that is not part of the patient record. Document in the patient's record an objective description of what you observed and follow-up actions taken without reference to the incident report/occurrence report. Reporting helps to identify high-risk trends in nursing care or daily unit operations that warrant correction. You complete the report even if an injury does not occur or is not apparent. The information from the reports helps nursing staff find solutions to prevent repeated incidents. The reports are an important part of the quality improvement program of a unit.

Adverse event reports are important sources of data for enhancing understanding of underlying causes of events that, when analyzed, can improve patient safety (ASHRM, 2014). Nurses are active participants in examining the cause of errors and redesigning systems to minimize the same type of errors in the future. By focusing on systems rather than individual failures, there is greater opportunity to improve patient safety (QSEN, 2014). For example, a patient is administered the wrong medication by a nurse. A review of the event focuses primarily on the medication process as opposed to blaming the nurse for the error.

Delegation and Collaboration
The skill of adverse event reporting cannot be delegated to nursing assistive personnel (NAP). The nurse instructs the NAP to:
- Report to the nurse any event such as a fall, incorrect treatment, or adverse reaction.
- Report to the nurse any pertinent information about the event so a report can be completed.

Equipment
- Adverse event report form or screen
- Black pen or digital technology

Procedural Steps
1. Identify the electronic patient record using at least two identifiers (e.g., name and birthday or name and medical record number) according to agency policy (Office of the National Coordination for Health Information Technology, 2014).

2. Use clinical reasoning skills to systematically and carefully determine what was involved in the event. Either report the event as witnessed or determine from NAP specifically what occurred. Record the exact sequence of events involved, including time and type of event; injury to patient, nurse, or other staff; and observation of factors that possibly contributed to the event (e.g., wet floor discovered in area of patient fall). Notify risk management per agency protocol.

Clinical Decision Point *Prepare the report on any questionable event. Do not avoid reporting because of concerns that punitive actions will occur if reports are filed.*

3. Assess extent of any injury to patient or others, including patient's subjective report and objective physical examination findings.
4. If the adverse event involves an injury, take steps to restore individual's safety such as stabilizing patient's position after a fall and assessing for further injuries.
5. When patient sustains an injury, call the health care provider immediately.
6. When visitor or staff member sustains an injury, refer to emergency department or appropriate treatment setting.
7. Complete adverse event report form.

Clinical Decision Point *Document on report form as quickly as possible. The closer to the event, the more accurate the recording.*

   a. Record time of event and describe exactly what occurred or was observed, using objective findings and observations. Use language that does not allow for subjective interpretation. Do not include personal opinions or feelings. Document victim's interpretation of event by using quotes.
   b. Objectively describe patient's or staff member's condition when event was discovered or observed.
   c. Describe measures taken by any caregivers at time of event.
   d. Send completed report to designated department.
8. When patient is involved, document events of incident in patient's chart.
   a. Only enter objective description of what happened.
   b. Record any assessment and intervention activities initiated as a result of event.
   c. Do not duplicate all information from report.
   d. Do not record that report was completed.
9. Submit the report properly with the risk-management department or designated people.

BOX 4.5

Examples of Serious Reportable Events Occurring Within a Health Care Agency

- Surgery or other invasive procedure performed on the wrong patient
- Patient death or serious injury associated with use of restraints or bedrails
- Patient death or serious injury associated with use or function of a device in patient care in which device is used for or functions other than intended
- Patient death or serious injury associated with a fall
- Patient death or serious injury associated with electrical shock

- Unintended retention of foreign object in a patient after surgery or invasive procedure
- Patient death or serious injury associated with elopement
- Patient death or serious injury associated with medication error
- Patient death or serious injury associated with unsafe administration of blood products
- Stage 3 or 4 pressure injury acquired after admission to a health care agency

Data from National Quality Forum: *List of serious reportable events,* nd, http://www.qualityforum.org/Topics/SREs/List_of_SREs.aspx. Accessed July 20, 2015.

HOME CARE DOCUMENTATION

The home care field continues to grow with shorter hospitalizations and increasing numbers of older adults requiring home care services. Medicare has specific guidelines for establishing eligibility for home care reimbursement (Centers for Medicare & Medicaid Services, 2015a). Documentation when caring for a patient at his or her home has different implications than in other areas of nursing. One primary difference is that the patient and family rather than the nurse witness the majority of care. In addition, documentation systems need to provide the entire health care team with the necessary information to work together effectively (Box 4.6). The documentation is both the quality control and the justification for reimbursement from Medicare, Medicaid, or private insurance companies.

Computerized patient records are evolving in the home care setting. The electronic health record facilitates clarity, continuity of care, and comprehensiveness because of increased standardization of language (Sockolow et al., 2014).

LONG-TERM HEALTH CARE DOCUMENTATION

Increasing numbers of older adults and disabled people in the United States require care in long-term health care agencies. Nursing personnel face documentation challenges much different from those in the acute care setting (Peterson, 2014). The federally mandated Long-Term Care Facility Resident Assessment Instrument provides standardized protocols for assessment and care planning and promotes quality improvement within and among agencies (Centers for Medicare & Medicaid Services, 2015b).

BOX 4.6

Forms for Home Care Documentation

The usual forms used to document home care include the following:
- Patient assessment
- Referral source information/intake form
- Discipline-specific care plans
- Health care provider's plan of treatment
- Medication sheet
- Clinical progress notes
- Miscellaneous (conference notes, verbal order forms, telephone calls)
- Discharge summary
- Reports to third-party payers

Each resident in long-term care is assessed with the Long-Term Care Facility Resident Assessment Instrument mandated by the Omnibus Budget Reconciliation Act of 1989 (OBRA) (Centers for Medicare & Medicaid Services, 2015b). A registered nurse is responsible for coordinating the plan of care. Documentation supports the assessment and planning process for patients using a multidisciplinary approach. Communication among health care providers, including nurses, social workers, recreational therapists, and dietitians, is essential in the documentation process. The fiscal support for long-term care residents depends on the justification of nursing care as demonstrated in sound documentation of the services rendered. The overall goal is a system of clinical documentation that identifies potential or actual problems and provides improved actions for each problem, which results in improved care for residents (Wysocki et al., 2015).

PROCEDURAL GUIDELINE 4.4 *Guidelines for Meaningful Use of an Electronic Health Record (EHR)*

As part of the American Recovery and Reinvestment Act (ARRA) of 2009, a meaningful use initiative was established with goals to improve clinical outcomes, increase efficiencies in health care, and develop a robust health care system database for research (HealthIT.gov, 2015; Wilson and Newhouse, 2012). Meaningful use means that health care providers effectively use electronic health records (EHRs) to improve patient care (HealthIT.gov, 2015). Final guidelines from CMS declared three implementation stages for meaningful use: (1) data collection and sharing; (2) care coordination and clinical decision making; and (3) clinical outcomes (CMS, 2013).

When health care agencies participate in meaningful use initiatives, health care providers use certified EHRs to record universal patient data, engage patients and families in care, and transmit critical patient data at care transition points (HealthIT. gov, 2015). An example of a care transition is a patient discharge from a hospital to a long-term care facility. CMS mandates that specific patient data collected from the sending facility is sent to the new provider when a transition occurs. Examples of data sent include history of allergies, cognitive status, functional status, immunizations, medications, and smoking history (Fuchs, 2014).

Continued

PROCEDURAL GUIDELINE 4.4 *Guidelines for Meaningful Use of an Electronic Health Record (EHR)—cont'd*

Medication reconciliation, the process of assessing the patient's current medications to medications actually prescribed at a care transition point, minimizes medication errors and adverse events (Andreoli et al., 2014). The EHR provides efficiencies for all health care providers performing medication reconciliation (Shuster and Sage, 2012). Medication reconciliation is 1 of 17 mandated core objectives in the second stage of the Meaningful Use initiative (CMS, 2013). Listed as a National Patient Safety goal (TJC, 2015c), medication reconciliation is a complex process requiring interprofessional collaboration (Vogelsmeier et al., 2013). By using a standardized process to assess a patient's medications at a care transition point, medication discrepancies such as omissions, duplications, contraindications, and vague information can be reduced (Ruggiero et al., 2015; TJC, 2015d). Although some agencies may assign other disciplines as the accountable discipline for medication reconciliation, the nurse plays an active collaborative role in the process (Vogelsmeier, 2014).

Delegation and Collaboration

The skill of using an EHR for medication reconciliation cannot be delegated to nursing assistive personnel (NAP). The nurse instructs the NAP to:
- Report to the nurse any pertinent information the patient or family caregiver reports about their medications.

Equipment
- Admission medication list
- Current medication list
- Discharge medication list
- Medication reconciliation work screen or worksheet (if implemented by agency)
- EHR

Procedural Steps
1. Use an organized format for medication reconciliation. A medication background, assessment, and reconciliation (MBAR) worksheet may effectively reduce medication

errors for patients transitioning from long-term to acute care (Blank et al., 2012).
2. Identify the electronic patient record using at least two identifiers (e.g., name and birthday or name and medical record number) according to agency policy (Office of the National Coordination for Health Information Technology, 2014).
3. Gather information from electronic documentation sources such as admission medications, active medications, and/or discharge medications.
4. Include two nurses to complete the medication reconciliation at time of care transition. Assess the current medications ordered to the medications prescribed for the care transition. If being discharged from a facility, assess the medications on admission and current medications to the discharge medications (Ruggiero et al., 2015).
5. Discrepancies are assessed by the two nurses.

Clinical Decision Point *If discrepancies still exist after nurse review, a nurse-to-physician reconciliation occurs.*

6. If being discharged from a facility, reconcile the medication list before giving information to the patient. Provide the patient with the written reconciled list of medications.
7. Teach the patient how to keep his or her medication list current.
8. Educate the patient about the medications and importance of sharing his or her current medication list at every health care visit.
9. **Use Teach-Back:** "I want to be sure you understand how to update your medication list. What steps will you use to keep your medication list current?" Revise your instruction now or develop a plan for revised patient or family caregiver teaching if patient or family caregiver is not able to teach back correctly.

◆ CLINICAL DEBRIEF

A 55-year-old retired teacher will be discharged this evening from the ambulatory care unit following his surgical hernia repair. His admission medication list includes hydrochlorothiazide 12.5-mg tablet orally once per day; fluoxetine 40-mg tablet orally once daily in the morning.

Immediately after surgery he rates his pain as 10 on a scale of 0-10, and he is medicated with hydromorphone 1 mg IV at 0930.

1. Based on his 'admission medication list, which medications do you expect to find on the discharge medication list?
2. At 1400, he rates his surgical pain as 9 on a scale of 0-10. He receives two Percocet 10/325 (oxycodone and acetaminophen) tablets orally for his pain at 1410. Thirty minutes later, he rates his pain as 2 on a scale of 0-10. At discharge the medication list reads: hydrochlorothiazide 12.5-mg tablet orally once per day and fluoxetine 40-mg tablet orally once daily in the morning. What are your nursing actions?
3. Using SBAR, show how you would communicate with the physician about the medication omission.

◆ REVIEW QUESTIONS

1. The patient falls on the unit. Which actions will the nurse perform? (Select all that apply.)
   1. Assess extent of any injury to the patient
   2. Document the adverse event report in the electronic health record (EHR)
   3. Identify the patient using at least two identifiers
   4. Complete an adverse event report on the basis of your initial reaction
   5. Document your clinical assessment in the EHR
2. During a hand-off report, the nurse will: (Select all that apply.)
   1. Use the patient's first and last name as the two identifiers.
   2. Provide background information about the patient.
   3. Recommend the priority of care for the next shift.
   4. Include in the assessment the patient's response to pain medications.
   5. Exclude the patient from the hand-off report.

3. The patient is being transitioned from the hospital to a long-term care facility. Place the following criteria in correct order for an SBAR report.

1. Medical history, allergies, code status, isolation, significant interventions, pain management, responses to interventions, report of abnormal studies, who was notified, any interventions, intravenous [IV] access

2. Admission date, chief complaint, and diagnosis

3. Review of systems: neurological, respiratory, cardiac, gastrointestinal, genitourinary, musculoskeletal, peripheral vascular, skin, hematological, endocrine, and psychosocial

4. Patient's daily goals, consultations, planned treatments, upcoming tests or surgery, discharge planning, and patient education

ⓔ *Visit the Evolve site for a complete list of Clinical Debrief and Review Questions answers.*

REFERENCES

American Society for Healthcare Risk Management (ASHRM): Serious safety events, 2014, http://www.ashrm.org/search?q=adverse+events&site=ASHRM&client=default_FE. Accessed July 23, 2015.

An D: Cochrane review brief: discharge planning from hospital to home, *Online J Issues Nurs* 20(2):2015.

Andreoli L, et al: Medication reconciliation: a prospective study in an internal medicine unit, *Drugs Aging* 31(5):387, 2014.

Appari A, et al: Meaningful use of electronic health record systems and process quality of care: evidence from a panel data analysis of US acute-care hospitals, *Health Serv Res* 48(2pt1):369, 2013.

Barry M: Issues up close: hand-off communication: assuring the transfer of accurate patient information, *Am Nurse Today* 9(1):30, 2014.

Blank L, et al: Bridging the gap in transitional care: a closer look at medication reconciliation, *Geriatr Nurs* 33(5):406, 2012.

Boyd M, et al: Read-back improves information transfer in simulated clinical crises, *BMJ Qual Safe* 23(12):989, 2014.

Centers for Medicare & Medicaid Services (CMS): Eligible professional guide to STAGE 2 of the EHR incentive programs, 2013, http://www.cms.gov/Regulations-and-Guidance/Legislation/EHRIncentivePrograms/Downloads/Stage2_Guide_EPs_9_23_13.pdf. Accessed July 18, 2015.

Centers for Medicare & Medicaid Services (CMS): Homecare PPS, 2015a, https://www.cms.gov/Medicare/Medicare-Fee-for-Service-Payment/HomeHealthPPS/index.html?redirect=/HomeHealthPPS/. Accessed July 15, 2015.

Centers for Medicare & Medicaid Services (CMS): MDS 3.0 RAI Manual, 2015b, http://www.cms.gov/Medicare/Quality-Initiatives-Patient-Assessment-Instruments/NursinghomeQualityInits/MDS30RAIManual.html. Accessed July 14, 2015.

Center for Nursing Classification and Clinical Effectiveness: *Nursing Intervention Classification (NIC)*, 2013a, http://www.nursing.uiowa.edu/cncce/nursing-interventions-classification-overview. Accessed July 18, 2015.

Center for Nursing Classification and Clinical Effectiveness: *Nursing Outcome Classification (NOC)* 2013b. http://www.nursing.uiowa.edu/cncce/nursing-outcomes-classification-overview. Accessed July 18, 2015.

Cornell P, et al: Impact of SBAR on nurse shift reports and staff rounding, *Medsug Nurs* 23(5):335, 341, 2014.

Dontje K, et al: Understanding patient perceptions of the electronic personal health record, *J Nurse Pract* 10(10):825, 2014.

Englebright J, et al: Defining and incorporating basic nursing care actions into the electronic health record, *J Nurs Scholarsh* 46(1):50, 2014.

Fengping L, et al: Electronic health records and improved nursing management of chronic obstructive pulmonary disease, *Patient Prefer Adherence* 9:499, 2015.

Foster-Hunt T, et al: Information structure and organisation in change of shift reports: an observational study of nursing hand-offs in a paediatric intensive care unit, *Intensive Crit Care Nurs* 31(3):156, 2015.

Fuchs J: Stage 2 meaningful use–implications for ambulatory care nursing, *AAACN Viewpoint* 36(4):10, 2014.

Gardner LA, Sparnon EM: Work-arounds slow electronic health record use, *AJN* 114(4):65, 2014.

Graham J, et al: Nurses' discharge planning and risk assessment: behaviours, understanding and barriers, *J Clin Nurs* 22(15/16):2339, 2013.

Harmon C, et al: Then and now: nurses' perceptions of the electronic health record, *Online J Nurs Inform* 19(1):5, 2015.

Healthcare Information and Management Systems Society (HIMSS): Electronic record, 2015a, http://www.himss.org/library/ehr/. Accessed July 12, 2015.

Healthcare Information and Management Systems Society (HIMSS): What is health informatics? 2015b, http://www.himss.org/ResourceLibrary/genResourceDetailPDF.aspx?ItemNumber=27767. Accessed July 12, 2015.

HealthIT.gov: Meaningful use definition and objectives, 2015, http://www.healthit.gov/providers-professionals/meaningful-use-definition-objectives. Accessed July 20, 2015.

Institute of Medicine (IOM): *Health IT and patient safety: building safer systems for better care (e-book)*, Washington, DC, 2012, IOM.

Joint Commission Center for Transforming Healthcare: Hand-off communications, nd, http://www.centerfortransforminghealthcare.org/projects/detail.aspx?Project=1. Accessed July 16, 2015.

NANDA International: *Nursing diagnoses: definitions and classification 2015-2017*, West Sussex, UK, 2014, Wiley Blackwell.

National Quality Forum: List of SRES, 2015, http://www.qualityforum.org/Topics/SREs/List_of_SREs.aspx. Accessed July 20, 2015.

Nunes S, et al: The experience of an information system for nursing practice: the importance of nursing records in the management of a care plan, *CIN, Comput Inform Nurs* 32(7):330, 2014.

Nursing Informatics: *Scope and standards of practice*, ed 2, Silver Spring, MD, 2014, American Nurses Association.

Office of the National Coordination for Health Information Technology: Self-assessment patient identification, 2014, http://www.healthit.gov/sites/safer/files/guides/safer_patientidentification_sg006_form.pdf. Accessed July 16, 2015.

Park H: Identifying core NANDA-I nursing diagnoses, NIC interventions, NOC outcomes, and NNN linkages for heart failure, *Int J Nurs Knowl* 25(1):30, 2014.

Perry J, et al: Assessment of the impact on time to complete medical record using an electronic medical record versus a paper record on emergency department patients: a study, *Emerg Med J* 31(12):980, 2014.

Peterson A: Nursing home medical records: part 2: documentation review, *J Legal Nurs Consult* 25(2):42, 2014.

Plemmons S, et al: Measurable outcomes from standardized nursing documentation in an electronic health record, *ANIA-CARING Newsletter* 27(2):7, 2012.

Quality, Safety, Education for Nurses (QSEN): Pre-licensure KSAS, 2014, http://qsen.org/competencies/pre-licensure-ksas/#safety. Accessed November 8, 2015.

Ruggiero J, et al: Discharge time out: an innovative nurse-driven protocol for medication reconciliation, *Medsurg Nurs* 24(3):170, 2015.

Rutten FL, et al: Patient perceptions of electronic medical records use and ratings of care quality, *Patient Relat Outcome Meas* 5:17, 2014.

Shuster K, Sage R: Improving medication reconciliation with standards, presented at NCDPD & HIMSS, 2012, http://files.himss.org/HIMSSorg/Content/files/Pharmacy_Informatics_Town%20Hall_December2012.pdf. Accessed July 28, 2015.

Simpson K: Electronic health records, *MCN Am J Matern Child Nurs* 40(1):68, 2015.

Sockolow P, et al: Impact of homecare electronic health record on timeliness of clinical documentation, reimbursement, and patient outcomes, *Appl Clin Inform* 5(2):445, 2014.

Spivey J: Where do you want to give report?, *Dimens Crit Care Nurs* 33(5):278, 2014.

The Joint Commission (TJC): *Comprehensive accreditation manual for hospitals: the official handbook*, Oakbrook Terrace, IL, 2015a, The Commission.

The Joint Commission (TJC): Facts about the official "do not use list," 2015b, http://www.jointcommission.org/facts_about_do_not_use_list. Accessed July 26, 2015.

The Joint Commission (TJC): *National Patient Safety Goals*, Oakbrook Terrace, IL, 2015c, The Commission. http://www.jointcommission.org/standards_information/npsgs.aspx.

The Joint Commission (TJC): Sentinel event data— root causes by event type, 2015d, http://www.jointcommission.org/Sentinel_Event_Statistics. Accessed July 19, 2015.

Trossman S: Stopping the revolving door, *Am Nurs* 47(1):9, 2015.

US Department of Health and Human Services (USDHHS): Standards for privacy of individuals, Health Insurance Portability and Accountability Act of 1996, *Fed Reg* 60053:1999. http://www.hhs.gov/ocr/privacy/hipaa/administrative/privacyrule/index.html. Accessed July 10, 2015.

Vogelsmeier A: Identifying medication order discrepancies during medication reconciliation: perceptions of nursing home leaders and staff, *J Nurs Manag* 22(3):369, 2014.

Vogelsmeier A, et al: Medication reconciliation: a qualitative analysis of clinicians' perceptions, *Res Social Adm Pharm* 9(4):419, 2013.

Wilson M, Newhouse R: Medication reconciliation across the continuum of care: a meaningful use mandate, *J Nurs Adm* 42(9):396, 2012.

Wysocki A, et al: Functional improvement among short-stay nursing home residents in the MDS 3.0, *J Am Med Dir Assoc* 16(6):470, 2015.

5 | Vital Signs

OBJECTIVES

Mastery of content in this chapter will enable the nurse to:
- Identify when it is appropriate to assess each vital sign.
- Accurately assess a patient's oral, rectal, axillary, tympanic membrane, and temporal artery temperatures.
- Describe factors that cause variations in body temperature, pulse, respirations, blood pressure, and oxygen saturation.
- Discuss factors in selecting temperature measurement sites.
- Accurately assess a patient's radial and apical pulses.
- Explain implications of a pulse deficit.
- Accurately assess a patient's respirations.
- Accurately measure a patient's blood pressure using techniques of auscultation and palpation.

- Discuss benefits and disadvantages of using an automatic blood pressure machine.
- Describe factors in selecting an extremity to measure blood pressure.
- Accurately assess a patient's oxygenation status using pulse oximetry.
- Identify ranges of acceptable vital sign values for infant, child, and adult.
- Correctly record vital signs.
- Appropriately delegate vital sign measurements to nursing assistive personnel.

MEDIA RESOURCES

- evolve http://evolve.elsevier.com/Perry/skills
- Review Questions
- Audio Glossary
- ▶ Video Clips

- Animations
- **NSO** Nursing Skills Online
- Clinical Debrief and Review Questions Answers
- Case Studies

PURPOSE

Vital signs, temperature, pulse, blood pressure, respirations and oxygen saturation reflect the physiological status of the body and its response to physical, environmental, and psychological stressors. Pain, a subjective symptom, is often referred to as a vital sign. You will frequently perform an assessment of a patient's level of comfort and pain during vital sign measurements (see Chapter 16).

Vital signs reveal both sudden changes in a patient's condition and changes that occur progressively over time. Any difference between a patient's normal baseline measurement and present vital signs may indicate the need for nursing therapies and necessary medical interventions.

STANDARDS OF CARE

- James et al., 2014—Evidence-Based Guideline for the Management of High Blood Pressure in Adults: Report From the Panel Members Appointed to the Eighth Joint National Committee—Hypertension Guidelines and Standards for Measurement
- The Joint Commission, 2016—Patient Identification

PRINCIPLES FOR PRACTICE

- Vital signs are included in a routine physical assessment (see Chapter 6).

When to Take Vital Signs

- On admission to a health care facility
- In a hospital or care facility on a routine schedule according to a health care provider's order or standards of practice of agency
- When assessing patient during home care visits
- Before, during, and after a surgical or invasive diagnostic procedure
- Before, during, and after the administration of medications or application of therapies that affect cardiovascular, respiratory, or temperature-control functions
- Before, during, and after a transfusion of any type of blood products
- Before, during, and after nursing interventions influencing a vital sign (e.g., before and after patient previously on bed rest ambulates, before and after he or she performs range-of-motion exercises)
- When patient reports specific symptoms of physical distress (e.g., feeling "funny" or "different")
- When patient's general physical condition changes (e.g., loss of consciousness, increased intensity of pain)

- Always obtain a baseline measurement of vital signs on first contact with a patient to provide a means for comparison with later vital sign measurements.
- Frequency of vital sign measurements depends on the specific patient's condition (Box 5.1). You apply clinical judgment to decide which vital sign to measure, when to obtain measurements, and the frequency of assessments.

PATIENT-CENTERED CARE

- Vital sign measurements can require removing clothing or exposing areas considered inappropriate or offensive to patients from other cultures. You must be sensitive to each patient's need for privacy and observe cultural norms. Provide privacy when performing apical pulse assessment (Giger, 2013).
- Always inform patients about their vital sign measurements. Many patients monitor their own vital signs at home and can be valuable partners in letting you know which values are normal for them.
- Procedures that are normally noninvasive sometimes produce anxiety because of cultural variables of touch, privacy, and gender.
- When reporting findings, patients from cultures with paternalistic values rely on a male elder to receive information on their behalf.
- Consult the health care provider and family decision maker regarding giving information to the patient about abnormal vital signs.
- Collectivistic ethnic groups may demonstrate their caring for ill members by protecting them from bad news about their health and well-being (Giger, 2013). Assess to determine if this applies to the patient for whom you care.

EVIDENCE-BASED PRACTICE

Obtaining an accurate and reliable blood pressure requires consideration of measurement conditions.

- Deep breathing during blood pressure measurement decreases systolic and diastolic blood pressure nearly 5 mm Hg (Zheng et al., 2012).
- Talking, especially when communicating sensitive or stressful information, increases systolic and diastolic blood pressure up to 6 mm Hg (Zheng et al., 2012).
- Two studies established that placing a blood pressure cuff over a sleeved arm in either hypertensive (Pinar et al., 2010) or normotensive (Ki et al., 2013) patients had no effect on blood pressure measurements.

SAFETY GUIDELINES

- A nurse caring for a patient is responsible for measuring vital signs. Nurses analyze vital signs to interpret their significance and make decisions about appropriate interventions.
- Equipment must be clean, functional, properly calibrated, and appropriate for the patient's size, age, condition, and characteristics.
- It is your responsibility to know each patient's usual range of vital signs. A patient's usual values may differ from the acceptable range for that age or physical state. They serve as a baseline for comparison with later findings; thus you detect changes in condition over time.
- You are also responsible for knowing a patient's medical history, therapies, and prescribed medications. Some illnesses or treatments cause predictable vital sign changes. Most medications affect at least one of the vital signs.
- Control or minimize environmental factors that affect vital signs. For example, assessing a patient's temperature in a warm, humid room may yield a value that is not a true indicator of his or her condition.
- Use an organized, systematic (step-by-step) approach when taking vital signs to ensure accurate findings.
- Based on a patient's condition, collaborate with the health care provider to decide the minimum frequency of vital sign assessment for each patient. Following surgery or treatment intervention, measure vital signs more frequently to detect complications. In a clinic or outpatient setting take vital signs before the health care provider examines the patient and after any invasive procedures. As a patient's physical condition worsens, it is important to monitor the vital signs as often as every 5 to 15 minutes. You are responsible for judging whether more frequent assessments are necessary.
- Analyze the results of vital sign measurements and incorporate all the clinical findings about a patient in determining nursing diagnoses. Do not interpret vital signs in isolation. You need to know related physical signs or symptoms and be aware of the patient's ongoing health status.
- Verify, communicate, and document significant changes in vital signs. Baseline measurements allow you to identify changes in vital signs. When vital signs appear abnormal, it helps to have another nurse repeat the measurement. Inform the health care provider when vital signs become abnormal and report any changes to the nurse in charge.

✦ SKILL 5.1 Measuring Body Temperature

NSO *Nursing Skills Online Vital Signs Module / Lessons 1 and 2* *Video Clip*

Body temperature is the difference between the amount of heat produced by body processes and the amount lost to the external environment. The core temperature, or temperature of the deep body tissues, is under control of the hypothalamus and remains within a narrow range. Skin or body surface temperature fluctuates dramatically as it rises and falls with the changing temperature of the surrounding environment.

The body tissues and cells function best within a relatively narrow temperature range, from 36° to 38°C (96.8° to 100.4°F), but no single temperature is normal for all people. For healthy young adults the average oral temperature is 37°C (98.6°F). In clinical practice nurses learn the temperature range of individual patients. An acceptable temperature range for adults depends on age, gender, range of physical activity, hydration status, and state of health (Fig. 5.1).

Many factors affect body temperature, but physiological and behavioral control mechanisms act to maintain a constant core temperature. For example, the mechanism of peripheral vasodilation increases blood flow to the skin, which increases the amount of heat radiated to the environment. Control mechanisms have failed when heat produced by the body is not equal to heat lost to the environment. For example, patients without sweat gland function are unable to tolerate warm temperatures because they cannot adequately cool themselves. Fever occurs when heat-loss mechanisms are unable to keep pace with excess heat production, resulting in an abnormal rise in body temperature. When an individual has a febrile condition (i.e., pyrexia), initiate temperature-control measures such as controlling environmental temperatures, removing external coverings, and administering ordered antipyretics to achieve better temperature control.

The purpose of measuring body temperature is to obtain a representative average temperature of core body tissues. Average usual temperature varies, depending on the measurement site used. Research findings from numerous studies are contradictory; however, it is generally accepted that rectal temperatures are usually 0.5°C (0.9°F) higher than oral temperatures. Axillary and tympanic membrane temperatures are usually 0.5°C (0.9°F) lower than oral temperatures. Sites reflecting core temperature are more reliable indicators of body temperature than sites reflecting surface temperatures (Mazerolle et al., 2011) (Box 5.2).

To ensure accurate temperature readings you need to measure each site correctly. Use the same site when repeated measurements are necessary or when comparing temperature measurements over time. Each site has advantages and disadvantages (Box 5.3). You need to determine the safest and most accurate site for a patient.

Several types of thermometers are commonly available to measure body temperature (Box 5.4). The mercury-in-glass thermometer, once the standard device found in the clinical setting, is now prohibited because of the potential mercury hazards. However, mercury-in-glass thermometers can still be found in patients' homes.

Delegation and Collaboration

The skill of temperature measurement can be delegated to nursing assistive personnel (NAP). The nurse instructs the NAP by:
- Communicating the appropriate route, device, and frequency of temperature measurement.
- Explaining any precautions needed in positioning the patient (e.g., for rectal temperature measurement).
- Reviewing the usual temperature values and significant changes to report to the nurse.

Equipment

- Thermometer (selected on the basis of site used; see Box 5.3)
- Soft tissue or wipe
- Alcohol swab
- Water-soluble lubricant (for rectal measurements only)
- Pen and vital sign flow sheet, record form, or electronic health record (EHR)
- Clean gloves (optional), plastic thermometer sleeve, disposable probe or sensor cover
- Towel

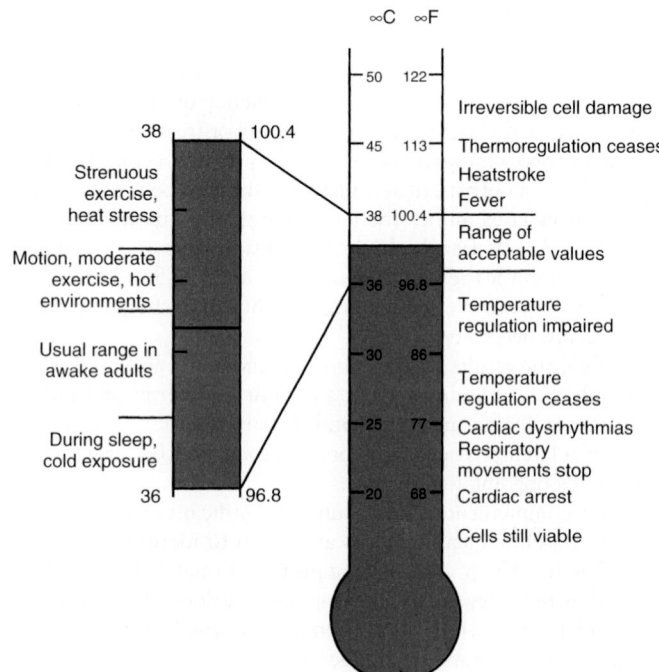

FIG 5.1 Ranges of normal temperature values and physiological consequences of abnormal body temperature. (*Modified from Thibodeau GA, Patton KT: Anatomy and physiology, ed 7, St Louis, 2010, Mosby.*)

BOX 5.2

Core and Surface Temperature Measurement Sites

Core Site	Surface Site
• Rectum	• Skin
• Tympanic membrane	• Oral cavity
• Temporal artery	• Axilla
• Esophagus	
• Pulmonary artery	
• Urinary bladder	

BOX 5.3

Advantages and Limitations of Select Temperature Measurement Sites

Oral
Advantages
- Easily accessible—requires no position change
- Comfortable for patient
- Provides accurate surface temperature reading
- Reflects rapid change in core temperature
- Reliable route to measure temperature for intubated patients

Limitations
- Causes delay in measurement if patient recently ingested hot/cold fluids or foods, chewed gum, or smoked
- Not used with patients who have had oral surgery or facial trauma, are unable to position in mouth, or have shaking chills or history of seizures
- Not used with infants; small children; or confused, unconscious, or uncooperative patients
- Risk for body fluid exposure

Tympanic Membrane
Advantages
- Easily accessible site
- Obtained without disturbing, waking, or repositioning patient
- Used for patients with tachypnea without affecting breathing
- Sensitive to core temperature changes
- Very rapid measurement (2 to 5 seconds)
- Unaffected by oral intake of food or fluids or smoking
- Used in newborns to reduce infant handling and heat loss (Ozdemir et al., 2011)

Limitations
- More variability of measurement than with other core temperature devices
- Requires removal of hearing aids before measurement
- Requires disposable sensor cover with only one size available
- Readings possibly distorted with otitis media and cerumen impaction
- Not used with patients who have had surgery of the ear or tympanic membrane
- Does not accurately measure core temperature changes during and after exercise
- Affected by ambient temperature devices such as incubators, radiant warmers, and facial fans
- Anatomy of ear canal makes it difficult to correctly position in neonates, infants, and children younger than 3 years of age
- Inaccuracies reported because of incorrect positioning of handheld unit

Rectal
Advantages
- Argued to be reliable when oral temperature is difficult or impossible to obtain

Limitations
- Lags behind core temperature during rapid temperature changes
- Not used for patients with diarrhea or those who have had rectal surgery, rectal disorders, bleeding tendencies, or neutropenia
- Requires positioning and is often source of patient embarrassment and anxiety
- Risk for body fluid exposure
- Requires lubrication
- Not used for routine vital signs in newborns
- Readings influenced by impacted stool

Axilla
Advantages
- Safe and inexpensive
- Reliable in stable and preterm infants (Charafeddine et al., 2014)

Limitations
- Long measurement time
- Requires continuous positioning
- Poorly reflects core temperature (Haugan et al., 2012; Reynolds et al., 2014).
- Not recommended for detecting fever in infants and young children
- Requires exposure of thorax, which can result in temperature loss, especially in newborns
- Affected by exposure to the environment, including time it takes to place thermometer
- Underestimates core temperature

Skin
Advantages
- Inexpensive
- Provides continuous reading
- Safe and noninvasive
- Used for neonates

Limitations
- Measurement lags behind other sites during temperature changes, especially during hyperthermia
- Impaired adhesion from diaphoresis or sweat
- Affected by environmental temperature
- Cannot be used for patients with allergy to adhesives

Temporal Artery
Advantages
- Easy to access without position change
- Very rapid measurement
- Comfortable with no risk of injury to patient or nurse
- Eliminates need to disrobe or unbundle
- Can be used for premature infants, newborns, and children (Reynolds et al., 2014)
- Reflects rapid change in core temperature
- Sensor cover not required

Limitations
- Inaccurate with head covering or hair on forehead
- Affected by skin moisture such as diaphoresis or sweating

BOX 5.4

Types of Thermometers

Electronic Thermometer (Fig. 5.2)
- Thermometer is a rechargeable battery-powered display unit with a thin wire cord and a temperature-processing probe covered by a disposable cover.
- Within 1 minute after placement the thermometer displays a digital temperature reading.
- Separate probes are available for oral and axillary temperature measurement (blue tip) and rectal temperature measurement (red tip).

Tympanic Membrane Thermometer
- The probe consists of an otoscope-like speculum with an infrared sensor tip that detects heat radiated from the tympanic membrane of the ear (Fig. 5.3).
- Within seconds after placing in the ear canal and depressing the scan button, a digital reading appears on the display unit. A sound signals when the peak temperature has been measured.

Temporal Artery Thermometer
- An infrared scanner is swept across the forehead, lifted, and then placed behind the ear where a woman would normally place perfume. If the patient is diaphoretic, a scan just behind the ear verifies the measurement accuracy (Fig. 5.4).
- Within seconds after scanning, a digital reading appears on the display unit.

Chemical Dot Single-Use or Reusable Thermometer
- Thermometer consists of thin strips of plastic with a temperature sensor at one end and chemically impregnated dots formulated to change color at different temperatures (Fig. 5.5).
- Chemical dots on thermometer change color to reflect temperature reading, usually within 60 seconds.
- It is useful for screening temperatures, especially in infants, during invasive procedures, for a patient on protective isolation, and in orally intubated critical care patients.
- It is not appropriate for monitoring fever in acutely ill patients or for temperature therapies.
- It can be used at axillary or rectal site if covered by a plastic sheath with a placement time of 3 minutes.
- Home disposable thermometers are useful for temperature screening but are not as accurate as nondisposable electronic thermometers (Counts et al., 2014).

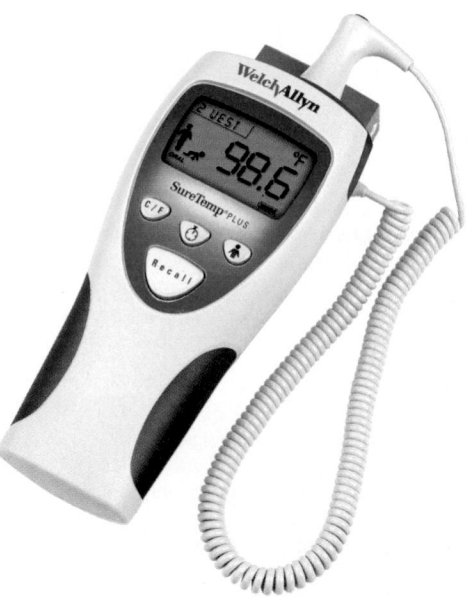

FIG 5.2 Electronic thermometer with disposable plastic probe cover. *(Photo courtesy Welch Allyn.)*

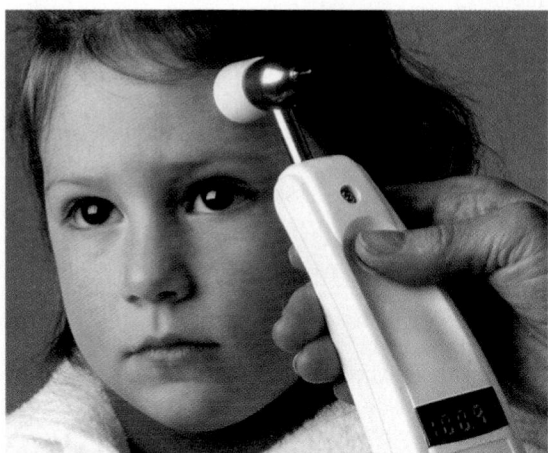

FIG 5.4 A temporal artery thermometer measures the heat from blood flowing through the superficial temporal artery. *(Photo courtesy Exergen.)*

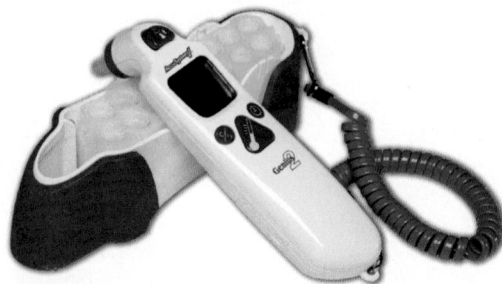

FIG 5.3 Tympanic membrane thermometer with disposable plastic probe cover. *(Copyright ©Covidien. All rights reserved.)*

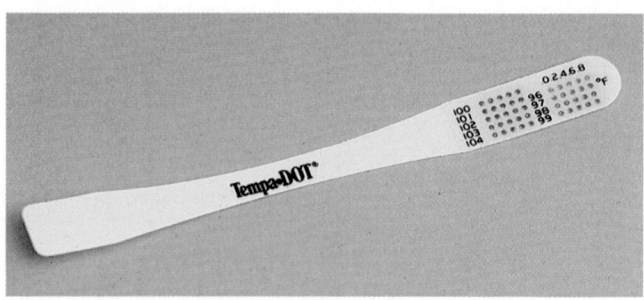

FIG 5.5 Chemical dot, disposable, single-use thermometer.

STEP	RATIONALE

ASSESSMENT

1. Identify patient using at least two identifiers (e.g., name and birthday or name and medical record number) according to agency policy.

Ensures patient safety. Complies with The Joint Commission standards and improves patient safety (TJC, 2016).

2. Determine need to measure patient's body temperature:

    a. Note patient's risks for temperature alterations:

- Expected or diagnosed infection
- Open wounds or burns
- White blood cell count below 5,000/mm³ or above 12,000/mm³
- Immunosuppressive drug therapy
- Injury to hypothalamus
- Exposure to temperature extremes
- Blood product infusion
- Hypothermia or hyperthermia therapy
- Postoperative status

Certain conditions place patients at risk for temperature alterations and require more frequent temperature measurement and nursing assessment.

    b. Assess for other signs and symptoms that accompany temperature alteration:

- *Hyperthermia:* Decreased skin turgor, dry mucous membranes; tachycardia; hypotension; decreased venous filling; concentrated urine
- *Heatstroke:* Body temperature of 40°C (104°F) or more (Goforth and Kazman, 2015); hot, dry skin; tachycardia; hypotension; excessive thirst; muscle cramps; visual disturbances; confusion or delirium
- *Hypothermia:* Pale skin; skin cool or cold to touch; bradycardia and dysrhythmias; uncontrollable shivering; reduced level of consciousness; shallow respirations

Physical signs and symptoms alert you to alterations in body temperature.

    c. Assess for factors that normally influence temperature:

Allows you to accurately assess for presence and significance of temperature alteration.

- Age

Older adults have narrower range of temperature than younger adults.

Clinical Decision Point *No single temperature is normal for all people. A temperature within an acceptable range in an adult may reflect a fever in an older adult. Undeveloped temperature-control mechanisms in infants and children cause temperature to rise and fall rapidly.*

- Exercise

Muscle activity increases metabolism, which increases heat production and raises temperature.

- Hormones

Women have wider temperature fluctuations than men because of menstrual cycle hormonal changes, because body temperature varies during menopause, and because women have thicker layer of subcutaneous fat.

- Stress

Stress elevates temperature.

- Environmental temperature

Infants and older adults are more sensitive to environmental temperature changes.

- Medications

Some drugs impair or promote sweating, vasoconstriction, or vasodilation or interfere with ability of hypothalamus to regulate temperature.

- Daily fluctuations

Body temperature normally changes 0.5° to 1°C (0.9° to 1.8°F) during 24-hour period. Temperature is lowest during early morning. Most patients have maximum temperature elevation between 5 PM and 7 PM; temperature falls gradually during night.

3. Determine appropriate measurement site and device for patient (see Box 5.3). Use disposable thermometer for patient on isolation precautions.

Determines if patient's status contraindicates selection of a specific method or site.

4. Determine previous baseline temperature and measurement site (if available) from patient's record.

Allows you to assess for change in condition. Provides comparison with future temperature measurements.

5. Assess patient's knowledge of procedure.

Encourages cooperation; minimizes risks and anxiety. Identifies teaching needs.

STEP	RATIONALE

NURSING DIAGNOSES

- Hyperthermia
- Hypothermia
- Ineffective thermoregulation
- Risk for hyperthermia
- Risk for imbalanced body temperature
- Risk for perioperative hypothermia

Related factors/Risk factors are individualized based on patient's condition or needs.

PLANNING

1. Expected outcomes following completion of procedure:
   - Body temperature is within acceptable range for patient's age-group.
   - Body temperature returns to baseline range following therapies for abnormal temperature.

   Thermoregulation is maintained.

   Environmental factors that alter temperature are controlled.

2. Explain to patient how you will measure temperature and importance of maintaining proper position until reading is complete.

   Promotes patient cooperation and increases compliance. Patients are often curious about their temperatures and should be cautioned against prematurely removing thermometer to read results.

3. Collect and bring appropriate supplies to patient's bedside.

   Ensures an organized approach for body temperature measurement

4. Verify that patient has not had anything to eat or drink and has not chewed gum or smoked within the past 20 minutes (if having oral temperature measured).

   Oral food and fluids, smoking, and gum can alter oral temperature measurement.

IMPLEMENTATION

1. Perform hand hygiene.

   Reduces transmission of microorganisms.

2. Help patient to comfortable position that provides easy access to temperature measurement site.

   Ensures patient's comfort and accuracy of temperature reading.

3. Obtain temperature reading.
   a. **Oral temperature (electronic):**
      (1) *Optional:* Apply clean gloves when there is risk for exposure to respiratory secretions or facial or mouth wound drainage.

      An oral probe cover is removable without physical contact; thus does not require gloves.

      (2) Remove thermometer pack from charging unit. Attach oral thermometer probe stem (blue tip) to thermometer unit. Grasp top of probe stem, being careful not to apply pressure on ejection button.

      Charging provides battery power. Ejection button releases plastic cover from probe stem.

      (3) Slide disposable plastic probe cover over thermometer probe stem until cover locks in place (see illustration).

      Soft plastic cover will not break in patient's mouth and prevents transmission of microorganisms between patients.

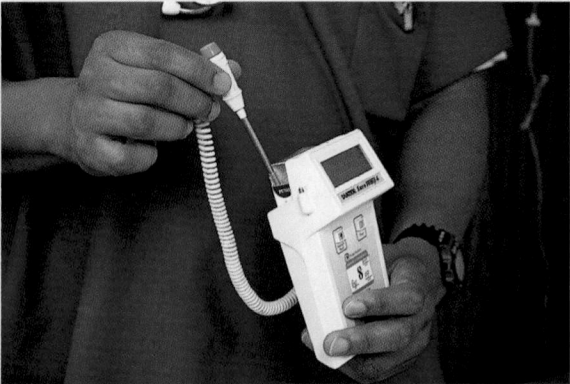

STEP 3a(3) Nurse inserts electronic thermometer probe stem into probe cover. Cover snaps in place.

   (4) Ask patient to open mouth; gently place thermometer probe under tongue in posterior sublingual pocket lateral to center of lower jaw (see illustration).

   Heat from superficial blood vessels in sublingual pocket produces temperature reading. With electronic thermometer, temperatures in right and left posterior sublingual pocket are significantly higher than in area under front of tongue.

STEP	RATIONALE

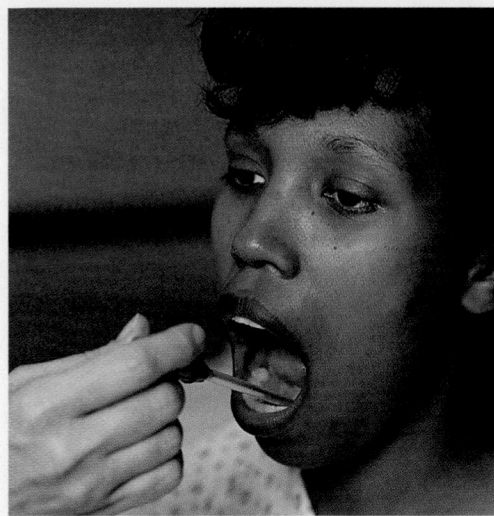

STEP 3a(4) Probe placed under tongue in posterior sublingual pocket.

(5) Ask patient to hold thermometer probe with lips closed.

Maintains proper position of thermometer during recording.

(6) Leave thermometer probe in place until audible signal indicates completion and patient's temperature appears on digital display; remove thermometer probe from under patient's tongue.

Probe must stay in place until signal occurs to ensure accurate reading.

(7) Push ejection button on thermometer probe stem to discard plastic probe cover into appropriate receptacle.

Reduces transmission of microorganisms.

(8) If wearing gloves, remove, dispose in appropriate receptacle, and perform hand hygiene.

Reduces transmission of microorganisms.

(9) Return thermometer probe stem to storage position of thermometer unit.

Protects probe stem from damage. Returning thermometer probe stem automatically causes digital reading to disappear.

b. Rectal temperature (electronic):

(1) Draw curtain around bed and/or close room door. Help patient to side-lying or Sims' position with upper leg flexed. Move aside bed linen to expose only anal area. Keep patient's upper body and lower extremities covered with sheet or blanket.

Maintains patient's privacy, minimizes embarrassment, and promotes comfort.

(2) Apply clean gloves. Cleanse anal region when feces and/or secretions are present. Remove soiled gloves and reapply clean gloves.

Maintains standard precautions when exposed to items soiled with body fluids (e.g., feces).

(3) Remove thermometer pack from charging unit. Attach rectal thermometer probe stem (red tip) to thermometer unit. Grasp top of probe stem, being careful not to apply pressure on ejection button.

Ejection button releases plastic cover from probe stem.

(4) Slide disposable plastic probe cover over thermometer probe stem until cover locks in place.

Soft plastic probe cover prevents transmission of microorganisms between patients.

(5) Using a single-use package, squeeze a liberal amount of lubricant on tissue. Dip probe cover of thermometer, blunt end, into lubricant, covering 2.5 to 3.5 cm (1 to 1½ inches) for adult.

Lubrication minimizes trauma to rectal mucosa during insertion. Tissue avoids contamination of remaining lubricant in container.

(6) With nondominant hand separate patient's buttocks to expose anus. Ask patient to breathe slowly and relax.

Fully exposes anus for thermometer insertion. Relaxes anal sphincter for easier thermometer insertion.

(7) Gently insert thermometer into anus in direction of umbilicus 3.5 cm (1½ inches) for adult. Do not force thermometer.

Ensures adequate exposure against blood vessels in rectal wall.

STEP	RATIONALE

(8) If you feel resistance during insertion, withdraw immediately. Never force thermometer.

Prevents trauma to mucosa.

Clinical Decision Point *If you cannot adequately insert thermometer into rectum or resistance is felt during insertion, remove thermometer and consider alternative method for obtaining temperature.*

(9) Once positioned, hold thermometer probe in place until audible signal indicates completion and patient's temperature appears on digital display; remove thermometer probe from anus (see illustration).

Probe must stay in place until signal occurs to ensure accurate reading.

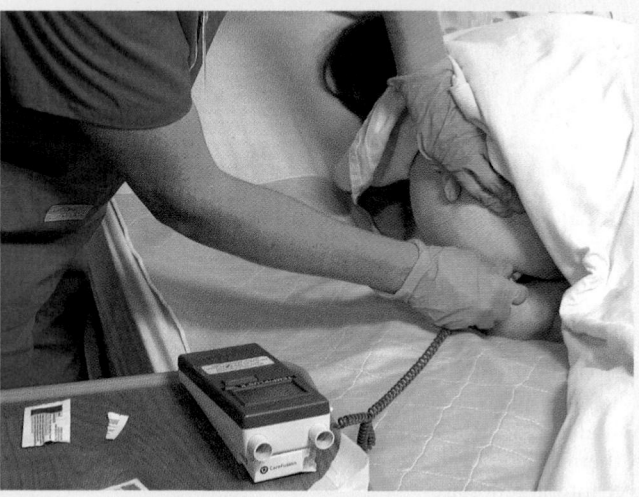

STEP 3b(9) Probe inserted into anus.

(10) Push ejection button on thermometer stem to discard plastic probe cover into appropriate receptacle. Wipe probe stem with alcohol swab, paying particular attention to ridges where probe stem connects to probe.

Reduces transmission of microorganisms.

(11) Return thermometer stem to storage position of recording unit.

Protects probe stem from damage. Returning thermometer stem automatically causes digital reading to disappear.

(12) Wipe patient's anal area with soft tissue to remove lubricant or feces and discard tissue. Help patient to assume a comfortable position.

Provides for comfort and hygiene.

(13) Remove and dispose of gloves in appropriate receptacle. Perform hand hygiene.

Reduces transmission of microorganisms.

c. Axillary temperature (electronic):

(1) Draw curtain around bed and/or close room door. Help patient to supine or sitting position. Move clothing or gown away from shoulder and arm.

Maintains patient's privacy, minimizes embarrassment, and promotes comfort. Exposes axilla for correct thermometer probe placement.

(2) Remove thermometer pack from charging unit. Attach oral thermometer probe stem (blue tip) to thermometer unit. Grasp top of thermometer probe stem, being careful not to apply pressure on ejection button.

Charging provides battery power. Ejection button releases plastic cover from probe stem.

(3) Slide disposable plastic probe cover over thermometer stem until cover locks in place.

Soft plastic probe cover prevents transmission of microorganisms between patients.

(4) Raise patient's arm away from torso. Inspect for skin lesions and excessive perspiration; if needed, dry axilla or select alternative site. Insert thermometer probe into center of axilla (see illustration), lower arm over probe and place arm across patient's chest.

Maintains proper position of thermometer against blood vessels in axilla.

STEP	RATIONALE

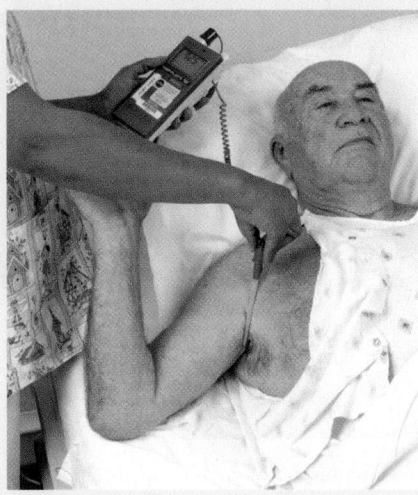

STEP 3c(4) Insert thermometer probe into center of axilla.

Clinical Decision Point *Do not use axilla if skin lesions are present because local temperature is sometimes altered and area may be painful to touch.*

STEP	RATIONALE
(5) Once thermometer probe is positioned, hold it in place until audible signal indicates completion and patient's temperature appears on digital display; remove thermometer probe from axilla.	Thermometer probe must stay in place until signal occurs to ensure accurate reading.
(6) Push ejection button on thermometer stem to discard plastic probe cover into appropriate receptacle.	Reduces transmission of microorganisms.
(7) Return thermometer stem to storage position of recording unit.	Returning thermometer stem to storage position automatically causes digital reading to disappear. Protects stem from damage.
(8) Help patient to assume comfortable position, replacing linen or gown.	Restores comfort and sense of well-being.
(9) Perform hand hygiene.	Reduces transmission of microorganisms.
d. Tympanic membrane temperature:	
(1) Help patient to assume comfortable position with head turned toward side, away from you. If patient has been lying on one side, use upper ear. Obtain temperature from patient's right ear if you are right-handed. Obtain temperature from patient's left ear if you are left-handed.	Ensures comfort and facilitates exposure of auditory canal for accurate temperature measurement. Heat trapped in ear facing down causes false-high temperature reading. The less acute the angle of approach, the better the probe seal.
(2) Note if there is an obvious presence of cerumen (earwax) in patient's ear canal.	Cerumen impedes lens cover of speculum. Switch to other ear or select alternative measurement site.
(3) Remove thermometer handheld unit from charging base, being careful not to apply pressure to ejection button.	Charging base provides battery power. Removal of handheld unit from base prepares it to measure temperature. Ejection button releases plastic probe cover from thermometer tip.
(4) Slide disposable speculum cover over otoscope-like lens tip until it locks in place. Be careful not to touch lens cover.	Soft plastic probe cover prevents transmission of microorganisms between patients. Lens cover should not have dust, fingerprints, or cerumen obstructing optical pathway.
(5) Insert speculum into ear canal following manufacturer instructions for tympanic probe positioning (see illustration):	Correct positioning of probe with respect to ear canal allows maximal exposure of tympanic membrane.
(a) Pull ear pinna backward, up, and out for an adult. For children less than 3 years of age, pull pinna down and back; point covered probe toward midpoint between eyebrow and sideburns. For children older than 3 years, pull pinna up and back (Hockenberry and Wilson, 2015).	Ear tug straightens external auditory canal, allowing maximum exposure of tympanic membrane and therefore correctly positioning speculum (Hockenberry and Wilson, 2015).

STEP	RATIONALE

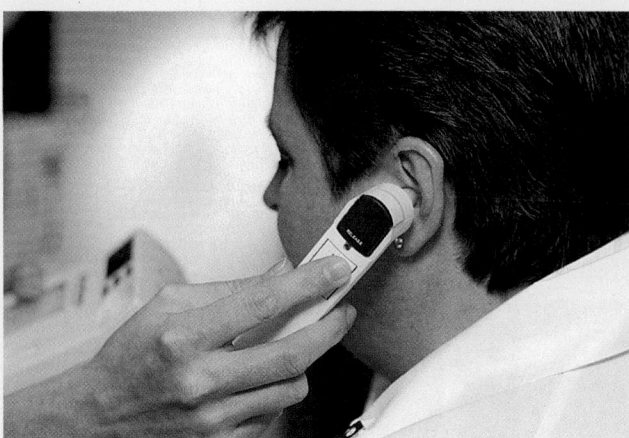

STEP 3d(5) Tympanic membrane thermometer with probe cover placed in patient's ear.

(b) Move thermometer in figure-eight pattern.	Some manufacturers recommend movement of speculum tip in figure-eight pattern that allows sensor to detect maximum tympanic membrane heat radiation.
(c) Fit speculum tip snug in canal, pointing toward nose.	Gentle pressure seals ear canal from ambient air temperature, which alters readings as much as 2.8°C (5°F).
(6) Once positioned, press scan button on handheld unit. Leave speculum in place until audible signal indicates completion and patient's temperature appears on digital display.	Pressing scan button causes detection of infrared energy. Speculum probe tip must stay in place until device has detected infrared energy noted by audible signal.
(7) Carefully remove speculum from auditory meatus. Push ejection button on handheld unit to discard speculum cover into appropriate receptacle.	Reduces transmission of microorganisms. Automatically causes digital reading to disappear.
(8) If temperature is abnormal or second reading is necessary, replace probe cover and wait 2 minutes before repeating in same ear or repeat measurement in other ear. Consider an alternative temperature site or instrument.	Lens cover must be free of cerumen to maintain optical path. Time allows ear canal to regain usual temperature.
(9) Return handheld unit to thermometer base.	Protects sensor tip from damage.
(10) Help patient assume comfortable position.	Restores comfort and sense of well-being.
(11) Perform hand hygiene.	Reduces transmission of microorganisms.
e. Temporal artery temperature:	
(1) Ensure that forehead is dry; dry with towel if needed.	Moisture interferes with thermometer sensor.
(2) Place sensor firmly on patient's forehead.	Flush contact avoids measurement of ambient temperature.
(3) Press red scan button with your thumb. Slowly slide thermometer straight across forehead while keeping sensor flat and firmly on skin (see Fig. 5.4). Keeping scan button depressed, lift sensor after sweeping forehead and touch sensor on neck just behind earlobe. Read temperature when clicking sound during scanning stops. Release scan button.	Thermometer continuously scans for highest temperature when scan button is depressed. Area behind earlobe is less affected by diaphoresis and verifies temperature.
(4) Gently clean sensor with alcohol swab, return to storage unit, and perform hand hygiene.	Prevents transmission of microorganisms.
4. Inform patient of temperature reading and record measurement.	Promotes participation in care and understanding of health status.
5. Return thermometer to charger.	Maintains battery charge of thermometer unit.

STEP	RATIONALE

EVALUATION

1. If you are assessing temperature for the first time, establish it as baseline if it is within acceptable range.

2. Compare temperature reading with patient's previous baseline and acceptable temperature range for patient's age-group.

3. If patient has fever, take temperature approximately 30 minutes after administering antipyretics and every 4 hours until temperature stabilizes.

4. **Use Teach-Back**: "I want to be sure I explained how to check your child's temperature at home. Show me how to swipe his forehead using the thermometer." Revise your instruction now or develop a plan for revised patient or family caregiver teaching if patient or family caregiver is not able to teach back correctly.

Used to compare future temperature measurements.

Body temperature fluctuates within narrow range; comparison reveals presence of abnormality. Improper placement or movement of thermometer can cause inaccuracies. Second measurement confirms initial findings of abnormal body temperature.

Determines if temperature begins to fall in response to therapy.

Determines patient's and family caregiver's level of understanding of instructional topic.

Unexpected Outcomes	Related Interventions
1. Patient has temperature 1°C (1.8°F) or more above usual range.	• Initiate measures to lower body temperature: • Cool room environment. • Reduce external covering on patient's body to promote heat loss but do not induce shivering. • Keep clothing and bed linen dry. • Apply hypothermia blanket as ordered. • Limit physical activity and sources of emotional stress. • Administer antipyretics as ordered. • Increase fluid intake to at least 3 L daily (unless contraindicated). • Initiate measures to stimulate appetite and provide nutrients to meet increased energy needs. • Prevent or control spread of infection. • Provide wound care (see Chapter 40). • Perform pulmonary hygiene (see Chapter 24). • Promote adequate urinary elimination (see Chapter 34).
2. Patient has temperature 1°C (1.8°F) or more below usual range.	• Initiate measures to raise body temperature: • Apply warm blankets and, unless contraindicated, offer warm liquids. • Apply hyperthermia blankets if ordered • Remove wet clothing or linen.
3. Unable to obtain temperature.	• Reassess correct placement of temperature probe or sensor. • Choose alternative temperature measurement site. • Obtain alternative temperature measurement device.

Recording and Reporting

- Record temperature and route on vital sign flow sheet or in nurses' notes in electronic health record (EHR) or chart.
- Report abnormal findings to nurse in charge or health care provider.
- Document your evaluation of patient and family caregiver learning.

Special Considerations
Teaching

- Identify patient's ability to initiate preventive health measures and recognize alteration in body temperature. Educate patient and family caregiver about measures to prevent body temperature alterations.

- Educate patients about risk factors for hypothermia and frostbite: fatigue; malnutrition; hypoxemia; cold, wet clothing; alcohol intoxication.
- Educate patients about risk factors for heatstroke: strenuous exercise in hot, humid weather; tight-fitting clothing in hot environments; exercising in poorly ventilated areas; sudden exposures to hot climates; poor fluid intake before, during, and after exercise.
- Educate patients regarding importance of taking and continuing antibiotics as directed until course of treatment for infection is completed.

Pediatric

- Infants and young children may lose more heat to the environment because of their increased body surface area/volume ratios.

- Critically ill children sometimes have cool skin but a high core temperature because of poor perfusion to the skin.
- Use axillary temperatures for screening purposes only; axillary temperature cannot be relied on to detect a fever.
- Children may assume prone position for rectal temperature measurement.
- With children who cry or become restless, it is best to take temperature as the last vital sign.

Gerontological

- The temperature of older adults is at the lower end of the acceptable temperature range: 36°C (96.8°F).
- Temperatures considered within normal range often reflect a fever in an older adult.
- Adults without teeth or older adults with poor muscle control may be unable to close their mouth tightly enough to obtain accurate oral temperature readings.
- Older adults are very sensitive to environmental temperature changes because their thermoregulatory systems are not as efficient.
- Oral temperature measurement is more reliable in older adults because cerumen tends to be drier and cilia become stiff,

contributing to buildup of cerumen impaction, which interferes with accurate tympanic temperature measurement.

- A decrease in sweat gland reactivity in the older adult results in a higher threshold for sweating at high temperatures, which can lead to hyperthermia.
- With aging a loss of subcutaneous fat reduces the insulating capacity of the skin.
- Older adults are at high risk for hypothermia because of diminished sensation to cold, abnormal vasoconstrictor responses, and impaired shivering.

Home Care

- Assess temperature and ventilation of patient's environment to determine existence of any environmental conditions that influence patient's temperature.
- In the home some patients continue to use mercury-in-glass thermometers. Assess safe storage of these thermometers to protect from breakage and mercury spills. Educate patient and family caregiver on proper use of the thermometer, mercury hazards, and proper disposal of any mercury-containing devices. Suggest alternative temperature measurement devices for home use.

◆ SKILL 5.2   Assessing Radial Pulse

NSO *Nursing Skills Online Vital Signs Module / Lesson 3* 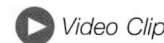 *Video Clip*

The ejection of blood from the heart distends the walls of the aorta. Because of the force of the blood exiting the heart, aortic distention creates a pulse wave that travels rapidly toward the extremities. When the pulse wave reaches a peripheral artery, you can feel it by palpating the artery lightly against underlying bone or muscle. The pulse is the palpable bounding of the blood flow. The number of pulsing sensations occurring in 1 minute is the pulse rate.

Assessing a patient's peripheral pulses determines the integrity of the cardiovascular system. An abnormally slow, rapid, or

irregular pulse indicates the inability of the heart to deliver adequate blood to the body; a pulse deficit may be present. The strength or amplitude of a pulse reflects the volume of blood ejected against the arterial wall with each heart contraction. If the volume decreases, the pulse often becomes weak and difficult to palpate. In contrast, a full bounding pulse is an indication of increased volume.

The integrity of peripheral pulses indicates the status of blood perfusion to the area distributed by the pulse (Table 5.1). For

---

TABLE 5.1

Pulse Sites

Site	Location	Rationale for Selection
Temporal	Over temporal bone of head, above and lateral to eyebrow	Easily accessible site to assess pulse in children
Carotid	Along medial edge of sternocleidomastoid muscle in neck	Easily accessible site to assess character of peripheral pulse; used during physiological shock or cardiac arrest when other sites are not palpable
Apical	Fourth to fifth intercostal space at left midclavicular line	Site used to auscultate apical pulse
Brachial	Groove between biceps and triceps muscles at antecubital fossa	Site used to auscultate upper-extremity blood pressure; assesses status of circulation to lower arm
Radial	Radial or thumb side of forearm at wrist	Common site to assess character of peripheral pulse; assesses status of circulation to hand
Ulnar	Ulnar side of forearm at wrist	Site used to assess status of circulation to ulnar side of hand; used to perform Allen's test
Femoral	Below inguinal ligament, midway between symphysis pubis and anterior superior iliac spine	Site used to assess character of pulse during physiological shock or cardiac arrest when other pulses are not palpable; assesses status of circulation to leg
Popliteal	Behind knee in popliteal fossa	Site used to auscultate lower-extremity blood pressure; assesses status of circulation to lower leg
Posterior tibial	Inner side of each ankle, below medial malleolus	Site used to assess status of circulation to foot
Dorsalis pedis	Along top of foot between extension tendons of great and first toe	Site used to assess status of circulation to foot

example, assessment of the right femoral pulse determines whether blood flow to the right leg is adequate. If a peripheral pulse distal to an injured or treated area of an extremity feels weak on palpation, the volume of blood reaching tissues below the affected area may be inadequate, and surgical intervention may be necessary.

You can assess any artery for pulse rate, but the radial and carotid arteries are commonly used because they are easy to palpate (Fig. 5.6). When a patient's condition suddenly worsens, the carotid site is recommended for finding a pulse quickly. Assessment of other peripheral pulse sites such as the brachial or femoral artery is unnecessary when routinely obtaining vital signs. Other peripheral pulses are assessed when a complete physical (see Chapter 6) is conducted or when the radial artery is not available for assessment because of surgery, trauma, or impaired blood flow.

Delegation and Collaboration

The skill of radial pulse measurement can be delegated to nursing assistive personnel (NAP) if a patient's condition is stable. The skill cannot be delegated when a patient's condition is unstable because the patient is at high risk for acute or serious cardiac problems or when the nurse is evaluating a patient's response to a treatment or medication. The nurse instructs the NAP by:

- Indicating the appropriate site for measuring pulse rate; frequency of measurement; and factors related to the patient history such as risk for abnormally slow, rapid, or irregular pulse.

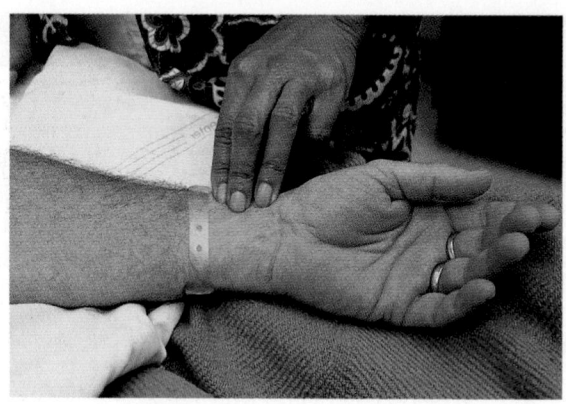

FIG 5.6 Palpating radial pulse.

- Reviewing patient's usual pulse rate and significant changes to report to the nurse.
- Reviewing the specific changes or abnormalities to report to the nurse for further assessment.

Equipment

- Wristwatch with second hand or digital display
- Pen and vital sign flow sheet in chart or electronic health record (EHR)

STEP	RATIONALE

ASSESSMENT

1. Identify patient using at least two identifiers (e.g., name and birthday or name and medical record number) according to agency policy.

Ensures patient safety. Complies with The Joint Commission standards and improves patient safety (TJC, 2016).

2. Determine need to assess radial pulse:

  a. Assess for any risk factors for pulse alterations:

    - History of heart disease
    - Cardiac dysrhythmia
    - Onset of sudden chest pain or acute pain from any site
    - Invasive cardiovascular diagnostic tests
    - Surgery
    - Sudden infusion of large volume of intravenous (IV) fluid
    - Internal or external hemorrhage
    - Administration of medications that alter cardiac function

Certain conditions place patients at risk for pulse alterations. A history of peripheral vascular disease often alters pulse rate and quality.

  b. Assess for signs and symptoms of altered cardiac function such as presence of dyspnea, fatigue, chest pain, orthopnea, syncope, palpitations, edema of dependent body parts, cyanosis, or pallor of skin (see Chapter 6).

Physical signs and symptoms often indicate alteration in cardiac function, which affects radial pulse rate and rhythm.

  c. Assess for signs and symptoms of peripheral vascular disease such as pale, cool extremities; thin, shiny skin with decreased hair growth; thickened nails.

Physical signs and symptoms indicate alteration in local arterial blood flow.

  d. Assess for factors that influence radial pulse rate and rhythm: age, exercise, position changes, fluid balance, medications, temperature, sympathetic stimulation (e.g., caffeine or nicotine).

Can anticipate factors that alter pulse, ensuring accurate interpretation.

Dysrhythmics, cardiotonics, antihypertensives, vasodilators, and vasoconstrictors affect pulse rate and rhythm.

3. Determine patient's previous baseline pulse rate (if available) from patient's record.

Allows you to assess for change in condition. Provides comparison with future pulse measurements.

4. If you anticipate need for patient or family caregiver to monitor heart rate at home, assess their knowledge of the procedure and rationale for measurement.

Determines need for patient or family caregiver instruction.

STEP	RATIONALE

NURSING DIAGNOSES

- Activity intolerance
- Decreased cardiac output
- Deficient fluid volume

- Deficient knowledge regarding pulse assessment

- Ineffective peripheral tissue perfusion

Related factors are individualized based on patient's condition and needs.

PLANNING

1. Expected outcomes following completion of procedure:
   - Radial pulse is palpable, within usual range for patient's age.
   - Rhythm is regular.
   - Radial pulse is strong, firm, and elastic.
2. Explain to patient that you will assess radial pulse rate (heart rate [HR]). Encourage patient to relax as much as possible. If patient has been active, wait 5 to 10 minutes before assessing pulse. If patient has been smoking or ingesting caffeine, wait 15 minutes before assessing pulse.
3. Collect appropriate equipment and bring to patient's bedside

Usual range for adults is 60 to 100 beats/min.

Cardiac status is stable.
Radial artery is patent.
Anxiety, activity, caffeine, and smoking elevate heart rate. Assessing radial pulse rate at rest allows for objective comparison of values.

Ensures an organized approach for assessing a radial pulse.

IMPLEMENTATION

1. Perform hand hygiene.
2. If necessary, draw curtain around bed and/or close door.

3. Help patient to assume a supine or sitting position.
4. If patient is supine, place his or her forearm straight alongside or across lower chest or upper abdomen (see illustration A). If sitting, bend patient's elbow 90 degrees and support lower arm on chair or on your arm. Place tips of first two or middle three fingers of hand over groove along radial or thumb side of patient's inner wrist (see illustration B). Slightly extend or flex wrist with palm down until you note strongest pulse.

Reduces transmission of microorganisms.
Maintains privacy and minimizes embarrassment. Helps patient relax.
Provides easy access to pulse sites.
Fingertips are most sensitive parts of hand to palpate arterial pulsation. Your thumb has pulsation that interferes with accuracy.

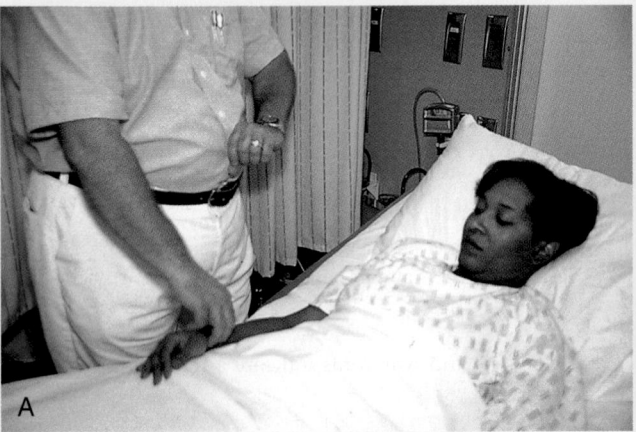 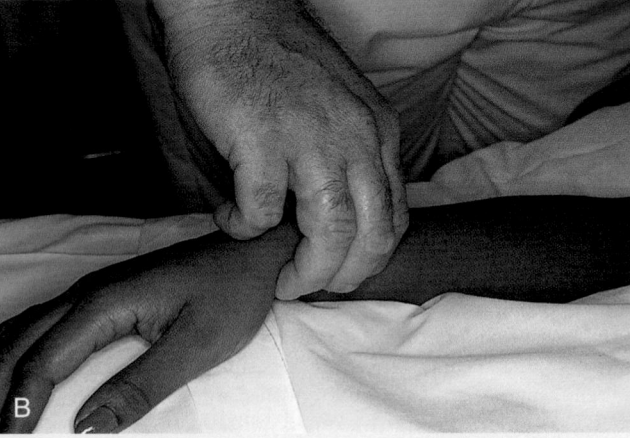

STEP 4 A, Pulse check with patient's forearm at side with wrist extended. **B,** Hand placement for pulse check.

5. Lightly compress pulse against radius, losing pulse initially; relax pressure so pulse becomes easily palpable.
6. Determine strength of pulse. Note whether thrust of vessel against fingertips is bounding (4+); full increased, strong (3+); expected (2+); barely palpable, diminished (1+); or absent, not palpable (0).

Pulse assessment is more accurate when using moderate pressure. Too much pressure occludes pulse and impairs blood flow.
Strength reflects volume of blood ejected against arterial wall with each heart contraction. Accurate description of strength improves communication among nurses and other health care providers.

STEP	RATIONALE

7. After palpating a regular pulse, look at watch second hand and begin to count rate. Count the first beat after the second hand hits the number on the dial; count as one, then two, and so on.

Rate is determined accurately only after pulse has been palpated. Timing begins with zero. Count of one is first beat palpated after timing begins.

8. If pulse is regular, count rate for 30 seconds and multiply total by 2.

A 30-second count is accurate for rapid, slow, or regular pulse rates.

9. If pulse is irregular, count rate for a full 60 seconds. Assess frequency and pattern of irregularity.

Inefficient contraction of heart fails to transmit pulse wave, resulting in irregular pulse. Longer time ensures accurate count.

10. When pulse is irregular, compare radial pulses bilaterally.

A marked difference between pulses indicates that arterial flow is compromised to one extremity and as a nurse you need to take action.

11. Help patient return to comfortable position.

Promotes comfort and sense of well-being.

12. Discuss findings with patient.

Promotes participation in care and understanding of health status.

13. Perform hand hygiene.

Reduces transmission of microorganisms.

EVALUATION

1. If assessing pulse for first time, establish radial pulse as baseline if it is within acceptable range.

Used to compare future pulse assessments.

2. Compare pulse rate and character with patient's previous baseline and acceptable range for patient's age.

Allows for assessment of change in patient's condition and presence of cardiac alteration.

3. **Use Teach-Back:** "I want to be sure I explained why it is important to check your pulse at home. Tell me why it is important to check your pulse when you have a pacemaker." Revise your instruction now or develop a plan for revised patient or family caregiver teaching if patient or family caregiver is not able to teach back correctly.

Determines patient's and family caregiver's level of understanding of instructional topic.

Unexpected Outcomes

1. Patient has weak, thready, or difficult-to-palpate radial pulse.

Related Interventions

- Assess both radial pulses and compare findings.
- Observe for symptoms associated with ineffective tissue perfusion, including pallor and cool skin distal to weak pulse.
- Assess for swelling in surrounding tissues or any encumbrance (e.g., dressing or cast) that may impede blood flow.
- Obtain Doppler or ultrasound stethoscope to detect low-velocity blood flow (see Chapter 6).
- Have another nurse assess pulse.

2. An adult patient's pulse rate is less than 60 beats/min (bradycardia) or more than 100 beats/min (tachycardia).

- Identify related data, including fever, pain, fear or anxiety, recent exercise, low blood pressure, blood loss, or inadequate oxygenation.
- Observe for signs and symptoms associated with abnormal cardiac function, including dyspnea, fatigue, chest pain, orthopnea, syncope, palpitations, edema of body parts, cyanosis, or pallor of skin.
- Auscultate apical pulse (see Skill 5.3).
- Confer with health care provider and be prepared to order/obtain electrocardiogram.

3. Patient has irregular pulse.

- Auscultate apical pulse (see Skill 5.3).
- Assess for pulse deficit: (a) nurse auscultates apical pulse while second provider palpates radial pulse; (b) nurse begins 60-second pulse count by calling out loud when to begin counting pulses; (c) the two pulse rates are compared. If pulse count differs by more than 2, a deficit exists; assess for other signs and symptoms of decreased cardiac output (see Chapter 6).

Recording and Reporting

- Record pulse rate and assessment site on vital sign flow sheet or in nurses' notes in electronic health record (EHR) or chart.
- Document measurement of pulse rate after administration of specific therapies in nurses' notes in EHR or chart.
- Document your evaluation of patient and family caregiver learning.
- Report abnormal findings to nurse in charge or health care provider.

Special Considerations
Teaching

- Patients taking certain prescribed cardiotonic or antidysrhythmic medications need to learn to assess their own pulse rates to detect side effects of medications.
- Patients undergoing cardiac rehabilitation need to learn to assess their own pulse rates to determine their response to exercise.
- Teach patients taking heart medications or starting a prescribed exercise regimen how to monitor carotid pulse rate.

Pediatric

- Radial artery is difficult to assess in an infant. Apical, femoral, or brachial pulse is best site for assessing pediatric heart rate and rhythm until 2 years of age.
- Children often have a sinus dysrhythmia, which is an irregular heartbeat that speeds up with inspiration and slows down with expiration.
- Breath holding in a child temporarily lowers pulse rate.

Gerontological

- Older adults have a reduced heart rate with exercise because of a decreased responsiveness to catecholamines.
- It takes longer for the heart rate to rise in the older adult to meet sudden increased demands that result from stress, illness, or excitement. Once elevated, the pulse rate of an older adult takes longer to return to normal resting rate.
- Peripheral vascular disease is more common among older adults, making radial pulse assessment difficult.

Home Care

- Patients taking certain prescribed cardiac medications should learn to assess their own pulse rates to detect side effects of medications.

◆ SKILL 5.3   Assessing Apical Pulse

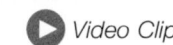 **NSO** *Nursing Skills Online Vital Signs Module / Lesson 3* ▶ *Video Clip*

The apical pulse is the most reliable noninvasive way to assess cardiac function. The apical pulse rate is the assessment of the number and quality of apical heart sounds in 1 minute. A single apical pulse is the combination of two heart sounds, S_1 and S_2. S_1 is the sound of the tricuspid and mitral valves closing at the end of ventricular filling, just before systolic contraction begins. S_2 is the sound of the pulmonic and aortic valves closing at the end of the systolic contraction. As you listen for sound waves with a stethoscope, you will hear the characteristic "lub-dub" as a single pulsation.

A stethoscope (Fig. 5.7) is a closed cylinder that amplifies sound waves as they reach the surface of the body. The five major parts of the stethoscope are the earpieces, binaurals, tubing, bell, and diaphragm. The plastic or rubber earpieces should fit snugly and comfortably in your ears. Binaurals should be angled and strong enough so the earpieces stay firmly in place without causing discomfort. The earpieces follow the contour of the ear canal, pointing toward the face when the stethoscope is in place.

The polyvinyl tubing should be flexible and 30 to 45 cm (12 to 18 inches) in length; longer tubing decreases sound transmission. Stethoscopes can have one or two tubes. At the end of the tubing is the chest piece, consisting of a bell and diaphragm that you rotate into position, depending on which part you choose to use.

The diaphragm is the larger, circular, flat-surfaced part of the chest piece. It transmits high-pitched sounds created by high-velocity movement of air and blood. Position the diaphragm to make a tight seal against a patient's skin. Exert enough pressure to complete the seal, leaving a temporary red ring on the patient's skin after you remove the diaphragm.

The bell is the cone-shaped part of the chest piece, usually surrounded by a rubber ring to avoid chilling the patient during placement. It transmits low-pitched sounds created by the low-velocity movement of blood. Hold the bell lightly against the skin for sound amplification.

Some stethoscopes have one chest piece that combines features of the bell and diaphragm. When you apply light pressure, the chest piece is a bell, whereas exerting more pressure converts the bell into a diaphragm. With the earpieces in your ears tap lightly on the diaphragm and note which side you hear most clearly. This determines which side of the chest piece is functioning.

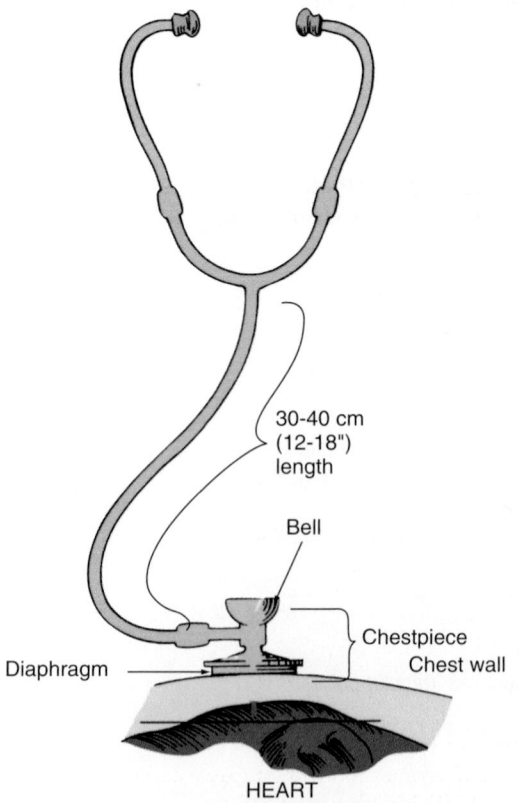

FIG 5.7 Acoustic stethoscope.

Delegation and Collaboration

The skill of apical pulse measurement cannot be delegated to nursing assistive personnel (NAP). Often you measure the apical pulse when you suspect an irregularity in the radial pulse or when a patient's condition requires a more accurate assessment.

Equipment

- Stethoscope
- Wristwatch with second hand or digital display
- Pen and vital sign flow sheet in chart or electronic health record (EHR)
- Alcohol swab

STEP	RATIONALE

ASSESSMENT

1. Identify patient using at least two identifiers (e.g., name and birthday or name and medical record number) according to agency policy.

Ensures patient safety. Complies with The Joint Commission standards and improves patient safety (TJC, 2016).

2. Determine need to assess apical pulse:

   a. Assess for any risk factors for apical pulse alteration: heart disease, onset of sudden chest pain or acute pain from any site, invasive cardiovascular diagnostic tests, surgery, sudden infusion of large volume of intravenous (IV) fluid, internal or external hemorrhage, administration of medications that alter heart function.

Certain conditions place patients at risk for pulse alterations.

   b. Assess for signs and symptoms of altered cardiac function such as dyspnea, fatigue, chest pain, orthopnea, syncope, palpitations, edema of dependent body parts, cyanosis, or pallor of skin (see Chapter 6).

Physical signs and symptoms indicate alteration in cardiac output or stroke volume.

   c. Assess for factors that normally influence apical pulse rate and rhythm:

Allows you to anticipate factors that alter apical pulse, ensuring an accurate interpretation.

    • Age

Infant's heart rate (HR) at birth ranges from 100 to 160 beats/min at rest; by age 2 pulse rate slows to 70 to 120 beats/min; by adolescence rate varies between 60 and 90 beats/min and remains so throughout adulthood (Hockenberry and Wilson, 2015).

    • Exercise

Physical activity increases HR; a well-conditioned patient may have a slower-than-usual resting HR that returns more quickly to resting rate after exercise.

    • Position changes

HR increases temporarily when changing from lying to sitting or standing position.

    • Medications

Antidysrhythmics, sympathomimetics, and cardiotonics affect rate and rhythm of pulse; large doses of narcotic analgesics can slow HR; general anesthetics slow HR; central nervous system stimulants such as caffeine can increase HR.

    • Temperature

Fever or exposure to warm environments increases HR; HR declines with hypothermia.

    • Sympathetic stimulation

Emotional stress, anxiety, or fear stimulates sympathetic nervous system, which increases HR.

2. Determine previous baseline apical rate (if available) from patient's record.

Allows nurse to assess for change in condition.

3. Determine any report of latex allergy. If patient has latex allergy, ensure that stethoscope is latex free.

Reduces risk of allergic reaction to stethoscope.

4. Determine if patient takes apical heart rate at home. Assess patient's knowledge and skill level.

Determine level and type of instruction required by patient or family caregiver.

NURSING DIAGNOSES

- Activity intolerance
- Decreased cardiac output
- Deficient knowledge regarding heart rate monitoring
- Ineffective peripheral tissue perfusion
- Risk for latex allergy response

Related factors/Risk factors are individualized based on patient's condition or needs.

PLANNING

1. Expected outcomes following completion of procedure:
   - Apical HR is within acceptable range.
   - Rhythm is regular.

Adults average 60 to 100 beats/min.
Cardiovascular status is stable.

STEP	RATIONALE
2. Explain to patient that you will assess apical pulse rate. Encourage patient to relax and not speak. If patient has been active, wait 5 to 10 minutes before assessing pulse. If he or she has been smoking or ingesting caffeine, wait 15 minutes before assessing pulse.	Anxiety, activity, caffeine, and smoking elevate HR. Patient's voice interferes with nurse's ability to hear sound when measuring apical pulse. Assessing apical pulse rate at rest allows for objective comparison of values.
3. Collect and bring appropriate supplies to patient's bedside.	Ensures an organized approach for assessing radial pulse.

IMPLEMENTATION

1. Perform hand hygiene.	Reduces transmission of microorganisms.
2. If necessary, draw curtain around bed and/or close door.	Maintains privacy and minimizes embarrassment. Helps patient relax.
3. Help patient to supine or sitting position. Move aside bed linen and gown to expose sternum and left side of chest.	Exposes part of chest wall for selection of auscultatory site. Stethoscope diaphragm must touch skin for best sounds.
4. Locate anatomical landmarks to identify point of maximal impulse (PMI), also called apical *impulse* (see Chapter 6). The heart is located behind and to left of sternum with base at top and apex at bottom. Find angle of Louis just below suprasternal notch between sternal body and manubrium; it feels like a bony prominence (see illustration A). Slip fingers down each side of angle to find second intercostal space (ICS) (see illustration B). Carefully move fingers down left side of sternum to fifth ICS and laterally to left midclavicular line (MCL) (see illustration C). A light tap felt within area 1 to 2.5 cm (½ to 1 inch) of PMI is reflected from apex of heart (see illustration D).	Use of anatomical landmarks allows correct placement of stethoscope over apex of heart. This position enhances ability to hear heart sounds clearly. If unable to palpate PMI, reposition patient on left side. In presence of serious heart disease, you may locate PMI to left of MCL or at sixth ICS. PMI may not be palpated in obese adults or patients with severe pulmonary disease that has changed shape of thorax.

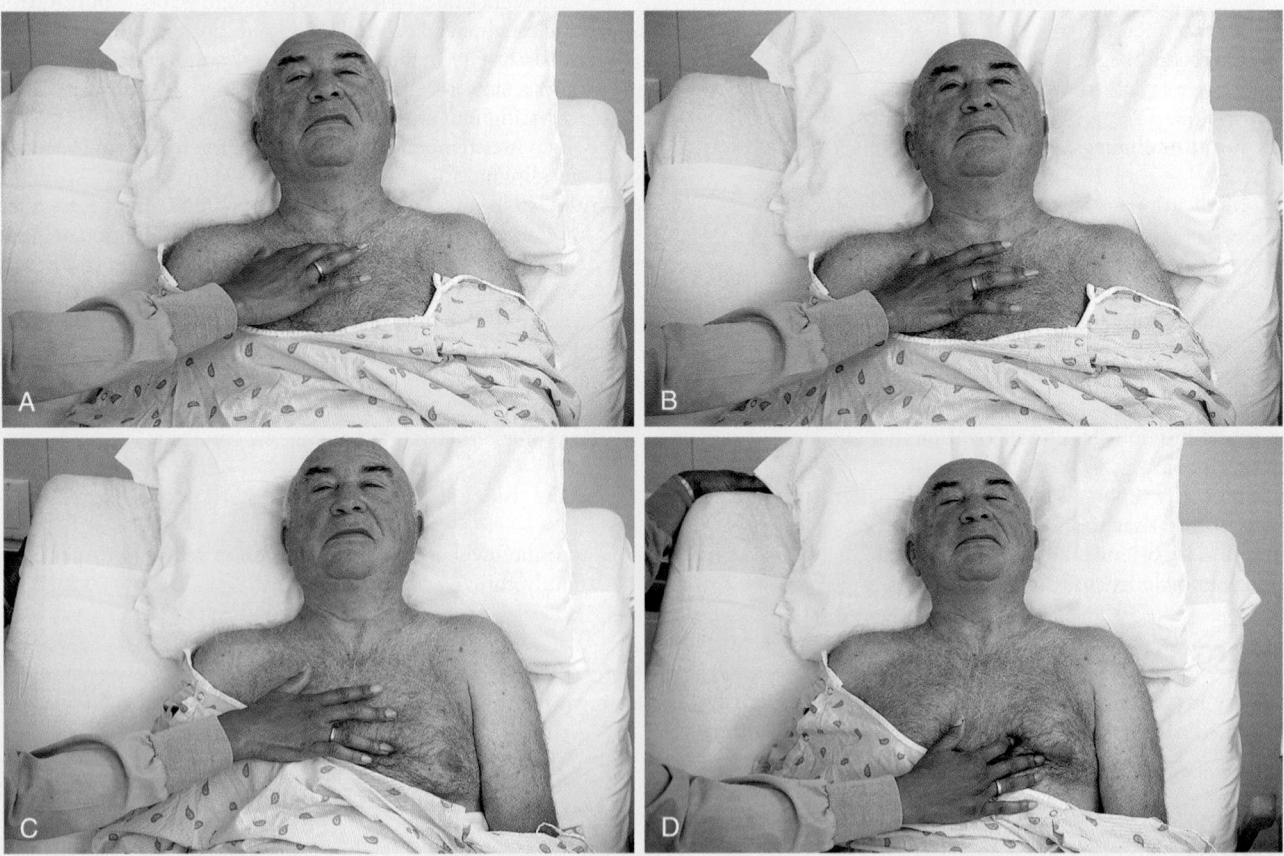

STEP 4 A, Nurse locates sternal notch. **B,** Nurse locates second intercostal space. **C,** Nurse locates fifth intercostal space. **D,** Nurse locates point of maximal impulse at fifth intercostal space at left midclavicular line.

STEP	RATIONALE

5. Place diaphragm of stethoscope in palm of hand for 5 to 10 seconds.

Warming of metal or plastic diaphragm prevents patient from being startled and promotes comfort.

6. Place diaphragm of stethoscope over PMI at fifth ICS, at left MCL, and auscultate for normal S_1 and S_2 heart sounds (heard as "lub-dub") (see illustrations).

Allow stethoscope tubing to extend straight without kinks that would distort sound transmission. Normal sounds S_1 and S_2 are high pitched and best heard with diaphragm.

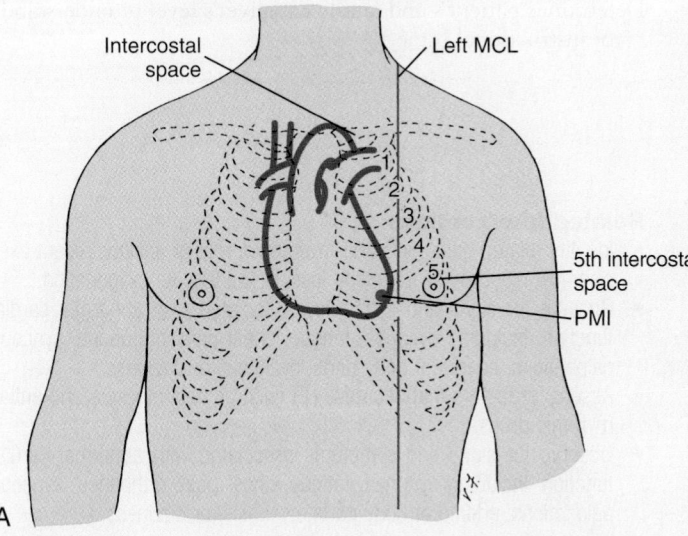

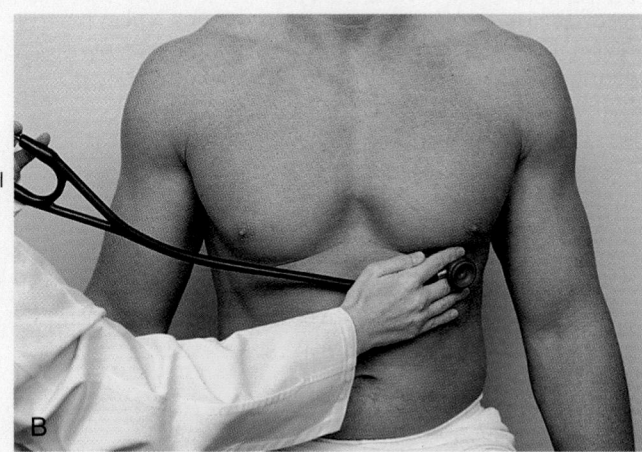

STEP 6 A, Location of point of maximal impulse (PMI) in adult. **B,** Listening to PMI in adult.

7. When you hear S_1 and S_2 with regularity, use second hand of watch and begin to count rate: when sweep hand hits number on dial, start counting with zero, then one, two, and so on.

Apical rate is determined accurately only after you are able to auscultate sounds clearly. Timing begins with zero. Count of one is first sound auscultated after timing begins.

8. If apical rate is regular, count for 30 seconds and multiply by 2.

You can assess regular apical rate within 30 seconds.

9. If HR is irregular or patient is receiving cardiovascular medication, count for a full 1 minute (60 seconds).

Irregular rate is more accurately assessed when measured over longer interval.

10. Note regularity of any dysrhythmia (S_1 and S_2 occurring early or late after previous sequence of sounds) (e.g., every third or every fourth beat is skipped).

Regular occurrence of dysrhythmia within 1 minute indicates inefficient contraction of heart and potential alteration in cardiac output.

11. Replace patient's gown and bed linen; help him or her return to comfortable position.

Restores comfort and promotes sense of well-being.

Clinical Decision Point *If apical rate is abnormal or irregular, repeat measurement or have another nurse conduct measurement. Original measurement may be incorrect. Second measurement confirms initial findings of an abnormal HR.*

12. Discuss findings with patient.

Promotes participation in care and understanding of health status.

13. Perform hand hygiene.

Reduces transmission of microorganisms.

14. Clean earpieces and diaphragm of stethoscope with alcohol swab routinely after each use.

Stethoscopes are frequently contaminated with microorganisms. Regular disinfection can control nosocomial infections (Longtin et al., 2014).

STEP	RATIONALE

EVALUATION

1. If assessing pulse for first time, establish apical rate as baseline if it is within an acceptable range.

2. Compare apical rate and character with patient's previous baseline and acceptable range of HR for patient's age.

3. **Use Teach-Back:** "I want to be sure I explained why it is important to check your heart rate at home. Tell me which medication you are taking that would decrease your heart rate." Revise your instruction now or develop a plan for revised patient or family caregiver teaching if patient or family caregiver is not able to teach back correctly.

Used to compare future pulse assessments.

Allows you to assess for change in patient's condition and for presence of cardiac alteration.

Determines patient's and family caregiver's level of understanding of instructional topic.

Unexpected Outcomes

1. Adult patient's apical pulse is greater than 100 beats/min (tachycardia).

2. Patient's apical pulse is less than 60 beats/min (bradycardia).

3. Patient's apical rhythm is irregular.

Related Interventions

- Identify related data, including fever, pain, fear or anxiety, recent exercise, low blood pressure, blood loss, or inadequate oxygenation.
- Observe for signs and symptoms associated with abnormal cardiac function, including dyspnea, fatigue, chest pain, orthopnea, syncope, palpitations, edema of body parts, cyanosis, or dizziness.
- Assess for factors that decrease HR such as beta blockers and antiarrhythmic drugs.
- Observe for signs and symptoms associated with abnormal cardiac function, including dyspnea, fatigue, chest pain, orthopnea, syncope, palpitations, edema of body parts, cyanosis, or dizziness.
- Have another nurse assess apical pulse.
- Report findings to nurse in charge and/or health care provider. It may be necessary to withhold prescribed medications that alter HR until health care provider can evaluate need to alter dosage.
- Assess for pulse deficit (see Skill 5.2): (a) nurse auscultates apical pulse while second provider palpates radial pulse; (b) nurse begins 60-second pulse count by calling out loud when to begin counting pulses; (c) if pulse count differs by more than 2, assesses for other signs and symptoms of decreased cardiac output (see Chapter 6).
- Report findings to nurse in charge and/or health care provider, who may order an electrocardiogram to detect cardiac conduction alteration.

Recording and Reporting

- Record apical pulse rate and rhythm on vital sign flow sheet or in nurses' notes in electronic health record (EHR) or chart. If apical pulse not found at fifth ICS and left MCL, document location of PMI.
- Document measurement of apical pulse rate after administration of specific therapies in appropriate area in EHR per agency policy.
- Report abnormal findings to nurse in charge or health care provider.
- Document your evaluation of patient and family caregiver learning.

Special Considerations

Teaching

- Teach family caregivers of patients taking prescribed cardiotonic or antidysrhythmic medications how to assess apical pulse rates to detect side effects of medications.

Pediatric

- The PMI of an infant is usually located at the third to fourth ICS near the left sternal border.

- In infants and children younger than 2 years, an apical pulse is more reliable and is counted for 1 full minute because of possible irregularities in rhythm.
- Breath holding in an infant or child temporarily lowers apical pulse rate.

Gerontological

- The PMI can be difficult to palpate in some older adults because the anterior-posterior diameter of the chest increases with age and the heart becomes repositioned because of left ventricular enlargement.
- When assessing older-adult women with sagging breast tissue, gently lift the breast tissue and place the stethoscope at the fifth ICS or the lower edge of the breast.
- Heart sounds are sometimes muffled or difficult to hear in older adults because of an increase in air space in the lungs.
- The older adult normally has a decreased HR at rest.

Home Care

- Assess home environment to determine which room affords a quiet environment for auscultation of apical rate.

◆ SKILL 5.4 Assessing Respirations

NSO *Nursing Skills Online Vital Signs Module / Lesson 4* *Video Clip*

Respiration is the exchange of oxygen (O_2) and carbon dioxide (CO_2) between cells of the body and the atmosphere. Three processes of respiration are: ventilation (i.e., mechanical movement of gases into and out of the lungs); diffusion (i.e., movement of oxygen and carbon dioxide between the alveoli and the red blood cells); and perfusion (i.e., distribution of red blood cells to and from the pulmonary capillaries). You assess ventilation by observing the rate, depth, and rhythm of respiratory movements. Accurate assessment of respirations depends on recognizing normal thoracic and abdominal movements. Normal breathing is both active and passive. On inspiration the diaphragm contracts, and the abdominal organs move down to increase the size of the chest cavity. At the same time the ribs and sternum lift outward to promote lung expansion. On expiration the diaphragm relaxes upward, and the ribs and sternum return to their relaxed position (Fig. 5.8). During quiet breathing the chest wall gently rises and falls. The body uses more energy during inspiration than during expiration. Expiration is an active process only during exercise, voluntary hyperventilation, and certain disease states.

Delegation and Collaboration

The skill of counting respirations can be delegated to nursing assistive personnel (NAP) unless the patient is considered unstable (i.e., complaints of dyspnea). The nurse instructs the NAP by:
• Communicating the frequency of measurement and factors related to patient history or risk for increased or decreased respiratory rate or irregular respirations.

• Reviewing any unusual respiratory values and significant changes to report to the nurse.

Equipment

• Wristwatch with second hand or digital display
• Pen and vital sign flow sheet in chart or electronic health record (EHR)

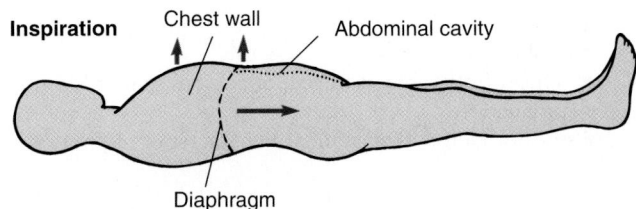

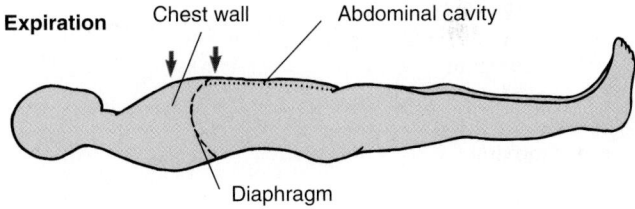

FIG 5.8 Diaphragmatic and chest wall movement during inspiration and expiration.

STEP	RATIONALE

ASSESSMENT

1. Identify patient using at least two identifiers (e.g., name and birthday or name and medical record number) according to agency policy.
2. Determine need to assess patient's respirations:
   a. Assess for risk factors of respiratory alterations:
   • Fever
   • Pain and anxiety
   • Diseases of chest wall or muscles
   • Constrictive chest or abdominal dressings
   • Presence of abdominal incisions
   • Gastric distention
   • Chronic pulmonary disease (emphysema, bronchitis, asthma)
   • Traumatic injury to chest wall with or without collapse of underlying lung tissue
   • Presence of chest tube
   • Respiratory infection (pneumonia, acute bronchitis)
   • Pulmonary edema and emboli
   • Head injury with damage to brainstem
   • Anemia

Ensures patient safety. Complies with The Joint Commission standards and improves patient safety (TJC, 2016).

Certain conditions place patient at risk for ventilatory alterations detected by changes in respiratory rate, depth, and rhythm.

STEP	RATIONALE

b. Assess for signs and symptoms of respiratory alterations such as:

- Bluish or cyanotic appearance of nail beds, lips, mucous membranes, and skin
- Restlessness, irritability, confusion, reduced level of consciousness
- Pain during inspiration
- Labored or difficult breathing
- Orthopnea
- Use of accessory muscles
- Adventitious breath sounds (see Chapter 6)
- Inability to breathe spontaneously
- Thick, frothy, blood-tinged, or copious sputum production

Physical signs and symptoms indicate alterations in respiratory status.

c. Assess for factors that influence character of respirations:

Allows you to anticipate factors that influence respirations, ensuring a more accurate interpretation.

- Exercise

Respirations increase in rate and depth to meet need for additional oxygen and rid body of carbon dioxide.

- Anxiety

Anxiety causes increase in respiration rate and depth because of sympathetic nervous system stimulation.

- Acute pain

Pain alters rate and rhythm of respirations; breathing becomes shallow. Patient inhibits or splints chest wall movement when pain is in area of chest or abdomen.

- Smoking

Chronic smoking changes pulmonary airways, resulting in increased respiratory rate at rest when not smoking.

- Medications

Narcotic analgesics, general anesthetics, and sedative hypnotics depress rate and depth; amphetamines and cocaine increase rate and depth; bronchodilators cause dilation of airways, which ultimately slows respiratory rate.

- Body position

Standing or sitting erect promotes full ventilatory movement and lung expansion; stooped or slumped posture impairs ventilatory movement; lying flat prevents full chest expansion.

- Neurological injury

Damage to brainstem impairs respiratory center and inhibits rate and rhythm.

- Hemoglobin function

Decreased hemoglobin levels lower amount of oxygen carried in blood, which results in increased respiratory rate to increase oxygen delivery. An increase in altitude lowers amount of saturated hemoglobin, which increases respiratory rate and depth.

3. Assess pertinent laboratory/clinical values:

a. *Arterial blood gases (ABGs):* Normal ranges (values vary slightly among agencies):
- pH, 7.35–7.45
- $PaCO_2$, 35–45 mm Hg
- HCO_3, 22–28 mEq/L
- PaO_2, 80–100 mm Hg
- SaO_2, 95%–100%

ABG values measure arterial blood pH, partial pressure of oxygen and carbon dioxide, and arterial oxygen saturation, which reflect patient's ventilation and oxygenation status.

b. *Pulse oximetry (SpO₂):* Normal SpO_2 ≥95%–100%; less than 90% is a clinical emergency (see Procedural Guideline 5.2).

SpO_2 less than 90% is often accompanied by changes in respiratory rate, depth, and rhythm.

c. *Complete blood count (CBC):* Normal CBC for adults (values vary within agencies):
- Hemoglobin: 14–18 g/100 mL, males; 12–16 g/100 mL, females
- Hematocrit: 42%–52%, males; 37%–47%, females
- Red blood cell count: 4.7–6.1 million/mm³, males; 4.2–5.4 million/mm³, females

CBC measures red blood cell count; volume of red blood cells; and concentration of hemoglobin, which reflects patient's capacity to carry oxygen.

4. Determine previous baseline respiratory rate (if available) from patient's record.

Assesses for change in condition. Provides comparison with future respiratory measurements.

STEP	RATIONALE

NURSING DIAGNOSES

- Activity intolerance
- Impaired gas exchange
- Impaired spontaneous ventilation
- Ineffective airway clearance
- Ineffective breathing pattern

Related factors are individualized based on patient's condition or needs.

PLANNING

1. Expected outcomes following completion of procedure:
- Respiratory rate is within acceptable range.
- Respirations are regular and of normal depth.

Adults average 12 to 20 breaths/min.
Respiratory status is stable.

2. If patient has been active, wait 5 to 10 minutes before assessing respirations.

Exercise increases respiratory rate and depth. Assessing respirations while patient is at rest allows for objective comparison of values.

3. Assess respirations after pulse measurement in an adult.

Inconspicuous assessment of respirations immediately after pulse assessment prevents patient from consciously or unintentionally altering rate and depth of breathing.

4. Be sure that patient is in comfortable position, preferably sitting or lying with head of bed elevated 45 to 60 degrees.

Sitting erect promotes full ventilatory movement. Position of discomfort causes patient to breathe more rapidly.

Clinical Decision Point *Assess patients with difficulty breathing (dyspnea) such as those with heart failure or abdominal ascites or in late stages of pregnancy in the position of greatest comfort. Repositioning may increase the work of breathing, which increases respiratory rate.*

IMPLEMENTATION

1. Perform hand hygiene.

Prevents transmission of microorganisms.

2. Draw curtain around bed and/or close door.

Maintains privacy.

3. Be sure that patient's chest is visible. If necessary, move bed linen or gown.

Ensures clear view of chest wall and abdominal movements.

4. Place patient's arm in relaxed position across abdomen or lower chest or place your hand directly over patient's upper abdomen.

A similar position used during pulse assessment allows respiratory rate assessment to be inconspicuous. Patient's or your hand rises and falls during respiratory cycle.

5. Observe complete respiratory cycle (one inspiration and one expiration).

Rate is accurately determined only after viewing a complete respiratory cycle.

6. After observing a cycle, look at second hand of watch and begin to count rate: when sweep hand hits number on dial, begin time frame, counting one with first full respiratory cycle.

Timing begins with count of one. Respirations occur more slowly than pulse; thus timing does not begin with zero.

7. If rhythm is regular, count number of respirations in 30 seconds and multiply by 2. If rhythm is irregular, less than 12, or greater than 20, count for 1 full minute.

Respiratory rate is equivalent to number of respirations per minute. Suspected irregularities require assessment for at least 1 minute (Box 5.5).

8. Note depth of respirations by observing degree of chest wall movement while counting rate. In addition, assess depth by palpating chest wall excursion or auscultating posterior thorax after you have counted rate (see Chapter 6). Describe depth as shallow, normal, or deep.

Character of ventilatory movement reveals specific disease states restricting volume of air from moving into and out of lungs.

9. Note rhythm of ventilatory cycle. Normal breathing is regular and uninterrupted. Do not confuse sighing with abnormal rhythm.

Character of ventilations reveals specific types of alterations. Periodically people unconsciously take single deep breaths or sighs to expand small airways prone to collapse.

Clinical Decision Point *Any irregular respiratory pattern or periods of apnea (cessation of respiration for several seconds) are symptoms of underlying disease in the adult, and you need to report this to the health care provider or nurse in charge. Further assessment and immediate intervention are often necessary.*

10. Replace bed linen and patient's gown.

Restores comfort and promotes sense of well-being.

11. Perform hand hygiene.

Reduces transmission of microorganisms.

STEP	RATIONALE

12. Discuss findings with patient.

Promotes participation in care and understanding of health status.

EVALUATION

1. If assessing respirations for first time, establish rate, rhythm, and depth as baseline if within acceptable range.

Used to compare future respiratory assessment.

2. Compare respirations with patient's previous baseline and usual rate, rhythm, and depth.

Allows you to assess for changes in patient's condition and presence of respiratory alterations.

3. Correlate respiratory rate, depth, and rhythm with data obtained from pulse oximetry and ABG measurements if available.

Evaluations of ventilation, perfusion, and diffusion are interrelated.

4. Use Teach-Back: "I want to be sure I explained why you will be reminded to take deep breaths after surgery. Tell me why deep breathing is important." Revise your instruction now or develop a plan for revised patient or family caregiver teaching if patient or family caregiver is not able to teach back correctly.

Determines patient's and family caregiver's level of understanding of instructional topic.

Unexpected Outcomes

1. Adult patient's respiratory rate is below 12 breaths/min (bradypnea) or above 20 breaths/min (tachypnea). Breathing pattern is sometimes irregular (see Box 5.5). Depth of respirations is increased or decreased. Patient complains of dyspnea.

2. Patient demonstrates Kussmaul's, Cheyne-Stokes, or Biot's respirations (see Box 5.5).

Related Interventions

- Assess for related factors, including obstructed airway, abnormal breath sounds, productive cough, restlessness, anxiety, and confusion (see Chapter 6).
- Help patient to supported sitting position (semi- or high-Fowler's) unless contraindicated.
- Provide oxygen as ordered (see Chapter 23).
- Assess for environmental factors that influence patient's respiratory rate such as secondhand smoke, poor ventilation, or gas fumes.
- Notify health care provider or nurse in charge if alteration continues.
- Notify health care provider for additional evaluation and possible medical intervention.

BOX 5.5

Alterations in Breathing Pattern

Alteration	Description
Apnea	Respirations cease for several seconds. Persistent cessation results in respiratory arrest.
Biot's respiration	Irregular respirations vary in depth and are interrupted by periods of apnea.
Bradypnea	Rate of breathing is regular but abnormally slow (fewer than 12 breaths/min).
Cheyne-Stokes respiration	Respiratory rate and depth are irregular, characterized by alternating periods of apnea and hyperventilation. Respiratory cycle begins with slow, shallow breaths that gradually increase to abnormal rate and depth. The pattern reverses; breathing slows and becomes shallow, climaxing in apnea before respiration resumes.
Hyperpnea	Respirations are increased in depth; occurs normally during exercise.
Hyperventilation	Rate and depth of respirations increase. Hypocarbia, an abnormally low level of carbon dioxide in the blood, may occur.
Hypoventilation	Respiratory rate is abnormally low; depth of ventilation may be depressed. Hypercarbia, an abnormally elevated level of carbon dioxide in the blood, may occur.
Kussmaul's respiration	Respirations are abnormally rapid and deep but regular; common in diabetic ketoacidosis.
Tachypnea	Rate of breathing is regular but abnormally rapid (more than 20 breaths/min).

Recording and Reporting

- Record respiratory rate, depth, and rhythm on vital sign flow sheet or in nurses' notes in electronic health record (EHR) or chart.
- Document measurement of respiratory rate after administration of specific therapies in nurses' notes in EHR or chart.
- Document your evaluation of patient and family caregiver learning.
- Record type and amount of oxygen therapy, if used, in nurses' notes in EHR or chart.
- Report abnormal findings to nurse in charge or health care provider.

Special Considerations

Teaching

- Patients who demonstrate decreased ventilation (e.g., after surgery) often benefit from learning deep-breathing and coughing exercises (see Chapter 37).
- Instruct family caregiver to contact home care nurse or health care provider if unusual fluctuations in respiratory rate occur.

Pediatric

- Assess respiratory rates before other vital signs or assessments if you are able to view movement of chest wall or abdomen. This allows assessment of rate and rhythm before child becomes anxious because of stranger anxiety or fear of other assessment procedures.
- Average respiratory rate (breaths per minute) for newborns is 30 to 60; infant (6 months to 1 year) is 30; toddler (2 years) is 25 to 32; and child from 3 to 12 years is 20 (Hockenberry and Wilson, 2015).
- Children up to age 7 breathe abdominally; thus respirations are observed by abdominal movement.
- An irregular respiratory rate and short apneic spells are normal for newborns.
- You can simply observe infant or young child while chest and abdomen are exposed.
- Use cardiorespiratory monitors for infants or newborns who are at risk for respiratory compromise or sustained apnea.

Gerontological

- Aging causes ossification of costal cartilage and downward slant of ribs, resulting in more rigid rib cage, which reduces chest wall expansion. Kyphosis and scoliosis, frequent in older adults, may also restrict chest expansion.
- Depth of respirations tends to decrease with aging.
- Change in lung function with aging results in respiratory rates generally higher in older adults, with a range of 16 to 25 breaths/ min.
- Some older adults depend more on accessory abdominal muscles than weakened thoracic muscles during respiration.

Home Care

- Assess for environmental factors in the home that influence patient's respiratory rate such as secondhand smoke, poor ventilation, or gas fumes.

◆ SKILL 5.5 Assessing Arterial Blood Pressure

NSO *Nursing Skills Online Vital Signs Module / Lesson 5*

Blood pressure (BP) is the force exerted by blood against the vessel walls. The peak pressure or systolic pressure occurs when the ventricular contraction of the heart forces blood under high pressure into the aorta. When the ventricles relax, the blood remaining in the arteries exerts a minimal or diastolic pressure against the arterial walls at all times.

The standard unit for measuring BP is millimeters of mercury (mm Hg). The most common technique of measuring BP is auscultation with a sphygmomanometer and stethoscope. As the sphygmomanometer cuff is deflated, the five different sounds heard over an artery are called *Korotkoff phases*. The sound in each phase has unique characteristics (Fig. 5.9). BP is recorded with the systolic reading (first sound) before the diastolic (beginning of the fifth sound). The difference between systolic and diastolic pressure is the pulse pressure. For a BP of 120/80, the pulse pressure is 40.

Hypertension

Hypertension is a major factor underlying death from heart attack and stroke in the United States and Canada. The Joint National Committee on Prevention, Detection, Evaluation, and Treatment of High Blood Pressure (James et al., 2014) has set criteria for determining categories of hypertension (Table 5.2). Prehypertension is a designation for patients at high risk for developing hypertension. In these patients early intervention by adoption of healthy lifestyles reduces the risk of or prevents hypertension. Hypertension is defined as systolic BP (SBP) of 140 mm Hg or greater, diastolic BP (DBP) of 90 mm Hg or greater, or taking antihypertensive medication (James et al., 2014). The diagnosis of hypertension in adults requires the average of two or more readings taken at each of two or more visits after an initial screening.

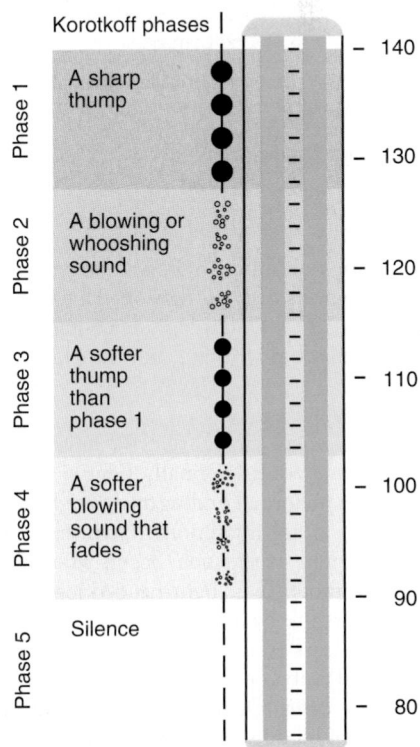

FIG 5.9 The sounds auscultated during blood pressure measurement can be differentiated into five phases. In this example the blood pressure is 140/90 mm Hg.

TABLE 5.2

Classification of Blood Pressure for Adults Ages 18 Years and Older*

Category	Systolic (mm Hg)		Diastolic (mm Hg)
Normal	<120	and	<80
Prehypertension	120–139	or	80–89
Stage 1	140–159	or	90–99
Stage 2	≥160	or	≥100

From James P, et al: 2014 Evidence-based guideline for the management of high blood pressure in adults: report from the panel members appointed to the Eighth Joint National Committee (JNC8), *JAMA* 311:507, 2014.

*Based on the average of two or more readings taken at each of two or more visits after an initial screening. Patient is not taking antihypertensive drugs and is not acutely ill. When systolic and diastolic blood pressures fall into different categories, the higher category should be selected to classify the individual's blood pressure status. For example, 160/92 mm Hg should be classified as stage 2 hypertension.

TABLE 5.3

Recommendations for Blood Pressure Follow-Up

Initial Blood Pressure	Follow-Up Recommended*
Normal	Recheck in 2 years.
Prehypertension	Recheck in 1 year.[†]
Stage 1 hypertension	Evaluate therapy within 1 month (James et al., 2014).
Stage 2 hypertension	Evaluate therapy within 1 month (James et al., 2014). For those with higher pressure (e.g., >180/110 mm Hg), evaluate and treat immediately or within 1 week, depending on clinical situation and complications.

*Modify follow-up scheduling according to reliable information about past blood pressure measurements, other cardiovascular risk factors, or target organ damage.
[†]Provide advice about lifestyle modifications.

One BP recording revealing a high systolic or diastolic BP does not qualify as a diagnosis of hypertension. However, if you assess a high reading (e.g., 150/90 mm Hg), encourage the patient to return for another checkup within 2 months (Table 5.3).

Hypotension

Hypotension occurs when the systolic BP falls to 90 mm Hg or below. Although some adults normally have a low BP, for most people a low BP is an abnormal finding associated with illness (e.g., hemorrhage or myocardial infarction). Orthostatic hypotension, also referred to as *postural hypotension*, occurs when a normotensive person develops symptoms (e.g., light-headedness or dizziness) and a drop in systolic pressure by at least 20 mm Hg or a drop in diastolic pressure by at least 10 mm Hg within 3 minutes of rising to an upright position (Shibao et al., 2013). A loss of consciousness may occur in severe cases. Orthostatic changes in vital signs are effective indicators of blood volume depletion. Some medications cause orthostatic hypotension, especially in young patients and older adults. Orthostatic hypotension is a risk factor for fall, especially among older adults with hypertension (Angelousi et al., 2014).

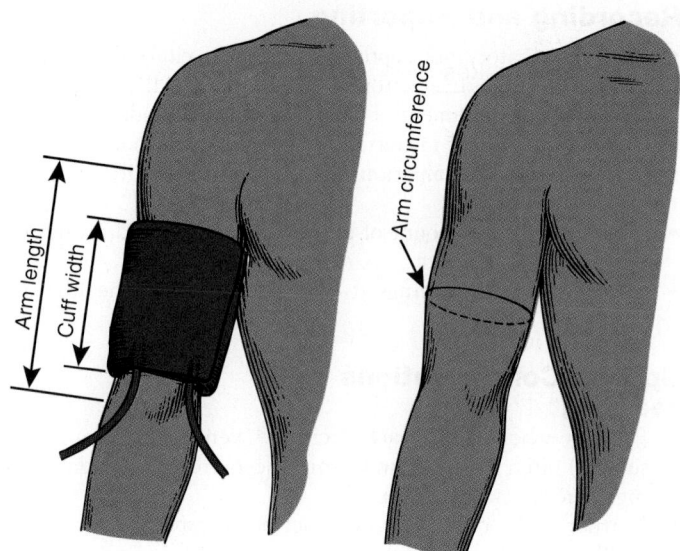

FIG 5.10 Guidelines for proper blood pressure cuff size. Cuff width equals 20% more than upper arm diameter or 40% of circumference around upper arm and two thirds of upper arm length.

Blood Pressure Equipment

You measure arterial BP either directly (invasively) or indirectly (noninvasively). The direct method requires electronic monitoring equipment and the insertion of a thin catheter into an artery. The risks associated with invasive BP monitoring require a patient to be in an intensive care setting.

The more common noninvasive method requires use of a sphygmomanometer and stethoscope. A sphygmomanometer includes a pressure manometer, an occlusive cloth or disposable vinyl cuff that encloses an inflatable rubber bladder, and a pressure bulb with a release valve that inflates the bladder. The aneroid pressure manometer has a glass-enclosed circular gauge containing a needle that registers millimeter calibrations. Before using the aneroid manometer, make sure that the needle is pointing to zero. The release valve of the sphygmomanometer that holds the pressure constant must be clean and freely movable in either direction.

Cloth or disposable vinyl compression cuffs contain an inflatable bladder and come in several different sizes. The size selected is proportional to the circumference of the limb that you are assessing. Ideally the width of the cuff should be 40% of the circumference (or 20% wider than the diameter) of the midpoint of the limb on which the cuff is to be used (Fig. 5.10). The bladder enclosed within the cuff should encircle at least 80% of the upper arm (James et al., 2014). Many adults require a large adult cuff. A regular-size cuff holds a bladder in the width of 12 to 13 cm (4.8 to 5.2 inches) and the length of 22 to 23 cm (8.5 to 9 inches). An improperly fitting cuff produces inaccurate BP measurements (Box 5.6).

Electronic or automatic BP machines consist of an electronic sensor positioned inside a BP cuff attached to an electronic processor (see Procedural Guideline 5.1). Electronic devices have limitations but are useful when frequent measurements are necessary (Box 5.7).

Delegation and Collaboration

The skill of BP measurement can be delegated to nursing assistive personnel (NAP) unless the patient is considered unstable (i.e., hypotensive). The nurse instructs the NAP by:

BOX 5.6

Common Mistakes in Blood Pressure Assessment

Error	Effect
Bladder or cuff too wide	False-low reading
Bladder or cuff too narrow or too short	False-high reading
Cuff wrapped too loosely or unevenly	False-high reading
Deflating cuff too slowly	False-high diastolic reading
Deflating cuff too quickly	False-low systolic and false-high diastolic reading
Arm below heart level	False-high reading
Arm above heart level	False-low reading
Arm not supported	False-high reading
Stethoscope that fits poorly or impairment of examiner's hearing, causing sounds to be muffled	False-low systolic and false-high diastolic reading
Stethoscope applied too firmly against antecubital fossa	False-low diastolic reading
Inflating too slowly	False-high diastolic reading
Repeating assessments too quickly	False-high systolic reading
Inaccurate inflation level	False-low systolic reading
Multiple examiners using different sounds for diastolic readings	False-high systolic and false-low diastolic reading

BOX 5.7

Advantages and Limitations of Assessing Blood Pressure Electronically

Advantages
- Ease of use
- Efficient when frequent repeated measurements are indicated
- Stethoscope not required
- Allows blood pressure to be recorded more frequently, as often as every 15 seconds with accuracy

Limitations
- Expensive
- Requires source of electricity
- Requires space to position machine
- Sensitive to outside motion interference and cannot be used in patients with seizures, tremors, or shivers or patients unable to cooperate
- Not accurate for patients with irregular heart rate or hypotension or in conditions with reduced blood flow (e.g., hypothermia)
- Accuracy standards for electronic blood pressure machine manufacturers are voluntary
- Vulnerable to error among older adults and obese patients

- Explaining the appropriate limb to use for measurement, BP cuff size, and equipment (manual or electronic) to be used.
- Communicating the frequency of measurement and factors related to the patient's history such as risk for orthostatic hypotension.
- Reviewing the patient's usual BP values and significant changes or abnormalities to report to the nurse.

Equipment

- Aneroid sphygmomanometer
- Cloth or disposable vinyl pressure cuff of appropriate size for patient's extremity
- Stethoscope
- Alcohol swab
- Pen and vital sign flow sheet in chart or electronic health record (EHR)

STEP	RATIONALE

ASSESSMENT

1. Identify patient using at least two identifiers (e.g., name and birthday or name and medical record number) according to agency policy.

Ensures patient safety. Complies with The Joint Commission standards and improves patient safety (TJC, 2016).

2. Determine need to assess patient's BP:
   a. Assess risk factors for BP alterations:
   - History of cardiovascular disease
   - Renal disease
   - Diabetes mellitus
   - Circulatory shock (hypovolemic, septic, cardiogenic, or neurogenic)
   - Acute or chronic pain
   - Rapid intravenous (IV) infusion of fluids or blood products
   - Increased intracranial pressure
   - Postoperative status
   - Toxemia of pregnancy

Certain conditions place patients at risk for BP alteration.

STEP	RATIONALE
b. Assess for signs and symptoms of BP alterations. In patients at risk for high BP (HBP), assess for headache (usually occipital), flushing of face, nosebleed, and fatigue in older adults. Hypotension is associated with dizziness; mental confusion; restlessness; pale, dusky, or cyanotic skin and mucous membranes; and cool, mottled skin over extremities.	Physical signs and symptoms indicate alterations in BP. Hypertension is often asymptomatic until pressure is very high.
c. Assess for factors that influence BP:	Allows you to anticipate factors that influence respirations, ensuring a more accurate interpretation.
• Age	Acceptable values for BP vary throughout life (see Pediatric and Gerontological Considerations).
• Gender	During and after menopause women often have higher BPs than men of same age.
• Daily (diurnal) variation	BP varies throughout day; pressure is highest during the day between 10:00 AM and 6:00 PM and lowest in early morning.
• Position	BP falls as person moves from lying to sitting or standing position; normally postural variations are minimal.
• Exercise	Increases in oxygen demand by body during activity increases BP.
• Weight	Obesity is an independent predictor of hypertension.
• Sympathetic stimulation	Pain, anxiety, or fear stimulates sympathetic nervous system, causing BP to rise.
• Medications	Antihypertensives, diuretics, beta-adrenergic blockers, vasodilators, calcium channel blockers, angiotensin-converting enzyme (ACE) inhibitors, angiotensin receptor blockers (ARBs), and antidysrhythmics lower BP; opioids and general anesthetics also cause a drop in BP.
• Smoking	Smoking results in vasoconstriction, a narrowing of blood vessels. BP rises acutely and returns to baseline approximately 15 minutes after stopping smoking (James et al., 2014).
• Ethnicity	Incidence of hypertension is higher in African-Americans than in European Americans. African-Americans tend to develop more severe hypertension at an earlier age and have twice the risk for the complications of hypertension (i.e., stroke and heart attack). Hypertension-related deaths are also higher among African-Americans.
3. Determine best site for BP assessment. Avoid applying cuff to extremity when IV fluids are infusing, an arteriovenous shunt or fistula is present, or breast or axillary surgery has been performed on that side. In addition, avoid applying cuff to traumatized or diseased extremity or one that has a cast or bulky bandage. Use lower extremities when brachial arteries are inaccessible.	Inappropriate site selection may result in poor amplification of sounds, causing inaccurate readings. Application of pressure from inflated bladder temporarily impairs blood flow and can further compromise circulation in extremity that already has impaired blood flow.
4. Determine previous baseline BP and site (if available) from patient's record. Determine any report of latex allergy.	Assesses for change in condition. Provides comparison with future BP measurements. If patient has latex allergy, verify that stethoscope and BP cuff are latex free.
5. Assess patient's knowledge of procedure and any BP alteration that exists.	Encourages cooperation; minimizes risks and anxiety. Identifies teaching needs.

NURSING DIAGNOSES

- Decreased cardiac output
- Deficient fluid volume
- Excess fluid volume
- Ineffective tissue perfusion
- Risk for falls

Related factors/Risk factors are individualized based on patient's condition or needs.

STEP	RATIONALE

PLANNING

1. Expected outcome following completion of procedure:
   • BP is within acceptable range for patient's age.

Cardiovascular status is stable.

2. Explain to patient that you will assess BP. Have patient rest at least 5 minutes before measuring lying or sitting BP and 1 minute before measuring standing. Ask patient not to speak while you are measuring BP.

Reduces anxiety that falsely elevates readings. Exercise causes false elevations in BP. Deep breathing lowers BP. Talking to a patient during assessment increases BP (Zheng et al., 2012).

3. Be sure that patient has not exercised, ingested caffeine, or smoked for 30 minutes before assessment of BP.

Smoking increases BP immediately and lasts up to 15 minutes. The effects of coffee or caffeine increase BP up to 3 hours (James et al., 2014).

4. Select appropriate cuff size (see Fig. 5.10) and ensure that other equipment is in patient's room.

Use of improper-size cuff causes false-low or false-high reading (Mourad et al., 2013) (see Box 5.6).

IMPLEMENTATION

1. Perform hand hygiene

Reduces transmission of microorganisms.

2. Have patient assume sitting or lying position. Be sure that room is warm, quiet, and relaxing. Close room curtains.

Maintains patient's comfort during measurement. Patient's perceptions that physical or interpersonal environment is stressful affect BP.

3. Assess BP by auscultation:

  a. *Upper extremity:* With patient sitting or lying, position his or her forearm at heart level with palm turned up (see illustration). If sitting, instruct patient to keep feet flat on floor without legs crossed. If supine, patient should not have legs crossed. If the patient cannot be placed in prone position, position him or her supine with knee slightly bent.

If arm is extended and not supported, patient will perform isometric exercise that can increase diastolic pressure. Placement of arm above level of heart causes false-low reading, 2 mm Hg for each inch above heart level.

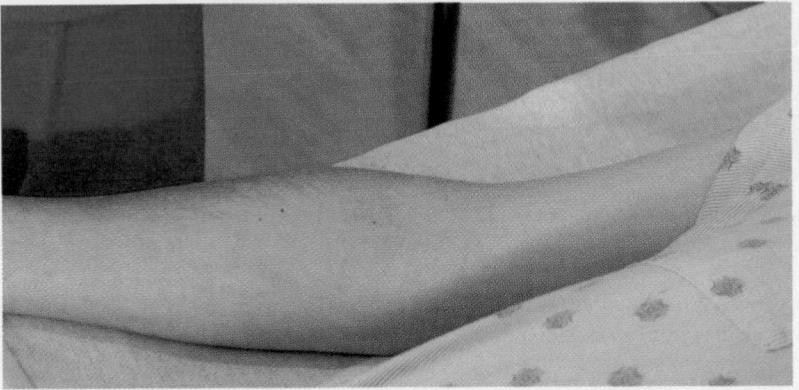

STEP 3a Patient's forearm supported on bed.

  Lower extremity: With patient prone, position patient so knee is slightly flexed.

Leg crossing can falsely increase BP.

  b. Expose extremity (arm or leg) fully by removing constricting clothing. Cuff may be placed over a sleeve as long as stethoscope rests on skin (Ki et al., 2013).

Ensures proper cuff application.

  c. Palpate brachial artery (arm, see illustration A) or popliteal artery (leg). With cuff fully deflated, apply bladder of cuff above artery by centering arrows marked on cuff over artery (see illustration B). If cuff does not have any center arrows, estimate center of bladder and place this center over artery. Position cuff 2.5 cm (1 inch) above site of pulsation (antecubital or popliteal space). With cuff fully deflated, wrap it evenly and snugly around upper arm (see illustration C) or leg (see illustration D).

Brachial artery is along groove between biceps and triceps muscles above elbow at antecubital fossa. Popliteal artery is just below patient's thigh, behind knee.

Placing bladder directly over artery ensures that you apply proper pressure during inflation. Loose-fitting cuff causes false-high readings.

STEP	RATIONALE

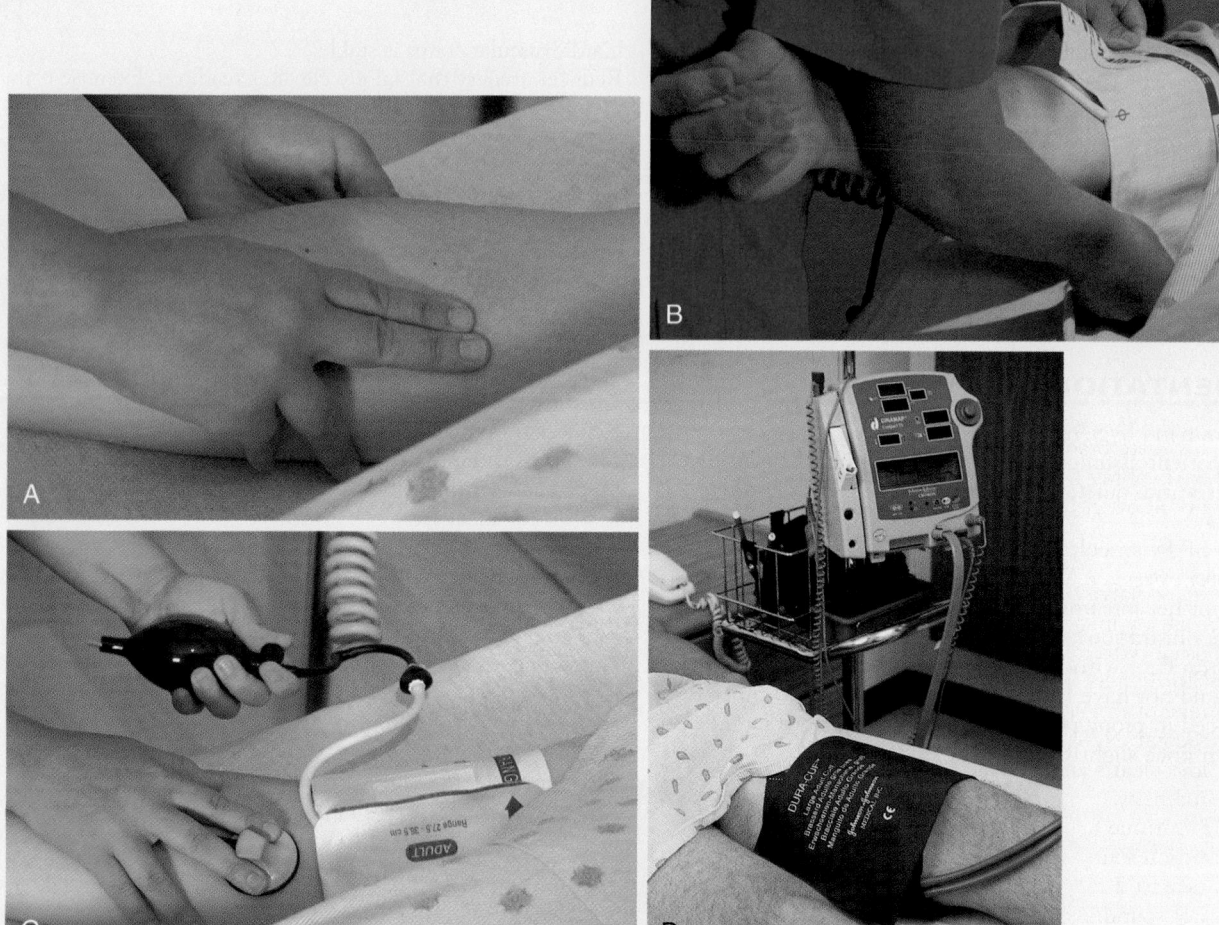

STEP 3c A, Palpating brachial artery. **B,** Aligning blood pressure cuff arrow with brachial artery. **C,** Blood pressure cuff wrapped around upper arm. **D,** Blood pressure cuff applied around thigh.

d. Position manometer gauge vertically at eye level. You should be no farther than 1 meter (approximately 1 yard) away.

Looking up or down at scale can result in distorted readings.

e. Measure BP using two-step method:

(1) Relocate brachial or popliteal pulse. Palpate artery distal to cuff with fingertips of nondominant hand while inflating cuff rapidly to pressure 30 mm Hg above point at which pulse disappears. Slowly deflate cuff and note point when pulse reappears. Deflate cuff fully and wait 30 seconds.

Estimating prevents false-low readings. Determine maximal inflation point for accurate reading by palpation. If unable to palpate artery because of weakened pulse, use ultrasonic stethoscope (see Chapter 6). Completely deflating cuff prevents venous congestion and false-high readings.

(2) Place stethoscope earpieces in ears and be sure that sounds are clear, not muffled.

Ensure that each earpiece follows angle of ear canal to facilitate hearing.

(3) Relocate artery and place bell or diaphragm chest piece of stethoscope over it. Do not allow chest piece to touch cuff or clothing.

Proper stethoscope placement ensures best sound reception. Stethoscope improperly positioned causes muffled sounds that often result in false-low systolic and false-high diastolic readings. The bell provides better sound reproduction, whereas the diaphragm is easier to secure with fingers and covers a larger area.

STEP	RATIONALE
(4) Close valve of pressure bulb clockwise until tight. Quickly inflate cuff to 30 mm Hg above patient's estimated systolic pressure.	Tightening valve prevents air leak during inflation. Rapid inflation ensures accurate measurement of systolic pressure.
(5) Slowly release pressure bulb valve and allow manometer needle to fall at rate of 2 to 3 mm Hg/second.	Too-rapid or too-slow a decline causes inaccurate readings (Zheng et al., 2011).
(6) Note point on manometer when you hear first clear sound. Sound will slowly increase in intensity.	First sound reflects systolic BP.
(7) Continue to deflate cuff gradually, noting point at which sound disappears in adults. Note pressure to nearest 2 mm Hg. Listen for 20 to 30 mm Hg after last sound and allow remaining air to escape quickly.	Beginning of last or fifth sound is indication of diastolic pressure in adults (Kaplan et al., 2015). In children distinct muffling of sounds indicates diastolic pressure (Kaplan et al., 2015).
f. Measure BP using one-step method:	
(1) Place stethoscope earpieces in ears and be sure that sounds are clear, not muffled.	Earpieces should follow angle of ear canal to facilitate hearing.
(2) Relocate brachial or popliteal artery and place bell or diaphragm chest piece of stethoscope over it. Do not allow chest piece to touch cuff or clothing.	Proper stethoscope placement ensures optimal sound reception. Stethoscope improperly positioned causes muffled sounds that often result in false readings. Bell provides better sound reproduction, whereas diaphragm is easier to secure with fingers and covers larger area.
(3) Close valve of pressure bulb clockwise until tight. Quickly inflate cuff to 30 mm Hg above patient's usual systolic pressure.	Tightening valve prevents air leak during inflation. Inflation above systolic level ensures accurate measurement of systolic pressure.
(4) Slowly release pressure bulb valve and allow manometer needle to fall at rate of 2 to 3 mm Hg/second. Note point on manometer when you hear first clear sound. Sound will slowly increase in intensity.	Too-rapid or too-slow decline in mercury level causes inaccurate readings (Zheng et al., 2011). First sound reflects systolic pressure.
(5) Continue to deflate cuff gradually, noting point at which sound disappears in adults. Note pressure to nearest 2 mm Hg. Listen for 10 to 20 mm Hg after last sound and allow remaining air to escape quickly.	Beginning of fifth sound is indication of diastolic pressure in adults (Kaplan et al., 2015). In children distinct muffling of sounds indicates diastolic pressure (Kaplan et al., 2015).
4. The American Heart Association recommends average of two sets of BP measurement, 2 minutes apart. Use second set of BP measurements as baseline. If readings are different by more than 5 mm Hg, additional readings are necessary.	Two sets of BP measurements help to prevent false-positive readings based on patient's sympathetic response (alert reaction). Averaging minimizes effect of anxiety, which often causes first reading to be higher than subsequent measures (Kaplan et al., 2015).
5. Remove cuff from patient's arm or leg unless you need to repeat measurement.	Continuous cuff inflation causes arterial occlusion, resulting in numbness and tingling of patient's arm/leg.
6. If this is first assessment of patient, repeat procedure on other arm or leg.	Comparison of BP in both arms or legs detects circulatory problems. (Normal difference of 5 to 10 mm Hg exists between arms.) Use arm with higher pressure for repeated measurements (Frese et al., 2011).
7. Assess systolic BP by palpation:	
a. Follow Steps 3a through 3d of auscultation method.	
b. Locate and then continually palpate brachial, radial, or popliteal artery with fingertips of one hand. Inflate cuff to pressure 30 mm Hg above point at which you can no longer palpate pulse.	Ensures accurate detection of true systolic pressure once pressure valve is released.

STEP	RATIONALE

Clinical Decision Point *If unable to palpate artery because of weakened pulse, use a Doppler ultrasonic stethoscope (Fig. 5.11).*

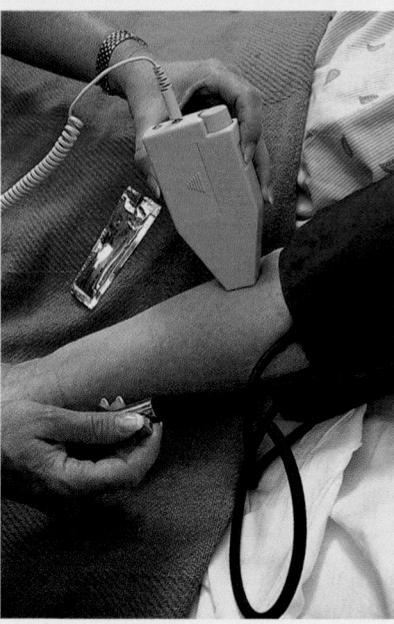

FIG 5.11 Doppler ultrasonic stethoscope over brachial artery to measure blood pressure.

STEP	RATIONALE
c. Slowly release valve and deflate cuff, allowing manometer needle to fall at rate of 2 mm Hg/second. Note point on manometer when pulse is again palpable.	Too-rapid or too-slow a decline results in inaccurate readings (Zheng et al., 2011). Palpation helps identify systolic pressure only.
d. Deflate cuff rapidly and completely. Remove cuff from patient's extremity unless you need to repeat measurement.	Continuous cuff inflation causes arterial occlusion, resulting in numbness and tingling of extremity.
8. Help patient return to comfortable position and cover upper arm or leg if previously clothed.	Restores comfort and provides sense of well-being.
9. Discuss findings with patient.	Promotes participation in care and understanding of health status. Makes patient accountable for follow-up assessment. Systolic BP in leg is 10 to 40 mm Hg higher than arm, but diastolic BP is same.
10. Clean earpieces and diaphragm of stethoscope with alcohol swab as needed. Wipe cuff with agency-approved disinfectant if used between patients. Perform hand hygiene.	Reduces transmission of microorganisms. Controls transmission of microorganisms when nurses share stethoscope.

EVALUATION

1. If assessing BP for first time, establish baseline BP if it is within acceptable range.	Used to compare future BP measurements.
2. Compare BP reading with patient's previous baseline and usual BP for patient's age.	Allows you to assess for change in condition. Provides comparison with future BP measurements.
3. **Use Teach-Back:** "I want to be sure I explained why it is important to stand up slowly since you have high BP. Tell me which of your medications might make you dizzy if you stand up too fast." Revise your instruction now or develop a plan for revised patient or family caregiver teaching if patient or family caregiver is not able to teach back correctly.	Determines patient's and family caregiver's level of understanding of instructional topic.

STEP	RATIONALE
Unexpected Outcomes 1. Patient's BP is above acceptable range.	**Related Interventions** • Repeat measurement in other extremity and compare findings. • Verify correct size and placement of BP cuff. • Have another nurse repeat measurement in 1 to 2 minutes. • Observe for related symptoms that are not apparent unless BP is extremely high, including headache, facial flushing, nosebleed, and fatigue in older patient. • Report BP to nurse in charge or health care provider to initiate appropriate evaluation and treatment. • Administer antihypertensive medications as ordered.
2. Patient's BP is not sufficient for adequate perfusion and oxygenation of tissues.	• Compare BP value to baseline. • Position patient in supine position to enhance circulation and restrict activity that decreases BP further. • Assess for signs and symptoms associated with hypotension, including tachycardia; weak, thready pulse; weakness; dizziness; confusion; and cool, pale, dusky, or cyanotic skin. • Assess for factors that contribute to low BP, including hemorrhage, dilation of blood vessels resulting from hyperthermia, anesthesia, or medication side effects. • Report BP to nurse in charge or health care provider to initiate appropriate evaluation and treatment. • Increase rate of IV infusion or administer vasoconstriction drugs if ordered.
3. Unable to obtain BP reading.	• Determine that no immediate crisis is present by obtaining pulse and respiratory rate. • Assess for signs and symptoms of decreased cardiac output; if present, notify nurse in charge or health care provider immediately. • Use alternative sites or procedures to obtain BP: use Doppler ultrasonic instrument (see Chapter 6); palpate systolic BP.
4. Patient experiences orthostatic hypotension.	• Maintain patient safety. • Return patient to safe position in bed or chair.

Recording and Reporting

- Record BP and site assessed on vital sign flow sheet or in nurses' notes in electronic health record (EHR) or chart.
- Document measurement of BP and any signs or symptoms of BP alterations after administration of specific therapies in nurses' notes in EHR or chart.
- Document your evaluation of patient and family caregiver learning.
- Report abnormal findings to nurse in charge or health care provider.

Special Considerations
Teaching

- Educate patient about risks for hypertension. People with family history of hypertension, premature heart disease, lipidemia, or renal disease are at significant risk. Obesity, cigarette smoking, heavy alcohol consumption, high blood cholesterol and triglyceride levels, and continued exposure to stress from psychosocial and environmental conditions are factors linked to hypertension (James et al., 2014).
- Primary prevention of hypertension includes lifestyle modifications (e.g., lose weight, exercise daily, reduce sodium and saturated fat intake, and maintain adequate intake of dietary potassium and calcium). Cigarette smoking is a significant risk factor; thus encourage patients to avoid tobacco in any form (James et al., 2014).

- Instruct primary caregiver to take BP at same time each day and after patient has had a brief rest. Take BP sitting or lying down; use same position and arm each time you take pressure.
- Instruct primary caregiver that, if the BP is difficult to hear, it is probably caused by one of the following: cuff too loose, not large enough, or too narrow; stethoscope not over arterial pulse; cuff deflated too quickly or too slowly; or cuff not pumped high enough for systolic readings.

Pediatric

- BP measurement is not a routine part of assessment in children younger than 3 years.
- BP measurement can frighten children. Prepare child for squeezing feeling of inflated BP cuff by comparing sensation to elastic band on finger or a tight hug on the arm.
- Obtain BP in child before performing anxiety-producing tests or procedures.
- BP sounds are difficult to hear in children because of low frequency and amplitude. Using the bell of a pediatric stethoscope is often helpful.

Gerontological

- Older adults, especially frail older adults, have lost upper-arm mass, requiring special attention to selection of BP cuff size.
- Skin of older adults is more fragile and susceptible to cuff pressure when measurements are frequent. More frequent

assessment of skin under cuff or rotation of measurement sites is recommended.

- Older adults have an increase in systolic pressure related to decreased vessel elasticity.
- Older adults often experience a fall in BP after eating.
- Instruct older adults to change position slowly and wait after each change to avoid postural hypotension and prevent injuries.

Home Care

- Assess home noise level to determine the room that provides the quietest environment for assessing BP.

- Instruct patient in the importance of an appropriate-size BP cuff for home use.
- Assess family's financial ability to afford a sphygmomanometer for performing BP evaluations on a regular basis. Recommend electronic devices or aneroid sphygmomanometers that have proven to be accurate according to standard testing and appropriate-size cuffs. Finger BP monitors are inaccurate (James et al., 2014).

PROCEDURAL GUIDELINE 5.1   *Noninvasive Electronic Blood Pressure Measurement*

NSO *Nursing Skills Online Vital Signs Module / Lesson 5*

Many different styles of electronic blood pressure machines are available to determine blood pressure automatically (Fig. 5.12). Electronic machines rely on an electronic sensor to detect the vibrations caused by the rush of blood through an artery. Although electronic blood pressure machines are fast, you must consider their advantages and limitations (see Box 5.7). The devices are used when frequent assessment is required such as in critically ill or potentially unstable patients, during or after invasive procedures, or when therapies require frequent monitoring. However, automatic blood pressure measurements are often inaccurate when patients have an irregular heart rate or extremely low or high blood pressure. Always verify an assessment of an abnormal blood pressure by an electronic machine with a sphygmomanometer and stethoscope.

Delegation and Collaboration

The skill of blood pressure measurement using an electronic blood pressure machine can be delegated to nursing assistive

personnel (NAP) unless the patient is considered unstable (i.e., hypotensive). The nurse instructs the NAP by:
- Explaining the frequency and extremity to use for measurement.
- Reviewing how to select appropriate-size blood pressure cuff for designated extremity and appropriate cuff for the machine.
- Reviewing patient's usual blood pressure and reporting significant changes or abnormalities to the nurse.

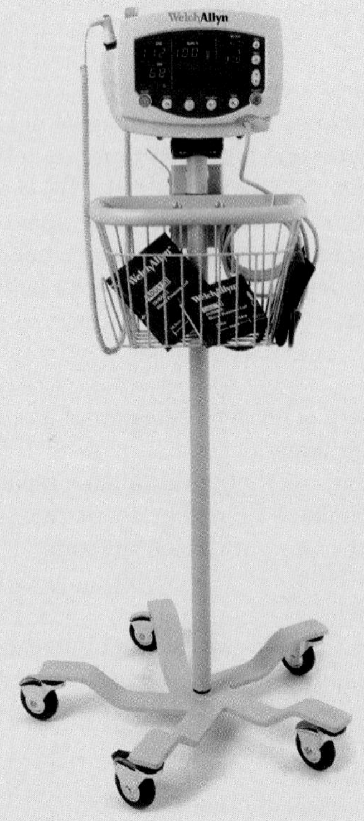

Equipment

- Electronic blood pressure machine
- Blood pressure cuff of appropriate size as recommended by manufacturer
- Pen and vital sign flow sheet in chart or electronic health record (EHR).

Procedural Steps

1. Identify patient using at least two identifiers (e.g., name and birthday or name and medical record number) according to agency policy (TJC, 2016).
2. Assess need to measure blood pressure (see Skill 5.5, Assessment Step 2) and determine patient's baseline blood pressure.
3. Determine appropriateness of using electronic blood pressure measurement. Patients with irregular heart rate, peripheral vascular disease, seizures, tremors, and shivering are not candidates for the device (Suokhrie et al., 2013).
4. Perform hand hygiene. Determine best site for cuff placement; inspect condition of extremities.
5. Collect and bring appropriate equipment to patient's bedside. Select appropriate cuff size for patient extremity (Table 5.4) and appropriate cuff for machine. Electronic blood pressure cuff and machine must be matched by manufacturer and are not interchangeable.

FIG 5.12 Noninvasive electronic blood pressure machine. (*Photo courtesy Welch Allyn.*)

TABLE 5.4	
Correct Blood Pressure Cuff Size for Electronic Monitor*	
Cuff Size	**Limb Circumference (cm)**
Small adult	17–25
Adult	23–33
Large adult	31–40
Thigh	38–50

*A 12- to 24-foot cord is required for adult blood pressure monitoring.

PROCEDURAL GUIDELINE 5.1 *Noninvasive Electronic Blood Pressure Measurement—cont'd*

6. Help patient to comfortable position, either lying or sitting. Plug device into electric outlet and place it near patient, ensuring that connector hose between cuff and machine reaches.

7. Locate on/off switch and turn on machine to enable device to self-test computer systems.

8. Remove constricting clothing to ensure proper cuff application.

9. Prepare blood pressure cuff by manually squeezing all the air out of the cuff and connecting it to connector hose.

10. Wrap flattened cuff snugly around extremity, verifying that only one finger can fit between cuff and patient's skin. Make sure that "artery" arrow marked on outside of cuff is placed correctly (see illustration).

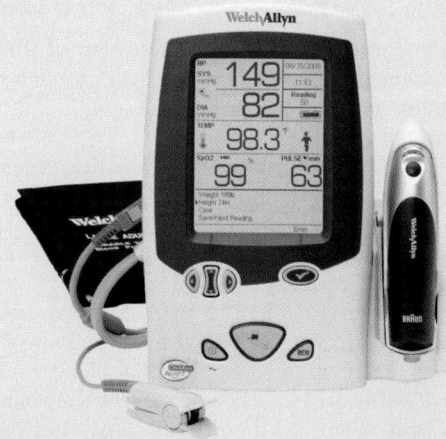

STEP 13 Digital electronic blood pressure display. *(Image courtesy Welch Allyn.)*

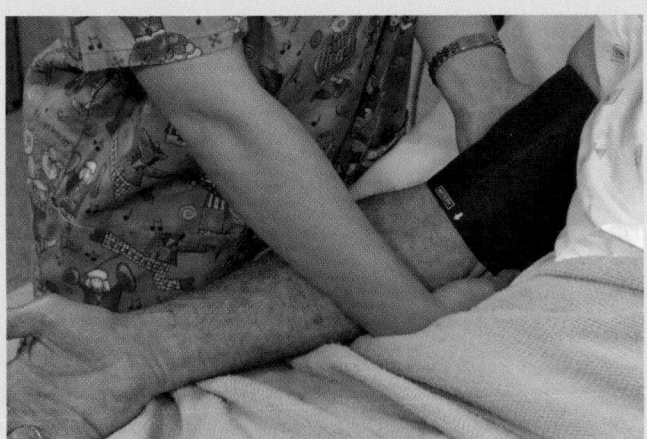

STEP 10 Aligning blood pressure cuff arrow with brachial artery.

11. Verify that connector hose between cuff and machine is not kinked. Kinking prevents proper inflation and deflation of cuff.

12. Following manufacturer directions, set frequency control for automatic or manual and press the start button. The first blood pressure measurement pumps cuff to a peak pressure of approximately 180 mm Hg. After this pressure is reached, the machine begins a deflation sequence that determines the blood pressure. The first reading determines peak pressure inflation for additional measurements.

13. When deflation is complete, digital display provides most recent values and flash time in minutes that have elapsed since the measurement occurred (see illustration).

Clinical Decision Point *If unable to obtain blood pressure with electronic device, verify machine connections (e.g., plugged into working electrical outlet, hose-cuff connections tight, machine on, correct cuff). Repeat electronic blood pressure; if unable to obtain, use auscultatory technique (see Skill 5.5).*

14. Set frequency of measurements and upper and lower alarm limits for systolic, diastolic, and mean blood pressure readings. Intervals between measurements can be set from 1 to 90 minutes. A nurse determines frequency and alarm limits on the basis of patient's acceptable range of blood pressure, nursing judgment, and health care provider order.

15. Obtain additional readings at any time by pressing the start button. Pressing the cancel button immediately deflates the cuff.

16. If frequent measurements are required, the cuff may be left in place. Remove it at least every 2 hours to assess underlying skin integrity and, if possible, alternate measurement sites. Patients with abnormal bleeding tendencies are at risk for microvascular rupture from repeated inflations. When patient no longer requires frequent blood pressure monitoring, remove and clean cuff according to agency policy to reduce transmission of microorganisms.

17. Discuss findings with patient. Perform hand hygiene.

18. Compare electronic blood pressure readings with auscultatory measurements to verify accuracy of electronic device.

19. Record blood pressure and site assessed on vital sign flow sheet or in nurses' notes in electronic health record (EHR) or chart; record any signs or symptoms of blood pressure alterations in narrative form in nurses' notes; report abnormal findings to nurse in charge or health care provider.

20. **Use Teach-Back:** "I want to be sure I explained why you need to keep your arm straight while the machine is taking your blood pressure. Tell me why it is important to remain still." Revise your instruction now or develop a plan for revised patient or family caregiver teaching if patient or family caregiver is not able to teach back correctly.

PROCEDURAL GUIDELINE 5.2 *Measuring Oxygen Saturation (Pulse Oximetry)*

NSO *Nursing Skills Online Airway Management Module / Lesson 6* ▶ *Video Clip*

Pulse oximetry is the noninvasive measurement of arterial blood oxygen saturation, the percent to which hemoglobin is filled with oxygen. A pulse oximeter is a probe with a light-emitting diode (LED) connected by cable to an oximeter. The LED emits light wavelengths that are absorbed differently by the oxygenated and deoxygenated hemoglobin molecules. The more hemoglobin saturated by oxygen, the higher the oxygen saturation. Normally oxygen saturation (SpO_2) is greater than 95%. A saturation less than 90% is a clinical emergency (WHO, 2011)

Pulse oximetry measurement of SpO_2 is simple and painless and has few of the risks associated with more invasive measurements of oxygen saturation such as arterial blood gas sampling. A vascular, pulsatile area is needed to detect the change in the transmitted light when making measurements with a finger or earlobe probe. Conditions that decrease arterial blood flow such as peripheral vascular disease, hypothermia, pharmacological vasoconstrictors, hypotension, or peripheral edema affect accurate determination of oxygen saturation in these areas. For patients with decreased peripheral perfusion, you can apply a forehead sensor. Factors that affect light transmission such as outside light sources or patient motion also affect the measurement of oxygen saturation. Carbon monoxide in the blood, jaundice, and intravascular dyes can influence the light reflected from hemoglobin molecules.

In adults you can apply reusable and disposable oximeter probes to the earlobe, finger, toe, bridge of the nose, or forehead (Box 5.8). Pulse oximetry is indicated in patients who have an unstable oxygen status or are at risk for impaired gas exchange.

Delegation and Collaboration
The skill of SpO_2 measurement can be delegated to nursing assistive personnel (NAP). The nurse instructs the NAP by:
- Communicating specific factors related to the patient that can falsely lower SpO_2.
- Informing NAP about appropriate sensor site and probe.
- Notifying frequency of SpO_2 measurements for a specific patient.
- Instructing to notify nurse immediately of any reading lower than SpO_2 of 95% or value for specific patient.
- Instructing to refrain from using pulse oximetry to obtain heart rate because oximeter will not detect an irregular pulse.

Equipment
- Oximeter
- Oximeter probe appropriate for patient and recommended by oximeter manufacturer
- Acetone or nail-polish remover if needed
- Pen and vital sign flow sheet in chart or electronic health record (EHR)

Procedural Steps
1. Identify patient using at least two identifiers (e.g., name and birthday or name and medical record number) according to agency policy (TJC, 2016).
2. Determine need to measure patient's oxygen saturation. Assess risk factors for decreased oxygen saturation (e.g.,

---

BOX 5.8

Characteristics of Pulse Oximeter Sensor Probes and Sites

Finger Probe
- Easy to apply, conforms to various sizes

Earlobe Probe
- Clip-on smaller and lighter, although more positional than finger probe
- Yields strong correlation with oxygen saturation
- Good when uncontrollable or rhythmic movements (e.g., hand tremors during exercise) are present
- Vascular bed least affected by decreased blood flow

Forehead Sensor
- Greater accuracy during decreased perfusion (Nesseler et al., 2012)
- Reliable for patients on vasoactive medications
- Detects desaturation quicker than other sites (Yont et al., 2011)
- Does not require a pulsatile vascular bed
- Good when uncontrollable or rhythmic movements (e.g., hand tremors) are present
- Requires headband to secure sensor

Disposable Sensor Pad
- Can be applied to a variety of sites: earlobe of adult, nose bridge, palm or sole of infant
- Less restrictive for continuous oxygen saturation monitoring
- Expensive
- Contains latex
- Skin under adhesive may become moist and harbor pathogens
- Available in variety of sizes; pad can be matched to infant weight

---

acute or chronic compromised respiratory problems, change in oxygen therapy, chest wall injury, recovery from anesthesia).

3. Perform hand hygiene. Assess for signs and symptoms of alterations in oxygen saturation (e.g., altered respiratory rate, depth, or rhythm; adventitious breath sounds [see Chapter 6]; cyanotic nails, lips, mucous membranes, or skin; restlessness; difficulty breathing).

4. Determine if patient has a latex allergy; disposable adhesive sensors are made of latex.

5. Assess for factors that influence measurement of SpO_2 (e.g., oxygen therapy, respiratory therapy such as postural drainage and percussion; hemoglobin level, hypotension, temperature, nail polish [Chan et al., 2013], and medications such as bronchodilators).

6. Review patient's medical record for health care provider's order or consult agency procedure manual for standard of care for measurement of SpO_2.

7. Determine previous baseline SpO_2 (if available) from patient's record.

PROCEDURAL GUIDELINE 5.2 *Measuring Oxygen Saturation (Pulse Oximetry)—cont'd*

8. Perform hand hygiene. Determine most appropriate patient-specific site (e.g., finger, earlobe, bridge of nose, forehead) for sensor probe placement by measuring capillary refill (see Chapter 6). If capillary refill is greater than 2 seconds, select alternative site.
  - Site must have adequate local circulation and be free of moisture.
  - A finger free of black or brown nail polish is preferred (Chan et al., 2013).
  - If patient has tremors or is likely to move, use earlobe or forehead. Motion artifact is the most common cause of inaccurate readings (Chan et al., 2013).
  - If patient's finger is too large for the clip on probe, as may be the case with obesity or edema, the clip-on probe may not fit properly; obtain a disposable (tape-on) probe.

9. Arrange equipment at the bedside.

10. Position patient comfortably. Instruct him or her to breathe normally.

11. Attach sensor to monitoring site (see illustration). If using finger, remove fingernail polish from digit with acetone or polish remover. Instruct patient that clip-on probe will feel like a clothespin on the finger but will not hurt.

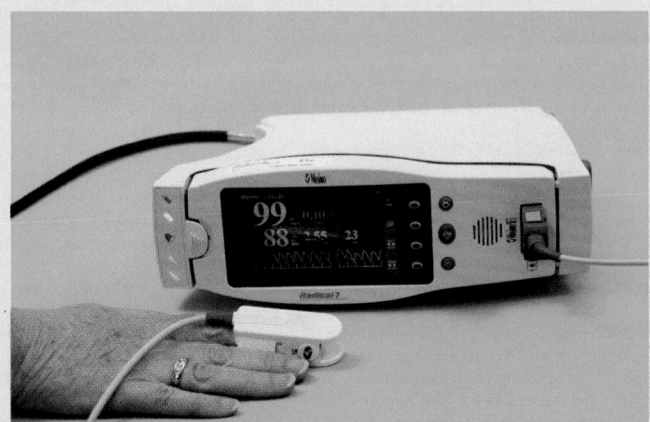

STEP 11 Oximeter sensor attached to finger.

Clinical Decision Point *Do not attach probe to finger, ear, or bridge of nose if area is edematous or skin integrity is compromised. Do not use earlobe and bridge of nose sensors for infants and toddlers because of skin fragility. Do not attach sensor to fingers that are hypothermic. Select ear or bridge of nose if adult patient has a history of peripheral vascular disease. Do not use disposable adhesive sensors if patient has a latex allergy. Do not place sensor on same extremity as electronic blood pressure cuff because blood flow to finger will be interrupted temporarily when cuff inflates and cause inaccurate reading that can trigger alarms (Skirton et al., 2011).*

12. Once sensor is in place, turn on oximeter by activating power. Observe pulse waveform/intensity display and audible beep. Correlate oximeter pulse rate with patient's radial pulse.

13. Leave sensor in place 10 to 30 seconds or until oximeter readout reaches constant value and pulse display reaches full strength during each cardiac cycle. Inform patient that oximeter alarm will sound if sensor falls off or patient moves it. Read SpO$_2$ on digital display.

14. If you plan to monitor SpO$_2$ continuously, verify SpO$_2$ alarm limits preset by manufacturer at a low of 85% and a high of 100%. Determine limits for SpO$_2$ and pulse rate as indicated by patient's condition. Verify that alarms are on. Assess skin integrity under sensor probe every 2 hours; relocate sensor at least every 4 hours and more frequently if skin integrity is altered or tissue perfusion compromised.

15. If you plan intermittent or spot-checking of SpO$_2$, remove probe and turn oximeter power off. Clean sensor and store sensor in appropriate location.

16. Discuss findings with patient. Perform hand hygiene.

17. Compare SpO$_2$ with patient's previous baseline and acceptable SpO$_2$.

18. Record SpO$_2$ on vital sign flow sheet in chart or EHR; indicate type and amount of oxygen therapy used by patient during assessment; record any signs or symptoms of alterations in oxygen saturation in narrative form in nurses' notes in EHR or chart.

19. Report abnormal findings to nurse in charge or health care provider.

20. **Use Teach-Back:** "I want to be sure I explained why you need to keep the probe on your finger. Tell me why this measurement is important and how moving your finger affects reading." Revise your instruction now or develop a plan for revised patient or family caregiver teaching if patient or family caregiver is not able to teach back correctly.

◆ CLINICAL DEBRIEF

Mr. Augsten is a 56-year-old unmarried university professor who is admitted from the trauma unit following a motorcycle-automobile accident. Mr. Augsten has a fractured left humerus and pelvis. Although he was wearing a helmet, he suffered a concussion. When doing your admission assessment, you note a cast on his left arm and an intravenous (IV) line in his right antecubital fossa. His sister is present and tells you that Mr. Augsten is on a beta-blocker for mild hypertension. He received IV opioids (morphine sulfate 15 mg) in the emergency department and is very sleepy. He awakens only to touch.

1. Which admission vital signs can you assign to the nursing assistive personnel (NAP)? Which directions do you provide the NAP regarding obtaining routine vital signs for this patient?
2. An hour after admission the patient has stabilized. One hour later the NAP reports that the radial pulse rate for Mr. Augsten is 54 beats/min. You note that the emergency department nurse recorded a heart rate of 108. What might explain the change in heart rate? Which interventions should you consider at this time?
3. Two hours after admission the NAP reports a respiratory rate of 12, oxygen saturation 90, blood pressure 112/60, pulse 92. You repeat and confirm these vital signs and note that the patient is very difficult to rouse. Using SBAR, show how you would communicate with the health care team about this patient.

◆ REVIEW QUESTIONS

1. Which of the following conditions would create a falsely elevated blood pressure measurement? (Select all that apply.)
    1. Arm positioned above heart level
    2. Deflating the cuff too slowly
    3. Inflating the cuff too fast
    4. Loose-fitting cuff
    5. Using an adult cuff on a toddler
2. Which of the sites below is used to auscultate the heart rate at the point of maximal impulse (PMI)?

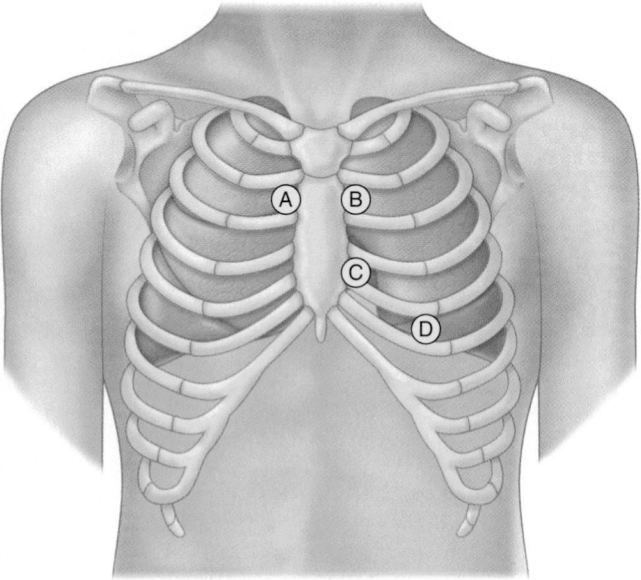

    1. A
    2. B
    3. C
    4. D

3. Which of the following conditions can cause an error in SpO_2 measurement? (Select all that apply.)
    1. Probe placed on finger with clear pink nail polish
    2. Finger probe on patient with a temperature of 35°C (95°F)
    3. Ear probe on patient with a temperature of 38.5°C (101.3°F)
    4. Foot probe on infant who is actively moving
    5. Forehead probe on patient who is perspiring

ⓔ *Visit the Evolve site for a complete list of Clinical Debrief and Review Questions answers.*

REFERENCES

Angelousi A, et al: Association between orthostatic hypotension and cardiovascular risk, cerebrovascular risk, cognitive decline and falls as well as overall mortality: a systematic review and meta-analysis, *J Hypertens* 32:1562, 2014.

Chan E, et al: Pulse oximetry: understanding its basic principles facilitates appreciation of its limitations, *Respir Med* 107:789, 2013.

Charafeddine L, et al: Axillary and rectal thermometry in the newborn: Do they agree? *BMC Res Notes* 31(7):584, 2014.

Counts D, et al: Evaluation of temporal artery and disposable digital oral thermometers in acutely ill patients, *Med Surg Nurs* 23(4):239, 2014.

Frese EM, et al: Blood pressure measurement guidelines for physical therapists, *Cardiopulm Phys Ther J* 22(2):5, 2011.

Giger JN: *Transcultural nursing: assessment and intervention*, ed 6, St Louis, 2013, Mosby.

Goforth C, Kazman J: Exertional heat stroke in navy and marine personnel: a hot topic, *Crit Care Nurse* 35(1):52, 2015.

Haugan B, et al: Can we trust the new generation of infrared tympanic thermometers in clinical practice? *J Clin Nurs* 22:698, 2012.

Hockenberry MJ, Wilson D: *Wong's nursing care of infants and children*, ed 10, St Louis, 2015, Mosby.

James P, et al: 2014 Evidence-based guideline for the management of high blood pressure in adults: report from the panel members appointed to the Eighth Joint National Committee (JNC8), *JAMA* 311:507, 2014.

Kaplan N, et al: Overview of hypertension in adults, UpToDate, 2015, http://www.uptodate.com/contents/overview-of-hypertension-in-adults. Accessed March 12, 2015.

Ki J, et al: Differences in blood pressure measurements obtained using an automatic oscillometric sphygmomanometer depending on clothes-wearing status, *Korean J Fam Med* 34:145, 2013.

Longtin Y, et al: Contamination of stethoscopes and physicians' hands after a physical examination, *Mayo Clin Proc* 89(3):291, 2014.

Mazerolle SM, et al: Is oral temperature an accurate measurement of deep body temperature? A systematic review, *J Athl Train* 46(5):566, 2011.

Mourad J, et al: Impact of miscuffing during home blood pressure measurement on the prevalence of masked hypertension, *Am J Hypertens* 26:1205, 2013.

Nesseler N, et al: Pulse oximetry and high-dose vasopressors: a comparison between forehead reflectance and finger transmission sensors, *Intensive Care Med* 38:1718, 2012.

Ozdemir H, et al: A comparison of different methods of temperature measurements in sick newborns, *J Trop Pediatr* 57:418, 2011.

Pinar R, et al: The effect of clothes on sphygmomanometric blood pressure measurement in hypertensive patients, *J Clin Nurs* 19:1861, 2010.

Reynolds M, et al: Are temporal artery temperatures accurate enough to replace rectal temperature measurement in pediatric ED patients? *J Emerg Nurs* 40:46, 2014.

Shibao C, et al: Evaluation and treatment of orthostatic hypotension, *J Am Soc Hypertens* 7:317, 2013.

Skirton H, et al: A systematic review of variability and reliability of manual and automated blood pressure readings, *J Clin Nurs* 20:614, 2011.

Suokhrie L, et al: Differences in automated and manual blood pressure measurement in hospitalized psychiatric patients, *J Psychosoc Nurs Ment Health Serv* 51(3):32, 2013.

The Joint Commission (TJC): 2016 National Patient Safety Goals, 2016, http://www.jointcommission.org/standards_information/npsgs.aspx. Accessed March 12, 2016.

World Health Organization (WHO): *Pulse oximetry training manual*, 2011, World Health Organization. http://www.who.int/patientsafety/safesurgery/pulse_oximetry/who_ps_pulse_oximetry_training_manual_en.pdf. Accessed March 12, 2016.

Yont GH, et al: Comparison of oxygen saturation values and measurement times by pulse oximetry in various parts of the body, *Appl Nurs Res* 24(4):e39, 2011.

Zheng D, et al: How important is the recommended slow cuff pressure deflation rate for blood pressure measurement? *Ann Biomed Eng* 39:2584, 2011.

Zheng D, et al: Effect of respiration, talking and small body movements on blood pressure measurement, *J Human Hypertens* 26:458, 2012.

6 | Health Assessment

OBJECTIVES

Mastery of content in this chapter will enable the nurse to:
- Discuss the purposes of health assessment.
- Describe the techniques used with each physical assessment skill.
- Describe proper patient positioning during each phase of the examination.
- Describe how to conduct a physical examination on patients from diverse cultures.
- List techniques to promote a patient's physical and psychological comfort during an examination.
- Make environmental preparations before an assessment.
- Identify data to collect from the nursing history before an examination.
- Discuss normal physical findings for patients across the life span.
- Discuss ways to incorporate health promotion and health teaching into an assessment.
- Identify self-screening assessments commonly performed by patients.
- Identify preventive screenings and the appropriate age(s) for each screening.
- Use physical assessment techniques and skills during routine nursing care.
- Document assessment findings on appropriate forms.
- Communicate abnormal findings to appropriate personnel.

MEDIA RESOURCES

- evolve http://evolve.elsevier.com/Perry/skills
- Review Questions
- Audio Glossary
- ▶ Video Clips
- Animations
- Case Studies
- Clinical Debrief and Review Questions Answers

PURPOSE

Systematic physical assessments are regularly performed by nurses to assess the status of a patient's health and his or her perception of health. The information gathered is documented in the patient's database.

STANDARDS OF CARE

- Agency for Healthcare Research and Quality (AHRQ), 2014—Prevention of Skin Cancer
- The American Cancer Society (ACS), 2015a, 2015b, 2015c, 2015d, 2015e—Cancer Prevention and Early Detection
- The Joint Commission (TJC), 2016—National Patient Safety Goals

PRINCIPLES FOR PRACTICE

- Use ongoing objective and comprehensive assessment to promote continuity of care.
- An admission assessment involves a detailed review of a patient's condition and includes a nursing history and behavioral and physical examination.
- Use open-ended questions and be sure that patients have exhausted their descriptions. For example, as a patient is describing a symptom, you can say "go on" to encourage more information sharing.
- Use critical thinking skills for evaluation and interpretation of findings.
- Initial assessment and examination provide a baseline for a patient's functional status and serve as a comparison for future

assessment findings. In addition, the information is useful in making clinical decisions about the management of a patient's health problems.

- Ensure patient safety and confidentiality.

PATIENT-CENTERED CARE

- Conduct a patient-centered interview to learn about problems from the patient's perspective.
- Show respect to patients and their families in seeking their involvement in the patient's plan of care.
- Have patients explain their symptoms by allowing them to offer details.
- After gathering data, group significant findings into patterns of data (clusters) that reveal actual or potential nursing diagnoses (Table 6.1).
- Be open to constant informing, communicating, and educating patients and family caregivers regarding patient care.
- Integrate health promotion and education into physical assessment activities. It is an ideal time to offer individualized patient teaching and to encourage promotion of health practices such as breast (Box 6.1) and genital (see Box 6.6) self-examination.
- A patient should understand any symptoms with which he or she presents and symptoms for which to look in detecting problems. For example, educate patients about the American Cancer Society (ACS) guidelines (2015b, 2015f) for early detection of breast and genital cancers.
- Ensure that patient is comfortable and free from pain.
- Provide emotional support.
- Respect patients' cultural diversity and beliefs when completing a physical assessment (Drenkard, 2014).
- Communicate respect through proper use of distance, attention, eye contact, tone, and loudness of voice.
- Use a professional interpreter familiar with a patient's culture and language.
- Obtain information about health risks common to a cultural group. Certain diseases are prevalent in some groups.

- Use gender-congruent health care providers to perform a physical assessment.
- Ask permission before you touch a patient.
- Drape a patient thoroughly and use the bedside screen or curtains.

EVIDENCE-BASED PRACTICE

Agencies such as the Agency for Healthcare Research and Quality (AHRQ), the ACS, and the US Preventative Services Task Force (USPSTF) conduct ongoing research and develop practice guidelines regarding prevention and management of certain diseases such as skin cancer. The ACS (2015e) recommends that people engage in regular skin self-examination (SSE) and protect themselves from ultraviolet rays. Risk factors for melanoma include fair skin that freckles or burns easily, red or blond hair, blue or green eyes, long-term treatment with ultraviolet light, and a first-degree relative having melanoma.

- Complete monthly skin examination, reporting any skin changes to their health care provider (AHRQ, 2014).
- Instruct patient to inform health care provider about any new moles, sores that do not heal, or any change in the color, size and shape of existing skin lesions (ACS, 2015e).
- People with high risk factors or previous skin cancers should have an annual comprehensive skin assessment by a dermatologist (ACS, 2015e).
- Stay in the shade and wear wraparound sunglasses.
- Use sunscreen liberally and reapply every 2 hours. When applying an SPF 30 sunscreen correctly, 1 hour in the sun is the same as 2 minutes totally unprotected.
- Apply sunscreen under makeup or bug repellent.
- Wear protective clothing (dark colors). Wear a hat with a 2 to 3 inch brim.
- Do not use tanning beds and sunlamps.

SAFETY GUIDELINES

- Prioritize an assessment on the basis of a patient's presenting signs and symptoms or health care needs. For example, when a patient develops sudden shortness of breath, first assess the lungs and thorax. If a patient is acutely ill, you may choose to assess only the involved body systems. Use judgment to ensure that an examination is relevant and inclusive.
- Organize an examination. Compare both sides of the body for symmetry. If a patient becomes fatigued, offer rest periods. Perform painful or intrusive procedures near the end of an examination.
- Use a head-to-toe approach following the sequence of inspection, palpation, percussion, and auscultation (except during abdominal assessment). This sequence facilitates an effective assessment.
- Encourage a patient's active participation. Patients usually know about their physical condition. Often a patient can let you know when certain findings are normal or when there have been changes.
- Follow standard precautions for infection control. During an assessment you may have contact with body fluids and discharge. Always wear clean gloves when there are breaks in the skin, lesions, or wounds or when having contact with mucous membranes. In some circumstances you will need to wear a gown and face/eye protection.

TABLE 6.1			
Development of Individualized Nursing Diagnoses			
Assessment Method	**Findings**	**Patterns**	**Nursing Diagnosis**
Inspection of skin	Skin along sacral area is intact. There is a 3-cm area of redness around coccyx; skin blanches on palpation. No skin lesions are observed.	There is tissue injury area around coccyx.	Risk for impaired skin integrity
Palpation of skin	Skin is moist from diaphoresis. There is tenderness to palpation at sacral area. Skin turgor is elastic.	Skin moisture promotes maceration.	
Historical data	Patient suffered fractured left leg. Patient is immobilized because of left leg traction.	Continued pressure is exerted over sacrum.	

BOX 6.1

Breast Self-Examination

According to the American Cancer Society (ACS) (2015b), screening refers to tests and examinations used to find a disease such as cancer in people who do not have any symptoms. Although research does not support a clear benefit of regular breast self-examination (BSE), it is important for all women to be familiar with their breasts' normal appearance and feel. A BSE is optional for women starting in their 20s (ACS, 2015b). Women should be told about the benefits and limitations of BSE and report any breast changes to their health professional right away.

Breast self-exam plays a small role in finding breast cancer compared with finding a breast lump by chance or simply being aware of what is normal for each woman. Some women feel very comfortable doing BSE regularly (usually monthly after their period), which involves a systematic step-by-step approach to examining the look and feel of their breasts. Other women are more comfortable simply looking at and feeling their breasts in a less systematic approach (e.g., while showering or getting dressed or doing an occasional thorough examination (ACS, 2015b). Familiarity makes it easier to notice any changes in the breast from one month to another. Early discovery of a change from what is "normal" is the main idea behind BSE.

For women who menstruate, the best time to do BSE is 2 or 3 days after a period ends, when the breasts are least likely to be tender or swollen. For women who no longer menstruate, pick a day such as the first day of the month to remind yourself to do BSE.

Procedure

1. Stand before a mirror. Inspect both breasts for anything unusual such as skin redness; any discharge from the nipples; puckering, dimpling, or scaling of the skin.

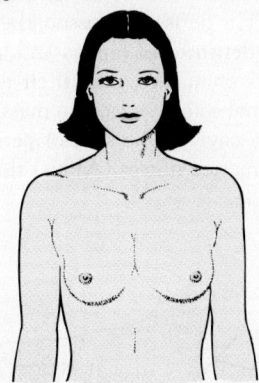

2. While in front of the mirror, press hands firmly on hips, look at your breasts, observing for any changes in size, shape, contour, dimpling, or redness or scaliness of the nipple or breasts tissue. Pressing down on your hips contracts the chest wall muscles and enhances and breast changes.

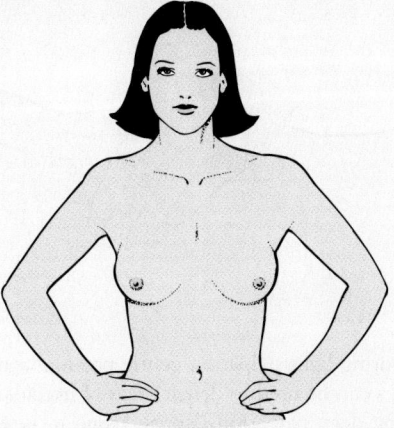

3. Examine your right breast. Lie down on your back and place your right arm behind your head. When you lie down versus standing, the breast tissue spreads evenly over the chest wall and is as thin as possible, making it much easier to feel all the breast tissue.

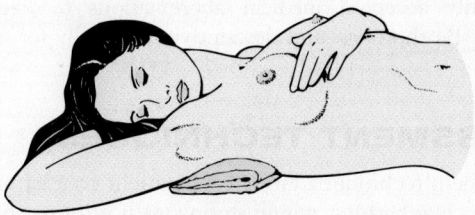

4. Use finger pads of the three middle fingers on your left hand to feel for lumps in the right breast. Use overlapping dime-sized circular motions of the finger pads to feel the breast tissue. Use three different types of pressure: light pressure to feel tissue closest to the skin, medium pressure to feel a little deeper, and firm pressure to feel tissue close to the chest and ribs. It is normal to feel a firm ridge in the lower curve of each breast. If you feel anything out of the ordinary, tell your health care provider.

5. Using your finger pads, move around the breast in an up-and-down pattern starting at an imaginary line drawn straight down your side from your underarm and moving across the breast to the middle of the chest bone (sternum or breastbone). Be sure to check the entire breast area, going down until you feel only ribs and up to the neck or collarbone (clavicle).

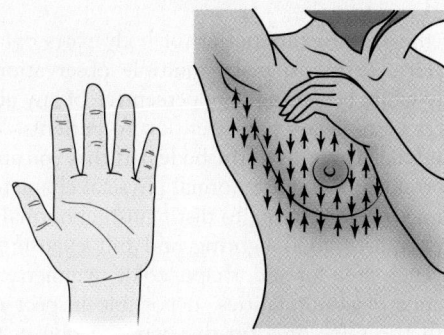

6. Repeat examination in the left breast, putting your left arm behind your head, and examine the left breast (see Steps 3-5).

7. Instruct patient to call the health care provider if she finds a lump or other abnormality.

8. **Use Teach-Back:** "I want to be sure I explained to you how to do a breast self-examination. Show me how to examine both of your breasts." Document your evaluation of patient learning. Revise your instruction now or develop a plan for revised patient teaching if patient is not able to teach back correctly.

From American Cancer Society (ACS): *American Cancer Society recommendations for early breast cancer detection in women without breast symptoms,* Atlanta, 2015, The Society. http://www.cancer.org/cancer/breastcancer/moreinformation/breastcancerearlydetection/breast-cancer-early-detection-acs-recs, accessed October 26, 2015; Ball JW et al: *Seidel's guide to physical examination,* ed 8, St Louis, 2015, Mosby.

- Consider the possibility of latex allergy. The incidence of serious allergic reaction to latex has increased dramatically (Ball et al., 2015).
- Record quick notes to facilitate accurate documentation. Inform a patient that you will be recording the data.
- Record a summary of the assessment using appropriate medical terminology and in the sequence that findings are gathered. Use commonly accepted medical abbreviations to keep notes concise. Be thorough and descriptive, especially for abnormal findings.

ASSESSMENT TECHNIQUES

Use assessment techniques during each patient contact, including activities such as bathing, administering medications, other therapies, or while talking with a patient. This practice will help you learn to become more observant and better able to identify changes quickly.

Inspection, palpation, percussion, auscultation, and olfaction are the five basic assessment techniques. Each skill allows you to collect a broad range of physical data about patients. Nurses need experience to recognize normal variations among patients and ranges of normal for an individual. Remember, cultural diversity is one factor that influences both normal variations and potential alterations that you may find during an assessment. It is important to take the time needed to carefully assess each body part. Hurrying causes you to overlook significant signs and make incorrect conclusions about a patient's condition.

Inspection

Inspection is the visual examination of body parts or areas. An experienced nurse learns to make multiple observations almost simultaneously while becoming very perceptive of any abnormalities. The secret is to always pay attention to patients. Watch all movements and look carefully at the body part that you are inspecting. It is important to recognize normal physical characteristics of patients of all ages before trying to distinguish abnormal findings.

Inspection requires good lighting and full exposure of body parts. Inspect each area for size, shape, color, symmetry, position, and the presence of abnormalities. If possible inspect each area compared with the same area on the opposite side of the body. When necessary, use additional light such as a penlight to inspect body cavities such as the mouth and throat. *Do not hurry. Pay attention to detail.* Verify and clarify all abnormalities with subjective patient data. In other words, ask the patient for further information about each abnormality or change such as whether the change is recent.

Palpation

Palpation uses the sense of touch. Through palpation the hands make delicate and sensitive measurements of specific physical signs. It detects resistance, resilience, roughness, texture, temperature, moisture, and mobility. You often use it with or after visual inspection. You will use different parts of the hand to detect specific characteristics. For example, the dorsum (back) of the hand is sensitive to temperature variations. The pads of the fingertips detect subtle changes in texture, shape, size, consistency, and pulsation of body parts. The palm of the hand is especially sensitive to vibration. You measure position, consistency, and turgor by lightly grasping a body part with the fingertips.

Help a patient relax and assume a comfortable position because muscle tension during palpation impairs the ability to palpate correctly. Asking a patient to take slow, deep breaths enhances muscle

relaxation. Palpate tender areas last because they could cause a patient to become tense and impede the assessment. Ask a patient to point out areas that are more sensitive and note any nonverbal signs of discomfort. Patients appreciate clean, warm hands; short fingernails; and a gentle approach. Palpation is either light or deep and is controlled by the amount of pressure applied with the fingers or hand. Light palpation precedes deep palpation. Consider a patient's condition, the area being palpated, and the reason for using palpation. For example, when a patient is admitted to the emergency department after an automobile accident, consider the factors surrounding the patient's injury and inspect the chest wall carefully before performing any palpation around the area of the ribs.

For light palpation apply pressure slowly, gently, and deliberately, depressing approximately 1 cm ($\frac{1}{2}$ inch) (Fig. 6.1A). Check tender areas further, using light, intermittent pressure. After light palpation you may use deeper palpation to examine the condition of organs (Fig. 6.1B). Depress the area that you are examining by approximately 2 cm (0.8 inch). Caution is the rule. Bimanual palpation involves one hand placed over the other while applying pressure. The upper hand exerts downward pressure as the other hand feels the subtle characteristics of underlying organs and masses. Seek the help of a qualified instructor before attempting deep palpation.

Percussion

Percussion involves tapping the body with the fingertips to vibrate underlying tissues and organs. The vibration travels through body tissues, and the character of the resulting sound reflects the density of underlying tissue. The denser the tissue, the quieter is the sound. By knowing various densities of organs and body parts, you learn how to locate organs or masses, map their edges, and determine their size. An abnormal sound suggests a mass or substance such as air or fluid in a body cavity. The skill of percussion is used more often by advanced practice nurses (APNs) than by nurses in daily practice at the bedside.

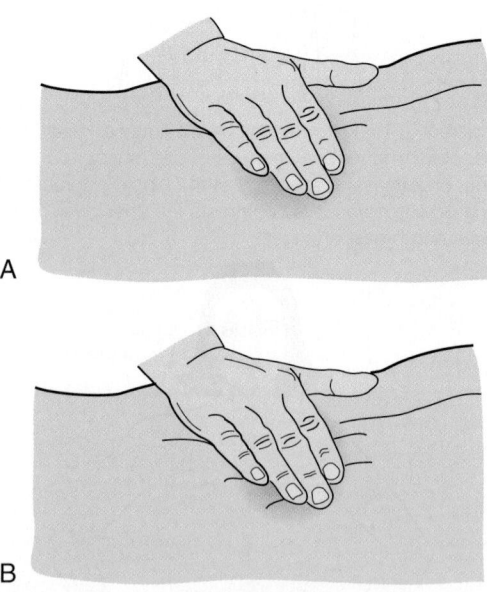

A

B

FIG 6.1 A, During light palpation gentle pressure against underlying skin and tissues can be used to detect areas of irregularity and tenderness. **B,** During deep palpation depress tissue to assess condition of underlying organs. (*From Ball JW et al: Seidel's guide to physical examination, ed 8, St Louis, 2015, Mosby.*)

The most commonly used percussion technique is the indirect technique. You perform the indirect technique by placing the middle finger of your nondominant hand firmly against the body surface. With palm and fingers remaining off the skin, the tip of the middle finger of the dominant hand strikes the base of the distal joint of the finger (Fig. 6.2). Use a quick, sharp stroke, keeping the forearm stationary. Relax the wrist to deliver the proper blow. Once the finger has struck, the wrist snaps back. If the blow is not sharp, if the hand is held loosely, or if the palm rests on the body surface, the sound is softened; and you will not detect the presence of underlying structures. A light, quick blow produces the clearest sounds. Table 6.2 describes the five different percussion sounds.

Auscultation

Auscultation is listening with a stethoscope to sounds produced by the body. To auscultate correctly, listen in a quiet environment for both the presence of sound and its characteristics. To be successful in auscultation, you must first recognize normal sounds from each body structure, including the passage of blood through an artery, heart sounds, and movement of air through the lungs. These sounds vary according to the location in which they can be heard most easily. Likewise you become familiar with areas that normally do not emit sounds. Practice listening to many normal sounds so you can recognize abnormal sounds when they arise.

To auscultate you need good hearing acuity, a good stethoscope, and knowledge of how to use the stethoscope properly (Box 6.2). Nurses with hearing disorders may purchase stethoscopes with

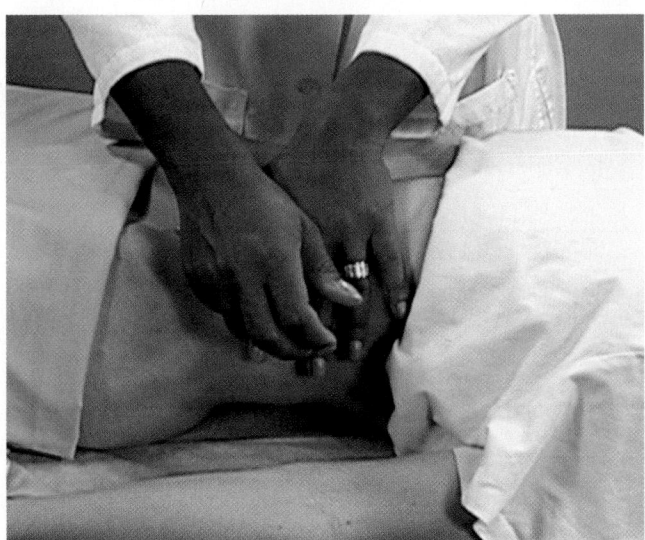

FIG 6.2 Percussion technique: tapping the interphalangeal joint. *(From Ball JW et al: Seidel's guide to physical examination, ed 8, St Louis, 2015, Mosby.)*

greater sound amplification and may need to ask colleagues to verify some findings through auscultation. It is essential to place the stethoscope directly on a patient's skin because clothing obscures and changes sound. Through auscultation the nurse notes that there are four characteristics of sound:

- *Frequency:* Number of sound wave cycles generated per second by a vibrating object. The higher the frequency, the higher the pitch of a sound and vice versa.
- *Loudness:* Amplitude of a sound wave. Auscultated sounds are described as loud or soft.
- *Quality:* Sounds of similar frequency and loudness from different sources. Terms such as *blowing* or *gurgling* describe quality of sound.
- *Duration:* Length of time that sound vibrations last. Duration of sound is short, medium, or long. Layers of soft tissue dampen the duration of sounds from deep internal organs.

A nurse cannot be successful at auscultation without knowing how to use a stethoscope properly. Chapter 5 describes the parts of the acoustic stethoscope and use of the bell and diaphragm.

Olfaction

Olfaction uses the sense of smell to detect abnormalities that go unrecognized by any other means. Some alterations in body function and certain bacteria create characteristic odors (Table 6.3).

PREPARATION FOR ASSESSMENT

Preparation of the environment, equipment, and patient facilitates a smooth assessment. Provide patients privacy to promote their comfort and the efficiency of an examination. In a health care agency close the door and pull privacy curtains. In the home examine the patient in the bedroom. A comfortable environment includes a warm, comfortable temperature; a loose-fitting gown or pajamas for a patient; adequate direct lighting; control of outside noises; and precautions to prevent interruptions by visitors or other health care personnel. If possible, place the bed or examination table at waist level so you can assess a patient easily. During an examination you must protect a patient from falls and injury and return the bed to a safe height at the completion of the assessment (TJC, 2016).

Preparing the Patient

Prepare patients both physically and psychologically for accurate assessments. A tense, anxious patient may have difficulty understanding, following directions, or cooperating with your instructions. To prepare a patient:

- Provide privacy.
- Implement comfort measures (e.g., positioning, hygiene) and provide the opportunity to empty the bowel or bladder (a good time to collect needed specimens).

TABLE 6.2					
Sounds Produced by Percussion					
Sound	**Intensity**	**Pitch**	**Duration**	**Quality**	**Common Location**
Tympany	Loud	High	Moderate	Drumlike	Gastric air bubble, puffed-out cheek
Resonant	Loud	Low	Long	Hollow	Healthy lung
Hyperresonant	Very loud	Low	Longer than resonance	Booming	Emphysematous lung
Dull	Soft to moderate	Moderate to high	Moderate	Thudlike	Over liver
Flat	Soft	High	Short	Very dull	Over muscle

Using a Stethoscope

1. Place earpieces in both ears with tips of earpieces turned toward the face. *Lightly* blow against the diaphragm (flat side of chest piece). Now place the earpieces in both ears with the tips turned toward the back of the head and again blow against the diaphragm. Compare comfort in the ears and amplification of sounds with earpieces in both directions. After you have learned the right fit for the loudest amplification, wear the stethoscope the same way each time. Earpieces should fit snugly and comfortably.

2. If the stethoscope has both a diaphragm (flat side) and a bell (bowl shaped with a rubber ring), put earpieces in ears and lightly blow against the diaphragm. The chest piece can be turned to allow sound to be carried through either side (bell or diaphragm). If sound is faint, lightly blow into the bell. Then turn the chest piece and blow again against both the diaphragm and the bell. The diaphragm is used for higher-pitched heart sounds, bowel sounds, and lung sounds. The bell is used for lower-pitched heart sounds and vascular sounds.

3. With earpieces in place and using the diaphragm, move the diaphragm lightly over the hair on your arm. The bristling sound mimics a sound heard in the lungs. When listening for significant sounds, hold the diaphragm still and firmly make a tight seal against the skin to eliminate extraneous sounds.

4. Place the diaphragm over the front of your chest directly on your skin and listen to your own breathing, comparing the bell and the diaphragm. Repeat the process while listening to your own heartbeat. Ask someone to speak in a conversational tone and note how the speech detracts from hearing clearly. When using a stethoscope, both you and the patient should remain quiet.

5. With the earpieces in your ears, gently tap the tubing. Note that it generates extraneous sounds. When listening to a patient, maintain a position that allows the tubing to extend straight and hang free. Movement may allow it to rub or bump objects, creating extraneous sounds. Kinked tubing muffles sounds.

6. *Care of a stethoscope:* Remove earpieces regularly and clean or remove cerumen (earwax). Keep the bell and diaphragm free of dust, lint, and body oils. Keep the tubing away from your body oils. Avoid draping the stethoscope around the neck next to the skin. To clean, wipe the entire stethoscope (e.g., diaphragm, tubing) with alcohol or soapy water. Be sure to dry all parts thoroughly. Follow manufacturer recommendations.

7. *Infection control:* Harmful bacteria, even antibiotic-resistant microorganisms, can be transferred from patient to patient when using portable equipment such as stethoscopes (Shiferaw et al., 2013). Follow agency infection control guidelines, especially contact precautions, to decrease this risk. Clean a stethoscope (diaphragm/bell) with a disinfectant before reuse on another patient. Using a disinfectant such as isopropyl alcohol (with or without chlorhexidine), benzalkonium, and sodium hypochlorite is effective in reducing the number of bacterial colonies. Earpieces of stethoscopes are also sources of transferable bacteria when you inadvertently touch your ears and then care for a patient. Potential pathogens could contaminate earpieces. Using hand hygiene before and after patient contact decreases the risk of transmitting microorganisms from your ear to your patient (Shiferaw et al., 2013).

Assessment of Characteristic Odors

Odor	Site or Source	Potential Causes
Alcohol	Oral cavity	Ingestion of alcohol; diabetes mellitus
Ammonia	Urine	Urinary tract infection, renal failure
Body odor	Skin, particularly in areas where body parts rub together (e.g., under arms, beneath breasts, perineal area) Wound site Vomitus	Poor hygiene, excess perspiration (hyperhidrosis), foul-smelling perspiration (bromhidrosis) Wound abscess; infection Abdominal irritation, contaminated food
Feces	Rectal area Vomitus/oral cavity (fecal odor)	Bowel obstruction Fecal incontinence; fistula
Fetid, sweet odor	Tracheostomy or mucus secretions	Infection of bronchial tree (*Pseudomonas* bacteria)
Foul-smelling stools in infants	Stool	Malabsorption syndrome
Halitosis	Oral cavity	Poor dental or oral hygiene, gum disease; sinus infection
Musty odor	Casted body part	Infection inside cast
Stale urine	Skin	Uremic acidosis
Sweet, fruity ketones	Oral cavity	Diabetic acidosis
Sweet, heavy, thick odor	Draining wound	*Pseudomonas* (bacterial) infection

- Minimize a patient's anxiety and fear by conveying an open, receptive, and professional approach. Using simple terms, thoroughly explain what will be done, what the patient should expect to feel, and how he or she can cooperate. Even if a patient appears unresponsive, it is still important to explain your actions.
- Provide access to body parts while draping areas that are not being examined.

- Reduce distractions. Turn down volume or turn off radio or television.
- Eliminate drafts, control room temperature, and provide warm blankets.
- Help patients assume positions during assessments so body parts are accessible and patients stay comfortable (Table 6.4). A patient's ability to assume positions depends on physical

TABLE 6.4

Positions for Physical Assessment

Position	Areas Assessed	Rationale	Limitations
Sitting	Head and neck, back, posterior thorax and lungs, anterior thorax and lungs, breasts, axillae, heart, vital signs, upper extremities	Sitting upright provides full expansion of lungs and better visualization of symmetry of upper body parts.	Physically weakened or developmentally disabled patient is sometimes unable to sit. Use supine position with head of bed elevated instead.
Supine	Head and neck, anterior thorax and lungs, breasts, axillae, heart, abdomen, extremities, pulses	This is most normally relaxed position. It provides easy access to pulse sites.	If patient becomes short of breath easily, raise head of bed.
Dorsal recumbent	Head and neck, anterior thorax and lungs, breasts, axillae, heart, abdomen	Position is for abdominal assessment because it promotes relaxation of abdominal muscles.	Patients with painful disorders are more comfortable with knees flexed.
Lithotomy	Female genitalia and genital tract	This position provides maximal exposure of genitalia and facilitates insertion of vaginal speculum.	Lithotomy position is embarrassing and uncomfortable; thus examiner minimizes time that patient spends in it. Keep patient well draped. Patients with arthritis or other joint deformities may be unable to tolerate the position.
Sims'	Rectum and vagina	Flexion of hip and knee improves exposure of rectal and genitourinary areas.	Joint deformities hinder patient's ability to bend hip and knee.
Prone	Musculoskeletal system	This position is for assessing extension of hip joint, skin, and buttocks.	Patients with respiratory difficulties do not tolerate this position well.
Lateral recumbent	Heart	This position aids in detecting murmurs.	Patients with respiratory difficulties do not tolerate this position well.
Knee-chest	Rectum	This position provides maximal exposure of rectal area.	This position is embarrassing and uncomfortable. Patients with arthritis or other joint deformities may be unable to assume it.

strength and limitations. Some positions are uncomfortable or embarrassing; keep a patient in position no longer than is necessary.

- Pace assessment according to an individual's physical and emotional tolerance.
- Use a relaxed tone of voice and facial expressions to put a patient at ease.

- Encourage a patient to ask questions and report discomfort felt during the examination.
- Have a third person of patient's gender in the room during assessment of genitalia. This prevents a patient from accusing you of behaving in an unethical manner.
- At conclusion of an assessment, ask the patient if there are any concerns or questions.

PHYSICAL ASSESSMENT OF VARIOUS AGE-GROUPS

Children and Adolescents

- Routine assessments of children focus on health promotion and illness prevention, particularly for care of well children with competent parenting and no serious health problems (Hockenberry and Wilson, 2015). Focus on growth and development, sensory screening, dental examination, and behavioral assessment.
- Children who are chronically ill, disabled, in foster care, or foreign-born adopted may require additional assessments because of unique health needs or risks.
- When obtaining histories of infants and children, gather all or part of the information from parents or guardians.
- Parents may think that the examiner is testing or judging them. Offer support during examination and do not pass judgment.
- Call children by their preferred name and address parents as "Mr. and Mrs. Brown" rather than by first names.
- Open-ended questions often allow parents to share more information and describe more of the child's problems.
- Older children and adolescents respond best when treated as adults and individuals and often can provide details about their health history and severity of symptoms.
- The adolescent has a right to confidentiality. After talking with parents about historical information, arrange to be alone with the adolescent to speak privately and perform the examination.

Older Adults

- Do not assume that aging is always accompanied by illness or disability. Older adults are able to adapt to change and maintain functional independence (Touhy and Jett, 2015).
- A thorough assessment of an older adult provides critical information that can be used to maximize independence.
- Provide adequate space for an examination, particularly if a patient uses a mobility aid.
- Plan the history and examination, taking into account an older adult's energy level, physical limitations, pace, and adaptability. You may need more than one session to complete the assessment (Touhy and Jett, 2015).
- Measure performance under the most favorable conditions. Take advantage of natural opportunities for assessment (e.g., during bathing, grooming, mealtime) (Touhy and Jett, 2015).
- Sequence an examination to keep position changes to a minimum. Be efficient throughout the examination to limit patient movement.
- Be sure that an examination of an older adult includes review of mental status.

◆ SKILL 6.1 General Survey

The general survey begins a review of a patient's primary health problems, and it includes assessment of vital signs, height and weight, general behavior, and appearance. It provides information about characteristics of an illness, a patient's hygiene, skin condition and body image, emotional state, recent changes in weight, and developmental status. The survey reveals important information about a patient's behavior that influences how you communicate instructions and continue an assessment.

Delegation and Collaboration

The skill of completing the general survey cannot be delegated to nursing assistive personnel (NAP). The nurse directs the NAP to:
- Measure the patient's height and weight.

- Obtain vital signs (not the initial set, but subsequent measurements if patient is stable).
- Monitor oral intake and urinary output.
- Report a patient's subjective signs and symptoms to the nurse.

Equipment

- Stethoscope
- Sphygmomanometer and cuff
- Thermometer
- Digital watch or wristwatch with second hand
- Tape measure
- Clean gloves (use nonlatex if necessary)
- Tongue blade
- Appropriate electronic record or documentation form

STEP	RATIONALE

ASSESSMENT

1. When beginning a physical examination identify patient using at least two identifiers (e.g., name and birthday or name and account number) according to agency policy.	Ensures correct patient. Complies with The Joint Commission standards and improves patient safety (TJC, 2016).
2. Note if patient has had any acute distress: difficulty breathing, pain, anxiety. If such signs are present, defer general survey until later and focus immediately on affected body system.	Signs establish priorities regarding which part of examination to conduct first.
3. Review graphic sheet for previous vital signs and consider factors or conditions that may alter values (see Chapter 5).	Provides baseline and historical data about patient's vital signs.
4. Determine patient's primary language. If you identify need for an interpreter, determine availability of a professional interpreter. It is best to have an interpreter of the same gender who is older and mature. Have interpreter translate verbatim if possible.	Facilitates patient understanding and promotes accuracy of information provided by patient.

STEP	RATIONALE

5. After reviewing history, confirm primary reason patient has sought health care.

Keeps assessment focused on patient to ensure that his or her expectations are addressed.

6. Identify patient's normal height, weight, and body mass index. If sudden gain or loss in weight has occurred, determine amount of weight change and period of time in which it occurred. Assess if patient has recently been dieting or following an exercise program. Use growth chart for children under 18 years of age.

Generally a body mass index of 25 to 29.9 for men and women is overweight, whereas 30 and over is obese (Ball et al., 2015). Fluid retention is one factor that must be ruled out. A person's weight can fluctuate daily because of fluid loss or retention (1 L of water weighs 1 kg [2.2 lbs]).

7. Ask if patient has noticed any changes in condition of skin (e.g., dryness, changes in color or lack of pigment, changes in moles or new skin lesions).

Skin changes can indicate underlying illnesses (e.g., dry skin may be associated with hypothyroidism, changes in moles may indicate early signs of skin cancers) (see Table 6.5).

8. Review patient's past fluid intake and output (I&O) records.

Fluid and electrolyte balance affects health and function in all body systems. Intake includes all liquids taken orally, by feeding tube, and parenterally. Liquid output includes urine, diarrhea stool, vomitus, drainage from fistulas and gastric suction, and drainage from postsurgical tubes such as chest tubes or Jackson-Pratt drains.

9. Identify patient's general perceptions about personal health.

Assessment of patient's general appearance coupled with patient's own perceptions may reveal specific problem areas.

10. Assess for history of latex allergy, which may include contact dermatitis or systemic reactions. Ask if patient has risk factors such as food allergies (papaya, avocado, banana, peach, kiwi, or tomato); has high latex exposure (housekeepers, food handlers, health care worker); or must avoid products containing latex (rubber bands, adhesive tape, certain paints or carpets).

Gloves are worn during certain aspects of the assessment. Repeated exposure to latex may result in more serious reactions, including asthma, itching, and anaphylaxis (Ball et al., 2014; Ball et al., 2015).

NURSING DIAGNOSES

- Anxiety
- Bathing self-care deficit
- Deficient fluid volume
- Excess fluid volume
- Fear

- Imbalanced nutrition: less than body requirements
- Impaired physical mobility
- Impaired skin integrity
- Ineffective breathing pattern

- Ineffective peripheral tissue perfusion
- Latex allergy response
- Obesity
- Pain (acute, chronic)

Related factors are individualized based on patient's condition or needs.

PLANNING

1. Expected outcomes following completion of procedure:
   - Patient demonstrates alert, cooperative behavior without evidence of physical or emotional distress during assessment.
   - Patient provides appropriate subjective data related to physical condition.

You use calm and confident approach during assessment. Patient has no abnormal findings.

Patient is able to cooperate with assessment.

2. *Prepare patient:* Tell patient that you will be doing routine process to check for areas of concern. Ask patient to tell you if any area that you examine hurts when touched.

Understanding promotes patient's cooperation. Pain is an important finding during assessment.

3. Perform hand hygiene. Assemble necessary equipment. Position patient initially, either sitting or lying supine with head of bed elevated.

Reduces transmission of infection. Promotes efficiency of examination.

IMPLEMENTATION

1. Throughout assessment note patient's verbal and nonverbal behaviors. Determine patient's level of consciousness (LOC) and orientation by observing and talking to him or her (Box 6.3).

Behaviors may reflect specific physical abnormalities. Dementia and LOC influence ability to cooperate.

2. Obtain temperature, pulse, respirations, and blood pressure unless taken within last 3 hours or if serious potential change is noted (e.g., change in LOC or difficulty breathing) (see Chapter 5). Inform patient of vital signs.

Vital signs provide important information regarding physiological changes related to oxygenation and circulation.

STEP	RATIONALE
3. Note patient's gender and race and ask his or her age. Note patient's external physical features.	Gender influences type of examination performed and manner in which you make assessments. Different physical characteristics and predisposition to illnesses are related to gender and race.
4. If uncertain whether patient understands a question, rephrase or ask a similar question.	Inappropriate response from a patient may be caused by language barriers or deterioration of mental status, preoccupation with illness, or decreased hearing acuity.
5. If patient's responses are inappropriate, ask short, to-the-point questions regarding information patient should know (e.g., "Tell me your name." "What is the name of this place?" "Tell me where you live." "What day is this?" "What month is this?" or "What season of the year is this?").	Measures patient's orientation to person, place, and time. You may note this in documentation as "Oriented × 3." If disoriented in any way, include subjective and/or objective data rather than just documenting "disoriented."
6. If patient is unable to respond to questions of orientation, offer simple commands (e.g., "Squeeze my fingers" or "Move your toes.").	LOC exists along a continuum ranging from full responsiveness, to inability to consciously initiate meaningful behaviors, to unresponsiveness to stimuli.
7. Assess affect and mood: Note if verbal expressions match nonverbal behavior and if appropriate to situation.	Reflects patient's mental and emotional status, consciousness, and feelings.
8. Watch patient interact with spouse or partner, older-adult child, or caregiver. Be alert for indications of fear, hesitancy to report health status, or willingness to let caregiver control assessment interview. Does partner or caregiver have a history of violence, alcoholism, or drug abuse? Is person unemployed, ill, or frustrated with caring for a patient? Note if patient has any obvious physical injuries.	Suspect abuse in patients who have suffered obvious physical injury or neglect, show signs of malnutrition, or have ecchymosis (bruises) on extremities or trunk. Health care providers are often the first to identify evidence of abuse because patients may not be able to tell family or friends. Partners or caregivers may have history of abusive or addictive behaviors.

Clinical Decision Point *Be discreet in how you conduct the interview. Ask direct questions about abuse in private. It is often necessary to delay assessment to a later time when the partner or caregiver is not present. Asking a partner or caregiver to leave during an assessment creates an awkward situation, but inquiring about possible abuse in front of an abuser puts a patient at risk for further abuse. Patients are more likely to reveal any problems when the suspected abuser is absent from the room.*

9. Observe for signs of abuse: a. *Child:* Blood on underclothing, pain in genital area, difficulty sitting or walking, pain on urination, vaginal or penile discharge, itching or unusual color in genital area, physical injury inconsistent with parent's or caregiver's account of how injury occurred.	Indicates child sexual abuse (Ball et al., 2015; Hockenberry and Wilson, 2015). Suggests child physical abuse.
b. *Female patient:* Injury or trauma inconsistent with reported cause or obvious injuries to head, face, neck, breasts, abdomen, and genitalia (e.g., black eyes, abrasions, bruises/welts, broken nose, lacerations, broken teeth, strangulation marks, burns, human bites, orbital fractures, fractured skull).	Suggests intimate partner violence (Ball et al., 2015). These signs also apply to male patient being abused by female partner.

BOX 6.3

Characteristics of Dementia

Cognition
- Memory impaired: trouble recalling recent conversations, events, and appointments
- Frequently misplaces objects

Speech/Language
- Struggles to find words
- Conversation possibly incoherent

Activity
- Unchanged from usual behavior
- Difficulty performing tasks that require many steps

Mood and Affect
- Depressed
- Apathetic
- Uninterested

Delusions/Hallucinations
- Can be some delusions
- No hallucinations

Modified from Ball JW et al: *Seidel's guide to physical examination*, ed 8, St Louis, 2015, Mosby.

STEP	**RATIONALE**
c. *Older adult:* Injury or trauma inconsistent with reported cause, injuries in unusual locations (e.g., neck or genitalia), pattern injuries (left when an object with which a person is struck leaves an imprint), parallel injuries (e.g., bilateral ecchymosis on upper arms suggesting that patient was held and shaken), burns (shaped like cigarette, iron, rope), fractures, poor hygiene, and poor nutrition.	Indicates elder abuse/neglect (Ball et al., 2015; Touhy and Jett, 2015). Prolonged interval between injury and time patient sought medical care also indicates older adult abuse or neglect.

Clinical Decision Point *A pattern of findings indicating abuse usually mandates a report to a social service center (refer to state guidelines). Obtain immediate consultation with health care provider, social worker, and other support staff to facilitate placement in a safer environment.*

10. Assess posture and position, noting alignment of shoulders and hips while patient stands and/or sits. Observe whether patient is slumped, erect, or has bent posture (see illustration).	Reveals musculoskeletal problem, mood, or presence of pain.

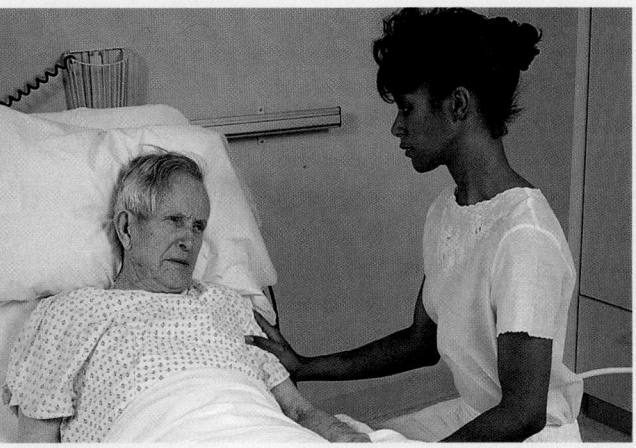

STEP 10 Observe patient's position and posture.

11. Assess body movements. Are they purposeful? Are there tremors of extremities? Are any body parts immobile? Are movements coordinated or uncoordinated?	May indicate neurological or muscular problem or emotional stress (see Skill 6.7).
12. Assess speech. Is it understandable and moderately paced? Is there association with patient's thoughts?	Alterations reflect neurological impairment, injury or impairment of mouth, improperly fitting dentures, differences in dialect or language, and some mental illnesses.
13. Observe hygiene and grooming for presence or absence of makeup, type of clothes (hospital or personal), and cleanliness. Hair, teeth, and nails are good places to assess for hygiene status.	Grooming may reflect activity level before examination, resources available to purchase grooming supplies, patient's mood, and self-care practices. It may also reflect culture, lifestyle, economic status, and personal preferences.
a. Observe color, distribution, quantity, thickness, texture, and lubrication of hair.	Changes in hair may reflect hormonal changes, changes from aging, poor nutrition, or use of certain hair-care products.
b. Inspect condition of nails (hands and feet). Note color, length, symmetry, cleanliness, and shape. Nails are normally transparent, smooth, and well rounded, with smooth, intact cuticle.	Changes indicate inadequate nutrition or grooming practices, nervous habits, or systemic diseases.
c. Assess presence or absence of body odor.	Body odor may result from physical exercise, deficient hygiene, or physical or mental abnormalities. Inadequate oral hygiene or unhealthy teeth cause bad breath.
14. Inspect exposed areas of skin and ask if patient has noted any changes, including:	Determines presence of abnormalities and cancerous lesions. Melanoma is an aggressive form of skin cancer; detection and prompt treatment are critical (Box 6.4).
a. Pruritus, oozing, bleeding	Itching could result from dry skin. Oozing could indicate infection, and bleeding may indicate a blood disorder.
b. Appearance of mole (nevus), bump, or nodule; change in sensation; itchiness, tenderness, or pain	These are key indicators that a lesion may be cancerous.
c. Petechiae (pinpoint-size red or purple spots on skin caused by small hemorrhages in skin layers)	Petechiae may indicate serious blood clotting disorder, drug reaction, or liver disease.

STEP	RATIONALE
15. Inspect skin surfaces. Compare color of symmetrical body parts, including areas unexposed to sun. Look for any patches or areas of skin color variation.	Changes in color can indicate pathological alterations (Table 6.5).

Clinical Decision Point *Be alert for basal cell carcinomas such as an open sore that does not heal, a shiny nodule, a pink or reddish growth, or scarlike area. These are often seen in sun-exposed areas and frequently occur in sun-damaged skin.*

STEP	RATIONALE
16. Carefully inspect color of face, oral mucosa, lips, conjunctiva, sclera, palms of hands, and nail beds.	Abnormalities are easier to identify in areas of body where melanin production is lowest.

Clinical Decision Point *When assessing the skin of a patient with bandages, cast, restraints, or other restrictive devices, note report of pain or tingling and areas of pallor, decreased temperature, decreased movement, and impaired sensation, which may indicate impaired circulation. Immediate release of pressure from the restrictive device may be necessary.*

STEP	RATIONALE
17. Use ungloved fingertips to palpate skin surfaces to feel texture and moisture of intact skin.	Changes in texture may be first indication of skin rashes in dark-skinned patients. Hydration, body temperature, and environment may affect skin. Older adults are prone to xerosis, presenting as dry, scaly skin (Touhy and Jett, 2015).

BOX 6.4

Malignant Melanoma Mnemonics

The ABCDE Rule of Melanoma

Here is a simple way to remember the characteristics that should alert you to the possibility of malignant melanoma.

A. *Asymmetry* of lesion: One side different than the other
B. *Borders:* Irregular (uneven, lumpy edges)
C. *Color:* Blue/black or variegated; pigmentation not uniform; variations/multiple colors (tan, black) with areas of pink, white, gray, blue, or red
D. *Diameter* greater than 6 mm
E. *Evolving:* Change in size, shape, color; itching or bleeding

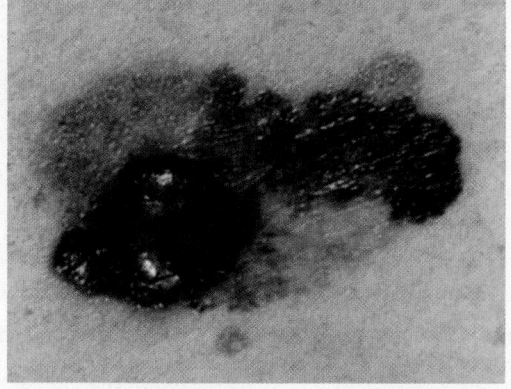

Figure from Ball JW et al: *Seidel's guide to physical examination,* ed 8, St Louis, 2015, Mosby.

TABLE 6.5

Skin Color Variations

Color	Condition	Cause	Assessment Location
Bluish (cyanosis)	Increased amount of deoxygenated hemoglobin (associated with hypoxia and is a late sign of decreased oxygen levels)	Heart or lung disease, cold environment	Nail beds, lips, base of tongue, skin (severe cases)
Pallor (decrease in color)	Reduced amount of oxyhemoglobin Reduced visibility of oxyhemoglobin resulting from decreased blood flow	Anemia Shock	Face, conjunctivae, nail beds, palms of hands Skin, nail beds, conjunctivae, lips
Loss of pigmentation	Vitiligo	Congenital autoimmune condition causing lack of pigment	Patchy areas on skin over face, hands, arms
Yellow-orange (jaundice)	Increased deposit of bilirubin in tissues	Liver disease, destruction of red blood cells	Sclerae, mucous membranes, skin
Red (erythema)	Increased visibility of oxyhemoglobin caused by dilation or increased blood flow	Fever, direct trauma, blushing, alcohol intake	Face; area of trauma; and areas at risk for pressure such as sacrum, shoulders, elbows, and heels
Tan-brown	Increased amount of melanin	Suntan, pregnancy	Areas exposed to sun: face, arms; areolae, nipples

STEP	RATIONALE
a. Stroke skin surfaces lightly with fingertips to detect texture of surface of skin. Note whether skin is smooth or rough, thick or thin, or tight or supple and if localized areas of hardness or lesions are present.	Localized texture changes result from trauma, surgical wounds, or lesions.
b. Palpate any areas that appear irregular in texture.	Allows detection of localized areas of hardness and/or tenderness within subcutaneous skin layers.
c. Using dorsum (back) of hand, palpate for temperature of skin surfaces. Compare symmetrical body parts. Compare upper and lower body parts. Note distinct temperature difference and localized areas of warmth.	Skin on dorsum of hand is thin, which allows detection of subtle temperature changes. Cool skin temperature often indicates decreased blood flow. A stage 1 pressure injury may cause warmth and erythema (redness) of an area. Environmental temperature and anxiety may also affect skin temperature.

Clinical Decision Point *In patients who receive routine injections (e.g., insulin, heparin), localized areas of hardness may be palpated over injection sites. Develop a plan to rotate injection sites systematically. Site rotation prevents local skin changes from repeated injections (Lewis et al., 2017).*

18. Apply clean gloves. Inspect character of any secretions; note color, odor, amount, and consistency (e.g., thin and watery, thick and oily). Remove gloves. Perform hand hygiene.	Description of secretions helps to indicate type of lesion, presence of infection, or wound healing.
19. Assess skin turgor by grasping fold of skin on sternum, forearm, or abdomen with fingertips. Release skinfold and note ease and speed with which skin returns to place (see illustration).	With reduced turgor skin remains suspended or "tented" for a few seconds before slowly returning to place, indicating decreased elasticity and possible dehydration. With altered turgor, provide measures for prevention of pressure injuries (see Chapter 39).

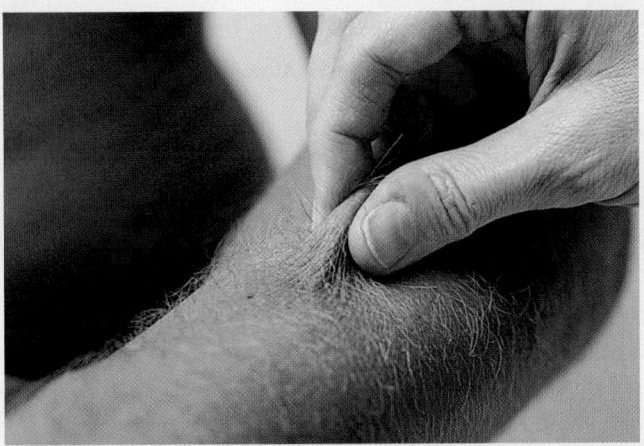

STEP 19 Checking skin turgor.

20. Assess condition of skin for pressure areas, paying particular attention to regions at risk for pressure (e.g., sacrum, greater trochanter, heels, occipital area, clavicles). If you see areas of redness, place fingertip over area, apply gentle pressure, and release. Look at skin color.	Normal reactive hyperemia (redness) is visible effect of localized vasodilation, the normal response of the body to lack of blood flow to underlying tissue. Affected area of skin normally blanches with fingertip pressure. If area does not blanch, suspect tissue injury.

Clinical Decision Point *When assessing darkly pigmented skin, visual inspection techniques to identify skin problems are ineffective. Skin inspection techniques for individuals with darkly pigmented skin must include assessment of temperature, edema, and changes in tissue consistency as compared with the surrounding skin (WOCN, 2016).*

Clinical Decision Point *With evidence of normal reactive hyperemia, reposition patient and develop a turning schedule if he or she is dependent.*

21. When you detect a lesion, use adequate lighting to inspect color, location, texture, size, shape, and type (Box 6.5). Also note grouping (e.g., clustered or linear) and distribution (e.g., localized or generalized).	Observation of skin lesions allows for accurate description and identification.
a. Apply gloves if lesion is moist or draining. Gently palpate any lesion to determine mobility, contour (e.g., flat, raised, or depressed), and consistency (e.g., soft or hard).	Gentle palpation prevents rupture of underlying cysts. Gloves reduce transmission of microorganisms.

STEP	RATIONALE

BOX 6.5

Types of Skin Lesions

Macule: Flat, nonpalpable change in skin color; smaller than 1 cm (0.4 inch) (e.g., freckle, petechia)

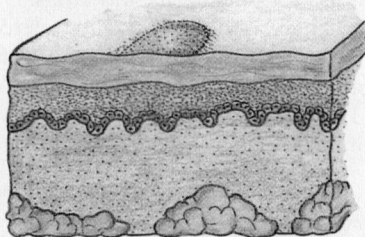

Vesicle: Circumscribed elevation of skin filled with serous fluid; smaller than 0.5 cm (0.2 inch) (e.g., herpes simplex, chickenpox)

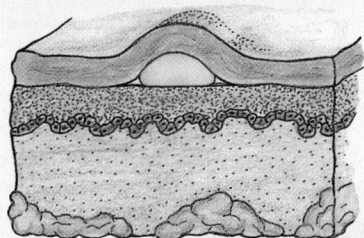

Papule: Palpable, circumscribed, solid elevation in skin; smaller than 0.5 cm (0.2 inch) (e.g., elevated nevus)

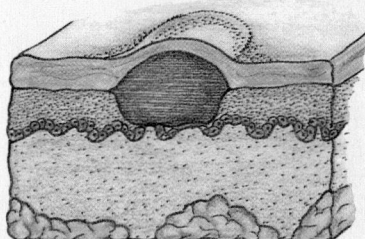

Pustule: Circumscribed elevation of skin similar to vesicle but filled with pus; varies in size (e.g., acne, staphylococcal infection)

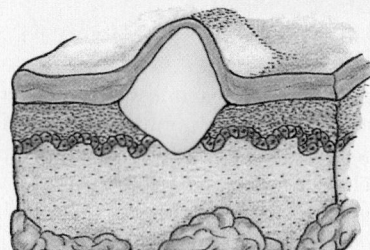

Nodule: Elevated solid mass, deeper and firmer than papule; 0.5 to 2 cm (0.2 to 0.8 inch) (e.g., wart)

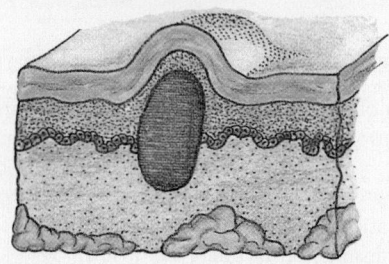

Ulcer: Deep loss of skin surface that may extend to dermis and frequently bleeds and scars; varies in size (e.g., venous stasis ulcer)

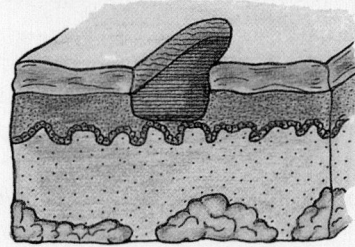

Tumor: Solid mass that may extend deep through subcutaneous tissue; larger than 1 to 2 cm (0.4 to 0.8 inch) (e.g., epithelioma)

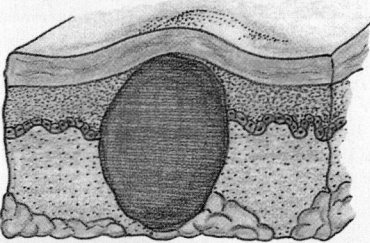

Atrophy: Thinning of skin with loss of normal skin furrow, with skin appearing shiny and translucent; varies in size (e.g., arterial insufficiency)

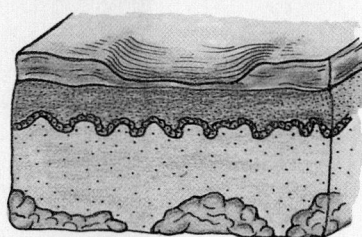

Wheal: Irregularly shaped, elevated area or superficial localized edema; varies in size (e.g., hive, mosquito bite)

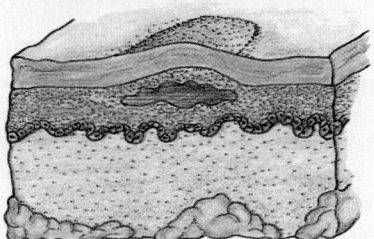

STEP	RATIONALE
b. Note if patient reports tenderness with or without palpation.	Tenderness may indicate inflammation or pressure on body part.
c. Measure size of lesion (height, width, depth) with centimeter ruler.	Provides for baseline to assess changes in lesion over time.
22. Remove gloves. Discard used supplies and gloves in proper receptacle. Help patient to comfortable position. Perform hand hygiene.	Prevents transmission of infections.

EVALUATION

1. Observe throughout assessment for evidence of physical or emotional distress, which may alter assessment data.

Interaction during assessment reveals emotional problems. Maneuvers used during physical examination reveal presence of physical problems.

2. Compare assessment findings with previous observations.

Determines if change has occurred.

3. Ask patient if there is information about physical condition that you have not discussed.

Some patients think that they are bothering you by asking questions unless opportunity for questions is provided.

4. **Use Teach-Back:** State to patient, "I want to be sure I explained everything about the bleeding mole I found on your back during assessment. Tell me why it is important to see a dermatologist." Revise your instruction now or develop a plan for revised patient or family caregiver teaching if patient or family caregiver is not able to teach back correctly.

Determines patient's and family caregiver's level of understanding of instructional topic.

Unexpected Outcomes	Related Interventions
1. Patient demonstrates acute distress (e.g., shortness of breath, acute pain, severe anxiety).	• Respond immediately to identified need (e.g., repositioning, oxygen, or medication as appropriate). • Obtain vital signs. • Notify health care provider.
2. Patient has abnormal skin condition (e.g., change in color of a mole, dry texture, reduced turgor, lesions, or erythema).	• Identify contributing factors and prevent continued irritation or damage as appropriate.
3. Patient is unwilling or unable to provide adequate information relating to identified concerns.	• Seek information from family caregivers if present. • Review patient's record for baseline data.

Recording and Reporting

- Record patient's vital signs on vital sign flow sheet in the electronic health record (EHR) or chart.
- Record description of alterations in patient's general appearance in the EHR or chart.
- Describe patient's behaviors using objective terminology. Include patient's self-report of signs and symptoms.
- Document your evaluation of patient and family caregiver learning.
- Report abnormalities and acute symptoms to nurse in charge or health care provider.

Special Considerations
Teaching

- During general survey inform patient about normal range of vital signs for age and physical condition and normal weight for height and body frame.
- If patient is on established diet, discuss any problems that he or she has preparing a diet or selecting food. The best form of weight reduction is to achieve gradual weight loss by increasing exercise and decreasing caloric intake. Refer to clinical dietitian for specific information.

Pediatric

- Measurement of physical growth is a key element in evaluation of a child's health status. These physical growth parameters include height, length, weight, skinfold thickness, and arm and head circumference (Hockenberry and Wilson, 2015). Use growth charts specific to child's age and condition.
- Weigh infants nude. Weigh children in light underclothes or gown.
- A child's interactions with parents provide valuable information regarding the child's behavior.

Gerontological

- An older adult's presenting signs and symptoms are sometimes deceiving. An older adult has a diminished physiological reserve that sometimes masks the usual, or "classic," signs and symptoms of a disease. In older adults signs and symptoms are often blunted or atypical (Touhy and Jett, 2015).
- Common skin changes with aging include dryness, thinning, decreased elasticity, and prominent small blood vessels. Common lesions include seborrheic keratosis (pigmented raised, warty lesion); cherry angioma (bright, ruby-red round papules); cutaneous tags (soft pinkish-tan to light-brown pedunculated

lesions); and solar lentigines (gray-brown, irregular macular lesions on sun-exposed areas) (Ball et al., 2015).

- Inspection of the feet is critically important in the presence of impaired circulation, impaired vision, and diabetes mellitus. Common foot conditions include ulceration, fungal infection, corns, calluses, bunions, plantar warts, and hammertoe.

Home Care

- In the home the focus may be on the patient's ability to perform basic self-care tasks. Be sure that the home assessment builds on all health concerns identified in other settings.
- The home health nurse takes a small portable scale to monitor weight changes.

✦ SKILL 6.2   Head and Neck Assessment

Examination of the head and neck includes assessment of the head, eyes, ears, nose, mouth, and sinuses. Assessment uses inspection, palpation, and auscultation, with inspection and palpation often used simultaneously.

Delegation and Collaboration

The skill of assessing the head and neck cannot be delegated to nursing assistive personnel (NAP). The nurse directs the NAP to:

- Observe for nasal discharge and nasal bleeding.
- Report any findings found during routine care (e.g., oral care, bathing) to the nurse for further assessment.

Equipment

- Stethoscope
- Clean gloves (use nonlatex if necessary)
- Tongue blade
- Pen light

STEP	RATIONALE

ASSESSMENT

1. Assess for history of headache, dizziness, pain, or stiffness.

Headaches and dizziness are signs of stress, a symptom of another underlying problem such as high blood pressure or a result of injury.

2. Determine if patient has history of eye disease, diabetes mellitus, or hypertension.

Common conditions predispose patients to visual alterations requiring health care provider referral.

3. Ask if patient has experienced blurred vision, flashing lights, halos around lights or reduced visual field.

These common symptoms indicate visual problems.

4. Ask if patient has experienced ear pain, itching, discharge, vertigo, tinnitus (ringing in the ears), or change in hearing.

These signs and symptoms indicate infection or hearing loss.

5. Review patient's occupational history.

Patient's occupation can create a risk of injury, potential for eye fatigue, or prolonged noise exposure.

6. Ask if patient has history of allergies, nasal discharge, epistaxis (nosebleeds), or postnasal drip.

History is useful in determining source of nasal and sinus drainage.

7. Determine if patient smokes or chews tobacco.

Tobacco users have greater risk for mouth and throat cancer (ACS, 2015g).

NURSING DIAGNOSES

- Deficient knowledge regarding the need for head and neck assessment
- Impaired oral mucous membranes
- Ineffective health maintenance
- Risk for injury

Related factors/Risk factors are individualized based on patient's condition or needs.

PLANNING

1. Expected outcomes following completion of procedure:
   - Patient recognizes warning signs and symptoms of eye, ear, sinus, and mouth disease.
   - Patient takes appropriate safety precautions for occupational injury related to head and neck.
   - Patient exhibits good visual acuity, normal hearing, moist and intact oral mucosa, and head and neck without masses or lesions.

Awareness of warning signs improves adherence to reporting problems to health care provider.

Awareness of safety precautions improves adherence to healthful behaviors.

Patient has no abnormal findings.

STEP	RATIONALE
2. Prepare patient. Tell him or her that you will be completing routine examination of head and neck to check for areas of concerns.	Understanding promotes patient's cooperation.
3. Anticipate teaching topics so during examination you can teach patient about common symptoms of eye, ear, sinus, and mouth problems and occupational health safety.	Enables you to incorporate teaching during examination.
4. Perform hand hygiene. Assemble necessary equipment.	Reduces transmission of infection. Promotes efficiency of examination.

IMPLEMENTATION

1. Position patient sitting upright if possible.	Provides for more thorough examination of head and neck structures.
2. Inspect head. Note head position and facial features. Look for symmetry.	Head tilting to one side may indicate hearing or visual loss. Neurological disorders such as paralysis often affect facial symmetry.
3. Assess eyes (include discussion of signs and symptoms related to eye diseases).	
a. Inspect position of eyes, color, condition of conjunctiva, and movement.	Asymmetrical positioning may reflect trauma or tumor growth. Differences in color are sometimes congenital; changes in color of conjunctiva may be result of local infection or symptomatic of another abnormality (e.g., pale conjunctiva is associated with anemia).
b. Assess patient's near vision (ability to read newspaper or magazines) and far vision (ability to follow movement, read clock, watch television, or read signs at a distance).	Patient with visual acuity or visual field loss indicates need for supporting self-care measures (e.g., feeding, bathing, hygiene, dressing) and teaching.
c. Inspect pupils for size, shape, and equality (see illustration).	Normal pupils are round, regular, and equal in size and shape.

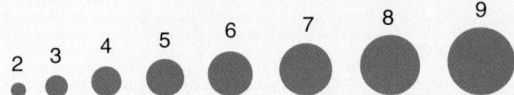

STEP 3c Pupil sizes in millimeters.

d. Test pupillary reflexes. To test reaction to light, dim room lights. If you cannot dim lights, cup hand over eye to temporarily shield light. As patient looks straight ahead, move penlight from side of patient's face and direct light on pupil. Observe pupillary response of both eyes, noting briskness and equality of reflex (see illustrations A and B).	Darkened room normally ensures brisk response of pupils to light. Pupil that is illuminated constricts. Pupil in other eye should constrict equally (consensual light reflex).

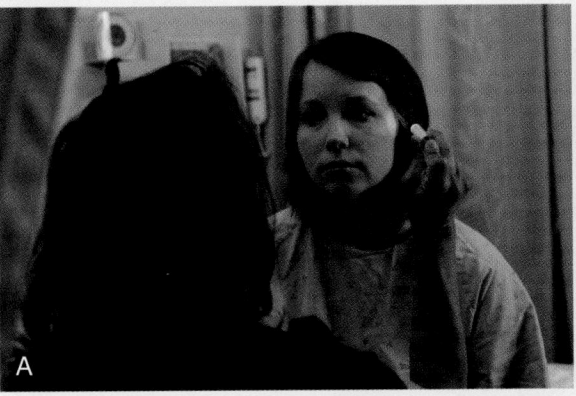 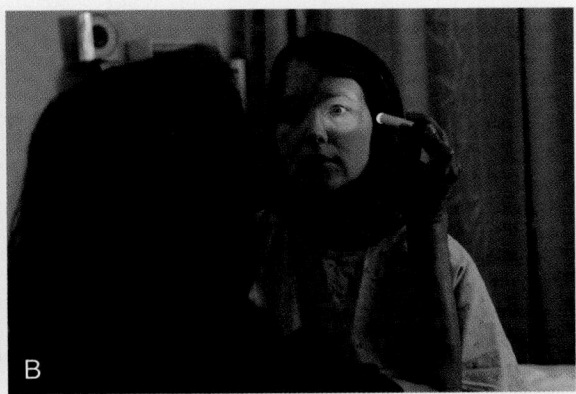

STEP 3d A, Holding penlight to side of patient's face. **B,** Illumination of pupil causes pupillary constriction.

STEP	RATIONALE

(1) Test for accommodation by asking patient to focus on distant object, which dilates the pupil. Then have patient shift to near object about 7 to 8 cm (3 to 3.2 inches) from nose and observe for pupil constriction and convergence of eyes. **NOTE:** You can also ask patient to follow an object (e.g., finger, pen) with eyes from far to near point.

Absence of constriction, convergence, or an asymmetrical response requires further ophthalmological assessment (Ball et al., 2015).

4. Assess hearing. Note patient's response to questions and presence/use of hearing aid. If you suspect patient has hearing loss, ask him or her to repeat random words that you state. Use one- or two-syllable words. Repeat, gradually increasing voice intensity until patient correctly repeats the words.

Patients normally hear three to six sounds clearly when whispered (Ball et al., 2015). For patient with obvious hearing impairment, speak clearly and concisely, stand so patient can see your face, stand toward patient's good ear, use low pitch, and avoid yelling.

Clinical Decision Point *If hearing deficit is present, have a qualified nurse inspect patient's ears because impaired hearing may be the result of impacted cerumen, external otitis, or swelling in ear canal because of allergic reactions to materials in hearing aids.*

5. Inspect nose externally for shape, skin color, alignment, drainage, and presence of deformity or inflammation. Note color of mucosa and any lesions, discharge, swelling, or presence of bleeding. If drainage appears infectious, consult with health care provider about obtaining a specimen.

Character of discharge and inflammation indicates allergy or infection. Perforation and erosion of septum and puffiness and/or increased vascularity of mucosa indicate habitual drug use.

6. In patients with nasogastric (NG), nasointestinal (NI), or nasotracheal tube, inspect nares for excoriation, inflammation, or discharge. Using penlight, look up into each naris. Stabilize tube as needed.

Swallowing or coughing reflex causes movement of tubes against nares, and pressure against tissues and mucosa can result in tissue injury.

7. Inspect sinuses by palpating gently over frontal and maxillary areas. Use thumbs to apply pressure up and under eyebrows to assess frontal sinuses. Use thumbs to apply pressure over maxillary sinuses, about 0.4 cm (1 inch) below eyes.

Infection, allergy, or drug use sometimes causes tenderness.

8. Assess mouth (include discussion about signs and symptoms of oral cancer).

   a. Apply clean gloves. Inspect lips for color, texture, hydration, and lesions. Have females remove lipstick.

Normal lips are pink, moist, symmetrical, and smooth.

   b. Inspect teeth and note position and alignment. Note color of teeth and presence of dental caries, tartar, and extraction sites.

Reveals quality of hygiene and discoloring effects of cola, coffee, and tobacco. Teeth are normally smooth, white, and shiny.

   c. Inspect mucosa and gums. Determine if patient wears dentures or retainers and if they are comfortable. Remove dentures to visualize and palpate gums. Use tongue blade to lightly depress tongue and inspect oral cavity with penlight (see illustration). Inspect oral mucosa, tongue, teeth, and gums for color, hydration, texture, and obvious lesions.

Dentures and retainers can cause chronic irritation. Normal mucosa is glistening, pink, smooth, and moist. Precancerous lesions can go unnoticed and progress rapidly.

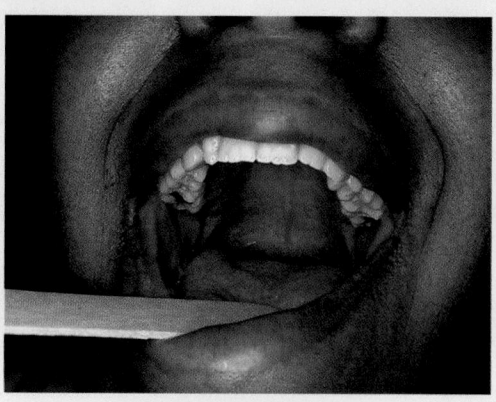

STEP 8c Inspect mouth.

STEP	RATIONALE

d. If oral lesions are present, palpate gently with gloved hand for tenderness, size, and consistency. Remove gloves. Perform hand hygiene.

Cancerous lesions tend to be hard and nontender.

9. Inspect and palpate the neck:

Assesses function of all neck structures, including neck muscles; lymph nodes; thyroid glands; and trachea.

a. Ask patient if there is history of neck pain or difficulty moving neck.

May indicate muscle strain, head injury, local nerve injury, or swollen lymph nodes.

b. Neck muscles: Inspect neck for bilateral symmetry of muscles. Ask patient to flex and hyperextend neck and turn head side to side.

Detects muscle weakness, strain, and range of motion (ROM).

c. Lymph nodes:

Lymph nodes are sometimes enlarged from infection or various diseases such as cancer.

(1) With patient's chin raised and head tilted slightly, inspect area where lymph nodes are distributed and compare both sides (see illustration).

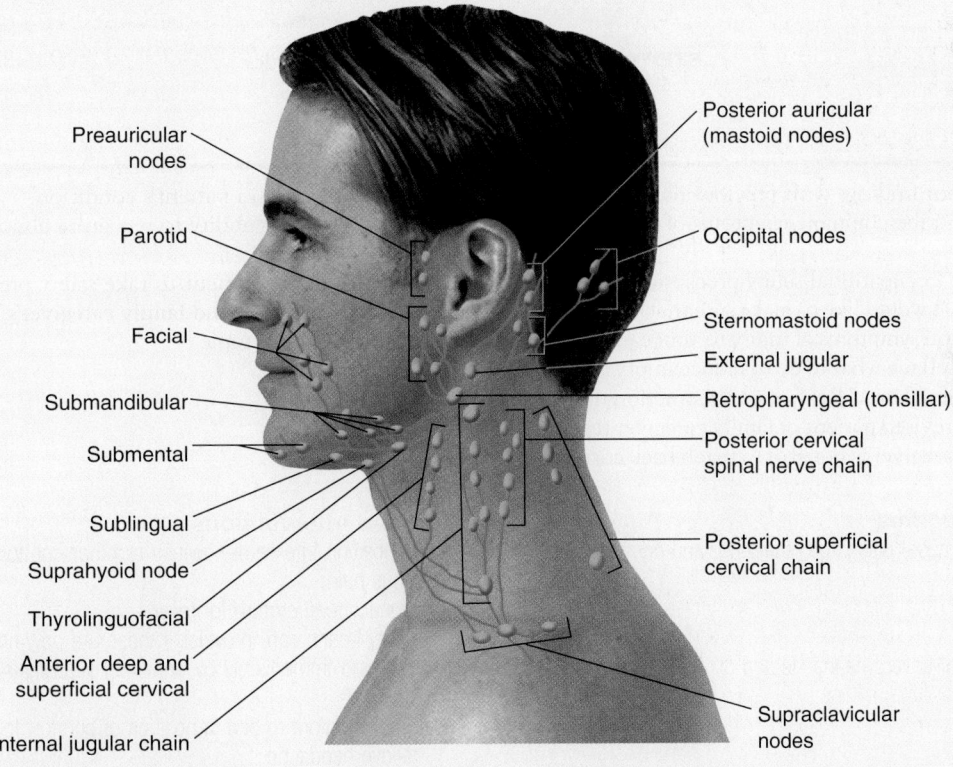

STEP 9c(1) Palpable lymph nodes of head and neck. (*From Ball JW et al: Seidel's guide to physical examination, ed 8, St Louis, 2015, Mosby.*)

(2) To examine lymph nodes, have patient relax with neck flexed slightly forward. To palpate, face or stand to side of patient and use pads of middle three fingers of hand (see illustration). Palpate gently in rotary motion for superficial lymph nodes.

This position relaxes tissues and muscles.

(3) Note if lymph nodes are large, fixed, inflamed, or tender.

Large, fixed, inflamed, or tender lymph nodes indicate local infection, systemic disease, or neoplasm.

10. Help patient to comfortable position. Perform hand hygiene.

Reduces transmission of infection.

STEP	RATIONALE

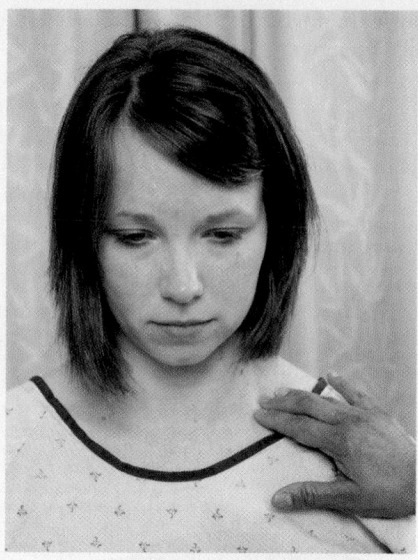

STEP 9c(2) Palpation of cervical lymph nodes.

EVALUATION

1. Compare assessment findings with previous observations.	Identifies changes in patient's condition.
2. Ask patient to describe common symptoms of eye, ear, sinus, or mouth disease.	Measures patient's ability to recognize abnormalities.
3. Ask patient to list occupational safety precautions.	Knowledge allows patient to take safety precautions.
4. **Use Teach-Back:** "I would like to make sure that you know some of the signs and symptoms of injury to your ears due to your occupation. Tell me what to do to reduce injury and potential hearing problems." Revise your instruction now or develop a plan for revised patient or family caregiver teaching if patient or family caregiver is not able to teach back correctly.	Determines patient's and family caregiver's level of understanding of instructional topic.

Unexpected Outcomes	Related Interventions
1. Patient has yellow nasal discharge, sneezing, and complaint of sinus pain.	• Reposition into semi-Fowler's or other comfortable position to relieve sinus pain. • Monitor temperature for fever. • Notify health care provider if these are new findings.
2. Patient complains of severe headache and dizziness when standing.	• Respond immediately by obtaining vital signs, especially blood pressure. • Return patient to bed in position of comfort to minimize dizziness and relieve headache. • Identify contributing factors (e.g., stress, pain, or elevated blood pressure). • Notify health care provider.
3. Patient has mouth sore that bleeds easily, lump or thickening in cheek, or white or red patch in mucosa.	• Notify health care provider.

Recording and Reporting

- Record all findings, including any abnormal findings such as hearing or visual loss, pain and its location, current infection, and character of drainage in nurses' notes in electronic health record (EHR) or chart.
- Document your evaluation of patient and family caregiver learning.
- Report any unexpected findings or changes to charge nurse or health care provider.

Special Considerations
Teaching

- Explain the common visual changes associated with aging, including reduced acuity (presbyopia), loss of or a reduction in peripheral vision, reduced tearing, and sensitivity to glare or bright lights. Inform patients when to seek help from an eye-care professional.
- Teach the visually impaired patient and family caregivers how to adjust room arrangements at home to promote safer

ambulation. Self-help aids are available to help patient function independently with daily activities.

Pediatric

- Some infants resist eye examination by closing eyes. Using distraction encourages eye opening (Hockenberry and Wilson, 2015).
- Headaches in children are usually caused by loss of sleep, poor nutrition, eye fatigue, and allergies. Children as young as 3 years of age can develop severe migraine headaches, but the symptoms are vague and difficult to diagnose (Hockenberry and Wilson, 2015).

Gerontological

- Older adults commonly have loss of peripheral vision caused by changes in the lens.
- Teach patients older than age 65 to have regular hearing checks.
- Measuring visual acuity helps determine level of assistance that patient requires with daily living activities and ability of patient to safely ambulate and function independently within the home.

✦ SKILL 6.3   Thorax and Lung Assessment

Assessment of the thorax and lungs requires review of the ventilatory and respiratory functions of the lungs. It is a critical part of assessment because alterations can be life threatening. Changes in respiration can occur quickly as a result of immobility, infection, certain analgesic and sedative medications, and fluid overload. Use data from all body systems to determine the nature of pulmonary alterations. You will use inspection, palpation, and auscultation during the examination.

Before assessing the thorax and lungs, know the landmarks of the chest (Fig. 6.3A-C). These landmarks help you identify findings and use assessment skills correctly. A patient's nipples, angle of Louis at the sternum, suprasternal notch, costal angle, clavicles, and vertebrae are key landmarks. Keep a mental image of the location of the lobes of the lung and the position of each rib (Fig. 6.4A-C).

Locating the position of each rib is critical to visualizing the lobe of the lung being assessed. To begin, locate the angle of Louis on the anterior chest by palpating the "speed bump" at the manubriosternal junction, where the second rib connects with the sternum. The angle is often visible and palpable. Count the ribs and intercostal spaces (between the ribs) from this point. The number of each intercostal space corresponds with that of the rib just above it. The spinous processes of the third thoracic vertebra and the fourth, fifth, and sixth ribs help to locate the lung lobes laterally. The lower lobes project laterally and anteriorly (see Fig. 6.4B). Posteriorly the tip or inferior margin of the scapula lies approximately at the level of the seventh rib (see Fig. 6.4C).

During the examination you use auscultation to listen to breath sounds with a stethoscope. You can hear these sounds best when the person breathes deeply through the mouth. Adventitious sounds (abnormal sounds) result from air passing through fluid, mucus, or narrowed airways or from an inflammation between the pleural linings. The four types of adventitious sounds are crackles, rhonchi, wheezes, and pleural friction rubs (Table 6.6). Note the location and characteristics of the sounds, diminished breath sounds, or absence of breath sounds. Determine where in the respiratory cycle the abnormal sounds are heard.

Delegation and Collaboration

The skill of assessing the lungs and thorax cannot be delegated to nursing assistive personnel (NAP). The nurse directs the NAP to:
- Measure the patient's respirations after vital signs confirm that patient is stable.
- Report respiratory distress, difficulty breathing, and changes in rate and depth.
- Keep head of bed elevated for a patient who has respiratory difficulties.

Equipment

- Stethoscope

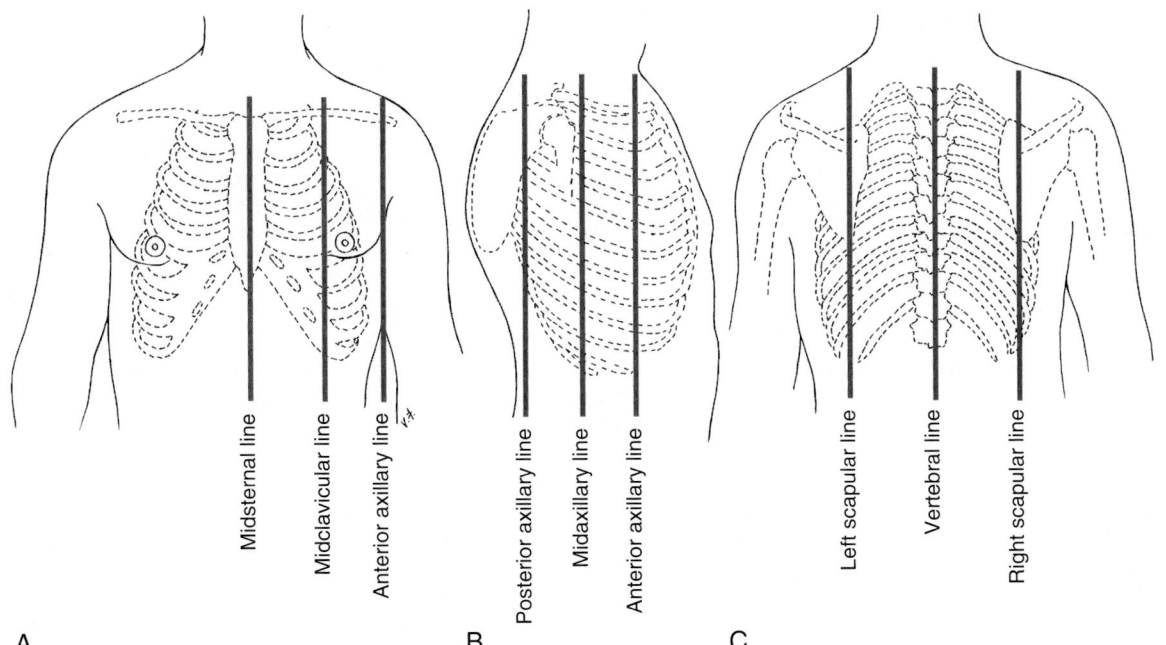

Midsternal line | Midclavicular line | Anterior axillary line

Posterior axillary line | Midaxillary line | Anterior axillary line

Left scapular line | Vertebral line | Right scapular line

A   B   C

FIG 6.3 Anatomical landmarks and order of progression for examination of thorax. **A,** Anterior thorax. **B,** Lateral thorax. **C,** Posterior thorax.

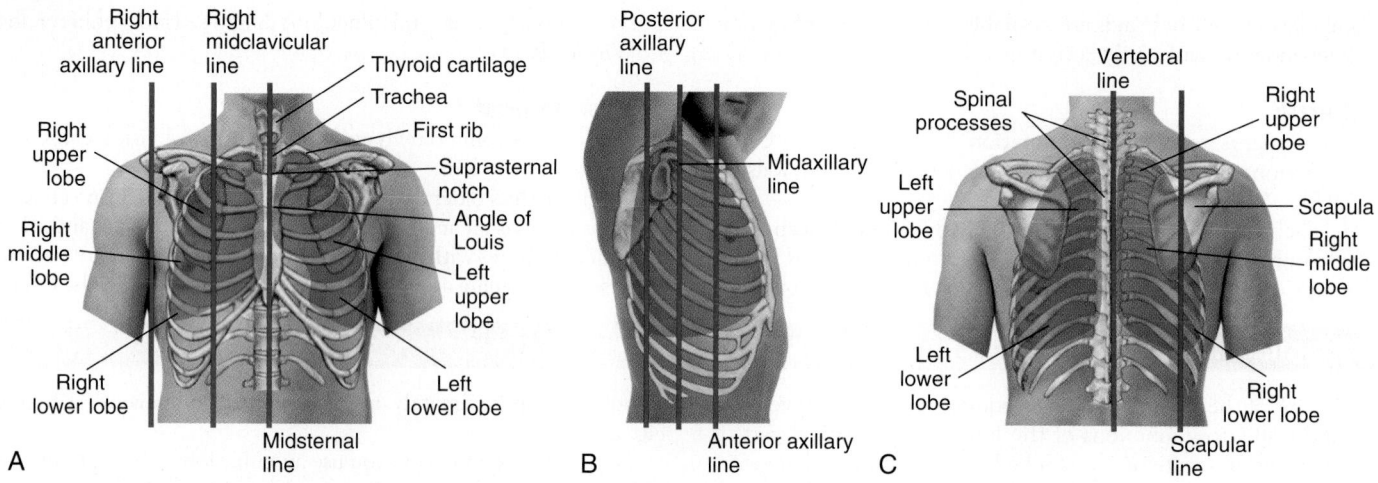

FIG 6.4 Position of lung lobes in relation to anatomical landmarks. **A,** Anterior position. **B,** Lateral position. **C,** Posterior position. *(From Seidel HM et al: Mosby's guide to physical examination, ed 7, St Louis, 2011, Mosby.)*

TABLE 6.6

Adventitious Breath Sounds

Sound	Site Auscultated	Cause	Character
Crackles	Most common in dependent lobes: right and left lung bases	Random, sudden reinflation of groups of alveoli; also related to increase in fluid in small airways	Fine, short, interrupted crackling sounds heard during end of inspiration, expiration, or both; may or may not change with coughing; sound like crushing cellophane Medium crackles: lower, moister sounds heard during middle of inspiration; not cleared with coughing Coarse crackles: loud bubbly sounds heard during inspiration; not cleared with coughing
Rhonchi (sonorous wheeze)	Heard primarily over trachea and bronchi; if loud enough, can be heard over most lung fields	Fluid or mucus in larger airways causing turbulence; muscular spasm	Loud, low-pitched, continuous sounds heard more during expiration; sometimes cleared by coughing Sound like blowing air through fluid with a straw
Wheezes (sibilant wheeze)	Heard over all lung fields but more distinct over posterior lung fields	High-velocity airflow through severely narrowed or obstructed bronchus	High-pitched, musical sounds such as a squeak heard continuously during inspiration or expiration; usually louder on expiration Not cleared with coughing
Pleural friction rub	Heard over anterior lateral lung field (if patient is sitting upright)	Inflamed pleura, parietal pleura rubbing against visceral pleura	Has grating quality heard best during inspiration; does not clear with coughing; heard loudest over lower lateral anterior surface

Data from Ball JW et al: *Seidel's guide to physical assessment*, ed 8, St Louis, 2015, Mosby.

STEP	RATIONALE

ASSESSMENT

1. Assess history of tobacco or marijuana use, including type of tobacco, duration (number of years), and amount in pack-years. Pack-years equal number of years smoking times number of packs per day (e.g., 4 years × ½ pack per day equals 2 pack-years). If patient has quit, determine length of time since smoking stopped.

Smoking is major cause of lung cancer, heart disease, and chronic lung disease (emphysema and chronic bronchitis). Risk factors for lung cancer include history of smoking for over 20 years, exposure to environmental pollution, and secondhand smoke (ACS, 2015a, 2015g).

2. Ask if patient experiences any of the following: *persistent cough* (productive or nonproductive), sputum production, *blood-streaked sputum, chest pain,* shortness of breath, orthopnea, dyspnea during exertion, activity intolerance, or *recurrent attacks of pneumonia or bronchitis.*

Symptoms of respiratory alterations help to localize objective physical findings. (Warning signals for lung cancer are in italics.)

3. Determine if patient works in environment containing pollutants (e.g., asbestos, arsenic, coal dust, or chemical irritants) or requiring exposure to radiation. Does patient have exposure to secondhand cigarette smoke?

Patients with chronic respiratory disease, particularly asthma, have symptoms aggravated by change in temperature and humidity, irritating fumes or smoke, emotional stress, and physical exertion.

4. Review history for known or suspected human immunodeficiency virus (HIV) infection, substance abuse, low income, residence or employment in nursing home or shelter, homelessness, recent imprisonment, being a family member of patient with tuberculosis (TB), and immigration to the United States from a country where TB is prevalent (CDC, 2013).

These are known risk factors for exposure to and/or development of TB.

5. Ask if patient has history of persistent cough, hemoptysis (bloody sputum), unexplained weight loss, fatigue, night sweats, and/or fever.

These are signs and symptoms for both TB and HIV infection.

6. Does patient have history of chronic hoarseness?

Hoarseness indicates laryngeal disorder or abuse of cocaine or opioids (sniffing).

7. Assess for history of allergies to pollen, dust, or other airborne irritants and to any foods, drugs, or chemical substances.

Allergic response is associated with wheezing on auscultation, dyspnea, cyanosis, and diaphoresis.

8. Review family history for cancer, TB, allergies, or chronic obstructive pulmonary disease (COPD).

Familial history places patient at risk for lung disease.

NURSING DIAGNOSES

- Fatigue
- Impaired gas exchange
- Ineffective airway clearance
- Ineffective breathing pattern
- Pain (acute, chronic)
- Risk for infection

Related factors/Risk factors are individualized based on patient's condition or needs.

PLANNING

1. Expected outcomes following completion of procedure:
   - Respirations are passive, diaphragmatic or costal, and regular (12 to 20/min in adult) with symmetrical expansion.

Characteristics of normal respirations.

   - Breath sounds are clear to auscultation and equal bilaterally.

Air flows without interference or obstruction. Corresponding sides should sound the same.

   - Patient is able to describe factors that predispose to lung disease.

Awareness of risks can improve patient adherence to healthy behavior.

   - Patient assumes appropriate posture for best breathing.

Patient can learn about benefits of good posture as examination maneuvers are performed.

2. Anticipate teaching topics so during the examination you can teach patient about any risk factors for lung disease.

Allows you to incorporate teaching during assessment process.

3. Perform hand hygiene. Assemble necessary equipment.

Reduces transmission of infection. Promotes efficiency of examination.

STEP	RATIONALE

IMPLEMENTATION

1. Position and prepare patient for examination:

a. Position patient sitting upright. For bedridden patient elevate head of bed 45 to 90 degrees. If unable to tolerate sitting, use supine and side-lying positions.

Promotes full lung expansion during examination. Patients with chronic respiratory disease may need to sit up throughout examination because of shortness of breath. May require help of another caregiver to position unresponsive patients.

b. Remove gown or drape first from posterior chest, keeping front of chest and legs covered. As examination progresses, remove gown from area being examined.

Avoids unnecessary exposure and provides full visibility of thorax. Allows direct placement of diaphragm or bell on patient's skin, which enhances clarity of sounds.

c. Explain all steps of procedure, encouraging patient to relax and breathe normally through mouth.

Anxiety alters respiratory function. Breathing through mouth decreases extraneous sounds from air passing through nose.

2. Posterior thorax:

a. If possible, stand behind patient. Inspect thorax for shape and symmetry. Note any deformities, position of spine, slope of ribs, retraction of intercostal spaces (ICS) during inspiration and bulging of ICS during expiration, and symmetrical expansion during inspiration. Note anteroposterior diameter.

Allows for identification of impairment in chest expansion and any symptoms of respiratory distress. Normal chest contour is symmetrical. In a child the shape of chest is almost circular, with anteroposterior (AP) diameter in 1:1 ratio. In an adult AP is one third to one half of side-to-side diameter. Chronic lung disease causes ribs to be more horizontal and increases AP diameter, resulting in "barrel chest." Patients with breathing problems assume postures that improve ventilation.

Clinical Decision Point *When a patient holds the chest wall during breathing, it indicates localized chest pain. Assess the nature of pain, including onset, severity, precipitating factors, quality, region, and radiation.*

b. Determine rate and rhythm of breathing (see Chapter 5). Examine thorax as a whole. Have patient relax.

This is a good time to count respirations, with patient relaxed and unaware of inspection. Awareness could alter respirations.

c. Systematically palpate posterior chest wall, costal spaces, and ICS, noting any masses, pulsations, unusual movement, or areas of localized tenderness (see illustration). If patient voices pain or tenderness, avoid deep palpation. If there is a suspicious mass, palpate lightly for shape, size, and qualities of lesion (see Skill 6.1). Do not palpate painful areas deeply.

Palpation assesses further characteristics and confirms or supplements findings from inspection. Localized swelling or tenderness indicates trauma to ribs or underlying cartilage. A fractured rib fragment could be displaced.

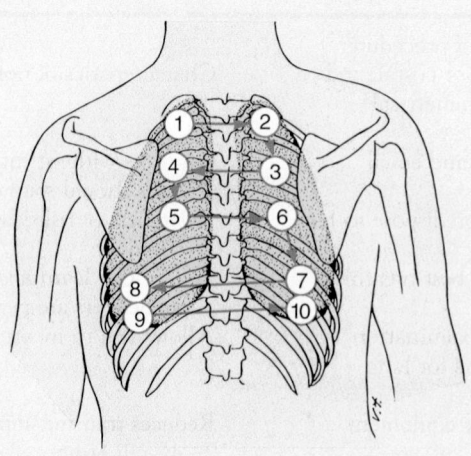

STEP 2c Pattern for assessment of posterior thorax.

STEP	RATIONALE

d. Assess chest expansion by standing behind patient and placing thumbs along spinal processes at tenth rib, with palms lightly contacting posterolateral surfaces (see illustration A). Keep thumbs about 5 cm (2 inches) apart, with thumbs pointing toward spine and fingers pointing laterally. Press hands toward patient's spine to form small skinfold between thumbs. After exhalation patient takes deep breath. Note movement of thumbs (see illustration B) and symmetry of chest wall movement. Normally symmetrical separation of thumbs occurs during chest excursion 3 to 5 cm (1½ to 2 inches).

Palpation of chest expansion assesses depth of patient's breathing. This technique is a good measure to evaluate patient's ability to perform deep-breathing exercises. Limited movement on one side indicates that patient is voluntarily splinting during ventilation because of pain. Avoid allowing hands to slide over skin, which gives false measure of excursion.

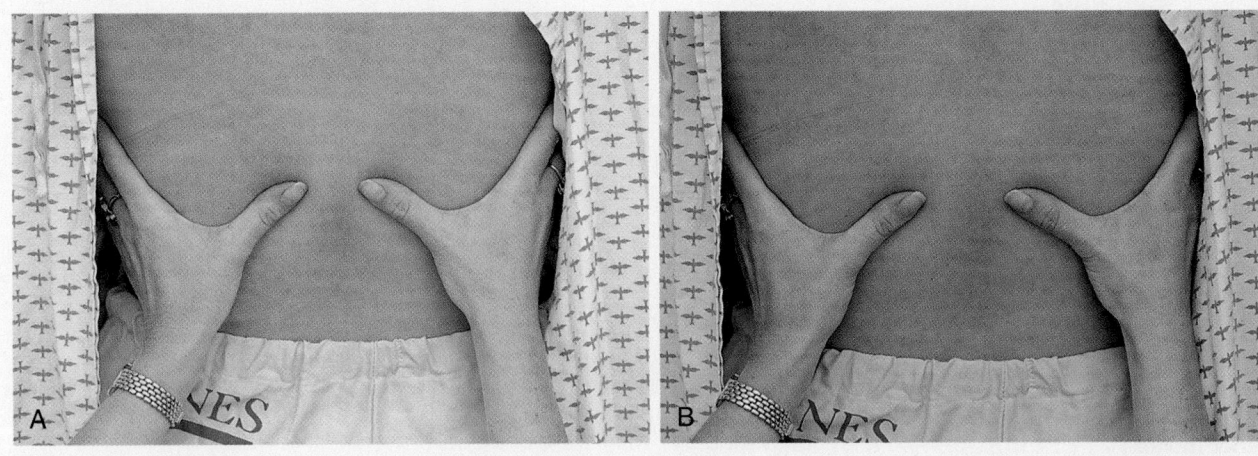

STEP 2d A, Position of hands for palpation of posterior thorax excursion. **B,** As patient inhales, movement of chest excursion separates nurse's thumbs.

e. Auscultate breath sounds. Instruct patient to take slow, deep breaths with mouth slightly open. For an adult, place diaphragm of stethoscope firmly on chest wall over intercostal spaces (see illustration). Listen to an entire inspiration and expiration at each stethoscope position (see pattern in Step 2c). If sounds are faint, as in obese patients, ask person to breathe harder and faster temporarily. Systematically compare breath sounds over right and left sides, listening for normal and adventitious sounds.

Assesses movement of air through tracheobronchial tree (Table 6.7). Recognition of normal airflow sounds allows detection of sounds caused by mucus or airway obstruction. Characterize sounds by length of inspiratory and expiratory phases.

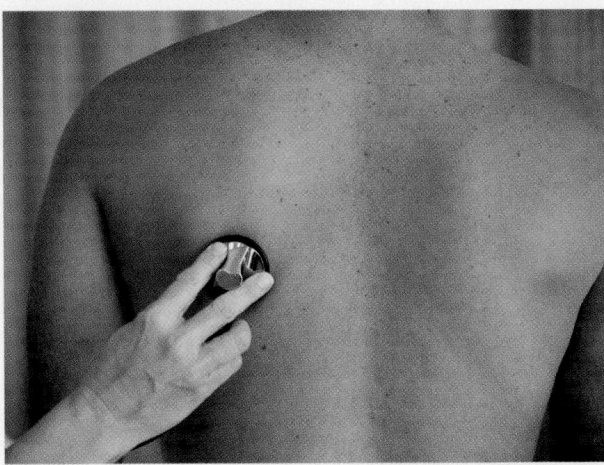

STEP 2e Auscultation with a stethoscope. (*From Ball JW et al: Seidel's guide to physical examination, ed 8, St Louis, 2015, Mosby.*)

STEP	RATIONALE

TABLE 6.7

Normal Breath Sounds

Type	Description	Location	Origin
Bronchial	Loud and high-pitched sounds with hollow quality Expiration lasts longer than inspiration (3:2 ratio).	Best heard over trachea	Created by air moving through trachea close to chest wall
Bronchovesicular	Medium-pitched and blowing sounds of medium intensity Inspiratory phase equal to expiratory phase	Best heard posteriorly between scapulae and anteriorly over bronchioles lateral to sternum at first and second intercostal spaces	Created by air moving through large airways
Vesicular	Soft, breezy, and low-pitched sounds Inspiratory phase 3 times longer than expiratory phase	Best heard over periphery of lung (except over scapula)	Created by air moving through smaller airways

f. If you auscultate adventitious sounds, have patient cough. Listen again with stethoscope to determine if sound has cleared with coughing. See Table 6.7 for a description of adventitious breath sounds.

Coughing may clear adventitious sounds. Rhonchi often are eliminated or altered by coughing. Crackles and wheezes are not.

3. Lateral thorax:

a. Instruct patient to raise arms and inspect chest wall for same characteristics as reviewed for posterior chest.

Improves access to lateral thoracic structures.

b. Extend palpation and auscultation of posterior thorax to lateral sides of chest, except for excursion measurement (see illustration).

Locates abnormalities in lateral lung fields.

4. Anterior thorax:

a. Inspect accessory muscles while patient is breathing: sternocleidomastoid, trapezius, and abdominal muscles, noting effort to breathe.

Extent to which accessory muscles are used reveals degree of effort to breathe. Accessory muscles move little with normal passive breathing. Patients who require great effort and rely on these muscles may produce a grunting sound.

b. Inspect width or spread of costal angle made by costal margins and tip of sternum. Angle is usually larger than 90 degrees between margins.

Indicates congenital, acquired, or traumatic alterations that may influence patient's chest expansion.

c. Observe patient's breathing pattern, observing symmetry and degree of chest wall and abdominal movement. Respiratory rate and rhythm are more often assessed on anterior chest wall.

Assesses patient's effort to breathe: symmetrical, passive movement indicates no respiratory distress. Male patient's breathing is diaphragmatic; whereas female's is more costal.

d. Palpate anterior thoracic muscles and ribs for lumps, masses, tenderness, or unusual movement, following a systematic pattern across and down (see illustration).

Localized swelling or tenderness indicates trauma to underlying ribs or cartilage.

e. Palpate anterior chest excursion. Place hands over each lateral rib cage, with thumbs approximately 5 cm (2 inches) apart and angled along each costal margin. As patient inhales deeply, thumbs should symmetrically move apart 3 to 5 cm (1½ to 2 inches), with each side expanding equally.

Assesses depth of patient's breathing and ability to perform deep-breathing exercises. Certain abnormalities are evident if expansion is not symmetrical.

f. With patient sitting, auscultate anterior thorax following same pattern as in Step 4d. Begin above clavicles; move across and then down as during palpation. Compare right and left sides. Give special attention to lower lobes, where mucus commonly gathers.

A systematic pattern of assessment comparing sides helps to identify abnormal sounds.

5. Clean and store stethoscope. Perform hand hygiene.

Reduces transmission of infection.

STEP	RATIONALE

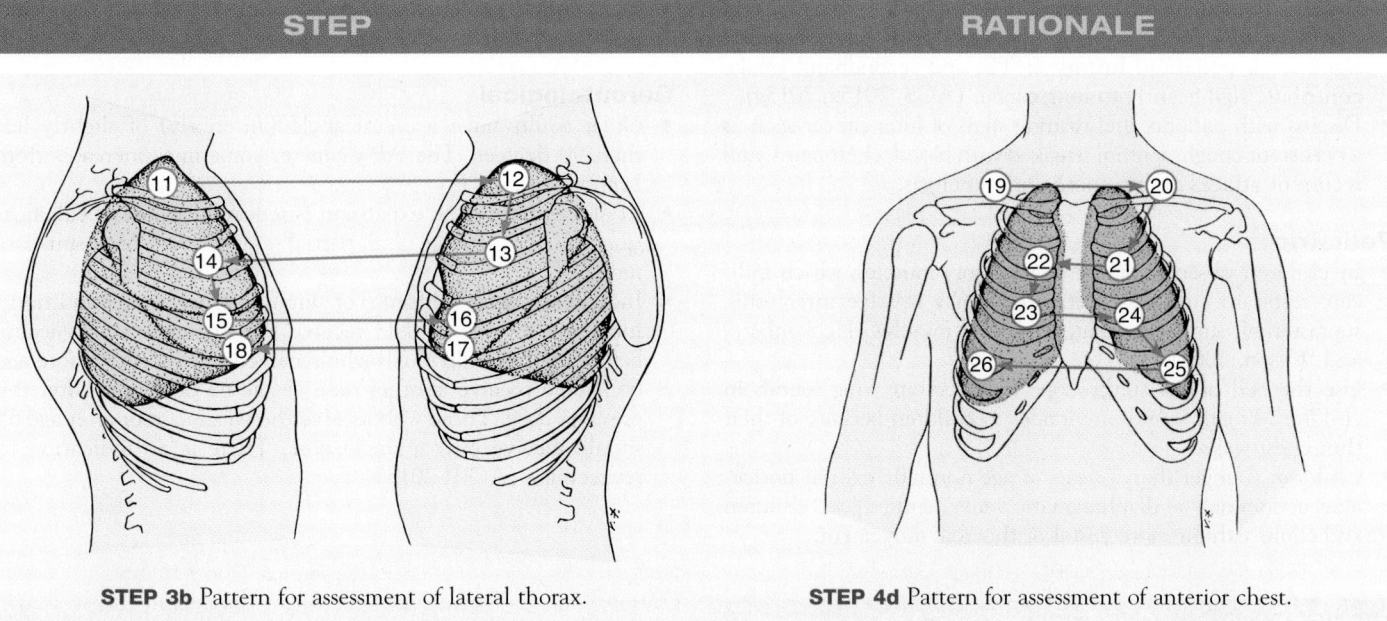

STEP 3b Pattern for assessment of lateral thorax.   **STEP 4d** Pattern for assessment of anterior chest.

EVALUATION

1. Compare respiratory findings with assessment characteristics for thorax and lungs.

   Determines presence of abnormalities.

2. Have patient identify factors leading to lung disease.

   Demonstrates learning.

3. **Use Teach-Back:** "I would like to make sure that you understand some of the risk factors your occupation poses for lung disease. Tell me what are the specific risks to your lungs from some of the chemical exposure in your hair salon?" Revise your instruction now or develop a plan for revised patient or family caregiver teaching if patient or family caregiver is not able to teach back correctly.

   Determines patient's and family caregiver's level of understanding of instructional topic.

Unexpected Outcomes	Related Interventions
1. Patient has copious mucus production; audible inspiratory wheezing; or congested cough with thick mucus.	• Help patient cough by splinting chest; teach to inhale slowly through nose, exhale, and cough; encourage expectoration of mucus. • Auscultate breath sounds before and after cough to evaluate cough effectiveness. • Auscultate lungs for adventitious sounds. • Encourage increased oral intake (if permitted). • If unable to clear airway by coughing, suctioning may be indicated. • Monitor vital signs. • Notify health care provider.
2. Respirations are rapid or slow and irregular (see Chapter 5), and bulging of intercostal spaces is present.	• Position patient more upright if appropriate. • Auscultate lungs for adventitious sounds. • Notify health care provider.
3. Chest excursion is reduced. Depth of breathing is reduced by pain, postural deformity, or fatigue.	• Reposition patient more comfortably. • Administer analgesic if appropriate.

Recording and Reporting

• Record patient's respiratory rate and character; breath sounds, including type, location, and presence on inspiration, expiration, or both; changes noted after coughing; and other physical assessment findings in nurses' notes in electronic health record (EHR) or chart.

• Report abnormalities immediately to the health care provider.

• Document your evaluation of patient and family caregiver learning.

Special Considerations
Teaching

• Educate patients about risks of cigarette smoking. Smoking accounts for at least 30% of all cancer deaths and 80% of lung cancer deaths (ACS, 2015g). Individuals who stop smoking have the potential to live longer than those who continue to smoke. The probability of these individuals dying from lung cancer or other related causes continues to decline with further abstinence.

- Explain to patients that exposure to radiation, arsenic, and asbestos from occupational, medical, and environmental sources; air pollution; history of TB; and secondhand smoke contribute significantly to lung cancer (ACS, 2015a, 2015g).
- Discuss with patients the warning signs of lung cancer such as a persistent cough, sputum streaked with blood, chest pains, and recurrent attacks of pneumonia or bronchitis.

Pediatric
- In children observe for use of accessory muscles, which indicate respiratory distress. Retractions may involve intercostal, suprasternal, supraclavicular, or sternal muscles (Hockenberry and Wilson, 2015).
- Use the bell of the stethoscope to auscultate lung sounds in children. Breath sounds are louder in children because of their thin chest walls.
- Children younger than 7 years of age normally exhibit noticeable abdominal or diaphragmatic movement. Older children and adults exhibit more costal or thoracic movement.

- Head bobbing and nasal flaring in infants are signs of significant respiratory distress (Hockenberry and Wilson, 2015).

Gerontological
- Older adults have a costal angle (anteriorly) of slightly less than 90 degrees. The AP diameter sometimes increases from kyphosis.
- In older adults chest expansion is reduced because of calcification of rib cartilage and partial contraction of inspiratory muscles.
- Individuals with chronic or immunosuppressed conditions, including asthma, should receive the pneumococcal vaccine before age 64. Individuals who received the vaccine before age 65 should receive another dose at age 65 or 5 years after the previous dose. Those who receive the vaccine at or after age 65 should receive only a single dose. There is no indication to revaccinate (ACIP, 2015).

✦ SKILL 6.4   Cardiovascular Assessment

A patient who presents with signs or symptoms of heart (cardiac) problems such as chest pain may be suffering a life-threatening condition requiring immediate attention. In this situation you act quickly and perform the parts of the examination that are absolutely necessary. This will reveal baseline heart function and any risks for heart disease. Patients tend to seek information about heart disease because it remains a leading cause of death in the United States. The heart, neck vessels, and peripheral circulation are assessed together because the systems work in unison. Then you can conduct a more thorough assessment when the patient is more stable.

Your assessment can determine the integrity of the circulatory system. Inadequate tissue perfusion results in an inadequate delivery of oxygen and nutrients to cells, a condition called *ischemia*. This is caused by constriction of vessels or occlusion (blockage) from clot formation. The effects of ischemia depend on the duration of the problem and the metabolic needs of the tissues. Ischemia results in pain. If lack of oxygen to tissues is unrelieved, tissue necrosis (death) occurs. An embolus is a blood clot that breaks loose and travels through the circulation. If the clot obstructs circulation to the lungs or brain, it can be life threatening.

You begin assessment of the heart after examining the lungs because the patient is already in a suitable position with the chest exposed. Assessment then proceeds to the neck vessels and ends with evaluating peripheral circulation. The skills of inspection, palpation, auscultation, and percussion are used during the examination.

Delegation and Collaboration
The skill of completing a comprehensive cardiovascular assessment cannot be delegated to nursing assistive personnel (NAP). The nurse directs the NAP to:
- Count peripheral pulses after vital signs confirm that patient is stable.
- Recognize skin temperature and color changes of affected extremities and report any changes to the nurse.
- Recognize changes in peripheral pulses and report any changes to the nurse.

Equipment
- Stethoscope
- Doppler stethoscope (optional)
- Conducting gel (if a Doppler stethoscope is used)
- Clean gloves (use nonlatex if appropriate)

STEP	RATIONALE

ASSESSMENT

1. Assess patient for history of smoking, alcohol intake, caffeine intake (e.g., coffee, tea, soft drinks, energy drinks, and chocolate) and use of "recreational" drugs. Determine exercise habits and dietary patterns and intake.

   These contribute to risk factors for cardiovascular disease. In addition, caffeine and alcohol cause tachycardia. Insufficient exercise and intake of fatty and salty foods increase risk for cardiovascular disease.

2. Determine if patient is taking medications for cardiovascular function (e.g., antiarrhythmics, antihypertensives, beta-blockers, antianginals) and if he or she knows their purpose, dosage, and side effects.

   Allows you to assess patient's adherence to and understanding of drug therapies. Medications for cardiovascular function cannot be taken intermittently.

3. Ask if patient has experienced dyspnea, chest pain or discomfort, palpitations, excess fatigue, cough, leg pain or cramps, edema of the feet, cyanosis, fainting, and orthopnea. Ask if symptoms occur at rest or during exercise.

   These are the cardinal symptoms of heart disease. Cardiovascular function is sometimes adequate during rest but not during exercise.

STEP	RATIONALE
4. If patient reports chest pain, determine onset (sudden or gradual), precipitating factors, quality, region, and severity and if it radiates. Anginal pain is usually a deep pressure or ache that is substernal and diffuse, radiating to one or both arms, neck, or jaw.	Symptoms reveal acute coronary syndrome or coronary artery disease (CAD).
5. Assess family history for heart disease, diabetes mellitus, high cholesterol and/or lipid levels, hypertension, stroke, or rheumatic heart disease.	Family history of these conditions increases risk for heart and vascular disease.
6. Ask patient about a history of any preexisting heart conditions (e.g., heart failure, congenital heart disease, CAD, dysrhythmias, or murmurs), heart surgery, or vascular disease (e.g., hypertension, phlebitis, varicose veins).	Knowledge reveals patient's level of understanding of condition. Preexisting condition influences which examination techniques to use and expected findings.
7. Determine if patient experiences leg cramps; numbness or tingling in extremities; sensation of cold hands or feet; pain in legs; or swelling or cyanosis of feet, ankles, or hand.	These are signs and symptoms of vascular disease.
8. If patient experiences leg pain or cramping in lower extremities, ask if it is relieved by walking or standing for long periods or if it occurs during sleep.	Relationship of symptoms to exercise clarifies if problem is vascular or musculoskeletal. Pain caused by vascular condition tends to increase with activity. Musculoskeletal pain is usually not relieved when exercise ends.
9. Ask women if they wear tight-fitting underwear or hosiery. Ask both men and women if they wear tight-fitting trouser socks and sit or lie in bed with legs crossed.	Tight hosiery around lower extremities and crossing legs can impair venous return, promoting clot formation.

NURSING DIAGNOSES

- Activity intolerance
- Decreased cardiac output
- Deficient knowledge regarding the need for a cardiovascular assessment
- Ineffective peripheral tissue perfusion
- Pain (acute, chronic)
- Risk for peripheral neurovascular dysfunction

Related factors/Risk factors are individualized based on patient's condition or needs.

PLANNING

1. Expected outcomes following completion of procedure:	
• Heart rate is 60 to 100 beats/min (adolescent through adult), without extra sounds or murmurs.	Indicates normal rate and sinus rhythm.
• Point of maximal impulse (PMI) is palpable at fifth intercostal space at left midclavicular line in children older than 7 years of age and adults.	Indicates normal heart position.
• Patient describes changes in own behavior that could improve cardiovascular function.	Instruction about cardiovascular disease risks may improve patient's health behavior habits.
• Patient describes schedule, dosage, purpose, and benefits of medications being taken for cardiovascular function.	Information related to health benefits may improve adherence to therapy.
• Blood pressure is within normal limits for patient (see Chapter 5).	This is one indicator of normal cardiovascular function.
• Carotid pulse is localized, strong, elastic, and equal bilaterally. No change occurs during inspiration or expiration; without carotid bruit.	This indicates a patent vessel.
• Jugular veins distend when patient lies supine and flatten when patient is in sitting position.	Venous pressure is normal.
• Peripheral pulses are equal and strong (2+); extremities are warm and pink, with capillary refill less than 2 seconds. There is no dependent edema. Peripheral hair growth is symmetrical and evenly distributed, and the skin is free of lesions.	Peripheral circulation is intact.
2. Anticipate teaching topics so during the examination you can teach patient about risks for heart and vascular disease.	Allows you to incorporate teaching during examination.
3. Perform hand hygiene. Prepare necessary supplies.	Reduces transmission of infection. Promotes efficient examination.

STEP	RATIONALE

IMPLEMENTATION

1. Help patient be as relaxed and comfortable as possible.

An anxious or uncomfortable patient can have mild tachycardia, which alters findings.

2. Have patient assume semi-Fowler's or supine position.

Provides adequate visibility and access to left thorax and mediastinum. Patient with heart disease often experiences shortness of breath while lying flat.

3. Explain procedure. Avoid facial gestures reflecting concern.

Patients with previously normal cardiac history may become anxious if you show concern.

4. Be sure that room is quiet.

Subtle, low-pitched heart sounds are difficult to hear.

5. Assess the heart:

    a. Form mental image of exact location of the heart (see illustration). Base of heart is the upper part, and apex is the bottom tip. Surface of right ventricle constitutes most of the anterior surface of the heart.

Visualization improves ability to assess findings accurately and determines possible source of abnormalities.

    b. Find angle of Louis, felt as ridge in sternum approximately 5 cm (2 inches) below suprasternal notch (between sternal body and manubrium). Slip fingers down each side of angle to feel adjacent ribs. Intercostal spaces (ICS) are just below each rib.

Provides you with landmarks to locate and assess heart sounds.

    c. Find the following anatomical landmarks (see illustration):

Familiarity with landmarks allows you to describe findings more clearly and ultimately may improve assessment.

        (1) Aortic area is at second ICS, right of patient's sternum, close to sternal border (*1*).

Listening to heart sounds from too far away from sternal border decreases ability to hear them clearly.

        (2) Pulmonic area is at second ICS, left of patient's sternum, close to sternal border (*2*).

        (3) Second pulmonic area is found by moving down left side of sternum to third ICS, close to sternal border (*3*), also referred to as *Erb's point*.

        (4) Tricuspid area (*4*) is located at fourth left ICS along sternum, close to sternal border.

        (5) Mitral area is found by moving fingers laterally to patient's left to locate fifth ICS at left midclavicular line (*5*).

        (6) Epigastric area (*6*) is at inferior tip of sternum.

    d. Stand to patient's right to inspect and palpate precordium with patient supine. Note any visible pulsations and more exaggerated lifts. Closely inspect area of apex. Palpate for pulsations (placing proximal half of four fingers together and then alternating with ball of hand at all anatomical landmarks).

Reveals size and symmetry of heart. Apical impulse may be visible at midclavicular line in fifth intercostal space. Apical impulse (PMI) may become visible only when patient sits up, bringing heart closer to anterior wall. Obesity obscures ability to visualize PMI. There should be no pulsations or vibrations. A thrill is a continuous palpable sensation, such as purring of a cat. A thrust is the upward lift felt when palpating the chest wall.

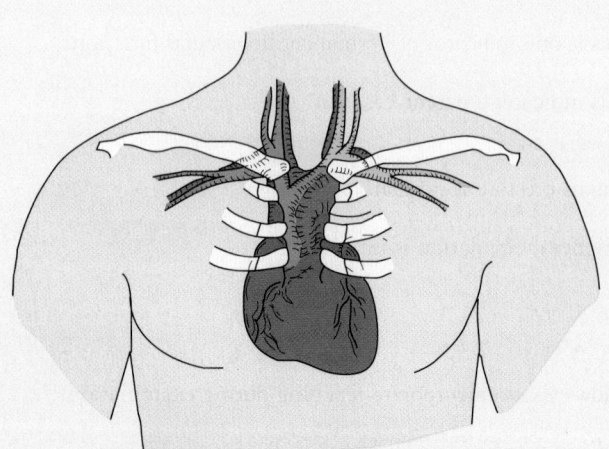

STEP 5a Anatomical position of heart.

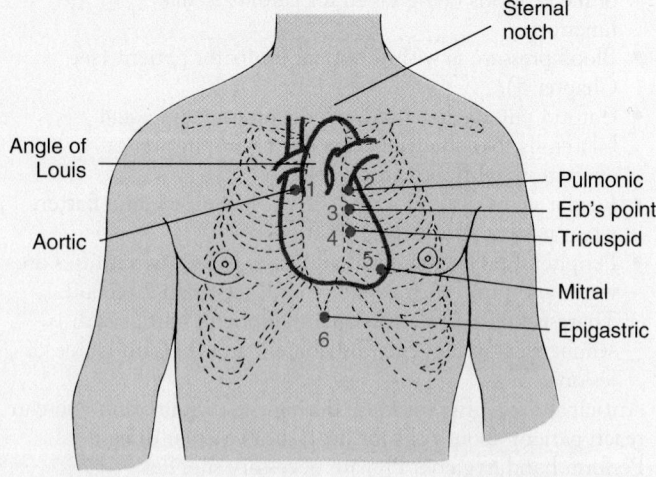

STEP 5c Anatomical sites for assessment of cardiac function.

STEP	**RATIONALE**

e. Locate PMI by palpating with fingertips along the fifth ICS in midclavicular line (see illustration). Note light, brief pulsation in area 1 to 2 cm (½ to 1 inch) in diameter at the apex.

In presence of serious heart disease, PMI is located to left of midclavicular line related to enlarged left ventricle. In chronic lung disease PMI may be to right of midclavicular line as a result of right ventricular enlargement.

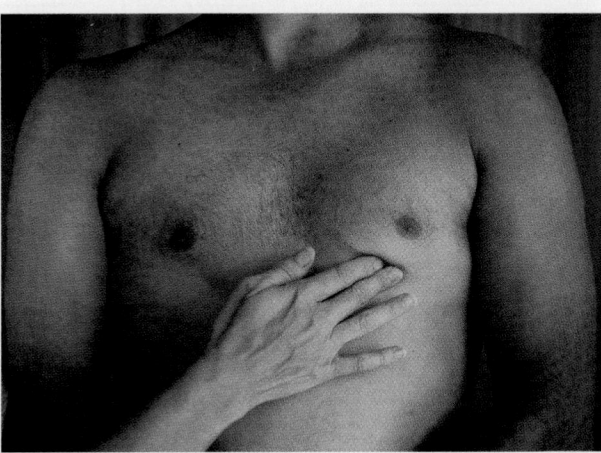

STEP 5e Palpation of point of maximal impulse. *(From Ball JW et al: Seidel's guide to physical examination, ed 8, St Louis, 2015, Mosby.)*

Clinical Decision Point *Presence of a palpable thrill is not normal and indicates a disruption of blood flow caused by a defect in closure of a heart valve or atrial septal defect. A stronger than expected impulse is a heave or lift, which indicates increased cardiac output or left ventricular hypertrophy. Report to health care provider.*

f. If palpating PMI is difficult, turn patient onto left side.

Maneuver moves heart closer to chest wall.

g. Inspect epigastric area and palpate abdominal aorta.
NOTE: You should feel a localized strong beat.

Rules out reduced blood flow or diffuse pulse, which indicates abnormality.

h. Auscultate heart sounds:

(1) Have patient sit up and lean slightly forward; then have him or her lie supine; and end examination with patient in left lateral recumbent position (see illustration A to C). In female patient it may be necessary to lift left breast to hear heart sounds more effectively.

Different positions help to clarify type of sounds heard. Sitting position is best to hear high-pitched murmurs (if present). Supine is common position to hear all sounds. Left lateral recumbent is best position to hear low-pitched sounds.

(2) While auscultating sounds at each anatomical landmark, ask patient not to speak but to breathe comfortably. Begin with diaphragm of stethoscope; alternate with bell. Use very light pressure for bell. Inch stethoscope along; avoid jumping from one area to another. Do not try to hear all heart sounds at once.

Auscultation requires you to isolate each heart sound at all auscultation sites, especially in patients with soft heart sounds.

(3) Begin at apex or PMI; move systematically to aortic area, pulmonic area, Erb's point, tricuspid area, and mitral area (see illustration in Step 5c). (NOTE: Some examiners use reverse sequence.) S_1 is loudest at apex and is simultaneous with carotid pulse. NOTE: Helpful mnemonic for remembering heart sound locations: **A P**ig **E**ats **T**oo **M**uch (Aortic, Pulmonic, Erb's point, Tricuspid, Mitral).

At normal slow rates S_1 is high pitched and dull in quality and sounds like a "lub." This sound precedes systolic phase of heart contraction.

(4) Listen for S_2 at each site. This sound is loudest at the aortic area. Heart sounds vary by pitch, loudness, and duration, depending on auscultatory site (Table 6.8).

Normal sounds S_1 and S_2 are high pitched and best heard with diaphragm. S_2 precedes diastolic phase and sounds like "dub."

(5) After both sounds are heard clearly as "lub-dub," count each combination of S_1 and S_2 as one heartbeat. Count number of beats for 1 minute.

Determines apical pulse rate.

STEP	RATIONALE

TABLE 6.8

Heart Sounds According to Auscultatory Area

	Aortic	Pulmonic	Second Pulmonic	Mitral	Tricuspid
Pitch	$S_1 < S_2$	$S_1 < S_2$	$S_1 < S_2$	$S_1 > S_2$	$S_1 = S_2$
Loudness	$S_1 < S_2$	$S_1 < S_2$	$S_1 < S_2$*	$S_1 > S_2$†	$S_1 > S_2$
Duration	$S_1 > S_2$	$S_1 > S_2$	$S_1 > S_2$	$S_1 > S_2$	$S_1 > S_2$

*S_1 is relatively louder in second pulmonic area than in aortic area.
†S_1 may be louder in mitral area than in tricuspid area.
Modified from Ball JW et al: *Seidel's guide to physical examination*, ed 8, St Louis, 2015, Mosby.

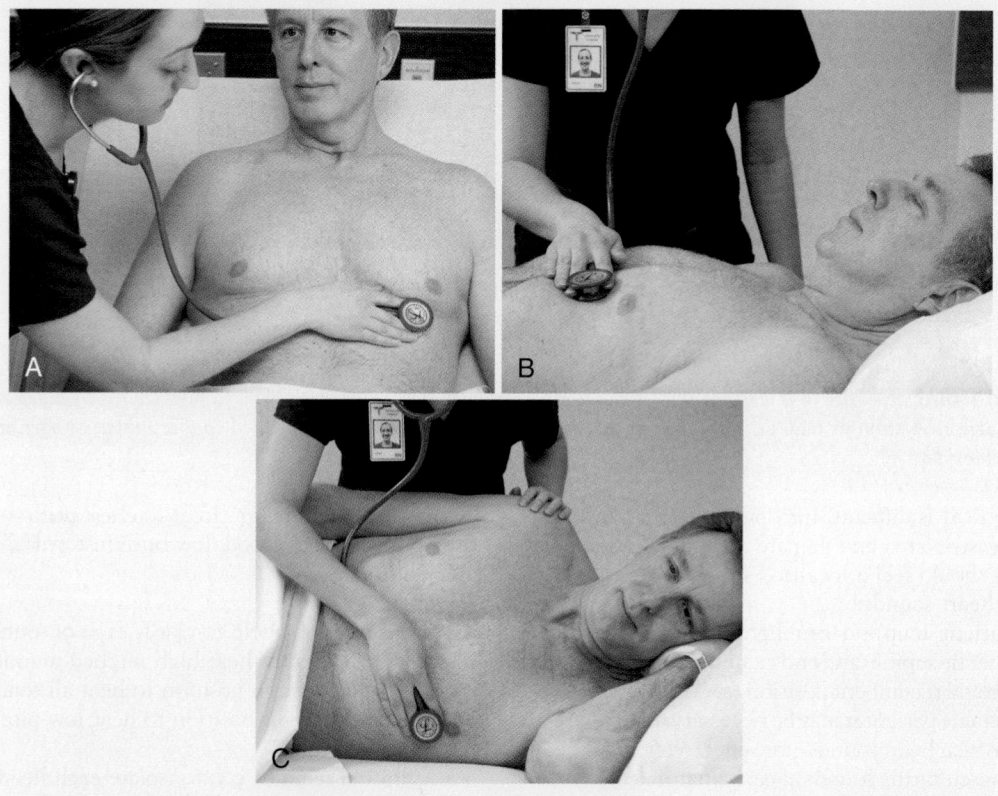

STEP 5h(1) Patient positions for auscultation of heart sounds. **A,** Sitting. **B,** Supine. **C,** Left lateral.
(*From Ball JW et al:* Seidel's guide to physical examination, *ed 8, St Louis, 2015, Mosby.*)

(6) Assess heart rhythm by noting time between S_1 and S_2 (systole) and then time between S_2 and the next S_1 (diastole). Listen to full cycle at each auscultation area. Note regular intervals between each sequence of beats. There should be a distinct pause between S_1 and S_2.

Failure of heart to beat at regular intervals is a dysrhythmia, which interferes with ability of heart to pump effectively.

(7) When heart rate is irregular, compare apical and radial pulses (Table 6.9). Auscultate apical pulse and then immediately palpate radial pulse. Also, you can ask a colleague to assess radial pulse while you simultaneously assess apical pulse.

Determines if pulse deficit (radial pulse is slower than apical) exists. Deficit indicates that ineffective contractions of heart fail to send pulse waves to periphery.

i. Auscultate for extra heart sounds at each site. Note pitch, loudness, duration, timing, location on chest wall, and where it is heard in cardiac cycle.

Abnormal sounds include murmurs. Characteristics of murmurs help to identify contributing factors.

TABLE 6.9

Abnormalities in Rates and Rhythms

Type	Findings	Description
Atrial fibrillation	Rapid, random contractions of atria cause irregular ventricular beats >100 beats/min and atrial beats at 200–350 beats/min.	Atria discharge very rapidly, with some impulses not reaching ventricles. This condition occurs in rheumatic heart disease and mitral stenosis. It causes reduced cardiac output.
Sinus arrhythmia	Pulse rate changes during respiration, increasing at peak of inspiration and decreasing during expiration.	Blood is momentarily trapped in lungs during inspiration, causing a fall in stroke volume of heart.
Sinus bradycardia	Pulse rhythm is regular, but rate is <60 beats/min.	Sinoatrial node fires less frequently. This is common in well-conditioned athletes and with use of antiarrhythmic medications.
Sinus tachycardia	Pulse rhythm is regular, but rate is accelerated to >100 beats/min.	Exercise, emotional stress, and caffeine or alcohol ingestion are common factors that cause increased firing of sinoatrial node.
Premature ventricular contraction	Premature beat occurs before regularly expected heart contraction. Underlying rhythm can be any rate.	Ventricle contracts prematurely because of electrical impulse bypassing normal conduction pathway. It may occur so early that it is difficult to detect as second beat. It may be followed by a pause.

(1) Use stethoscope bell and listen for low-pitched extra heart sounds such as S_3 and S_4 gallops, clicks, and rubs. S_3, or a ventricular gallop, occurs just after S_2 at end of ventricular diastole. It sounds like "lub-dub-ee" or "Ken-tuc-ky." S_4, or an atrial gallop, occurs just before S_1 or ventricular systole. It sounds like "dee-lub-dub" or "Ten-nes-see."

Premature rush of blood into a ventricle that is stiff or dilated or an atrial contraction pushing against a ventricle that is not accepting blood causes gallops.

(2) With patient leaning forward or lying on left side, listen for friction rubs as "squeaky" or rubbing sounds.

Rubs result from lungs or inflamed visceral and parietal layers of the pericardium of the heart rubbing against one another.

j. Auscultate for heart murmurs over each auscultation site.

Murmurs are sustained swishing or blowing sounds heard at beginning, middle, or end of systole or diastole. Increased blood flow through a normal valve, forward flow through a stenotic valve or into a dilated vessel or chamber, or backward flow through a valve that fails to close causes murmurs.

(1) When you detect a murmur, listen carefully to note where you hear it best. Note intensity of the murmur.

Intensity is related to rate of blood flow through the heart or amount of blood regurgitated.

(2) Note if murmur is low, medium, or high in pitch, using bell for low-pitched sounds.

Pitch depends on velocity of blood flow through the valves.

6. Assess neck vessels:

a. To assess carotid arteries, have patient remain in sitting position.

Allows easier mobility of neck to expose artery for inspection and palpation.

b. Inspect neck on both sides for obvious arterial pulsations. Sometimes a pulse wave can be seen.

Carotids are the only sites to assess quality of pulse wave (see illustration). Experience is required to evaluate wave in relation to events of cardiac cycle.

c. Palpate each carotid artery separately with index and middle fingers around medial edge of sternocleidomastoid muscle. Ask patient to raise chin slightly, keeping head straight (see illustration) or slightly away from artery. Note rate and rhythm, strength, and elasticity of artery. Also note if pulse changes as patient inhales and exhales.

If both arteries were occluded simultaneously, patient could lose consciousness from reduced circulation to brain. Turning head improves access to artery. A change indicates a sinus arrhythmia.

Clinical Decision Point *Do not palpate or massage the carotid artery vigorously. Stimulation of carotid sinus causes a reflex drop in heart rate and blood pressure.*

d. Place bell of stethoscope over each carotid artery, auscultating for blowing sound (bruit) (see illustration). Ask patient to exhale and hold breath for a few heartbeats so respiratory sounds do not interfere with auscultation (Ball et al., 2015).

Narrowing of lumen of carotid artery by arteriosclerotic plaques causes disturbance in blood flow. Blood passing through narrowed section creates turbulence and emits blowing or swishing sound. Normally you do not hear a bruit.

STEP	RATIONALE

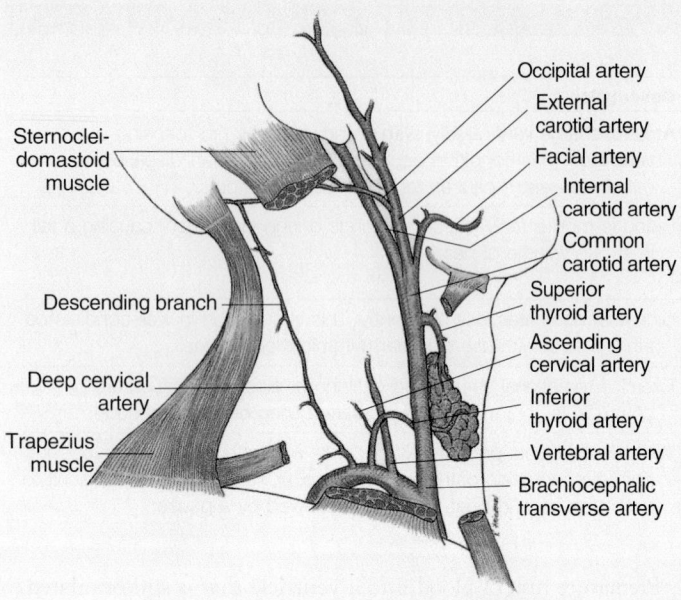

STEP 6b Anatomical position of carotid artery.

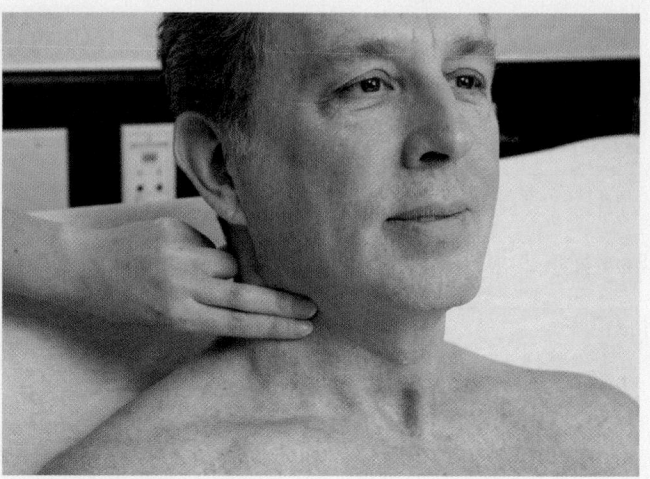

STEP 6c Palpate each carotid artery separately.

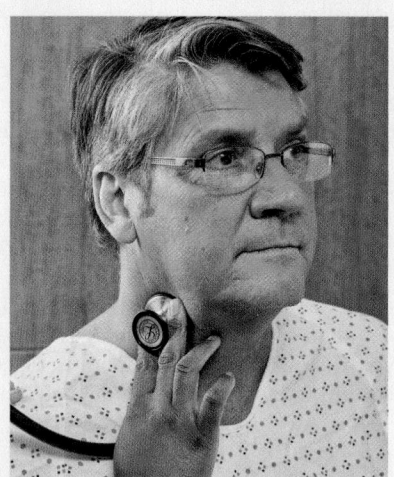

STEP 6d Auscultation for carotid artery bruit. *(From Ball JW et al: Seidel's guide to physical examination, ed 8, St Louis, 2015, Mosby.)*

7. Peripheral vascular assessment:
   a. Inspect lower extremities for changes in color and condition of skin (Table 6.10). Note skin and nail texture, hair distribution, venous patterns, edema, and scars or impaired skin integrity. Compare skin color with patient lying and standing.

   Changes may reflect impaired peripheral circulation.

   b. Palpate edematous areas, noting mobility, consistency, and tenderness.

   Helps to determine extent of edema.

   c. Assess for pitting edema by pressing area firmly with one finger for 5 seconds and releasing. Depth of indentation determines severity (see illustration).
      2 mm: 1+ edema
      4 mm: 2+ edema
      6 mm: 3+ edema
      8 mm: 4+ edema

   Limb edema is classic sign of deep vein thrombosis (DVT), although this can be seen in other conditions; therefore, if DVT is suspected. diagnostic tests must be performed (Patel et al., 2014).

STEP	**RATIONALE**

TABLE 6.10

Signs of Venous and Arterial Insufficiency

Assessment Criterion	Venous	Arterial
Pain	Aching; increases in evening and with dependent position	Burning, throbbing, cramping; increases with exercise
Paresthesia	None	Numbness, tingling, decreased sensation
Temperature	Normal to touch	Cool to touch
Color	Normal or cyanotic	Pale; worsened by elevation of extremity; dusky red when extremity is lowered
Capillary refill	Not applicable	>2 seconds
Pulse	Present	Decreased or absent
Skin changes	Brown pigmentation around ankles	Thin, shiny skin; decreased hair growth; thickened nails
Ulcerations	Shallow ulcers around ankles (chronic venous stasis); edema apparent	Deep, well defined at site of trauma or tips of toes

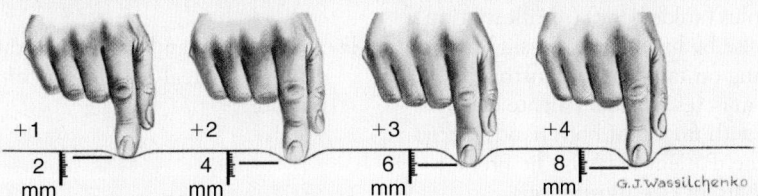

STEP 7c Assessing for pitting edema. *(From Seidel HM et al: Mosby's guide to physical examination, ed 7, St Louis, 2011, Mosby.)*

   d. Use tape measure to measure circumference of extremity.

Measuring circumference establishes baseline for future comparison.

   e. Check capillary refill by grasping patient's fingernail or toenail and noting color of nail bed. Apply gentle, firm pressure to nail bed. Release quickly, watching for color change. Circulation is restored and normally returns to pink color in less than 2 seconds.

Capillary refill is measured in seconds; less than 2 seconds is brisk; whereas greater than 4 seconds is sluggish.

Cold environmental temperature with vasoconstriction and vascular disease can delay refill. Local pressure from cast or bandage also slows refill.

   f. Ask if patient experiences pain or tenderness and gently palpate for heat, firmness, or localized swelling of calf muscle, all of which are signs of phlebitis or DVT.

The most frequent cause of DVT is immobilization such as in postoperative patients and in individuals after an airplane flight lasting over 8 hours. Other factors that contribute to DVT are chronic illness such as strokes and lengthy surgeries (Patel et al., 2014).

Clinical Decision Point *Homans' sign (pain in calf on dorsiflexion of foot) is no longer considered a reliable indicator for the presence or absence of DVT (Ball et al., 2015) and should not be considered a reliable test. Trauma to a vein or muscle, reduced mobility, and increased blood clotting are reliable risk factors. If calf is swollen, tender, or red, notify patient's health care provider for further assessment and evaluation. If there is a strong suspicion of DVT, testing for Homans' sign is contraindicated. If a clot is present, it may become dislodged from its original site during this test. This could result in a pulmonary embolism.*

   g. Palpate peripheral arteries.

     (1) Start at most distal part of each extremity. Palpate each peripheral artery for equality, comparing side to side; elasticity of vessel wall (depress and release artery, noting ease with which it springs back to shape); and strength of pulse (force of blood against arterial wall) using the following rating scale (Ball et al., 2015):

Comparison of both arteries allows you to determine any localized obstruction or disturbance in blood flow. Pulses should be symmetrical side to side. If asymmetry is noted, look for other factors related to impaired circulation.

     0   Absent, not palpable
     1+ Diminished, pulse barely palpable, weak and thready, and easy to obliterate
     2+ Normal pulse, easy to palpate
     3+ Full, easy to palpate, increases
     4+ Strong, bounding against fingertips; cannot be obliterated

STEP	RATIONALE
(2) Palpate radial pulse by lightly placing tips of first and second fingers in groove formed along radial side of forearm, lateral to flexor tendon of wrist (see illustration).	Pulse is relatively superficial and should not require deep palpation.
(3) Palpate ulnar pulse by placing fingertips along ulnar side of forearm (see illustration).	Palpated when arterial insufficiency to hand is expected or when you assess for radial occlusion (e.g., during arterial blood gas sampling), which may affect circulation to hand.
(4) Palpate brachial pulse by locating groove between biceps and triceps muscles above elbow at antecubital fossa (see illustration). Place tips of first two fingers in muscle groove.	Artery runs along medial side of extended arm, requiring moderate palpation. If difficult to palpate, hyperextend arm to bring pulse site closer to the surface.
(5) Have patient lie supine with feet relaxed and palpate dorsalis pedis pulse. Gently place fingertips between great and first toe; slowly move fingers along groove between extensor tendons of great and first toe until pulse is palpable (see illustration).	Artery lies superficially and does not require deep palpation. Pulse may be congenitally absent.
(6) Palpate posterior tibial pulse by having patient relax and extend feet slightly. Place fingertips behind and below medial malleolus (ankle bone) (see illustration).	Artery is easily palpable with foot relaxed.
(7) Palpate popliteal pulse by having patient slightly flex knee with foot resting on table or bed. Instruct patient to keep leg muscles relaxed. Palpate deeply into popliteal fossa with fingers of both hands placed just lateral to midline. Patient may also lie prone to achieve exposure of artery (see illustration).	Flexion of knee and muscle relaxation improves accessibility of artery. Popliteal pulse is one of the more difficult pulses to palpate.

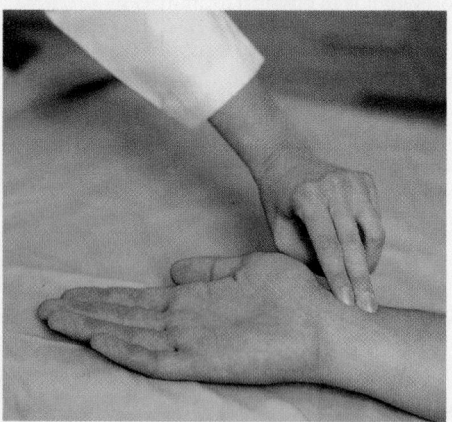

STEP 7g(2) Palpation of radial pulse.

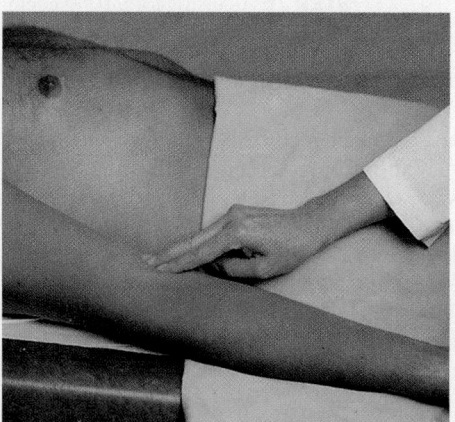

STEP 7g(4) Palpation of brachial pulse.

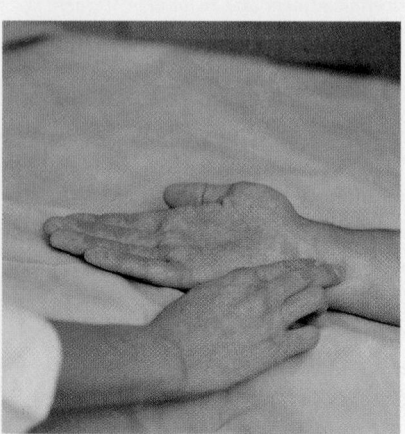

STEP 7g(3) Palpation of ulnar pulse.

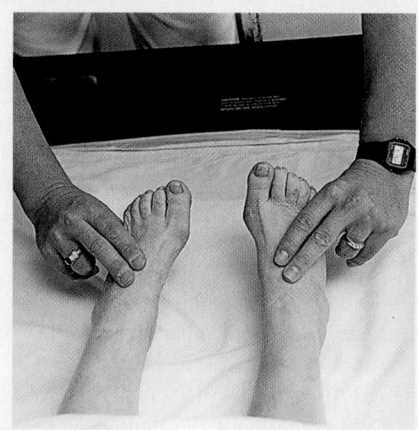

STEP 7g(5) Palpation of dorsalis pedis pulses.

STEP	**RATIONALE**
(8) Apply clean gloves. With patient supine, palpate femoral pulse by placing first two fingers over inguinal area below inguinal ligament, midway between pubic symphysis and anterosuperior iliac spine (see illustration).	Supine position prevents flexion in groin area, which interferes with artery access.
h. If pulses are difficult to palpate or are not palpable, use a Doppler instrument over pulse site:	Doppler amplifies sounds, allowing you to hear low-velocity blood flow through peripheral arteries.
(1) Apply conducting gel to patient's skin over pulse site or onto transducer tip of probe. Turn Doppler on.	
(2) Gently apply ultrasound probe to skin, changing Doppler angle until pulsation is audible. Adjust volume as needed (see illustration). Wipe off gel from patient and Doppler.	
7. Remove gloves and discard used supplies and gloves in proper receptacle. Help patient to comfortable position. Perform hand hygiene.	Reduces transmission of infection.

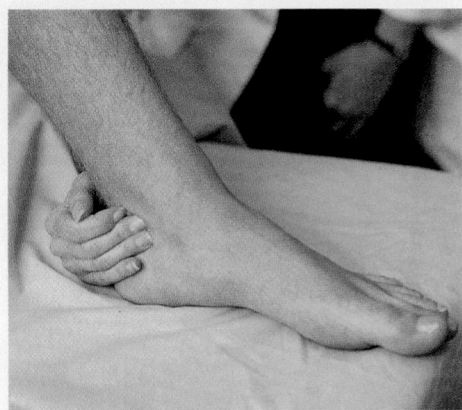

STEP 7g(6) Palpation of posterior tibial pulse.

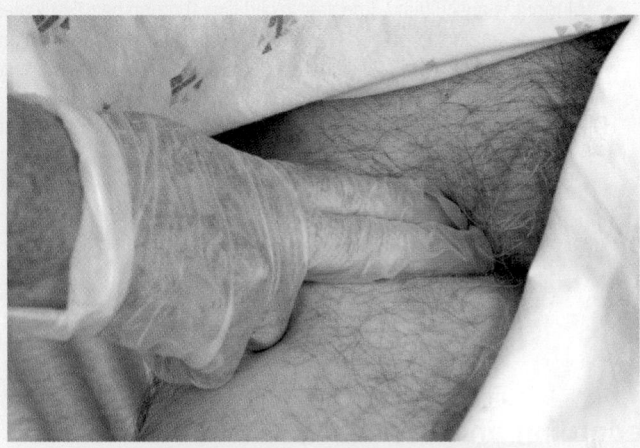

STEP 7g(8) Palpation of femoral pulse.

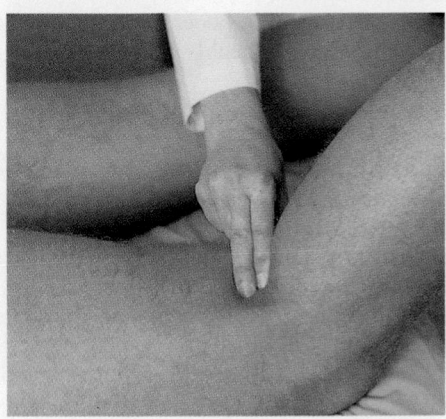

STEP 7g(7) Palpation of popliteal pulse with patient prone.

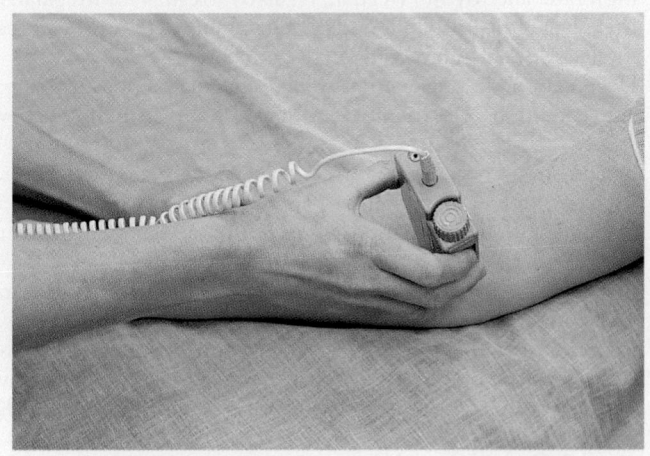

STEP 7h(2) Use of Doppler to assess brachial pulse.

EVALUATION

1. Compare findings with normal assessment characteristics of heart and vascular system.	Determines presence of abnormalities.
2. If heart sounds are not audible or pulses are not palpable, ask another nurse to confirm assessment.	Validates abnormal assessment findings.
3. Ask patient to describe behaviors that increase risk for heart and vascular disease.	Demonstrates learning.

STEP	RATIONALE
4. Compare pulses and capillary refill bilaterally with previous assessment.	Demonstrates change from baseline measures.
5. **Use Teach-Back:** "I would like to make sure you understand some of the risks and behaviors that can lead to heart disease. Tell me how your lack of exercise affects your risk for heart disease." Revise your instruction now or develop a plan for revised patient or family caregiver teaching if patient or family caregiver is not able to teach back correctly.	Determines patient's and family caregiver's level of understanding of instructional topic.

Unexpected Outcomes	Related Interventions
1. Findings differ from previous assessments, including: • Pulsations, vibrations, or both are palpable. These are result of valvular problem, murmur, or both. • Extra heart sounds S_3 or S_4 are auscultated. Extra sounds indicate atrial or ventricular gallop. • Murmur is auscultated. Impaired blood flow through heart indicates need for immediate medical attention. Some murmurs are benign. • JVP is elevated. This is sign of right-sided heart failure or fluid overload.	• Prepare to obtain or help with electrocardiogram (ECG).
2. Heart rate is irregular, with rate less than 60 beats/min or more than 100 beats/min.	• Check blood pressure. If low, dysrhythmia is contributing to inadequate cardiac output. • Observe for sensations or reports of dizziness or feeling "faint." • Prepare to obtain ECG.
3. Pulse deficit is noted. There is risk for inadequate cardiac output.	• Obtain vital signs.

Recording and Reporting

- Document quality (clear or muffled), intensity (weak or pounding), rate, and rhythm (regular, regularly irregular, or irregularly irregular) of heart sounds and peripheral pulses in nurses' notes in electronic health record (EHR) or chart.
- Document additional cardiac findings, jugular venous pressure, and condition of extremities in nurses' notes in EHR or flow sheet.
- Document activity level and subjective data related to fatigue, shortness of breath, and chest pain.
- Document your evaluation of patient and family caregiver learning.
- Report immediately to health care provider any irregularities in heart function and indications of impaired arterial blood flow.
- Report to health care provider changes in peripheral circulation, which may indicate circulatory compromise, which may result in permanent nerve damage or tissue death if untreated.

Special Considerations
Teaching

- Explain risk factors for heart disease: high dietary intake of saturated fat or cholesterol, lack of regular aerobic exercise, smoking, excess weight, stressful lifestyle, hypertension, and family history of heart disease.
- Refer patient (if appropriate) to resources available for controlling or reducing risks (e.g., nutrition counseling, exercise class, and stress-reduction programs).
- Encourage patient to discuss with health care provider the need for periodic C-reactive protein (CRP) testing. CRP levels assess a patient's cardiovascular disease risk.

- Help patient to find resources to help quitting smoking because this lowers the risk for coronary heart disease and coronary vascular disease (ACS, 2014). Nicotine in cigarette smoke causes vasoconstriction.
- Patients who are at risk benefit from taking a daily low dose of aspirin. Consult health care provider before starting therapy.

Pediatric

- PMI is at fourth intercostal space at left midclavicular line in children younger than 7 years of age (Hockenberry and Wilson, 2015).
- Capillary refill in infants is usually less than 1 second.
- It is not uncommon for children to have third heart sounds (S_3). Sinus arrhythmia occurs normally in many infants and children (Hockenberry and Wilson, 2015).
- Children have louder, higher-pitched heart sounds because of their thin chest walls.

Gerontological

- PMI may be difficult to find in an older adult because anteroposterior diameter of the chest deepens.
- Accidental massage of the carotid sinus during palpation of the carotid artery is a particular problem for older adults, causing a sudden drop in heart rate from vagal nerve stimulation.
- Older adults with hypertension benefit from regular monitoring of blood pressure (daily, weekly, or monthly). Home monitoring kits are available. Teach patient how to use them correctly.

Abdominal assessment is complex because of the multiple organs located within and near the abdominal cavity. This area of the body is associated with many health complaints; and many people are embarrassed by bowel or bladder dysfunction, reproductive problems, or urinary elimination problems. Abdominal pain is one of the most common symptoms that patients report when seeking medical care. It can be caused by alterations in organs such as the stomach, gallbladder, or intestines; or the pain may be the result of spinal or muscular injury. An accurate assessment requires matching the patient's history with a careful assessment of the location of physical symptoms (Table 6.11).

To perform an effective abdominal assessment you need to know the location and function of the underlying structures involved, including the lower pelvis, kidneys, rectum, genitalia, liver, gallbladder, stomach, spleen, appendix, pancreas, intestines, and reproductive organs (Fig. 6.5). An abdominal assessment is routine after abdominal surgery, for any patient who has undergone invasive diagnostic tests of the gastrointestinal (GI) tract, and for

patients with abnormalities affecting GI function. The order of an abdominal assessment differs from that of other assessments. You begin with inspection and follow with auscultation. It is important to auscultate before palpation and percussion because these maneuvers alter the frequency and character of bowel sounds.

Delegation and Collaboration

The skill of abdominal assessment cannot be delegated to nursing assistive personnel (NAP). The nurse directs the NAP to:
- Report the development of abdominal pain and changes in the patient's bowel habits or dietary intake to the nurse.

Equipment
- Stethoscope
- Tape measure
- Examination light
- Water-based marking pen
- Drapes

TABLE 6.11

Common Causes of Abdominal Pain

Condition	Physical Alteration	Physical Signs and Symptoms
Appendicitis	Obstruction of appendix associated with inflammation, perforation, and peritonitis Patient often lies on back or side with knees flexed to decrease pain	Sharp pain directly over the irritated peritoneum 2–12 hours after onset. Often pain localizes in right lower quadrant between anterior iliac crest and umbilicus. Associated with rebound tenderness. Accompanied by anorexia, nausea, and vomiting.
Celiac disease	Damage to small intestine mucosa from ingestion of barley, rye, oats, and wheat	Foul-smelling diarrhea, abdominal distention, and symptoms of malnutrition may be present.
Cholecystitis	Obstruction of cystic duct causing inflammation or distention of gallbladder	*Murphy's sign:* Apply gentle pressure below right subcostal arch and liver margin. Sharp pain and increased respiratory rate occur when patient takes a deep breath (Ball et al., 2015).
Constipation	Disruption in normal bowel pattern, which may occur with opioid use or inadequate fiber and fluid intake	Generalized discomfort accompanied by distention and palpation of a hard mass in the left lower quadrant. Nausea and vomiting may begin after several days.
Crohn's disease	Chronic inflammatory disease of the ileum	Steady colicky pain in the right lower quadrant, with cramping, tenderness, flatulence, nausea, fever, and diarrhea. Often associated with bloody stools, weight loss, weakness, and fatigue. A tender mass of thickened intestine may be palpated in right lower quadrant.
Gastroenteritis	Inflammation of the stomach and intestinal tract	Generalized abdominal discomfort accompanied by anorexia, nausea, vomiting, diarrhea, abdominal cramping.
Pancreatitis	Inflammation of the pancreas associated with alcoholism, drug reaction, and gallbladder disease	Steady severe epigastric pain close to umbilicus radiates to back. Associated with abdominal rigidity and vomiting. Pain is unrelieved by vomiting, worsens by lying supine.
Paralytic ileus	Obstruction of the small bowel that occurs after abdominal surgery, from abdominal radiation, or from use of anticholinergic medications	Generalized severe abdominal distention, nausea, and vomiting; decreased/absent bowel sounds.
Peptic ulcers (gastric and duodenal)	Damage of gastrointestinal (GI) mucosa at any area of the GI tract May be caused by bacterial infection (*Helicobacter pylori*) or nonsteroidal antiinflammatory drugs (NSAIDs) Thought to be unrelated to stress Aggravated by smoking and excessive alcohol use	*Gastric ulcer:* Dull epigastric pain, localized midline. Early satiety; not usually relieved by food or antacids. *Duodenal ulcer:* Pain is episodic, lasting 30 minutes to 2 hours. It is located midline in epigastric region, may radiate around costal border to back; described as aching, burning, or gnawing. Typically occurs 1–3 hours after meals and at night (12 midnight to 3 AM). Often relieved by food/antacid. *Both (dyspepsia syndrome):* Complaints of fullness, epigastric discomfort, vague feeling of nausea, abdominal distention, and bloating; anorexia; weight loss.

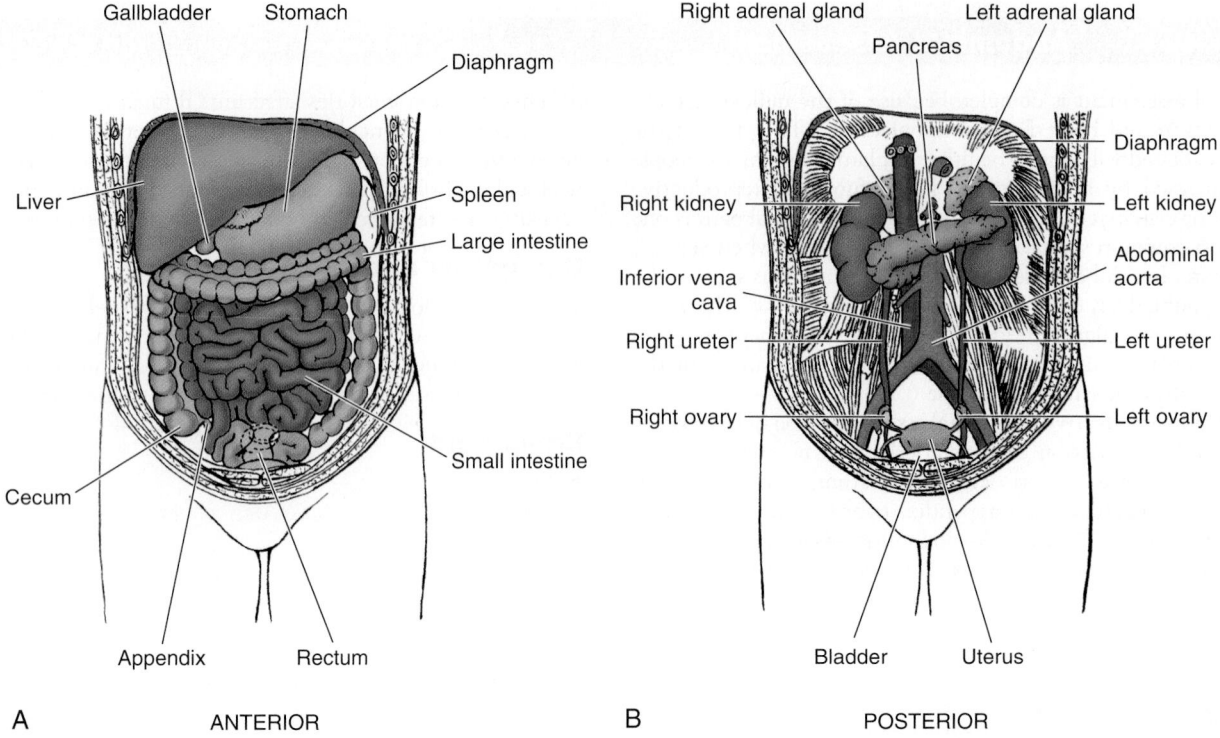

FIG 6.5 Location of organs in abdomen. **A,** Anterior. **B,** Posterior. (*Modified from Mosby's expert 10-minute physical examinations, ed 2, St Louis, 2005, Mosby.*)

STEP	RATIONALE

ASSESSMENT

1. If patient has abdominal or low back pain, assess the character of pain in detail (location, onset, frequency, precipitating factors, aggravating factors, type of pain, severity, course).

Knowing pattern of characteristics of pain helps determine its source.

2. Carefully observe patient's movement and position such as lying still with knees drawn up, moving restlessly to find a comfortable position, or lying on one side or sitting with knees drawn up to chest.

Positions assumed by patient reveal nature and source of pain (e.g., peritonitis, kidney stone, appendicitis). Patients with peritonitis lie still because movement aggravates pain. Supine position worsens acute pancreatitis pain; flexed knee, curved-back position brings relief. Patients with appendicitis lie on side or back with knees flexed in attempt to decrease muscle strain on abdominal wall.

3. Assess patient's normal bowel habits: frequency of stools; character of stools; recent changes in character of stools; measures used to promote elimination such as laxatives, enemas, and dietary intake; and eating and drinking habits.

Data compared with information from physical assessment may help identify cause and nature of elimination problems.

4. Determine if patient has had abdominal surgery, trauma, or diagnostic tests of GI tract.

Surgery or trauma to abdomen may result in altered position of underlying organs. Diagnostic tests may change character of stool.

5. Assess if patient has had recent weight changes or intolerance to diet (nausea, vomiting, cramping, especially in past 24 hours).

Changes may indicate alterations in upper GI tract (e.g., stomach or gallbladder) or lower colon.

6. Assess for difficulty in swallowing, belching, flatulence, bloody emesis (hematemesis), black or tarry stools (melena), heartburn, diarrhea, or constipation.

Indicative of GI alterations.

7. Determine if patient takes antiinflammatory medications (e.g., aspirin, steroids, and nonsteroidal antiinflammatory drugs [NSAIDs]), or antibiotics.

These medications may cause GI upset or bleeding.

STEP	RATIONALE
8. Review family history of cancer, kidney disease, alcoholism, hypertension, or heart disease.	Information may reveal risk for significant abdominal alterations. Chronic alcohol ingestion causes GI and liver problems.
9. Review patient's history for health care occupation, hemodialysis, intravenous drug use, household or sexual contact with hepatitis B virus (HBV) carrier, sexually active heterosexual person (more than one sex partner in previous 6 months), sexually active homosexual or bisexual man, international traveler in area of high HBV prevalence.	These are risk factors for HBV exposure. Abdominal findings for hepatitis include jaundice, hepatomegaly, anorexia, abdominal and gastric discomfort, tea-colored urine, and clay-colored stools (Lewis et al., 2017).

NURSING DIAGNOSES

- Constipation
- Deficient knowledge regarding need for an abdominal assessment
- Diarrhea
- Imbalanced nutrition: less than body requirements
- Imbalanced nutrition: more than body requirements
- Ineffective health maintenance
- Nausea
- Pain (acute, chronic)

Related factors are individualized based on patient's condition or needs.

PLANNING

STEP	RATIONALE
1. Expected outcomes following completion of procedure:	
• Abdomen is soft and symmetrical, with smooth and even contour. No mass, distention, or tenderness is palpable. There are no forceful visible pulsations.	These are normal abdominal assessment findings.
• Bowel sounds are active and audible in all four quadrants.	Indicates normal peristaltic activity.
• No costovertebral angle (CVA) tenderness is present.	Indicates no inflammation of kidney.
• Patient denies discomfort or worsening of existing discomfort following examination.	Proper examination procedures have been implemented.
• Patient is able to list warning signs of colorectal cancer.	Demonstrates learning.
2. Anticipate teaching topics during the examination that you can teach patient about warning signs of colorectal cancer.	Allows you to incorporate instruction during physical assessment.
3. Perform hand hygiene. Prepare necessary supplies.	Reduces transmission of infection. Ensures efficiency during examination.

IMPLEMENTATION

STEP	RATIONALE
1. Prepare patient for abdominal assessment:	
a. Ask if patient needs to empty bladder or defecate.	Palpation of full bladder causes discomfort and feeling of urgency and makes it difficult for patient to relax.
b. Keep upper chest and legs draped.	Maintains patient's comfort during examination, promoting relaxation.
c. Be sure that room is warm.	Promotes patient's comfort. Reduces risk of patient tensing abdominal muscles.
d. Have patient lie supine or in dorsal recumbent position with arms down at sides and knees slightly bent. Place small pillow under patient's knees.	Placing arms under head or keeping knees fully extended causes abdominal muscles to tighten. Tightening of muscles prevents adequate palpation.
e. Move sheet or blanket to expose area from just above xiphoid process down to symphysis pubis.	Provides full visualization of abdomen.
f. Maintain conversation during assessment except during auscultation. Explain steps calmly and slowly.	Patient's ability to relax during assessment improves accuracy of findings. Talking interferes with hearing bowel sounds.
g. Ask patient to point to tender areas.	Assess painful areas last. Manipulation of body part increases patient's pain and anxiety and makes remainder of assessment difficult to complete.

STEP	RATIONALE

2. Abdominal assessment:

   a. Identify landmarks that divide abdominal region into quadrants. Boundary begins at tip of xiphoid process to symphysis pubis with line crossing and intersecting umbilicus, dividing abdomen into four equal sections (see illustration).

      Location of findings by common reference point helps successive examiners confirm findings and locate abnormalities.

   b. Inspect skin of surface of abdomen for color, scars, venous patterns, rashes, lesions, silvery white striae (stretch marks), and artificial openings (stomas). Observe skin lesions for characteristics described in Skill 6.1.

      Scars reveal evidence that patient has had past trauma or surgery. Striae indicate stretching of tissue from growth, obesity, pregnancy, ascites, or edema. Venous patterns reflect liver disease (portal hypertension). Artificial openings indicate bowel or urinary diversion (see Chapters 34 and 35).

   c. If you note bruising, ask if patient self-administers injections (e.g., heparin or insulin).

      Frequent injections may cause bruising and hardening of underlying tissues.

Clinical Decision Point *Bruising may also indicate physical signs of abuse, accidental injury, or bleeding disorder. When bruising is noted, additional information may be needed from the patient.*

   d. Inspect contour, symmetry, and surface motion of abdomen. Note any masses, bulging, or distention. (Flat abdomen forms a horizontal plane from xiphoid process to symphysis pubis. Round abdomen protrudes in convex sphere from horizontal plane. Concave abdomen sinks into muscular wall. All are normal.)

      Changes in symmetry or contour reveal underlying masses, fluid collection, or gaseous distention. Everted umbilicus (protruding outward) indicates distention. Hernia also causes umbilicus to protrude upward.

   e. If abdomen appears distended, note if distention is generalized. Look at flanks on each side.

      Distention may be caused by the nine F's (fat, flatus, feces, fluids, fibroid, full bladder, false pregnancy, fatal tumor, and fetus) (Ball et al., 2015). If gas causes distention, flanks do not bulge. If fluid causes distention, flanks bulge. Tumor may cause more unilateral bulging or distention. Pregnancy causes symmetrical bulge in lower abdomen.

   f. If you suspect distention, measure size of abdominal girth by placing tape measure under patient and around abdomen at level of umbilicus (see illustration). Use marking pen to indicate where tape measure was applied.

      Consecutive measurements show any increase or decrease in abdominal distention. Make all subsequent measurements at same level of umbilicus to provide objective means to evaluate changes. Use water-based pen to make mark on abdomen for subsequent measurements.

   g. If patient has a nasogastric (NG) or nasointestinal (NI) tube connected to suction, turn off momentarily.

      Sound of suction obscures bowel sounds.

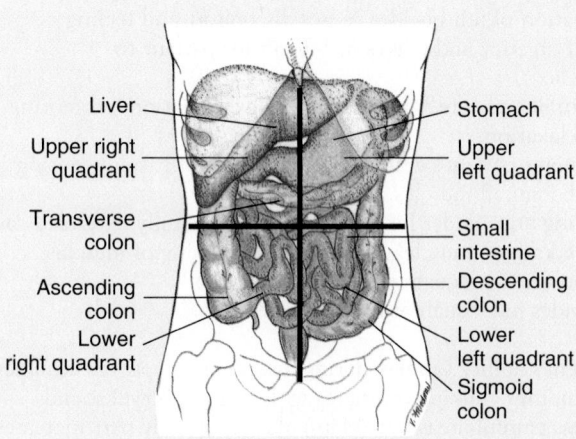

STEP 2a Division of abdomen into quadrants.

Liver — Upper right quadrant — Transverse colon — Ascending colon — Lower right quadrant

Stomach — Upper left quadrant — Small intestine — Descending colon — Lower left quadrant — Sigmoid colon

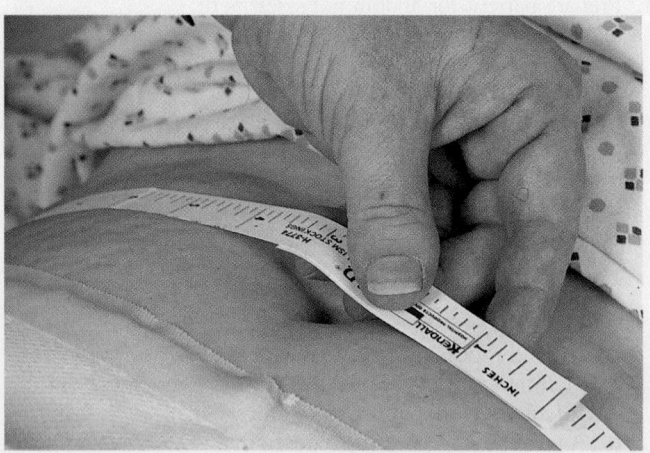

STEP 2f Measuring abdominal girth at level of umbilicus.

STEP	RATIONALE
h. To auscultate bowel sounds, place diaphragm of stethoscope lightly over each of four abdominal quadrants. Ask patient not to talk. Listen until you hear repeated gurgling or bubbling sounds in each quadrant (minimum of once in 5 to 20 seconds). Describe sounds as normal, hyperactive, hypoactive, or absent. Listen 5 minutes over each quadrant before deciding that bowel sounds are absent.	Normal bowel sounds occur irregularly every 5 to 15 seconds. Absence of sounds indicates cessation of gastric motility. Hyperactive bowel sounds not related to hunger or recent meal may indicate diarrhea or early intestinal obstruction. Hypoactive or absent bowel sounds indicate paralytic ileus or peritonitis. It is common for bowel sounds to be hypoactive after surgery for 24 hours or more, especially following abdominal surgery.

Clinical Decision Point *Nausea and vomiting, increasing distention, and inability to pass flatus may accompany severe paralytic ileus.*

i. Place bell of stethoscope over epigastric region of abdomen and each quadrant. Auscultate for vascular (whooshing) sounds.	Determines presence of turbulent blood flow (bruit) through thoracic or abdominal aorta, which may indicate an aneurysm.

Clinical Decision Point *If aortic bruit is auscultated, suggesting presence of an aneurysm, stop assessment and notify health care provider immediately. Percussion or palpation over abdominal bruit could cause rupture of an already weakened vessel wall in the presence of an abdominal aneurysm.*

j. With patient supine, gently percuss each of four abdominal quadrants systematically. Note areas of tympany and dullness.	Reveals presence of air or fluid in stomach and intestines. Normal percussion is tympanic because of swallowed air in GI tract. Presence of fluid or underlying masses is revealed by dull percussion.
k. Ask patient if abdomen feels unusually tight and determine if this is a recent development.	Continued sensation of fullness helps to detect distention. Feeling of fullness after heavy meal causes only temporary distention. Tightness is not felt with obesity.
l. With patient sitting, gently but firmly percuss over each CVA along scapular lines (see illustration A). Use ulnar surface of fist indirectly by placing nondominant hand flat against CVA and percussing with dominant hand or percuss directly against patient's skin (see illustration B). Note if patient experiences pain.	Determines presence of kidney inflammation.

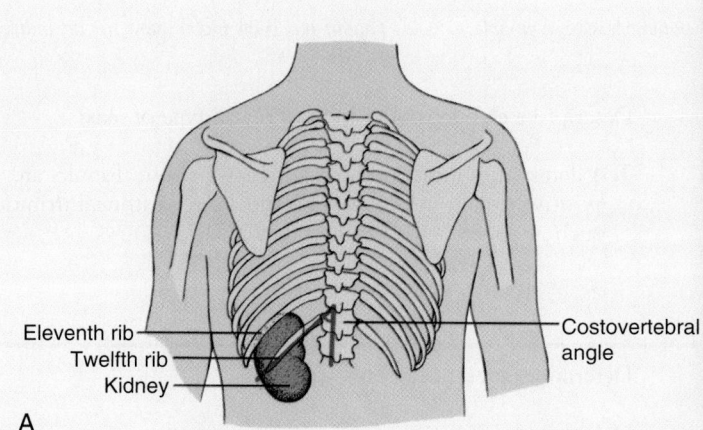
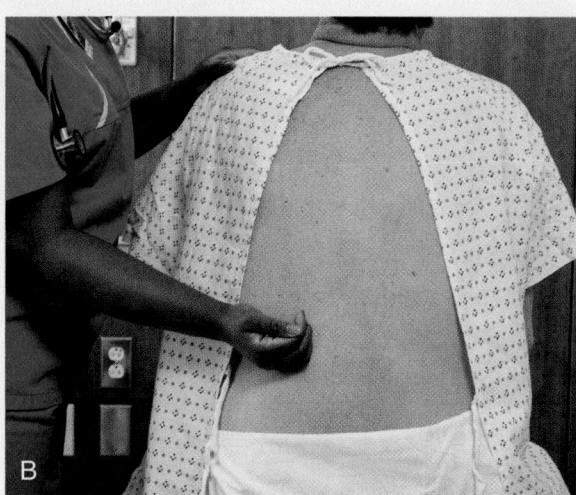

STEP 2l A, Position of kidney in relation to costovertebral angle. **B,** Direct percussion of kidney for costovertebral angle tenderness. (**A** *From Seidel HM et al:* Mosby's guide to physical examination, *ed 6, St Louis, 2006, Mosby;* **B** *From Ball JW et al:* Seidel's guide to physical examination, *ed 8, St Louis, 2015, Mosby.*)

Eleventh rib
Twelfth rib
Kidney

Costovertebral angle

A

STEP	RATIONALE

m. Lightly palpate over each abdominal quadrant, laying palm of hand with fingers extended and approximated lightly on abdomen. Keep palm and forearm horizontal. Pads of fingertips depress skin no more than 1 cm (½ inch) in gentle dipping motion (see illustration). Palpate painful areas last.

Detects areas of localized tenderness, degree of tenderness, and presence and character of underlying masses or fluid. Palpation of sensitive area causes guarding (voluntary tightening of underlying abdominal muscles).

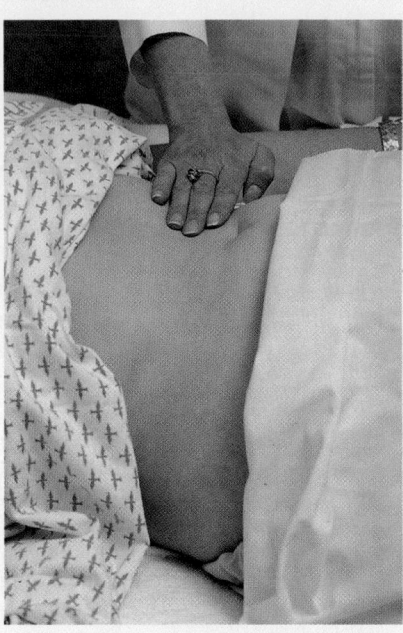

STEP 2m Light palpation of abdomen.

(1) Note muscular resistance, distention, tenderness, and superficial masses or organs while observing patient's face for signs of discomfort.

(2) Note if abdomen is firm or soft to touch.

Patient's verbal and nonverbal cues may indicate discomfort from tenderness. Firm abdomen indicates active obstruction with buildup of fluid or gas.

Soft abdomen is normal or reveals that obstruction is resolving.

n. Just below umbilicus and above symphysis pubis, palpate for smooth, rounded mass. While applying light pressure, ask if patient has sensation of need to void.

Detects presence of dome of distended bladder.

Clinical Decision Point *Routinely check for distended bladder if patient has been unable to void, patient has been incontinent, or an indwelling Foley catheter is not draining well or has been removed recently.*

o. If masses are palpated, note size, location, shape, consistency, tenderness, mobility, and texture.

Descriptive characteristics help to reveal type of mass.

p. When tenderness is present, press one hand slowly and deeply into involved area and let go quickly. Note if pain is aggravated.

Test determines if rebound tenderness is present. Results are positive if pain increases. This indicates peritoneal irritation such as appendicitis (Ball et al., 2015).

EVALUATION

1. Compare assessment findings with previous assessment characteristics to identify changes.

Determines presence of abnormalities.

2. Ask patient to describe signs and symptoms of colorectal cancer.

Demonstrates learning.

3. **Use Teach-Back:** "I would like to make sure that you understand the signs and symptoms of colorectal cancer. Tell me three changes in how your bowel functions that might be signs of colorectal cancer." Revise your instruction now or develop a plan for revised patient or family caregiver teaching if patient or family caregiver is not able to teach back correctly.

Determines patient's and family caregiver's level of understanding of instructional topic.

STEP	RATIONALE
Unexpected Outcomes	**Related Interventions**
1. Abdomen protrudes symmetrically with skin taut; patient complains of tightness, and/or bowel sounds are absent. GI motility has ceased. Patient is vomiting. Signs suggest an obstruction.	• Keep patient on nothing by mouth (NPO) status and encourage ambulation. • Notify health care provider. • Gastric decompression following insertion of NG tube sometimes may be necessary. • Patient may need to be NPO.
2. Hyperactive bowel sounds are evident with GI motility. Commonly they result from anxiety, diarrhea, overuse of laxatives, inflammation of bowel, or reaction of intestines to certain foods.	• Contact health care provider to consider ordering antidiarrheal medication.
3. Rebound abdominal tenderness is palpated.	• Avoid palpating area a second time. • Notify health care provider. • Keep patient NPO.
4. Bladder is palpable over symphysis pubis and distended.	• Facilitate voiding by placing patient in sitting position or encouraging him or her to bear down (if not contraindicated); run water within hearing distance or have patient place hand in basin of warm water. • Use bladder scan to determine extent of bladder fullness (see Chapter 34). • If unable to void, urinary catheterization is necessary (see Chapter 34).

Recording and Reporting

• Document appearance of abdomen, quality of bowel sounds, presence of distention, abdominal circumference, and presence and location of tenderness in nurses' notes in electronic health record (EHR) or chart.

• Document evaluation of patient and family caregiver learning.

• Record patient's ability to void and defecate, including description of output in the EHR or chart.

• Report serious abnormalities such as absent bowel sounds, presence of a mass, or acute pain to nurse in charge and health care provider.

Special Considerations
Teaching

• Explain that factors such as diet, regular exercise, limited use of over-the-counter drugs causing constipation, establishment of regular elimination schedule, and adequate fluid intake promote normal bowel elimination.

• If patient is a health care worker or has contact with blood or body fluids of affected people, encourage him or her to receive series of three HBV vaccine doses.

Pediatric

• Most common palpable abdominal mass in child is feces, usually palpated in right lower quadrant (Hockenberry and Wilson, 2015).

• Have a child stand erect and then lie supine during inspection of abdominal surface. Normal abdomen of infants and young children is cylindrical in erect position and flat in supine position. School-age children may have a rounded abdomen until 13 years of age when standing.

• In infants and children skin of abdomen is usually taut and without wrinkles or creases.

• Infants and children until the age of 7 years are abdominal breathers.

• Some children perceive superficial palpation as tickling. Drawing attention to their laughter only causes it to increase. Have the children help by placing their hand on top of yours or have them place their hand on their abdomen with their fingers separated and then palpate between their fingers.

Gerontological

• Older adults often lack abdominal tone; underlying organs are more easily palpable.

• Constipation along with nausea, flatulence, and heartburn is common.

• Stress to older adults importance of adequate fluid intake; regular exercise; and a diet with at least four servings daily of fresh fruit, vegetables, and high-fiber food to promote normal defecation.

◆ SKILL 6.6 Genitalia and Rectum Assessment

The best time to examine a patient's external genitalia is while performing routine hygiene measures or preparing to insert or care for a urinary catheter. An examination of female and male external genitalia is part of preventive health screenings. Male patients need to learn how to perform self-examinations of the genitalia to detect testicular cancer (Box 6.6). You examine adolescent and young adults because of the growing incidence of sexually transmitted infections (STIs). The average age of menarche among girls has declined, and most male and female teenagers are sexually active by age 19 (Hockenberry and Wilson, 2015). You can easily combine rectal and anal assessments with this examination because the patient assumes a lithotomy or dorsal recumbent position.

Delegation and Collaboration

The skill of assessing the genitalia and rectum cannot be delegated to nursing assistive personnel (NAP). The nurse directs the NAP to:

• Report changes in patient's genitourinary function and presence of drainage in the perineal area.

Equipment

• Examination light
• Clean gloves (use nonlatex if necessary)
• Drapes

Genital Self-Examination

All men 15 years and older should perform this examination monthly. Perform the examination during or after a warm bath or shower when the scrotal sac is relaxed. Call your health care provider if you find a lump or any other abnormality.

Genital Examination

1. Perform the examination after a warm bath or shower when the scrotal skin is less thick.
2. Stand naked in front of a mirror, hold the penis in your hand, and examine the head. Pull back the foreskin if uncircumcised to expose the glans.
3. Inspect and palpate the entire head of the penis in a clockwise motion, looking carefully for any bumps, sores, or blisters.
4. Look for any genital warts.
5. Look at the opening (urethral meatus) at the end of the penis for discharge.

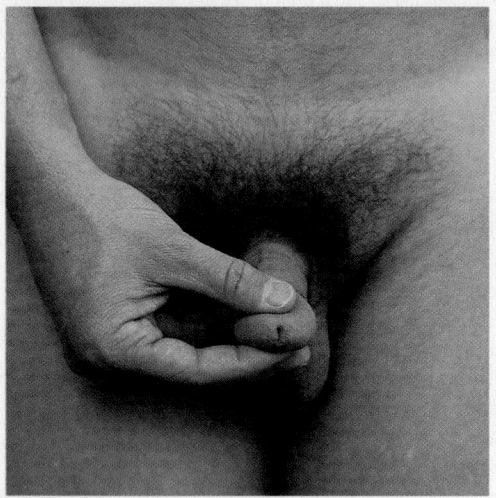

6. Look along the entire shaft of the penis for the same signs.
7. Separate pubic hair at the base of the penis and carefully examine the skin underneath.

Testicular Examination

1. Look for swelling or lumps in the skin of the scrotum while looking in the mirror.
2. Use both hands, placing the index and middle fingers under the testicles and the thumb on top.
3. Gently roll the testicle, feeling for hard lumps; smooth, rounded bumps; or thickening

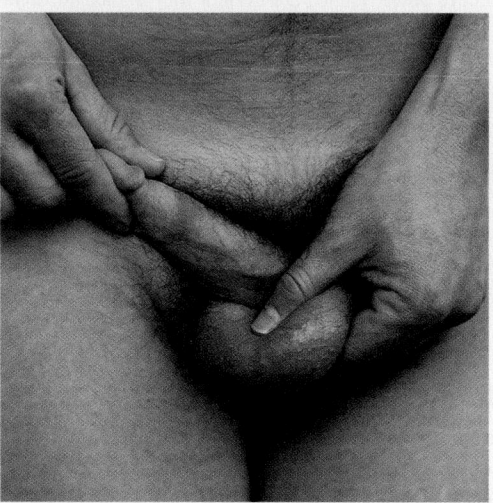

4. Find the epididymis (feels like a small "bump" on the upper or middle outer side of the testis).
5. Feel for small, pea-size lumps on the front and side of the testicle. The lumps are usually painless and are abnormal.
6. Instruct patient to call the health care provider if abnormalities are noted.
7. **Use Teach-Back:** "I want to be sure I explained to you how to do a genital and testicular self-examination. Describe for me the steps you will follow to examine your own genitals for cancer." Document your evaluation of patient learning. Revise your instruction now or develop a plan for revised patient teaching if patient is not able to teach back correctly.

Data from American Cancer Society (ACS): *Overview guide for testicular cancer,* Atlanta, 2015, The Society. http://www.cancer.org/cancer/testicularcancer/detailedguide/testicular-cancer-detection. Accessed May 28, 2016.
Illustrations from Ball JW et al: *Seidel's guide to physical examination,* ed 8, St Louis, 2015, Mosby.

STEP	RATIONALE

ASSESSMENT

1. Assessment: female patients:

   a. Determine if patient has signs and symptoms of vaginal discharge, painful or swollen perianal tissues, or genital lesions.

   These signs and symptoms are consistent with an STI or other pathological condition.

   b. Determine if patient has symptoms or history of genitourinary problems, including burning during urination (dysuria), frequency, urgency, nocturia, hematuria, or incontinence.

   Urinary problems are associated with gynecological disorders, including STIs.

   c. Ask if the patient has had signs of bleeding outside of normal menstrual cycle or after menopause or unusual vaginal discharge.

   These are warning signs for cervical and endometrial cancer or vaginal infection.

STEP	RATIONALE
d. Determine if patient has received human papillomavirus (HPV) vaccine.	The CDC (2015) recommends that all 11- or 12-year-old girls get the three doses of HPV vaccine (Gardasil or Cervarix) to protect against cervical cancer. Gardasil also protects against most genital warts and some cancers of the vulva, vagina, and anus. Girls and young women ages 13 through 26 should get HPV vaccine if they have not received any or all doses when they were younger. CDC also recommends Gardasil for all boys ages 11 or 12 years and for males ages 13 through 21 years who did not get any or all of the three recommended doses when they were younger. All men should confer with their doctor about vaccination.
e. Determine if patient has history of HPV (condyloma acuminatum, herpes simplex, or cervical dysplasia); had first pregnancy before age of 17; smokes cigarettes; is obese; eats diet low in fruits and vegetables; has had multiple full-term pregnancies.	These are risk factors for cervical cancer (ACS, 2015c; USPSTF, 2012).
f. Determine if patient is older than 63; is obese; has history of ovarian dysfunction, breast or endometrial cancer, or endometriosis; has family history of reproductive cancer; has history of infertility or nulliparity; or uses estrogen (alone) as hormone replacement therapy.	These are risk factors for ovarian cancer (ACS, 2015d).
g. Determine if patient is postmenopausal, obese, or infertile; had early menarche or late menopause; has history of hypertension, diabetes mellitus, gallbladder disease, or polycystic ovary disease; has family history of endometrial, breast, or colon cancer; or has a history of estrogen-related exposure (estrogen-replacement therapy, tamoxifen use).	These are risk factors for endometrial cancer (ACS, 2015d).
h. Determine patient's knowledge of risk factors and signs of cervical and other gynecological cancers.	Provides baseline for patient education.
2. Assessment of male patients:	
a. Review normal elimination pattern, including frequency of voiding; history of nocturia; character and volume of urine; daily fluid intake; symptoms of burning, urgency, and frequency; difficulty starting stream; and hematuria.	Urinary problems are directly associated with genitourinary problems because of anatomical structure of men's reproductive and urinary systems.
b. Ask if patient has noted penile pain or swelling, genital lesions, or urethral discharge.	These are signs and symptoms of STIs.
c. Determine if patient has noted heaviness, painless enlargement, or irregular lumps of testis.	These signs and symptoms are early warning signs for testicular cancer.
d. Determine if patient reports any enlargement in inguinal area and assess if intermittent or constant, associated with straining or lifting, and painful. Assess whether coughing, lifting, or straining at stool causes pain.	Signs and symptoms indicate potential inguinal hernia.
e. Ask if patient has experienced weak or interrupted urine flow, inability to urinate, difficulty starting or stopping urine flow, polyuria, nocturia, hematuria, or dysuria. Determine if patient has continuing pain in lower back, pelvis, or upper thighs.	These are warning signs of prostatic cancer (ACS, 2015f). Symptoms also may indicate infection or prostate enlargement.
f. Assess patient's knowledge of risk factors and signs of prostate and testicular cancer.	Provides baseline for patient education.
3. Assessment of all patients:	
a. Determine whether patient has rectal bleeding, black or tarry stools (melena), rectal pain, or change in bowel habits (constipation or diarrhea).	These are warning signs of colorectal cancer (Short et al, 2015) or other gastrointestinal (GI) alterations.
b. Determine whether patient has personal or strong family history of colorectal cancer, polyps, or chronic inflammatory bowel disease. Ask if patient is over age 50.	These are risk factors for colorectal cancer (Short et al, 2015).

STEP	RATIONALE

c. Inquire about dietary habits, including high fat intake, diet high in processed or red meats, diet high in meats cooked at high temperatures (frying, broiling, grilling), or deficient fiber content (inadequate fruits and vegetables).

Colon cancer is often linked to dietary intake of fat, red meat, high cooking temperatures, or insufficient fiber intake (Short et al, 2015).

d. Determine if patient is obese, physically inactive, smokes, has type 2 diabetes, or consumes alcohol.

These are risk factors for colorectal cancer (Short et al, 2015).

e. Assess medication history for use of laxatives or cathartic medications.

Repeated use causes diarrhea and eventual loss of intestinal muscle tone.

f. Assess for use of codeine or iron preparations.

Codeine causes constipation. Iron turns stool black and tarry.

g. Assess patient's knowledge of risks and signs of colorectal cancer.

Provides baseline for patient education.

NURSING DIAGNOSES

- Deficient knowledge regarding need for a genital and rectal assessment
- Ineffective health maintenance
- Pain (acute, chronic)
- Readiness for enhanced immunization status

Related factors are individualized based on patient's condition or needs.

PLANNING

1. Expected outcomes following completion of procedure:
- Patient denies discomfort or worsening of existing discomfort following examination.

Proper examination procedures have been implemented.

- Patient is able to list warning signs of colorectal cancer: female patient: cervical, endometrial, and ovarian cancer; male patient: testicular and prostate cancer.

Demonstrates learning.

- Patient is able to discuss guidelines for HPV immunization.

Demonstrates learning.

2. Anticipate teaching topics so during the examination you can teach patient about warning signs of colorectal cancer.

Prepares you for incorporating teaching into assessment activities.

3. Perform hand hygiene. Prepare necessary supplies.

Reduces transmission of infection.

IMPLEMENTATION

1. Prepare patient for assessment:
a. Ask if patient needs to empty bladder or defecate.

Palpation of full bladder causes discomfort and feeling of urgency and makes it difficult for patient to relax.

b. Keep upper chest and legs draped and keep room warm.

Maintains patient's comfort during examination, promoting relaxation.

c. Position patient:
(1) Female should lie in dorsal recumbent position with arms down at sides and knees slightly bent. Place small pillow under her knees.

Placing arms under head or keeping knees fully extended causes tightening of abdominal muscles.

(2) Male should lie supine with chest, abdomen, and lower legs draped; or have him stand during examination.

d. Apply clean gloves.

2. Female genitalia examination. (Use this time to discuss woman's risk for STIs and signs and symptoms of cervical, ovarian, and endometrial cancers.)
a. Expose perineal area, repositioning sheet as needed.

b. Inspect surface characteristics of perineum and retract labia majora; observe for inflammation, edema, lesions, or lacerations. Note if there is any vaginal discharge. Presence of discharge may indicate need for a culture.

Skin of perineum is smooth, clean, and slightly darker than other skin. Mucous membranes are dark pink and moist. Labia majora are symmetrical; may be dry or moist. Normally there is no vaginal discharge.

STEP	RATIONALE
3. Male genitalia examination. (Use this time to discuss man's risk for STIs and signs and symptoms of testicular cancer.)	
a. Expose perineal area. Observe genitalia for rashes, excoriations, or lesions.	Normally skin is clear without lesions.
b. Inspect and palpate penile surfaces (see also Box 6.6).	
(1) Inspect corona, prepuce (foreskin), glans, urethral meatus, and shaft. Retract foreskin in uncircumcised males. Observe for discharge, lesions, edema, and inflammation. Return foreskin to normal position.	Glans should be smooth and pink along all surfaces. Urethral meatus is slitlike and normally positioned at tip of glans. Foreskin should retract easily. Area between foreskin and glans is common site for venereal lesions.
c. Inspect and palpate testicular surfaces.	
(1) Inspect size, color, shape, and symmetry; also gently palpate for lesions and edema.	Left testicle is normally lower than right. Scrotal skin is usually loose, surface is coarse, and skin color is more deeply pigmented than body skin.
d. Palpate testes (see also Box 6.6).	
(1) Note size, shape, and consistency of tissue.	Testes are normally ovoid and approximately 2 to 4 cm (0.8 to 1.6 inches) in size, feel smooth and rubbery, and are free from nodules. Most common symptom of testicular cancer is irregular, nontender fixed mass.
(2) Ask if patient experiences tenderness with palpation.	Testes are normally sensitive but not tender.
5. Assess rectum.	
a. Female patient remains in dorsal recumbent position or assumes side-lying (Sims') position.	These positions allow for optimum visualization of the rectum.
b. Male patient stands and bends forward with hips flexed and upper body resting across examination table; examine nonambulatory patient in Sims' position.	
c. View perianal and sacrococcygeal areas by gently retracting buttocks with your nondominant hand.	Perianal skin is smooth, more pigmented, and coarser than skin covering buttocks.
d. Inspect anal tissue for skin characteristics, lesions, external hemorrhoids (dilated veins that appear as reddened skin protrusion), inflammation, rashes, and excoriation.	Anal tissues are moist and hairless; voluntary sphincter holds anus closed.
6. Remove and discard gloves. Discard disposable supplies. Help patient to comfortable position. Perform hand hygiene.	Reduces transmission of infection.

EVALUATION

1. Compare assessment findings with previous assessment characteristics to identify changes.	Determines presence of abnormalities.
2. Ask patient to list warning signs of colorectal cancer: female patient: cervical, endometrial, and ovarian cancer; male patient: testicular and prostate cancer.	Demonstrates learning.
3. Ask patient to identify guidelines for HPV vaccination.	Demonstrates learning.
4. Use Teach-Back:	Determines patient's level of understanding of instructional topic.
Male patient: "I would like to make sure that you understand the warning signs of colorectal, testicular, and prostate cancer. Tell me some of the signs and symptoms of testicular cancer." Revise your instruction now or develop a plan for revised patient teaching if patient is not able to teach back correctly.	
Female patient: "I would like to make sure that you understand the warning signs of colorectal, cervical, endometrial, and ovarian cancer. Tell me some of the signs and symptoms of cervical cancer." Revise your instruction now or develop a plan for revised patient teaching if patient is not able to teach back correctly.	

STEP	RATIONALE

Unexpected Outcomes

1. Patient has vaginal/penile drainage and burning sensation during voiding. Women may have vaginal bleeding between menstrual periods. Symptoms may suggest STI.

Related Interventions

- Notify health care provider.
- Prepare to collect a culture of the discharge.
- Provide additional education.

Recording and Reporting

- Record results of assessment in nurses' notes in electronic health record (EHR) or chart.
- Record patient's ability to void, including description of output, in the EHR or chart.
- Document evaluation of patient learning.
- Report any abnormalities such as presence of a mass or acute pain to nurse in charge and health care provider.

Special Considerations

Teaching

- Discuss the guidelines of the ACS (2015a) for early detection of colorectal cancer for both men and women. The ACS (2015a) recommends the following examination schedules beginning at age 50:
  - Tests that detect polyps and cancer; one of the following: (1) flexible sigmoidoscopy (every 5 years), (2) colonoscopy (every 10 years), (3) double-contrast barium enema (every 5 years), (4) computed tomographic colonoscopy (every 5 years).
  - Tests that primarily detect cancer: (1) guaiac-based fecal occult blood test (gFOBT), or fecal immunochemical test (FIT) with high sensitivity for cancer (every year), (2) stool deoxyribonucleic acid (DNA) (interval unclear).
- Discuss warning signs of colorectal cancer, including long-term progressive weight loss, change in bowel habits, and blood in stools.
- Discuss dietary planning and healthy lifestyle choice to maintain or improve colon health.

Female Health Teaching

- Teach patient about purpose and recommended frequency of Papanicolaou (Pap) smears and gynecological examinations.
- Explain warning signs of STIs: pain or burning on urination, pain during sex, pain in pelvic area, bleeding between menstruation, itchy rash around vagina, and abnormal vaginal discharge.
- Teach measures to prevent STIs (e.g., male partner's use of condoms, restricting number of sexual partners, avoiding sex with people who have several other partners, and perineal hygiene measures).
- Reinforce the importance of performing perineal hygiene (as appropriate).

Male Health Teaching

- Explain warning signs of STIs: pain on urination and during sex, abnormal penile discharge, swollen lymph nodes, or rash or ulcer on skin or genitalia.
- Teach measures to prevent STIs: use of condoms, avoiding sex with infected partner, avoiding sex with people who have multiple partners, and using regular perineal hygiene. Tell patients with an STI to inform their sexual partners of the need to have an examination. Instruct patient to seek treatment as soon as possible if partner becomes infected with an STI.
- Teach patient how to perform genital self-examination (see Box 6.6).

Pediatric

- When examining the testes in a male infant, avoid stimulating the cremasteric reflex, which causes the testes to pull higher into the pelvic cavity.

◆ SKILL 6.7   Musculoskeletal and Neurological Assessment

You use the skills of inspection and palpation during the musculoskeletal and neurological assessment. During the general survey you inspect gait, posture, and body position. A more thorough assessment of major bone, joint, and muscle groups and sensory, motor, and cranial nerve (CN) function is indicated in the presence of abnormalities. The assessment can be performed as you examine other body systems. For example, while assessing head and neck structures assess neck range of motion (ROM) and examine select CNs. Integrate assessment into routine activities of care (e.g., while bathing or positioning the patient). Assessment of these systems is important when a patient reports pain, loss of sensation, or impairment of muscle function. Prolonged illness or immobility may result in muscle weakness and atrophy. Neurological assessment is often conducted simultaneously because muscles may be weakened as a result of nerve involvement.

Delegation and Collaboration

The skill of assessing musculoskeletal and neurological function cannot be delegated to nursing assistive personnel (NAP). The nurse directs the NAP to:

- Report patients' problems with gait, balance, ROM, and muscle strength.
- Be informed of patients at risk for falls (unsteady gait, foot dragging, weakness of lower extremities).
- Help patients with muscular weakness with transfer and ambulation.

Equipment

- Cotton balls or cotton-tipped applicators
- Penlight
- Tape measure
- Tongue blade
- Tuning fork
- Reflex hammer

STEP	RATIONALE

ASSESSMENT

1. Review patient history for use of alcohol intake of more than two drinks/day; inadequate intake of protein, vitamin D, or calcium; thin and light body frame; family history of osteoporosis; white or Asian ancestry; sedentary lifestyle; long-term use of certain medications (e.g., corticosteroids, lithium, or heparin); and certain medical conditions (e.g., diabetes, hyperthyroidism) (Ball et al., 2015).

These factors increase risk for osteoporosis.

2. Determine if patient has been screened for osteoporosis.

Women age 65 and older need routine screening for osteoporosis. There is insufficient evidence that men require this screening (Jeremiah et al., 2015).

3. Ask patient to describe history of changes in bone, muscle, or joint function (e.g., recent fall, trauma, lifting heavy objects, bone or joint disease with sudden or gradual onset) and location of alteration.

History helps in assessing nature of musculoskeletal problem. It is estimated that 9.9 million Americans have osteoporosis and an additional 43.1 million have osteopenia (NOF, 2014).

4. Assess height and weight (see Skill 6.1). Note if there is a decrease in women older than 50 by subtracting current height from recall of maximum adult height.

Body mass index less than 22 is a risk factor, and loss of height more than 7.5 cm (3 inches) is one of the first clinical signs of osteoporosis (Touhy and Jett, 2015).

5. Assess nature and extent of patient's musculoskeletal pain: location, duration, severity, predisposing and aggravating factors, relieving factors, and type of pain. If patient reports pain or cramping in lower extremities, ask if walking relieves or aggravates it. Assess distance walked and characteristics of pain before, during, and after activity.

Pain frequently accompanies alterations in bone, joints, or muscle. It has implications for comfort and also ability to perform activities of daily living (ADLs). Pain caused by certain vascular conditions tends to increase with activity.

6. Determine if patient uses analgesics, antipsychotics, antidepressants, nervous system stimulants, or recreational drugs.

These medications alter level of consciousness (LOC) or cause behavioral changes. Abuse sometimes causes tremors, ataxia, and changes in peripheral nerve function.

7. Determine if patient has recent history of seizures/convulsions: clarify sequence of events (aura, loss of muscle tone, falling, motor activity, loss of consciousness); character of any symptoms; and relationship to time of day, fatigue, or emotional stress.

Seizure activity often originates from central nervous system (CNS) alteration. Characteristics of seizure help determine its origin.

8. Screen patient for headache, tremors, dizziness, vertigo, numbness or tingling of body part; visual changes; weakness; pain; or changes in speech.

These symptoms commonly result from CNS dysfunction. Identifying patterns aids in diagnosis.

9. Discuss with spouse, family member, or friends any recent changes in patient's behavior (e.g., increased irritability, mood swings, memory loss, change in energy level).

Behavioral changes may result from intracranial pathology.

10. Determine if patient has noticed change in vision (cranial nerve I), hearing (cranial nerve VIII), smell, taste (cranial nerve VII), or touch.

Major sensory nerves originate from brainstem. These symptoms help to localize nature of problem during cranial nerve examination.

11. If patient displays sudden acute confusion (delirium), review history for drug toxicity (e.g., anticholinergics, digoxin, antihistamines, antipsychotics, benzodiazepines, opioid analgesics, sedative/hypnotics, steroids); serious infections, metabolic disturbances (e.g., diabetes mellitus); heart failure; and severe anemia.

Delirium is one of most common mental disorders in older people (Touhy and Jett, 2015), but it also occurs in children.

12. Review history for head or spinal cord injury, meningitis, congenital anomalies, neurological disease, or psychiatric counseling.

These neurological symptoms or behavioral changes help to focus assessment on possible cause.

STEP	RATIONALE

NURSING DIAGNOSES

- Activity intolerance
- Impaired physical mobility
- Impaired walking
- Ineffective peripheral tissue perfusion

- Pain (acute, chronic)
- Risk for injury
- Risk for peripheral neurovascular dysfunction

- Risk for trauma
- Self-care deficit (bathing/hygiene, dressing/grooming, feeding, or toileting)

Related factors/Risk factors are individualized based on patient's condition or needs.

PLANNING

1. Expected outcomes following completion of procedure:
  - Patient demonstrates erect posture; strong grasp; steady gait, with arms swinging freely at side.

    Indicates normal alignment, gait, and neuromuscular muscle strength.

  - There is bilateral symmetry of extremities in length, circumference, alignment, position, and skinfolds.
  - Full active ROM is present in all joints, with good muscle tone and absence of contractures, spasticity, or muscular weakness.

    Indicates normal ROM of joints.

  - Patient is alert and oriented to person, place, and time. Behavior and appearance appropriate for condition/situation.

    Indicates normal cerebral function.

  - Patient demonstrates normal pupil reaction to light and accommodation (see Skill 6.2); external ocular muscles (EOMs) intact; facial sensation intact; symmetrical facial expressions; soft palate and uvula midline and rise on phonation; gag reflex intact; speech clear without hoarseness; no difficulty swallowing.

    Indicates normal functioning of CNs III, IV, V, VI, VII, IX, and X.

  - Patient distinguishes between sharp and dull sensations and light touch on symmetrical areas of extremities. Position sense intact to lower extremities.

    Indicates normal function of sensory nerves.

  - Gait is coordinated, steady with appropriate stance and swing phases. Romberg test negative.

    Indicates normal cerebellar and motor system functioning.

2. Perform hand hygiene. Prepare necessary supplies.

  Reduces transmission of infection.

IMPLEMENTATION

1. Prepare patient:
  a. Integrate musculoskeletal and neurological assessments during other parts of physical assessment or during nursing care (e.g., when patient moves in bed, rises from chair, or walks).

    You can conduct assessment as patient performs activities or goes through movements required during complete physical examination. Integration with care conserves patient's energy and allows observation of patient performing more naturally.

  b. Plan time for short rest periods during assessment.

    Movement of body parts and various maneuvers may tire patient. Always plan rest periods with older adult and very ill patients.

2. Assess musculoskeletal system. (Discuss any risks patient may have for falls or other injuries.)
  a. Observe ability to use arms and hands for grasping objects (e.g., pen, utensils).

    Assesses coordination and muscle strength.

  b. To assess hand grasp strength, cross your hands and have patient grasp index and middle fingers of both of your hands and squeeze them as hard as possible (see illustration).

    It is common for patient's dominant hand to be slightly stronger than nondominant hand. By crossing your hands, patient's right hand grasps your right hand. This helps with recall of which is patient's right/left hand.

STEP	RATIONALE

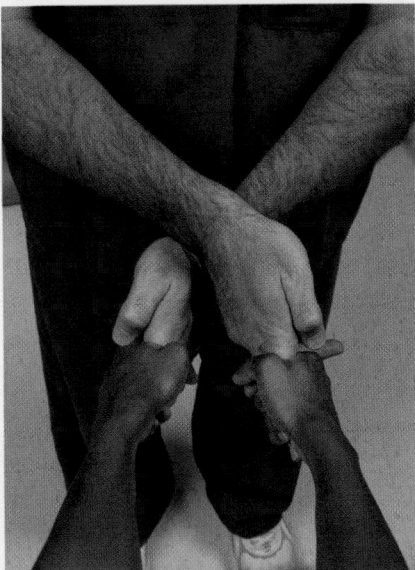

STEP 2b Assessing strength of hand grasps, comparing sides.

c. To assess strength of lower arms or legs, ask patient first to contract the muscle you indicate by extending or flexing the joint. Then have patient resist as you apply force against that muscle contraction. Have patient maintain pressure until told to stop. Compare symmetrical muscle groups. Note weakness and compare right with left.

Compares strength of symmetrical muscle groups. Upper and lower extremities on dominant side are usually stronger. Rate muscle strength on scale of 0 to 5 as follows:

0   No voluntary contraction
1   Slight contractility, no movement
2   Full ROM, passive
3   Full ROM, active
4   Full ROM against gravity, some resistance
5   Full ROM against gravity, full resistance

Each joint or muscle group requires different position for measurement.

d. Observe body alignment for sitting, supine, prone, or standing positions. Muscles and joints should be exposed and free to move to allow for accurate measurement.

e. Inspect gait as patient walks. Have patient use his or her assistive device (e.g., cane, walker) if appropriate. Observe for foot dragging, shuffling or limping, balance, presence of obvious deformity in lower extremities, and position of trunk in relation to legs.

Gait is more natural if patient is unaware of your observation. Assesses for neuromusculoskeletal disorder.

f. Perform timed get-up-and-go test: Have adult wear regular footwear, sit back in comfortable chair, and use normal assist devices, if needed. Have watch with a second hand. On the word "Go," begin timing as you have the patient stand from a sitting position without using chair arms for support, stand still momentarily, walk 10 feet (3 meters) in a line, turn around and return to chair; and sit back in chair without using chair arms for support. Observe gait and ability to stand.

The timed get-up-and-go test is an assessment that should be conducted as part of routine evaluation of older adults. The test helps to detect a person's risk for falls. Normally a person completes the task in less than 10 seconds; over 20 seconds is abnormal.

g. Stand behind patient and observe postural alignment (position of hips relative to shoulders). Look sideways at cervical, thoracic, and lumbar curves (see illustration).

Abnormal curves of posture include kyphosis (hunchback, exaggerated posterior curvature of thoracic spine), lordosis (swayback, increased lumbar curvature), and scoliosis (lateral spinal curvature). Postural changes indicate muscular, bone, or joint deformity; pain; or muscular fatigue. Head should be held erect.

STEP 2g Observe spinal deformities. **A,** Kyphosis. **B,** Lordosis. **C,** Scoliosis. **D,** Scoliosis with patient bending forward.

h. Make a general observation of extremities. Look at overall size, gross deformity, bony enlargement, alignment, and symmetry.	General review pinpoints areas requiring in-depth assessment.
i. Gently palpate bones, joints, and surrounding tissue in involved areas. Note any heat, tenderness, edema, or resistance to pressure.	Reveals changes resulting from trauma or chronic disease. Do not attempt to move joint when fracture is suspected or joint is apparently "frozen" by lack of movement over a long period of time.
j. Ask patient to put major joint through its full ROM (Table 6.12). Patients with deformities, reduced mobility, joint fixation, or weakness require passive ROM assessment. Observe equality of motion in same body parts:	Assessment of patient's normal ROM provides baseline for assessing later changes after surgery or inactivity.
(1) *Active motion:* (Patient needs no support or help and is able to move joint independently.) Teach patient to move each joint through its normal range. Sometimes it is necessary to demonstrate and ask patient to mimic your movements.	Identifies muscle strength and detects limited ROM.
(2) *Passive motion:* (Joint has full ROM, but patient does not have strength to move it independently.) Have patient relax and move same joints passively until end of range is felt. Support extremity at joint. Do not force joint if there is pain or muscle spasm.	Determines ability to perform joint motion in presence of muscle weakness. Forcing joint causes injury and pain.
k. Palpate joint for swelling, stiffness, tenderness, and heat; note any redness.	Indicates acute or chronic inflammation. ROM causes pain or injury.
l. Assess muscle tone in major muscle groups. Normal tone causes mild, even resistance to movement through entire ROM.	If muscle has increased tone (hypertonicity), any sudden movement of joint is met with considerable resistance. Hypotonic muscle moves without resistance. Muscle feels flabby.
3. Neurological assessment	
a. Assess LOC and orientation by asking patient to identify name, location, day of week, and year; note behavior and appearance. This can be completed during general survey.	A fully conscious patient responds to questions spontaneously. As consciousness declines patient may show irritability, shortened attention span, or unwillingness to cooperate. As consciousness continues to deteriorate patient becomes disoriented to name, time, and place. Behavior and appearance reveal information about patient's mental status.

STEP	RATIONALE

TABLE 6.12

Assessing Range of Motion*

Body Part	Assessment Procedure	ROM
Upper Extremities		
Neck	Bend head forward and then backward. Bend neck side to side. Turn head to look over each shoulder.	Flexion, lateral flexion, rotation
Shoulders	Raise both arms to vertical position level at sides of head. Bring arm across upper chest to touch opposite shoulder. Place both hands behind neck, with elbows out to sides. Place both hands behind small of back. Have patient make small circles with hands, with arms extended at shoulder level.	Flexion Adduction External rotation and abduction Internal rotation Circumduction
Elbows	Bend and straighten elbows. Place hands at waist with elbows flexed.	Flexion and extension Internal rotation
Wrists	Flex and extend wrist (bend and straighten). Bend wrist to radial and then ulnar side. Turn palm upward and then downward.	Flexion and extension Radial and ulnar deviation Supination and pronation
Hands	Make a fist with both hands; open hand. Extend and spread fingers and thumb outward; bring back together.	Flexion and extension Adduction and abduction
Lower Extremities		
Hips (with patient supine)	With knees extended, raise one leg upward. Cross leg over other leg. Swing legs laterally. With knee flexed, hold ankle and rotate leg inward and outward.	Flexion and extension: Expect 90 degrees flexion Abduction: Expect 45 degrees Adduction: Expect 30 degrees Internal and external rotation: Expect 40–45 degrees
Knees (with patient sitting)	Raise foot, keeping knee in place.	Extension: Expect full extension and up to 15 degrees hyperextension
Ankles	With foot held off floor, point toes downward and bring them back toward knee.	Plantar flexion: Expect 45 degrees Dorsiflexion: Expect 20 degrees
Toes	Turn foot (sole) inward and sole outward. Bend toes down and back.	Inversion and eversion: Expect to reach 5 degrees Flexion and hyperextension: Expect to reach 40 degrees

AROM, Active range of motion; *PROM,* passive range of motion; *ROM,* range of motion.
*This may be done actively by the patient (AROM) or passively by the nurse (PROM).

   b. Assess CNs:
     (1) For CNs III (oculomotor), IV (trochlear), and VI (abducens), assess extra ocular movements (EOMs). Ask patient to look straight ahead without moving head and follow movement of your finger through six cardinal positions of gaze; measure pupillary reaction to light reflex and accommodation (see Skill 6.2) using penlight.

These CNs are those most likely to be affected by increasing intracranial pressure (ICP), which causes change in response or size of pupil; pupils may change shape (more oval) or react sluggishly. ICP impairs movements of EOMs. Accommodation is ability of eye to adjust vision from near to far.

     (2) For CN V (trigeminal), apply light sensation with cotton ball to symmetrical areas of face.

Sensations should be symmetrical; unilateral decrease or loss of sensation may be caused by CN V lesion.

     (3) For CN VII (facial) note facial symmetry. Have patient frown, smile, puff out cheeks, and raise eyebrows.

Expressions should be symmetrical; Bell's palsy causes drooping of upper and lower face; CVA causes asymmetry.

     (4) For CNs IX (glossopharyngeal) and X (vagus), have patient speak and swallow. Ask him or her to say "ah" while using tongue blade and penlight. Check for midline uvula and symmetrical rise of uvula and soft palate. Use tongue blade and place on posterior tongue to elicit gag reflex.

Damage to CN IX causes impaired swallowing; damage to CN X causes loss of gag reflex, hoarseness, nasal voice. When palate fails to rise and uvula pulls toward normal side, this indicates a unilateral paralysis.

   c. Assess extremities for sensation. Perform all sensory testing with patient's eyes closed so he or she is unable to see when or where a stimulus strikes skin. Use minimal stimulation initially, increasing gradually until patient is aware of it.

For all sensory stimulus testing, patient should note minimal differences side to side, correctly describe the sensation (sharp or dull, hot or cold), and recognize side of the body tested and location.

STEP	RATIONALE
(1) *Pain:* Ask patient to indicate when sharp or dull sensation is felt as you alternately apply sharp and dull ends of a broken tongue blade to skin surface. Apply in symmetrical areas of extremities.	Patient should be able to distinguish sharp or dull sensations. Impaired sensations indicate disorders of spinal cord or peripheral nerve roots.
(2) *Light touch:* Apply light wisp of cotton to different points along surface of skin in symmetrical areas of extremities.	Patient should be able to distinguish when touched.
(3) *Position:* Grasp finger or toe, holding it by its sides with your thumb and index finger. Alternate moving finger or toe up and down. Ask patient to state when finger is up or down. Repeat with toes.	Patient should be able to distinguish movements of a few millimeters. Decreased/absent position sense may occur in spinal anesthesia, paralysis, or other neurological disorders.
d. Assess motor and cerebellar function:	
(1) *Gait:* Have patient walk across room, turn, and come back. Similarly note use of assistive devices. This is good time to instruct on proper use of assistive devices.	Neurological and musculoskeletal disorders impair gait and balance.
(2) *Romberg's test:* Have patient stand with feet together, arms at sides, both with eyes open and eyes closed (for 20 to 30 seconds). Protect patient's safety by standing at side; observe for swaying.	Romberg's test should be negative; slight swaying is considered normal.
e. Assess deep tendon reflexes (DTRs):	
(1) In patients with back pain or surgery, CVA, or spinal cord compression, it is appropriate to monitor DTRs (Ball et al., 2015). This requires an advanced level of skill. In most settings this is not part of routine physical assessment.	Muscle spasticity and hyperactive reflexes may result from disorders such as stroke and paralysis. Diminished DTRs and muscle weakness may suggest electrolyte abnormalities or lower motor neuron disorders (e.g., amyotrophic lateral sclerosis [ALS] or Guillain-Barré syndrome).
(2) For each reflex tested, compare sides and assign a grade on the following scale: 0 No response 1+ Sluggish or diminished response 2+ Normal, active or expected response 3+ More brisk than expected; slightly hyperactive 4+ Very brisk; hyperactive, with clonus.	Grade indicates extent of neuron dysfunction. Clonus is described as repeated spasms of muscular contraction and relaxation.
(3) *Knee reflex:* Palpate patellar tendon just below patella. Tap pointed end of reflex hammer briskly on tendon (see illustration).	Knee reflex is the most common DTR assessment performed. The normal response is knee extension.
(4) *Plantar response (Babinski's reflex):* Using handle end of reflex hammer, stroke lateral aspect of sole from heel to ball of foot.	Toes should flex inward and downward (see illustration).

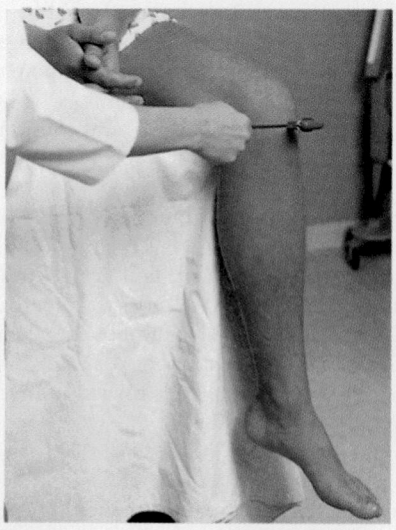

STEP 3e(3) Assessing knee reflex. Knee should extend.

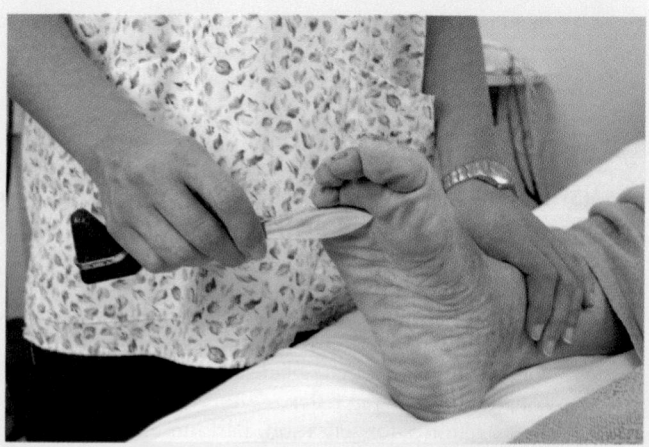

STEP 3e(4) Assessing plantar response. Toes should flex inward and downward.

STEP	RATIONALE
(5) After stroking soles of feet, if Babinski's reflex is present, great toe dorsiflexes, accompanied by fanning of the other toes.	Indicates CNS dysfunction. Dorsiflexion of great toe and fanning of the others are normal in child younger than age 2 (Hockenberry and Wilson, 2015).
4. Dispose of supplies. Perform hand hygiene.	Reduces transmission of infection.

EVALUATION

1. Compare muscle strength and ROM with previous physical assessment.	Determines presence of abnormalities.
2. Compare neurological status with previous physical assessment.	Determines presence of abnormalities.
3. Evaluate level of patient's discomfort following procedure, using appropriate pain scale.	Determines if manipulation of musculoskeletal structures intensifies patient's discomfort.
4. **Use Teach-Back:** "I want to be sure you understand the reasons why you are at risk for falling that we discussed during your exam. Tell me two reasons why you are at risk for falling." Revise your instruction now or develop a plan for revised patient or family caregiver teaching if patient or family caregiver is not able to teach back correctly.	Determines patients' and family caregiver's level of understanding of instructional topic.

Unexpected Outcomes	Related Interventions
1. Joints are prominent, swollen, and tender with nodules or overgrowth of bone in distal joints, indicating signs of arthritis.	• Teach patient proper ROM. • Determine patient's knowledge regarding use of antiinflammatory medications and nonpharmacological measures (see Chapter 16).
2. ROM is reduced in one or more major joints: shoulder, elbow, wrist, fingers, knee, hip.	• Assess further for pain during movement with joint unstable, stiff, painful, or swollen or with obvious deformity. • Notify health care provider. • Reduce mobility in extremity until cause of abnormal joint motion is determined.
3. Patient demonstrates weakness in one or more major muscle groups or has difficulty with gait or ability to walk and sit during get-up-and-go test, indicating a fall risk.	• Place patient on fall precautions. • Provide patient safety when ambulating (see Chapter 12). • Notify health care provider.
4. Patient has changes in mental status and pupillary response or other neurological deficits.	• Notify health care provider immediately. • Continue to assess patient's vital signs and LOC closely. • Place on fall precautions.

Recording and Reporting

- Record posture, gait, muscle strength, and ROM in nurses' notes in electronic health record (EHR) or chart.
- Record LOC, orientation, pupillary response, sensation, and reflex responses in nurses' notes in EHR or chart.
- Document evaluation of patient and family caregiver learning.
- Report to nurse in charge or health care provider acute pain or sudden muscle weakness, change in LOC, or change in size or pupillary reaction, which require immediate treatment.

Special Considerations
Teaching

- Teach patient about correct postural alignment. Consult with physical therapist to provide patient with exercises for improving posture.
- To reduce bone demineralization, teach older-adult patient about a proper weight-bearing exercise program (e.g., walking, low-impact aerobics) to be followed 3 or more times a week.
- Encourage intake of calcium to meet the recommended daily allowance. Increased vitamin D aids calcium absorption (400 to 800 international units daily). Recommendation for daily calcium supplements for adults over age 50: 1200 mg/day. Instruct patient to take no more than 500 mg of calcium supplements at one time (Touhy and Jett, 2015).
- Explain to patients with low back pain that they can benefit from modification of work-related risk factors (e.g., lifting heavy weights, use of protective equipment), regular aerobic exercise, exercises that strengthen the back and increase trunk flexibility, and learning how to lift properly.
- Explain measures to ensure safety (e.g., use of ambulation aids or safety bars in bathrooms or stairways) for patients with sensory or motor impairments.

Pediatric

- Examine infants carefully for musculoskeletal anomalies resulting from genetic or fetal insults. An examination includes review of posture, generalized movement, symmetry and skin creases of the extremities, muscle strength, and hip alignment.

- Normally the back of a newborn is rounded or **C** shaped from the thoracic and pelvic curves.
- Scoliosis, lateral curvature of the spine, is an important childhood problem, especially in females, usually identified at puberty. (For closer examination have child stand erect wearing only underclothes. Observe from behind, looking for asymmetry of shoulders and hips. Then observe from the back as child bends forward.) Uneven dress hems or trouser hems or uneven fit of clothing at the waist is an indication of scoliosis.
- Watching a child during play reveals information about musculoskeletal function.
- Children ages 13 to 19 years need 1300 mg of calcium daily with 400 international units of vitamin D (Hockenberry and Wilson, 2015).

Gerontological

- Teach older adults about fall prevention. Make modifications in the home environment to reduce the risk of falls (see Chapter 43).
- Teach older adults and those with osteoporosis about proper body mechanics, ROM exercises, and moderate weight-bearing exercises (e.g., swimming, walking) to minimize trauma.
- Functional assessment is a measurement of older person's ability to perform ADLs (Ball et al., 2015). When patient is unable to perform self-care easily, determine need for assistive devices (e.g., zippers on clothing instead of buttons, elevation of chairs to minimize bending of knees and hips).
- Older adults tend to assume a stooped, forward-bent posture with hips and knees somewhat flexed, arms bent at the elbows, and level of arms raised.

PROCEDURAL GUIDELINE 6.1 *Monitoring Intake and Output*

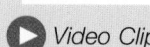 *Video Clip*

Measuring and recording intake and output (I&O) during a 24-hour period is part of the assessment database for fluid and electrolyte balance (Table 6.13). You are responsible for accurate recording of all intake (liquids taken orally, by enteral feedings, and parenterally) and output (urine, diarrhea, vomitus, gastric suction, and drainage from surgical tubes). Monitoring a patient on I&O requires cooperation and help from the patient and family caregivers. Accuracy is critical as physicians will use findings in prescription of medications and intravenous (IV) fluids.

Monitor I&O for patients with a fever or edema, receiving or diuretic therapy, or on restricted IV fluids. It is also important when a patient has electrolyte losses associated with vomiting, diarrhea, gastrointestinal drainage, or extensive open wounds such as burns. Total and evaluate I&O at the end of each shift or at specified times such as every 8 hours. Significant alterations are apparent by comparing 24-hour totals over several days. Because fluid imbalance occurs at any time, be aware of I&O for all patients, even when documentation is not required.

Delegation and Collaboration

The skills of assessing I&O totals at the end of each shift; comparing 24-hour totals over several days; and monitoring and recording intravenous (IV) therapy, wound or chest tube drainage, and tube feedings cannot be delegated to nursing assistive personnel (NAP). The nurse emphasizes maintaining standard precautions related to body fluids, accurately measuring and recording I&O,

and using the metric system with standard containers. The nurse directs the NAP to:

- Measure and record oral intake, urinary output, liquid diarrheal stools, vomitus, and wound drainage device output.
- Report changes in patient's condition such as alteration in intake or changes in color, amount, or odor of output.

Equipment

- Sign to alert personnel of I&O measurement
- Daily I&O record form or computer graphic
- Graduated measuring container
- Bedpan, urinal, bedside commode, or urine "hat" (a receptacle that fits under the toilet seat)
- Clean gloves
- Mask, eye protection, and gown (optional)

Procedural Steps

1. Identify patients with conditions that increase fluid loss (e.g., fever, diarrhea, vomiting, surgical wound drainage, chest tube drainage, gastric suction, major burns, or severe trauma).
2. Identify patients with impaired swallowing, unconscious patients, and patients with impaired mobility.
3. Identify patients on medications that influence fluid balance (e.g., diuretics and steroids).

TABLE 6.13

Adult Average Fluid Gains and Losses

Fluid Intake and Output	Volume (mL)	Fluid Intake and Output	Volume (mL)
Fluid Intake		**Fluid Output**	
Oral fluids	1100–1400	Kidneys	1200–1500
Solid foods	800–1000	Skin	500–600
Oxidative metabolism	300	Lungs	400
		Gastrointestinal	100
Total Gains	2200–2700	**Total Losses**	2200–2700

From Hall JE: *Guyton and Hall textbook of medical physiology*, ed 13, Philadelphia, 2016, Saunders.

PROCEDURAL GUIDELINE 6.1 *Monitoring Intake and Output—cont'd*

4. Assess signs and symptoms of dehydration and fluid overload (e.g., bradycardia versus tachycardia, hypotension versus hypertension, and reduced skin turgor versus edema).
5. Weigh patients daily using the same scale, the same time of day, and with comparable clothing.
6. Monitor laboratory reports:
   • Urine specific gravity (normal is 1.010 to 1.030)
   • Hematocrit (Hct) (normal range is 38% to 47% for females and 40% to 54% for males).
7. Assess patient's and family's knowledge of purpose and process of I&O measurement.
8. Explain to patient and family the reasons that I&O are important.
9. Perform hand hygiene.
10. Measure and record all fluid intake:
    a. Liquids with meals, gelatin, custards, ice cream, popsicles, sherbets, ice chips (recorded as 50% of measured volume [e.g., 100 mL of ice chips equals 50 mL of water]). Convert household measures to the metric system: 1 oz equals 30 mL; therefore 12 oz (soda can) equals 360 mL.
    b. Count liquid medicines such as antacids and fluids with medications as fluid intake.
    c. Calculate fluid intake from tube feedings (see Chapter 32).
    d. Calculate fluid intake from parenteral fluids, blood components, and total parenteral nutrition solutions (see Chapters 29, 30, and 33).

Clinical Decision Point *Record intake as soon as you measure it to maintain accuracy. If more than one patient is in the same room, each must have urine receptacles labeled with name and bed location.*

11. Instruct patient and family member to call you or the NAP to empty contents of urinal, urine hat, or commode each time patient uses it. Have patient and family monitor incontinence, vomiting, and excessive perspiration and report it to the nurse.
12. Inform patient and family that Foley catheter drainage bag and wound, gastric, or chest tube drainage are closely monitored, measured, and recorded and who is responsible for this. Each patient must have a graduated container clearly marked with name and bed location and used only for the patient indicated.
13. Apply clean gloves. Measure drainage at the end of the shift or as indicated, using appropriate containers and noting color and characteristics. If splashing is anticipated, wear mask, eye protection, and/or gown.
    a. Measure urine drainage using a "hat" into which patient voids or a graduated container (see illustration).
    b. Observe color and characteristics of urine in Foley tubing and drainage bag. Sometimes a measuring device is part of the drainage bag (see illustration). Otherwise measure with a graduated container.

c. Measure chest tube drainage by marking and recording the time on the collection chamber at specified intervals (see illustration) (see Chapter 27). Chest tube collection devices are changed when they become full.
d. Measure Jackson-Pratt/Hemovac drainage with a medicine cup (see illustration) (see Chapter 40).
e. Measure gastric drainage or larger drainage pouches by opening clamp and pouring into graduated cup with a 240-mL capacity (see illustration).

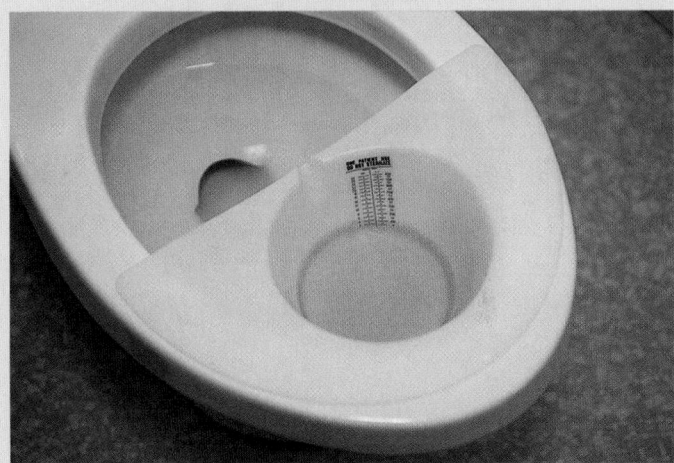

STEP 13a Urine "hat."

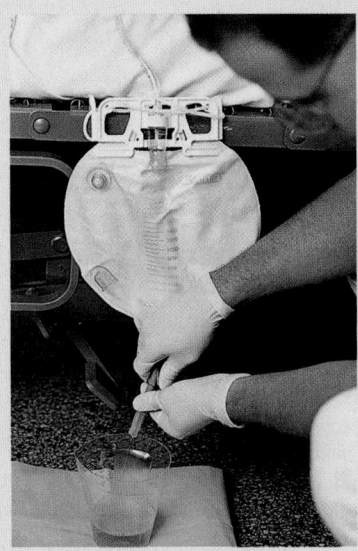

STEP 13b Device for monitoring hourly urine output.

Continued

PROCEDURAL GUIDELINE 6.1 *Monitoring Intake and Output—cont'd*

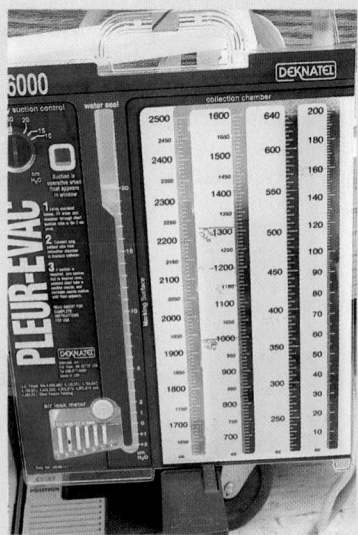

STEP 13c Collection chamber for measuring chest tube drainage.

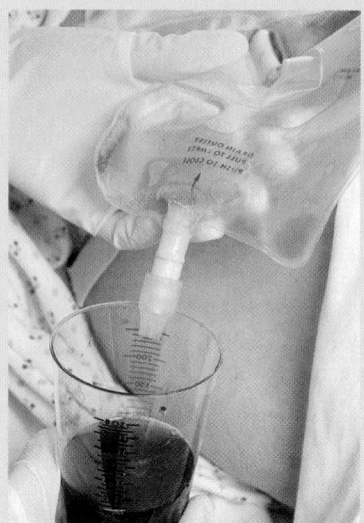

STEP 13e Measuring drainage from large drainage pouch.

14. Remove gloves and dispose of them in appropriate receptacle. Perform hand hygiene.
15. Note I&O balance or imbalance and report to health care provider any urine output less than 30 mL/hr or significant changes in daily weight.
16. Document on I&O forms or electronic record.

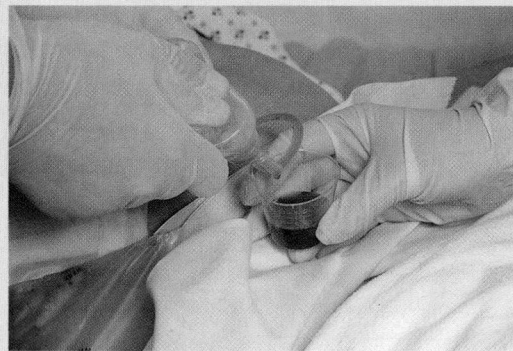

STEP 13d Measuring wound drainage through Jackson-Pratt drain.

◆ CLINICAL DEBRIEF

You are performing your morning assessment on a 69-year-old male patient 3 days postcoronary artery bypass surgery (CABG). When asked about pain, the patient states, "My heart hurts. I feel short of breath and very hot."

1. Which body systems would you assess on the patient and why?
2. You check his last recorded temperature, which was 1 hour ago, and it reads 37.7°C (100°F; you check it again and it is now 38.3°C (101°F). What could cause this change in temperature?
3. On auscultation of his heart you hear a "squeaky" or rubbing sound. Which cardiac abnormality do you suspect?
4. Your assessment of vital signs reveals BP 140/86, T 101° F, HR 90, RR 22, oxygen saturation 91%. How would you document your assessment findings using SBAR, and what should be your next step?

◆ REVIEW QUESTIONS

1. Which of the following are characteristics of malignant melanoma? (Select all that apply.)

1. An irregularly shaped lesion
2. A lesion with lumpy edges
3. A small papule with a dry, rough scale
4. A pearly papule with a central crater and a waxy border
5. A lesion with blue/black or variegated color
6. A lesion of greater than 6 mm in size

2. In conducting a general survey of a patient, the nurse knows that the survey should include which of the following? (Select all that apply.)

1. Appearance
2. Obtaining peripheral pulses
3. Measuring chest expansion
4. Conducting a detailed history
5. Behavior
6. Pupillary response
7. Posture

3. You are about to begin an abdominal assessment on your patient. Place the following sequence in order.
1. Auscultation
2. Inspection
3. Palpation
4. Percussion

ⓔ *Visit the Evolve site for a complete list of Clinical Debrief and Review Questions answers.*

REFERENCES

Advisory Committee on Immunization Practices (ACIP): Advisory Committee on Immunization Practices recommended immunization schedule for adults aged 19 years or older, *Ann Intern Med* 162:214, 2015.

Agency for Healthcare Research and Quality (AHRQ) National Guideline Clearinghouse: *Prevention of skin cancer*, 2014. http://www.guideline.gov/content.aspx?id=48130&search=skin+cancer. Accessed May 30, 2016.

American Cancer Society (ACS): *Guide to quitting smoking*, 2014, http://www.cancer.org/healthy/stayawayfromtobacco/guidetoquittingsmoking/index. Accessed May 30, 2016.

American Cancer Society (ACS): *Cancer prevention and early detection: facts and figures 2015-2016*, Atlanta, 2015a, The Society. http://www.cancer.org/acs/groups/content/@research/documents/webcontent/acspc-045101.pdf. Accessed May 30, 2016.

American Cancer Society (ACS): *American Cancer Society recommendations for early breast cancer detection in women without breast symptoms*, Atlanta, 2015b, The Society. http://www.cancer.org/cancer/breastcancer/moreinformation/breastcancerearlydetection/breast-cancer-early-detection-acs-recs. Accessed May 28, 2016.

American Cancer Society (ACS): *Cervical cancer prevention and early detection*, Atlanta, 2015c, The Society. http://www.cancer.org/cancer/cervicalcancer/. Accessed May 30, 2016.

American Cancer Society (ACS): *Ovarian cancer*, Atlanta, 2015d, The Society. http://www.cancer.org/cancer/ovariancancer/index. Accessed May 30, 2016.

American Cancer Society (ACS): *Skin cancer prevention and early detection*, Atlanta, 2015e, The Society. http://www.cancer.org/acs/groups/cid/documents/webcontent/003184-pdf.pdf. Accessed May 30, 2016.

American Cancer Society (ACS): *Overview guide for testicular cancer*, Atlanta, 2015f, The Society. http://www.cancer.org/cancer/testicularcancer/overviewguide/testicular-cancer-overview-found-early. Accessed May 28, 2016.

American Cancer Society (ACS): *Who should be screened for lung cancer?*, Atlanta, 2015g, The Society. http://www.cancer.org/news/features/who-should-be-screened-for-lung-cancer. Accessed May 28, 2016.

Ball JW, et al: *Child health nursing: partnering with children and families*, ed 3, New Jersey, 2014, Pearson Prentice Hall.

Ball JW, et al: *Seidel's guide to physical examination*, ed 8, St Louis, 2015, Mosby.

Centers for Disease Control and Prevention (CDC): *Tuberculosis (TB)*, 2013, http://www.cdc.gov/tb/topic/basics/default.htm. Accessed May 30, 2016.

Centers for Disease Control and Prevention (CDC): *HPV vaccines: vaccinating your preteen or teen*, 2015, http://www.cdc.gov/hpv/parents/vaccine.html. Accessed May 30, 2016.

Drenkard K: *Patient-centered care*, American Association of Colleges of Nursing, QSEN, 2014 Consortium, http://www.aacn.nche.edu/qsen/workshop-details/san-antonio/KD-PCC.pdf. Accessed May 30, 2016.

Hockenberry JN, Wilson D: *Wong's nursing care of infants and children*, ed 10, St Louis, 2015, Elsevier.

Jeremiah M, et al: Diagnosis and management of osteoporosis, *Am Fam Physician* 92(4):261, 2015.

Lewis S, et al: *Medical-surgical nursing: assessment and management of clinical problems*, ed 10, 2017, Elsevier.

National Osteoporosis Foundation (NOF): *Clinician's guide to prevention and treatment of osteoporosis*, Washington, DC, 2014, National Osteoporosis Foundation. http://link.springer.com/article/10.1007/s00198-014-2794-2. Accessed May 30, 2016.

Patel K, et al: *Deep venous thrombosis*, 2014, http://emedicine.medscape.com/article/1911303-overview. Accessed May 30, 2016.

Shiferaw T, et al: Bacterial contamination and bacterial profile of stethoscopes, *Ann Clin Microbiol Antimicrob* 12:39, 2013.

Short MW, et al: Colorectal cancer and screening and surveillance, *Am Fam Physician* 91(2):93, 2015.

The Joint Commission (TJC): *2016 National Patient Safety Goals*, Oakbrook Terrace, IL, 2016, TJC. http://www.jointcommission.org/standards_information/npsgs.asp. Accessed May 28, 2016.

Touhy T, Jett K: *Ebersole and Hess' toward healthy aging*, ed 9, St Louis, 2015, Mosby.

US Preventative Services Task Force (USPSTF): *Cervical cancer: screening*, 2012, http://www.uspreventiveservicestaskforce.org/Page/Document/UpdateSummaryFinal/cervical-cancer-screening. Accessed May 30, 2016.

Wound Ostomy and Continence Nurses (WOCN) Society: *Guideline for prevention and management of pressure ulcers*, WOCN clinical practice guideline series, Mt. Laurel, NJ, 2016, The Society.

7 | Specimen Collection

OBJECTIVES

Mastery of content in this chapter will enable the nurse to:
- Explain the rationale for the collection of each specimen.
- Identify special conditions necessary for collection of each specimen.
- Provide patient education to promote patient cooperation during specimen collection.
- Identify measures to minimize anxiety and promote safety during specimen collection.
- Discuss nursing responsibilities for processing a specimen after collection.
- Document appropriate information in a patient's electronic health record (EHR) or written record after collection of a specimen.

- Use correct technique for collecting clean-voided, timed, and catheterized urine specimens.
- Use correct technique for collecting specimens and cultures for blood and other body fluids.
- Use correct technique to perform venipuncture.
- Use infection control practices during specimen collection techniques.
- Use correct technique to perform arterial puncture for blood gas measurement.
- Identify nursing responsibility for reporting laboratory results to the health care provider.

MEDIA RESOURCES

- evolve http://evolve.elsevier.com/Perry/skills
- Review Questions
- ▶ Video Clips

- Audio Glossary
- **NSO** Nursing Skills Online
- Clinical Debrief and Review Questions Answers

PURPOSE

Laboratory test results aid in the diagnosis of health care problems, provide information about the stage and activity of a disease process, and measure a patient's response to therapy. Nurses are accountable for correctly collecting specimens, monitoring patient outcomes, and ensuring that these tests are collected and shared with the interprofessional team in a timely manner.

STANDARDS OF CARE

- The Joint Commission (TJC), 2016—Patient Identification

- Occupational Safety & Health Administration (OSHA), 2015—Bloodborne Pathogen Standards

PRINCIPLES FOR PRACTICE

- Proficiency and judgment in obtaining specimens minimize patient discomfort, promote patient safety, and ensure accuracy and quality of diagnostic procedures.
- Everyone who handles body fluids is at risk for exposure. The use of hand hygiene and clean gloves or personal protective equipment is necessary to protect yourself and patients. Proper labeling in a container marked as biohazard protects laboratory personnel and others who may come in contact with the specimen (OSHA, 2015).
- Each agency may establish its own values for each test, which are printed on the agency laboratory forms. When questions arise, consult the agency procedure manual or call the laboratory.

PATIENT-CENTERED CARE

- Patients often experience embarrassment or discomfort when giving a sample of body excretions or secretions, especially urine, urogenital, or stool samples. It is important to handle excretions or secretions discretely and provide a patient with as much privacy as possible. Given clear instructions, patients are able to obtain their own specimens of urine, stool, and sputum without unnecessary exposure (Pagana and Pagana, 2015).
- Consider both cultural and language barriers when delegating specimen collection to patients and family caregivers. Language barriers make it difficult to explain the purpose of tests and collection techniques. Be sure to provide repeated return demonstrations to ensure that patient or family caregiver understands how to perform a procedure (Raingruber, 2014).
- Whenever possible, use gender-congruent caregivers when collecting vaginal, rectal, and urinary specimens from patients whose cultural values demand modesty and distinct separation of gender roles.

EVIDENCE-BASED PRACTICE

- Hemolysis of blood specimens causes delayed treatment of patients and increases health care costs (Lippi, et al., 2014).
- Venipuncture is recommended over the use of obtaining a blood sample from an intravenous (IV) site to prevent hemolysis when possible (Wollowitz, et al., 2013).
- Hemolysis may result from vigorously shaking a blood sample, which invalidates the test.
- Promptly deliver blood specimens to the laboratory for processing to prevent hemolysis.

SAFETY GUIDELINES

- Adapt to patient's need and ability to safely perform and/or participate in specimen collection procedures.
- Verify the type of procedure scheduled and the procedure site with the patient.
- Follow standard precautions (see Chapter 9) when collecting specimens of blood or body fluids.
- Properly label all specimens with patient's identification, date and time the specimen is obtained, name of the test, and source of the specimen/culture for each container (TJC, 2016).
- Deliver specimens to the laboratory within the recommended time or ensure that they are stored properly for later transport.
- Follow procedures for special conditions (e.g., iced specimens, special containers with preservatives) required for transport of specimens. Specific required prerequisite conditions include fasting and nothing by mouth (NPO) and may need to be completed before the collection of a specimen (Pagana and Pagana, 2015).
- Know agency policy regarding infection control practices for transportation of all specimen containers of body substances.
- Follow procedures for medications or dietary intake that may result in some deviations from normal values.
- Follow precautions for collecting specimens from patients who are in protective isolation.

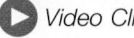 **SKILL 7.1** **Urine Specimen Collection: Midstream (Clean-Voided) Urine; Sterile Urinary Catheter**

▶ *Video Clip* **NSO** *Nursing Skills Online Specimen Collection Module / Lessons 1 and 2*

A urinalysis provides information about kidney or metabolic function, nutrition, and systemic diseases. Urine collection uses a variety of methods, depending on the purpose of the urinalysis and the presence or absence of a urinary catheter. Guidelines for assessment, planning, and evaluation are similar, regardless of the method of collection. Routine urinalysis includes measurement of nine or more elements, including urine pH, protein and glucose levels, ketones, specific gravity, white blood cell (WBC) count, and presence of bacteria and/or blood (Pagana and Pagana, 2015).

Types of Urine Tests and Specimens

- A *random urine specimen for routine urinalysis* is collected using a specimen "hat" (Fig. 7.1), which you place under a toilet seat to collect voided urine. You then place approximately 120 mL of urine in a specimen container, properly labeled, and send to the laboratory.

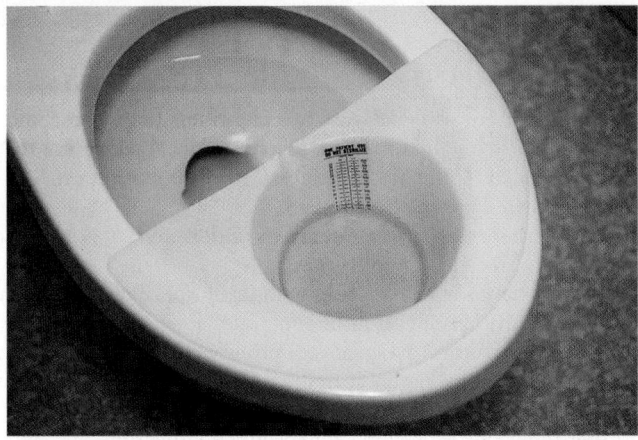

FIG 7.1 Specimen hat.

- A *culture and sensitivity (C&S) of urine* is performed to identify if bacteria are present (culture) and determine the most effective antibiotic for treatment (sensitivity). You collect specimens for C&S either as a clean-voided midstream specimen or under sterile technique from a urinary catheter. Urine collected by this method may also be analyzed for the same components as a routine urinalysis.
- A *timed urine specimen for quantitative analysis* requires urine to be collected over 2 to 72 hours. The 24-hour timed collection (see Procedural Guideline 7.1) is most common and allows for measurement and quantitative analysis of elements such as amino acids, creatinine, hormones, glucose, and adrenocorticosteroid excretion.
- *Chemical properties of urine* are tested by immersing a specially prepared test strip of paper (Chemostrip) into a clean urine specimen. The test detects the presence of glucose, ketones, protein, or blood not normally present in the urine (see Procedural Guideline 7.2). When the screening test for the presence of substances in the urine is positive, additional laboratory tests are used to determine a patient's diagnosis or measure the effectiveness of treatment.

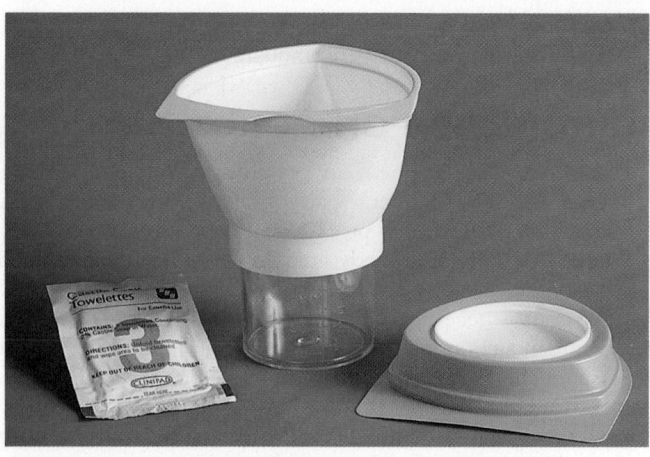

FIG 7.2 Clean-voided specimen collection kit.

Delegation and Collaboration

The skill of collecting urine specimens can be delegated to nursing assistive personnel (NAP). The nurse instructs the NAP to:
- Obtain the specimens at a specified time when appropriate.
- Position patient as necessary when mobility restrictions are present
- Report to the nurse if the urine is not clear (e.g., contains blood, cloudiness, or excess sediment).
- Report to the nurse when a patient is unable to initiate a stream or has pain or burning on urination.

Equipment

- Completed identification labels with appropriate patient identifiers
- Completed laboratory requisition, including patient identification, date, time, name of test, and source of culture
- Small plastic biohazard bag for delivery of specimen to laboratory (or container specified by agency)

Clean-Voided Urine Specimen
- Commercial kit for clean-voided urine (Fig. 7.2) containing:
  - Sterile cotton balls or antiseptic towelettes
  - Antiseptic solution (chlorhexidine or povidone-iodine solution)
  - Sterile water or normal saline
  - Sterile specimen container
  - Urine cup
- Clean gloves
- Soap, water, washcloth, and towel
- Bedpan (for nonambulatory patient), specimen hat (see Fig. 7.1) (for ambulatory patient)

Sterile Urine Specimen From Urinary Catheter
- 20-mL Luer-Lok for routine urinalysis or 3-mL safety Luer-Lok syringe for culture
- Alcohol, chlorhexidine, or other disinfectant swab
- Clamp or rubber band
- Specimen container (nonsterile for routine urinalysis; sterile for culture)
- Clean gloves

STEP	RATIONALE

ASSESSMENT

STEP	RATIONALE
1. Identify patient using at least two identifiers (e.g., name and birthday or name and medical record number) according to agency policy. Compare identifiers with information on patient's MAR or medical record.	Ensures correct patient. Complies with The Joint Commission standards and improves patient safety (TJC, 2016).
2. Assess patient's or family caregiver's understanding of purpose of test and method of collection.	Information allows you to clarify misunderstanding; promotes patient cooperation.
3. Assess patient's ability to help with urine specimen collection; able to position self and hold container.	This determines degree of help patient requires.
4. Assess for signs and symptoms of urinary tract infection (UTI) (frequency, urgency, dysuria, hematuria, flank pain, fever; cloudy, malodorous urine).	These are indicators of UTI.
5. Refer to agency procedures for specimen collection methods.	Agency policies may vary regarding collection and/or handling of specimens.

STEP	RATIONALE

NURSING DIAGNOSES

- Deficient knowledge regarding specimen collection
- Risk for infection

Related factors/Risk factors are individualized based on patient's condition or needs.

PLANNING

1. Expected outcomes following completion of procedure:
   - Specimen free of contaminants is collected.

   - Patient discusses procedure for specimen collection.
   - Patient discusses purpose and benefits of specimen collection.

Proper collection technique prevents substances from changing normal characteristics of urine.

Procedure is performed safely.
Evaluates patient's learning.

IMPLEMENTATION

1. Perform hand hygiene, check labels, and complete laboratory requisition for specimen container.

   Reduces transfer of microorganisms. Organizes procedure.

2. Provide privacy for patient; close curtains around bed or close room door. Allow mobile patients to collect specimen in bathroom.

   Privacy allows patient to relax and produce specimen more easily.

3. Collect clean-voided urine specimen.
   a. Apply clean gloves. Give patient cleaning towelette or towel, washcloth, and soap to clean perineum or help with cleaning perineum. Help bedridden patient onto bedpan to facilitate access to perineum. Remove and dispose of gloves.

   Patients prefer to wash their own perineal areas when possible. Cleaning prevents contamination of specimen after urine passes from urethra.

   b. Using aseptic technique, open outer package of commercial specimen kit.

   Maintains sterility of equipment.

   c. Apply clean gloves.

   Prevents contact of microorganisms on your hands.

   d. Pour antiseptic solution over cotton balls (unless kit contains prepared antiseptic towelettes).

   Cotton ball or towelette is used to clean perineum.

   e. Open specimen container, maintaining sterility of inside specimen container, and place cap with sterile inside up. Do not touch inside of cap or container.

   Contaminated specimen is most frequent reason for inaccurate reporting of urine C&S.

   f. Use aseptic technique to help patient or allow patient to independently clean perineum and collect specimen. Amount of help needed varies with each patient. Inform patient that antiseptic solution will feel cold.

   Maintains patient's dignity and comfort.

   (1) *Male:*
       (a) Hold penis with one hand; using circular motion and antiseptic towelette, clean meatus, moving from center to outside 3 times with different towelettes (see illustration). Have uncircumcised male patient retract foreskin for effective cleaning of urinary meatus and keep retracted during voiding. Return foreskin when done.

       Reduces number of microorganisms at urethral meatus and moves from areas of least to most contamination. Return of foreskin prevents stricture of penis.

       (b) If agency procedure indicates, rinse area with sterile water and dry with cotton balls or gauze pad.

       Prevents contamination of specimen with antiseptic solution.

       (c) After patient initiates urine stream into toilet or bedpan, have him pass urine specimen container into stream and collect 90 to 120 mL of urine (Pagana and Pagana, 2015) (see illustration).

       Initial urine flushes out microorganisms that normally accumulate at urinary meatus and prevents transfer into specimen.

   (2) *Female:*
       (a) Either nurse or patient spreads labia minora with fingers of nondominant hand.

       Provides access to urethral meatus.

STEP	RATIONALE

(b) With dominant hand clean urethral area with antiseptic swab (cotton ball or gauze). Move from front (above urethral orifice) to back (toward anus). Use fresh swab each time; clean 3 times; begin with labial fold farthest from you, then labial fold closest, and then down center (see illustration).

Prevents contamination of urinary meatus with fecal material. Cleaning down center last decreases contamination from labia.

(c) If agency procedure indicates, rinse area with sterile water and dry with cotton ball.

Prevents contamination of specimen with antiseptic solution.

(d) While continuing to hold labia apart, patient initiates urine stream into toilet or bedpan; after stream is achieved, pass specimen container into stream and collect 90 to 120 mL of urine (Pagana and Pagana, 2015) (see illustration).

Initial stream flushes out resident microorganisms that accumulate at urethral meatus and prevents transfer into specimen.

g. Remove specimen container before flow of urine stops and before releasing labia or penis. Patient finishes voiding into bedpan or toilet. Offer to help with personal hygiene as appropriate.

Prevents contamination of specimen with skin flora. Prevents sediment from bladder getting into specimen.

h. Replace cap securely on specimen container, touching only outside.

Retains sterility of inside of container and prevents spillage of urine.

i. Clean urine from exterior surface of container.

Prevents transfer of microorganisms to others.

4. Collect urine from indwelling urinary catheter.

a. Explain that you will use syringe without need to remove urine through catheter port and that patient will not experience any discomfort.

Minimizes anxiety when you manipulate catheter and aspirate urine with syringe from catheter port.

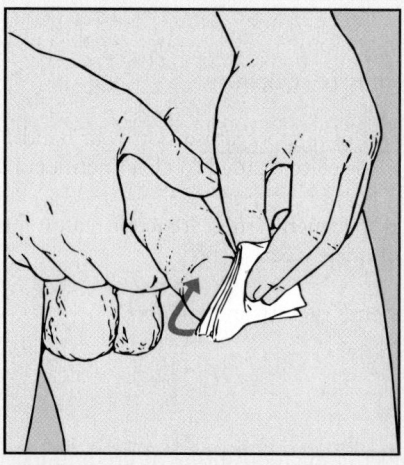

STEP 3f(1)(a) Cleaning technique (male).

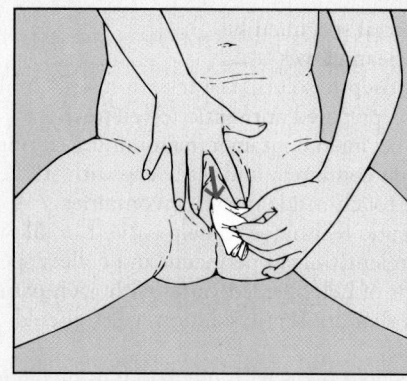

STEP 3f(2)(b) Clean from front to back, holding labia apart.

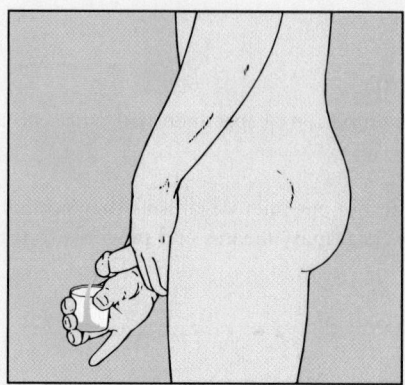

STEP 3f(1)(c) Collecting midstream urine specimen (male).

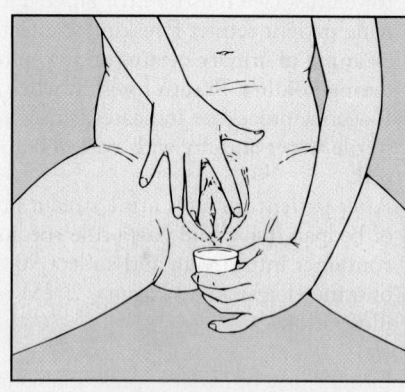

STEP 3f(2)(d) Collecting midstream urine specimen (female).

STEP	RATIONALE
b. Explain that you will need to clamp catheter for 10 to 15 minutes before obtaining urine specimen and that urine cannot be obtained from drainage bag.	Allows urine to accumulate in catheter. Urine in drainage bag is not considered sterile.
c. Apply clean gloves. Clamp drainage tubing with clamp or rubber band for as long as 15 minutes below site chosen for withdrawal (see illustration).	Permits collection of fresh sterile urine in catheter tubing rather than draining into bag.
d. After 15 minutes, position patient so catheter sampling port is easily accessible. Location of port is where catheter attaches to drainage bag tube (see illustration). Clean port for 15 seconds with disinfectant swab and allow to dry.	Prevents entry of microorganisms into catheter.
e. Attach needleless Luer-Lok syringe to built-in catheter sampling port (see illustration). Some needleless ports use blunt plastic valve or slip-tip syringe inserted into port diaphragm.	Guideline recommends use of Luer-Lok needleless system. Needleless system prevents injury by needlestick.
f. Withdraw 3 mL for culture or 20 mL for routine urinalysis.	Allows collection of urine without contamination. Proper volume is needed to perform test.
g. Transfer urine from syringe into clean urine container for routine urinalysis or into sterile urine container for culture.	Prevents contamination of urine during transfer procedure.
h. Place lid tightly on container.	Prevents contamination of specimen by air and loss by spillage.
i. Unclamp catheter and allow urine to flow into drainage bag. Ensure that urine flows freely.	Allows urine to drain by gravity and prevents stasis of urine in bladder.

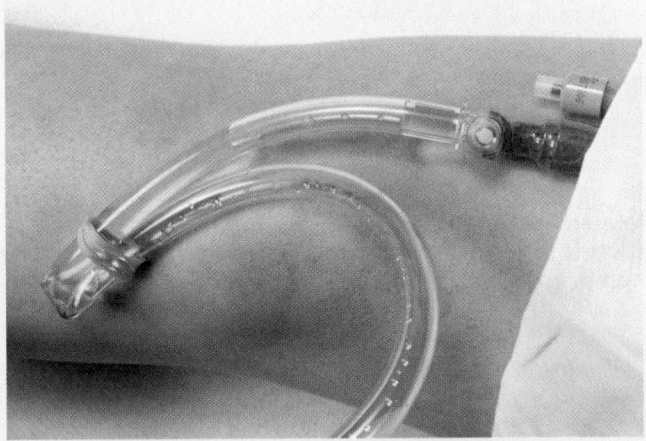

STEP 4c Rubber band used to clamp drainage tube.

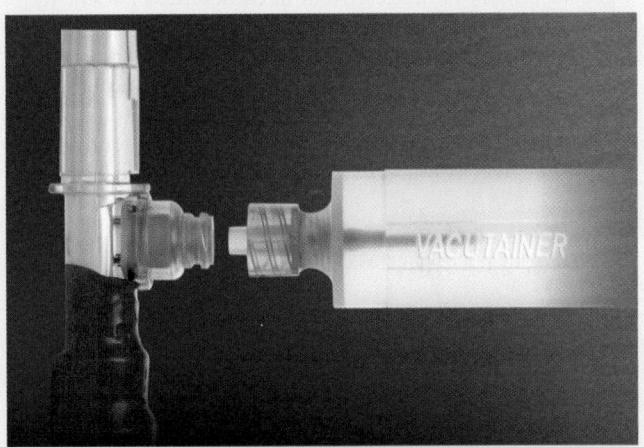

STEP 4d Port with syringe attached.

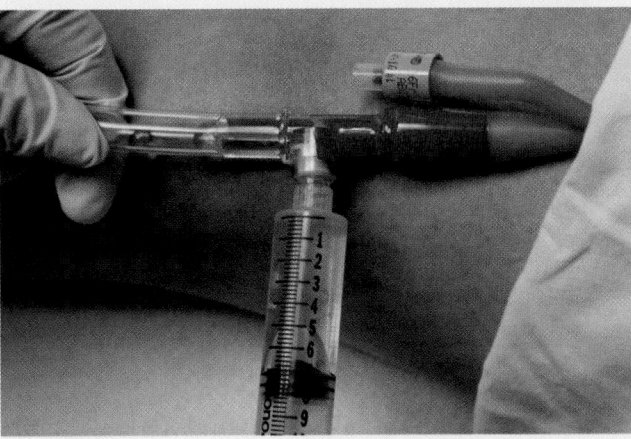

STEP 4e Access urinary catheter port with Luer-Lok syringe or syringe with blunt plastic valve.

STEP	RATIONALE
5. Securely attach label to container (not lid). In patient's presence, confirm label identifiers (two identifiers, specimen source, and collection date and time). If patient is female, indicate if she is menstruating.	Ensures that specimen is identified correctly for proper diagnosis (TJC, 2016).
6. Dispose of soiled supplies. Remove and dispose of gloves and perform hand hygiene.	Prevents transmission of microorganisms.
7. Send specimen and completed requisition to laboratory within 20 minutes. Refrigerate specimen if delay cannot be avoided.	Delay of analysis may significantly alter test results (Pagana and Pagana, 2015).

EVALUATION

1. Inspect clean-voided specimen for contamination with toilet paper or stool.	Contaminants prevent specimen from being used.
2. Evaluate patient's urine C&S report for bacterial growth.	Routine cultures identify organism(s), and sensitivity study identifies antimicrobial medications that may be effective against pathogen.
3. Observe urinary drainage system in catheterized patient to ensure that it is intact and patent.	System must remain closed to remain sterile.
4. **Use Teach-Back:** "I want to be sure I explained the way to obtain a clean-voided specimen. Please repeat the steps back to me." Revise your instruction now or develop a plan for revised patient or family caregiver teaching if patient or family caregiver is not able to teach back correctly.	Determines patient's and family caregiver's level of understanding of instructional topic.

Unexpected Outcomes
1. Urine specimen is contaminated with stool or toilet paper.

2. Patient is unable to void, or urine does not collect in drainage tube.
3. Urine culture reveals bacterial growth (determined by colony count of more than 10,000 organisms per milliliter).

4. Lumen leading to balloon that holds catheter in place is punctured.

Related Interventions
- Repeat patient instruction and specimen collection. If unable to obtain specimen through clean voiding, patient may need catheterization (see Skill 34-1).
- Offer fluids if permitted to enhance urine production.
- Report findings to health care provider.
- Administer medications as ordered.
- Monitor patient for fever and dysuria.
- Notify health care provider.
- Prepare for removal of existing catheter and insertion of new catheter.

Recording and Reporting

- Record collection of specimen in nurses' notes in electronic health record (EHR) or chart or per agency policy; note method used to obtain specimen, date and time collected, type of test ordered, appearance, odor and color of urine, and time sent to laboratory.
- Document your evaluation of patient and family caregiver learning.
- Report any abnormal findings to health care provider.

Special Considerations
Teaching
- Discuss signs and symptoms of UTI with patient and family caregiver if appropriate.
- Explain significance of cleaning genital area before collecting specimen.

Pediatric
- Use clean technique and apply a sterile plastic urine-collecting bag (Fig. 7.3) that adheres to the perineum of an infant or a non–toilet-trained child (Hockenberry and Wilson, 2015).

Gerontological
- Older adults may need help in positioning to obtain specimen. In confused patients NAP may be necessary to help the patient collect a specimen (Touhy and Jett, 2014).

Home Care
- Instruct a patient collecting a sample at home to keep it on ice until it reaches the laboratory to minimize bacterial growth before applying it to a culture medium in the laboratory setting.

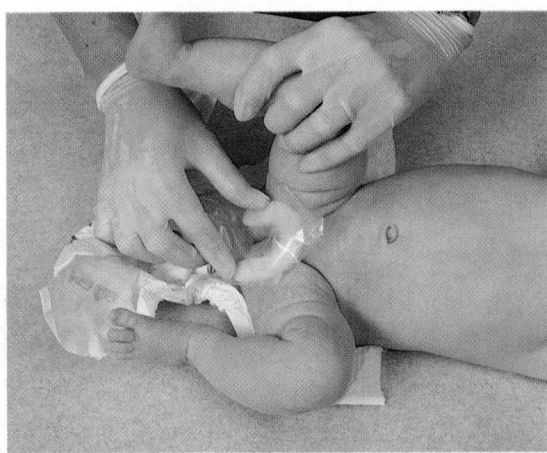

FIG 7.3 Application of urine collection bag. (*From Warekois RS, Robinson R:* Phlebotomy worktext and procedures manual, *ed 3, St Louis, 2012, Mosby.*)

PROCEDURAL GUIDELINE 7.1 *Collecting a Timed Urine Specimen*

Some tests of renal function and urine composition require urine to be collected over 2 to 72 hours. The 24-hour timed collection is used most often and measures elements such as amino acids, creatinine, hormones, glucose, and adrenocorticosteroids. A timed urine collection provides a means to measure the concentration or dilution of urine.

To ensure the accuracy of a 24-hour timed urine specimen, the patient and staff must work together to collect all voided urine in a 24-hour period. Obtain an appropriate container with or without preservative from the laboratory. The type of analysis for the 24-hour timed specimen determines the need for any preservative. You may place the specimen container in the patient's bathroom or the "soiled" utility room. Post a sign to remind the patient and staff that a test is in progress. Label the specimen container with all appropriate identification information and the number of containers sequentially if more than one container is needed. Documentation and collection of all urine is necessary for an accurate test result.

Delegation and Collaboration
The skill of collecting a timed urine specimen can be delegated to nursing assistive personnel (NAP). The nurse informs the NAP about:
- When timed collection begins, proper method to store the collected urine, where to place signs that a timed urine collection is in progress, and saving all urine.
- Reporting when blood, mucus, or foul odors are present in the urine specimen or if there is a break in the collection procedure.

Equipment
- Large collection bottle with cap that usually contains a chemical preservative
- Bedpan, urinal, specimen hat, bedside commode, or pediatric potty-chair
- Graduated measuring container for intake and output (I&O) measurement
- Large basin to hold collection bottle surrounded by ice if immediate refrigeration is required
- Specimen identification label and completed laboratory requisition (with appropriate patient identifiers and specimen information)
- Instructional signs that remind patient and staff of timed urine collection

- Clean gloves
- Plastic biohazard plastic bag or container (see agency policy)

Procedural Steps
1. Identify patient using two identifiers (e.g., name and birthday or name and medical record number) according to agency policy. Compare identifiers with information on patient's MAR or medical record (TJC, 2016).
2. Explain the reason for specimen collection, how patient can help, and that urine must be free of feces and toilet tissue.
3. Place specimen collection container in the bathroom and, if indicated, in a pan of ice. Post signs to remind staff, family and visitors, and patient of timed urine collection on patient's door and toileting area. If patient leaves unit, be sure that personnel in receiving area collect and save all urine.
4. If possible, have patient drink two to four glasses of water about 30 minutes before times of collection to facilitate ability to void at the appropriate time for test to begin.
5. Perform hand hygiene and apply clean gloves. Discard the first voided specimen as the test begins. Indicate time test began on laboratory requisition. For accurate results the patient must begin the test with an empty bladder. Begin collecting all urine for designated time.
6. Measure volume of each voiding if I&O are to be recorded. Place all voided urine in labeled specimen bottle with appropriate additives.
7. Unless instructed otherwise, keep specimen bottle in specimen refrigerator or container of ice in bathroom to prevent decomposition of urine.
8. Encourage patient to drink two glasses of water 1 hour before timed urine collection ends. Encourage patient to empty bladder during last 15 minutes of urine collection period.
9. Perform hand hygiene and apply clean gloves. Collect final specimen at end of collection period. Label specimen (two identifiers, specimen source, collection date and time, number of bottle) in patient's presence, attach appropriate requisition, and send to laboratory. Remove gloves and perform hand hygiene.
10. Remove signs. Tell patient that specimen collection period is completed.

PROCEDURAL GUIDELINE 7.2 *Urine Screening for Glucose, Ketones, Protein, Blood, and pH*

▶ *Video Clip*

Tests for chemical properties of urine are part of the routine urinalysis completed in the laboratory or as a point-of-care test performed at the bedside or in the home. The use of a Multistix reagent test strip may simultaneously assess for up to nine chemical properties: specific gravity, pH, protein, glucose, ketones, blood bilirubin, urobilinogen, leukocytes, and nitrates. The test is easy to perform and causes no pain. This type of screening is used when more detailed laboratory testing is not available (e.g., health care provider's office, clinic, or long-term care setting). The use of urine testing for managing blood glucose is no longer recommended but continues to be useful in detecting presence of ketones in patients with diabetes (ADA, 2013a). Capillary blood monitoring is an accurate assessment of serum glucose levels (Pagana and Pagana, 2015).

Delegation and Collaboration

The skill of urine screening for chemical properties can be delegated to nursing assistive personnel (NAP). The nurse informs the NAP to:

* Obtain the specimen correctly (e.g., before meals, following a "double-voided" specimen).
* Report the results of the test or any odor, blood, or mucus in the urine specimen.

Equipment

* Bedpan, urinal, specimen hat, bedside commode, or pediatric potty-chair
* Container for urine from catheter
* Watch with second hand or digital counter
* Reagent test strip (check expiration date on container)
* Test strip color chart
* Paper towel
* Clean gloves
* Small biohazard plastic bag for delivery of specimen to laboratory (or container specified by agency)

Procedural Steps

1. Identify patient using two identifiers (e.g., name and birthday or name and medical record number) according to agency policy. Compare identifiers with information on patient's MAR or medical record (TJC, 2016).
2. Determine if double-voided specimen is needed for glucose testing. If required, ask patient to void, discard, and then drink a glass of water.
3. Perform hand hygiene and apply clean gloves. Ask patient to collect a fresh, random urine specimen. If patient is catheterized, remove a 5-mL specimen from the catheter port (see Skill 7.1).
4. Immerse end of reagent strip into urine container. Remove the strip immediately and tap it gently against the side of the container to remove excess urine.

5. Hold strip in horizontal position to prevent mixing of chemical reagents (see illustration).

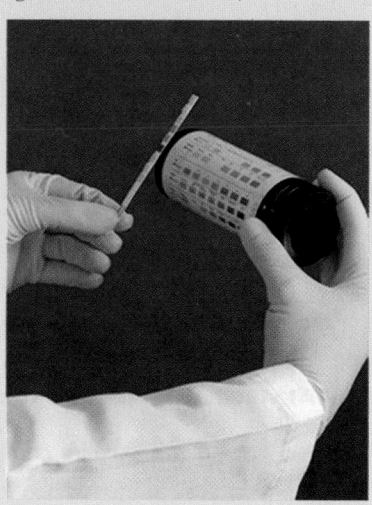

STEP 5 Testing urine using reagent strip.

6. Precisely time the number of seconds specified on container and compare color of strip with color chart on container (Table 7.1).
7. When appropriate, discuss test results with patient. Discard urine. Remove and discard gloves; perform hand hygiene.
8. Record results immediately on appropriate testing flow sheet. Report reading to health care provider.

TABLE 7.1		
Color Chart for Reagent Strip		
Test	**When to Read**	**Range of Results**
pH	Anytime	4.6–8.0
Protein	Anytime	None or up to 8 mg/100 mL
Glucose	10 seconds (qualitative) 30 seconds (quantitative)	(–) to +4 (–) to +4 (270)
Ketones	15 seconds	(–) to +3 (large)
Blood	25 seconds	(–) to +3 (large)

✦ SKILL 7.2 Measuring Occult Blood in Stool

 Video Clip **NSO** *Nursing Skills Online Specimen Collection Module / Lesson 3*

Hemoccult testing is useful for screening for the presence of occult (not visible) blood in the stool for conditions such as colon cancer, bleeding gastrointestinal (GI) ulcers, and localized gastric or intestinal irritation. Use caution; a false-positive result may occur if a patient has ingested red meat within 3 days of testing or is taking certain medications (e.g., iron). A false-negative may result if that patient is taking vitamin C (Pagana and Pagana, 2015). The test measures microscopic amounts of blood in the stool. Normally a person loses small amounts of blood daily in the feces as a result of minor abrasions of the nasopharyngeal or oral mucosa. If greater than 50 mL of blood enters the feces from the upper GI tract, the blood causes melena (darkening of feces). When blood is present, further testing is indicated to determine the source of the bleeding.

Patients are often instructed on how to collect stool specimens for the test in the home. Only a small amount of stool is needed to perform the test successfully. The most common guaiac tests are the Hemoccult slides and the Hematest tablets. A new deoxyribonucleic acid (DNA) stool sample test promises to be twice as sensitive as the current guaiac testing for precancerous benign and malignant tumors. The DNA stool sample test identifies nonbleeding polyps with abnormal DNA (Pagana and Pagana, 2015).

Delegation and Collaboration

The skill of testing stool for occult blood can be delegated to nursing assistive personnel (NAP). The nurse informs the NAP to:
- Report immediately if any blood is detected and not to discard stool from a positive test so the nurse may repeat the testing.

Equipment

- Soap, water, washcloth, and towel
- Paper towel
- Clean gloves
- Wooden applicators

Hemoccult Test
- Cardboard Hemoccult slide (Fig. 7.4)
- Hemoccult developing solution

Hematest
- Hematest tablets (must be protected from moisture, heat, and light)
- Guaiac paper
- Clean container of tap water

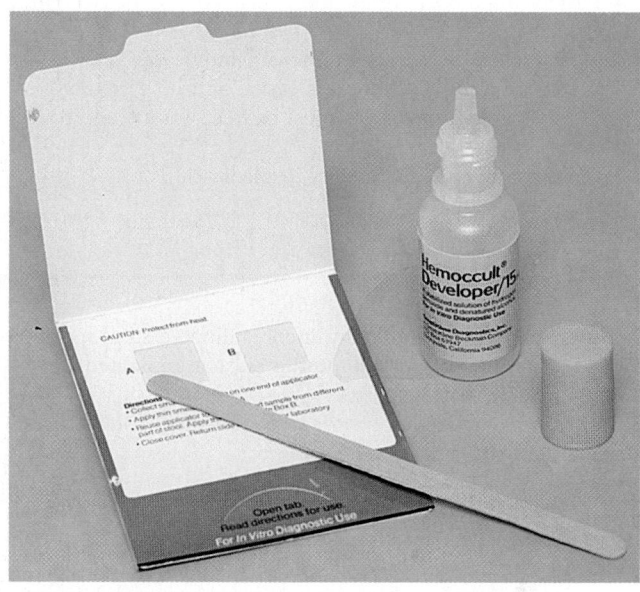

FIG 7.4 Hemoccult testing kit for measuring occult blood.

STEP	RATIONALE

ASSESSMENT

STEP	RATIONALE
1. Identify patient using at least two identifiers (e.g., name and birthday or name and medical record number) according to agency policy. Compare identifiers with information on patient's MAR or medical record.	Ensures correct patient. Complies with The Joint Commission standards and improves patient safety (TJC, 2016).
2. Assess patient's or family caregiver's understanding of need for stool test.	Provides information on which to base necessary health teaching.
3. Assess patient's ability to cooperate with procedure and collect specimen.	To avoid embarrassment, patients often prefer to collect own stool specimen. Some patients require help.
4. Assess patient's medical history for GI disorders (e.g., history of bleeding, colitis, or hemorrhoids).	You can institute routine screening. Hemorrhoids can cause bleeding that may be misinterpreted as upper GI bleeding.
5. Review patient's medications for drugs that contribute to GI bleeding.	Anticoagulants increase risk for bleeding in GI tract, even from minor trauma to mucosa. Long-term use of steroids, nonsteroidal antiinflammatory drugs (NSAIDs), and acetylsalicylic acid (aspirin) can irritate mucosa and result in bleeding (Pagana and Pagana, 2015).
6. Refer to health care provider's orders for medication or dietary modifications or restrictions before test.	Specimens will be positive if contaminated by menstrual blood, hemorrhoid blood, or povidone-iodine. Diets rich in meats, green leafy vegetables, poultry, and fish may produce false-positive results.

STEP	RATIONALE

NURSING DIAGNOSES

- Anxiety
- Bowel incontinence
- Constipation
- Deficient knowledge regarding collection and testing of stool specimen
- Diarrhea

Related factors are individualized based on patient's condition or needs.

PLANNING

1. Expected outcomes following completion of procedure:
   - Test for occult blood is negative.

   - Patient discusses purpose and benefits of testing stool for blood.
2. Explain procedure to patient and/or family caregiver. Discuss reason for specimen collection and how patient can help. Explain that feces must be free of urine and toilet tissue.
3. Arrange for any needed dietary or medication restrictions.

Patient has only small amount of blood in feces because of normal nasopharyngeal and oral mucosa abrasions.
Validates learning.

Patient who understands procedure is more likely to cooperate and may be able to obtain specimen independently. Also prevents accidental disposal of specimen.

Ensures accuracy of test results.

IMPLEMENTATION

1. Perform hand hygiene
2. Apply clean gloves. Obtain uncontaminated stool specimen and place in clean, dry container not contaminated with urine, water, or toilet tissue.
3. Use tip of wooden applicator to obtain small part of feces.
4. Measure for occult blood.
   a. Perform Hemoccult slide test:
      (1) Open flap of Hemoccult slide. Apply thin smear of stool on paper in first box.
      (2) Obtain second fecal specimen from different part of stool and apply thinly to second box of slide (see illustration).

      (3) Close slide cover and turn slide over to reverse side. Open cardboard flap and apply 2 drops of Hemoccult developing solution on each box of guaiac paper (see illustration).

Reduces transmission of microorganisms.
Prevents transmission of microorganisms. Allows for accurate testing when specimen is not contaminated with other products.
Small specimen is sufficient for measuring blood content.

Guaiac paper inside box is sensitive to fecal blood content.

Occult blood from upper GI tract is not always dispersed equally throughout stool. Findings of occult blood are more conclusive for GI bleeding when entire specimen is found to contain blood.
Developing solution penetrates underlying fecal specimen. Change in color of guaiac paper indicates blood.

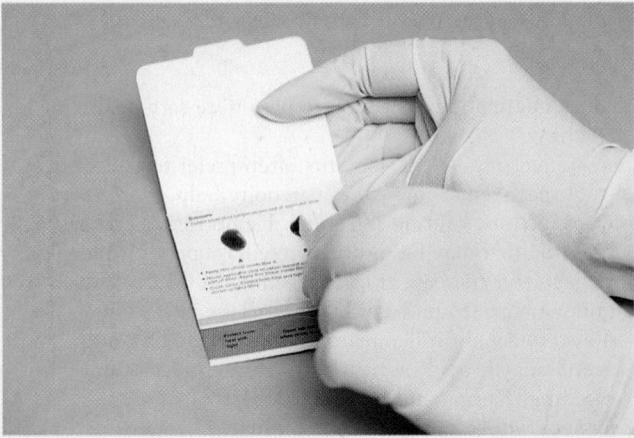

STEP 4a(2) Applying stool specimen to both spots on Hemoccult slide.

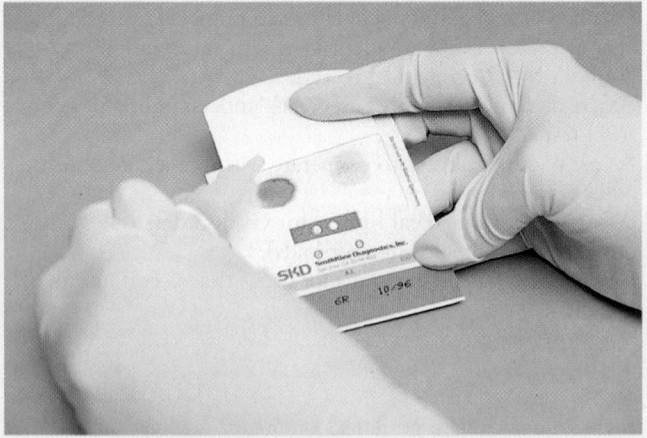

STEP 4a(3) Applying developing solution.

STEP	RATIONALE
(4) Read results of test after 30 to 60 seconds. Note color changes.	Ensures correct results. Bluish discoloration indicates occult blood (guaiac positive). No change in color of guaiac paper indicates negative results.
(5) Dispose of test slide in proper receptacle.	Reduces transfer of microorganisms.
b. Perform test using Hematest tablets:	Tablet contains solid form of developing solution.
(1) Place stool on guaiac paper. Then place Hematest tablet on top of stool specimen. Apply 2 to 3 drops of tap water to tablet, allowing water to flow onto guaiac paper.	Tap water dissolves Hematest tablet and thus dispenses developing solution over specimen and guaiac paper.
(2) Observe color of guaiac paper within 2 minutes.	Bluish discoloration is guaiac positive. Do not read color after 2 minutes. False findings may occur.
(3) Dispose of tablet and paper in proper receptacle.	Reduces transfer of microorganisms.
5. Wrap wooden applicator in paper towel, grasp in nondominant hand, remove gloves over wrapped applicator. Discard in proper receptacle. Perform hand hygiene.	Reduces transfer of microorganisms.

EVALUATION

1. Note color changes in guaiac paper.	Reveals blood in feces.
2. Use Teach-Back: "You will need to check your stool two more times for blood when you go home. I want to be sure I explained the procedure correctly. Tell me the steps you will use to collect this specimen." Revise your instruction now or develop a plan for revised patient or family caregiver teaching if patient or family caregiver is not able to teach back correctly.	Determines patient's and family caregiver's level of understanding of instructional topic.

Clinical Decision Point *Single positive test result does not confirm bleeding or indicate colorectal cancer. To confirm positive results, test must be repeated while patient is on meat-free, high-residue diet with more in-depth diagnosis (Van Leeuwen et al., 2015).*

3. Note character of stool specimen.	Certain abnormal constituents of stool may be visible.

Unexpected Outcomes	Related Interventions
1. Test for occult blood is positive.	• Continue to monitor patient.
	• Notify health care provider.

Recording and Reporting

- Record results of test and include stool characteristics in nurses' notes in electronic health record (EHR) or chart.
- Document your evaluation of patient and family caregiver learning.
- Report positive test results to health care provider.

Special Considerations
Pediatric

- Children of school age and older are concrete thinkers and often very curious. They may ask many questions about the test.

Answer questions honestly and at child's level of understanding. Allow child to watch, if desired, while performing test (Hockenberry and Wilson, 2015).

- Testing reagent is often poisonous; thus keep it out of reach of the small child.

Home Care

- Many patients or family caregivers are instructed to collect specimens at home and return them to the clinic or health care provider's office. Be sure they know infection control principles.

✦ **SKILL 7.3** **Measuring Occult Blood in Gastric Secretions (Gastroccult)**

NSO *Nursing Skills Online Specimen Collection Module / Lesson 4*

Analysis of gastric secretions or emesis can detect blood that is not always visible. Gastroccult testing helps to reveal bleeding in the esophagus or stomach. The test can verify the presence of blood when red or black coloration of the gastric contents is noted or when the gastric contents or emesis has the appearance of coffee grounds. The test measures microscopic amounts of blood in the gastric secretions. It is a useful diagnostic tool for conditions such as upper gastrointestinal (GI) ulcers or bleeding. Because the test is easy to perform, patients are often taught how to test emesis in the home.

Delegation and Collaboration

The skill of Gastroccult testing can be delegated to nursing assistive personnel (NAP) for test on emesis. You cannot delegate the skill of Gastroccult testing to NAP if the specimen is collected from a nasogastric (NG) or nasoenteral (NE) tube. The nurse informs the NAP to:

- Report immediately if blood or coffee-ground emesis is visible in NG or NE tube secretions.
- Save specimen for repeat testing.

Equipment

- Facial tissues
- Emesis basin
- Wooden applicator or 3-mL syringe
- Bulb or catheter tip syringe
- Cardboard Gastroccult test slide
- Gastroccult developing solution
- Clean gloves

STEP	RATIONALE
ASSESSMENT	
1. Identify patient using at least two identifiers (e.g., name and birthday or name and medical record number) according to agency policy. Compare identifiers with information on patient's MAR or medical record.	Ensures correct patient. Complies with The Joint Commission standards and improves patient safety (TJC, 2016).
2. Assess patient's or family caregiver's understanding of need for test.	Provides nurse with information on which to base necessary health teaching.
3. Assess patient's medical history for bleeding or GI disorders.	You can institute routine screening.
4. Assess patient's medical history for GI disorders (e.g., history of bleeding, colitis).	Anticoagulants increase risk for bleeding in GI tract, even from minor trauma to mucosa. Long-term use of steroids, nonsteroidal antiinflammatory drugs (NSAIDs), and acetylsalicylic acid (aspirin) can irritate mucosa.

NURSING DIAGNOSES

- Anxiety
- Deficient knowledge regarding occult blood testing
- Fear

Related factors are individualized based on patient's condition or needs.

PLANNING	
1. Expected outcomes following completion of procedure:	
• Test for occult blood is negative.	Patient has only small or no amount of blood in gastric secretions.
• Patient discusses purpose and benefits of testing gastric contents for blood.	Validates learning.
2. Explain procedure to patient and/or family caregiver. Discuss why specimen collection is necessary.	Patient who understands procedure is more likely to be less anxious and more cooperative.

IMPLEMENTATION	
1. Perform hand hygiene.	Reduces transmission of microorganisms.
2. Verify NG tube placement (see Chapter 32).	Ensures aspiration of gastric contents.
3. Obtain specimen by disconnecting suction or gravity drainage tube from NG or NE tube. Using a bulb or catheter tip syringe, aspirate 5 to 10 mL of fluid from NG or NE tube.	Only small amount of specimen is needed for testing.

STEP	RATIONALE

Clinical Decision Point *Observe specimen. If you find red blood or coffee-ground material, report these findings immediately to health care provider.*

4. To obtain sample of emesis, use 3-mL syringe or wooden applicator to obtain sample from emesis basin.	Small specimen is sufficient for measuring blood content.
5. *Perform Gastroccult test:*	
a. Using wooden applicator or syringe, apply 1 drop of gastric sample to Gastroccult blood test slide.	Sample must cover test paper for test reaction to occur.
b. Apply 2 drops of commercial developer solution over sample and 1 drop between positive and negative performance monitors (see illustration).	

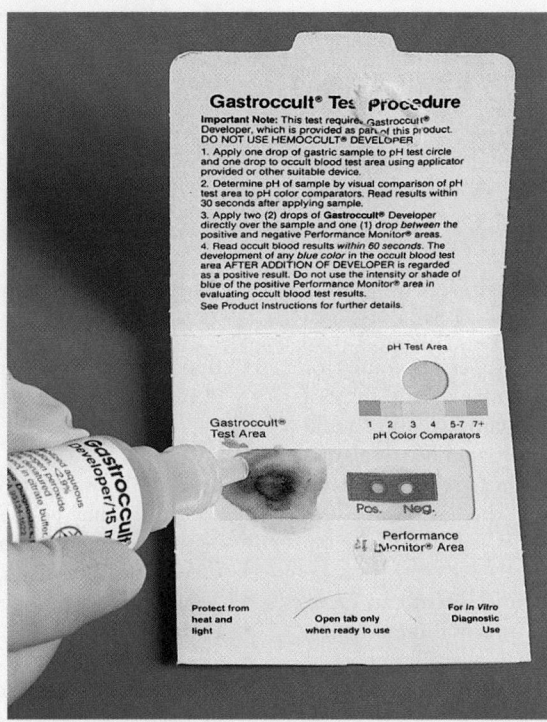

STEP 5b Applying developing solution to Gastroccult test area.

c. Verify that performance monitor turns blue in 30 seconds.	Indicates proper function of testing paper.
d. After 60 seconds compare color of gastric sample with that of performance monitor.	If sample turns blue, test is positive for occult blood. If sample turns green, it is negative for occult blood.
e. Dispose of test slide, wooden applicator, and syringe in proper receptacle. If needed, reconnect enteral tube to drainage system or suction. Remove gloves. Perform hand hygiene.	Reduces transmission of microorganisms.

EVALUATION

1. Note character of gastric secretions.	Blood may be visible, or coffee-ground material denoting blood may be observed.
2. Note color changes in guaiac paper.	Reveals blood in gastric secretions.
3. **Use Teach-Back:** "I want to be sure I explained the purpose and procedure for obtaining a specimen of your gastric secretions. Please state the necessary steps you will use to obtain this specimen." Revise your instruction now or develop a plan for revised patient or family caregiver teaching if patient or family caregiver is not able to teach back correctly.	Determines patient's and family caregiver's level of understanding of instructional topic.

STEP	RATIONALE

Unexpected Outcomes
1. Test for occult blood is positive.

Related Interventions
- Continue to monitor patient.
- Notify health care provider.

Recording and Reporting

- Record results of test and presence of any unusual characteristics of gastric contents in nurses' notes in electronic health record (EHR) or chart.
- Document your evaluation of patient and family caregiver learning.
- Report positive test results to health care provider.

Special Considerations
Pediatric

- Children of school age and older are concrete thinkers, are often very curious, and may ask many questions about test. Answer questions honestly and at child's level of understanding. Allow child to watch, if desired, while test is performed (Hockenberry and Wilson, 2015).

Home Care
- Many patients or family caregivers can perform the Gastroccult test on emesis. Be sure they know infection control principles.

◆ SKILL 7.4 **Collecting Nose and Throat Specimens for Culture**

When patients have signs and symptoms of upper respiratory or sinus infection, a nose or throat culture is a simple diagnostic tool to identify the presence and type of microorganisms. You should obtain cultures before antibiotic therapy is initiated because antibiotics may interrupt the growth of the organisms in the laboratory. If a patient is receiving antibiotics, notify the laboratory and identify which specific antibiotics he or she is receiving (Pagana and Pagana, 2015).

Collection of a specimen from the nose and throat can cause discomfort and gagging because of sensitive mucosal membranes. It is important to collect a throat culture before mealtime or at least 1 hour after eating or drinking to decrease the chance of inducing vomiting.

Delegation and Collaboration

The skill of obtaining specimens from the nose and throat cannot be delegated to nursing assistive personnel (NAP). The nurse informs the NAP to:

- Report shortness of breath, difficulty breathing, and other signs of respiratory distress.

Equipment

- Two sterile swabs in sterile culture tubes (flexible wire swab with cotton tip may be used for nose cultures)
- Nasal speculum (*optional*)
- Emesis basin or clean container (*optional*)
- Tongue blades and penlight
- Facial tissues/gauze
- Clean gloves
- Completed identification labels with proper patient identifiers
- Completed laboratory requisition (date, time, name of test, patient identification, source of culture)
- Small biohazard plastic bag for delivery of specimen to laboratory (or container specified by agency)

STEP	RATIONALE

ASSESSMENT

1. Identify patient using at least two identifiers (e.g., name and birthday or name and medical record number) according to agency policy. Compare identifiers with information on patient's MAR or medical record.

   Ensures correct patient. Complies with The Joint Commission standards and improves patient safety (TJC, 2016).

2. Assess patient's understanding of purpose for procedure and ability to cooperate. You may need help to obtain throat cultures from confused, combative, or unconscious patients.

   Provides basis to determine need for health teaching and assistance.

3. Inspect condition of nares and drainage from nasal mucosa and sinuses.

   Reveals physical signs that indicate infection or allergic irritation. Clear drainage usually indicates allergy. Yellow, green, or brown drainage usually indicates infection.

STEP	RATIONALE
4. Determine if patient experiences postnasal drip, sinus headache or tenderness, nasal congestion, sore throat, or exposure to others with similar symptoms.	Symptoms help reveal nature of problem.
5. Apply clean gloves. Assess condition of posterior pharynx (see Chapter 6).	Reveals local inflammation or lesions of pharynx.
6. Assess patient for signs of infection, including fever, chills, and/or fatigue.	Infection originating within nasopharynx can become systemic, requiring antibiotic therapy.
7. Review health care provider's orders to determine if nose, throat, or both cultures are needed.	Prevents exposing patient to unnecessary discomfort of repeated cultures.

NURSING DIAGNOSES

- Acute pain
- Chronic pain
- Deficient knowledge regarding specimen collection
- Risk for infection

Related factors/Risk factors are individualized based on patient's condition or needs.

PLANNING

1. Expected outcomes following completion of procedure:	
• There is no bacterial growth in specimens.	Absence of bacterial infection.
• Patient does not experience bleeding of nasal mucosa.	Procedure is atraumatic.
• Specimen is not contaminated.	Evidenced by results of laboratory analysis.
• Patient discusses purpose of nose and throat cultures.	Validates learning.
2. Plan to do culture before mealtime or at least 1 hour after eating.	Procedure often induces gagging; timing decreases patient's chances of vomiting.
3. Explain procedure to patient and/or family caregiver. Discuss reason for specimen collection and how patient can help.	Understanding procedure usually decreases anxiety and promotes cooperation.
4. Explain that patient may have tickling sensation or gagging during swabbing of throat. Nasal swab may create urge to sneeze. Each procedure only takes a few seconds to complete.	Helps patient relax.

IMPLEMENTATION

1. Ask patient to sit erect in bed or chair facing you. Acutely ill patient or young child may lie back against bed with head of bed raised to 45-degree angle in semi-Fowler's position.	Provides easy access to nasal or oral structures.
2. Perform hand hygiene. Have swab in tube ready for use. Loosen top so swab can be removed easily.	Reduces transmission of microorganisms. Allows you to grasp swab easily without danger of contamination. Most commercial tubes have tops that fit securely over end of swab. Allows touching outer tops without contaminating swab stick.
3. **Collect throat culture**	
a. Apply clean gloves.	Reduces transmission of microorganisms.
b. Instruct patient to tilt head backward. For patients in bed, place pillow behind shoulders.	Facilitates visualization of pharynx.
c. Ask patient to open mouth and say "ah." To visualize pharynx, depress tongue with tongue blade and note inflamed areas of pharynx or tonsils. Depress anterior third of tongue only and illuminate with penlight as needed.	Permits exposure of pharynx, relaxes throat muscles, and minimizes gag reflex. Area to be swabbed should be visualized clearly.

Clinical Decision Point *Do not attempt throat culture in a pediatric patient if you suspect acute epiglottitis because trauma from swab might cause increase in edema, resulting in occlusion of airway (Hockenberry and Wilson, 2015).*

d. Insert swab without touching lips, teeth, tongue, cheeks, or uvula.	Prevents contamination with organisms from oral cavity (Pagana and Pagana, 2015).

STEP	RATIONALE

   e. Gently but quickly swab tonsillar area side to side, making contact with inflamed or purulent sites (see illustration).

These areas contain most microorganisms.

   f. Carefully withdraw swab without touching oral structures.

Collects microorganisms from throat tissues without contamination from mouth and tongue.

4. Collect nasal culture

   a. Apply clean gloves.

Reduces transmission of microorganisms.

   b. Encourage patient to blow nose and then check nostrils for patency with penlight. Select nostril with greatest patency.

Clears nasal passages of mucus containing resident bacteria.

   c. In sitting position have patient tilt head backward. Patients in bed should have small pillow behind shoulders.

Provides access to nasal passages and facilitates visualization of nasal septum and sinuses.

   d. Gently insert nasal speculum in one nostril *(optional)*.

Allows retraction of mucosa for easier swab insertion.

   e. Carefully pass swab into nostril until it reaches that part of mucosa that is inflamed or containing exudate. Rotate swab quickly. **NOTE:** If you need to obtain nasopharyngeal culture, use special swab on flexible wire that can be flexed downward to reach nasopharynx.

Swab should remain sterile until it reaches area to be cultured. Rotating swab covers all surfaces where exudate is present.

   f. Remove swab without touching sides of speculum or nasal canal.

Prevents contamination of swab by resident bacteria.

   g. Carefully remove nasal speculum (if used) and place in basin. Offer patient facial tissue.

Minimizes period of time that patient experiences discomfort.

5. Insert swab into culture tube. Use gauze to protect your fingers while crushing ampule at bottom of tube to release culture medium (see illustrations).

Placing tip within culture medium maintains life of bacteria for testing.

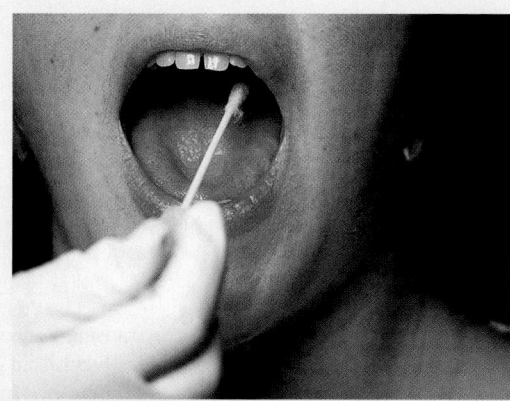

STEP 3e Collecting specimen from posterior pharynx.

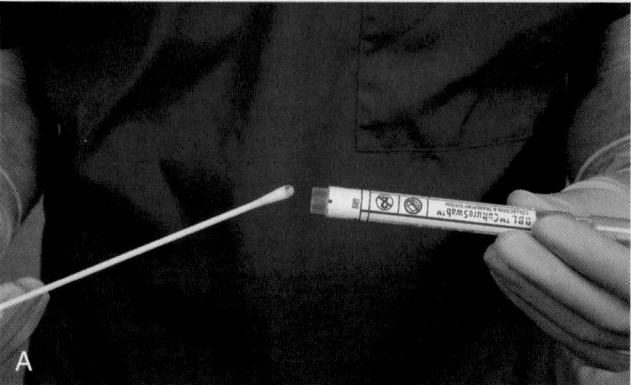
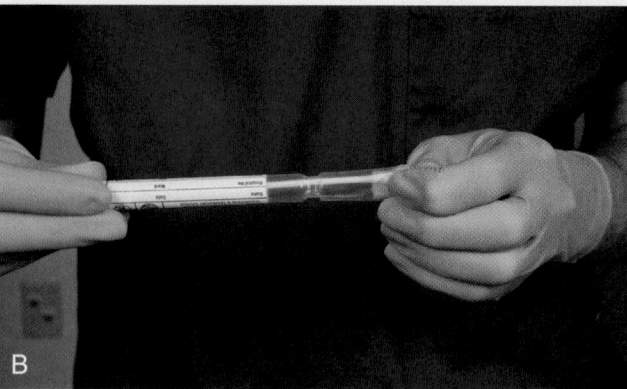

STEP 5 Activating culture tube. **A,** Place swab into tube. **B,** Crush end of tube to release liquid medium.

STEP	RATIONALE
6. Place tip of swab into liquid medium and place top securely on top of tube.	Preserves specimen for testing.
7. Securely attach completed identification label and laboratory requisition to culture tube and confirm identifiers, specimen source, and collection date and time in front of patient (see agency policy). Note on laboratory requisition if patient is taking antibiotic or if specific organism is suspected (e.g., *Bordetella pertussis*).	Incorrect identification of specimen could result in diagnostic or therapeutic errors.
8. Enclose specimen in plastic biohazard bag (according to agency policy) and send immediately to laboratory.	Specimen not sent to laboratory immediately or refrigerated allows growth of organisms and inaccurate results.
9. Return patient to position of comfort. Remove and dispose of gloves and perform hand hygiene.	Provides for patient comfort. Reduces transmission of microorganisms.

EVALUATION

1. Check laboratory record for results of culture test.	Results reveal type of organisms in nose or pharynx and antibiotics most likely to be effective.
2. **Use Teach-Back:** "I want to be sure I explained the purpose and procedure for obtaining a throat culture. Please tell me why we are obtaining this culture?" Revise your instruction now or develop a plan for revised patient or family caregiver teaching if patient or family caregiver is not able to teach back correctly.	Determines patient's and family caregiver's level of understanding of instructional topic.

Unexpected Outcomes	Related Interventions
1. Nose and throat cultures reveal bacterial growth.	• Notify health care provider of findings. • Administer medications as ordered.
2. Patient experiences minor nasal bleeding.	• Apply mild pressure and ice pack over bridge of nose. • Notify health care provider of patient's condition.
3. Specimen is contaminated.	• Repeat specimen collection.

Recording and Reporting

- Describe appearance of nasal and oral mucosal structure and record specimen collection, date, time, and disposition in nurses' notes in electronic health record (EHR) or chart.
- Document your evaluation of patient and family caregiver learning.
- Report unusual test results to health care provider.

Special Considerations
Teaching
- Teach patient that procedure may cause slight discomfort and gagging is common.
- Discuss reason for time delay in receiving culture results.

Pediatric
- Allowing young children to visualize and examine speculum decreases their fear.

- Immobilization of child's head and arms is important when obtaining specimen. You should do this in a firm, gentle, kind manner. Ask another nurse to help if necessary.
- Ask parents to act as coach and suggest that they hold their child on their lap. Do not ask parents to restrain child (Hockenberry and Wilson, 2015).
- Showing tongue blade and penlight to child and demonstrating how to say "ah" helps to decrease anxiety.
- School-age child will be more cooperative if given opportunity to ask questions about procedure and results.

Gerontological
- Some older adults need help in keeping mouth open to obtain specimen.
- Some older adults have poor dentition. Take care not to break a tooth and consider removal of dentures.

◆ **SKILL 7.5**   **Obtaining Vaginal or Urethral Discharge Specimens**

Normally drainage from the vagina or urethra is thin, nonpurulent, whitish or clear, and small in amount. Factors such as poor hygiene practices can cause an accumulation of discharge. If a patient develops an increased amount of discharge or if there is a change in the character of discharge from the vagina or urethra, medical follow-up is necessary.

Patients most commonly requiring cultures of vaginal or urethral discharge have signs and symptoms of sexually transmitted infection (STI) or urinary tract infection. Patients suspected of having an STI may be embarrassed by their condition. Show respect and understanding toward a patient. When collecting vaginal or urethral specimens, work quickly and calmly, maintaining the patient's privacy at all times.

Delegation and Collaboration

The skill of obtaining vaginal or urethral discharge specimens cannot be delegated to nursing assistive personnel (NAP).

Equipment

- Sterile swab in sterile culture tube (commercially available culture tubes have swab and tube with ampule containing special transport medium)

- Sheet, blanket, or paper drape
- Clean gloves
- Penlight or gooseneck lamp
- Completed identification labels with proper patient identifiers
- Completed laboratory requisition (date, time, name of test, patient identification, source of culture)
- Small biohazard plastic bag for delivery of specimen to laboratory (or container specified by agency)

STEP	RATIONALE

ASSESSMENT

1. Identify patient using at least two identifiers (e.g., name and birthday or name and medical record number) according to agency policy. Compare identifiers with information on patient's MAR or medical record.

   Ensures correct patient. Complies with The Joint Commission standards and improves patient safety (TJC, 2016).

2. Assess patient's understanding of need for culture and ability to cooperate with procedure.

   Provides you with information on which to base necessary health teaching.

3. Perform hand hygiene and apply clean gloves. Assess condition of external genitalia and urethra, meatus, and vaginal orifice. Observe for redness; swelling; complaint of tenderness; and discharge that is whitish, mucoid, or purulent or a whitish discharge such as cottage cheese. Remove and discard gloves and perform hand hygiene. **NOTE:** This step may be done during collection.

   Reduces transmission of microorganisms. Assessment findings and specimen test results reveal nature of problem.

4. Ask patient about dysuria, localized pruritus of genitalia, or lower abdominal pain.

   Symptoms of urinary tract or vaginal infection.

5. If symptoms suggest STI, gather and record patient's sexual history.

   Determines sexual activity and if there has been sexual contact with a person known to have an STI. If culture results are positive, tell patient to receive treatment and have sexual partners evaluated (Pagana and Pagana, 2015).

6. Refer to health care provider's order to determine if culture is to be vaginal or urethral.

   Patient may require one or both types of cultures.

NURSING DIAGNOSES

- Acute pain
- Anxiety

- Deficient knowledge regarding specimen collection

- Risk for infection

Related factors/Risk factors are individualized based on patient's condition or needs.

PLANNING

1. Expected outcomes following completion of procedure:
   - Specimen is not contaminated.

     Results on laboratory test will reveal whether skin cells or mucosal cells have contaminated specimen.

   - Vaginal or urethral cultures do not reveal growth of microorganisms.

     Evidence of absence of infection.

2. Explain procedure to patient and/or family caregiver. Discuss reason for specimen collection and how patient can help. Instruct female patient not to douche 24 hours before culture is obtained. Male is not to urinate 1 hour before urethral culture is obtained.

   Patient who understands procedure is less anxious and more likely to cooperate. Douching of vaginal canal would remove discharge containing pathogens. Urinating by male washes secretions out of urethra (Pagana and Pagana, 2015).

STEP	RATIONALE

IMPLEMENTATION

1. Perform hand hygiene. Apply clean gloves.	Reduces transmission of microorganisms.
2. Draw bedside curtains or close room door. Place "Do Not Enter" sign on door (if available).	Provides privacy for patient and demonstrates respect for patient's well-being.
3. Help patient to proper position, raise gown, and drape body parts to be exposed:	Provides easy access to perineal area. Draping minimizes exposure of body parts, minimizing anxiety.
a. *Female:* Dorsal recumbent position with sheet draped over each leg and genitalia.	
b. *Male:* Sitting on chair or bed or lying supine with sheet draped across lower trunk and genitalia.	
4. Direct light source onto perineum (may not be needed for male patient).	Allows better visualization of external urethral or vaginal structures.
5. Open culture tube and hold swab in dominant hand.	Provides for easier manipulation of swab during culture collection.
6. Instruct patient to deep breathe slowly.	Helps patient relax. Tensing of muscles around pelvic floor may cause discomfort during swabbing.
7. Obtain specimens.	
a. Female:	
(1) With nondominant hand, fully separate labia to expose vaginal orifice.	Exposes perineum and ensures that specimen is of vaginal discharge.
(2) Touch tip of swab into discharge pool, being careful not to touch skin or mucosa along perineum or vaginal canal. If no discharge is visible, gently insert swab 1 to 2.5 cm ($\frac{1}{3}$ to 1 inch) into vaginal orifice and rotate before removal.	Discharge contains greatest concentration of microorganisms.
(3) To expose urethral meatus use nondominant hand to pull gently on labia minora upward and back to separate.	Allows better visualization of urethral orifice.
(4) Use clean swab; gently apply to tip of meatus where discharge is visible. Avoid touching labia.	Discharge contains greatest concentration of microorganisms.

Clinical Decision Point *If discharge near vagina appears different from discharge along perineum, collect separate specimens from each area because, if two organisms are present, they could be cross-contaminated on a single swab. Label specimen with area of patient's body that you swabbed.*

b. Male:	
(1) Grasp patient's penis proximal to glans with nondominant hand; if male is uncircumcised, gently retract foreskin.	Provides clear exposure of urethral meatus.
(2) Use dominant hand to hold swab. Apply gently to area of discharge at urinary meatus.	Discharge contains greatest number of microorganisms.
(3) If no discharge is apparent, health care provider may order swab to be introduced into urinary meatus. Hold male genitalia firmly but gently.	Excess manipulation can cause erection.
(4) Return foreskin to natural position.	Tightening of foreskin around shaft of penis can cause localized discomfort, edema, and potential necrosis.
8. Return each swab to culture tube and secure top.	Retains microorganisms within tube.
9. If using commercial culture tube, wrap ampule with gauze to prevent injury to your fingers while crushing. Immediately squeeze end of tube to crush ampule (see Skill 7.4). Push tip of swab into fluid medium.	Medium supports life of microorganisms until culture is analyzed.
10. Remove and discard gloves. Perform hand hygiene.	Reduces transmission of microorganisms.
11. Label each culture tube with identification label, affix completed requisition, and confirm identifiers in front of patient (TJC, 2016).	Incorrect specimen identification could lead to diagnostic or therapeutic error.
12. Send specimen to laboratory immediately or refrigerate.	Bacteria multiply quickly. Prompt analysis ensures accurate results.
13. Help patient to comfortable position, help with personal hygiene, and remove and discard drape.	Reinforces patient's sense of self-esteem. Reduces transmission of microorganisms.

STEP	RATIONALE

EVALUATION

1. Review laboratory results for evidence of pathogens.	Results will reveal type of organisms present. Certain organisms are common to vaginal tract. Urethra should be free of microorganisms.
2. Continue to monitor whether discharge is present; if so, observe color and amount.	Characteristics of discharge indicate specific type of infection.
3. **Use Teach-Back:** "I want to be sure I explained the purpose and procedure for obtaining a vaginal culture. Please tell me the steps of this procedure." Revise your instruction now or develop a plan for revised patient or family caregiver teaching if patient or family caregiver is not able to teach back correctly.	Determines patient's and family caregiver's level of understanding of instructional topic.

Unexpected Outcomes
1. Vaginal or urethral cultures reveal growth of pathogenic microorganisms.
2. Specimen is contaminated with feces or epidermal cells.

Related Interventions
- Notify health care provider of findings and follow new orders.
- Continue to monitor patient.
- Repeat specimen collection.

Recording and Reporting

- Record types of cultures obtained and date and time sent to laboratory in nurses' notes in electronic health record (EHR) or chart.
- Document your evaluation of patient and family caregiver learning.
- Report laboratory results to health care provider.

Special Considerations
Teaching

- Discuss sexuality and safe sex practices with patient if appropriate.
- Patients with urethral or vaginal discharge often require instruction about perineal hygiene measures.

- If topical treatments (e.g., suppositories) are ordered, teach patient proper administration of medication (see Chapter 21).

Pediatric
- A second nurse can help with specimen collection from an infant or young child by gently holding child's legs apart in froglike position. Have parent present to encourage cooperation.
- Parents should understand that obtaining vaginal specimen will not affect virginity of child.

PROCEDURAL GUIDELINE 7.3 *Collecting a Sputum Specimen by Expectoration*

Sputum is mucus produced by cells of the lungs, bronchi, and trachea. You collect a specimen either by having a patient cough and expectorate into a sterile specimen container or by suctioning into a sterile sputum trap (see Skill 7.6). In a healthy patient sputum production is minimal; a disease state can increase the amount and character of sputum. Sputum specimens are collected to identify cancer cells, for culture and sensitivity (C&S), and for acid-fast bacillus to diagnose pulmonary tuberculosis.

Delegation and Collaboration
The skill of collecting a sputum specimen by expectoration can be delegated to nursing assistive personnel (NAP). The nurse instructs the NAP to:
- Immediately report the presence of blood in the sputum or changes in patient's vital signs.

Equipment
- Completed identification labels with appropriate patient identifiers

- Completed laboratory requisition, including appropriate patient identification, date, time, name of test, and source of culture
- Small biohazard plastic bag for delivery of specimen to laboratory (or container as specified by agency)
- Sterile specimen container with cover
- Clean gloves
- Facial tissues
- Emesis basin (*optional*)
- Toothbrush (*optional*)
- Disinfectant swab (*optional*)

Procedural Steps
1. Identify patient using at least two identifiers (e.g., name and birthday or name and medical record number) according to agency policy. Compare identifiers with information on patients MAR or medical record (TJC, 2016).

PROCEDURAL GUIDELINE 7.3 *Collecting a Sputum Specimen by Expectoration—cont'd*

2. Provide opportunity to clean or rinse mouth with water. Patient should not use mouthwash or toothpaste because the products may alter culture results.
3. Perform hand hygiene and apply clean gloves. Provide sputum cup and instruct patient not to touch the inside of the container.
4. Have the patient take three to four deep, slow breaths with full exhalation. Then take full inhalation followed immediately by a forceful cough, expectorating sputum directly into specimen container.
5. Repeat until 5 to 10 mL of sputum (not saliva) has been collected.

6. Secure lid on container tightly. If any sputum is present on outside of container, wipe it off with disinfectant.
7. Offer patient tissues after patient expectorates, dispose of tissues, and offer mouth care.
8. Remove and dispose of gloves. Perform hand hygiene.
9. Securely attach properly completed identification label and laboratory requisition to side of specimen container (not lid). Confirm identifiers in patient's presence.
10. Enclose specimen in a plastic biohazard bag.
11. Send specimen to laboratory immediately.

◆ SKILL 7.6   **Collecting a Sputum Specimen by Suction**

 Video Clip

Sputum is produced by cells lining the respiratory tract. Although production is minimal in the healthy state, disease states can increase the amount or change the character of sputum. Examination of sputum aids in the diagnosis and treatment of several conditions, ranging from simple bronchitis to lung cancer.

Suctioning is often indicated to collect sputum from patients unable to spontaneously expectorate a sample for laboratory analysis. Sometimes suctioning provokes violent coughing, which can induce vomiting and constriction of pharyngeal, laryngeal, and bronchial muscles. In addition, it may cause hypoxemia or vagal overload, causing cardiopulmonary compromise and increased intracranial pressure.

Delegation and Collaboration

The skill of collecting sputum specimens by suction cannot be delegated to nursing assistive personnel (NAP). The nurse instructs the NAP to:
• Notify the nurse if the patient expectorates bloody sputum.

Equipment

• Completed identification labels with proper patient identifiers
• Completed laboratory requisition, including patient identification, date, time, name of test, and source of culture
• Suction device (wall or portable)
• Sterile suction catheter (size 14, 16, or 18 Fr [not large enough to cause trauma to nasal mucosa]) or suction catheter with sleeve (see Chapter 25).
• Sterile gloves and clean gloves
• Sterile water in container
• In-line specimen container or sputum trap
• Small plastic bag for delivery of specimen to laboratory (or a container as specified by agency)
• Oxygen therapy equipment if indicated
• Protective eyewear
• Disinfectant wipe

STEP	RATIONALE

ASSESSMENT

1. Identify patient using at least two identifiers (e.g., name and birthday or name and medical record number) according to agency policy. Compare identifiers with information on patient's MAR or medical record.

Ensures correct patient. Complies with The Joint Commission standards and improves patient safety (TJC, 2016).

2. Check health care provider's orders for type of sputum analysis and specifications (e.g., amount of sputum, number of specimens, time of collection, method to obtain). Specimens for acid-fast bacillus (AFB) require three consecutive morning samples.

Specific test dictates when or how frequently specimens are collected. Ideal time to collect sputum is early morning because bronchial secretions tend to accumulate during the night. Bacteria also accumulate as secretions pool.

3. Assess patient's level of understanding of procedure and its purpose.

Provides baseline to establish teaching plan.

4. Assess when patient last ate meal (or had tube feeding).

It is best to obtain specimen 1 to 2 hours after or 1 hour before meal to minimize gagging, which can cause vomiting and aspiration.

5. Determine type of help needed by patient to obtain specimen.

Positioning, postural drainage, and deep-breathing and coughing exercises may improve ability to cough productively. Suctioning is often indicated when patient is unable to cough and expectorate.

STEP	RATIONALE
6. Assess patient's respiratory status, including respiratory rate, depth, pattern, and color of mucous membranes.	Active coughing may alter respiratory status. Respiratory status can depend on amount of sputum in tracheobronchial tree.

NURSING DIAGNOSES

- Deficient knowledge regarding specimen collection procedures
- Ineffective airway clearance
- Ineffective breathing pattern
- Risk for aspiration
- Risk for infection

Related factors/Risk factors are individualized based on patient's condition or needs.

PLANNING

1. Expected outcomes following completion of procedure:	
• Patient's respirations are same rate and character before and after procedure.	Specimen collection did not alter respiratory status.
• Patient maintains comfort level and experiences minimal anxiety.	Suctioning tends to cause anxiety.
• Sputum is not contaminated by saliva or oropharyngeal flora.	Sputum must originate from tracheobronchial tree for accurate results.
• Patient discusses purpose and benefit of sputum collection.	Validates learning.
2. Explain steps of procedure and purpose. Instruct patient to breathe normally during suctioning to prevent hyperventilation.	Promotes understanding and cooperation.

IMPLEMENTATION

1. Close curtains or room door.	Provides privacy.
2. Position patient in high- or semi-Fowler's position for suctioning.	Promotes full lung expansion and facilitates ability to cough.

Clinical Decision Point *If patient has surgical incision or localized area of discomfort, have him or her place pillow or hands firmly over affected area. Splinting of painful area minimizes muscular stretching and discomfort during coughing and thus makes cough more productive.*

3. Perform hand hygiene and apply clean glove to nondominant hand. Prepare suction machine or device and determine if it functions properly.	Adequate amount of suction is necessary to aspirate sputum.
4. Connect suction tube to adapter on sputum trap. Open sterile water (see Chapter 25).	Establishes suction that passes through sputum trap to aspirate specimen.
5. Using sterile technique, apply sterile glove to dominant hand or use clean glove if suction catheter has plastic sleeve.	Tracheobronchial tree is sterile body cavity. Allows you to manipulate suction catheter without contamination.
6. With gloved hand connect sterile suction catheter to rubber tubing on sputum trap.	Aspirated sputum will go directly to trap instead of to suction tubing.
7. Lubricate suction catheter tip with sterile water (*with suction off*).	Lubrication allows for easier insertion of catheter.
8. Gently insert tip of suction catheter through nasopharynx, endotracheal tube, or tracheostomy tube without applying suction (see Chapter 25).	Minimizes trauma to airway as catheter is inserted.
9. Gently and quickly advance catheter into trachea. Warn patient to expect to cough.	Entrance of catheter into larynx and trachea triggers cough reflex.
10. As patient coughs, apply suction for 5 to 10 seconds, collecting 2 to 10 mL of sputum.	Ensures collection of sputum from deep within tracheobronchial tree. Suctioning longer than 10 seconds can cause hypoxia and mucosal damage.
11. Release suction and remove catheter; turn off suction.	Suction can damage mucosa if applied during withdrawal.
12. Detach catheter from specimen trap and dispose of catheter in appropriate receptacle.	Decreases risk for spreading microorganisms.
13. Secure top on specimen container tightly. For sputum trap, detach suction tubing and connect rubber tubing on sputum trap to plastic adapter (see illustration).	Contains microorganisms within container, preventing exposure to personnel handling specimen.

STEP	RATIONALE

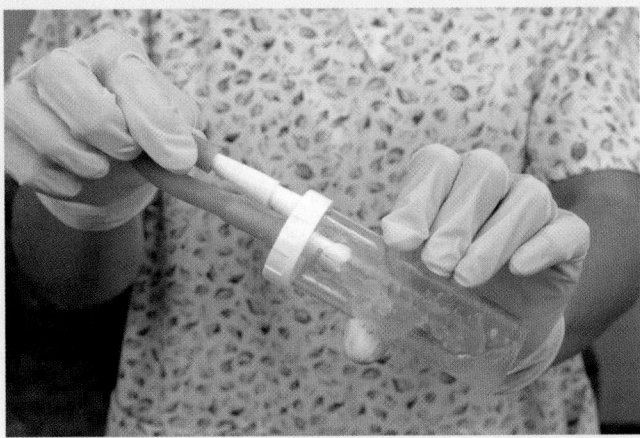

STEP 13 Closing sputum specimen trap.

STEP	RATIONALE
14. If any sputum is present on outside of container, wipe it off with disinfectant.	Prevents spread of infection to people handling specimen.
15. Offer patient tissues after suctioning. Dispose of tissues in emesis basin or appropriate container.	Maintains cleanliness and comfort.
16. Remove and dispose of gloves. Perform hand hygiene.	Reduces transmission of microorganisms.
17. Label specimen with identification label on side of specimen container (not lid). Confirm identifiers in front of patient (TJC, 2016). Place specimen in small plastic bag (or container specified by agency) and attach requisition.	Incorrect identification could lead to diagnostic or therapeutic error. Plastic bag or container reduces risk for health care worker's exposure to sputum.
18. Send specimen immediately to laboratory or refrigerate.	Bacteria multiply quickly. Prompt analysis ensures accurate results.
19. Offer patient mouth care if desired.	Promotes comfort.

EVALUATION

1. Observe patient's respiratory status throughout procedure, especially during suctioning. If under distress, measure oxygen saturation with pulse oximeter.	Excessive coughing or prolonged suctioning can alter respiratory pattern and cause hypoxia. Determines oxygenation status.
2. Note anxiety or discomfort in patient.	Procedure can be uncomfortable. If patient becomes short of breath, anxiety will develop.
3. Observe character of sputum: color, consistency, odor, volume, viscosity, and/or presence of blood.	Characteristics may indicate disease entities.
4. Refer to laboratory reports for test results.	Indicates if abnormal cells or microorganisms are present in sputum.
5. **Use Teach-Back:** "I want to be sure I explained the purpose and procedure for obtaining a sputum specimen. Please tell me how I will obtain this sputum specimen." Revise your instruction now or develop a plan for revised patient or family caregiver teaching if patient or family caregiver is not able to teach back correctly.	Determines patient's and family caregiver's level of understanding of instructional topic.

STEP	RATIONALE

Unexpected Outcomes

1. Patient becomes hypoxic with increased respiratory rate and effort and shortness of breath.

2. Patient remains anxious or reports discomfort from suction catheter.

3. Patient reports pain when coughing to produce sputum.

Related Interventions

- Discontinue suctioning immediately.
- Administer oxygen (if ordered).
- Notify health care provider of patient's condition.
- Continue to monitor patient's vital signs and pulse oximetry.
- Discontinue procedure until stable.
- Administer oxygen (if ordered).
- Notify health care provider of patient's change in condition.
- Continue to monitor patient's vital signs and pulse oximetry.
- Encourage patient who is recovering from surgical procedure to splint incision before coughing.
- Obtain order for pain medication as needed (prn).
- Inform health care provider of changes in patient's condition.

Recording and Reporting

- Record in nurse's notes in electronic health record (EHR) or chart the method used to obtain specimen, date and time collected, type of test ordered, and transport to laboratory in nurses' notes. Describe characteristics of sputum specimen. Describe patient's tolerance of procedure.
- Report unusual sputum characteristics to nurse in charge or health care provider.
- Document your evaluation of patient and family caregiver learning.
- When laboratory reports are available, report abnormal findings to health care provider. If AFB sputum culture is positive, initiate appropriate isolation techniques.
- Most agencies require nurses to note on specimen requisition if patient is receiving antibiotics.

Special Considerations
Teaching

- Demonstrate proper splinting technique for postoperative patients.
- If aerosol treatment is indicated, teach patient purpose of procedure, explaining that it will stimulate coughing and sputum expectoration.

Pediatric

- Children need very clear instructions or demonstration for deep breathing. Infants and young children will be unable to cooperate; aerosol treatment may be indicated.
- Use smaller catheter size for young children. It may be possible to elicit a cough by tickling the back of the throat with the suction catheter.

◆ SKILL 7.7 Obtaining Wound Drainage Specimens

NSO *Nursing Skills Online Specimen Collection Module / Lesson 5*

When caring for a patient with a wound, assess the condition of the wound and observe for the development of infection. Localized inflammation, tenderness, and warmth at the wound site and purulent drainage are signs and symptoms of wound infection. Identification of the causative organism confirms an infection and provides guidelines for accurate treatment. A specimen of wound drainage is analyzed to determine the type and number of pathogenic microorganisms.

Always collect a wound culture sample from fresh exudate from the center of a wound, not the skin edge, after removing old drainage. Collect the specimen before irrigating the wound; remove any antibiotic ointment and wait several hours before obtaining the specimen (Pagana and Pagana, 2015). Resident colonies of bacteria on the skin grow in wound exudate and may not be the true causative organisms of infection. Use separate techniques to collect specimens for measuring aerobic versus anaerobic microorganisms. Aerobic organisms grow in superficial wounds exposed to the air. Anaerobic organisms grow deep within body cavities, where oxygen is not normally present.

Delegation and Collaboration

The skill of obtaining wound drainage specimens cannot be delegated to nursing assistive personnel (NAP). The nurse instructs the NAP to:

- Report foul odor, increase in drainage, and increase in temperature or patient reports discomfort.

Equipment

- Culture tube with swab and transport medium for aerobic culture
- Anaerobic culture tube with swab (tubes contain carbon dioxide or nitrogen gas)
- 5- to 10-mL safety syringe and 19-gauge needle
- Two pairs of clean gloves and sterile gloves

- Protective eyewear
- Antiseptic swab
- Sterile dressing materials (determined by type of dressing)
- Paper or plastic disposable bag
- Completed specimen identification label with proper patient identifiers

- Completed laboratory requisition (date, time, name of test, patient identification, and source of culture)
- Small plastic biohazard bag for delivery of specimen to laboratory (or container specified by agency)

STEP	RATIONALE

ASSESSMENT

1. Identify patient using at least two identifiers (e.g., name and birthday or name and medical record number) according to agency policy. Compare identifiers and information on patient's MAR or medical record.

Ensures correct patient. Complies with The Joint Commission standards and improves patient safety (TJC, 2016).

2. Assess patient's understanding of need for wound culture and ability to cooperate with procedure.

Use data to develop teaching plan. Wound is painful site. Collection of specimen may cause anxiety or fear.

3. Assess patient for signs of fever, chills, or excessive thirst. Note in medical record laboratory results if white blood cell (WBC) count is elevated.

Signs and symptoms indicate systemic infection.

4. Ask patient about extent and type of pain at wound site using a scale of 0 to 10. If patient requires analgesic before dressing changes, give medication 30 minutes before beginning procedure to reach peak effect.

Pain at wound site often increases with infection.

5. Determine when dressing change is scheduled (see Chapter 39 and 41). Perform wound assessment as part of actual procedure.

6. Review health care provider's orders for aerobic or anaerobic culture.

Specimens are taken from different sites and placed in different containers, depending on type of culture.

7. Perform hand hygiene and apply clean gloves. Remove old dressings covering wound. Fold soiled sides of dressing together and dispose properly. Remove gloves and perform hand hygiene. Apply sterile gloves to palpate wound. Observe for swelling, separation of wound edges, inflammation, and drainage. Palpate gently along wound edges and note tenderness or drainage. Remove and discard gloves and perform hand hygiene.

Gloves minimize exposure to microorganisms
Signs indicate wound infection.

NURSING DIAGNOSES

- Acute pain
- Anxiety
- Chronic pain

- Deficient knowledge regarding wound drainage culture procedure
- Impaired tissue integrity

- Risk for infection
- Risk for injury

Related factors/Risk factors are individualized based on patient's condition or needs.

PLANNING

1. Expected outcomes following completion of procedure:
   - Wound culture does not reveal bacterial growth.
   - Culture swab is free of contamination from skin bacteria.
   - Patient discusses purpose and procedure for specimen collection.

Wound remains free of pathogenic microorganisms.
Test results indicate type of cells present.

Validates learning.

2. Determine if analgesia is necessary. Administer analgesic 30 minutes before dressing change and/or specimen collection.

Minimizes discomfort during procedure. Provides patient-centered care.

3. Explain reason for wound culture and how it will be collected.

Promotes understanding and cooperation and eases anxiety.

4. Explain that patient may feel tickling sensation when wound is swabbed.

Anticipation of expected sensations minimizes anxiety.

STEP	RATIONALE

IMPLEMENTATION

1. Close bedside curtains or door to room.

   Provides privacy.

2. Perform hand hygiene and apply clean gloves.

   Provides baseline for condition of wound.

3. Clean area around wound edges with antiseptic swab or sterile saline as ordered. Wipe from edges outward. Remove old exudate.

   Removes skin flora, preventing possible contamination of specimen.

4. Discard swab and remove and dispose of soiled gloves in appropriate receptacle. Perform hand hygiene.

   Reduces spread of infection.

5. Open packages containing sterile culture tube and dressing supplies. *Apply sterile gloves.*

   Provides sterile field for picking up and handling sterile supplies.

6. Obtain cultures.

   a. Aerobic culture

   (1) Take swab from culture tube, insert tip into wound in area of drainage, and rotate swab gently. Remove swab and return to culture tube (wrap outside of ampule with gauze to prevent injury to your fingers). Crush ampule of medium and push swab into fluid.

   Swab should be coated with fresh secretions from within wound. Medium keeps bacteria alive until analysis is complete.

   b. Anaerobic culture

   (1) Take swab from special anaerobic culture tube, swab deeply into draining body cavity, and rotate gently. Remove swab and return to culture tube.

   Specimen is taken from deep cavity where oxygen is not present. Carbon dioxide or nitrogen gas keeps organisms alive until analysis is complete. Air injected into tube would cause organisms to die.

   Or

   (2) Insert tip of syringe (without needle) into wound and aspirate 5 to 10 mL of exudate. Attach 19-gauge needle, expel all air, and inject drainage into special culture tube.

   Sterile large-bore needle (19-gauge) allows exudate to be transferred from sterile syringe into special culture tube without contamination.

7. Remove and dispose of gloves. Perform hand hygiene.

   Reduces transfer of microorganisms.

8. Place correct specimen label on each culture tube. Verify identifiers in front of patient (TJC, 2016). **NOTE:** Indicate on specimen if patient is receiving antibiotics.

   Ensures correct results for correct patient.

9. Send specimens to laboratory immediately.

   Bacteria multiple rapidly. Prompt analysis ensures accurate results.

10. Clean wound per health care provider's order. Apply new sterile dressing (see Chapters 39 and 41) using aseptic technique. Secure dressing with tape or ties.

    Protects wound from further contamination; aids in absorbing drainage and debridement of wound.

11. Remove and dispose of gloves and soiled supplies in appropriate receptacle according to agency policy. Perform hand hygiene.

    Reduces transmission of microorganisms.

12. Help patient to comfortable position.

    Promotes patient's ability to relax.

EVALUATION

1. Obtain laboratory report for results of cultures.

   Report indicates if pathogenic organisms are identified.

2. Observe character of wound drainage.

   Characteristics can reveal abnormal status and infection.

3. Observe edges of wound for redness and bleeding.

   Indicates trauma to healing tissue.

4. **Use Teach-Back:** "I want to be sure I explained the purpose and procedure for obtaining a wound specimen. Please state the steps of the procedure." Revise your instruction now or develop a plan for revised patient or family caregiver teaching if patient or family caregiver is not able to teach back correctly.

   Determines patient's and family caregiver's level of understanding of instructional topic.

STEP	RATIONALE
Unexpected Outcomes	**Related Interventions**
1. Wound cultures reveal bacterial growth.	• Monitor patient for fever, chills, or excessive thirst, which indicate systemic infection.
	• Inform health care provider of findings.
2. Wound culture is contaminated from superficial skin cells.	• Monitor patient for fever and pain.
	• Inform health care provider of findings.
	• Repeat collection of specimen as ordered.
3. Patient reports increased pain.	• Provide analgesia.
	• Notify health care provider.

Recording and Reporting

- Record types of specimens obtained, source, and time and date sent to laboratory and describe appearance of wound and characteristics of drainage in nurses' notes in electronic health record (EHR) or chart.
- Report any evidence of infection to the health care provider.
- Document your evaluation of patient and family caregiver learning.
- Record patient's tolerance of procedure and response to analgesics.

Special Considerations
Teaching

- Instruct patient to inform you if procedure causes pain or if you need to stop because unable to tolerate pain.

- Teach patient to assess status of wound for changes and signs and symptoms of infection.

Pediatric

- If procedure is to be performed on a child and is anticipated to be painful, some agencies prefer performing it in area other than child's room to maintain feeling that child's room is safe place (Hockenberry and Wilson, 2015).
- It is often helpful to have an additional nurse or other adult available to help with specimen collection in a young child or infant.

Home Care

- Teach patient antiseptic practices (e.g., handwashing, disposal of dressings, and clean technique for applying dressing).

◆ SKILL 7.8 Collecting Blood Specimens and Culture by Venipuncture (Syringe and Vacutainer Method)

NSO *Nursing Skills Online Caring for Central Vascular Access Devices (CVAD) Module / Lesson 3*

Blood tests are one of the most common diagnostic aids in the care and evaluation of patients. Tests allow health care providers to screen patients for early signs of physical illness, monitor changes in acute or chronic diseases, and evaluate responses to therapies.

In some agencies you are responsible for collecting blood specimens; however, many agencies have specially trained phlebotomists who are responsible for drawing venous blood. Be familiar with your agency policies and procedures and your state Nurse Practice Act regarding guidelines for drawing blood samples.

The three methods of obtaining blood specimens are (1) venipuncture, (2) skin puncture, and (3) arterial puncture. All procedures require sterile technique. Venipuncture is the most common method of obtaining blood specimens. This method involves inserting a hollow-bore needle into the lumen of a large vein to obtain a specimen using either a needle and syringe or a Vacutainer device that allows the drawing of multiple samples. Because veins are major sources of blood for laboratory testing and routes for intravenous (IV) fluid or blood replacement, maintaining their integrity is essential. You need to be skilled in venipuncture to avoid unnecessary injury to veins.

Skin puncture, also called *capillary puncture*, is the least traumatic method of obtaining a blood specimen. A sterile lancet or needle is used to puncture a vascular area on a finger or earlobe in an adult or child. You place a drop of blood on a test slide, wick a

drop of blood to a test slide, or collect it within a thin glass capillary tube for laboratory analysis. Changes in health care economics and delivery result in the increased use of skin puncture. Point-of-care (POC) clinical laboratory tests at the bedside most frequently use skin puncture (Pagana and Pagana, 2015).

Blood cultures aid in detection of bacteria in the blood. It is important that at least two culture specimens be drawn from two different sites. Because bacteremia may be accompanied by fever and chills, blood cultures should be drawn when these symptoms are present (Pagana and Pagana, 2015). Bacteremia exists when both cultures grow the infectious agent. Only one culture growing bacteria is considered contamination. Draw all cultures before antibiotic therapy begins because the antibiotic may interrupt the growth of an organism in the laboratory. If the patient is receiving antibiotics, notify the laboratory and inform them of specific antibiotics the patient is receiving (Pagana and Pagana, 2015).

Delegation and Collaboration

The skill of collecting blood specimens by venipuncture can be delegated to specially trained nursing assistive personnel (NAP). In some agencies phlebotomists obtain the venipuncture samples. Agency and government regulations and policies differ regarding personnel who may draw blood specimens. The nurse informs the NAP to:

- Report any patient discomfort or signs of excessive bleeding from the puncture site to the nurse.

Equipment
All Procedures
- Chlorhexidine or antiseptic swab (check agency policy for use of 70% alcohol or other antiseptic solutions)
- Clean gloves
- Small pillow or folded towel
- Sterile 2 × 2–inch gauze pads
- Tourniquet
- Adhesive bandage or adhesive tape
- Completed identification labels with proper patient identifiers
- Completed laboratory requisition (appropriate patient identification, date, time, name of test, and source of culture)
- Small plastic biohazard bag for delivery of specimen to laboratory (or container specified by agency)
- Sharps container

Venipuncture With Syringe
- Sterile safety needles (20- to 21-gauge for adults; 23- to 25-gauge for children)

- Sterile 10- to 20-mL Luer-Lok safety syringes
- Needle-free blood transfer device
- Appropriate blood specimen tubes

Venipuncture With Vacutainer
- Vacutainer and safety access device with Luer-Lok adapter
- Sterile double needles (20- to 21-gauge for adults; 23- to 25-gauge for children)
- Appropriate blood specimen tubes

Blood Cultures
- Sterile double needles (20- to 21-gauge for adults; 23- to 25-gauge for children)
- Two 20-mL sterile syringes
- Anaerobic and aerobic culture bottles (check agency policy)

Central Venous Catheter Collection
- Two empty 10-mL sterile syringes
- Sterile 10-mL normal saline flushes
- Vacutainer and safety access device Luer-Lok adapter
- Appropriate blood specimen tubes

STEP	RATIONALE

ASSESSMENT

STEP	RATIONALE
1. Identify patient using at least two identifiers (e.g., name and birthday or name and medical record number) according to agency policy. Compare identifiers with information on patient's MAR or medical record.	Ensures correct patient. Complies with The Joint Commission standards and improves patient safety (TJC, 2016).
2. Determine whether patient understands purpose of procedure and ability to cooperate.	Provides data for you to establish teaching plan and provides emotional support. Some patients' past experiences increase anxiety.
3. Determine if special conditions need to be met before specimen collection (e.g., patient allowed nothing by mouth [NPO], specific time for collection in relation to medication given, need to ice specimen).	Some tests require meeting specific conditions to obtain accurate measurement of blood elements (e.g., fasting blood sugar, drug peak and trough level, timed endocrine hormone levels).
4. Assess patient for possible risks associated with venipuncture: anticoagulant therapy, low platelet count, bleeding disorders (history of hemophilia). Review medication history.	Patient history may include abnormal clotting abilities caused by low platelet count, hemophilia, or medications that increase risk for bleeding and hematoma formation.
5. Assess patient for contraindicated sites for venipuncture: presence of IV infusion, hematoma at potential site, arm on side of mastectomy, or hemodialysis shunt.	Drawing specimens from such sites can result in false test results or may injure patient. Samples taken from vein near IV infusion may be diluted or contain concentrations of IV fluids. Postmastectomy patient may have reduced lymphatic drainage in arm on operative side, increasing risk for infection from needlesticks. Never use arteriovenous shunt to obtain specimens because of risks for clotting and bleeding. Hematoma indicates existing injury to vessel wall.
6. Identify presence of tape sensitivities or latex or povidone-iodine (Betadine) allergies.	Requires voiding exposure to these items.
7. Before drawing blood cultures, assess for systemic signs and symptoms of bacteremia, including fever and chills.	Three blood culture samples should be drawn at least 1 hour apart beginning at the earliest signs of sepsis (Pagana and Pagana, 2015).
8. Review health care provider's orders for type of tests.	Multiple samples are often needed. Health care provider's order is required.

Clinical Decision Point *Some specimens have special collection requirements before or after specimen collection; examples follow:*
- *Cryoglobulin levels: Use prewarmed test tubes.*
- *Ammonia and ionized calcium levels: Place tube in ice for delivery to laboratory.*
- *Lactic acid levels: Do not use tourniquet.*
- *Vitamin levels: Avoid exposure of test tube to light.*

STEP	RATIONALE

NURSING DIAGNOSES

- Anxiety
- Deficient knowledge regarding blood specimen collection process
- Fear
- Risk for infection
- Risk for injury

Related factors/Risk factors are individualized based on patient's condition or needs.

PLANNING

STEP	RATIONALE
1. Expected outcomes following completion of procedure:	
• Venipuncture site shows no evidence of continued bleeding or hematoma at venipuncture site after specimen collection.	Indicates that hemostasis is achieved.
• Patient denies anxiety or discomfort.	Explanation relieves anxiety; procedure is performed quickly. Removal of painful stimulus lessens anxiety.
• An adequate sample is collected for testing (see agency policy or laboratory manual).	Appropriate laboratory analysis can be conducted.
• Patient discusses purpose, procedure, and benefits of venipuncture.	Validates learning.
2. Explain procedure to patient: describe purpose of tests; explain how sensation of tourniquet, alcohol swab, and needlestick will feel.	Anticipatory guidance helps to reduce anxiety.

IMPLEMENTATION

STEP	RATIONALE
1. Bring equipment to bedside and organize.	Facilitates procedure.
2. Close bedside curtain or room door. Perform hand hygiene.	Provides for privacy. Reduces transmission of infection.
3. Raise or lower bed to comfortable working height.	Reduces strain on your back muscles and improves access to venipuncture site.
4. Help patient to supine or semi-Fowler's position with arms extended to form straight line from shoulders to wrists. Place small pillow or towel under upper arm. (*Option:* Lower arm briefly so it fills veins in hand and lower arm with blood.)	Helps to stabilize extremity because arms are most common sites of venipuncture. Supported position in bed reduces chance of injury to patient if fainting occurs.
5. Apply tourniquet so it can be removed by pulling an end with single motion.	Tourniquet blocks venous return to heart from extremity, causing veins to dilate for easier visibility.
a. Position tourniquet 5 to 10 cm (2 to 4 inches) above venipuncture site selected (antecubital fossa site is most often used).	
b. Cross tourniquet over patient's arm (see illustration). May place it over gown sleeve to protect skin.	Older adult's skin is very fragile.
c. Hold tourniquet between your fingers close to arm. Tuck loop between patient's arm and tourniquet so you can grasp free end easily (see illustration).	Pull free end to release tourniquet after venipuncture.

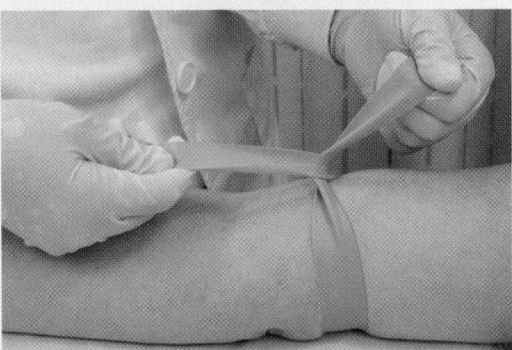

STEP 5b Cross tourniquet over arm.

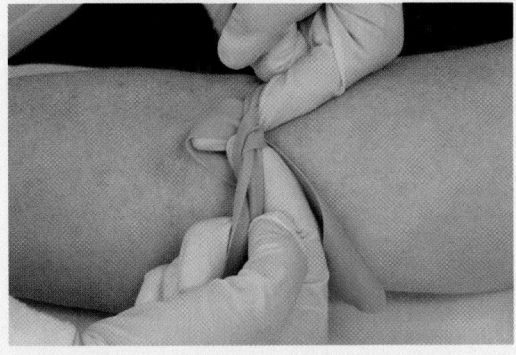

STEP 5c Tuck loop between patient's arm and tourniquet.

STEP	RATIONALE

Clinical Decision Point *Palpate distal pulse (e.g., radial) below tourniquet. If pulse is not palpable, remove tourniquet, wait 60 seconds, and reapply it more loosely. If tourniquet is too tight, pressure will impede arterial blood flow.*

6. Do not keep tourniquet on patient longer than 1 minute.	Prolonged tourniquet application causes stasis, localized acidemia, and hemoconcentration (Pagana and Pagana, 2015).
7. Quickly inspect extremity for best venipuncture site, looking for straight, prominent vein without swelling or hematoma. Of three veins located in antecubital area, median cubital vein is preferred (see illustration).	Straight and intact veins are easiest to puncture.
8. Apply clean gloves. Palpate selected vein with finger (see illustration). Note if vein is firm and rebounds when palpated or if it feels rigid or cordlike and rolls when palpated. Avoid vigorously slapping vein, which can cause vasospasm.	Patent, healthy vein is elastic and rebounds on palpation. Thrombosed vein is rigid, rolls easily, and is difficult to puncture.
9. Obtain blood specimen. **a. Syringe method**	
(1) Have syringe with appropriate needle securely attached.	Needle must not dislodge from syringe during venipuncture.
(2) Clean venipuncture site with antiseptic swab, with first swab moving back and forth on horizontal plane, another swab on vertical plane, and last in circular motion from site outward for about 5 cm (2 inches) for 30 seconds. Allow to dry.	Antimicrobial agent cleans skin surface of resident bacteria so organisms do not enter puncture site. Allowing antiseptic to dry completes its antimicrobial task and reduces "sting" of venipuncture. Alcohol left on skin can cause hemolysis of sample and retraction of tissue away from puncture site.
(a) If drawing sample for blood alcohol level or blood cultures, use only antiseptic swab rather than alcohol swab.	Ensures accurate test results.
(3) Remove needle cover and inform patient that "stick" lasts only a few seconds.	Patient has better control over anxiety when prepared for what to expect.

Clinical Decision Point *Observe needle for defects such as burrs, which can cause increased discomfort and damage to patient's vein (McCall and Tankersley, 2012).*

(4) Place thumb or forefinger of nondominant hand 2.5 cm (1 inch) below site and gently pull skin taut. Stretch skin steadily until vein is stabilized.	Stabilizes vein and prevents rolling during needle insertion.
(5) Hold syringe and needle at 15- to 30-degree angle from patient's arm with bevel up.	Reduces chance of penetrating both sides of vein during insertion. Bevel up decreases chance of contamination by not dragging bevel opening over skin and allows point of needle to first puncture skin, reducing trauma.

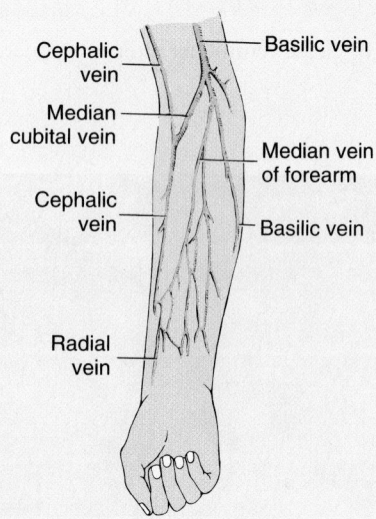

STEP 7 Location of antecubital veins.

Cephalic vein — Basilic vein
Median cubital vein
Median vein of forearm
Cephalic vein — Basilic vein
Radial vein

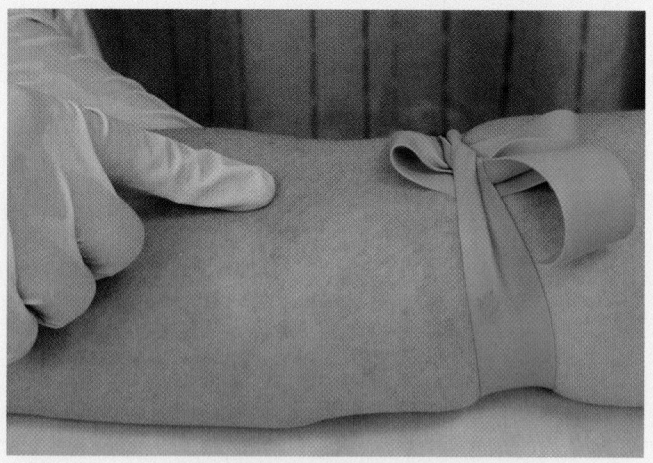

STEP 8 Palpate vein.

STEP	RATIONALE
(6) Slowly insert needle into vein, stopping when "pop" is felt as needle enters vein (see illustration).	Prevents puncture through vein to opposite side.
(7) Hold syringe securely and pull back gently on plunger.	Syringe held securely prevents needle from advancing. Pulling on plunger creates vacuum needed to draw blood into syringe. If plunger is pulled back too quickly, pressure may collapse vein.
(8) Observe for blood return (see illustration).	If blood flow fails to appear, needle may not be in vein.
(9) Obtain desired amount of blood, keeping needle stabilized.	Test results are more accurate when required amount of blood is obtained. You cannot perform some tests without minimal blood requirement. Movement of needle increases discomfort.
(10) After obtaining specimen, release tourniquet.	Reduces bleeding at site when needle is withdrawn.
(11) Apply 2 × 2–inch gauze pad without applying pressure. Quickly but carefully withdraw needle from vein and apply pressure following removal of needle (see illustration). Check for hematoma.	Pressure over needle can cause discomfort. Careful removal of needle minimizes discomfort and vein trauma. Hematoma may cause compression injury (McCall and Tankersley, 2012).
(12) Activate safety cover and immediately discard needle in appropriate container.	Prevents needlestick injury.
(13) Attach blood-filled syringe to needle-free blood transfer device. Attach tube and allow vacuum to fill tube to specified level. Remove and fill other tubes as appropriate (see illustration). Gently rotate each tube back and forth 8 to 10 times.	Additives prevent clotting. Shaking can cause hemolysis of red blood cells (RBCs).

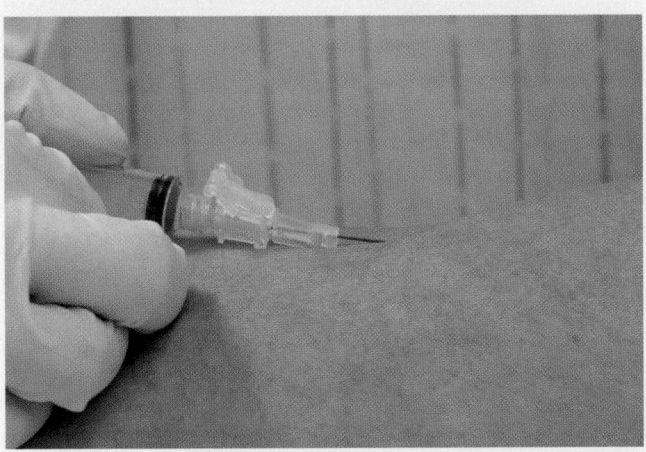

STEP 9a(6) Insert needle into vein.

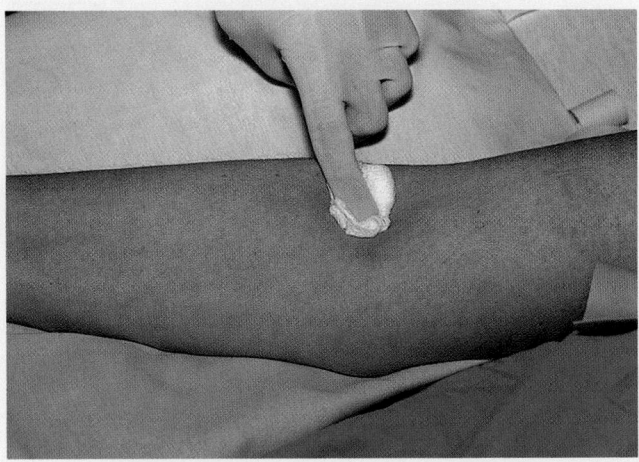

STEP 9a(11) Apply gauze to puncture site.

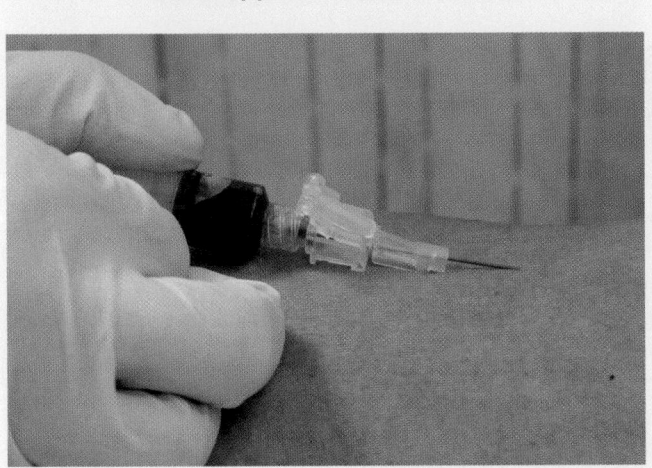

STEP 9a(8) Observe for blood return.

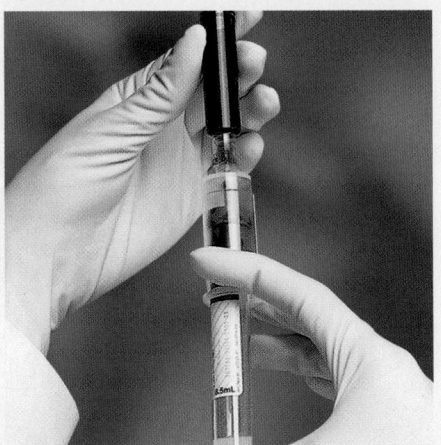

STEP 9a(13) Attach blood-filled syringe to needle-free blood transfer device.

STEP	RATIONALE

b. Vacutainer system method

(1) Attach double-ended needle to Vacutainer tube (see illustration).

Long end of needle is used to puncture vein. Short end fits into blood tubes.

(2) Have proper blood specimen tube resting inside Vacutainer device but do not puncture rubber stopper.

Puncturing causes loss of tube vacuum.

(3) Clean venipuncture site by following Steps 9a(2) and 9a(2)(a) for antiseptic swab. Allow to dry.

Cleans skin surface of resident bacteria so organisms do not enter puncture site. Drying maximizes effect of antiseptic.

(4) Remove needle cover and inform patient that "stick" will occur, lasting only a few seconds.

Patient has better control over anxiety when prepared about what to expect.

(5) Place thumb or forefinger of nondominant hand 2.5 cm (1 inch) *below* site and gently pull skin taut. Stretch skin down until vein stabilizes.

Helps to stabilize vein and prevent rolling during needle insertion.

(6) Hold Vacutainer needle at 15- to 30-degree angle from arm with bevel up.

Smallest and sharpest point of needle will puncture skin first. Reduces chance of penetrating sides of vein during insertion. Keeping bevel up causes less trauma to vein.

(7) Slowly insert needle into vein (see illustration).

Prevents puncture on opposite side.

(8) Grasp Vacutainer securely and advance specimen tube into needle of holder (do not advance needle in vein).

Pushing needle through stopper breaks vacuum and causes flow of blood into tube. If needle in vein advances, vein may become punctured on other side.

(9) Note flow of blood into tube, which should be fairly rapid (see illustration).

Failure of blood to appear indicates that vacuum in tube is lost or needle is not in vein.

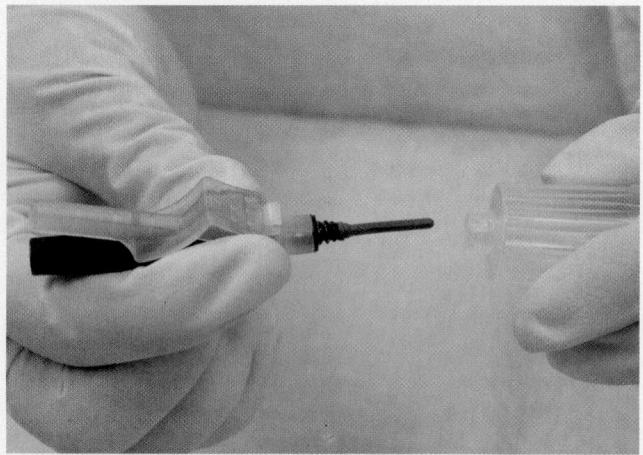

STEP 9b(1) Attach double-ended needle to Vacutainer tube.

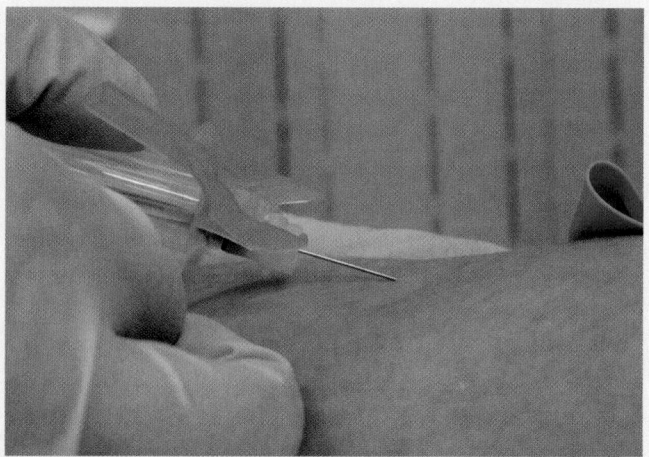

STEP 9b(7) Insert Vacutainer needle into vein.

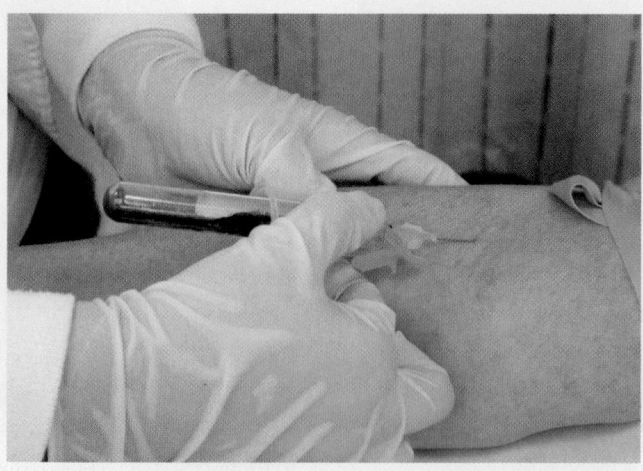

STEP 9b(9) Blood flowing into tube.

STEP	RATIONALE

(10) After filling specimen tube, grasp Vacutainer firmly and remove tube. Insert additional specimen tubes as needed. Gently rotate each tube back and forth 8 to 10 times.

Vacuum in tube stops flow at amount to be collected. Grasping prevents needle from advancing or dislodging. Tube should fill completely because additives in certain tubes are measured in proportion to filled tube. Ensures proper mixing with additive to prevent clotting.

(11) After last tube is filled and removed from Vacutainer, release tourniquet.

Reduces bleeding at site when needle is withdrawn.

(12) Apply 2 × 2–inch gauze pad over puncture site without applying pressure and quickly but carefully withdraw needle with Vacutainer from vein.

Pressure over needle can cause discomfort. Careful removal of needle minimizes discomfort and vein trauma.

(13) Immediately apply pressure over venipuncture site with gauze or antiseptic pad for 2 to 3 minutes or until bleeding stops. Observe for hematoma. Tape gauze dressing securely.

Direct pressure minimizes bleeding and prevents hematoma formation. Hematoma may cause compression and nerve injury. Pressure dressing controls bleeding.

(14) Dispose of syringe, needle, gauze, and other supplies in appropriate containers.

Safe disposal of supplies exposed to body fluids prevents transfer of microorganisms.

c. Blood culture

(1) Clean venipuncture site as in Step 9a(2) with antiseptic swab or follow agency policy. Allow to dry.

Antimicrobial agent cleans skin surface so organisms do not enter puncture site or contaminate culture. Drying ensures complete antimicrobial action and decreases stinging.

(2) Clean bottle tops of culture bottles for 15 seconds with agency-approved cleaning solution. Allow to dry.

Ensures that bottle top is sterile.

(3) Collect 10 to 15 mL of venous blood using syringe method (see Step 9a) in 20-mL syringe from two different venipuncture sites.

Two blood cultures must be collected from two different sites to confirm culture growth (Pagana and Pagana, 2015).

(4) With each specimen activate safety guard and discard needle. Replace with new sterile needle before injecting each blood sample into culture bottle.

Maintains sterile technique and prevents contamination of specimen.

(5) If both aerobic and anaerobic cultures are needed, fill anaerobic bottle first.

Anaerobic organisms may take longer to grow (Pagana and Pagana, 2015).

(6) Gently mix blood in each culture bottle.

Mixes medium and blood.

d. Central venous catheter (CVC) collection

(1) Select appropriate port on IV catheter (see illustration). Turn off all IV pumps and clamp lumens.

If more than one lumen, select distal lumen if possible. Prevents dilution of sample with medication or total parenteral nutrition (TPN).

(2) Wipe all Luer-Lok caps with alcohol-wipe antiseptic solution or remove Luer-Lok alcohol-impregnated cap (Dual Cap System) (see illustration). Attach 10-mL saline prefilled syringe to selected port. Release clamp. Aspirate gently for blood return. Flush with 5 to 10 mL normal saline (NS) (check agency policy). Do not use syringe smaller than 10 mL. Remove syringe.

Luer-Lok–impregnated caps recommended by INS (2011). 70% isopropyl alcohol-impregnated Luer-Lok cap (DualCap System) eliminates issue of wiping CVC ports adequately. Aspirating and flushing ensures patency of selected lumen and catheter in vein.

Pressure from small syringe may damage catheter.

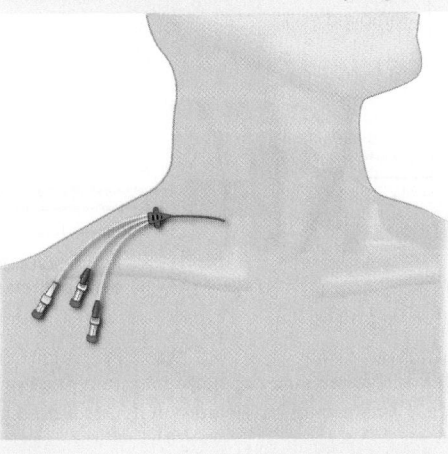

STEP 9d(1) Triple-lumen central venous catheter; select appropriate distal lumen port.

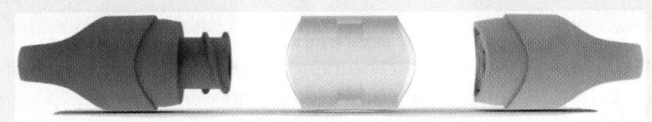

STEP 9d(2) DualCap system. Disinfects and protects both IV catheter needleless Luer access and end of IV tubing.

STEP	RATIONALE
(3) Wipe port with alcohol wipe. For **syringe method** attach syringe to selected port, aspirate 5 mL of blood, and discard. Reclamp catheter. Wipe port, attach 10- to 20-mL Luer-Lok syringe, unclamp catheter, and aspirate desired amount of blood. Reclamp catheter and remove syringe. Clean catheter port with alcohol. To transfer blood from syringe to specimen tube, use Vacutainer holder with Luer-Lok attachment. Insert appropriate specimen tube into Vacutainer holder. Attach syringe to Luer-Lok attachment and fill desired tubes.	Discard ensures that blood sample is not contaminated with IV fluids, medication, or other products. Tubes have vacuum and automatically fill to necessary amount.
(4) For **Vacutainer method,** clamp catheter and attach needleless connecter to Vacutainer holder. Place blood tube into Vacutainer holder. Disinfect injection or access cap with alcohol. Insert Vacutainer needleless connection into injection or access cap, unclamp catheter, and advance blood tube into holder to activate blood flow. Allow blood to fill tube, clamp catheter, and discard first tube in appropriate biohazard container. Attach specimen tubes to Vacutainer with Luer-Lok adapter, unclamp catheter, and obtain blood specimens (see illustration).	Tubes have vacuum and automatically fill to necessary amount.
(5) After all specimens are collected, clamp catheter. Remove Vacutainer holder and needleless connection from injection or access cap and disinfect with alcohol.	Reduces risk for contamination by bloodborne pathogens.
(6) Attach 10-mL prefilled NS syringe and flush with 5 to 10 mL NS using push, pause method. Ensure positive pressure for lumen. Cap with spring automatically has positive pressure; thus syringe can be removed, and lumen locked (see illustration). For caps without positive pressure, hold syringe plunger steady at completion of flush, lock off lumen with slide clamp, and remove syringe. Reattach alcohol-impregnated cap.	Push, pause creates turbulence that helps to clear lumen. Positive pressure prevents blood from flowing into tip of catheter and forming clot.
(7) Blood tubes contain additives; gently rotate back and forth 8 to 10 times.	Additives mix with blood to prevent clotting. Shaking can cause hemolysis of RBCs, producing inaccurate test results.

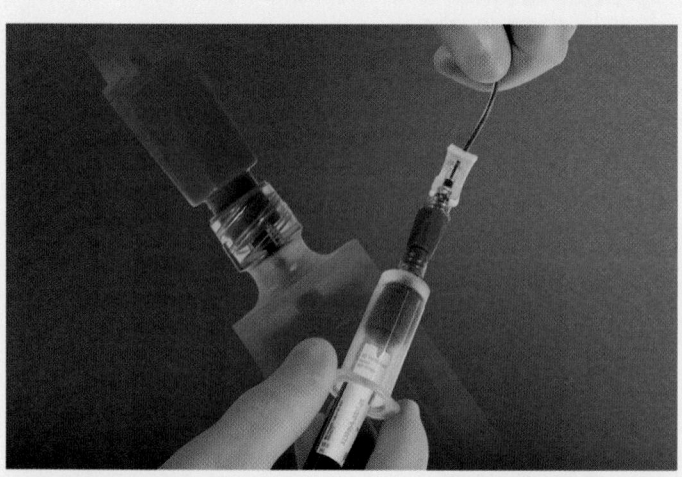

STEP 9d(4) Male Luer-Lok Vacutainer adapter attaches to port; blood draws directly into specimen tubes. (*Courtesy and copyright ©Becton Dickinson.*)

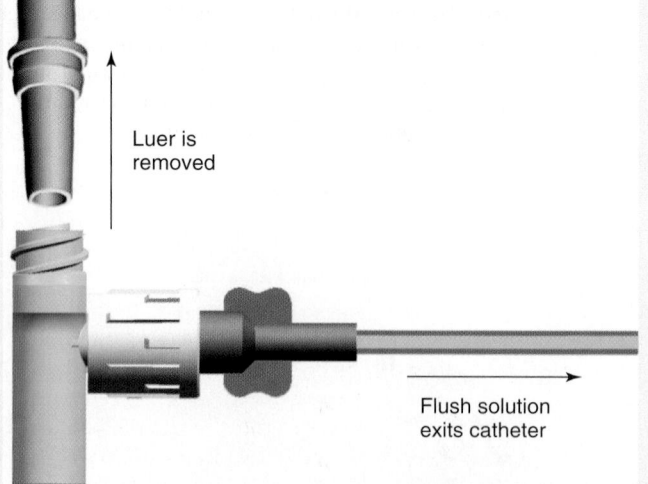

STEP 9d(6) Positive-pressure cap helps maintain patency of vascular access device. (*With permission, courtesy ICU Medical, San Clemente, CA.*)

STEP	RATIONALE
10. Check tubes for any sign of external contamination with blood. Decontaminate with 70% alcohol if necessary.	Prevents cross-contamination. Reduces risk for exposure to pathogens present in blood.
11. Remove gloves and perform hand hygiene after specimen is obtained and any spillage is cleaned.	Reduces risk for exposure to bloodborne pathogens.
12. Help patient to comfortable position.	
13. Securely attach properly completed identification label to each tube and affix proper requisition. Verify identifiers in front of patient (TJC, 2016).	Incorrect identification of specimen could result in diagnostic or therapeutic errors.
14. Place specimens in plastic biohazard bag and send to laboratory. Cultures must be sent to laboratory within 30 minutes (Pagana and Pagana, 2015).	Minimizes spread of microorganisms.
15. Perform hand hygiene.	Reduces transfer of microorganisms.

EVALUATION

1. Inspect venipuncture site for homeostasis.
2. Determine if patient remains anxious or fearful.

3. Check laboratory report for test results.
4. **Use Teach-Back:** "I want to be sure I explained the purpose and procedure for obtaining a blood specimen. Tell me why we are collecting this blood specimen." Revise your instruction now or develop a plan for revised patient or family caregiver teaching if patient or family caregiver is not able to teach back correctly.

Determines if bleeding has stopped or hematoma has formed.
Some patients require more blood tests in future. Address concerns and let patient express anxiety.
Reveals constituents of blood specimen.
Determines patient's and family caregiver's level of understanding of instructional topic.

Unexpected Outcomes	Related Interventions
1. Hematoma forms at venipuncture site.	• Apply pressure using 2 × 2–inch gauze dressing. • Continue to monitor patient for pain and discomfort.
2. Bleeding at site continues.	• Apply pressure to site; patient may also apply pressure. • Monitor patient.
3. Signs and symptoms of infection at venipuncture site occur.	• Notify health care provider. • Notify health care provider.

Recording and Reporting

• Record in electronic health record (EHR) or chart the method used to obtain blood specimen, date and time collected, type of test ordered, disposition of specimen, and description of venipuncture site.
• Document your evaluation of patient and family caregiver learning.
• Report any STAT or abnormal test results to health care provider.

Special Considerations
Teaching

• Instruct patient to briefly apply pressure to venipuncture site. Patients with bleeding disorders or those undergoing anticoagulant therapy should apply pressure for at least 5 minutes.
• Instruct patient to notify nurse or health care provider if persistent or recurrent bleeding or expanding hematoma develops at venipuncture site.

Pediatric

• Explain procedure to child at developmentally appropriate age and provide atraumatic care (Hockenberry and Wilson, 2015).

• Because children often fear that loss of their blood is a threat to their lives, explain to them that their blood is continually being produced. An adhesive bandage gives them assurance that their blood will not leak out through puncture site (Hockenberry and Wilson, 2015).
• At times it is advantageous to draw children's blood specimens in a treatment room instead of in bed or room to maintain feeling that their room is a safe place (Hockenberry and Wilson, 2015).
• When performing venipuncture on children, explore sources for vein access: scalp, antecubital fossa, saphenous, and hand veins.
• Application of eutectic mixture of local anesthetics (EMLA) cream to the venipuncture site may be ordered before the stick to reduce pain in infants and young children (Hockenberry and Wilson, 2015).
• Vacutainers are not recommended in children under 2 years of age because of possible vein collapse with their use.

Gerontological

• Older adults have fragile veins that are easily traumatized during venipuncture. Sometimes application of warm compresses may help to obtain samples. Using small-bore catheter may be beneficial.

✦ SKILL 7.9   Blood Glucose Monitoring

Blood glucose monitoring (BMG) is an essential component of any diabetes self-management program (ADA, 2013b; Lecklider, 2015). The procedure is less painful than venipuncture, and the ease of the skin puncture method makes it possible for patients to perform this procedure at home. The development of reagent strips, home glucose monitors, and the skin puncture method has revolutionized home-management care of patients with diabetes mellitus.

Blood glucose reflectance meters are lightweight and run on batteries (e.g., AccuChek III, OneTouch) (Fig. 7.5). After a drop of blood from the skin puncture is dropped or wicked onto a reagent strip, the meter provides an accurate measurement of blood glucose level in 5 to 50 seconds. Point-of-care (POC) blood glucose testing meters must be cleaned and disinfected after each patient use (USFDA, 2015).

The meters differ in several ways, including amount of blood needed for each test, testing speed, overall size, ability to store test results in memory, cost of the meter, and cost of test strips (Diabetes Forecast, 2013). Some larger meters are voice activated, which provides support for the older adult or patient with visual impairments. Most meters now allow for the use of alternative site or forearm capillary testing. Improved technology introduced a method for glucose measurement now available on the market. A minimally invasive glucose meter uses a very small, fine plastic sensor inserted through the abdomen and provides continuous readings of blood glucose levels (Fig. 7.6). A disadvantage is that the patient must wear the meter at all times for continuous blood glucose monitoring (CBM). Initiatives and clinical trials are under way to develop noninvasive glucose testing that evaluates intermittent blood glucose levels (Lecklider, 2015).

Testing of glycosylated hemoglobin (HbA1$_c$) evaluates the amount of glucose available in the bloodstream over the 120-day life span of a red blood cell. HbA1$_c$ provides an accurate long-term index of a patient's average blood glucose level drawn by venous puncture (Pagana and Pagana, 2015).

Delegation and Collaboration

Assessment of a patient's condition cannot be delegated to nursing assistive personnel (NAP). When the patient's condition is stable, the skill of obtaining and testing a sample of blood for blood glucose level can be delegated to NAP. The nurse informs the NAP by:

- Explaining appropriate sites to use for puncture and when to obtain glucose levels.
- Reviewing expected blood glucose levels and when to report unexpected glucose levels to the nurse.

Equipment

- Antiseptic swab
- Cotton ball
- Lancet device, either self-activating or button activated
- Blood glucose meter (e.g., Accucheck III, OneTouch)
- Blood glucose test strips appropriate for meter brand used
- Clean gloves
- Paper towel

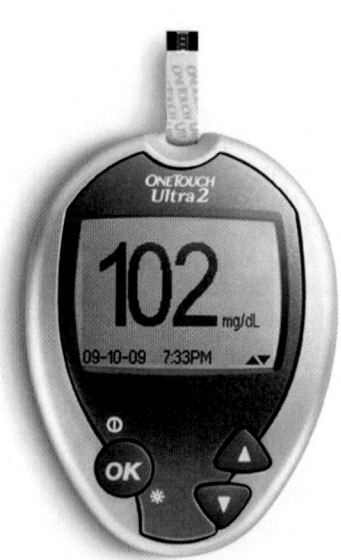

FIG 7.5 Blood glucose monitor. (*Courtesy LifeScan, Milpitas, CA.*)

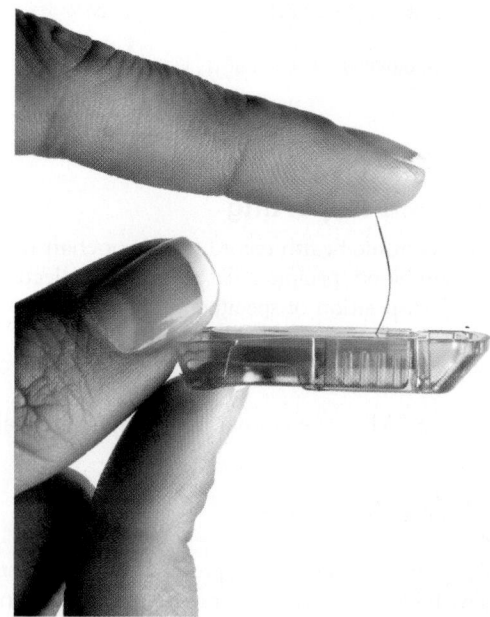

FIG 7.6 Tiny sensor implanted under skin transmits continuous reading to receiver. (*Courtesy DexCom.*)

STEP	RATIONALE

ASSESSMENT

1. Identify patient using at least two identifiers (e.g., name and birthday or name and medical record number) according to agency policy. Compare identifiers with information on patient's MAR or medical record.

Ensures correct patient. Complies with The Joint Commission standards and improves patient safety (TJC, 2016).

2. Assess patient's understanding of procedure and purpose of blood glucose monitoring. Determine if patient understands how to perform test and its importance in glucose control.

Provides baseline for developing teaching plan.

3. Determine if specific conditions need to be met before or after sample collection (e.g., fasting, postprandial, after certain medications, before insulin doses).

Dietary intake of carbohydrates and ingestion of concentrated glucose preparations alter blood glucose levels.

4. Determine if risks exist for performing skin puncture (e.g., low platelet count, anticoagulant therapy, bleeding disorders).

Abnormal clotting mechanisms increase risk for local ecchymosis and bleeding.

5. Assess area of skin to be used as puncture site. Inspect fingers or forearms for edema, inflammation, cuts, or sores. Avoid areas of bruising and open lesions. Avoid using hand on side of mastectomy.

Sides of fingers are commonly selected because they have fewer nerve endings.

Measurements from alternative sites are meter specific and may be different from those at traditional sites. Puncture site should not be edematous, inflamed, or recently punctured because these factors cause increased interstitial fluid and blood to mix and also increase risk for infection.

6. Review health care provider's order for time or frequency of measurement.

Health care provider determines test schedule on basis of patient's physiological status and risk for glucose imbalance.

7. For patient with diabetes who performs test at home, assess ability to handle skin-puncturing device. Patient may choose to continue self-testing while in hospital.

Patient's physical health may change (e.g., vision disturbance, fatigue, pain, disease process), preventing him or her from performing test.

NURSING DIAGNOSES

- Anxiety
- Deficient knowledge regarding blood glucose monitoring
- Ineffective health maintenance

Related factors are individualized based on patient's condition or needs.

PLANNING

1. Expected outcomes following completion of procedure:
- Puncture site shows no evidence of bleeding or tissue damage.

Hemostasis is achieved. Lancet or needle did not puncture skin too deeply.

- Blood glucose measurements are accurate.

Normal fasting glucose is 70 to 110 mg/dL, indicating good metabolic control (Pagana and Pagana, 2015). Values may vary slightly; check agency policy.

- Patient can verbalize procedure for self-monitoring blood glucose.

Demonstrates psychomotor learning.

- Patient explains test results.

Validates knowledge.

2. Explain procedure and purpose to patient and/or family caregiver. Offer patient and family caregiver opportunity to practice testing procedures. Provide resources/teaching aids for patient and family caregiver.

Promotes understanding and cooperation.

IMPLEMENTATION

1. Perform hand hygiene. Instruct adult to perform hand hygiene, including forearm (if applicable) with soap and water. Rinse and dry.

Promotes skin cleansing and vasodilation at selected puncture site. Reduces transmission of microorganisms.

2. Position patient comfortably in chair or in semi-Fowler's position in bed.

Ensures easy accessibility to puncture site. Patient assumes position when self-testing.

3. Remove reagent strip from vial and tightly seal cap. Check code on test strip vial. Use only test strips recommended for glucose meter. Some newer meters do not require code and/or have disk or drum with 10 or more test strips.

Protects strips from accidental discoloration caused by exposure to air or light. Code on test strip vial must match code entered into glucose meter.

STEP	RATIONALE
4. Insert strip into meter (refer to manufacturer directions (see illustration). Do not bend strip. Meter turns on automatically.	Some machines must be calibrated; others require zeroing of timer. Each meter is adjusted differently.
5. Remove unused reagent strip from meter and place on paper towel or clean, dry surface with test pad facing up (see manufacturer directions).	Moisture on strip can alter accuracy of final test results.
6. Meter displays code on screen that must match code from test strip vial. Press proper button on meter to confirm matching codes. Meter is ready for use.	Codes must match for meter to operate. Meters have different messages that confirm that meter is ready for testing and blood can be applied.
7. Perform hand hygiene and apply clean gloves. Prepare single-use lancet or multiple-use lancet device.	Reduces transmission of microorganisms.
NOTE: Some meters recommend that this step be completed before preparing test strip. Remove cap from lancet device; insert new lancet. Some lancet devices have disk or cylinder that rotates to new lancet.	Never reuse a lancet because of risk of infection.
a. Twist off protective cover on tip of lancet. Replace cap of lancet device.	
b. Cock lancet device, adjusting for proper puncture depth.	Each patient varies as to depth of insertion needed for lancet to produce blood drop.
8. Obtain blood sample.	
a. Wipe patient's finger or forearm lightly with antiseptic swab and allow to dry. Choose vascular area for puncture site. In stable adults select lateral side of finger. Avoid central tip of finger, which has denser nerve supply (Pagana and Pagana, 2015).	Removes microorganisms from skin surface. Side of finger is less sensitive to pain.
b. Hold area to be punctured in dependent position. Do not milk or massage finger site.	Increases blood flow to area before puncture. Milking may hemolyze specimen and introduce excess tissue fluid (Pagana and Pagana, 2015).
c. Hold tip of lancet device against area of skin chosen for test site (see illustration). Press release button on device. Some devices allow you to see blood sample forming. Remove device.	Placement ensures that lancet enters skin properly.
d. With some devices a blood sample begins to appear. Otherwise gently squeeze or massage fingertip until round drop of blood forms (see illustration).	Adequate-size blood sample is needed to test glucose.

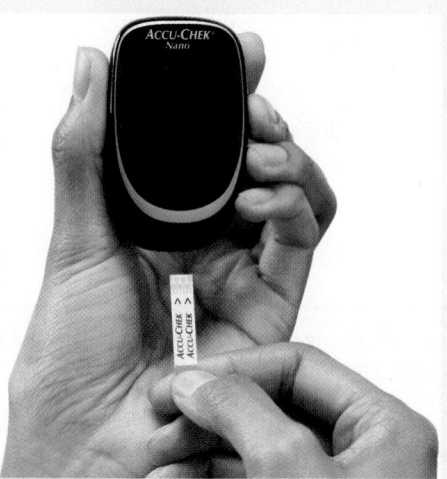

STEP 4 Load test strip into meter. (*Courtesy Accucheck Glucometer.*)

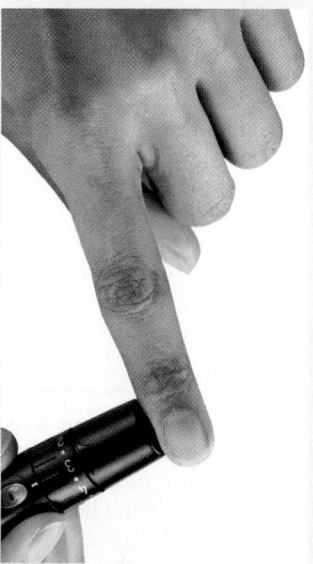

STEP 8c Prick side of finger with lancet. (*Courtesy Accucheck Glucometer.*)

STEP	RATIONALE
9. Obtain test results.	Exposure of blood to test strip for prescribed time ensures proper results.
a. Be sure that meter is still on. Bring test strip in meter to drop of blood. Blood will be wicked onto test strip (see illustration). Follow specific meter instructions to be sure that you obtain adequate sample.	Blood enters strip, and glucose device shows message on screen to signal that enough blood is obtained.

Clinical Decision Point *Do not scrape blood onto the test strips or apply it to wrong side of test strip. This prevents accurate glucose measurement.*

STEP	RATIONALE
b. Blood glucose test result will appear on screen (see illustration). Some devices "beep" when completed.	
10. Turn meter off. Some meters turn off automatically. Dispose of test strip, lancet, and gloves in proper receptacles.	Meter is battery powered. Proper disposal reduces risk for needlestick injury and spread of infection.
11. Perform hand hygiene.	Reduces transmission of microorganisms.
12. Discuss test results with patient and encourage questions and eventual participation in care if this is a new diabetes mellitus diagnosis.	Promotes participation and adherence to therapy.

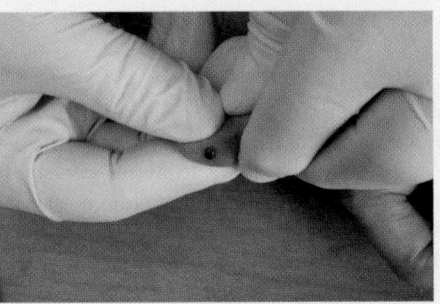

STEP 8d Gently squeeze puncture site until drop of blood forms.

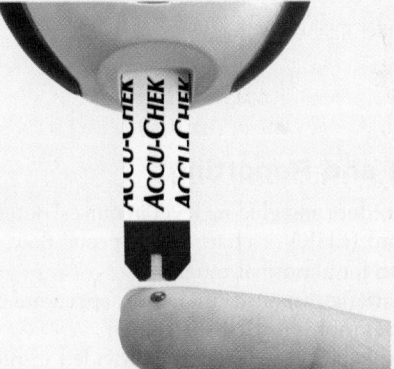

STEP 9a Touch test strip to blood drop. Blood wicks into test strip. (*Courtesy Accucheck Glucometer.*)

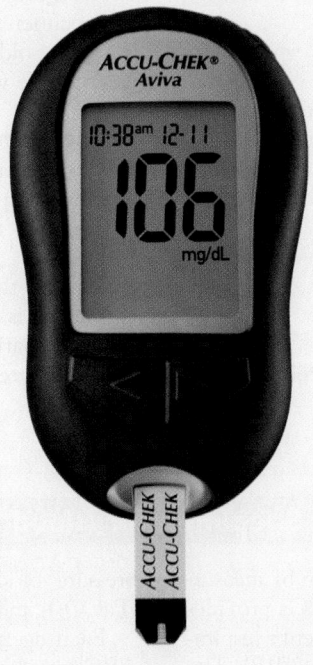

STEP 9b Results appear on meter screen. (*Courtesy Accucheck Glucometer.*)

| STEP | RATIONALE |

EVALUATION

1. Inspect puncture site for bleeding or tissue injury.
2. Compare glucose meter reading with normal blood glucose levels and previous test results.
3. **Use Teach-Back:** "I want to be sure I explained the way to obtain a blood glucose reading. Show me the steps you will use to obtain your blood glucose measurement. Revise your instruction now or develop a plan for revised patient or family caregiver teaching if patient or family caregiver is not able to teach back correctly.

Site can be source of discomfort and infection.
Determines if glucose level is normal.

Determines patient's and family caregiver's level of understanding of instructional topic.

Unexpected Outcomes	**Related Interventions**
1. Puncture site is bruised or continues to bleed.	• Apply pressure. • Notify health care provider if bleeding continues. • Continue to monitor patient.
2. Blood glucose level is above or below target range.	• Check if there are medication orders for deviations in glucose level. • Notify health care provider. • Administer insulin or carbohydrate source as ordered, depending on glucose level.
3. Glucose meter malfunctions.	• Review instructions for troubleshooting glucose meter. • Repeat test.

Recording and Reporting

- Record procedure and glucose level in nurses' notes in electronic health record (EHR) or chart or on special flow sheet. Record action taken for abnormal range.
- Describe patient response, including appearance of puncture site, in nurses' notes in EHR or chart.
- Describe explanations or teaching provided in nurses' notes in EHR or chart.
- Document your evaluation of patient and family caregiver learning.
- Record and report abnormal blood glucose levels.

Special Considerations
Teaching
- Provide information on where patient with diabetes mellitus can obtain testing supplies. When possible, teach with the same meter that patient will use at home.
- Provide patient with information on where to obtain help if glucose meter has malfunctioned.
- Stress importance of the timing of blood glucose levels, particularly in patients with diabetes mellitus.

Pediatric
- Allow young children to choose puncture site; heel and great toe are common puncture sites in infants.

- Heel warming helps to obtain specimen from a neonate.
- Infection or abscess of the heel and necrotizing osteochondritis are the most serious complications of heelstick puncture in infants. To avoid osteochondritis make sure that puncture is not deeper than 2 mm and is made at the outer aspect of the heel (Hockenberry and Wilson, 2015).
- Allow young child with parent to demonstrate technique; incorporate a play activity for further understanding.

Gerontological
- Warming fingertips with warm water may facilitate obtaining specimen.
- Some older adults have vision or dexterity problems that interfere with performing self-fingersticks.

Home Care
- Provide information on correct disposal of sharps in nonpermeable and puncture-resistant container.
- Suggest that patient attend diabetic support group if needed.
- Be sure that patient's family caregiver can perform test when patient is ill or is unable to manipulate devices.
- Teach patient and family caregiver to record findings or how to retrieve results from the memory of the glucose meters.

◆ SKILL 7.10   Obtaining an Arterial Specimen for Blood Gas Measurement

You assess effectiveness of oxygenation and ventilation by measuring arterial blood gases (ABGs). Measurement of ABGs provides valuable information in assessing and managing a patient's respiratory and metabolic disturbances (Pagana and Pagana, 2015). The parameters measured in an ABG include arterial blood pH, partial pressure of oxygen (PaO_2), partial pressure of carbon dioxide ($PaCO_2$), and arterial oxygen saturation (SaO_2).

Each agency has a policy regarding who is allowed to obtain ABG samples. Many agencies allow nurses in specialty areas (e.g., critical care) to obtain them; others specify a certified respiratory therapist, and some require institutional certification of this skill.

Delegation and Collaboration

The skill of obtaining an ABG sample cannot be delegated to nursing assistive personnel (NAP). The nurse informs the NAP to:
- Report any bleeding from arterial puncture site.
- Report any changes in patient vital signs, level of consciousness, or restlessness.

Equipment

- Commercial blood gas kit or individual supplies, including:
- 3-mL heparinized syringe
- 23- or 25-gauge needle with safety guard
- Filter cap (allows expelling of air and retains blood)
- Alcohol swabs (2)
- 2 × 2–inch gauze pad
- Tape
- Heparin (1 : 1000 solution)
- Cup or plastic bag with crushed ice
- Clean gloves
- Protective eyewear
- Completed identification labels with proper patient identifiers
- Completed laboratory requisition with date, time, name of test, patient identification, and source of specimen
- Small plastic biohazard bag for delivery of specimen to laboratory (or container specified by agency)

STEP	RATIONALE

ASSESSMENT

1. Identify patient using at least two identifiers (e.g., name and birthday or name and medical record number) according to agency policy. Compare identifiers with information on patient's MAR or medical record.	Ensures correct patient. Complies with The Joint Commission standards and improves patient safety (TJC, 2016).
2. Assess for factors that influence ABG measurements:	Allows you to eliminate factors that interfere with accurate measurement.
a. Hypoventilation or hyperventilation	Hypoventilation can cause retention of CO_2, and hyperventilation can cause decreased CO_2 levels (Hockenberry and Wilson, 2015).
b. Body temperature	Change in body temperature as little as 17°C 1°F can alter ABG values (Hockenberry and Wilson, 2015).
3. Identify medications that may influence ABG measurement (e.g., anticoagulants, diuretics).	Certain medications increase risk for bleeding at puncture site or may cause hemoconcentration.
4. Assess respiratory status, including rate, depth, rhythm, adventitious sounds, and use of accessory muscles.	Physical signs and symptoms may indicate need for ABG sample.
5. Review criteria for choosing site for ABG sample.	Prevents causing compromised circulation from puncture.

Clinical Decision Point *Factors that contraindicate use of arterial site include amputation, contractures, localized infection, dressing or cast, mastectomy, or arteriovenous shunts.*

a. Assess collateral blood flow. *Perform Allen test.*	Allen test assesses collateral circulation before performing arterial puncture on radial artery. Positive Allen test ensures that there is collateral circulation to hand in case thrombosis of radial artery occurs following puncture (Pagana and Pagana, 2015).
(1) Have patient make tight fist and raise hand above heart.	Removes as much blood from hand as possible.
(2) Apply direct pressure to both radial and ulnar arteries (see illustration).	Obstructs arterial blood flow to hand.

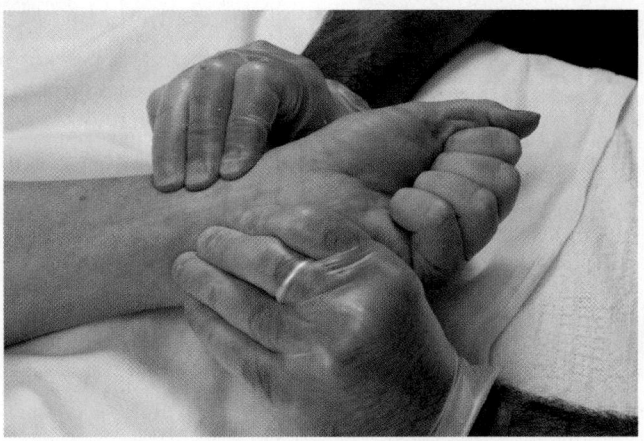

STEP 5a(2) Apply pressure to radial and ulnar arteries.

STEP	RATIONALE
(3) Have patient lower and open hand (see illustration).	Fingers and hand should be pale and blanched, indicating lack of arterial blood flow.
(4) Release pressure over ulnar artery; observe color of fingers, thumbs, and hand (see illustration).	Flushing identifies that circulation through ulnar artery is good and that ulnar artery alone is capable of providing blood supply to entire hand. Therefore you can use radial artery for puncture.

Clinical Decision Point *If there is no flushing in 15 seconds, Allen test is negative and you should repeat it on the other arm or choose another artery for puncture (Pagana and Pagana, 2015).*

b. Assess accessibility of vessel.	Palpating, stabilizing, and performing venipuncture of superficial artery is easier. Superficial arteries are located at distal ends of extremities.
c. Assess tissue surrounding artery.	Muscle, tendon, and fat have decreased sensation to pain. Bony periosteum and nerves are highly sensitive to pain.
d. Assess that arteries are not directly adjacent to veins.	Helps reduce chance of venous puncture and possibility of inaccurate samples.
6. Assess arterial sites for use in obtaining specimen.	Arterial blood may be obtained from areas where strong pulses are palpable (i.e., radial, brachial, or femoral artery) (Pagana and Pagana, 2015).

Clinical Decision Point *Previous puncture sites or preexisting conditions may eliminate potential sites (see agency policy). Artery should be easily accessible.*

a. Radial artery	Safest, most accessible site for puncture. Is superficial, is not adjacent to large veins, usually has adequate collateral circulation by ulnar artery, and is relatively painless if periosteum is avoided. Used when Allen's test is positive.
b. Brachial artery	Has reasonable collateral blood flow, is less superficial, is more difficult to palpate and stabilize, carries increased risk for venous puncture, and results in increased discomfort for patient if brachial nerve is punctured. Used when radial artery is inaccessible or Allen's test is negative.
c. Femoral artery	Nurses without specialized training should not use this artery. Has no adequate collateral flow if obstructed below inguinal ligament, is difficult to stabilize, is deep, and is directly adjacent to femoral vein. Is best artery to use in emergency (e.g., cardiac arrest or hypovolemic shock when pulses are difficult to palpate).
7. Review baseline ABG values for patient.	Provides baseline for comparison and evaluation of therapies.
8. Determine patient's knowledge about ABG procedure.	Obtaining blood specimen is painful. Patient who is knowledgeable will be more cooperative.

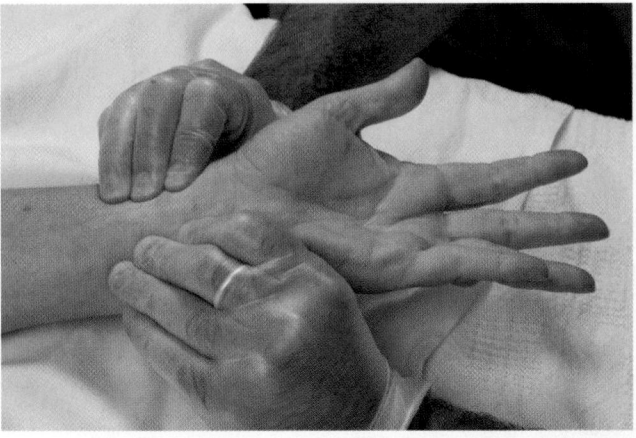

STEP 5a(3) Patient opening hand; note color.

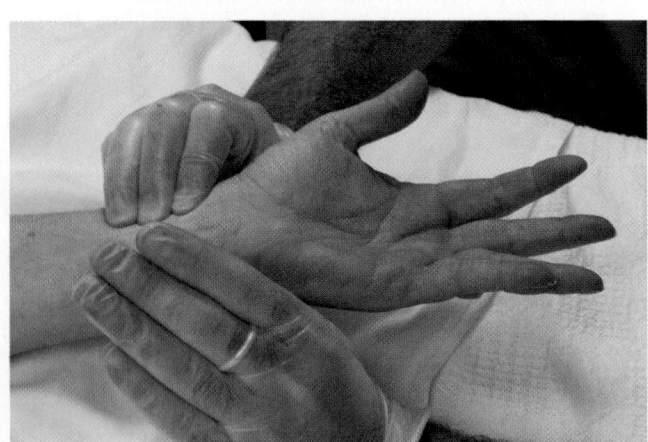

STEP 5a(4) Release pressure over ulnar artery and note color of hand.

STEP	RATIONALE

NURSING DIAGNOSES

- Anxiety
- Deficient knowledge regarding arterial blood gases

- Impaired gas exchange
- Ineffective airway clearance
- Ineffective breathing pattern

- Ineffective peripheral tissue perfusion
- Risk for injury

Related factors/Risk factors are individualized based on patient's condition or needs.

PLANNING

1. Expected outcomes following completion of procedure:
   - Patient's ABG values are within normal range.
   - Patient's extremity distal to puncture remains warm and pink, has adequate capillary refill, and is free of pain.
   - Patient denies anxiety, and respiratory rate remains within baseline.
   - Patient correctly discusses ABG procedure.
2. Prepare heparinized syringe (if not in commercial kit).
   a. Aspirate 0.5 mL sodium heparin (1000 units/mL) into syringe from vial or ampule.
   b. Withdraw plunger entire length of syringe. Maintain asepsis.
   c. Eject all heparin in barrel out of syringe.

3. Explain steps and purpose of procedure to patient.

Indicates adequate oxygenation.
Indicates adequate arterial circulation to extremity.

Anxiety increase respiratory rate, which can alter ABG results.

Indicates learning.
Heparin mixes with specimen to prevent clotting.
Prevents blood sample from clotting before reaching laboratory. Excessive heparin can affect pH of arterial sample.
Coats inside of barrel of syringe with heparin.
In hub of syringe 0.15 to 0.25 mL of sodium heparin remains; 0.05 mL of sodium heparin adequately anticoagulates 1 mL of blood; 0.15 mL adequately anticoagulates 3 mL without affecting pH level.
Reduces anxiety and promotes understanding and cooperation.

IMPLEMENTATION

1. Perform hand hygiene.
2. Palpate selected radial, femoral, or brachial site with fingertips.
3. Using radial artery, elevate patient's wrist with small pillow and ask him or her to extend fingers downward. Stabilize artery by slight hyperextension of wrist.
4. Apply clean gloves. Clean area of maximal impulse with alcohol swab or antiseptic swab (check agency or manufacturer recommendation). Wipe in circular motion away from site or use back-and-forth strokes. Allow to dry.
5. Hold 2 × 2 inch–gauze pad with same fingers used to palpate artery.
6. Use corner of sterile gauze pad or alcohol wipe to point to chosen site.
7. Hold needle bevel up and insert at 45-degree angle into artery. Prepare patient for needlestick because radial sticks are painful.
8. Stop advancing needle when blood is noted returning into hub of needle or syringe.
9. Allow arterial pulsations to pump 2 to 3 mL of blood into heparinized syringe slowly (see illustration).
10. When sampling is complete, hold 2 × 2–inch gauze pad over puncture site, withdraw syringe and needle, and activate safety guard over needle.
11. Apply pressure over and just proximal to puncture site with pad (see illustration).

12. Maintain continuous pressure on and proximal to site for 3 to 5 minutes (approximately 15 minutes if patient is undergoing anticoagulant therapy or has bleeding disorder) (Pagana and Pagana, 2015). Have another nurse remove safety needle and attach filter cap to syringe (see Step 15 below) if prolonged pressure is needed.

Reduces transmission of infection.
Determines area of maximal impulse for puncture site.

Flexes wrist and positions radial artery closer to surface. Reduces mobility of artery and makes insertion of needle easier.
Reduces number of resident bacteria on surface of skin. Drying maximizes antibacterial effects.

Keeps gauze pad accessible for covering puncture site when necessary.
Maintaining location of artery improves likelihood of successful puncture.
Angle allows for better arterial flow into needle. Prepared patient will be less likely to withdraw arm.

Quick return of blood indicates that arterial flow is obtained. Prevents puncturing through both sides of artery.
Allowing pulsations to help fill syringe reduces presence of air bubbles in sample. Bubbles alter ABG results.
Pad minimizes pulling of skin as needle is withdrawn.
Decreases contamination from blood and accidental needlestick.
Insertion of needle into artery is just proximal to insertion site through skin. Gauze absorbs any blood that might ooze from site.
To avoid hematoma formation, apply and hold pressure or apply a pressure dressing to arterial puncture site for 3 to 5 minutes (Pagana and Pagana, 2015). Prevents delay in preparing syringe in ice.

STEP	RATIONALE

13. Visually inspect site for signs of bleeding or hematoma formation.

Determines if continued need exists to exert pressure. Because artery rather than vein has been accessed, monitor puncture site for bleeding.

14. Palpate artery below or distal to puncture site.

Determines if pulse quality has changed, indicating alteration in arterial flow.

15. Take syringe, remove safety needle, and discard needle in appropriate biohazard container. Attach filter cap to syringe (available in kit) to expel air or cover tip of syringe with 2 × 2–inch sterile gauze to expel air (see agency procedure). Some kits may have all supplies, including syringe with heparin, needle with safety needle cap, and filter cap that allows air to vent and not blood (see illustration).

Decreases chance of contamination from room air. Air bubbles in specimen can falsely elevate or decrease results, depending on patient's blood gas concentration (Van Leeuwen et al., 2015).

16. Prepare syringe for laboratory analysis (according to agency policy).

   a. Place patient identification label on syringe in front of patient; confirm identifiers (TJC, 2016).

Ensures proper identification of sample.

   b. Place syringe in cup of crushed ice (check agency policy).

Failure to place ABG sample can affect results of pH, PaO_2, and $PaCO_2$ (Pagana and Pagana, 2015)

   c. Attach properly labeled laboratory requisition to blood gas sample. Add appropriate patient data (e.g., hemoglobin, mode and flow of supplemental oxygen, and patient's body temperature) (check agency policy).

Prevents mislabeled specimens.

Hemoglobin level, supplemental oxygen, and hypothermia or hyperthermia affects partial pressure of oxygen (PaO_2) or partial pressure of carbon dioxide ($PaCO_2$) values.

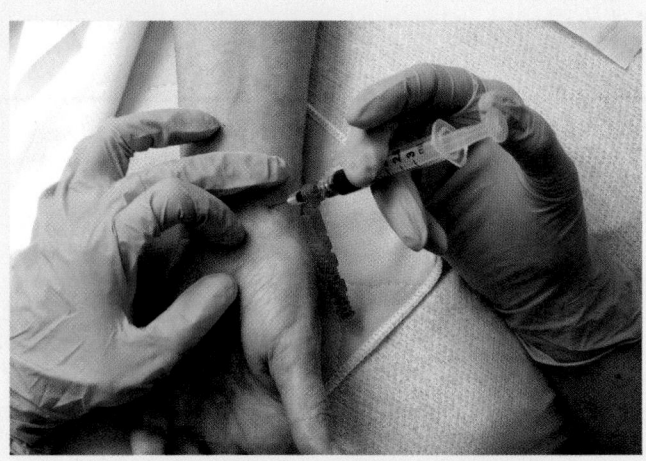

STEP 9 Blood flowing into syringe.

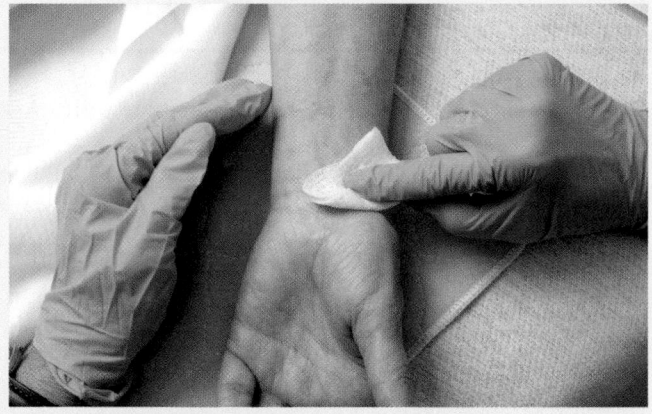

STEP 11 Apply firm pressure to arterial puncture site.

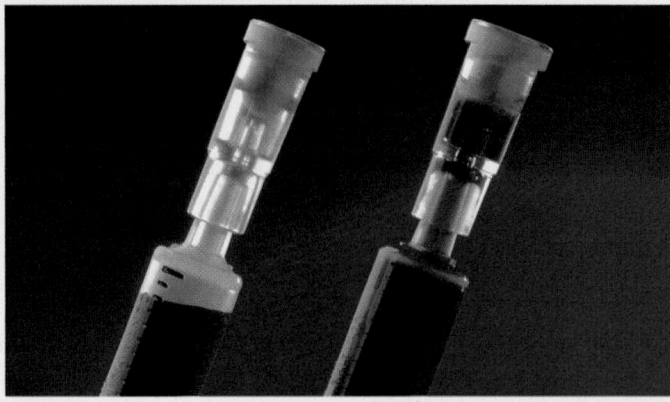

STEP 15 Filter-Pro Air Bubble Removal Device expels air safely from syringe without accidentally expelling blood and aerosolizing sample. (*With permission from Smiths Medical, Carlsbad, CA.*)

STEP	RATIONALE
17. Place sample in biohazard bag. Send sample to laboratory immediately.	Prevents alteration in gas tensions resulting from metabolic processes that continue after blood is drawn.
18. Remove gloves and perform hand hygiene.	Reduces transmission of microorganisms.

EVALUATION

1. Inspect puncture site and area distal to puncture site for complications.	An artery can be obstructed, or important structures anatomically juxtaposed to an artery can be penetrated (Pagana and Pagana, 2015).
2. Review results of sample as soon as possible.	Identifies any abnormality and expedites initiation of treatment.
3. **Use Teach-Back:** "I want to be sure I explained the way I will obtain your arterial blood gas specimen. Tell me the steps I will use to obtain this specimen." Revise your instruction now or develop a plan for revised patient or family caregiver teaching if patient or family caregiver is not able to teach back correctly.	Determines patient's and family caregiver's level of understanding of instructional topic.

Unexpected Outcomes	Related Interventions
1. Patient has abnormal ABG values.	• Continue to monitor patient. • Notify health care provider of findings and obtain further orders.
2. Patient has hematoma formation at puncture site.	• Continue to monitor patient. • Notify health care provider.
3. Puncture site is bruised or continues to bleed.	• Apply pressure. • Notify health care provider if bleeding continues.

Recording and Reporting

- Record results of Allen test, location and condition of puncture site, patient's tolerance of procedure, and disposition of specimen to laboratory in nurses' notes in electronic health record (EHR) or chart.
- Report ABG results to health care provider as soon as available.
- Report patient's fraction of inspired oxygen concentration (FiO_2) and any ventilator settings (e.g., tidal volume [V_t], respiratory frequency [RF], mode of ventilation).
- Document your evaluation of patient and family caregiver learning.
- Record results of test in nurses notes in EHR or chart.

Special Considerations
Teaching

- Teach patient to report numbness, burning, and/or tingling during and after in hand that had radial artery puncture.

Pediatric

- In neonatal and pediatric patients you can use capillary blood gas. Procedures are similar to those for obtaining heelsticks.
- When dealing with neonatal patients, especially premature infants, normal values for ABGs often differ from those of adults.
- Arterial blood samples from punctures are painful and cause crying and breath holding that affect the accuracy of ABG values (decreases PaO_2) (Hockenberry and Wilson, 2015).

Gerontological

- Pay special attention during interpretation of ABGs for patients with chronic pulmonary conditions. In these patients compensatory mechanisms may allow normal pH in face of markedly elevated $PaCO_2$.

✦ CLINICAL DEBRIEF

1. An 88-year-old female is admitted from home to the health care agency. She has an indwelling Foley catheter. Her urine is dark and cloudy. She is pulling at her Foley catheter, temperature 38.4°C (101.2°F), blood pressure 88/50, pulse 128, and she is restless and confused. On the basis of these findings, which laboratory specimens would you expect to obtain?

2. A male patient was diagnosed with type 1 diabetes mellitus 2 years ago. He was admitted with diabetes ketoacidosis (DKA) related to an upper respiratory infection related to his past history of chronic obstructive pulmonary disease (COPD). He stated that he quit taking his insulin because he was nauseated and vomiting. You observed that he has multiple puncture sites that are reddened on the central tip of his fingers. He states that his fingertips are sore. He is expected to be discharged to home the next day. Which instructions will you provide to the patient to help in his self-management of type 1 diabetes mellitus?

3. He was to be discharged today, but during the night he developed shortness of breath. He has received multiple respiratory treatments over the past 3 hours, yet you observe that his work-of-breathing has increased dramatically. Using SBAR, show how you would communicate with the health care team.

✦ REVIEW QUESTIONS

1. A urine specimen for culture and sensitivity is being collected from a male patient. Which steps would be used to obtain an accurate specimen? (Select all that apply.)
   1. Check two patient identifiers.
   2. Help patient to perform pericare before the sterile part of the procedure.
   3. Wipe head of the penis back and forth 3 times with each swab.
   4. Collect 10 to 20 mL for the sample.
   5. Have patient initially void into a bedpan or clean container.
   6. Have patient hold penis above the sterile specimen cup without touching the container.

2. The nurse is preparing to obtain a throat culture on a 22-year-old female. Which step(s) would facilitate obtaining an accurate specimen? (Select all that apply.)
   1. Placing patient in a sitting position or with head elevated at a 45-degree angle
   2. Having patient lean head forward
   3. Inserting swab without touching lips, teeth, tongue, or cheeks
   4. Swabbing the tonsillar area
   5. Swabbing the uvula
   6. Having patient blow her nose

3. Place the following steps for collecting a sterile urine specimen for a culture and sensitivity from a Luer-Lok catheter port in the correct order.
   1. Attach Luer-Lok syringe to Luer-Lok port.
   2. Clamp drainage tube with clamp or rubber band for 15 minutes.
   3. Clean catheter entry port and wait for disinfectant to dry.
   4. Unclamp catheter and allow urine to flow into drainage bag.
   5. Aspirate 3 mL of urine into syringe attached to Luer-Lok.

ⓔ *Visit the Evolve site for a complete list of Clinical Debrief and Review Questions answers.*

REFERENCES

American Diabetes Association (ADA): *DKA (ketoacidosis) & ketones*, 2013a, http://www.diabetes.org/living-with-diabetes/complications/ketoacidosis-dka.html. Accessed April 1, 2016.

American Diabetes Association (ADA): *Checking your blood glucose*, 2013b, http://www.diabetes.org/living-with-diabetes/treatment-and-care/blood-glucose-control/checking-your-blood-glucose.html. Accessed April 1, 2016.

Diabetes Forecast: *Blood glucose meters*, Alexandria, VA, 2013, American Diabetes Association.

Hockenberry MJ, Wilson D: *Wong's nursing care of infants and children*, ed 10, St Louis, 2015, Mosby.

Infusion Nurses Society (INS): *Infusion nursing: standards of practice*, Norwood, MA, 2011, Lippincott Williams & Wilkins.

Lecklider T: Monitoring blood glucose levels, *Eval Engineering* 54(8):22, 2015.

Lippi G, et al: Blood collection from intravenous lines: is one drawing site better than others, *Lab Med* 45(2):172, 2014.

McCall R, Tankersley C: *Phlebotomy essentials*, ed 5, Philadelphia, 2012, Lippincott Williams & Wilkins.

Occupational Safety & Health Administration (OSHA): *Bloodborne pathogen standard 29CFR1910.1030*, 2015, https://www.osha.gov/pls/oshaweb/owadisp.show_document?p_table=STANDARDS&p_id=10051. Accessed April 1, 2016.

Pagana K, Pagana T: *Mosby's diagnostic and laboratory test reference*, ed 12, St Louis, 2015, Mosby.

Raingruber B: *Contemporary health promotion in nursing practice*, Burlington, MA, 2014, Jones & Bartlett Learning.

The Joint Commission (TJC): *2016 National Patient Safety Goals*, Oakbrook Terrace, IL, 2016, The Commission, http://www.jointcommission.org/standards_information/npsgs.aspx. Accessed April 1, 2016.

Touhy T, Jett K: *Ebersole and Hess' Gerontological nursing and healthy aging*, ed 4, St Louis, 2014, Mosby.

United States Food and Drug Administration (USFDA): *Blood glucose monitoring devices*, 2015, http://www.fda.gov/medicaldevices/productsandmedicalprocedures/invitrodiagnostics/glucosetestingdevices/default.htm. Accessed April 1, 2016.

Van Leeuwen A, et al: *Davis's comprehensive handbook of laboratory and diagnostic tests with nursing implications*, ed 6, Philadelphia, 2015, FA Davis.

Wollowitz A, et al: Use of butterfly needles to draw blood is independently associated with marked reduction in hemolysis compared to intravenous catheters, *Acad Emerg Med* 20:1151–1155, 2013.

8 | Diagnostic Procedures

OBJECTIVES

Mastery of content in this chapter will enable the nurse to:
- Identify the physiological indications for diagnostic procedures.
- Describe the health care team collaboration and teamwork required before, during, and after procedures, including delegation to nursing assistive personnel (NAP).
- Perform appropriate physical and psychosocial assessments before, during, and after diagnostic procedures.

- Assist health care providers with angiogram, cardiac catheterization, intravenous pyelogram, bone marrow aspiration/biopsy, lumbar puncture, paracentesis, thoracentesis, bronchoscopy, and endoscopy.
- Explain nursing responsibilities related to the use of intravenous sedation during diagnostic/surgical procedures.

MEDIA RESOURCES

- evolve http://evolve.elsevier.com/Perry/skills
- Review Questions

- Audio Glossary
- Clinical Debrief and Review Questions Answers

PURPOSE

Diagnostic procedures are performed at patients' bedsides or in specially equipped rooms within a hospital or outpatient care setting. Before beginning, check the agency protocol specific to the procedure you will be performing or with which you are assisting. As a nurse you are responsible for assessing a patient's knowledge of a procedure; preparing the patient; providing a safe environment and emotional support throughout the procedure; providing pre-procedure and postprocedure assessment, care, and documentation; and providing discharge teaching. The health care provider is responsible for providing the patient with an explanation of the test/procedure, risks, benefits, treatment options, and outcomes before the procedure as part of the *informed consent* process.

STANDARDS OF CARE

American Society of Anesthesiologists (ASA), 2014—Intravenous Sedation

The Joint Commission (TJC), 2016—National Patient Safety Goals

PRINCIPLES FOR PRACTICE

- It is crucial for nurses to ensure that patients requiring diagnostic testing understand their testing and postprocedural care requirements.
- Some tests require intravenous (IV) sedation along with the diagnostic procedure such as a gastrointestinal endoscopy; others require contrast media or aspirations.
- Diagnostic procedures pose some risk for the patient. It is important that you understand the diagnostic procedure, including why it is needed, which preprocedural assessments are needed, expected outcomes, your role during the procedure, potential risks, actions appropriate in the event or unexpected outcomes, and appropriate postprocedural nursing care, to help ensure patient safety.
- IV sedation is used for diagnostic or surgical procedures that do not require complete or general anesthesia. Sedation classifications include "minimal," "moderate," or "deep" sedation/analgesia, depending on the depth of sedation (ASA, 2014a).
- Objective scales such as the American Society of Anesthesiologists (ASA) physical status classification system are used to

determine if patients are at risk for undesirable outcomes. Use of an objective scale can reduce the risk for complications by determining when it is prudent to involve an anesthesiologist to help manage the care of a complicated patient condition (ASA, 2014b).

- These scales incorporate evidence-based guidelines to reduce the risk for sedation-induced complications such as cardiac arrhythmias, respiratory failure, renal failure, neurological disorders related to the use of paralytic agents, or bleeding disorders resulting from hepatic failure.

PATIENT-CENTERED CARE

- Any diagnostic procedure can create a sense of powerlessness for patients. The unknown (e.g., not knowing what a test may reveal or not completely understanding what a test involves or feels like) can also create fear and anxiety.
- It is important to involve patients in a discussion of what a test involves and give them opportunity to ask questions. Learn what their concerns are because you may be able to alleviate them. For example, if a patient worries about being physically exposed during a procedure, communicate with procedure staff to see if there is a way to minimize exposure and use more draping.
- When a patient is chronically ill or fatigued or has decreased functional status, plan the diagnostic testing schedule to provide rest periods between multiple tests performed on the same day.
- Provide reassurance to a patient throughout a procedure. Most of these procedures cause moderate discomfort, and the patient tolerates them better if you remain at his or her side and explain each step.

EVIDENCE-BASED PRACTICE

Patients undergoing lumbar puncture (LP) are at risk for experiencing oversedation and site complications of postprocedure headaches (PPHs) and excessive loss of cerebral spinal fluid (CSF). In addition, the procedure itself can be painful for the patient; therefore research has focused on ways to make the patient more comfortable during and after an LP and on risk factors of LP.

- Although an epidural blood patch may be effective in treating PPHs in some patients, it is not effective in preventing these headaches, and it leads to intracranial hypertension (Kranz et al., 2014).
- Pain management can be achieved in children by reducing IV opioids when using an adjunctive eutectic mixture of local anesthetics (EMLA) pain reliever in conjunction with propofol (Whitlow et al., 2015).
- Rest, fluids (including caffeinated beverages), and analgesics have been considered effective measures for managing headache pain, although little evidence supports extensive rest and fluids (Destrebecq et al., 2014).
- A recent updated review of the literature concluded that there was no evidence suggesting that routine bed rest after LP is beneficial for the prevention of PPH onset. The role of fluid supplementation in the prevention of PPH also remained unclear (Arevalo-Rodriguez et al., 2016).
- A variety of factors contribute to postprocedure complications, including puncture needle size; excessive bed rest; epidural injections of saline; and numerous patient characteristics, including age, gender, pregnancy, body mass index, and previous LP history (Destrebecq, et al., 2014).

SAFETY GUIDELINES

Before a Procedure

- It is essential to be sure that patient undergoes the correct procedure. Ensure proper identification of a patient by using a minimum of two identifiers, verifying the correct procedure (and site, when applicable). This includes verbal verification and written/computerized documentation of the preceding information on patient arrival, again in the procedure room, and just before starting a procedure (TJC, 2016).
- Assess for completion of relevant documentation (e.g., history and physical, signed procedure consent form, nursing assessment, and preanesthesia assessment) necessary for performing a safe procedure.
- Identify any medications for which uninterrupted dosing is required (e.g., anticonvulsants, antibiotics, and certain cardiac medications). If the procedure requires a patient to have nothing by mouth (NPO), discuss medications with the health care provider to decide if the patient should take any medications before the procedure. When insulin or oral hypoglycemic medications are given to patients before procedures, arrange to have either the patient's meal or other nutritional support available on completion of the procedure.
- Verify that informed consent was obtained before administering any sedatives. The health care provider performing the procedure is responsible for obtaining informed consent from a patient. In some agencies after the health care provider discusses the procedure and obtains verbal consent, the registered nurse obtains the patient's signature on the consent form. (Check agency policy to determine if a consent form is required and the expectations of the nurse in this process.) *When there is no evidence of informed consent in the patient medical record, hold any preprocedure medications that may alter the patient's level of consciousness and notify the health care provider performing the procedure and staff in any receiving area.*
- Make sure that emergency equipment (e.g., oxygen, suction, defibrillator) is available in the procedure area and has been checked to ensure function.
- Confirm presence and date of expiration for sedation reversal agents.

During a Procedure

- When a procedure involves the use of radiation:
  - Minimize the amount of radiation exposure by using protective shielding devices such as a lead apron and goggles, radioprotective gloves, and/or thyroid shield.
  - Monitor staff radiation exposure with the use of a dosimeter if necessary.
  - Remain positioned as far away from the radiographic equipment as possible while performing required patient care.
- Monitor physiological parameters indicated by the procedure.
- Position patients carefully to avoid musculoskeletal or neurological injury.
- Label any specimens obtained during a procedure properly.

After the Procedure

- Assess for possible procedural complications and conduct appropriate assessments for early detection.
- Monitor oxygen saturation and vital signs to detect sedation failure and adverse effects (e.g., vomiting, hypoxic events) (ACR, 2015; ASA, 2014b).
- Know the use, side effects, and complications of the sedative and reversal agents to be administered.

- Be able to recognize cardiac dysrhythmias.
- Institute fall precautions until patient has recovered from effects of sedatives.

- Timely and complete neurovascular checks are critical to identify postprocedure limb ischemia or other arterial complications.

♦ **SKILL 8.1** **Intravenous Moderate Sedation**

Certain diagnostic or therapeutic procedures require patients to receive intravenous (IV) moderate sedation. Moderate sedation/analgesia produces a minimally depressed level of consciousness induced by the administration of pharmacological agents during which a patient retains a continuous and independent ability to maintain protective reflexes and a patent airway and is aroused by physical or verbal stimulation. Moderate sedation improves a patient's cooperation with a procedure, allows a rapid return to his or her preprocedure status, and minimizes the risk for injury. It often raises a patient's pain threshold and provides amnesia concerning the actual procedural events. In addition, no interventions are required during a procedure to maintain a patent airway, and spontaneous ventilation is adequate (ASA, 2014a).

Deep sedation is one risk associated with moderate sedation when a patient's level of consciousness depresses past the point at which he or she cannot maintain a patent airway. Because of this risk, the use of IV moderate sedation is closely controlled and normally restricted to physicians and registered nurses (RNs) who receive specialized training or credentialing (Antonelli et al., 2013; Bui and Urman, 2013). Know the agency policy for recommended and maximum doses of medications and monitoring and documentation requirements when using IV sedation.

The most common types of medications used to achieve moderate sedation include benzodiazepines and opiates. Benzodiazepines reduce anxiety and promote muscle relaxation. Midazolam also produces an amnesic effect. Opiates such as morphine sulphate or fentanyl help control pain while achieving sedation. Propofol, a safe, rapid-acting hypnotic, is also commonly used and may offer a faster recovery time than the combination of benzodiazepines and opiates (Ellett, 2010; Muller and Wehrmann, 2011).

Patient risks during IV sedation include hypoventilation, airway compromise, hemodynamic instability, and/or altered levels of consciousness that include an overly depressed level of consciousness or agitation and combativeness. Emergency equipment appropriate for the patient's age and size (see Chapter 28) and a staff competent in airway management, oxygen delivery, and use of resuscitation equipment are essential. During a procedure patients need continuous monitoring (recorded at least every 5 minutes) of heart and respiratory rate and rhythm, blood pressure, oxygen saturation, and level of consciousness (ACR, 2015). End-tidal carbon dioxide (CO_2) is also becoming a common parameter for monitoring sedation tolerance (Conway et al., 2015). Monitoring continues after the procedure.

Delegation and Collaboration

The skill of assisting with IV moderate sedation, including the preprocedure assessment, cannot be delegated to nursing assistive personnel (NAP). In most agencies an RN or health care provider assesses and monitors a patient's level of sedation, airway patency, and level of consciousness. Roles in monitoring depend on scope-of-practice guidelines as determined by state regulations (see agency policy).

Equipment

- Personal protective equipment (PPE): Gloves, mask, head cover, gown, eye protection
- Sedation as prescribed: Benzodiazepines, opiates, propofol, and fentanyl
- Emergency equipment: Crash cart, cardiac monitor/defibrillator, and endotracheal intubation/airway management equipment in various sizes and appropriate for patient's age
- Equipment for insertion of a peripheral IV catheter (see Chapter 29)
- Oxygen and airway supplies: Bag and mask device, oral/nasopharyngeal airways
- Suction equipment (see Chapter 25)
- Sphygmomanometer or noninvasive blood pressure monitor
- Pulse oximeter or end-tidal CO_2 monitor
- Electrocardiogram (ECG) monitor
- Appropriate reversal drugs (e.g., flumazenil for reversal of benzodiazepines, naloxone for reversal of opiates) and labels for each
- Pain medication (opioids) for procedures anticipated to cause discomfort such as dizziness, disorientation, nausea, vomiting,

---

STEP	RATIONALE

ASSESSMENT

1. Identify patient using at least two identifiers (e.g., name and birthday or name and medical record number) according to agency policy. Compare identifiers with information in patient's MAR or medical record.

Ensures correct patient. Complies with The Joint Commission standards and improves patient safety (TJC, 2016).

2. Verify type of procedure scheduled and procedure site with patient.

Ensures correct procedure for correct patient.

3. Verify that a preprocedure medication reconciliation and history and physical (H&P) examination were completed.

Accrediting agencies such as the TJC (2016) require a documented preprocedure medication history and H&P before administration of procedural IV sedation.

4. Verify that informed consent was obtained before administering any sedatives.

Federal regulations, many state laws, and accreditation agencies require informed consent for procedure.

STEP	RATIONALE
5. Assess patient's past history of adverse reaction to IV sedation (e.g., hemodynamic instability, nausea or vomiting, airway compromise, altered level of consciousness).	Patients with history of these reactions are at higher risk for procedural complications if IV sedation is used.
6. Verify patient's ASA Physical Status Classification (Box 8.1).	ASA recommends that patients receiving classification of 3 or higher have anesthesia consultation before receiving IV sedation (ASA, 2014a).

Clinical Decision Point *Consultation with an anesthesiologist is often required by the agency if a patient has an ASA classification of 3 to 6 or history of or evidence for difficult intubation, sleep apnea, or complications related to sedation/anesthesia.*

STEP	RATIONALE
7. Assess patient for history of airway abnormalities, liver failure, lung disease, heart failure, hypotonia, morbid obesity, severe gastroesophageal reflux, and history of adverse reaction to sedatives (ACR, 2015)	Risk factors that increase likelihood of adverse event (ACR, 2015).
8. Assess patient's current or past history for substance abuse or liver/kidney disease.	A history of substance abuse and/or liver/kidney disease usually requires dose adjustment of sedative agents.
9. Verify that patient has not ingested food or fluids, except for oral medications, for at least 4 hours.	Because risk of moderate sedation is loss of airway protection, empty stomach reduces risk for aspiration.
10. Determine if patient is allergic to latex, antiseptic, tape, or anesthetic solutions.	Allergic reactions to latex or tape range from mild skin reaction to anaphylaxis. Common allergic reactions to local anesthetic agents include central nervous system (CNS) depression, respiratory difficulty, and hypotension.
11. Assess patient's level of understanding of procedure, including any concerns.	Determines extent of instruction or level of support required.
12. Assess baseline heart rate, breath sounds, respiratory rate, blood pressure, level of consciousness, pain level, and oxygen saturation (SpO$_2$).	Establishes baseline for comparison during and after procedure.
13. Determine patient's height and weight.	Needed to calculate drug dosages.
14. Assess patient's baseline status via designated scoring system of agency. A variety of tools are available for scoring, including the "Aldrete score" (Aldrete, 2007; Table 8.1).	Establishes baseline for comparison after procedure.

BOX 8.1

ASA Physical Status Classification System

ASA 1 = Normal healthy patient
ASA 2 = Patient with mild systemic disease
ASA 3 = Patient with severe systemic disease
ASA 4 = Patient with severe systemic disease that is a constant threat to life
ASA 5 = Moribund patient who is not expected to survive without the operation
ASA 6 = Declared brain-dead patient whose organs are being removed for donor purposes
"E" is added if the procedure is performed as an emergency.

From American Society of Anesthesiologists: *ASA Physical Status Classification System*, 2014, http://www.asahq.org/quality-and-practice-management/standards-and-guidelines/search?q=ASA%20physical%20status. Accessed August 26, 2016.

TABLE 8.1

Aldrete Scoring System

		Score
Activity (moving voluntarily on command)	4 extremities	2
	2 extremities	1
	0 extremities	0
Respiration	Able to breathe deeply and cough freely	2
	Dyspnea, shallow or limited breathing	1
	Apneic	0
Circulation	BP ± 20 mm Hg of presedation level	2
	BP ± 20–50 mm Hg of presedation level	1
	BP ± 50 mm Hg of presedation level	0
Consciousness	Fully awake	2
	Arousable on having name called	1
	Not responding	0
Color	Normal	2
	Pale, dusky, blotchy, jaundiced, or other change	1
	Cyanotic	0

From Aldrete JA: The post-anesthesia recovery score revisited, *J Clin Anesth* 7:89, 1995; Aldrete JA: Post-anesthetic recovery score, *J Am Coll Surg* 205(5):3, 2007.
BP, Blood pressure.

STEP	RATIONALE

NURSING DIAGNOSES

- Acute pain
- Anxiety
- Deficient knowledge regarding procedure
- Risk for aspiration
- Risk for injury

Related factors/Risk factors are individualized based on patient's condition or needs.

PLANNING

1. Expected outcomes following completion of procedures:
   - Adhere to Universal Protocol (Box 8.2).
   - Patient's airway remains patent.

   - Patient's level of comfort is equivalent to score of 4 or less on pain scale of 0 to 10.
2. Explain to patient that IV sedation will cause relaxation and amnesia but that he or she will be awake during procedure. If patient will not be able to verbalize because of nature of procedure, teach him or her agreed-on nonverbal signals such as "yes," "no," and "pain."
3. Explain that close monitoring of vital signs and frequent checks to determine that patient is awake are normal and do not mean that there are problems.
4. Explain to patient major steps of procedure.
5. Position patient as needed for procedure.

Maintains patient safety (TJC, 2016)
Moderate sedation is monitored successfully without progression to deep sedation.
Procedure managed to minimize patient's pain.

Encourages cooperation and minimizes risks and anxiety about procedure.

Reduces patient anxiety during procedure.

Reduces patient anxiety during procedure.

IMPLEMENTATION

1. Establish peripheral IV access (CDC, 2011) (see also Chapter 29).
2. Implement Universal Protocol in presence of appropriate health care team members (as applicable) and in accordance with agency policy (see Box 8.2).
3. During diagnostic procedure, monitor heart rate and SpO_2 continuously via pulse oximetry equipment. Some agencies also use end-tidal CO_2 monitoring (capnography) (Conway et al., 2015). Monitor patient's airway patency, respiratory rate and depth, blood pressure, and level of consciousness and responsiveness every 5 minutes (ACR, 2015). Keep oxygen and suction equipment nearby.
4. Observe for verbal or nonverbal evidence of pain, facial grimacing, and eye opening.
5. Assess level of sedation using Modified Ramsay Sedation Scale (Table 8.2) or other criteria adopted by agency.

Provides access for administration of sedation and any emergency medications (as needed).
Ensures patient safety by correctly identifying correct patient with correct procedure.

Vital signs, oximetry, and capnography provide comparison with patient's baseline status.
Oxygen and suction equipment may be required in an emergent situation.

Physical responses indicate level of sedation.

Determines patient's level of sedation. Numeric rating scale offers consistent assessment and accurate judgment of patient's changing status and verbal/physical stimulation.

Clinical Decision Point *Report a Ramsay sedation score higher than 3 (responsive to commands only) to the health care provider (see Table 8.2).*

6. Reposition patient as needed without interrupting diagnostic procedure.

Prevents pressure- and position-related injuries (ACR, 2015)

BOX 8.2

The Joint Commission Universal Protocol

- Verification of correct person, correct site, and correct procedure occurs.
- Procedure site is marked before moving to procedure area.
- A "time-out" is performed immediately before starting procedures.
- When patient is in preprocedure area (immediately before moving him or her to procedure room), a checklist (e.g., paper, electronic, or other medium such as a wall-mounted white board) is used to review and verify that required items are available and accurately matched to the patient.

From The Joint Commission: *2016 National Patient Safety Goals*, 2016, The Commission. http://www.jointcommission.org/standards_information/npsgs.aspx. Accessed August 26, 2016.

STEP	RATIONALE

TABLE 8.2

Modified Ramsay Sedation Scale

Minimal sedation (anxiolysis)	1	Anxious and agitated or restless or both
	2	Cooperative, oriented, and tranquil
Moderate sedation/analgesia (conscious sedation)	3	Responds to commands spoken in a normal voice
Deep sedation/analgesia	4	Brisk response to a light forehead tap or loud auditory stimulus
	5	Sluggish response to a light forehead tap or loud auditory stimulus
	6	No response to a light forehead tap or loud auditory stimulus

Data from American Society of Anesthesiologists (ASA): Continuum of depth of sedation: definition of general anesthesia and levels of sedation/analgesia, Committee of Origin: Quality Management and Departmental Administration, The Society, 2014, http://www.asahq.org/~/media/Sites/ASAHQ/Files/Public/Resources/standards-guidelines/continuum-of-depth-of-sedation-definition-of-general-anesthesia-and-levels-of-sedation-analgesia.pdf. Accessed April 4, 2016; and Sessler C, et al: Evaluating and monitoring analgesia and sedation in the critical care unity, *Crit Care* 12(suppl 3):S2, 2008.

EVALUATION

1. Monitor patient throughout procedure using the Modified Ramsay Sedation Scale (or other criteria adopted by the agency).

   Provides data to verify patient's expected return to baseline status.

2. After procedure: Use Aldrete score (see Table 8.1) and monitor level of consciousness, respiratory rate, SpO$_2$, blood pressure, heart rate and rhythm, and pain score according to agency policy (ACR, 2015) (e.g., every 5 minutes for at least 30 minutes, then every 15 minutes for an hour, and then every 30 minutes until patient meets discharge criteria).

   Enables prompt detection of any airway compromise or protective reflexes caused by delayed action of medications.

3. Ask patient to repeat back what he or she understands regarding procedure or any postprocedure patient instructions, including medication orders and instructions.

   Verifies patient understanding of procedure or discharge education.

4. Have patient's "designated driver" explain any postprocedure education and sign appropriate documents.

   Patients who receive conscious sedation are restricted from driving for 24 to 48 hours, depending on procedure, type of sedation, and postprocedure restrictions.

5. **Use Teach-Back:** "I want to be sure I explained your postprocedure medications to you. Tell me what you know about the medications you will be taking once you're home." Revise your instruction now or develop a plan for revised patient or family caregiver teaching if patient or family caregiver is not able to teach back correctly.

   Determines patient's and family caregiver's level of understanding of instructional topic.

Unexpected Outcomes

1. Oversedation, evidenced by decreasing SpO$_2$ (cyanosis, slow shallow respirations with periods of apnea), tachycardia, sedation score of 4 (exhibiting brisk response to light glabellar tap or loud auditory stimulus) or higher on Modified Ramsay Sedation Scale or less than 8 on Aldrete scale.

Related Interventions

- Support patient's breathing via positioning and manual bagging.
- Immediately notify health care provider.
- Be prepared to administer reversal agents. Naloxone is for reversal of opioids, and flumazenil is for reversal of benzodiazepines.

Clinical Decision Point *Naloxone or nalmefene can be used as reversal agents. Although reversal of opioid sedation/respiratory depression with these drugs has been associated with significant complications, including pulmonary edema, tachycardia, hypertension, and even death, this is unlikely to occur when they are used to reverse the acute effects of opioid administration (Tobias and Leder, 2011).*

2. Patient develops cardiac instability evidenced by irregular heart rate, change in pulse rate, or change in blood pressure.

- Initiate oxygen therapy, ensure IV access, and obtain ECG as ordered.
- Immediately notify health care provider.

Recording and Reporting

- Document vital signs, SpO$_2$, end-tidal CO$_2$, and sedation level at baseline, then every 5 minutes during the procedure, and every 15 minutes for at least 30 minutes after the procedure according to agency policy.
- Record dosage, route, and time of administration for drugs given during and after the procedure, including reversal agents, in nurses' notes in electronic health record (EHR) or chart.
- Record significant patient reactions during the procedure. Include IV fluids and blood products if administered.
- Immediately report to patient's health care provider any respiratory distress, cardiac compromise, or unexpected altered mental status.

- Document discharge teaching, medication reconciliation, discontinuation of IV access, final/discharge assessment, and to whom/how discharged (e.g., designated driver, ambulance/transporter, nursing home).
- Document your evaluation of patient and family caregiver learning.

Special Considerations
Teaching

- Explain that it is unlikely for patients to remember the procedure because of the amnesic effect of the sedative(s).
- Before the procedure, instruct patient to arrange for transportation home after the procedure because (at most agencies) patient will not be permitted to drive for 24 hours after receiving sedation.
- Provide patients and family caregivers with discharge instructions that include complications that may occur; how to manage complications; and physical signs and symptoms to report to the health care provider, including contact information and postprocedure medication reconciliation and instructions.

Pediatric

- Children are more likely than adults to sustain a serious complication resulting from anesthesia. Such complications are often linked to either the cardiovascular or respiratory system. For this reason the American Academy of Pediatrics recommends that personnel who are able to manage a child's airway be present for the procedure (AAP, 2015).
- A preprocedure medical evaluation is required. To safely administer sedation to a pediatric patient, consider anatomical and physiological variations, preprocedure assessments, and pharmacological techniques (AAP, 2015).
- During the preprocedure assessment answer the parent's questions in a relaxed and confident manner. When communicating with children, take into account the child's developmental stage.

Gerontological

- Closely monitor the effects of medications on patient's respiratory status and pulse. These drugs interfere with breathing or increase or decrease heart rate as a result of reduced drug clearance through the kidneys or liver (Schlitzkus et al., 2015).
- Physical limitations of the patient, including hearing and vision loss, contribute to frustration and confusion, compounding the sense of loss of control.
- As a result of aging liver, some medications are not metabolized as rapidly as they might be in younger patients.

Home Care

- Instruct patient to avoid making any legally binding decisions until at least 24 hours after the procedure.

◆ **SKILL 8.2**   **Contrast Media Studies: Arteriogram (Angiogram), Cardiac Catheterization, and Intravenous Pyelogram**

Contrast media studies involve visualization of blood vessels and internal organs by intravascular injection of a radiopaque medium. An arteriogram (angiogram) permits visualization of the vasculature and arterial system of an organ (Fig. 8.1). Arteriography is usually performed by an interventional radiologist to diagnose arterial or venous occlusions; stenosis; emboli; thromboses; aneurysms; tumors; congenital malformations; or trauma to the brain, heart, lung, kidneys, or lower extremities.

Cardiac catheterization is a specialized form of angiography performed by an interventional cardiologist. An intravenous (IV) or intraarterial catheter introducer is inserted into the left or right side of the heart via a major peripheral vessel, usually the femoral artery and/or vein. The test studies pressures within the heart, cardiac volumes, valvular function, and patency of coronary arteries. Cardiac catheterizations are performed in specially equipped laboratories (Fig. 8.2). A contrast medium is injected, and the structures and functions of the heart and lungs are assessed.

Cardiac catheterizations are contraindicated in patients who would refuse needed surgery, are allergic to iodine contrast media, are uncooperative or cannot lie still during the entire procedure,

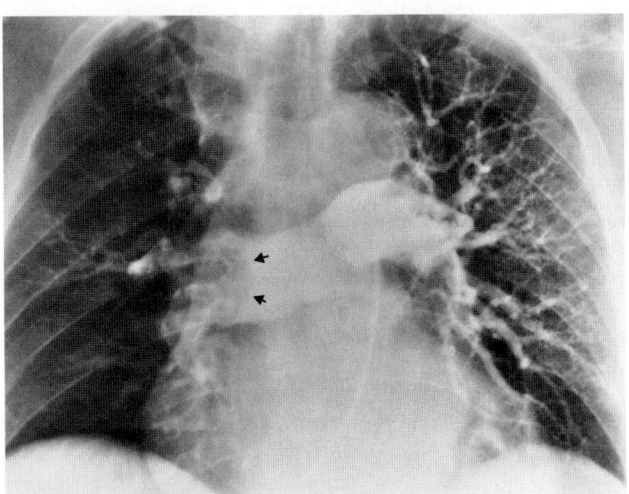

FIG 8.1 Pulmonary arteriogram shows obstruction (*arrows*) of right pulmonary artery. (*From Eisenberg R, Johnson N: Comprehensive radiographic pathology, ed 4, St Louis, 2007, Mosby.*)

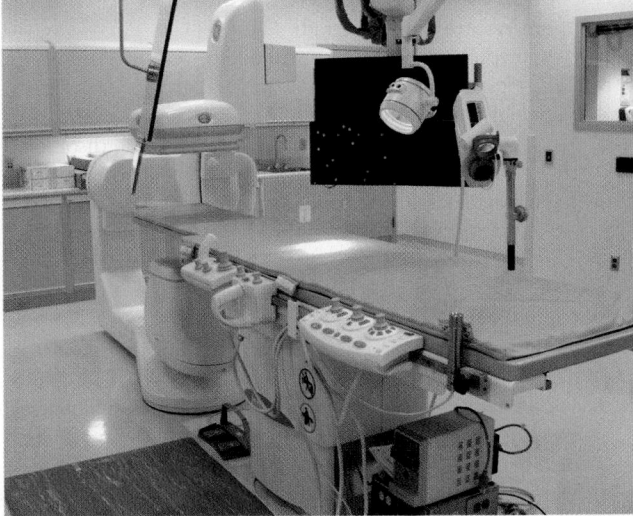

FIG 8.2 Cardiac catheterization laboratory. (*Image used with permission, Flagstaff Medical Center, Northern Arizona Healthcare. All rights reserved.*)

or are susceptible to dye-induced renal failure. People at particular risk for renal issues or contrast-induced nephrotoxicity (CIN) are those with preexisting renal dysfunction, diabetes mellitus, congestive heart failure, hypertension or hypotension, advanced age, anemia, or multiple myeloma (Ludwig and Keller, 2014). Interventions to help prevent dye-induced renal failure are controversial and include ensuring that the patient is well hydrated with bicarbonate solution or sodium chloride with or without prophylactic N-acetylcysteine (Ludwig and Keller, 2014). In addition, statins and vasodilators have also been explored as agents to reduce dye-induced renal failure (Ludwig and Keller, 2014). IV pyelography (IVP) is a venographic examination of the flow of radiopaque contrast medium through the kidneys, ureters, and bladder to identify obstruction, hematuria, stones, bladder injury, or renal artery occlusion. Dye is injected into a peripheral vein, and serial radiographs are taken over the subsequent 30 minutes.

Delegation and Collaboration

The skill of helping with angiography and IVP can be delegated to nursing assistive personnel (NAP) if the patient is stable and no IV sedation is used. The registered nurse (RN) directs the NAP about:

* When to obtain and report vital signs, urinary output, and weight.
* Which signs and symptoms to report to the nurse.
* Accompanying the patient to the procedure room and helping specially trained and licensed radiology personnel with the specific angiography procedure.

The skill of assisting with cardiac catheterization can be delegated to specially trained NAP with a nurse continuously present. The nurse provides continuous patient assessment and monitoring for serious complications. The NAP helps with patient transport, positioning, and obtaining supplies.

Equipment

* Personal protective equipment (PPE): Mask, sterile gown, head cover, eye protection, and sterile gloves
* Sterile packs containing catheters/equipment for performing procedures
* Equipment for peripheral IV access
* Medications such as sedatives (e.g., diazepam, midazolam, propofol) for IV sedation, or analgesics for relaxation and pain control
* Emergency equipment: Oxygen, endotracheal intubation/airway management equipment, emergency cart, cardiac monitor/defibrillator, sedative reversal agents
* Pulse oximeter, end-tidal carbon dioxide (CO_2) monitor, blood pressure (BP) equipment

STEP	RATIONALE

ASSESSMENT

1. Identify patient using at least two identifiers (e.g., name and birthday or name and medical record number) according to agency policy. Compare identifiers with information on patient's MAR or medical record.

Ensures correct patient. Complies with The Joint Commission standards and improves patient safety (TJC, 2016).

2. Verify type of procedure scheduled and procedure site with patient.

Ensures correct procedure and patient (TJC, 2016).

3. Verify that informed consent was obtained before administering any sedatives.

Federal regulations, many state laws, and accreditation agencies require informed consent for procedure.

4. Determine if patient is taking anticoagulants, aspirin, or any nonsteroidal medication.

Some medications increase risk for bleeding and are often stopped before procedure.

5. Assess patient for history of any allergies to iodine dye, shellfish, or latex and whether patient has had previous reaction to contrast agent (Westermann-Clark et al., 2015). If so, notify cardiologist or radiologist.

Allergic individuals may be at a mildly increased risk for developing adverse reactions to radiocontrast media (Westermann-Clark et al., 2015). Hypoallergenic contrast medium is sometimes used.

6. Review medical record for contraindications:
   a. *All contrast media:* Pregnancy unless benefits of test outweigh risks to fetus.

Radioactive iodinated contrast media crosses blood-placental barrier.

   b. *Angiography:* Anticoagulant therapy, bleeding disorders, thrombocytopenia, dehydration, uncontrolled hypertension, renal insufficiency, and pregnancy.

Anticoagulants and bleeding disorders interfere with patient's blood-clotting abilities and may cause blood loss.
Dehydration and renal insufficiency are contraindications to use of ionic radiographic contrast media because patient has impaired ability to excrete contrast media via kidneys.

   c. *Cardiac catheterization:* History of severe cardiomyopathy, severe dysrhythmias, uncontrolled heart failure (HF).

Introduction of catheter into myocardium increases risk for dysrhythmias (Pagana et al., 2015)

   d. *IVP:* History of dehydration, known renal insufficiency (with blood urea nitrogen [BUN] level >40 mg/100 mL or creatinine >2 mg/dl) (Pagana et al., 2015)

Iodinated dye is sometimes nephrotoxic and worsens existing renal disease.

   e. Determine whether patient took metformin hydrochloride within previous 48 hours. If so, notify health care provider immediately.

Metformin hydrochloride may or may not be discontinued 1 day before procedure and 2 days after catheterization because of the possibility of causing lactic acidosis and acute nephropathy (Maden et al., 2013).

STEP	RATIONALE
7. Assess patient's bleeding and coagulation status (e.g., complete blood count [CBC], platelets, prothrombin time [PT], activated partial thromboplastin time [aPTT]/ international normalized ratio [INR]) and patient's renal function (e.g., BUN, creatinine levels) before procedure. Assess electrolytes (sodium and potassium).	Abnormal laboratory findings may contraindicate procedure because of potential complications of hemorrhage and/or renal failure. Report elevated BUN or creatinine levels because such patients are at risk for renal failure induced by contrast media (Pagana et al., 2015). Abnormal electrolytes may reveal possible electromechanical problems.
8. Obtain vital signs and peripheral pulses. For arterial procedures mark patient's peripheral pulses before procedure. For cardiac catheterization also auscultate heart and lungs and obtain weight.	Provides baseline data and locations for comparison with findings during and after procedure.
9. Assess patient's hydration status, including condition of mucous membranes, and recent 24-hour intake.	Severe dehydration can lead to renal failure (Pagana et al., 2015)
10. Assess patient's level of understanding of procedure, including any concerns.	Determines extent of instruction or level of support required.
11. Determine type of arteriogram scheduled (e.g., carotid, femoral, brachial). If cardiac catheterization, verify if test is for right or left heart or both. For IVP ask if study is for one or both kidneys.	Enables you to anticipate patient teaching needs and postprocedure interventions.
12. Determine and document last time of ingested food, drink, or medications.	Prevents possible aspiration because patient is sedated. Excessive hydration causes dilution of contrast medium, making structures more difficult to visualize. Patients should be NPO for 2 to 8 hours before procedure (Pagana et al., 2015).

Clinical Decision Point *Exceptions occur for patients at risk for contrast media–induced renal impairment who are specifically instructed to drink increased fluids in the hours before the procedure or those instructed by the health care provider to take medications before the procedure. Good preprocedure hydration reduces the risk for renal impairment caused by contrast media (Pagana et al., 2015).*

STEP	RATIONALE
13. Review health care provider's orders for preprocedure medications, hydration, antihistamines, and IV sedation:	Increased sedation is necessary in anxious or confused patients. Increased hydration is often required for renal insufficiency and antihistamines for possible allergic reaction.
a. Atropine	Decreases salivary secretions and increases heart rate when bradycardia is present.
b. Diphenhydramine	Used prophylactically to block histamine and decrease allergic response.
c. Preprocedural sedative	Decreases anxiety and promotes relaxation.

NURSING DIAGNOSES

- Acute pain
- Anxiety
- Decreased cardiac output

- Deficient knowledge regarding procedure
- Fear

- Risk for infection
- Risk for injury

Related factors/Risk factors are individualized based on patient's condition or needs.

PLANNING

1. Expected outcomes following completion of procedure:	
• Patient does not experience any procedure or postprocedure complications such as significant changes in vital signs, diminished or absent peripheral pulses, allergic response, or decreased or absent urine output.	Procedure performed without complication.
• Patient's level of comfort is equal to score of 4 or less on pain scale of 0 to 10. Expected discomfort includes soreness at catheter insertion site and possible backache.	Patient tolerates procedure.
• Patient tolerates increased fluid intake and urinates sufficiently (at least 30 mL/hr or 0.5 mL/kg/hr) to excrete radiographic dye.	Adequate renal function.
• Patient recovers from IV sedation without respiratory complications or change in level of consciousness.	Appropriate level of sedation.

STEP	RATIONALE
2. Explain to patient purpose of and what will happen during procedure.	Helps to minimize patient's anxiety.
3. Remove all of patient's jewelry, metal objects, and body piercings.	Eliminates objects that interfere with radiography visualization of vessels and could be conductive material during electrocautery.
4. Preprocedure preparation: a. *For IVP:* Verify that patient has completed necessary bowel preparation of orally administered evacuation preparation 24 hours before test and evacuation enema 8 hours before test (check agency policy).	An evacuated lower intestine and bowel improve visualization of urinary structures.
b. *For cardiac catheterization:* Determine whether hair at site of catheter insertion needs clipping or preparation with antiseptic just before procedure. Allow antiseptic to dry. Do not shave site.	Reduces risk for site-related infection. Drying promotes maximal antibacterial activity. Shaving results in increased chance for infection.
5. For cardiac catheterization it is common to verify availability of emergent cardiac surgery because of risk for complete coronary artery occlusion from dislodged plaque or inadvertent perforation of vasculature. Also verify patient's ASA classification before procedure (see Box 8.1).	Prepares backup plan for possible procedural outcomes that would require emergency surgery.

IMPLEMENTATION

1. Have patient empty bladder or bowels before procedure.	Ensures that patient will not need to void during procedure.
2. Prepare cardiac monitor, pulse oximeter, and/or end-tidal CO_2 monitor.	Provides easy access to equipment for monitoring patient status during and after procedure.
3. Perform hand hygiene and apply appropriate protective equipment.	Reduces transmission of microorganisms.
4. Provide IV access using large-bore cannula. Remove gloves.	Provides access for delivery of IV fluids and/or drugs.
5. Help patient assume a comfortable supine position on x-ray table. Some patients undergoing IVP may be in supine or in a slight Trendelenburg's position. Immobilize extremity that will be injected. Pad any bony prominences.	For arterial procedures, patient may need to maintain position for 1 to 3 hours. Padding the bony prominences reduces the risk for impaired skin integrity.
6. Take "time-out" to verify patient's name, type of procedure to be performed, and procedure site with patient.	"Time-out" verification just before starting an invasive procedure includes health care provider and all involved personnel and is a safety precaution to prevent wrong patient, wrong site, and wrong procedure errors (TJC, 2016).
7. Monitor vital signs, pulse oximetry (SpO_2), end-tidal CO_2; and, for arterial procedures, palpate peripheral pulses.	Data provide comparison with baseline to determine patient's response to procedure.
8. Inform patient that during injection of dye it is common to experience some chest pain and a severe hot flash that is quite uncomfortable but lasts only a few seconds.	Dye causes feeling of warmth, flushing, or metallic taste shortly after injection.
9. Physician cleanses arterial puncture site for catheter insertion (femoral, radial, carotid, or brachial) with antiseptic.	Reduces transmission of microorganisms.
10. All health care team members apply mask and goggles, sterile gown, head cover, and sterile gloves. Drape patient with sterile drapes, leaving puncture site exposed.	Maintains surgical asepsis.
11. Physician anesthetizes skin overlying arterial puncture site.	Provides local anesthetic to area of incision or puncture.
12. For arterial procedures physician does the following: a. Punctures artery, inserts introducer (think plastic tube) into artery, inserts guidewire through introducer and advances, and inserts flexible catheter over guidewire and advances into heart. Introducers allow for use of various procedure catheters, depending on need (e.g., balloon angioplasty, stent placement, ablation).	Permits access to artery and coiling of catheter in artery.
b. Advances catheter to desired artery or cardiac chamber, removes guidewire, and injects contrast medium through catheter.	Permits radiographic visualization of structures, aneurysms, occlusions, or anomalies.

STEP	RATIONALE
13. During dye injection specialized machinery takes rapid sequence of x-ray films.	Permits radiographic records of visualization of dye through artery and any abnormalities present.
14. If iodinated dye is used, observe patient for signs of anaphylaxis, including respiratory distress, palpitation, itching, and diaphoresis.	Allergic reactions can be life threatening.
15. During cardiac catheterization RN helps with measuring cardiac volumes and pressure.	Provides data related to cardiac output, central venous pressure (CVP), ventricular pressures, and pulmonary artery pressure.

Clinical Decision Point *Be prepared to end the cardiac catheterization procedure early in the event of severe unrelieved chest pain, neurological symptoms of a cerebrovascular accident, cardiac dysrhythmias, or hemodynamic changes (Pagana et al., 2015).*

16. Nurse administering IV sedation monitors levels of sedation, level of consciousness, and vital signs (see Skill 8.1).	Proper IV sedation does not cause loss of consciousness.
17. Physician withdraws catheter and applies manual pressure to puncture site until homeostasis occurs (5 to 15 minutes or longer).	Five to fifteen minutes of manual pressure is often enough to stop active site bleeding. However, certain amount of bed rest is needed to achieve reliable hemostasis. Check agency policy for postprocedure bed rest requirements. This may vary from 2 to 6 hours when no arteriotomy closure device is used.
a. *Option:* Physician may choose to use an arteriotomy closure device (ACD), which can be categorized as either passive-closure device (helps with compression such as clamps/tamping devices, assisted or enhanced coagulation, and sealants) or active-closure device (immediate closure with suture devices, clips, and collagen plug devices).	Use of ACDs is reasonable after invasive cardiovascular procedures performed via femoral artery to achieve faster hemostasis, shorter duration of bed rest, and possibly improved patient comfort. Use of devices should be weighed against risk of complications (Krishnasamy et al., 2015; Schulz-Schüpke et al., 2014)

Clinical Decision Point *Before removing catheter sheath, check health care provider's orders for instructions for treating a vasovagal reaction. Manual pressure applied to the groin/femoral area can stimulate the baroreceptors and cause a vasovagal reaction in which the patient becomes bradycardic and hypotensive. Vasovagal reactions are usually brief and self-limiting. When applying pressure to the groin after sheath removal, be alert for a vasovagal reaction and prepared to treat it by lowering the head of the bed to the flat position and giving a bolus of IV fluids.*

18. If a percutaneous coronary intervention (PCI) such as a percutaneous transluminal coronary angioplasty (PTCA) or directional coronary atherectomy (DCA) was performed during cardiac catheterization, a femoral introducer/sheath is often left in place and removed in several hours.	Postinterventional sheaths provide emergency access to vasculature in event that coronary artery becomes occluded, allowing time for anticoagulants to wear off.
19. Remove and discard gloves. Perform hand hygiene.	Reduces transmission of microorganisms.
20. Postprocedure	
a. For arterial procedures:	
(1) Keep affected extremity immobilized for 2 to 6 hours after removal of sheath (see agency policy). Use orthopedic bedpan for female patient as needed for bowel or bladder evacuation while on bed rest.	There is evidence of no benefit relating to bleeding and hematoma formation in patients who have more than 3 hours of bed rest following transfemoral diagnostic cardiac catheterization. There is evidence of benefit relating to decreased incidence and severity of back pain after 3 hours of bed rest. Inconclusive evidence suggests that bed rest for 2 hours following transfemoral cardiac catheterization may be sufficient (Abdollahi et al., 2015).
(2) Emphasize need to lie flat for 6 to 12 hours (and possibly overnight if sheath is left in groin).	Helps to prevent disruption of hemostasis.
b. Encourage patient to drink fluids after procedure.	Facilitates elimination of contrast material and prevents renal damage (Pagana et al., 2015).

EVALUATION

1. Evaluate patient's body position and comfort during procedure.	Position can cause stress on insertion site and patient's musculoskeletal structures.
2. Monitor vital signs and SpO_2 and assess for signs of cardiac complications every 15 minutes for 1 hour, every 30 minutes for 2 hours, or until vital signs are stable.	Verifies patient's physiological status and evaluates effect of procedure. Signs of cardiac complications include chest pain or pressure, new dysrhythmias, and/or shortness of breath.

STEP	RATIONALE

3. Monitor for complications:
   a. Perform neurovascular checks by palpating peripheral pulses on affected extremity and comparing right and left extremities for skin color, temperature, and sensation. Use Doppler ultrasonic stethoscope to locate pulses that are not palpable (see Chapter 6).

   Enables prompt detection of circulatory impairment caused by intravascular clotting or bleeding at procedure site. Signs of reduced circulation include diminishing distal pulses and/or coolness, mottling, pallor, pain, numbness, and tingling in affected extremity.

   b. With vital signs assess vascular access site for bleeding and hematoma.

   Verifies expected sealing of puncture.

   c. Auscultate heart and lungs and compare with preprocedure findings.

   Evaluates patient response to procedure.

   d. Observe patient for possible delayed reaction to iodine dye (if used)—dyspnea, hives, tachycardia, and rash (Pagana and Pagana, 2014).

   Reaction may occur up to 6 hours after injection of dye.

4. Evaluate level of sedation, level of consciousness, and SpO_2. Use Aldrete scale (see Table 8.1).

   Determines patient's response to IV sedation.

5. Assess postprocedure laboratory values—CBC, prothrombin time, aPTT, INR, electrolytes, BUN/creatinine.

   Detects changes in laboratory values that indicate onset of complications such as bleeding.

6. Have patient rate discomfort on pain scale of 0 to 10.

   Pain is early sign of complications.

7. **Use Teach-Back:** "I want to be sure I explained what to watch for regarding signs of an allergic reaction after this procedure. Tell me what feelings would make you think you might be having an allergic reaction." Revise your instruction now or develop a plan for revised patient or family caregiver teaching if patient or family caregiver is not able to teach back correctly.

   Determines patient's and family caregiver's level of understanding of instructional topic.

Unexpected Outcomes

1. Vasovagal response occurs (at time of femoral puncture or after procedure with femoral pressure). Symptoms include feeling faint, dizzy, and light-headed and possible momentary loss of consciousness. Bradycardia is caused by stimulation of vagus nerve via baroreceptors.

2. Evidence of oversedation:
   - Prolonged reduced level of consciousness.

3. Pedal pulses are nonpalpable bilaterally 2 hours after arteriogram with change in skill color and temperature.

4. Hematoma or hemorrhage is present at catheter insertion site.

5. Patient has allergic reaction to contrast medium with symptoms of flushing, itching, and urticaria.

6. Renal toxicity from contrast medium occurs:
   Urine output less than 30 mL/hr or 0.5 mL/kg/hr.

7. Patient experiences retroperitoneal bleeding (when femoral access site is used):
   - Low back pain radiating to both sides of body (hallmark sign)
   - Tachycardia

Related Interventions

- Support airway (through positioning).
- Lower table or head of bed to flat position or to Trendelenburg's position if ordered.
- Be prepared to administer bolus of IV fluid (normal saline).
- See Skill 8.1.

- Assess pulse with Doppler.
- Immediately notify health care provider.
- Apply pressure over insertion site.
- Monitor catheter site every 15 to 30 minutes for 2 to 3 hours; follow agency protocol.
- Notify health care provider if interventions do not stop bleeding or if patient has symptoms of acute blood loss (hypotension, tachycardia, decreased level of consciousness).
- Monitor vital signs and observe for symptoms of anaphylaxis.
- Notify health care provider.
- Follow specific postprocedure orders related to findings.
- Prepare to administer antihistamine or epinephrine if ordered.
- Place on strict intake and output (I&O) monitoring.
- Monitor closely for signs of fluid overload.
- Review electrolyte, urea nitrogen, and creatinine levels.
- Prepare patient for emergency surgery.
- Monitor vital signs every 5 to 15 minutes.
- Monitor distal pulses hourly.

Recording and Reporting

- Record patient's status: vital signs, SpO_2/end-tidal CO_2, status of peripheral pulses for equality and symmetry, blood pressure for hypotension, temperature and color of catheterized extremity, condition of IV site, and level of patient responsiveness in electronic health record (EHR) or chart. Record any drainage from puncture site, appearance of dressing, and condition of puncture site.

- Report to health care provider any vital sign change, excessive bleeding or increasing hematoma at puncture site, decreased or absent peripheral pulses, persistent pain, altered neurological status, dysrhythmias, decreased SpO_2 or increased end-tidal CO_2, or decreased responsiveness after sedation.

- Document your evaluation of patient and family caregiver learning.

Special Considerations

Teaching

- See Skill 8.1, Teaching Considerations.
- Prepare patient to stay in the hospital if complications occur or if an intervention necessitates prolonged postprocedure vascular checks.

Pediatric

- Infants and children are particularly susceptible to the diuretic effects of radiocontrast dyes because of their small body size and immature renal/hepatic systems. In addition, those with congenital cardiac anomalies develop compensatory erythrocytosis and thus experience complications from dehydration very quickly. Emphasize to the parent(s) or caregiver the importance of fluid intake with the child after the procedure. Urinary output should exceed 1 mL/kg/hr (Hockenberry and Wilson, 2015).

Gerontological

- Physical exposure and low room temperature contribute to hypothermia in frail older adults who are unable to communicate that they are cold. Use heated blankets or forced-air heat to maintain core temperature at comfortable, safe levels (Lewis et al., 2017).
- In older adults slight alterations in vital signs or behavior are signs for impending problems; therefore close monitoring is important.

Home Care

- On discharge provide patient with written instructions to contact the health care provider (or affiliated emergency department) if the following occur after arteriogram or cardiac catheterization:
  - Bleeding from the catheterization puncture site; apply gentle pressure with a clean gauze or cloth
  - Formation of a knot or lump under the skin that increases in size
  - Worsening of a bruise or its movement down the extremity rather than disappearing
  - Pain at puncture site or in the extremity used for the catheterization
  - Extremity is pale and cool to the touch where arterial puncture is made
  - Appearance of redness, swelling, or warmth of the affected extremity
- It is helpful to have patient repeat these instructions back to you and to acknowledge clear understanding.
- After arteriogram or cardiac catheterization, instruct patient not to drive or climb stairs for 24 hours; to avoid sports, strenuous activity/housework, and lifting (e.g., groceries, children) for 3 days; and to avoid taking baths until wound is healed.
- On discharge after an IVP, instruct patient to:
  - Drink at least 64 ounces (1 to 2 L) of water to help flush the contrast media through the kidneys.
  - Watch for signs of a delayed reaction to the contrast medium for 24 hours after the procedure and call the health care provider or go to the nearest emergency department.

◆ SKILL 8.3	**Assisting With Aspirations: Bone Marrow Aspiration/Biopsy, Lumbar Puncture, Paracentesis, and Thoracentesis**

Aspirations are sterile invasive procedures involving the removal of body fluids or tissue for diagnostic procedures (Table 8.3). The nurse helps the health care provider during an aspiration procedure. Informed consent is required for these invasive procedures.

Bone marrow aspiration is the removal of a small amount of the liquid organic material in the medullary canals of selected bones. The sternum and the posterior superior iliac crests are the most common in adults. In children the anterior or posterior iliac crests are used, and in infants the proximal tibia is used (Hockenberry and Wilson, 2015; Pagana et al., 2015). A biopsy is the removal of a core of marrow cells for laboratory analysis. Both aspiration and biopsy diagnose and differentiate leukemia, certain malignancies, anemia, and thrombocytopenia. The marrow is examined in a laboratory to reveal the number, size, shape, and development of red blood cells (RBCs) and megakaryocytes (platelet precursors). Bone marrow cultures help differentiate infectious diseases such as tuberculosis (TB) or histoplasmosis. This procedure takes approximately 20 minutes to perform. Potential complications of bone marrow aspiration or biopsy include bleeding, especially if coagulopathy is present; infection; and, less commonly, organ puncture.

A lumbar puncture (LP), called a *spinal puncture* or *tap*, involves the introduction of a needle into the subarachnoid space of the spinal column. The purpose of the test is to measure pressure in the subarachnoid space; obtain cerebrospinal fluid (CSF) for visualization and laboratory examination; and inject anesthetic, diagnostic, or therapeutic agents. CSF is examined in a laboratory to help diagnose spinal cord tumors, central nervous system (CNS) infections, hemorrhage, and degenerative brain disease. The procedure takes approximately 30 minutes to perform.

The major contraindication for LP is evidence of increased intracranial pressure (ICP). The LP causes a sudden release of pressure and possible herniation of the brain structures through the foramen magnum. This herniation compresses the brainstem, which contains the vital cardiac, respiratory, and vasomotor centers; and sudden death results. In elective LP preprocedure computed tomography results are reviewed for evidence of brain shift to rule out ICP. Spinal punctures are contraindicated in patients who are suspected of having it.

Abdominal paracentesis involves aspiration of peritoneal fluid from the abdomen. Cytological analysis of the aspirate determines presence of bacteria, blood, glucose, and protein to help diagnose the causes of an abdominal effusion. Paracentesis may also be a palliative measure to provide temporary relief of abdominal and respiratory discomfort caused by severe ascites. Lavage paracentesis, in which a lavage of solution is instilled and then withdrawn, is done to detect the presence of bleeding, as in cases of blunt abdominal trauma or tumor cells when cancer is suspected. Although not contraindicated, paracentesis is performed with caution in patients with coagulopathies, with portal hypertension accompanied by abdominal collateral circulation, and in those who are pregnant. The procedure takes approximately 30 minutes to perform.

TABLE 8.3

Summary of Aspiration Procedures

Aspiration Procedure	Preparation/Assessment Specific to Test	Position and Site	Special Considerations
Bone marrow aspiration	Assess complete blood count for abnormalities.	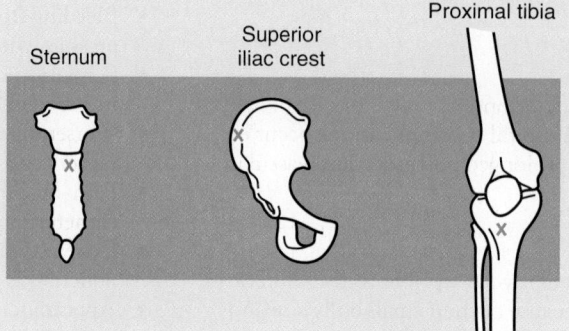 Sternum Superior iliac crest Proximal tibia "X" marks site of aspiration. *(From Ignatavicius DD, Workman ML: Medical-surgical nursing: patient-centered collaborative care, St Louis, ed 6, 2010, Saunders.)* 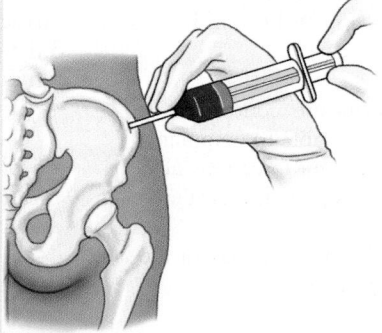 Bone marrow aspiration from the iliac crest. *(From Ignatavicius DD, Workman ML: Medical-surgical nursing: patient-centered collaborative care, St Louis, ed 7, 2013, Saunders.)*	Patients with arthritis or orthopnea may have difficulty assuming the positions. Pressure is applied to the site following procedure.
Lumbar puncture	Assess neurological status, including movement, sensation, and muscle strength of legs to provide a baseline for comparison.	Lateral decubitus position 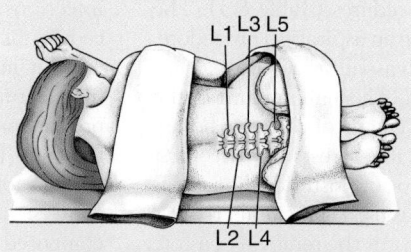 L1 L3 L5 L2 L4 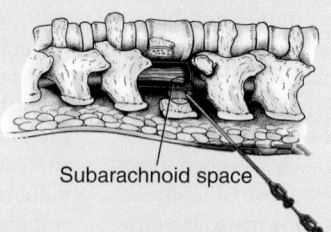 Subarachnoid space *(From Ignatavicius DD, Workman ML: Medical-surgical nursing: patient-centered collaborative care, ed 7, St Louis, 2013, Saunders.)*	*Risk for spinal headache:* Instruct patient to remain flat and logroll according to health care provider's orders. Observe for excessive drainage at site. Fluid loss at site can predispose patient to headache and infection.

TABLE 8.3

Summary of Aspiration Procedures—cont'd

Aspiration Procedure	Preparation/Assessment Specific to Test	Position and Site	Special Considerations
Paracentesis	Assess bladder for distention and determine last voiding. Weigh patient, inspect and palpate abdomen, and measure abdominal girth at largest point. Mark location.	*(From Pagana KD, Pagana TJ: Mosby's manual of diagnostic and laboratory tests, ed 5, St Louis, 2014, Mosby.)*	After fluid is removed, pressure on diaphragm is released, and breathing becomes much easier. *Risk for trauma:* Have patient empty urinary bladder before procedure.
Thoracentesis	Assess respiratory rate and depth, symmetry of chest on inspiration and expiration, cough, and sputum. Help patient remain still during procedure to prevent trauma to visceral pleura. Patient will need to hold breath and avoid coughing during procedure.	Area for needle insertion Ribs Parietal pleura Visceral pleura Lung tissue (parenchyma) Pleural effusion Syringe Diaphragm	Monitor blood pressure for hypotension if large quantity of fluid is removed. *Risk for pneumothorax:* Observe for sudden shortness of breath, tracheal deviation, anxiety, altered vital signs, and decreased oxygen saturation.

Thoracentesis is performed to analyze or remove pleural fluid or instill medications intrapleurally. Cytological studies of specimens reveal presence of blood, glucose, amylase, lactate dehydrogenase (LD), and cellular composition. Cytological specimens are also examined for malignancy, differentiated between transudative and exudative characteristics, and cultured for pathogens. The following cause transudate in the pleural space: ascites, cirrhosis (hepatic), heart failure, hypertension (pulmonary, systemic), nephritis, and nephrosis. Therapeutic thoracentesis relieves pain, dyspnea, and signs of pleural pressure. The test takes approximately 30 minutes to perform.

Delegation and Collaboration

The skill of helping with aspirations can be delegated to nursing assistive personnel (NAP) if the patient is stable (check agency policy). However, assessment of the patient's condition must be completed by the nurse and cannot be delegated. The nurse directs the NAP about:

- Proper positioning of the patient during the procedure.
- When to take and report vital signs.
- Which signs and symptoms experienced by the patient would be of immediate concern.

Equipment

- Personal protective equipment: Masks, goggles, gowns, head cover, sterile gloves for all health care personnel performing the procedure
- Test tubes, sterile specimen containers, laboratory requisitions, and labels
- Analgesia (if ordered)

- Antiseptic solution
- 4 × 4–inch sterile gauze pads, tape, Band-Aid
- Sphygmomanometer, pulse oximeter/end-tidal CO_2 monitor
- Aspiration tray: Most agencies provide trays specific to the aspiration procedure. Standard tray includes antiseptic solution (e.g., povidone-iodine; chlorhexidine); gauze sponges (4 × 4–inch); sterile towels; local anesthetic solution (e.g., lidocaine 1%); two 3-mL sterile syringes with 16- to 27-gauge needles.

Additional Equipment for Specific Aspirations

- Bone marrow aspiration: Two bone marrow needles with inner stylet (Fig. 8.3)
- LP: Manometer to measure spinal pressure and at least four test tubes
- Paracentesis: Intravenous (IV) fluids as ordered, vacuum bottles to collect fluid, stopcock with extension tubing, sterile collection containers, measuring tape
- Thoracentesis: Vacuum bottles to collect fluid, stopcock with extension tubing

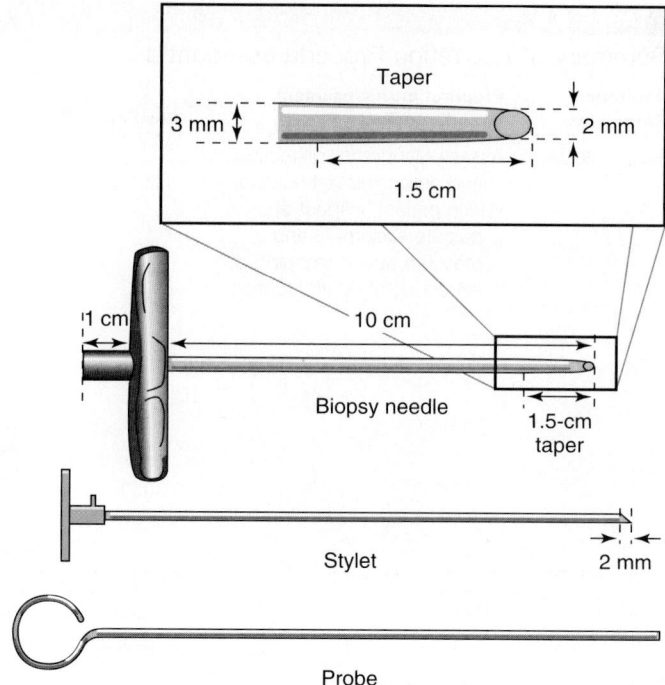

FIG 8.3 Bone marrow biopsy needle showing shape and size. (*From Monahan F et al: Phipps' medical-surgical nursing: health and illness perspectives, ed 8, St Louis, 2007, Mosby.*)

STEP	RATIONALE

ASSESSMENT

1. Identify patient using at least two identifiers (e.g., name and birthday or name and medical record number) according to agency policy. Compare identifiers with information on patient's MAR or medical record.

   Ensures correct patient. Complies with The Joint Commission standards and improves patient safety (TJC, 2016).

2. Verify type of procedure scheduled, purpose, and procedure site with patient and medical record.

   Ensures correct patient and procedure (TJC, 2016).

3. Verify that informed consent was obtained before administering any analgesia or antianxiety agents.

   Federal regulations, many state laws, and accreditation agencies require informed consent for procedures.

4. Review medical record for contraindications.
   a. *Lumbar puncture (LP):* Increased intracranial pressure (ICP), spinal deformities, and clotting disorders.
   b. *Paracentesis:* Clotting disorders, intestinal obstructions, and pregnancy.
   c. *Bone marrow biopsy:* Patient cannot maintain position during procedure.
   d. *Thoracentesis:* Patient cannot maintain position during procedure.

   Factors can cause hemorrhage, and ICP may cause brainstem herniation.
   Paracentesis in pregnant woman may injure fetus.

5. Determine patient's ability to assume position required for procedure and ability to remain still (see Table 8.3). Discuss with health care provider need for premedication for anxious patients.

   Movement during procedure can cause complications such as bleeding and injury to nerves or tissue. Required position depends on site used for aspiration.

6. Before procedure: Obtain vital signs, oxygen saturation (SpO_2)/end-tidal carbon dioxide (CO_2) value, and weight. For paracentesis obtain abdominal girth measurement. (Use ink pen to mark measurement location for abdominal girth measurement.) For LP assess lower extremity movement, sensation, and muscle strength.

   Provides baseline for comparison with vital signs during and after procedure. Patients will have decreased abdominal girth and lose weight after paracentesis.

7. Instruct patient to empty bladder.

   Reduces risk for bladder trauma during paracentesis. Promotes patient comfort.

STEP	RATIONALE
8. Assess patient's coagulation status: use of anticoagulants, complete blood count (CBC), platelet count, clotting factors, activated partial thromboplastin time (aPTT)/international normalized ratio (INR), and prothrombin time (PT).	Invasive procedures are contraindicated in patients with coagulation disorders because of risk for bleeding (Pagana et al., 2015).
9. Determine whether patient is allergic to antiseptic, latex, or anesthetic solutions.	Precautions can be taken to decrease chance of allergic reactions.
10. Assess patient's level of understanding of procedure, including any concerns.	Determines extent of instruction and level of support required.
11. Assess baseline pain level, using scale of 0 to 10.	Determines need for preprocedure analgesia. Pain control helps patients maintain proper position and tolerate aspiration procedure.

NURSING DIAGNOSES

- Acute pain
- Anxiety
- Deficient knowledge regarding procedure

- Fear
- Impaired gas exchange
- Impaired mobility

- Ineffective breathing pattern
- Risk for infection
- Risk for injury

Related factors/Risk factors are individualized based on patient's condition or needs.

PLANNING

1. Expected outcomes following completion of procedure:	
• Patient describes purpose of procedure.	Demonstrates understanding and improves likelihood of cooperation.
• Patient assumes and maintains required position and remains still throughout procedure.	Correct position facilitates safe and timely completion of procedure.
• There is no bleeding at needle insertion site.	Precautions during procedure prevent bleeding.
• Amount of aspirate is sufficient to perform laboratory testing.	
• Patient's level of comfort equals score of 4 or less on pain scale of 0 to 10.	Procedure performed with minimal discomfort to patient.
• Vital signs, SpO$_2$, and end-tidal CO$_2$ remain within normal limits during and after aspiration procedure.	Removal of abdominal (ascites) or pleural fluid increases lung expansion and improves gas exchange.
• Patient undergoing paracentesis has reduced abdominal girth and improved respirations.	Fluid successfully removed from peritoneal space.
2. Explain steps of skin preparation, anesthetic injection, needle insertion, position required.	Anticipation of expected sensations and procedural activities reduces anxiety.
3. If ordered, premedicate for pain 30 minutes before procedure. *Option:* In some cases patients will receive antianxiety medications.	Pain and anxiety control helps patient to remain in position, minimizes discomfort from needle insertion, and decreases anxiety.
4. Before thoracentesis verify recent chest x-ray film examination.	Provides preprocedure baseline to determine location of pleural fluid.

IMPLEMENTATION

1. Perform hand hygiene.	Reduces transmission of microorganisms.
2. Set up sterile tray or open supplies to make accessible for health care provider.	Maintains integrity of sterile field and promotes prompt completion of procedure.
3. Take "time-out" to verify patient's name, type of procedure scheduled, and procedure site with patient and health care team.	"Time-out" verification just before starting procedure includes physician and all personnel and is safety precaution to prevent wrong patient, wrong site, and wrong procedure errors (TJC, 2016).
4. Help patient maintain correct position. Reassure patient while explaining procedure.	Decreases chance of complications occurring during procedure. Explanations increase patient comfort and relaxation.
a. Bone marrow	
• *Adults:* For sternal biopsy place in supine position. For iliac crest biopsy place in prone or lateral recumbent position.	Provides best access to bone containing marrow.

STEP	RATIONALE
• *Children:* For iliac crest biopsy place in prone or lateral recumbent position.	
b. LP Position in lateral recumbent (fetal) position with head and neck flexed (see Table 8.3).	Provides full curvature and flexion of spinal column to allow maximal space between vertebrae.
c. Paracentesis Position in bed in semi-Fowler's position or sitting upright on side of bed or in chair with feet supported (see Table 8.3).	Position uses gravity to cause fluid to accumulate in lower abdominal cavity, where it is drained more easily.
d. Thoracentesis Place in orthopneic position (upright position with arms and shoulders raised and supported on padded over-bed table) (see Table 8.3). If patient is unable to tolerate, help to side-lying position with affected lung positioned upward.	Expands intercostal space for needle insertions.

Clinical Decision Point *Emphasize the importance of remaining immobile during procedure to prevent trauma, especially with the LP. Sudden movement is a risk for spinal cord nerve root damage. Sudden movement during paracentesis or thoracentesis risks damage of the abdominal or pulmonary structures. Also instruct patient not to cough, sneeze, or breathe deeply during the procedures because these actions increase the risk for needle displacement and damage of other structures.*

STEP	RATIONALE
5. Explain to patient that pain may occur when lidocaine (local anesthetic) is injected into tissues. Pressure may also occur when tissue or fluid is aspirated.	Aspiration is painful but lasts for only a few moments. If patient is having bone marrow aspirate, deep pressure feeling is frequently experienced as bone marrow is withdrawn (Pagana et al., 2015).
6. Physician applies sterile gloves, mask, gown, and goggles; cleans patient's skin with antiseptic solution; and drapes site with sterile drape.	Removes surface bacteria from skin at area of puncture site. Creates sterile field.
7. Physician injects local anesthetic and allows time for anesthesia to occur.	Provides optimal effect of local anesthesia.
8. Physician inserts needle or trocar into spinal space or body cavity involved (see Table 8.3). To aspirate tissue or body fluids for specimen analysis, syringe is attached to trocar or needle, and aspirate is placed into specimen container.	Success depends on positioning, accurate insertion site, and patient remaining still.
9. Nurse assesses patient's condition during procedure, including respiratory status, vital signs if indicated, and any complaints of pain.	Identifies any changes that indicate complication.

Clinical Decision Point *Increased or worsening abdominal or thoracic pain is significant in paracentesis and thoracentesis. Severe abdominal pain indicates a possible bowel perforation following a paracentesis. Following a thoracentesis abdominal pain results from diaphragmatic, liver, or spleen perforation. Inspiratory chest pain results from perforation of the lung.*

STEP	RATIONALE
10. Note characteristics of aspirate:	
a. *Bone marrow aspirate:* Marrow may appear red or yellow.	Normal marrow.
b. *LP:* Record opening pressure; observe fluid for color, cloudiness, or blood.	Normal CSF is clear and colorless. Cloudiness is result of protein, which indicates an infection.
c. *Paracentesis:* Fluid may appear yellow, cloudy, bile-stained green, or blood tinged. Peritoneal lavage fluid may appear bright red.	Blood-tinged fluid is caused by traumatic tap. In patient with abdominal trauma bloody lavage identifies active bleeding.
d. *Thoracentesis:* Pleural fluid may appear clear yellow, puslike, or cloudy.	Clear yellow is normal. Transudate and exudates are typically yellow, straw color. Blood-tinged fluid indicates malignancy, pulmonary infarction, or severe inflammation. Puslike fluid indicates infection (empyema); milky fluid indicates chylothorax (i.e., leak from thoracic duct resulting in lymphatic drainage in pleural cavity).
11. Properly label specimens in presence of patient and transport to laboratory in proper containers. Label specimens in order of collection.	Ensures that correct laboratory results are assigned to right patient. Test tubes are numbered in sequence of collection (e.g., 1 through 4).

STEP	RATIONALE
12. Physician removes needle/trocar and applies pressure over insertion site until drainage ceases. If necessary, help with direct pressure and application of gauze dressing.	Helps in homeostasis and secures insertion site.
13. All health care team members in procedure remove protective equipment, discard in appropriate receptacle, and perform hand hygiene.	Reduces transmission of infection.

EVALUATION

1. Monitor level of consciousness, vital signs, and SpO_2/end-tidal CO_2. Check agency policy; sometimes vital signs are obtained every 15 minutes for 2 hours.	Verifies patient's physiological status in response to procedure or any potential complications.
2. Inspect dressing over puncture site for bleeding, swelling, tenderness, and erythema. Inspect area under patient for bleeding. Avoid disrupting healing clot at site if pressure dressing is present.	Determines further blood loss from puncture site. Infection is potential complication, especially if patient is leukopenic (Pagana et al., 2015).
3. Evaluate pain score to determine if patient's level of comfort is equivalent to a score of 4 or less on pain scale of 0 to 10.	Determines if patient is having increased pain to warrant postprocedure analgesia.
4. Following paracentesis, measure abdominal girth and respirations and compare to preprocedure measurements.	Determines amount of change in abdominal size and ability to ventilate.
5. **Use Teach-Back:** "I want to be sure that I explained what to expect regarding how you may feel after this procedure. Tell me what you know about what to expect." Revise your instruction now or develop a plan for revised patient or family caregiver teaching if patient or family caregiver is not able to teach back correctly.	Demonstrates patient's and family caregiver's level of understanding of instructional topic.

Unexpected Outcomes
1. Oversedation occurs.
2. Site complications occur:
   a. *Bone marrow:* Tenderness or erythema at site.

   b. *LP:*
      (1) Postprocedure headache (PPH) is evidenced by headache, blurred vision, and tinnitus.

      (2) Excess loss of CSF is indicated by decreased level of consciousness, hearing loss, dilated pupils, and decreased ICP.
   c. *Paracentesis:* Leakage of fluid from site and acute abdominal pain occur.

   d. *Thoracentesis:* Pneumothorax is evidenced by sudden dyspnea, tachypnea, and asymmetrical chest excursion.

Related Interventions
- See Skill 8.1.
- Notify health care provider and obtain further orders.
- Administer analgesic as ordered.
- Continue to monitor site.

- Monitor fluid loss.
- Physician may inject blood patch into epidural space.
- Medicate for pain as ordered.
- Maintain airway.
- Transfer to intensive care unit (ICU) per physician order.
- Reinforce dressing; may also be instructed to place sterile collection bag over site.
- Monitor vital signs and SpO_2.
- Assess abdomen for bowel sounds.
- Administer oxygen.
- Monitor vital signs and SpO_2.
- Anticipate chest x-ray film examination and possible chest tube insertion.

Recording and Reporting

- Record name of procedure; preprocedure preparation; location of puncture site; amount, consistency, and color of fluid drained or specimen obtained; duration of procedure; patient's tolerance (e.g., vital signs, SpO_2) and comfort level; laboratory tests ordered and specimen sent; type of dressing; postprocedure activities (e.g., chest x-ray film examination); and other procedure-specific assessments (e.g., extremity assessment, abdominal girth, level of consciousness) in nurses' notes in electronic health record (EHR) or chart.

- Immediately report to health care provider any change in vital signs and SpO_2, unexpected pain/discomfort, and any excessive drainage from dressing over puncture site.
- Document your evaluation of patient and family caregiver learning.

Special Considerations
Teaching
- Instruct patient that some people experience tenderness at the puncture site for several days after the study and that mild analgesia often helps to relieve some of the discomfort.

Pediatric

- Conscious or unconscious sedation is commonly used. If using unconscious sedation, an anesthesiologist or nurse anesthetist is needed for the procedure.
- Prepare preschool children before the procedure; make a game out of having child recall the next procedural step, which can serve as a distraction (Hockenberry and Wilson, 2015).

Gerontological

- Older adults with arthritis need help to stay in the required position.

- Older adults have reduced elastic lung recoil, weaker cough efficiency, and decreased chest expansion. Restlessness may indicate hypoxia following thoracentesis.
- Be aware that older adults may have specific fears and anxiety related to postprocedure falling and fatigue.

Home Care

- Teach patients and family caregivers about specific postprocedure complications and when to report them to the health care provider.
- If patient is transferred to long-term care facility, ensure thorough communication between agencies regarding results of procedure and patient condition.

◆ SKILL 8.4   Care of a Patient Undergoing Bronchoscopy

Bronchoscopy is the examination of the tracheobronchial tree through a lighted tube containing mirrors. A flexible fiberoptic bronchoscope has lumens that allow both visualization and simultaneous administration of oxygen (Fig. 8.4). The fiberoptic bronchoscope is used for obtaining sputum, foreign bodies, and biopsy specimens. Laser ablation of endotracheal lesions may also be performed through the bronchoscope.

Bronchoscopy may be an emergency or elective procedure and may be performed for diagnostic or therapeutic reasons. The main purposes of this procedure include aspirating excessive sputum or

mucus plugs that airway suctioning cannot remove; visualizing the tracheobronchial tree for assessment of abnormalities of the mucosa, abscesses, aspiration pneumonia, strictures, and tumors; obtaining deep-tissue biopsy and sputum specimens; and/or removing foreign bodies. This procedure is contraindicated in patients who cannot tolerate interruption of high-flow oxygen unless intubated. Potential complications of bronchoscopy include fever, infection, hypoxemia, bronchospasm and/or laryngospasm, pneumothorax, aspiration, dysrhythmias and hypotension, hemorrhage (after biopsy), and cardiac arrest (Kar et al., 2015).

The procedure is performed at the bedside or in a specially equipped endoscopy room. Usually a pulmonary specialist or surgeon performs it in approximately 30 to 45 minutes.

Delegation and Collaboration

The skill of helping with a bronchoscopy cannot be delegated to nursing assistive personnel (NAP). The nurse directs the NAP to:

- Measure follow-up postprocedure vital signs (after nurse's RN's initial assessment).
- Help position the patient appropriately (based on procedure and patient limitations).
- Immediately report to the nurse if patient has possible respiratory distress or is coughing up blood after the procedure.

Equipment

- Personal protective equipment: Mask, gown, gloves, head cover, and goggles for all health care providers
- Bronchoscopy tray, if available from central supply, which includes flexible fiberoptic bronchoscope (see Fig. 8.4); 4 × 4–inch gauze sponges; local anesthetic spray (lidocaine); sterile tracheal suction catheters; diazepam, midazolam, or other sedative for intravenous (IV) sedation
- Oxygen, resuscitative equipment
- Pulse oximeter/end-tidal carbon dioxide (CO_2) monitor, cardiac monitor
- Sterile gloves
- Sterile water-soluble lubricating jelly (**NOTE:** Petroleum-based lubricants are not used because of the hazard of aspiration and subsequent pneumonia.)
- Emesis basin
- Suction machine and connecting tube
- Blood pressure equipment

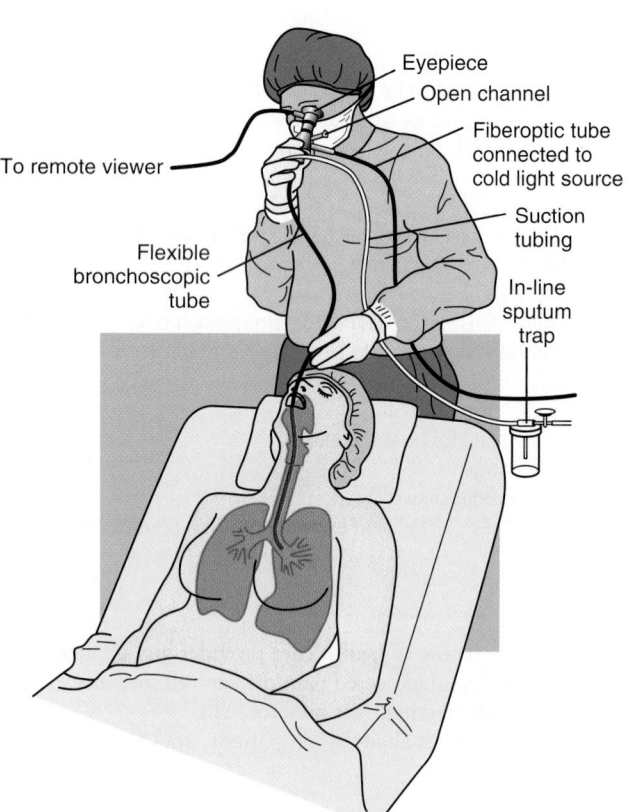

FIG 8.4 Flexible fiberoptic bronchoscopy.

STEP	RATIONALE

ASSESSMENT

1. Identify patient using at least two identifiers (e.g., name and birthday or name and medical record number) according to agency policy. Compare identifiers with information on patient's MAR or medical record.

Ensures correct patient. Complies with The Joint Commission standards and improves patient safety (TJC, 2016).

2. Verify type of procedure scheduled and procedure site with patient.

Ensures procedure and correct patient. Complies with The Joint Commission standards and improves patient safety (TJC, 2016).

3. Verify that informed consent was obtained before administration of any sedatives.

Federal regulations, many state laws, and accreditation agencies such as The Joint Commission require informed consent for procedure.

4. Assess patient's history for inability to tolerate interruption of high-flow oxygen unless intubated.

Determines need for oxygen administration during procedure.

5. Obtain baseline vital signs, pulse oximetry (SpO_2) and end-tidal CO_2 values.

Baseline data provide for comparison with findings during and after procedure.

6. Assess type of cough, sputum produced, heart and lung sounds.

Provides for comparison with respiratory status during and after procedure.

7. Determine purpose of procedure: for sputum aspiration, assessment, tissue biopsy, or removal of foreign body.

Anticipates equipment needs of physician and type of information to convey to patient during teaching.

8. Determine whether patient is allergic to local anesthetic used for spraying throat (usually lidocaine).

Allergy causes laryngeal edema or laryngospasm.

9. Assess need for preprocedure medication (usually atropine and opioid or sedative).

Atropine decreases secretions and inhibits vagally stimulated bradycardia; opioids or sedatives relieve anxiety and decrease discomfort.

10. Assess time patient last ingested food/fluids or medications. Patient must be NPO for at least 8 hours before a bronchoscopy; however, some medications may be taken before procedure by physician order.

Reduces risk for aspiration.

11. Assess patient's level of understanding of procedure, including any concerns.

Determines extent of instruction and level of support required.

NURSING DIAGNOSIS

- Anxiety
- Deficient knowledge regarding procedure
- Fear

- Impaired gas exchange
- Ineffective airway clearance
- Ineffective breathing pattern

- Risk for aspiration
- Risk for infection
- Risk for injury

Related factors/Risk factors are individualized based on patient's condition or needs.

PLANNING

1. Expected outcomes following completion of procedure:
- Patient recovers from sedation without respiratory complications or change in level of consciousness.

Sedation adequate, and patient tolerates procedure.

- Patient's level of comfort is equivalent to score of 4 or less on pain scale of 0 to 10.

Minimal trauma caused by bronchoscope.

- Physician is able to observe, suction, and obtain specimens from tracheobronchial tree.

Indicates that purpose of procedure was achieved.

- Patient explains procedure and assumes appropriate position.

Demonstrates patient's understanding.

2. Administer atropine, opioid, or antianxiety agent 30 minutes before procedure.

Ensures that medication takes effect before procedure.

3. Explain procedure to patient.

Reduces anxiety and increases cooperation.

4. Remove and safely store patient's dentures and/or eyeglasses.

Minimizes chance of airway obstruction.

STEP	RATIONALE

IMPLEMENTATION

1. Assess current IV access or establish new IV access with large-bore cannula (see Chapter 29).

   Provides immediate access for IV fluids or medications if emergency occurs.

2. Help patient assume position desired by physician: usually semi-Fowler's.

   Provides maximal visualization of lower airway and adequate lung expansion.

3. Take "time-out" to verify patient's name, type of procedure scheduled, and procedure site with patient and health care team.

   "Time-out" verification just before starting procedure includes physician and all personnel and is safety precaution to prevent wrong patient, wrong site, and wrong procedure errors (TJC, 2016).

4. Perform hand hygiene and apply protective equipment. Position tip of suction catheter for easy access to patient's mouth.

   Reduces transmission of microorganisms. Removes secretions to reduce risk for aspiration.

5. Physician usually sprays nasopharynx and oropharynx with topical anesthetic. Lidocaine is commonly used 10 to 15 minutes before procedure. When a patient is intubated or has tracheostomy, anesthetic spray is usually not needed.

   Provides swift anesthesia of oropharynx.

6. Instruct patient not to swallow local anesthetic; provide emesis basin for expectorating it.

   Reduces unintended anesthesia of esophagus.

7. Another physician or staff member attaches bronchoscope to machine light source.

   Enhances visualization during procedure.

8. Physician applies goggles, mask, and sterile gloves; introduces bronchoscope into mouth to pharynx; passes through glottis and into trachea and bronchi (see Fig. 8.4). More anesthetic spray may be used at glottis to prevent cough reflex. For intubated patients flexible bronchoscope is introduced through their endotracheal tube.

   Bronchoscope must be passed through upper airway structures to promote visualization of lower airways. Trachea and bronchi are observed for lesions and obstructions. Adaptor accompanies bronchoscope and is used for bag-valve mask or ventilator use.

9. Physician suctions mucus and performs bronchial washing with cytological specimens taken with wire brush or curette. Biopsy specimens may also be obtained.

   Cytological specimens are obtained to diagnose carcinoma.

10. Help patient through procedure by providing explanations, verbal reassurance, and support.

    Although premedicated and drowsy, remind patient not to change position and to cooperate. Reinforce that patient will be able to breathe during procedure.

11. Assess patient's pulse, blood pressure, respirations, SpO_2, end-tidal CO_2, and breathing capacity during procedure; observe degree of restlessness, capillary refill, and color of nail beds.

    Bronchoscope can cause feelings of suffocation and vasovagal response and laryngospasm. Because airway is partially occluded, patient can develop hypoxia during procedure.

12. Note characteristics of suctioned material. Expect small amount of blood mixed with aspirate because of tissue trauma.

    Information used to record and report and make further patient observations.

13. Using gloved hand, wipe patient's mouth and nose to remove lubricant after bronchoscope is removed.

    Promotes hygiene and comfort.

14. Instruct patient not to eat or drink until tracheobronchial anesthesia has worn off and gag reflex has returned, usually in 2 hours. Use tongue depressor to touch pharynx to test for presence of gag reflex.

    Prevents aspiration.

15. Remove protective equipment, discard, and perform hand hygiene.

    Reduces transmission of microorganisms.

EVALUATION

1. Monitor vital signs, SpO_2, and end-tidal CO_2.

   Verifies physiological response to procedure.

2. Observe character and amount of sputum. Physician may order serial sputum collection for 24 hours for cytological examination.

   Evaluates for complication of bronchial perforation, indicated by severe hemoptysis.
   Slight blood-tinged sputum is normal after this procedure.

3. Observe respiratory status closely; palpate for facial or neck crepitus.

   Detects early sign of bronchial or esophageal perforation.

STEP	RATIONALE
4. Assess for return of gag reflex. It usually returns in approximately 2 hours.	Helps prevent aspiration pneumonia, which is risk until gag reflex returns.
5. **Use Teach-Back:** "I want to be sure I explained what are considered postprocedure normal and abnormal symptoms. Tell me what you know about these symptoms." Revise your instruction now or develop a plan for revised patient or family caregiver teaching if patient or family caregiver is not able to teach back correctly.	Demonstrates patient's and family caregiver's level of understanding of instructional topic.

Unexpected Outcomes	Related Interventions
1. Vasovagal response caused by stimulation of baroreceptors during bronchoscope insertion, causing symptoms of: • Feeling nauseous, faint, dizzy, and/or light-headed. • Diaphoresis with slow, steady pulse. • Unconsciousness for few seconds.	• Lower head of table. • Continue vital signs monitoring. • Lower head of table. • Support airway (positioning/suctioning).
2. Laryngospasm and bronchospasm as evidenced by: • Sudden, severe shortness of breath.	• Call physician immediately. • Support airway (positioning). • Prepare emergency resuscitation equipment. • Anticipate possible cricothyrotomy.
3. Hypoxemia as evidenced by: • Gradual shortness of breath. • Decreasing level of consciousness.	• Monitor SpO$_2$. • Maintain airway and breathing. Notify physician immediately.
4. Hemorrhage as evidenced by: • Acute blood loss • Hypotension and tachycardia • Decreasing level of consciousness	• Notify physician immediately. • Monitor vital signs. • Be prepared to administer IV fluids.
5. Oversedation	• See Skill 8.1.

Recording and Reporting

- Record procedure(s) performed (e.g., biopsy); character of sputum; duration of procedure, patient's tolerance and, if any, complications; and the collection and disposition of specimen(s) in nurses' notes in electronic health record (EHR) or chart. Document time of gag reflex return.
- Report bleeding or respiratory distress following the procedure or any changes in vital signs beyond patient's normal limits to physician immediately. Report results of procedure to appropriate health care personnel.
- Document your evaluation of patient and family caregiver learning.

Special Considerations
Teaching
- Before the procedure instruct patient to perform good mouth care to decrease risk for introducing bacteria into lungs during the procedure.
- In some cases patients may receive IV sedation (see Skill 8.1, Teaching Considerations).
- If ordered, teach patient how to perform controlled coughing techniques for obtaining serial sputum samples (see Chapter 7).

Pediatric
- In children the procedure is most frequently performed under general anesthesia to remove foreign bodies from the larynx or

trachea. Follow-up care after the foreign body is removed includes chest physiotherapy, monitoring for respiratory distress, and education of parents.
- Children are at higher risk for hypoxemia than adults because their bronchus is smaller and the bronchoscope decreases the available breathing space (Pagana et al., 2015).

Gerontological
- Physical exposure and room temperature contribute to hypothermia in frail older adults who are unable to communicate that they are cold. Use warmed blankets or forced-air heat to maintain core temperature at comfortable, safe levels (Lewis et al., 2017).
- Postprocedure restlessness often indicates hypoxemia or pain. Thoroughly assess pulmonary capacity before administering opioids, which may depress the respiratory centers.

Home Care
- Instruct ambulatory care patients to notify the physician if the following symptoms develop: fever, chest pain or discomfort, dyspnea, wheezing, or hemoptysis.
- Throat discomfort is managed with throat lozenges or warm saline gargles.

◆ **SKILL 8.5** **Care of a Patient Undergoing Endoscopy**

Endoscopy allows direct visualization of an internal organ or structure by means of a long, flexible fiberoptic scope. The tip of the scope has a light source and camera lens that allows visualization of the lining of the gastrointestinal (GI) structures on a large display screen (Fig. 8.5A–C). For visualization of the upper GI tract, esophagoscopy, gastroscopy, gastroduodenojejunoscopy (GDJ), or duodenoscopy is performed; or more frequently esophagogastroduodenoscopy (EGD), which permits visualization of the esophagus, stomach (Fig. 8.6), and duodenum in one examination. Besides direct observation, endoscopy enables biopsy of suspicious tissue, polyp removal, and performance of many other procedures such as direct visual guidance for fine-needle aspiration biopsies and dilation and stenting of strictures. For visualization of the hepatobiliary tree and pancreatic ducts, an endoscopic retrograde cholangiopancreatography (ERCP) is performed. For visual examination of the lower GI tract, proctoscopy, sigmoidoscopy, or colonoscopy is performed. Typically these patients receive intravenous (IV) moderate sedation.

Risks of endoscopic procedures include intestinal perforation, hemorrhage, peritonitis, aspiration, respiratory depression, and/or myocardial infarction secondary to vasovagal response. Both upper and lower GI endoscopic examinations may be performed in a specially equipped endoscopic unit or at the patient's bedside.

Delegation and Collaboration

The skill of helping with endoscopy cannot be delegated to nursing assistive personnel (NAP). The nurse directs the NAP about:
• How to help with patient positioning.

Equipment

• Personal protective equipment: Mask, gown, gloves, head cover, goggles for all health care personnel
• Endoscopy tray
• Fiberoptic endoscope and camera
• Solutions for biopsy specimens
• Local anesthetic spray
• Tracheal suction equipment (see Chapter 25)
• Blood pressure equipment
• Sterile water-soluble jelly
• Sterile gloves for physician

• Emesis basin
• IV fluid and equipment for IV start (*optional*)
• Diazepam, midazolam, or other sedative for IV sedation (*optional*)
• Sedative reversal agents
• Carbon dioxide source to inflate colon (for lower GI procedures)
• Oxygen, resuscitative equipment, SpO$_2$/end-tidal carbon dioxide (CO$_2$) monitor

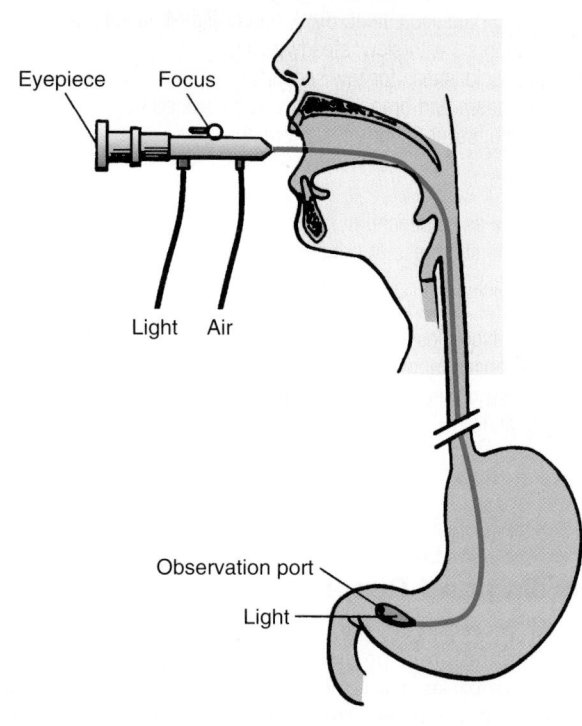

FIG 8.6 Stomach may be visualized by means of a fiberscope. (*From Ignatavicius DD, Workman ML: Medical-surgical nursing: patient-centered collaborative care, St Louis, ed 6, 2010, Saunders.*)

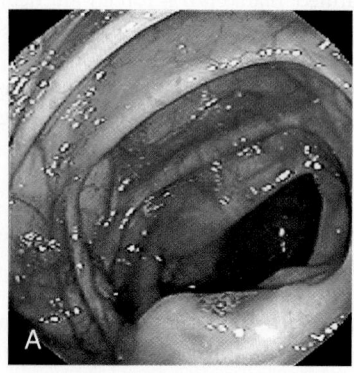
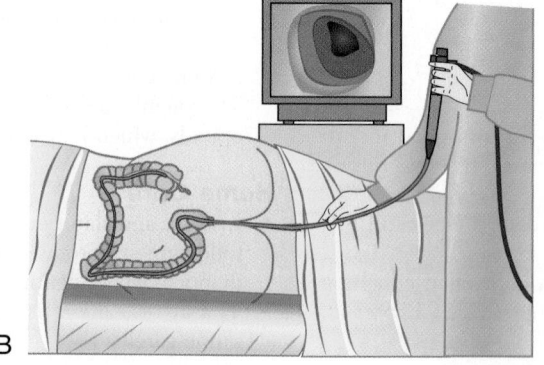
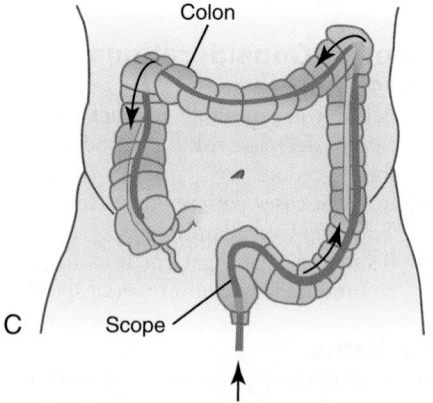

FIG 8.5 A, Scope view of healthy colon. **B,** Overview of colonoscopy process. **C,** Path of scope through colon.

STEP	RATIONALE

ASSESSMENT

1. Identify patient using at least two identifiers (e.g., name and birthday or name and medical record number) according to agency policy. Compare identifiers with information in patient's MAR or medical record.

Ensures correct patient. Complies with The Joint Commission standards and improves patient safety (TJC, 2016).

2. Verify type of procedure scheduled and procedure site with patient.

Ensures correct procedure and patient. Complies with The Joint Commission standards and improves patient safety (TJC, 2016).

3. Verify that informed consent was obtained before administering sedation.

Federal regulations, many state laws, and accreditation agencies such as The Joint Commission require informed consent for procedure.

4. Determine if GI bleeding is present. Observe character of emesis, stool, and nasogastric (NG) tube drainage for frank blood or material that looks like coffee grounds.

Test is contraindicated in patients with severe upper GI bleeding because viewing lens becomes covered with blood clots, preventing visualization (Pagana and Pagana, 2014).

5. Obtain vital signs and SpO_2/end-tidal CO_2 values.

Baseline data provide for comparison with findings during and after procedure.

Clinical Decision Point *If patient is bleeding actively, physician may order lavage of the stomach and aspiration to clear clots before procedure is attempted.*

---

6. Determine purpose of procedure: biopsy, examination, or coagulation of bleeding sites.

Anticipates appropriate equipment needs.

7. Verify that patient was NPO for at least 8 hours for endoscopy of upper GI tract.

Introduction of endoscope increases risk for vomiting resulting from stimulation of gag reflex. Empty stomach reduces risk for aspiration of stomach contents.

8. For lower GI studies (proctoscopy, sigmoidoscopy, or colonoscopy), verify that patient followed clear liquid diet for 2 days and has completed any ordered bowel-cleansing regimen.

An empty intestinal tract promotes endoscopic insertion and clear visualization of interior walls.

9. Assess patient's level of understanding and previous experience with procedure, including any concerns.

Determines extent of instruction and level of support required.

NURSING DIAGNOSES

- Anxiety
- Deficient knowledge regarding procedure
- Fear
- Impaired gas exchange
- Ineffective breathing pattern
- Risk for aspiration
- Risk for infection
- Risk for injury

Related factors/Risk factors are individualized based on patient's condition or needs.

PLANNING

1. Expected outcomes following completion of procedure:
   - Patient does not aspirate and has no postprocedure bleeding.

   Indicates absence of complications and tolerance of procedure.

   - Patient's level of comfort is equivalent to score of 4 or less on pain scale of 0 to 10.

   Provides reliable detection of increasing pain so postprocedure analgesia is given.

   - Patient is without respiratory complications or change in level of consciousness.

   Recovers from sedation.

   - Patient describes purposes and steps of procedure.

   Documents patient understanding.

2. Prepare patient:
   a. Explain steps of procedure, including sensations to expect.

   Relieves anxiety and answers patient's questions.

   b. Administer pain medication or preprocedure medication.

   Promotes relaxation and reduces anxiety.

IMPLEMENTATION

1. Perform hand hygiene and apply protective equipment.

Reduces transmission of microorganisms.

2. Remove patient's eyeglasses, dentures, or other dental appliances.

Prevents damage to eyeglasses or damage/dislodgement of dental structures during intubation phase.

STEP	RATIONALE
3. Take "time-out" to verify patient's name, type of procedure scheduled, and procedure site with patient and health care team.	"Time-out" verification just before starting procedure includes physician and all personnel and is safety precaution to prevent wrong patient, wrong site, and wrong procedure errors (TJC, 2016)
4. Ensure that IV line is patent and administer IV sedation as ordered (see Skill 8.1).	Provides route for emergency medications and creates immediate conscious sedation.
5. Help patient assume proper position for procedure and apply appropriate drape.	Improves efficiency of procedure and ability of physician to visualize site. Drape provides comfort and minimizes exposure.
a. *Upper GI procedures:* Help patient maintain left lateral Sims' position.	Sims' position allows easy passage of upper or lower endoscope. Provides airway clearance if patient gags and vomits gastric contents.
b. *Lower GI procedures:* Help patient maintain left lateral decubitus position. Drape patient for privacy.	Left lateral decubitus position provides access to lower GI tract.
6. Physician performs hand hygiene and puts on protective equipment.	Reduces transmission of microorganisms.
7. **Upper GI procedures:**	
a. Help physician spray nasopharynx and oropharynx with local anesthetic.	Topical anesthetic decreases gag reflex caused by passage of endoscope, thus improving safety and comfort.
b. Administer atropine if ordered.	Reduces quantity of secretions, therefore reducing risk for aspiration.
c. Position tip of suction cannula for easy access in patient's mouth.	Drains oral secretions to reduce risk for aspiration.
8. **Lower GI procedures:**	
a. Prepare lubricant for fiberoptic endoscope.	Facilitates passage of tubing.
9. Physician slowly passes endoscope into mouth or through anus to view esophagus, stomach, colon, or rectum and advances to desired depth while visualizing lining of structures.	Provides visualization of all structures to detect polyps, cancerous lesions, or areas of inflammation and stricture.
10. Physician insufflates air through endoscope into upper GI tract or carbon dioxide into lower GI tract in case of colonoscopy.	Distends GI structures for better visualization. Carbon dioxide insufflation produces less postprocedure abdominal cramping than air insufflation because it is more readily absorbed.
11. Help patient throughout procedure.	
a. Anticipate needs and promote comfort.	Patient is unable to speak after tube is passed into throat.
b. Tell patient what is happening as each part of procedure is carried out (e.g., abdominal cramping).	Reassures patient about procedure and how long it will last.
c. For upper GI procedures, suction if there are excessive oral secretions or vomitus.	Prevents aspiration of oral secretions or gastric contents.
12. Place tissue specimens in proper laboratory containers or on proper slides. Seal as needed. Date, time, and initial all specimen containers before sending to laboratory.	Ensures proper specimen preservation and labeling and preparation of specimens for microscopic examination.
13. Help patient return to comfortable position.	Promotes relaxation.
14. Help to dispose of equipment and perform hand hygiene.	Reduces transmission of infection.
15. In recovery, after sedation resolves, inform patient not to eat or drink until gag reflex returns.	Reduces risk for aspiration.

EVALUATION

1. Monitor vital signs and oxygen saturation according to agency policy, which can be every 15 minutes for 2 hours.	Change in vital signs may indicate new bleeding in GI tract or oversedation.
2. Assess for levels of sedation and consciousness (see Skill 8.1).	Determines patient's response to IV sedation.
3. Ask patient to describe level of comfort using pain scale of 0 to 10. Observe for pain.	Monitors for sudden abdominal pain, which can indicate rupture of abdominal organs.
4. Evaluate emesis or aspirate for frank or occult blood (see Chapter 7).	Monitors for GI bleeding.
5. Assess for return of gag reflex, usually in 2 to 4 hours. Provide oral hygiene when gag reflex returns.	Determines when effects of anesthetic have disappeared. Gag reflex prevents aspiration.

STEP	RATIONALE
6. **Use Teach-Back:** "I want to be sure I explained the postprocedure diet and activity limitations. Tell me what you know about postprocedure dietary and activity limitations." Revise your instruction now or develop a plan for revised patient or family caregiver teaching if patient or family caregiver is not able to teach back correctly.	Determines patient's and family caregiver's level of understanding of instructional topic.

Unexpected Outcomes	Related Interventions

1. Vasovagal response caused by stimulation of baroreceptors during endoscope insertion as evidenced by:
  • Feeling nauseous, faint, dizzy, and/or light-headed.
  • Diaphoresis with slow, steady pulse.
  • Few seconds of unconsciousness.
	• Lower head of table.
	• Support airway.

2. For upper GI procedures: Laryngospasm and bronchospasm as evidenced by: • Sudden, severe shortness of breath.	• Call physician immediately. • Support airway (positioning). • Prepare emergency resuscitation equipment. • Anticipate possible cricothyrotomy.

3. For upper GI procedures: Hypoxemia as evidenced by:
  • Gradual shortness of breath.
  • Decreasing level of consciousness.
	• Monitor SpO$_2$.
	• Maintain airway and breathing.
	• Notify physician immediately.

4. Pulmonary aspiration as evidenced by: • Dyspnea, tachypnea, decreasing levels of oxygen saturation.	• Support airway. • Follow specific postprocedural orders related to findings. • Monitor oxygen saturation.
5. Abdominal pain, fever, or bleeding, indicating damage to intestinal wall.	• Continue to monitor vital signs. • Notify physician of findings.
6. Oversedation with decreasing level of consciousness.	• See Skill 8.1.

Recording and Reporting

- Record the procedure, duration, patient's tolerance, complications and interventions, and collection and disposition of specimen in nurses notes' electronic health record (EHR) or chart.
- Report onset of bleeding, abdominal pain, dyspnea, and vital sign changes to physician.
- Document your evaluation of patient and family caregiver learning.

Special Considerations
Teaching

- Upper GI endoscopy:
  - Explain method for endoscope insertion. Prepare patient for a slight feeling of not being able to breathe. Assure him or her that this feeling is common but that air is delivered through the endoscope and suffocation will not occur.
  - Teach patient simple hand signals for pain or discomfort because he or she will not be able to speak after the endoscope is positioned in the esophagus.
- Lower GI procedures (colonoscopy, sigmoidoscopy, proctoscopy):
  - Explain that it is normal to experience increased flatus and abdominal cramping.
  - Small amounts of blood in the stool are common if a biopsy was taken.

Pediatric

- Introduction of the endoscope in infants and small children who have a narrow and collapsible airway may result in respiratory distress.

Gerontological

- Older adults frequently have reduced drug clearance from decreased glomerular filtration rate (GFR) and nephron activity or decreased hepatic function. It is important to monitor the effects of medications given to older adults (Brenes-Salazar et al., 2015).
- Because of age-related changes in older adults, the gastric mucosa is thinner, which increases the incidence of irritation, ulceration, and perforation (Brenes-Salazar et al., 2015).
- Physical exposure and room temperature contribute to hypothermia in frail older adults who are unable to communicate that they are cold. Use warmed blankets or forced-air heat to maintain core temperature at comfortable, safe levels (Lewis et al., 2017).
- Some older adults experience dehydration, electrolyte imbalance, and exhaustion from pretest preparation. If the procedure is done on an ambulatory care basis, it is helpful to have someone stay with the patient for at least 24 hours.

Home Care

- Explain that patient might have hoarseness or a sore throat after an upper GI procedure. Patient can have ice chips or anesthetic lozenges after gag reflex returns.
- Instruct patient or family caregiver to notify physician if patient has a fever, abdominal pain, rigid abdomen, and rectal bleeding or stool in blood.

◆ CLINICAL DEBRIEF

A 67-year-old African-American is a retired executive. He lives with his wife and son in a single-family home and has recently experienced what he describes as "mild discomfort" in his chest when he exercises. He is scheduled for a cardiac catheterization under moderate sedation. Currently he is taking warfarin. The order for the procedure faxed from the health care provider's office lists "new-onset chest pain" as the clinical indication for the procedure.

1. Which laboratory data would you review as part of your preparation of for his procedure?

2. He has arrived in the waiting area of the catheterization laboratory; you are the nurse assigned to this case. Describe the steps you would take to perform patient verification safety procedures for the patient.

3. The patient's cardiac catheterization procedure is finished, and he is now in the recovery area. The right femoral site was used for catheter insertion. Using SBAR, show how you would communicate with the health care team about this patient.

◆ REVIEW QUESTIONS

1. Place the steps listed here in the correct order for helping a patient who is undergoing a lumbar puncture.
   1. Help patient maintain lateral recumbent position with head and neck flexed.
   2. Properly label specimen in presence of patient.
   3. Assess patient's condition during procedure.
   4. Take "time-out" to verify patient's name, type of procedure scheduled, and procedure site.
   5. Explain to patient that pain may occur when lidocaine (local anesthetic) is injected into the site.
   6. Record the opening intracranial pressure; observe fluid for color.

2. A patient underwent a bronchoscopy and is now entering the recovery area. The patient develops sudden, severe shortness of breath. You should take which of the following sets of actions? (Select all that apply.)
   1. Support the patient's airway and monitor SpO_2.
   2. Call physician immediately and prepare for possible resuscitation.
   3. Measure vital signs and ensure that the patient has patent intravenous (IV) access.
   4. Observe for blood-tinged mucus and suction airway.
   5. Anticipate the need for a possible cricothyrotomy

3. Which patients would be unable to undergo an angiogram? (Select all that apply.)
   1. 44-year-old female who is taking warfarin
   2. 52-year-old male suspected of having an abdominal aneurysm
   3. 77-year-old female suspected of having an arterial occlusion of the renal artery
   4. 65-year-old female who actually is 30 weeks' pregnant
   5. 36-year-old male who has a history of uncontrolled hypertension

ⓔ *Visit the Evolve site for a complete list of Clinical Debrief and Review Questions answers.*

REFERENCES

Abdollahi AA, et al: Effect of positioning and early ambulation on coronary angiography complications: a randomized clinical trial, *J Caring Sci* 4(2):125, 2015.

Aldrete JA: Post-anesthetic recovery score, *J Am Coll Surg* 205(5):3, 2007.

American Academy of Pediatrics (AAP) Section on Anesthesiology and Pain Medicine, Tobias JD, et al, editors: *Procedural sedation for infants, children, and adolescents*, New York, 2015, Bantam.

American College of Radiology (ACR): *ACR-SIR practice parameter for sedation/analgesia*, 2015, The American College of Radiology. http://www.acr.org/~/media/F194CBB800AB43048B997A75938AB482.pdf. Accessed August 26, 2016.

American Society of Anesthesiologists (ASA): *Continuum of depth of sedation: definition of general anesthesia and levels of sedation/analgesia*, 2014a, Committee of Origin: Quality Management and Departmental Administration, The Society. http://www.asahq.org/~/media/Sites/ASAHQ/Files/Public/Resources/standards-guidelines/continuum-of-depth-of-sedation-definition-of-general-anesthesia-and-levels-of-sedation-analgesia.pdf. Accessed August 26, 2016.

American Society of Anesthesiologists (ASA): *Standards for post-anesthesia care*, 2014b. Available at http://www.asahq.org/quality-and-practice-management/standards-and-guidelines. Accessed August 26, 2016.

Antonelli MT, et al: Procedural sedation and implications for quality and risk management, *J Healthc Risk Manag* 33(2):3, 2013.

Arevalo-Rodriguez I, et al: Posture and fluids for preventing post-dural puncture headache, *Cochrane Database Syst Rev* (3):CD009199, 2016.

Brenes-Salazar JA, et al: Clinical pharmacology relevant to older adults with cardiovascular disease, *J Geriatr Cardiol* 12(3):192, 2015.

Bui AH, Urman RD: Clinical safety considerations for moderate and deep sedation, *J Med Pract Manage* 29(1):35, 2013.

Centers for Disease Control and Prevention (CDC): *Guidelines for the prevention of intravascular catheter-related infections*, 2011, http://www.cdc.gov/hicpac/bsi/bsi-guidelines-2011.html. Accessed August 26, 2016.

Conway A, et al: Capnography monitoring during procedural sedation and analgesia: a systematic review protocol, *Syst Rev* 4(92):2015.

Destrebecq A, et al: Post-lumbar puncture headache: a review of issues for nursing practice, *J Neurosci Nurs* 46(3):180, 2014.

Ellett ML: A literature review of the safety and efficacy of using propofol for sedation in endoscopy, *Gastroenterol Nurs* 33(2):111, 2010.

Hockenberry MJ, Wilson D: *Wong's nursing care of infants and children*, ed 10, St Louis, 2015, Mosby.

Kar KÖ, et al: Sedation for fiberoptic bronchoscopy: review of the literature, *Tuberk Toraks* 63(1):42, 2015.

Kranz PG, et al: Rebound intracranial hypertension: a complication of epidural blood patching for intracranial hypotension, *AJNR Am J Neuroradiol* 35(6):1237, 2014.

Krishnasamy VP, et al: Vascular closure devices: technical tips, complications, and management, *Tech Vasc Interv Radiol* 18(2):100, 2015.

Lewis S, et al: *Medical-surgical nursing: assessment and management of clinical problems*, ed 10, St Louis, 2017, Elsevier.

Ludwig U, Keller F: Prophylaxis of contrast-induced nephrotoxicity, *Biomed Res Int* 2014. http://www.hindawi.com/journals/bmri/2014/308316/. Accessed August 26, 2016.

Maden B, et al: An overview of diabetes and its impact on cath lab care, *Cath Lab Digest* 2013. http://www.cathlabdigest.com/articles/Overview-Diabetes-Its-Impact-Cath-Lab-Care. Accessed April 1, 2016.

Muller M, Wehrmann T: How best to approach endoscopic sedation? *Nat Rev Gastroenterol Hepatol* 8(9):481, 2011.

Pagana KD, Pagana TJ: *Mosby's manual of diagnostic and laboratory tests*, ed 5, St Louis, 2014, Mosby.

Pagana KD, et al: *Mosby's diagnostic and laboratory test reference*, ed 12, St Louis, 2015, Mosby.

Schlitzkus LL, et al: Perioperative management of elderly patients, *Surg Clin North Am* 95(2):391, 2015.

Schulz-Schüpke S, et al: Comparison of vascular closure devices vs manual compression after femoral artery puncture, *JAMA* 312(19):1981, 2014.

The Joint Commission (TJC): *2016 National Patient Safety Goals*, 2016, The Commission. http://www.jointcommission.org/standards_information/npsgs.aspx. Accessed August 26, 2016.

Tobias JD, Leder M: Procedural sedation: a review of sedative agents, monitoring, and management of complications, *Saudi J Anaesth* 5(4):395, 2011.

Westermann-Clark E, et al: Debunking myths about "allergy" to radiocontrast media in an academic institution, *Postgrad Med* 127(3):295, 2015.

Whitlow PG, et al: Topical analgesia treats pain and decreases propofol use during lumbar punctures in a randomized pediatric leukemia trial, *Pediatr Blood Cancer* 61(1):85, 2015.

9 | Medical Asepsis

OBJECTIVES

Mastery of content in this chapter will enable the nurse to:
- Discuss how to apply critical thinking in the prevention of the transmission of infection.
- Explain the difference between medical and surgical asepsis.
- Identify nursing care measures intended to break the chain of infection.
- Describe how each element of the infection chain contributes to infection.
- Describe the factors that influence nursing staff compliance with hand hygiene.
- Perform proper procedures for hand hygiene.
- Perform correct isolation precautions.

MEDIA RESOURCES

- evolve http://evolve.elsevier.com/Perry/skills
- Review Questions
- ▶ Video Clips
- Audio Glossary
- **NSO** Nursing Skills Online
- Clinical Debrief and Review Questions Answers

PURPOSE

Infection prevention and control practices reduce or eliminate sources and transmission of infection. These prevention and control practices are designed to protect patients and health care providers from disease. Medical asepsis, or clean technique, includes procedures used for reducing the number of organisms and preventing their transfer.

STANDARDS OF CARE

- Centers for Disease Control and Prevention (CDC), 2007—Guideline for Isolation Precautions; Preventing Transmission of Infectious Agents in Healthcare Settings
- Centers for Disease Control and Prevention (CDC), 2008—Guideline for Hand Hygiene in Healthcare Settings
- Centers for Disease Control and Prevention (CDC), 2010b—Respiratory Protection in Health Care Settings
- The Joint Commission (TJC), 2016—2016 National Patient Safety Goals

PRINCIPLES FOR PRACTICE

- Hand hygiene practices are major principles of infection control and are essential to safe patient care.
- Patients in all health care settings are at risk of becoming colonized or infected as a result of an impaired immune response, exposure to an increased number of pathogenic organisms, and performance of invasive procedures (Fluten, 2014).
- Know a patient's susceptibility to infection. Age, nutritional status, stress, disease processes, and forms of medical therapy place patients at risk (Roach, 2014).
- Health care–associated infections (HAIs) result from delivery of health services in a health care setting that were not present at the time of admission. A hospital is one of the most likely settings for acquiring an HAI because staff, patients, and environmental factors support a high population of pathogens that are resistant to antibiotics. Health care workers transmit many HAIs by direct contact during the delivery of care (Ellingson et al., 2014).
- Recognize elements of the chain of infection and initiate measures to prevent the onset and spread of infections. The presence of a pathogen does not mean that an infection will occur. Infection occurs in a cycle, often referred to as the *chain of infection*. An infection develops if this chain remains intact (Fig. 9.1). In patient care it is important to use infection control practices to break an element of the chain so as not to transmit infection (Table 9.1). The six elements in the chain are:
  - An infectious agent or pathogen.
  - A reservoir or source for pathogen growth.
  - A portal of exit from the reservoir.
  - A mode of transmission.
  - A portal of entry to the host.
  - A susceptible host.
- Medical asepsis, or clean technique, includes procedures that reduce the number of organisms and prevent their transfer.
- Principles of hand hygiene, barrier techniques, and routine environmental cleaning are examples of medical asepsis. These principles are common in the health care and home environment (e.g., washing hands before preparing food).

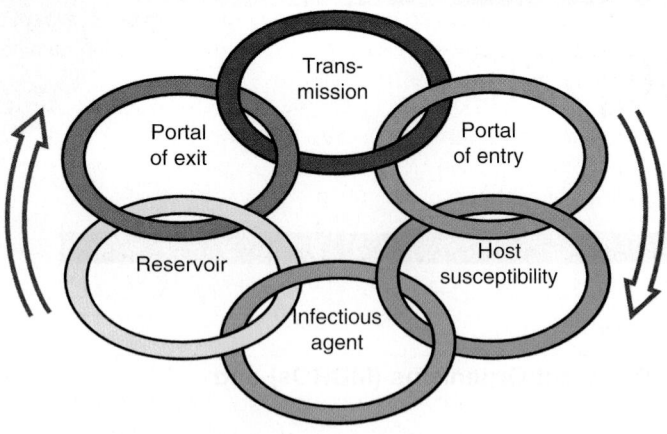

FIG 9.1 Chain of infection.

PATIENT-CENTERED CARE

- Nurses are responsible for educating patients and their families about infection control, including information concerning signs and symptoms of infection, modes of transmission, methods of prevention, knowledge of the infectious process, disease transmission, and critical thinking skills associated with use of aseptic techniques and barrier protection.
- Infection can require isolation. This may lead to loneliness or changes in self-concept or body image.
- Know the cultural views and preferences of your patients. Some may choose to rely on alternative health care practices
- When a patient from another culture requires isolation, use caution to be sure that the patient and family caregiver understand the therapeutic purpose of isolation (Campinha-Bacote, 2011). For example, the isolation of a loved one may be considered disrespectful and uncaring behavior in collectivistic cultures.

TABLE 9.1

Breaking the Chain of Infection

Element of Infection Chain	Medical Asepsis Practices
Infectious agent (pathogenic organism capable of causing disease)	Clean contaminated objects. Clean, disinfect, and sterilize.
Reservoir (site or source of microorganism growth)	Perform hand hygiene before and after patient contact with appropriate antiseptic (e.g., chlorhexidine), or soap and water. Control sources of body fluids and drainage. Bathe patient with soap and water, chlorhexidine, or disposable bath. Change soiled dressings. Dispose of soiled tissues, dressings, or linen in moisture-resistant bags. Place syringes, uncapped hypodermic needles, and intravenous needles in designated puncture-proof containers. Keep table surfaces clean and dry. Do not leave bottled solutions open for prolonged periods. Keep solutions tightly capped. Keep surgical wound drainage tubes and collection bags patent. Empty and dispose of drainage suction bottles according to agency policy.
Portal of exit (means by which microorganisms leave a site)	Respiratory • Avoid talking, sneezing, or coughing directly over wound or sterile dressing field. • Cover nose and mouth when sneezing or coughing. • Wear mask if suffering respiratory tract infection. Urine, feces, emesis, and blood • Wear clean gloves when handling blood and body fluids. • Wear gowns and eyewear if there is a chance of splashing fluids. • Handle all laboratory specimens as if infectious.
Transmission (means of spread)	Reduce microorganism spread: • Perform hand hygiene. • Use personal set of care items for each patient. • Avoid shaking bed linen or clothes; dust with damp cloth. • Avoid contact of soiled item with uniform. • Discard any item that touches the floor. • Follow standard precautions or select transmission-based isolation precautions.
Portal of entry (site through which microorganism enters a host)	Skin and mucosa • Maintain skin and mucous membrane integrity; lubricate skin, offer frequent hygiene, turn and position. • Cover wounds as needed. • Clean wound sites thoroughly. • Dispose of used needles in puncture-proof container. Urinary • Keep all drainage systems closed and intact, maintaining downward flow.
Host (patient)	Reduce susceptibility to infection. Provide adequate nutrition. Ensure adequate rest. Promote body defenses against infection. Provide immunizations.

EVIDENCE-BASED PRACTICE

- Bundled interventions such as ongoing education, reminders (e.g., posters), administrative support, wall-mounted alcohol dispensers, and pocket-size bottles improve hand hygiene practices (Schweizer et al., 2014).
- Handwashing with plain soap sometimes results in paradoxical increases in bacterial counts on the skin (WHO, 2009, 2016). A systematic review supports the WHO-5 Moments for Hand Hygiene; and compliance with hand hygiene practices among health care providers is increased through goal setting, incentives, and accountability (Luangasanatip et al., 2015).
- Alcohol-based products are more effective for standard handwashing or hand antisepsis than soap or antiseptic soaps (WHO, 2009). Moreover, brisk alcohol-based rinses or gels containing emollients cause substantially less skin irritation and dryness than plain or antimicrobial soaps (CDC, 2008; Haas, 2015).
- Soap and water are still necessary for hand hygiene if hands are visibly soiled or when caring for patients infected with *Clostridium difficile* (CDC, 2016; Edmonds et al., 2013).

SAFETY GUIDELINES

- Hand hygiene with an appropriate alcohol-based hand antiseptic or soap and water is an essential part of patient care and infection prevention and is fundamental to patient safety (CDC, 2008).

- Always know a patient's susceptibility to infection. Age, nutritional status, stress, disease processes, and forms of medical therapy can place patients at risk.
- Recognize the elements of the chain of infection and initiate measures to prevent its onset and spread.
- Health care workers should not wear artificial nails and extenders because of bacterial buildup.
- Fingernails should not be longer than 0.625 cm (¼ inch) in length, and nail polish should not be chipped. There are no recommendations regarding nail polish color (Cook, 2011).
- Consistently incorporate the basic principles of medical asepsis into patient care.
- Ensure that patients, family caregivers, and health care workers follow "cough hygiene practices" and cover the mouth and nose when coughing or sneezing, use tissues to contain respiratory secretions, dispose of tissues in the waste receptacle, and wash their hands.
- Use clean gloves when you anticipate contact with body fluids, nonintact skin, or mucous membranes when there is a risk of drainage.
- Use barrier protection (e.g., gown, mask, and eye protection) when there is a splash risk.
- Protect fellow health care workers from exposure to infectious agents through proper use and disposal of equipment.
- Be aware of body sites where HAIs are most likely to develop (e.g., urinary or respiratory tract). This enables you to direct preventive measures.

◆ SKILL 9.1 Hand Hygiene

▶ *Video Clip* [NSO] *Nursing Skills Online Infection Control Module / Lessons 1 and 2*

The most important and basic technique in preventing and controlling transmission of infection is hand hygiene. Hand hygiene is a general term that applies to handwashing, antiseptic hand wash, antiseptic hand rub, or surgical hand antisepsis. Handwashing refers to washing hands with plain soap and water. An antiseptic hand wash is defined as washing hands with water and soap or other detergents containing an antiseptic agent. An antiseptic hand rub means applying an antiseptic hand rub product to all surfaces of the hands to reduce the number of microorganisms present. Surgical hand antisepsis is the use of an antiseptic hand wash or antiseptic hand rub before surgery by surgical personnel to eliminate transient and reduce resident hand flora (see Chapter 38).

The decision to perform hand hygiene depends on four factors: (1) the intensity or degree of contact with patients or contaminated objects, (2) the amount of contamination that may occur with the contact, (3) the patient or health care worker's susceptibility to infection, and (4) the procedure or activity to be performed (Haas, 2015). It is a critical responsibility for all health care workers to follow these guidelines for hand hygiene (Al-Tawfiq et al., 2013; CDC, 2008; WHO, 2009):

- Wash hands with either plain soap and water or an antibacterial soap and water when they are visibly dirty or soiled with blood or other body fluids, before eating, and after using the toilet.
- Wash hands if exposed to spore-forming organisms such as *Clostridium difficile*.
- If hands are not visibly soiled, use an alcohol-based hand rub for routinely decontaminating hands in the following clinical situations:

- Before and after having direct contact with patients
- Before applying sterile gloves and inserting an invasive device such as indwelling urinary catheters and intravenous peripheral vascular catheters
- After contact with body fluids or excretions, mucous membranes, and nonintact skin
- After contact with wound dressings (if hands are not visibly soiled)
- When moving from a contaminated body site to a clean body site during patient care
- After contact with inanimate objects (e.g., medical equipment) in the immediate vicinity of a patient
- After removing gloves

Delegation and Collaboration

The skill of hand hygiene is performed by all caregivers. Hand hygiene is not optional.

Equipment

- Antiseptic hand rub
  - Alcohol-based waterless antiseptic containing emollients
- Handwashing
  - Easy-to-reach sink with warm running water
  - Antimicrobial or regular soap
  - Paper towels or air dryer
  - Disposable nail cleaner (optional)

STEP	RATIONALE

ASSESSMENT

1. Inspect surface of hands for breaks or cuts in skin or cuticles. Cover any skin lesions with a dressing before providing care. If lesions are too large to cover, you may be restricted from direct patient care.

   Open cuts or wounds can harbor high concentrations of microorganisms. Agency policy may prevent nurses from caring for high-risk patients if open lesions are present on hands (WHO, 2009).

2. Inspect hands for visible soiling.

   Visible soiling requires handwashing with soap and water.

3. Inspect condition of nails. Natural tips should be no longer than 0.625 cm (¼ inch) long. Be sure that fingernails are short, filed, and smooth.

   Subungual areas of hand harbor high concentrations of bacteria. Long nails and chipped or old polish increase the number of bacteria residing on hands (CDC, 2008). Artificial nail applications increase microbial load on hands (Felembam, 2012).

NURSING DIAGNOSES

This skill is required for patients with a variety of nursing diagnoses.

Related factors are individualized based on patient's condition or needs.

PLANNING

1. Expected outcomes following completion of procedure:
   - Hands and areas under fingernails are clean and free of debris.

     Transient bacteria have been removed.

IMPLEMENTATION

1. Push wristwatch and long uniform sleeves above wrists. Avoid wearing rings. If worn, remove during hand hygiene.

   Provides complete access to fingers, hands, and wrists. The skin underneath rings carries higher bacterial count; bacteria include gram-negative bacilli, enterobacteria, and *Staphylococcus aureus* (Messano, 2013).

2. **Antiseptic hand rub**

   a. According to manufacturer directions, dispense ample amount of product into palm of one hand (see illustration).

      Use enough product to cover hands thoroughly.

   b. Rub hands together, covering all surfaces of hands and fingers with antiseptic (see illustration).

      Provides enough time for product to work.

   c. Rub hands together until alcohol is dry. Allow hands to dry completely before applying gloves.

      Ensures complete antimicrobial action.

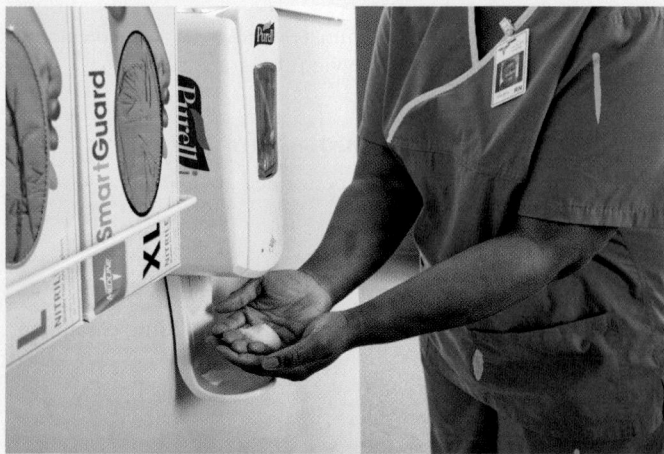

STEP 2a Apply waterless antiseptic to hands.

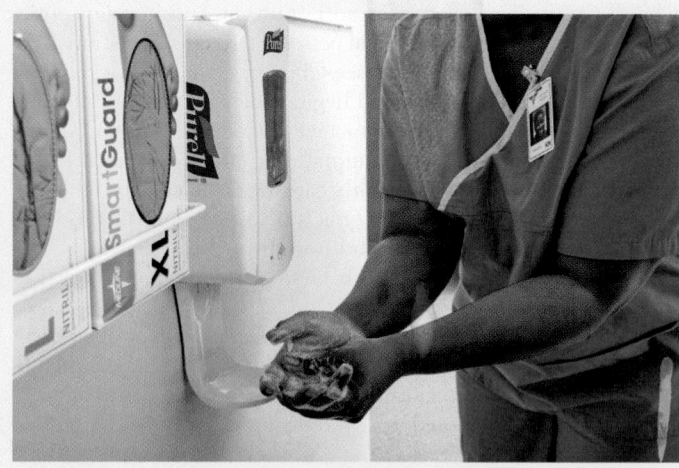

STEP 2b Rub hands thoroughly.

STEP	RATIONALE

3. Handwashing using regular or antimicrobial soap:

a. Stand in front of sink, keeping hands and uniform away from sink surface. (If hands touch sink during handwashing, repeat sequence.)

Inside of sink is contaminated area. Reaching over sink increases risk of touching edge, which is contaminated.

b. Turn on water. Turn on faucet (see illustration) or push knee pedals laterally or press pedals with foot to regulate flow and temperature.

Knee pads within operating room and treatment areas are preferred to prevent hand contact with faucet. Faucet handles are likely to be contaminated with organic debris and microorganisms (AORN, 2014).

c. Avoid splashing water against uniform.

Microorganisms travel and grow in moisture.

d. Regulate flow of water so temperature is warm.

Warm water removes less of protective oils on hands than hot water.

e. Wet hands and wrists thoroughly under running water. Keep hands and forearms lower than elbows during washing.

Hands are most contaminated parts to wash. Water flows from least to most contaminated area, rinsing microorganisms into sink.

f. Apply 3 to 5 mL of antiseptic soap and rub hands together (see illustration).

Ensure that all surfaces of hands and fingers are cleaned.

Clinical Decision Point *If a patient is critically ill, chlorhexidine baths are more effective for infection prevention (Raines and Rosen, 2016).*

g. Perform hand hygiene using plenty of lather and friction for at least 15 seconds. Interlace fingers and rub palms and back of hands with circular motion at least 5 times each. Keep fingertips down to facilitate removal of microorganisms.

Soap cleans by emulsifying fat and oil and lowering surface tension. Friction and rubbing mechanically loosen and remove dirt and transient bacteria. Interlacing fingers and thumbs ensures that all surfaces are cleaned. Adequate time is needed to expose skin surfaces to antimicrobial agent.

h. Areas underlying fingernails are often soiled. Clean them with fingernails of other hand and additional soap or with disposable nail cleaner.

Area under nails can be highly contaminated, which increases risk for transmission of infection from nurse to patient.

i. Rinse hands and wrists thoroughly, keeping hands down and elbows up (see illustration).

Rinsing mechanically washes away dirt and microorganisms.

j. Dry hands thoroughly from fingers to wrists with paper towel, single-use cloth, or warm air dryer.

Drying from cleanest (fingertips) to least clean (wrist) avoids contamination. Drying hands prevents chapping and roughened skin. Do not tear or cut skin under or around nail.

k. If used, discard paper towel in proper receptacle.

Prevents transfer of microorganisms.

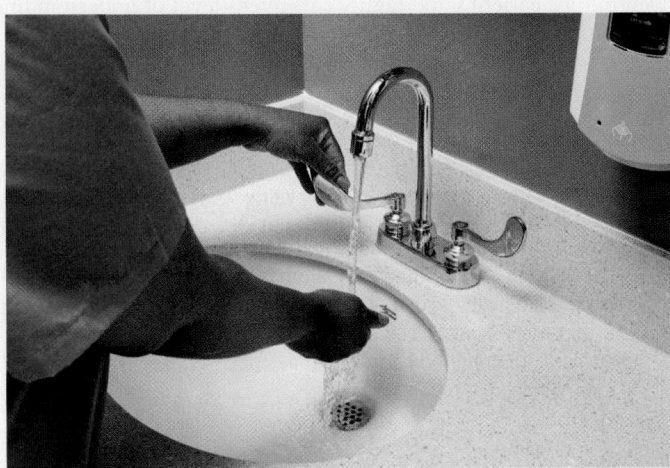

STEP 3b Turn on water.

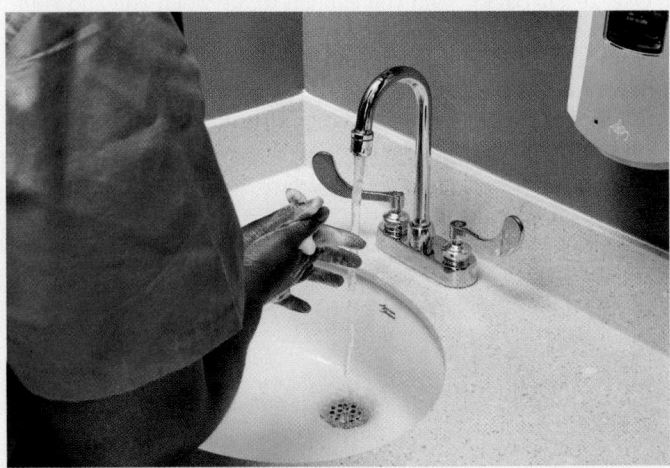

STEP 3f Lather hands thoroughly.

STEP	RATIONALE

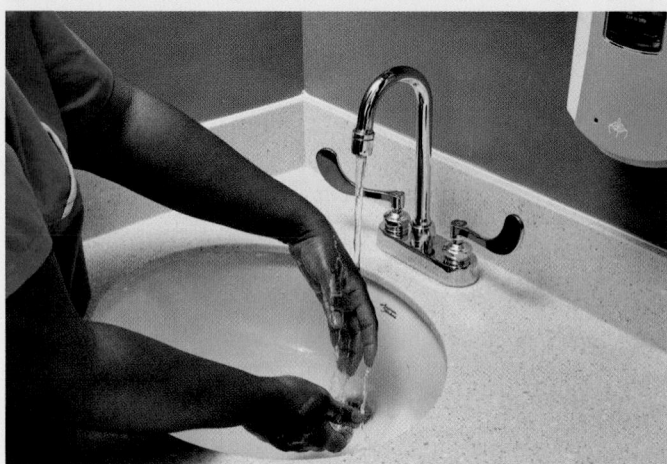

STEP 3i Rinse hands.

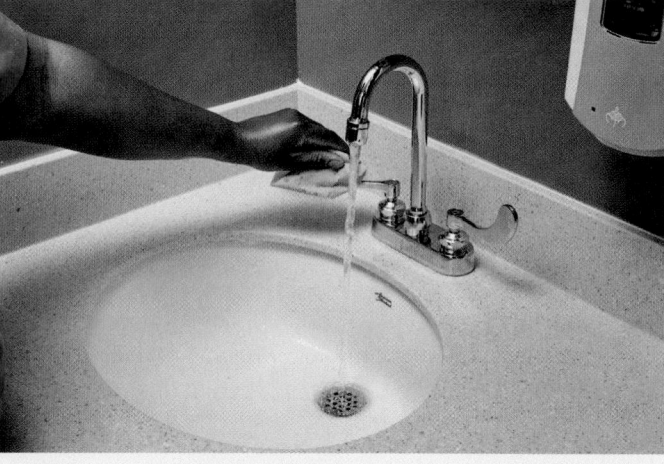

STEP 3l Turn off faucet.

l. To turn off hand faucet, use clean, dry paper towel; avoid touching handles with hands (see illustration). Turn off water with foot or knee pedals (if applicable).

m. If hands are dry or chapped, use small amount of lotion or barrier cream dispensed from individual-use container.

Wet towel and hands allow transfer of pathogens from faucet by capillary action.

Helps to minimize skin dryness. There is risk of organism growth in lotion; therefore only apply after patient care activities are complete.

EVALUATION

1. Inspect surface of hands for obvious signs of dirt or other contaminants.
2. Inspect hands for dermatitis or cracked skin.

3. **Use Teach-Back:** "Can you explain to me when you and your family caregiver perform hand hygiene and the different kinds of ways you can wash your hands?" Revise your instruction now or develop a plan for revised patient or family caregiver teaching if patient or family caregiver is not able to teach back correctly.

Determines if hand hygiene is adequate.

Breaks in skin integrity increase risk for transmission of microorganisms.

Determines patient's and family caregiver's level of understanding of instructional topic.

Unexpected Outcomes
1. Hands or areas under fingernails remain soiled.
2. Repeated use of soaps or antiseptics causes dermatitis or cracked skin.

Related Interventions
- Repeat handwashing with soap and water.
- Rinse and dry hands thoroughly after using soap and water; avoid excessive amounts of soap or antiseptic; try various products.
- Use approved hand lotions or barrier creams. Small individual-use containers are preferred because large containers have been found to harbor pathogens.

Special Considerations
Teaching Considerations

- Instruct patient and family caregiver in proper techniques and situations for hand hygiene.
- When patients are educated about the risks for infections, they play an important role in improving hand hygiene compliance in health care settings by reminding visitors and health care workers to perform hand hygiene.

Gerontological Considerations

- The impact of infections is greater in older adults. Hand hygiene by staff attending older adults is of utmost importance and should be an ongoing continuing-education requirement.

Home Care

- Evaluate patient and family caregiver to determine their understanding of the transmission of microorganisms and their ability and motivation to perform hand hygiene correctly.
- Evaluate the hand hygiene facilities in the home to determine the possibility of contamination, proximity of the facilities to the patient, and ability to maintain supplies and equipment.

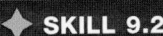 **SKILL 9.2** **Caring for Patients Under Isolation Precautions**

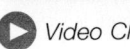 *Video Clip*

When a patient has a known or suspected source of colonization or infection, health care workers follow specific infection prevention and control practices to reduce the risk of cross-contamination to other patients. Certain procedures performed at a patient's bedside require the application of personal protective equipment (PPE) such as a mask, cap, eyewear, gown, or gloves. Standard precautions require you to wear clean gloves before coming in contact with mucous membranes, nonintact skin, blood, body fluids, or other infectious material. You wear clean gloves routinely when performing a variety of procedures (e.g., nasogastric tube insertion). Masks are worn when there is the risk of splash during a procedure or when certain sterile procedures such as changing a central line dressing are performed. Protective eyewear and masks become important when there is a risk for splash of blood or other body fluids to the eyes or mouth.

Assess the need for PPE for each task you plan and for all patients, regardless of their diagnoses. Because of increased attention to the prevention of bloodborne pathogens and tuberculosis (TB) (Box 9.1), the Centers for Disease Control and Prevention (CDC) (2009, 2011) and the Occupational Safety and Health Administration (OSHA) (2011) have stressed the importance of barrier protection. The Hospital Infection Control Practices Advisory Committee (HICPAC) of the CDC (2009) published revised guidelines for isolation precautions. The guidelines contain recommendations for respiratory hygiene/cough etiquette as part of standard precautions.

Standard precautions, or tier one precautions, are for the care of all patients, regardless of risk or presumed infection status (Box 9.2). Standard precautions are the primary strategies for prevention of infection transmission and apply to contact with blood, body fluids, nonintact skin, respiratory secretions, mucous membranes, and equipment or surfaces contaminated with these potentially infectious materials.

The second tier (Table 9.2) includes precautions designed for care of patients who are known or suspected to be infected, or colonized, with microorganisms transmitted by the contact, droplet, or airborne route (Brisko, 2015; CDC, 2007) or by contact with contaminated surfaces (see Table 9.2). The three

BOX 9.1
Special Tuberculosis Precautions

The Centers for Disease Control and Prevention (CDC) published guidelines for preventing tuberculosis (TB) transmission in health care agencies in response to a resurgence of TB in the United States associated with the increasing incidence of human immunodeficiency virus (HIV) infection, TB infection transmission in health care settings, and increasing immigration from countries with a high incidence of TB (CDC, 2012).

- Current CDC guidelines for preventing and controlling TB focus on early detection of infection, preventing close contact with patients with active TB disease, and applying effective infection control measures in health care settings. Suspect TB in any patient with respiratory symptoms lasting longer than 3 weeks accompanied by other suspicious symptoms such as unexplained weight loss, night sweats, fever, and a productive cough often streaked with blood.
- Consider the potential for infectious pulmonary or laryngeal TB from documented positive acid-fast bacilli (AFB) smear or culture, cavitation on chest x-ray film, or history of recent TB exposure.
- Isolation for patients with suspected or confirmed TB includes placing the patient on airborne precautions in a single-patient negative-pressure room.
- Health care workers who care for patients with suspected or confirmed TB must wear special respirators (e.g., N95 or P100) (CDC, 2010b). These respirators are high-efficiency particulate masks that have the ability to filter particles at a 95% or better efficiency (CDC, 2010b; OSHA, 2011).
- The CDC now recommends the use of the QuantiFERON-TB Gold test (QFT-GIT) or the T-SPOT (CDC, 2011), a blood test, in place of the traditional TB skin test. The advantages of the QFT-GIT test are that it does not boost responses measured by subsequent tests and the results are not subject to reader bias.

types of transmission-based precautions—airborne, droplet, and contact—may be combined for diseases that have multiple routes of transmission (e.g., chickenpox). Whether used either singly or in combination, you use them in addition to standard precautions.

BOX 9.2

Centers for Disease Control and Prevention Isolation Guidelines

Standard Precautions (Tier One) for Use With All Patients

- Standard precautions apply to blood, blood products, all body fluids, secretions, excretions (except sweat), nonintact skin, and mucous membranes.
- Perform hand hygiene before, after, and between direct contact with patients. (Examples of between-contact activities are cleaning hands after a patient care activity, moving to a non–patient care activity, and cleaning hands again before returning to perform patient contact.)
- Perform hand hygiene after contact with blood, body fluids, mucous membranes, nonintact skin, secretions, excretions, or wound dressings; after contact with inanimate surfaces or articles in a patient room; and immediately after gloves are removed.
- When hands are visibly soiled or contaminated with blood or body fluids, wash them with either a nonantimicrobial soap or an antimicrobial soap and water.
- When hands are not visibly soiled or contaminated with blood or body fluids, use an alcohol-based hand rub to perform hand hygiene.
- Wash hands with nonantimicrobial soap and water if contact with spores (e.g., *Clostridium difficile*) is likely to have occurred.
- Do not wear artificial fingernails or extenders if duties include direct contact with patients at high risk for infection and associated adverse outcomes.

- Wear gloves when touching blood, body fluids, secretions, excretions, nonintact skin, mucous membranes, or contaminated items or surfaces is likely. Remove gloves and perform hand hygiene between patient care encounters and when going from a contaminated to a clean body site.
- Wear personal protective equipment (PPE) when the anticipated patient interaction indicates that contact with blood or body fluids may occur.
- A private room is unnecessary unless the patient's hygiene is unacceptable (e.g., uncontained secretions, excretions, or wound drainage).
- Discard all contaminated sharp instruments and needles in a puncture-resistant container. Health care agencies must make available needleless devices. Any needles should be disposed of uncapped, or a mechanical safety device must be activated for recapping.
- Respiratory hygiene/cough etiquette: Have patients cover the nose/mouth when coughing or sneezing; use tissues to contain respiratory secretions and dispose in nearest waste container; perform hand hygiene after contacting respiratory secretions and contaminated objects/materials; contain respiratory secretions with procedure or surgical mask; sit at least 91.4 cm (3 feet) away from others if coughing.

Modified from Centers for Disease Control and Prevention (CDC), Hospital Infection Control Practices Advisory Committee: Guidelines for isolation precautions in hospitals, *MMWR Morb Mortal Wkly Rep* 57/RR-16:39, 2007.

TABLE 9.2

Centers for Disease Control and Prevention Isolation Guidelines: *Transmission-Based Precautions (Tier Two) for Use With Specific Types of Patients*

Category	Infection/Condition	Barrier Protection
Airborne precautions (droplet nuclei smaller than 5 microns)	Measles, chickenpox (varicella), disseminated varicella zoster, pulmonary or laryngeal tuberculosis	Private-room, negative-pressure airflow of at least 6 to 12 exchanges per hour via HEPA filtration; mask or respiratory protection device, N95 respirator (depending on condition)
Droplet precautions (droplets larger than 5 microns; being within 3 feet of patient)	Diphtheria (pharyngeal), rubella, streptococcal pharyngitis, pneumonia or scarlet fever in infants and young children, pertussis, mumps, *Mycoplasma* pneumonia, meningococcal pneumonia or sepsis, pneumonic plague	Private-room or cohort patients; mask or respirator (refer to agency policy)
Contact precautions (direct patient or environmental contact)	Colonization or infection with multidrug-resistant organisms such as VRE and MRSA, *Clostridium difficile*, shigella, and other enteric pathogens; major wound infections; herpes simplex; scabies; varicella zoster (disseminated); respiratory syncytial virus in infants, young children or immunocompromised adults	Private-room or cohort patients (see agency policy), gloves, gowns; patients may leave their room for procedures or therapy if infectious material is contained or covered and placed in a clean gown and hands cleaned
Protective environment	Allogeneic hematopoietic stem cell transplants	Private room; positive airflow with ≥12 air exchanges per hour; HEPA filtration for incoming air; mask to be worn by patient when out of room during times of construction in area

Modified from Centers for Disease Control and Prevention (CDC), Hospital Infection Control Practices Advisory Committee: Guidelines for isolation precautions in hospitals, *MMWR Morb Mortal Wkly Rep* 57/RR-16:39, 2007.
HEPA, High-efficiency particulate air; *MRSA*, methicillin-resistant *Staphylococcus aureus*; *VRE*, vancomycin-resistant enterococcus.

Delegation and Collaboration

The skill of caring for patients on isolation precautions can be delegated to nursing assistive personnel (NAP). However, the nurse must assess the patient's status and isolation indications. The nurse instructs the NAP about:

- Reason patient is on isolation precautions.
- Precautions for bringing equipment into the patient's room.
- Special precautions regarding individual patient needs such as transportation to diagnostic tests.

Equipment

- Personal protective equipment (PPE) determined by type of isolation required: clean gloves, mask, eyewear or goggles, face shield, and gown (gowns may be disposable or reusable, depending on agency policy)
- Other patient care equipment (as appropriate) (e.g., hygiene items, medications, dressing supplies, sharps container, disposable blood pressure [BP] cuff)

- Soiled linen bag and trash receptacle
- Sign for door indicating type of isolation and/or for visitors to come to the nurses' station before entering room
- TB isolation
  - Room with negative airflow
  - N95 or P100 respirator.

STEP	RATIONALE

ASSESSMENT

1. Assess patient's medical history for possible indications for isolation (e.g., risk factors for TB, major draining wound, or purulent productive cough). Review precautions for specific isolation system, including appropriate barriers to apply (see Table 9.2).

   Mode of transmission for infectious microorganism determines type and degree of precautions followed. Ensures adequate protection.

2. Review laboratory test results (e.g., wound culture, acid-fast bacillus [AFB] smears, changes in white blood cell [WBC] count).

   Reveals type of microorganism for which patient is being isolated, body fluid in which it was identified, and whether patient is immunosuppressed.

3. Review agency policies and isolation precautions necessary for type of isolation ordered and consider types of care measures that you will perform while in patient's room (e.g., medication administration or dressing change).

   Allows you to organize care items for procedures and time spent in patient's room.

4. Review nursing care plan notes or confer with colleagues regarding patient's emotional state and reaction/adjustment to isolation. Also assess patient's understanding of purpose of isolation.

   Provides opportunity to plan for patient's need for emotional support and teaching.

5. Assess whether patient has known latex allergy. If allergy is present, refer to agency policy and resources available to provide full latex-free care.

   Protects patient from serious allergic response.

NURSING DIAGNOSES

- Deficient knowledge regarding purpose of isolation
- Impaired social interaction
- Ineffective protection
- Risk for infection

Related factors/Risk factors are individualized based on patient's condition or needs.

PLANNING

1. Expected outcomes following completion of procedure:
   - Patient asks for information about disease transmission.

     Active interaction reveals patient's willingness and/or ability to communicate and be taught and understand information.

   - Patient explains purpose of isolation.

     Instruction about precautions improves patient's ability to cooperate in care.

IMPLEMENTATION

1. Perform hand hygiene (see Skill 9.1).

   Reduces transmission of microorganisms.

2. Prepare all equipment to be taken into patient's room. In many cases dedicated equipment such as stethoscopes, BP equipment, and thermometers should remain in room until patient is discharged. If patient is infected or colonized with resistant organism (e.g., vancomycin-resistant enterococcus, methicillin-resistant *Staphylococcus aureus*), equipment remains in room and is thoroughly disinfected before removal (see agency policy).

   Prevents you from making more than one trip into room. The CDC recommends use of dedicated noncritical patient care equipment (CDC, 2007).

STEP	RATIONALE

3. Prepare for entrance into isolation room. Ideally, before applying PPE, step into patient's room and stay by door. Introduce yourself and explain care that you are providing. If this is not possible, apply PPE outside of the room.

Proper preparation ensures protection from microorganism exposure. Allows patient to see you without PPE and without exposing yourself to risk of infection transmission.

   a. Apply gown, being sure that it covers all outer garments. Pull sleeves down to wrist. Tie securely at neck and waist (see illustration).

Prevents transmission of infection; protects you when patient has excessive drainage or discharges.

   b. Apply either surgical mask or fitted respirator around mouth and nose (type and fit-testing depend on type of isolation and agency policy). You must have a medical evaluation and be fit-tested before using a respirator.

Prevents exposure to airborne microorganisms or microorganisms from splashing of fluids.

   c. If needed, apply eyewear or goggles snugly around face and eyes. If you wear prescription glasses, side shields may be used.

Protects you from exposure to microorganisms that may occur during splashing of fluids.

   d. Apply clean gloves. (NOTE: Wear unpowdered, latex-free gloves if you, patient, or another health care worker has latex allergy.) Bring glove cuffs over edge of gown sleeves (see illustration).

Reduces transmission of microorganisms.

4. Enter patient's room. Arrange supplies and equipment. (NOTE: If equipment will be reused, place on clean paper towel.)

Prevents extra trips entering and leaving room. Minimizes contamination of care items.

5. Explain purpose of isolation and precautions for patient and family caregiver to take. Offer opportunity to ask questions. If patient is on TB precautions, instruct to cover mouth with tissue when coughing and to wear disposable surgical mask when leaving room.

Improves patient's and family caregiver's ability to participate in care and minimizes anxiety. Identifies opportunity for planning social interaction and diversional activities. Reduces TB microorganism transmission.

6. Assess vital signs (see Chapter 5).

   a. If patient is infected or colonized with resistant organism (e.g., vancomycin-resistant enterococci [VRE], methicillin-resistant *S. aureus* [MRSA]), equipment remains in room, including stethoscope and BP cuff (CDC, 2010a).

Decreases risk of infection being transmitted to another patient.

   b. If stethoscope is to be reused, clean earpieces and diaphragm or bell with 70% alcohol or agency-approved germicide. Set aside on clean surface.

Systematic disinfection of stethoscopes with 70% alcohol or approved germicide minimizes chance of spreading infectious agents between patients (CDC, 2009).

   c. Use individual or disposable thermometers and BP cuffs when available.

Prevents cross-contamination.

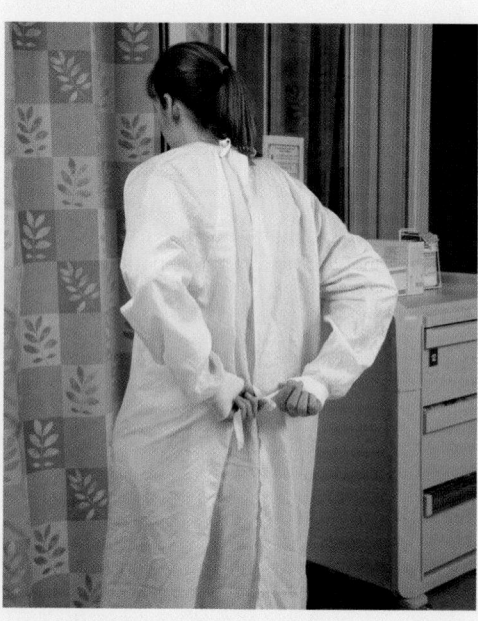

STEP 3a Tie isolation gown at waist.

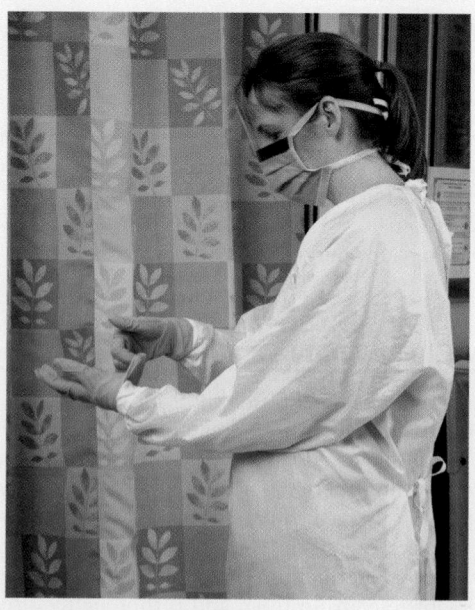

STEP 3d Apply gloves over gown sleeves.

STEP	RATIONALE

Clinical Decision Point *If disposable thermometer indicates a fever, assess for other signs/symptoms. Confirm fever using an alternative thermometer. Do not use electronic thermometer if patient is suspected or confirmed* Clostridium difficile *(Cohen et al., 2010).*

7. Administer medications (see Chapters 20, 21, and 22).

   a. Give oral medication in wrapper or cup.
       Handle and discard supplies to minimize transfer of microorganisms.

   b. Dispose of wrapper or cup in plastic-lined receptacle.
   c. Wear gloves when administering an injection.
       Reduces risk of exposure to blood.
   d. Discard needleless syringe or safety sheathed needle into designated sharps container.
       Needleless devices should be used to reduce risk of needlesticks and sharps injuries to health care workers.

8. Administer hygiene, encouraging patient to ask any questions or express concerns about isolation. Provide informal teaching at this time.
       Hygiene practices further minimize transfer of microorganisms. Quality time should be spent with patient when in room.

   a. Avoid allowing isolation gown to become wet; carry washbasin outward away from gown; avoid leaning against wet tabletop.
       Moisture allows organisms to travel through gown to uniform.

Clinical Decision Point *When there is a risk for excess soiling, wear a gown impervious to moisture.*

   b. Help patient remove own gown; discard in leak-proof linen bag.
       Reduces transfer of microorganisms.

   c. Remove linen from bed; avoid contact with isolation gown. Place in leak-proof linen bag.
       Handle linen soiled by patient's body fluids to prevent contact with clean items.

   d. Provide clean bed linen.
   e. Change gloves and perform hand hygiene if gloves become excessively soiled and further care is necessary. Reglove.

9. Collect specimens (see Chapter 7).

   a. Place specimen container on clean paper towel in patient's bathroom and follow procedure for collecting specimen of body fluids.
       Container will be taken out of patient's room; prevents contamination of outer surface.

   b. Follow agency procedure for collecting specimen of body fluids (see Chapter 7).

   c. Transfer specimen to container without soiling outside of container. Place container in plastic bag and place label on outside of bag or per agency policy. Label specimen in front of patient (TJC, 2016). Perform hand hygiene and reglove if additional procedures are needed.
       Specimens of blood and body fluids are placed in well-constructed containers with secure lids to prevent leaks during transport. Proper labeling prevents diagnostic error.

   d. Check label on specimen for accuracy. Send to laboratory (warning labels are often used, depending on agency policy). Label containers of blood or body fluids with biohazard sticker (see illustration).
       Ensures that health care providers who transport or handle containers are aware of infectious contents.

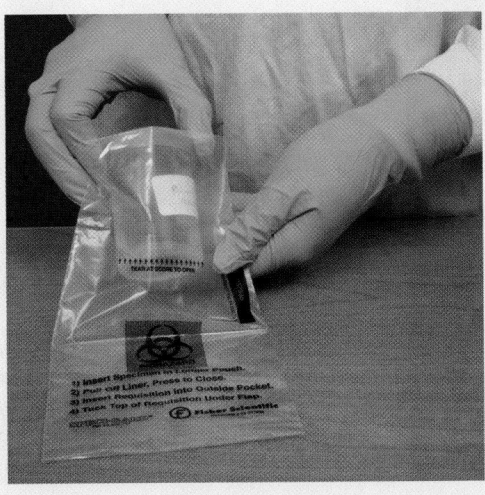

STEP 9d Place specimen container in biohazard bag.

STEP	RATIONALE

10. Dispose of linen, trash, and disposable items.
    a. Use sturdy moisture-impervious bags to contain soiled articles. Use double bag if necessary for heavily soiled linen or heavy wet trash.
    b. Tie bags securely at top in knot (see illustration).

Linen or refuse should be contained totally to prevent exposure of personnel to infectious material.

11. Remove all reusable pieces of equipment. Clean any contaminated surfaces with hospital-approved disinfectant (CDC, 2009) (see agency policy).

All items must be properly cleaned, disinfected, or sterilized for reuse.

12. Resupply room as needed. Have staff colleague hand new supplies to you.

Limiting trips of personnel into and out of room reduces your and patient's exposure to microorganisms.

13. Leave isolation room. Order of removal of PPE depends on what you wear in room. This sequence describes steps to take if all barriers were worn. PPE worn in room must be removed before leaving room.

Order of removal minimizes exposure to any infectious material on barriers.

    a. Remove gloves. Remove one glove by grasping cuff and pulling glove inside out over hand. Hold removed glove in gloved hand (see illustration). Slide fingers of ungloved hand under remaining glove at wrist. Peel glove off over first glove. Discard gloves in proper container.

Technique prevents contact with outer surface contaminated of glove.
Change gloves between exposures to body sites and patient equipment. Inadequate glove changes and hand hygiene can lead to contamination, increasing the risk of health care–associated infections (HAIs) (Haas, 2015).

    b. Remove eyewear, face shield, or goggles. Handle by headband or earpieces. Discard in proper container.

Outside of goggles is contaminated. Hands have not been soiled.

    c. Untie neck strings and then untie back strings of gown. Allow gown to fall from shoulders (see illustration); touch inside of gown only. Remove hands from sleeves without touching outside of gown. Hold gown inside at shoulder seams and fold inside out into bundle; discard in laundry bag.

Hands do not come in contact with soiled front of gown.

    d. Remove mask. If mask secures over ears, remove elastic from ears and pull mask away from face. For tie-on mask, untie *bottom* mask string and then top strings, pull mask away from face (see illustration A), and drop into trash receptacle (see illustration B). (Do not touch outer surface of mask.)

Ungloved hands are not contaminated by touching only elastic or mask strings. Prevents top part of mask from falling down over uniform.

Clinical Decision Point *If patient is on TB precautions, place reusable mask in labeled paper bag for storage, being careful not to crush mask (check agency policy for number of times reusable masks can be used).*

    e. Perform hand hygiene.
    f. Retrieve wristwatch and stethoscope (unless items must remain in room).

Reduces transmission of microorganisms.

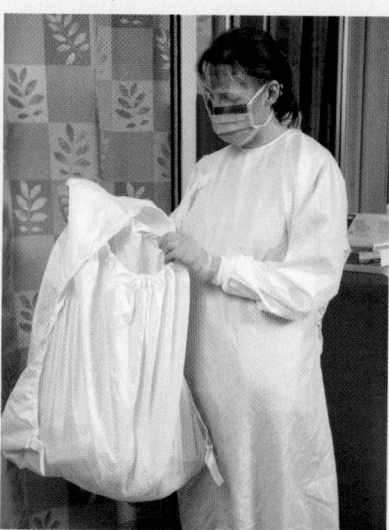

STEP 10b Tie bag securely.

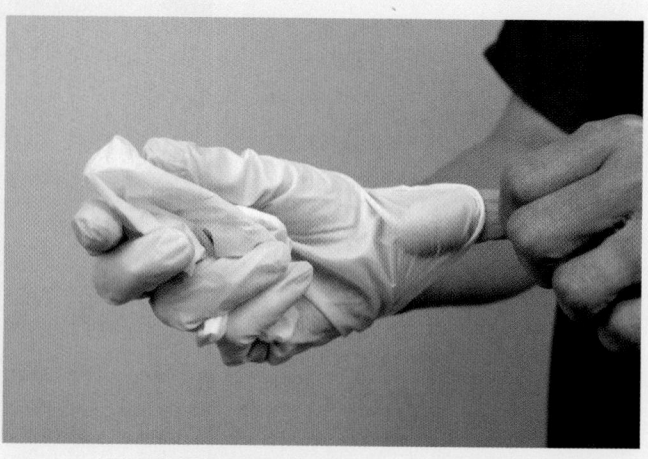

STEP 13a Remove gloves.

STEP	RATIONALE

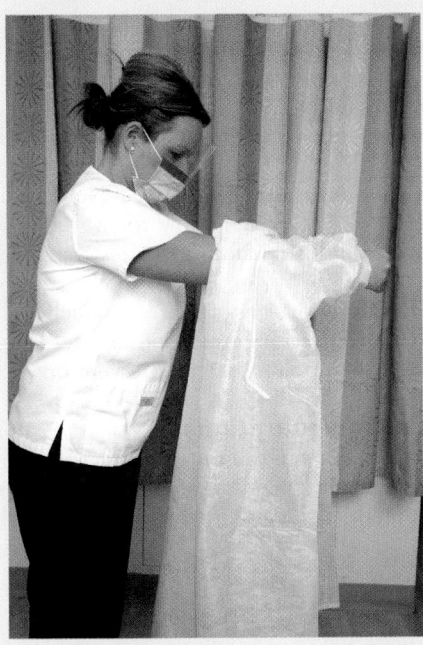

STEP 13c Remove gown by allowing it to fall from shoulders.

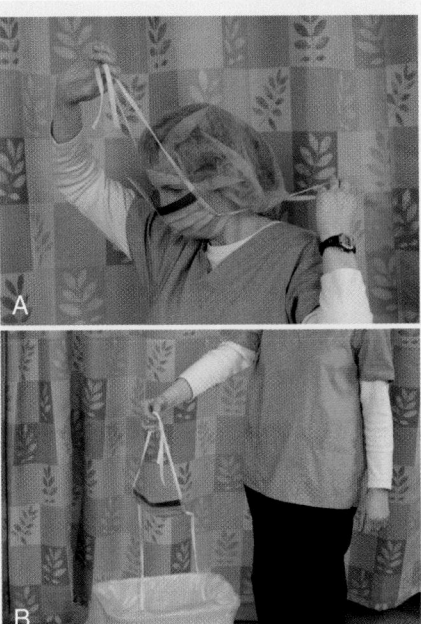

STEP 13d A, Pull mask away from face. **B,** Drop into trash receptacle.

g. Explain to patient when you plan to return to room. Ask whether patient requires any personal care items. Offer books, magazines, audiotapes.

Diversions can help to minimize boredom and feeling of social isolation.

h. Dispose of all contaminated supplies and equipment in manner that prevents spread of microorganisms to other people (see agency policy). Perform hand hygiene.

i. Leave room and close door if necessary. Close door if patient is on airborne precautions or in negative-airflow room.

Maintains negative-airflow environment and reduces transmission of microorganisms.

EVALUATION

1. Observe patient's and family caregiver's use of isolation precautions when visiting.

Promptly identifies any improper use of precaution.

2. While in room, ask if patient has had sufficient chance to discuss health problems, course of treatment, or other topics important to him or her.

Measures patient's perception of adequacy of discussions with caregivers.

3. **Use Teach-Back:** "I want to be sure I explained when these precautions are needed. Can you tell when these isolation precautions must be used?" Revise your instruction now or develop a plan for revised patient or family caregiver teaching if patient or family caregiver is not able to teach back correctly.

Determines patient's and family caregiver's level of understanding of instructional topic.

Unexpected Outcomes

1. Patient avoids social and therapeutic discussions.

2. Patient or health care worker may have an allergy to latex gloves.

Related Interventions

- Confer with family caregiver and/or significant other and determine best approach to reduce patient's sense of loneliness and depression.
- Notify health care provider/employee health and treat sensitivity or allergic reaction appropriately.
- Use latex-free gloves for future care activities.

Recording and Reporting

- Document procedures performed and patient's response to social isolation. Also document any patient or family education performed and reinforced on flow sheet or in nurses' notes in electronic health record (EHR) or chart.
- Document type of isolation in use and the microorganisms (if known).

Special Considerations
Teaching Considerations

- Teach visitors and family caregivers how to follow the recommended isolation precautions when visiting a patient.

Pediatric Considerations

- Isolation creates a sense of separation from family and loss of control. Strange environment adds to the confusion that a child feels during isolation. Preschoolers are unable to understand cause-effect relationship for isolation. Older children may be able to understand cause but still fantasize.
- Children require simple explanations (e.g., "You need to be in this room to help you get better.") Show all barriers to a child.

Actively involve parents in any explanations. Nurses let child see their faces before applying masks so child does not become frightened.

Gerontological Considerations

- Isolation can be a particular concern for older adults, especially those who have signs and symptoms of confusion or depression. Many times patients become more confused when they are confronted with a nurse using barrier precautions or when they are left in a room with the door closed. Nurses must assess need for closing door (negative-airflow room) along with safety of patient and additional safety measures that may need to be taken.
- Assess older adults for signs of depression such as loss of appetite or decrease in verbal communications. If necessary, report to the health care team for appropriate interventions.

Home Care Considerations

- Although isolation precautions followed in the hospital are not directly applicable to home care, caregivers should be aware of potential sources of contamination in the home (see Box 9.2).

PROCEDURAL GUIDELINE 9.1 *Caring for Patients With Multidrug-Resistant Organisms (MDROs) and* Clostridium difficile

Multidrug-resistant organisms (MDROs) such as methicillin-resistant *Staphylococcus aureus* (MRSA) and vancomycin-resistant enterococcus (VRE) have become increasingly common as a cause of colonization and health care–associated infections (HAIs). MRSA is a frequently identified pathogen associated with increased mortality. In recent reports MRSA caused upward of 19% of health care–associated bloodstream infections (Becker and Kahl, 2015). VRE, another MDRO, poses a greater risk to immune-compromised and debilitated patients (Archibald, 2015). *Clostridium difficile* (*C. difficile*) infection is one of the most common and costly HAIs (CDC, 2016; Edmonds et al., 2013). In most instances patient susceptibility to *C. difficile* infection requires prior treatment with antibiotics. Unlike MRSA and VRE, *C. difficile* is more difficult to eliminate from the environment because it is a spore-forming organism, meaning that it can remain on surfaces in its dormant state for long periods of time. No matter which MDRO is involved, the most common means of transmission is by way of a health care worker's hands. To reduce the risk of cross-contamination among patients, use contact precautions in addition to standard precautions when caring for these patients.

Delegation and Collaboration

Assessment of a patient's status and type of care required cannot be delegated to nursing assistive personnel (NAP). Basic care procedures performed using contact precautions can be delegated to NAP. The nurse instructs the NAP to:

- Clarify personal precautions used under contact precautions.
- Explain the type of changes in patient status to report to the nurse.

Equipment

- Clean gloves, gown, protective eyewear, surgical mask (based on patient's clinical condition)
- Basic care items (e.g., medication equipment, hygiene items)

Procedural Steps

1. Perform hand hygiene.
2. Prepare all equipment needed in patient's room.
3. Before entering room apply gown, being sure that it covers all outer garments. Pull sleeves down to wrists. Tie securely at neck and waist.
4. Apply clean gloves.
5. Explain purpose of contact precautions to patient and family caregivers.
6. Provide personal care and treatments.
7. Leave room after telling patient when you will return and asking if he or she has questions concerning his or her care.
8. Remove gloves and discard per agency policy.
9. Untie neck and waist ties on gown. Remove gown, allowing it to fall from shoulders. Discard in appropriate receptacle per agency policy.
10. Perform hand hygiene. If patient is being treated for *C. difficile* infection, clean hands with soap and water. Alcohol-based hand rubs are not effective against the spores of *C. difficile*.

◆ CLINICAL DEBRIEF

A 78-year-old man is admitted from the nursing home to an acute hospital. He is confused and has a fever, and his urinary output is decreased. After greeting the patient, the nurse begins to conduct a physical assessment.

As the nurse turns the patient to check the condition of his skin, she notices moisture on the skin. As she looks more closely, she realizes that the moisture is from an open, oozing 2 × 2–cm lesion on the patient's sacral area.

1. What should the nurse do next?
2. A few hours later the nurse prepares to enter the patient's room. Wearing gloves, she assesses the wound and quickly checks the position and function of the indwelling urinary catheter. She performs hand hygiene before leaving the patient's room. Critique the nurse's approach. Did she use correct technique?
3. Two days later the patient is complaining of increased pain at wound sight. On further assessment the nurse sees that the wound is now 3 × 3 cm; is red; and has thick, yellow drainage. Use SBAR to communicate this finding to the health care team.

REVIEW QUESTIONS

1. Which of the following are true statements in relation to hand hygiene? (Select all that apply.)
   1. The percentage of health care workers using hand hygiene has been decreasing over the last few years.
   2. The incidence of health care–associated infections has decreased because of hand hygiene.
   3. There must be a mode of transmission for an infection to occur.
   4. Soap and water must be used when hands are visibly soiled.
   5. Hand hygiene can be antiseptic hand wash, antiseptic hand rub, or handwashing.
2. A nurse is taking care of a patient on airborne precautions for tuberculosis. Which would be an appropriate intervention? (Select all that apply.)
   1. Place patient in a private room.
   2. Explain why the patient across the hall is not on precautions.
   3. Wear gloves when giving an intramuscular injection.
   4. Educate patient regarding his or her isolation.
   5. Wear a surgical mask into the room to take vital signs.
3. The nurse is having a complication of dermatitis related to repeated handwashing. Which intervention could be used to help the nurse with the situation? (Select all that apply.)
   1. Use personal hypoallergenic soap instead of soap provided.
   2. Use only approved hand lotions or barrier creams.
   3. Rinse and dry hands thoroughly after every handwashing.
   4. Quickly wash hands when needed to avoid excess damage to skin.
   5. Wear gloves and change them frequently instead of washing hands.

ⓔ *Visit the Evolve site for a complete list of Clinical Debrief and Review Questions answers.*

REFERENCES

Al-Tawfiq JA, et al: Promoting and sustaining a hospital wide, multifaceted hand hygiene program resulted in significant reduction in health care associated infections, *Am J Infect Control* 41(6):482, 2013.

Archibald L: Enterococci. In Grota P, editor: *APIC text of infection control and epidemiology*, ed 4, Washington, DC, 2015, Association for Professionals in Infection Control and Epidemiology (APIC).

Association of Operating Room Nurses (AORN): *Standards, recommended practices, and guidelines*, Denver, 2014, The Association.

Becker K, Kahl B: Staphylococci. In Grota P, editor: *APIC text of infection control and epidemiology*, ed 4, Washington, DC, 2015, Association for Professionals in Infection Control and Epidemiology (APIC).

Brisko V: Isolation precautions. In Grota P, editor: *APIC text of infection control and epidemiology*, ed 4, Washington, DC, 2015, Association for Professionals in Infection Control and Epidemiology (APIC).

Campinha-Bacote J: Delivering patient-centered care in the midst of a cultural conflict: the role of cultural competence, *OJIN* 16(2):5, 2011. http://www .nursingworld.org/MainMenuCategories/ANAMarketplace/ANAPeriodicals/ OJIN/TableofContents/Vol-16-2011/No2-May-2011/Delivering-Patient-Centered-Care-in-the-Midst-of-a-Cultural-Conflict.html. Accessed March 12, 2016.

Centers for Disease Control and Prevention (CDC): *2007 Guideline for isolation precautions: preventing transmission of infectious agents in healthcare settings*, 2007 (last update 2010), http://www.cdc.gov/hicpac/2007IP/2007isolation Precautions.html. Accessed March 12, 2016.

Centers for Disease Control and Prevention (CDC), Hospital Infection Control Practice Advisory Committee, and the HICPAC/SHEA/APIC/IDSA Hand Hygiene Task Force: *Guideline for hand hygiene in health-care settings*, Atlanta, 2008, Centers for Disease Control and Prevention.

Centers for Disease Control and Prevention (CDC): Hospital Infection Control Practices Advisory Committee: *Guidelines for isolation precautions in hospitals*, *MMWR Morb Mortal Wkly Rep* 57:RR–16, 2009.

Centers for Disease Control and Prevention (CDC): *Healthcare-associated infections (HAIs) elimination, methicillin-resistant Staphylococcus aureus (MRSA) infections*, 2010a, http://www.cdc.gov/HAI/pdfs/toolkits/MRSA_toolkit_white_020910_v2.pdf. Accessed March 12, 2016.

Centers for Disease Control and Prevention (CDC): *Respiratory protection in health care settings*, 2010b, http://www.cdc.gov/tb/publications/factsheets/prevention/rphcs.pdf. Accessed March 12, 2016.

Centers for Disease Control and Prevention (CDC): *Tuberculosis (TB): treatment*, 2011, http://www.cdc.gov/tb/topic/treatment/default.htm. Accessed March 12, 2016.

Centers for Disease Control and Prevention (CDC): *Tuberculosis (TB): basic TB facts*, 2012, http://www.cdc.gov/tb/topic/basics/default.htm. Accessed March 12, 2016.

Centers for Disease Control and Prevention: *Healthcare-associated infections (HAIS): Clostridium difficile infection*, 2016, http://www.cdc.gov/HAI/organisms/cdiff/Cdiff_infect.html. Accessed March 12, 2016.

Cohen SH, et al: Clinical practice guidelines for *Clostridium difficile* infection in adults: update by the Society for Healthcare Epidemiology of America (SHEA) and the Infectious Diseases Society of America (IDSA), *Infect Control Hosp Epidemiol* 31(5):341, 2010.

Cook K: The hands have it! Hand hygiene in the OR, *OR Nurse* 5(6):14, 2011.

Edmonds S, et al: Effectiveness of hand hygiene for removal of *Clostridium difficile* spores from hands, *Infect Control Hosp Epidemiol* 34(3):302, 2013.

Ellingson K, et al: Strategies to prevent health care–associated infections through hand hygiene, *Infect Control Hosp Epidemiol* 35(6):937, 2014.

Felembam O, et al: Hand hygiene practices of home visiting community nurses: perceptions, compliance, techniques, and contextual factors of practice using the World Health Organization's five moments for hand hygiene, *Home Health Nurse* 30(3):152, 2012.

Fluten D: Risk factors facilitating transmission of infectious agents. In Grota P, editor: *APIC text of infection control and epidemiology*, ed 4, Washington DC, 2014, Association for Professionals in Infection Control and Epidemiology (APIC).

Haas J: Hand hygiene. In Grota P, editor: *APIC text of infection control and epidemiology*, ed 4, Washington, DC, 2015, Association for Professionals in Infection Control and Epidemiology (APIC).

Luangasanatip N, et al: Comparative efficacy of interventions to improve hand hygiene in hospital: systematic review and network meta-analysis, *BMJ* 351:h3728, 2015.

Messano GA: Bacterial and fungal contamination of dental hygienists' hands with and without finger rings, *Acta Stomatologica Naissi* 29:1260, 2013.

Occupational Safety and Health Administration (OSHA): *Infectious disease: final rule*, 29 CFR Part 1910, *Fed Reg* 75:87, 2011.

Raines K, Rosen K: The effects of chlorhexidine bathing on rates of nosocomial infections among the critically ill populations: an analysis of current clinical research and recommendations for practice, *Dimens Crit Care Nurs* 35(2):84, 2016.

Roach R: Geriatrics. In Grota P, editor: *APIC text of infection control and epidemiology*, ed 4, Washington, DC, 2014, Association for Professionals in Infection Control and Epidemiology (APIC).

Schweizer MI, et al: Searching for an optimal hand hygiene bundle: a meta-analysis, *Clin Infect Dis* 58(2):248, 2014.

The Joint Commission (TJC): *2016 National Patient Safety Goals*, Oakbrook Terrace, IL, 2016, The Commission. http://www.jointcommission.org/standards_information/npsgs.aspx. Accessed March 12, 2016.

WHO guidelines on hand hygiene care, Geneva, Switzerland, 2009, World Health Organization (WHO) Press.

World Health Organization (WHO): *Five moments for hand hygiene*, 2016, http://who.int/gpsc/tools/Five_moments/en/. Accessed March 2016.

10 | Sterile Technique

OBJECTIVES

Mastery of content in this chapter will enable the nurse to:
- Discuss settings where surgical aseptic techniques are necessary.
- Describe conditions when surgical asepsis is necessary.
- Identify the principles of surgical asepsis.
- Explain the importance of organization and caution when using surgical aseptic techniques.

- Apply and remove a cap, mask, and protective eyewear correctly.
- Identify individuals at risk for a latex allergy.
- Perform the following skills: preparing a sterile field, applying sterile gloves using open-glove method, and applying a sterile drape correctly.

MEDIA RESOURCES

- evolve http://evolve.elsevier.com/Perry/skills
- Review Questions
- ▶ Video Clips

- Audio Glossary
- **NSO** Nursing Skills Online
- Clinical Debrief and Review Questions Answers

PURPOSE

Sterile technique and aseptic practices maintain an area that is free from pathogenic organisms, serve to isolate an operative area from the unsterile environment, and maintain a sterile field for surgery and invasive procedures. Proper sterile asepsis minimizes patient exposure to infection-causing agents, therefore reducing the patient's risk for infection. These techniques are common in the operating room, labor and delivery area, and major diagnostic areas, but they are also used at the bedside (e.g., when inserting an IV or urinary catheter).

STANDARDS OF CARE

Association of Perioperative Registered Nurses (AORN), 2016—Guidelines for Perioperative Practice

Centers for Disease Control and Prevention, 2007—Guidelines for Isolation Precautions

Infusion Nurses Society (INS), 2016—Infusion Therapy Standards of Practice

The Joint Commission (TJC), 2016—National Patient Safety Goals

PRINCIPLES OF PRACTICE

- The majority of sterile technique practices are used in the operating room (OR) or diagnostic procedure areas, including applying a mask, protective eyewear, and a cap; performing a surgical hand scrub; applying a sterile gown; and applying sterile gloves.
- As with medical asepsis, proper hand hygiene with an appropriate cleaner or antiseptic is required before initiating any sterile procedure.
- Surgical aseptic technique is also used at the bedside in the following situations: during procedures that require intentional puncture of the skin or insertion of devices into an area of the body that is normally sterile (e.g., sterile dressing change) or in a situation in which skin integrity is compromised because of incision or burn (Box 10.1).
- When sterile procedures are carried out in the OR or procedure area, health care providers must follow a series of steps to maintain sterile asepsis: applying a mask, protective eyewear, and cap; performing a surgical hand scrub; and applying sterile gown and gloves.
- When sterile procedures such as a sterile dressing change are carried out at the bedside, the health care provider must perform hand hygiene and apply sterile gloves. When the risk of splash is present, other personal protective equipment (PPE) is required.
- When completing a sterile procedure at the bedside, communicate with the patient about which steps are being taken to prevent infection, including which actions the patient should avoid to keep the field sterile. These actions include avoiding sudden body movements, refraining from touching sterile supplies, and avoiding coughing or talking over sterile area.

BOX 10.1

Principles of Surgical Asepsis

1. All items used within a sterile field must be sterile.
2. A sterile barrier that has been permeated by punctures, tears, or moisture must be considered contaminated.
3. Once a sterile package is opened, a 2.5-cm (1-inch) border around the edges is considered unsterile.
4. Tables draped as part of a sterile field are considered sterile only at table level.
5. If there is any question or doubt about the sterility of an item, the item is considered to be unsterile.
6. Sterile people or items contact only sterile areas; unsterile people or items contact only unsterile areas.
7. Movement around and in the sterile field must not compromise or contaminate the field.
8. A sterile object or field out of the range of vision or an object held below a person's waist is contaminated.
9. A sterile object or field becomes contaminated by prolonged exposure to air; stay organized and complete any procedure as soon as possible.

PATIENT-CENTERED CARE

- Whether performed in a hospital, ambulatory care setting, the patient's home, or health care provider's office, invasive procedures such as starting an intravenous (IV) line or inserting a urinary catheter pose a risk for infection. It is your responsibility to protect patients from infection by adhering strictly to the principles of surgical asepsis when performing invasive procedures or when helping with such a procedure and to intervene to stop it when a break in sterile technique occurs. The Joint Commission (TJC) encourages nurses to "speak up" in these instances (TJC, 2016).
- Take into consideration the patient's cultural background or beliefs when sterile asepsis is required. Individualized patient-centered education for patients and families before any aseptic procedure reduces fears and misconceptions about sterile asepsis attire. This also provides an opportunity for patients and families to ask questions and express their concerns regarding surgical attire.

EVIDENCE-BASED PRACTICE

- Recommendations such as patient-centered education, insertion of devices only when necessary, using sterile technique, and removing devices that are no longer needed have decreased the number of health care–associated infections (HAIs). However, 1 in 25 hospital patients still has at least one health care–associated infection (CDC, 2015).
- Prevention of contamination of a sterile work area is an overall goal to reduce HAIs. This can be done by minimizing traffic; comprehensive cleaning and disinfecting; changing skin preparation; administering antibiotics; and removing watches, jewelry, and artificial nails (Barnes, 2015).
- Use of additional antiseptics such as chlorhexidine reduce bacterial count on the patient's skin (AORN, 2016)
- Most health care agencies have policies against artificial nails, including extensions or tips, gels and acrylic overlays, and resin wraps (Wood and VanWicklin, 2015). The subungual area (under a fingernail) of the hand and the 'lifting' of the product from the nail bed contain a high concentration of bacteria, more specifically coagulase-negative staphylococci, gram-negative rods, and fungal growth. These organisms are not removed effectively after hand hygiene.

SAFETY GUIDELINES

- Follow standard precautions with all patients (CDC, 2007; TJC, 2016).
- Review agency policies and procedures before conducting a sterile procedure.
- Assess the potential for splash and/or transmission of infection before choosing the barrier to be used such as masks or protective eyewear.
- Nurses use barrier techniques to decrease the transmission of microorganisms from health care personnel and the environment to a patient.
- Remain organized while performing any sterile procedure; keep bedside surfaces free of clutter.
- Remember that hand hygiene is essential before and after initiating any sterile procedure to reduce HAIs (CDC, 2013).
- Apply the principles of surgical asepsis when conducting any sterile procedure.

◆ **SKILL 10.1** Applying and Removing Cap, Mask, and Protective Eyewear

NSO *Nursing Skills Online Infection Control Module / Lesson 1*

Although masks and caps are usually worn in surgical procedure areas (e.g., the operating room [OR]), certain aseptic procedures performed at a patient's bedside also require the application of additional personal protective equipment (PPE), such as eyewear, gown, and gloves. For example, it may be agency policy for a nurse to wear a mask during the changing of a central line dressing or insertion of a peripherally inserted central catheter (PICC). Other policies might require that a nurse wear a mask and a cap to secure hair during dressing changes on a patient with extensive burns or a central line (INS, 2016). When there is a risk of splattering blood or body fluid, there is also the need to apply protective eyewear (OSHA, 2012). This skill summarizes how to apply a mask, cap, and protective eyewear, which are not considered sterile. The additional application of clean or sterile gloves depends on the type of procedure being performed.

Assess a patient's potential for acquiring an infection and the splash risk before deciding whether to apply a mask (e.g., Does the patient have a large open wound? Is he or she immunosuppressed? Is there a splash risk from his or her wound?). If you wear a mask, change it when it becomes moist or soiled (e.g., splattered with blood). Wear eyewear when there is a risk of body fluids splashing into your eyes.

Delegation and Collaboration

The skill of applying and removing cap, mask, and protective eyewear is required of all caregivers when working in areas in which sterile procedures are performed. However, the procedures performed at a patient's bedside that require cap, mask, or eyewear generally cannot be delegated to nursing assistive personnel (NAP). The skill of applying PPE can be delegated to nursing assistive personnel (NAP). The nurse instructs the NAP to:

- Be available to hand off equipment or help with patient positioning during a sterile procedure.
- If the procedure is to use sterile technique, educate the NAP regarding the sterile field.

Equipment

- Surgical mask (different types are available for people with different skin sensitivities)
- Surgical cap (**NOTE:** Use in OR or if agency policy requires. Use to secure hair if there is a possibility of contamination of a sterile field.)
- Hairpins, rubber bands, or both
- Protective eyewear (e.g., goggles or glasses with appropriate side shields) *Option:* Clean or sterile gloves (applied after cap, mask, or eyewear are applied). See Chapter 9 and Skill 10.3.

STEP	RATIONALE

ASSESSMENT

1. Review type of sterile procedure to be performed and consult agency policy for use of mask/caps/protective eyewear.	Not all sterile procedures require mask, cap, or protective eyewear. Ensures that nurse and patient are properly protected.
2. If you or other health care providers have symptoms of a respiratory infection, either avoid participating in procedure or apply a mask.	A greater number of pathogenic microorganisms reside within the respiratory tract when infection is present.
3. Assess patient's risk for infection (e.g., older adult, neonate, or immunocompromised patient).	Some patients are at a greater risk for acquiring an infection; thus use additional protective barriers.

NURSING DIAGNOSES

- Ineffective protection
- Risk for infection

Related factors/Risk factors are individualized based on patient's condition or needs.

PLANNING

1. Expected outcome following completion of procedure: • Patient does not develop signs of localized infection (e.g., redness, tenderness, edema, drainage) or systemic infection (e.g., fever, change in white blood cell [WBC] count) 24 hours after procedure.	Indicates lack of microorganism transfer to patient and sterile field.
2. Prepare equipment and inspect packaging for integrity and exposure to sterilization.	Ensures availability of equipment and sterility of supplies before procedure begins.

IMPLEMENTATION

1. Perform hand hygiene (see Chapter 9)	Reduces transient microorganisms on skin.
2. *Option:* In cases in which you are performing or assisting with a procedure at a patient's bedside, apply a clean gown if there is a risk of splatter or soiling. Apply the gown with opening to the back. Be sure that it covers all outer garments. Pull sleeves down to wrist. Tie securely at neck and wrist.	Proper draping prevents transmission of infections when patient has excessive drainage or discharges.
3. Apply a cap.	
a. If hair is long, comb back behind ears and secure.	Cap must cover all hair entirely.
b. Secure hair in place with pins.	Long hair should not fall down or cause cap to slip and expose hair.
c. Apply cap over head as you would apply hairnet. Be sure that all hair fits under edges of cap (see illustration).	Loose hair hanging over sterile field or falling dander contaminates objects on sterile field.
4. Apply a mask.	
a. Find top edge of mask, which usually has thin metal strip along edge.	Pliable metal fits snugly against bridge of nose.
b. Hold mask by top two strings or loops, keeping top edge above bridge of nose.	Position prevents contact of hands with clean facial part of mask. Mask covers all of nose.

STEP	**RATIONALE**

c. Tie two top strings at top of back of head, over cap (if worn), with strings above ears (see illustration). Alternatively place loops over ears.

Position of ties at top of head provides tight fit. Strings over ears may cause irritation.

d. Tie two lower ties snugly around neck with mask well under chin (see illustration).

Tying prevents escape of microorganisms through sides of mask as you talk and breathe.

e. Gently pinch upper metal band around bridge of nose.

Pinching prevents microorganisms from escaping around nose and eyeglasses from steaming up.

5. Apply protective eyewear.

a. Apply protective glasses, goggles, or face shield comfortably over eyes and check that vision is clear (see illustration).

Positioning affects clarity of vision.

b. Be sure that face shield fits snugly around forehead and face.

Snug fitting ensures that eyes are fully protected.

6. If performing a sterile procedure, apply sterile gown (see Skill 10.3) at this time. After applying cap, mask, and eyewear, you will apply clean gloves for nonsterile procedures and sterile gloves (see Skill 10.3) for sterile procedures. Pull up clean gloves to cover each wrist (see illustration). **NOTE:** Provide a latex-free environment if patient or health care worker has a latex allergy.

7. Remove protective barriers.

a. Remove gloves first if worn (see Chapter 9 or Skill 10.3). Remove gloves by grasping cuff and pulling glove inside out over hand. Hold removed glove in hand. Slide fingers of ungloved hand under remaining glove at wrist (see illustration). Peel glove off over first glove. Discard gloves in proper container

Proper removal prevents contamination of hair, neck, and facial area.

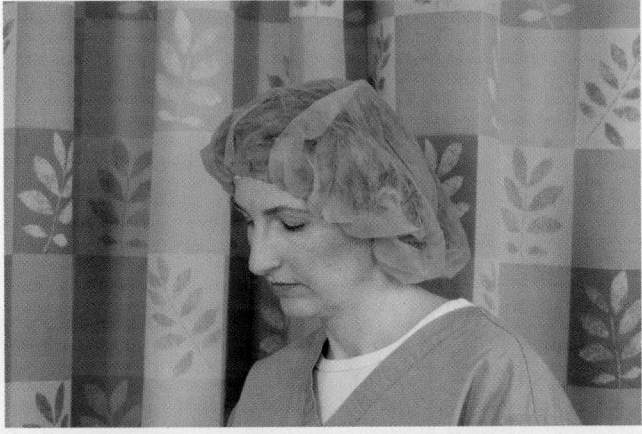

STEP 3c Apply cap over head, covering all hair.

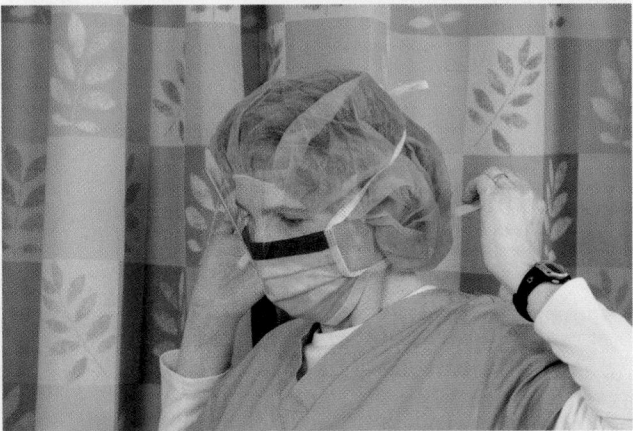

STEP 4d Tie bottom strings of mask.

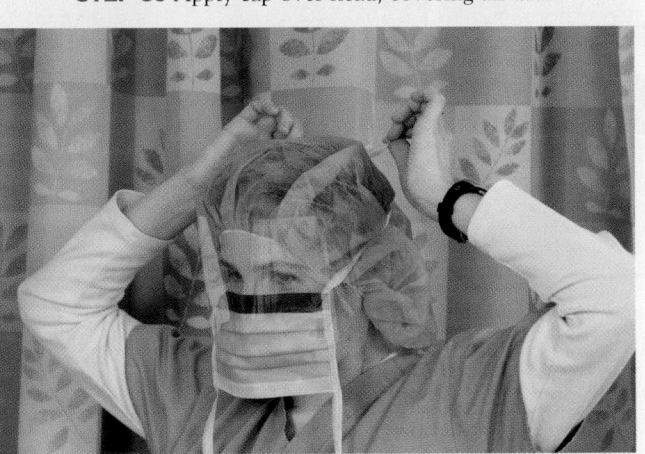

STEP 4c Tie top strings of mask.

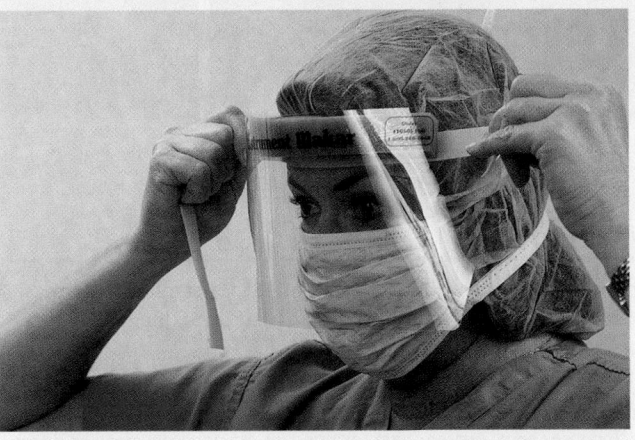

STEP 5a Apply face shield over cap.

STEP	RATIONALE
b. Remove eyewear. Avoid placing hands over soiled lens. NOTE: If wearing a face shield, remove it before removing mask.	Proper removal prevents transmission of microorganisms.
c. Remove gown by unfastening neck ties and pulling away from neck and shoulders. Touching only inside of gown, turn gown inside out, roll, or fold into a bundle and discard.	Front and sleeves of gown are contaminated. This method of disposal prevents transmission of infection.
d. Untie bottom strings of mask. First hold strings, untie top strings, and pull mask away from face while holding strings. Remove mask from face and discard in proper receptacle (see illustrations).	Proper removal prevents top part of mask from falling down over uniform. If mask falls and touches uniform, uniform will be contaminated.
e. Grasp outer surface of cap and lift from hair.	Proper removal minimizes contact of hands with hair. Routine reduces transmission of infection.
f. Discard cap in proper receptacle and perform hand hygiene.	

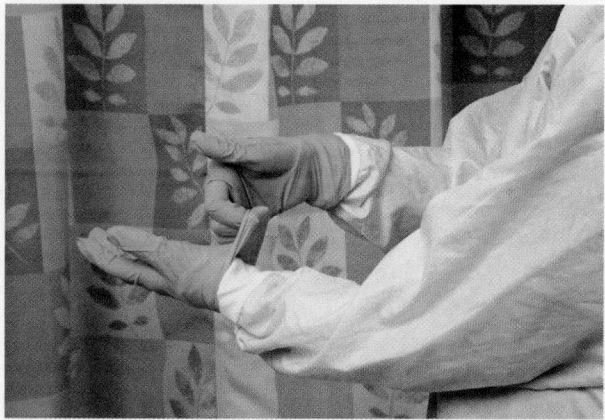

STEP 6 Apply gloves over gown sleeves.

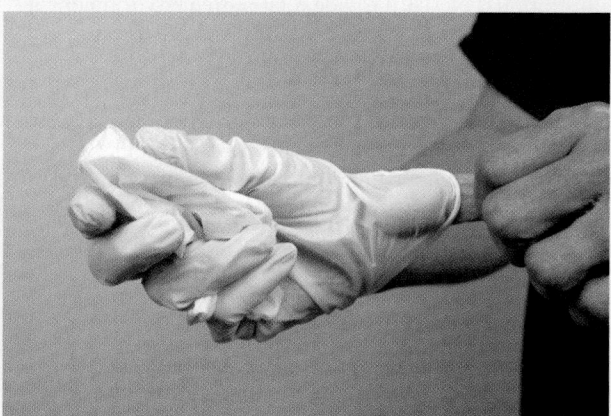

STEP 7a Remove second glove while holding soiled glove.

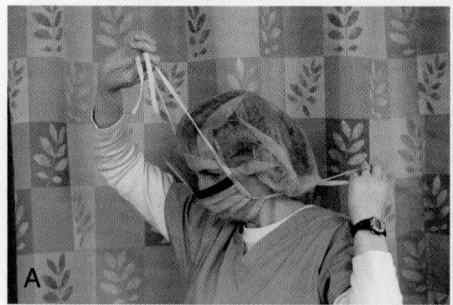 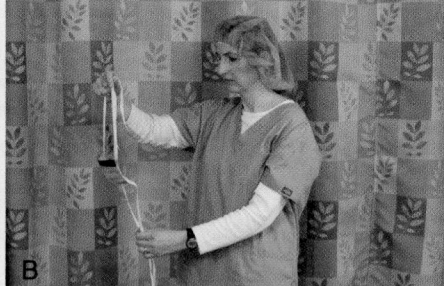 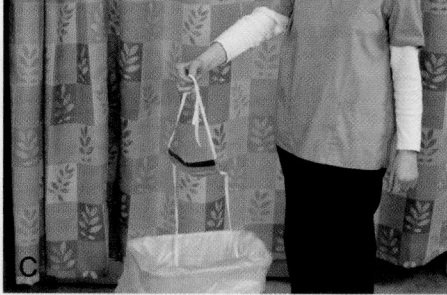

STEP 7d A, Untie top mask strings. **B,** Remove mask from face. **C,** Discard mask.

EVALUATION

1. Following the procedure, assess patient for signs of systemic infections or local area of body treated for drainage, tenderness, edema, or redness.

Assessment rules out presence of localized infection.

Unexpected Outcomes
1. Redness, heat, edema, pain, or purulent drainage develops at wound or treatment site, indicating possible infection.

Related Interventions
• Notify health care provider of change in condition of affected area and initiate appropriate treatments as ordered.

Recording and Reporting
- It is unnecessary to document use of PPE.

Special Considerations
Home Care
- Instruct family caregiver about specifics of when to use PPE and how to dispose of properly.

- Determine ability of family caregiver to use equipment safely.
- Observe for the signs and symptoms of infection.

| ◆ **SKILL 10.2** | **Preparing a Sterile Field** |

▶ *Video Clip* **NSO** *Nursing Skills Online Infection Control Module / Lesson 3*

When performing sterile aseptic procedures, you need a sterile work area in which objects can be handled with minimal risk for contamination. A sterile field provides a sterile surface for placement of sterile equipment. Sterile drapes establish a sterile field around a treatment site such as a surgical incision, venipuncture site, or site for introduction of an indwelling urinary catheter. Sterile drapes also provide a work surface for placing sterile supplies and manipulating items with sterile gloves. After a sterile kit is opened, the inside surface of the cover can be used as a sterile field. Once you create a sterile field, you are responsible for performing the procedure and making sure that the field is not contaminated.

Delegation and Collaboration
Surgical technicians may prepare a sterile field (see agency policy); however, nursing assistive personal (NAP) cannot. The nurse can direct the NAP to:

- Help with patient positioning and obtain any necessary supplies.

Equipment
- Sterile pack (commercial or institution wrapped)
- Sterile drape or kit that is to be used as a sterile field
- Sterile gloves (*optional*)
- Sterile solution and equipment specific to a procedure
- Waist-high table/countertop surface
- Appropriate personal protective equipment (PPE): gown, mask, cap, protective eyewear (see agency policy)

STEP	RATIONALE

ASSESSMENT

1. Identify patient using at least two identifiers (e.g., name and birthday or name and medical record number) according to agency policy.

   Ensures correct patient. Complies with The Joint Commission standards and improves patient safety (TJC, 2016).

2. Verify in agency policy and procedure manual that procedure requires surgical aseptic technique.

   Some procedures require medical rather than surgical aseptic technique.

3. Assess patient's comfort, positioning, oxygen requirements, and elimination needs before preparing for procedure.

   Certain procedures that require a sterile field may last a long time. Anticipates patient's needs so patient can relax and avoid any unnecessary movement that might disrupt procedure.

4. Instruct patient (and family if present) not to touch work surface or equipment during procedure.

   Instruction prevents contamination of sterile field.

5. Assess for latex allergies.

   A review may reveal latex allergies and determine the need to use latex-free supplies.

6. Check sterile package integrity for punctures, tears, discoloration, moisture, or any other signs of contamination. If using commercially packaged supplies or those prepared by agency, check for sterilization indicator (marker that changes color when exposed to heat or steam).

   Inspection of packaging ensures that only sterile items are presented to sterile field (AORN, 2016).

7. Anticipate number and variety of supplies needed for procedure.

   Not all sterile kits contain sufficient amounts or types of supplies. Failure to have necessary supplies causes you to leave sterile field, increasing risk for contamination.

NURSING DIAGNOSES

- Ineffective protection
- Risk for infection

Related factors/Risk factors are individualized based on patient's condition or needs.

STEP	RATIONALE

PLANNING

1. Expected outcomes following completion of procedure:
   • Sterile field is not contaminated.
   • Patient is not exposed to microorganisms.
2. Complete all other nursing interventions (e.g., medication administration, suctioning patient) before beginning procedure.

3. Ask visitors to step out briefly during procedure. Instruct staff helping with procedure not to move.
4. Arrange equipment at bedside.

5. Position patient comfortably for specific procedure to be performed. If a body part is to be examined or treated, position patient so area is accessible. Have NAP help with positioning as needed.
6. Explain to patient purpose of procedure and importance of sterile technique.

Correct surgical aseptic practice is performed.
Lack of exposure prevents likelihood of infection transmission.
Prepare sterile fields as close as possible to time of use to reduce potential for contamination (AORN, 2016).

Traffic or movement can increase potential for contamination through spread of microorganisms by air currents.
Ensures availability before procedure and prevents break in sterile technique. (**NOTE:** Povidone-iodine and chlorhexidine are not considered sterile solutions and require separate work surfaces for preparation.)
Patient should be able to lie still in one position comfortably during procedure. Movement can contaminate sterile field.

Explanation ensures patient's ability to cooperate with procedure. Performing patient teaching before procedure reduces need to talk during procedure, which can cause air-droplet contamination of sterile area.

IMPLEMENTATION

1. Apply PPE as needed (consult agency policy) (see Skills 10.1 and 10.3).
2. Select a clean, flat, dry work surface above waist level.

3. Perform hand hygiene (see Chapter 9).

4. Prepare sterile work surface.
   a. Use sterile commercial kit or pack containing sterile items.
      (1) Place sterile kit or pack on the prepared work surface.
      (2) Open outside cover (see illustration) and remove package from dust cover. Place on work surface.

PPE controls spread of airborne microorganisms.

A sterile object placed below a person's waist is considered contaminated.
Hand hygiene reduces number of microorganisms on hands, thus reducing transmission to patient. Do not allow rinse water to run down arms onto clean hands (i.e., arms are considered dirty).

Sterile object placed above waist level is considered sterile.

Inner kit remains sterile.

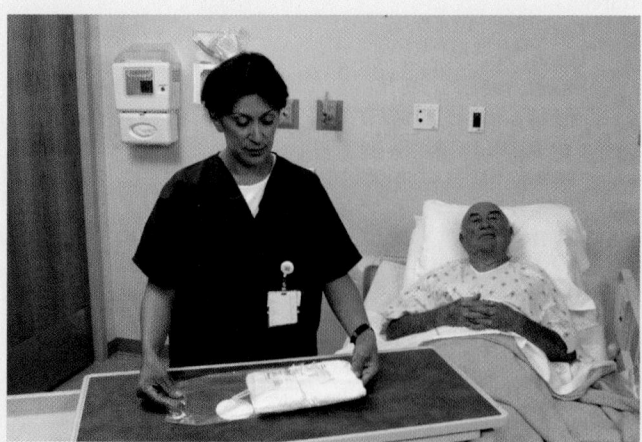

STEP 4a(2) Open outside cover of sterile kit.

STEP	RATIONALE
(3) Grasp outer surface of tip of outermost flap.	Outer surface of package is considered unsterile. There is a 2.5-cm (1-inch) border around any sterile drape or wrap that is considered contaminated and can be touched with clean fingers.
(4) Open outermost flap away from body, keeping arm outstretched and away from sterile field (see illustration).	Reaching over sterile field contaminates it.
(5) Grasp outside surface of edge of first side flap.	Outer border is considered unsterile.
(6) Open side flap, pulling to side, allowing it to lie flat on table surface. Keep arm to side and not over sterile surface (see illustration).	Drape or wrapper should lie flat so it does not accidentally rise up and contaminate inner surface or sterile contents.
(7) Repeat Step (6) for second side flap (see illustration).	
(8) Grasp outside border of last and innermost flap (see illustration). Stand away from sterile package and pull flap back, allowing it to fall flat on table. Kit is ready to be used.	Outer border is considered unsterile. Never reach over a sterile field.
b. Open sterile linen-wrapped package.	
(1) Place package on clean, dry, flat work surface above waist level.	Sterile items placed below waist level are considered contaminated.
(2) Remove sterilization tape seal and unwrap both layers following same steps (see Steps 4a [2] through 4a [8]) as for sterile kit (see illustration).	Linen-wrapped items have two layers. The first is a dust cover. The second layer must be opened to view chemical indicator.
(3) Use opened package wrapper as sterile field.	Inner surface of wrapper is considered sterile.

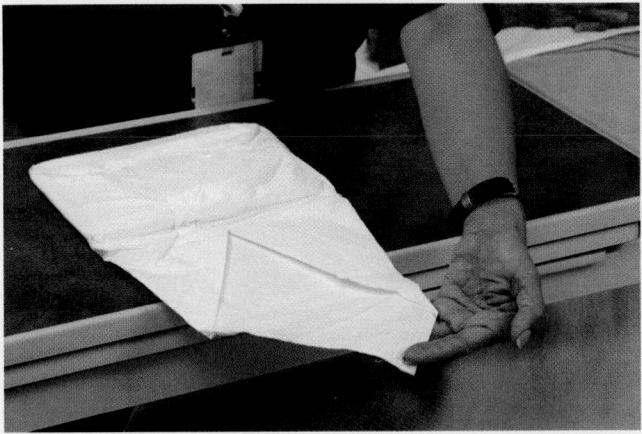

STEP 4a(4) Open outermost flap of sterile kit away from body.

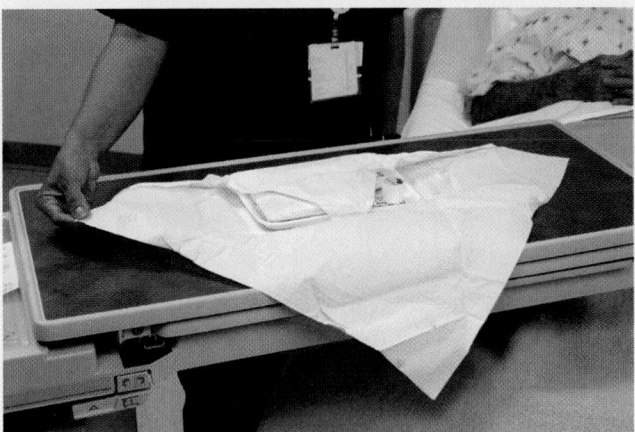

STEP 4a(7) Open second side flap, pulling to side.

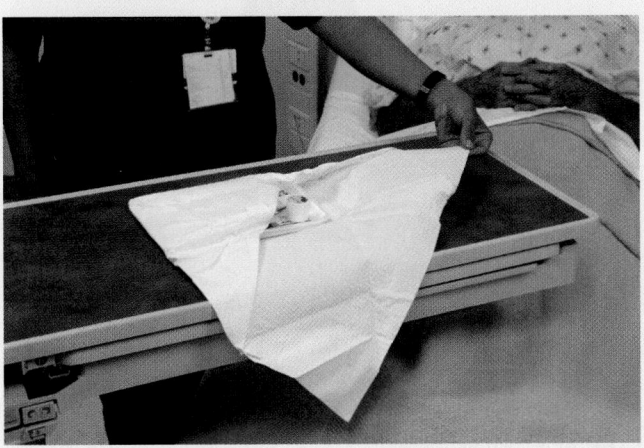

STEP 4a(6) Open first side flap, pulling to side.

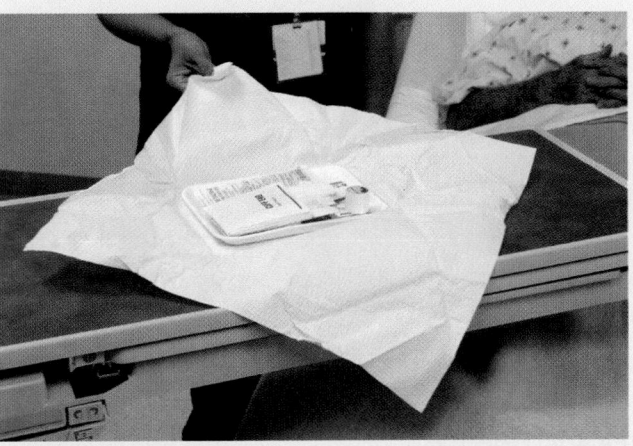

STEP 4a(8) Open last and innermost flap.

STEP	RATIONALE

c. Prepare sterile drape.

(1) Place pack containing sterile drape on flat, dry surface and open as described (see Steps 4a [2] through 4a[8]) for sterile package.

Packaged drape remains sterile.

(2) Apply sterile gloves (*optional*, see agency policy). You may touch outer 2.5-cm (1-inch) border of drape without wearing gloves.

Sterile object remains sterile only when touched by another sterile object. Gloves are not necessary as long as fingers grasp the 2.5-cm (1-inch) unsterile border of the drape.

(3) Using fingertips of one hand, pick up folded top edge of drape along 2.5 cm (1-inch) border. Gently lift drape up from its wrapper without touching any object. Discard wrapper with other hand.

If sterile object touches any nonsterile object, it becomes contaminated.

(4) With other hand, grasp an adjacent corner of drape and hold it straight up and away from body. Allow drape to unfold, keeping it above waist and work surface and away from body (see illustration). (Carefully discard wrapper with other hand.)

An object held below a person's waist or above chest is contaminated.

Drape can now be placed properly with two hands.

(5) Holding drape, position bottom half over top half of intended work surface (see illustration).

Proper positioning prevents nurse from reaching over sterile field.

(6) Allow top half of drape to be placed over bottom half of work surface (see illustration).

Proper positioning creates flat, sterile work surface for placement of sterile supplies.

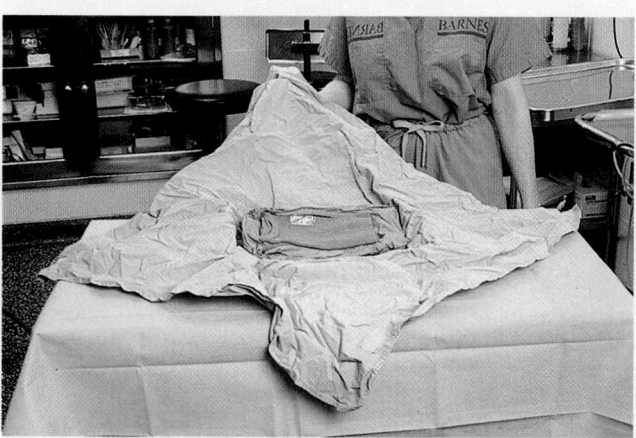

STEP 4b(2) Open sterile linen-wrapped package.

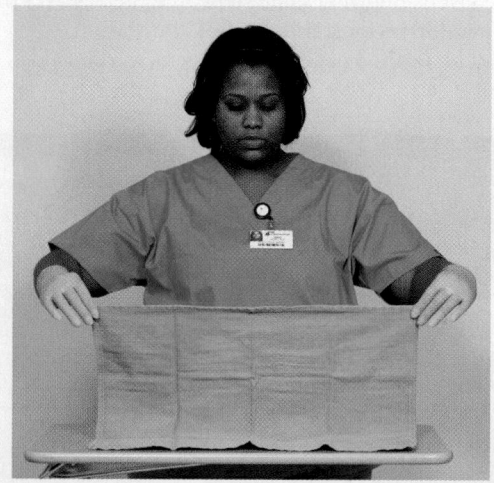

STEP 4c(5) Position bottom half of sterile drape over top half of work space.

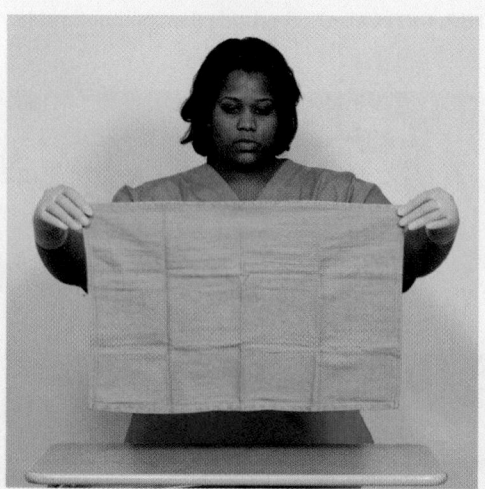

STEP 4c(4) Grasp corners of sterile drape, then hold up and away from body.

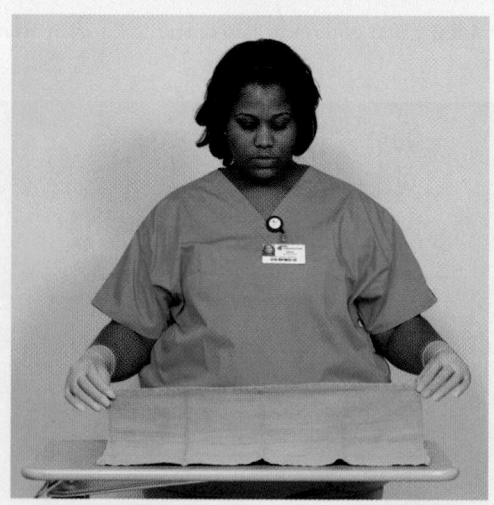

STEP 4c(6) Allow top half of drape to be placed over bottom half of work surface.

STEP	RATIONALE

5. Add sterile items to sterile field.

a. Open sterile item (following package directions) while holding outside wrapper in nondominant hand.

Use of nondominant hand frees dominant hand for unwrapping outer wrapper.

b. Carefully peel wrapper over nondominant hand.

Item remains sterile. Inner surface of wrapper covers hand, making it sterile.

c. Be sure that the wrapper does not fall down onto the sterile field. Place the item onto the field at an angle (see illustration). **Do not hold arms over sterile field.**

Secured wrapper edges prevent flipping wrapper and contaminating contents of sterile field (AORN, 2016).

Clinical Decision Point *Do not flip or toss objects onto sterile field.*

d. Dispose of outer wrapper.

Disposal prevents accidental contamination of sterile field.

6. Pour sterile solutions.

a. Verify contents and expiration date of solution.

Verification ensures proper solution and sterility of contents.

b. Place receptacle for solution near table/work surface edge. Sterile kits have cups or plastic molded sections into which fluids can be poured.

Proper placement prevents reaching over sterile field during pouring of solution.

c. Remove sterile seal and cap from bottle in upward motion.

Upward movement prevents contamination of bottle lip.

d. With solution bottle held away from field and bottle lip 2.5 to 5 cm (1 to 2 inches) above inside of sterile receiving container, slowly pour needed amount of solution into container. Hold bottle with label facing palm of hand (see illustration).

Edge and outside of bottle are considered contaminated. Slow pouring prevents splashing. Sterility of contents cannot be ensured if cap is replaced.

Prevents label from becoming wet and illegible.

Clinical Decision Point *When liquids permeate sterile field or barrier, it is called strike through, resulting in contamination of the sterile field.*

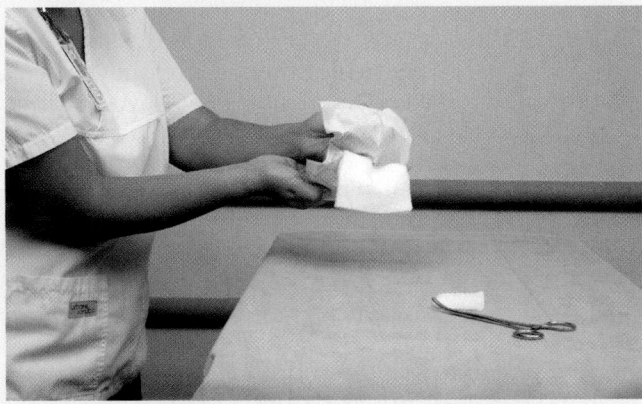

STEP 5c Add items to sterile field.

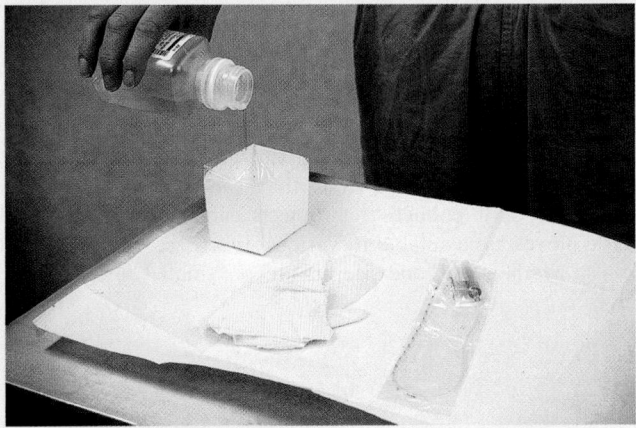

STEP 6d Pour solution into receiving container on sterile field.

EVALUATION

1. Observe for breaks in sterile technique.

A break in sterile field requires you to set up new sterile field.

Unexpected Outcomes	Related Interventions
1. Sterile field comes in contact with contaminated object or liquid splatters onto drape, causing strike through.	• Discontinue field preparation and start over with new equipment.
2. Sterile item falls off sterile field.	• Open another package containing new sterile item and add to field unless field becomes contaminated, in which case a new sterile field would need to be established.

Recording and Reporting

• No recording or reporting is required for this set of skills. Record sterile procedure performed and patient status on flow sheet or in nurses' notes in electronic health record (EHR) or chart.

Special Considerations
Home Care

• Most care procedures in the home setting involve clean technique. In the event that a sterile environment is ordered, patient and family caregiver need to be aware of the principles that apply to the sterile environment. For example, teach family caregiver how to correctly use package wrapper as a sterile drape/barrier when applying a sterile dressing or the correct procedure for removing sterile item from package.

• Assess patient's and family caregiver's understanding and ability to provide a sterile environment when needed to perform a specific procedure.

✦ SKILL 10.3   Sterile Gloving

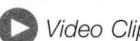 Video Clip   **NSO** Nursing Skills Online Infection Control Module / Lesson 4

Sterile gloves help prevent the transmission of pathogens by direct and indirect contact. Nurses apply sterile gloves before performing sterile procedures such as inserting urinary catheters or applying sterile dressings. Sterile gloves do not replace hand hygiene.

It is important to verify if the patient or health care providers have a latex allergy. When allergies are present, select latex-free gloves. Repeated exposure to latex can lead to a latex allergy; in which case latex-free gloves would need to be used. Box 10.2 lists risk factors for a latex allergy. Latex proteins enter the body through skin or mucous membranes, intravascularly, or via inhalation. Reactions to latex range from mild to severe (Box 10.3).

Gloves must be the proper size. The gloves should not stretch so tightly over the fingers that they can tear easily, yet they need to be tight enough that objects can be picked up easily. Sterile gloves are available in various sizes (e.g., 6, 6½, 7). They are also available in "one size fits all" or "small," "medium," and "large."

Delegation and Collaboration

Assisting with skills that include the application and removal of sterile gloves may be delegated to nursing assistive personnel (NAP). However, most procedures that require the use of sterile gloves cannot be delegated to NAP. The nurse instructs the NAP about:

• The reason for using sterile gloves for a specific procedure.

Equipment

• Package of proper-size sterile gloves, latex or synthetic nonlatex. If patient has a latex allergy, ensure that gloves are latex free and powder free.

BOX 10.2

Individuals at Risk for Latex Allergy

• Spina bifida
• Multiple surgeries or medical procedures
• High latex exposure (e.g., health care workers, housekeepers, food handlers, tire manufacturers, workers in industries that use gloves routinely)
• Rubber industry workers
• Personal or family history of allergies.
• There is a connection between an allergy to latex and an allergy to avocados, bananas, chestnuts, kiwis and passion fruits. These foods have some of the identical allergens that are found in latex.

Mayo Clinic: Diseases and conditions: latex allergy: 2014, http://www.mayoclinic.org/diseases-conditions/latex-allergy/basics/risk-factors/con-20024233. Accessed January 2016.

BOX 10.3

Levels of Latex Reactions

The three types of common latex reactions (in order of severity) are as follows:

1. *Irritant dermatitis:* Skin reaction isolated to the area of contact.
   a. Acute reaction: Red, dry, itchy and irritated
   b. Chronic reaction: Dry, thick skin, crusting and possibly cracking or peeling, resulting in open sores
2. *Type IV delayed hypersensitivity:* Allergic reaction to chemicals used in latex processing.
   a. Acute reaction: Dry, red, rash, itchy, hives, small blisters
   b. Chronic reaction: Dry, thickened skin, crusting, scabbing sores, vesicles, peeling (appears 4-96 hours after exposure)
3. *Type I immediate hypersensitivity:* Could be life-threatening, and reactions can start as soon as 2-3 minutes after contact up to several hours.
   a. Acute reaction: Hives, swelling, runny nose, nausea, abdominal cramps, dizziness, low blood pressure, bronchospasm, anaphylaxis (shock)

Centers for Disease Control and Prevention, Frequently asked questions: contact dermatitis and latex allergy, 2013, http://www.cdc.gov/oralhealth/infectioncontrol/faq/latex.htm. Accessed January 2016.

STEP	RATIONALE

ASSESSMENT

1. Consider the type of procedure to be performed and consult agency policy on use of sterile gloves. In some institutions double gloving has been recommended for the OR (Childs, 2013).

Ensures proper use of sterile gloves when needed. Evidence supports the use of double gloving and double gloving with an indicator glove system to decrease the risk of percutaneous injury and therefore is an effective barrier to bloodborne pathogen exposure (AORN, 2016).

2. Consider patient's risk for infection (e.g., preexisting condition and size or extent of area being treated).

Knowledge of risk directs you to follow added precautions (e.g., use of additional protective barriers) if necessary.

3. Select correct size and type of gloves and examine glove package to determine if it is dry and intact with no water stains.

Torn or wet package is considered contaminated. Signs of water stains on package indicate previous contamination by water.

4. Inspect condition of hands for cuts, hangnails, open lesions, or abrasions. In some settings you are allowed to cover any open lesion with a sterile, impervious transparent dressing (check agency policy). In some cases presence of such lesions may prevent you from participating in a procedure.

Cuts, abrasions, and hangnails tend to ooze serum, which possibly contains pathogens. Breaks in skin integrity permit microorganisms to enter and increase the risk for infection for both patient and nurse (AORN, 2016).

5. Assess patient for the following risk factors before applying latex gloves:

Risk factors determine level of patient's risk for latex allergy.

   a. Previous reaction to the following items within hours of exposure: adhesive tape, dental or face mask, golf club grip, ostomy bag, rubber band, balloon, bandage, elastic underwear, intravenous (IV) tubing, rubber gloves, condom

Items are known to lead to latex allergy.

   b. Personal history of asthma, contact dermatitis, eczema, urticaria, rhinitis

Patients with a history of these conditions are at higher risk of having a reaction.

   c. History of food allergies, especially avocado, banana, peach, chestnut, raw potato, kiwi, tomato, papaya

Patients with a history of food allergies are at higher risk of developing a reaction.

   d. Previous history of adverse reactions during surgery or dental procedure

Previous history suggests allergic response.

   e. Previous reaction to latex product

Previous reaction suggests allergic response.

NURSING DIAGNOSES

- Ineffective protection
- Risk for infection
- Risk for injury

Related factors/Risk factors are individualized based on patient's condition or needs.

PLANNING

1. Expected outcomes following completion of procedure:
   - Patient does not develop signs or symptoms of infection after procedure.

Lack of signs of infection indicates that microorganisms are not introduced into sterile body cavities or sites (such as skin or urinary tract).

   - Patient does not develop latex sensitivity or latex allergy reaction.

Patient at risk for latex allergy is not exposed to latex proteins.

Clinical Decision Point *Synthetic nonlatex gloves (latex free/powder free) must be used when patients are at risk or if nurse has sensitivity or allergy to latex.*

IMPLEMENTATION

1. Apply sterile gloves.
   a. Perform thorough hand hygiene. Place glove package near work area.

Hand hygiene reduces number of bacteria on skin surfaces and transmission of infection. Proximity to work area ensures availability before procedure.

   b. Remove outer glove package wrapper by carefully separating and peeling apart sides (see illustration).

Proper removal prevents inner glove package from accidentally opening and touching contaminated objects.

   c. Grasp inner package and lay on clean, dry, flat surface at waist level. Open package, keeping gloves on inside surface of wrapper (see illustration).

Sterile object held below waist is contaminated. Inner surface of glove package is sterile.

STEP	RATIONALE
d. Identify right and left glove. Each glove has a cuff approximately 5 cm (2 inches) wide. Glove dominant hand first.	Proper identification of gloves prevents contamination by improper fit. Gloving of dominant hand first improves dexterity.
e. With thumb and first two fingers of nondominant hand, grasp glove for dominant hand by touching only inside surface of cuff.	Inner edge of cuff will lie against skin and thus is not sterile.
f. Carefully pull glove over dominant hand, leaving a cuff and being sure that cuff does not roll up wrist. Be sure that thumb and fingers are in proper spaces (see illustration).	If outer surface of glove touches hand or wrist, it is contaminated.
g. With gloved dominant hand, slip fingers underneath cuff of second glove (see illustration).	Cuff protects gloved fingers. Sterile touching sterile prevents glove contamination.
h. Carefully pull second glove over fingers of nondominant hand (see illustration).	Contact of gloved hand with exposed hand results in contamination.

Clinical Decision Point *Do not allow fingers and thumb of gloved dominant hand to touch any part of exposed nondominant hand. Keep thumb of dominant hand abducted back.*

i. After second glove is on, interlock hands together and hold away from body above waist level until beginning procedure (see illustration).	Ensures smooth fit over fingers and prevents contamination.

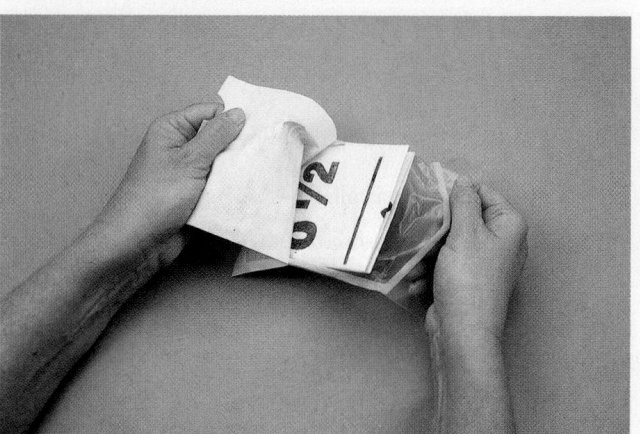

STEP 1b Open outer glove package wrapper.

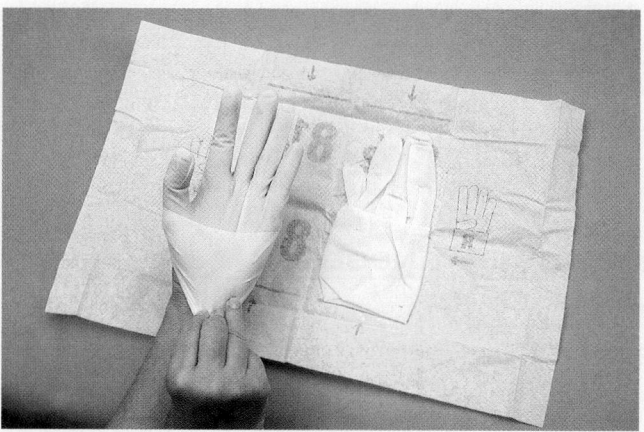

STEP 1f Pick up glove at cuff of dominant hand and insert fingers. Pull glove completely over dominant hand (example is for left-handed person)

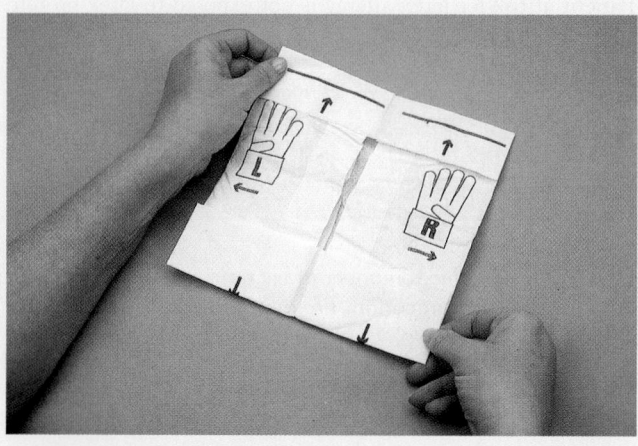

STEP 1c Open inner glove package on work surface.

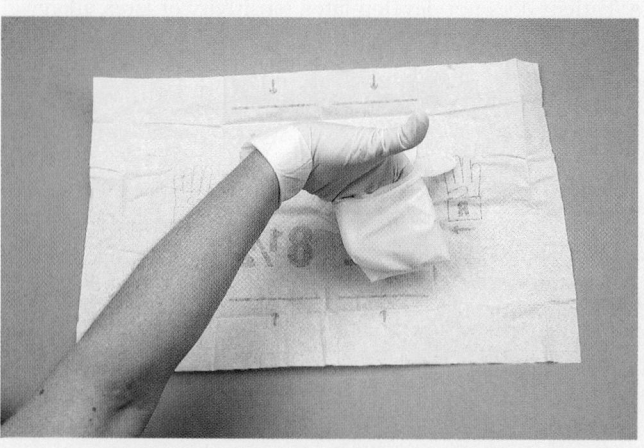

STEP 1g Pick up glove for nondominant hand.

STEP	RATIONALE

2. Perform procedure.
3. Remove gloves.
   a. Grasp outside of one cuff with other gloved hand; avoid touching wrist.
   b. Pull glove off, turning it inside out, and place it in gloved hand.
   c. Take fingers of bare hand and tuck inside remaining glove cuff (see illustration). Peel glove off inside out and over previously removed glove. Discard both gloves in receptacle.
   d. Perform thorough hand hygiene.

Procedure minimizes contamination of underlying skin.

Outside of glove does not touch skin surface.

Fingers do not touch contaminated glove surface.

Hand hygiene protects health care worker from contamination resulting from any unseen tears or pinholes in gloves; also removes powder from hands to prevent skin irritation.

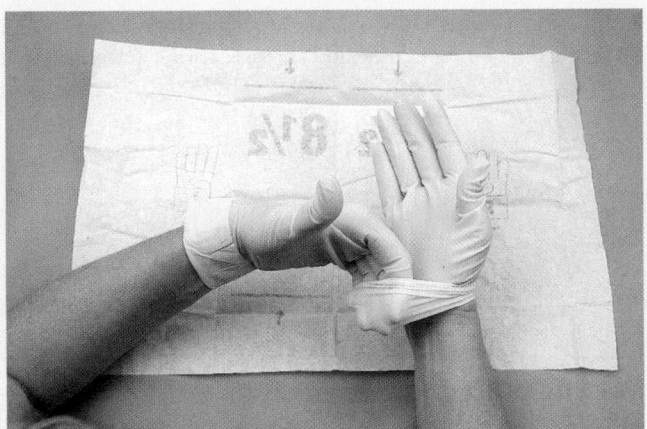

STEP 1h Pull second glove over nondominant hand.

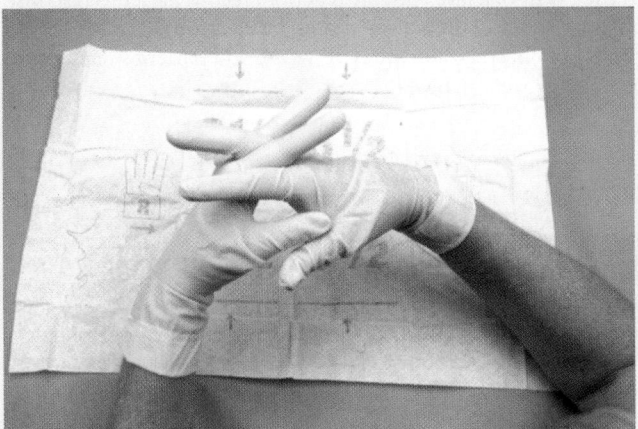

STEP 1i Interlock gloved hands.

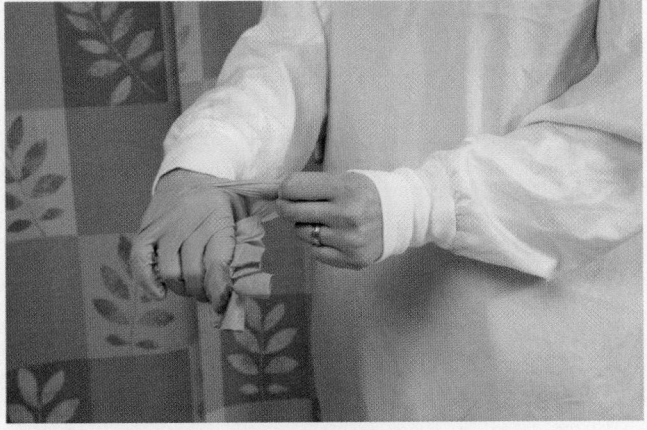

STEP 3c Remove second glove by turning it inside out.

EVALUATION

1. Assess patient for signs of infection, focusing on area treated.
2. Assess patient for signs of latex allergy.

Improper technique contributes to development of an infection.
Assessment establishes baseline for patient's reaction to latex.

Unexpected Outcomes

1. Patient develops localized signs of infection (e.g., urine becomes cloudy or odorous; wound becomes painful, edematous, or reddened with purulent drainage).
2. Patient develops systemic signs of infection (e.g., fever, malaise, increased white blood cell count).
3. Patient develops allergic reaction to latex (see Box 10.3).

Related Interventions

- Contact health care provider and implement appropriate treatments as ordered.

- Contact health care provider and implement appropriate treatments as ordered.
- Immediately remove source of latex.
- Bring emergency equipment to bedside. Have epinephrine injection ready for administration, and be prepared to initiate IV fluids and oxygen.

Recording and Reporting

- It is not necessary to record application of gloves. Record specific procedure performed and patient's response and status.
- In the event of a latex allergy reaction, record patient's response on flow sheet or in nurses' notes in electronic health record (EHR) or chart. Note type of response and patient's reaction to emergency treatment.

Special Considerations
Teaching

- Nurse or patient with a known latex allergy should wear a medical alert bracelet or tag and carry a wallet card stating "latex allergy."
- Individuals with known latex allergies should carry a quick-acting oral antihistamine and an epinephrine autoinjector at all times.

◆ CLINICAL DEBRIEF

A 78-year-old blind woman is being admitted for a cholecystectomy (removal of gallbladder). You enter her room to begin a series of procedures: inserting an indwelling urinary catheter, irrigating a nasogastric tube, suctioning the oral cavity, and measuring her blood pressure.

1. Which procedure requires use of sterile gloves?
2. The health care provider is planning to insert a central venous line. You obtained the necessary equipment, prepared a sterile drape, and opened the sterile pack. You removed the outer wrapper and placed the item on the sterile field. While doing this, you noticed that the item touched the drape 5 cm (2 inches) from the border of the drape. What would you do next?
3. The patient tells you that she develops dermatitis when she uses rubber gloves while doing the dishes and develops a rash when she eats bananas or tomatoes. How would you use SBAR (Situation-Background-Assessment-Recommendation) to communicate this information to the rest of the health care team?

◆ REVIEW QUESTIONS

1. When opening a sterile pack, which action compromises the sterility of the contents? (Select all that apply.)
   1. Positioning the contents of the pack at the very edge of the drape
   2. Holding or moving the object below the waist
   3. Opening the pack just before the procedure
   4. Allowing minimal movement around the sterile field
   5. Obtaining a nonlatex catheter for the procedure
2. When performing a sterile procedure at the bedside, the NAP can help by helping the nurse _____ the patient.
3. Which of the following procedures requires sterile (aseptic) technique? (Select all that apply.)
   1. Urinary catheterization
   2. Insertion of a feeding tube
   3. Tracheal suctioning
   4. Lumbar puncture
   5. Insertion of a rectal suppository
   6. Sitz bath

Ⓔ *Visit the Evolve site for a complete list of Clinical Debrief and Review Questions answers.*

REFERENCES

Association of periOperative Registered Nurses (AORN): *Guidelines for perioperative practice*, Denver, 2016, AORN.

Barnes S: Infection prevention: the surgical care continuum, *AORN J* 101(5):512, 2015.

Centers for Disease Control and Prevention (CDC): 2007 *Guideline for isolation precautions: preventing transmission of infectious agents in healthcare settings*, http://www.cdc.gov/hicpac/2007IP/2007isolationPrecautions.html. Accessed January, 2016.

Centers for Disease Control and Prevention (CDC): *Frequently asked questions: contact dermatitis and latex allergy*, 2013, http://www.cdc.gov/oralhealth/infectioncontrol/faq/latex.htm. Accessed January, 2016.

Centers for Disease Control and Prevention (CDC): *Health care associated infections*, 2015, http://www.cdc.gov/hai/surveillance/index.html. Accessed May 21, 2016.

Childs T: Use of double gloving to reduce surgical personnel's risk of exposure to bloodborne pathogens: an integrative review, *AORN J* 98(6):585, 2013.

Infusion Nurses Society: Infusion therapy standards of practice, *J Intraven Nurs* 39(Suppl 1):1S, 2016.

Occupational Safety and Health Administration (OSHA): Blood-borne pathogens, *Fed Reg* 77:19934, 2012.

The Joint Commission (TJC): *National Patient Safety Goals*, Oakbrook Terrace, IL, 2016, The Commission. http://www.jointcommission.org/topics/patient_safety.aspx. Accessed January, 2016.

Wood A, VanWicklin SA: Ultraviolet (UV)-cured nail polish, *AORN J* 101(6):702, 2015.

11 | Safe Patient Handling, Transfer, and Positioning

OBJECTIVES

Mastery of content in this chapter will enable the nurse to:
- Describe principles of safe patient handling, transfer, and positioning.
- Explain the importance of using mechanical lifts and other assist devices when moving, positioning, and transferring patients.
- Perform an assessment for determining the type of approach to use and amount of help needed to transfer and position patients safely.
- Describe transfer and positioning procedures to follow to ensure patient and nurse safety.
- Describe positioning techniques for the supported Fowler's, supine, prone, 30-degree lateral side-lying, and Sims' positions.
- Describe the procedures for helping a patient move up in bed, helping a patient to a sitting position, logrolling a patient, and transferring a patient from a bed to a chair.

MEDIA RESOURCES

- evolve http://evolve.elsevier.com/Perry/skills
- Review Questions
- ▶ Video Clips
- Audio Glossary
- **NSO** Nursing Skills Online
- Clinical Debrief and Review Questions Answers

PURPOSE

Health care agencies are required to provide employees with safety information and training to use when transferring, positioning, and lifting patients. Relying on proper body mechanics and manual lifting techniques alone is not effective for reducing health care workers' musculoskeletal injuries. A comprehensive safe patient-handling program that combines management commitment with employee involvement, polices, and proper mechanical equipment availability and training is needed (OSHA, nd). Workers might need to move, roll, steady, and position patients while using lifting equipment. However, because most musculoskeletal injuries in hospital settings are cumulative, any steps taken to minimize the potential for musculoskeletal injuries during patient handling tasks benefit health care workers. Refer to the policies and procedures of the agency in which you work. Many patients have conditions resulting in immobility or require limitations in activity imposed by their treatment plan. It is an important nursing role to safely and correctly position and move patients effectively to reduce the risks related to immobilization such as skin breakdown, pneumonia, and deep vein thrombosis. When performing the skills in this chapter, it is essential to use safe patient-handling techniques.

STANDARDS OF CARE

- Occupational Safety & Health Administration (OSHA), 2014—Guidelines for Back Safety
- American Nurses Association (ANA), 2013a, b—Safe Patient Handling
- Occupational Safety & Health Association, 2015—Worker Safety in Hospitals
- The Joint Commission, 2016—Patient Safety Goals

PRINCIPLES FOR PRACTICE

- Body mechanics is the coordinated effort of the musculoskeletal and nervous systems to maintain balance, posture, and body alignment during lifting, bending, moving, and performing activities of daily living (ADLs).
- The use of safe patient transfer and positioning techniques helps patients achieve an optimal level of independence without resultant injury to health care providers.
- Teaching the use of safe patient-handling equipment in combination with proper body mechanics is more effective than either one in isolation (Krill et al., 2012; Pelczarski, 2012).
- Key principles in determining the proper handling techniques to use for patients are knowing if a patient is weight bearing and the patient's weight and height, strength, and ability to cooperate and provide help (Nelson and Baptiste, 2006).
- Patients who are at high risk for complications from improper positioning and injury during transfer include those with poor nutrition, poor circulation, loss of sensation, alterations in bone formation or joint mobility, and impaired muscle development.

PATIENT-CENTERED CARE

- Ultimately it is a patient's choice to increase his or her mobility and activity level. Consider a patient's knowledge, cultural beliefs, and attitudes about the loss of independent activity and the willingness to participate in activity when developing a plan of care.
- Use simple language when you provide patients information about the complications of immobility and their unique risks.
- Consider the circumstances surrounding a patient's loss of independent activity and mobility to ensure that a plan of care is realistic and attainable.
- Understand to what extent the patient chooses to have a family caregiver involved to learn transfer and positioning techniques for home care.

EVIDENCE-BASED PRACTICE

Evidence has grown with regard to techniques necessary to reduce workplace injuries within health care settings.

- Inpatient health care settings have some of the highest rates of injury and illness among all industries. In 2014, US hospitals recorded 294,000 nonfatal work-related injuries and illnesses—a total case rate of 6.2 work-related injuries and illnesses for every 100 full-time employees, almost twice as high as the rate for private industry as a whole (3.2 per 100 full-time employees) (Bureau of Labor Statistics, 2014).
- OSHA has provided guidelines for how to complete an ergonomics hazard assessment on the basis of patient population, patient-handling tasks, and physical environment (OSHA, 2014; 2015). It is critical to train health care staff about devices, equipment, and handling policies (OSHA, 2014; 2015).
- Most organizations have developed "no-lift" policies that discourage manual lifting and require the use of safe handling of equipment and devices as needed (ANA, 2013a;b).
- Knowledge about safe, efficient transfer and positioning techniques (Box 11.1) and proper use of assistive equipment and devices promotes safe patient transfer without injury to a patient or health care worker (ANA, 2013a;b).

Principles of Safe Body Mechanics When Transferring and Positioning Patients

Mechanical lifts and lift teams are essential when patient is unable to help. When a patient is able to help, remember these principles:

- The lower the center of gravity, the greater the stability of the nurse.
- The equilibrium of an object is maintained as long as the line of gravity passes through its base of support.
- Facing the direction of movement prevents abnormal twisting of the spine.
- Dividing balanced activity between arms and legs reduces the risk for back injury.
- Leverage, rolling, turning, or pivoting requires less work than lifting.
- When friction is reduced between the object to be moved and the surface on which it is moved, less force is required to move it.

SAFETY GUIDELINES

- Know how physiological influences on body alignment and mobility affect patients throughout the life span. Inactive older adults are at risk for muscle atrophy, loss of bone mass, contractures of joints, and pressure injury (Touhy and Jett, 2014).
- Control the factors that can indirectly affect body mechanics by making the environment safe. Cluttered hallways and bedside areas increase a patient's risk of falling (see Chapter 43).
- Assess a patient's range of motion. Contractures or spasticity limit joint and muscle mobility; take care not to position a patient's limb in an unnatural position. This could result in injury or dysfunction of the affected limb (see Chapter 12).
- Determine a patient's level of sensory perception (vision and hearing) because this affects his or her ability to cooperate during transfer and lifting procedures (see Chapter 6).
- Loss of sensation increases vulnerability to the hazards of immobility because of the inability to sense pain or the need for repositioning.
- Use assistive equipment and devices to transfer and position patients safely (Sherwood and Barnsteiner, 2012).

◆ SKILL 11.1   **Using Safe and Effective Transfer Techniques**

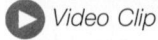 *Video Clip* **NSO** *Nursing Skills Online Safety Module / Lesson 3*

Safe and effective transfer is a nursing skill for assisting dependent patients or patients with restricted mobility attain positions to regain or maintain optimal independence. For example, transferring from a bed to a chair promotes physical activity to maintain and improve joint motion, increase strength, promote circulation, relieve pressure on the skin, and improve urinary and respiratory functions (see Chapter 12). It also benefits a patient psychologically by increasing social activity and mental stimulation and providing a change in environment (Huether and McCance, 2016).

Consider an individual patient's clinical problems during a transfer. For example, a patient who has been immobile for several days or longer may be weak or dizzy or may develop orthostatic hypotension (a drop in blood pressure) when transferred to a chair. To ensure safe patient transfers, always use a gait or transfer belt or

an appropriate lift and get help from a colleague (Freeman et al., 2011; Largo et al., 2012).

Delegation and Collaboration

The skill of effective transfer techniques can be delegated to trained nursing assistive personnel (NAP). The nurse is responsible to initially assess patient's readiness and ability to transfer. The nurse directs the NAP by:

- Helping and supervising when moving patients who are transferred for the first time after prolonged bed rest, extensive surgery, critical illness, or spinal cord trauma.
- Explaining the patient's mobility restrictions, changes in blood pressure to monitor for, or sensory alterations that may affect safe transfer.

- Explaining what to observe for and report back to the nurse such as dizziness or the patient's ability to help.

Equipment

- Transfer belt
- Sling (as needed)
- Nonskid shoes, bath blankets, pillows
- Slide board (friction-reducing board)
- Bedside chair with arms
- Stretcher: Position next to bed, lock brakes on stretcher, lock brakes on bed
- Mechanical/hydraulic lift: Use frame, canvas strips or chains, and hammock or canvas strips; stand-assist lift device
- Sphygmomanometer and stethoscope
- Clean gloves (if risk of soiling)

STEP	RATIONALE

ASSESSMENT

1. Identify patient using at least two identifiers (e.g., name and birthday or name and medical record number, according to agency policy).

   Ensures correct patient. Complies with The Joint Commission standards and improves patient safety (TJC, 2016)

2. Perform hand hygiene.

   Reduces transmission of microorganisms.

3. Review medical record or directly assess physical capacity of a patient to transfer and help with transfer (see Chapter 6). Assess the following:

   Determines patient's ability to tolerate and help with transfer and whether special adaptive techniques or safe handling devices are necessary.

   a. Muscle strength (legs and upper arms) through active range of motion

   Immobile patients have decreased muscle strength, tone, and mass. Affects ability to bear weight, raise body, and thus help with transfer.

   b. Joint mobility and contracture formation

   Immobility or inflammatory processes (e.g., arthritis) may lead to contracture formation and impaired joint mobility.

   c. Paralysis or paresis (spastic or flaccid)

   Patient with central nervous system (CNS) damage may have bilateral paralysis (requiring transfer by swivel bar, sliding bar, mechanical lift) or unilateral paralysis, which requires belt transfer to strong side. Weakness (paresis) requires stabilization of knee while transferring. Flaccid arm must be supported with sling during transfer.

   d. Bone continuity (trauma, amputation) or calcium loss from long bones

   Patients with trauma to one leg or hip may be non–weight bearing when transferred. Amputees may use sliding board to transfer. Osteoporosis increases risk for injury.

4. Refer to medical record for most recent recorded weight and height for patient.

   These factors are used to determine if mechanical transfer device or friction-reducing device is needed for transfer.

5. Assess for history of presence of weakness, dizziness, or postural hypotension (when sitting or standing).

   Determines risk for fainting or falling during transfer. The move from supine to vertical position with a decrease of 20 mm Hg or more in systolic blood pressure results in orthostatic hypotension (Lewis et al., 2017).

6. Assess medical record for patient's level of fatigue and activity tolerance during previous transfers. Assess endurance by noting patient's participation in activities of daily living (ADLs).

   Estimates ability of patient to participate in transfer. Planned rest periods before transfer may enhance function.

7. Assess patient's proprioceptive function (awareness of posture and changes in equilibrium):

   Determines stability of patient's balance for transfer.

   a. Ability to maintain balance while sitting in bed or on side of bed

   Determines risk for fainting or falling during transfer.

   b. Tendency to sway or position self to one side

   Patients with brain dysfunction may have proprioceptive losses. This may cause them to lean to one side or lose balance during transfer.

8. Assess patient's sensory status, including adequacy of vision and hearing and presence of peripheral sensation loss (see Chapter 6).

   Determines influence of sensory loss on ability to make transfer. Visual field loss decreases patient's ability to see in direction of transfer. Peripheral sensation loss decreases proprioception. Patients with visual and hearing losses need transfer techniques adapted to deficits.

Clinical Decision Point *Patients with hemiplegia may "neglect" one side of the body (inattention to or unawareness of one side of body or environment), which distorts perceptions of the visual field.*

STEP	RATIONALE
9. Assess patient for pain (e.g., joint discomfort, muscle spasm) and measure level of pain using scale of 0 to 10. Offer prescribed analgesic 30 minutes before transfer.	Pain reduces patient's motivation and ability to be mobile. Pain relief before transfer enhances patient participation (Christo et al., 2011).
10. Assess patient's cognitive status:	Determines patient's ability to follow directions and help during transfer.
a. Ability to follow verbal instructions	May indicate that patient is at risk for injury.
b. Short-term memory	Patient with short-term memory deficit may have difficulty with transfer, initial learning, or consistent performance.
c. Recognition of physical deficits and limitations to movement	Patient's knowledge of deficits can help you plan a safe transfer.
11. Assess patient's level of motivation such as his or her eagerness versus unwillingness to be mobile.	Altered psychological states often reduce patient's desire to engage in activity.
12. Assess previous mode of transfer (if applicable).	Determines mode of transfer and help required to provide continuity.
13. Just before transfer assess patient's vital signs.	Vital sign changes such as increased pulse and respiration may indicate activity intolerance (see Chapter 5). Patient with low blood pressure may not tolerate sudden position change and is at risk for orthostatic hypotension. Provides baseline to determine tolerance to transfer.
14. Refer to safe-handling algorithm (available in most agencies) to determine if a lift device or mechanical transfer device is needed and the number of people needed to help with transfer. Do not start procedure until all required caregivers are available.	Ensures safe patient handling, reducing risk of injury to patient and caregivers.

NURSING DIAGNOSES

- Activity intolerance
- Acute or chronic pain
- Acute confusion

- Risk for falls
- Impaired physical mobility

- Impaired skin integrity
- Risk for injury

Related factors/Risk factors are individualized based on patient's condition or needs.

PLANNING

1. Expected outcomes following completion of procedure:	
• Patient sits on side of bed without dizziness, weakness, or orthostatic hypotension.	Precautions during transferring prevent vascular compromise.
• Patient tolerates increased activity.	Gradual increase in number of transfers and period of time out of bed increases tolerance and endurance.
• Patient can bear more weight.	Repeated transfers usually result in improved endurance and greater independence of patient.
• Patient transfers without injury.	Proper techniques avoid injury.
• Patient transfers with minimal discomfort.	Transfer procedures performed correctly.
2. Explain to patient (in simple language) how you are going to prepare for transfer technique and safety precautions to be used. Explain benefits and reasons for getting up in a chair. Do so in a way that matches patient's beliefs and values regarding recovery or maintaining health (Shieh et al., 2015).	Provides for clearer understanding by patient. Motivates patient to be involved in transfer.
3. Close room curtains or door.	Provides for patient privacy.
4. Get additional caregivers and/or necessary lift or transfer device to perform transfer.	Safe-handling algorithms (see agency policy) determine number of caregivers and type of devices needed to transfer a patient if lifting is required.

STEP	RATIONALE

IMPLEMENTATION

1. Perform hand hygiene.
2. Help patient from supine to sitting position on edge of bed with bed positioned so top of mattress is even with your elbows. (See Chapter 12, Procedural Guideline 12-4, Step 14 with illustrations.)

Reduces transmission of microorganisms.
Reduces strain on your back.

3. Allow patient to sit on side of bed for a few minutes. Have patient alternately flex and extend feet, move lower legs up and down. Ask if he or she feels dizzy; if so, check blood pressure. Have patient relax and take a few deep breaths until dizziness subsides and balance is gained. If dizziness lasts more than 60 seconds, return patient to bed (Myszenski, 2014). Recheck blood pressure.

Allows patient's circulation to equilibrate to reduce chance of orthostatic hypotension.

Clinical Decision Point *Remain in front of patient until he or she regains balance and continue to provide physical support to weak or cognitively impaired patient.*

4. **Transfer patient from bed to chair:**
   a. Have chair in position at 45-degree angle with one side against bed, facing foot of bed.

   Positions chair with easy access for transfer.

   b. Place bed in low position or to point where patient's feet are comfortably on the floor.

   Provides patient stability when transferring.

   c. If patient has partial weight bearing with upper body strength or caregiver must lift more than 15.9 kg (35 lbs), use mechanical lift or transfer aid with minimum of two or three caregivers (see illustration). Follow manufacturer lift guidelines to apply.

   The use of mechanical lift devices is strongly recommended to transfer a patient to reduce risk for musculoskeletal injury (Degelau et al., 2014; OSHA, 2014; 2015; Pelczarski, 2012).

Clinical Decision Point *If patient demonstrates weakness or paralysis of one side of the body, place chair on his or her strong side.*

   d. If patient has partial weight bearing, is cooperative and able to stand, and has upper body strength, use stand-and-pivot technique with one caregiver.
      (1) Apply transfer belt (see illustration). Be sure that it completely circles waist. Place belt low and be sure that it is snug. Avoid placing belt over any intravenous lines, incisions, or drainage tubes.

   Transfer belt allows you to maintain stability of patient during transfer and reduces risk for falling (Degelau et al., 2014; OSHA, 2014).

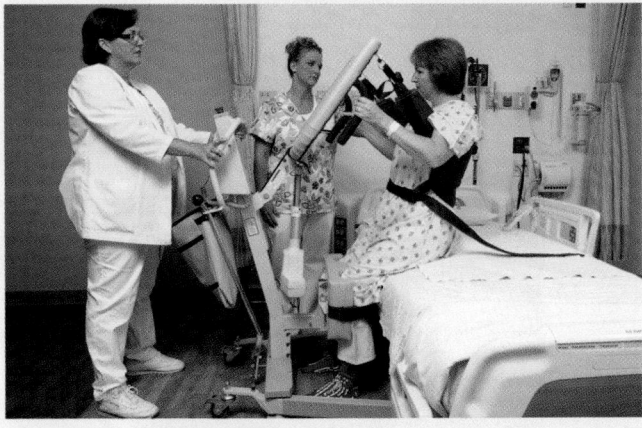

STEP 4c Patient grasps handles as nurse turns on motorized lift.

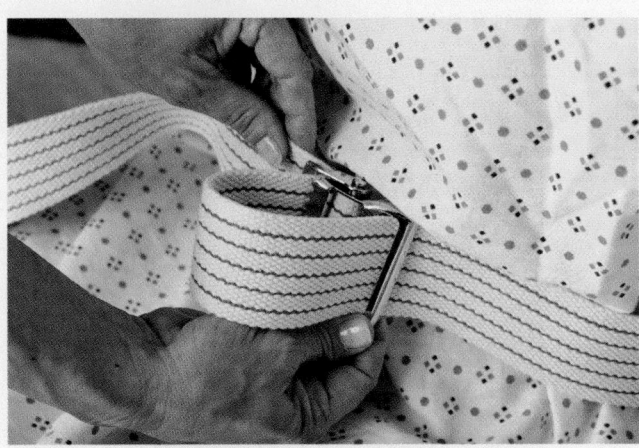

STEP 4d(1) Application of transfer belt.

STEP	RATIONALE
(2) If not already in place, help patient apply stable, nonskid shoes/socks. Place patient's weight-bearing or strong leg forward on floor, with weak foot back.	Nonskid soles decrease risk for slipping during transfer. Always have patient wear shoes during transfer; bare feet increase risk for falls. Patient will stand on stronger, or weight-bearing, leg.
(3) Spread your feet apart. Flex hips and knees, aligning knees with patient's knees.	Ensures balance with wide base of support. Flexing knees and hips lowers your center of gravity to object to be raised; aligning knees with those of patient allows for stabilization of knees when patient stands.
(4) Grasp transfer belt, keeping your palms up, along patient's sides (see illustration).	Transfer belt allows you to move patient at center of gravity. Patients should never be lifted by or under their arms.
(5) Rock patient up to standing position on count of three while straightening hips and legs and keeping knees slightly flexed (see illustration). While rocking patient in back-and-forth motion, make sure that your body weight is moving in the same direction as patient's to ensure that you and patient are moving in same direction simultaneously. Unless contraindicated, patient may be instructed to use hands to push up if applicable.	Rocking motion gives patient's body momentum and requires less muscular effort to lift him or her.
(6) Maintain stability of patient's weakened leg with your knee.	Ability to stand can often be maintained in weak limb with support of knee to stabilize.
(7) Pivot on foot farthest from chair.	Maintains support of patient while allowing adequate space for patient to move.
(8) Instruct patient to use armrests on chair for support and ease into chair (see illustration).	Increases patient stability.
(9) Flex hips and knees while lowering patient into chair.	Prevents injury from poor body mechanics.
(10) Assess patient for proper alignment in sitting position. Provide support for weakened extremity. You can use a sling or lap board to support an injured or flaccid arm. Stabilize leg with bath blanket or pillow.	Prevents injury to patient from poor body alignment.

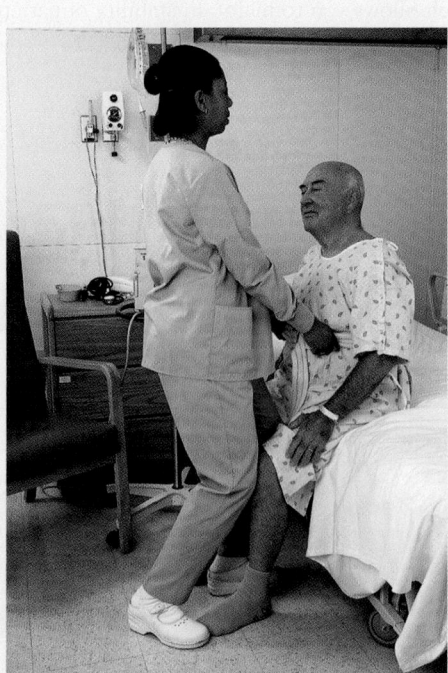

STEP 4d(4) Nurse flexes hips and knees, aligns knees with patient's knee, and grasps transfer belt palms up.

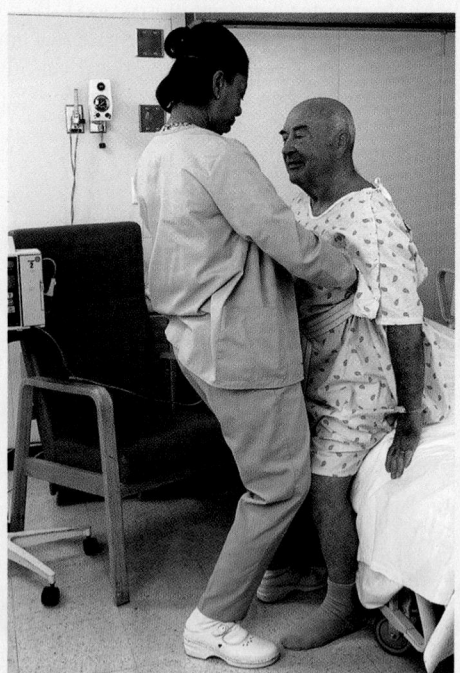

STEP 4d(5) Nurse rocks patient (who is able to help) to standing position.

STEP	RATIONALE

(11) Proper alignment for sitting position: head is erect, and vertebrae are in straight alignment. Body weight is evenly distributed on buttocks and thighs. Thighs are parallel and in horizontal plane. Both feet are supported on floor, and ankles are comfortably flexed. A 2.5- to 5-cm (1- to 2-inch) space is maintained between edge of seat and popliteal space on posterior surface of knee.

Prevents stress on intravertebral joints. Prevents increased pressure over bony prominences and reduces damage to underlying musculoskeletal system.

e. **If patient is not able to cooperate (regardless of ability to bear weight) or has no upper body strength, use ceiling or floor hydraulic lift to transfer patient from bed to chair.**

Research supports use of mechanical lifts to prevent musculoskeletal injuries (ANA, 2013a, b). Use of ceiling-mounted lifts is a popular choice because of availability of lift in each patient's room (see illustration).

(1) Bring mechanical floor lift to bedside or lower ceiling lift and position properly.

Ensures safe elevation of patient off bed.

(2) Position chair near bed and allow adequate space to maneuver the lift.

Prepares environment for safe use of lift and subsequent transfer.

(3) Raise bed to high position with mattress flat. Lower side rail on side near chair.

Allows you to use proper body mechanics.

(4) Have second nurse positioned at opposite side of bed.

Maintains patient safety, preventing fall from bed.

(5) Roll patient on side away from you.

Positions patient for placement of lift sling.

(6) Place hammock or canvas strips under patient to form sling. With two canvas pieces, lower edge fits under patient's knees (wide piece), and upper edge fits under patient's shoulders (narrow piece).

Two types of seats are supplied with mechanical/hydraulic lift: hammock style is better for patients who are flaccid, weak, and need support; canvas strips can be used for patients with normal muscle tone. Hooks should face away from patient's skin. Place sling under patient's center of gravity and greatest part of body weight.

(7) Roll patient back toward you as second nurse pulls hammock (straps) through.

Ensures that sling is in proper position before lift.

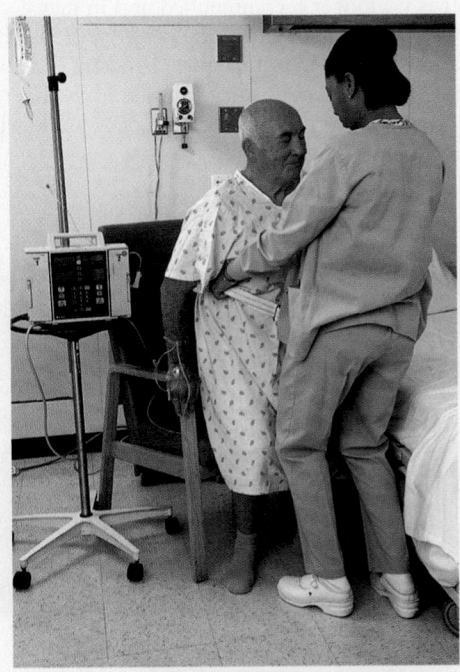

STEP 4d(8) Patient uses armrests and is guided to sit in chair.

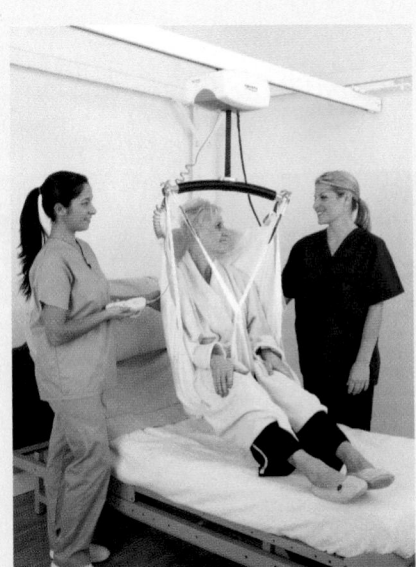

STEP 4e Ceiling lift. (*Courtesy Waverly Glen Systems, a Prism Medical Co.*)

STEP	RATIONALE
(8) Return patient to supine position. Be sure that hammock or straps are smooth over bed surface. Sling should extend from shoulders to knees (hammock) to support patient's body weight equally.	Completes positioning of patient on mechanical/hydraulic sling.
(9) Remove patient's glasses if appropriate.	Swivel bar is close to patient's head and could break eyeglasses.
(10) Place horseshoe base of floor lift under patient's bed (on side with chair).	Positions lift efficiently and promotes smooth transfer.
(11) Lower horizontal bar to sling level by following manufacturer directions. Lock valve if required.	Positions hydraulic lift close to patient. Locking valve prevents injury to patient.
(12) Attach hooks on strap (chain) to holes in sling. Short chains or straps hook to top holes of sling; longer chains hook to bottom of sling (see manufacturer directions).	Secures hydraulic lift to sling.
(13) Elevate head of bed to Fowler's position.	Positions patient in sitting position.
(14) Have patient fold arms over chest.	Prevents injury to patient's arms during transfer.
(15) Pump hydraulic handle using long, slow, even strokes until patient is raised off bed (see illustration). For ceiling lift turn on control device to move lift.	Ensures safe support of patient during elevation.
(16) Use lift to raise patient off bed and use steering handle to pull lift from bed as you and other nurse maneuver patient to chair. Have second nurse alongside patient.	Lifts patient off the bed safely; nurse's position reduces any risk of patient falling from sling.
(17) Roll base of lift around chair. Release check valve slowly and lower patient into chair (see manufacturer directions) (see illustration).	Positions lift in front of chair into which patient is to be transferred. Safely guides patient into back of chair as seat descends.
(18) Close check valve as soon as patient is down in chair and straps can be released.	If valve is left open, boom may continue to lower and injure patient.
(19) Remove straps and roll mechanical/hydraulic lift out of patient's path.	Prevents damage to skin and underlying tissues.
(20) Check patient's sitting alignment and correct if necessary.	Prevents injury from poor posture.
5. Perform lateral transfer from bed to stretcher:	The three-person lift for horizontal transfer from bed to stretcher is no longer recommended and in fact is discouraged (OSHA, 2014; Waters et al., 2011). Physical stress can be decreased significantly by using slide board or friction-reducing board positioned under drawsheet beneath patient. In addition, patient is more comfortable with this method.

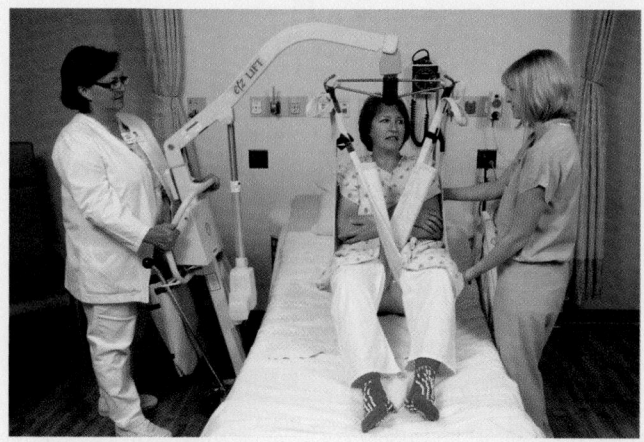

STEP 4e(15) Patient lifted in hydraulic lift above bed.

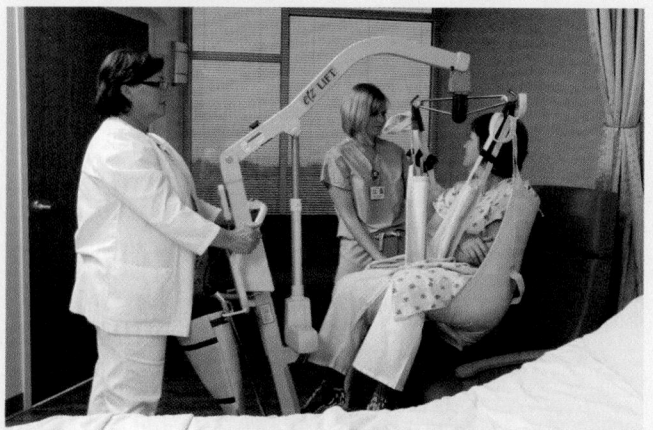

STEP 4e(17) Use of hydraulic lift lowers patient into chair.

STEP	RATIONALE
a. Determine if patient can assist.	Patient's level of strength and weight determine level of help required for safe transfer. During any patient-transferring task, if any caregiver is required to lift more than 15.9 kg (35 lbs) of patient's weight, patient is considered fully dependent, and an assist device is used (OSHA 2014, 2015).
(1) If patient can assist, caregiver is only needed to stand by for safety, with stretcher and bed locked as patient moves to stretcher.	
(2) If patient is partially or not at all able to help and is <200 lbs, use friction-reducing device or lateral transfer board.	
(3) If patient is partially or not at all able to help and is >200 lbs, use a ceiling lift with supine sling or a mechanical lateral-transfer device with three caregivers.	
b. Lateral transfer with friction- reducing device— slide board (see illustration) or air assisted device:	Maintains alignment of spinal column. Ensures that bed does not move inadvertently.
(1) Apply clean gloves if there is risk of soiling. Lower head of bed as much as patient can tolerate. Be sure to lock bed brakes.	Reduces transmission of microorganisms.
(2) Cross patient's arms on chest.	Prevents injury to arms during transfer.
(3) Lower side rails. To place slide board under patient, position two nurses on side of bed toward which patient will be turned. Position third nurse on other side of bed.	Distributes weight equally between nurses.
(4) Fanfold drawsheet on both sides.	Provides strong handles to grip drawsheet without slipping.
(5) On count of three logroll patient onto side toward the two nurses. Turn patient as one unit with smooth, continuous motion.	Maintains body in alignment, preventing stress on any part.
(6) Place slide board under drawsheet (see illustration). *Option:* Apply air-assisted device.	Prevents friction from contact of skin with board.
(7) Gently roll patient back onto slide board.	
(8) Line up stretcher so surface is ½ inch lower than bed. Lock brakes on stretcher. Instruct patient not to move.	Ensures that stretcher does not move inadvertently during transfer.
(9) Two nurses position themselves on side of stretcher while third nurse positions self on side of bed without stretcher. All three nurses place feet widely apart with one foot slightly in front of the other and grasp friction-reducing device.	

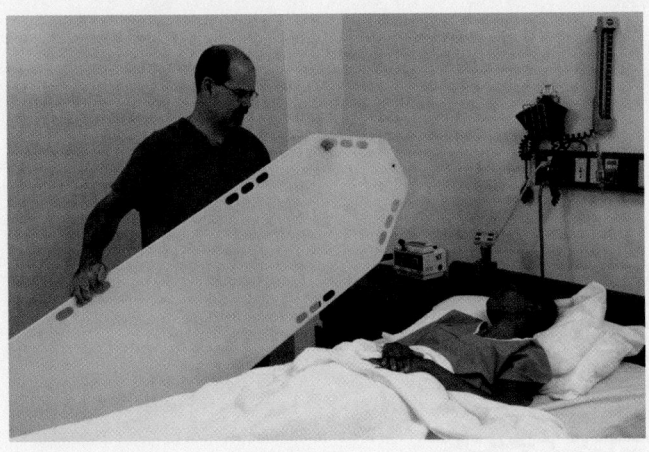

STEP 5b Slide board.

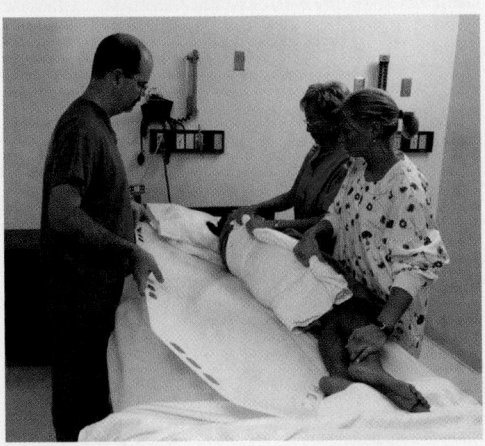

STEP 5b(6) Caregivers placing slide board under drawsheet.

STEP	RATIONALE

Clinical Decision Point *A nurse may also be positioned at the head of patient's bed to protect and support his or her head and neck if patient is weak or unable to help.*

(10) Holding fan-folded drawsheet and one nurse counting to three, the two nurses pull drawsheet across slide board, positioning patient onto stretcher (see illustration A). The third nurse holds slide board in place. *Option:* Inflate air-assisted device and slide patient across bed onto stretcher (see illustrations B and C).

Slide board remains stationary, provides slippery surface to reduce friction, and allows patient to transfer easily to stretcher.

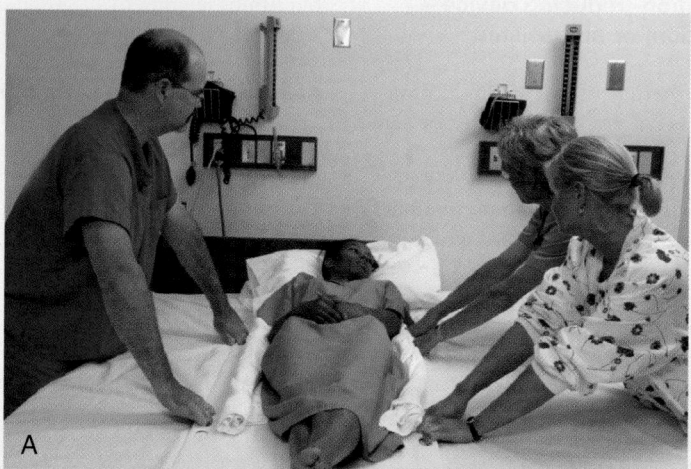

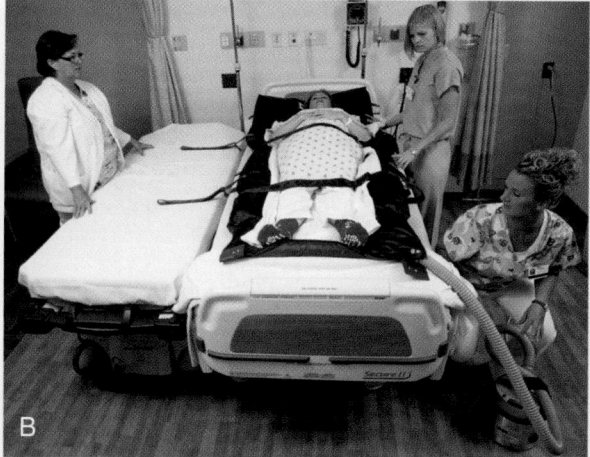
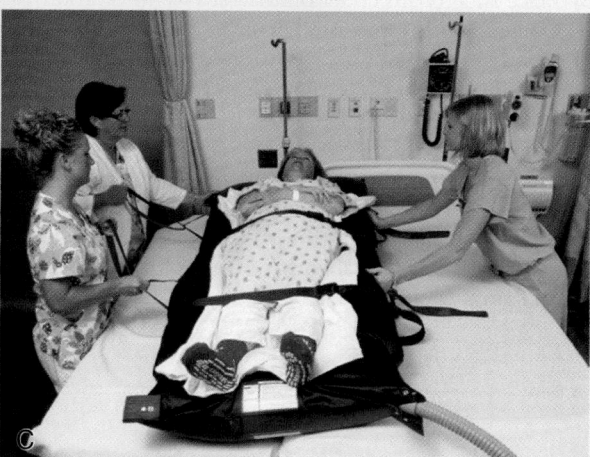

STEP 5b(10) A, Transfer of patient to stretcher using slide board. **B,** Inflating air-assisted transfer device. **C,** Transfer of patient using air-assisted transfer device.

(11) Position patient in center of stretcher. Raise head of stretcher if not contraindicated. Raise stretcher side rails. Cover patient with blanket.

Provides for patient comfort.

6. Remove and dispose of gloves (if used) and perform hand hygiene.

Reduces transmission of microorganisms.

STEP	RATIONALE

EVALUATION

1. Monitor vital signs. Ask if patient feels dizzy or tired. Ask him or her to rate pain on pain scale.

   Evaluates patient's response to postural changes and activity.

2. Note patient's behavioral response to transfer.

   Reveals level of motivation and self-care potential.

3. **Use Teach-Back:** "I want to be sure I explained the steps we are going to use to transfer you to the chair. Tell me the steps you can take to make the transfer safe?" Revise your instruction now or develop a plan for revised patient or family caregiver teaching if patient or family caregiver is not able to teach back correctly.

   Determines patient's and family caregiver's level of understanding of instructional topic.

Unexpected Outcomes	Related Interventions
1. Patient is unable to comprehend or is unwilling to follow directions for transfer.	• Reassess continuity and simplicity of your instruction. • If patient is tired or in pain, allow for rest period before transferring. • Consider medicating for pain if indicated). • Consider using hydraulic lift.
2. Patient sustains injury on transfer.	• Evaluate incident that led to injury (e.g., inadequate assessment, change in patient status, improper use of equipment). • Complete incident report according to agency policy.
3. Patient is unable to stand for time required to transfer to chair.	• Consider use of lateral transfer slide board (see Procedural Guideline 11.1) or hydraulic lift.

Recording and Reporting

• Record procedure, including pertinent observations: weakness, ability to follow directions, weight-bearing ability, balance, ability to pivot, number of personnel needed to help, assist device used, amount of help (muscle strength) required, and patient's response in nurses' notes in electronic health record (EHR) or chart.

• Document your evaluation of patient and family caregiver learning.

• Report transfer ability and help needed to next shift or other caregivers. Report progress or remission to rehabilitation staff (physical therapist, occupational therapist).

Special Considerations
Teaching

• Teach patient and family caregiver the importance of increasing activity out of bed.

• Instruct family caregiver on how to assess a patient's tolerance to increased activity.

Pediatric

• Whenever possible, transporting a child by stretcher, stroller, or wheelchair outside confines of room increases environmental stimuli and provides social contact with others (Hockenberry and Wilson, 2015).

• Children confined to bed for any length of time such as those in traction need to have dependent skin surfaces assessed at least 3 times in a 24-hour period.

Gerontological

• A health concern that threatens the function of an older adult is the risk for falls (Touhy and Jett, 2014). Concern increases when an older adult enters a hospital. Assess the patient for the risk for falls on admission and implement a protocol to prevent falls (Lewis et al., 2017) (see Chapter 14).

Home Care

• Have family caregiver practice and demonstrate transfer skills in hospital to achieve success before taking patient home. Alternatively have patient (if living alone) practice transfer skills in bed that will be used at home. Teach patient to transfer to a chair with arms for ease of rising and sitting. Home should be free of hazards (e.g., throw rugs, electric cords in walkways, slippery floors). If wheelchair is used as chair, access must be possible through all doors, and space for transfer must be available in bedroom and bathroom (see Chapter 43).

• Aids that enhance transfer ability are shower stools, elevated commodes, handrails on tub, and nonskid shower surface. Medical supply stores provide excellent information and catalogs of such supplies.

PROCEDURAL GUIDELINE 11.1 *Wheelchair Transfer Techniques*

Transferring a patient from a bed to a wheelchair encompasses most of the same principles discussed in Skill 11.1. The following procedural guideline focuses on the safety precautions that need to be considered when a weight-bearing patient is using a wheelchair. This is common when hospitalized patients are taken by wheelchair to procedures. Several additional steps must be taken to maintain safety of a patient and the nurse to prevent injury when transferring from or to a wheelchair (Pierson and Fairchild, 2013). Check wheelchair locks, wheels, and footplates for proper functioning before use.

Delegation and Collaboration
The skill of transferring a patient to or from a wheelchair can be delegated to nursing assistive personnel (NAP). The nurse directs NAP by:
- Assessing and supervising when moving patients who are transferring for the first time after prolonged bed rest, extensive surgery, critical illness, or spinal cord trauma.
- Explaining the patient's mobility restrictions, changes in blood pressure, or sensory alterations that may affect safe transfer.

Equipment
- Transfer belt, nonskid shoes, wheelchair, transfer board

Procedural Steps
1. Perform hand hygiene.
2. Review medical record to assess patient's weight, height, and strength; cognition; level of pain; and balance during previous transfer. Or complete a full assessment (see Skill 11.1) to determine patient's ability to help with transfer.
3. Explain to patient the steps you will be taking to help in transfer.
4. **Transferring patient from a wheelchair to bed (patient is cooperative and weight bearing) using pivot technique.**
   a. Adjust the height of the bed to the level of the seat of the wheelchair.
   b. Position wheelchair at a 45-degree angle next to the bed midway between the head and foot of the bed, with the wheelchair facing toward the foot of the bed. Remove the armrest nearest the side of the bed.
   c. Lock the wheelchair. Locks are located above the rims of the wheels. Push handle forward to lock.
   d. Raise the footplates.
   e. Place a transfer belt on patient. Be sure that it completely circles patient's waist. Place the belt low and be sure that it is snug. Avoid placing the belt over any intravenous lines, incisions, or drainage tubes.
   f. Have patient place hands on armrests and stand by as you have him or her move to the front of the wheelchair.
   g. Stand slightly in front of patient to guard and protect him or her throughout the transfer.
   h. Instruct patient to stand at a count of three as you place both hands (palms up) under transfer belt while bending your knees.
   i. Allow patient to stand a few seconds to ensure that he or she is not dizzy and has good balance. Pivot with patient as he or she turns to face away from the side of the bed. Then have patient sit on the edge of the mattress.
   j. With patient sitting on the edge of the bed, place your arm nearest the head of the bed under his or her shoulder while supporting the head and neck. Place your other arm under patient's knees. Bend your knees and keep your back straight.
   k. Tell patient to help lift the legs when you begin to move. On a count of three, standing with a wide base of support, raise patient's legs as you pivot his or her body and lower the shoulders onto the bed. Remember to keep your back straight.
   l. Help patient return to a comfortable position in bed.
5. **Transferring patient from a wheelchair to bed (patient is non–weight bearing and unable to stand but is cooperative and has upper body strength) using transfer board.**
   a. Position patient in wheelchair at a 45-degree angle next to the bed midway between the head and foot of the bed, with the wheelchair facing toward the foot of the bed.
   b. Remove the armrest nearest the side of the bed.
   c. Lock the wheelchair. Locks are located above the rims of the wheels. Push handle forward to lock.
   d. Raise the footplates.
   e. If not already applied, place a transfer belt on patient. Be sure that it completely circles patient's waist. Place the belt low and be that sure it is snug. Avoid placing the belt over any intravenous lines, incisions, or drainage tubes.
   f. If possible, have the seat of the wheelchair level with the top of the bed mattress. Position a transfer board by placing it across the bed to the chair so patient can slide across it. Be sure the board overlaps the chair and mattress so that it will not slip out of place.
   g. Stand in front of patient and have him or her move to the front of the wheelchair.
   h. Place your legs on the outside of patient's legs. Be sure that patient's feet are on the floor. Grasp the transfer belt (palms up) along both of patient's sides. Have patient place one hand on the slide board and the other on the mattress surface.
   i. Bend your knees and on a count of three have patient use the arms to slide across the board from the chair to the bed. If patient is struggling to move across the board, try to have him or her lean the head and shoulders opposite to the way he or she want the hips to move.
   j. Have patient sit on edge of bed.
   k. Follow Steps 4 j–l when helping patient to comfortable position in bed.
6. Perform hand hygiene.
7. Monitor vital signs after patient has been transferred. Ask if patient feels dizzy or fatigued.
8. Note patient's behavioral response to transfer.
9. **Use Teach Back:** "I want to be sure I explained what to do as I move you from the chair to the bed. Tell me how you can help move to the bed." Revise your instruction now or develop a plan or revised patient or family caregiver teaching if patient or family caregiver is not able to teach back correctly.
10. Document patient's ability to tolerate transfer.

✦ SKILL 11.2   Moving and Positioning Patients in Bed

NSO *Nursing Skills Online Safety Module / Lesson 3* ▶ *Video Clip*

Correctly positioning patients in bed is crucial for maintaining their body alignment and comfort; preventing injury to their musculoskeletal and integumentary systems; and providing sensory, motor, and cognitive stimulation. A patient with impaired mobility, decreased sensation, impaired circulation, or lack of voluntary muscle control can suffer damage to the musculoskeletal and integumentary systems while lying down. Proper positioning with correct body alignment minimizes these risks. The term *body alignment* refers to the condition of the joints, tendons, ligaments, and muscles in various body positions. When the body is aligned, whether standing, sitting, or lying, no excessive strain is placed on these structures. Caregivers are at risk for injury during positioning of patients in bed. It is important to follow an agency's safe-handling algorithms and use appropriate repositioning devices.

Delegation and Collaboration

The skills of moving and positioning patients in bed and maintaining correct body alignment can be delegated to nursing assistive personnel (NAP). The nurse directs the NAP by:

- Explaining about any moving and positioning restrictions (e.g., avoid prone position, patient has one-sided weakness) and type of safe patient-handling devices needed.
- Designating specific times throughout the shift that NAP must reposition the patient.
- Providing information regarding patient's individual needs for body alignment (e.g., patient with spinal cord injury), ability to help, and number of other caregivers needed to help.

Equipment

- Pillows, drawsheet
- Appropriate safe patient handling assistive device (e.g., friction-reducing device, ceiling lift, or mechanical floor lift)
- Therapeutic boots/splints (optional)
- Trochanter roll
- Sandbag
- Hand rolls
- Clean gloves

STEP	RATIONALE

ASSESSMENT

STEP	RATIONALE
1. Identify patient using at least two identifiers (e.g., name and birthday or name and medical record number, according to agency policy).	Ensures correct patient. Complies with The Joint Commission standards and improves patient safety (TJC, 2016).
2. Perform hand hygiene.	Prevents transmission of microorganisms.
3. Assess patient's range of motion (ROM) (see Chapters 6 and 12) and current body alignment while patient is lying down.	Provides baseline data for later comparisons. Determines ways to improve position and alignment.
4. Assess for risk factors that contribute to complications of immobility:	Increased risk factors require patient to be repositioned more frequently.
a. *Reduced sensation:* Cerebrovascular accident (CVA), spinal cord injury, or neuropathy	With reduced sensation, patient has difficulty moving and poor awareness of involved body part. Patient is unable to position body part and protect it from pressure.
b. *Impaired mobility:* Traction, arthritis, CVA, spinal cord injury, hip fracture, joint surgery, or other contributing disease processes	Traction, bone fractures, surgery, or arthritic changes of affected extremity result in decreased ROM. Loss of function caused by CVA or spinal injury can lead to contractures.
c. *Impaired circulation:* Arterial insufficiency	Decreased circulation predisposes patient to pressure injury.
d. *Age:* Very young, older adult	Premature and young infants require frequent turning because their skin is fragile. Normal physiological changes associated with aging predispose older adults to greater risks for developing complications of immobility.
5. Assess patient's level of consciousness.	Determines need for special aids or devices. Patients with altered levels of consciousness may not understand instructions and may be unable to help with positioning.
6. Assess patient for presence of pain; rate on scale of 0 to 10.	Pain reduces patient's motivation and ability to be mobile. Pain relief before transfer enhances patient participation (Christo et al., 2011).
7. Assess condition of patient's skin, especially over bony prominences.	Provides baseline to determine effects of positioning.
8. Refer to medical record for most recent recorded weight and height for patient.	Factors needed to determine if mechanical lift, mechanical transfer device, or friction-reducing device is needed for moving patient up in bed.

STEP	RATIONALE
9. Assess patient's physical ability to help with moving and positioning, which may be affected by age, level of consciousness, disease process, strength, ROM, and coordination.	Enables you to use patient's mobility, strength, and coordination during positioning. Determines need for additional help. Ensures patient and nurse safety.
10. Assess for sensory loss (vision and hearing) (see Chapter 6).	Deficits affect patient's ability to cooperate during repositioning procedures.
11. Apply clean gloves (as needed) to assess for presence of incisions, drainage tubes, and equipment (e.g., traction). Empty drainage bags before positioning. Remove and dispose of gloves. Perform hand hygiene.	Alters positioning procedure and type of position in which to place patient. Eliminates barriers to moving patient.
12. Assess motivation of patient and ability of family caregivers to participate in moving and positioning if patient to be discharged home.	Indicates whether instruction is necessary before discharge.
13. Check health care provider's orders before positioning patient.	Some positions may be contraindicated in certain situations (e.g., spinal cord injury; hip fracture; respiratory difficulties; certain neurological conditions; presence of incisions, drains, or tubing).

NURSING DIAGNOSES

- Activity intolerance
- Acute confusion
- Impaired physical mobility
- Impaired skin integrity
- Risk for impaired skin integrity

Related factors/Risk factors are individualized based on patient's condition or needs.

PLANNING

1. Expected outcomes following completion of procedure:	
• Patient retains ROM.	Correct positioning allows patient to achieve optimal joint mobility and alignment.
• Patient's skin shows no evidence of breakdown.	Frequent position changes decrease occurrence of skin breakdown.
• Patient's comfort level increases.	Proper positioning reduces stress on joints.
• Patient's level of independence in completing activities of daily living (ADLs) increases.	Maintaining good body alignment and joint mobility increases patient's overall mobility. Patient with inadequate joint mobility may need help to carry out ADLs.
2. If patient perceives level of pain to be enough to avoid movement, offer an analgesic 30 minutes (if ordered) before repositioning.	Will lessen discomfort when positioning extremities. **Note:** The frequency of an analgesic may not be available as frequently as a patient will require turning.
3. Remove all pillows and devices used in previous position.	Reduces interference from bedding during positioning procedure.
4. Get additional caregivers and/or necessary lift or transfer device to perform positioning.	Safe-handling algorithms (see agency policy) determine number of caregivers and type of devices needed to position a patient if lifting is required.
5. Explain positioning procedure to patient using plain language.	Helps to decrease anxiety and increase cooperation.

IMPLEMENTATION

1. Perform hand hygiene.	Reduces transmission of microorganisms.
2. Close door to room or bedside curtains.	Provides for patient privacy.
3. Raise level of bed to comfortable working height, level with your elbows.	Raises level of work toward nurse's center of gravity and reduces risk for back injuries.
4. **Assist patient to move up in bed:**	This is not a one-person task unless patient can help completely (OSHA, 2014). Pulling patients who've migrated in bed carries an extremely high risk of caregiver injury (Wiggermann, 2014)
a. Determine if the patient can assist.	Determines degree of risk in repositioning patient and technique required to safely help patient.
(1) Patient is fully able to assist:	Promotes patient independence.
(a) Stand at bedside to help with positioning of tubing and equipment as patient moves.	

STEP	**RATIONALE**

(b) Have patient place feet flat on mattress, grasp either side rails or overhead trapeze and, on a count of 3, lift hips up and push legs so body moves up in bed.

(2) Patient is partially able to assist:

  (a) Encourage patient to help using friction-reducing device (e.g., slide board).

  (b) Patient weighs <200 lbs: use friction-reducing sheet or slide board and two or three caregivers.

  (c) Patient weighs >200 lbs: use friction-reducing device and at least three caregivers.

    i. Using a friction-reducing device (three nurses). Position patient supine with head of bed flat. A nurse stands on each side of bed.

    ii. Remove pillow from under head and shoulders and place it at head of bed.

    iii. Turn patient side to side to place friction-reducing device under drawsheet on bed, with device extending from shoulders to thighs/ankles.

    iv. Return patient to supine position.

    v. Have two caregivers grasp drawsheet (one on each side of bed) firmly and have third nurse hold onto end of friction-reducing device.

    vi. Place feet apart with forward-backward stance. Flex knees and hips. On count of three, shift weight from front to back leg and move patient and drawsheet to desired position up in bed.

(3) Patient unable to assist:

  (a) Use appropriate number of caregivers and appropriate safe-handling devices (e.g., supine sling with ceiling lift or floor-based lift and two or more caregivers).

Rationale column:

Repositioning device reduces friction as patient is moved up in bed.

Prevents friction from contact of skin with board.

Slide board remains stationary, provides slippery surface to reduce friction, and allows patient to move up in bed easily.

Positions patient smoothly without exerting shear against skin and without risk of injury to nurses.

Repositioning patients manually is associated with high risk of musculoskeletal injury (Wiggermann, 2014).

Clinical Decision Point *Protect patient's heels from shearing force by having another caregiver lift heels while moving patient up in bed.*

5. Position patient in bed in one of the following positions. Ensure correct body alignment. Protect pressure areas.

  a. Determine if patient can assist.

  b. Begin with patient lying supine and move up in bed following Steps 4a (1)–(3).

  c. Position patient in supported semi-Fowler's (see illustration) or Fowler's position:

Rationale column:

Prevents injury to patient's musculoskeletal system and integument.

Even positioning patient side to side requires use of safe-handling techniques.

Determines degree of risk in repositioning patient and the technique required to safely help patient.

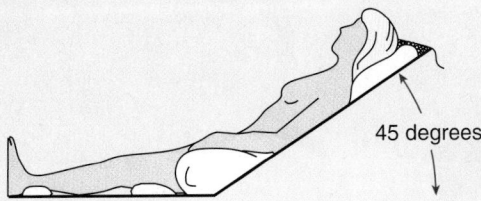

45 degrees

STEP 5c Supported semi-Fowler's position.

  (1) With patient lying supine, elevate head of bed 45 to 60 degrees if not contraindicated.

  (2) Rest head against mattress or on small pillow.

Rationale column:

Increases comfort, improves ventilation, and increases patient's opportunity to socialize or relax.

Prevents flexion contractures of cervical vertebrae.

STEP	RATIONALE
(3) Use pillows to support arms and hands if patient does not have voluntary control or use of hands and arms.	Prevents shoulder dislocation from effect of downward pull of unsupported arms, promotes circulation by preventing venous pooling, and prevents flexion contractures of arms and wrists.
(4) Position small pillow at lower back.	Supports lumbar vertebrae and decreases flexion of vertebrae.
(5) Place small pillow or roll under thigh.	Prevents hyperextension of knee and occlusion of popliteal artery from pressure from body weight.
(6) Support calves with pillows.	Heels should not be in contact with bed to prevent prolonged pressure of mattress on heels. This is sometimes referred to as *floating* heels.
d. Position hemiplegic patient in supported semi-Fowler's or Fowler's position:	
(1) Elevate head of bed 45 to 60 degrees.	Increases comfort, improves ventilation, and increases patient's opportunity to relax. Adjust head of bed according to patient's condition. For example, those with increased risk for pressure injury remain at 30-degree angle (see Chapter 39).
(2) Position patient in Fowler's position as anatomically straight as possible.	Counteracts tendency to slump toward affected side. Improves ventilation and cardiac output; decreases intracranial pressure. Improves patient's ability to swallow and helps prevent aspiration of food, liquids, and gastric secretions.
(3) Position head on small pillow with chin slightly forward. If patient is totally unable to control head movement, avoid hyperextension of neck.	Prevents hyperextension of neck. Too many pillows under head may cause or worsen neck flexion contracture.
(4) Provide support for involved arm and hand by placing arm away from patient's side and supporting elbow with pillow.	Paralyzed muscles do not automatically resist pull of gravity as they do normally. As a result, shoulder subluxation, pain, and edema may occur.
(5) Place rolled blanket (trochanter roll) firmly alongside patient's legs.	Ensures proper alignment. Prevents external rotation of hips, which contributes to contractures.
(6) Support feet in dorsiflexion with therapeutic boots or splints.	Prevents plantar flexion contractures or footdrop by positioning patient's ankle in neutral dorsiflexion. Positions foot so heel is aligned in opening of splint to prevent pressure. Other therapeutic boots or splints are manufactured with thick padding to cushion heel and prevent pressure injury.
e. Position patient in supported supine position:	
(1) Place patient supine with head of bed flat.	Necessary for properly aligning patient.
(2) Place small rolled towel under lumbar area of back.	Provides support for lumbar spine.
(3) Place pillow under upper shoulders, neck, and head.	Maintains correct alignment and prevents flexion contractures of cervical vertebrae.
(4) Place trochanter rolls or sandbags parallel to lateral surface of patient's thighs.	Reduces external rotation of hip.
(5) Place patient's feet in therapeutic boots or splints.	Maintains feet in dorsiflexion. Prevents plantar flexion contractures or footdrop.
(6) Place pillows under pronated forearms, keeping upper arms parallel to patient's body (see illustration).	Reduces internal rotation of shoulder and prevents extension of elbows. Maintains correct body alignment.

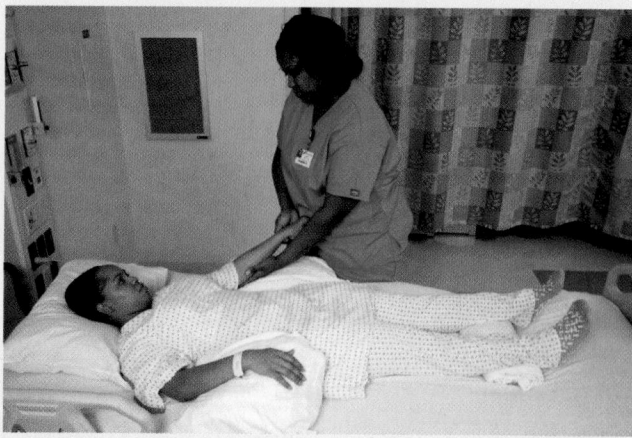

STEP 5e(6) Supported supine position with pillows in place.

STEP	RATIONALE
(7) Place hand rolls in patient's hands. Consider physical therapy referral for use of hand splints.	Reduces extension of fingers and abduction of thumb. Maintains thumb slightly adducted and in opposition to fingers.
f. Position hemiplegic patient in supine position:	
(1) Place head of bed flat.	Necessary for positioning in supine position.
(2) Place folded towel or small pillow under shoulder of affected side.	Decreases possibility of pain, joint contracture, and subluxation. Maintains mobility in muscles around shoulder to permit normal movement patterns.
(3) Keep affected arm away from body with elbow extended and palm up. Position affected hand in one of recommended positions for flaccid or spastic hand. (Alternative is to place arm out to side, with elbow bent and hand toward head of bed.)	Maintains mobility in arm, joints, and shoulder to permit normal movement patterns. (Alternative position counteracts limitation of ability of arm to rotate outward at shoulder [external rotation]. External rotation must be present to raise arm overhead without pain.)
(4) Place folded towel under hip of involved side.	Diminishes effect of spasticity in entire leg by controlling hip position.
(5) Flex affected knee 30 degrees by supporting it on pillow or folded blanket.	Slight flexion breaks up abnormal extension pattern of leg. Extensor spasticity is most severe when patient is supine.
(6) Support feet with soft pillows at right angle to leg.	Maintains foot in dorsiflexion and prevents footdrop. Pillows prevent stimulation to ball of foot by hard surface, which has tendency to increase muscle tone in patient with extensor spasticity of lower extremity.
g. Position patient in 30-degree lateral (side-lying) position (one nurse):	This position is recommended to prevent development of pressure injury by reducing direct contact of trochanter with support surface (see Chapter 39).
(1) Lower head of bed completely or as low as patient can tolerate.	Provides position of comfort for patient and removes pressure from bony prominences on back.
(2) Lower side rail and position patient on side of bed opposite direction toward which patient is to be turned. Move upper trunk, supporting shoulders first; then move lower trunk, supporting hips.	Provides room for patient to turn to side.
(3) Raise side rail and go to opposite side of bed.	
(4) Flex patient's knee that will not be next to mattress. Keep foot on mattress. Place one hand on patient's upper bent leg near hip and other hand on patient's shoulder.	Use of leverage makes turning to side easy.
(5) Roll patient onto side toward you.	Rolling decreases trauma to tissues. In addition, patient is positioned so leverage on hip makes turning easy.
(6) Place pillow under patient's head and neck.	Maintains alignment. Reduces lateral neck flexion. Decreases strain on sternocleidomastoid muscle.
(7) Place hands under patient's dependent shoulder and bring shoulder blade forward.	Prevents patient's weight from resting directly on shoulder joint.
(8) Position both arms in slightly flexed position. Support upper arm with pillow level with shoulder; other arm, by mattress.	Decreases internal rotation and adduction of shoulder. Supporting both arms in slightly flexed position protects joint. Ventilation improves because chest is able to expand more easily.
(9) Place hands under dependent hip and bring hip slightly forward so angle from hip to mattress is approximately 30 degrees.	The 30-degree lateral position reduces pressure on trochanter; designed to prevent pressure injury.
(10) Place small tuck-back pillow behind patient's back. (Make by folding pillow lengthwise. Smooth area is slightly tucked under patient's back.)	Provides support to maintain patient on side.
(11) Place pillow under semiflexed upper leg level at hip from groin to foot (see illustration).	Flexion prevents hyperextension of leg. Maintains leg in correct alignment. Prevents pressure on bony prominences.

STEP	RATIONALE

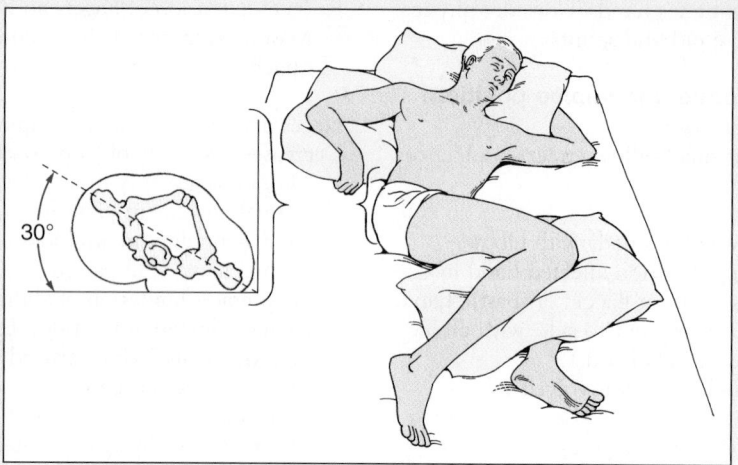

STEP 5g(11) Thirty-degree lateral position with pillows in place.

(12) Place sandbags parallel to plantar surface of dependent foot. May use ankle-foot orthotic on feet if available.	Maintains dorsiflexion of foot.
h. Position patient in Sims' (semi-prone) position:	
(1) Lower head of bed completely.	Provides for proper body alignment while patient is lying down.
(2) Place patient supine on side of bed opposite direction toward which he or she is to be turned. Move upper trunk, supporting shoulders first, followed by moving lower trunk, supporting hips.	Prepares patient for position.
(3) Move to other side of bed and turn patient on side. Position in lateral position, lying partially on abdomen, with dependent shoulder lifted out and arm placed at patient's side.	
(4) Place small pillow under patient's head.	Maintains proper alignment and prevents lateral neck flexion.
(5) Place pillow under flexed upper arm, supporting arm level with shoulder.	Prevents internal rotation of shoulder. Maintains alignment.
(6) Place pillow under flexed upper legs, supporting leg level with hip.	Prevents internal rotation of hip and adduction of leg. Flexion prevents hyperextension of leg. Reduces mattress pressure on knees and ankles.
(7) Place sandbags parallel to plantar surface of foot (see illustration).	Maintains foot in dorsiflexion. Prevents plantar flexion contractures or footdrop.

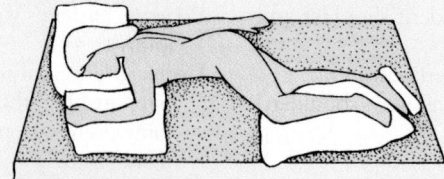

STEP 5h(7) Sandbag supporting right foot in dorsiflexion.

i. Logroll patient (three nurses):

Clinical Decision Point *A registered nurse supervises and helps the NAP when there is a health care provider's order to logroll a patient. Patients with a spinal cord injury or who are recovering from neck, back, or spinal surgery often need to keep the spinal column in straight alignment to prevent further injury.*

STEP	RATIONALE
(1) Place small pillow between patient's knees.	Prevents tension on spinal column and adduction of hip.
(2) Cross patient's arms on chest.	Prevents injury to arms.
(3) Position two nurses on side toward which patient is to be turned and one nurse on side where pillows are to be placed (see illustration).	Distributes weight equally between nurses during turning.
(4) Fanfold drawsheet alongside of patient who will be turning.	Provides strong handles to grip drawsheet without slipping.
(5) With one nurse grasping drawsheet at lower hips and thighs and the other nurse grasping drawsheet at patient's shoulders and lower back, roll patient as one unit in a smooth, continuous motion on count of three (see illustration).	Maintains proper alignment by moving all body parts at the same time, preventing tension or twisting of spinal column.
(6) Nurse on opposite side of bed places pillows along length of patient for support (see illustration).	Maintains patient in side-lying position.
(7) Gently lean patient as a unit back toward pillows for support.	Ensures continued straight alignment of spinal column, preventing injury.

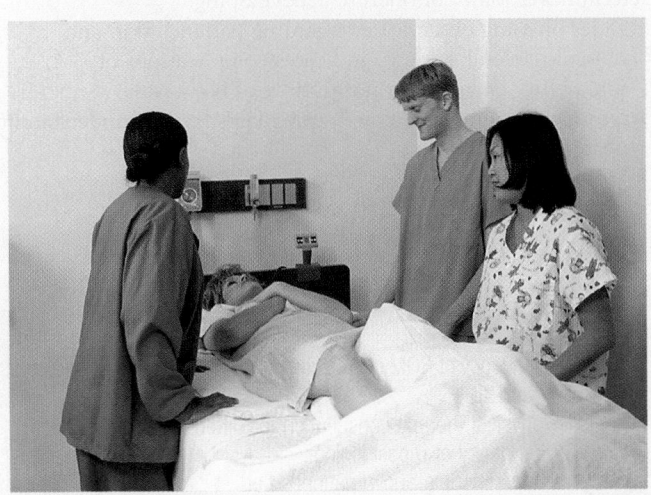

STEP 5i(3) Preparing patient for logrolling.

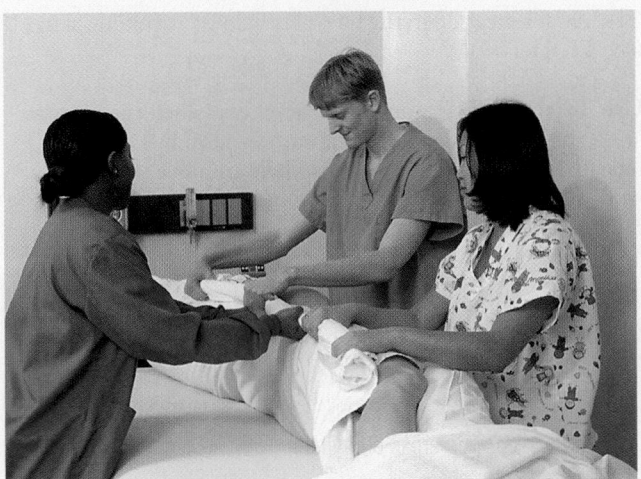

STEP 5i(5) Logrolling patient onto side.

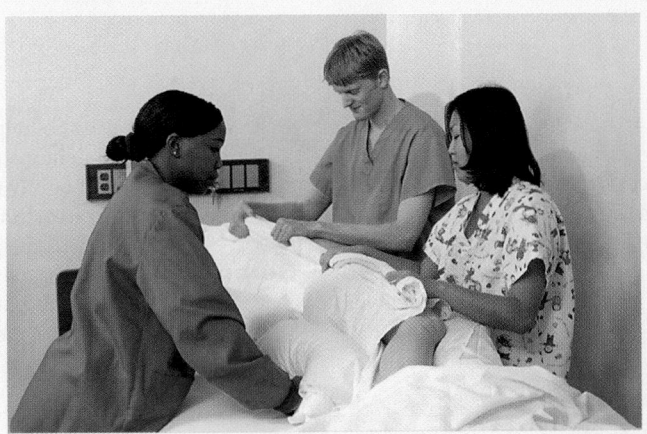

STEP 5i(6) Placing pillows along patient's back for support.

STEP	RATIONALE
6. Perform hand hygiene.	Reduces transmission of microorganisms. 

EVALUATION

1. Assess patient's body alignment, position, and level of comfort. Patient's body should be supported by adequate mattress, and vertebral column should be without observable curves.	Determines effectiveness of positioning. Additional supports (e.g., pillows, bath blankets) may be added or removed to promote comfort and correct body alignment.
2. Measure ROM.	Determines if joint contracture is developing.
3. Observe for areas of erythema or breakdown involving skin (see Chapter 39).	Provides ongoing observation regarding patient's skin and musculoskeletal systems. Indicates complications of immobility or improper positioning of body part.
4. Use Teach-Back: "I want to be sure I explained the steps we are going to use to move and position you in bed. Can you repeat the steps you can follow to help us move you up in bed?" Revise your instruction now or develop a plan for revised patient or family caregiver teaching if patient or family caregiver is not able to teach back correctly.	Determines patient's and family caregiver's level of understanding of instructional topic.

Unexpected Outcomes	Related Interventions
1. Joint contractures develop or worsen.	• Increase frequency of ROM exercises to affected and immobilized areas (see Chapter 12). • Consider physical therapy consultation for different positioning.
2. Skin shows localized areas of erythema and breakdown.	• Increase frequency of repositioning. • Place turning schedule above patient's bed.
3. Patient avoids moving.	• Medicate with analgesia as ordered by health care provider to ensure patient's comfort before moving. • Allow pain medication to take effect before repositioning.

Recording and Reporting

- Record time and position change of patient throughout shift, observations (e.g., condition of skin, joint movement, patient's ability to help with positioning), and whether positioning devices needed in nurses' notes in electronic health record (EHR) or chart.
- Document your evaluation of patient and family caregiver learning.
- Report observations at change of shift and document in nurses' notes in electronic health record (EHR) or chart.

Special Considerations
Teaching

- Teach family caregiver how to position patient, especially when caring for infant, young child, or confused or unconscious patient.

- Teach patient ways to help with positioning and provide opportunity for return demonstration.
- Teach patient and family caregiver signs and symptoms of pressure injury and contractures.

Gerontological

- Reposition older adult patients at least every 1 to 2 hours and maintain a regular program of ROM exercises (Touhy and Jett, 2014).

◆ CLINICAL DEBRIEF

A 37-year-old man who may have suffered a spinal cord injury in a motor vehicle accident is admitted to the health care agency. He has sustained multiple deep lacerations on his face and trunk and facial fractures of the maxillary and zygomatic bones. He has a cervical collar in place. He rates his pain at 9 on a scale of 0 to 10. He weighs approximately 88 kg (193.6 lbs). You are preparing to transfer him to a stretcher. The emergency department nurse was extremely busy and was unable to provide a complete report.

1. Which other information would you obtain about this patient before safely transferring him to a stretcher?

2. The nursing assistive personnel (NAP) states that the patient wants to be turned and that he will be glad to reposition him without help. The health care provider's (HCP's) orders are for logrolling until computed tomography (CT) scan is completed and injury to the neck and spine is ruled out. What is the appropriate, safe action in response to turning the patient? Explain your answer.

3. The patient's pain continues to be at a level of 7 after receiving pain medication, his heart rate is 118 compared to a baseline of 82. The patient states, "I can't take this pain anymore." He refuses to go to radiology for his procedure. Write an SBAR for communicating this situation.

◆ REVIEW QUESTIONS

1. A patient is to sit up in a chair for breakfast 1 day after abdominal surgery per the health care provider's orders. Which of the following would you select to ensure a safe transfer while facilitating cooperation from the patient? (Select all that apply.)
   1. Offer pain medication 30 minutes before transferring patient.
   2. Assess presence of weakness, dizziness, and muscle strength.
   3. Determine need for safe patient-handling device.
   4. Tell the NAP to transfer patient to the chair.
   5. Follow orders to transfer patient even though he or she is refusing.

2. Place the following in correct sequence that facilitates safe transfer from a wheelchair to bed.
   1. Position wheelchair at a 45-degree angle next to bed.
   2. Stand by as you have patient move to front of wheelchair.
   3. Raise footplates and apply transfer belt.
   4. Lock wheelchair.
   5. Position self slightly in front of patient.
   6. Have patient stand as you place both hands under transfer belt and pivot to side of bed.
   7. Adjust height of bed to level of wheelchair seat.

3. Place the following in correct sequence that reflects safe use of a mechanical/hydraulic lift to transfer patients from bed to chair.
   1. Release check valve slowly and lower patient into chair.
   2. Roll patient back toward you as second nurse pulls hammock (straps) through holes.
   3. Position chair near bed and allow adequate space to maneuver lift.
   4. Attach hooks on strap to holes in sling.
   5. Roll patient onto side toward second nurse and position sling under patient.
   6. Use lift to raise patient off bed and steering handle to pull lift from bed and maneuver to chair.
   7. Place horseshoe base of floor lift under patient's bed and lower horizontal bar to sling level.
   8. Roll patient supine onto canvas seat.

ℯ *Visit the Evolve site for a complete list of Clinical Debrief and Review Questions answers.*

REFERENCES

American Nurses Association (ANA): *Safe patient handling and mobility interprofessional standards,* Silver Spring, MD, 2013a, American Nurses Association.

American Nurses Association (ANA): *ANA leads initiative to develop national safe patient handling standards,* Silver Springs, MD, 2013b, American Nurses Association.

Bureau of Labor Statistics, U.S. Department of Labor: *The Economics Daily,* Hospital workers suffered 294,000 nonfatal workplace injuries and illnesses in 2014 on the Internet at http://www.bls.gov/opub/ted/2016/hospital-workers-suffered-294000-nonfatal-workplace-injuries-and-illnesses-in-2014.htm, Accessed July 03, 2016.

Christo P, et al: Effective treatment for pain in the older patient, *Curr Pain Headache Rep* 15(1):22, 2011.

Degelau J, et al, Institute for Clinical Systems Improvement (ICSI): *Prevention of falls (acute care): health care protocol,* Bloomington, MN, 2014, Institute for Clinical Systems Improvement.

Freeman R, et al: Consensus statement on the definition of orthostatic hypotension, neutrally mediate syncope and the postural tachycardia syndrome, *Auton Neurosci* 161(1–2):46, 2011.

Hockenberry MJ, Wilson D: *Wong's nursing care of infants and children,* ed 10, St Louis, 2015, Mosby.

Huether SE, McCance KL: *Understanding pathophysiology,* ed 6, St Louis, 2016, Mosby.

Krill C, et al: Empowering staff nurses to use research to change practice for safe patient handling, *Nurs Outlook* 60(3):152, 2012.

Largo J, et al: Diastolic blood pressure drop after standing as a clinical sign for increased mortality in older falls clinic patients, *J Hypertens* 30(6):1195, 2012.

Lewis S, et al: *Medical-surgical nursing: assessment and management of clinical problems,* ed 10, St Louis, 2017, Elsevier.

Myszenski A: *The essential role of lab values and vital signs in clinical decision making and patient safety for the acutely ill patient,* PhysicalTherapy.com, 2014, http://www.physicaltherapy.com/articles/essential-role-lab-values-and-2336. Accessed March 11. 2016.

Nelson A, Baptiste AS: Evidence-based practices for safe patient handling and movement, *Orthop Nurs* 25(6):366, 2006.

Occupational Safety & Health Association (OSHA): *Safe patient handling—preventing musculoskeletal disorders in nursing homes,* OSHA Publication 3108, 2014, https://www.osha.gov/Publications/OSHA3708.pdf. Accessed March 11, 2016.

Occupational Safety & Health Administration (OSHA): *Worker safety in hospitals,* OSHA Publication, 2015, https://www.osha.gov/dsg/hospitals/. Accessed March 11, 2016.

Occupational Safety & Health Administration (OSHA): *Safe patient handling,* nd, https://www.osha.gov/dsg/hospitals/documents/3.1_Mythbusters_508.pdf. Accessed March 11, 2016.

Pelczarski KM: Back in action, *Health Facil Manage* 25(8):21, 2012.

Pierson M, Fairchild S: *Principles & techniques of patient care,* ed 5, St Louis, 2013, Saunders.

Sherwood G, Barnsteiner J: *Quality and safety in nursing,* Oxford, UK, 2012, Wiley-Blackwell.

Shieh C, et al: Association of self-efficacy and self-regulation with nutrition and exercise behaviors in a community sample of adults, *J Community Health Nurs* 32(4):199, 2015.

The Joint Commission (TJC): *2016 National Patient Safety Goals,* Oakbrook Terrace, IL, 2016, The Commission. http://www.jointcommission.org/standards_information/npsgs.aspx. Accessed March 11, 2016.

Touhy T, Jett K: *Ebersole and Hess's gerontological nursing and healthy aging,* ed 4, St Louis, 2014, Mosby.

Waters T, et al: AORN ergonomic tool 1: lateral transfer of a patient from a stretcher to an OR bed, *AORN J* 93(3):223, 2011.

Wiggermann N: The sliding patient: how to respond to and prevent migration in bed: migration can cause negative patient outcomes and caregiver injuries related to repositioning, *Am Nurse Today* 9(9):2014.

12 | Exercise and Mobility

OBJECTIVES

Mastery of content in this chapter will enable the nurse to:
- Discuss implications for preventing deconditioning and deep vein thrombosis in hospitalized inpatients.
- Describe the evidence that supports early activity and exercise in patient care.
- Explain how to plan a safe exercise program for a patient.
- Discuss indications for performing range-of-motion exercises.
- Discuss the risks for patients to develop deep vein thrombosis
- Identify complications that may develop in a patient wearing either elastic stockings or a sequential compression device.

- Identify significant assessment data to be noted before assisting with exercise and ambulation.
- Demonstrate correctly assisting with ambulation, assisting with ambulation with the use of an assistive device, assisting with range-of-motion exercises, and applying elastic stockings and sequential compression device.
- Develop teaching plans for safety in the home while using an ambulation aid, applying and monitoring effects of elastic stockings and sequential compression devices, and performing range-of-motion.

MEDIA RESOURCES

- evolve http://evolve.elsevier.com/Perry/skills
- Review Questions
- Case Studies

- ▶ Video Clips
- Audio Glossary
- Clinical Debrief and Review Questions Answers

PURPOSE

Regular physical activity and exercise contribute to patients' physical and emotional well-being (Edelman et al., 2013; Esposito and Fitzpatrick, 2011). This is a principle that you, as a nurse, should apply in the care of patients in all settings. Functional decline (e.g., the loss of the ability to perform self-care or activities of daily living), may result not only from illness or adverse treatment effects but also can be the result of deconditioning. Deconditioning is associated with inactivity and can result in generalized weakness and impaired aerobic capacity within a short period of time (Gorman et al., 2014). Deconditioning results in numerous physical changes and is a particular risk for hospitalized patients who spend most of their time in bed, even when they are able to walk. Nurses can play an important role in increasing the overall activity of hospitalized patients to minimize the effects of deconditioning. In addition to deconditioning, patients with limited mobility are at risk for developing thromboembolic disease and deep vein thrombosis (Box 12.1). The promotion of early exercise and mobility in the inpatient setting

and as a daily therapy for patients in outpatient settings is basic to competent nursing practice.

STANDARDS OF CARE

Agency for Healthcare Research and Quality (AHRQ), 2015—Preventing Hospital-Acquired Venous Thromboembolism and Prophylaxis

The Joint Commission, 2016—National Patient Safety Goals

American Association of Critical Care Nurses, 2015—Early Progressive Mobility Protocol

Quality and Safety Education for Nurses (QSEN): Pre-Licensure KSAs, 2014—Patient-Centered Care.

PRINCIPLES FOR PRACTICE

- Older adults are at greater risk for a reduction of muscle mass, strength, and power and for developing orthostatic hypotension, syncope, confusion, increased risk for fractures, and

Risk Factors for Deep Vein Thrombosis

- Injury to a vein, often caused by:
  - Fractures.
  - Severe muscle injury.
  - Major surgery (e.g., involving the abdomen, pelvis, hip, or legs).
- Slow blood flow, often caused by:
  - Confinement to bed (e.g., caused by a medical condition or after surgery).
  - Limited movement (e.g., a cast on a leg to help heal an injured bone).
  - Sitting for a long time, especially with crossed legs.
  - Paralysis.
- Increased estrogen, often caused by:
  - Birth control pills.
  - Hormone replacement therapy, sometimes used after menopause.
  - Pregnancy, for up to 6 weeks after giving birth.
- Certain chronic medical illnesses such as:
  - Heart disease, lung disease, cancer and its treatment, inflammatory bowel disease (Crohn's disease or ulcerative colitis).
- Other factors include:
  - Previous DVT or PE.
  - Family history of DVT or PE.
  - Age (risk increases as age increases).
  - Obesity.
  - A catheter located in a central vein.

From Centers for Disease Control and Prevention (CDC): *Venous thromboembolism (blood clots)*, 2015, http://www.cdc.gov/ncbddd/dvt/facts.html. Accessed March 20, 2016.
DVT, Deep vein thrombosis; pulmonary embolism.

functional incontinence as a result of decreased mobility from bed rest (Touhy and Jett, 2014).

- Early mobility and activity reduce impairment in cardiovascular and metabolic functioning, risk for pulmonary complications and development of pressure injury, and elimination alterations.
- Changes in a patient's mobility and activity can result from a variety of health problems (e.g., musculoskeletal, cardiovascular, and neurological) and therapeutic reasons (e.g., prescribed bed rest or reduced activity from sedation). Direct nursing measures to maintain and/or restore optimal mobility and decrease the hazards associated with immobility.
- It is important to act aggressively and implement early activity and mobility once patients are physiologically stable and able to respond to verbal stimulation (AACN, 2015).
- When caring for patients with reduced mobility, consider that there may be profound psychosocial and developmental effects. Immobilization often leads to emotional, intellectual, sensory, and sociocultural alterations. For young and older adults, immobility may alter employment, family role functions, and social interactions. Such changes can lead to altered self-concept, lowered self-esteem, and depression.

PATIENT-CENTERED CARE

- Respect patient preferences for degree of active engagement in the care process (e.g., activity and exercise [QSEN, 2014]). Assess each patient's expectations concerning activity and exercise and determine his or her perception of what is normal or acceptable.

- Always assess a patient's level of physical and emotional comfort before implementing activity or exercise therapies (QSEN, 2014). Patients with pain, nausea, or fatigue have little motivation to engage in physical activity. Patients who are anxious or afraid of injury often resist participation.
- When helping with exercises or ambulation, keep in mind that these activities may place patients in positions that can be embarrassing. Provide a garment that protects a patient's privacy. Many cultures emphasize modesty, and patients from these cultures may not participate in treatment measures for fear of being exposed.

EVIDENCE-BASED PRACTICE

- It is estimated that more than half of all patients hospitalized are at increased risk for the development of venous thromboembolism. Current evidence supports early nonpharmacological interventions in addition to pharmacological prophylaxis to prevent VTE (Pai and Douketis, 2016; Zisberg et al., 2015):
  - Early ambulation
  - Mechanical methods of VTE prevention (e.g., intermittent pneumatic compression, graduated compression stockings, venous foot pump)
  - Continuation of prophylaxis until the patient is ambulatory or discharged
  - Pharmacological prophylaxis for patients at low risk for bleeding who have at least one risk factor for the development of VTE (e.g., prolonged immobility ≥3 days, age ≥60 years of age, previous VTE)
  - A formal program in health care agencies for VTE prevention
- Immobility and the resultant deconditioning of hospitalized patients have led to greater efforts within hospitals to adopt evidence-based early progressive mobility protocols.
  - Zisberg et al. (2015) studied 684 patients (age 70 and older) admitted to a hospital with a nondisabling condition. Functional decline at discharge was reported by 282 participants (41.2%), and 317 (46.3%) participants reported functional decline at 1 month after discharge. In-hospital low mobility accounts for immediate and 1-month posthospitalization functional decline (Zisberg et al., 2015). These are potentially modifiable hospitalization risk factors for which exercise programs can be targeted.
  - In a systematic review of the literature, Adler and Malone (2012) found evidence supporting early mobilization and physical therapy as safe and effective interventions that can have a significant impact on functional outcomes in the critical care setting. In the ICU and immediate post-acute environment, the mobilization of critically ill but stable patients who have required a period of mechanical ventilation can be done safely with minimal risk to patients.
  - In a systematic review examining the effects of early mobility protocols on postoperative thoracic and abdominal surgery patients, the researchers concluded that the outcomes achieved are unclear (Castelino et al., 2016). Important questions that need to be studied include: At what frequency and intensity should patients mobilize after surgery? What mobilization targets should be used? And do patients treated with an early mobilization protocol have better postoperative outcomes compared with patients who mobilize at will? More research is needed in this area, but early mobilization is becoming a more common practice.

SAFETY GUIDELINES

- Obtain and become familiar with any type of assistive device to be used. Know how to properly prepare and use a device so you can teach patients or family caregivers how to use it safely and correctly.
- Prepare patients. Make sure that their vital signs are stable, they are rested and not overly tired, and their pain is under control. Obtain extra personnel to help as needed; use safe patient-handling devices and flat, nonskid shoes/socks for the patient.

- Address a patient's fear of falling if present. Ask patients how they feel about walking, whether they have fallen recently, and how you intend to remove risks for falling.
- Use appropriate clinical guidelines (see agency protocols) for advancing a patient's activity level. Consult with a physical therapist.
- Know a patient's home care plan. A patient may need to continue the exercise regimen or use an assistive device at home.

◆ SKILL 12.1 Promoting Early Activity and Exercise

Recently concerted effort has been made in hospitals to increase inpatients' activity and mobility levels as soon as possible to prevent deconditioning and other complications of immobilization. The American Association of Critical Care Nurses (AACN) (2015) now recommends an early progressive mobility protocol for critical care patients (refer to agency policy for protocols). When patients are transferred out to general nursing units, early mobility protocols should continue. This is often a challenge because staff nurses on general units often have difficulty routinely ambulating patients because of overall patient care demands, access to equipment, or unfamiliarity with transfer skills (see Chapter 11). Some hospitals have designated special mobility teams or mobility assistants to engage patients in early ambulation and activity.

A goal of the Healthy People 2020 initiative is to improve health, fitness, and quality of life through daily physical activity (Healthy People 2020, 2015). This goal is based on guidelines that suggest that regular physical activity can improve the health and quality of life of Americans of all ages, regardless of the presence of a chronic disease or disability (USDHHS, 2008a, b). As a nurse you may work in outpatient settings with the opportunity to plan health promotion activities. It is crucial to educate patients and family caregivers about the importance of regular physical activity

and exercise and how these activities can be incorporated into daily routines.

Delegation and Collaboration

The skill of promoting early activity and exercise for inpatients can be delegated to nursing assistive personnel (NAP) trained in transfer and assisted ambulation skills. In the outpatient setting education regarding activity and exercise cannot be delegated. Within inpatient settings the nurse directs the NAP by:

- Explaining the level of progressive mobility a patient has achieved.
- Explaining any restrictions in range-of-motion (ROM) exercises to perform (see Procedural Guideline 12.1).
- Explaining if there are any weight-bearing precautions or if patient needs to use assist device.
- Explaining criteria to use to stop assisted ambulation or sitting if patient cannot tolerate activity.

Equipment

- Inpatient—Pulse oximeter, gait belt, appropriate assist devices (see Skill 12.2)
- Outpatient—Depends on type of exercise recommended (e.g., 2.2 kg (5-lb) weights, resistance bands)

STEP	RATIONALE

ASSESSMENT

1. Identify patient using at least two identifiers (e.g., name and birthday or name and medical record number) according to agency policy.

Ensures correct patient. Complies with The Joint Commission standards and improves patient safety (2016).

2. Review patient's medical history for conditions that could influence or contraindicate mobility/exercise (e.g., dysrhythmias, recent myocardial infarction, stroke, paralyzed extremity, neuromuscular disease, peripheral neuropathy, current pregnancy). Review health care provider's order for early mobility or exercise program. Obtain physician clearance for outpatient exercise.

Examples of conditions that may contraindicate or require adjustments to activity. Patients should have medical clearance to begin activity/exercise program.

3. Gather baseline assessment of vital signs and oxygen saturation (if available).

Allows you to later evaluate patient's response to activity/exercise.

4. Assess patient's pain level; ask patient to rate pain on scale of 0 to 10.

Determines if there is need for an analgesic before mobilizing or ambulating inpatient. In outpatient settings, data will allow you to counsel patient as to best time to try more strenuous exercise.

STEP	RATIONALE
5. Assess patient's beliefs, values, and perceptions regarding current health status and confidence in being capable of performing exercise.	Perceived self-efficacy is a judgment of capability. The outcomes that people anticipate depend largely on their judgments of how well they will be able to perform in given situations (Bandura, 2006).
6. Implement Inpatient Early Mobility Protocol—to begin in intensive care unit (ICU) (AACN, 2015).	Protocol established for ICU patients; however, different levels of mobility can be continued when patient transfers out of ICU.

Clinical Decision Point NOTE: *Each agency (or even each ICU) may have different screening criteria based on the population that it commonly sees.*

STEP	RATIONALE
7. Perform safety screening (MOVE).	
M: Assess patient's myocardial stability.	Ensures cardiac stability. Exercise can initiate ischemic attack or worsen dysrhythmias.
• No evidence of active myocardial ischemia has occurred over last 24 hours.	
• No dysrhythmia requiring new antidysrhythmic drug has occurred over last 24 hours.	
O: Assess oxygenation status, must be adequate on:	Activity assessment criteria allow for early ambulation (Hopkins et al., 2016).
• FiO$_2$ ≤0.6.	
• PEEP (on ventilator) <10 cm H$_2$O.	
• *Option:* heart rate <120/min at rest, respiratory rate <28 (Hopkins et al., 2016).	
V: Minimal vasopressors	Change in vasopressor dose could lead to side effects such as tachycardia, dysrhythmias, and blood pressure changes such as orthostatic hypotension (Burchum and Rosenthal, 2016).
• No increase of any vasopressor has occurred for last 2 hours.	
E: Patient engages to voice of caregiver.	Patient must be alert and responsive, able to follow directions.
• Patient responds appropriately to verbal stimulation/commands.	
8. Outpatient assessment	
a. Identify patient's activity/exercise history:	Provides information on patient's motivation or willingness to exercise regularly.
• Which type of regular daily exercise do you perform at home?	Allows you to plan exercise that compliments and advances patient's activity level.
• Do you exercise or play a sport at least 3 times a week?	
• On a scale of 0 to 5 with 0 being no daily exercise and 5 strenuous regular exercise daily, how would you rate yourself?	
• How long have you been exercising regularly?	
b. Ask patient to what extent he or she enjoys exercising and what his or her beliefs are about ability to exercise.	Factors positively associated with adult physical activity (Healthy People 2020, 2015).
c. Determine if patient has social support from peers, family, or spouse.	Factors positively associated with adult physical activity (Healthy People 2020, 2015).
d. Determine if patient has access to facility or area to exercise. Is neighborhood considered safe?	Absence of facility or sense of safety discourages activity/exercise.
e. Consider these factors in your assessment: patient's age, income level, time available to exercise, rural resident, overweight, being disabled.	Factors negatively associated with adult participation in activity (Healthy People 2020, 2015)
f. Have patient rate level of quality of life based on current activity level.	Serves as baseline to measure long-term benefits of exercise.

NURSING DIAGNOSIS

- Activity intolerance
- Acute pain
- Chronic pain
- Impaired bed mobility
- Impaired physical mobility
- Readiness for enhanced health management

Related factors are individualized based on patient's condition or needs.

STEP	RATIONALE

PLANNING

1. Expected outcomes following completion of procedure:
- Inpatient: Patient will progress from sitting on edge of bed to sitting in chair 20 minutes 3 times a day (TID).
- Inpatient: Patient will gradually increase ambulation distance during hospital stay.
- Outpatient: Patient will identify and develop an exercise and activity program to perform.
- Outpatient: Patient will demonstrate adherence to exercise/activity plan at home.
- Patient will report a perceived improvement in overall mobility and quality of life (**NOTE:** Some institutions may use a scale for measurement).

Early mobility protocol is designed with progressive levels of exercise to promote improved patient function, reduce length of hospital stay, and improve patients' perceived quality of life.

Relevant and appropriate exercise plan increases adherence.

2. Inpatient: Consult with physical therapy (PT) regarding role in protocol to provide planned active resistance exercise for patients. If PT is available in home health, consult on types of exercises suited for outpatient's mobility restrictions.

Progressive resistance exercise (PRE) is method of increasing ability of muscles to generate force.

3. All patients: Explain benefits and reasons for activity/exercise. Do so in a way that matches patient's beliefs and values regarding recovery or maintaining health.

Exercise self-efficacy is an important predictor of the adoption and maintenance of exercise behaviors. Self-efficacy is the belief and conviction that one can perform a given activity successfully (Fletcher and Banasik, 2001; Shieh et al., 2015).

4. Inpatient: Explain precautions that will be taken to prevent falls during ambulation (gait belt, assisted walking, monitoring for dizziness).

Patients may have a fear of falling. Explanation may relieve anxiety.

5. Inpatient: As patient progresses to ambulating, try to schedule ambulation around patient's other activities.

Avoids overexertion of patient. Organizes nursing care activities.

IMPLEMENTATION

1. Inpatient Early Progressive Mobility Protocol (AACN, 2015)

Each patient starts at a different level, depending on his or her medical status and ability to participate in mobility.

Level 1
- Initiate passive ROM exercises TID (see Procedural Guideline 12.1). Turn patient every 2 hours.
- Help patient to sitting position in bed (e.g., stretcher chair or elevating head of bed to 45 degrees) and maintain for 20 minutes TID.
- Obtain a PT consultation if patient is alert to determine if strengthening exercises are indicated.

This level is designed for patients who are medically unstable to tolerate activity and/or have bed rest orders because of a medical condition.

Level 2
- Continue passive ROM exercises TID.
- Turn patient every 2 hours.
- Help patient to sitting position in bed and maintain for 20 minutes TID.
- Initiate sitting patient on edge of bed or lift patient to chair.
- Obtain PT consultation for mobility/strengthening program (e.g., active resistance exercise).

Patient begins to progress, he or she is starting to be able to sit independently on edge of bed or tolerate sitting up in a chair.

Principles of active resistance exercise: (1) to perform small number of repetitions until fatigue, (2) to allow sufficient rest between exercises for recovery, and (3) to increase resistance as ability to generate force increases. There is some evidence that PRE improves endurance and ability to generate muscle force, which can carry over into an improved ability to do everyday tasks (Taylor et al., 2005).

STEP	RATIONALE
Level 3	Patient progresses to transfer training, prewalking activities. Patient can still be in ICU during this phase or on nursing unit.
• Continue passive ROM exercises TID.	
• Turn every 2 hours.	
• Help patient to sitting position in bed and maintain for 20 minutes TID; sitting on edge of bed unsupported (but supervised).	
• Active transfer to chair with the patient sitting up in chair 20 minutes TID.	
• PT to continue with strengthening program as ordered.	
Level 4	Patients can still be in ICU during this phase or out on general nursing unit. Progression of mobility (amount of help required and distance walked) should occur until hospital discharge.
Continue passive ROM TID.	
• Turn every 2 hours.	
• Active transfer to chair with patient sitting up in chair 20 minutes TID sitting on edge of bed unsupported (but supervised).	
• PT to continue with strengthening program.	
• Initiate ambulation. Apply gait belt (if needed). Have patient ambulate (marching in place, walking in halls) (see Procedural Guideline 12.4 and Skill 12.2). NOTE: Ambulation time/distance should increase daily during hospitalization.	
2. Outpatient exercise and activity promotion	
a. Initiate an exercise program that contains any of the following components:	Warmup directs needed blood flow to muscles and prepares body for exercise. Warming up is important for preventing injury. Flexibility exercises help prevent tightness of muscles and improve joint ROM. Loss of ROM or muscle tightness can impede a person's function. Cool downs help body recover from exercises.
• Warm-up (5–10 minutes)	
• Strengthening exercises	
• Endurance exercises	
• Balance exercises	
• Flexibility exercises	
Consider consulting PT to help develop complete exercise program that would fit needs of your patient. A good overview of exercise programs can be found at http://health.gov/paguidelines/guidelines/.	
b. Recommend strength training for adults.	Strength training has been shown to improve strength and bone density and can be beneficial for older adult.
c. AHA (2015) recommends aerobic exercise at least 150 minutes per week of moderate exercise or 75 minutes per week of vigorous exercise (or combination of moderate and vigorous activity). This includes activities (e.g., climbing stairs; playing sports; or aerobic activities such as walking, jogging, swimming, or biking).	Designed to improve overall cardiovascular health.
d. Recommend balance exercises for older adults to decrease risk of falls. Have patient be sure to have something sturdy nearby on which to hold (wall or chair) if he or she becomes unsteady.	Helps to improve person's balance while standing or sitting and may decrease risk of falls.
• Perform exercises: standing on one foot, walking heel to toe, balance walking, back leg raises, side leg raises. Have patient do strength exercises (back leg raises, side leg raises) 2 or more days per week, but not on any 2 days in a row (NIH, 2015).	
e. Recommend patient perform cool down (5 to 10 minutes) after exercising:	Exercises help muscles relax and become more flexible.
• Quadriceps stretch	
• Hamstring/calf stretch	
• Chest and arm stretch	
• Neck, upper back, and shoulder stretch	

STEP	RATIONALE

EVALUATION

1. Measure vital signs and oxygen saturation during activity/ exercise and compare findings with baseline.	Determines patient's exercise tolerance.

Clinical Decision Point *Terminate physical activity when (Adler and Malone, 2012):*
- *Heart rate is greater than a 20% decrease in resting value or less than 40 beats/min or greater than 130 beats/min.*
- *Oxygen saturation shows greater than 4% drop from baseline or less than 88%–90%.*
- *Blood pressure: Systolic pressure is greater than 180 mm Hg or greater than 20% decrease in systolic/diastolic or orthostatic hypotension.*
- *Respirations: Less than 5 breaths/min or greater than 40 breaths/min*

Terminate exercise if dizziness last 60 seconds or fainting or diaphoresis occurs; change in breathing pattern occurs with increase in accessory muscle use, extreme fatigue, or severe dyspnea with respiratory rate greater than baseline by >20/min (Myszenski, 2014).

2. Evaluate patient's pain severity using 0 to 10 pain scale.	Exercises can increase muscle discomfort.
3. Monitor number of steps or estimated distance during walking.	Provides objective measure of ambulation progression.
4. After patient has reached Level 4 of inpatient mobility protocol or after outpatient has been exercising over 2 to 3 months, evaluate level of confidence in performing exercises.	Determines self-efficacy and likelihood of continued participation in exercise.
5. **Use Teach-Back:** "We've talked about doing a warmup and cool down as part of your exercise plan. Tell me why each is important." Revise your instruction now or develop a plan for revised patient or family caregiver teaching if patient or family caregiver is not able to teach back correctly.	Determines patient's and family caregiver's level of understanding of instructional topic.

Unexpected Outcomes	**Related Interventions**
1. Patient has abnormal vital sign response or decrease in oxygen saturation requiring termination of exercise. (In home setting be sure that patient or family caregiver knows patient's normal pulse range and when to terminate exercise.)	• Return patient to chair or bed immediately using safe patient-handling principles. • Notify health care provider. • Continue to monitor vital signs until patient's condition stabilizes.
2. Patient develops chest pain/discomfort during exercise.	• Return patient to chair or bed immediately using safe patient-handling principles. • Notify health care provider. • Prepare for possible electrocardiogram. • Continue to monitor vital signs until patient's condition stabilizes. • In home setting have caregiver call 911.

Recording and Reporting

- Record in the inpatient medical record or clinic record results of patient screening, type of exercise implemented, preexercise and postexercise assessments, and patient's tolerance in nurses' notes in electronic health record (EHR) or chart.
- Document your evaluation of patient and family caregiver learning.
- Report to health care provider any signs or symptoms indicative of exercise intolerance.

Special Considerations
Home Care

- Teach outpatient or family caregiver how to measure carotid or radial pulse, what a normal range is for patient, how to monitor exercise tolerance, and when to notify health care provider about problems.
- Have patient or family caregiver keep diary to record exercise activities, progression, and patient response.

PROCEDURAL GUIDELINE 12.1 *Performing Range-of-Motion Exercises*

Range of motion (ROM) refers to the distance or amount of freedom a joint can be moved in a certain direction (e.g., rotating, bending, or twisting). ROM exercises may be active, passive, or active assisted. They are active if a patient is able to move the limb against gravity; active assisted when a caregiver is needed to help the patient move the limb against gravity; and passive when the exercises are performed by a caregiver. Always encourage patients to be as active and independent as possible in every aspect of activities of daily living (ADLs). Incorporate active ROM exercises in a patient's ADLs (Table 12.1) and incorporate passive ROM into bathing and feeding activities. Collaborate with patients to develop schedules for ROM activities.

Delegation and Collaboration

The skill of performing ROM exercises can be delegated to trained nursing assistive personnel (NAP). Patients with spinal

PROCEDURAL GUIDELINE 12.1 *Performing Range-of-Motion Exercises—cont'd*

cord injuries, burns, or orthopedic trauma usually require ROM exercises by professional nurses or physical therapists. The nurse directs the NAP to:

- Perform exercises slowly and provide adequate support to each joint being exercised.
- Not exercise joints beyond the point of resistance or to the point of fatigue or pain.
- Be aware of a patient's individual limitations or preexisting conditions such as arthritis that affect ROM.

Equipment
- No mechanical or physical equipment needed
- Clean gloves *(option)*

Procedural Steps
1. Identify patient using at least two identifiers (e.g., name and birthday or name and medical record number) according to agency policy (TJC, 2016).
2. Review patient's chart for physical assessment findings that could affect the performance of ROM exercises (e.g., pain in joint, skin integrity or presence of wound near joint, presence of deformity; level of consciousness and ability to attend); health care provider's orders (e.g., any ROM restrictions for medical reasons); medical diagnosis, medical history, and progress.
3. Obtain data on patient's baseline joint function. Observe for obvious limitations in joint mobility, redness, or warmth over joints; joint tenderness; deformities, or edema.
4. Determine patient's or family caregiver's readiness to learn (e.g., desire to learn, perceived ability to perform exercise, perceived benefit of exercise). Explain in plain language reason for the ROM exercises and describe and demonstrate exercises to be performed.
5. Assess patient's level of comfort (on a scale of 0 to 10 with 10 being the worst pain) before exercises. Determine if patient would benefit from pain medication before beginning ROM exercises; then administer analgesic 30 min before exercise.
6. Perform hand hygiene and apply clean gloves if wound drainage or skin lesions are present.
7. Help patient to a comfortable position, preferably sitting or lying down.
8. When performing passive ROM exercises (Table 12.2), support joint by holding distal part of extremity or using cupped hand to support joint (see illustration).
9. Complete exercises in head-to-toe sequence. Repeat each movement 5 times during exercise period. Inform patient how these exercises can be incorporated into ADLs (see Table 12.1).

Clinical Decision Point *When resistance is noted within a joint, do not force joint motion. Consult with health care provider or physical therapist.*

10. Observe patient performing ROM activities.
11. Remove gloves, if worn. Perform hand hygiene.
12. Measure joint motion as needed to determine level of improvement.

13. Evaluate patient during exercise by having him or her rate the severity of pain on a pain scale.
14. **Use Teach-Back:** "Let's review what I discussed about ways to practice ROM at home. Tell me some exercises you can do at home." Revise your instruction now or develop a plan for revised patient or family caregiver teaching if patient or family caregiver is not able to teach back correctly.
15. Document exercises performed and patient's tolerance in nurses' notes in electronic health record (EHR) or chart.

TABLE 12.1

Incorporating Active Range-of-Motion Exercises Into Activities of Daily Living

Joint Exercised	Activity of Daily Living	Movement
Neck	Nodding head "yes"	Flexion
	Shaking head "no"	Rotation
	Moving right ear to right shoulder	Lateral flexion
	Moving left ear to left shoulder	Lateral flexion
Shoulder	Reaching to turn on overhead light	Flexion, extension
	Reaching to bedside stand for book	Hyperextension
	Rotating shoulders toward chest	Internal rotation
	Rotating shoulders toward back	External rotation
Elbow	Eating, bathing, shaving, grooming	Flexion, extension
Wrist	Eating, bathing, shaving, grooming	Flexion, extension, zulnar/radial deviation
Fingers and thumb	All activities requiring fine-motor coordination (e.g., writing, eating, painting)	Flexion, extension, abduction, adduction, opposition
Hip	Walking	Flexion, extension, hyperextension
	Moving to side-lying position	Flexion, extension, abduction
	Moving from side-lying position	Extension, adduction
	Rolling feet inward	Internal rotation
	Rolling feet outward	External rotation
Knee	Walking	Flexion, extension
	Moving to and from side-lying position	Flexion, extension
Ankle	Walking	Dorsiflexion, plantar flexion
	Moving toe toward head of bed	Dorsiflexion
	Moving toe toward foot of bed	Plantar flexion
Toes	Walking	Extension, hyperextension
	Wiggling toes	Abduction, adduction

Continued

PROCEDURAL GUIDELINE 12.1 *Performing Range-of-Motion Exercises—cont'd*

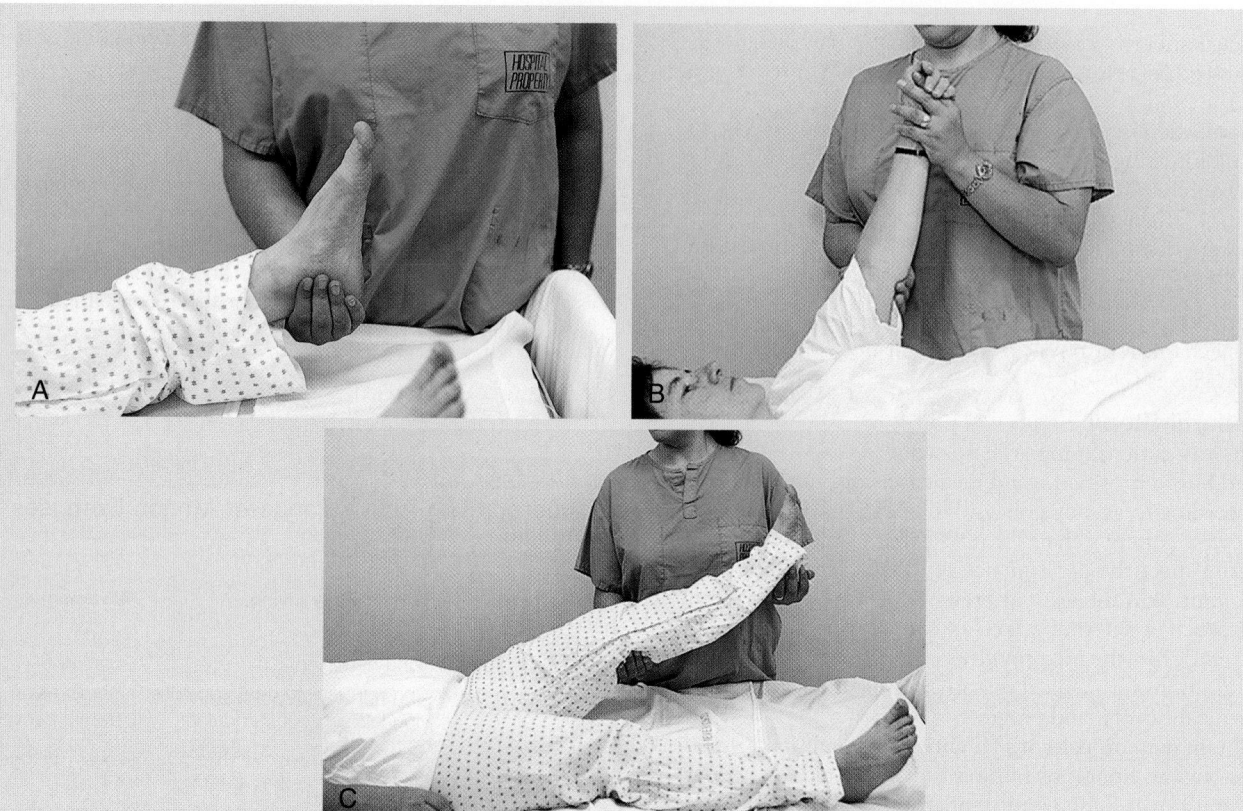

STEP 8 A, Support joint by holding distal and proximal areas adjacent to joint. **B,** Support joint by cradling distal part of extremity. **C,** Use cupped hand to support joint.

TABLE 12.2

Range-of-Motion Exercises

Body Part	Type of Joint	Type of Movement	Range (Degrees)	Primary Muscles
Neck, cervical spine	Pivotal	Flexion: Bring chin to rest on chest.	45	Sternocleidomastoid
		Extension: Return head to erect position.	45	Trapezius
		Hyperextension: Bend head back as far as possible.	10	Trapezius
		Lateral flexion: Tilt head as far as possible toward each shoulder.	40–45	Scalenes
		Rotation: Turn head as far as possible in circular movement.	180	Sternocleidomastoid, upper trapezius

PROCEDURAL GUIDELINE 12.1 *Performing Range-of-Motion Exercises—cont'd*

TABLE 12.2

Range-of-Motion Exercises—cont'd

Body Part	Type of Joint	Type of Movement	Range (Degrees)	Primary Muscles
Shoulder	Ball and socket	Horizontal flexion: swing arm horizontally forward	130	Coracobrachialis, deltoid, pectoralis major
		Horizontal extension: Swing arm horizontally backward	45	Latissimus dorsi, teres major, triceps brachii
		Abduction: Bring arm up sideways	180	Supraspinatus, deltoid, trapezius, and serratus anterior
		Adduction: Bring arm toward midline of the body	45	Pectoralis major, triceps, teres major
		Shoulder extension: Move arm behind body, keeping elbow straight.	0–60	Latissimus dorsi, teres major, deltoid
		Circumduction: Move arm in full circle (circumduction is combination of all movements of ball-and-socket joint).	360	Deltoid, coracobrachialis, latissimus dorsi, teres major
Elbow	Hinge	Flexion: Bend elbow so lower arm moves toward its shoulder joint and hand is level with shoulder.	150	Biceps brachii, brachialis, brachioradialis
		Extension: Straighten elbow by lowering hand.	150	Triceps brachii
Forearm	Pivotal	Supination: Turn lower arm and hand so palm is up.	70–90	Supinator, biceps brachii
		Pronation: Turn lower arm so palm is down.	70–90	Pronator teres, pronator quadratus

Continued

PROCEDURAL GUIDELINE 12.1 *Performing Range-of-Motion Exercises—cont'd*

TABLE 12.2

Range-of-Motion Exercises—cont'd

Body Part	Type of Joint	Type of Movement	Range (Degrees)	Primary Muscles
Wrist	Condyloid	Flexion, move palm toward inner aspect of forearm.	80–90	Flexor carpi ulnaris, flexor carpi radialis
		Extension: Move fingers and hand posterior to midline.	70–80	Extensor carpi radialis brevis, extensor carpi radialis longus, extensor carpi ulnaris
		Hyperextension: Bring dorsal surface of hand back as far as possible.		Extensor carpi radialis brevis, extensor carpi radialis longus, extensor carpi ulnaris
		Radial deviation: Bend wrist medially toward thumb.	Up to 30	Flexor carpi radialis brevis, extensor carpi radialis brevis, extensor carpi radialis longus
		Ulnar deviation: Bend wrist laterally toward fifth finger.	30	Flexor carpi ulnaris, extensor carpi ulnaris
Fingers	Condyloid hinge	Flexion: Make fist.	90	Lumbricales, interosseus volaris, interosseus dorsalis
		Extension: Straighten fingers.	90	Extensor digiti quinti proprius, extensor digitorum communis, extensor indicis proprius
		Hyperextension: Bend fingers back as far as possible.	30–60	
		Abduction: Spread fingers apart.	30	Extensor digitorum / Interosseus dorsalis
		Adduction: Bring fingers together.	30	Interosseus volaris
Thumb	Saddle	Flexion: Move thumb across palmar surface of hand.	90	Flexor pollicis brevis
		Extension: Move thumb straight away from hand.	90	Extensor pollicis longus, extensor pollicis brevis
		Abduction: Extend thumb laterally (usually done when placing fingers in abduction and adduction).	30	Abductor pollicis brevis and longus
		Adduction: Move thumb back toward hand.	30	Adductor pollicis obliquus, adductor pollicis transversus
		Opposition: Touch thumb to each finger of same hand.		Opponens pollicis, opponens digiti minimi
Hip	Ball and socket	Flexion: Move leg forward and up.	110–120	Psoas major, iliacus, sartorius
		Extension: Move leg back beside other leg.	90–120	Gluteus maximus, semitendinosus, semimembranosus

PROCEDURAL GUIDELINE 12.1 *Performing Range-of-Motion Exercises—cont'd*

TABLE 12.2

Range-of-Motion Exercises—cont'd

Body Part	Type of Joint	Type of Movement	Range (Degrees)	Primary Muscles
		Abduction: Move leg laterally away from body.	30–50	Gluteus medius, gluteus minimus
		Adduction: Move leg back toward midline position and beyond if possible.	20–30	Adductor longus, adductor brevis, adductor magnus
		Internal rotation: Turn foot and leg toward other leg.	45	Gluteus medius, gluteus minimus, tensor fasciae latae
		External rotation: Turn foot and leg away from other leg.	45	Obturatorius internus, obturatorius externus, quadratus femoris, piriformis, gemellus superior and inferior, gluteus maximus
		Circumduction: Move leg in circle.	120–130	Psoas major, gluteus maximum, gluteus medius, adductor magnus
Knee	Hinge	Flexion: Bring heel back toward back of thigh.	120–130	Biceps femoris, semitendinosus, semimembranosus, sartorius
		Extension: Return leg to floor.	120–130	Rectus femoris, vastus lateralis, vastus medialis, vastus intermedius
Ankle	Hinge	Dorsal flexion: Move foot so toes are pointed upward.	20–30	Tibialis anterior
		Plantar flexion: Move foot so toes are pointed downward.	45–50	Gastrocnemius, soleus
Foot	Gliding	Inversion: Turn sole of foot medially.	35 or less	Tibialis anterior, tibialis posterior
		Eversion: Turn sole of foot laterally.	10 or less	Peroneus longus, peroneus brevis

Continued

PROCEDURAL GUIDELINE 12.1 *Performing Range-of-Motion Exercises—cont'd*

TABLE 12.2

Range-of-Motion Exercises—cont'd

Body Part	Type of Joint	Type of Movement	Range (Degrees)	Primary Muscles
Toes	Condyloid	Flexion: Curl toes downward.	30–60	Flexor digitorum, lumbricalis pedis, flexor hallucis brevis
		Extension: Straighten toes.	30–60	Extensor digitorum longus, extensor digitorum brevis, extensor hallucis longus
		Abduction: Spread toes apart.	15 or less	Abductor hallucis, interosseus dorsalis
		Adduction: Bring toes together.	15 or less	Adductor hallucis, interosseus plantaris

PROCEDURAL GUIDELINE 12.2 *Monitoring a Patient on a Continuous Passive Motion Machine*

The continuous passive motion (CPM) machine is designed to exercise various joints such as the hip, ankle, knee, shoulder, and wrist. It is used most commonly after knee surgery. However, questions have been raised about CPM benefits (Maniar et al., 2012). A recent review of research involving knee arthroplasty surgery show that the CPM probably improves the ability of a patient to bend the knee slightly but may not ease pain or improve function (Harvey et al., 2014). It is usually prescribed from the first to fourth day following surgery for 1.5 to 24 hours a day, depending on a surgeon's preference and patient's condition (Harvey et al., 2014; Lewis et al., 2017). An initial setting is typically 20 to 30 degrees of flexion and full extension at two cycles per minute. The purpose of the CPM machine is to keep a joint mobilized to improve range of motion (ROM), reduce swelling, and ultimately prevent contractures and improve function. Although the value of the therapy has been questioned, it continues to be used, and you must be able to monitor patients safely on the device.

The electronically controlled CPM machine has Velcro straps to secure an extremity. When the device is turned on, the frame slides slowly back and forth, gently moving the joint through a preset ROM. The CPM machine can weigh up to 11.3 kg (25 lbs). Using two caregivers to lift the machine reduces the risk for caregiver back strain and prevents risk of damage to a patient's extremity.

Delegation and Collaboration
The skill of applying the CPM machine cannot be delegated to nursing assistive personnel (NAP). The nurse directs the NAP to:
- Immediately report to the nurse any increase in patient's pain when on CPM.
- To notify nurse of any skin breakdown observed when CPM is off.

Equipment
- CPM machine
- Padding
- Clean gloves

Procedural Steps
1. Review medical record and assess nature of patient's condition and ROM limits prescribed by health care provider. Be sure that order designates cycles per minute and time on machine.
2. Assess CPM machine for electrical safety. If you suspect a problem, notify the electrical safety department in your agency.
3. Assess setup of machine before placing on bed: check stability of frame, flexion/extension controls, padding of exposed metal parts or hard surfaces, and on/off switch.
4. Identify patient using at least two identifiers (e.g., name and birthday or name and medical record number) according to agency policy (TJC, 2016).
5. Perform hand hygiene.
6. Establish a baseline by assessing patient's pain on a scale of 0 to 10 (10 being the worst pain) before and during use.
7. Assess patient's heart rate, blood pressure, and respirations to establish baseline for exercise tolerance.
8. Assess patient's knowledge about CPM and ability and willingness to learn about the CPM machine.
9. Explain procedure and demonstrate CPM machine, turning machine on for patient to observe a cycle before placing on bed.
10. Help patient to comfortable supine position.

Clinical Decision Point *Before placing patient in a CPM device, attend to his or her elimination needs and, if ordered, provide an analgesic 30 minutes before a new treatment begins.*

11. Apply clean gloves if wound drainage is present.
12. Place elastic compression stockings on patient (if ordered) to promote venous return (see Procedural Guideline 12.3).
13. Place CPM machine on bed. Set limits of flexion and extension as ordered. Set speed control to slow or moderate range as ordered; turn machine on for it to run one full cycle.

PROCEDURAL GUIDELINE 12.2 *Monitoring a Patient on a Continuous Passive Motion Machine—cont'd*

14. Stop CPM machine when in extension. Place padding on CPM machine.
15. Support patient's affected joint while placing extremity in CPM machine frame.
16. Adjust CPM machine to patient's extremity. Lengthen and shorten appropriate sections of frame while centering patient's extremity on it. Align patient's joint with mechanical joint of CPM.
17. Secure patient's extremity on CPM machine with Velcro straps (see illustration). Apply loosely.

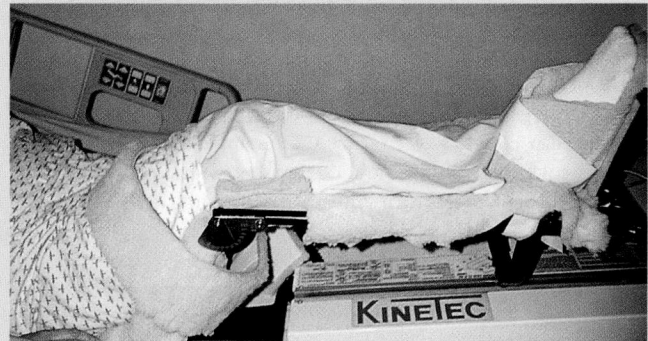

STEP 17 Patient's extremity properly placed and secured on CPM machine.

18. Press power switch to start machine. When it reaches flexed position, stop it and check degree of flexion. Then observe patient and affected extremity for two full cycles.

19. Ask if patient feels comfortable; evaluate pain severity on pain scale.
20. Be sure that CPM on/off power switch is within patient's reach. Instruct patient to turn CPM machine off if malfunctioning or if he or she is experiencing pain. Instruct him or her to notify nurse immediately.
21. Discard gloves and perform hand hygiene.
22. **Use Teach-Back:** "I want to be sure you understand what the CPM machine is supposed to do for you. In your own words, tell me the purpose of the CPM machine." Revise your instruction now or develop a plan for revised patient or family caregiver teaching if patient or family caregiver is not able to teach back correctly.
23. Inspect bony prominences and areas of skin in contact with machine at least every 2 hours; looking for breakdown.
24. Check patient's alignment and positioning at least every 2 hours.
25. Continue to evaluate patient for presence of pain. If patient is on a continuous cycle, provide analgesic at next scheduled dose.
26. Observe patient and CPM machine with each increase in flexion and extension.
27. Record in the nurses' notes in electronic health record (EHR) or chart patient's tolerance for CPM machine, rate of cycles per minute, degree of flexion and extension used, condition of extremity and skin, condition of operative site if present, and length of time CPM machine is in use.
28. Report immediately to nurse in charge or health care provider any resistance to ROM; increased pain; swelling, heat, or redness in joint.

PROCEDURAL GUIDELINE 12.3 *Applying Graduated Compression (Elastic) Stockings and Sequential Compression Device*

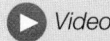 *Video Clip*

The development of deep vein thrombosis (DVT) is a hazard of immobility. Common risk factors include conditions that influence the Virchow's triad: hypercoagulability (e.g., clotting disorders, fever, dehydration); venous wall abnormalities (e.g., orthopedic surgery, varicose veins); and blood flow stasis (e.g., immobility, obesity, pregnancy) (Lewis et al., 2017). Signs of DVT include swelling in the affected leg (rarely swelling in both legs); warm, cyanotic skin; and pain in the leg that often starts in the calf and can feel like cramping or soreness. If a DVT is suspected, keep patient calm and quiet in bed and notify the health care provider.

If patients are at high risk for DVT, mechanical thromboprophylaxis (use of elastic stockings or intermittent sequential compression devices [SCDs]) is still a recommended form of therapy (AHRQ, 2015; Pai and Douketis, 2016; Sachdeva et al, 2014), especially in surgical patients after surgery.

Anticoagulant medication is the best approach for preventing DVTs; however, early ambulation, wearing compression stockings or intermittent SCDs, and using foot pumps are equally important (AHRQ, 2015; Pai and Douketis, 2016). All intermittent compression systems have a simple objective (i.e., to squeeze blood

from the underlying deep veins, which, assuming that the valves are competent, will be displaced proximally). On deflation of the cuff, the veins will refill and, because of the intermittent nature of the system, will ensure periodic flow of blood through the deep veins as long as there is a supply (Morris and Woodcock, 2004). Compression stockings appear to function more by preventing distention of veins. Reduction of edema and leg pain during the course of the day is accomplished while wearing elastic stockings (Carvalho et al., 2015). (SCDs pump blood into deep veins, thus removing pooled blood and preventing venous stasis. A venous plexus foot pump promotes venous return by pumping blood through compression, mimicking the natural action of walking (Fig. 12.1). The combination of stockings and foot compression has been shown to be more effective than stockings alone in both DVT and pulmonary embolism incidence (Morris and Woodcock, 2004).

Delegation and Collaboration

The skill of applying and maintaining graduated compression stockings and intermittent SCDs may be delegated to nursing assistive personnel (NAP). The nurse initially determines the size

Continued

PROCEDURAL GUIDELINE 12.3 *Applying Graduated Compression (Elastic) Stockings and Sequential Compression Device—cont'd*

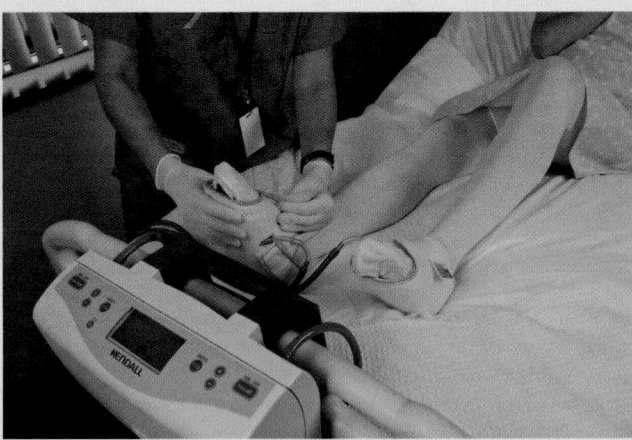

FIG 12.1 Venous plexus foot pump with bedside controls. *(Courtesy Tyco Healthcare Group LP.)*

of elastic stockings and assesses the patient's lower extremities for any signs and symptoms of a DVT or impaired circulation. The nurse directs the NAP to:

- Remove the SCD sleeves before allowing a patient to get out of bed.
- Report to the nurse if a patient's calf appears larger than the other or is red or hot, if the patient complains of calf pain, or if there are signs of allergic reactions to elastic (redness, itching, or irritation).

Equipment
- Tape measure
- Powder or cornstarch (optional)
- Graduated compression stockings
- SCD insufflator with air hoses attached, adjustable Velcro compression stockings/SCD sleeve
- Hygiene supplies

Procedural Steps
1. Review medical record for order for SCDs or graduated compression stocking.
2. Identify patient using at least two identifiers (e.g., name and birthday or name and medical record number) according to agency policy (TJC, 2016).
3. Assess patient for risk factors for developing DVT (see Box 12.1) (CDC, 2015).
4. Assess for contraindications for use of elastic stockings or SCDs:
   a. Dermatitis or open skin lesions on area to be covered by stockings/SCD
   b. Recent skin graft to lower leg
   c. Decreased arterial circulation in lower extremities as evidenced by cyanotic, cool extremities and/or gangrenous conditions affecting the lower limb(s)
   d. If signs/symptoms of a DVT are present, do not manipulate the leg to apply stockings.
5. Assess condition of patient's skin (area to be covered by stockings) and circulation to the legs. Palpate pedal pulses, note any palpable veins, and inspect skin over lower extremities for edema, skin discoloration, warmth, presence of lesions.
6. Obtain health care provider's order.
7. Assess patient's or family caregiver's knowledge of previous use of elastic or sequential compression stockings.
8. Explain procedure and reason for applying elastic stockings/SCDs.
9. Position patient in supine position.
10. Perform hand hygiene. Bathe patient's legs as needed. Dry thoroughly. Perform hand hygiene.
11. **Apply graduated compression stocking:**
    a. Use tape measure to measure patient's leg to determine proper elastic stocking size (follow package directions).
    b. *Option:* Apply a small amount of powder or cornstarch to legs provided patient does not have sensitivity.
    c. Turn elastic stocking inside out: place one hand into stocking, holding heel of stocking. Take other hand and pull stocking inside out until reaching the heel (see illustration).

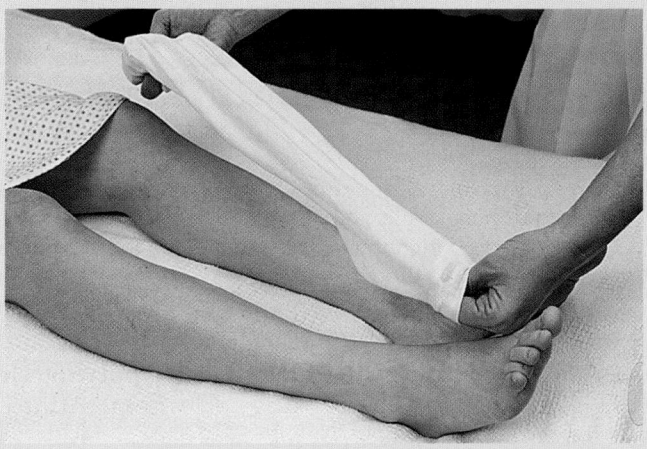

STEP 11c Turn stocking inside out; hold heel and pull through.

    d. Place patient's toes into foot of elastic stocking up to the heel, making sure that stocking is smooth (see illustration).

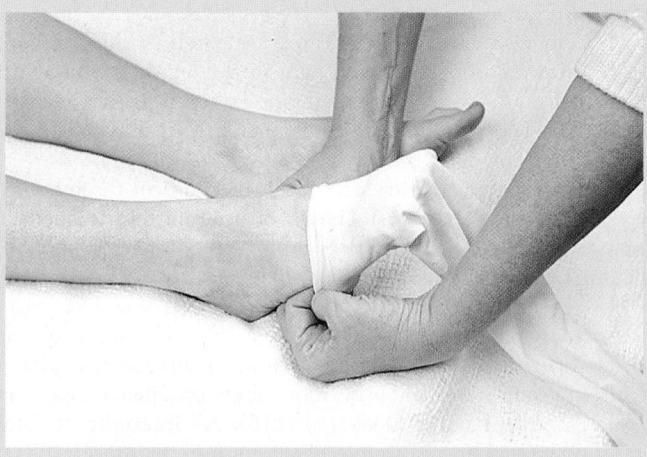

STEP 11d Place toes into foot of stocking.

PROCEDURAL GUIDELINE 12.3 *Applying Graduated Compression (Elastic) Stockings and Sequential Compression Device—cont'd*

e. Slide remaining part of stocking over patient's foot, making sure that toes are covered. Make sure that foot fits into toe-and-heel position of stocking. Stocking will now be right side out (see illustration).

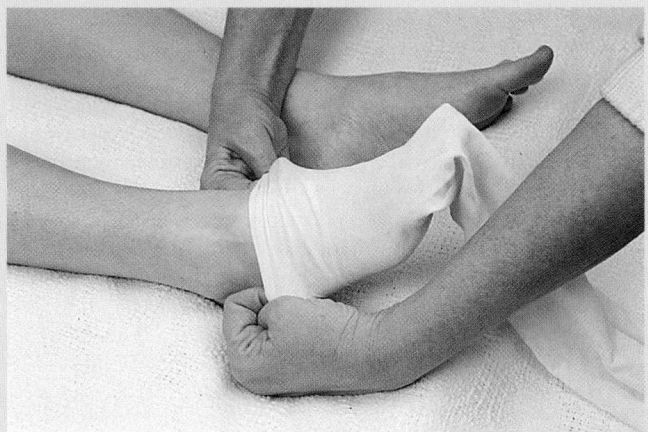

STEP 11e Slide remaining part of stocking over foot.

f. Slide stocking up over patient's calf until sock is completely extended. Be sure that stocking is smooth and that no ridges or wrinkles are present (see illustration).

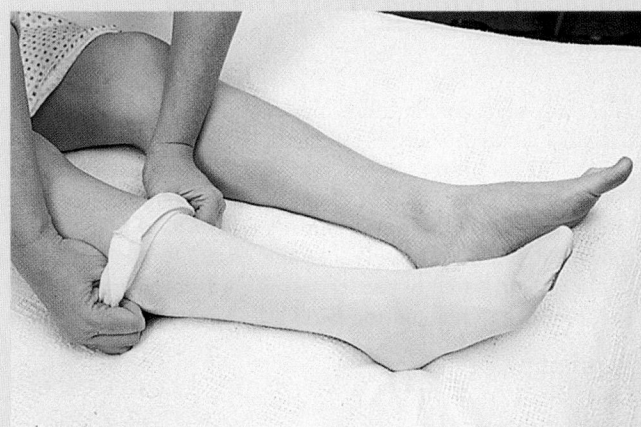

STEP 11f Slide sock up leg until completely extended.

g. Instruct patient not to roll stockings partially down, to avoid wrinkles and crossing legs, and to elevate legs while sitting.

12. Apply SCD sleeve(s):
   a. Remove SCD sleeve from plastic cover; unfold and flatten on bed.
   b. Arrange SCD sleeve under patient's leg according to leg position indicated on inner lining of sleeve.
   c. Place patient's leg on SCD sleeve. Back of ankle should line up with ankle marking on inner lining of sleeve.
   d. Position back of knee with popliteal opening on inner sleeve (see illustration).

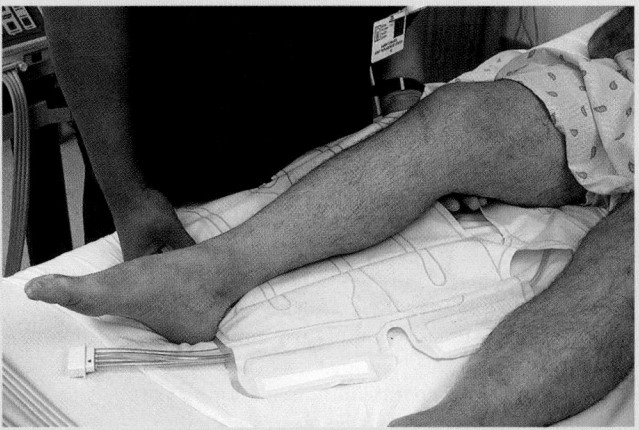

STEP 12d Position back of patient's knee with popliteal opening.

e. Wrap SCD sleeve securely around patient's leg. Check fit of SCD sleeve by placing two fingers between patient's leg and sleeve (see illustration).

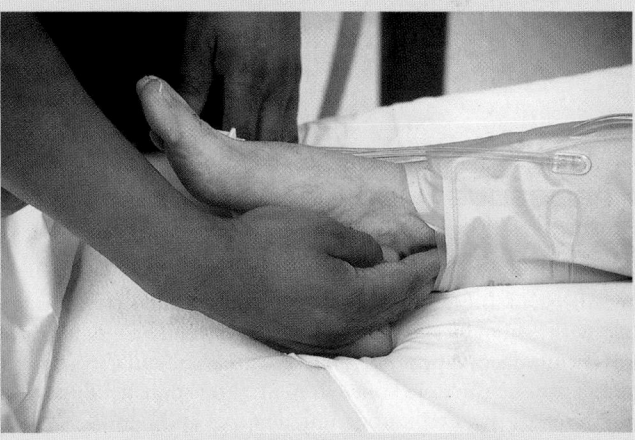

STEP 12e Check fit of SCD sleeve.

f. Attach SCD sleeve connector to plug on mechanical unit. Arrows on connector line up with arrows on plug from mechanical unit (see illustration).

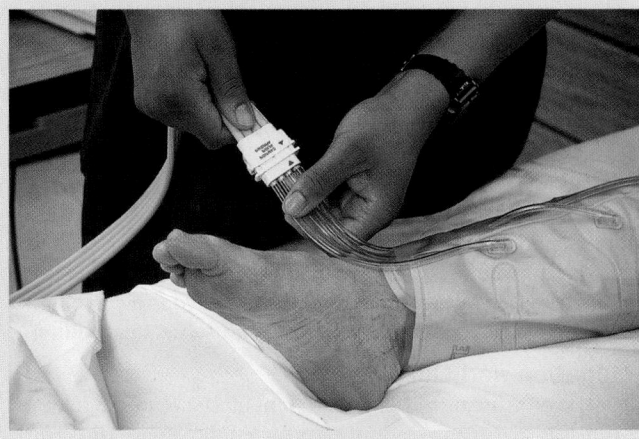

STEP 12f Align arrows when connecting plug to mechanical unit.

Continued

PROCEDURAL GUIDELINE 12.3 *Applying Graduated Compression (Elastic) Stockings and Sequential Compression Device—cont'd*

g. Turn on mechanical unit. Green light indicates that unit is functioning. Monitor functioning SCD through one full cycle of inflation and deflation.

13. Position patient comfortably and perform hand hygiene.

Clinical Decision Point *Caution patient not to exit bed and walk with SCDs in place. Have patient call for help.*

14. Remove compression stockings or SCD sleeves at least once per shift (e.g., long enough to inspect skin for irritation or breakdown and determine patient's comfort level).

15. Evaluate skin integrity and circulation to patient's lower extremities as ordered (see agency policy).

16. Educate patient/family caregiver about how to care for elastic stockings (keep two pair and wash one daily) and precautions to take to prevent DVT at home (CDC, 2015):
- Stay active and move around as much as possible.
- When sitting for long periods of time such as when traveling for more than 4 hours:
  - Get up and walk around every 2 to 3 hours.
  - Drink plenty of water.

- Exercise your legs while you're sitting by raising and lowering your heels while keeping your toes on the floor, raising and lowering your toes while keeping your heels on the floor, tightening and releasing your leg muscles.
- Wear loose-fitting clothes.

17. Use Teach-Back: "I want to be sure you understand why you have elastic stockings. Tell me in your own words the reasons why you are wearing these stockings?" Revise your instruction now or develop a plan for revised patient or family caregiver teaching if patient or family caregiver is not able to teach back correctly.

18. Document condition of lower extremities, application of stockings/SCD, patient education, and patient response in nurses' notes in electronic health record (EHR) or chart.

PROCEDURAL GUIDELINE 12.4 *Assisting With Ambulation (Without Assist Devices)*

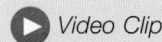 *Video Clip*

Patients who are immobile for even a short time often require help with ambulation. Ambulating patients early is important in preventing deconditioning. The benefits of ambulation include maintenance of muscle tone, strength, and joint flexibility and function of the respiratory, circulatory, and gastrointestinal systems. Use a gait belt when you help a patient ambulate to increase patient safety and decrease a patient's fall risk.

When helping a patient up and out of bed or a chair, there is a risk for orthostatic hypotension. Orthostatic hypotension or postural hypotension is a drop in blood pressure that occurs when a patient changes from a horizontal to a vertical position. A drop in blood pressure greater than 20 mm Hg in systolic pressure or 10 mm Hg in diastolic pressure with symptoms of dizziness, light-headedness, nausea, tachycardia, pallor, and fainting indicates orthostatic hypotension (Lewis et al., 2017). When a patient moves from a lying to a sitting position, dangling on the side of the bed (sitting on the edge of the bed with patient moving legs back and forth) and making sure the legs can touch the floor can minimize onset of orthostatic hypotension by allowing the circulatory system to equilibrate. After dangling, have patient stand; if he or she tolerates standing without dizziness, proceed with ambulation. Use safety precautions before and during ambulation to control for orthostatic hypotension and subsequent falling.

Delegation and Collaboration
The skill of assisting patients with ambulation can be delegated to nursing assistive personnel (NAP). The nurse directs the NAP to:

- Have a patient dangle following lying in bed and check patient's blood pressure before ambulation.
- Immediately return a patient to the bed or chair if he or she is nauseated, dizzy, pale, or diaphoretic and report these signs and symptoms to the nurse immediately.
- Apply safe, nonskid shoes/socks and ensure that the environment is free of clutter and there is no moisture on the floor before ambulating patient.

Equipment
- Gait belt
- Nonskid shoes/socks

Procedural Steps
1. Review medical record for patient's most recent activity experience, including distance ambulated, use of any assistive device, tolerance to activity, balance, and gait. Note any medications, chronic illnesses, presence of foot/leg deformity, or a history of falling, all of which may influence patient's ability to ambulate independently.

2. Review most recently recorded weight for patient; this may reveal need for help from another care provider.

3. Review medical record for any history of or risks for orthostatic hypotension; identify medications or conditions that may place patient at risk.

4. Review health care provider's order for activity; note any mobility or weight-bearing restrictions.

PROCEDURAL GUIDELINE 12.4 *Assisting With Ambulation (Without Assist Devices)—cont'd*

5. Determine the best time to ambulate, considering other scheduled activities such as bathing or other medical procedures.

6. Check patient's environment for any barriers or safety risks. When walking, it is helpful within a hospital or rehabilitation center to walk in an area where handrails are on the walls and chairs are near.

7. Identify patient using at least two identifiers (e.g., name and birthday or name and medical record number) according to agency policy (TJC, 2016).

8. Perform hand hygiene.

9. Assess patient's physical readiness to ambulate:
   a. Assess baseline resting heart rate, blood pressure, oxygen saturation (when available), and respirations.
   b. If patient's strength and endurance have been affected by illness or deconditioning, assess range of motion (ROM) and muscle strength (see Chapter 6) of lower extremities while in bed.
   c. Ask if patient feels excessively tired or is currently experiencing any pain. Determine source and severity of pain (using a 0-to-10 pain-rating scale). This may delay ambulation. Offer an analgesic 30 minutes before ambulation to improve patient's tolerance to exercise.

Clinical Decision Point *Do not administer an analgesic that could make the patient feel dizzy.*

10. Assess patient's level of response to commands. Is he or she able to understand instructions and cooperate during ambulation? Also assess patient's views and perceptions regarding current state of health and willingness to participate in activity.

11. Assess patient for any visual, hearing, or perceptual deficit that may affect his or her ability to follow instructions.

12. If this is the first time ambulating or if patient has been unsteady in past, have a chair or wheelchair positioned close to path you choose for ambulation. You want to be able to move patient quickly into a safe sitting position if he or she becomes unstable.

13. Explain to patient (in simple language) how you are going to prepare for ambulation (i.e., transfer technique and safety precautions to be used). Explain the benefits and reasons for activity/exercise. Do so in a way that matches patient's beliefs and values regarding recovery or maintaining health (Fletcher and Banasik, 2001; Shieh et al., 2015).

14. **Assist patient from a supine position to side of bed:**
   a. With patient in supine position in bed, raise head of bed 30 degrees and place bed in low position, level with your hips. Place nonskid shoes/socks on patient.
   b. While standing on side of bed where patient will sit, turn patient onto his or her side facing you.
   c. Stand opposite patient's hips. Turn diagonally to face patient and far corner of foot of bed.
   d. Place your feet apart in wide base of support with foot closer to head of bed in front of other foot.

   e. Place your arm nearer to head of bed under patient's lower shoulder, supporting his or her head and neck. Place your other arm over and around patient's thighs (see illustration).

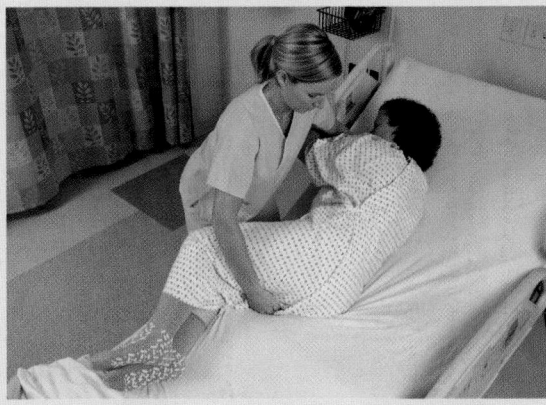

STEP 14e Nurse places arm over patient's thighs, other arm under patient's shoulder.

   f. Move patient's lower legs and feet over side of bed. Pivot weight onto your rear leg as you allow patient's upper legs to swing downward (see illustration). At same time, continue to shift weight to your rear leg and elevate patient's trunk to the upright position.

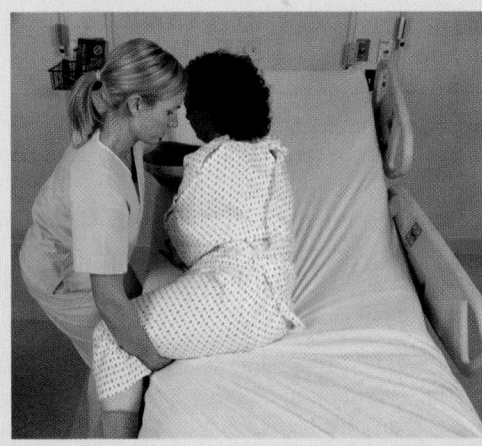

STEP 14f Nurse shifts weight to rear leg and elevates patient to sitting position.

15. Allow patient to sit on side of bed for a few minutes. Have patient alternately flex and extend feet and move lower legs up and down (see illustration). Ask if patient feels dizzy; if so, check the blood pressure. Have patient relax and take a few deep breaths until dizziness subsides and balance is gained. If dizziness lasts more than 60 seconds, return patient to the lying position in bed (Myszenski, 2014). Recheck blood pressure.

Continued

PROCEDURAL GUIDELINE 12.4 *Assisting With Ambulation (Without Assist Devices)*—cont'd

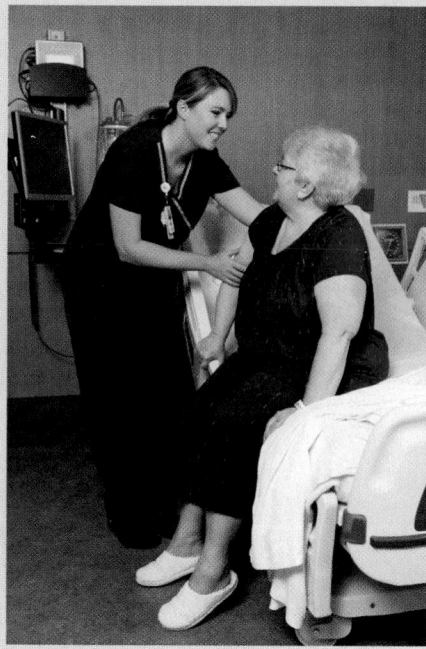

STEP 15 Patient sits on side of bed.

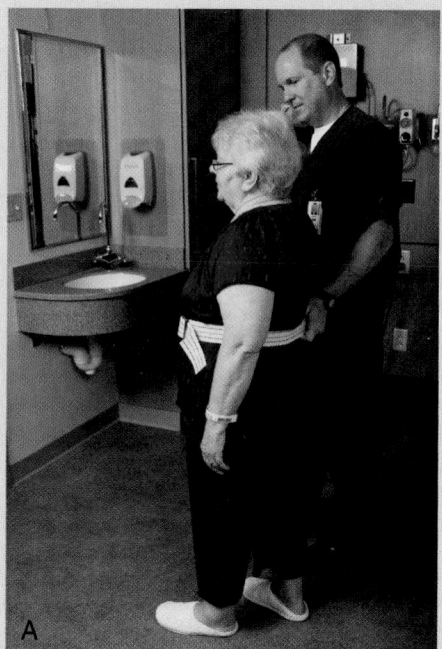

A

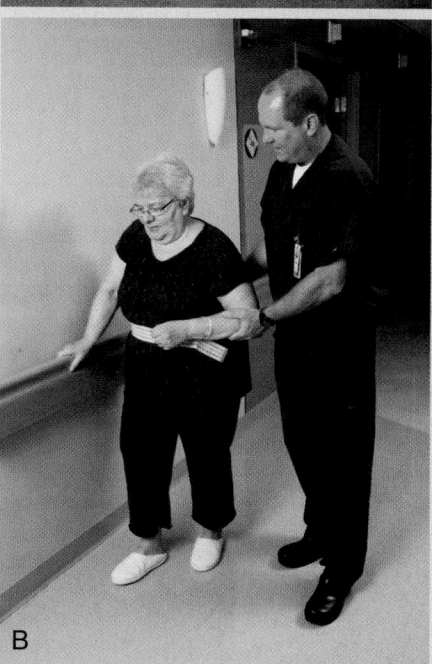

B

STEP 23 A, Nurse grasps gait belt firmly. **B,** Helps patient by providing support under patient's flexed arm.

16. Apply gait belt around patient's waist. Be sure that it completely circles the waist. Place belt low and be sure that it is snug. Avoid placing it over any intravenous (IV) lines, incisions, or drainage tubes. You may need to adjust it once patient stands. Hold onto belt along patient's back with your palm facing up. The gait belt controls patient's center of mass during mobility, controls descent if a fall occurs, and reduces the chance of grabbing patient's upper extremities.

17. Help patient into standing position at bedside. Have patient stand fully erect with shoulders back and looking ahead (not at floor). At this time assess his or her ability to bear weight and balance.

18. If patient is unsteady, place him or her in chair or return to bed immediately and obtain additional help.

19. If patient has an IV line, place IV pole on same side as patient's arm where the infusion is located. Instruct patient where to hold and push the pole while walking.

20. If a Foley catheter is present, empty drainage bag before ambulating patient. You or patient will carry bag below the level of patient's bladder. Sometimes you can pin the bag in the proper position on patient's gown. Be sure that there is no tension on the tubing.

21. Decide with patient how far or how long to ambulate to set mutual goal. Walk a distance that patient can tolerate (see mobility protocols of agency). Plan to increase ambulation time/distance during successive walks, as patient is able to tolerate.

22. Stand on patient's strong side and slightly behind. If assistive device (e.g., cane, walker) is used (see Skill 12.2), stand on patient's weak side and slightly behind.

23. Grasp gait belt firmly with palm facing up (see illustration). Take a few steps, supporting patient with one hand on the gait belt and the other under the elbow of patient's flexed arm (see illustration). *Option:* Use ambulation lift or ceiling lift with a gait harness for a more dependent patient who is now walking for first time after being in bed.

24. Have patient take a few steps forward. Then assess his or her strength and balance before continuing.

25. When ambulating down hallway, position patient between yourself and the wall. Encourage use of handrail (if present).

PROCEDURAL GUIDELINE 12.4 *Assisting With Ambulation (Without Assist Devices)*—cont'd

26. Observe how patient walks (posture, gait, balance, coordination) and evaluate his activity tolerance to ambulation (i.e., measure pulse and respirations and compare with baseline).

27. If patient starts to fall (see illustrations):
- **a.** Grasp patient's gait belt with both hands around his or her waist with palms up.
- **b.** Stand with feet apart for a broad base of support (see illustration A).
- **c.** Extend one leg, pull patient against you, and let him or her slide down your leg as you ease him or her to the floor (see illustration B). *Caution:* If patient is obese, do not risk personal injury.
- **d.** Bend your knees and lower your body as patient slides to floor (see illustration C).
- **e.** Stay with patient until help arrives.

28. Once patient has completed his or her walk, return him or her to a bed or chair and help to assume a comfortable position. Perform hand hygiene.

29. Record time or distance ambulated, any changes in vital signs, and patient's tolerance (symptoms such as pain and fatigue) in nurses' notes in electronic health record (EHR) or chart.

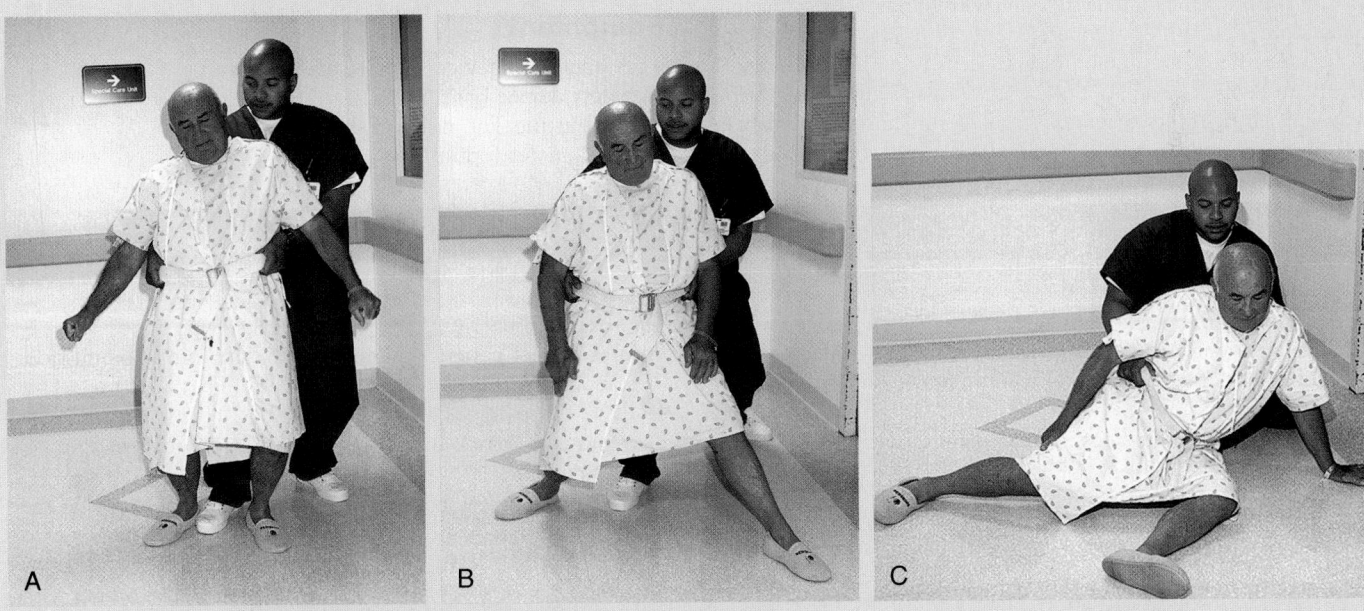

STEP 27 A, Grasp gait belt and stand with feet apart to provide broad base of support. **B,** Extend one leg and let patient slide against it to floor. **C,** Bend knees to lower body as patient slides to floor.

◆ SKILL 12.2   Assisting With Use of Canes, Walkers, and Crutches

An assistive device is any device that is designed, made, or adapted to help a person perform a particular task or function. For example, canes, crutches, and walkers are assistive devices for walking. An assistive device increases stability during ambulation; supports weak extremities; or reduces the load on weight-bearing structures such as hips, knees, or ankles. These devices range from standard canes, which provide balance and minimal physical support, to crutches and walkers, which are used by patients with weight-bearing limitations on one or more of their legs.

A licensed physical therapist should be consulted to help choose the proper assistive device, fit the device, and instruct the patient on the correct technique. Selection of an appropriate device depends on a patient's age, diagnosis, muscular coordination, weight-bearing status, and ease of maneuverability. Use of assistive devices may be temporary (e.g., during recovery from a fractured extremity or orthopedic surgery) or permanent (e.g., a patient with paralysis or permanent weakness of the lower extremities). As a nurse, you help patients use their devices correctly during ambulation. When helping a patient with an assistive device ambulate, always have a gait belt on the patient and stand slightly behind and off to the side of the patient (on his or her weak side).

Canes are lightweight, easily movable devices that extend about waist high and are made of wood or metal. They help to maintain balance by widening the base of support. There are three types of canes. The standard crook cane has a half circle handle and provides the least support for patients requiring only minimal assistance to walk. The tripod cane (pyramid cane) has three legs, and the quad cane has four legs; the additional legs provide a wider base of support. These types of canes are useful for patients with unilateral or partial leg paralysis. They also have the advantage of standing alone, freeing the arms to help a patient rise from a chair.

A crutch is a wooden or metal staff that reaches from the ground almost to the axilla. Crutches remove weight from one leg. They are used by patients who must transfer more weight to their arms than is possible with canes. There are two types of crutches: axillary and Lofstrand. Patients of all ages often use axillary crutches short term for various weight-bearing limitations on the lower extremities. A Lofstrand crutch has a handgrip and a metal band that fits around a patient's forearm. Both the metal band and the handgrip are adjusted to fit a patient's height. This type of crutch is useful for patients with a permanent disability such as paraplegia. The metal armband stabilizes and helps to guide the crutch. It also allows patients to use their hands for other activities such as opening doors without dropping the crutches. Second, the anterior opening of the band allows patients to free themselves of the crutches if a fall occurs.

A walker is a lightweight, movable device that stands about waist high, consisting of a metal frame with handgrips; four widely placed sturdy legs, and one open side. It provides a wide base of support and the greatest stability and security during walking. A walker can be used by a patient who is weak, has a weight-bearing limitation on a lower extremity, or has problems with balance. Most of the walkers that are being used today are wheeled walkers.

These walkers have two wheels on the front posts of the walker, making them easier to use and requiring less energy. This design is safer to use for patients with balance disorders because a patient keeps all four posts on the floor at all time. In contrast, a standard walker (has no wheels, only the four posts) requires a patient to have the balance to lift up the walker to advance it.

Delegation and Collaboration

The skill of assisting patients with ambulation can be delegated to nursing assistive personnel (NAP). The nurse should conduct the initial assessment when patient is ambulating for the first time. The nurse directs the NAP to:

- Have a patient dangle following lying in bed before ambulation.
- Immediately return a patient to the bed or chair if he or she is nauseated, dizzy, pale, or diaphoretic and report these signs and symptoms to the nurse immediately.
- Apply safe, nonskid shoes on patient and ensure that the environment is free of clutter and there is no moisture on the floor before ambulating patient.

Equipment

- Ambulation device (crutch, walker, cane)
- Safety device (gait belt)
- Well-fitting, flat, nonskid shoes for patient
- Goniometer (optional)

STEP	RATIONALE

ASSESSMENT

STEP	RATIONALE
1. Identify patient using at least two identifiers (e.g., name and birthday or name and medical record number) according to agency policy.	Ensures correct patient. Complies with The Joint Commission standards and improves patient safety (TJC, 2016).
2. Complete assessment steps in Procedural Guideline 12.4, Steps 1-5, 7-11.	Determines patient's ability to ambulate with a device and readiness for learning necessary gaits and precautions.
3. Determine patient's or family caregiver's understanding of type of device to be used in ambulating.	Allows patient to verbalize concerns. Patients who have been immobile may be hesitant to ambulate. Family caregiver may be hesitant to learn how to help with ambulation.
4. Assess degree of assistance that patient needs. Physical therapy (PT) will also make this recommendation.	For safety, another person may be needed initially to help with patient ambulation. Allow patient as much independence as possible.

NURSING DIAGNOSES

- Activity intolerance
- Deficient knowledge regarding use of assist device
- Fatigue

- Impaired physical mobility
- Risk for falls
- Risk for injury

- Ineffective health management
- Readiness for enhanced health management

Related factors/Risk factors are individualized based on patient's condition or needs.

PLANNING

STEP	RATIONALE
1. Expected outcomes following completion of procedure:	
• Patient ambulates using assistive device without injury.	Appropriate level of assistance with device ensures patient's safety.
• Patient is able to ambulate without excessive fatigue or dizziness and with return of vital signs to baseline 3 to 5 minutes after rest.	Assistive device chosen requires minimal exertion. Patient tolerates exercise.
• Patient demonstrates correct use of assist device, gait pattern, and weight-bearing status.	Demonstrates learning and physical ability to use device.

STEP	RATIONALE

2. Explain to patient how you are going to prepare for ambulation (e.g., transfer technique out of bed and safety precautions to be used while walking). Explain benefits and reasons for activity/exercise. Do so in a way that matches patient's educational level and beliefs and values regarding recovery or maintaining health.

Exercise self-efficacy is an important predictor of the adoption and maintenance of exercise behaviors. Self-efficacy is a belief and conviction that one can successfully perform a given activity (Fletcher and Banasik, 2001; Shieh et al., 2015).

3. Explain and demonstrate specific gait technique to patient or family caregiver.

Teaching and demonstration enhance learning, reduce anxiety, and encourage cooperation.

4. Check for appropriate height and fit of assist device. If physical therapist has seen patient, the device should be at appropriate height. **NOTE:** *this is usually done when patient is standing at side of bed and is stable.*

Ensures that patient is able to ambulate successfully without injury using device.

   a. *Cane measurement:* Cane should extend from greater trochanter of the hip to floor while cane is held 15 cm (6 inches) from foot. Allow 15- to 30-degree elbow flexion. Cane handle should fit comfortably in palm of hand.

If cane is too short, patient has difficulty supporting weight and is bent over and uncomfortable. As weight is taken on by hands and affected leg is lifted off floor, complete extension of elbow is needed.

   b. *Crutch measurement:* Includes three areas: patient's height, distance between crutch pad and axilla, and angle of elbow flexion. Use one of two methods:

Promotes optimal support and stability.

     (1) *Standing:* Position crutches with crutch tips at 15 cm (6 inches) to side and 15 cm in front of patient's feet (tripod position). Crutch pads should be 5 cm (1½ to 2 inches) (3.75 to 5 cm) or 2–3 finger widths) under axilla (American College of Foot and Ankle Surgeons, 2016) (see illustration).

Radial nerve passes under axillary area superficially. If crutch is too long, it places pressure on axilla and radial nerve. Injury to radial nerve causes paralysis of elbow and wrist extensors, commonly called *crutch palsy.* In addition, if crutch is too long, shoulders are forced upward, and patient cannot push body off the ground. If ambulation device is too short, patient is bent over and uncomfortable.

     (2) *Supine:* Crutch pad is approximately 5 cm (2 inches) or two-to-three finger widths under axilla with crutch tips positioned 15 cm (6 inches) lateral to patient's heel (see illustration).

     (3) Height of handgrip must be adjusted so patient's elbow is flexed 15 to 30 degrees or it sits at approximately height of wrist crease. Both height of crutch and handgrip dimensions are adjustable on a well-made crutch.

Low handgrips cause radial nerve damage. High handgrips cause elbow to be sharply flexed, decreasing strength and stability of arms. This allows patient to fully extend the elbow when taking a step.

   c. *Walker measurement:* When patient relaxes arms at side of body and stands up straight, top of walker should line up with crease on inside of wrist (AAOS, 2015). Elbows should flex about 15 to 30 degrees when standing inside walker, with hands on handgrips.

Walker should be at proper height so patient does not bend forward. Patient must have sufficient strength to be able to move walker.

5. Make sure that ambulation device has rubber tips.

Prevents device from slipping.

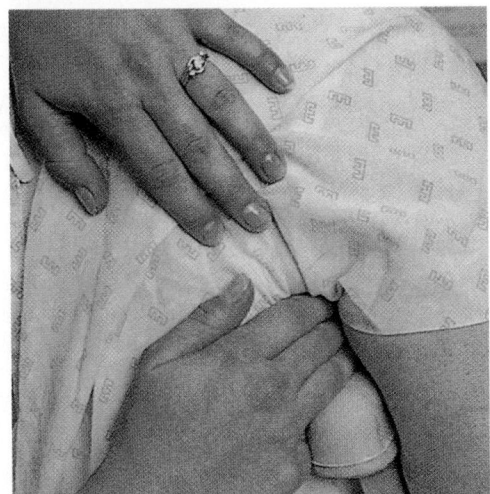

STEP 4b(1) Crutch pad is 2 to 3 finger widths under axilla.

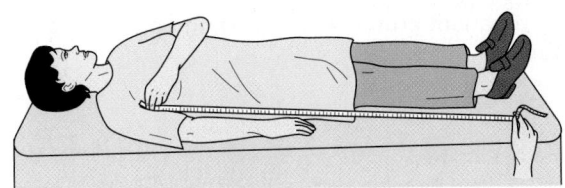

STEP 4b(2) Measuring length of crutch with patient in bed.

STEP	RATIONALE

Clinical Decision Point *Remove obstacles from pathways, including throw rugs (in the home), fall pads, and electrical cords; and wipe up any spills immediately. Avoid crowds. Crowds increase the risk of the crutch, cane, or walker being kicked or jarred and patient losing balance.*

IMPLEMENTATION

STEP	RATIONALE
1. Perform hand hygiene.	
2. If using crutches, have patient report any tingling or numbness in upper torso.	Helps to indicate that crutches are being used incorrectly or that they are wrong size.
3. Help patient from lying position to side of bed (see Procedural Guideline 12.4, Step 13) or up from chair.	Ensures that patient is stable and ready to ambulate.
4. Allow patient to sit on edge of bed for a few minutes. Have patient alternately flex and extend feet, move lower legs. Ask if he or she feels dizzy. Have patient relax and take a few deep breaths until dizziness subsides and balance is gained.	Determines ability to tolerate standing. If dizziness lasts more than 60 seconds, may indicate orthostatic hypotension; return patient to bed (Myszenski, 2014). Recheck blood pressure.
5. Apply gait belt around patient's waist. Be sure that it completely circles patient's waist. Place belt low and be sure that it is snug. You may need to adjust belt once patient stands. You hold belt along patient's back with your palms facing up as patient walks.	Belt controls patient's center of mass during mobility, controls descent if a fall occurs, and reduces chance of grabbing patient's upper extremities.
6. Help patient stand at bedside. Reassess height of device to make sure that it is correct size. Have patient stand fully erect with shoulders back and looking ahead (not at floor). At this time assess patient's ability to bear weight (e.g., Does patient have discomfort, unsteady stance?) and balance.	Ensures that patient begins ambulation with correct posture and position.
7. If patient is unsteady, seat him or her in chair or return to bed immediately.	Patient may require strengthening exercises or evaluation of balance by PT.
8. Decide with patient how far to ambulate.	Determines mutual goal.
9. Implement ambulation around patient's other activities.	Taking scheduled rest periods between activities reduces patient fatigue.
10. **Help patient walk with cane (steps are the same with standard, tripod, or quad cane):**	
a. Have patient hold cane on strong side. Direct patient to place cane forward 10 to 15 cm (4 to 6 inches) and slightly to the side of the foot, keeping body weight on both legs. Allow approximately 15- to 30-degree elbow flexion.	Offers most support when on stronger side of body. Cane and weaker leg work together with each step.
b. To begin, have patient move cane forward about 15 to 25 cm (6 to 10 inches), keeping body weight on both legs.	Distributes body weight equally.
c. Instruct patient to advance involved leg forward, even with the cane. The cane and affected leg swing and strike the ground at the same time.	Body weight is supported by cane and strong leg.
d. Have patient advance strong leg 15 to 25 cm (6 to 10 inches) past cane.	Aligns patient's center of gravity. Returns patient body weight to equal distribution.
e. Have patient move involved leg forward, even with strong leg, which can go as far forward as bad leg or slightly past it.	
f. Repeat sequences as patient tolerates. Once comfortable, have patient advance cane and weak leg together.	
11. **Help patient crutch walk by using appropriate crutch gait:**	To use crutches, patient supports self with hands and arms; therefore ability to balance body in upright position and stamina are necessary. Type of crutch gait depends on patient's weight-bearing status.

STEP	RATIONALE

a. Four-point gait:

This is most stable crutch gait. It provides at least three points of support at all times. Patient must be able to bear weight on both legs. Patient moves each leg alternately with each opposing crutch so three points of support are on floor all the time. Often used when patient has some form of paralysis, (e.g., children with spastic cerebral palsy) (Hockenberry and Wilson, 2015). May also be used for arthritic patients.

(1) Begin in tripod position (see illustration). Have patient place the crutch tips about 4 to 6 inches (10 to 15 cm) to the side and in front of each foot (American College of Foot and Ankle Surgeons, 2016). Have patient place weight on handgrips, not under arms.

Improves balance by providing wide base of support. Patient should have posture of erect head and neck, straight vertebrae, and extended hips and knees.

(2) Move right crutch forward 10 to 15 cm (4 to 6 inches) (see illustration A).

Crutch and foot position is similar to arm and foot position during normal walking.

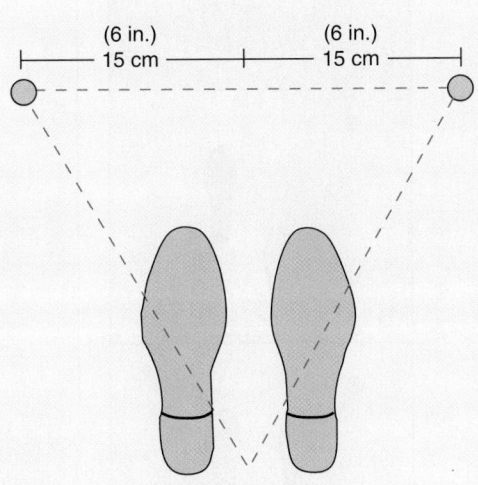

STEP 11a(1) Tripod position.

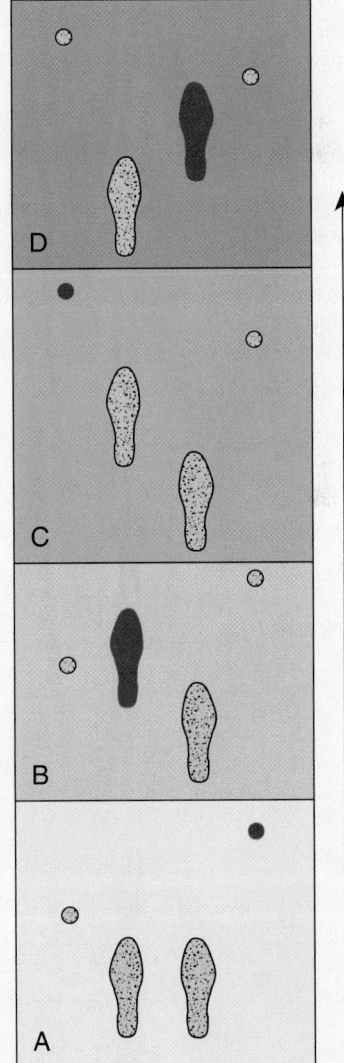

STEP 11a(2) Four-point gait. Solid feet and crutch tips show foot and crutch tip movement in each of four phases. (Read from bottom to top.) **A,** Right tip moves forward. **B,** Left foot moves toward left crutch. **C,** Left crutch tip moves forward. **D,** Right foot moves toward right crutch.

STEP	RATIONALE

(3) Move left foot forward to level of left crutch (see illustration B).

(4) Move left crutch forward 10 to 15 cm (4 to 6 inches) (see illustration C).

(5) Move right foot forward to level of right crutch (see illustration D).

(6) Repeat above sequence.

b. Three-point gait (see illustrations):

Requires patient to bear all weight on one foot. Weight is borne on strong leg and then on both crutches. Affected leg does not touch ground during early phase of three-point gait. May be useful for patient with broken leg or sprained ankle.

Improves patient's balance by providing wide base of support.

(1) Begin in tripod position (see illustration A), with patient standing on weight-bearing foot.

(2) Advance both crutches and involved leg, keeping foot of involved leg off floor (see illustration B).

(3) Move weight-bearing leg forward, stepping on floor (see illustration C).

(4) Repeat sequence.

c. Two-point gait (see illustrations):

Requires at least partial weight bearing on each foot. Is faster than four-point gait. Requires more balance because only two points support body at one time.

Improves patient's balance by providing wide base of support.

Crutch movements are similar to arm movement during normal walking; patient moves crutch at same time as opposing leg.

(1) Begin in tripod position (see illustration A).

(2) Move left crutch and right foot forward (see illustration B).

(3) Move right crutch and left foot forward (see illustration C).

(4) Repeat sequence.

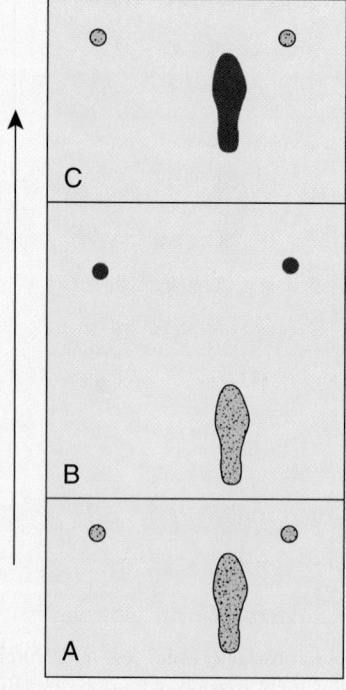

STEP 11b Three-point gait with weight borne on unaffected right leg. Solid foot and crutch tips show weight bearing in each phase **A** to **C.** (Read from bottom to top.)

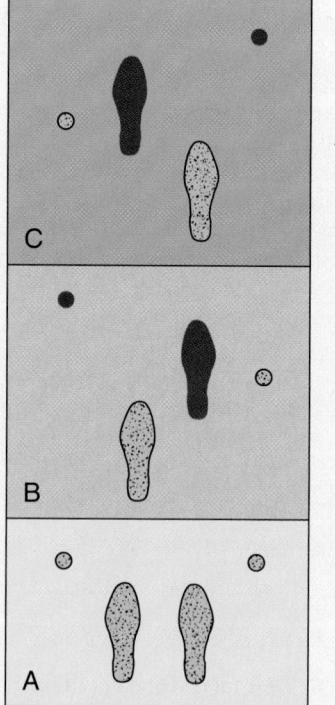

STEP 11c Two-point gait. Solid areas indicate weight-bearing leg and crutch tips **A** to **C.** (Read from bottom to top.)

STEP	RATIONALE
d. Swing-to gait:	Used by patients whose lower extremities are paralyzed or who wear weight-supporting braces on their legs.
(1) Begin in tripod position.	This is the easier of two swinging gaits. It requires ability to partially bear body weight on both legs.
(2) Move both crutches forward.	
(3) Lift and swing legs to crutches, letting crutches support body weight.	
(4) Repeat two previous steps.	
e. Swing-through gait:	Requires that patient have ability to bear partial weight on both feet.
(1) Begin in tripod position.	Improves patient's balance by providing wide base of support.
(2) Move both crutches forward.	Initial placement of crutches increases patient's base of support so, when body swings forward, patient is moving center of gravity toward additional support provided by crutches.
(3) Lift and swing legs through and beyond crutches.	
(4) Repeat previous steps.	
12. Helping patient climb up stairs with a railing with crutches (partial weight bearing, one leg):	Climbing stairs with use of a railing is safest way for patient with crutches to ascend stairs.

Clinical Decision Point *There is a risk for falling using this technique. Monitor patient's balance carefully. See option below.*

STEP	RATIONALE
a. Have patient begin in tripod position. Stand on weight-bearing leg.	Improves patient's balance by providing wide base of support.
b. Patient transfers body weight to crutch.	Prepares patient to transfer weight to strong leg when ascending first stair.
c. Have patient hold handrail with one hand (strong leg next to railing). As the nurse, you carry crutch positioned next to handrail. Patient holds other crutch.	Ensures patient safety.
d. Have patient support his or her weight evenly between the handrail and crutch.	Achieves balance.
e. Patient next places some weight on crutches and then steps up with first step with weight-bearing foot. Have patient get his or her balance.	
f. Patient then straightens uninvolved knee and lifts his or her body weight, bringing crutches and affected leg up the stair.	
g. Repeat sequence of steps until patient reaches top of stairs. Observe patient's balance and level of fatigue.	
h. Option: Have patient sit on the lower stair. If distance and reach allow, place the crutches at the top of the staircase. If this isn't possible, have patient place crutches as far up the stairs as he or she can. Then patient will move them to the top as he or she progresses up the stairs (American College of Foot and Ankle Surgeons, 2016).	Reaching for inaccessible crutches could lead to a fall. Moving up by seat avoids risks of losing balance and tripping on stairs.
(1) In the seated position, have patient reach behind with both arms.	
(2) Then have patient use arms and weight-bearing foot/leg to lift up one step.	
(3) Repeat this process one step at a time	
13. Helping patient descend stairs with a railing with crutch (partial weight bearing, one leg):	

STEP	RATIONALE

Clinical Decision Point *There is a risk for falling using this technique. Monitor patient's balance carefully. See option below.*

a. Begin in tripod position.

b. Patient transfers body weight to strong leg and aligns with crutches.

c. Have patient hold handrail with one hand (involved leg next to railing). You, as the nurse, carry crutch positioned next to handrail. Patient holds other crutch.

d. Have patient bend his or her strong knee while moving crutch and involved leg down a step.

e. Patient then supports his or her weight evenly between handrail and crutch. Be sure that patient has good balance.

f. Have patient slowly bring involved leg down step. Caution patient not to hop.

g. **Option:** Have patient sit on the top step. Place crutches down the stairs by sliding them to the lowest possible point on the stairway. Then continue to move them down as patient progresses down the stairs (American College of Foot and Ankle Surgeons, 2016).

   (1) In the seated position, have patient reach behind with both arms.

   (2) Have patient use arms and weight-bearing foot/leg to lift self down one step.

   (3) Repeat this process one step at a time

14. Helping patient ambulate with walker:

a. Have patient stand straight in center of walker and grasp handgrips on upper bars.

b. Have patient move walker comfortable distance forward, about 15 to 20 cm (6 to 8 inches). Patient then takes step forward with involved leg first and follows through with good leg. Instruct patient not to advance leg past the front bar of walker. If patient has equal strength in both legs, it makes no difference which leg advances first.

c. If patient is unable to bear weight on involved leg, have him or her slowly hop to center of walker using strong leg, supporting weight on hands.

d. Instruct patient not to try to climb stairs with walker unless he or she has specific walker for steps.

15. After patient ambulates, help him or her back to bed or chair and help assume comfortable position.

16. Perform hand hygiene.

Rationale column:

Improves patient's balance by providing wide base of support.

Prepares patient to release support of body weight maintained by crutches.

Hopping could injure leg and create risk for fall.

Reaching for inaccessible crutches could lead to a fall. Moving down by seat avoids risk of losing balance and falling down stairs.

Patients who are able to bear partial weight use walkers. Patient balances self before attempting to walk.

Provides broad base of support between walker and patient. Patient then moves center of gravity toward walker. Keeping all four feet of walker on floor is necessary to prevent tipping walker.

Patient should use handrails as alternative. Using walker could cause a fall.

Prevents transmission of infection.

EVALUATION

1. After ambulation, obtain patient's vital signs, observe skin color, and ask about his or her comfort and energy levels.

   Evaluates how patient tolerated procedure and whether there was progress in ambulation. Assesses stage of patient's illness and degree of convalescence when evaluating process.

2. Evaluate patient's subjective statements regarding experience.

   Evaluates activity tolerance.

3. Evaluate patient's gait pattern: observe body alignment in standing position and balance during gait.

   Determines if patient is using supportive aids for ambulation correctly. Keep in mind patient's previous manner of ambulating when assessing gait.

STEP	RATIONALE
4. Use Teach-Back "You have done well walking with your walker. We reviewed with your wife how to place a gait belt. I talked about why it is important for your wife to use a gait belt to help you at first. Can both of you tell me why a gait belt is important." Revise your instruction now or develop a plan for revised patient or family caregiver teaching if patient or family caregiver is not able to teach back correctly.	Determines patient's and family caregiver's level of understanding of instructional topic.

Unexpected Outcomes	Related Interventions
1. Patient is unable to ambulate because of fear of falling, physical discomfort, upper body muscles that are too weak to use ambulation device, or lower extremities that are too weak to support body.	• Consult with PT about possible exercise program to strengthen muscles or other alternative methods that patient can use for ambulation. • Provide analgesic for discomfort. • Discuss with patient fears or concerns about walking using assist device.
2. Patient sustains an injury.	• Notify health care provider. • Return patient to bed if injury stable. • Document per institution/agency policy.
3. When using cane or walker, patient bends over and does not stand straight.	• Reinforce correct posture.

Recording and Reporting

• Record in the medical record assessment findings, type of assist device and gait patient used, amount of help required, distance walked, and activity tolerance in the electronic health record (EHR) or chart.
• Document your evaluation of patient and family caregiver learning.
• Immediately report any injury sustained during attempts to ambulate, alteration in vital signs, or inability to ambulate to nurse in charge or health care provider.

Special Considerations
Teaching

• Instruct the patient with exercises such as squeezing a rubber ball, raising and lowering both arms in a slow and rhythmic manner while holding weights, chair pushups, and pull-ups, which help to strengthen the upper extremities.
• Teach patients who use a walker to examine the frame daily. When inspecting a walker, patient should observe for signs of bending or deformation of the frame, protruding screws that can scratch, and loose or missing screws that weaken the joints of the frame. Assess handgrips for any cracks or signs of being loose.
• Teach patients to use the arms of a chair rather than the assistive device to give them leverage when getting up from a chair; the device is likely to tip if used for this purpose.
• Blistering or soreness of the hands can result from continual pressure between the hand and the handle of a crutch. Advise patient to release pressure intermittently and wear gloves or pad the handle to reduce friction.
• Instruct patient that, if wearing shoes with varying heel sizes, the crutches, canes, and walkers may need to be adjusted to maintain the proper height.
• Caution patients when using an assistive device: **Don't** look down. Look straight ahead as you normally do when you walk.

Don't walk on slippery surfaces. Avoid snowy, icy, or rainy conditions. **Don't** put *any* weight on the affected foot if your doctor has so advised (American College of Foot and Ankle Surgeons, 2016).

Pediatric

• For rehabilitation of a small child who has not yet learned to walk or who is unsteady, special crutches with three or four legs provide the needed stability to allow the child to maintain an upright posture and learn to walk (Hockenberry and Wilson, 2015).
• Another option for children who are just learning to walk would be front- or rear-rolling walkers.

Gerontological

• The National Institute on Aging's Go4Life campaign has many resources for walking and other kinds of physical activity for older adults. It also has tips for care providers on how to motivate patients (https://go4life.nia.nih.gov/).

Home Care

• Teach patient how to use the ambulation aid on various terrains (e.g., carpet, stairs, rough ground, inclines). Teach him or her how to maneuver around obstacles such as doors and how to use the aid when transferring to and from a chair, toilet, and tub.
• Teach family caregivers how to help and what to observe to ensure that an assistive device is used correctly.

Long-Term Care

• Conduct safety and maintenance checks of ambulation devices on a routine basis.
• Perform periodic assessments to ensure that the patient is using the ambulation device properly.

◆ CLINICAL DEBRIEF

A 72-year-old woman was transferred out of the intensive care unit (ICU) following an auto accident and has progressed through Levels 1 and 2 of an early mobility protocol to Level 3, where she will sit in a chair for 20 minutes. She had a fractured right hip that was repaired in surgery and has multiple bruises causing discomfort in her right shoulder and chest area. During surgery she had significant blood loss. She has been in the ICU for 3 days. Her heart rate since being hospitalized has ranged from 72 to 94, BP 118–146/72–84, and respirations 18 to 26. The nurse is helping the patient with active range-of-motion (ROM) exercises before getting her to sit on the side of the bed.

1. What should be included in the nurse's assessment before getting the patient up to sit in a chair?

2. The health care provider ordered graduated compression stockings for the patient to wear. Which risk factors does she have for developing a deep vein thrombosis?

3. The patient is about to move to a Level 4 in the mobility protocol. She received an analgesic 30 minutes ago. The nurse completes assessment of vital signs: BP 138/80; R 26, P 88, oxygen saturation 96%. The patient has been sitting in a chair for 15 minutes, and her pain score is a 4 before ambulation. The nurse begins to help Mrs. Daniels walk down the hallway for the first time. She walks approximately 20 feet and develops sudden chest pain and dizziness. The nurse returns the patient to a nearby chair immediately. Her vital signs are BP 110/60, P 130, R 32. Write an SBAR for this situation

◆ REVIEW QUESTIONS

1. Place the following steps for a four-point crutch gait in the correct order.

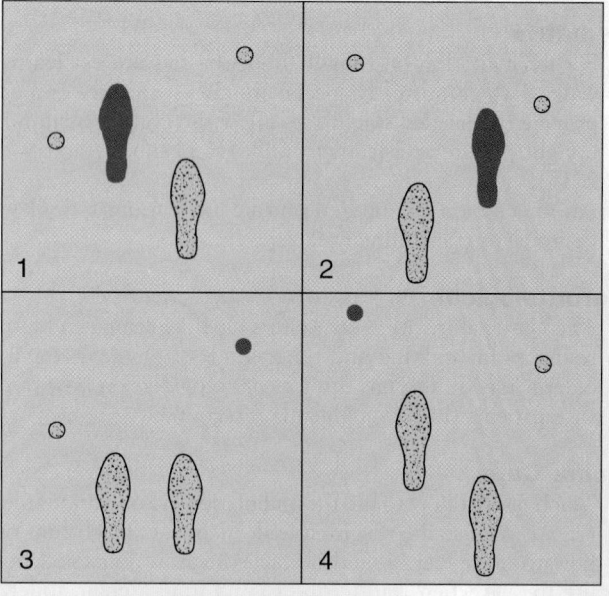

2. Which tips should you recommend to patients for preventing deep vein thrombosis in the home environment? (Select all that apply.)
1. Avoid sitting for any period of time over 2 to 3 hours.
2. Limit fluid intake during traveling.
3. Wear loose-fitting clothes if traveling more than 4 hours.
4. When sitting, always keep your legs crossed
5. Perform foot exercises when flying in a plane for more than 4 hours.

3. A patient is placed on an early progressive mobility protocol. After helping him or her sit in a chair for 15 minutes, which patient data indicate to the nurse that the patient needs to return to bed immediately? (Select all that apply.)
1. Patient is dizzy for 15 seconds.
2. Respiratory rate increases over baseline by 4/min.
3. Systolic blood pressure (BP) falls 30 mm Hg below baseline systolic level.
4. Patient expresses severe fatigue.
5. Patient becomes diaphoretic.

🄔 *Visit the Evolve site for a complete list of Clinical Debrief and Review Questions answers.*

REFERENCES

Adler J, Malone D: Early mobilization in the intensive care unit: a systematic review, *Cardiopulm Phys Ther J* 23(1):5, 2012.

Agency for Healthcare Research and Quality (AHRQ): *Preventing hospital-acquired venous thromboembolism prophylaxis*, 2015, http://www.ahrq.gov/sites/default/files/wysiwyg/professionals/quality-patient-safety/patient-safety-resources/resources/vtguide/vteguide.pdf. Accessed July 4, 2016.

American Academy of Orthopaedist Surgeons (AAOS): *How to use crutches, canes, and walkers*, 2015, http://orthoinfo.aaos.org/topic.cfm?topic=A00181. Accessed March 23, 2016.

American Association of Critical Care Nurses (AACN): *Implementing the ABCDE bundle at the bedside—early progressive mobility protocol*, 2015, http://www.aacn.org/wd/practice/content/actionpak/withlinks-ABCDE-ToolKit.content?menu=practice. Accessed March 23, 2016.

American College of Foot and Ankle Surgeons: *Instructions for using crutches*, 2016 http://www.acfas.org/footankleinfo/crutches.htm. Accessed July 9, 2016.

American Heart Association (AHA): *American Heart Association recommendations for physical activity in adults*, 2015, http://www.heart.org/HEARTORG/GettingHealthy/PhysicalActivity/FitnessBasics/American-Heart-Association-Recommendations-for-Physical-Activity-in-Adults_UCM_307976_Article.jsp#.VkjC8aSFOpo. Accessed March 23, 2016.

Bandura A: Guide for constructing self-efficacy scales. In Urdan T, Pajares F, editors: *Self-efficacy beliefs of adolescents*, Charlotte, NC, 2006, Information Age Publishing.

Burchum JR, Rosenthal LD: *Lehne's pharmacology for nursing care*, ed 9, St Louis, 2016, Elsevier.

Carvalho CA, et al: Reduction of pain and edema of the legs by walking wearing elastic stockings, *Int J Vasc Med* 2015. http://www.hindawi.com/journals/ijvm/2015/648074/. Accessed March 23, 2016.

Castelino T, et al: The effect of early mobilization protocols on postoperative outcomes following abdominal and thoracic surgery: A systematic review, *Surgery* 159:991–1003, 2016.

Centers for Disease Control and Prevention (CDC): *Venous thromboembolism*, 2015, http://www.cdc.gov/ncbddd/dvt/facts.html. Accessed March 23, 2016.

Edelman CL, et al: *Health promotion throughout the life span*, ed 8, St Louis, 2013, Mosby.

Esposito E, Fitzpatrick J: Registered nurses' beliefs of the benefits of exercise, their exercise behaviour, and their patient teaching regarding exercise, *Int J Nurs Pract* 17:351, 2011.

Fletcher JS, Banasik JL: Exercise self-efficacy, *Clin Excell Nurse Pract* 5(3):134, 2001.

Gorman G, et al: Physical activity, exercise, and aging, *Wellbeing* 4(7):1–19, 2014.

Harvey LA, et al: Continuous passive motion following total knee arthroplasty in people with arthritis, *Cochrane Database Syst Rev* (2):CD0024260, 2014.

Healthy People 2020: *Physical activity*, Office of Disease Prevention and Health Promotion, 2015, http://www.healthypeople.gov/2020/topics-objectives/topic/physical-activity. Accessed March 23, 2016.

Hockenberry MJ, Wilson D: *Wong's nursing care of infants and children*, ed 10, St Louis, 2015, Mosby.

Hopkins R, et al: Implementing a mobility program to minimize post-intensive care syndrome, *AACN Adv Crit Care* 27(2):187, 2016.

Lewis S, et al: *Medical-surgical nursing: Assessment and management of clinical problems*, ed 10, St Louis, 2017, Elsevier.

Maniar RN, et al: To use or not to use continuous passive motion post-total knee arthroplasty presenting functional assessment results in early recovery, *J Arthroplasty* 27(2):193, 2012.

Morris RJ, Woodcock JP: Evidence-based compression: prevention of stasis and deep vein thrombosis, *Ann Surg* 239(2):162, 2004.

Myszenski A: *The essential role of lab values and vital signs in clinical decision making and patient safety for the acutely ill patient*, Physical Therapy.com, 2014, http://www.physicaltherapy.com/articles/essential-role-lab-values-and-2336. Accessed March 23, 2016.

National Institutes of Health (NIH): *NIH senior health: exercises*, 2015, http://nihseniorhealth.gov/exerciseandphysicalactivityexercisestotry/balanceexercises/01.html. Accessed March 23, 2016.

Pai M, Douketis J: *Prevention of venous thromboembolic disease in acutely ill hospitalized medical adults*, UpToDate, 2016. Available at http://www.uptodate.com/contents/1346. Accessed July 4, 2016.

Quality and Safety Education for Nurses (QSEN): *Pre-licensure KSAs*, 2014, http://qsen.org/competencies/pre-licensure-ksas/. Accessed March 23, 2016.

Sachdeva A, et al: Graduated compression stockings for prevention of deep vein thrombosis, *Cochrane Database Syst Rev* (12):CD001484, 2014.

Shieh C, et al: Association of self-efficacy and self-regulation with nutrition and exercise behaviors in a community sample of adults, *J Community Health Nurs* 32(4):199, 2015.

Taylor NF, et al: Progressive resistance exercise in physical therapy: a summary of systematic reviews, *Phys Ther* 85(11):1208, 2005.

The Joint Commission (TJC): 2016 *National Patient Safety Goals*, Oakbrook Terrace, IL, 2016, The Commission. http://www.jointcommission.org/standards_information/npsgs.aspx. Accessed March 23, 2016.

Touhy T, Jett K: *Ebersole and Hess' gerontological nursing and healthy aging*, ed 4, St Louis, 2014, Mosby.

US Department of Health and Human Services (USDHHS), Office of Disease Prevention and Health Promotion: *Physical activity guidelines for Americans*, Washington, 2008a, HHS.

US Department of Health and Human Services (USDHHS), Office of Disease Prevention and Health Promotion: *Physical activity guidelines advisory committee report*, Washington, 2008b, HHS.

Zisberg A, et al: Hospital-associated functional decline: the role of hospitalization processes beyond individual risk factors, *J Am Geriatr Soc* 63(1):55, 2015.

13 | Support Surfaces and Special Beds

OBJECTIVES

Mastery of content in this chapter will enable the nurse to:

- Identify the different types of support surfaces and specialty beds used for pressure redistribution.
- Explain why preventive nursing care is still essential when using support surfaces and specialty beds.
- Describe guidelines for placing patients on support surfaces and specialty beds.

- Compare and contrast differences between mattress overlays and mattress replacements.
- Describe mechanisms by which skin breakdown can occur on a special bed, a support surface mattress, or wheelchair seat cushion.
- Describe the steps for correct placement of a patient on a special bed or a support surface mattress.

MEDIA RESOURCES

- evolve http://evolve.elsevier.com/Perry/skills
- Review Questions

- Audio Glossary
- Clinical Debrief and Review Questions Answers

PURPOSE

Despite increasing technological advances in health care, pressure injuries remain a major problem that affects patient comfort, length of stay in a health care agency, and health care costs. Although an interprofessional team approach is key to reducing pressure injuries, nurses are at the forefront of their prevention and treatment in health care settings (Doughty and McNichol, 2016).

STANDARDS OF CARE

- Clinical Guidelines Committee of the American College of Physicians, 2015—Risk Assessment and Prevention of Pressure Ulcers
- Doughty and McNichol: Wound, Ostomy, and Continence Nurses Society, 2016—Core Curriculum for Wound Management
- Wound, Ostomy and Continence Nurses Society, 2016—Guidelines for Prevention and Management of Pressure Ulcers (Injuries)

PRINCIPLES FOR PRACTICE

- Factors contributing to pressure injury formation are both extrinsic (e.g., pressure, moisture, friction, and shear) and intrinsic (e.g., malnutrition, loss of sensation, impaired mobility, aging skin, impaired mental status, infection, incontinence, and low arteriolar pressure) (Serpa and Santos, 2014). Pressure injuries are localized injuries to the skin and/or underlying tissue, usually over a bony prominence, as a result of pressure or

pressure in combination with shear and/or friction. Pressure injuries occur in any age-group or ethnic population, regardless of socioeconomic status (WOCN, 2016).

- The major cause of pressure injuries is unrelieved pressure. The greater the pressure and the longer it is applied, the greater the likelihood for pressure injury development. When external pressure on the tissues exceeds 32 mm Hg (the capillary closing pressure), the network of capillaries collapses. This interrupts the supply of oxygen and nutrients to the cells and the removal of metabolic waste products. As a result, there is tissue ischemia and, if unrelieved, tissue death or necrosis.
- Support surfaces are one important aspect of pressure injury prevention. Support surfaces are specialized devices (e.g., mattress overlays, mattress replacements, integrated bed systems, seat cushions, or seat cushion overlays) that redistribute pressure and are designed for management of tissue loads, microclimate, shear, and/or other therapeutic functions (McNichol et al., 2015; NPUAP, 2014). Microclimate is the mean skin temperature and skin moisture between the patient's skin and the support surface (WOCN, 2016). They are used in acute, rehabilitative, long-term, and home care settings. Support surfaces reduce pressure by redistributing it over a larger surface area. The extent to which a support surface reduces pressure is characterized in two ways. The first is preventive, in which pressure is not consistently reduced below 32 mm Hg (e.g., foam, air, or gel overlay). The second is therapeutic, in which pressure is consistently reduced below 32 mm Hg (e.g., powered overlay air mattress or low-air-loss mattress).
- Preventive surfaces are for patients at risk for skin breakdown and partial-thickness injury.

- Therapeutic surfaces are for patients at high risk for pressure injury development or for those with existing pressure injuries (WOCN, 2016; NPUAP, 2014). Support surfaces are one intervention for redistributing pressure; they are used in conjunction with other pressure injury risk-reduction strategies (see Chapter 39) (Anton, 2013; Higelin, 2014).
- Individuals at high risk for pressure injury should be placed on a pressure redistribution support surface (McNichol et al., 2015; WOCN, 2016). Use specialized support surfaces (e.g., foam, air, or gel mattresses; beds; and cushions) to reduce pressure (Moore and Cowman, 2014; Qaseem et al., 2015).
- Pressure-redistribution surfaces are classified as nonpowered (formerly called *static*) support surfaces or powered (formerly called *dynamic*) support surfaces (NPUAP, 2014). Nonpowered support surfaces include mattresses or mattress overlays filled with air, water, gel, foam, or a combination of any of these. Powered support surfaces change the pressure beneath a patient, reducing the duration of any applied pressure. Many studies have reported the benefits demonstrated by pressure-redistribution surfaces in the prevention of pressure injuries (McInnes et al., 2015; Slade, 2013).
- Several support surfaces also reduce friction, shear, and moisture. Support surfaces with a slick surface help decrease friction and shear. Surfaces with porous covers allow airflow, which reduces moisture, resulting in decreased risk for skin maceration. Table 13.1 provides a comparison of support surfaces.

TABLE 13.1

Support Surfaces

Category and Mechanism of Action	Indications for Use	Advantages	Disadvantages
Support Surfaces and Overlays			
Foam Overlay (Available as an Overlay or in a Full Mattress)			
Reduces pressure; the cover (top) can reduce friction and shear. Base height of 7.5–10 cm (3–4 inches); see manufacturer guidelines regarding amount of body weight supported	Use for moderate- to high-risk patients	One-time charge No setup fee Cannot be punctured Available in various sizes (e.g., bed, chair, operating room table) Little maintenance Does not need electricity	Elevated body temperature Hot and may trap moisture Limited life span Plastic protective sheet needed for incontinent patients or patients with draining wounds Not indicated for those with existing stage 3 or 4 pressure injuries
Water Overlay (Available as an Overlay or in a Full Mattress)			
Reduces pressure and pressure points because surface provides flotation with pressure reduction by redistributing patient's weight evenly over entire support surface	Use for high-risk patients	Readily available Some control over motion sensations Easy to clean	Easily punctured Heavy Fluid motion may make procedures (e.g., dressing changes, CPR) difficult Maintenance needed to prevent microorganism growth Patient transfers out of bed are difficult Difficult to raise and lower head of bed
Gel Overlay			
Reduces pressure and pressure points because surface provides flotation by redistributing patient's weight evenly over entire support surface	Use for moderate- to high-risk patients Use for patients who are wheelchair dependent	Low maintenance Easy to clean Multiple-patient use Impermeable to needle punctures	Heavy Expensive Lacks airflow for moisture control Variable friction control
Nonpowered Air-Filled Overlay			
Reduces pressure by lowering mean interface pressure between patient's tissue and mattress	Use for moderate- to high-risk patients Use for patients who can reposition themselves	Easy to clean Multiple-patient use Low maintenance Potential repair of some air-filled products Durable	Damaged by punctures from needles and sharps Requires routine monitoring to determine adequate inflation pressure Patient transfers out of bed are difficult
Low-Air-Loss Overlay (Available as an Overlay or in a Full Mattress)			
Maintains constant and slight air movement against patient's skin; also assists in managing the heat and humidity (microclimate) of the skin	Use for moderate- to high-risk patients	Easy to clean Maintains constant inflation Deflates to facilitate transfer and CPR Moisture control Fabric covering overlay is air permeable, bacteria impermeable, and waterproof Reduces shear and friction Setup provided by manufacturer	Damaged by needles and sharps Noisy Requires electricity, but some are available with short backup battery In home may need to purchase backup generator in case of loss of electrical power

Continued

TABLE 13.1

Support Surfaces—cont'd

Category and Mechanism of Action	Indications for Use	Advantages	Disadvantages
Specialty Beds			
Air-Fluidized Bed			
Bedframe contains silicone-coated beads and provides pressure redistribution by the fluid-like medium that is created by forcing air through beads, resulting in immersion and envelopment of the patient.	Use for high-risk patients Use for patients with stage 3 or 4 pressure injuries or burns	Less frequent turning or repositioning Improved patient comfort Quickly becomes firm for CPR or other treatments when device is turned "off" Reduces shear, friction, and edema to site May facilitate management of copious wound drainage or incontinence Setup provided by manufacturer	Continuous circulation of warm, dry air may increase patient risk for dehydration Possible increase in room temperature Patient may experience disorientation Patient transfer difficult Heavy Expensive May not be wide enough for use with obese patients or patients with contractures Patient cannot lie prone because of risk of suffocation
Low-Air-Loss Bed			
Bedframe with series of connected air-filled pillows. The flow of air controls the amount of pressure in each pillow and assists in managing the heat and humidity (microclimate) of the patient's skin.	Use for patients who need pressure relief, those who cannot be repositioned frequently, or those who have skin breakdown on more than one surface Contraindicated in patients with unstable spinal column	Can raise and lower head and foot of bed Easy transfer in and out of bed Less frequent turning schedule Pillows can be transferred to stretcher with patient Setup provided by manufacturer	Portable motor is noisy Bed surface material is slippery; patients can easily slide down mattress or out of bed when being transferred
Kinetic Therapy			
Provides continuous passive motion to promote mobilization of pulmonary secretions and low air loss, which provides pressure relief	Use primarily for patients needing spinal stabilization Should not be used when the patient is hemodynamically unstable	Reduces pulmonary complications associated with restricted mobility Reduces risk for urinary stasis and urinary tract infections Reduces venous stasis	Does not reduce shear or moisture Cannot be used with cervical or skeletal traction Possible motion sickness initially Possible sensations of claustrophobia

CPR, Cardiopulmonary resuscitation.
Data from Doughty D, McNichol L: *Wound, Ostomy and Continence Nurses Society (WOCN): Core curriculum: wound management*, Philadelphia, 2016, Wound, Ostomy, and Continence Society; Wound, Ostomy and Continence Nurses Society (WOCN): *Guideline for prevention and management of pressure ulcers*, WOCN clinical practice guideline series, ed 2, Mt. Laurel, NJ: 2016, Author.

- Frequent repositioning, which temporarily relieves pressure, is the backbone of prevention protocols. No bed or mattress totally eliminates the need for competent nursing care. It is your responsibility to use appropriate turning schedules for patients in bed or in a chair. Use lift teams and lifting devices to transfer patients from a regular bed to a special support surface (see Chapter 11). Although useful, turning devices still injure soft tissues, requiring a nurse to be especially observant for signs of pressure formation.

PATIENT-CENTERED CARE

- When making decisions about the best support surface for a patient, you must first complete thorough patient assessment, including individual needs, health care provider needs, and location of the patient.

- Ultimately the features of the support surface must match a patient's unique needs.
- Always describe to a patient and family caregivers which interventions will be instituted and allow time for questions as needed.
- Some cultural groups may hesitate to question or ask for help, especially when they have limited English communication.
- Educate patient and family caregivers on all of the features of the support surface, provide for demonstration, and observe return demonstration of these features.

EVIDENCE-BASED PRACTICE

Pressure injuries can be partially controlled by an appropriate support surface. Evidence suggests that pressure redistribution devices can reduce the incidence of pressure injuries by 60% (Doughty and McNichol, 2016).

- Pressure reduction and relief are major nursing interventions for the prevention of pressure injuries (Doughty and McNichol, 2016; McInnes et al., 2015).
- Pressure-redistribution surfaces need to serve as adjuncts and not replacements for repositioning protocols (Doughty and McNichol, 2016).
- There is insufficient evidence to support one specific pressure redistribution surface/design over another for the prevention of pressure injuries (WOCN, 2016; McInnes et al., 2015; Qaseem et al., 2015).
- Some surfaces such as Australian sheepskin and foam mattress overlays have been shown to reduce pressure injuries in at-risk patients (McInnes et al., 2013; AMDA, 2013).
- High-specification foam mattress compared with a standard hospital mattress with foam overlay is effective in decreasing the incidence of pressure injuries in high-risk patients (WOCN, 2016).
- Encourage patients to be up as soon as medically possible in a specialty chair or wheelchair equipped with a tailored support surface for pressure relief.
- Measure seat cushions so they are properly fitted to the person's body type and chair size to prevent friction and pressure.
- Pressure distribution surfaces should be used in the operating room for individuals assessed to be at high risk for pressure injury development, especially in older adult and bariatric patients. Pressure redistribution has been associated with a decreased incidence of postoperative pressure injuries (WOCN, 2016; Broome et al., 2015).

SAFETY GUIDELINES

- Perform complete assessment to determine patient's risk for pressure injuries. A complete patient assessment includes use of appropriate pressure injury risk scales, which include factors such as presence of shear and friction and a patient's mobility and continence status (see Chapter 39).
- Select a support surface based on patient's risk for developing pressure injuries, such as impaired mobility, need for microclimate control, reduction of shear, and size and weight of patient.
- Know the reason for and extent of a patient's reduced mobility. A patient who is not easy to reposition or who has pressure injuries involving multiple surfaces benefits from pressure-redistribution support devices.
- The use of incontinence pads increases peak pressure by 20% to 25%. Have an incontinence-management plan in place (Norton et al., 2011).
- Continue to provide basic prevention care measures against the hazards of immobility (e.g., regular skin assessment, turning, correct positioning, or range-of-motion exercises).
- Use safe patient-handling techniques and proper body mechanics when positioning or working with patients (see Chapter 11).
- Follow all safety measures to prevent injury to patients from accidental falls or improper positioning when placing them on special beds or mattresses.
- Educate family caregivers about the advantages/disadvantages and methods of operation of all support devices to ensure their proper use in all settings.
- Collaborate and consult with health care professionals who have expertise in this area.

PROCEDURAL GUIDELINE 13.1 *Selection of a Pressure-Redistribution Support Surface*

Delegation and Collaboration
The selection of a pressure-redistribution support device cannot be delegated to nursing assistive personnel (NAP).

Equipment
- Pressure injury risk assessment tool (see agency policy) (see Chapter 39)
- Body chart, tape measure, and/or camera to document existing areas of impaired skin integrity
- Documentation form or electronic health record
- Skin-care products

Procedural Steps
1. Assess patient's risk for skin breakdown using a risk assessment tool (e.g., Braden Scale score ≤18 indicates patient is at risk).
2. Assess patient's existing pressure injuries, including location, stage, areas of blistering, abnormal reactive hyperemia, and abrasion.
3. Consider patient weight and weight distribution and the following risk factors/comorbidities: advanced age, fever, poor dietary intake of protein, diastolic pressure <60 mm Hg, hemodynamic instability, generalized edema, and anemia (WOCN, 2016).
4. Assess patient's level of comfort using a pain scale of 0 to 10.

5. Determine the need for a pressure-reduction surface from assessment data. Place "at-risk" patients on a pressure-reduction surface, high-specification foam mattress and not on a standard hospital mattress (WOCN, 2016; NPUAP, 2014).
6. Identify patient factors when selecting an appropriate surface (Fig. 13.1):
   a. Braden Scale score ≤18.
   b. Does patient need pressure redistribution (e.g., you cannot reposition the patient, or there is an existing pressure injury)?
   c. Is the surface needed for short- or long-term care? A short-term surface is usually needed for an acute illness and hospitalization. A long-term surface is usually needed for extended or home care.
   d. What is the potential comfort level achieved by the surface? If patient is sensitive to noise, a device with a loud motor will increase his or her discomfort.
   e. Are patient and family caregivers cooperative and adherent to repositioning? In addition, are they aware that a support surface should never replace repositioning? Is adequate help available for repositioning? In a home setting a support surface is often necessary when the family caregiver or patient is

Continued

PROCEDURAL GUIDELINE 13.1 *Selection of a Pressure-Redistribution Support Surface—cont'd*

WOCN Society's Evidence- and Consensus-Based Support Surface Algorithm

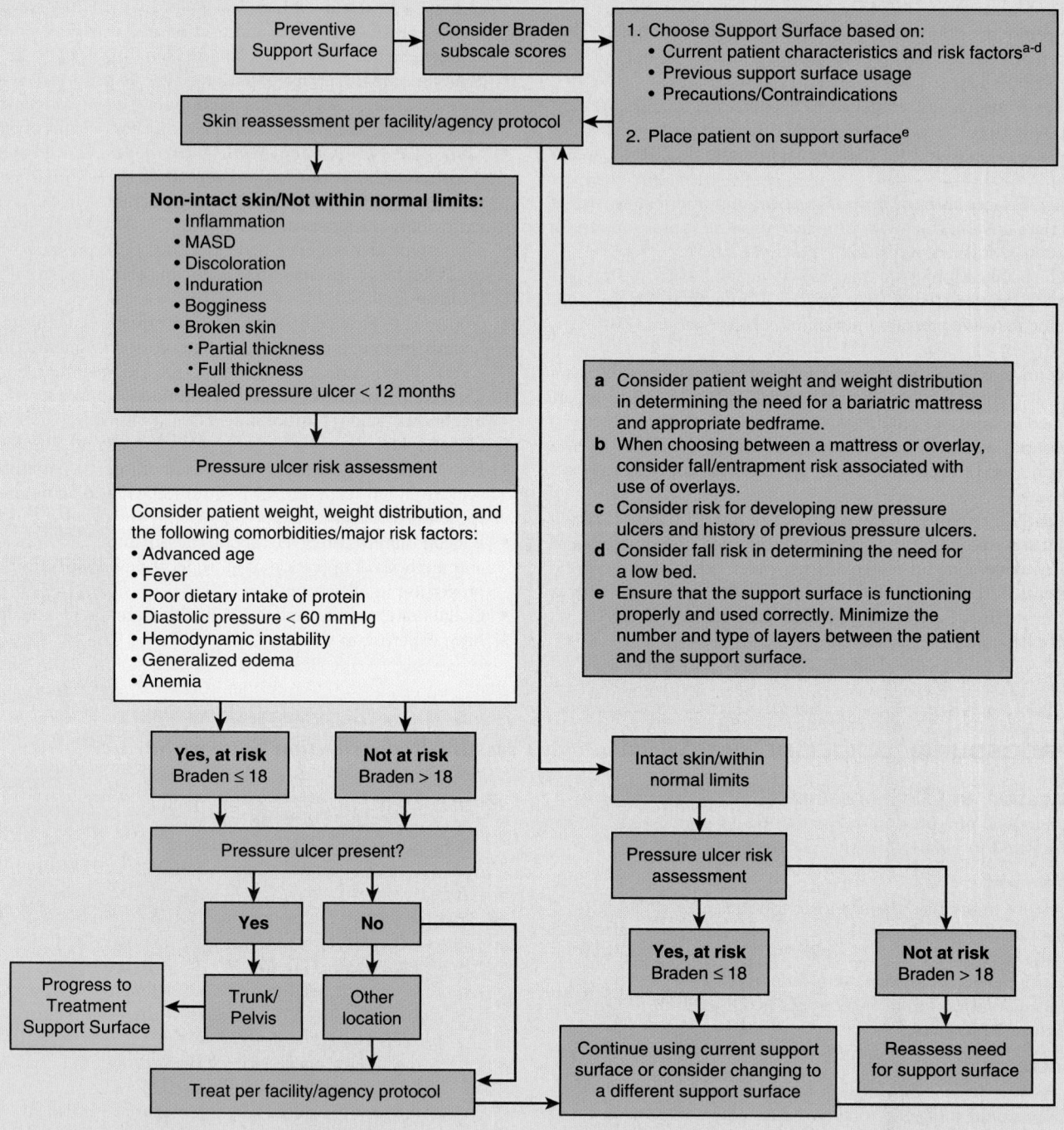

FIG 13.1 Flow diagram for ordering specialty beds.

unable to reposition independently or help with repositioning.

f. Does the support surface have a potential to interfere with patient's independent functioning? The height of the overlay and its soft edge may affect patient's ability to transfer, and a high-air-loss bed is not appropriate for a patient who needs to get in and out of bed frequently.

g. What are patient's financial limitations?

h. If patient is using the device in the home, what are the environmental limitations? Will the home and existing electrical service accommodate the surface selected? Can the family caregivers in the home manage the surface?

i. How durable is the product? Is the surface easily subjected to puncture? How easily can the surface be cleaned?

j. Does patient need pressure-relief surfaces in a chair/wheelchair? Has the family or caregiver been instructed on appropriate inflation of the device?

7. Choose the appropriate surface (see Table 13.1).

PROCEDURAL GUIDELINE 13.1 *Selection of a Pressure-Redistribution Support Surface—cont'd*

a. Pressure redistribution devices redistribute the pressure/load over the control area of the patient's body to reduce the overall pressure and avoid areas of localized pressure (WOCN, 2016). Surfaces providing pressure redistribution include therapeutic mattress replacements, nonpowered and powered (e.g., moving) surfaces, low-air-loss beds and mattresses, and air-fluidized beds (Doughty and McNichol, 2016). Pressure-redistribution surfaces are also used in the operating room for individuals who are at high risk or for lengthy procedures (Broome et al., 2015).

b. Use a nonpowered support surface if patient can assume a variety of positions without bearing weight on a pressure injury without bottoming out. Bottoming out makes the support surface ineffective because it is inadequate for patient's weight and the body sinks too deeply into the surface.

Clinical Decision Point *Hand checks are a satisfactory but subjective method for assessing for "bottoming out" of static air overlay mattresses. According to NPUAP, the hand check method is inappropriate for replacement mattresses and integrated bed systems (bedframe and support surfaces) (WOCN, 2016; Call et al., 2015).*

c. Select a powered support surface when patient cannot assume a variety of positions without bearing weight on a pressure injury, if patient fully compresses the nonpowered support surface, or if the pressure injury does not show evidence of healing. Alternating or powered mattresses are associated with lower incidence of pressure injuries compared with standard mattresses (Doughty and McNichol, 2016).

d. High-specification foam is effective in decreasing the incidence of pressure injuries in fairly high-risk patients, including older adults and patients with fractures of the neck and femur (WOCN, 2016; Doughty and McNichol, 2016; McInnes et al., 2015).

e. Patients with stage 3 or 4 pressure injuries on multiple turning surfaces often benefit from an air-fluidized bed (Doughty and McNichol, 2016).

f. There is limited evidence that low-air-loss beds reduce the incidence of pressure injuries in intensive care (Doughty and McNichol, 2016).

g. When excess moisture is a potential risk, a support surface that provides airflow is important in drying the skin and reducing the incidence of pressure injuries (WOCN, 2016; NPUAP, 2014).

8. Check agency policy regarding implementing a support surface.

a. Obtain a health care provider's order. This is usually required for a patient to obtain third-party reimbursement.

b. Consult with agency case manager or social worker to help with patient's financial eligibility and terms and length of third-party reimbursement for the surface.

c. Consult with agency home care or discharge planning if the device is anticipated for long-term use. Specific procedures and evaluations are needed for continuity of surface when patient is transferred to extended care or discharged home.

9. Perform hand hygiene. Apply clean gloves. Inspect condition of skin regularly according to agency policy to evaluate changes in skin and effectiveness of therapy.

10. Inspect existing pressure injuries for evidence of healing.

11. Observe for side effects associated with specific pressure-reducing surface (e.g., nausea, dizziness).

12. Document pressure injury risk assessment and skin assessment in patient's electronic health record (EHR) or chart.

13. Document the support surface selected and patient response to the surface (see specific skills for recording and reporting details) in patient's EHR or chart.

✦ SKILL 13.1 Placing a Patient on a Support Surface

There are numerous support surfaces to reduce pressure on tissues overlying bony prominences. These devices are recommended for preventive measures for patients with reduced mobility and risk for developing pressure injuries. Most of the devices are easy to apply and keep clean. The extent to which the devices actually reduce pressure and prevent skin breakdown is highly variable.

Support surfaces are categorized as mattress (or wheelchair) overlays (Fig. 13.2), mattress replacements, or specialty beds. An overlay rests on top of a hospital mattress and uses foam, air, water, gel, or combinations of these products to provide pressure relief. Mattress overlays and mattress replacements are either nonpowered (e.g., foam, gels) or powered (e.g., alternating-pressure surfaces).

A flotation pad is made of a silicone or polyvinyl-chloride gel enclosed in a vinyl-covered square. The pad serves as an artificial layer of fat to protect bony surfaces such as the sacrum and greater trochanters. These flotation pads are available for the bed or wheelchair (Fig. 13.3).

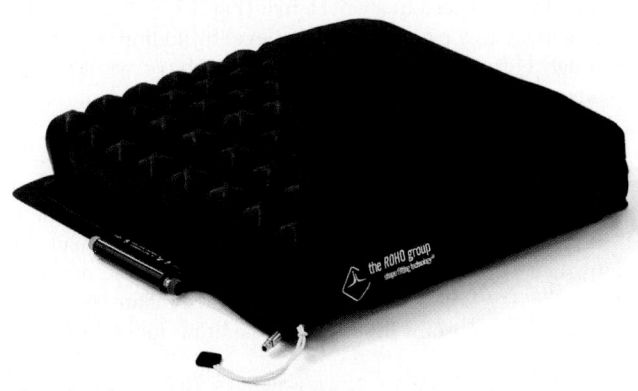

FIG 13.2 ROHO cushion for wheelchair. (©*ROHO Group. Reprinted with permission. All rights reserved.*)

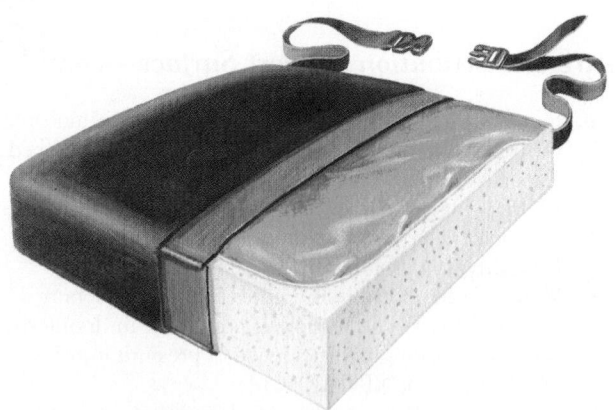

FIG 13.3 Gel cushion for wheelchair. (©*Skil-Care Corp. Reprinted with permission. All rights reserved.*)

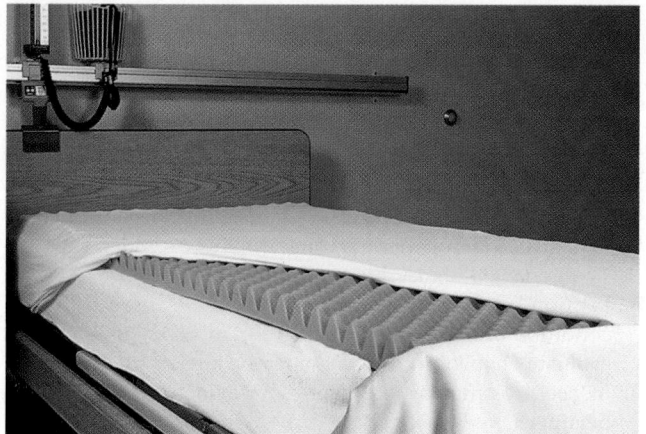

FIG 13.4 Egg-crate foam overlay is primarily for comfort.

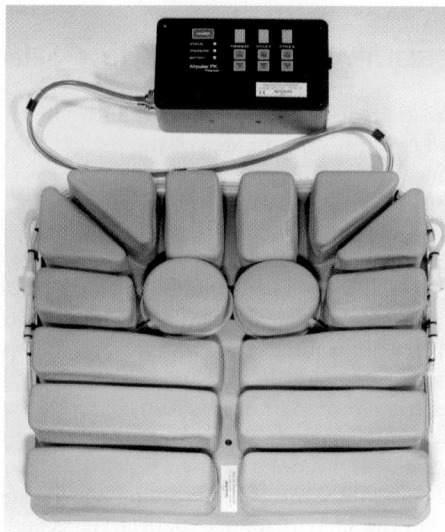

FIG 13.5 Air-filled cushion for wheelchair. (©*Aquila Corporation, Reprinted with permission. All rights reserved.*)

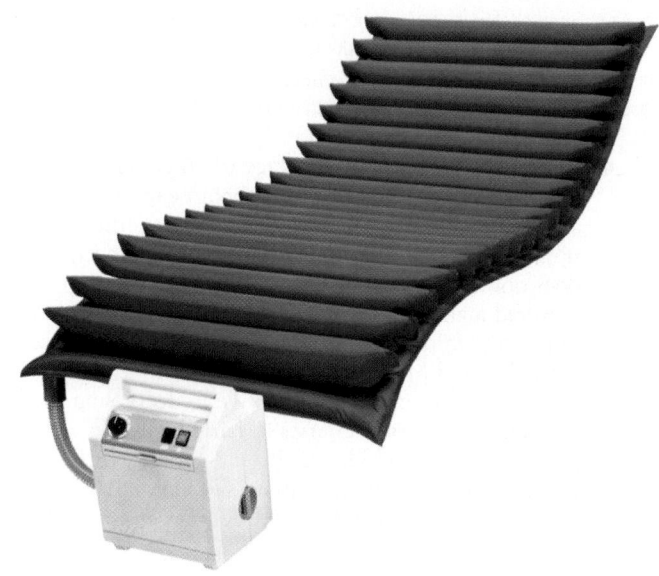

FIG 13.6 Dynamic air mattress overlay. (©*2002 Hill-Rom Services. Reprinted with permission. All rights reserved.*)

There are two types of foam mattresses. One is the foam mattress overlay, which has a flat smooth surface; foam rubber peaks (egg-crate, Fig. 13.4); or a cut surface. Place one on top of a bed mattress and place a sheet over the foam mattress pad overlay to prevent soiling and provide ease of cleaning. The second type is the high-specification foam specialty mattress, which completely replaces the hospital mattress and is covered by a loose-fitting cover intended to protect the mattress and minimize friction and shear. Some of the newer foam mattresses have memory and an increased life span. The memory foam molds to the shape of the body and reduces pressure to the area in contact with the foam.

One type of air mattress is fully integrated into the hospital bed or designed to be placed in a wheelchair (Fig. 13.5). You can adjust this bed surface to a patient's comfort level by adding or removing air through buttons within the patient's reach, or you can automatically adjust pressures to a patient's position and movement when in the automatic mode. Always use a bedsheet to cover an air mattress to prevent skin from touching the plastic surface.

Air mattress overlays are either nonpowered or powered and consist of interconnected air cells or cushions inflated by the use of a motorized blower (Fig. 13.6). More complex air mattresses contain several layers of tubes or support cells. These mattresses use a pressure-cycling device to intermittently inflate and deflate or to maintain a constant inflation and slight air movement in the mattress.

A nonpowered support surface is inflated with a simple air blower after placing the mattress on a bed. An integrated air mattress connects with a pressure-cycling device that intermittently inflates

and deflates sections of the mattress, creating a cycling effect that minimizes pressure on bony prominences (Fig. 13.7).

Replacement mattresses have foam, gel, air, or fluid sections that you can customize to the needs of a specific patient with moderate-to-high risk for skin breakdown. Another available option is an air-integrated replacement mattress instead of the conventional mattress. These mattresses may also be fully integrated into the bed. Air mattresses are usually for patients with moderate-to-high risk for skin breakdown. You must deflate air mattresses before initiating cardiopulmonary resuscitation (CPR). Many agencies have purchased replacement mattresses to replace their standard hospital mattresses because of improved skin and wound outcomes.

Another preventive intervention is a low-pressure seat cushion (Fig. 13.8) overlaid on a wheelchair or a dry, nonpowered flotation mattress system (Fig. 13.9) that you overlay on a bed. Through a system of controlled dynamics, a cushion maintains low pressures

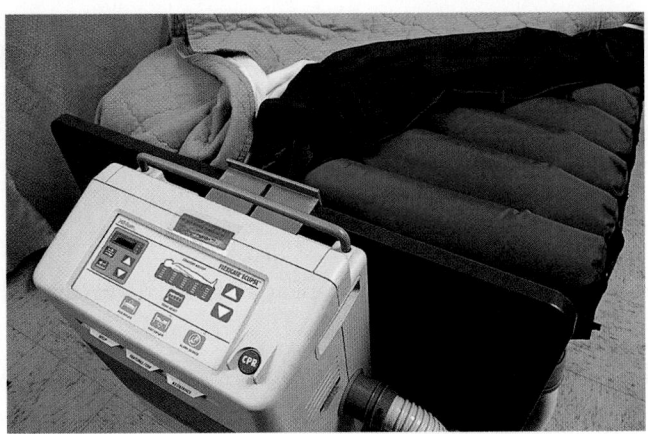

FIG 13.7 Motor for integrated air mattress.

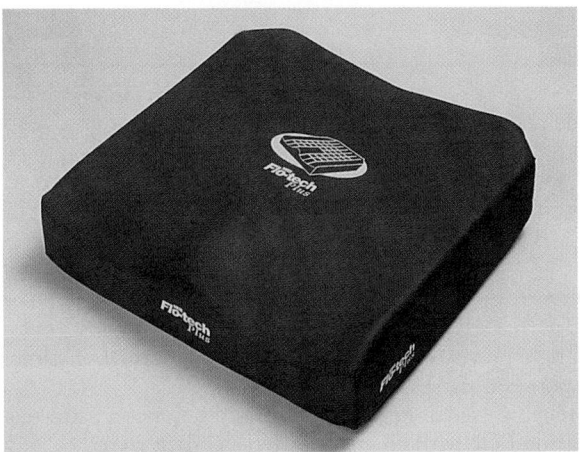

FIG 13.8 Low-pressure seat cushion. (*Reproduced with permission from Medical Support Systems Ltd.*)

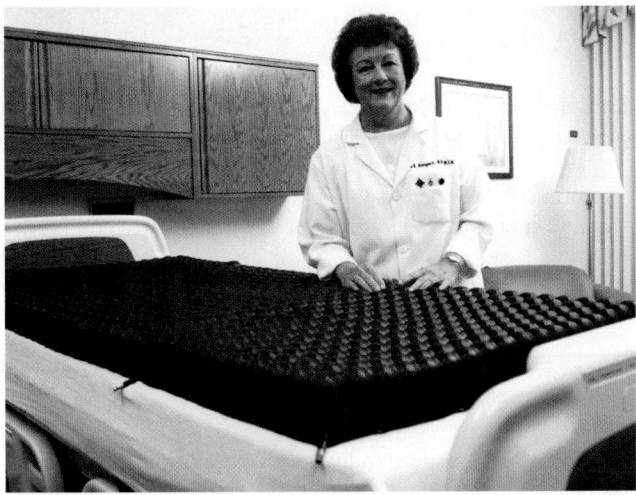

FIG 13.9 ROHO dry flotation mattress for bed. (*©The ROHO Group. Reprinted with permission. All rights reserved.*)

Delegation and Collaboration

The skill of placing a patient on a support surface can be delegated to nursing assistive personnel (NAP). However, you must first complete the assessment, determine the need for a support surface, and select the specific surface. Some types of support surfaces require that a manufacturer representative set up and maintain the support system. The nurse directs the NAP to:

- Notify the nurse of any changes in a patient's skin; the nurse then evaluates condition of the skin.
- Continue to regularly turn and reposition a patient and seek help for patient position changes as necessary in bed or wheelchair.
- Monitor the normal functioning of the support device such as inflation and deflation cycles and report to the nurse any changes in these cycles or leakage of air, water, or gel.

Equipment

- Pressure injury risk-assessment tool (see agency policy) (see Chapter 39)
- Mattress and/or chair overlay support surface of choice: foam overlays, air mattress overlay, bed with integrated surface, air-integrated replacement mattress
- Sheet(s)
- Clean gloves (if soiled linen is being handled)
- Standard bedframe (with mattress) if overlay is to be used (*optional*)

by distributing pressure across a patient's body surface, reducing friction and shear.

Support surfaces aid in reducing pressure on a patient's skin but do not replace regular repositioning, meticulous skin assessment and skin care, or range-of-motion exercises. The decision to place a patient on a pressure-redistribution surface and the selection of this surface is a nursing responsibility (see Procedural Guideline 13.1).

STEP	RATIONALE

ASSESSMENT

1. Identify patient using at least two identifiers (e.g., name and birthday or name and medical record number) according to agency policy.

2. Perform hand hygiene.

3. Determine patient's risk for pressure injury formation using a valid assessment tool (e.g., Braden Scale) and assess for risk factors for pressure injuries (e.g., nutritional deficits, shear stress, friction, alterations in mobility and sensory perception, moisture, and abnormal serum albumin and hemoglobin levels) (see Chapter 39).

Ensures correct patient. Complies with The Joint Commission standards and improves patient safety (TJC, 2016).

Reduces transmission of microorganisms.
Risk assessment tools provide an objective measure of risk consistent over time (Doughty and McNichol, 2016).

STEP	RATIONALE

Clinical Decision Point *Patients with unstable conditions do not always tolerate turning or positioning required for thorough assessment or the application of a support surface mattress.*

4. Perform skin assessment (see Chapters 6 and 39). Inspect condition of skin, especially over dependent sites and bony prominences.	Provides baseline to determine change in skin integrity or in existing pressure injury.
5. Assess patient's level of comfort using a pain scale of 0 to 10.	Provides baseline to determine patient's response to therapy and comfort needs.

Clinical Decision Point *Some patients experiencing pain need pain medication before application of support surface of choice or transfer to another bed (WOCN, 2016; NPUAP, 2014).*

6. Assess patient's understanding of purpose of support surface.	Misconceptions affect patient's cooperation in use of mattress.
7. Verify health care provider's order for type of support surface.	Health care provider's order is usually required to ensure third-party payment of support surface.

NURSING DIAGNOSES

- Deficient knowledge regarding use of support surface mattress
- Impaired physical mobility
- Impaired skin integrity
- Ineffective peripheral tissue perfusion
- Pain (acute, chronic)
- Risk for impaired skin integrity
- Risk for infection

Related factors/Risk factors are individualized based on patient's condition or needs.

PLANNING

1. Expected outcomes following completion of procedure:	
• Patient's skin is without erythema or mottling.	Mottling represents hypoxia, which is an abnormal physiological response in tissues under pressure.
• Existing pressure injury shows signs of healing.	Skin remains free of new pressure injuries. Support surface does not interfere with circulation to dependent areas.
• Patient expresses improved level of comfort.	Equalized pressures have eliminated localized areas of discomfort.
• Patient is removed from therapeutic surface when risk for pressure injuries decreases.	Provides for efficient, cost-effective care while maintaining high-quality outcomes.
2. Explain purpose of mattress and method of application to patient and family caregiver.	Reduces anxiety and promotes cooperation.

IMPLEMENTATION

1. Close room door or bedside curtain.	Provides patient privacy and considerate care during application of mattress to bed or transfer to alternative bed.
2. Perform hand hygiene. Apply clean gloves (if linens are soiled or wet). Get help to position patient and/or mattress as needed.	Prevents transmission of microorganisms. Assistance from other caregivers reduces risk for friction and shear in transfer to new surface.
3. Apply support surface to bed or prepare alternative bed (bed may be occupied or unoccupied). Keep sharp objects away from air mattress or air-surface bed.	
a. Replacing mattress:	
(1) Apply mattress to bedframe after removing standard hospital mattress.	Hospital mattress needs to be stored. In some instances mattress replacements are standard procedure.
(2) Apply sheet over mattress. Keep linens between surfaces to a minimum.	Sheet reduces soiling. Multiple layers decrease surface effectiveness in reducing pressure (Doughty and McNichol, 2016).
b. Preparing an air mattress/overlay:	
(1) Apply deflated mattress flat over surface of bed mattress. (There may be directions on pad indicating which side to place up.)	Provides smooth, even surface.
(2) Bring any plastic strips or flaps around corners of bed mattress.	Secures air mattress in place.

STEP	RATIONALE
(3) Attach connector on air mattress to inflation device. Inflate mattress to proper air pressure determined by air pump or blower.	Mattresses vary as to requiring one-time or continuous inflation cycle. Check inflation daily. Manufacturer directions indicate desired air pressure designed to distribute patient's body weight evenly. Directions are included with each mattress.
(4) Place sheet over air mattress, being sure to eliminate all wrinkles.	Prevents soiling of mattress; reduces direct contact of skin with plastic surface. Wrinkles can cause pressure.

Clinical Decision Point *Avoid placing excessive linens and incontinence pads on top of support surface. This can interfere with functioning of support surface (WOCN, 2016; NPUAP, 2014).*

STEP	RATIONALE
(5) Check air pumps to be sure that pressure cycle alternates.	Alternating airflow mattress produces intermittent cycling, inflating only parts of mattress at any one time. Intermittent cycle continually alternates pressure against skin and soft tissue.
(6) Help patient transfer in and out of bed.	Mattress surface is less firm and slippery. This makes it difficult for some patients to transfer from bed to chair/stretcher.
c. Using an air-surface bed: **(1)** Obtain and place linen on bed.	In some instances an air-surface bed is available in patient rooms. If not, an ordering system exists to obtain one as needed (see agency policy).
(2) Place switch in "prevention" mode.	In "prevention" mode, surface pressures change automatically with patient position to equalize pressure and eliminate points of pressure.

Clinical Decision Point *Most pressure-relieving beds in the hospital and home care are equipped with a CPR switch to instantly lower head section from an elevated position and deflate the mattress to provide a firm surface for chest compressions (Fig. 13.10). Note this on the patient's record.*

STEP	RATIONALE
4. Position patient comfortably as desired over support surface. Reposition routinely.	Location of existing pressure injury might influence type of positioning (Doughty and McNichol, 2016).
5. Remove and dispose of gloves and perform hand hygiene.	Reduces transmission of microorganisms.

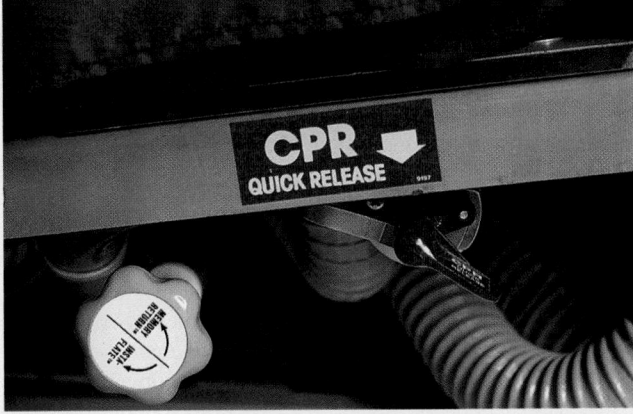

FIG 13.10 Cardiopulmonary resuscitation switch deflates low-air-loss bed to provide hard surface.

EVALUATION

1. Reassess patient's risk for pressure injury formation at routine intervals.	Documents change in status, which is critical for evaluating continued need for therapeutic surface.
2. Inspect and compare condition of patient's skin every 8 hours or according to agency policy to determine changes in skin integrity, pressure injury status, and effectiveness of support surface.	Determines if pressure sores develop or if condition of existing sores changes.
3. Ask patient to rate comfort on a scale of 0 to 10.	If pressure-relief mattress is effective, patient generally experiences less discomfort.
4. Evaluate functioning of support surface periodically.	Regular inspection of mechanical components of mattress ensures proper functioning (WOCN, 2016).
5. Use Teach-Back: "I want to be sure I explained why you are on this special bed. Tell me why we placed you on this type of bed." Revise your instruction now or develop a plan for revised patient or family caregiver teaching if patient or family caregiver is not able to teach back correctly.	Determines patient's and family caregiver's level of understanding of instructional topic.

STEP	RATIONALE
Unexpected Outcomes	**Related Interventions**
1. Patient develops localized areas of abnormal reactive hyperemia for longer than 30 minutes, mottling, swelling, and tenderness with evidence of breakdown.	• Modify skin-care regimen. • Increase frequency of skin assessment. • Increase types of pressure-relief interventions. • Check for proper inflation of support surface. • Revise turning schedule. • Consult with skin-care expert. • Notify health care provider.
2. Existing pressure areas fail to heal or increase in size or depth.	• Modify skin-care regimen. • Revise turning schedule. • Consult with skin-care expert. • Notify health care provider.
3. Patient expresses discomfort while on support surface.	• Evaluate need for analgesia or mild sedation. • Evaluate need to modify support surface. • Reposition patient more frequently. • Unless contraindicated, provide back massage. Do not massage reddened areas or bony prominences because massage to these areas contributes to skin breakdown (Doughty and McNichol, 2016).

Recording and Reporting

- Record type of support surface applied, extent to which patient tolerated procedure, and condition of patient's skin in nurses' notes in electronic health record (EHR) or chart and/or skin assessment flow sheet.
- Document your evaluation of patient and family caregiver learning.
- Report evidence of pressure injury formation to nurse in charge or health care provider.

Special Considerations
Teaching

- Explain risks of immobility and pressure injury formation to patient and family caregivers (see Chapter 39).
- Instruct in proper use of body mechanics, positioning, and pressure relief methods.
- Explain purpose and function of the pressure-redistribution surface. Include reminder that the surface augments care and does not replace the need for turning and pressure-relief maneuvers.
- Explain precautions regarding sharp objects and fire hazards.

Pediatric

- Various pain assessment tools have been developed specifically for use in children (see Chapter 16).

- Parents can support children in being able to express their pain and treatment preferences (Hockenberry and Wilson, 2015).

Gerontological

- Implement preventive measures because aging skin is drier, thinner, and less pressure sensitive, increasing the risk for skin breakdown.
- Adding mattress overlays changes the bed height. Use care when transferring and teaching family caregiver to transfer a patient from bed to chair.

Home Care

- Most of the devices may be adapted for home use on a standard twin bed or hospital bed.
- Base selection on patient needs and environmental audit. For example, a patient on total bed rest who smokes is not an ideal candidate for a foam mattress because of the potential for fire; a patient with pets that sleep in the bed is not suited for an air-filled mattress because of the risk for puncture.
- Address concerns in the home setting related to need for a back-up generator or other plan to maintain the support surface during power outages.

◆ SKILL 13.2   Placing a Patient on a Special Bed

Air-suspension beds are designed for patients who are immobile or confined to bed. The air-suspension bed supports a patient's weight on air-filled cushions. There are two types of systems: low-air-loss and high-air-loss. A low-air-loss system minimizes pressure and reduces shear. In this type of system, air flow is provided to assist in managing the heat and humidity (microclimate) of the patient's skin (WOCN, 2016). If a patient has large stage 3 or 4 pressure injuries on multiple turning surfaces of the skin, a low-air-loss bed or air-fluidized bed may be indicated. If wounds are not healing, a change in support surface is indicated and should be matched to patient's needs (Doughty and McNichol, 2016).

High-air-loss beds provide for selective drying and do not increase insensible fluid losses. For patients requiring high air loss under a body part (e.g., under the buttocks), you can substitute high-air-loss cushions. It is also possible to adapt the air-suspension beds to individual patient needs with specialty cushions for positioning, foot support, and lateral arm supports.

Another adaptation of the air-suspension bed is the kinetic low-air-loss bed (Fig. 13.11). This bed is used in intensive care areas and has the ability to provide a pressure-relief surface while rotating approximately 30 to 35 degrees continuously. Do not use this surface with a patient who has an unstable spine or who is in traction.

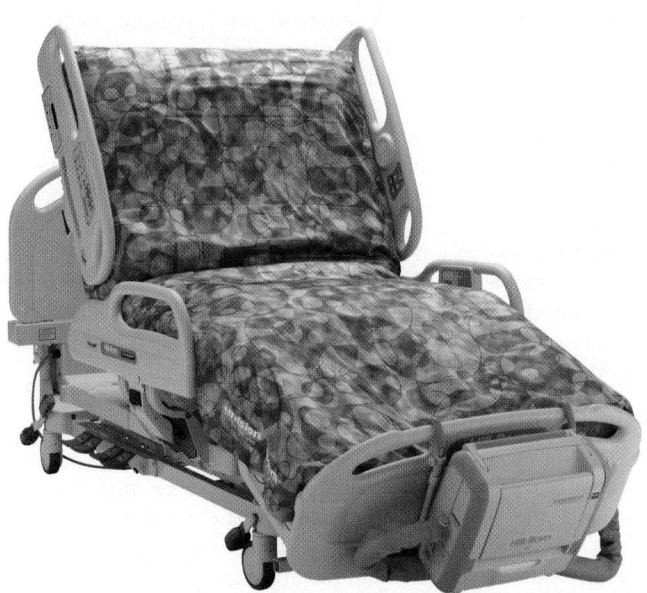

FIG 13.11 Low-air-loss bed. (©2002 Hill-Rom Services. Reprinted with permission. All rights reserved.)

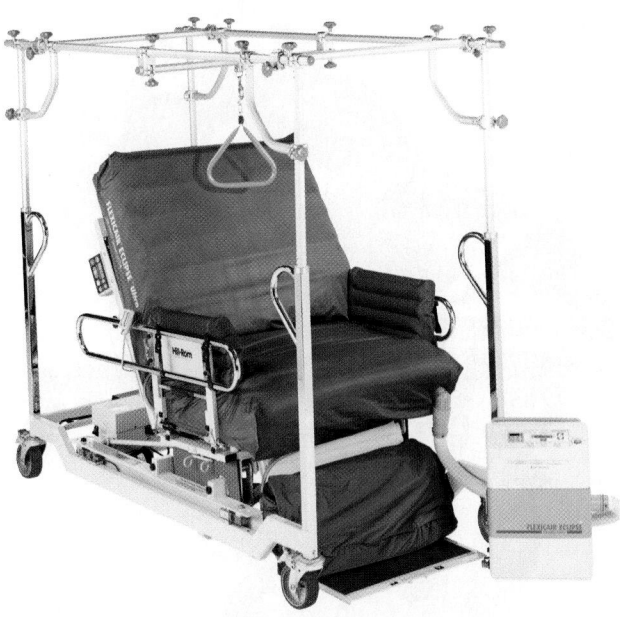

FIG 13.13 Bariatric bed with low-air-loss mattress replacement. (©2008 Hill-Rom Services. Reprinted with permission. All rights reserved.)

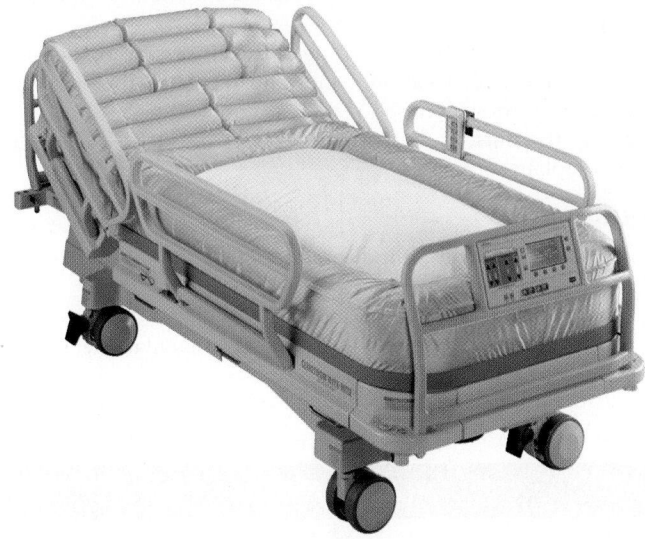

FIG 13.12 Combination air-fluidized, low-air-loss bed. (©2008 Hill-Rom Services. Reprinted with permission. All rights reserved.)

An air-fluidized or combination bed is a powered device designed to distribute a patient's weight evenly over its support surface (Fig. 13.12). In this type of system, pressure redistribution occurs by a fluid-like media that is created by forcing air through beads (microspheres). The contact pressure of the patient's body against the filter sheet stays at 11 to 16 mm Hg. The bed minimizes pressure and reduces shearing force and friction through the principle of fluidization. Fluidization is created by forcing a gentle flow of temperature-controlled air upward through a mass of fine ceramic microspheres (WOCN, 2016). The patient lies directly on a polyester filter sheet that allows air to pass through but does not allow the microspheres to escape. Patients feel as though they are floating on a surface such as a warm waterbed.

Air-fluidized beds are useful in the care of patients who require minimal movement to prevent skin damage by shearing force and for patients who experience significant pain when being turned or positioned (e.g., burn patients, those who have undergone extensive skin grafts or have existing pressure injuries, and victims of multiple trauma). Patients tend to perspire and lose body fluids while on the bed because the surface of the filter sheet warms. As patients perspire, moisture is quickly absorbed into the circulating microspheres. Diaphoresis often goes undetected; thus insensible fluid loss is not always evident until a patient develops fluid and electrolyte imbalances. Therefore you need to monitor the patient's fluid balance status carefully.

Head-of-bed position changes are not possible with some conventional fluidized beds. Use foam wedges to elevate the head. Combinations of fluidized-low-air-loss beds that allow head-of-bed elevation are also available. These beds use air to lift the upper body while the lower body stays on a fluidized bed surface. The weight of the bed structure makes transport extremely difficult. A pediatric version of this bed is available.

A valuable resource in the care of a morbidly obese patient (a person who weighs more than 100 lbs above ideal weight) is the bariatric bed (Fig. 13.13). The bariatric bed is capable of allowing upright or sitting positions, patient transport, and in-bed scale use. It is equipped with hand controls that allow self-positioning and facilitate independence for an obese patient. The full-function hand controls also allow you to change the bed position and thus facilitate care while reducing risk for staff injury when moving a patient. The in-bed scale provides you with a means of obtaining accurate weights and thus improves health care and patient dignity. The bed is slightly wider than a standard hospital bed; yet it is within the guidelines for standard door width, which allows movement into and out of a room without difficulty. Because the bariatric bed is capable of supporting weights up to 386 kg (850 lbs), it provides a stable balanced surface that limits hospital liability should the standard bedframe collapse or the electric motor burn out.

A full or double-wide bariatric bed can accommodate a patient up to 454 kg (1000 lbs). However, when using this bed, you must assemble it in the patient's room and not use it for transfers because it is too large to fit through standard hospital doorways.

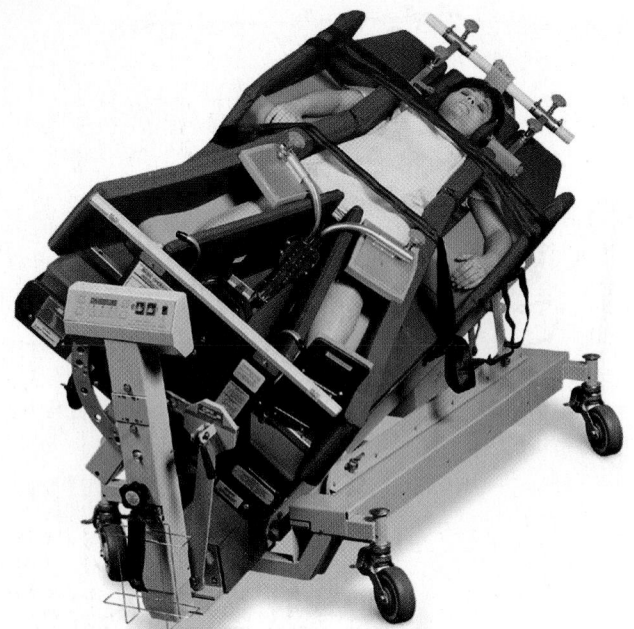

FIG 13.14 Rotokinetic bed. (*RotoRest, Courtesy Kinetic Concepts, San Antonio, TX.*)

A limitation of this bed is the lack of pressure reduction or relief in the mattress. An at-risk obese patient needs to have some type of pressure-redistribution mattress placed on the bariatric bed. Choices for pressure redistribution include air or gel type of mattresses and low-air-loss replacement systems. These beds also have cardiopulmonary resuscitation (CPR) switches, which permit an immediate hard surface for chest compressions.

The Rotokinetic bed helps maintain skeletal alignment while providing constant rotation (Fig. 13.14). It is used in the care of patients with spinal cord injuries or multiple traumas. The support structure of the bed outlines the body parts and maintains proper alignment when secured properly. This bed improves skeletal alignment with constant side-to-side rotation up to 90 degrees.

It rotates from side to side at a 60- to 90-degree angle every 7 minutes. You may adjust turning angles to meet a patient's needs. Constant rotation reduces pressure injury development and stimulates body systems. It is recommended that the bed stay in the rotation mode for at least 20 hours a day. There is an emergency lever that can quickly interrupt rotation when needed. To initiate CPR, return the bed to the horizontal position and lock in place.

The constant motion often leads to sensory distress for patients, especially older adults. This is associated with the constant kinetic stimulation, the limited visual field, and inner ear disequilibrium. Be aware of these complications and provide necessary emotional support.

Delegation and Collaboration

The skill of placing a patient on a specialty bed can be delegated to nursing assistive personnel (NAP). However, first the nurse completes the assessment, determines the need for a support surface, and selects the specific surface. Some types of support surfaces require that the manufacturer representative set up and maintain the support system. The nurse directs the NAP to:

- Notify the nurse of any changes in the patient's skin.
- Continue to turn and reposition the patient regularly and seek help for patient position changes as necessary. This is not always necessary for patients who are placed on a lateral-rotation air-suspension bed.
- Monitor the normal functioning of the air-suspension bed such as inflation and deflation cycles and report to the nurse any changes in these cycles.
- Notify the nurse if the patient becomes disoriented or restless or complains of nausea.

Equipment

- Disposable bed pads, if indicated
- Clean gloves (*optional*)
- Foam positioning wedges if indicated
- Special sheet (if appropriate, supplied by manufacturer)
- Mechanical lift (if indicated)

STEP	RATIONALE

ASSESSMENT

1. Identify patient using two identifiers (e.g., name and birthday or name and medical record number) according to agency policy.	Ensures correct patient. Complies with The Joint Commission standards and improves patient safety (TJC, 2016).
2. Perform hand hygiene.	Reduces transmission of microorganisms.
3. Determine patient's risk for pressure injury formation using a valid assessment tool (e.g., Braden Scale) and assess for risk factors for pressure injuries (e.g., nutritional deficits, shear stress, friction, alterations in mobility and sensory perception, moisture, and abnormal serum albumin and hemoglobin levels) (see Chapter 39).	Risk assessment tools provide an objective measure of risk consistent over time (Doughty and McNichol, 2016).
4. Identify patients who will benefit from air-suspension therapy or air-fluidized therapy (e.g., immobilized or burn patients).	Determines that patient receives correct type of bed for his or her needs.

Clinical Decision Point *Patients with unstable conditions do not always tolerate turning or positioning required for thorough assessment or the application of a support surface mattress.*

5. Inspect condition of skin, especially over dependent sites and bony prominences. Note appearance of existing pressure injury and determine stage of injury (see Chapter 39).	Provides baseline to determine patient's response to therapy and comfort needs.

STEP	RATIONALE
6. Assess patient's level of comfort using a pain scale of 0 to 10.	Provides baseline to determine patient's response to therapy and comfort needs.

Clinical Decision Point *Some patients experiencing pain need pain medication before application of support surface of choice or transfer to another bed (WOCN, 2016; NPUAP, 2014).*

STEP	RATIONALE
7. Verify health care provider's order for type of support surface.	Health care provider's order is usually required to ensure third-party payment of support surface.
8. Review patient's serum electrolyte levels if available.	Movement of air through mattress increases patient's risk for dehydration (Doughty and McNichol, 2016).
9. Determine if patient needs frequent weights.	Scales are available in some air-suspension beds and as underbed units for patients who need to be weighed frequently or those who cannot be moved for weighing.
10. Assess risk of complications from air-fluidized beds.	
a. Dehydration	Patients may become dehydrated with use of this bed because of insensible fluid loss.
b. Aspiration	Inability to elevate head of bed is limited to placing foam wedges under patient's head and shoulders.
c. Difficulty with patient positioning	Repositioning is limited to use of foam wedges.
d. Level of orientation	Patients may be at risk for developing delirium from dehydration and floating sensation with air-fluidized bed.

NURSING DIAGNOSES

- Deficient knowledge regarding use of support surface mattress
- Deficient fluid volume
- Impaired physical mobility
- Impaired skin integrity
- Ineffective peripheral tissue perfusion
- Pain (acute, chronic)
- Risk for impaired skin integrity

Related factors/Risk factors are individualized based on patient's condition or needs.

PLANNING

1. Expected outcomes following completion of procedure:	
• Patient's skin is without erythema or mottling.	Mottling represents hypoxia, which is an abnormal physiological response in tissues under pressure.
• Existing pressure injury shows signs of healing.	Skin remains free of new pressure injuries. Support surface does not interfere with circulation to dependent areas.
• Patient expresses improved level of comfort.	Equalized pressures have eliminated localized areas of discomfort.
• Patient is removed from therapeutic surface when risk for pressure injuries decreases.	Provides for efficient, cost-effective care while maintaining high-quality outcomes.
2. Explain purpose of mattress and method of application to patient and family caregiver.	Reduces anxiety and promotes cooperation.
3. Review instructions provided by manufacturer.	Promotes safe and correct use of bed.
4. Obtain additional personnel needed to transfer patient to bed.	Ensures safety by having sufficient personnel for transfer.
5. For patients with moderate-to-severe pain, pre-medicate approximately 30 minutes before transfer to bed.	Promotes patient's comfort and ability to cooperate during transfer to bed. Decreases patient's energy expenditure (Doughty and McNichol, 2016).

IMPLEMENTATION

1. Close room door or bedside curtain.	Provides patient privacy and considerate care during application of mattress to bed or transfer to alternative bed.
2. Perform hand hygiene. Apply clean gloves (if linens are soiled or wet). Get help to position patient and/or mattress as needed.	Prevents transmission of microorganisms. Assistance from other caregivers reduces risk for friction and shear in transfer to new surface.
3. Transfer patient to bed using appropriate transfer techniques (see Chapter 11). Bed surface is sometimes slippery; thus do not attempt transfers without help.	Appropriate safe patient-handling techniques maintain alignment and reduce risk of injury during procedure. Manufacturer representative adjusts bed to patient's height and weight.

STEP	RATIONALE
4. Once patient has been transferred, turn bed on by depressing switch; regulate temperature.	Releasing Instaflate or turning on bed allows pressure cushions to adjust automatically to preset levels to minimize pressure, friction, and shear.
5. Position patient and perform range-of-motion exercises as appropriate.	Promotes comfort and reduces contracture formation.
6. To turn patient, position bedpans, or perform other therapies, turn on Instaflate or other setting. Once you have completed the procedure, release Instaflate. With air-fluidized bed, use foam wedges to position patient as needed.	Instaflate firms bed surface to facilitate turning and handling patient. Patient does not receive pressure relief while bed is in this mode.
7. Use special features of bed as needed.	
a. Scales	Facilitates ability to obtain routine weights.
b. Portable transport units to maintain inflation when primary power is interrupted	Provides for continuous pressure reduction.
c. Specialty cushions for positioning, providing pressure relief, reducing moisture, preventing patient from sliding down in bed, or relieving weight from orthopedic devices	Reduces pressure, friction, and shearing forces.
d. Lateral rotation (Fig. 13.15), which allows approximately 30 degrees of turning	Underinflation or improper functioning of certain overlays may result in tissue damage. Likewise, overinflation can result in too firm a surface and create pressure damage.

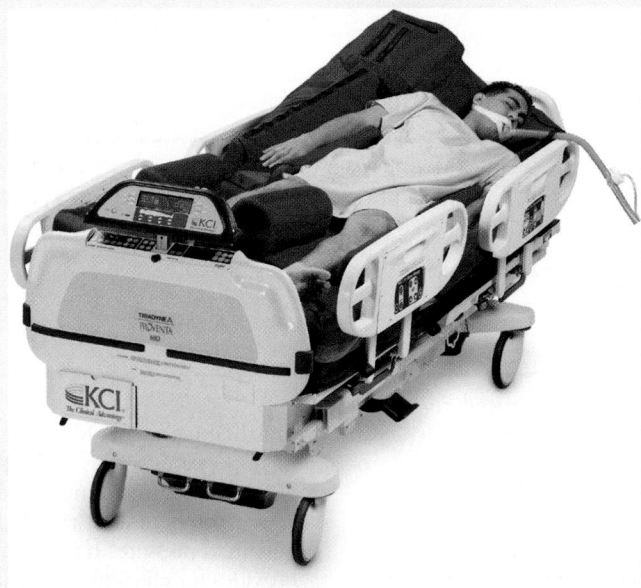

FIG 13.15 Lateral rotation bed. (*Tria Dyne™ Therapy System. Courtesy KCI Licensing, Inc., 2013.*)

Clinical Decision Point *A patient should never be placed in prone position on an air-fluidized bed because of the chance of suffocation.*

8. Assess effectiveness of pressure-relief mattress or seat cushion by placing hand beneath support surface under a bony prominence.	Helps reduce risk and prevent pulmonary and urinary complications of reduced mobility (Doughty and McNichol, 2016).
9. Remove and dispose of gloves and perform hand hygiene.	Reduces transmission of microorganisms.

EVALUATION

1. Reassess patient's risk for pressure injury formation at routine intervals.	Documents change in status, which is critical for evaluating continued need for therapeutic surface.
2. Inspect and compare condition of patient's skin every 8 hours or according to agency policy to determine changes in skin integrity, pressure injury status, and effectiveness of support surface.	Determines if pressure sores develop or if condition of existing sores changes.
3. Ask patient to rate comfort on a scale of 0 to 10.	If pressure-relief mattress is effective, patient generally experiences less discomfort.

STEP	RATIONALE
4. Evaluate functioning of support surface periodically.	Regular inspection of mechanical components of mattress ensures proper functioning.
5. Use Teach-Back: "I want to be sure I explained why this bed is turned laterally. Tell me why we placed you laterally and how you might feel." Revise your instruction now or develop plan for revised patient or family caregiver teaching if patient or family caregiver is not able to teach back correctly.	Determines patient's and family caregiver's level of understanding of instructional topic.

Unexpected Outcomes	Related Interventions
1. Existing areas of skin breakdown or pressure areas fail to heal or increase in size and depth.	• Modify skin-care regimen. • Increase frequency of skin assessment. • Change types of pressure-relief interventions. • Check for proper inflation of support surface. • Revise turning schedule. • Consult with skin-care expert. • Notify health care provider.
2. Patient becomes nauseated.	• Provide short-term antiemetic such as prochlorperazine. If using lateral rotation, obtain antiemetic order around the clock. • If using lateral rotation, decrease cycle frequency. • Notify health care provider.

Recording and Reporting

- Record transfer of patient to bed, amount of help needed for transfer, tolerance of procedure, and condition of skin in nurses' notes in electronic health record (EHR) or chart and/or skin assessment flow sheet.
- Document your evaluation of patient and family caregiver learning.
- Report changes in condition of skin, level of orientation, and electrolyte levels to health care provider.

Special Considerations

Teaching

- Explain function and purpose of specialty bed.
- Explain the need to continue to change position at intervals to diminish the effects of immobility.
- Explain the need for adequate fluid intake because bed surface sometimes causes dehydration.

Pediatric

- The air-suspension bed is used commonly with older children and for children with significant burns. Make sure that instructions are age appropriate and include any restrictions such as raising the head of the bed.
- Parents need to know that the child will have some dizziness or nausea when first placed on the air-fluidized or other specialty bed. This is because of the flotation sensation and will disappear as the child becomes adjusted to the bed.

Gerontological

- Some hospitalized older adults experience misperceptions of their environment that are intensified by the constant flotation of these types of beds. Proprioception abnormalities affecting older adults are the result of nervous system and muscle changes (Doughty and McNichol, 2016).

Home Care

- The air-fluidized bed weighs between 772 and 954 kg (1700 and 2100 lbs); therefore, the company leasing the bed needs to inspect the home for accessibility and structural support.
- Consult with social worker or case manager to determine third-party reimbursement. Thorough documentation of skin condition is essential in obtaining reimbursement.
- A version of the air-fluidized bed is available for home use for rent or purchase; the bed rental company is responsible for proper cleaning.
- Instruct family caregiver in importance of maintaining patient hydration and skin care.
- Instruct family caregiver regarding steps to take in the event of a power failure. This may include purchasing a back-up generator for the home.

Long-Term Care

- Nurses and NAPs need to be instructed on proper use and inflation of the bed.
- Post signs and have protocols in place for procedures in the event of the need to perform CPR (e.g., how to deflate the bed to provide a flat surface for compressions).

◆ CLINICAL DEBRIEF

You are assigned to admit a 48-year-old male who was involved in a motor vehicle accident that resulted in quadriplegia (causing loss of sensation and movement below the neck). The patient is unable to change positions or transfer without help. He also has a language barrier, and communicating instructions about his care is difficult. The nurse has arranged for the services of a qualified interpreter to help breach the language barrier.

Following consultation with physical therapy and social service, the health care provider orders an air-suspension bed with lateral rotation because he has some blistering over bony prominences and his impaired mobility and sensation increase his risk for developing pressure injuries. The patient begins experiencing a small amount of nausea and restlessness when placed on the air-suspension bed initially.

1. When this patient complains of sudden dizziness, the nurse checks his blood pressure and notes that on lateral rotation he develops orthostatic hypotension. What should the nurse's initial actions be?
2. While conducting a skin assessment, the nurse notices skin breakdown over the coccyx and left hip, even though this patient has received meticulous skin care and routine repositioning. What is the appropriate nursing action to take first?
3. The patient continues to complain of nausea and dizziness on the air-suspension bed.

Using SBAR, show how you would communicate with the health care team about this patient.

◆ REVIEW QUESTIONS

1. The patient is discharged to home with home health care. He has been ordered a Roho cushion and is taught to self-adjust the inflation during the day when he is in his wheelchair. The family caregiver notes that the patient has small areas of continuing redness on his ischia. Which interventions are indicated? The family caregiver should: (Select all that apply.)
   1. Report the situation to the nurse or case manager immediately.
   2. Instruct the patient to not change the chair cushion inflation.
   3. Check for proper inflation of the cushion.
   4. Reinflate the cushion appropriately while the patient is sitting on it and wait to reevaluate the skin condition later.
   5. Increase frequency of checking the patient's skin.
2. Place the following steps for applying an air mattress overlay in the correct order:
   1. Check air pumps to be sure that pressure cycle alternates.
   2. Bring any plastic strips or flaps around corners of bed mattress.
   3. Apply deflated mattress flat over surface of bed mattress.
   4. Place sheet over air mattress, being sure to eliminate all wrinkles.
   5. Attach connector on air mattress to inflation device and inflate to proper pressure.
3. For which of the following complications should the nurse assess when caring for a patient on an air-fluidized bed? (Select all that apply.)

1. Back pain from lack of firm support
2. Dehydration from the amount of warm circulating air
3. Problems moving the patient out of bed because of the body submersion
4. Lack of healing of the pressure injury because of high skin/bed pressures
5. Difficulty moving the bed to another location because of its weight

ⓔ *Visit the Evolve site for a complete list of Clinical Debrief and Review Questions answers.*

REFERENCES

American Medical Directors Association (AMDA): *Pressure ulcers in long-term care setting*, Columbia, MD, 2013, National Guidelines Clearinghouse.

Anton PM: Maintaining skin integrity. In Mauk KL, editor: *Rehabilitation nursing: a contemporary approach to practice*, Sudbury, MA, 2013, Jones & Bartlett.

Broome C, et al: Nursing care of the super bariatric patient: challenges and lessons learned, *Rehabil Nurs* 40:92, 2015.

Call E, et al: *Hand check method: is it an effective method to monitor support surfaces for bottoming out? A National Pressure Ulcer Advisory Position Statement*, 2015, http://www.npuap.org/wp-content/uploads/2012/01/Hand-Check-Position-Statement-June-2015.pdf. Accessed September 2, 2016.

Doughty D, McNichol L: *Wound, Ostomy, and Continence Nurses Society (WOCN) Core curriculum: wound management*, Philadelphia, 2016, Wound, Ostomy, and Continence Society.

Higelin S: Pressure ulcers. In Mauk KL, editor: *Gerontological nursing: competencies for care*, Sudbury, MA, 2014, Jones & Bartlett.

Hockenberry MJ, Wilson J: *Wong's nursing care of infants and children*, ed 10, St Louis, 2015, Mosby.

McInnes E, et al: Preventing pressure ulcers: are pressure-redistributing support surfaces effective? A Cochrane Systematic review and meta-analysis, *Int J Nurs Stud* 49(3):345, 2013.

McInnes E, et al: Support surfaces for pressure ulcer prevention, *Cochrane Database Syst Rev* 9:CD00173, 2015.

Moore Z, Cowman S: Risk assessment tools for the prevention of pressure ulcers, *Cochrane Database Syst Rev* 2:1, 2014.

National Pressure Ulcer Advisory Panel Support Surfaces Standard Initiative (NPUAP): *Pressure ulcer treatment recommendations: clinical practice guidelines*, Washington, DC, 2014, National Pressure Ulcer Advisory Panel.

Norton L, et al: Beds: practical pressure management for surfaces/mattresses, *Adv Skin Wound Care* 24(7):325, 2011.

Qaseem A, et al: Risk assessment and prevention of pressure ulcers: a clinical practice guideline from the American College of Physicians, *Ann Intern Med* 162(5):359, 2015.

Serpa L, Santos V: Validity of the Braden Nutrition Subscale in predicting pressure ulcer development, *J Wound Ostomy Continence Nurs* 41(5):436, 2014.

Slade S: *Pressure area care: prevention, evidence summary*, South Australia, 2013, The Joanna Briggs Institute.

The Joint Commission (TJC): *2016 National Patient Safety Goals*, Oakbrook Terrace, IL, 2016, The Commission. http://www.jointcommission.org/standards_information/npsgs.aspx. Accessed March 13, 2016.

Wound, Ostomy and Continence Nurses Society (WOCN): *Guideline for prevention and management of pressure ulcers*, WOCN clinical practice guideline series, ed 2, Mt. Laurel, NJ, 2016, Author.

14 | Patient Safety

OBJECTIVES

Mastery of content in this chapter will enable the nurse to:

- Discuss the importance of national standards for patient safety.
- Discuss current evidence in the area of fall prevention.
- Discuss the importance of a nursing assessment in providing for patient safety.
- Describe nursing interventions specific for reducing patients' risks for falls.

- Describe steps in the design of a restraint-free environment.
- Describe nursing interventions taken in the event of a fire, electrical shock, or chemical spill.
- Discuss precautions used to prevent injury in patients who are restrained.
- Describe nursing interventions for a patient who experiences generalized seizures.
- Describe methods to evaluate safety interventions.

MEDIA RESOURCES

- evolve http://evolve.elsevier.com/Perry/skills
- Review Questions
- ▶ Video Clips

- Audio Glossary
- **NSO** Nursing Skills Online
- Clinical Debrief and Review Questions Answers

PURPOSE

Reducing the risk of harm associated with the delivery of health care is a national health care policy priority (Nabhan et al., 2012; NQF, 2015). Health care provided in a safe environment, in which nurses practice safety-related skills, reduces the risk for illness and injury and contains the costs of health care by preventing extended lengths of treatment and/or hospitalization, improving or maintaining a patient's functional status, and increasing the patient's sense of well-being.

STANDARDS OF CARE

- National Quality Forum, 2015—Fall Screening and Management
- The Joint Commission, 2016—Patient Identification, National Patient Safety Goals
- QSEN, 2014—Patient-Centered Care, Patient Safety and Quality Improvement
- Neuro Critical Care Society, 2012—Guidelines for Care of Patients in Status Epilepticus

PRINCIPLES FOR PRACTICE

- The integration of evidence-based practice (EBP) into nursing skills and procedures promotes a safer health care environment and improves patient outcomes.

- A nurse must be responsible for incorporating critical thinking skills when using the nursing process, assessing each patient and his or her environment for hazards that threaten safety, and planning and intervening appropriately to maintain a safe environment.
- Safe patient care is a priority with a focus on reducing the incidence of adverse health care–associated conditions and reducing harm from inappropriate care (NQF, 2015).
- The Quality and Safety Education for Nurses (QSEN) initiative identifies skills for safety competency, including demonstrating effective use of technology and standardized practices; demonstrating effective use of strategies to reduce risk of harm to self or others; using appropriate strategies to reduce reliance on memory; and communicating observations or concerns related to hazards and errors to patients, families, and the health care team (QSEN, 2014).
- As a health care provider it is essential to share information about any patient injury, learn from errors, and participate in the trending and evaluation of those errors (Speroni et al., 2013).

PATIENT-CENTERED CARE

- Patient-centered is defined by QSEN (2014) as recognizing a patient as the source of control and full partner in providing compassionate and coordinated care based on respect for patient's preferences, values, and needs. By partnering with patients and families (e.g., not only involving them in decisions about their care, but also gaining the benefit of their help and insights to better plan and deliver care safely), patients can achieve better outcomes (AHA, 2015).

- Being hospitalized or living in an assisted-living facility places patients at risk for injury in an unfamiliar and confusing environment. Normal life cues such as a bed without side rails and the direction one usually takes to the bathroom are absent. Thought processes and coping mechanisms are affected by physical and psychological illness and the accompanying emotions. Thus patients are more vulnerable to injury.

- For patients of diverse cultural backgrounds, vulnerability to injury may be intensified. It is a nurse's responsibility to diligently protect all patients, regardless of their cultural background. Most adverse events are related to failures of communication. Health care providers must be particularly attentive to communication during assessment. For example, a nurse must use approaches that recognize a patient's cultural background (e.g., an interpreter or simple language) so appropriate questions can be raised to clearly reveal health behaviors and risks.

- You enhance a patient's safety by considering him or her in light of the whole person and seeing each care situation through "the patient's eyes" and not just your perspective. The following include some specific patient-centered safety guidelines:
  - Nurses should support patients emotionally and empower them to express their values and preferences and ask questions without being inhibited (Bhutani et al., 2013).
  - When restraints are needed, clarify their meaning to the patient and family. Some patients may view restraining an older adult to be disrespectful. Similarly some survivors of war or persecution view restraints as imprisonment or punishment.
  - Collaborate with family members in accommodating a patient's cultural perspectives regarding restraints. Removing restraints when family members are present shows respect and caring for a patient.
  - Be familiar with agency restraint protocol. Identify potential areas for negotiation with a patient's and family's preferences such as using a mitten versus arm restraints.
  - Inform patients and family members of the reasons a patient is at fall risk. It is important for patients to know their risks, the options that exist to promote safety, and the consequences of not following precautions.

EVIDENCE-BASED PRACTICE

Significant research continues in the area of fall prevention, both in community and health care settings.

- Young neurological patients with impaired gait and balance or medium-to-severe motor disability are at an increased risk of falling. Patients who are relatively independent and still involved in challenging activities have an increased exposure to fall risk. Improperly fitted canes and walkers, wheelchair characteristics, and environmental hazards are significant environmental risk factors (Saverino et al., 2014).

- In long-term care settings, multifactorial interventions (using multiple fall prevention strategies) significantly reduce falls and the number of recurrent fallers (Vlaeyen et al., 2015).

- Older adults should be screened routinely for relevant risk factors for falling. These individuals will most likely benefit

from a fall prevention program targeted to their risk factors (e.g., frailty, polypharmacy, multi-morbidity, vitamin D status, and home hazards). Not all fall prevention strategies are useful for all patients (Pfortmueller et al., 2014).

- Single exercise interventions (e.g., Tai Chi) can significantly reduce numbers of falls among older adults with and without cognitive impairment in institutional or noninstitutional settings (El-Khoury et al., 2013). Such programs also reduce the rate of falls that lead to medical care (El-Khoury et al., 2013).

- Vitamin D and calcium supplementation, home visits, and adjustments within the living environment can reduce the risk of falls among older adults in noninstitutional settings (Guo et al., 2014). Including an occupational therapist or physical therapist in a home-hazard assessment may have added benefit.

- Exercise programs designed to prevent falls in older adults, including planned group exercise, also seem to prevent injuries caused by falls, including the most severe ones. Such programs also reduce the rate of falls leading to medical care (El-Khoury et al., 2013).

- The Agency for Healthcare Research and Quality (AHRQ, 2013c) cites factors for health care organizations to consider when implementing best practices for fall prevention. Some factors that make fall prevention challenging include the following:
  - Fall prevention must be balanced with other priorities for a patient. A patient is usually not in the health care agency because of falls; therefore attention naturally is directed elsewhere. Yet a fall in a sick patient can be disastrous and prolong the recovery process.
  - Fall prevention must be balanced with the need to mobilize patients. It may be tempting to leave patients in bed to prevent falls, but they need to transfer and ambulate to maintain their strength and avoid complications of bed rest.
  - Fall prevention is one of many activities needed to protect patients from harm during their health care agency stay. Health care staff must consider how to prevent falls while maintaining focus on other priorities such as infection control.
  - Fall prevention is interprofessional. Nurses, physicians, pharmacists, physical therapists, occupational therapists, patients, and families need to cooperate to prevent falls.
  - Fall prevention needs to be individualized. Each patient has a different set of fall risk factors; thus care must address each patient's unique needs thoughtfully.

SAFETY GUIDELINES

- Accurate patient identification is crucial to safety before any procedures. Use at least two ways to identify patients (TJC, 2016).

- Safety begins with a patient's immediate environment (Fig. 14.1). Always keep a bed in the low position and a bed alarm activated and use necessary fall prevention strategies. The call-light/bed-control system allows patients to adjust bed positions and signal caregivers for help. Explain to patients and visiting family members how to operate a call system correctly and then use teach-back to confirm understanding and have them demonstrate use of device.

- Always be alert to conditions within a patient's environment that pose risks for patient injury (e.g., personal care items out of reach, hazards along walking paths, liquid spilled on the floor, poorly functioning equipment).

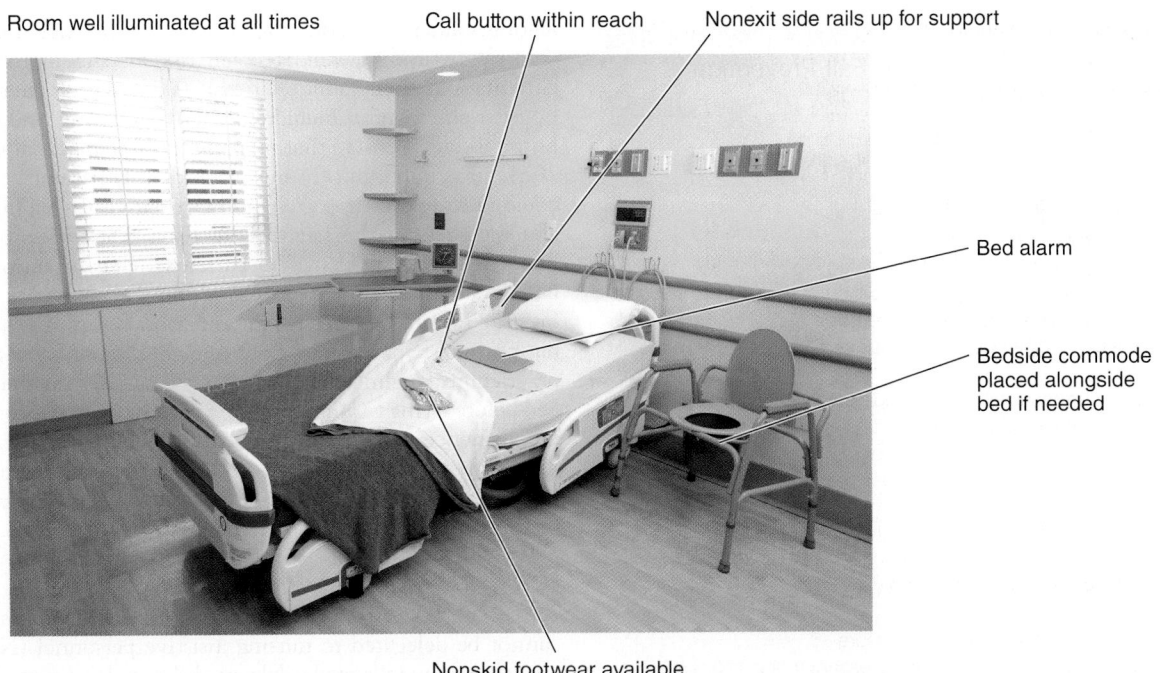

Room well illuminated at all times Call button within reach Nonexit side rails up for support

Bed alarm

Bedside commode placed alongside bed if needed

Nonskid footwear available

FIG 14.1 Safe patient room environment with bed in low position, bed alarm activated, nonskid floor mat and call light in place, and bedside commode positioned along bedside.

- Follow agency policy and procedure in the agency where you work. Do not use work-arounds when performing skills or procedures. A work-around occurs when a person improvises or works around intended work practices.

- Communicate clearly to other health care providers the plan of care, including procedures to be performed, procedures completed, and patient response. Communicate all important test results to the right staff person in a timely manner (TJC, 2015).

◆ SKILL 14.1 Fall Prevention in Health Care Agencies

NSO *Nursing Skills Online Safety Module / Lessons 1 and 2*

Patient falls are a recurrent problem in health care agencies. Each year approximately 700,000 to 1,000,000 people in the United States fall in hospitals (AHRQ, 2013a). A fall may result in fractures, bruises, lacerations, or internal bleeding, leading to increased diagnostic tests and treatments, extended hospital stays, and discharge to rehabilitation or long-term care instead of home. Research shows that approximately one third of falls can be prevented (AHRQ, 2013a). Fall prevention involves identifying and managing a patient's underlying fall risk factors and optimizing the physical design and environment of the health care agency.

Falls are multifactorial. Individual intrinsic factors such as co-morbidities, muscle weakness, and urinary incontinence increase the risk of falling in a hospital and community setting (de Jong et al., 2013; Spoelstra et al., 2012). Transient factors that can change over time such as postural hypotension, polypharmacy, and use of high-risk medications also are fall risks (Chang et al., 2011). Extrinsic fall risks such as the environment of a health care agency (e.g., poor lighting, slippery flooring, and improper use of assist devices) also contribute to falls (de Jong et al., 2013). As a nurse your role is to assess these factors in each patient and determine the most suitable preventive interventions that match the patient's risks and behavior.

The Centers for Medicare and Medicaid Services (CMS) have identified select serious adverse events as "Never Events" (e.g., adverse events that should never occur in a health care setting)

(DHHS, 2008). One of these "Never Events" is hospital-acquired injury from external causes (e.g., fractures, head injury, crushing injury), as in the case of falls. The CMS denies hospitals higher payment for any hospital-acquired condition resulting from or complicated by the occurrence of a "Never Event."

Fall prevention is not simple. There is no conclusive evidence for any particular set of interventions that will consistently prevent falls. Spoelstra et al. (2012) identified interventions that have shown some success in reducing hospital fall rates:

- Developing a culture of safety, including ongoing staff education and feedback on fall incidents
- Using validated fall risk assessments that are predictive of falls in hospitals where used
- Individualizing multifactorial interventions (Box 14.1)
- Conducting postfall follow-up and quality improvement
- Having a fall risk program integrated with electronic health records (EHR)

Another area of risk includes wheelchair-related falls involving older adults and people with disabilities. Patients fall from wheelchairs as a result of unlocked brakes, overreaching, sliding, tipping the chair, and unassisted transfers. Wheelchair-related injuries from falls include fractures, concussions, dislocations, amputations, and serious head and spinal injuries. An example of a wheelchair characteristic that increases risk for falls is having smaller and harder front wheels that cause a chair to tip when striking uneven

Components of Evidence-Based Fall Prevention Interventions in Health Care Settings

- Correction of environmental hazards
- Identification armbands and bed and door signs for high-risk patients
- Bedrails and bed height kept at the lowest level
- Nurse call bell explained and within reach
- Unsafe footwear replaced and/or nonskid footwear provided
- Individualized patient and caregiver education and written instructions (preferably prescribed on the basis of risk factors)
- Staff assignments in close proximity (assigned to patients in adjacent rooms)
- Improving staff communication by including nonlicensed staff
- Improving patient hand-off communication
- Advising patients on changing position slowly
- Encouraging patients to use eye glasses, hearing aids, footwear, and mobility devices
- Nurse toilet and turn or comfort and care safety rounds (conducted hourly)
- Supervision and assistance with transfer and toilet use
- Toileting before pain medication
- Medical referral for abnormal blood pressure
- Medication review for sedatives, antidepressants, diuretics, and polypharmacy
- Ophthalmology referral for poor eyesight and optician visit if lost glasses

Adapted from Spoelstra SL et al: Fall prevention in hospitals: an integrative review, *Clin Nurs Res* 21(1):92, 2012.

terrain. Caregivers are also at risk for injury by not handling patients correctly or not asking for help. Injuries can occur while caregivers transfer patients who are agitated, fearful, unsteady, or too weak to transfer. Tripping over the front foot or leg rest and leaning over the back of the wheelchair to engage or disengage the wheel lock are common sources of injury.

The Joint Commission (TJC) Center for Transforming Healthcare aims to prevent inpatient falls with injury. Seven hospitals in the United States worked with the center and successfully reduced total number of falls and falls with injury by creating awareness among staff, empowering patients to take an active role in their own safety, using a validated fall risk assessment tool, engaging patients and their families in the fall safety program, providing hourly rounding that includes proactive toileting, and engaging all hospital staff to ensure that no patient walks unaccompanied (TJC, 2014). It is important for nurses to identify patients' fall risks and communicate these risks to patients, their visiting family members, and members of the health care team. Patient-centered care is important, with nurses making patients their partners in recognizing fall risks and taking preventive action. Fall prevention strategies must be targeted to specific patient risks. For example, if a patient has postural hypotension, a nurse might choose a low bed and the practice of dangling the patient for 5 minutes on the side of the bed before trying to ambulate. Or a patient with a history of urinary incontinence might be given a bedside commode to use. Remember that patient situations change. Preventing falls and fall-related injuries requires diligent ongoing nursing assessment and engagement of the entire health care team.

Delegation and Collaboration

The skill of assessing and communicating a patient's risk for falling cannot be delegated to nursing assistive personnel (NAP). Skills used to prevent falls can be delegated. The nurse directs the NAP by:
- Explaining a patient's mobility limitations and specific fall prevention measures needed to minimize risks.
- Teaching specific environmental safety precautions to use (e.g., bed locked in low position, call light within reach).
- Explaining patient behaviors (e.g., disorientation, wandering, anxiety) that are precursors to falls and that should be reported immediately.

Equipment

- Validated fall risk assessment tool (TJC, 2014)
- Hospital bed with side rails; *option:* low bed
- Wedge cushion
- Call-light intercom system
- Gait belt for assisting with ambulation
- Wheelchair and seat belt (as needed)
- Additional safety devices (e.g., bed alarm pad, wedge cushion)

STEP	RATIONALE

ASSESSMENT

1. Identify patient using at least two identifiers (e.g., name and birthday or name and medical record number) according to agency policy.

   Ensures correct patient. Complies with The Joint Commission standards and improves patient safety (TJC, 2016).

2. Assess for fall risks using a validated fall risk assessment tool specific and sensitive to population being screened: patient's age (over 65), presence of co-morbidities, altered memory and cognition, incontinence or urinary frequency/urgency, reduced hearing and vision, orthostatic hypotension, arthritis, impaired gait, weak lower extremities, poor balance, fatigue, need for transfer assistance, and decreased peripheral sensation (Pfortmueller et al., 2014; Spoelstra et al., 2012). Also assess for risk for injury during fall (e.g., vitamin D level, osteoporosis, bleeding tendency).

   A variety of physiological factors predispose patients to fall and injury from falling. There are a variety of fall risk assessment tools. Those with a greater number of risk factors are less likely to be sensitive because all patients will be found at risk. Tools based on the risk factors of a population (e.g., elderly, oncology, or neurological patient) are more likely sensitive to predicting falls.

Clinical Decision Point *Do not ask patient to provide a self-report of balance, gait, or ability to ambulate. Ask patient to walk a short distance and observe each factor.*

STEP	RATIONALE
3. Assess level of patient's pain using a rating scale that ranges from 0 to 10.	Pain has been shown to be a risk factor for falls (de Jong et al., 2013).
4. Determine if patient has a history of recent falls or other injuries within the home. Assess previous falls using the acronym SPLATT (Touhy and Jett, 2014). • Symptoms at time of fall • Previous fall • Location of fall • Activity at time of fall • Time of fall • Trauma after fall	Symptoms are helpful in identifying cause for falls. Onset, location, and activity associated with a fall provide further details about causative factors and how to prevent future falls.
5. Review patient's medications (including over-the-counter [OTC] medications and herbal products) for use of antidepressants, sedatives and hypnotics (especially benzodiazepines), anxiolytics, beta-blockers, diuretics, antihypertensives, neuroleptics, anti-Parkinson drugs, hypoglycemics, nonsteroidal antiinflammatories, opioids, antipsychotics, and laxatives. Assess for polypharmacy (e.g., over four medications, duplicate medications, drugs inappropriate for condition) (de Jong et al., 2013).	Effects of certain medications and use of multiple medications increase risk for falls and injury (Chang et al., 2011; Kojima et al., 2011).

Clinical Decision Point *If patient is on multiple medications, confer with health care provider and pharmacist about possibility of reducing or adjusting doses.*

STEP	RATIONALE
6. Assess patient for fear of falling: consider those over 70 years of age, female, lower income, or single and have poor perceived general health (Kiel, 2016).	Fear of falling is interrelated with incidence of falls, change in way patient walks, curtailment of activities, immobility, functional dependence, falls with serious injury (Greenberg, 2012).
7. Perform the "timed get up and go (TUG)" test if patient is able to ambulate. At a minimum, observe patient walk in room (with or without help). Steps for TUG dual assessment: • Give patient verbal instructions to stand up from a chair, walk 10 feet (3 meters) as quickly and safely as possible (cross a line marked on the floor), turn around, walk back, and sit down. • Have patient rise from straight-back chair without using arms for support. • Begin counting. • Look for unsteadiness in patient's gait. • Have patient return to chair and sit down without using arms for support. Check time elapsed. • For accuracy, a patient should have one practice trial that is not included in the score. Patient must use the same assistive device each time he or she is tested to be able to compare scores.	The TUG test is a simple and quick clinical, performance-based measure of lower-extremity function, mobility, and fall risk, useful even with healthy adults (Herman et al., 2011). It is a revision of the original get up and go test (Podsiadlo and Richardson, 1991). It quantifies a patient's functional mobility. Observing a patient walk allows you to determine if gait and posture are normal. The TUG test is a measure of physical and cognitive performance. Ability to follow simple instructions measures cognitive function. An older adult who takes ≥12 seconds to complete the TUG test is at high risk for falling (CDC, 2015). Balance function is scored on a five-point scale: 1 = Normal, 2 = Very slightly abnormal, 3 = Mildly abnormal, 4 = Moderately abnormal, 5 = Severely abnormal (Mathias et al., 1986). A score of 3 or more on the balance scale indicates that patient is at risk of falling (Mathias et al., 1986). **NOTE:** The TUG test has been found to have limited ability to predict falls in community-dwelling elderly and should not be used in isolation to identify individuals at high risk of falls in this setting (Barry et al., 2014).
8. Assess condition of equipment (e.g., legs on bedside commode, tips of walker)	Equipment in poor repair increases risk for fall.
9. Assess patient's medical history for osteoporosis, being on anticoagulants, history of previous fracture, cancer, and recent chest or abdominal surgery.	Factors increase likelihood of injury from fall.
10. Use patient-centered approach to determine what patient knows about risks for falling and steps that he or she can take to prevent falls.	Knowledge of fall risks influences one's ability to take necessary precautions in reducing falling. Matching interventions with factors that patient perceives as relevant may increase success in preventing falls.
11. If patient is assessed to be a fall risk, apply color-coded wristband (see illustration). Some agencies institute fall risk signs on doors.	Color-coded yellow bands are easily recognizable.

STEP	RATIONALE

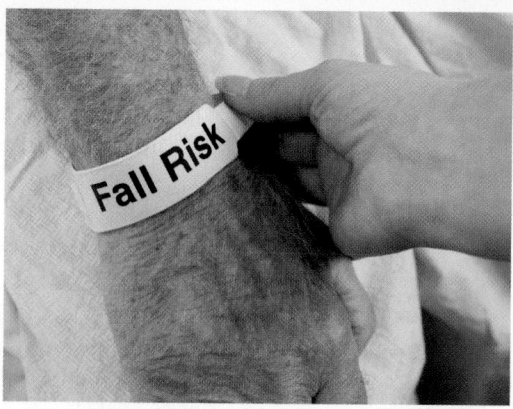

STEP 11 Fall risk armband alerts health care staff to patient's risk of falling.

12. If patient is in a wheelchair, assess his or her level of comfort, fatigue, boredom, mental status, or level of engagement with others.	These factors can cause patient to make an attempt to exit wheelchair without help.

NURSING DIAGNOSES

- Activity intolerance
- Acute or chronic pain
- Impaired memory
- Impaired physical mobility
- Impaired transfer ability
- Impaired urinary elimination
- Impaired walking
- Risk for falls
- Risk for injury
- Risk for trauma

Related factors/Risk factors are individualized based on patient's condition or needs.

PLANNING

1. Expected outcomes following completion of procedure:	
• Patient's environment is free of hazards	Hazards predispose to tripping and falls.
• Patient and/or family caregiver is able to identify fall risks.	Patient awareness of risks promotes cooperation and understanding of fall prevention plan.
• Patient and/or family caregiver verbalizes understanding of fall prevention interventions.	Includes patient and family caregiver in decisions about preventive strategies.
• Patient does not experience a fall or injury.	Fall precautions show success in preventing falls.
2. Gather equipment and perform hand hygiene.	Organizes care. Reduces transmission of microorganisms.
3. Explain what you plan to do. Specifically discuss reasons that patient is at risk for falling. Include family caregivers (as appropriate) in discussion. Provide privacy. Be sure that patient is comfortable.	Reduces patient anxiety and promotes cooperation. Results in fall prevention measures that are patient centered and not just routine. Younger patients are very independent and often believe that they are not likely to fall.

IMPLEMENTATION

1. Conduct hourly rounds on all patients to determine status of pain, need to toilet, and need to relocate personal items for easy reach; provide pain relief intervention.	Provides nurses with surveillance mechanism to purposefully keep patients safe and comfortable by proactively meeting their needs. Research associating rounds to fall reduction needs to be more rigorous (Hempel et al., 2013).
2. Adjust bed to low position with wheels locked (see illustration). Place nonslip padded floor mats at exit side of bed.	Height of bed allows ambulatory patient to get in and out of bed easily and safely. Pads provide nonslippery surface on which to stand.
3. Encourage use of properly fitted skid-proof footwear. *Option:* Place nonslip padded floor mat on exit side of bed.	Prevents falls from slipping on floor.
4. Orient patient to surroundings, call light, and routines to expect in plan of care.	Orientation to room and plan of care provides familiarity with environment and activities to anticipate.
a. Provide patient's hearing aid and glasses. Be sure that each is functioning/clean. If patient complains of visual or hearing problems, refer to appropriate health care provider.	Enables patient to remain alert to conditions in environment.

STEP	RATIONALE

b. Place call-light/bed-control system in an accessible location within patient's reach. Explain and demonstrate how to turn system on and off at bedside and in bathroom (see illustration). Have patient perform return demonstration.

Knowledge of location and use of call light is essential for patient to be able to call for help quickly. Reaching for an object when in bed can lead to an accidental fall.

c. Explain to patient/family member when and why to use call system (e.g., report pain, get out of bed, go to bathroom). Provide clear instructions to patient/family member regarding mobility restrictions.

Increases likelihood that patient will call for help and of nurse being able to respond to patient's needs in a timely way.

5. Safe use of side rails:

a. Explain to patient and family caregivers reason for using side rails: moving and turning self in bed.

Promotes cooperation.

b. Check agency policy regarding side rail use.

(1) Dependent, less mobile patients: In two–side rail bed, keep both rails up. (**NOTE:** Rails on newer hospital beds allow for room at foot of bed for patient to safely exit bed.) In four-side rail bed, leave two upper rails up.

Side rails are restraint devices if they immobilize or reduce ability of a patient to move his or her arms, legs, body, or head freely.

(2) Patient able to get out of bed independently: In four–side rail bed, leave two upper side rails up. In two–side rail bed, keep only one rail up.

Allows for safe exit from bed.

6. Make patient's environment safe:

a. Remove excess equipment, supplies, and furniture from rooms and halls.

Reduces likelihood of falling or tripping over objects.

b. Keep floors free of clutter and obstacles (e.g., intravenous [IV] pole, electrical cords), particularly path to bathroom.

Reduces likelihood of falling or tripping over objects.

c. Coil and secure excess electrical, telephone, and any other cords or tubing.

Reduces risk of entanglement.

d. Clean all spills promptly. Post sign indicating wet floor. Remove sign when floor is dry (usually done by housekeeping).

Reduces risk of falling on slippery, wet surfaces.

e. Ensure adequate glare-free lighting; use a night-light at night.

Glare may be problem for older adults because of vision changes.

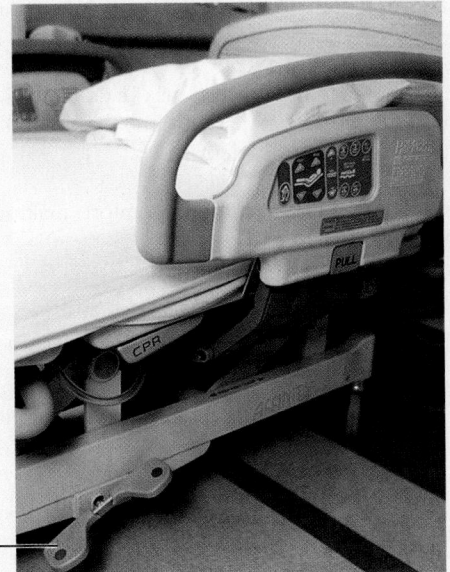

Brake lock

STEP 2 Hospital bed should be kept in lowest position with wheels locked and side rails up (as appropriate).

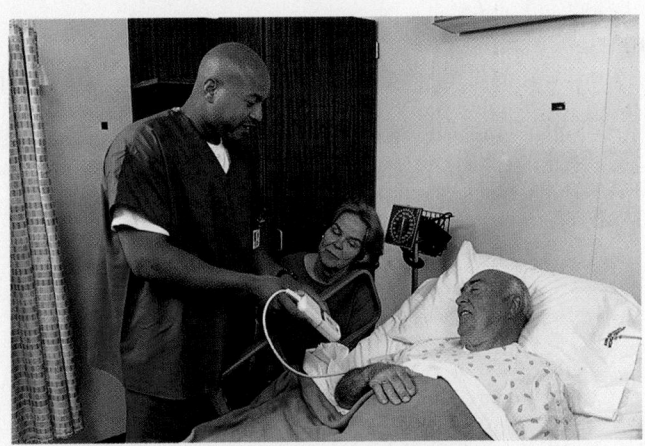

STEP 4b Nurse demonstrates use of call light to patient.

STEP	RATIONALE
f. Have assistive devices (e.g., cane, walker, bedside commode) on exit side of bed. Have chair back of commode placed against wall of room if possible.	Provides added support when transferring out of bed. Stabilizes commode.
g. Arrange personal items (e.g., water pitcher, telephone, reading materials, dentures) within patient's easy reach and in logical way.	Facilitates independence and self-care; prevents falls related to reaching for hard-to-reach items.
h. Secure locks on beds, stretchers, and wheelchairs.	Prevents accidental movement of devices during patient transfer.
7. Provide comfort measures, offer ordered analgesics for patients experiencing pain.	Pain can be a factor causing patients to exit bed; thus pain relief is essential. However, be cautious as opioids increase fall risk.
8. Interventions for patients at moderate-to-high risk for falling (based on fall risk assessment):	
a. Prioritize call-light responses to patients at high risk, using team approach with all staffing knowing responsibility to respond.	Ensures rapid response by health care provider when patient calls for help.
b. Establish elimination schedule, using bedside commode when appropriate.	Proactive toileting keeps patients from being unattended with sudden urge to use toilet.

Clinical Decision Point *Toileting is a common event leading to a patient's fall (Berry and Kiel, 2016).*

STEP	RATIONALE
c. Stay with patient during toileting (standing outside bathroom door).	Patients often try to get up to stand and walk back to their beds from the bathroom without help.
d. Place patient in geri chair or wheelchair with wedge cushion. Use wheelchair only for transport, not for sitting an extended time.	Maintains alignment and comfort and makes it difficult to exit chair.
e. Use low bed that has low height above floor and apply floor mats.	Reduces fall-related injuries.
f. Activate bed alarm for patient.	Alarm activates when patient rises off sensor. Alarm sounds alert to staff.
g. Confer with physical therapy on feasibility of gait training, strength and balance training, and regular weight-bearing activities.	Exercise can reduce falls, fall-related fractures, and several risk factors for falls in individuals with low bone density and older adults (Schubert, 2011). Strength and balance training has been shown to reduce the rate of injurious falls in older adults (Uusi-Rasi et al., 2015).
h. Use sitters or restraints only when alternatives are exhausted.	A sitter is a nonprofessional staff member or volunteer who stays in a patient room to closely observe patients who are at risk for falling. Restraints should be used only as final option (see Skill 14.2).
9. When ambulating patient, have patient wear a gait belt or walking sling and walk along his or her side (see Chapter 12).	Safe patient-handling techniques (e.g., use of walking sling/gait belt) allows for safe patient ambulation and prevention of injury to you and patient.
10. Safe use of wheelchair:	
a. Be sure that wheelchair is correct fit for patient: Patient thighs are level while sitting, feet flat on floor; back of chair comes up to mid shoulder, elbows rest on armrests without leaning over or tucking arms in, and two fingers of space between patient and side of chair.	Correctly fitted chair promotes comfort, making it less likely for patient to try to exit it.
b. Transfer patient to wheelchair.	
(1) Determine level of help needed to transfer patient to wheelchair. Position wheelchair on same side of bed as patient's strong or unaffected side (see Chapter 11).	Patient's condition may require more than a one-person assist. Positioning of chair facilitates patient's ability to help in transfer.
(2) Place wedge cushion in chair (see illustration).	Prevents patient from slipping out of chair.
(3) Securely lock brakes on both wheels when transferring patient into or out of wheelchair.	Keeps chair steady and secure.
(4) Raise footplates before transfer to chair; then lower footplates, placing patient's feet on them after he or she is seated.	Prevents tripping over footplate.

STEP	RATIONALE
(5) Have patient sit with buttocks well back in seat. *Option:* Apply quick-release seat belt.	Prevents patient from sliding out of chair.
(6) Back wheelchair into and out of elevator or door, leading with large rear wheels first (see illustration).	Prevents smaller front wheels from catching in crack between elevator and floor, causing chair to tip.
c. Manage patient's pain and do not allow him or her to sit in wheelchair an extended amount of time; provide alternative sitting option.	Reduces restlessness and discomfort that can lead to wheelchair exit.
11. Remove unnecessary supplies. Perform hand hygiene.	Reduces transmission of microorganisms.

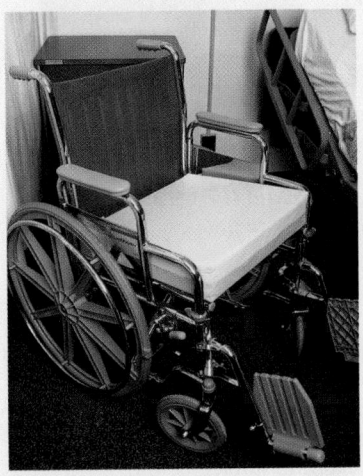

STEP 10b(2) Wheelchair with footplates raised and wedge cushion in place.

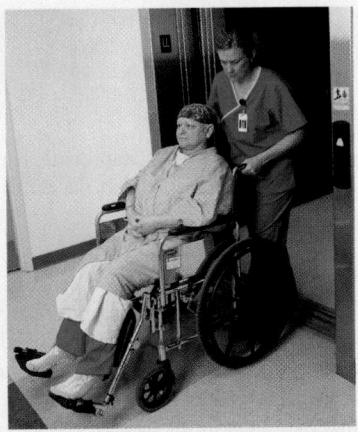

STEP 10b(6) Nurse backing wheelchair into elevator.

EVALUATION

1. Ask patient/family caregiver to identify patient's fall risks.	Demonstrates learning.
2. Ask patient/family caregiver to describe fall prevention interventions that are implemented.	Demonstrates learning.
3. Evaluate patient's ability to use assistive devices such as walker or bedside commode.	Adjustments in devices may become necessary.
4. Evaluate for changes in motor, sensory, and cognitive status and review if any falls or injuries have occurred.	May require different interventions to be added. Fall outcomes determine success of plan.
5. Use Teach-Back: "I want to be sure I explained clearly to you (example) why you are more likely to fall than other patients. Tell me some of those reasons." Revise your instruction now or develop plan for revised patient or family caregiver teaching if patient or family caregiver is not able to teach back correctly.	Determines patient's and family caregiver's level of understanding of instructional topic.

Unexpected Outcomes	**Related Interventions**
1. Patient/family caregiver unable to identify fall risks or fall prevention strategies.	• Reinforce identified risks with patient and review safety measures with family caregiver.
2. Patient starts to fall while ambulating with nurse or other caregiver.	• Put both arms around patient's waist or grasp gait belt.
	• Stand with feet apart to provide broad base of support.
	• Extend one leg and let patient slide against it to floor (Fig. 14.2A).
	• Bend knees and lower body as patient slides to floor (see Fig. 14.2B).
	• Call for assistance.
3. Patient found after falling.	• Assess patient for injury and stay with him or her until help arrives.
	• Notify primary health care provider and family caregiver.
	• Complete an agency occurrence or sentinel event report (see agency policy)
	• Evaluate patient's environment and risk factors; revise fall prevention plan as needed.

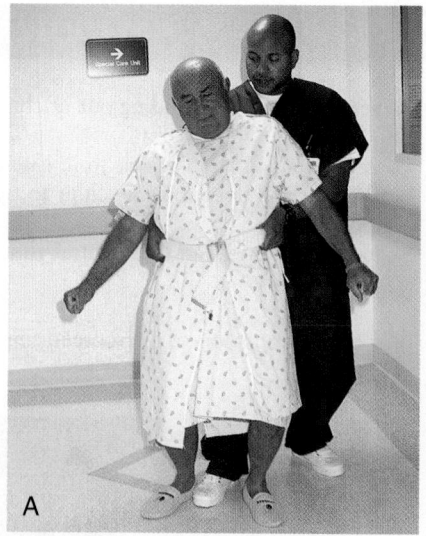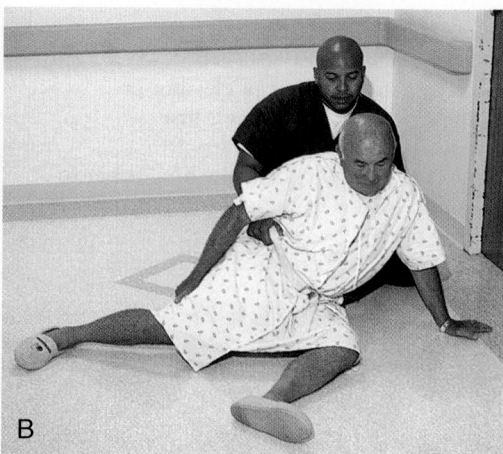

FIG 14.2 A, Stand with feet apart to provide broad base of support; extend one leg against which patient can slide to floor. **B,** Bend knees and lower body as patient slides to floor.

Recording and Reporting

- Record fall risk assessment findings, specific interventions used to prevent falls, and patient's response to teach-back in care plan on flow sheet or in nurses' notes in electronic health record (EHR) or chart.
- Report to health care personnel specific risks to patient's safety and measures taken to minimize risks.
- Document your evaluation of patient and family caregiver learning.
- If a fall occurs, document a description of the fall as given by patient or you as witness. Be sure to include baseline assessment, any injuries noted, tests or treatments given, follow-up care, and additional safety precautions taken after fall. Complete an agency adverse event report.

Special Considerations
Teaching

- The website for the Centers for Disease Control and Prevention (CDC, 2013) has educational resources on fall prevention for older adults and family caregivers at http://www.cdc.gov/Features/OlderAmericans/.
- Encourage patients to have annual vision and hearing examinations. Adaptive devices such as a hearing aid or glasses are sometimes necessary or need modification.
- Emphasize to patients the need to always look ahead when ambulating and use good posture.
- Teach patients how to use assistive devices and keep them in good repair.

Pediatric

- Encourage parents to follow these CDC (2016) recommendations for the home:
  - *Play safely.* Be sure that playground equipment that a child uses is designed and maintained properly and that there is a safe, soft landing surface below.
  - *Make your home safer.* Use home safety devices such as guards on windows that are above ground level, stair gates, and guard rails.
  - *Keep sports safe.* Be sure that a child wears protective gear such as wrist guards, knee and elbow pads, and a helmet for biking or skating when playing active sports.
  - *Supervision is key.* Supervise young children at all times around fall hazards, whether at home or out to play.
- Keep side rails of hospital beds down to allow toddlers and preschoolers easy exit and decrease the need to crawl over the rails (Hockenberry and Wilson, 2015).
- When caring for infants, keep a hand on a child when you turn away from the bedside.

Gerontological

- Interventions to improve balance confidence has shown benefits, including multicomponent behavioral group interventions and exercise (including tai chi), which increases lower body strength and dynamic balance (Bula et al., 2011).

Home Care
- See Chapter 43.

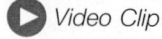 **SKILL 14.2**   **Designing a Restraint-Free Environment**

▶ *Video Clip*   **NSO** *Nursing Skills Online Safety Module / Lesson 1*

A physical restraint is any manual method, physical or mechanical device (such as full set of side rails), material, or equipment that immobilizes or reduces the ability of a patient to move his or her arms, legs, body, or head freely (TJC, 2015). Chemical restraints are medications such as anxiolytics and sedatives used to manage a patient's behavior and are not a standard treatment or dosage for a patient's condition. A restraint does not include devices such as orthopedically prescribed devices, surgical dressings or bandages, protective helmets, or other methods that involve physically holding a patient to conduct routine physical examinations or tests, protecting the patient from falling out of bed, or permitting a patient to participate in activities without the risk of physical harm (TJC, 2015).

Because physical and chemical restraints restrict a patient's physical activity or normal access to the body, serious and often fatal complications can develop, especially when patients try to get out of restraints. Current federal and state regulations have standards for restraint use (see Skill 14.3). Creating a restraint-free environment allows you to have interventions in place to reduce wandering and risk of patient falls. *A restraint-free environment is the first goal of care for all patients.*

Patients at risk for falls or wandering present special safety challenges. Wandering is the meandering, aimless, or repetitive locomotion that exposes a patient to harm and is often in conflict with boundaries, limits, or obstacles (NANDA, 2014). It is a common problem in patients who are confused or disoriented (e.g., patients with dementia). Interrupting a wandering patient can increase his or her distress. Wandering is a persistent problem in long-term care settings. Common strategies to manage wandering include environmental adaptations, use of signaling tags, distraction, social interaction, regular exercise, and circular design of a patient care unit. More frequent observation of patients, involvement of family during visitation, and frequent reorientation are also helpful measures.

Delegation and Collaboration

The skills of assessing patient behaviors and orientation to the environment and determining the type of restraint-free interventions to use cannot be delegated to nursing assistive personnel (NAP). Actions for promoting a safe environment can be delegated to NAP. The nurse directs the NAP about:

- Using specific diversional or activity measures for making the environment safe.
- Applying appropriate alarm or monitoring devices.
- Reporting patient behaviors and actions (e.g., confusion, getting out of bed unassisted, combativeness) to the nurse.

Equipment

- Visual or auditory stimuli (e.g., calendar, clock, radio, photos, MP3 player, television)
- Diversional activities (e.g., puzzle, game, audiobooks, DVD)
- Wedge cushion
- Wrap-around belt
- *Options:* Electronic bracelet or pressure pad alarm sensor; bed enclosure system

STEP	RATIONALE

ASSESSMENT

1. Assess patient's medical history for dementia, depression, and following conditions: are considered dangerous to self or others; are gravely disabled as result of mental disorder; lack cognitive ability (either permanently or temporarily) to make relevant decisions; or have physical limitations that increase their risk.

Wandering is commonly associated with these conditions (Cipriani et al., 2014, Stewart et al., 2014).

2. Assess patient's behavior (e.g., orientation, level of consciousness, ability to understand and follow directions, combative behaviors, restlessness, agitation), balance, gait, vision, hearing, bowel/bladder routine, level of pain, electrolyte and blood count values, and presence of orthostatic hypotension.

Accurate assessment identifies patients with safety risks and the physiological causes for patient behaviors that prompt caregivers to use restraints. Ensures proper selection of nonrestraint interventions.

3. Review over-the-counter (OTC) and prescribed medications (see Skill 14.1) that pose risk for falling. Assess for interactions and untoward effects.

Medication interactions or side effects often contribute to falling or altered mental status.

4. Assess patient's or family caregiver's knowledge of condition and prescribed treatments.

Knowledge of treatment protocols and rationales increases patient's cooperation.

5. For patients who wander or have known dementia, assess for cognitive decline using Mini-Mental State Examination (MMSE) (see Chapter 6).

Determines cause and nature of wandering, which leads to effective intervention selection.

6. Assess degree of wandering behavior using Algase Wandering Scale Version 2 (AWS-V2) (Martin et al., 2015; Nelson and Algase, 2007).

The AWS-V2 is a valid and reliable measure overall and for persistent walking, spatial disorientation, and eloping behavior subscales.

7. For patient with dementia, ask family or friends about his or her usual communication style and cues to indicate pain, fatigue, hunger, need to urinate or defecate.

Enables you to use best method to determine patient needs, which often prompt wandering when need is unmet.

8. Inspect condition of any therapeutic medical devices.

Patients who become restless, agitated, or confused will attempt to remove medical devices and then become candidates for physical restraint.

STEP	RATIONALE

NURSING DIAGNOSES

- Deficient knowledge regarding need for restraint-free environment
- Risk for falls
- Risk for injury
- Risk for trauma
- Wandering

Related factors/Risk factors are individualized based on patient's condition or needs.

PLANNING

1. Expected outcomes following completion of procedure:
   - Patient is injury free and/or does not inflict injury on others while in restraint-free environment.
   - Patient does not remove a therapeutic medical device.

Restraints and/or alternatives are successful in reducing agitation and preventing injury.

IMPLEMENTATION

STEP	RATIONALE
1. Orient patient and family caregiver to surroundings, introduce to staff, and explain all treatments and procedures. Be sure that patient is able to read your name badge.	Promotes patient understanding and cooperation.
2. Assign same staff to care for patient as often as possible. Encourage family and friends to stay with patient. In some agencies volunteers are effective companions.	Increases familiarity with individuals in patient's environment, decreasing anxiety and restlessness. Companions are helpful and prevent patient from being alone.
3. Place patient in room that is easily accessible to caregivers, close to nurses' station.	Allows for frequent observation to reduce falls in high-risk patients.
4. Be sure that patient is wearing glasses, hearing aid, or other sensory-aid devices and that all are functioning.	Improves patient's level of orientation to environment.
5. Provide visual and auditory stimuli meaningful to patient (e.g., clock, calendar, radio/MP3 player [with patient's choice of music], television, and family pictures).	Orients patient to day, time, and physical surroundings. You must individualize stimuli for this to be effective.
6. Anticipate patient's basic needs (e.g., toileting, relief of pain, relief of hunger) as quickly as possible; conduct hourly rounds (TJC, 2014).	Providing basic needs in timely fashion decreases patient discomfort, anxiety, restlessness, and incidence of falls.
7. Provide scheduled ambulation, chair activity, and toileting (e.g., ask patient every hour during rounds about toileting needs). Organize treatments so patient has uninterrupted periods throughout the day.	Regular opportunity to void avoids risk of patient trying to reach bathroom alone. Provides for sleep and rest periods. Constant activity overstimulates patients.
8. Position intravenous (IV) catheters, urinary catheters, and tubes/drains out of patient view. Use camouflage by wrapping IV site with bandage or stockinette. Place undergarments on patient with urinary catheter or cover abdominal feeding tubes/drains with loose abdominal binder.	Maintains medical treatment and reduces patient access to tubes/lines.
9. Decrease wandering: Eliminate stressors from environment such as cold at night, changes in daily routines, and extra visitors.	Reduced stress allows patient's energy to be channeled more appropriately.
10. Use stress-reduction techniques such as back rub, massage, and guided imagery (see Chapter 16).	Reduces level of anxiety and restlessness.
11. Use diversional activities: puzzles, games, music therapy, pet therapy, activity apron, performing purposeful activity (e.g., folding towels, drawing/coloring). Be sure that it is an activity in which patient has interest. Involve family member caregiver (if appropriate).	Meaningful diversional activities provide distraction, help to reduce boredom, and provide tactile stimulation. Minimize occurrences of wandering.
12. Position patient on wedge cushion and apply wraparound belt (see illustration).	Cushion prevents slipping in chair and makes it difficult for patient to get out of chair without help. Wraparound belt allows patient to lift flap for self-release.

STEP	**RATIONALE**

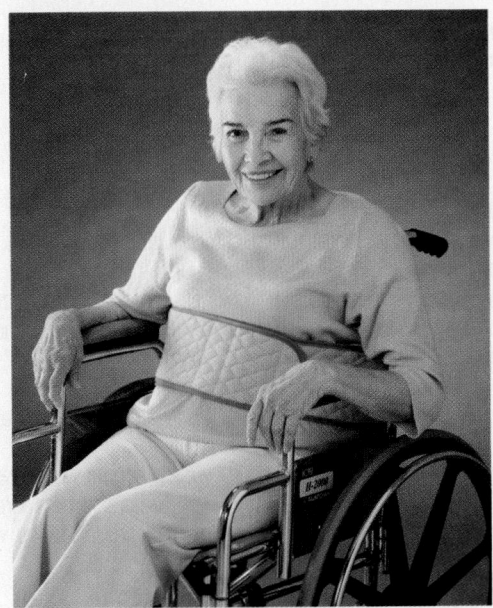

STEP 12 Wraparound belt. (*Courtesy Posey Company, Arcadia, CA.*)

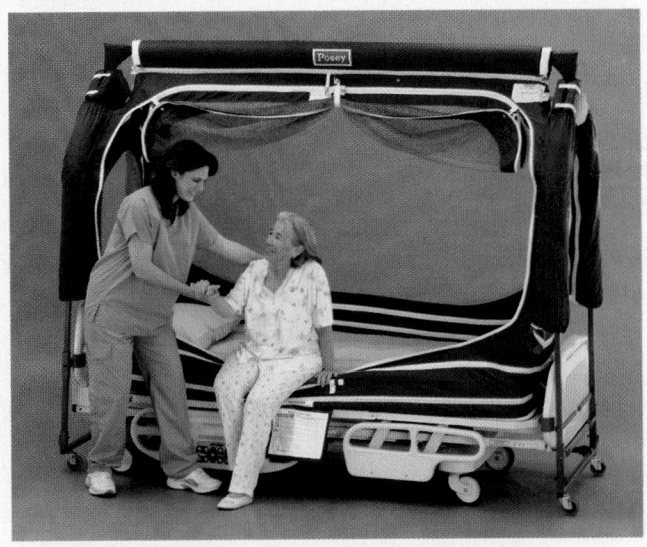

STEP 15 Bed enclosure system.

13. Use pressure-sensitive bed or chair pad with alarms:

    a. Explain use of device to patient and family caregiver.
    b. When in bed, position device so it is correctly positioned under patient's mid-to-low back or buttocks.

    c. Test alarm by applying and releasing pressure.

14. Place electronic monitoring bracelet on wrist of patient with dementia.

15. Place wandering patient in bed enclosure system (see illustration).

16. Consult with physical, speech, and occupational therapy for activities that provide stimulation and exercise.

17. Minimize invasive treatments (e.g., tube feedings, blood sampling) as much as possible.

Alarms alert staff to patient who is standing or rising from bed or chair without help.

Alarm activates sooner if placed under patient's back. By the time buttocks are off, sensor patient may be almost out of bed.
Ensures that alarm is audible through call-light system.
Tag in bracelet contains radio-frequency circuit that communicates with detection sensor usually installed at an exit door or elevator. Distance between tag and monitor is constantly measured with an alarm, which sounds when predetermined distance is exceeded.
Restraint alternative that allows patient freedom of movement within protected environment.
Involvement in meaningful and purposeful activities reduces tendency to wander. Exercise improves balance and coordination.
Stimuli increase patients' restlessness.

EVALUATION

1. Monitor patient's behavior routinely.

2. Observe patient for any injuries.
3. Observe patient's behavior toward staff, visitors, and other patients.

Will determine if agitation, wandering, or attempt to remove medical devices has been prevented.
Patient should be injury free.
Ensures that patient's behavior does not cause injury to others.

STEP	RATIONALE
4. Use Teach-Back: "We've talked about what we are doing to reduce your husband's wandering. Tell me ways you can help. I want to be sure you understand." Revise your instruction now or develop plan for revised family caregiver teaching if family caregiver is not able to teach back correctly.	Determines family caregiver's level of understanding of instructional topic.

Unexpected Outcomes

1. Patient displays behaviors that increase risk for injury to self or others.

2. Patient sustains injury or is agitated and places others at risk for injury.

3. Patient wanders away from health care agency.

Related Interventions

- Review episodes for pattern (e.g., activity, time of day) that indicates alternatives that would eliminate behavior.
- Discuss with all caregivers and family alternative interventions.
- Notify health care provider. Complete incident or occurrence report according to agency policy.
- Identify alternative measures for safety or behavioral control.
- Apply physical restraint (see Skill 14.3) only after all other interventions are unsuccessful.
- Be prepared to follow agency policy, which should include: whom to notify; who will search for patient; which areas will be searched and their priority; who will notify authorities, if necessary; who will notify family members; who will coordinate search efforts.

Recording and Reporting

- Record restraint alternatives used, patient behaviors that relate to cognitive status, and interventions to mediate these behaviors in nurses' notes in electronic health record (EHR) or chart.
- Document your evaluation of family caregiver learning.

Special Considerations
Teaching

- Teach family caregiver ways to involve patient in their visits, keeping patient appropriately stimulated.
- Teach the family caregiver how to adapt the home environment (see Chapter 43) to minimize wandering.

Gerontological

- Keep older adults active and ambulatory to increase endurance and function.
- Reminiscence helps older adults remain oriented.

Home Care

- Patients at risk for self-injury or violence to others need intensive supervision. Family members and home health caregivers need to recognize this and take appropriate preventive measures.
- Have family caregiver set up an area in the home where it is safe for an older adult to wander.

◆ SKILL 14.3   Applying Physical Restraints

▶ *Video Clip*   **NSO** *Nursing Skills Online Safety Module / Lesson 2*

In health care settings restraints are most commonly used to prevent the disruption of therapy. Restraint use is more common in critical care settings, where patients who are seriously ill often unknowingly attempt to remove endotracheal tubes, intravenous (IV) catheters, urinary catheters, and feeding tubes (AHRQ, 2013b). Unplanned removal of endotracheal tubes has been found to be associated with agitation, inadequate sedation, and reduced patient surveillance by health care staff (Kiekkas et al., 2013). Nurses often pursue orders for restraints when they are concerned that disruption of therapy can significantly injure patients. There are approaches to use to better secure medical devices and prevent accidental removal without using restraints (Box 14.2). The use of physical and chemical restraints in long-term care has been associated with concerns about patient behaviors (e.g., wandering and aggression) and fall risks and a shortage of nurse staffing (fewer staff to monitor patient safety).

The Centers for Medicare and Medicaid (CMS, 2015a) and The Joint Commission (TJC, 2015) have standards for reducing the use of restraints in health care settings and using them only with extreme caution. In 2011 the National Quality Forum (NQF) released its National Voluntary Consensus Standards for Public Reporting of Patient Safety Events (NQF, 2011). The NQF has endorsed a select list of serious reportable events, one of which is patient death or serious disability associated with the use of restraints or bedrails while being cared for in a health care agency.

The CMS (2015b) released revisions to the interpretive guidelines for the safe use of restraints in hospitals and defining patients' rights and choices regarding restraints. It requires that a restraint be used only under the following circumstances: (1) to ensure the immediate physical safety of the patient, a staff member, or others; (2) when less restrictive interventions have been ineffective; (3) in accordance with a written modification to the patient's plan of care; (4) when it is the least restrictive intervention that will be effective to protect a patient, staff member, or others from harm; (5) in accordance with safe and appropriate restraint techniques as determined by hospital policies; and (6) when it is discontinued at the earliest possible time.

Strategies for Reducing Accidental Removal of Medical Devices

Endotracheal Tube
- Verification of security of system used to anchor tube (see Chapter 25)
- Appropriate sedation and analgesia protocols to reduce agitation

Nasogastric Tube
- If being used for feeding, consult with nutritionist and speech therapist for swallow evaluation to consider gastrostomy feeding or other appropriate feeding measures.
- Anchor tubing by taping technique or commercial holder (see Chapter 32).

Intravenous Lines
- Use commercial holder for anchoring.
- Provide long-sleeved robes or commercial sleeves for arms to cover IV catheter site.
- Consider saline lock and cover with gauze (see Chapter 29).
- Tape or secure IV line under gown.
- Keep IV bag out of visual field.

Bladder Indwelling Catheter
- Consider intermittent catheterization (see Chapter 34).

Adapted from Agency for Healthcare Research and Quality (AHRQ): National guidelines clearinghouse: physical restraints and side rails in acute and critical care settings. In AHRQ: *Evidence-based geriatric nursing protocols for best practice*, Rockville, MD, 2013b, AHRQ. http://www.guideline.gov/content.aspx?id=43934. Accessed March 26, 2016.
IV, Intravenous.

Restraints are a temporary way to keep patients safe. However, there is no evidence that they prevent falls, reduce wandering, or prevent medical devices from being pulled out. Research has shown that patients suffer fewer injuries if left unrestrained (Knox and Holloman, 2012). The use of mechanical or physical restraints requires a licensed health care provider's order and must be based on a face-to-face patient assessment. A patient's or family caregiver's informed consent is necessary in the long-term care setting.

The use of restraints is associated with serious complications, including pressure injuries, hypostatic pneumonia, constipation, incontinence, and death. The Food and Drug Administration (FDA) regulates restraints as medical devices and requires manufacturers to label them "prescription only." Most patient deaths in the past have resulted from strangulation from a vest or jacket restraint. Numerous agencies no longer use vest restraints. For these reasons this text does not describe their use.

Delegation and Collaboration

The skills of assessing a patient's behavior and level of orientation, the need for restraints, the appropriate restraint type, and the ongoing assessments required while a restraint is in place cannot be delegated to nursing assistive personnel (NAP). Applying and routinely checking a restraint can be delegated to NAP. TJC (2009) requires training in first aid for anyone who monitors patients in restraints. The nurse directs the NAP by:
- Reviewing correct placement of the restraint and how to routinely check the patient's circulation, skin condition, and breathing.
- Reviewing when and how to change a patient's position and provide range-of-motion (ROM) exercises, toileting, and skin care.
- Instructing NAP to notify nurse immediately if there is a change in level of patient agitation, skin integrity, circulation of extremities, or patient's breathing.

Equipment
- Proper restraint (e.g., belt, wrist, mitten)
- Padding (if needed)

STEP	RATIONALE

ASSESSMENT

1. Identify patient using at least two identifiers (e.g., name and birthday or name and medical record number) according to agency policy.

Ensures correct patient. Complies with The Joint Commission standards and improves patient safety (TJC, 2016).

2. Assess for underlying cause(s) of agitation and cognitive impairment leading to patient-initiated medical device removal (Bradas et al., 2012):
   a. Assess for life-threatening physiological impairments.

Physiological alterations might lead to accidental patient-initiated medical device removal (AHRQ 2013b; Bradas et al., 2012). Identification of conditions might lead to more appropriate medical or pharmacological treatment, eliminating need for restraints (see Skill 14.2).

   b. Assess for respiratory, neurological, fever and sepsis, hypoglycemia and hyperglycemia, alcohol or substance withdrawal, and fluid and electrolyte imbalance.
   c. Notify health care provider of change in mental status and compromised physiological status.
   d. Obtain baseline or premorbid cognitive function from family caregivers.

Family caregivers provide excellent source of information for patient's behavior patterns and past history.

   e. Establish whether patient has history of dementia or depression.
   f. Review medications that cause risk for falling to identify drug-drug interactions, adverse effects.
   g. Review current laboratory values.

STEP	RATIONALE
3. Assess patient's current behavior (e.g., confusion, disorientation, agitation, restlessness, combativeness, inability to follow directions or repeated removal of tubing, dressing, or other therapeutic devices). Does patient create a risk to other patients?	If patient's behavior continues despite treatment or restraint alternatives, use of restraint is indicated. You will use the least restrictive type of restraint.
4. If restraint alternatives failed earlier, confer with health care provider. Review agency policies and state laws regarding restraints. Obtain current health care provider's order. Order must include purpose, type, location, and time or duration of restraint. Determine if signed consent for use of restraint is necessary (long-term care). Orders may be renewed according to time limits for a maximum of 24 consecutive hours (TJC, 2015).	A health care provider's order for least restrictive type of restraint is required. (TJC, 2015).

Clinical Decision Point *A licensed independent health care provider responsible for the care of the patient evaluates the patient in person within 1 hour of the initiation of restraint used for the management of violent or self-destructive behavior that jeopardizes the physical safety of the patient, staff, or others. A registered nurse or a physician assistant may conduct the in-person evaluation if he or she is trained in accordance with the requirements and consults with the above health care provider after the evaluation as determined by hospital policy (TJC, 2015). Always use the least restrictive restraint possible (e.g., mitts, elbow extenders) (AHRQ, 2013b; CMS, 2015b).*

5. Review manufacturer instructions for restraint application before entering patient's room. Determine most appropriate size restraint.	You need to be familiar with all devices used for patient care and protection. Incorrect application of restraint device results in patient injury or death.

NURSING DIAGNOSES

- Risk for injury
- Risk for trauma

Risk factors are individualized based on patient's condition or needs.

PLANNING

1. Expected outcomes following completion of procedure:	
• Patient maintains intact skin integrity, pulses, temperature, color, and sensation of restrained body part.	Restraints applied and monitored correctly.
• Patient is free from injury.	Restraints removed in a timely manner.
• Patient's therapy (e.g., intravenous [IV] tube, catheters) is uninterrupted.	Disruption of therapy causes patient injury, pain, or discomfort and increases risk of infection.
• Patient maintains self-esteem and sense of dignity.	Physical restraints have detrimental effect on psychosocial well-being of patient.
• Restraint is discontinued as soon as possible.	Limits period of time patient is at risk for injury.
2. Gather equipment and perform hand hygiene.	Promotes organization and reduces transmission of microorganisms.
3. Explain what you plan to do and why. Provide privacy.	Reduces patient anxiety and promotes cooperation.

IMPLEMENTATION

1. Adjust bed to proper height and lower side rail on side of patient contact. Be sure that patient is comfortable and in proper body alignment.	Allows you to use proper body mechanics and prevents injury during restraint application. Positioning prevents contractures and neurovascular injury while restraint is in place.
2. Inspect area where restraint is to be placed. Note if there is any nearby tubing or device. Assess condition of skin, sensation, adequacy of circulation, and range of joint motion.	Restraints sometimes compress and interfere with functioning of devices or tubes. Assessment provides baseline to monitor patient's response to restraint.
3. Pad skin and bony prominences (as necessary) that will be under restraint.	Reduces friction and pressure from restraint to skin and underlying tissue.

STEP	RATIONALE

4. Apply proper-size restraint. **NOTE:** Refer to manufacturer directions.

   a. *Mitten restraint:* Thumbless mitten device restrains patient's hands. Place hand in mitten, being sure that Velcro strap is around wrist and not forearm (see illustration).

Prevents patient from dislodging or removing medical device, removing dressings, or scratching but allows greater movement than wrist restraint. It is considered a restraint alternative if untethered and patient is physically and cognitively able to remove it.

   b. *Elbow restraint (freedom splint):* Restraint consists of rigidly padded fabric that wraps around arm and is closed with Velcro. The upper end has a clamp that hooks to sleeve of patient's gown or shirt (see illustration). Insert arm so elbow joint rests against padded area, keeping joint extended.

Commonly used with infants and children to prevent elbow flexion (e.g., with IV line placed in antecubital fossa). Restraint keeps elbow extended, making it difficult to remove or disrupt a medical device.

   c. *Belt or body restraint:* Have patient in sitting position in bed. Apply belt over clothes, gown, or pajamas. Be sure to place restraint at waist, not chest or abdomen. Slot in belt may be positioned in front for limited movement or rear for increased movement. Remove wrinkles or creases in clothing. Bring ties through slots in belt. Help patient lie down in bed. Have patient roll to side and avoid applying belt too tightly. Ensure that straps secured to bedframe are snug so belt does not slide to sides of bed (see illustrations). *Option:* Apply restraint net if intent is to limit patient turning.

Restrains center of gravity and prevents patient from rolling off stretcher, sitting up while on stretcher, or from falling out of bed. Tight application interferes with ventilation if belt moves up over abdomen or chest.

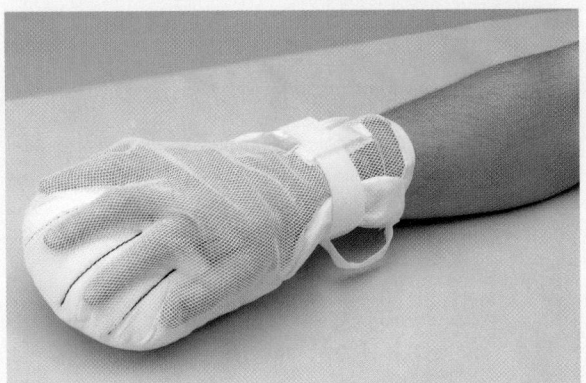

STEP 4a Mitten restraint. (*Courtesy Posey Company, Arcadia, CA.*)

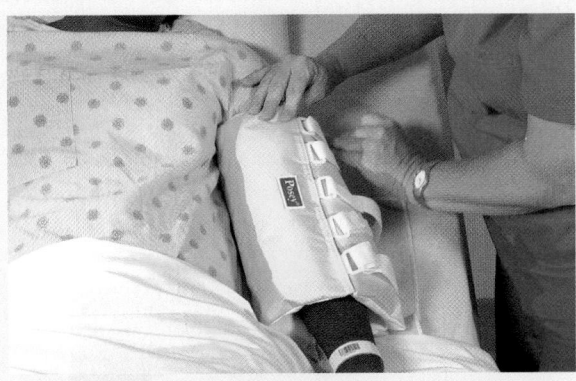

STEP 4b Freedom elbow restraint.

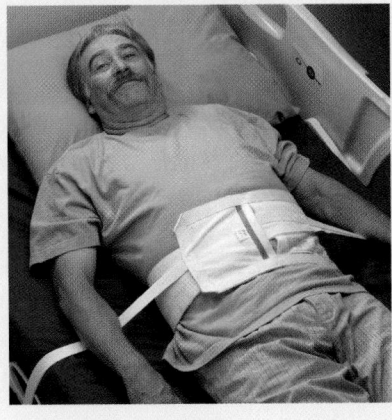 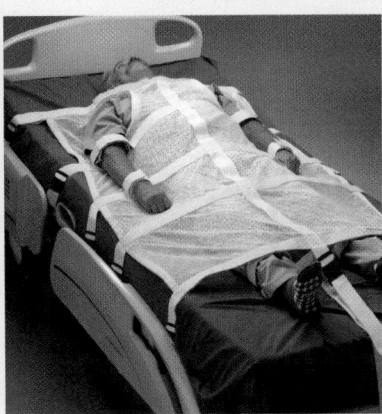

STEP 4c A, Properly applied belt restraint allows patient to turn in bed. **B,** *Option:* Restraint with net limits patient's ability to turn.

STEP	RATIONALE
d. *Extremity (ankle or wrist) restraint:* Restraint made of soft quilted material or sheepskin with foam padding. Wrap limb restraint around wrist or ankle with soft part toward skin and secure snugly (not tightly) in place by Velcro strap (see illustration). Insert two fingers under secured restraint (see illustration).	Restraint designed to immobilize one or all extremities. Maintain immobilization of extremity to protect patient from fall or accidental removal of therapeutic device (e.g., IV tube, Foley catheter). Tight application interferes with circulation and potentially causes neurovascular injury.

Clinical Decision Point *Patient with wrist and ankle restraints is at risk for aspiration if positioned supine. Place patient in lateral position or with head of bed elevated rather than supine.*

5. Attach restraint straps to part of bedframe that moves when raising or lowering head of bed. Be sure that straps are secure. *Do not attach to side rails.* Attach restraint to chair frame for patient in chair or wheelchair, being sure that buckle is out of patient's reach.	Properly positioned strap does not tighten and restrict circulation when bed is raised or lowered.
6. Secure restraints on bedframe with quick-release buckle (see illustration). *Do not tie strap in a knot.* Be sure that buckle is out of patient reach.	Allows for quick release in emergency.
7. Double-check and insert two fingers under secured restraint one more time. Assess proper placement of restraint, including skin integrity, pulses, skin temperature and color, and sensation of restrained body part.	Provides baseline to later evaluate if injury develops from restraint.
8. Remove restraint at least every 2 hours (TJC, 2015) or more frequently as determined by agency policy. Reposition patient, provide comfort and toileting measures, and evaluate patient condition each time. If patient is violent or noncompliant, remove one restraint at a time and/or have staff assistance while removing restraints.	Provides opportunity to attend to patient's basic needs and determine need for continuation.

Clinical Decision Point *Do not leave a patient who is violent or aggressive unattended while restraints are off.*

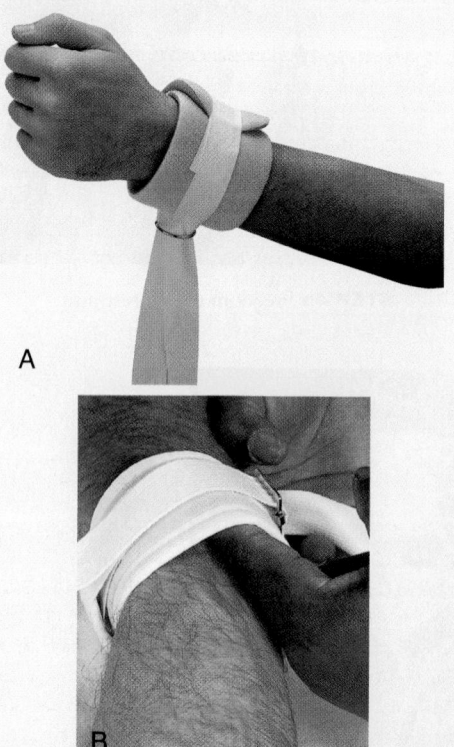

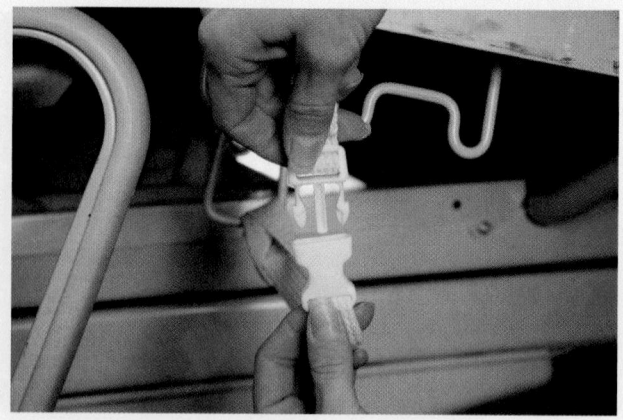

STEP 4d A, Extremity restraint. **B,** Check restraint for constriction by inserting two fingers under restraint.

STEP 6 Quick-release buckle makes it easier to disconnect and evacuate patients in an emergency.

STEP	RATIONALE

9. Secure call-light or intercom system within patient's reach.

Allows patient, family, or caregiver to get help quickly.

10. Leave bed or chair with wheels locked. Keep bed in lowest position.

Prevents bed or chair from moving if patient tries to get out. If patient falls with bed in lowest position, this reduces chance of injury.

11. Perform hand hygiene.

Reduces transmission of microorganisms.

EVALUATION

1. After application, evaluate patient for signs of injury every 15 minutes (e.g., circulation, vital signs, ROM, physical and psychological status, and readiness for discontinuation). Perform visual checks if patient is too agitated to approach (TJC, 2015).

Frequent evaluation prevents injury to patient and ensures removal of restraint at earliest possible time. Frequency of monitoring guides staff in determining appropriate intervals for evaluation based on patient's needs and condition, type of restraint used, risk associated with use of chosen intervention, and other relevant factors.

2. Evaluate patient's need for toileting, nutrition and fluids, hygiene, and elimination and release restraint at least every 2 hours.

Prevents injury to patient and attends to basic needs.

3. Evaluate patient for any complications of immobility.

Early detection of skin irritation, restricted breathing, or reduction in mobility prevents serious adverse events.

4. The licensed health care provider or registered nurse trained according to CMS requirements needs to evaluate patient within either 1 or 4 hours after initiation of restraints, depending on Medicare status of hospital (see agency policy).

Determines patient's immediate situation, reaction to restraints, medical and behavioral condition, and need to continue or terminate restraints.

5. After 24 hours, before writing a new order, health care provider who is responsible for patient's care must see and reassess patient.

Ensures that restraint application continues to be medically appropriate.

6. Observe IV catheters, urinary catheters, and drainage tubes to determine that they are positioned correctly and that therapy remains uninterrupted (see Box 14.2).

Reinsertion is uncomfortable and increases risk for infection or interrupts therapy.

7. Observe patient's behavior and reaction to presence of restraint.

Restraints can increase restlessness and agitation, resulting in harm.

8. **Use Teach-Back:** "We've talked about the reason we're using restraints on your father. Tell me that reason. I want to be sure you understand." Revise your instruction now or develop a plan for revised family caregiver teaching if family caregiver is not able to teach back correctly.

Determines family caregiver's level of understanding of instructional topic.

Unexpected Outcomes	Related Interventions
1. Patient experiences impaired skin integrity.	• Evaluate need for continued use of restraint and if alternatives can be used. • If restraint still needed, be sure that it is applied correctly and provide adequate padding. • Check skin under restraint for abrasions and remove restraints more often. Provide appropriate skin care and change wet or soiled restraints.
2. Patient becomes more confused or agitated.	• Determine cause of behavior and eliminate if possible; consult with health care provider. • Determine need for more or less sensory stimulation and make any stimulation meaningful. • Reorient as needed and try restraint-free options.
3. Patient has neurovascular injury (e.g., cyanosis, pallor, and coldness of skin or complains of tingling, pain, or numbness).	• Remove restraint immediately, stay with patient, and have health care provider notified. • Protect extremity from further injury.

Recording and Reporting

- Record nursing interventions and restraint alternatives tried on restraint flow sheet or in nurses' notes in electronic health record (EHR) or chart.
- Document your evaluation of family caregiver learning.
- Record purpose for restraint, type and location, time applied, time ending the restraint, and routine observations made every 15 minutes (e.g., skin color, pulses, sensation, vital signs, behavior) in the flow sheets or nurses' notes.
- Record patient's level of orientation and behavior after restraint application. Record times patient was evaluated, attempts to use alternatives, and patient's response when restraint was removed.

Special Considerations
Teaching

- Explain thoroughly to patient and family caregiver the use of restraints. Caution family caregiver against removing, repositioning, or retying restraint.

Pediatric

- Limit the use of restraints to clinically appropriate and adequately justified situations (e.g., examination or treatment that involves the head and neck) after using all appropriate alternatives. Remain with infant while restrained and remove restraint immediately after treatment is completed.

- When a child needs to be restrained for a procedure, it is best if the person applying the restraint is not the child's parent or guardian.
- When an infant or small child requires a restraint, a mummy wrap using a blanket or sheet effectively controls his or her movements (Hockenberry and Wilson, 2015).

Gerontological

- Restrained older adults often respond with anger, fear, depression, humiliation, demoralization, discomfort, and resignation.
- Consider the risks associated with restraints (e.g., pressure injuries, impaired strength and balance) for older adults (Touhy and Jett, 2014). All of the complications of immobility are amplified, leading to greater risk for functional decline.

Home Care

- A health care provider's order is needed for use of a restraint in the home. Provide clear, detailed instructions to the family caregiver, with a return demonstration of restraint application. Do not send a restraint home with family caregiver unless a device is necessary to protect patient from injury. Carefully assess the family caregiver for competency and understanding of intent for using restraint.

PROCEDURAL GUIDELINE 14.1 *Fire, Electrical, and Chemical Safety*

From 2006 to 2010 US fire departments responded to an estimated average of 6240 structure fires in or on health care properties per year with almost half (46%) at nursing homes and almost one quarter (23%) in hospitals or hospices (Ahrens, 2012). Most fires involve cooking equipment, but in hospital settings fires are typically electrical or anesthetic related. Smoking-related fires pose a significant risk because of unauthorized smoking in beds or bathrooms. In the home setting oxygen-related fires is a risk for patients requiring oxygen therapy (see Chapter 23). Health care agencies routinely check and maintain all electrical devices. Every biomedical device (e.g., suction machine, infusion pump) must have a safety inspection sticker with an expiration date applied to it. Electrical equipment in good working order requires a three-prong electrical plug for proper grounding. If a patient brings an electrical device to a hospital, an engineer must inspect the device for safe wiring and function before use. Always discourage patients from bringing nonessential electrical devices (e.g., hair dryers or electric toothbrushes) into a health care agency. Many patients with disabilities use battery chargers for mobility equipment function. These devices need to be inspected by hospital engineers as well. Prevention is the key to fire safety. Always comply with agency smoking policies, use equipment correctly, and keep combustible materials away from heat sources.

Chemicals in many medications (e.g., chemotherapy drugs), anesthetic gases, cleaning solutions, and disinfectants are potentially toxic. They injure the body after skin or mucous membrane (e.g., eyes) contact, ingestion, or vapor inhalation. Health care agencies provide employees access to a safety data sheet (SDS) (previously called material safety data sheet) for each hazardous chemical in the workplace (United States Department of Labor, 2015). An SDS form contains information about the properties of the particular chemical and handling the substance in a safe manner (Box 14.3).

BOX 14.3

Information Required on OSHA Safety Data Sheets

- **Identification**—Product identifier; manufacturer or distributor name, address, phone number; emergency phone number; recommended use; restrictions on use
- **Hazard(s)**—All hazards regarding the chemical; required label element
- **Composition/information on ingredients**—Chemical ingredients; trade secret claims
- **First-aid measures**—Symptoms/effects, acute, delayed; required treatment
- **Fire-fighting measures**—Suitable extinguishing techniques, equipment; chemical hazards from fire
- **Accidental release measures**—Emergency procedures; protective equipment; proper methods of containment and cleanup
- **Handling and storage**—Precautions for safe handling and storage, including incompatibilities
- **Exposure controls/personal protection**—OSHA's Permissible Exposure Limits (PELs) and any other exposure limit used or recommended by the chemical manufacturer, importer, or employer and appropriate engineering controls; personal protective equipment (PPE)
- **Physical and chemical properties**—Lists characteristics of chemical
- **Stability and reactivity**—Lists chemical stability and possibility of hazardous reactions
- **Toxicological information**—Routes of exposure; related symptoms, acute and chronic effects; numerical measures of toxicity

Adapted from United States Department of Labor: *OSHA quickcard: hazard communication safety data sheets*, 2015, https://www.osha.gov/Publications/HazComm_QuickCard_SafetyData.html. Accessed March 26, 2016. *OSHA*, Occupational Safety & Health Administration.

PROCEDURAL GUIDELINE 14.1 *Fire, Electrical, and Chemical Safety—cont'd*

Delegation and Collaboration

The skill of fire, electrical, and chemical safety can be delegated to nursing assistive personnel (NAP). A nurse leads the health care team in an emergency response. In the event of fire a nurse collaborates with the fire department. In the event of an electrical or chemical event the team collaborates with the safety officer of the agency. The nurse directs the NAP to:

- Identify patients requiring the most help to evacuate or protect.
- Be aware of any risks for chemical exposure.

Equipment
Fire
- Appropriate fire extinguisher for fire: type A, B, C, or ABC

Chemical
- Appropriate personal protective equipment: clean gloves, mask, gown
- SDS form

Procedural Steps

1. Review agency policies for rapid response to fire, electrical, and chemical emergency. Know your responsibilities such as initiating fire alarm and patient evacuation.
2. Know the location of fire alarms, emergency equipment (e.g., fire extinguishers), SDS forms, emergency eyewash stations, and emergency exit routes.
3. Assess patient's mental status and ability to ambulate, transfer, or move to anticipate the procedures that will be needed to evacuate him or her.
4. Be alert to situations that increase the risk of fire (e.g., a patient on oxygen charging a cell phone while in bed). Regularly check a patient room for electrical or fire hazards.
5. Know which patients are on oxygen. Oxygen delivery may be shut off in the event of a severe fire.
6. Inspect equipment for current maintenance sticker. Check electrical equipment for basic safety features (i.e., intact cords and plugs, intact casing). Know agency process for tagging and reporting broken or unsafe equipment.
7. **Fire safety:**
   a. Follow the acronym *RACE*.
      (1) **R**escue patient from immediate injury by removing from area or shielding from fire to avoid burns.
      (2) **A**ctivate fire alarm immediately. Follow agency policy for alerting staff to respond. (In many situations perform Steps (1) and (2) simultaneously by using call system to alert staff while you help patients at risk.)
      (3) **C**ontain the fire by:
         (a) Closing all doors and windows.
         (b) Turning off oxygen and electrical equipment.
         (c) Placing wet towels along base of doors.
      (4) **E**vacuate patients:
         (a) Direct ambulatory patients to walk by themselves to a safe area. Know the fire exits and emergency evacuation route.
         (b) If patient is on life support, maintain respiratory status manually (Ambu bag) until you remove him or her from fire area.

(c) Move bedridden patients by stretcher, bed, or wheelchair.
(d) For patients who cannot walk or ambulate use these options:
   (i) Place on blanket and drag patient out of area of danger.
   (ii) *Use two-person swing:* Place patient in sitting position and have two staff members form a seat by clasping forearms together. Lift patient into "seat" and carry out of area of danger (see illustrations A and B).

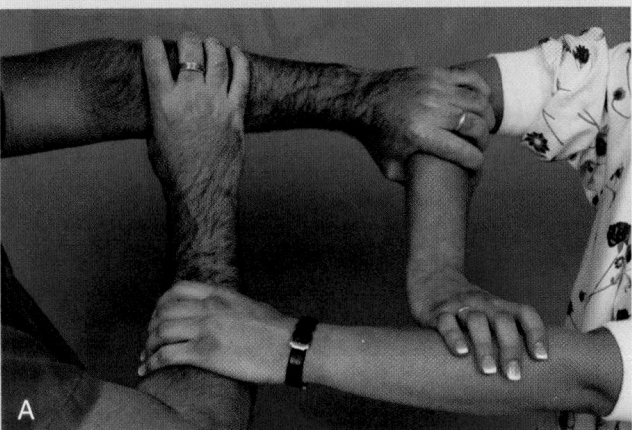

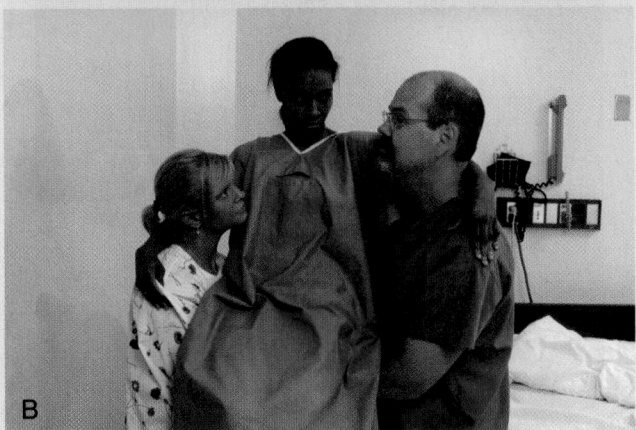

STEP 7a(4)(d)ii A, Hands positioned to form two-person evacuation swing. **B,** Patient seated firmly on swing and holding shoulders of nurses for evacuation.

Clinical Decision Point *Consider the patient's weight and size when choosing an evacuation carry. Use safe patient-handling techniques. Have a staff member help to avoid injury.*

   (e) If fire department personnel are on the scene, they will help with evacuation of patients.
   b. Extinguish fire using appropriate fire extinguisher: type A for ordinary combustibles (e.g., wood, cloth, paper, most plastics), type B for flammable liquids (e.g., gasoline, grease, paint, anesthetic gas), type C for

Continued

PROCEDURAL GUIDELINE 14.1 *Fire, Electrical, and Chemical Safety—cont'd*

electrical equipment, type ABC for any type of fire (most common extinguisher in use). To use an extinguisher, follow the acronym *PASS*.

(1) *P*ull the pin (see illustration A).
(2) *A*im nozzle at base of fire (see illustration B).
(3) *S*queeze extinguisher handles (see illustration C).
(4) *S*weep from side to side to coat area evenly.

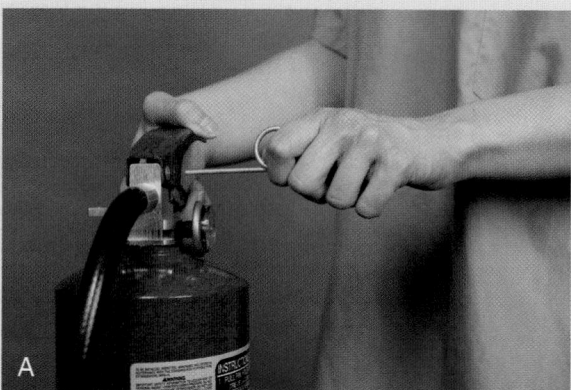

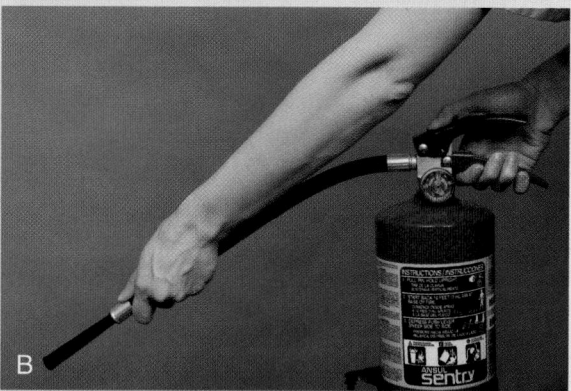

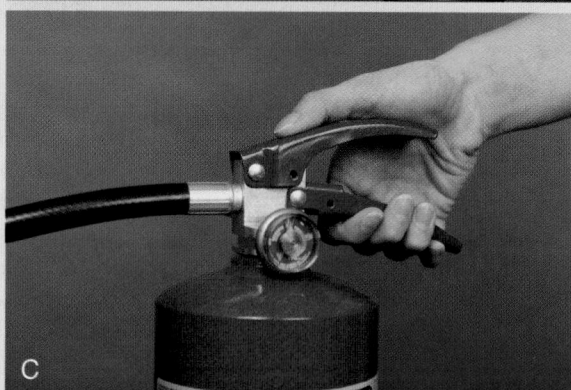

STEP 7b(1) A, Pull safety pin from fire extinguisher. **B,** Aim nozzle of hose at base of fire. **C,** Squeeze handle while sweeping side to side with nozzle.

c. Most agencies have fire doors that are held open by magnets and close automatically when a fire alarm sounds. Fire doors should never be blocked.

8. Electrical safety:
  a. If patient receives an electrical shock, immediately turn off power to electrical source and assess for presence of a pulse. *Caution:* When disengaging electrical source, check for presence of water on floor.

Clinical Decision Point *Do not touch a person who is being shocked while he or she is still engaged with the electrical source. If unable to turn off power, call emergency number for help.*

  b. Once the source of electricity is disconnected, provide appropriate assistance. If patient is pulseless, institute emergency resuscitation (see Chapter 28).
  c. Notify emergency personnel and patient's health care provider.
  d. If patient has a pulse and remains alert and oriented, obtain vital signs and assess the skin for signs of thermal injury.

9. Chemical safety:
  a. Attend to any person exposed to a chemical. Treat chemical splashes to the eyes immediately; flush eyes with water using clean, lukewarm tap water for 15 to 20 minutes; stand under a shower or place head under running faucet. Remove contact lenses if flushing does not remove them (see Chapter 19).
  b. Notify people in the immediate area of the spill and evacuate all nonessential personnel from area.
  c. Refer to SDS; if spilled material is flammable, turn off electrical and heat sources.
  d. Avoid breathing vapors of spilled material; apply appropriate respirator.
  e. Use appropriate personal protective equipment (refer to SDS) to clean up a spill.
  f. Dispose of any materials used in cleanup as hazardous waste.

10. Follow agency policy for reporting a sentinel event. Documentation will likely be made as a sentinel event report and not in nurses' notes in electronic health record (EHR) or chart.

◆ **SKILL 14.4** Seizure Precautions

Seizures are sudden, abnormal, electrical discharges in the brain causing alterations in behavior, sensation, or consciousness. Seizures that appear to begin everywhere in the brain at once are classified as generalized seizures, whereas seizures beginning in one location of the brain are classified as partial seizures (Johns Hopkins Medicine, 2015). There are three phases to a seizure:

- **Aura**—the start of a partial seizure. If the aura is the only phase a patient experiences, the patient has had a simple partial seizure. If the seizure spreads and affects consciousness, it is a complex partial seizure. If the seizure spreads to the rest of the brain, it becomes a generalized seizure.
- **Ictus**—meaning *attack* Ictus is another word for the physical seizure involving a series of muscle contractions, called *tonic* and *clonic contractions.*
- **Postictal**—meaning *after the attack.* Postictal refers to the aftereffects of a seizure (e.g., arm numbness, altered consciousness, partial paralysis).

Status epilepticus involves 5 minutes or more of either continuous clinical or electrographic (shown on an electroencephalogram [EEG]) seizure activity or recurrent seizure activity without recovery between seizures (Brophy et al., 2012). It is a medical emergency. Status epilepticus can be convulsive (rhythmic jerking of the extremities) or nonconvulsive (activity on EEG).

Traditionally patients who have a seizure are immediately placed in the side-lying position to prevent aspiration of oral secretions. This is still a standard of practice. However, the patient should be rolled gently into this position and only if possible without injuring any body part (Smith et al., 2015). Refer to your agency policy for positioning guidelines.

The current practice guidelines for patients with status epilepticus include the following (Brophy et al., 2012; Smith et al., 2015):

- Within first 2 minutes establish and protect the airway when patient loses consciousness.
- Provide noninvasive airway protection and gas exchange with head positioning, keeping the airway patent and administering oxygen (see Chapters 23 and 25).
- Measure vital signs: oxygen saturation, blood pressure, and heart rate immediately and every 2 minutes.

- Establish an intravenous (IV) route for emergency medications.
- When seizure begins to subside, intubation (insertion of an artificial airway) should be attempted only if gas exchange is compromised or if patient is believed to have increased intracranial pressure.

Delegation and Collaboration

The skill of assessing a patient's risk for seizures cannot be delegated to nursing assistive personnel (NAP). However, the skills for making a patient's environment safe and the ongoing care of patients on seizure precautions can be delegated. The nurse directs NAP about:

- The patient's prior seizure history and factors that may trigger a seizure.
- Taking immediate action in the event of a seizure by protecting the patient from falling or injury, not trying to restrain the patient, and not placing anything into the mouth.
- Informing the nurse immediately when seizure activity develops.
- Observing the patient's seizure pattern.

Equipment

- Seizure pads for side rails and headboard
- Suction machine and oral Yankauer suction catheter
- Oral airway
- Oxygen via nasal cannula or face mask
- Equipment for vital signs, pulse oximetry and blood glucose testing (see Chapter 5)
- Equipment for IV insertion (see Chapter 29)
- Emergency antiepileptic medications:
  - For emergent condition, IV lorazepam, midazolam for intramuscular (IM) administration (also nasal or buccal), rectal diazepam; for urgent treatment, oral valproate sodium or phenytoin, IV midazolam (Brophy et al., 2012; Smith et al., 2015)
- Clean gloves
- Equipment for vital signs, pulse oximetry, and blood glucose monitoring

STEP	RATIONALE

ASSESSMENT

1. Assess patient's seizure history (e.g., new diagnosis, seizure within last year), knowledge of precipitating factors (e.g., emotional stress, sleep deprivation), frequency of seizures, presence of aura (e.g., metallic taste, perception of breeze blowing on face, or noxious odor), body parts affected, and sequence of events if known. Use family as resource if necessary.

Knowledge about seizure history and nature of seizures allows you to eliminate triggers that cause seizure, anticipate onset of seizure activity, and take appropriate safety measures.

2. Assess for medical and surgical conditions, including history of head trauma, electrolyte disturbances (e.g., hypoglycemia, hyperkalemia), heart disease, excess fatigue, alcohol or caffeine consumption. Also assess for any bleeding tendencies.

Common conditions that lead to seizures or worsen existing seizure condition. Bleeding conditions could predispose patient to injury during seizure.

3. Assess medication history (e.g., antidepressants and antipsychotics). Assess for patient's adherence to anticonvulsants and therapeutic drug levels if test results available.

Certain medications lower seizure threshold. Seizure medications must be taken as prescribed and not stopped suddenly. Stopping or changing dose may precipitate seizure activity.

STEP	RATIONALE

4. Inspect patient's environment for potential safety hazards (e.g., extra furniture or equipment). Keep bed in low position, side rails up at head of bed.

Protects patient from injury sustained by striking head or body on furniture or equipment.

5. Assess patient's individual and cultural perspective about the meaning of seizures and their treatment.

Some cultures follow different caring practices for a person with seizures.

NURSING DIAGNOSES

- Deficient knowledge regarding seizure precautions
- Noncompliance
- Risk for aspiration
- Risk for injury
- Risk for ineffective airway clearance
- Situational low self-esteem

Related factors/Risk factors are individualized based on patient's condition or needs.

PLANNING

1. Expected outcomes following completion of procedure:
   - Patient remains free of traumatic injury while experiencing seizure.
   - Patient's airway remains patent during seizure activity.

   - Patient does not experience lowered sense of self-esteem following seizure episode.
2. Inform patient and appropriate family caregiver that patient is on seizure precautions.

Seizure precautions prevent patients from incurring injury from a fall or seizure.
Airway occlusion and aspiration are potential complications of seizure activity.
Loss of bowel or bladder control is common in generalized seizures, causing patient to feel embarrassment or shame.
May help to relieve patient and family caregiver anxiety.

IMPLEMENTATION

1. For patients with history of seizures, keep bed in lowest position with side rails up (see agency policy). Pad rails if patient is at risk for head injury. Have oral suction and oxygen equipment ready for use.

Modifications to environment minimize risk of injury from seizure activity or related fall. Use padded side rails only when patient is at risk for head injury (see illustration).

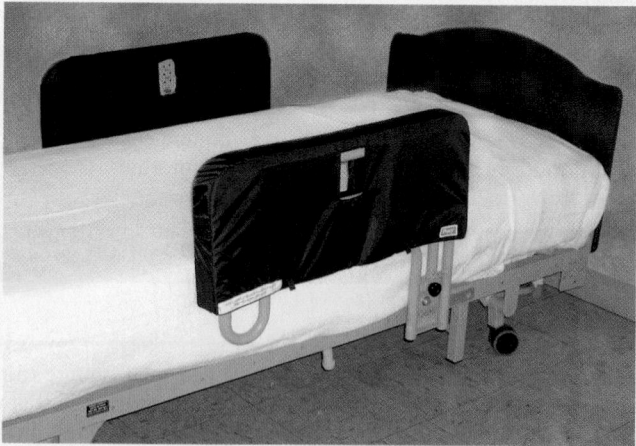

STEP 1 Padded side rails for patients at risk for head injury.

2. Place patient with history of seizures in room close to nurse's station or room with video monitor.

Improves likelihood of quick response with emergency equipment.

3. **Partial or general seizure response:**
   a. Position patient safely.
   (1) If patient is standing or sitting, guide him or her to floor and protect head by cradling in your lap or place pillow under head. Position patient so as to keep head tilted to maximize breathing (if able). Try to position patient on side *but do not force.* Do not lift patient from floor to bed during seizure.

Position protects patient from aspiration and traumatic injury, especially head injury.

STEP	RATIONALE
(2) If patient is in bed, turn him or her onto side (*do not force*) and raise side rails.	
b. Note time seizure began and call for help immediately to have staff member bring emergency cart to bedside and clear surrounding area of furniture. Provide airway protection and gas exchange by positioning head. Have health care provider notified immediately.	Timing and description of seizure may help in ultimate identification of type of seizure. Establishing and protecting airway when patient loses consciousness must occur in first 2 minutes (Brophy et al., 2012).
c. Keep patient in side-lying position (if possible), supporting head and keeping it flexed slightly forward.	Position prevents tongue from blocking airway and promotes drainage of secretions, reducing risk of aspiration.
d. Do not restrain patient; if patient is flailing limbs, hold them loosely. Loosen restrictive clothing/gown to aid breathing.	Prevents musculoskeletal injury. Promotes free ventilatory movement of chest and abdomen.
e. *Never force any object into patient's mouth* such as fingers, medicine, tongue depressor, or airway when teeth are clenched.	Prevents injury to mouth and possible aspiration.

Clinical Decision Point *Injury can result from forcible insertion of a hard object into the mouth. Soft objects break and become aspirated. Insert a bite block or oral airway in advance if you recognize the possibility of a generalized seizure.*

STEP	RATIONALE
f. If possible, provide privacy. Have staff control flow of visitors in area.	Embarrassment is common after a seizure, especially if others witnessed it.
g. Observe sequence and timing of seizure activity. Note type of seizure activity (tonic, clonic, staring, blinking); whether more than one type of seizure occurs; sequence of seizure progression; level of consciousness; character of breathing; presence of incontinence; presence of autonomic signs of lip smacking, mastication, or grimacing; rolling of eyes.	Continued observation helps to document, diagnose, and treat seizure disorder.
h. As patient regains consciousness, assess vital signs and reorient and reassure him or her. Explain what happened and answer patient's questions. Stay with patient until fully awake.	Informing patients of type of seizure activity experienced helps them to participate knowledgeably in their care. Some patients remain confused for period of time after seizure or become violent.
4. Status epilepticus is a medical emergency.	
a. Follow Steps 3a to 3c to stabilize airway and call emergency team.	Ensures rapid response and management of airway and breathing.
b. Assist health care provider with intubation (introduction of endotracheal tube or oral airway) (see Chapter 25) if oxygen saturation is compromised or elevated intracranial pressure is suspected (**NOTE:** Apply clean gloves if timing allows). Physician on team will intubate patient when jaw is relaxed (between seizure activity).	Medical emergency requires rapid response. Airway establishes oxygenation (Brophy et al., 2012; Smith et al., 2015).
c. Access and administer oxygen; turn on suction equipment; keep airway patent with oral suctioning (if possible).	Maintains oxygenation.

Clinical Decision Point *Never place hands in patient's mouth during a seizure. The patient may accidentally bite your fingers. Do not force any type of airway into mouth.*

STEP	RATIONALE
d. Have another nurse on team measuring blood pressure, heart rate, respirations, and oxygen saturation immediately and then every 2 minutes and have team member perform fingerstick to check blood glucose (Brophy et al., 2012; Smith et al., 2015).	Necessary to monitor and support baseline vital signs and determine if patient is hypoglycemic (common cause of seizure).
e. Member of team will prepare for and insert IV catheter (if one is not in place) with 0.9% sodium chloride infusing and administer IV antiseizure medications (see Chapter 29).	Provides route for IV medication to stop seizure and for fluid resuscitation (Brophy et al., 2012; Smith et al., 2015).
f. As seizure begins to subside, suction patient's airway if secretions have accumulated. If oral airway was inserted, be sure that it remains in correct position. Continue oxygen administration.	Maintains open airway and oxygenation.

STEP	RATIONALE
g. Keep patient in side-lying position of comfort in bed with side rails up and bed in lowest position.	Provides for continued safety to reduce risk of aspiration of secretions as patient regains consciousness and lessens risk of fall with injury if patient tries to exit bed.
5. As patient regains consciousness, reorient and reassure. Explain what happened and provide quiet, nonstimulating environment (e.g., lights low, minimal care interruptions). Place call-light or intercom system within reach. Instruct patient not to get out of bed without help.	Provides for continued safety. Patients are often confused and lethargic following seizure (postictal). At risk for falls if they attempt to get out of bed.
6. Clean up patient care area; dispose of used supplies. Perform hand hygiene.	Reduces transmission of microorganisms.

EVALUATION

1. Check vital signs and oxygen saturation every 15 minutes during postictal phase and maintain patent airway.	Determines patient's cardiopulmonary status and response to seizure episode.
2. Recheck blood glucose per health care provider order.	Determines if normal blood glucose level has been reached.
3. Examine patient for injury, including oral cavity (broken teeth, laceration of tongue or mucosa) and extremities.	Determines presence of any traumatic injuries resulting from seizure activity.

Clinical Decision Point *If onset of seizure was not witnessed and you suspect that patient fell and struck head, treat as a closed head injury or spinal injury. Place a cervical collar on patient before attempting to turn or reposition.*

4. Evaluate patient's mental status after seizure (level of consciousness, confusion, hallucinations). Encourage him or her to verbalize feelings.	Temporary mental status changes are common following seizure. Therapeutic interaction enables patient to recognize feelings associated with having a seizure disorder.
5. Help health care provider as needed conduct neurological examination of patient and collect any ordered blood tests (see Chapter 7).	Evaluates for any intracranial lesions, bleeding and life-threatening metabolic condition (Brophy et al., 2012; Smith et al., 2015).

Unexpected Outcomes	Related Interventions
1. Patient suffers traumatic injury.	• Continue to protect patient from further injury.
	• Notify health care provider immediately.
	• Administer prescribed treatments.
	• Reassess patient's environment to ensure that environment is free of safety hazards.
	• Complete agency adverse event report.
2. Patient aspirates oral secretions.	• Turn onto side, insert oral airway (if possible; see Chapter 25), and apply suction to remove material in oral pharynx and maintain patent airway.
	• Administer oxygen as needed per order.

Recording and Reporting

- Record in nurses' notes in electronic health record (EHR) or chart what you observed before, during, and after seizure. Provide detailed description of the type of seizure activity and sequence of events (e.g., presence of aura [if any], level of consciousness, vital signs and oxygen saturation, color, movement of extremities, incontinence, patient's status immediately following seizure, and time frame of events).
- Record treatments administered: establishment of IV line, fluid infusing, stabilization of airway.
- Alert health care provider immediately as seizure begins. Status epilepticus is an emergency situation requiring immediate medical therapy.

Special Considerations
Teaching

- Inform an adult with an unprovoked first seizure that his or her seizure recurrence risk is greatest early within the first 2 years (21%–45%). The patient's physician is likely to order immediate antiepileptic drug (AED) therapy to reduce recurrence risk within the first 2 years (Krumholz et al., 2015).
- Patients need to know that antiseizure medications help control epilepsy. Warn them to take prescribed medications regularly. They should never stop medications suddenly because this precipitates seizures.
- Advise patient to avoid alcohol, which is often incompatible with anticonvulsive medications and intensifies central nervous system depression.

- Proper oral hygiene and frequent dental care are necessary when patient takes phenytoin long term because gingival hyperplasia is a side effect.
- Encourage patient to wear a medical alert bracelet or carry identification card noting presence of seizure disorder and listing medications taken.
- Fatigue, stress, and illness can potentiate seizures. Teach patients to eat a balanced diet regularly, get adequate sleep, and consult their health care provider promptly when ill.
- A seizure disorder usually imposes driving limitations. It is recommended that a waiting period of 1 seizure-free year elapses before patient attempts to drive or operate dangerous equipment (see individual state law).

Pediatric

- Teach parents for what to observe in their child's seizure.
- Child should wear a medical alert bracelet noting presence of a seizure disorder.
- Encourage children with severe atonic seizures (abrupt loss of muscle tone, often dropping to floor) to wear helmets to protect them when they fall.

Gerontological

- Older adults often have symptoms that make it difficult to recognize a seizure disorder. Confusion lasting several days,

receptive and expressive speech problems, and unusual behaviors are often the result of a seizure.
- Older adults metabolize some antiseizure medications more slowly, allowing drugs to accumulate and possibly result in toxicity. Consult a pharmacist for specific information.
- If patient has dentures, do not try to remove them during a seizure. If they loosen, tilt head slightly forward and remove after seizure.

Home Care

- Instruct family caregiver about steps to take when patient experiences a seizure.
- Assess patient's home for environmental hazards that could increase the risk of injury in the event of a fall.
- Until a seizure condition is well controlled (usually for at least 1 year), make sure that patient does not take a tub bath or engage in activities such as swimming unless a knowledgeable family member is present.
- Refer patient to the Epilepsy Foundation or a community resource for support groups.

◆ CLINICAL DEBRIEF

A 72-year-old male patient was admitted to an acute medicine division. He has diabetes mellitus, heart disease, and arthritis and has been admitted for acute pneumonia. His home medications include an oral hypoglycemic (glyburide), a nonsteroidal antiinflammatory drug (NSAID), and a laxative. He has symptoms of fever 39.4°C (103°F), productive cough with dark yellow mucus, and chest pain when breathing and coughing. His appetite has been poor. He has an intravenous (IV) line running with D₅NS at 80 mL/h. He reports feeling very tired. The nurse observes him having difficulty standing up from the bed and needing help to walk to the nearby bedside commode. The health care provider orders a colonoscopy to investigate the new development of blood in his stool and abdominal cramping. The patient is placed on nothing by mouth (NPO) status until after the colonoscopy. It has been 7 hours since the test was ordered, and the patient has not eaten.

1. Identify the factors that place the patient at risk for falling and recommend three fall prevention strategies appropriate for this patient.
2. The nurse enters the room to find the patient lying in bed, unresponsive to verbal command with tonic and clonic movement of his extremities. What is the first step the nurse should take and why? What likely caused the seizure?
3. The patient begins to awaken from the seizure. He knows his name but is confused about date and time. He asks, "What happened?" Blood glucose is at 60. How would the nurse report the patient's clinical situation using SBAR?

◆ REVIEW QUESTIONS

1. A 42-year-old patient is on an orthopedic floor following a compound fracture of the lower leg. The patient's leg is in a splint enclosed with an Ace bandage. The nurse enters the room and discovers fire in the bedside trash can. Place in the correct order the actions that should be taken by the nurse.

   1. The nurse turns off the oxygen source at the head of the bed.
   2. The nurse gets help from a staff member, transfers the patient into a wheelchair, and moves him to a different room.
   3. The nurse moves the patient's bed away from the trash can.
   4. The nurse hits the emergency button in the room and instructs the secretary to report a fire emergency.

2. The nurse is caring for an 82-year-old woman with progressive dementia. The nurse is concerned about the patient being at risk for wandering. Which of the following interventions would be appropriate for this patient? (Select all that apply.)

   1. Determine from family the patient's usual communication style and cues to indicate hunger or need to go to bathroom.
   2. Provide a diversional activity that family reports patient enjoys.
   3. Place patient in a bed enclosure.
   4. Use soft wrist restraints for the patient when restlessness increases.
   5. Control room temperature and reduce number of care routines.

3. A nurse is assessing a 70-year-old patient who reports she fell a month ago at home but did not sustain an injury. Which of the following would the nurse assess about the previous fall? (Select all that apply.)

   1. The medications the patient is currently taking
   2. The location of the fall in the home
   3. The patient's medical conditions
   4. The activity the patient was engaged in just before the fall
   5. Whether the patient had dizziness or weakness just before falling

ⓔ *Visit the Evolve site for a complete list of Clinical Debrief and Review Questions answers.*

REFERENCES

Agency for Healthcare Research and Quality (AHRQ): *Preventing falls in hospitals*, Rockville, MD, 2013a, AHRQ. http://www.ahrq.gov/professionals/systems/hospital/fallpxtoolkit/. Accessed March 26, 2016.

Agency for Healthcare Research and Quality (AHRQ): National Guidelines Clearinghouse: physical restraints and side rails in acute and critical care settings. In *Evidence-based geriatric nursing protocols for best practice*, Rockville MD, 2013b, AHRQ. http://www.guideline.gov/content.aspx?id=43934. Accessed March 26, 2016.

Agency for Healthcare Research and Quality (AHRQ): *Which fall prevention practices do you want to use?*, Rockville, MD, 2013c, AHRQ. http://www.ahrq.gov/professionals/systems/hospital/fallpxtoolkit/fallpxtk3.html. Accessed March 26, 2016.

Ahrens M: *Fires in healthcare facilities*, 2012, National Fire Protection Association. http://www.nfpa.org/research/reports-and-statistics/fires-by-property-type/health-care-facilities/fires-in-health-care-facilities. Accessed March 26, 2016.

American Hospital Association (AHA): *Resources: strategies for leadership: patient- and family-centered care*, 2015. http://www.aha.org/advocacy-issues/quality/strategies-patientcentered.shtml. Accessed March 26, 2016.

Barry E, et al: Is the timed get up and go test a useful predictor of risk of falls in community-dwelling older adults: a systematic review and meta-analysis, *BMC Geriatr* 14:14, 2014.

Berry S, Kiel D: Falls: prevention in nursing care facilities and the hospital setting, *UpToDate* 2016. http://www.uptodate.com/contents/falls-prevention-in-nursing-care-facilities-and-the-hospital-setting. Accessed June 30, 2016.

Bhutani J, et al: Achieving patient-centered care: communication and cultural competence, *Indian J Endocrinol Metab* 17(1):187, 2013.

Bradas CM, et al: *Nursing standard of practice protocol: physical restraints and side rails in acute and critical care settings*, 2012, Hartford Institute for Geriatric Nursing. https://consultgeri.org/geriatric-topics/physical-restraints. Accessed March 26, 2016.

Brophy GM, et al: Guidelines for the evaluation and management of status epilepticus, *Neurocrit Care* 17(1):3, 2012.

Bula CJ, et al: Interventions aiming at balance confidence improvement in older adults: an updated review, *Gerontology* 57(3):276, 2011.

Centers for Disease Control and Prevention (CDC): *Injury prevention & control: protect the ones you love: child injuries are preventable*, 2016. http://www.cdc.gov/safechild/Falls/index.html. Accessed June 30, 2016.

Centers for Disease Control and Prevention (CDC): *Preventing falls among older adults*, 2013, CDC. http://www.cdc.gov/Features/OlderAmericans/. Accessed March 26, 2016.

Centers for Disease Control and Prevention (CDC): *The timed get up and go test (TUG)*, 2015. http://www.cdc.gov/steadi/pdf/tug_test-a.pdf. Accessed March 26, 2016.

Centers for Medicare and Medicaid Services (CMS): *Survey protocol, regulations and interpretive guidelines for critical access hospitals*, Bethesda, MD, 2015a, US Department of Health and Human Services. https://www.cms.gov/Regulations-and-Guidance/Guidance/Manuals/downloads/som107ap_w_cah.pdf. Accessed June 30, 2016.

Centers for Medicare and Medicaid Services (CMS): *Guidance to surveyors appendix m*, Bethesda, MD, 2015b, US Department of Health and Human Services. https://www.cms.gov/Regulations-and-Guidance/Guidance/Manuals/downloads/som107ap_m_hospice.pdf. Accessed June 30, 2016.

Chang CM, et al: Medical conditions and medications as risk factors of falls in inpatient older people: a case-control study, *Int J Geriatr Psychiatry* 26(6):602, 2011.

Cipriani G, et al: Wandering and dementia, *Psychogeriatrics* 14(2):135, 2014.

de Jong MR, et al: Drug-related falls in older patients: implicated drugs, consequences, and possible prevention strategies, *Ther Adv Drug Saf* 4(4):147, 2013.

Department of Health and Human Services (DHHS) Office of Inspector General: *Adverse events in hospitals: overview of key issues*, OEI-06-07-00470, Washington, DC, 2008, DHHS.

El-Khoury F, et al: The effect of fall prevention exercise programmes on fall-induced injuries in community-dwelling older adults: systematic review and meta-analysis of randomised controlled trials, *BMJ* 347:f6234, 2013.

Greenberg SA: Analysis of measurement tools of fear of falling for high-risk, community-dwelling older adults, *Clin Nurs Res* 21(1):113, 2012.

Guo J, et al: Interventions to reduce the number of falls among older adults with/without cognitive impairment: an exploratory meta-analysis, *Int J Geriat Psychol* 29(7):661, 2014.

Hempel S, et al: Hospital fall prevention: a systematic review of implementation, components, adherence, and effectiveness, *J Am Geriatr Soc* 61(4):483, 2013.

Herman T, et al: Properties of the "timed get up and go test": more than meets the eye, *Gerontology* 57(3):203, 2011.

Hockenberry MJ, Wilson D: *Wong's nursing care of infants and children*, ed 10, St Louis, 2015, Mosby.

Johns Hopkins Medicine: *Health library: epilepsy and seizures*, 2015. http://www.hopkinsmedicine.org/healthlibrary/conditions/adult/nervous_system_disorders/epilepsy_and_seizures_85, p00779/. Accessed March 26, 2016.

Kiekkas P, et al: Unplanned extubation in critically ill adults: clinical review, *Nurs Crit Care* 18(3):123, 2013.

Kiel D: Falls in older persons: risk factors and patient evaluation, *UpToDate* 2016. http://www.uptodate.com/contents/falls-in-older-persons-risk-factors-and-patient-evaluation. June 30, 2016.

Knox DK, Holloman GH: Use and avoidance of seclusion and restraint: Consensus statement of the American Association for Emergency Psychiatry Project BETA Seclusion and Restraint Workgroup, *West J Emerg Med* 13(1):35, 2012.

Kojima T, et al: Association of polypharmacy with fall risk among geriatric outpatients, *Geriatr Gerontol Int* 11(4):438, 2011.

Krumholz A, et al: Evidence-based guideline: management of an unprovoked first seizure in adults, *Neurology* 84:1705, 2015.

Martin E, et al: French validation of the Revised Algase Wandering Scale for Long-Term Care, *Am J Alzheimers Dis Other Demen* 30(8):762, 2015.

Mathias S, Nayak US, et al: Balance in elderly patients: the "get-up and go" test, *Arch Phys Med Rehabil* 67(6):387, 1986.

Nabhan M, et al: What is preventable harm in healthcare? A systematic review of definitions, *BMC Health Serv Res* 25(12):128, 2012.

National Quality Forum (NQF): *National voluntary consensus standards for public reporting of patient safety events*, 2011. http://www.qualityforum.org/Publications/2011/02/National_Voluntary_Consensus_Standards_for_Public_Reporting_of_Patient_Safety_Event_Information.aspx. Accessed March 26, 2016.

National Quality Forum (NQF): *Patient safety 2015—the opportunity*, National Quality Forum, 2015, http://www.qualityforum.org/ProjectDescription.aspx?projectID=77836. Accessed March 26, 2016.

Nelson AL, Algase DL: *Evidence-based protocols for managing wandering behavior*, New York, 2007, Springer Publishing.

NANDA-I International (NANDA): *Nursing diagnoses: definitions and classification, 2015-2017*, ed 10, Oxford, 2014, Wiley-Blackwell.

Pfortmueller CA, et al: Reducing fall risk in the elderly: risk factors and fall prevention, a systematic review, *Minerva Med* 105(4):275, 2014.

Podsiadlo D, Richardson S: The timed "get up & go": a test of basic functional mobility for frail elderly persons, *J Am Geriatr Soc* 39(2):142, 1991.

Quality and Safety Education for Nurses (QSEN) Institute: *Pre-licensure KSAs*, 2014. http://qsen.org/competencies/pre-licensure-ksas/. Accessed March 26, 2016.

Saverino A, et al: The risk of falling in young adults with neurological conditions: a systematic review, *Disabil Rehabil* 36(12):963, 2014.

Schubert TE: Evidence-based exercise prescription for balance and falls prevention: a current review of the literature, *J Geriatr Phys Ther* 34(3):100, 2011.

Smith G, et al: Epilepsy update: part 2: nursing care and evidence-based treatment, *AJN* 115(6):34, 2015.

Speroni KG, et al: What causes near-misses and how are they mitigated?, *Nursing* 43(4):19, 2013.

Spoelstra SL, et al: Fall prevention in hospitals: an integrative review, *Clin Nurs Res* 21(1):92, 2012.

Stewart TV, et al: Practice patterns, beliefs, and perceived barriers to care regarding dementia: a report from the American Academy of Family Physicians (AAFP) national research network, *J Appl Biomater Funct Mater* 27(2):275, 2014.

The Joint Commission (TJC): *Provision of care, treatment and services: restraint/seclusion for hospitals that use TJC for deemed status purposes*, Chicago, 2009, Author.

The Joint Commission (TJC): Center for Transforming Healthcare aims to prevent inpatient falls with injury, *Joint Commission Online* 2014. http://www.jointcommission.org/assets/1/23/jconline_April_30_141.PDF. Accessed March 26, 2016.

The Joint Commission (TJC): *2015 Comprehensive accreditation manual for hospitals: the official handbook*, Oakbrook Terrace, IL, 2015, The Commission.

The Joint Commission (TJC): *2016 National Patient Safety Goals*, Oakbrook Terrace, IL, 2016, The Commission. http://www.jointcommission.org/standards_information/npsgs.aspx. Accessed March 26, 2016.

Touhy T, Jett K: *Ebersole and Hess' gerontological nursing & health care*, ed 4, St Louis, 2014, Elsevier.

United States Department of Labor: *OSHA quickcard: hazard communication safety data sheets*, 2015. https://www.osha.gov/Publications/HazComm_QuickCard_SafetyData.html. Accessed March 26, 2016.

Uusi-Rasi K, et al: Exercise and vitamin D in fall prevention among older women: a randomized clinical trial, *JAMA Intern Med* 175(5):703, 2015.

Vlaeyen E, et al: Characteristics and effectiveness of fall prevention programs in nursing homes: a systematic review and meta-analysis of randomized controlled trials, *J Am Geriat Soc* 63(2):211, 2015.

15 | Disaster Preparedness

OBJECTIVES

Mastery of content in this chapter will enable the nurse to:
- Describe elements of emergency preparedness and response.
- Discuss the characteristics of different types of disasters.
- Identify actions to take in the event of biological, chemical, and radiation exposure.

- Discuss guidelines for patient care in the event of a mass casualty incident.
- Describe psychosocial effects of disasters on patients.
- Describe psychosocial effects of disasters on nurses and other health care providers.

MEDIA RESOURCES

- evolve http://evolve.elsevier.com/Perry/skills
- Review Questions

- Audio Glossary
- Clinical Debrief and Review Questions Answers

PURPOSE

The terrorist attacks on the World Trade Center and Pentagon on September 11, 2001, forever changed the reality and sense of security felt by citizens of the United States. Recent natural disasters, including hurricanes Katrina in 2005 and Sandy in 2012, have further reinforced the need for public health education on disaster preparedness and response. Disasters can also be in the form of a disease outbreak such as the Ebola outbreak of 2014. All of these events increase the demand for disaster preparedness of health care providers who will educate the public and deliver care to diverse populations at times of crisis. Nurses play a key role in the coordination and implementation of an interprofessional approach to prepare for and respond to disaster. In addition, nurses and other professionals are also at risk for the physical and psychological effects of disasters. Information gathered from the many postdisaster evaluations that have occurred in recent years have provided a considerable body of knowledge and experience to improve the response of an entire health care team and the many agencies/individuals involved in a disaster response.

STANDARDS OF CARE

- American Nurses Association (ANA), 2015—Disaster Preparedness and Response
- American Red Cross, 2015—Preparedness and Response
- Centers for Disease Control and Prevention CDC, 2015—Emergency Preparedness and Response
- Federal Emergency Management Agency (FEMA), 2016—Plan & Prepare

PRINCIPLES FOR PRACTICE

- A disaster is any unexpected event, the effect of which leads to significant destruction and/or adverse consequences (Box 15.1).
- Surveillance of the public by the World Health Organization (WHO) focuses on diseases such as Ebola virus (EBV) disease and avian influenza (bird flu) for indications of mutations and increased transmission (Boxes 15.2 and 15.3).
- The most common forms of disaster are natural or manmade. If the public is not adequately protected, the spread of natural-borne disease can create a natural disaster.
- The Centers for Disease Control and Prevention (CDC) strategic plan *A National Strategic Plan for Public Health Preparedness and Response* focuses on the sustainability of public health resources and infrastructure (CDC, 2011).
- In the event of a biological, chemical, or radiation attack, the CDC strategic plan includes preparedness and prevention, detection and surveillance, diagnosis and characterization of agents, response, and communication.
- Detection and surveillance focus on an awareness of the environment, recognizing what is unusual or different and knowing what these differences possibly mean for the purpose of mitigation or prevention (DHS, 2011).
- Traditional modes of communication will likely be interrupted in the event of a mass casualty incident (MCI); part of disaster preparedness involves back-up plans such as the use of two-way radios and satellite phones.
- Through the clinician outreach and communication activity (COCA) resource, the CDC helps health care providers respond

BOX 15.1

Disaster Definitions and Types

- **Disaster:** A catastrophic and/or destructive event (e.g., tsunamis, terrorist attacks) that disrupts normal functioning; may include any anticipated or unexpected event, the effects of which lead to significant destruction and/or adverse consequences
- **Mass casualty incident or event (MCI):** Any event or situation (e.g., bombing of a public area) that results in multiple casualties and/or deaths; exists when health care needs exceed health care resources
- **All-hazards event:** Multiple manmade or natural events with destructive capacity to cause multiple casualties
- **All-hazards preparedness:** The comprehensive preparedness necessary to manage casualties resulting from a disaster, regardless of etiology
- **Casualty:** Any individual who is ill, injured, missing, or killed as a result of an MCI
- **Medical disasters:** Catastrophic events (e.g., mass shootings) that result in human casualties that overwhelm the available health care resources
- **Natural/environmental disasters:** Catastrophic events that result from an ecological event that exceeds the capacity of the community (e.g., the impact of hurricanes or tornados on a community)
- **Manmade disasters:** Catastrophic events (e.g., wildfires) the principal direct cause of which is attributable to human action
- **Technological disasters:** Catastrophic events in which people, property, community infrastructure, and economic welfare are adversely affected by the disruption of technology (e.g., industrial accidents, unplanned release of nuclear waste)

BOX 15.2

Ebola Virus Disease (EVD)

- Transmitted to people from blood, secretions, organs, or other bodily fluids of infected animals such as chimpanzees, gorillas, fruit bats, monkeys, forest antelope, and porcupines found ill or dead or in the rain forest.
- Spreads by human-to-human contact via direct contact with the blood, secretions, organs, or other bodily fluids of infected people and with surfaces and materials.
- First discovered in 1976. Current West African outbreak is the largest and most complex. The most severely affected countries are Guinea, Liberia, and Sierra Leone.
- The incubation period is 2–21 days; humans are not infectious until they develop symptoms.
- Early symptoms include sudden onset of fever, fatigue, muscle pain, headache, and sore throat, followed by vomiting, diarrhea, rash, symptoms of impaired kidney and liver function, and in some cases both internal and external bleeding.
- Treatment includes supportive care; two vaccines currently are under trial in humans.
- Prevention and control focuses on reducing the risk of transmission and outbreak containment measures.
- Health care providers take standard precautions and apply extra infection control measures when caring for a patient with EVD.

Data from World Health Organization (WHO): *Ebola virus disease,* 2016, http://www.who.int/mediacentre/factsheets/fs103/en/. Accessed June 19, 2016.

BOX 15.3

Avian Influenza ("Bird Flu")

- There are two main avian influenza (AI) viruses that infect humans: AI (H5N1) and AI (H7N9). No cases of AI (H7N9) outside of China have been reported.
- AI is an infectious disease of birds that is highly contagious among poultry; it has also been documented in pigs, tigers, leopards, ferrets, and domestic cats. Believed to be transmitted primarily through close contact with live or dead diseased birds or contaminated surfaces; person-to-person transmission is rare.
- No evidence of disease spread through properly prepared eggs or poultry; a few human cases have been linked to consumption of food containing raw, contaminated poultry blood.
- Incubation period is 2 to 8 days, possibly as long as 17 days.
- Initial symptoms: high fever and flulike symptoms (i.e., fever, cough, sore throat, and muscle aches); diarrhea, vomiting, and abdominal pain; chest pain; and bleeding from the nose and gums.
- Additional early symptoms: respiratory distress, a hoarse voice, and crackling sounds on inhalation.
- Antiviral drugs (e.g., oseltamivir phosphate) can improve survival when administered within 48 hours of symptom onset.
- The US Food and Drug Administration approved a vaccine against one strain of the AI (H5N1) virus. The vaccine has been purchased by the federal government and is being held in the strategic national stockpile for distribution by public health officials if needed.

Data from World Health Organization (WHO): *Avian influenza fact sheet,* 2014, http://www.who.int/mediacentre/factsheets/avian_influenza/en/. Accessed June 19, 2016.

department store, Salvation Army), or care for the deceased (funeral homes).

- Disaster planning is an interprofessional and multiagency task. Average citizens, government agencies, and other health care workers play a vital role in addition to nurses in disaster preparedness.
- Disaster preparedness: Some states are enacting new laws that require disaster training as part of the continuing education requirement for licensure (ANA, 2015).
- Nurses may deliver care during emergencies in states where they are not licensed. The American Nurses Association (ANA, 2015) is continually working to create laws to protect providers.
- The National Terrorism Advisory System (NTAS) facilitates public awareness of disasters. The system provides government officials, first responders, and public citizens with information regarding the nature and degree of terrorist threat (Fig. 15.1) (DHS, 2016).
- Detection is the first goal in an MCI and includes (a) determining the presence of an MCI or public health emergency (PHE), (b) recognizing the cause of the incident, and (c) becoming aware of the environment or more specifically changes in the environment (e.g., an unusual pattern of patient presentation or unusual smells).
- Although many events have a clear cause, others have an insidious onset. Detection is sometimes simply the awareness of an unusual health care situation.
- Incident command is the need for an emergency system to be activated when a threat or hazard is suspected. For most individuals this means activating the 9-1-1 system.
- An incident command system (ICS) is used by all disciplines to help respond to an emergency situation (FEMA, 2015). See Fig. 15.2 for an example of a hospital ICS.
- In terms of a disaster, support means, "Give me what I need to get the job done." The earlier you ask for support, the better.

to emergencies by communicating relevant and timely information (CDC, 2015b).

- The CDC and the American Red Cross (2015) advocate preparedness and coordination of prompt, effective emergency efforts. This includes outreach to other agencies or groups through mutual aid agreements (e.g., willingness of an agency to provide shelter [school or church]), clothing (e.g.,

Alert Is Issued		
Elevated Threat Alert Warns of a credible terrorist threat against the United States		**Imminent Threat Alert** Warns of a credible, specific, and impending terrorist threat against the United States
Information Included in Alert		
Summary	Details, including affected areas	Duration of alert
How you can help	Steps to stay prepared	How to stay informed
Sunset Provision An individual threat alert is issued for a specific time period and then automatically expires. It may be extended if new information becomes available or the threat evolves.		

FIG 15.1 National Terrorism Advisory System overview. (*Department of Homeland Security—Adapted from data available at http://www.dhs.gov/xlibrary/assets/ntas/ntas-public-guide.pdf.*)

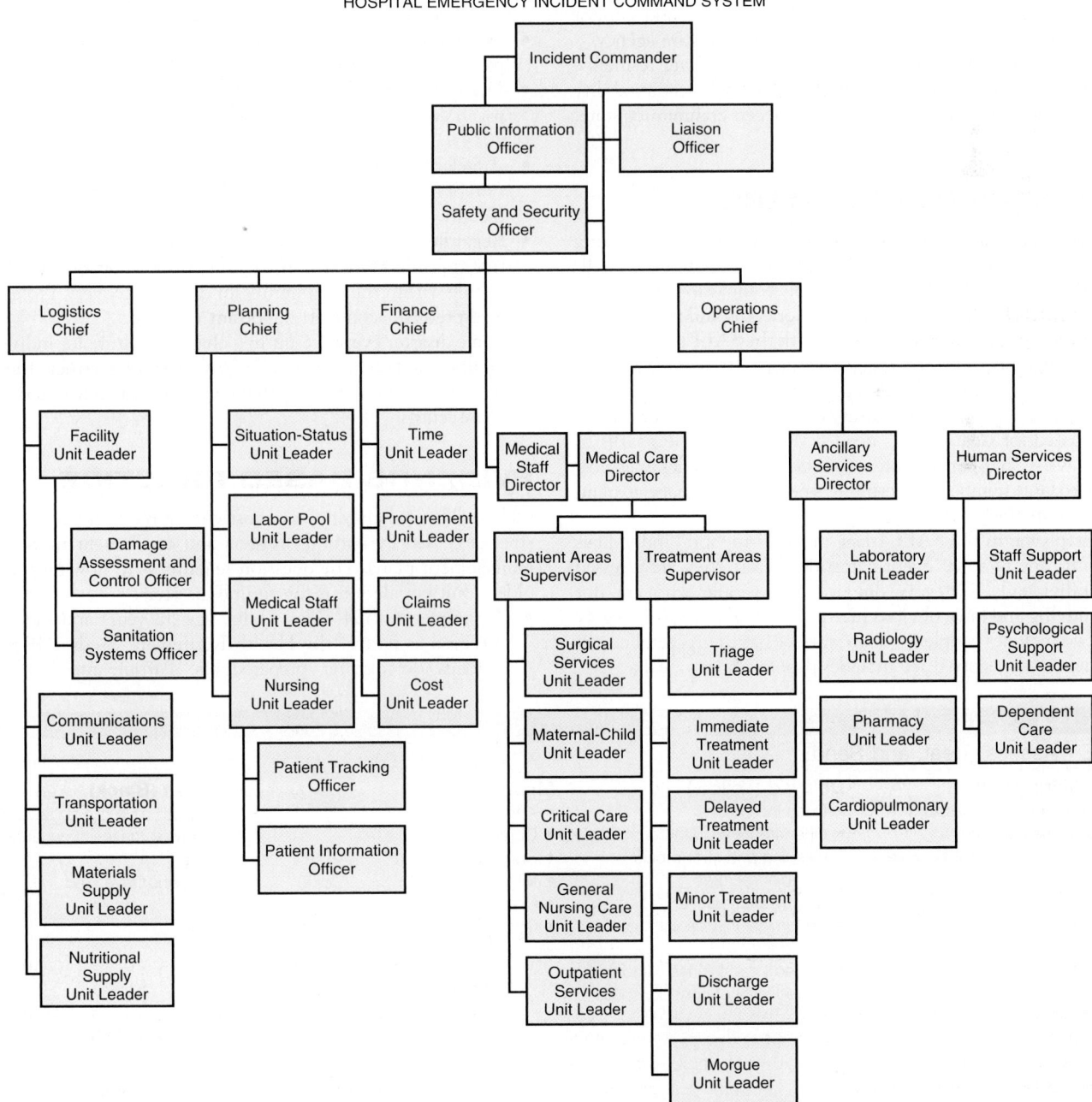

FIG 15.2 The hospital emergency incident command system prepares all response teams to work smoothly in a disaster situation.

- Support resources necessary during a disaster include human resources, agencies, facilities, supplies, and vehicles.
- Support is for the victims of disaster and all health care providers involved. Support is holistic, encompassing the body, mind, and spirit. Health care providers (including nurses, first responders, and physicians) are at risk for posttraumatic stress disorder (PTSD).
- Once local and federal authorities confirm the need for medicine and supplies, the CDC's strategic national stockpile (SNS) is accessed, and items are delivered to the state in need. Each state has a plan to receive and distribute SNS (CDC, 2015c).
- Health care providers care for the worried well (those injured and able to transport themselves to a hospital and those frightened by the events) and the sick and injured individuals already admitted to the hospital or emergency department (ED).
- First responders quickly distinguish between actual victims with exposure to the weapon of mass destruction (chemical, biological, or nuclear) that led to the MCI and the worried well.
- Health care providers offer a valuable resource and cannot spend time maintaining the security of a health care agency.
- Nurses provide public health education to empower resilience in communities by focusing on individual self-accountability and responsibility and knowing how to access community, state, and federal resources.

PATIENT-CENTERED CARE

- Triage, treat, and evacuate: Triage is the process of sorting individuals by the seriousness of their condition and the likelihood of their survival (Box 15.4). Apply compassion and respect in this process. Learn your patients' concerns and fears.
- Disaster triage can be accomplished with the SALT (Sort-Assess-Lifesaving interventions-Triage/treatment) triage system. All victims are first sorted into groups on the basis of mobility.
- They are then individually assessed, sorted into categories, and evacuated for treatment as needed (Fig. 15.3). The goal is to sort, assess, and perform lifesaving measures as quickly as possible to large numbers of victims. Using simple language, explain to patients the process of triage.
  - Step One in the SALT triage model is to "sort" individuals into one of three major categories before they are assessed individually. Category one includes people who are not moving and have obvious life-threatening injuries. Category two includes people who can wave or have purposeful movements. Category three includes people who can walk.

- Step Two of the SALT triage system involves individual assessment and further patient sorting into categories that include (1) those minimally injured, (2) people who will survive even with delayed treatment, (3) those who need immediate intervention, and (4) people expected to die. Lifesaving interventions will be administered according to which category the person is labeled.
- Step Three of SALT triage involves treatment and/or transport of victims. As with any emergency, reassessment is always necessary. During reassessment rescue workers consider patient conditions, resources, and scene safety.
- In an epidemic situation triage is also used to prevent secondary spread of the disease.
- During triage the focus may shift to psychological support of survivors or transport to specific facilities.
- Remain calm and assess a patient's immediate psychological response. Some patients present with dissociative symptoms such as disorientation, depression, anxiety, psychosis, and an inability to care for self.
- Community engagement is key to successfully controlling people's responses during disasters; establishing trust is essential.
- Physical injuries may be similar across cultures; however, the psychological responses will differ among cultures (Sterling, 2014).
- A lack of cultural considerations of victims leads to the impression of insensitivity and biases toward patients who are different racially, sexually, or ethnically.
- Regardless of cultural differences and perhaps language difficulties, it is important to convey compassion and work closely with people within the community for disaster recovery. Professional interpreters become an important resource.
- Some disaster events result in a changed culture for individuals, families, and communities. Once a disaster has struck, there can be a sense of vulnerability that causes increased fear and a sense of insecurity.

EVIDENCE-BASED PRACTICE

Older adults and children are most vulnerable to the physiological stresses caused by natural disasters and can benefit from disaster management plans. The question remains as to how prepared the older adult population is for natural disasters.

- A sample of 1304 older adults, age 50 years and older, were surveyed as part of the Health Retirement Study (HRS) with a focus on disaster preparedness. Participants were asked

---

BOX 15.4

IDME—Assess, Treat, and Send

Immediate (Red)	**Delayed (Yellow)**	**Minimal (Green)**	**Expectant (Black)**
• Unconscious or unresponsive	• Deep lacerations	• Abrasions	• Victims still alive but so severely injured as to have little chance of survival
• Altered mental status	• Open fractures with controlled bleeding and strong pulses	• Contusions	
• Experiencing hypoxia or near-hypoxia	• Multiple fractures	• Sprains	• Victims who have died
• Chest pain	• Finger amputations	• Minor lacerations	
• Chest wounds	• Abdominal injuries with stable vital signs	• No apparent injuries	
• Full-thickness burns over 20% to 60% of the body	• Closed head injuries without altered level of consciousness	• Other injuries of similar severity	
• Uncontrollable bleeding			
• Amputations above elbow or knee			
• Rapid or weak pulse			
• Open abdominal wounds			

IDME, Immediate, delayed, minimal, expectant.

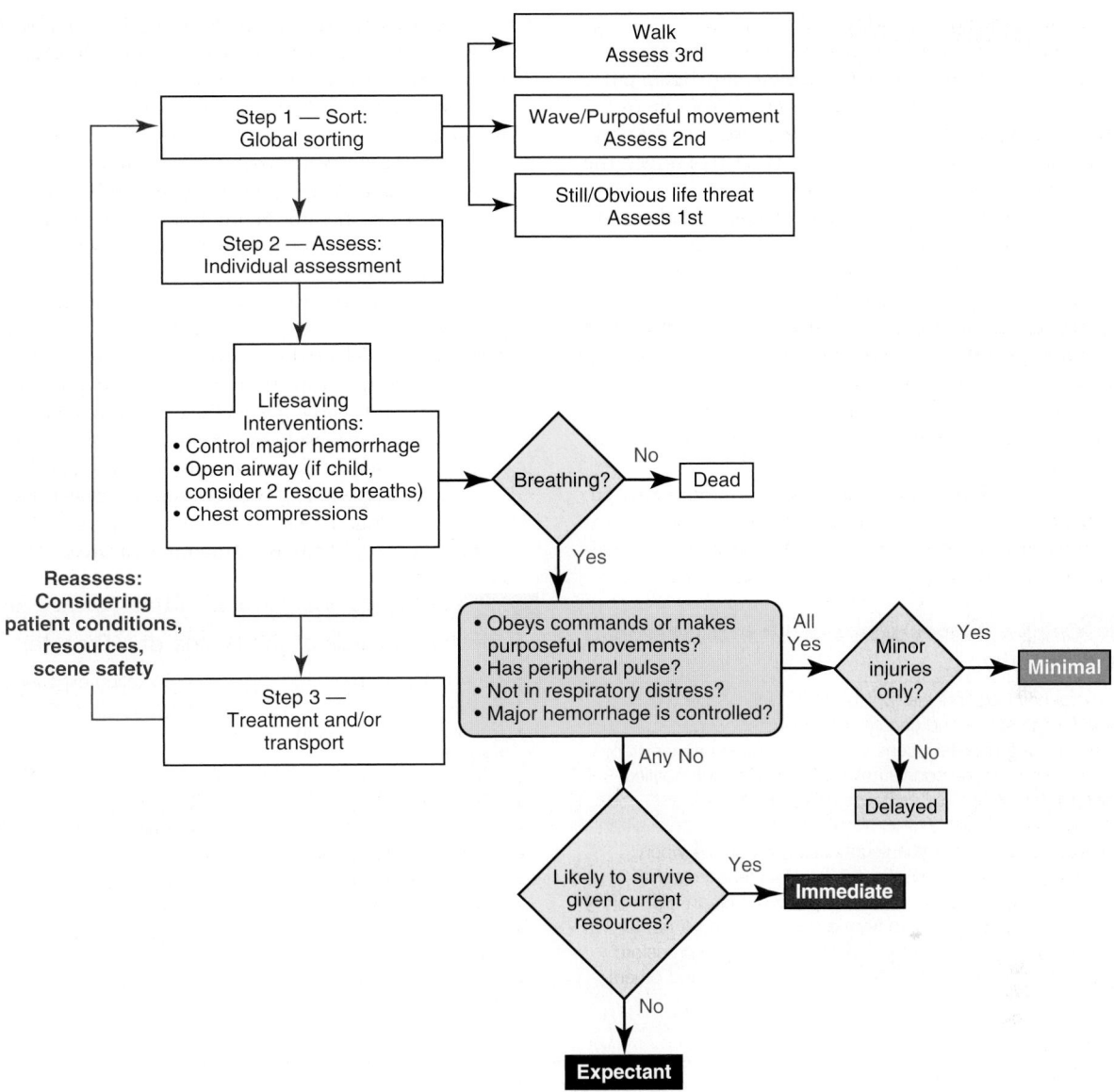

FIG 15.3 SALT Mass casualty triage algorithm (Sort, Assess, Lifesaving interventions, Treatment/ transport). (*US Department of Health and Human Services: Adapted from Lerner EB et al: Mass casualty triage: an evaluation of the science and refinement of a national guideline, Disaster Med Public Health Prep 5(2):129, 2011.*)

questions related to preparedness. Did they have an evacuation plan, including the ability to have an immediate exit in case of disaster? Did they have a 3-day emergency kit; a household member with a car and ability to drive and a recently checked, functioning smoke detector (Al-Rousan et al., 2014)? Significant findings included about 15% of the sample used a medical device that required externally supplied electricity; two thirds of the sample had no emergency plan and were not familiar with resources to help them; lower socioeconomic status was associated with lower disaster-preparedness scores (Al-Rousan et al., 2014).

- Although resources are available of which older adults are not aware, there remains a great need for their education and support for disaster preparedness and response.
- Children experience unique feelings after being exposed to a disaster and need support to recover from physical and psychological effects. Pfefferbaum and North (2013) reviewed relevant

literature and clinical experiences with the aim of highlighting two components for child disaster mental health assessment: screening and clinical evaluation.

- Screening helps identify children at heightened risk for psychiatric disorders. Providers must choose an appropriate assessment tool based on what is to be assessed: distress, symptoms, or diagnoses.
- "A full diagnostic evaluation is appropriate for children who are directly exposed to a disaster, those whose family members and (or) close associates are directly exposed, those who are identified as at risk for psychiatric disturbance through screening, and those with known prior trauma and (or) preexisting psychopathology" (Pfefferbaum and North, p. 139).
- PTSD can be difficult to assess in very young children because of their immature cognitive and language development.

SAFETY GUIDELINES

When considering all forms of disaster, there are basic safety guidelines for a nurse or other health care provider to follow:

- The first priority at any disaster scene is to protect yourself and other team members. The second priority is to protect the public, patients, and the environment (Box 15.5).
- It is essential that rescue and health care workers avoid becoming victims. This may go against your initial instinct to help others, but first responders must wait until a disaster scene is secured and all safety precautions are taken.
- Assessing hazards is more important than knowing the exact cause of a disaster; MCI can result in secondary hazards that come in many forms (Box 15.6).
- The potential for public alarm and major disruption of everyday life is enormous. Know crisis intervention and stress-management techniques.
- In an MCI the majority of people, whether contaminated, exposed, or not, will self-triage and go directly to a local hospital, bypassing triage and treatment. Plans are needed to transfer patients to other medical facilities.

- Personal protective equipment (PPE) minimizes the risk for contact with contaminated materials or individuals. Proper use of advanced forms of PPE requires training, fitting, and an understanding that not all PPE protects against all potential hazards.
- When used inappropriately, PPE becomes a hazard (e.g., dehydration, decreased vision, mobility, and ability to communicate). Some of these hazards result because, while using advanced forms of PPE, the user is unable to eat, drink, or go to the bathroom.
- PPEs are categorized by levels A to D for the level of safety provided.
  - Level A—Selected when the greatest level of skin, respiratory, and eye protection is required. It provides maximum protection because it offers a self-contained breathing apparatus, total encapsulating chemical-protective suit, coveralls, undergarments, chemical-resistant boots and gloves, hard hat, and disposable protective suit worn over the encapsulating suit (Fig. 15.4). Highly trained personnel use level A protection in heavily contaminated areas. If you are not

---

BOX 15.5

Safety and Security

- Trained emergency personnel (e.g., firefighters and police) are responsible for the safety and security of a disaster scene.
- Nurses stay out of a disaster scene unless well trained and invited. Call 9-1-1 if emergency personnel have not already been notified.
- Do not disturb the scene; key evidence could be lost or contaminated.
- A health care agency becomes a secondary disaster site when contaminated by the agent from the original disaster scene. For example, a patient has been exposed to mustard gas, an oily chemical that is difficult to remove from a patient's body. If not properly decontaminated, the victim contaminated by the mustard gas will inadvertently contaminate health care providers and others (CDC, 2013a).

BOX 15.6

Potential Hazards at the Scene of a Disaster

- Downed power lines
- Smoke/toxic gases
- Debris that can result in trauma
- Fractured/leaking gas lines
- Fire resulting in burns
- Structural collapse
- Blood and other body fluids
- Inclement weather
- Hazardous materials
- Nuclear, biological, or chemical exposure
- Flooding and the threat of drowning
- Radiation exposure
- Explosion, particularly secondary explosions
- Snipers
- Darkness
- Infection
- High-velocity projectiles and the pressure wave after an explosion
- Becoming incapacitated and unable to protect yourself or your patient

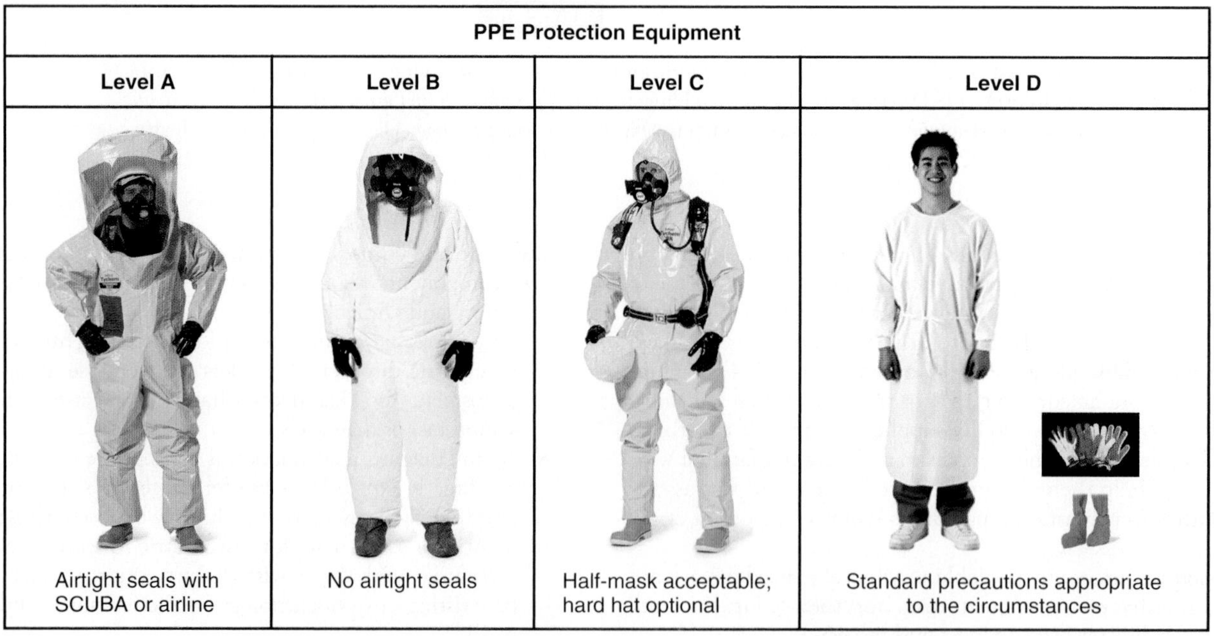

PPE Protection Equipment			
Level A	**Level B**	**Level C**	**Level D**
Airtight seals with SCUBA or airline	No airtight seals	Half-mask acceptable; hard hat optional	Standard precautions appropriate to the circumstances

FIG 15.4 The Occupational Safety and Health Administration (OSHA) defines personal protective equipment for the four levels of hazardous exposure. *PPE*, Personal protective equipment; *SCUBA*, self-contained underwater breathing apparatus.

wearing this type of protection and you are near an area where level A PPE is being used, get out or do not enter.

- Level B—Provides the highest level of respiratory protection but less skin protection. Used by trained responders, this PPE includes a self-contained breathing apparatus; hooded chemical-resistant suit; and face, boot, and glove protection. Level B protection also requires training and fitting.
- Level C—First responders (emergency personnel first on the scene) and hospital personnel are trained and fitted to use level C protection, which involves knowing the concentration and type of airborne substance(s) and the criteria for using air-purifying respirators. Level C constitutes the use of full-face or half-mask air-purifying respirators (National Institute for Occupational Safety and Health [NIOSH]-approved), hooded chemical-resistant clothing, and protective gloves and boots. Because of the garment protection worn with levels A, B and C, the user is at risk for dehydration and hyperthermia.

- Level D—Standard work uniforms or work clothes are appropriate and used for nuisance contamination only. The users must wear coveralls and chemical-resistant shoes; and, depending on the contaminant, gloves, goggles, mask, face shield, and hard hats may also be worn. There is no respiratory protection. It is important to take standard precautions when using level D protection. Depending on the circumstances, some health care providers also choose to use a fluid-impermeable gown, cap, eye protection, mask, gloves, and shoe covers (OSHA, 2011).
- The most recently labeled level of protection is BioPPE. BioPPE requires the use of standard work clothes along with contact and respiratory protection. Double gloving and an N95 mask (see Chapter 9) or a better respirator are recommended. BioPPE protection is not adequate when caring for patients exposed to toxic chemicals; however, it provides adequate protection against radiological and biological agents.
- Hand hygiene that includes washing with soap and water followed by use of an alcohol gel is important at all levels.

✦ SKILL 15.1 Care of a Patient After Biological Exposure

In a bioterrorism attack there is a deliberate release of viruses, bacteria, or other germs with the intent to cause illness or death (NIH, 2014). The use of biological agents is a considerable terrorist threat because they are easy to disperse and affect large numbers of people at a relatively low cost (Box 15.7). Incubation periods and common initial clinical symptoms make detection of a biological attack difficult. Some biological attacks are unannounced or covert, and the onset of symptoms is delayed by an incubation period (i.e., the time between exposure and onset of symptoms). Differing biological agents have incubation periods from 1 or 2 days to several weeks, during which some of these agents may be transmitted as an infected patient exposes others. The mode of transmission of the biological agent determines the severity of the disaster. Recognition of bioterrorism is a challenge because early signs and symptoms mimic the flu or produce a rash mistaken for a viral illness (Fig. 15.5A–B). Sometimes several biological agents are disseminated at the same time, further confusing the issue. To understand how to protect yourself from becoming a victim, you need to understand the mode of transmission and precautions to take for biosafety (Table 15.1).

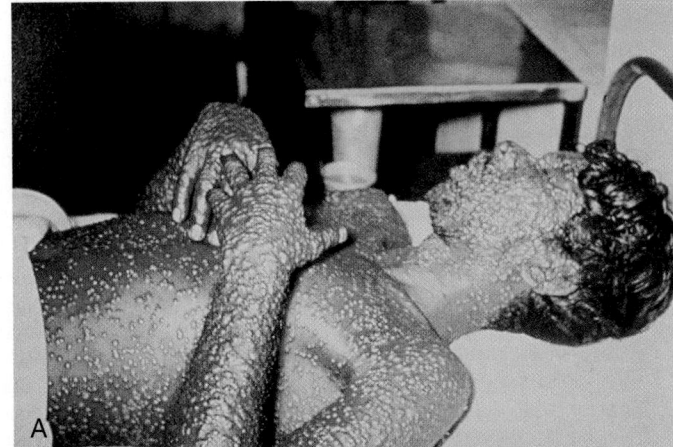

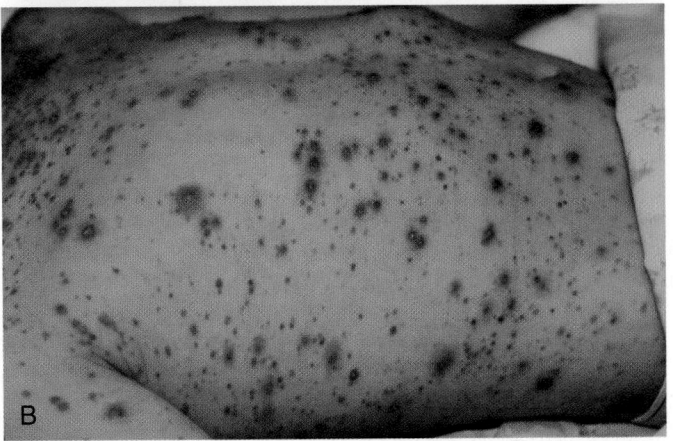

FIG 15.5 Differences in distribution of smallpox versus chickenpox. **A,** Man with smallpox. *(Courtesy CDC/NIP/Barbara Rice.)* **B,** Chickenpox covering patient torso. *(Courtesy David Effron, MD.)*

BOX 15.7

Potential Bioterrorism Agents/Diseases

- Anthrax (*Bacillus anthracis*)
- Botulism (*Clostridium botulinum* toxin)
- Brucellosis (*Brucella* species)
- *Chlamydia psittaci* (psittacosis)
- Ebola virus hemorrhagic fever
- Emerging infectious diseases such as Nipah virus and Hantavirus
- Epsilon toxin of *Clostridium perfringens*
- Escherichia coli O157:H7 (*E. coli*)
- Food safety threats (e.g., *Salmonella* species, *E. coli* O157:H7, Shigella)
- Plague (*Yersinia pestis*)
- Q fever (*Coxiella burnetii*)
- *Salmonella* species (salmonellosis)
- Staphylococcal enterotoxin B
- Tularemia (*Francisella tularensis*)
- Typhoid fever (*Salmonella typhi*)
- Variola major (smallpox)
- *Vibrio cholerae* (cholera)
- Viral encephalitis (alphaviruses [e.g., Venezuelan equine encephalitis, eastern equine encephalitis, western equine encephalitis])
- Water safety threats (e.g., *Vibrio cholerae, Cryptosporidium parvum*)

Data from Centers for Disease Control and Prevention (CDC): *Bioterrorism agents/diseases*, 2014, http://www.emergency.cdc.gov/agent/agentlist.asp. Accessed March 8, 2016.

TABLE 15.1

Summary of Selected Class A Biological Warfare Agents

Disease/Infectious Agent	Form and Incubation/Onset of Symptoms	Untreated Course of Disease		Probable Route of Contamination for Use as a Biological Warfare Agent	Treatment of Mass Casualties	Prophylaxis/Vaccine
		Early-Onset Symptoms	Late-Onset Symptoms			
Bacterial Biological Agents						
Anthrax *Bacillus anthracis*, a gram-positive bacillus that can remain stable in spore form	Inhalation or pulmonary (usually within 48 hours but may incubate for up to 60 days)	Febrile flulike symptoms (malaise, low-grade fever, dry cough, and headache)	Severe respiratory distress, hemodynamic failure, and death	Aerosol; no person-to-person transmission	Ciprofloxacin or doxycycline	Ciprofloxacin or, if susceptible, doxycycline; vaccine available but in short supply
	Cutaneous (1–12 days)	Local urticaria; painless papular lesions usually located on head, forearms, or hands	Papular lesions become vesicular, later developing black eschar and edema	Person-to-person transmission with direct contact with skin lesions		
	Gastrointestinal (1–7 days)	Abdominal pain, nausea, vomiting, and diarrhea	Gastrointestinal bleeding, fever; usually followed by toxic sepsis and death	Contaminated food and/or water		
Plague Acute, severe bacterial infection secondary to a gram-negative bacillus, *Yersinia pestis*	Bubonic Onset of symptoms dependent on route of transmission (1–6 days)	Swollen, tender lymph nodes (most notable femoral and inguinal), high fever, rapid pulse	Hypotension, extreme exhaustion, death	Aerosol and then human-to-human by droplet inhalation	Ciprofloxacin or doxycycline	Ciprofloxacin or doxycycline; no vaccine available at present time
	Pneumonic (1–6 days)	High fever, chills, tachycardia, headache	Fulminate pneumonia (foamy hemoptysis, tachypnea, and dyspnea), sepsis, and death			
Botulism Anaerobic gram-positive bacillus that produces a potent muscle-paralyzing neurotoxin	Foodborne (12–36 hours)	Nausea, vomiting, diarrhea	Symmetrical cranial nerve paralysis, descending flaccid paralysis (progressive paralysis of arms, respiratory muscles, and legs), and death	Contaminated food	Passive immunization (antitoxin); supportive care	Passive immunization (antitoxin); antitoxin available in short supply
	Inhalational (2 hours–8 days)	No fever, no changes in mental status	Symmetrical cranial nerve paralysis, descending flaccid paralysis (progressive paralysis of arms, respiratory muscles, and legs), and death	Inhalation of aerosolized toxin		
Typhoidal tularemia *Francisella tularensis*, an extremely infectious bacteria	Contaminated water or food or via aerosol distribution (1–14 days)	Flulike symptoms (headache, cough, fever and chills, malaise)	Pharyngeal ulcers, pleuritic chest pain, pneumonia, pericarditis, respiratory failure, sepsis, and death	Inhalation of aerosolized bacteria	Ciprofloxacin or doxycycline	Ciprofloxacin or doxycycline; vaccine available, only limited supply; vaccine offers incomplete protection

TABLE 15.1

Summary of Selected Class A Biological Warfare Agents—cont'd

Disease/Infectious Agent	Form and Incubation/Onset of Symptoms	Untreated Course of Disease		Probable Route of Contamination for Use as a Biological Warfare Agent	Treatment of Mass Casualties	Prophylaxis/Vaccine
		Early-Onset Symptoms	Late-Onset Symptoms			
Major Viral Biological Agent of Concern—Smallpox						
Smallpox variola virus	Distribution via airborne droplets, aerosols, and fomites (7–17 days; weaponized smallpox when delivered aerosolized has an incubation period of only 3–5 days)	Acute viral symptoms (high fever, myalgia, headache, and backache)	Continued viral symptoms, high fever, prostration, synchronous onset of rash progressing from macules to papules to vesicles, and eschar formation Vesicles more abundant on extremities and face, and all develop at the same time; pustules appear on palms of hands and soles of feet (unlike chickenpox)	Transmitted person to person by large droplets; therefore spread may be by inhalation of aerosolized virus, oral secretions, infected human vector exposure, or exposure to contaminated objects	Supportive therapy only (ventilator)	None; vaccine available in short supply

Delegation and Collaboration

The skill of assessing a patient exposed to a biological agent cannot be delegated to nursing assistive personnel (NAP). The nurse directs the NAP to:

- Use appropriate personal protective equipment (PPE) to prevent exposure during care activities.
- Use proper techniques for handling a body after death to prevent contamination.

Equipment

Choice of equipment depends on the route of transmission of the infectious agent. The following is a general list of supplies that might be used in the event of release of the most contagious biological agents.

- Biohazard bags with label
- Soap and water
- 0.5% diluted bleach or Environmental Protection Agency (EPA)–approved germicidal agent
- Negative-pressure room (high-efficiency particulate air [HEPA] filtration may be required) with anteroom
- Clean gloves
- Gown
- Shoe covers
- Head covers
- Mask
- Standard face mask
- N95 mask
- Face shield
- Equipment for physical examination
- Oxygen therapy
- Airway maintenance supplies
- Intravenous therapy supplies

STEP	RATIONALE

ASSESSMENT

1. Perform hand hygiene. Don proper PPE.

Proper PPE provides safety to personnel and helps prevent spread of infectious agent to health care provider.

2. Identify patient using at least two identifiers (e.g., name and birthday or name and medical record number) according to agency policy.

Ensures correct patient. Complies with The Joint Commission standards and improves patient safety (TJC, 2016).

3. Conduct focused health history and physical examination (e.g., skin assessment; pulmonary assessment—oxygen saturation, lung sounds, sputum character; cardiac—heart sounds; gastrointestinal (GI)—nausea, vomiting, diarrhea; neurological—movement of extremities, Glasgow Coma Scale, reflexes). Review history of patient's presenting symptoms and determine if pattern exists (see Chapter 6).

Symptom identification and clustering data help to accurately determine exposure to type of biological agent and patient's response.

STEP	RATIONALE
4. Measure patient's vital signs and include assessment of pain on a scale of 0 to 10.	Provides baseline to later evaluate patient's response to therapy.
5. Review results of diagnostic tests and consult with health care provider.	Initial signs and symptoms of exposure to biological agent suggest common disorders (e.g., flu). Further review of diagnostic findings helps to rule out other common disorders.
6. Assess patient for health risks (e.g., history of heart disease, pulmonary disease, cancer) that complicate effects of exposure to biological agent.	Patients with preexisting medical conditions often require additional treatment or are at greater risk for death.
7. Stay calm. Listen and assess patient's immediate psychological response after exposure. Some patients present with dissociative symptoms (e.g., feeling as though "not there" or sensing that everything is outside of the person): disorientation, depression, anxiety, psychosis, and inability to care for self. Even without direct exposure to a biological agent, many individuals, spurred by feelings of fear and doom, present for emergency services.	Aids in providing appropriate crisis intervention and stress management. Remaining calm and projecting confidence while assessing individuals for clinical symptoms reduce anxiety of the ill and worried well as they experience the general sense of panic associated with a biological event.
8. Identify and gather all patient contacts (names, addresses, and phone numbers) before the patient leaves the emergency department (ED).	All patient contacts need to be identified for proper follow-up by public health department. Often patients will self-triage and transport to ED.
9. Identify agency resources available (e.g., critical-incident stress-debriefing teams, counselors, psychiatric/mental health nurse practitioners).	Expert resources help to assess extent of psychological impact of disaster.

Clinical Decision Point *Consider that a biological event has occurred when large numbers of ill persons present who have unexplained yet similar symptoms; when there are unexplained deaths, particularly among young and healthy populations; when there is an unusual pattern associated with the symptoms (e.g., geographical, seasonal, patient population); when a patient fails to respond to traditional therapy; when a single patient presents with symptoms suggestive of an uncommon agent (e.g., anthrax or smallpox). Once you suspect a biological event, notify incident command immediately.*

NURSING DIAGNOSES

- Acute confusion
- Acute pain
- Anxiety/fear
- Decreased cardiac output
- Impaired gas exchange

- Impaired oral mucous membrane
- Impaired skin integrity
- Impaired swallowing
- Ineffective airway clearance
- Nausea

- Posttrauma syndrome
- Risk for imbalanced body temperature
- Risk for imbalanced fluid volume
- Risk for peripheral neurovascular dysfunction

Related factors/Risk factors are individualized based on patient's condition or needs.

PLANNING

1. Expected outcomes following completion of procedure:	
• Patient is comforted.	In some cases care is only palliative, with comfort as the focus. Do not underestimate the value of *comfort* as *care*.
• Patient's vital signs return to baseline.	When there are no underlying medical conditions and *if* the patient's disease process is responsive to treatment (when available), vital signs will normalize. However this may take days or weeks.
• Patient's work of breathing decreases.	Indicates improved gas exchange and cardiac output.
• Patient's skin integrity returns to baseline.	Antibiotic and antitoxin therapy will aid in resolution/healing of lesions over time.
• Patient's level of consciousness (LOC) returns to baseline.	Treatment measures restore neurological function and oxygenation status.
• Patient's mental health status returns to pretrauma level of functioning.	Crisis intervention successfully reduces patient's anxiety, fear, and dissociative symptoms.
2. Dispense timely and accurate information: accurate description of agent to which patient is exposed and implications to patient and family.	Information relieves anxiety and fear.

STEP	RATIONALE

IMPLEMENTATION

1. Continue wearing PPE applied before assessment. Follow transmission-based isolation precautions (see Chapter 9). (See Table 15.1 for route of contamination.) Use strict isolation with smallpox because of its communicability from person to person. Use airborne precautions, contact precautions, and a negative-pressure room for patients suspected of having smallpox.

Reduces transmission of microorganisms and the likelihood of additional secondary sites of contamination.

2. Decontaminate (see emergency policies). If you suspect anthrax, have patient remove clothing and place in labeled plastic biohazard bag. **CAUTION:** *Do not pull over patient's head; instead cut garments off.* Instruct patient to shower thoroughly with soap and water.

Handle clothing minimally to avoid agitation. Showering with soap and water helps decontaminate and reduce exposure (CDC, 2014a).

3. Administer appropriate antibiotics and/or antitoxins.

Various biological agents are commonly treated with ciprofloxacin and/or doxycycline.

4. Administer immunizations (in the event of smallpox).

The best treatment is prevention by immunization with vaccine before onset of symptoms. Vaccination within 3 days of exposure completely prevents the disease or significantly reduces its effect. Vaccination 4 to 7 days after exposure offers some protection from disease or decreases its severity (CDC, 2009).

5. Administer fluid and nutrition therapy.

Biological agents commonly cause GI disturbances that sometimes result in dehydration.

6. Administer oxygen therapy.

Various biological agents (e.g., pulmonary anthrax) commonly cause respiratory symptoms that result in altered gas exchange.

7. Provide supportive care (e.g., comfort measures, including pain management).

Some victims of a biological attack will not survive; palliative care is essential (see Chapter 17).

8. After leaving patient area, remove most heavily contaminated items first. Peel off gown and gloves, roll inside out, and dispose. Perform hand hygiene. Remove face shield from behind and dispose of safely. Remove goggles and mask from behind. Place goggles in container for reprocessing; dispose of mask safely. Perform hand hygiene.

Avoids contamination of self, others, and environment. Reduces transmission of microorganisms.

9. Counsel patient and family about acute and potential long-term psychological effects of exposure. Offer access to trained counselors. Support survivors of a disaster by identifying resources available.

Reaction of patients will include shock, fear, and immobilization. Long-term psychological effects can arise without proper counseling. Social support networks foster coping in the days following a disaster.

Clinical Decision Point *Collaborate with the health care provider and other rescue workers for an ongoing plan for managing patients exposed to a biological agent while caring for other patients who are already present in the health care agency seeking care for illness unrelated to the current mass casualty incident (MCI).*

EVALUATION

1. Observe for improved airway maintenance, breathing, circulation, LOC, and neurological functioning.

Evaluates patient's response to available treatment and/or supportive care.

2. Evaluate vital signs and level of pain.

Evaluates patient's response to treatment.

3. Inspect condition of patient's skin; note character of remaining lesions.

Evaluates patient's response to antibiotic therapy.

4. Query patient, "Tell me how you feel right now." Check level of orientation and ability to conduct conversation.

Evaluates patient for changes that suggest either improvement or deterioration of psychological status.

STEP	RATIONALE

Unexpected Outcomes

1. Patient's physical or psychological symptoms progress.

2. Patient death occurs.

3. Secondary contamination of rescue workers.

Related Interventions

- Notify health care provider.
- Notify mental health treatment team.
- Remain calm, offer reassurance, and protect self and others from physical harm.
- Continue to provide comfort care.
- When handling bodies, take into account continued risk for contamination; make sure that everyone is fully informed regarding proper procedure.
- Rescue workers immediately report symptoms to a health care provider or nursing supervisor.

Recording and Reporting

- Report suspected cases of a biological incident to health care provider or ED officer. In the event of an ED exposure to a communicable disease, the department will be locked down immediately. Public health officials (e.g., the emergency officer) will determine if the hospital should be locked down.
- Use disaster checklists to quickly record specific data regarding patient status, treatment administered, and response to treatment and/or comfort measures.
- Report any unexpected outcome to health care provider in charge.

Special Considerations
Teaching

- Preparation for an MCI goes a long way toward preventing casualties and chaos. Public education of the likelihood of a mass casualty biological event is necessary and includes information about types of biological agents, mode of transmission, symptoms, treatment, and locations of shelters and disaster treatment sites.
- Preparedness includes teaching individuals, families, and communities resilience and the ability to care for themselves when support services are not available or inaccessible.
- Health care providers need an opportunity to debrief after a disaster to help avoid psychological complications such as posttraumatic stress disorder.
- Encourage families to prepare for the unexpected (see Home Care).

Pediatric

- Children are one of the most vulnerable populations, and many facets influence the impact of disaster on children. These facets often include age, sex, family dynamics, and the level of and direct exposure to disaster (Hockenberry and Wilson, 2015).
- Children have both physical and emotional needs during disasters. They often show stress-related symptoms and may have temporary changes in behavior after a disaster (Hockenberry and Wilson, 2015).
- Many disasters result in the need to relocate, which creates stress and unique challenges in children. Stress may be increased by changes in children's cultural, psychological, and social environment. Reactions of their parents and other family members contribute to how well the child will cope with relocation and whether or not he or she will be able to stay connected with friends and familiar activities (Hockenberry and Wilson, 2015).

- Children are very vulnerable to the adverse effects of environmental chemicals and toxins because (1) pound for pound children take in larger doses of toxins through food, water, and air; (2) their organ systems are less mature and unable to remove some of the toxins; and (3) their life expectancy is longer, and long-term effects of exposure to toxins is unknown (Hockenberry and Wilson, 2015).
- Disasters disrupt infrastructure and may cause large-scale displacement, leading to unsafe water, lack of access to health care, and decreases in vector control and infectious agents (WHO, 2011). Outbreaks of communicable diseases have been reported after natural disasters, and children are more likely to develop infections secondary to immature immune systems (Hockenberry and Wilson, 2015).
- Keep families together after a disaster. Family togetherness offers reassurance to a child and lessens fears of being abandoned and unprotected (Hockenberry and Wilson, 2015).
- Media has an enormous influence over children and may impact development and behavior. Encourage parents to limit their children's exposure to media reports of the disaster and to watch television with them whenever possible to clarify information and answer questions (Hockenberry and Wilson, 2015).
- The death of a child is always traumatic; parents may have a compelling need to be present during pediatric resuscitation and at the time of death; ideally you should allow it. It is important for a nurse to be present to explain what is happening and facilitate the grieving process (Hockenberry and Wilson, 2015).

Gerontological

- Under disaster conditions triage older adults according to injuries, not age.
- Because older adults often have several concurrent illnesses, exposure to a biological agent often worsens these conditions and results in the need for more immediate care than an initial triage may suggest.
- Older adults may have impaired mobility, diminished sensory awareness, multiple chronic health conditions, and social and economic limitations that may impact their ability to prepare for, respond to, and adapt during MCIs (CDC, 2012).

Home Care

- Assemble a disaster kit before disaster strikes. FEMA (2016) and the American Red Cross (2015) offer free literature on establishing home care preparedness (Boxes 15.8 and 15.9).

BOX 15.8

Basic Disaster Supply Kit

- Water: 1 gallon of water per person per day (minimum of 3-day supply)
- Food: minimum of 3-day supply for evacuation/2-week supply for home
- Manual can opener
- Plastic resealable bags
- Utility knife
- Disposable cups, plates, and utensils
- Several flashlights
- Battery-powered or hand cranked radio
- Fresh batteries
- Matches in waterproof container
- First-aid kit
- Medications (7-day supply) and medical items
- Map of the area
- Emergency blanket
- Sanitation and hygiene items (e.g., hand sanitizer, toilet paper)
- Cell phone and chargers
- Copies of personal documents (e.g., birth certificates, deed to home, passport)
- Family and emergency contact

Additional Considerations

- Items for infants, seniors, or disabled people
- Pet-care items
- Entertainment items for small children
- Extra set of keys and identification
- Copies of medical prescriptions in plastic sealable bags

Additional Supplies for Sheltering-in-Place (in the Event of a Chemical or Radiological Hazard)

- Roll of duct tape and scissors
- Plastic sheeting precut to fit shelter-in-place room openings (10 square feet per person will provide sufficient air to prevent carbon dioxide buildup for up to 5 hours.)
- Additional supplies in preparation for a pandemic flu (Have a 2-week supply of basic items so you can survive without outside help or going out in public.)
- Thermometer, nonaspirin pain reliever, prescription medication
- Household-cleaning supplies (e.g., disinfectant sprays, bleach)
- Extra bath and hand soap

Data adapted from American Red Cross (ARC) and Centers for Disease Control and Prevention (CDC): *Plan and prepare*, 2015, http://www.redcross.org/prepare/location/home-family/get-kit. Accessed March 8, 2016.

BOX 15.9

Suggested Foods for a Disaster Supply Kit

Foods to use/replace within 1 year:

- Canned soups, canned nuts
- Canned fruits, fruit juices, vegetables
- Peanut butter, jelly
- Ready to eat cereals and uncooked instant cereals

If stored in proper conditions/containers, foods kept indefinitely:

- Dried corn, dried pasta
- Instant coffee, tea, cocoa
- White rice; bouillon products

Data from Centers for Disease Control and Prevention (CDC): *Emergency food supplies,* 2014, http://emergency.cdc.gov/preparedness/kit/food/. Accessed March 8, 2016.

- Individuals with special needs (e.g., hearing impairment, impaired mobility, special diets) and individuals without vehicles require additional planning to be prepared for a disaster.
- Post emergency telephone numbers by the telephone and teach children how and when to call 9-1-1.
- Family members need to establish a meeting place away from the home in case they cannot stay in their home or cannot reach their home during a disaster.
- Remain isolated and advise friends and relatives not to visit if family members are symptomatic.
- Instruct family to use the appropriate PPE needed to protect the family; this can include sheltering-in-place.
- Maintain strict hand hygiene for both well and symptomatic family members after using the bathroom, before eating and drinking, and after contact with pets.
- When a sick individual's symptoms worsen, transport to the nearest designated hospital.
- Change a sick person's clothing and bed linens frequently; wash them separately from those of other family members, using any commercial detergent.
- Disinfect surfaces with which the symptomatic person comes in contact. Use an appropriate disinfectant (e.g., Lysol), especially when soiled by blood or other body fluids.
- Family caregivers need to get plenty of rest, drink fluids frequently, and eat a healthy diet. If the caregiver develops symptoms, obtain appropriate medical care immediately.

◆ SKILL 15.2   Care of a Patient After Chemical Exposure

A chemical disaster is the dispersal of a toxic chemical agent into the environment. The mechanism of dispersal is not always known. In fact, the dispersal mechanism such as an explosion or fire can be a secondary terrorist attack designed to create greater fatalities. Explosions spread a toxic chemical in uncontrolled directions, creating more victims. Symptoms from chemical exposure are usually apparent within minutes, but some are delayed up to 24 hours. Early recognition of a chemical event is a priority because you will need to administer many chemical antidotes quickly. Toxic chemical incidents such as biological events are often unannounced or overt. Terrorists often intend for chemical agents to cause mass casualties and induce fear and/or mass hysteria.

Chemical events are generally confined to small areas, although larger dispersal of these agents may occur (e.g., via a crop duster). The nature and scale of contamination depends on the state of the agent used (e.g., gas versus liquid), characteristics of the chemical used (e.g., heavy or lighter than air), and where the event occurs (e.g., indoors, where ventilation systems affect dispersal; or outdoors, where wind and velocity affect speed and direction of dispersal). For safety reasons rescue workers should be upwind and uphill from a toxic chemical disaster scene to avoid exposure. The exception is when cyanide gas has been released. Cyanide is lighter than air and thus will travel uphill. It has the unique smell of bitter almonds. If you detect the smell, evacuate the area immediately, although exposure may have already occurred (CDC, 2013b).

Because symptoms are almost immediate, evacuate victims as quickly as possible from a contaminated zone to a decontamination zone. Special respiratory and skin PPE protects rescue workers. Before decontamination, victims are a potential source of contamination for rescue workers. Protect yourself against toxic chemical contamination when in contact with a contaminated patient.

TABLE 15.2

Summary of Selected Chemical Warfare Agents

Chemical Agent	Onset of Symptoms	Untreated Course of Chemical Exposure
"Lethal" agents—nerve agents (tabun, sarin, soman, and VX)	Symptoms are generally immediate.	Pinpoint pupils and shortly thereafter salivation, runny nose, dyspnea, chest tightness, nausea, muscle twitching, coma, seizures, and death
"Blood" agents—hydrogen cyanide	Rapid onset of symptoms though cyanide poisoning is often associated with the smell of bitter almonds.	Death caused by asphyxiation
"Blister" agents—mustard and lewisite	Symptoms may be immediate or delayed.	Skin irritation and blistering
"Choking" agents—phosgene and chlorine	Symptoms can be immediate or delayed up to 24 hours.	Coughing, choking, and disruption in pulmonary function that can lead to death

Secondary contamination is high with toxic chemical incidents. Table 15.2 summarizes chemical warfare agents, presenting symptoms, and untreated course of exposure.

The rapid chemical decontamination of victims of a toxic chemical incident is more important than determining the exact toxic chemical. When rapid decontamination is needed, trained personnel are required. Decontamination is either gross or technical, which generally occurs at a scene. A hospital provides decontamination when a contaminated individual presents for treatment. A nurse and all other health care personnel need to use appropriate precautions to avoid becoming victims.

Delegation and Collaboration

The skill of assessing and caring for a patient exposed to a chemical agent cannot be delegated to nursing assistive personnel (NAP). The nurse directs the NAP to:
- Use appropriate PPE to prevent chemical exposure.
- Use techniques for handling a body after death to prevent contamination.

Equipment

- Decontamination room or area (adult decontamination rooms may not meet the needs of children requiring decontamination; decontamination areas for ambulatory victims will not meet the needs of those who are not ambulatory)

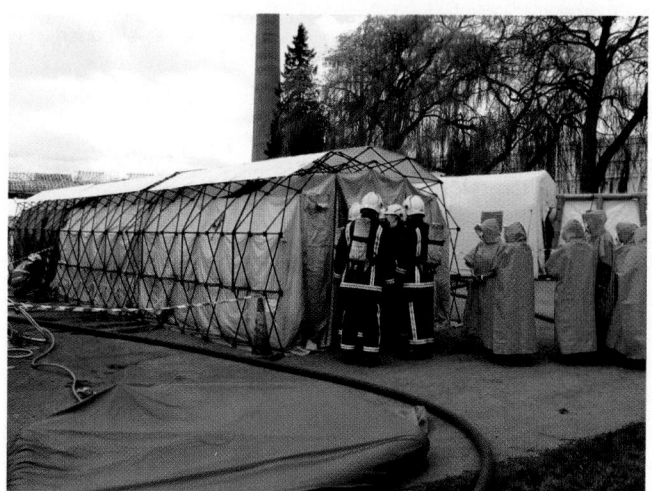

FIG 15.6 Inflatable decontamination shower for ambulatory victims. (*Courtesy Professional Protection Systems, Ltd.*)

- Scissors or a tool to cut off clothing
- Biohazard bags with labels
- Large volumes of water, decontamination shower (Fig. 15.6)
- Appropriate personal protective equipment (PPE)
- Equipment for physical examination

STEP	RATIONALE

ASSESSMENT

1. Perform hand hygiene. Don proper PPE.

   Provides safety to personnel and helps prevent spread of infectious agent to health care provider.

2. Identify patient using at least two identifiers (e.g., name and birthday or name and medical record number) according to agency policy.

   Ensures correct patient. Complies with The Joint Commission standards and improves patient safety (TJC, 2016).

3. Conduct focused physical assessment (see Chapter 6) (e.g., skin assessment; pulmonary assessment—oxygen saturation, lung sounds; cardiac—heart sounds; gastrointestinal—nausea, vomiting) (see Skill 15.1). Observe for presence of liquid on patient's skin, mucous membranes, or clothing and odor (e.g., chlorine), assessing the condition of skin to determine severity of exposure.

   Common conditions present when chemical exposure has occurred. Symptoms vary, depending on type of chemical used.

4. Assess patient for preexisting medical conditions that will complicate effects of toxic chemical exposure.

   These patients will likely require additional treatment and sometimes are at greater risk for death.

STEP	RATIONALE

Clinical Decision Point *Consider a toxic chemical event when large numbers of ill persons present who have unexplained yet similar symptoms. The primary objective for initial care is decontamination (i.e., the removal of harmful contaminants from the skin surface). You achieve this by removing clothing; scrubbing the skin; and hydrolysis, a process of chemical dilution using large volumes of water.*

5. Remain calm. Listen and assess patient's immediate psychological response after exposure. Some patients present with dissociative symptoms: disorientation, depression, anxiety, psychosis, and inability to care for self. Even without direct exposure to a chemical agent, many individuals, spurred by feelings of fear and doom, will present for emergency services and quickly overwhelm available emergency services.

Aids in being able to provide appropriate crisis intervention and stress management. Remaining calm and projecting confidence reduces anxiety of the ill and worried well as they experience the general sense of panic associated with chemical exposure.

6. Identify agency resources available (e.g., critical-incident stress-debriefing teams, counselors, psychiatric/mental health nurse practitioners).

Expert resources assess extent of psychological impact of disorders.

NURSING DIAGNOSES

- Acute confusion
- Acute pain
- Anxiety/fear
- Decreased cardiac output
- Impaired gas exchange
- Impaired oral mucous membrane
- Impaired skin integrity
- Impaired swallowing
- Impaired verbal communication
- Ineffective airway clearance
- Nausea
- Posttrauma syndrome
- Risk for imbalanced fluid volume
- Risk for peripheral neurovascular dysfunction

Related factors/Risk factors are individualized based on patient's condition or needs.

PLANNING

1. Expected outcomes following completion of procedure:
   - Patient is comforted.

   - Patient's vital signs return to baseline.

   - Patient's work of breathing decreases.
   - Patient's skin integrity returns to baseline, or no new injury develops.
   - Patient's level of consciousness (LOC) returns to baseline.

   - Patient's mental health status returns to a pretrauma level of functioning.

Because of fatal nature of many chemical agents, the only care available may be palliative.

When there are no underlying medical conditions and *if* patient's condition is responsive to treatment (when available), vital signs will return to normal within days or weeks.

Indicates improved gas exchange and cardiac output.

Minimizing exposure of skin to chemical agent reduces severity and extent of lesions.

Neurological stability is achieved by minimizing exposure to chemical and giving antitoxin quickly.

Crisis intervention successfully reduces patient's anxiety, fear, and dissociative symptoms.

2. Explain care to patient and family, including decontamination and treatment. Explain your role, orient to location and activities to perform, explain what patient has experienced, and ask, "How are you feeling right now?" Assure them that a medical professional will see them shortly.

Information helps to calm anxiety and fear.

IMPLEMENTATION

1. Continue wearing PPE applied during assessment. Prepare for decontamination.

Reduces transmission of and injury from toxic chemicals. Reduces likelihood of secondary toxic chemical contamination to untrained personnel attempting decontamination.

Clinical Decision Point *Only trained personnel using required PPE may decontaminate patients with toxic chemical contamination. Hold victim outside decontamination area until preparations are completed for decontamination. If patient is grossly contaminated, consider decontamination before entry into building.*

2. Provide for patient privacy by closing room curtains or door.

Prevents discomfort and embarrassment when clothing is removed.

STEP	RATIONALE
3. Decontaminate patient:	
a. Act quickly; avoid touching contaminated parts of clothing as much as possible.	Prevents your own contamination.
b. Remove all of patient's clothing. **CAUTION:** *Do not pull over patient's head; instead cut garments off.*	Cutting off clothing prevents contamination of head and hair.
c. Use large amounts of soap and water to wash patient thoroughly.	Leads to chemical dilution and in some cases prevents patient death.
d. If eyes are burning or vision is blurred, rinse eyes with plain water for 10 to 15 minutes. If patient wears contacts, remove and place with contaminated clothing; do not reinsert in eyes. Wash eyeglasses with soap and water; reapply when completed.	Flushes toxins from eye.
4. Dispose of patient's contaminated clothing in appropriate biohazard bag and seal. Place bag in another plastic bag and seal (see agency policy).	Reduces likelihood of secondary chemical contamination.
5. Initiate treatment for chemical agent using appropriate chemical agent protocol.	Appropriate chemical agent protocol varies with patient exposure (e.g., linesterase, mustard, nerve agent, chlorine, and lewisite) (Box 15.10).
6. Establish airway if needed; administer oxygen therapy (see Chapter 23).	Various chemical agents commonly cause respiratory problems that will result in altered gas exchange.
7. Control bleeding.	Various chemical agents cause extensive bleeding.
8. Establish intravascular access. Administer fluid and nutrition therapy (see Chapters 29 and 33).	Various chemical agents commonly cause gastrointestinal disturbances that can result in dehydration.
9. Provide supportive care (e.g., comfort measures, including pain management) (see Chapters 16 and 17).	Some victims will not survive; it is essential for a nurse to provide palliative symptom control.
10. Remove most heavily contaminated items first. Peel off gown and gloves, roll inside out, and dispose. Perform hand hygiene. Remove face shield from behind and dispose of safely. Remove goggles and mask from behind. Place goggles in container for reprocessing; dispose of mask safely. Perform hand hygiene.	Avoids contamination of self, others, and environment. Reduces transmission of microorganisms.
11. Counsel patient and family on both acute and potential long-term psychological effects of exposure. Offer access to trained counselors.	Reaction of patients to exposure includes shock, immobilization, and fear. Long-term psychological effects can arise without proper counseling.

Clinical Decision Point *Collaborate with the health care provider and other rescue workers for an ongoing plan to manage patients exposed to a toxic chemical agent. You will need to do this while also caring for other patients who are already present in the health care agency seeking care for illness unrelated to the current mass casualty incident (MCI).*

BOX 15.10

Examples of Chemical Exposure Protocols

Chlorine Protocol
1. Dyspnea?
   - Try bronchodilators
   - Admit to hospital
   - Oxygen by mask
   - Chest x-ray film examination
2. Treat other problems and reevaluate (consider phosgene)
3. Respiratory system OK?
   - Yes—Go to 5
4. Is phosgene poisoning possible?
   - Yes—Go to Phosgene Protocol on CDC website
5. Give supportive therapy: treat other problems or discharge

Mustard Protocol
1. Airway obstruction?
   - Yes—Tracheostomy
2. If there are large burns:
   - Establish intravenous line—Do not push fluids as for thermal burns
   - Drain vesicles—Unroof large blisters and irrigate area with topical antibiotics
3. Treat other symptoms appropriately:
   - Antibiotic eye ointment
   - Sterile precautions prn
   - Morphine prn

Data from the Centers for Disease Control and Prevention (CDC): *Emergency room procedures in chemical hazard emergencies: a job aid*, 2013a, http://www.cdc.gov/nceh/demil/articles/initialtreat.htm#CHLORINEPROTOCOL. Accessed March 8, 2016.

STEP	RATIONALE

EVALUATION

1. Observe status of airway maintenance, breathing, circulation, LOC, and neurological functioning. Assess vital signs.

Evaluates patient's physical response to available treatment and/or supportive care.

2. Ask patient to rate pain level on a scale of 0 to 10.

Determines if comfort measures are effective.

3. Inspect condition of skin; note extent of blistering.

Determines extent of healing.

4. Evaluate patient's level of orientation, ability to problem solve, and perception of condition.

Evaluates patient's psychological status and ability to make decisions.

Unexpected Outcomes

1. Secondary contamination of rescue workers occurs.

2. Patient's physical symptoms progress despite appropriate treatment.

3. Patient's psychological symptoms progress despite appropriate treatment. Patient exhibits anxiety, disorientation, and suicidal ideation.

4. Patient death occurs.

Related Interventions

- Rescue workers immediately remove their clothing, scrub their bodies, and use copious amounts of soap and water.
- Contain clothes in appropriate biohazard bags.
- Provide clean clothes.
- Notify health care provider in charge.
- Continue to provide comfort care.
- Notify mental health treatment team.
- Remain calm, offer reassurance, and protect self and others from physical harm.
- Continue to provide comfort measures.
- When handling bodies, there is continued risk for contamination; make sure that everyone is fully informed regarding proper procedures (see Skill 17.3). When delegating preparation of the deceased, always take into account the level of training of those managing the body.

Recording and Reporting

- Report suspected cases of a toxic chemical event to health care provider or emergency officer.
- Record in nurses' notes in electronic health record (EHR) or chart or in special checklist: patient's status, decontamination and treatment procedures, and response to treatment and/or comfort measures.
- Report any unexpected outcome to health care provider in charge.

Special Considerations
Teaching

- Preparation for an MCI goes a long way toward preventing casualties and chaos. Public education about the likelihood of a mass casualty chemical event is necessary. This education includes information regarding types of chemical agents, mode of dissemination, symptoms, and treatment.
- Education of the public includes locations of shelters and disaster treatment sites.
- Preparedness includes teaching individuals, families, and communities resilience and the ability to care for themselves when support services or not available or inaccessible.
- Health care providers need to debrief after a disaster to help avoid psychological complications such as posttraumatic stress disorder.
- See Skill 15.1 for family disaster plan and preparation.

Pediatric

- To avoid becoming a secondary victim, emergency responders need to consider potential contamination of children before picking them up and holding them. Often decontamination consists of providing fresh air and a large volume of low-pressure warm water. Observe children for potential hypothermia because they are more susceptible.
- Adult decontamination facilities are not always appropriate to meet the needs of children. The special PPE worn by rescue workers may frighten young children. The cleaning process and possible separation from uncontaminated parents will likely cause considerable stress and anxiety. Additional health care workers are often necessary to ensure that adequate decontamination has taken place. Verbal encouragement and praise are effective in facilitating the process.
- See Skill 15.1 for further pediatric considerations.

Gerontological

- See Skill 15.1 for gerontological considerations.

Home Care

- Keep upwind and uphill from the release of the toxic chemical unless it is cyanide.
- Use appropriate PPE to protect the family; this includes sheltering-in-place.
- See Skill 15.1 for further home care considerations.

◆ SKILL 15.3   Care of a Patient After Radiation Exposure

Radiological events differ from nuclear events. A radiological event is the dispersal of radioactive material via a "dirty bomb," by deliberate contamination of food or water supplies, or over the terrain. A nuclear event involves a device that releases nuclear energy in an explosive manner as a result of a nuclear chain reaction. Radiation affects the body in many ways, depending on the level of exposure. High levels of radiation exposure cause a person to develop acute radiation syndrome (ARS) with symptoms of nausea, vomiting, and diarrhea (CDC, 2014b).

Radiation comes in a variety of forms. Alpha particles are the least dangerous, traveling only a few centimeters. They do not penetrate materials easily and are harmful only if ingested. An individual's clothing blocks alpha particles from reaching the skin. Beta particles penetrate a short distance into the skin. Protective clothing is necessary for protection. Gamma rays pose the greatest health risk because the waves penetrate deeply, causing severe burns and internal injury. Lead shielding protects against gamma rays. Blasts caused by a nuclear explosion cause not only injury from radiation exposure but also traumatic injuries and burns. Some victims will present with many combined forms of injury requiring treatment. The sooner symptoms begin to appear, the greater a patient's exposure to the radiation. Early symptoms (i.e., within a few hours) suggest that an individual has received a lethal dose of radiation.

Nuclear incidents usually result in wide destruction requiring specialized equipment and resources at the scene to assess structural damage and levels of radioactivity. Radiological events usually cover much smaller areas, but they are often difficult to define. Specialized equipment and training are required to assess the source of radioactivity, determine the scope of contamination, and perform decontamination. The principles to follow to protect individuals from exposure include get inside, stay inside, and stay tuned (CDC, 2014c).

Delegation and Collaboration

The skill of assessment and care of a patient exposed to a radiological agent cannot be delegated to nursing assistive personnel (NAP). The nurse directs the NAP to:

- Use appropriate personal protective equipment (PPE) to prevent exposure.
- Use techniques for handling a body after death to prevent contamination.

Equipment

- Decontamination room or area (adult decontamination rooms do not always meet the needs of children requiring decontamination; decontamination of ambulatory victims will not meet the needs of those who are not ambulatory)
- Scissors or some other tool to cut off clothing
- Clothing containers; type depends on the kind of radiological exposure
- Appropriate PPE for use by personnel in area of radiation release
- Appropriate PPE for health care workers in hospital setting (i.e., surgical masks, N95 masks recommended if available)
- Radiation meter available to survey hands and clothing at frequent intervals
- Equipment for select specimen collection
- Equipment for physical examination

STEP	RATIONALE

ASSESSMENT

1. Perform hand hygiene. Don proper PPE.	Provides safety to personnel and helps prevent spread of infectious agent to health care provider.
2. Identify patient using at least two identifiers (e.g., name and birthday or name and medical record number) according to agency policy.	Ensures correct patient. Complies with The Joint Commission standards and improves patient safety (TJC, 2016).

Clinical Decision Point *Before assessment a specially trained technician conducts a radiation survey of the patient, initially scanning the face, hands, and feet with a radiation survey instrument. If meter results are positive, a thorough survey (5 to 8 minutes per person) is conducted.*

3. Assess patient's symptoms by performing a focused physical examination (see Skill 15.1).	Symptom identification and clustering data are first steps to determine patient's condition and response to radiation.
4. Measure patient's vital signs and include assessment of pain on a scale of 0 to 10.	Provides baseline to later evaluate patient's response to therapy.

Clinical Decision Point *Do not touch a wound if you suspect that radioactive fragments are present.*

5. Assess patient for preexisting medical conditions that will complicate effects of the radiological exposure. Symptoms of acute radiation syndrome include nausea, vomiting, headache, and diarrhea (CDC, 2014b).	Patients with preexisting medical conditions can require additional treatment or are at greater risk for death.
6. Determine patient's allergies, specifically allergy for iodine sensitivity.	Patients with iodine sensitivity need to avoid taking potassium iodide, the treatment of choice for radioactive iodine exposure.

STEP	RATIONALE

7. Assess individual psychological response to radiological event. Some patients present with dissociative symptoms (e.g., feeling as though "not there," sensing that experiences are outside the person): disorientation, depression, anxiety, psychosis, and an inability to care for self. Ask patient, "How do you feel now?" Determine level of orientation, ability to follow conversation.

Allows you to provide appropriate crisis intervention and stress management. Remaining calm and projecting confidence while assessing individuals for clinical symptoms versus feeling of panic goes a long way toward reducing the anxiety of the ill and worried well as they experience the general sense of panic associated with a radiological event.

8. Identify agency resources available (e.g., critical-incident stress-debriefing teams, counselors, psychiatric/mental health nurse practitioners).

Expert resources assess extent of psychological impact of disaster.

Clinical Decision Point *A radiological event is the event most feared by most individuals. Many are uneducated regarding the dangers of and differences among radiation materials. Health care agencies will likely have many anxious, frightened individuals who can potentially create a danger to the environment. Assess individual for sign of psychological distress. Early identification of symptoms and stress-management interventions can help prevent an individual or mass panic response (CDC, 2014b).*

NURSING DIAGNOSES

- Acute pain
- Anxiety
- Deficient fluid volume
- Diarrhea
- Fear
- Impaired tissue integrity
- Nausea
- Posttrauma syndrome
- Risk for infection

Related factors/Risk factors are individualized based on patient's condition or needs.

PLANNING

1. Expected outcomes following completion of procedure:
   - Patient is comforted.
   - Patient is successfully decontaminated.

   - Patient's vital signs return to baseline.

   - Patient is free of nausea and diarrhea.

   - Patient's skin integrity returns to baseline.

   - Patient's immune system (e.g., complete blood count [CBC]) returns to baseline.
   - Patient's work of breathing decreases.
2. Explain care to patient and family. Explain your role, orient to location and activities to perform, explain what patient has experienced, and ask, "How are you feeling right now?" Assure them that medical personnel will see them shortly.

In some cases the only care that is available is palliative.
Decontamination procedures remove radioactive materials from patient's skin.
When there are no underlying medical conditions and *if* the patient's disease process is responsive to treatment (when available), vital signs will return to normal within days or weeks.
Gastrointestinal (GI) alterations following radiation exposure typically respond to antidiarrheal and antiemetic medications.
Radiological burns are minimized through successful decontamination procedures.
Exposure to radiation is minimized successfully.

Indicates improved gas exchange and cardiac output.
Crisis intervention reestablishes patient's orientation and sense of reality.

IMPLEMENTATION

1. Perform hand hygiene.
2. Continue wearing PPE applied during assessment. Prepare for decontamination. *Only trained personnel use required PPE to decontaminate patients with radiological contamination.*
3. Provide for patient privacy by closing room curtains or door.
4. Decontaminate patient:
   a. Remove patient's clothing.
   b. Wash patient's skin thoroughly with water and soap, taking care not to abrade or irritate the skin. Use tepid decontamination water. Cover wounds with waterproof dressings to avoid spread of radioactivity (REMM, 2015a).

Reduces transmission of microorganisms.
Reduces likelihood of secondary radiological contamination to untrained personnel attempting decontamination.

Prevents anxiety or embarrassment when clothes are removed.

Normally eliminates up to 90% of contamination.
Use of large amounts of water is critical in decontamination.

Water that is too cold will close pores, and water that is too hot enhances absorption of radioactive materials (REMM, 2015a).

STEP	RATIONALE
c. Have radiation technician resurvey patient after washing. Rewash as necessary.	Determines if radiation residual is present.
d. Isolate and cover any area of skin that is still positive for radiation by using plastic bag or wrap.	Area is washed until no further reduction in contamination is achieved (verified by survey instrumentation) and then covered to reduce exposure of health care workers.
5. Bag and tag patient's contaminated clothing for further evaluation and place in appropriate biohazard container.	Reduces likelihood of secondary contamination when you use containers designed to contain radiological particles.

Clinical Decision Point *Collaborate with the health care provider and other rescue workers for an ongoing plan to manage patients exposed to radiological materials. You will need to do this while also caring for other patients who are already present in the health care agency seeking care for illness unrelated to the current nuclear or radiological event.*

STEP	RATIONALE
6. Prepare for possibly obtaining a CBC, urinalysis, fecal specimen, and swabs of body orifices (see Chapter 7).	CBC establishes baseline to determine patient's immunological status over time. A health care provider who suspects internal contamination will order collection of urine, feces, and body orifice swabs to analyze for radionuclides.
7. Treat symptoms according to ordinary treatment practices: provide intravenous fluid support, antidiarrheal therapies, antiemetic medications, and potassium iodide tablets.	Patient exposed to radiation is at risk for GI alterations and fluid imbalance. Treatment is directed at limiting or removing internal contamination, depending on type of radioactive material (CDC, 2014d).
8. Remove most heavily contaminated items first. Peel off gown and gloves, roll inside out, and dispose. Perform hand hygiene. Remove face shield from behind and dispose of safely. Remove goggles and mask from behind. Place goggles in container for reprocessing; dispose of mask safely. Perform hand hygiene.	Avoids contamination of self, others, and environment. Reduces transmission of microorganisms.
9. Counsel patient and family on psychological effects of exposure. Offer access to trained counselors.	Reaction of patients to exposure includes shock, immobilization, and fear. Long-term psychological effects can arise without proper counseling.

EVALUATION

1. Observe skin integrity, fluid balance, respiratory and GI status, level of consciousness, and neurological functioning. Look for improvement of other radiological agent-specific symptoms. Evaluate vital signs.	Evaluates patient's physical response to available treatment and/or supportive care.
2. Monitor CBC and other laboratory tests.	Determines patient's immune response.
3. Evaluate patient's level of consciousness, orientation, and ability to relate events. Ask if patient remembers what has occurred; observe affect.	Determines if psychological status has improved.

Unexpected Outcomes

1. Secondary contamination of rescue workers occurs.
2. Patient's symptoms progress despite appropriate treatment.

3. Patient's psychological state deteriorates with development of disorientation, suicidal ideation, violence toward others.

4. Patient death occurs.

Related Interventions

- Institute appropriate decontamination of worker.
- Notify health care provider in charge.
- Continue to provide comfort care.
- Notify mental health treatment team.
- Remain calm, offer reassurance, and protect self and others from physical harm.
- Continue to provide comfort care (see Chapter 17).
- When handling bodies, take into account continued risk for contamination; make sure that everyone is fully informed about proper procedure.
- If the deceased is known or suspected to be contaminated, all people handling the body will wear PPE and a personal dosimeter. A Disaster Mortuary Operations Response Teams (DMORTs) may need to be called to assist (REMM, 2015b)
- When delegating preparation of the deceased, take into account the level of training of those managing the body.

Recording and Reporting

- Record in nurses' notes in electronic health record (EHR) or chart patient's status and response to treatment and/or comfort measures.
- Report presence of open wound and any suspected radioactive fragment to health care provider in charge.
- Report any unexpected outcomes to health care provider.

Special Considerations

Teaching

- See Skill 15.1.

Pediatric

- Children are vulnerable to radiation because (1) their organ systems are more sensitive than those of adults, and (2) they have more years of life expectancy over which to develop complications from the radiological exposure.
- See Skills 15.1 and 15.2 for further pediatric considerations.

Gerontological

- Because some older adults have many concurrent illnesses, radiological agents can worsen these conditions and result in the older adult needing more immediate care than an initial triage had indicated.
- See Skill 15.1 for further gerontological considerations.

Home Care

- When a radiological or nuclear event becomes reality, listen to the radio or television for special instructions, including appropriate means for maintaining a safe shelter.
- Keep upwind and uphill from the release of the radioactive materials.
- See Skill 15.1 for further home care considerations.

◆ CLINICAL DEBRIEF

Victims of an explosion at a chemical plant are arriving in the emergency department (ED). Authorities state that the substance is unknown at this time, but there were reports by people in the area of a "funny smell" earlier in the day.

1. Which safety measures should the nurses take to avoid exposure to themselves and other patients in the ED?

2. The nurse on the scene has been asked to triage the remainder of victims using the SALT triage system. Place the following patients in order of highest to lowest priority. A 22-year-old with cyanosis, a respiratory rate of 35, and confusion; a 14-year-old with a diffuse red rash on the extremities; a 56-year-old with controlled bleeding of deep lacerations received from falling debris; a 41-year-old with full-thickness burns on 50% of the body.

3. One of the final victims to arrive in the ED is an 85-year-old man with a history of angina and prostate cancer. Mr. R. lives alone in an apartment in the retirement community; and, although he has audible wheezes on assessment, he is able to answer all questions clearly. Vital signs are as follows: P: 96 and irregular; R: 28; SaO₂: 88%. His electrocardiogram (ECG) on admission to the ED reveals a possible anterior wall myocardial infarction (MI). Using SBAR, show how you would communicate with the health care team about this patient's condition.

◆ REVIEW QUESTIONS

1. In the case of a biological exposure, the nurse can direct the nursing assistive personnel (NAP) to: (Select all that apply.)
   1. Conduct a focused health history.
   2. Handle the body after death.
   3. Review diagnostic test results.
   4. Gather and wear personal protective equipment (PPE).
   5. Administer a decontamination shower.

2. The nurse caring for a patient after radiation exposure suspects that the patient is suffering a psychological response. Which signs and symptoms is the nurse likely to observe? (Select all that apply.)
   1. Disorientation to place and time
   2. Heightened self-care practices
   3. Depression related to the exposure
   4. Inability to follow a conversation
   5. Planning for a family vacation

3. Your patient was exposed to a chemical agent and needs to be decontaminated. Place the following steps in correct order:
   1. Wash patient with soap and water.
   2. Dispose of contaminated clothing.
   3. Remove contaminated clothing.
   4. Administer intravenous (IV) fluids.
   5. Rinse eyes with plain water.
   6. Initiate treatment for chemical agent.

ⓔ *Visit the Evolve site for a complete list of Clinical Debrief and Review Questions answers.*

REFERENCES

Al-Rousan TM, et al: Preparedness for natural disasters among older US adults: a nationwide survey, *Am J Public Health* 104(3):506, 2014.

American Nurses Association (ANA): *Disaster preparedness and response*, 2015, http://www.nursingworld.org/disasterpreparedness. Accessed March 8, 2016.

American Red Cross: *Preparedness and response*, 2015, http://www.redcross.org/support/emergency-preparedness. Accessed March 8, 2016.

Centers for Disease Control and Prevention (CDC): *Questions and answers about smallpox vaccine*, 2009, http://emergency.cdc.gov/agent/smallpox/faq/characteristics.asp. Accessed March 8, 2016.

Centers for Disease Control and Prevention (CDC): *National strategic plan for public health preparedness and response*, 2011, http://www.cdc.gov/phpr/publications/A_Natl_Strategic_Plan_for_Preparedness.htm. Accessed March 8, 2016.

Centers for Disease Control and Prevention (CDC): *Identifying vulnerable older adults and legal options for increasing their protection during all-hazards emergencies: a cross-sector guide for states and communities*, 2012, http://www.cdc.gov/aging/emergency/pdf/guide.pdf. Accessed March 8, 2016.

Centers for Disease Control and Prevention (CDC): *Emergency room procedures in chemical hazard emergencies: a job aid*, 2013a, http://www.cdc.gov/nceh/demil/articles/initialtreat.htm. Accessed March 8, 2016.

Centers for Disease Control and Prevention (CDC): *Facts about cyanide*, 2013b, http://emergency.cdc.gov/agent/cyanide/basics/facts.asp. Accessed March 8, 2016.

Centers for Disease Control and Prevention (CDC): *Anthrax overview*, 2014a, http://www.cdc.gov/niosh/topics/anthrax/default.html. Accessed March 8, 2016.

Centers for Disease Control and Prevention (CDC): *Radiation emergencies and your health*, 2014b, http://emergency.cdc.gov/radiation/healthandsafety.asp. Accessed March 8, 2016.

Centers for Disease Control and Prevention (CDC): *Radiation emergencies: What should I do?* 2014c, http://emergency.cdc.gov/radiation/whattodo.asp. Accessed March 8, 2016.

Centers for Disease Control and Prevention (CDC): *Medical countermeasures (treatments) for radiation exposure and contamination*, 2014d, http://www.bt.cdc.gov/radiation/countermeasures.asp. Accessed March 8, 2016.

Centers for Disease Control and Prevention (CDC): *Emergency preparedness and response*, 2015a, http://emergency.cdc.gov/. Accessed March 8, 2016.

Centers for Disease Control and Prevention (CDC): *Clinician outreach and communication activity (COCA)*, 2015b, http://emergency.cdc.gov/coca/index.asp. Accessed March 8, 2016.

Centers for Disease Control and Prevention (CDC): *Strategic national stockpile (SNS)*, 2015c, http://www.cdc.gov/phpr/stockpile/stockpile.htm. Accessed March 8, 2016.

Department of Homeland Security (DHS): *If you see something say something campaign*, 2011, http://www.dhs.gov/files/reportincidents/see-something-say-something.shtm. Accessed March 8, 2016.

Department of Homeland Security (DHS): *National terrorism advisory system*, 2016, https://www.dhs.gov/ntas/advisory/ntas_16_0615_0001. Accessed June 20, 2016.

Federal Emergency Management Agency (FEMA): *Incident command system resources*, 2015, http://www.fema.gov/incident-command-system-resources. Accessed March 8, 2016.

Federal Emergency Management Agency (FEMA): *Plan & prepare*, 2016, http://www.fema.gov/plan-prepare. Accessed June 20, 2016.

Hockenberry M, Wilson D: *Wong's nursing care of infants and children*, ed 10, St Louis, 2015, Mosby.

National Institutes of Health (NIH): *Biodefense and bioterrorism*, 2014, http://www.nlm.nih.gov/medlineplus/biodefenseandbioterrorism.html. Accessed March 8, 2016.

Occupational Safety and Health Administration (OSHA): *OSHA fact sheet: personal protective equipment (PPE) reduces exposure to bloodborne pathogens*, 2011, www.osha.gov/OshDoc/data_BloodborneFacts/bbfact03.pdf. Accessed March 8, 2016.

Pfefferbaum B, North CS: Assessing children's disaster reactions and mental health needs: screening and clinical evaluation, *Can J Psychiatry* 58(3):135, 2013.

Radiation Emergency Medical Management (REMM): *Decontamination procedures*, 2015a, http://www.remm.nlm.gov/ext_contamination.htm. Accessed March 8, 2016.

Radiation Emergency Medical Management (REMM): *Management of the deceased*, 2015b, http://www.remm.nlm.gov/deceased.htm. Accessed March 8, 2016.

Sterling YM: Nursing 'caring' during catastrophic events: theoretical, research, and clinical insights, *Int J Human Caring* 18(1):60, 2014.

The Joint Commission (TJC): *2016 National Patient Safety Goals*, 2016, http://www.jointcommission.org/standards_information/npsgs.aspx. Accessed March 8, 2016.

World Health Organization (WHO): *Disaster risk management for health: communicable diseases*, 2011, http://www.who.int/hac/events/drm_fact_sheet_communicable_diseases.pdf. Accessed March 8, 2016.

16 | Pain Management

OBJECTIVES

Mastery of content in this chapter will enable the nurse to:
- Assess a patient's level of pain.
- Assess a patient's level of sedation.
- Describe how an initial pain assessment allows you to provide a patient basic comfort measures.
- Describe the process for delivering medication through a patient-controlled analgesia (PCA) device.
- Teach a patient how to use a PCA device.
- Monitor and manage a patient receiving epidural analgesia.

- Monitor and manage a patient receiving a local anesthetic infusion pump.
- Identify and discuss various nonpharmacological pain-relief measures.
- Monitor and manage a patient receiving nonpharmacological measures to relieve pain.
- Evaluate the effectiveness of pain-management techniques.

MEDIA RESOURCES

- evolve http://evolve.elsevier.com/Perry/skills
- Review Questions
- Case Studies

- ▶ Video Clips
- Audio Glossary
- Clinical Debrief and Review Questions Answers

PURPOSE

Pain is the most common reason that people seek health care; yet it is often underrecognized, misunderstood, and inadequately treated. Data from the 2012 National Health Interview Survey (NHIS) found that an estimated 25.3 million adults (11.2%) experience daily pain (i.e., they had pain every day for the 3 months before the survey (NIH, 2015b). A patient is the only one who knows whether pain is present and what the experience is like. Your role as a nurse is to recognize the unique nature of pain for each patient and help select appropriate therapies. The skills in this chapter emphasize the importance of using critical thinking along with an integrated approach that considers both pharmacological and nonpharmacological therapies in managing a patient's pain.

STANDARDS OF CARE

- The Joint Commission, 2016—Patient Identification
- American Pain Society (APS) and American Association of Pain Medicine (AAPM)—Opioids Guideline Panel-Part 1, 2009—Analgesic Administration and Evaluation
- American Society of Anesthesiologists (ASA) Task Force on Acute Pain Management: Practice Guidelines for Acute Pain

Management in the Perioperative Setting, 2012—Education of Patients Placed on Patient-Controlled Analgesia
- Rowbotham et al.; The Royal College of Anaesthetists—Best Practice in the Management of Epidural Analgesia in the Hospital Setting, 2010—Management of Epidural Infusions

PRINCIPLES FOR PRACTICE

- The Joint Commission requires that a patient's reports of pain are to be addressed and appropriately treated (Box 16.1).
- Patients' cognitive impairments represent special challenges to pain assessment. Carefully observe a patient's behavior and nonverbal responses to pain when he or she is unable to self-report (Box 16.2).
- The two types of pain that you observe in patients are acute (transient) and chronic (persistent), which includes cancer and noncancer pain.
- The most effective pain management combines pharmacological and nonpharmacological strategies. There are three types of analgesics: (1) nonopioids and nonsteroidal antiinflammatory drugs (NSAIDs); (2) opioids (traditionally called *narcotics*); and (3) adjuvants or coanalgesics (e.g., antidepressants and muscle relaxants) that enhance analgesics or have analgesic properties.

The Joint Commission Pain Standards

- The organization assesses and manages the patient's pain.
  - Patients can expect that their health care providers will involve them in their assessment and management of pain.
  - Both pharmacological and nonpharmacological strategies have a role in the management of pain.
- The organization either treats the patient's pain or refers the patient for treatment.
  - Strategies should reflect a patient-centered approach and consider the patient's current presentation; the health care providers' clinical judgment; and the risks and benefits associated with the strategies, including potential risk of dependency, addiction, and abuse.
- Record the assessment in a way that facilitates regular reassessment and follow-up.
- Educate providers/patients and families.
- Establish policies that support appropriate prescription or ordering of pain medicines.
- Include patient needs for symptom control in discharge planning.
- Collect data to monitor effectiveness and appropriateness of pain management.

From The Joint Commission: *Clarification of the pain management standard,* The Joint Commission, 2014, http://www.jointcommission.org/assets/1/18/ Clarification_of_the_Pain_Management__Standard.pdf. Accessed March 26, 2016.

Pain Assessment in Nonverbal Patients

Recommended Assessment Approaches

- Attempt a self-report of pain using simple yes/no responses or vocalizations or a numerical rating scale.
- Search for the potential cause of pain by using physical examination techniques (e.g., palpation).
- Assume that pain is present after ruling out other causes (infection or constipation).
- Identify pathological conditions or procedures that may cause pain.
- Observe patient behaviors (e.g., confusion, pacing, facial expressions, vocalizations, body movements such as guarding) that indicate pain. These vary based on patient's developmental level.
- Ask family caregivers or parent, for a proxy report of patient's pain.
- Attempt an analgesic trial if pathological conditions or procedures that may induce pain are present.

Using a Behavioral Pain Assessment Tool

- Use reliable and valid tools such as the Abbey Pain Scale, Pain Assessment in Advanced Dementia Scale (PAINAD), and Noncommunicative Patient's Pain Assessment Instrument (NOPPAIN) to recognize the presence or absence of pain and provide a rating of pain severity in older people with impaired cognition (Lukas et al., 2013).
- Select an appropriate scale for each patient (e.g., visual analogue scale or FACES scale); no one scale is required for all specific groups of patients.
- Vital signs are not sensitive indicators for the presence of pain.

Modified from Bell L: Pain assessment in the adult nonverbal or sedated patients, *Am J Crit Care* 19:356, 2010; Herr K, et al: *Pain in the nonverbal patient: position statement with clinical practice recommendations,* The American Society for Pain Management Nursing, 2011a, ASPMN; Lukas A, et al: Observer-rated pain assessment instruments improve both the detection of pain and the evaluation of pain intensity in people with dementia, *Eur J Pain* 17(10):1558, 2013.

- Timely analgesic administration before a patient's pain becomes severe is crucial for optimal relief. Pain is easier to prevent than treat.
- In most situations administration of pharmacological agents "around the clock" (ATC) rather than on an "as-needed" (prn) basis is preferable. The American Pain Society and the American Association of Pain Medicine (2009) supports ATC administration if pain is anticipated for most of the day.
- The current pharmacological approach to acute and chronic pain management is to provide *multimodal analgesia,* which combines drugs with at least two different mechanisms of action so pain control can be optimized.
- Make every effort to include complementary/integrative methods, which generally do not require a health care provider's order (check agency policy). Complementary strategies provide an opportunity for a patient to assume an active role in achieving a higher level of comfort and in some instances freedom from pain (NIH, 2015a).

PATIENT-CENTERED CARE

- Pain management should be patient centered, with nurses practicing patient advocacy, patient empowerment, compassion, and respect. Caring for patients in pain requires recognition that pain can and should be relieved.
- Teaching your patient and his or her family about pain treatment and having an attitude of dignity and caring will allow you to individualize a patient's pain control plan.
- Pain is unique to each individual. It is important to recognize all factors influencing a patient's pain and integrate them into an individualized plan for pain management. A timely, factual, and accurate pain assessment requires you to work closely with patients and their families. Be objective, listen carefully, and assess any symptoms that a patient expresses.
- Effective communication and caring are key to gathering all the information needed to accurately determine the character of a patient's pain and its impact. Knowing these factors will help you intervene effectively to manage your patient's pain.
- A patient's culture affects his or her recognition of pain, expression of pain, when to seek treatment, and which treatments are desirable. For example, research has shown that minority patients are at high risk for poor pain outcomes. When patients belong to a culture that is different from that of their health care provider, the provider faces additional challenges (compared with patients from the same culture) to successfully assess and manage the patients' pain (Narayan, 2010).
- Explore a patient's beliefs about pain/discomfort. For example, cultures with a holistic worldview of health and illness mix religious/spiritual, natural, and the supernatural in their belief systems. Use interpreters to explain pain tools and help patients report their pain as needed.
- The International Nurses Society on Addictions (IntNSA) and the American Society for Pain Management Nursing supports the position that every patient with pain, including those with substance-use disorders, has the right to be treated with dignity, respect, and high-quality pain assessment and management (Oliver et al., 2012).
- When patients have preexisting chronic painful conditions, a complete preoperative pain evaluation is an essential component to identify pain control interventions to manage perioperative and postoperative pain (ASA, 2012).

EVIDENCE-BASED PRACTICE

One of the more challenging conditions in pain management is chronic low back pain. In a systematic review by Kamper et al. (2015), 41 clinical trials involving patients who had duration of pain of more than 1 year and who often had failed previous treatment were examined. Patients received interprofessional rehabilitation, which involved a physical component and one or both of a psychological component or a social or work-targeted component. The strength of the 41 research studies varied in quality. The results showed that:

- Interdisciplinary biopsychosocial rehabilitation interventions were more effective than usual care (moderate-quality evidence) and physical treatments (low-quality evidence) in decreasing pain and disability in people with chronic low back pain.
- For work outcomes interdisciplinary rehabilitation seems to be more effective than physical treatment but not more effective than usual care.
- A biopsychosocial approach to care is an individual-centered model that considers the person, his or her health problem, and the social context:
  - *Biological* refers to the physical or mental health condition.
  - *Psychological* recognizes that personal/psychological factors also influence functioning.
  - *Social* recognizes the importance of the social context (e.g., work, family), pressures, and constraints on functioning.

SAFETY GUIDELINES

- Monitor patients who receive opioids (by any route) for signs and symptoms of oversedation and respiratory depression. Excess sedation (difficult to arouse) precedes respiratory depression, especially in opioid-naïve patients (i.e., patients who *are not* chronically receiving opioid analgesics on a daily basis) (AAPM, 2013). Using a standard sedation scale can prevent respiratory depression by observing and intervening for oversedation (Box 16.3).
- Monitor activities such as standing, ambulation, and transfer to a chair if patient has received an opioid. Assess patient's blood pressure, pulse, and respirations before initiating activity.
- If a patient has undergone an outpatient procedure, educate patient and family caregiver about precautions: patient cannot drive for 24 hours; caregiver may need to provide help with ambulation or take precautions to make home environment safe.

BOX 16.3

Sedation Scale*

S = Sleep, easy to arouse
1 = Awake and alert
2 = Slightly drowsy, easily aroused
3 = Frequently drowsy, arousable, drifts off to sleep during conversation
4 = Somnolent, minimal-or-no response to physical stimulation

Remember—sedation precedes respiratory depression.

From Pasero C, McCaffery M: *Pain assessment and pharmacological management,* St Louis, 2011, Mosby.
*Many institutional sedation scales include nursing actions to be taken for each level of sedation.

- Monitor for potential side effects of opioid analgesics and recommend or institute supportive measures (e.g., addition of stool softener or high-fiber diet for side effect of constipation).
- Epidural analgesia intravenous (IV) infusion lines should be labeled clearly and identified as such to prevent accidental connection with tubing of a different type (e.g., tube feeding, blood infusion line) (Rowbotham et al., 2010). Follow these guidelines (ISMP, 2013):
  - Limit access to epidural lines to health care providers with proper education and competence. There can be serious ramifications of misconnections, infections, occlusions, or misadministration of medications.
  - Trace an epidural catheter line from the access site into the patient's body all the way to the end source of an infusion or capped access port before you connect or reconnect tubing or administer a medication.
  - Communicate any practice changes, including dressing location, type of tubing and connectors, with all members of the health care team who are providing care to the patient.
- Patients currently receiving opioids for chronic pain often require higher doses of analgesics to alleviate new or increased pain. This is tolerance, not an early sign of addiction (AAPM, 2013) (Box 16.4). Confer with health care provider who might not be aware of at-home dosages. Be aware of individualized dosages and ensure that all caregivers are informed.
- Drug-drug interactions, including enhanced or reduced effects or side effects, often occur with the multiple drug use required by people with chronic pain. This practice is termed *rational polypharmacy* or *multimodal analgesia* (Manougian, 2010; Pasero and McCaffery, 2011).
- Know agency policy for frequency of pain assessment and timing for follow-up assessments. The first 24 hours on opioids requires frequent assessment, at least every 4 hours.

BOX 16.4

Terminology Related to the Use of Opioids in Pain Treatment

The American Society for Pain Management Nursing (ASPMN) has released a formal position statement: every patient with pain, including those with substance use disorders, has the right to be treated with dignity, respect, and high-quality pain assessment and management. Failure to identify and treat the concurrent conditions of pain and substance use disorders will compromise the ability to treat either condition effectively (Oliver et al., 2012). Common conditions involving use of opioids in pain treatment include the following:

Physical dependence: A state of adaptation that is manifested by a drug class–specific withdrawal syndrome produced by abrupt cessation, rapid dose reduction, decreasing blood level of an opioid, and/or administration of a drug that can act as an antagonist.

Addiction: A primary, chronic, neurobiological disease, with genetic, psychosocial, and environmental factors influencing its development and manifestations. Addictive behaviors include one or more of the following: impaired control over drug use, compulsive use, continued use despite harm, and craving.

Drug tolerance: A state of adaptation in which exposure to a drug induces changes that result in a diminution of one or more of the effects of the drug over time.

Approved by the Boards of Directors of the American Academy of Pain Medicine, The American Pain Society, and American Society of Addiction Medicine, February 2011, American Pain Society, 2011.

◆ SKILL 16.1   Pain Assessment and Basic Comfort Measures

An accurate and comprehensive pain assessment is necessary to identify the nature of pain, the patient's perception of pain, and the effects on his or her lifestyle, as well as offer clues to the cause of the pain. A thorough assessment will allow you to arrive at proper nursing diagnoses and select appropriate pain relief therapies. Effectively managing a patient's pain does not necessarily mean eliminating it, but it does mean getting it to an acceptable level for him or her. Pain management requires you to work with a patient and family to prevent pain whenever possible and identify an acceptable intensity of pain and level of other factors, especially sleep, that allow maximum patient function.

Use of the nursing process allows you to recognize distinct and unique differences in patient perceptions and responses to pain. The nursing process guides you in learning to know a patient and develop an individualized plan of care.

Delegation and Collaboration

Assessment of a patient's pain cannot be delegated to nursing assistive personnel (NAP). The NAP may screen patients for pain and provide selected nonpharmacological strategies (e.g., back rubs, heat or cold application) as instructed by the nurse. The nurse directs the NAP to:

- Eliminate environmental conditions that worsen pain (e.g., an excessively warm, noisy room).
- Provide maximum rest periods for patient; a written schedule for caregivers to follow is ideal.
- Turn and place patients in a position of comfort at least every 2 hours or remind patients to turn themselves. Encourages patient to use a pillow for splinting if needed.
- Observe for and report to the nurse behavioral signs of pain for patients who are unable to self-report (see Box 16.2).
- Ask a patient to describe pain using a pain-intensity scale chosen by patient and nurse.
- Report in a timely manner to nurse any patient reports of pain intensity above predetermined goal and nonverbal behaviors suggestive of pain.
- Screen for pain during patient transfer or other activity that might provoke pain.

Equipment

- Pain rating scale (check agency policy)

STEP	RATIONALE

ASSESSMENT

STEP	RATIONALE
1. Identify patient using at least two identifiers (e.g., name and birthday or name and medical record number) according to agency policy.	Ensures correct patient. Complies with The Joint Commission standards and improves patient safety (TJC, 2016).
2. Assess patient's risk for pain (e.g., those undergoing invasive procedures, anxious patients, those unable to communicate).	Allows you to anticipate patient's needs and intervene in timely manner, possibly preventing pain.
3. Ask patients if they are in pain. Observe for nonverbal indicators of pain; ask significant others if they believe patient is in pain (Herr et al., 2011a). Older adults and patients from various cultures may not admit to having pain. Try using other terms such as *hurt* or *discomfort*, or *use professional interpreter if language difference exists.*	There is no objective test to measure pain. Accept patient's self-report of pain (Pasero and McCaffery, 2011). Recognizes that cultural differences exist in how pain is expressed.
4. Perform hand hygiene. Examine site of patient's pain or discomfort when possible. Inspect (discoloration, swelling, drainage), palpate (change in temperature, area of altered sensation, painful area, areas that trigger pain), and assess range of motion of involved joints. Percussion and auscultation can help to identify abnormalities (e.g., underlying mass or lung crackles) and determine cause of pain (see Chapter 6). *When assessing abdomen, always auscultate first and then inspect and palpate.*	Reduces transmission of infection. Reveals nature of pain and directs you toward appropriate interventions.

5. Assess physical, behavioral, and emotional signs and symptoms of pain:
  a. Moaning, crying, whimpering, groaning, vocalizations
  b. Decreased activity
  c. Facial expressions (e.g., grimace, clenched teeth)
  d. Change in usual behavior (e.g., less active, irritable)
  e. Abnormal gait (e.g., shuffling) and posture (e.g., bent, leaning)
  f. Guarding a body part
  g. Diaphoresis
  h. When appropriate, assess for increased blood glucose level reflecting stress of unrelieved pain
	Signs and symptoms may reveal source and nature of pain. Nonverbal responses to pain are useful in assessing pain in patients who are cognitively impaired or nonverbal.
	
	The stress of unrelieved pain causes the endocrine system to release excessive amounts of hormones (especially cortisol) and decreased levels of insulin (Pasero and McCaffery, 2011).

STEP	RATIONALE
i. Decreased gastrointestinal (GI) motility, constipation, nausea, and vomiting	Signs and symptoms of pain originate from involvement of visceral organs with stimulation of the parasympathetic nervous system, which decreases gastrointestinal (GI) tract activity (Drew and St. Marie, 2011).
j. Insomnia, anorexia, and fatigue	
k. Depression, hopelessness, anger, fear, social withdrawal	Depression frequently occurs in patients with chronic pain and increases perception and intensity of pain (Drew and St. Marie, 2011).
l. Concomitant symptoms: symptoms that often occur with pain (e.g., headache, constipation). **NOTE:** Constipation is common with opioid use.	Multiple symptoms increase complexity in care of patient.

Clinical Decision Point *Physiological responses (e.g., tachycardia, hypertension) to acute pain are of short duration and return to normal within minutes. Be aware that with persistent pain a patient does not usually exhibit physical signs and symptoms. Never use physiological responses alone to determine pain therapy selected, even with acute pain (Pasero and McCaffery, 2011).*

STEP	RATIONALE
6. Assess characteristics of pain. Follow agency policy regarding frequency of assessment. Use the PQRSTU pain assessment.	Guides clinician in collecting complete information about patient's pain experience.
a. Provocative/Palliative factors (e.g., "What makes your pain better or worse?"): Consider patient's experience with over-the-counter (OTC) drugs (including herbals and topicals) that have helped to reduce pain in the past.	Identifies nature and source of pain and what patient uses to reduce discomfort. Combination of interventions is often most effective approach to pain relief.
b. Quality: Use open-ended questions such as "Tell me what your pain feels like."	Helps to determine underlying pain mechanism (e.g., somatic versus neuropathic pain).
c. Region/Radiation (e.g., "Show me everywhere your pain is."). Have patient use finger (if possible) to point out areas of pain.	Identify location of pain and possible causative factors for acute/transient pain.
d. Severity: Use valid pain rating scale appropriate to patient's age, language skills, developmental level, and comprehension (see illustrations). Ask patient to rate pain at rest, before any intervention, and when he or she is moving or engaged in care activity. In the case of patients with dementia or those who have no verbal skills, use observational pain assessment scales such as the Pain Assessment Checklist for Seniors with Limited Ability to Communicate (PACSLAC) and The Pain Assessment in Advanced Dementia Scale (PAINAD) (Touhy and Jett, 2014; Zwakhalen et al., 2006).	An appropriate pain rating scale is reliable, is easily understood, and reflects changes in pain intensity (Herr et al., 2011a).
e. Timing: Ask patient if pain is constant, intermittent, continuous, or a combination. Does pain increase during specific times of day, with particular activities, or in specific locations?	Environmental stimuli such as loud noises, bright lights, strong odors, or temperature extremes sometimes alter patient's response to pain.
f. How is pain affecting U (patient) regarding activities of daily living (ADLs), work, relationships, and enjoyment of life?	Provides important baseline information to later gauge effectiveness of interventions.
7. Assess patient's medical history and type of therapies successfully used to relieve pain (e.g., medications, OTC products, heat and cold therapies).	History provides information for type of therapies to use for patient's specific situation. Many patients do not mention using OTC products for fear of being criticized or because they do not want them taken away.
8. Assess patient's response to previous pharmacological interventions, especially ability to function (e.g., sleeping, eating, and other ADLs). Determine if any analgesic side effects are likely based on medication and patient's previous responses (e.g., itching or nausea).	Determines extent to which therapies have or have not been successful in the past (Gloth, 2011). Some side effects, especially itching that can occur with morphine, are often poorly tolerated by patient and indicate need to identify another analgesic.
9. Assess for allergies to medications, with focus on analgesics.	Some patients with asthma or an allergy to aspirin are also allergic to other nonsteroidal antiinflammatory drugs (NSAIDs) (Morales et al., 2015).

STEP	RATIONALE

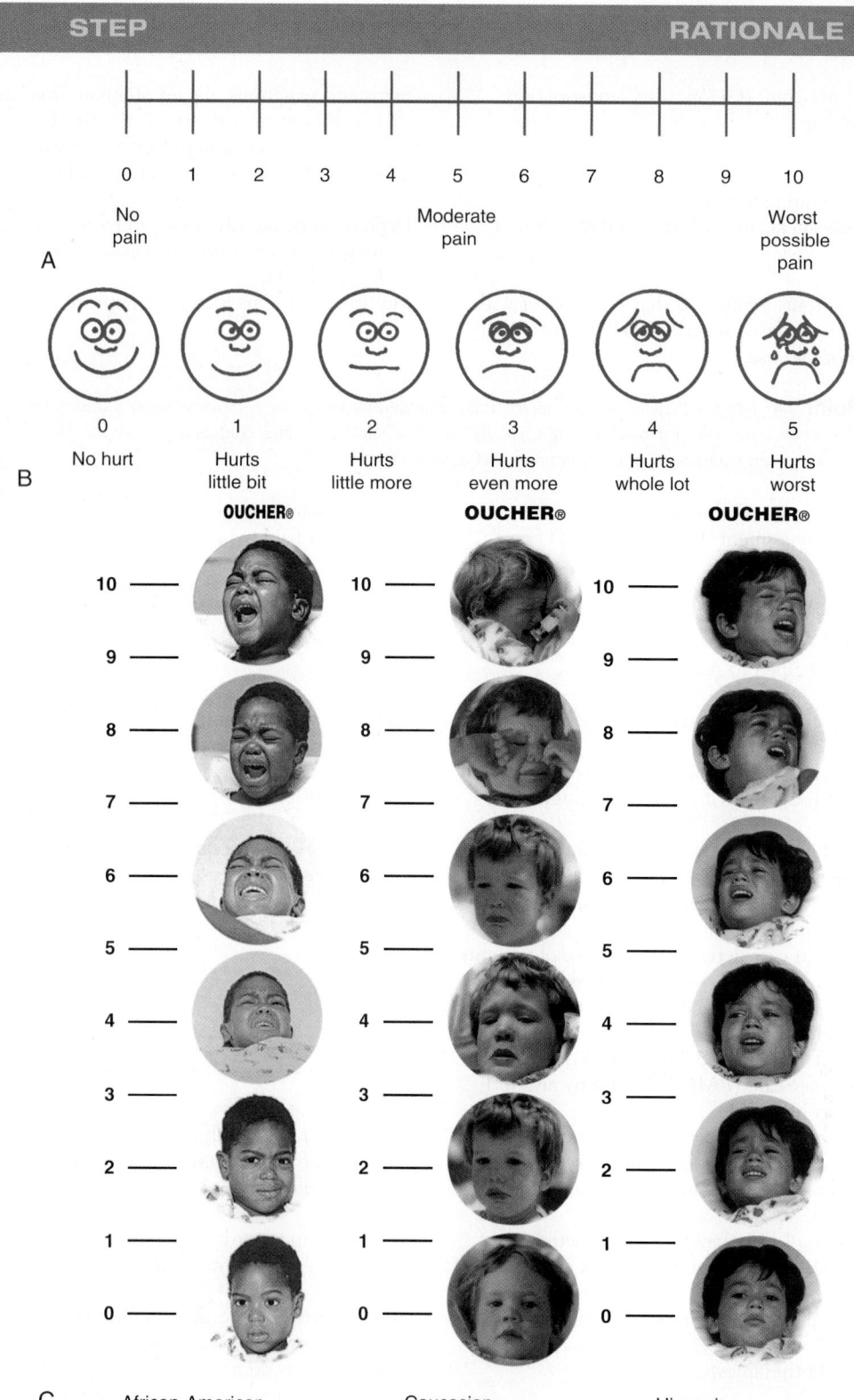

STEP 6d A, Pain rating scale. *From McCaffery M, Pasero C: Pain: clinical manual, ed 2, St Louis, 1999, Mosby.* **B,** Wong-Baker FACES pain rating scale. *From Wong DL et al.: Whaley and Wong's nursing care of infants and children, ed 7, St Louis, 2003, Mosby.* **C(1),** African-American version of Oucher pain scale. *Developed and copyrighted in 1990 by Mary J. Denyes, PhD, RN, Wayne State University, and Antonia M. Villarruel, PhD, RN, University of Michigan. Cornelia P. Porter, PhD, RN, and Charlotta Marshall, RN, MSN, contributed to the development.* **C(2),** Caucasian version of Oucher pain scale. *Developed and copyrighted in 1983 by Judith E. Beyer, PhD, RN, University of Missouri-Kansas City School of Nursing, Kansas City, MO.* **C(3),** Hispanic version of Oucher pain scale. *Developed and copyrighted in 1990 by Antonia M. Villarruel, PhD, University of Michigan, and Mary J. Denyes, PhD, RN, Wayne State University.*

STEP	RATIONALE

NURSING DIAGNOSES

- Activity intolerance
- Acute pain
- Anxiety
- Chronic pain

- Deficient knowledge regarding alternative pain therapies
- Disturbed sleep pattern
- Fatigue
- Fear

- Impaired physical mobility
- Ineffective coping
- Powerlessness
- Readiness for enhanced comfort
- Risk for constipation

Related factors/Risk factors are individualized based on patient's condition or needs.

PLANNING

STEP	RATIONALE
1. Expected outcomes following completion of procedure: • Patient verbalizes full or partial relief from pain. • Patient displays nonverbal behaviors such as relaxed face and absence of squinting. • Patient reports improvement in sleep, nutritional intake, physical activity, and personal relationships. **2.** Set pain-intensity goal with patient (when able).	Patient's self-report of pain is single most reliable indicator of pain (Pasero and McCaffery, 2011). Nonverbal behaviors can be valid and reliable indicators of pain and pain relief in the cognitively impaired (Herr et al., 2011a). Adequate pain relief usually permits patient to participate in usual ADLs. Pain is unique to each individual. Patient sets individual goal for tolerable pain severity.

IMPLEMENTATION

STEP	RATIONALE
1. Perform hand hygiene and apply clean gloves (if indicated).	Reduces transmission of microorganisms.
2. Prepare patient's environment. • Temperature suited to patient • Sound • Lighting • Eliminate unnecessary interruptions and coordinate care activities; allow for rest.	Temperature and sound extremes can enhance patient's perception of pain. Bright or very dim lighting can aggravate pain sensation. Fatigue increases pain perception.
3. Teach patient how to use pain rating scale. Explain range of intensity scores and how they relate to measure pain.	Accurate reporting by patient or family improves ongoing pain assessment, treatment, and evaluation.
4. Prepare and administer appropriate pain-relieving medications (nonopioids, opioids, co-analgesic or multimodal combination) per health care provider's order (see Chapter 20). Choice of medication depends on patient's condition. For example, postoperative pain is often treated initially with opioids or intravenous acetaminophen, which provides effective nonopioid analgesia for postoperative patients.	Nonopioids are effective for mild-to-moderate pain. Patients with chronic pain are typically prescribed multimodal therapy (more than one type of analgesic) for pain relief.
5. Remove or reduce painful stimuli. **a.** Help patient turn and reposition to comfortable position in good body alignment. **b.** Smooth wrinkles in bed linens. **c.** Loosen constrictive bandages (if appropriate to purpose of bandage) or loosen or remove devices (e.g., blood pressure cuff, elastic hose, or sequential stockings). **d.** Reposition underlying tubes or equipment. **e.** Use pillows as needed for alignment and positioning support (see illustration)	Reduction of pain stimuli and pressure receptors maximizes responses to pain-relieving interventions. Reduces stress on musculoskeletal system. Reduces pressure and irritation to skin. Bandage or device encircling extremity can restrict circulation and cause pain (see Chapter 41). Removes pressure on skin. Helps maintain position that reduces strain on muscles and pressure areas.
6. Teach patient how to splint over painful site using either a pillow or hand. **a.** Explain purpose of splinting.	Splinting reduces pain by minimizing muscle movement at time of stress. Promotes patient's cooperation.

STEP	RATIONALE

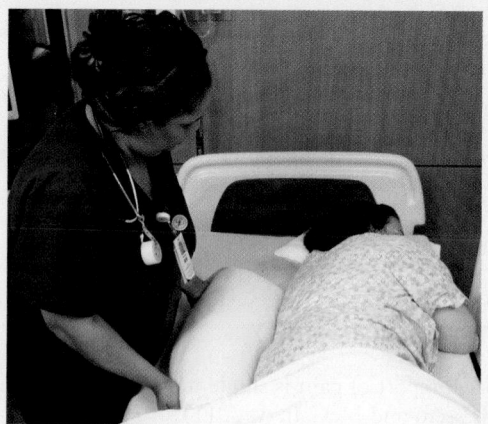

STEP 5e Positioning patient in side-lying lateral position for comfort.

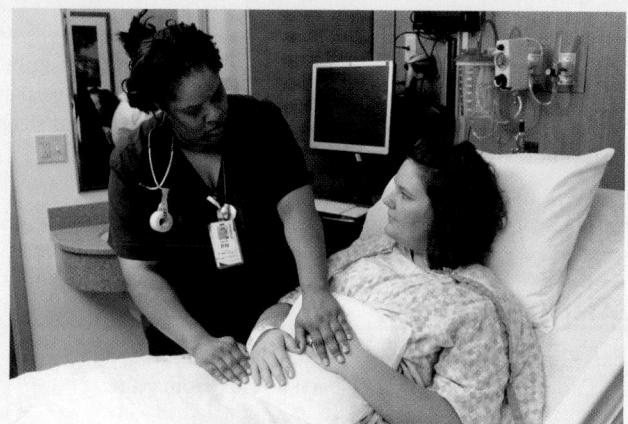

STEP 6b Patient shown how to splint painful area.

b. Place pillow or blanket over site of discomfort and help patient place hands firmly over area of discomfort (see illustration).	Splinting immobilizes painful area.
c. Have patient hold area firmly while coughing, deep breathing, and turning.	Splinting decreases movement and subsequent pain during activity.
7. Reduce or eliminate emotional factors that increase pain experiences (see Skill 16.5). Use biopsychosocial treatments: cognitive-behavioral and/or behavioral therapies.	Helps patients relax. Thoughts influence feelings, which change perception and behaviors, including a perception of pain relief (Baird et al., 2010). Psychological approaches to the management of chronic pain aim to achieve increased self-management, behavioral change, and cognitive change rather than directly eliminate locus of pain (Roditi and Robinson, 2011).
a. Offer information that reduces anxiety (e.g., explaining cause of pain if known).	
b. Offer patient opportunity to pray (if appropriate).	Serves as form of distraction.
c. Spend time to allow patient to talk about pain and answer questions. Listen attentively.	Conveys a sense of caring and interest in patient's welfare.
8. If used, remove and dispose of gloves. Perform hand hygiene.	Reduces transmission of microorganisms.

EVALUATION

1. Within 1 hour of an intervention (e.g., repositioning or after a medication reaches its peak effect), ask patient to describe level of relief using a scale of 0 to 10.	Evaluates effectiveness of pain-relieving interventions in timely manner (Pasero and McCaffery, 2011).
2. Compare patient's current pain with personally set pain-intensity goal.	Helps to determine appropriate changes to pain-management plan. Makes patient active participant in care.
3. Compare patient's ability to function and perform ADLs before and after pain interventions.	Contributes to determining effectiveness of pain-relieving interventions, especially in nonverbal patients (APS, 2009; Gloth, 2011; Herr et al., 2011a).
4. Observe patient's nonverbal behaviors.	Determines effectiveness of pain-relieving interventions (Herr et al., 2011a).
5. Evaluate for analgesic side effects.	Side effects of analgesics may be controlled by reducing dose, increasing time intervals, or administering other medications.
6. Use Teach-Back: "We discussed how splinting, turning on your nonsurgical side, and relaxation can relieve pain. Explain to me when you can use these approaches at home." Revise your instruction now or develop a plan for revised patient teaching if patient is not able to teach back correctly.	Determines patient's level of understanding of instructional topic.

STEP	RATIONALE

Unexpected Outcomes

1. Patient verbalizes continued pain that exceeds pain-intensity goal or displays nonverbal behavior reflecting worsening pain.

2. Patient experiences unexpected or adverse reaction to medication.

Related Interventions

- Repeat complete pain assessment.
- Implement different nonpharmacological pain-relief measures.
- Ask patient and family caregivers which alternatives might be helpful.
- Notify health care provider.
- Assess unexpected effects on patient.
- Notify health care provider immediately.
- Be prepared to administer antidote if indicated (e.g., antiemetic, antihistamine, opioid-reversing agent such as naloxone).
- Monitor for effectiveness of antidote; antidote may have shorter half-life than opioid; repeat dose of antidote may be needed.
- Complete adverse reaction documentation according to agency policy.

Recording and Reporting

- Record and report character of pain before an intervention, the pain-relief therapies used, any patient or family education provided, and patient response to interventions in nurses' notes in electronic health record (EHR) or chart.
- Document your evaluation of patient learning.
- Record and report inadequate pain relief (not reaching goal), a reduction in patient function, and adverse effects from pain interventions (pharmacological and nonpharmacological) in the EHR or chart.

Special Considerations
Teaching

- Review patient's and family's understanding of the pain rating scale used and how to use it when providing pain therapies.
- Explain to patient and family about the behavioral changes that may result from pain (e.g., change in activity level, splinting a body part, decreased social interaction).

- Ask patient and family about fear of addiction, a common primary concern, or other misconceptions that could undermine the patient's pain relief (Table 16.1).

Pediatric

- A numerical rating pain scale is a valid measure for assessing pain intensity in children with chronic pain (Ruskin et al., 2014).
- The absolute value of a pain-intensity score is not as important as the changes in scores in each individual child. In clinical use with individual patients, a change in pain of 2 of 10 (i.e., a change of one face) represents the least change that can be considered clinically significant when using a Faces Scale (Tomlinson et al., 2010).
- Some children are reluctant to report pain because they have misconceptions about the cause of their pain or they fear the consequences (e.g., another painful procedure or an injection).

TABLE 16.1

Misconceptions: Barriers to the Assessment and Treatment of Pain

Misconception	Correction
The best judge of the existence and severity of a patient's pain is the health care provider or nurse caring for the patient.	The patient's self-report is the most reliable indicator of the existence and intensity of pain.
Clinicians should use their personal opinions and beliefs about the truthfulness of a patient to determine his or her true pain status.	Allowing each clinician to act on personal beliefs presents the potential for different pain assessments by different clinicians, leading to different interventions from each clinician. This results in inconsistent and often inadequate pain management. A patient's self-report of pain is the standard for pain assessment.
Visible signs, either physiological or behavioral, always accompany pain and can be used to verify its existence and severity.	Even with severe pain, periods of physiological and behavioral adaptation occur, leading to periods of minimal-or-no observable signs of pain. Lack of pain expression does not necessarily mean lack of pain.
The pain rating scale preferred for use in daily clinical practice is the visual analogue scale (VAS).	The preferred pain rating scale depends on a patient's cognitive and physical ability, culture, developmental level, and availability.
Cognitively impaired older adults are unable to use pain rating scales.	When an appropriate pain rating scale is used and a patient is given sufficient time to process information and respond, many cognitively impaired older adults can use a pain rating scale.
If patients hurt enough, they will tell you.	Patients are often hesitant to report pain for fear of being labeled as complainers, hypochondriacs, or addicts.
Psychosocial interventions alone reduce or alleviate pain.	Nonpharmacological interventions are synergistic with medications but are not a substitute for pharmacological management of pain.

Modified from Pasero C, McCaffery M: *Pain: assessment and pharmacological management,* St Louis, 2011, Mosby.

- Infants and children experience pain but respond to it differently than adults. For example, they cry and thrash about, have sleep disturbances, have a shortened attention span, suck or rock, refuse to eat or play, or are quiet and withdrawn. Variations in pain response are related to the child's personality, developmental level, and previous pain experiences (Hockenberry and Wilson, 2015).
- Parents are helpful when assessing their child's pain and planning pain-relief therapies. Most parents know how their child exhibits pain and which pain-relief interventions have been successful.
- Children with verbal skills can rate their level of pain on the Wong-Baker FACES pain rating scale or the Oucher pain scale (deTovar et al., 2010).

Gerontological

- Older adults who are able to express themselves can use self-report pain scales. In addition, your assessment should include how the pain is affecting function, sleep, appetite, activity, mood, and relationships with others (Touhy and Jett, 2014).
- Some older adults may require more time (than younger adults) for you to explain a pain-assessment scale.
- Pain is not a natural occurrence of aging, although older adults are at risk for experiencing more pain-producing conditions.
- Nonverbal older adults experiencing pain typically receive fewer analgesics than similar patients who are able to report their pain (Herr et al., 2011b). Thus be sure that your assessment is thorough and evaluate a patient's response critically.

Home Care

- Consider home conditions such as type of bed and environmental stimuli. A supportive bed and quiet environment enhance sleep and promote pain management.
- Family caregivers are the main support for older people. Educate them about causes of painful conditions, common misconceptions about use of analgesics, type of pain medicines appropriate for patient, and how to support medication adherence.

✦ SKILL 16.2   Patient-Controlled Analgesia

 Video Clip

Patient-controlled analgesia (PCA) is an interactive method of pain management that permits patient control over pain through self-administration of opioids (usually morphine, hydromorphone, or fentanyl) with minimal risk of overdose. It is a safe method of analgesic administration for acute and chronic pain, including conditions such as postoperative pain, cancer, and end-of-life pain. The goal is to maintain a constant plasma level of analgesic to avoid the problems of prn dosing. Systemic PCA traditionally involves intravenous (IV) or subcutaneous drug administration.

PCA devices are programmed individually to automatically deliver a specific health care provider–prescribed continuous infusion (basal rate) of medication, a bolus dose (patient initiated), or both. PCA prevents overdosing in two ways: having control limits for the total dosage that can be administered each hour and having a timing control (lock-out period) that regulates the minimum interval (e.g., 10 minutes between doses) (Burchum and Rosenthal, 2016).

A patient depresses the button on a PCA device to deliver a regulated dose of analgesic. It is crucial that candidates for PCA be able to understand how, why, and when to self-administer a medication (APS and AAPM, 2009). Monitoring levels of sedation is essential with the use of PCA. This is especially true for most patients who are "opioid naïve" (i.e., those who have never taken opioids for any reason or who have not taken opioids in the past 5 weeks) (Pasero and McCaffery, 2011). In addition, oversedation is a risk in patients with obstructive sleep apnea (OSA) (brief cessation of respirations during sleep) or obese patients with short, thick, necks who commonly have undiagnosed sleep apnea. Assessment of patient sedation levels is critical (see Box 16.4).

The advantages of PCA include achieving more constant serum levels of an opioid and avoiding peaks and troughs of a large bolus. Patients receive better pain relief and fewer side effects from opioids because blood levels are maintained at a level of minimum effective analgesia concentration. Increased patient control and independence are other advantages for patients. Because PCA provides medication on demand, the total amount of opioid use can be reduced.

Concerns involving PCA use are patient related, pump failure, or health care provider errors. Patients may misunderstand how PCA therapy works, mistake the PCA button for a nurse call button, or have family members operate the demand button. A pump may fail to deliver a drug on demand, have a faulty alarm or low battery, or lack free-flow protection. Health care providers may incorrectly program a dose, concentration, or rate. Incorrect programming is the most common type of error. Other errors include failing to clamp or unclamp tubing, improperly loading syringe or cartridge, failing to monitor for side effects/overdose, and not responding to alarms. PCA requires careful monitoring; never try to operate it without fully understanding the particular model in use. Some agencies require a two–registered nurse (RN) check when initiating a PCA, changing the dose, or discontinuing its use.

Delegation and Collaboration

The skill of administration of PCA cannot be delegated to nursing assistive personnel (NAP). The nurse directs the NAP to:

- Notify the nurse if the patient complains of change in status, including unrelieved pain or oversedation.
- Notify the nurse if the patient has questions about the PCA process or equipment.
- Never administer a PCA dose for the patient and notify the nurse if anyone other than the patient is observed administering a dose for the patient.

Equipment

- PCA system and tubing
- Identification label and time tape (may come attached and completed by pharmacy)
- Needleless connector
- Alcohol swab
- Adhesive tape
- Clean gloves (when applicable)
- Equipment for vital signs and pulse oximeter, or capnography (CO_2) monitoring equipment

STEP	RATIONALE

ASSESSMENT

1. Check accuracy and completeness of medication administration record (MAR) or computer printout with health care provider's order for patient's name, name of medication, dose, frequency of medication (continuous or demand or both), and lockout period.

   Health care provider order required for administration of opioid medication. Ensures that patient receives right medications.

2. Review medication information in drug reference manual or consult with pharmacist if uncertain about any medications to be administered.

   Understanding medications before administering them prevents medication errors (Adhikari et al., 2014).

3. Perform hand hygiene. Assess severity and character of patient's pain (see Skill 16.1). Also assess patient's ability to manipulate PCA control and cognitive status for ability to understand purpose of PCA and how to use control device.

   Reduces transmission of microorganisms. Reveals source and nature of pain and factors that may increase pain. Determines patient's ability to use PCA safely and correctly.

4. Assess environment for factors that could contribute to pain (e.g., noise, room temperature).

   Elimination of irritating stimuli may help to reduce pain perception.

5. Assess for conditions that predispose patients to unwanted effects from opioids. Known, untreated, or unknown OSA poses a significant risk for respiratory depression (Craft, 2010). Use the STOP-BANG questionnaire to assess for OSA (Lockhart et al., 2013) (see agency policy).

   Assessment should be completed before surgery by anesthesia. Identification allows treatment teams (surgeon, respiratory therapy, anesthesia) to take appropriate precautions such as making continuous positive–airway pressure or bi-level positive–airway pressure ventilation devices available.

6. Apply clean gloves. Assess patency of intravenous (IV) access and surrounding tissue for inflammation or swelling (see Chapter 29).

   IV line needs to be patent for safe administration of pain medication. Confirmation of placement of IV catheter and integrity of surrounding tissues ensures that medication is safely administered.

7. If patient has had surgery, inspect incision, continuing to wear clean gloves. Gently palpate around area for tenderness. Use sterile gloves if necessary to place hand directly on incision. Remove gloves and perform hand hygiene.

   Reveals evidence of tissue trauma or damage, which stimulates peripheral pain receptors to transmit impulses to cortex to create conscious awareness of pain (Drew and St. Marie, 2011)

8. Check medical record for patient's history for drug allergies and typical reactions.

   Avoids placing patient at risk for allergic reaction.

Clinical Decision Point *Be aware that nausea is not an allergic reaction and it can be treated; pruritus alone is not an allergic reaction and is common to opioid use. Pruritus is treatable and does not rule out the use of PCA.*

9. Assess patient's knowledge and perceived effectiveness of previous pain-management strategies, especially previous PCA use.

   Response to pain-control strategies helps identify learning needs and affects patient's willingness to try therapy.

NURSING DIAGNOSES

- Acute pain
- Anxiety
- Chronic pain
- Deficient knowledge regarding use of PCA
- Fear
- Ineffective coping
- Impaired physical mobility

Related factors are individualized based on patient's condition or needs.

PLANNING

1. Expected outcomes following completion of procedure:
   - Patient verbalizes pain relief.
   - Patient rates pain lower on pain scale.
   - Patient exhibits relaxed facial expression and body position.
   - Patient remains alert and oriented.

   - Patient increasingly participates in self-care activities.
   - Patient correctly operates PCA device.

   Subjective measure of pain relief.
   Objective measure of pain relief.
   Nonverbal cues of pain relief.

   Indicates freedom from overly sedating effects of opioids. Sleepiness is usually from fatigue and not necessarily a sign of oversedation.

   Suggests successful pain relief.
   Demonstrates safe and appropriate use of PCA.

STEP	RATIONALE
2. Collect appropriate equipment. Draw curtains around patient's bed or close door to room.	Aids in organization. Maintains patient privacy.

IMPLEMENTATION

STEP	RATIONALE
1. Perform hand hygiene.	Reduces transmission of infection.
2. Obtain PCA analgesic in module prepared by pharmacy. Check label of medication 2 times; when removed from storage and when preparing for assembly.	Follows six rights of medication administration to be sure of correct medication. *This is the first and second check for accuracy.*
3. At bedside identify patient using at least two identifiers (e.g., name and birthday or name and medical record number) according to agency policy. Compare identifiers with information on patient's MAR or medical record.	Ensures correct patient. Complies with The Joint Commission standards and improves patient safety (TJC, 2016).
4. At bedside compare MAR or computer printout with name of medication on drug cartridge. Have second registered nurse (RN) confirm health care provider's order and correct setup of PCA. Second RN should check order and the device independently and not just look at existing setup.	Ensures that correct patient receives right medication. *This is the third check for accuracy.*
5. Before initiating analgesia, explain purpose and demonstrate function of PCA to patient and family caregiver as follows:	Allows patient participation in care and independence in pain control. Preoperative education about PCA therapy improves postoperative pain relief (D'Arcy, 2011; Pasero and McCaffery, 2011).
a. Explain type of medication in device.	
b. Explain that device safely administers self-initiated small but frequent amounts of medication when needed to provide comfort and minimizes side effects from analgesia.	
c. Explain that self-dosing aids in repositioning, walking or coughing, and deep breathing.	
d. Explain that device is programmed to deliver ordered type and dose of pain medication, lockout interval, and 1- to 4-hour dosage limits. Explain how lockout time prevents overdose.	
e. Demonstrate to patient how to push medication demand button (see illustration). Instruct family caregiver to not push PCA button to give medication.	
f. Instruct patient to notify nurse for possible side effects, problems in gaining pain relief, changes in severity or location of pain, alarm sounding, or questions.	
6. Apply clean gloves. Check infuser and patient-control module for accurate labeling or evidence of leaking.	Avoids medication error and injury to patient.
7. Position patient comfortably to be sure that venipuncture or central line site is accessible.	Ensures unimpeded flow of infusion.
8. Insert drug cartridge into infusion device (see illustration) and prime tubing.	Locks system and prevents air from infusing into IV tubing.
9. Attach needleless adapter to tubing adapter of patient-controlled module.	Needed to connect with IV line.
10. Wipe injection port of maintenance IV line vigorously with alcohol or antiseptic for 15 seconds and allow to dry.	Minimizes entry of surface microorganisms during needle insertion, reducing risk of catheter-related bloodstream infection.
11. Insert needleless adapter into injection port nearest patient (at Y-site of peripheral IV or central line or connect to its own IV site). There should not be a chance to use PCA tubing for administering IV push with another drug.	Establishes route for medication to enter main IV line. Needleless systems prevent needlestick injuries. Prevents medication interaction and incompatibility.

STEP	RATIONALE

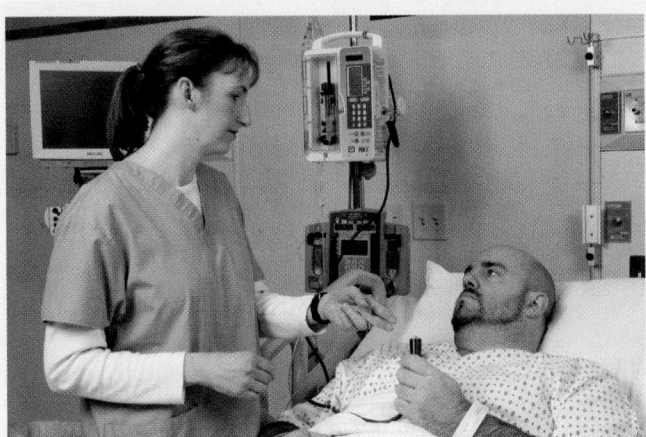

STEP 5e Patient learns how to press PCA device button.

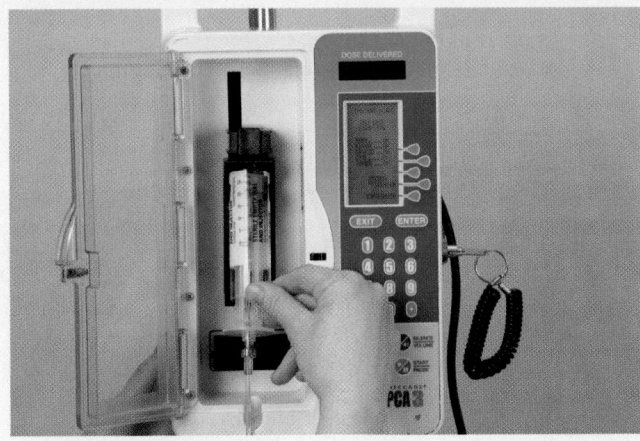

STEP 8 Nurse inserting drug cartridge into PCA device.

12. Secure connection and anchor PCA tubing with tape. Label PCA tubing.

Prevents dislodging of needleless adapter from port. Facilitates patient's ability to ambulate. Label prevents error from connecting tubing from different device to PCA.

13. Program computerized PCA pump as ordered to deliver prescribed medication dose and lockout interval. Have second nurse check setting. (**NOTE:** Recheck with oncoming RN during shift hand-off to ensure line reconciliation).

Ensures safe, therapeutic drug administration. With appropriate dose intervals (e.g., 10 min), usually an appreciable analgesic effect and/or mild sedation is achieved before patient can access the next dose; thus there is lower chance for oversedation and respiratory depression (Craft, 2010).

14. Administer loading dose of analgesia as prescribed. Manually give 1-time dose or turn on pump and program dose into pump.

Establishes initial level of analgesia.

15. Discard gloves and supplies in appropriate containers. Dispose of empty cassette or syringe in compliance with institutional policy. Perform hand hygiene.

Reduces transmission of microorganisms. The Federal Controlled Substances Act regulates control and dispensation of opioids for all institutions.

16. If experiencing pain, have patient demonstrate use of PCA system; if not, have patient repeat instructions given earlier.

Repeating instructions reinforces learning. Checking patient's understanding through return demonstration helps you determine patient's level of understanding and ability to manipulate device.

17. Be sure that venipuncture or central line site is protected and recheck before leaving patient.

Ensures patency of IV line.

18. **To discontinue PCA:**
    a. Check health care provider order for discontinuation. Obtain necessary PCA information from pump for documentation; note date, time, amount infused and amount of drug wasted and reason for wastage.

    Ensures correct documentation of a schedule II drug.

    Two RNs must witness wastage of opioids (narcotics) and sign record to meet requirements of the Controlled Substances Act for scheduled drugs.

    b. Perform hand hygiene and apply clean gloves. Turn off pump. Disconnect PCA tubing from primary IV line but maintain IV access.

    Reduces transmission of infection. Ensures continuation of IV infusion.

    c. Dispose of empty cartridge, tubing and gloves according to agency policy.

STEP	RATIONALE

EVALUATION

1. Use pain rating scale to evaluate patient's pain intensity following treatments and procedures according to agency policy.

2. Observe patient for nausea or pruritus.

3. Monitor patient's level of sedation, vital signs, and pulse oximetry or capnography every 1 to 2 hours for first 12 hours (APS and AAPM, 2009). Monitor more often at start, during first 24 hours, and at night when hypoventilation and hypoxia tend to occur (Ramachandran et al., 2011). Follow agency policy.

4. Have patient demonstrate dose delivery.

5. According to agency policy, evaluate number of attempts (number of times patient pushed button), delivery of demand doses (number of times drug actually given and total amount of medication delivered in particular time frame), and basal dose if ordered.

6. Observe patient initiate self-care.

7. **Use Teach-Back:** "I want to be sure I explained how PCA will help with your pain and how you should use the device. Tell me the steps you will use to activate the PCA." Revise your instruction now or develop a plan for revised patient teaching if patient is not able to teach back correctly.

Determines response to PCA dosing. Documenting "PCA in use" or "PCA effective" is not an adequate record of patient's pain level.

Common side effects of opioid.

Patient is at highest risk the first 24 hours of use. Excess sedation (difficult to arouse) precedes respiratory depression.

Evaluates skill in use of PCA.

Helps to evaluate effectiveness of PCA dose and frequency in relieving pain. Maintains compliance with Controlled Substances Act.

Demonstrates pain relief.

Determines patient's level of understanding of instructional topic.

Unexpected Outcomes	Related Interventions
1. Patient verbalizes continued or worsening discomfort or displays non-verbal behaviors indicative of pain.	• Perform complete pain reassessment. • Assess for possible complications other than pain. • Inspect IV site for possible catheter occlusion or infiltration. • Evaluate number of attempts and deliveries initiated by patient. • Check that maintenance of IV fluid is running continuously. • Evaluate pump for operational problems. • Consult with health care provider.
2. Patient is sedated and not easily aroused.	• Stop PCA. • Notify health care provider. • Elevate head of bed 30 degrees unless contraindicated. • Instruct patient to take deep breaths. • Apply oxygen at 2 L/min per nasal cannula (if ordered). • Assess vital signs, oxygen saturation, and/or capnography. • Evaluate amount of opioid delivered within past 4–8 hours. • Ask family members if they pressed button without patient's knowledge. • Review MAR for other possible sedating drugs. • Prepare to administer an opioid-reversing agent. • Observe patient frequently (APS, 2009).
3. Patient unable to manipulate PCA device to maintain pain control.	• Consult with health care provider regarding alternative medication route or possibly a basal (continuous) dose.

Recording and Reporting

• Record drug, concentration, dose (basal and/or demand), time started, lockout time, amount of IV solution infused, and remaining solution in the electronic health record (EHR) or chart. Many agencies have special PCA documentation forms.

• Record regular assessment of patient response to analgesia on PCA medication form, in nurses' notes in electronic health record (EHR) or chart, on pain-assessment flow sheet, or on other documentation according to agency policy. This includes vital signs, oximetry or capnography, sedation status, pain rating, and status of vascular access site.

• Document your evaluation of patient learning.

Special Considerations
Teaching

• Give instructions during pain-free or pain-reduced states and before initiating therapy. Instruct surgical patients before surgery.

• Encourage patients to push button on timing unit at the earliest indication of pain. Teach preemptive pain management.

• Explain regimen to family so they can support and coach patient (but not push button for patient).

• Inform patient of nonpharmacological pain-management strategies that supplement or enhance pharmacological intervention (see Skill 16.5).

- Inform patient and family that patient will not overdose with PCA if only the patient pushes the button.

Pediatric
- PCA is an effective means of pain control in children who can understand the concept. When selecting children for PCA use, consider a patient's developmental level, cognitive level, and motor skills. Ordinarily PCA use is safe and effective for patients as young as 5 years old (deTovar et al., 2010). From a developmental perspective, use of PCA is particularly effective with adolescents because it leads to feelings of control.
- Although controversial, some agencies have provided specific guidelines and training to allow parents and nurses to push the button for children too young or unable to use the device on their own. When this is allowed, the concept of patient control is negated, and the inherent safety of PCA needs to be monitored (Hockenberry and Wilson, 2015)

- Pharmacological pain support is safe and effective in pediatric patients when dose is calibrated according to child's weight (Klieber et al., 2011).

Gerontological
- Older patients sometimes appear more sensitive to analgesics and experience more opioid side effects (Gloth, 2011). Older adults' reduced renal and liver function slows opioid metabolism and excretion. This causes a faster peak effect and a longer duration of action of the opioid. Dosages should be started low and titrated upward slowly until pain relief is achieved (Drew and St. Marie, 2011; Gloth, 2011).
- If patient confusion occurs while using PCA, call to get orders to lower the dose, lengthen the lockout, or add a nonopioid analgesic to reduce the opioid dose; nurse-activated around-the-clock dosing is another alternative; refusing to medicate is not the answer; confusion may be caused by pain, not the medications (Pasero and McCaffery, 2011).

◆ **SKILL 16.3** | **Epidural Analgesia**

Epidural analgesia is highly effective for controlling acute pain during labor; after surgery; or after trauma to the chest, abdomen, pelvis or lower limbs. It has the potential to provide excellent pain relief, minimal side effects, and high patient satisfaction when compared with other methods of analgesia (Rowbotham et al., 2010). Patient-controlled epidural analgesia (PCEA) has been shown to provide excellent control of labor and postoperative pain when compared with intravenous (IV) patient-controlled analgesia (PCA) (Ferguson et al., 2009; Freeman et al., 2015). Use of PCEA is safe and efficient, and complications from this technique are rare. Epidural opioids reduce the total amount of opioid medication required to control pain and thus produce fewer opioid-related side effects (D'Arcy, 2011). However, if epidural analgesia is not managed correctly, it can cause serious complications; safe and effective management requires a coordinated interprofessional approach.

The epidural space is a potential space that contains a network of vessels, nerves, and fat located between the vertebral column and the dura mater, the outermost meninges covering the spinal cord (Fig. 16.1). Analgesics delivered into this space distribute by: (1) diffusion through the dura mater into the cerebrospinal fluid (CSF), where they act directly on the receptors in the dorsal horn of the spinal cord; (2) blood vessels in the epidural space, where they are delivered systemically; and/or (3) absorption by fat in the epidural space, creating a depot where the analgesia is slowly released systemically. An analgesic acts by binding to opiate receptors in the dorsal horn of the spinal column, thus blocking pain impulse transmission to the cerebral cortex.

Opioids and local anesthetics, separately or in combination, are used in epidural analgesia. Opioids are delivered close to their site of action (central nervous system) and thus require much smaller doses to achieve the same pain relief (D'Arcy, 2011). Common

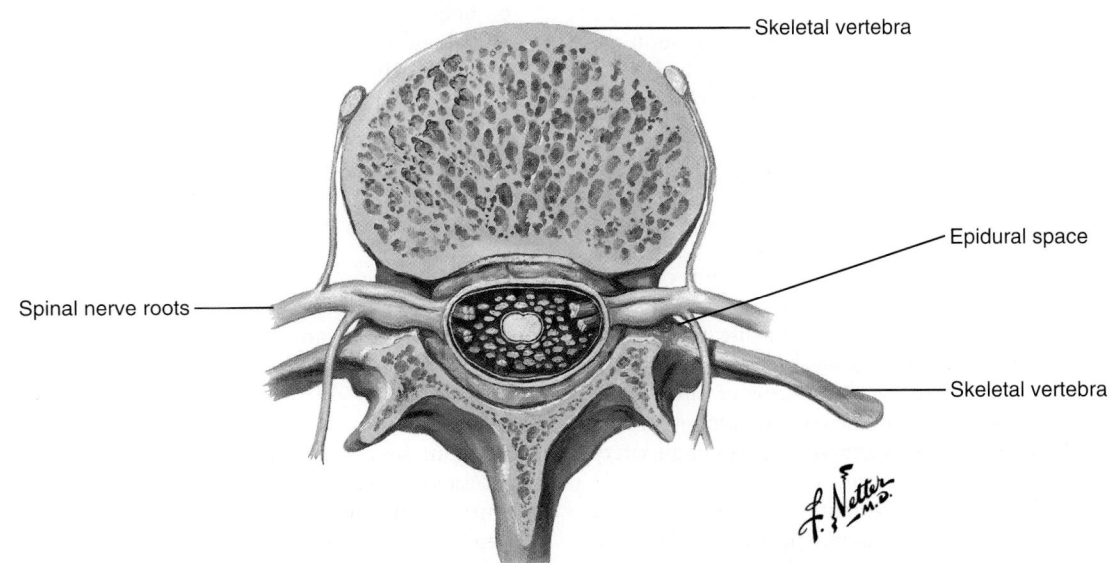

Skeletal vertebra

Epidural space

Spinal nerve roots

Skeletal vertebra

FIG 16.1 Anatomical drawing of epidural space. (*Reprinted from www.netterimages.com ©Elsevier, Inc. All rights reserved.*)

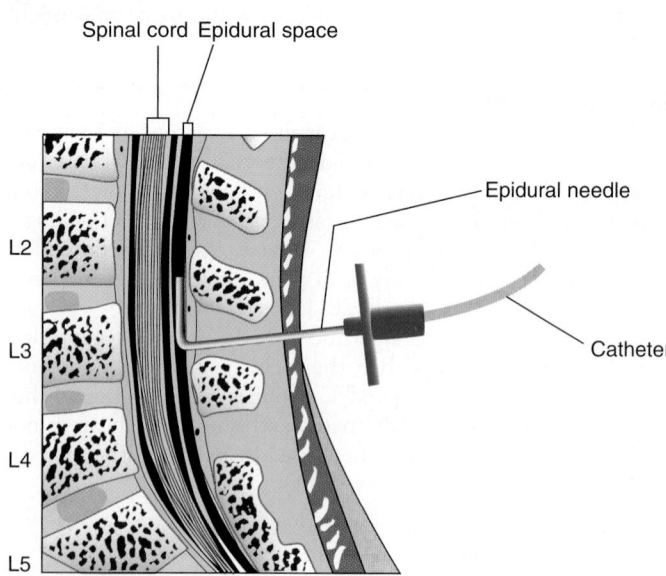

FIG 16.2 Placement of epidural catheter.

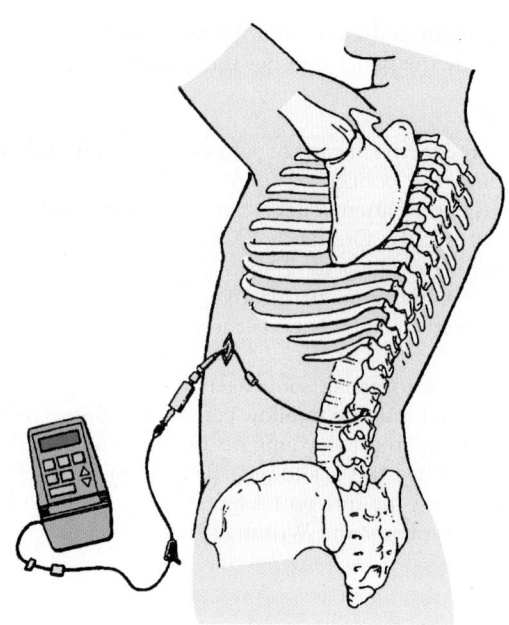

FIG 16.3 Epidural catheter attached to ambulatory infusion pump. *(Image courtesy Astra Zeneca Pharmaceuticals, Wilmington, DE. All rights reserved.)*

opioids given epidurally include morphine, hydromorphone, fentanyl, and sufentanil. These opioids differ by their lipophilic "fat-loving" and hydrophilic "water-loving" properties, which affect absorption rate and duration of action. Fentanyl and sufentanil are fat loving, causing them to have a quicker onset and shorter duration of action (2 hours). Morphine and hydromorphone are water-loving, resulting in longer onset and duration of action (24 hours).

A patient is placed in the lateral side-lying or sitting position with the shoulders and hips in alignment and the hips and head flexed during insertion of an epidural catheter. An anesthesia provider, using sterile technique, typically places a catheter into the epidural space below the second lumbar vertebra, where the spinal cord ends (Fig. 16.2). However, epidurals may also be placed at the thoracic level of the spinal cord. Temporary or short-term catheters are not sutured in place and exit from the insertion site on the back. A catheter intended for permanent or long-term use is "tunneled" subcutaneously and exits on the side of the body (Fig. 16.3) or on the abdomen. Tunneling reduces infection and catheter dislodgement. A sterile occlusive dressing covers the catheter exit site and is secured to the patient. An x-ray film confirms epidural catheter placement.

A health care provider administers epidural medication intermittently via a bolus, or a patient can inject intermittently on demand (PCEA) through a pump. An epidural infusion can also be given continuously via a controlled delivery system such as an implanted infusion pump (D'Arcy, 2011). The use of epidural opioids requires astute nursing observation and care; thus most institutions require specialized training for nurses who will manage epidural analgesia. Nursing students involved in helping with care of patients receiving epidural analgesia must understand all safety principles.

The catheter poses a threat to patient safety because of its anatomical location, its potential for migration through the dura, and its proximity to spinal nerves and vessels. Catheter migration into the subarachnoid space can produce dangerously high medication levels. Frequent complications include hypotension, respiratory depression, motor block, urinary retention, pruritus, and superficial infection around a catheter. **Do not administer other supplemental opioids or sedatives when patients are on an epidural.** The combined effect adds to the risk for respiratory depression. In many health care agencies anesthesia providers are the only health care providers who may initiate epidural opioid infusions or administer a medication bolus.

Delegation and Collaboration

The skill of epidural analgesia administration cannot be delegated to nursing assistive personnel (NAP). The nurse directs the NAP to:

- Observe the dressing over the insertion site when repositioning or ambulating patients to prevent catheter disruption.
- Avoid pulling patient up in bed while he or she is lying flat on the back, which can dislodge the epidural catheter.
- Report any catheter disconnection or leakage from dressing immediately.
- Immediately report to the nurse any change in patient status, comfort level, or loss of sensation or movement.

Equipment

- Clean gloves
- Sterile gloves (if removing epidural dressing)
- Prediluted preservative-free opioid as prescribed by health care provider for use in IV infusion pump (This is prepared by pharmacy.)
- Infusion pump and compatible tubing (Do not use Y-ports for infusion; some infusion pumps have color-coded tubing for intraspinal use.)
- Antibacterial filter
- Tape
- Label (for tubing and injection port)
- Equipment for vital signs and pulse oximetry or capnography (see agency policy)

STEP	RATIONALE

ASSESSMENT

1. Assess if patient has completed informed consent and is aware of risk and benefits of epidural analgesia (see agency policy) (Rowbotham et al., 2010).

   Epidural analgesia is a significant procedure that poses risks of serious and potentially fatal complications.

2. Verify health care provider's order against medication administration record (MAR) for name of medication, dosage, route, infusion method (bolus, continuous, or demand), and lockout settings. Recopy or reprint any portion of MAR that is difficult to read.

   The order sheet is the most reliable source and the only legal record of medications that patient is to receive. Ensures that right drug is administered to patient.

3. Perform hand hygiene. Assess level of patient's pain on scale from 0 to 10; assess character of patient's pain (see Skill 16.1). For cognitively impaired or non-English–speaking patients, assess nonverbal pain responses or seek help of professional interpreter.

   Establishes baseline pain level. Cognitively impaired patients or patients for whom English is a second language may have difficulty understanding the therapy, especially if PCEA is used. Nonverbal responses provide baseline pain assessment.

4. Check to see if patient recently received anticoagulants.

   Recent anticoagulation may contraindicate the placement of epidural catheter because of inability to apply pressure at insertion site and risk for bleeding (Pasero and McCaffery, 2011).

5. Assess if patient routinely takes herbal medications; document complete list.

   Some herbal medications interfere with the clotting mechanism (e.g., ginkgo biloba, ginseng, ginger). Currently there is no contraindication to their use (NIH, 2015a).

Clinical Decision Point *Contraindications to epidural analgesia include coagulopathies, abnormal clotting test results, compromised immunity, history of multiple abscesses, and sepsis. Additional contraindications include skeletal or spinal abnormalities (Pasero and McCaffery, 2011).*

6. Assess for history of drug allergies.

   Avoids placing patient at risk for allergic reaction.

7. Assess patient's sedation level by assessing level of wakefulness or alertness, ability to follow commands, and drowsiness (see Box 16.3).

   Establishes baseline before first dose. Assessment of sedation level is more reliable for detecting early opioid-induced respiratory depression than decreased respiratory rate. Sedation always precedes respiratory depression from opioids.

8. Assess rate, pattern, and depth of respirations; pulse oximetry or capnography; blood pressure and temperature (see Chapter 5).

   Establishes baseline of circulatory and oxygenation status. Opioids can cause hypotension. Infection is complication of epidurals, reflected by fever.

9. Assess initial motor and sensory function of lower extremities (see Chapter 6). Test sensation to touch in lower extremities. Have patient flex both feet and knees and raise each leg off bed. Pay special attention to patients with preexisting sensory or motor abnormalities.

   Establishes baseline. Ongoing monitoring of motor and sensory status ensures that neural blockage is not affecting function (D'Arcy, 2011).

Clinical Decision Point *For all patients on PCEA, assess for sensory and motor function before ambulation or transfer (D'Arcy, 2011).*

10. Perform hand hygiene. Inspect catheter insertion site for redness, warmth, tenderness, swelling, and drainage. Apply sterile gloves when removing occlusive dressing.

    Catheter sites are at risk for local infections. Purulent drainage is sign of infection. Clear drainage may indicate cerebrospinal fluid (CSF) leaking from punctured dura. Bloody drainage may indicate that catheter entered blood vessel.

11. Follow catheter tubing and check connection site with IV tubing. Verify that catheter is secured to patient's skin from back, side, or front. Be sure that catheter is connected securely to IV tubing. Remove gloves and perform hand hygiene.

    Prevents catheter dislodgement or migration. Tubing misconnections cause severe patient injury and death because tubes with different functions can be connected easily using Luer connectors or connections can be "rigged" (constructed) using adapters, tubing, or catheters (TJC, 2014). New IOS (International Organization for Standardization) tubing connector standards are being developed for manufacturers of IV tubing.

Clinical Decision Point *Note that in most health care settings pharmacy prepares and provides the medication/infusion bag.*

STEP	RATIONALE
12. Check patency of IV tubing. Check infusion pump for proper calibration and operation.	Kinked or clamped tubing interrupts analgesic infusion; may cause clotting at end of IV catheter and require replacement. Patent IV line allows IV access in case medications are needed to counteract adverse reactions.

Clinical Decision Point *Note that epidural infusions should be labeled "For Epidural Use Only." Infusion pumps should be configured specifically for epidural analgesia with preset limits for maximum infusion rate and bolus size; lock-out time should be standardized if used for PCEA (Rowbotham et al., 2010).*

NURSING DIAGNOSES

- Activity intolerance
- Acute pain
- Anxiety
- Chronic pain

- Deficient knowledge regarding epidural analgesia
- Impaired physical mobility

- Risk for infection
- Risk for injury

Related factors/Risk factors are individualized based on patient's condition or needs.

PLANNING

1. Expected outcomes following completion of procedure:

- Patient verbalizes pain relief within 30 to 60 minutes of initiating epidural infusion.

  Indicates that drug and dose are effective in relieving pain, catheter is intact, and equipment is functioning properly in compliance with health care provider's order.

- Patient has no headache during epidural infusion or after discontinuation.

  Indicates that catheter is in epidural space. No CSF leakage.

- Patient remains normotensive, and heart rate remains at or above baseline.

  Indicates absence of some of the circulatory side effects of epidural opioids.

- Patient is alert, oriented, and easily aroused.

  Indicates absence of excessive sedation/oversedation (see Box 16.3).

- Patient's respirations are regular, of adequate depth, and equal to or greater than 8 breaths/min. Pulse oximetry SpO_2 95% or greater; capnography end-tidal CO_2 5% or 35 to 37 mm Hg.

  Indicates adequate ventilation and reduced risk for respiratory depression from opioids.

- Patient voids without difficulty; averages a minimum of 30 mL/h.

  Indicates absence of urinary retention (potential opioid side effect).

- Patient has no or minimal pruritus and no paresthesias of lower extremities.

  Indicates absence of potential side effect of epidural medications.

- Epidural system remains intact and functioning.

  Infusion system is patent; no interruption in medication delivery to epidural space.

2. Explain purpose and function of epidural analgesia and expectations of patient during procedure (e.g., ask patient to call for help before getting out of bed). Demonstrate to patient how to use pump on demand (when appropriate).

Proper explanation enhances patient cooperation and helps with effective results.

3. Place patients receiving epidural analgesia close to the nurses' station.

Ensures close supervision during infusion (Rowbotham et al., 2010).

IMPLEMENTATION

1. Identify patient using at least two identifiers (e.g., name and birthday or name and medical record number) according to agency policy if you are preparing infusion. Compare identifiers with information on patient's MAR or medical record.	Ensures correct patient. Complies with The Joint Commission standards and improves patient safety (TJC, 2016).
2. Perform hand hygiene. Follow "six rights" for administration of medications (see Chapter 20). **NOTE:** *Pharmacy prepares medication for pump.* Check label of medication carefully with MAR or computer printout 2 times.	Reduces transmission of microorganisms. Ensures safe and appropriate medication administration. *This is the first and second check for accuracy.*

STEP	RATIONALE

3. When receiving patient during hand-off or when helping during insertion by anesthesia provider, apply an "epidural line" label to the epidural infusion tubing. Be sure that there are *no* Y *ports* on tubing. Epidural infusions should be labeled "For Epidural Use Only."

Labeling helps to ensure that analgesic is administered into correct line and the epidural space. Epidural infusion system between pump and patient should be considered closed, with no injection or Y ports (Rowbotham et al., 2010).

4. At the bedside compare MAR or computer printout with name of medication on drug container.

This is the third check for accuracy and ensures that right patient receives right medication.

5. Apply clean gloves. Administer infusion: Anesthesia provider typically starts or administers first dose. Thereafter nurse maintains infusion.
   a. **Continuous infusion:**

   (1) Attach container of diluted preservative-free medication to infusion pump tubing and prime tubing (see Chapter 22).

   Tubing filled with solution and free of air bubbles avoids air embolus.

   (2) Insert tubing into infusion pump (see Chapter 22) and attach distal end of tubing to antibacterial filter; then connect to epidural catheter using aseptic technique (Rowbotham et al., 2010).

   Pump propels fluid through tubing. Filter reduces entrance of microorganisms into infusion line.

   (3) Check infusion pump for proper calibration, setting, and operation. Many agencies have two nurses check settings.

   Ensures that patient is receiving proper dosing.

   (4) Tape all connections. Start infusion (see Chapter 22).

   Taping maintains secure closed system to prevent infection.

   b. Administer bolus dose of analgesic via infusion pump.
   (1) While helping anesthesia provider, perform Steps 5a(1) to 5a(4). Adjust infusion pump setting for preset limit for maximum bolus size. Initiate pump to deliver ordered bolus.

   Prevents accidental infusion of an overdose.

   c. Administer dose on demand.
   (1) While helping anesthesia provider, perform Steps 5a(1) to 5a(4). Set pump for lockout time (as ordered).
   (2) Have patient initiate demand dose as needed.

   Gives patient control over administration of analgesic.

6. Explain that nurses will monitor patient's response to epidural analgesic routinely. Also instruct patient on signs or problems to report to nurse (e.g., pruritus, inability to pass urine, change in sensation).

   Builds trust to encourage patient to be partner in care.

7. Keep an IV line patent for 24 hours after epidural analgesia has ended.

   Provides route for any emergency medications.

8. Remove and dispose of gloves. Perform hand hygiene.

   Reduces transmission of microorganisms.

9. Before removal of epidural catheter, check for presence of therapeutic anticoagulation. Check agency policy for removal while patient is receiving anticoagulation therapy.

   Removal of epidural catheter while patient is anticoagulated increases risk for spinal hematoma because of anticoagulation and inability to compress vessels.

EVALUATION

1. Evaluate patient's pain severity using a pain rating scale of 0 to 10 and evaluate character of pain.

   Evaluates effectiveness of epidural infusion.

2. Evaluate blood pressure and heart rate; respiratory rate, rhythm, depth, and pattern; pulse oximetry or capnography; and sedation level based on patient's clinical condition. Generally measured more frequently in first 12 hours of infusions (e.g., hourly) (see agency policy), after bolus infusions or changes of infusion rate, and in periods of cardiovascular or respiratory instability (Rowbotham et al., 2010).

   Oversedation occurs before respiratory depression and should be monitored closely to prevent respiratory depression. Postural hypotension, vasodilation, and heart rate changes may occur from pain or medication side effects (Pasero and McCaffery, 2011).

3. Help patient when changing positions.

   Protects patient in case of postural hypotension.

4. Evaluate catheter insertion site every 2 to 4 hours for redness, warmth, tenderness, swelling, or drainage. Note character of drainage (e.g., bloody, clear, or purulent).

   Bloody drainage may occur if catheter has migrated into a vessel. Report immediately and treat as emergency (Pasero and McCaffery, 2011).

STEP	RATIONALE
5. Inspect epidural site for disruption or displacement of catheter.	Could lead to infusion of medication into higher level of spinal cord.
6. Observe for pruritus, especially of face, head, neck, and torso. Inform patient that this is a side effect but is often not an allergic response.	Pruritus *alone* is rarely an allergy to opioids (Pasero and McCaffery, 2011).
7. Observe for nausea and vomiting and presence of headache. Note any nonverbal signs of headache (grimacing, massaging head).	Nausea from epidural analgesia worsens by movement. Headache and CSF fluid leakage may occur from a dural puncture.
8. Monitor intake and output. Evaluate for bladder distention and urinary frequency or urgency. Consult with health care provider for possible need for intermittent catheterization.	Prevents urinary retention.
9. Evaluate for motor weakness or numbness and tingling of lower extremities (paresthesias).	Reducing epidural dose (per order) may help eliminate unwanted motor and sensory deficits (Pasero and McCaffery, 2011).
10. **Use Teach-Back:** "We discussed the side effects or problems that you might have from the epidural medicine that is running. Which effects should you tell me about?" Revise your instruction now or develop a plan for revised patient or family caregiver teaching if patient or family caregiver is not able to teach back correctly.	Determines patient's and family caregiver's level of understanding of instructional topic.

Unexpected Outcomes

1. Patient states that pain is still present or has increased. Primary causes are insufficient drug dose or catheter blockage, breakage, or improper position.

2. Patient is sedated or not easily aroused.

3. Patient experiences periods of apnea; or respirations are less than 8 breaths/min, shallow, or irregular.

4. Patient reports sudden headache. Clear drainage is present on epidural dressing, or more than 1 mL of fluid is aspirated from catheter.

5. Patient experiences minimal urinary output, urinary frequency or urgency, bladder distention, pruritus, or nausea and vomiting.

Related Interventions

- Check all tubing, connections, medication doses, and pump settings.
- Confer with health care provider on adequacy of medication dose.

- Stop epidural infusion and elevate patient's head of bed 30 degrees (unless contraindicated). *Stay with patient and call for help.*
- Notify health care provider and prepare to administer opioid-reversing agent naloxone per health care provider's order.
- Monitor all vital signs, pulse oximetry, capnography, and sedation level continuously until patient is easily aroused.
- Instruct patient to take deep breaths.
- Stop epidural infusion, stay with patient and call for help. Notify health care provider.
- Prepare to administer opioid-reversing agent (naloxone) per health care provider's order (agency procedure manual may have protocol).
- Monitor at least every 30 minutes until respirations are at least 8 or more per minute and of adequate depth for 2 hours.
- Stop infusion or bolus dosing. Stay with patient and call for help
- Notify health care provider.
- Consult with health care provider about reducing dose of opioid and discuss treatment for side effects.

Reporting and Recording

- Record drug, dose, method of administration (bolus, demand, or continuous), and time given (if injection) or time begun and ended (if demand or continuous) on appropriate medication record in the electronic health record (EHR) or chart. Specify concentration and diluent.
- With continuous or demand infusion, obtain and record pump readout hourly for first 24 hours after infusion begins and then every 4 hours. Review pump settings and usage together with staff coming on the next shift.
- Record regular periodic assessments of patient's status in nurses' notes in electronic health record (EHR) or chart and/or on appropriate flow sheet, including vital signs, pulse oximetry/ capnography, intake and output (I&O), sedation level, pain severity score, neurological status, appearance of epidural site, presence

or absence of adverse reactions to medication, and presence or absence of complications resulting from placement and maintenance of epidural catheter (Pasero and McCaffery, 2011).
- Report any adverse reactions or complications to health care provider immediately.
- Document your evaluation of patient and family caregiver learning.

Special Considerations
Teaching

- Describe catheter placement and purpose to patient as appropriate. Drawing or showing pictures often helps.
- Teach patient and family caregivers the purpose, action, and signs and symptoms of adverse reactions to opioid or local anesthetic. Teach when and which signs and symptoms to report to a nurse.

- Teach patient to report pain level with acceptable (to patient) pain scale.
- Inform patient of other pain-management strategies that supplement or enhance pharmacological intervention (e.g., imagery, distraction, relaxation) (Allred et al., 2010; NIH, 2015a).
- Some patients may attempt to ambulate without help or overdo other activities. Caution them to begin slowly to avoid injury and to always call for nurse to help with any activity. Explain that the first attempt to ambulate may feel strange secondary to decreased sensation, but motor (leg) function should be unaffected.

Pediatric
- Apply EMLA cream to the epidural site a minimum of 60 minutes before catheter insertion.
- Dosing regimens for children must be adapted for age and weight, with maximum dosage clearly defined to minimize cumulative local anesthetic toxicity (Rowbotham et al., 2010).
- Hourly assessments are recommended, especially in the first 12 hours. There should be regular review of need for infusion, especially after 48 hours (Rowbotham et al., 2010).

Gerontological
- Older adults are at the same risk for complications and medication adverse effects as other adult patients.

Home Care
- Patients needing long-term therapy are discharged with a tunneled catheter. Before considering catheter placement and care in the home, assess patient's fine-motor skills, cognitive ability, stage of disease and prognosis, and degree of involvement of family caregiver.
- Teach patient and family caregiver proper dosage and administration of medication. Evaluating patient's technique for catheter care, administering medication, and reinforcing instructions are priorities.
- Teach patient and family caregiver aseptic technique for medication administration as needed and for all catheter care procedures, including dressing changes. Instruct patient to change dressing every week (policy varies with home care agency). Teach signs and symptoms of infection and instruct patient to report to nurse or health care provider immediately should signs and symptoms appear.
- Teach patient and family caregiver about signs and symptoms of adverse reactions to medication being used and interventions to alleviate mild side effects in the home.
- Give patient and family caregiver phone numbers of health care providers to contact in emergency and resources in the community.

♦ SKILL 16.4   Local Anesthetic Infusion Pump for Analgesia

During surgery for conditions such as hernia repair, knee arthroplasty, shoulder laparoscopy, breast reconstruction, and cholecystectomy, some surgeons insert a one-way catheter into the surgical site and attach it to an infusion pump (Fig. 16.4) (Rawlani et al., 2008; Wu et al., 2014). The pump delivers a local anesthetic (e.g., bupivacaine and ropivacaine or mepivacaine) directly into the wound bed to constantly "bathe" the specific nerve or nerve plexus responsible for pain at the surgical site, thus maintaining analgesia during and after surgery. Patients may still require oral analgesics, but the total dosage is often reduced (ISMP, 2011). The pump has a demand (4 to 6 mL/bolus) and a continuous (basal) rate (2 to 4 mL/h) feature. Continuous-flow reservoirs hold 100 mL, whereas patient-controlled units have a 60-mL reservoir. The device is 1-time use only and usually remains in a few days, allowing patients to control their postoperative pain with a local anesthetic infusion at home. Patients regain their mobility quickly, thus reducing the risk of developing postsurgical complications. Rarely is a pump removed during hospitalization. Patients and their family caregivers learn how to remove the catheter at home. Nursing care focuses on assessment of catheter site and connections, evaluation of local anesthetic side effects, and patient teaching.

Delegation and Collaboration

The skill of managing local anesthetic infusion pump analgesia cannot be delegated to nursing assistive personnel (NAP). The nurse directs the NAP to:
- Pay close attention to the insertion site when providing care to avoid dislocation.
- Report if the dressing becomes moist; report any catheter disconnection immediately.
- Notify nurse immediately of a change in patient's status or level of comfort.

Equipment
- Pump in place from surgery

Home Catheter Removal
- Clean gloves
- Sterile 4 × 4–inch gauze pads
- Band-Aid
- Tape
- Plastic bag

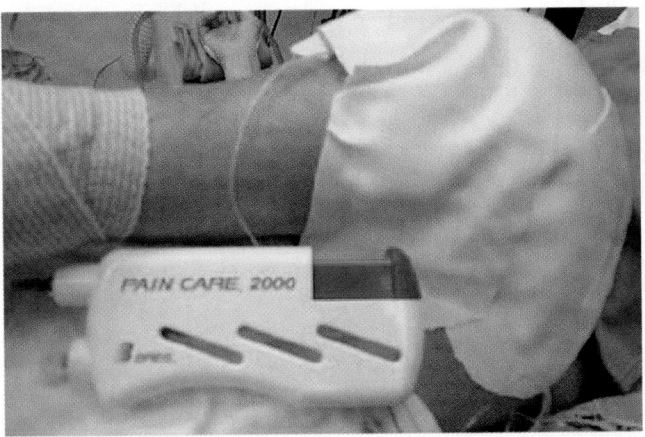

FIG 16.4 Local anesthetic infusion pump in use after shoulder surgery. (*Image courtesy Breg, Inc., Vista, CA, All rights reserved.*)

STEP	RATIONALE

ASSESSMENT

1. Identify patient using two identifiers (e.g., name and birthday or name and medical record number) according to agency policy. Compare identifiers with information on the patient's MAR or medical record.

   Ensures correct patient. Complies with The Joint Commission standards and improves patient safety (TJC, 2016).

2. Perform hand hygiene, apply clean gloves, and assess surgical dressing and site of catheter insertion. Dressing should be dry and intact.

   Determines if catheter is placed properly.

3. Be sure that catheter tubing is correctly labeled; then assess catheter connection. Be sure that it is secure. If catheter becomes detached, do *not* reattach or reinsert; instead notify surgeon immediately.

   Reattachment could lead to infection. Tubing misconnections could lead to infusion of inappropriate agents into surgical wound site.

4. Perform a complete pain assessment (see Skill 16.1).

   Provides baseline to determine efficacy of analgesia.

5. Review surgeon's operative report for position of catheter.

   Confirms catheter location with your own observation.

6. Read medication label on device and compare to MAR or health care provider's order.

   Provides information regarding type of anesthetic, concentration, volume, flow rate, date and time prepared.

7. Assess for presence of blood backing up in tubing. If blood is present, stop infusion and notify health care provider. Remove gloves and perform hand hygiene.

   Indicates possible displacement of catheter into blood vessel.

8. Determine level of extremity activity that patient can perform per health care provider's orders.

   Excessive activity can cause catheter displacement.

9. Confirm patient's allergies (should be completed preoperatively and intraoperatively). Assess for signs of local anesthetic toxicity: hypotension, dizziness, tremor, severe itching, swelling of skin or throat, irregular heartbeat, palpitations, confusion, ringing in ears, muscle twitching, numbness around mouth, metallic taste, seizures.

   Early identification of toxicity prevents or lessens possibility of complications. Local anesthetics can have serious systemic effects (ISMP, 2011).

10. Assess patient's and family caregiver's knowledge of infusion pump.

    Assesses level of teaching and support required.

NURSING DIAGNOSES

- Acute pain
- Anxiety
- Deficient knowledge regarding purpose of infusion pump
- Impaired physical mobility
- Risk for infection

Related factors/Risk factors are individualized based on patient's condition or needs.

PLANNING

1. Expected outcomes following completion of procedure:

   - Patient verbalizes full or partial relief from pain.

     Patient's self-report of pain is single most reliable indicator of pain.

   - Patient achieves reduction of nonverbal behaviors indicative of pain such as grimacing, clenching teeth, rocking.

     Nonverbal behaviors are valid and reliable indicators of pain in absence of self-report (Herr et al., 2011a).

   - Patient moves about in bed, sleeps and eats better, is more active, and communicates easily with family and friends.

     Adequate pain relief allows patient to participate in activities of daily living (ADLs).

   - Catheter is removed correctly without injury to patient.

     Patient and family caregiver are able to follow instructions for catheter removal.

IMPLEMENTATION

1. Perform hand hygiene. When repositioning or ambulating patient, use caution.

   Avoids catheter dislodgement.

STEP	RATIONALE
2. When preparing patient for discharge (depending on type of pump), it may be necessary for you to connect the catheter to a smaller pump for use at home. One example is a pump about the size of a baby bottle. When pump is connected, balloon inside pump is full of medication, and plunger is all the way to the top. As medication infuses, balloon inside pump shrinks, and plunger goes down.	
3. Teach patient or family caregiver what to observe and how to remove catheter at home (may also be done by home health nurse).	
a. Explain how to perform hand hygiene and apply clean gloves.	Decreases transmission of microorganisms.
b. Have patient assume relaxed position in bed or chair with lower extremity in normal alignment.	Relaxes joint muscles, reducing traction from muscle tension, and provides distraction.
c. Apply clean gloves. Have patient or family caregiver gently lift adhesive dressing covering catheter insertion site and remove any remaining tape.	Exposes catheter insertion site.
4. Teach patient or family caregiver how to remove catheter (may be done by home health nurse).	
a. Direct patient or family caregiver to place 4 × 4–inch gauze over site, grasp catheter as close as possible to where it enters skin, and gently pull it out with steady motion. This should cause little discomfort or resistance. A small amount of blood or fluid drainage is normal.	Prevents breakage of catheter.
b. Have patient or family caregiver look for mark on end of catheter tip. Hold new sterile gauze using pressure over the site for at least 2 minutes.	Indicates complete removal of catheter. Achieves hemostasis.
c. Wash skin to remove any surgical soap or adhesive near the site. Apply Band-Aid.	Cleanses insertion site.
d. Place catheter in plastic bag using standard precautions. Remind patient to bring to health care provider's office at first follow-up visit. Remove and dispose of gloves; perform hand hygiene.	Catheter will be inspected by surgeon to ensure that no breakage occurred. Reduces transmission of microorganisms.
e. Explain to patient that any remaining numbness should go away within 24 hours after catheter is removed.	Allows patient and caregiver to anticipate progress and recognize problems.
5. Remind patient or family caregiver of follow-up appointment with surgeon.	Increases patient adherence.

EVALUATION

1. Ask patient to rate pain intensity using appropriate scale at both rest and with activity.	Determines patient response to local infusion of medication.
2. Observe for signs of adverse drug reaction and report any signs immediately.	Local analgesics can result in systemic adverse effects if absorbed by veins (Pasero and McCaffery, 2011).
3. Observe patient's position, mobility, relaxation, participation in ADLs, and any nonverbal behaviors.	Indicates successful pain management.
4. Inspect condition of surgical dressing.	Wet dressing indicates possible catheter migration out of wound, especially if drainage is clear.
5. During follow-up visit inspect catheter exit site.	Determines if area has healed without infection.
6. **Use Teach-Back:** "It is important for you to remove the catheter at home correctly. Explain to me the steps to take to remove the catheter." Revise your instruction now or develop a plan for revised patient or family caregiver teaching if patient or family caregiver is not able to teach back correctly.	Determines patient's and family caregiver's level of understanding of instructional topic.

STEP	RATIONALE
Unexpected Outcomes	**Related Interventions**

Unexpected Outcomes

1. Patient verbalizes pain intensity greater than previously determined goal or demonstrates nonverbal behaviors indicative of pain. Catheter may be displaced or clogged, or surgical site may be developing complications.

2. Patient reports symptoms of local anesthetic adverse reaction (bleeding, arrhythmias, weakness or numbness of affected area, seizure, confusion, infection, drowsiness, ringing in ears), possible hypersensitivity to local anesthetic, displacement of catheter into vein, or pump failure (releasing too much drug into site).

Related Interventions

- Check reservoir for presence of medication.
- Check patency of tubing.
- Notify health care provider.

- Stop infusion (ISMP, 2011).
- Notify health care provider.

Reporting and Recording

- Record drug, concentration, date catheter inserted, and type of demand feature (continuous or demand) in MAR in the electronic health record (EHR) or chart.
- Record location of catheter, patient's pain rating, response to anesthetic, and additional comfort measures given in nurses' notes in electronic health record (EHR) or chart.
- Record additional analgesics necessary to control pain on MAR in the EHR or chart.
- Record any adverse reactions to local anesthetic (ISMP, 2011) in nurses' notes in electronic health record (EHR) or chart and report to health care provider.
- Report damp dressing and/or displaced catheter to surgeon.
- Document your evaluation of patient and family caregiver learning.

Special Considerations
Teaching

- Provide preoperative teaching about purpose and use of device before patient goes to operating room.
- If device is on demand (not continuous), instruct patient to depress button the frequency ordered by health care provider.
- Instruct patient to inform nurse if pain exceeds pain-intensity goal because additional oral and/or intravenous analgesics are available for breakthrough pain.

Pediatric

- Local continuous infusion pumps have been used for children undergoing orthopedic surgery. Instruct parents and the child as described under Home Care considerations. Explain special precautions not to dislodge the catheter.

Gerontological

- Continuous dosing is sometimes administered, but demand doses require a mentally competent adult (Herr et al., 2011b). In addition, take special precautions to protect the catheter.

Home Care

- Instruct patient and family caregiver to notify health care provider immediately if excessive fluid or bleeding on the dressing occurs; if patient has signs of anesthetic reaction, including arrhythmias, weakness, or numbness of affected area, seizure, confusion, drowsiness, ringing in the ears; or if signs of infection develop (redness and tenderness at catheter site, drainage, or fever). Provide written copy of instructions.
- Provide verbal and written instructions regarding how and when to discontinue device when at home. Remind patient to place catheter in a plastic bag and bring it to first follow-up visit with health care provider.
- Provide instructions regarding any restrictions to extremity movement after surgery.
- Home-health nurse may be ordered to remove pump via surgeon's order.

◆ SKILL 16.5   Nonpharmacological Pain Management

 Video Clip

Effective pain management does not always mean the elimination of pain. A variety of nonpharmacological therapies are available to directly lessen a patient's pain and provide additive relief when analgesics are administered. Nonpharmacological interventions can be used in any health care setting. These interventions are classified as complimentary or alternative therapies, and there is evidence of their efficacy in providing pain relief (NIH, 2015a). Use these interventions in combination with pharmacological interventions, not in place of them. Nonpharmacological techniques diminish the physical effects of pain, alter a patient's perception of pain, and provide a patient with a greater sense of control.

Nonpharmacological interventions are appropriate for patients who find such interventions appealing, express anxiety or fear, may benefit from avoiding or reducing drug therapy, and have

incomplete pain relief with pharmacological interventions alone. You will be able to help patients control their pain by teaching them to add a variety of nonpharmacological techniques for self-care (Box 16.5). Patients and families today are more aware of complementary techniques and should be encouraged to continue whatever has worked for them. Because everyone responds differently, finding new methods that work for a patient may take more time than finding pharmacological techniques.

Relaxation and Guided Imagery

Relaxation and guided imagery help to relieve acute and chronic pain, anxiety, and depression. Deep, slow breathing associated with relaxation performed alone or in combination with the focused concentration of guided imagery influences autonomic and pain

Nonpharmacological Strategies for Pain Management*

Relaxation and Power of the Mind
- Self-comfort
- Progressive muscle relaxation
- Autogenics training
- Breathing exercises
- Music relaxation
- Visual imagery
- Yoga

Put Your Body to Work
- Exercise
- Pacing
- Energy conservation
- Body mechanics

Spirituality and Reflection
- Engaging in religious practices
- Humor
- Setting aside time to focus on what *is*
- Sharing your stress with others
- Journaling
- Praying

What to Do When Pain Flares
- Cold and hot therapies
- Ball therapy
- Contrast baths
- Hand massage
- Herbals†

*Should be used along with analgesia medications.
†Contact health care provider before using herbals, which could interact with prescribed analgesics.

processing, essential features in the modulation of sympathetic arousal and pain perception (Busch et al., 2012). Relaxation has been shown to be effective in reducing postoperative pain from upper abdominal surgery and labor pain (Jones et al., 2012; Topcu and Findik, 2012). A patient's full participation and cooperation are necessary for relaxation techniques to be effective. Relaxation and guided imagery provide patients with self-control when pain occurs. In guided imagery a person draws on personal memories, dreams, and visions to create an image in the mind; concentrates on that image; and gradually becomes less aware of pain. Focus of the imagination helps patients change their perceptions about their disease, treatment, and healing ability, which helps relieve pain, tension, or stress. Choosing images that patients find pleasant requires a careful assessment. Otherwise you may mistakenly describe images of objects or things that a patient fears or dislikes (Baird et al., 2010). For example, a scene of rolling waves at the seashore is restful to one patient but may be frightening to another. The technique has been shown to be effective in improving the functional status and sense of self-efficacy for managing pain and other symptoms of fibromyalgia (Menzies et al., 2006).

Cutaneous Stimulation

Massage

A gentle massage, a form of cutaneous stimulation, is the application of touch and movement to muscles, tendons, and ligaments without manipulation of the joints. A proper massage not only blocks perception of pain impulses but also helps relax muscle tension and spasm that otherwise might increase pain. Massage therapy can produce a relaxation response that creates a calm state and enhances the ability to rest (Adams et al., 2010). Massage hastens the elimination of wastes stored in muscles, improves oxygenation of tissues, and stimulates the relaxation response in the nervous system. In a study involving a small sample of medical,

surgical, and obstetrics inpatients, massage was shown to reduce patients' actual pain levels; but the study also revealed a relationship among pain, relaxation, sleep, emotions, recovery, and the healing process (Adams et al., 2010). A superficial massage of the back, shoulders, and lower part of the neck is sometimes referred to as a backrub. Offering a backrub after a bath or before a patient prepares for sleep promotes relaxation and comfort. An effective backrub takes 3 to 6 minutes and is an important intervention for decreasing pain and improving sense of well-being.

Heat and Cold

Heat and cold applications are applied to the skin to relieve pain and promote healing by improving circulation and reducing edema. The selection of heat versus cold varies with a patient's preference and condition. The application of heat or cold in a health care agency or home health environment requires a health care provider's order. Although the physiological responses to heat and cold differ, superficial heat or cold applications provide comfort in conditions such as muscle spasms, strains, and localized joint pain (see Chapter 42 for a review of warm and cold therapy).

Distraction

Distraction is a technique that diverts an individual's attention away from mild or moderate pain sensation. It can be used alone to manage mild pain or with analgesics to manage brief bouts of severe pain such as pain related to procedures (ONS, 2015). By introducing meaningful stimuli, you help a patient consciously attend to only one stimulus, thus diverting the attention away from pain. There are internal and external distraction techniques. Internal techniques include having patients count, sing to themselves, pray, or repeat statements in their head such as "I can cope" (ONS, 2015). External distractions include changing a patient's activity, needlework, listening to music, reading, walking, playing a musical instrument, or watching a comedy program (NIH, 2015a). Therapeutic communication with a nurse is another example of distraction. When the distraction is removed, a patient may have a heightened awareness of pain.

Delegation and Collaboration

Assessment of a patient's pain cannot be delegated to nursing assistive personnel (NAP). The skill of nonpharmacological pain-management strategies can be delegated to NAP. The nurse directs the NAP by:
- Identifying and explaining which nonpharmacological measures work best for a patient.
- Explaining how to adapt strategies to patient restrictions (e.g., massage in side-lying versus prone position).
- Instructing to report worsening of a patient's pain.

Equipment

- Pain rating scale
- *Massage:* Lotion or oil (consider aroma therapy lotion), folded sheet, bath towel
- *Relaxation:* Patient's music preference, radio or CD player, relaxation tape and tape player
- *Distraction:* Based on patient preference (e.g., reading material, puzzles, video games)

STEP	RATIONALE

ASSESSMENT

1. Assess patient's language level and values he or she has regarding alternative pain-relief approaches. Identify descriptive terms that you will use when guiding patient through relaxation or guided imagery.

   Ensures that care is culturally appropriate. Establishes connection with patient to enhance your ability to guide relaxation.

2. Assess character of patient's pain (see Skill 16.1) and review findings to consider cause for pain.

   Establishes baseline to determine effects of intervention. Helps determine if nonpharmacological approaches are appropriate.

3. Assess facial expressions, nonverbal indications of discomfort (e.g., grimacing, frowning, voice tone), body position and movement (e.g., restlessness, muscle tension), and patient's self-report (see Skill 16.1).

   Serves as baseline to evaluate effectiveness of pain-relief measures.

   Overt signs and symptoms are usually not present with chronic pain. Physical signs and symptoms indicate change in comfort level.

4. Perform hand hygiene, apply gloves when drainage is present. Examine site of patient's pain or discomfort. Include inspection (discoloration, swelling, drainage), palpation (change in temperature, area of altered sensation, painful area, areas that trigger pain), and range of motion of involved joints (if applicable).

   Clinical observations may clarify information from patient. Site of discomfort may direct you to specific types of pain-relief measures.

5. Assess character of patient's respirations.

   Establishes baseline. Relaxation techniques focus on breathing.

6. Review health care provider's orders for pain relief (if required by agency).

   In some acute care settings a medical order is necessary to perform nonpharmacological therapies.

7. Assess patient's understanding of pain and willingness to receive nonpharmacological pain-relief measures.

   Participation increases effectiveness of pain-relief measure. If patient is reluctant to try activity, provide information about suggested therapy.

8. Assess preferred patient activities (e.g., puzzles, crocheting, game on electronic device, board games, music, or relaxation tape).

   Improves likelihood of distraction being effective.

9. Assess type of image patient would prefer to use in guided imagery.

   Prevents use of image that could frighten patient.

10. Review any restrictions in patient's mobility or positioning.

    Determines whether massage is appropriate and position to have patient assume.

NURSING DIAGNOSES

- Activity intolerance
- Acute pain
- Anxiety
- Chronic pain

- Deficient knowledge regarding nonpharmacological methods of pain control

- Ineffective coping
- Powerlessness

Related factors are individualized based on patient's condition or needs.

PLANNING

1. Expected outcomes following completion of procedures:
   - Patient demonstrates and describes pain-relief measures.

     Demonstrates patient understanding and learning.

   - Patient is relaxed and comfortable after technique as evidenced by slow, deep respirations; calm facial expressions; calm tone of voice; relaxed muscles; relaxed posture.

     Nonpharmacological strategies help patient relax and experience less discomfort. Physiological response to relaxation procedures and massage is deep relaxation.

   - Patient reports pain relief on 0 to 10 scale.

     Patient's subjective report is most reliable indicator of presence of pain.

2. Explain purpose of technique and what you expect of patient during activity. Explain how to use pain rating scale (Skill 16.1).

   Proper explanation of activity enhances patient participation. Accurate reporting of pain by patient improves your evaluation and treatment.

3. Set mutual pain-intensity goal with patient (when able) for rest and during routine care activities.

   Patient sets individual goal for tolerable pain severity.

STEP	RATIONALE

4. Plan time to perform technique when patient is able to concentrate (e.g., after voiding, awakening from nap).

Increases opportunity for success.

5. Administer an analgesic 30 minutes before implementing a nonpharmacological therapy.

Patient is able to gain a level of comfort needed to perform nonpharmacological therapies.

IMPLEMENTATION

1. Perform hand hygiene and prepare patient's environment.
Temperature suited to patient
Sound
Lighting
Minimize interruptions and coordinate care activities; allow for rest.

Reduces transmission of microorganisms.
Temperature and sound extremes can enhance patient's perception of pain.
Bright or very dim lighting can aggravate pain sensation.
Fatigue increases pain perception.

2. Massage:

Clinical Decision Point *Massage is contraindicated in cases of muscle, bone, or joint injury; bruised, swollen, or inflamed areas.*

a. Place patient in comfortable position such as prone or side-lying. Have patients with difficulty breathing lie on side of bed with head of bed elevated.

Enhances relaxation and exposes areas to be massaged.

b. Adjust bed to comfortable position for you; lower upper side rail on side where you are standing. Drape patient to expose only area that you will massage.

Ensures proper body mechanics and prevents strain on back.

c. Turn on music to patient's preference.

Promotes relaxation.

d. Ensure that patient is not allergic to lotion; warm lotion in hands or in basin of warm water. **NOTE:** If you massage head and scalp, delay use of lotion until completed.

Warm lotion is soothing, and warmth helps to produce local muscle relaxation.

e. Choose stroke technique based on desired effect or body part.

Ensures fuller relaxation of body part.

Clinical Decision Point *Use very gentle massage with patients who are unable to communicate because they cannot tell you if massage becomes uncomfortable.*

(1) Effleurage: massaging upward and outward from vertebral column and back again (see illustration).

Light, gliding stroke used without manipulating deep muscles smooths and extends muscles, increases nutrient absorption, and improves lymphatic and venous circulation.

(2) Pétrissage (see illustration).

Kneading tense muscle groups promotes relaxation and stimulates local circulation.

(3) Friction

Strong circular strokes bring blood to surface of skin, increasing local circulation and loosening tight muscle groups.

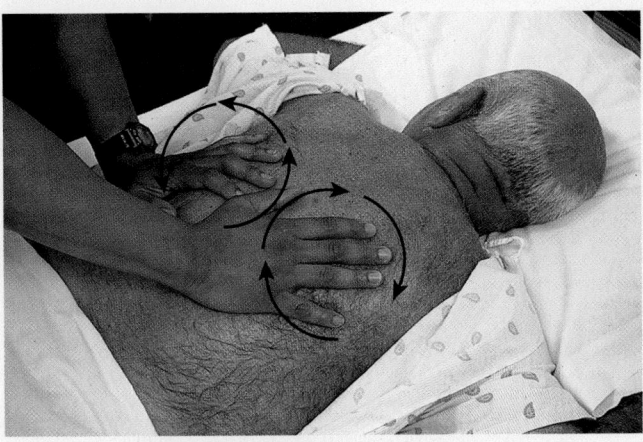

STEP 2e(1) Effleurage.

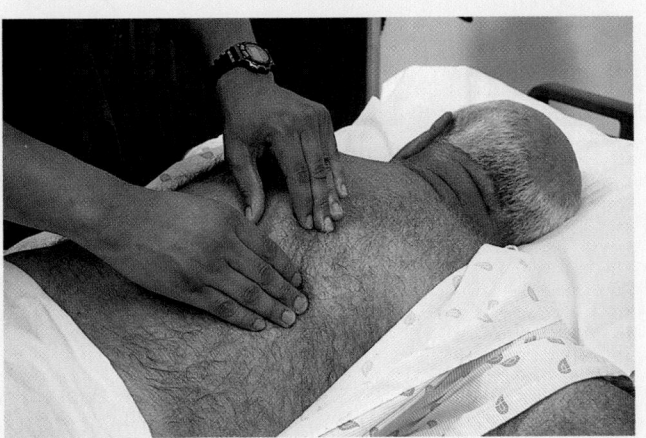

STEP 2e(2) Pétrissage.

STEP	RATIONALE

f. Encourage patient to breathe deeply and relax during massage.

Potentiates effects of massage.

g. Standing behind patient, stimulate scalp and temples.

h. Supporting patient's head, use friction to rub muscles at base of head.

Strong circular strokes (friction) stimulate local circulation and relaxation.

i. Reposition if needed. With patient in supine position, massage hands and arms as appropriate (Asadizker et al., 2011):

Releases tension in hands and arms. Studies indicate that anxious behaviors may be reduced significantly with hand massage (Asadizker et al., 2011).

  (1) Support hand and apply friction to palm using both thumbs.

  (2) Support base of finger and work each finger in corkscrew-like motion.

  (3) Complete hand massage using effleurage strokes from fingertips to wrist.

  (4) Knead muscles of forearm and upper arm between thumb and forefinger.

Encourages relaxation; enhances circulation and venous return.

j. After determining that patient has no neck injury or condition that contraindicates neck manipulation, massage neck as appropriate:

  (1) Place patient prone unless contraindicated.

Provides access to neck muscles.

  (2) Knead each neck muscle between thumb and forefinger.

Reduces tension that often localizes in neck muscles.

  (3) Gently stretch neck by placing one hand on top of shoulders and other at base of head. Gently move hands away from one another.

Helps relax muscle body.

k. Massage back as appropriate:

Patient with back injury, surgery, or epidural infusion should not receive back massage.

  (1) Assist patient to prone position unless contraindicated; side-lying position is option.

Provides access to muscle groups in back.

  (2) Do not allow hands to leave patient's skin.

Continuous contact with surface of skin is soothing and stimulates circulation to tissues.

Breaking contact with skin can startle patient.

  (3) Apply hands first to sacral area; massage in circular motion. Stroke upward from buttocks to shoulders. Massage over scapulas with smooth, firm stroke. Continue in one smooth stroke to upper arms and laterally along sides of back down to iliac crest (see illustration). Continue massage pattern for 3 minutes.

General, firm pressure applied to all muscle groups promotes relaxation.

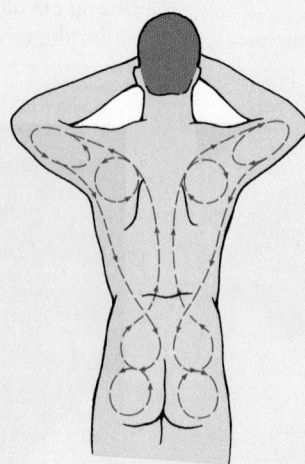

STEP 2k(3) Circular massage of the back.

STEP	RATIONALE
(4) Use effleurage along muscles of spine in upward and outward motion.	Massage follows distribution of major muscle groups.
(5) Use pétrissage on muscles of each shoulder toward front of patient.	Area often tightens because of tension.
(6) Use palms in upward and outward circular motion from lower buttocks to neck.	Brings blood to surface of skin.
(7) Knead muscles of upper back and shoulder between thumb and forefinger.	These muscles are thick and can be massaged vigorously.
(8) Use both hands to knead muscles up one side of back and then the other.	
(9) End massage with long, stroking effleurage movements.	Most soothing of massage movements.
l. Massage feet as appropriate:	
(1) Place patient in supine position.	Returns patient to comfortable anatomical position.
(2) Hold foot firmly. Support ankle with one hand or support sides of foot with each hand while performing massage.	Maintains joint stability during massage (Asadizker et al., 2011).
(3) Make circular motions with thumb and fingers around bones of ankle and top of foot.	All massage strokes help to relax muscles.
(4) Trace space between tendons with firm finger pressure, moving from toe to ankle.	
(5) Massage sides and top of each toe.	
(6) Use top of fist to make circular motions on bottom of foot.	
(7) Knead sides of foot between index finger and thumb.	
(8) Conclude with firm, sweeping motions over top and bottom of foot.	Too light strokes may tickle.
m. Tell patient that you are ending massage.	Informs and prepares patient to inhale and exhale deeply.
n. When procedure is complete, instruct patient to inhale deeply and exhale. Caution him or her to move slowly after resting a few minutes.	Returns patient to more awake and alert state. When deeply relaxed, patient may experience dizziness on arising too rapidly and need time for vessels to redistribute blood supply.
o. Wipe excess lotion or oil from patient's body with bath towel.	Excess lotion or oil can irritate skin and lead to breakdown.
p. Return bed to low position and raise side rails as appropriate when massage is finished. Perform hand hygiene.	Side rails cannot be used as a restraint.
3. Progressive relaxation with deep breathing:	
a. Have patient assume comfortable sitting position: sit with feet uncrossed or lie in supine position with small pillow under head.	Maximizes ability to relax.
b. Instruct patient to take several slow, deep, diaphragmatic breaths. It may help to have patient close his or her eyes.	Increased oxygen lessens anxiety and prevents shortness of breath with relaxation breathing technique. Avoids hyperventilation. Eye closure maintains patient focus on exercise.
c. Explain as follows: "The air coming in through your nose should move downward into your lower belly. Let your belly expand fully. Now breathe out through your mouth (or your nose, if that feels more natural). Alternate normal and deep breaths several times. Pay attention to how you feel when you breathe in and breathe out normally and when you breathe deeply. Shallow breathing feels tense and constricted, while deep breathing helps you relax."	Patient able to focus on exercise with your coaching. Becoming mindful of how body feels can enhance relaxation.

STEP	RATIONALE
d. Continue the exercise: "To practice, put one hand on your abdomen, just below your belly button. Feel your hand rise about an inch each time you breathe in and fall about an inch each time you breathe out. Your chest will rise slightly, too, along with your belly. Remember to relax your belly so that each time you breathe in, it expands fully. As you breathe out slowly, let yourself sigh out loud."	Allows patient to master slow deep breathing.
e. Observe patient and caution against hyperventilation.	Causes patient to eliminate more carbon dioxide than is produced, and consequently results in respiratory alkalosis and an elevated blood pH. Patient becomes dizzy and light-headed.
f. Coach patient to locate any area of muscle tension and alternate tightening and relaxing all muscle groups for 6 to 7 seconds, beginning at feet and working upward toward head.	Relaxation is an integrated response associated with diminished sympathetic nervous system arousal; decreased muscle tension is desired outcome.
(1) Instruct patient to tighten muscles during inhalation and relax muscles during exhalation.	Relaxation decreases pulse and respiration rates, and blood pressure and helps reduce anxiety (Baird et al., 2010).
(2) As each muscle group relaxes, ask patient to enjoy relaxed feeling and allow mind to drift and think how nice it is to be relaxed. Have patient breathe deeply.	Allows opportunity to enjoy feelings of relaxation.
(3) Calmly explain during exercise that patient may feel sensations of tingling, heaviness, floating, or warmth as relaxation occurs.	Prevents anxiety if sensation occurs without warning.
(4) Have patient continue slow deep breaths throughout exercise.	
(5) When finished, have patient inhale deeply, exhale, and then initially move about slowly after resting a few minutes.	Returns patient to more awake and alert state. Rising too rapidly can cause dizziness.
4. Guided imagery:	
a. Direct patient through guided imagery exercise while having him or her focus on an image. Example follows:	
(1) Instruct patient to imagine that inhaled air is ball of healing energy.	Developing specific images helps to remove pain perception.
(2) Imagine that inhaled air travels to area of pain.	Patient's ability to concentrate decreases pain perception.
b. Alternatively you may direct imagery.	
(1) Ask patient to imagine a pleasant place such as beach or mountains. Choose an image peaceful for patient.	Directs imagery after selection of restful place.
(2) Direct patient to experience all sensory aspects of restful place (e.g., for beach: warm breeze, warm sand between toes, warmth of sunshine, rhythmic sound of waves, smell of salt air, gulls gliding and swooping in air).	Helps patient concentrate and relax through stimulation of numerous senses (Baird et al., 2010). Make sure that it is something in their experience, not just yours.
(3) Direct patient to continue deep, slow, rhythmic breathing.	Promotes relaxation through muscle relaxation.
(4) Direct patient to count to three, inhale, and open eyes. Suggest that patient move about slowly initially.	
c. Provide patient time to practice exercise without interruption. Practice relaxation tapes are available almost everywhere; libraries are an excellent source.	Guided imagery requires an intense level of concentration that takes time to achieve.
5. Distraction	
a. Direct patient's attention away from pain by involving him or her in a distraction technique.	Redirection of attention can alter emotional or cognitive aspects of pain (Allred et al., 2010).
(1) Music: play selection for approximately 30 minutes in location where patient is comfortable. Set volume or loudness at comfortable level. Use music of patient's choosing. Emphasize listening to rhythm and adjust volume as pain increases or decreases.	Music creates positive psychological outcomes, including decreased anxiety and depression (Zhang et al., 2012).

STEP	RATIONALE
(2) Direct patient to give detailed account of an event or story; describe pleasant memories.	Stress details of event to enhance distraction from painful stimulus.
(3) Provide activity (e.g., puzzle, game boy, reading material) at time when patient is relaxed.	Engagement in activity requires level of comfort for participation.
(4) Engage patient in meaningful conversation; encourage participation of family members and visitors.	Visitors can help direct attention away from mild-to-moderate pain. Rarely is someone in severe pain able to use distraction.
6. Remove and dispose of any supplies. Perform hand hygiene.	Reduces transmission of microorganisms.

EVALUATION

1. Observe character of respirations, body position, facial expression, tone of voice, mood, mannerisms, verbalization of discomfort.
2. Ask patient to use pain rating scale to rate comfort level.
3. Observe patient perform pain-control measures.
4. **Use Teach-Back:** "I want to be sure I explained some techniques for reducing pain without using medication. Tell me what technique you might want to try." Revise your instruction now or develop a plan for revised patient or family caregiver teaching if patient or family caregiver is not able to teach back correctly.

Determines effectiveness of procedure, level of relaxation, degree of pain relief achieved, and which procedures were most effective.
Measures change in pain intensity.
Confirms learning.
Determines patient's and family caregiver's level of understanding of instructional topic.

Unexpected Outcomes
1. Patient is not able to concentrate on technique because pain intensity is unchanged or escalating or demonstrates nonverbal behaviors indicative of pain.

Related Interventions
- Evaluate character of pain and determine if further analgesia is necessary.
- Ensure that environment is conducive to learning and using technique.
- Consult with health care provider on increase in dose or alternate medication.
- Consider different technique or combination of complementary strategies.

Recording and Reporting

- Record in nurses' notes in electronic health record (EHR) or chart patient's assessment findings, procedure and technique(s) used, preparation given to patient, patient's response to procedure or technique, change in overall condition, and further comfort needs related to event. Incorporate pain-relief technique into nursing care plan.
- Report patient's response to nonpharmacological interventions to the staff at change of shift or in care plan meeting.
- Document your evaluation of patient and family caregiver learning.
- Report any unusual responses to techniques (e.g., uncontrolled or aggravated pain or muscle spasms) to nurse in charge or health care provider.

Special Considerations
Teaching

- Provide patient information about each nonpharmacological therapy, including purpose, rationale for how pain is relieved, and how patient can maximize benefits. If NAP performs massage, you still need to provide patient education.
- Some techniques require more practice before patients achieve results. Pharmacological intervention is sometimes required to lessen pain so patient can relax.
- Teach patient to rest between periods of activity at home and hospital because fatigue increases pain perception.
- Teach family caregiver how to perform massage (if not contraindicated) as part of home care.

Pediatric

- You can use nonpharmacological pain-management therapies successfully with children. Adapt distraction and relaxation strategies to the developmental level of the child (e.g., use a pacifier for an infant, offer reading or playing a recording of a favorite story for a preschooler, encourage a teenager to listen to music on a CD player with headphones) (Allred et al., 2010; Hockenberry and Wilson, 2015). Play therapists are usually available at large pediatric hospitals and are good resources for appropriate distraction techniques.
- Because children usually have an active imagination, relaxation is often a powerful adjuvant in pain control.
- Parents are very helpful in providing pain relief. For example, they provide comfort by their presence, conversation, and holding and cuddling their child.

Gerontological

- Visual, hearing, cognitive, and motor impairments make it difficult for older adults to be able to effectively use procedures such as distraction, relaxation, or guided imagery. Make certain that glasses, hearing aids, and other assistive devices are in place. Do not assume that complementary techniques will not work on the elderly (NIH, 2015a).
- An evidence-based practice protocol for pain management in older adults recommends these guidelines for nonpharmacological therapies (Horgas et al., 2012):
  - Tailor nonpharmacological techniques to the individual.
  - Cognitive behavioral strategies may not be appropriate for the cognitively impaired.
  - Physical pain-relief strategies focus on promoting comfort and altering physiological responses to pain and are generally safe and effective.

Home Care

- Family members need to collaborate on planning time to reduce noise and other stimuli in the home to promote patient's relaxation.

◆ CLINICAL DEBRIEF

A 56-year-old male account executive underwent a colectomy (removal of a portion of colon) this morning. He returns from the operating room with an epidural catheter connected to an intravenous pump set for a dose-on-demand. The anesthesia provider left orders for an initial bolus of 0.1% ropivacaine (10 mL) and fentanyl (100 mcg), which was administered in the recovery room. Patient-controlled epidural analgesia was instituted, delivering ropivacaine 0.1% with fentanyl 2 mcg/mL with a demand dosage set at 5 mL every 20 minutes. The patient has been able to follow instructions and self-administer analgesic doses correctly. The nurse caring for the patient knows to be observant for side effects of the epidural analgesic.

1. It is approximately 10 hours after surgery, and the patient has not been able to void. The nurse assesses him and finds that he likely has bladder distention. Considering his clinical situation, what are the options that explain the patient's symptoms?

2. The patient is scheduled to stand up at the bedside within 6 hours of returning from surgery. Describe measures the nurse can institute for him to enhance his ability to safely mobilize and then return to bed more comfortably.

3. The patient's epidural infusion is discontinued, and he is placed on an analgesic for moderate pain relief. The patient's vital signs are stable: BP 132/86, Pulse 84 reg, Resp 20, Temp 37.6°C. Epidural and surgical dressings are intact. Abdomen palpated with mild discomfort over bladder. Pain is at a level of 5. His wife is visiting and asks if there is a way she can be helpful in supporting her husband's recovery. Describe ways that his wife can help promote pain relief. Using SBAR, show how you would communicate with the health care team about this patient.

◆ REVIEW QUESTIONS

1. You are caring for a 72-year-old patient who has peripheral neuropathy causing ongoing nerve pain. In addition, the patient has discomfort in his back from osteoarthritis. Your assessment reveals that the patient has reduced hearing and is cognitively alert. Which of the following statements accurately describe guidelines for how to select pain-relief therapies for this patient? (Select all that apply.)
   1. A cognitive behavioral strategy would likely not be effective for this patient.
   2. Work with patient to determine the combination of analgesics and/or adjuvants ordered by the physician that is most effective in relieving pain.
   3. Explain to the patient that initial opioid dosages will be high and then tapered down to achieve pain relief.
   4. Be certain that patient's hearing aid is in place before practicing guided imagery.
   5. Plan a quiet time to provide patient a body massage.

2. You are caring for a patient who is receiving morphine by way of patient-controlled analgesia. You have just completed measuring the patient's respirations and pulse oximetry. You review the patient's medical record to identify his or her risk for oversedation. Which of the following factors increase a patient's risk for oversedation? (Select all that apply.)
   1. A patient who has received an opioid for pain within last 2 months
   2. A patient who is cognitively impaired
   3. A patient who has a history of obstructive sleep apnea
   4. A patient who has an allergy to opioids
   5. A patient who is opioid naïve

3. Fill in the rationale for each step that explains how to instruct a family caregiver in the proper approach for removing a local anesthetic catheter in the home.

Step	Rationale
Explain how to perform hand hygiene.	
Have patient or family caregiver gently lift the adhesive dressing covering the catheter insertion site, and remove any remaining tape.	
Direct patient or family caregiver to grasp the catheter as close as possible to where it enters the skin and gently pull it out.	
Hold pressure over the site for 5 minutes. Then apply a Band-Aid.	
Explain to patient that any remaining numbness should go away within 24 hours after the catheter is removed.	

ⓔ *Visit the Evolve site for a complete list of Clinical Debrief and Review Questions answers.*

REFERENCES

Adams R, et al: The effects of massage therapy on pain management in the acute care setting, *Int J Ther Massage Bodywork* 3(1):4, 2010.

Adhikari R, et al: A multi-disciplinary approach to medication safety and the implication for nursing education and practice, *Nurse Educ Today* 34(2):185, 2014.

Allred K, et al: The effect of music on postoperative pain and anxiety, *Pain Manage Nurs* 11(1):15, 2010.

American Academy of Pain Medicine (AAPM): *Use of opioids for the treatment of chronic pain*, 2013, http://www.painmed.org/files/use-of-opioids-for-the-treatment-of-chronic-pain.pdf. Accessed June 25, 2016.

American Pain Society (APS): *Principles of analgesic use in the treatment of acute and cancer pain*, ed 6, Glenview, IL, 2009, The Society.

American Pain Society (APS) and American Association of Pain Medicine (AAPM): Opioids guideline panel: Part 1, *J Pain* 10(2):113, e22, 2009.

American Society of Anesthesiologists (ASA): American Society of Anesthesiologists Task Force on Acute Pain Management: practice guidelines for acute pain management in the perioperative setting: an updated report, *Anesthesiology* 116(2):248, 2012.

Asadizker M, et al: The effect of foot and hand massage on postoperative cardiac surgery pain, *Int J Nurs Midwifery* 3(10):165, 2011.

Baird C, et al: Efficacy of guided imagery with relaxation for osteoarthritis symptoms and medication intake, *Pain Manage Nurs* 11(1):56, 2010.

Burchum JR, Rosenthal LD: *Lehne's pharmacology for nursing care*, ed 9, St Louis, 2016, Elsevier.

Busch V, et al: The effect of deep and slow breathing on pain perception, autonomic activity, and mood processing—an experimental study, *Pain Med* 13(2):215, 2012.

Craft J: Patient-controlled analgesia: is it worth the painful prescribing process?, *Proc (Bayl Univ Med Cent)* 23(4):434, 2010.

D'Arcy Y: New thinking about postoperative pain management, *OR Nurse* 5(6):29, 2011.

deTovar C, et al: Postoperative self-report of pain in children: interscale agreement, response to analgesic, and preference for a FACES scale and a visual analog scale, *Pain Res Manage* 15(3):163, 2010.

Drew DJ, St Marie BJ: Pain in critically ill patients with substance abuse disorder or long-term opioid use for chronic pain, *AACN Adv Crit Care* 22(3):238, 2011.

Ferguson S, et al: A prospective randomized trial comparing patient-controlled epidural analgesia to patient-controlled intravenous analgesia on postoperative pain control and recovery after major open gynecologic cancer surgery, *Gynecol Oncol* 114(1):111, 2009.

Freeman LM, et al: Patient-controlled analgesia with remifentanil versus epidural analgesia in labour: randomised multicentre equivalence trial, *BMJ* 350:H846, 2015.

Gloth M: Pharmacological management of persistent pain in older persons: focus on opioids and nonopioids, *J Pain* 12(3 Suppl):S14, 2011.

Herr K, et al: Pain assessment in the patient unable to self-report: position statement with clinical practice guidelines, *Pain Manag Nurs* 12(4):230, 2011a.

Herr K, et al: Pain assessment strategies in older patients, *J Pain* 12(3 Suppl):S3, 2011b.

Hockenberry MJ, Wilson D: *Wong's nursing care of infants and children*, ed 10, St Louis, 2015, Mosby.

Horgas AL, et al: Pain management. In Boltz M, et al, editors: *Evidence-based geriatric nursing protocols for best practice*, ed 4, New York, 2012, Springer.

Institute for Safe Medication Practices (ISMP): *Medication safety alert: process for handling elasomere pain-relief balls (On-Q Painbuster and others) requires safety improvements*, ISMP Acute Care Quarterly Action Agenda, 2011, http://www.ismp.org/Newsletters/acutecare/articles/20090716.asp. Accessed March 27, 2016.

Institute for Safe Medication Practices (ISMP): *ISMP articles on catheter misconnections: stay connected—FAQs about small-bore connectors and tubing misconnections*, 2013, http://www.ismp.org/newsletters/acutecare/articles/CatheterMisconnections.asp. Accessed March 27, 2016.

Jones L, et al: Pain management for women in labour: an overview of systematic reviews, *Cochrane Database Syst Rev* (3):CD009234, 2012.

Kamper SJ, et al: Interdisciplinary biopsychosocial rehabilitation for chronic low back pain: Cochrane systematic review and meta-analysis, *BMJ* 350:h4, 2015.

Klieber C, et al: Evidence-based pediatric pain management in emergency departments of a rural state, *J Pain* 12(8):900, 2011.

Lockhart E, et al: Obstructive sleep apnea screening and postoperative mortality in a large surgical cohort, *Sleep Med* 14(5):407, 2013.

Lukas A, et al: Observer-rated pain assessment instruments improve both the detection of pain and the evaluation of pain intensity in people with dementia, *Eur J Pain* 17(10):1558, 2013.

Manougian E: Why some patients require high-dose opioid therapy, *Practical Pain Manage* 10(6):1, 2010.

Menzies V, et al: Effects of guided imagery on outcomes of pain, functional status, and self-efficacy in persons diagnosed with fibromyalgia, *J Altern Complement Med* 12(1):23, 2006.

Morales DR, et al: NSAID-exacerbated respiratory disease: a meta-analysis evaluating prevalence, mean provocative dose of aspirin and increased asthma morbidity, *Allergy* 70(7):828, 2015.

Narayan MC: Culture's effects on pain assessment and management, *Am J Nurs* 110(4):38, 2010.

National Institutes of Health (NIH), National Center for Complementary and Integrative Health (NCCIH): *Selected results of NCCAM funded research on CAM research*, 2015a, https://nccih.nih.gov/research. Accessed March 27, 2016.

National Institutes of Health (NIH), National Center for Complementary and Integrative Health (NCCIH): *Americans are in pain: analysis of data on the prevalence and severity of pain from national survey*, 2015b, https://nccih.nih.gov/research/results/spotlight/081515. Accessed March 27, 2016.

Oliver J, et al: American society for pain management nursing position statement: pain management in patients with substance use disorders, *Pain Manag Nurs* 13(3):169, 2012.

Oncology Nursing Society: *Nonmedical treatments for pain*, 2015, http://www.cancer.org/treatment/treatmentsandsideeffects/physicalsideeffects/pain/non-medical-treatments-for-cancer-pain. Accessed March 27, 2016.

Pasero C, McCaffery M: *Pain assessment and pharmacological management*, St Louis, 2011, Mosby.

Ramachandran SK, et al: Life-threatening critical respiratory events: a retrospective study of postoperative patients found unresponsive during analgesic therapy, *J Clin Anesth* 13(3):207, 2011.

Rawlani V, et al: A local anesthetic pump reduces postoperative pain and narcotic and antiemetic use in breast reconstruction surgery: a randomized controlled trial, *Plast Reconstr Surg* 122(1):39, 2008.

Roditi D, Robinson ME: The role of psychological interventions in the management of patients with chronic pain, *Psychol Res Behav Manag* 4:41, 2011.

Rowbotham D, et al: *Best practice in the management of epidural analgesia in the hospital setting*, London, 2010, Faculty of Pain Medicine of The Royal College of Anaesthetists. https://www.aagbi.org/sites/default/files/epidural_analgesia_2011.pdf. Accessed June 27, 2016.

Ruskin D, et al: Assessing pain intensity in children with chronic pain: convergent and discriminant validity of the 0 to 10 numerical rating scale in clinical practice, *Pain Res Manag* 19(3):141, 2014.

The Joint Commission (TJC): Managing risk during transition to new ISO tubing connector standards, *Sentinel Event Alert* 53:2014. http://www .jointcommission.org/assets/1/6/SEA_53_Connectors_8_19_14_final.pdf. Accessed March 27, 2016.

The Joint Commission (TJC): *2016 National Patient Safety Goals (NPGs)*, 2016, TJC, http://www.jointcommission.org/standards_information/npsgs.aspx. Accessed March 27, 2016.

Tomlinson D, et al: A systematic review of FACES scales for the self-report of pain intensity in children, *Pediatrics* 126(5):e1168, 2010.

Topcu SY, Findik UY: Effect of relaxation exercises on controlling postoperative pain, *Pain Manage Nurs* 13(1):11, 2012.

Touhy T, Jett K: *Ebersole and Hess' gerontological nursing & healthy aging*, ed 4, St Louis, 2014, Mosby.

Wu CC, et al: Local anesthetic infusion pump for pain management following open inguinal hernia repair: a meta-analysis, *Int J Surg* 12(3):245, 2014.

Zhang JM, et al: Music interventions for psychological and physical outcomes in cancer: a systematic review and meta-analysis, *Support Care Cancer* 20(12):3043, 2012.

Zwakhalen SMG, et al: Pain in elderly people with severe dementia: a systematic review of behavioural pain assessment tools, *BMC Geriatr* 6:3, 2006.

17 | Palliative Care

OBJECTIVES

Mastery of content in this chapter will enable the nurse to:
- Discuss principles of palliative care.
- Describe hospice care.
- Describe approaches to physical symptom management at the end of life.
- Describe approaches to spiritual symptom management at the end of life.
- Describe physiological changes in impending death.
- Identify a nurse's role in assisting patients and families in grief and at the end of life.
- Describe the process of postmortem care.
- Discuss a nurse's role in facilitating autopsy and organ and tissue donation requests.

MEDIA RESOURCES

- evolve http://evolve.elsevier.com/Perry/skills
- Review Questions
- Case Studies
- Audio Glossary
- Clinical Debrief and Review Questions Answers

PURPOSE

Nurses have historically played a vital role in the care of patients and families facing serious, life-limiting illness and death. The World Health Organization (2015) defines palliative care as an approach that "improves the quality of life of patients and their families facing the problems associated with life-threatening illness, through the prevention and relief of suffering by means of early identification and impeccable assessment and treatment of pain and other problems, physical, psychosocial and spiritual." Palliative care may be provided in conjunction with other life-sustaining treatments such as surgery or chemotherapy. The goals of palliative care include comprehensive management of pain and other symptoms and psychosocial and spiritual support provided by an inter-professional team comprised of physicians, nurses, social workers, chaplains, and dietitians ((NCP, 2013) (Box 17.1). To be successful, it is important to provide a caring presence and apply therapeutic communication principles (Fig. 17.1).

At the end of life, palliative care may transition to hospice care. Hospice, an inter-professional, patient- and family-centered program of care, helps people live as well as possible through the dying process. Patients are eligible for hospice care as a Medicare or Medicaid benefit during the final phase of a terminal illness, usually the last 6 months of life. Because hospice is a philosophy of care, the services can be provided at home; in freestanding hospice facilities; or in nursing home, extended care, or acute care settings.

At the time of death nurses provide compassionate care to patients and family members by offering information, guidance, and support and facilitating communication. In addition, nurses provide postmortem care (e.g., care of the body after death) in a dignified manner, consistent with a patient's religious and cultural beliefs.

STANDARDS OF CARE

- National Consensus Project for Quality Palliative Care (NCP) Guidelines, 2013—Assessment and Management of Pain and Other Symptoms; Assessment and Management of Patient and Family Psychosocial Needs; Assessment and Management of Cultural, Religious and/or Spiritual Needs of Patient and Family; and Postmortem Care Provided to Patient in a Respectful and Culturally Sensitive Manner
- The Joint Commission, 2016—National Patient Safety Goals

PRINCIPLES FOR PRACTICE

- Expert palliative care involves helping patients reach peaceful deaths at the end of life.
- Providing palliative care requires holistic assessment of a patient, management of physical signs and symptoms, and providing psychosocial and spiritual support to patients and their families.
- Symptoms are experienced by a patient and can only be reported by the patient. Signs are observed by the nurse and may accompany the patient's symptoms (Nunn, 2014).
- Management of physical symptoms at the end of life can decrease psychosocial distress, thus improving overall quality of life (Nunn, 2014).

Goals of Palliative Care

- Provide patients relief from pain and other distressing symptoms
- Affirm life and regard dying as a normal process
- Aim to neither hasten or postpone death
- Integrate the psychological and spiritual aspects of patient care
- Offer a support system to help patients live as actively as possible until death
- Offer a support system to help the family cope during the patient's illness and in their own bereavement
- Enhance quality of life and positively influence the course of illness

Adapted from World Health Organization: WHO Definition of palliative Care, 2015, http://www.who.int/cancer/palliative/definition/en/. Accessed March 13, 2016.

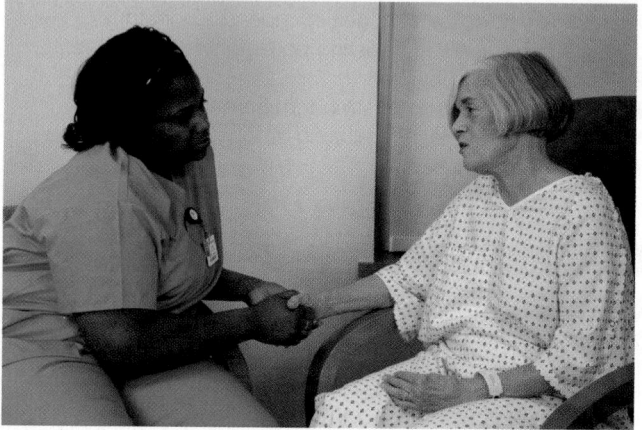

FIG 17.1 Nurses use their presence and therapeutic communication to assess how symptoms affect a patient's life.

- As a nurse, listen carefully to understand the significance of a loss to a patient or family member, identify concerns, and assess his or her ability to sustain hope and move forward in life.
- To receive hospice care at home, a family caregiver must be available to provide care when a patient is no longer able to function alone. Hospice team members offer 24-hour accessibility and coordinate care between the home and inpatient settings.
- As the time of a patient's death approaches, the hospice team provides intensive support to the patient and family. Hospice benefits include respite for family caregivers, limited hospitalization for acute symptom management, and bereavement care after death (Hospice Foundation of America, 2015).
- To nurture your capacity as a nurse to remain empathically engaged with patients and family members, you must also care for yourself physically, spiritually, and emotionally.
- Recognize your own attitudes, feelings, values, and expectations about death and the individual, cultural, and spiritual diversity existing in these beliefs and customs (ELNEC, 2015).

PATIENT-CENTERED CARE

- A patient-centered approach to palliative and end-of-life care engages a patient and family with an interprofessional team that provides education and supports the patient and family to be informed and make autonomous decisions regarding the patient's treatment (or discontinuation of treatment) (Brazil et al., 2012).

- The nursing care provided incorporates a patient's preferences and cultural and religious/spiritual needs and is delivered in a holistic manner.
- Patients are encouraged to set realistic goals and help identify ways to achieve them so they can maintain their usual routines and a sense of normalcy.
- When patients with advanced illness are no longer able to participate in making decisions, they can communicate their values and preferences in an advance directive. Advance directives specify medical interventions that a patient does not want in certain situations and are also used to communicate the care a patient would like to have (Ache et al., 2014; Brown and Vaughan, 2013).
- Medical terminology in an advance directive can be made clear to a patient when a nurse takes time to communicate the various options for care (Hinderer and Lee, 2014). If a patient has an advance directive, place a copy in the medical record and instruct him or her to give copies to their health care provider and family members (see agency policy).
- Cardiopulmonary resuscitation (CPR) (see Chapter 28) is used in cases of cardiac and/or pulmonary arrest. Adults in consultation with the health care team may consent to a "do not resuscitate" (DNR) status verbally or in writing. Assure patients who choose not to be resuscitated that they will continue to receive full palliative care and symptom relief.
- Cultural norms reflect family, gender, and community roles at the time of a patient's death. A patient's culturally influenced health care beliefs and practices, communication patterns, and family structures affect the dying process (Bullock, 2011; Fiorelli and Jenkins, 2012).
- Culture affects the meaning of pain and suffering, how one expresses grief, and ideas about an afterlife. Given the wide range of cultural beliefs, first engage in self-reflection on your own cultural and personal beliefs about loss and death. Gather knowledge on common end-of-life cultural or religious practices; then validate through nurse-patient discussions the relevance of these practices for a particular patient.
- Understand a patient's cultural background and know which family member may be the most important or appropriate person with whom to communicate about decision making at the end of life.

EVIDENCE-BASED PRACTICE

Research continues on the topic of end-of life care, with researchers exploring the prevalence of symptoms, patient and family caregiver coping, and family decision making. In a qualitative study involving patients with end-stage heart failure and chronic obstructive pulmonary disease, findings revealed that patients experienced high symptom burden and uncertainty about the future (Lowey et al., 2013). Among these patients, few enrolled in hospice because the patients believed they still had time. They hoped that their illnesses would remain stable. All expected that their doctors would tell them when their illnesses became life threatening.

There are few randomized controlled trials in palliative care. However in a study by Curtis et al. (2016), critical care patients with a predicted mortality of >30% and surrogates as their decision makers were randomized into two groups. One group (control) received standard communication and education. The second group (intervention) received a communication facilitator, who supported communication between clinicians and families, adapted communication to family needs, and mediated conflict. The study aimed to reduce family distress and the intensity (costs) of end-of-life care. Family members who were supported by the communication facilitator experienced decreased depressive symptoms at 6 months compared with the control group, but there were no significant differences between the two groups in psychological symptoms at 3 months or anxiety at 6 months. The intervention was not associated with intensive care unit (ICU) mortality, but decreased ICU costs among all patients. This was the first study to find a reduction in intensity of end-of-life care with similar or improved family distress.

Research supports the use of the following strategies for expert palliative care nursing:

- Patients and family members are most satisfied when they receive attentive, compassionate care. Novice nurses who are grounded in authentic, openhearted, holistic nursing care practices are capable of providing valuable care to patients at the end of life.
- Personalize your plan of care. Discuss priorities and preferences for care with patients and family members regularly because changes in a patient's condition may shift care preferences and needs.

SAFETY GUIDELINES

- Patients receiving palliative or hospice care are vulnerable and need nurse advocates who are comfortable discussing various

treatment options and levels of care (Jeffers, 2014). Nurses who learn about end-of-life care from trusted nursing educators may enter the profession prepared to address patient's questions regarding end-of-life issues.

- Patients at the end of life often receive opioids for symptom management. Nurses may be concerned with the ethical principle of double effect: administering an opioid such as morphine may decrease pain and dyspnea; however, a side effect may be respiratory depression, possibly leading to a hastened death. Research has shown that opioids should be administered to manage pain or other symptoms and are not likely to hasten death (Bailey et al., 2012; Macauley, 2012).
- Patients at the end of life or with dementia lose their capacity to report side effects, call for help, evaluate treatments, or make decisions. Among the risks is poor symptom management and patient falls. Apply effective communication with those with cognitive impairment and be aware of likely causes of anxiety, fear, and resistance to care when carrying out interventions (Regan et al., 2014).
- Proper patient identification, especially in communicating a patient's DNR or CPR status, ensures that caregivers will not initiate unwanted and unhelpful medical interventions. Know the methods of your agency for designating a patient's resuscitation status.

✦ **SKILL 17.1** **Supporting Patients and Families in Grief**

Grief experiences in situations of serious illness and at the end of life have profound physical, psychological, social, and spiritual effects on dying people, family members, friends, and caregivers. The grief associated with serious illness or death arises from fear of the unknown, pain, sadness about leaving loved ones behind, loss of control, or unresolved guilt.

Hospitalization, chronic illness, and disability involve multiple losses. Hospitalized patients lose privacy and control over normal routines. With chronic illness a person's body no longer functions as it once did, leading to a loss of self-esteem and social roles. Disability and threat of end of life creates financial insecurity and often threatens interpersonal relationships. Death separates people from the physical presence of a person in their lives.

Grief

Grief is the emotional response to a loss, based on personal experiences, psychological makeup, cultural expectations, and family and spiritual beliefs. Losses at the end of life may be financial, physical, emotional, social, or spiritual. Examples of these losses include role changes, altered self-image, loss of income, or emotional distress. The depth and duration of grief (e.g., one's inner emotional response to loss) depends on the type of loss and the person's perception of it. Coping with grief involves a period of mourning (e.g., the outward, social expressions of grief and the behavior associated with loss). Mourning behaviors and rituals help grieving individuals adapt to loss, receive social support, adjust expectations, and go forward in life. Most mourning rituals are culturally influenced, learned behaviors. Bereavement includes grief and mourning (e.g., the inner emotional responses and outward behaviors in response to loss) (Arizmendi and O'Connor, 2015; Widera and Block, 2012).

As a nurse you help patients by understanding types of grief. Normal or uncomplicated grief is evidenced by feelings, behaviors,

and reactions associated with loss such as sadness, anger, crying, resentment, and loneliness. Families may feel the presence of the lost person and yearn for his or her return. They may find it difficult to resume life as it was before their loss. An uncomplicated grief experience often helps a person mature and develop life perspective. Anticipatory grief occurs before an actual loss or death and involves gradual disengagement from what is being lost. For example, if a dying process is lengthy, the patient and family prepare for death before it occurs and sometimes, but not always, display fewer common grief responses at the time of death. Complicated grief (symptoms lasting 6 months or longer) occurs when a person experiences significant distress related to the loss. Criteria for a person experiencing complicated grief may include inability to accept the death of loved one, anger, depression, or inability to maintain social relationships and intense longing for the deceased (Guldin, 2014).

People do not experience grief in the same way. Some people do not report feeling distressed or depressed, and others feel distressed for a lifetime without negative consequences. Not all people want to process the emotional experience of grief and focus instead on resilience, growth, or positive outcomes after a loss.

Use basic knowledge of grief responses to support patients and their families and to address other common psychosocial and spiritual symptoms at the end of life. Patients and their families may talk openly about a patient's approaching death, and others choose not to acknowledge it. Health care providers, depending on their own personal and cultural understandings of grief and death, often avoid initiating conversations on these difficult topics. Provide opportunities for discussion, paying close attention to a patient's response and indications of a desire to talk further. Educating a patient and family about what to expect during the final days or hours can alleviate anxiety and promote a more positive death experience for all involved (Dosser and Kennedy, 2014; Moir et al., 2015).

Delegation and Collaboration

The skills of assessing patients' or family members' grief reactions and designing appropriate interventions cannot be delegated to nursing assistive personnel (NAP). The nurse directs the NAP to:

- Inform the nurse when a patient or family member exhibits behavior commonly associated with grief (e.g., crying, anger, withdrawal).

- Form supportive relationships with patients and families and inform the nurse when patients or family members have questions or concerns.
- Alert the nurse to the arrival of family members so the nurse can discuss the plan of care and offer support.

STEP	RATIONALE

ASSESSMENT

1. Sit near patient in a quiet, private location. Center yourself and establish a quiet presence. Establish eye contact. Be aware that use of eye contact in some cultures conveys disrespect or discomfort.	Presence expresses caring and creates healing moments (Arbour and Wiegand, 2014; McMahon and Christopher, 2011). Privacy protects confidentiality and promotes a sense of safety for patient when expressing thoughts and emotions.
2. Consider the influence of patient's cultural background on communication. Apply principles of plain language and health literacy during assessment (NCP, 2013).	Individual differences influence patient's grief response and communication style (Clabots, 2012; Selman et al., 2014).
3. Listen carefully to patient's story. Observe patient responses. Use open communication.	Develops trust in a caring relationship. Actively listening to patient's concerns and verbalizing patient's needs conveys empathy and compassion (Doherty and Thompson, 2014).
4. Determine meaning of the loss to patient: its type, suddenness, and when it occurred. Use open-ended questions such as: • "Tell me how your loss affects your family." • "You said your illness was unexpected. Describe how that made you feel?"	The type, meaning, suddenness, and time elapsed since the loss influence the grief experience and coping methods.
5. Combine knowledge of grief theory with observation of patient behaviors. Validate observations by sharing them with patient; paraphrase, clarify, or summarize, as in the following examples: • "You've mentioned several times that you feel hopeless." • "It seems that this is hard for you to talk about." • "You look sad. Is there something in particular that brought on your tears?"	Use information about type and stage of grief to guide discussion, not to judge patient's responses. Confirms accuracy of your observations and validates patient's feelings. Prompts patient to continue.
6. Encourage patient to describe the loss and its impact on daily life (e.g., "You said your diagnosis changed your life forever. Tell me more").	Listening to patient's description helps to minimize assumptions.
7. Ask patient to describe the coping strategies that he or she uses most often in difficult times (e.g., "What or who helps you in times of crisis?").	Familiar, effective coping strategies are often helpful in the current crisis, loss, or grief experience.
8. Assess family caregivers' unique needs and resources. Note if patient receives care at home and who gives the care.	Illness significantly affects family relationships. Although family members experience similar issues, their needs may differ.
9. Assess patient's spiritual needs, beliefs, and resources. Focus on aspects likely to be involved (e.g., trust, life purpose, faith/belief, and hope).	Identifies patient's spiritual beliefs and values. Enables patient autonomy by identifying beliefs and preferences for care or rituals related to faith and/or spirituality. Offers a greater understanding of patient's culture and values, leading to patient-centered care (Hodge, 2015).

NURSING DIAGNOSES

- Anxiety
- Compromised family coping
- Death anxiety
- Fear
- Grieving

- Hopelessness
- Ineffective denial
- Readiness for enhanced coping
- Readiness for enhanced family coping
- Readiness for enhanced hope

- Risk for caregiver role strain
- Risk for complicated grieving
- Risk for spiritual distress

ted factors/Risk factors are individualized based on patient's condition or needs.

STEP	RATIONALE

PLANNING

1. Expected outcomes following completion of procedures:
- Patient maintains relationships with significant people.
- Patient expresses grief in keeping with his or her cultural and religious practices.
- Patient uses effective coping strategies.
- Patient maintains normal life routines.

Patient in grief or loss retains connections with social network.
Patient receives support necessary to retain cherished values and ways of being.
Patient identifies sense of relief.
Patient adjusts to life-changing circumstances and maintains sense of control.

IMPLEMENTATION

1. Show an empathic understanding of patient's strengths and needs.

Promotes nurse-patient trust, caring, compassion, and empathy (Doherty and Thompson, 2014).

2. Offer information about patient's illness and treatment. Clarify misunderstandings or misinformation. Use culturally appropriate language and simple terms.

Misunderstanding adds to patient's uncertainty, anxiety, and suffering.

3. Encourage patient to sustain relationships with others to help maintain independence and receive necessary help. Include patient-identified support people in discussions.

Affiliation with others offers support and helps patient stay engaged in life.

4. Help patient achieve short-term goals (e.g., symptom relief, task completion, resolution of relational problems).

Helping patients identify and meet their personal goals contributes to their quality of life.

5. Provide frequent opportunities for patient and family members to express their fears and concerns. Be attentive to expressions of intense emotions.

Emotions change quickly and frequently during stress and complicate communication for nurses and patients.

6. Educate and support patient and family. Discuss procedures, plan of care, and anticipated changes. Use interprofessional team to support patient's needs and preferences.

Provides emotional support and comfort, decreases anxiety, and allows patient to rest. Advocating for patient encourages patient autonomy and incorporates patient preferences into plan of care (Arbour and Wiegand, 2014).

7. Instruct patient in relaxation strategies: mindfulness-based stress reduction, guided imagery, meditation, hand massage, healing touch (see Chapter 16).

Complementary therapies have been shown in select cases to relieve anxiety and effectively reduce stress, thus providing useful coping strategies (Hofmann et al., 2010).

8. Encourage visits with loved ones, life review with stories or photographs, or projects such as organizing photo albums or journal writing.

Reviewing positive and negative events in one's life allows a person to find meaning in their experiences, resolve conflicts, and come to a place of acceptance (Keall et al., 2015).

9. Facilitate patient's religious/spiritual practices and connections with religious community. Use prayer or music and provide a listening presence. Make a referral to a spiritual care provider if appropriate.

Spiritual interventions help patients maintain hope and connect with the core of their identity. Spiritual interventions can decrease anxiety, promote a sense of peace, and help patient find meaning in his or her life (Kisvetrova et al., 2013; Wynne, 2013).

EVALUATION

1. Note patient descriptions of relationships and activities with others.

Provides information on extent to which patient retains relational ties.

2. Observe patient's behaviors during ongoing interactions.

Demonstrates patient's ability to express grief and coping.

3. Elicit patient perceptions of benefit gained from use of coping interventions.

Evaluates efficacy of interventions.

4. Discuss progress toward performing routine activities at home.

Evaluates patient's achievement of desired goals or need for goal revision.

Unexpected Outcomes	**Related Interventions**
1. Patient does not acknowledge loss and shows signs of extreme sorrow, anger, withdrawal, or denial. 2. Family and patient relationships do not give patient needed support.	• Consider referral to grief specialist professional (e.g., nurse practitioner, psychologist, spiritual care provider). • Share and validate observations of family strain or patient concern over family interactions. • Consider family-patient discussion with health care team.

Recording and Reporting

- Record interventions used to support patient coping and note patient's verbal and nonverbal responses in nurses' notes in electronic health record (EHR) or chart.
- Report patient's grief reactions to members of the interprofessional team, noting behaviors that affect health outcomes such as treatment refusals or prolonged inactivity.

Special Considerations
Teaching

- Give family caregivers basic information about common grief responses and how to offer support. Coach them on ways to provide physical, emotional, and spiritual support to patient and one another (e.g., providing basic hygiene, listening attentively, avoiding false reassurances, allowing for the expression of difficult emotions, talking about normal family activities).

Pediatric

- Children's understanding of death, influenced by age and developmental level, differs from that of adults. Respect parents' wishes about when and what to tell children about illness or death. When discussing sensitive topics with children, encourage parents to offer caring explanations at a level a child is able to understand.

- Play therapy or drawing helps children express thoughts, emotions, or fears about illness or death.
- Be alert to all family members' grief reactions because they may feel guilt, resentment, or helplessness with the illness or death of a sibling, child, or grandchild. Facilitate communication with family members who must be separated from the child.
- Surrogate decision makers, usually the parents, need to make health care decisions for infants and young children. Some decisions are difficult because outcomes in children are often unpredictable.

Gerontological

- Losing a partner after a long and satisfying relationship is very difficult and is essentially a loss of self. The mourning is as much for oneself as for the individual (Touhy and Jett, 2014).
- Intense grief may cause a temporary decrease in cognitive function that can be manifested as confusion (Ward et al., 2007; Touhy and Jett, 2014).
- Many older adults have coexisting medical conditions that add to their symptom burden. They also have lived long enough to have experienced cumulative losses, including members of their family and support group, which complicates their grief experience.

◆ SKILL 17.2 Symptom Management at the End of Life

Quality palliative care offers vigilant symptom management while avoiding futile treatment (Luckett et al., 2014). The American Nurses Association (ANA) supports aggressive treatment of pain and suffering even if it hastens a patient's death (Fowler, 2015). It is crucial to have an interprofessional team approach to symptom assessment and treatment (NCP, 2013).

Patients living with life-limiting illness experience multiple, complex physical, emotional, and spiritual symptoms. Managing patients' symptoms at the end of life begins by understanding the impact that these symptoms have on patients' and their family's lives from their shared and individual point of view (Fig. 17.2). Ethnicity and culture are strongly related to attitudes toward life-sustaining treatments during terminal illness and the use of hospice services (Loggers et al., 2013). Consider these factors when you assess all symptoms and concerns thoroughly because a patient's fear of not being heard or believed compounds the magnitude of symptoms. Patients identify pain as their most common and severe symptom (see Chapter 16). In addition to the psychological and spiritual interventions discussed in Skill 17.1, nurses manage physiological symptoms at the end of life.

Delegation and Collaboration

Supportive care for symptom management can be delegated to nursing assistive personnel (NAP). However, the nurse must conduct the initial assessments of symptoms and determination of therapies. The nurse directs the NAP to:

- Notify the nurse if patient reports new symptoms or if existing symptoms worsen or change.
- Provide basic comfort care such as positioning, room temperature control, hygiene, and mouth care.

- Report possible adverse effects of drug therapy as instructed by the nurse.
- Speak to unconscious or dying patients because hearing is the last sense to diminish.

Equipment

- Personal care items most preferred by patient
- Comfort and hygiene products
- Clean gloves

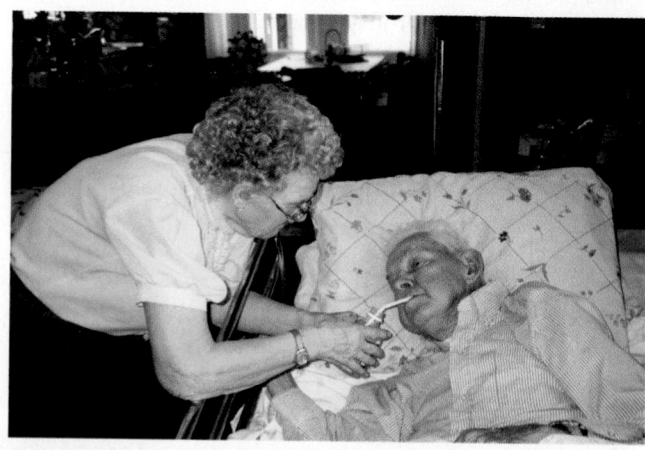

FIG 17.2 A patient-centered approach involves family and patients as partners in care.

STEP	RATIONALE

ASSESSMENT

1. Identify patient using at least two identifiers (e.g., name and birthday or name and medical record number) according to agency policy.

Ensures correct patient. Complies with The Joint Commission standards and improves patient safety (TJC, 2016).

2. Ask patients to describe symptoms in their own words. Use open-ended prompts such as "Describe your leg pain to me," or "Tell me about how you are sleeping since you started taking this medicine."

Symptoms are personal perceptions and only experienced by the patient (Nunn, 2014).

3. Allow sufficient time for patients to describe their symptoms and encourage them to say more:
   • "Is there anything else bothering you?"
   • "You've told me about your _____ pain. Do you have pain anywhere else?"

Ensures a more complete assessment. Prevents you from making assumptions about patient's symptoms, prematurely stopping the assessment process.

4. Assess patient's emotional health. Does the patient feel anxious, sad, depressed, bored, or understimulated? Use standardized tool to assess anxiety if available (ELNEC, 2015).

Emotional conditions have potential to worsen fatigue in patients with cancer (ACS, 2014)

5. Assess patient's pain severity on a pain scale of 0 to 10 (see Chapter 16). If patient cannot self-report pain, observe for these symptoms (ACS, 2014):

Consistent use of a standard pain scale helps assess changes in patient pain levels and evaluate effectiveness of pain interventions (Paice, 2015). Using a pain scale is recommended by the American Cancer Society (2014) as a helpful way to describe patients' responses to pain-relief measures.

   • Noisy breathing—labored, harsh, or rapid breaths
   • Making pained sounds—including groaning, moaning, or expressing hurt
   • Facial expressions—looking sad, tense, or frightened; frowning or crying
   • Body language—tension, clenched fists, knees pulled up, inflexibility, restlessness, or looking like he or she is trying to get away from the hurt area
   • Body movement—changing positions to get comfortable but can't

Patients unable to report or verbalize pain show nonverbal signs of pain.

6. Perform hand hygiene.

Reduces transmission of microorganisms.

7. Assess for feeling of breathlessness (does patient feel that he or she is getting enough air), respiratory rate, breathing patterns, and lung sounds. Assess for presence of airway secretions.

Dyspnea, air hunger, or shortness of breath results from metabolic or respiratory changes. Near the end of life, Cheyne-Stokes respirations are common and are characterized by alternating periods of apnea and hyperpnea.

8. Observe condition of skin, especially back, heels, and buttocks (see Chapter 6).

Decreased peripheral circulation and activity level contribute to skin breakdown.

9. Inspect patient's oral cavity, including mucosa, tongue, and teeth (see Chapter 6).

Dehydration, difficulty swallowing, and inflammation of mouth are common at end of life.

10. Assess bowel function (see Chapter 35).

Patients experience constipation because of decreased oral intake, immobility, and medications such as opioids (Clark and Currow, 2014). Patients who have diarrhea are at risk for dehydration.

   a. Determine usual bowel elimination pattern (frequency, character, usual time of day) and effectiveness of usual bowel-management routines.

   b. If patient is passing liquid stool, assess for presence of fecal impaction (see agency policy).

Watery stool leaking around blockage indicates fecal impaction.

   c. Review medication regimens, prescriptions, and over-the-counter drugs known to cause constipation (e.g., opioids, antacids).

Medications can alter bowel elimination patterns. Diarrhea results from infections, diseases, or medications (e.g., antibiotics or chemotherapy). Change in therapy might be necessary.

   d. Identify typical food and fluid intake over 1 week and patient's activity levels.

Oral intake and activity levels influence bowel elimination patterns.

11. Assess urinary elimination (see Chapter 34) and ability to control urination. If incontinent, assess for skin breakdown or patient discomfort.

Urinary incontinence results from patient's disease process, altered level of consciousness, or medications (diuretics, anticholinergics, opioids) (Baker and Ward-Smith, 2011).

STEP	RATIONALE

12. Assess patient's appetite, ability to swallow, and for presence of nausea or vomiting. Use standardized tool for assessment if available (ELNEC, 2015).

Medications, pain, depression, disease progression, or decreased blood flow to digestive organs near death often contribute to nausea, vomiting, and decreased appetite.

   a. Consider presence of nausea in patients receiving enteral feedings.

Patients who have decreased consciousness are unable to report nausea.

13. Assess daily food and fluid intake in relation to patient's condition and preferences.

Nutrition screening helps to identify deficits and allows for interventions to be carried out to improve nutritional status (Shaw and Eldridge, 2015).

14. Use descriptive scale to assess fatigue (e.g., scale with descriptors none, moderate, severe). Ask if fatigue limits patient's ability to perform desired activities.

Metabolic demands of a disease, anemia as a result of chemotherapy, treatments, and cumulative effects of other symptoms cause weakness and fatigue (ACS, 2014).

15. Assess for terminal delirium in patient near death (e.g., confusion, restlessness, and/or agitation, with or without day-night reversal).

Allows you to identify this condition and implement interventions to keep patient safe and decrease patient anxiety (Moyer, 2011).

   a. Consider if patient has pain, nausea, dyspnea, full bladder or bowel, poor sleep patterns, anxiety, or joint pain from immobility.

Risk factors for presence of delirium are common physical problems that need to be treated or ruled out as causative factors.

   b. Review medical record for hypercalcemia, hypoglycemia, hyponatremia, or dehydration.

Metabolic imbalances cause restlessness or delirium.

   c. Review patient's medications.

Unintended responses to medications result in changed activity states.

   d. Determine if patient has unresolved emotional or spiritual issues.

Spiritual distress contributes to restlessness or increased pain.

NURSING DIAGNOSES

- Activity intolerance
- Acute pain
- Anxiety
- Bowel incontinence
- Chronic pain

- Constipation
- Diarrhea
- Fatigue
- Impaired oral mucous membrane
- Impaired swallowing

- Ineffective breathing pattern
- Ineffective peripheral tissue perfusion
- Nausea
- Risk for constipation
- Total urinary incontinence

Related factors/Risk factors are individualized based on patient's condition or needs.

PLANNING

1. Expected outcomes following completion of procedure:
   - Patient reports acceptable level of pain.
   - Patient reports feeling warm and comfortable.

   Indicate s pain control.
   Warming interventions help reverse effects of reduced peripheral circulation.

   - Patient reports comfortable eating and drinking patterns.

   Optimal food and fluid intake are based on patient preferences and comfort.

   - Patient has soft, formed bowel movements.
   - Skin remains free of irritation or breakdown.

   Indicates adequate bowel function and peristaltic activity.
   Interventions to protect skin from bowel or urinary incontinence are effective.

   - Patient is not restless.
   - Patient reports less distress from fatigue.

   Therapies have calming effect.
   Energy conservation methods are effective; patient adjusts to changes in activity level.

   - Patient experiences less respiratory distress.

   Patient is less apprehensive and breathes easily.

IMPLEMENTATION

1. Perform hand hygiene.

   Reduces transmission of microorganisms.

2. Provide pain relief. Use multimodal interventions.

   Management of symptoms should be multimodal (NCP, 2013).

   a. Administer ordered analgesics and adjuvants. Confer with health care provider and recommend an around-the-clock (ATC) dosing schedule, especially if pain is anticipated for majority of day. A variety of extended- or controlled-release oral opioid formulations (dosing intervals of 8, 10, 12 or 24 hours) and transdermal patches (72 hours) are effective.

   Opioids should be given on a fixed dosage schedule ATC rather than prn, with doses given before pain returns (Burchum and Rosenthal, 2016). An ATC medication lessens the severity of end-of-dose pain, allowing a patient to sleep through the night and reduce "clock watching" for the next dose. Extended-release medications maintain constant serum opioid concentration, minimizing toxic and subtherapeutic concentrations (Burchum and Rosenthal, 2016).

STEP	RATIONALE
b. Provide nonpharmacological interventions such as mindfulness-based stress reduction, relaxation exercises, guided imagery (see Chapter 16).	Nonpharmacological measures supplement pain medication and can increase patient comfort (Hall, 2014; Nunn, 2014).
c. Provide patient and family education on causes and patterns of pain and safety of opioid use and explain interventions.	Encourages patient autonomy and reduces emotional distress, clarifying misinformation about opioid therapies.
d. Reassess patient's pain 1 hour after administration of pain medication or alternative therapy.	To determine if desired effect of medication or alternative treatment was achieved; if patient has reduced pain level.
3. Provide general comfort measures.	
a. Provide bath and skin care based on patient's preferences and hygiene needs (see Chapter 18). NOTE: Daily baths are not always desired or necessary at end of life if they cause discomfort, fatigue, or increased pain.	Clean skin promotes comfort.
b. Provide eye care and use artificial tears in patients with decreased consciousness (see Chapter 19).	Eye irritation causes pain. Blink reflex diminishes near death, causing drying of cornea.
c. Reposition frequently; do not position on tubes or other objects.	Prolonged, even slight pressure from weight of patient's body or objects causes skin injury.
4. Provide oral hygiene after meals and at bedtime while awake and more frequently in mouth-breathing or unconscious patients (see Chapter 18).	Oral mucosa integrity is needed for normal swallowing and to minimize anorexia and malnutrition. Mouth rinses remove oral debris and clean the mouth. Dehydration develops as patient experiences metabolic changes and fluid intake declines.
a. Use antifungal oral rinses as prescribed or sodium bicarbonate or normal saline rinses.	Patients near death breathe through the mouth, drying oral mucosa.
b. Moisten lips with nonpetroleum balm.	Prevents skin breakdown.
5. Initiate bowel-management regimen to reduce risk for constipation or diarrhea:	Interventions improve peristalsis in constipation, soften fecal mass, and decrease abdominal discomfort (Clark and Currow, 2014; Santucci and Battista, 2015).
a. Give patient whatever fluids he or she enjoys if medically tolerated. Near end of life, patient may refuse fluids. Do not force fluid intake.	Decreased blood flow to intestines at end of life causes anorexia.
b. Encourage regular physical activity (e.g., walking) if tolerated.	
c Administer daily stool softener or laxative, especially in patients using opioids for pain management.	
d. In case of diarrhea, provide low-residue diet; treat infections or discontinue medications if possible. Administer antidiarrheal medications. Patients with chronic diarrhea require rigorous skin care to promote comfort.	Treatments reduce incidence and severity of diarrhea, which can lead to dehydration.
6. Manage urinary incontinence with intervention appropriate for patient's conditions (e.g., condom catheter, adult incontinence pads [see Chapter 34]).	Urinary output declines near death, making it possible to manage incontinence without an indwelling catheter.

Clinical Decision Point *Consider an indwelling catheter only if skin integrity, patient preference, or fatigue from bed changes becomes an issue.*

STEP	RATIONALE
7. Offer patient favorite foods in amount and at time he or she desires. Do not overly encourage patient to eat.	Patients may be experiencing gastrointestinal (GI) distress, dry mouth, or other symptoms related to their disease process, which may contribute to decreased oral intake. In addition, patients nearing final hours of life decrease their oral intake as a result of slowing of bodily functions and/or altered level of consciousness (Gillespie and Raftery, 2014).
a. Treat nausea by administering antiemetics intravenously or rectally as prescribed. As nausea subsides, offer clear liquids and ice chips. Avoid caffeinated liquids, milk, and fruit juices.	GI mucosa tolerates clear liquids more readily. Certain liquids increase stomach acidity.

STEP	RATIONALE
8. Manage fatigue.	Taking rest breaks during activity will help conserve energy (Koornstra et al., 2014). Tired patients need help and monitoring to ensure patient safety.
a. Help patient identify valued or desired tasks and preferred time of day to perform tasks and determine how to conserve energy for only those tasks. Help with activities of daily living. Eliminate extra steps in activities.	
b. Explain care activities before performing and include patient in setting daily schedule.	Minimizes anxiety and maintains patient's autonomy and involvement.
c. Discuss with patient easy ways to incorporate exercise (e.g., yoga, walking, biking, and swimming) into daily activities.	Research has shown that, even for people with advanced-stage cancer, exercise can lessen pain and decrease anxiety, stress, depression, shortness of breath, and fatigue (Albrecht and Taylor, 2012; Koornstra et al., 2014).
9. Support patient's breathing efforts.	
a. Position for comfort in semi-Fowler's or Fowler's position.	Promotes maximal ventilation, lung expansion, and drainage of secretions.
b. Elevate head to facilitate postural drainage. Turn from side to side to mobilize and drain secretions. Suction only if necessary.	Deep airway suctioning causes discomfort and is not effective in reducing airway noise or secretion clearance (Bailey and Harmon, 2016).
c. Provide ordered antimuscarinic medications.	Anticholinergic medications reduce saliva and excessive secretions (Nunn, 2014), thus decreasing noisy respirations.
d. Stay with patients experiencing dyspnea or air hunger. Use interventions that patients perceive as relieving their shortness of breath (choice of oxygen-delivery modes, fan near face, body position). Administer opioids or anxiolytics as prescribed. Benzodiazepines may also be administered for anxiety related to dyspnea. Keep room cool with low humidity.	Sharing control with patients reduces anxiety that contributes to feelings of air hunger. Morphine is the drug of choice for dyspnea, decreasing respiratory rate and decreasing anxiety. Use of oxygen has little benefit unless patient feels better using it (Nunn, 2014; Quinn-Lee, et al., 2012).
10. Manage restlessness.	
a. Keep patient's room quiet with soft lighting and at comfortable temperature. Offer family members opportunities to maintain close contact. Encourage use of soft music, prayer, or reading from patient's favorite book.	Reduces unnecessary external stimulation and provides comforting space. Privacy allows family members chance to provide verbal assurances and touch. Presence of a family member to hold a hand provides a calming effect (Moyer, 2011).
b. Use least-sedating pharmacological options to control restlessness. Consult with interprofessional team about titrating a medication (e.g., lorazepam). Discontinue all nonessential medication. Use subcutaneous, transdermal, sublingual, or rectal medication delivery routes.	Reduce delirium without making patient unconscious. Control of restlessness relieves family's concern that patient is in pain or distress. Determine cause of delirium, if possible, to decrease use of medication (Bailey and Harmon, 2016).
11. Manage anxiety.	
a. Provide counseling and supportive therapy. Consult with prescribing health care provider for benzodiazepines, the drugs of choice. Offer available counseling services (e.g., pastoral care, psychologist, social work).	Counseling improves patient/family understanding of the disease and its expected course and identifies strengths and coping strategies.

Clinical Decision Point *Caution: The use of benzodiazepines in very elderly patients can result in a paradoxical agitation.*

EVALUATION

1. Ask patient to rate pain on scale of 0 to 10 (see Chapter 16) and evaluate pain characteristics. Assess behavior in nonverbal patients.	Determines extent of pain relief.
2. Ask patient to describe mouth comfort and inspect oral cavity.	Evaluates condition of oral cavity and ability to chew or swallow.
3. Evaluate frequency of defecation; after patient defecates, inspect feces.	Determines status of bowel function and character of stool.

STEP	RATIONALE
4. Observe skin condition.	Determines if skin tears or areas of pressure or maceration are present.
5. Ask patient to rate fatigue (scale from none to moderate to severe) and compare with baseline. Observe for fatigue or shortness of breath when patient performs activities.	Determines if patient is less distressed with activity.
6. Observe patient's respiratory patterns and ask if breathing is easy and comfortable.	Determines if respiratory distress is relieved.
7. Observe patient's behavior or ask family to report on it. Note level of restlessness.	Determines level of comfort and extent of restlessness.
8. **Use Teach-Back:** "I want to be sure I explained that we want to control your pain, and this requires you to describe it. Tell me what the numbers on the pain scale mean. Tell me when it is a good time to let me know about your pain before it gets too severe." Revise your instruction now or develop a plan for revised patient or family caregiver teaching if patient or family caregiver is not able to teach back correctly.	Determines patient's and family caregiver's level of understanding of instructional topic.

Unexpected Outcomes

1. One or several symptoms remain unresolved, with patient reporting little or no relief.
2. Patient becomes anxious, fearful, or exhausted as a result of continued symptoms.

Related Interventions

- Increase frequency of or change an intervention.
- Try combination therapies.
- Give patients therapy choices and try different interventions.
- Explain goals of therapies and possible reasons for symptoms.
- Answer call lights quickly and explain plan of care throughout the day.

Recording and Reporting

- Record detailed description of patient symptoms in nurses' notes in electronic health record (EHR) or chart and/or appropriate flow sheets. Use consistent descriptors for comparison over time.
- Document your evaluation of patient and family caregiver learning.
- Record type of interventions used and patient's response in nurses' notes in EHR or chart. Note successful interventions in the care plan.
- Report unexpected new symptoms or uncontrolled existing symptoms to health care provider.

Special Considerations
Teaching

- Involve family members in the patient's care (see Fig. 17.2). With proper instruction they can perform most symptom-management interventions, deliver personal care (e.g., bathing, oral hygiene), and administer medications in the home setting.
- Recognize a patient's transition to the active dying phase and communicate to the patient and family the expectation of imminent death. Educate the patient and family members about signs of imminent death (NCP, 2013)

Pediatric

- Allow young children to visit a dying parent or grandparent if desired. Encourage parents to express their concerns about how to talk about death and loss with their child.

- Teach parents how to recognize and assess pain in a nonverbal child.
- Encourage involvement of siblings of a child who is dying on the basis of their needs and readiness (Hockenberry and Wilson, 2015).

Gerontological

- Include older adults in conversations and accommodate communication limits (e.g., hearing deficits).
- Older adults need companionship and maintenance of self-esteem. Detached caregiver behaviors such as being slow to respond to physical discomforts, failing to keep room odor free, and speaking in hushed tones of voice are often perceived by the person as abandonment. Encourage a family member, friend, sitter, or hospice volunteer to stay with the patient during the night. Some older adults who have developed a lifestyle around aloneness prefer solitude. Be sensitive to patient's preferences (Touhy and Jett, 2014).
- Assessing and addressing pain in an older adult who is cognitively impaired or nonverbal is sometimes difficult and involves proactive symptom management.

Home Care

- Recommend that family members monitor their own energy levels and request respite care when they need relief. Suggest resources for help with meals, shopping, or staying with the patient while family goes out.

◆ SKILL 17.3 Care of a Body After Death

Nurses provide postmortem care in patient's homes and institutional settings. Treat the body after death with respect according to the cultural and religious practices of the family and in accordance with local law (NCP, 2013). Religious and cultural practices govern how to care for a body near or after death (Loggers et al., 2013) (Box 17.2).

Two legal considerations arise at the time of death. First, the 1986 Omnibus Budget Reconciliation Act (OBRA) legally requires that a patient's survivors be made aware of the option of organ and tissue donation. In most states citizens can sign the back of their driver's license if they wish to be an organ or tissue donor. However, a family member still usually gives consent for donation at the time of death. Patients may indicate their wish to donate organs and tissue in an advance directive.

In the case of vital organ donation (e.g., heart, lungs, liver, pancreas, or kidneys), a patient must remain on life support until the organs are surgically removed. A nurse's role in organ procurement includes helping to identify potential organ donors, providing care for the donor's body, and caring for the family throughout the donation process (Findlater and Thomson, 2015; Matzo and Hill, 2014). Family members often need help understanding what "brain death" (i.e., the irreversible absence of all brain function, including the brainstem) means for a person who has died. Patients appear to still be alive because life support keeps the deceased's organs functioning until they can be retrieved. Tissues such as eyes, bone, and skin are retrieved from deceased patients not on life support. Because of the sensitive nature of making requests for organ donation, professionals educated in organ procurement often assume that responsibility. They inform family members of their options for donation, provide information about costs (no cost to the family), and inform them that donation does not delay funeral arrangements.

Nurses also play a role in the donation request process. Facilitate the conversation by providing a private place and helping to identify the surrogate to be involved in the request. Sometimes you notify the local donor registry to determine if a patient qualifies for organ donation because certain medical conditions prohibit donation. Reinforce explanations of the procedure and inform the family about how you will care for the deceased's body. Above all, honor the family's cultural and religious practices and support their final decision. Donor families often report that donating organs helped them in their grief and that they felt positive about the experience.

The second procedure of legal and medical significance often performed after a death is an autopsy, or postmortem examination. An autopsy, the surgical dissection of a body after death, helps determine the exact cause and circumstances of a death, discovers the pathway of a disease, or provides research data. It is not performed in every death. State laws determine when autopsies are required, but they are usually performed in circumstances of unusual death (e.g., violent trauma; unexpected death in the home) and when death occurs within 24 hours of hospital admission (Matzo and Hill, 2014). Be available to answer questions and support the family's choices. Autopsies normally do not delay burial or change the appearance of the deceased, but there may be a cost to families.

Delegation and Collaboration

The skill of care of a body after death can be delegated to nursing assistive personnel (NAP). However, it is often easier for the nurse and NAP to work together in providing postmortem care. The nurse directs the NAP to:
- Follow agency policy in cases of autopsy or organ and tissue donation.
- Honor family cultural or religious rituals when performing postmortem care.
- Handle the body with dignity and respect for privacy.

Equipment
- Clean gloves and isolation gown
- Plastic bag for hazardous waste disposal
- Washbasin, washcloth, warm water, and bath towel
- Clean gown or disposable gown for body as indicated by agency policy
- Shroud kit with name tags
- Syringes for removing urinary catheter
- Scissors
- Small pillow or towel
- Paper tape, gauze dressings
- Paper bag, plastic bag, or other suitable receptacle for patient's belongings to be returned to family members
- Valuables envelope

BOX 17.2

Religious and Cultural Considerations in Care of the Body Near and After Death

Buddhism—People prefer a quiet place for death. Incense may be used. When the person has died, cover the body with a cotton sheet. Leave the deceased's mouth and eyes open. Others should not touch the body. Maintain strict silence after death. Autopsy and organ donation are permitted.

Christianity—Christian denominations have varying practices at time of death. Bible texts may be read near or at the time of death. Protestants receive the sacraments of Holy Communion or sometimes baptism. Roman Catholics often request sacraments of Penance, Anointing of the Sick, and Holy Communion at the end of life. Many Christian groups offer prayers and anointing and view death as "going home" to Jesus. There are no prescribed rituals for body preparation, and autopsy and organ donation are usually permissible.

Hinduism—People prefer to die at home or in a quiet setting. Because of a belief in reincarnation, efforts are made to resolve relationships before death. The head of a person nearing death should face the east with a lamp placed near the head. If the dying person is unable to chant his mantra, a family member can chant it into the right ear. Passages from the Bhagavad Gita are recited. Family members prefer to wash the body after death and are present to chant, pray, and use incense. Hindus prefer cremation of the body.

Islam—A Muslim reader recites verses from the Qur'an when the person is near death. Family members prepare the body, and non-Muslims should not touch it. Close the person's eyes after death and straighten the arms and legs. Autopsy or organ donation is generally not permissible, except as required by law.

Judaism—Death bed confessional, blessings, and readings from the Torah are traditional in Orthodox Judaism. A family member remains with the body until burial, which takes place within 24 hours, not on the Sabbath. A family member closes the deceased's eyes on death. Synagogue burial societies may prepare the body, which is wrapped in white linen. Organ donation prohibitions may exist in Orthodox Judaism, but not for all Jews. Autopsies may be considered if organs are not removed.

STEP	RATIONALE

ASSESSMENT

1. Ask health care provider to establish time of death and determine if he or she has requested an autopsy. If an autopsy is planned or a possible crime is involved, use special precautions to preserve evidence (see agency policy).

2. Determine if family members or significant others are present and if they have been informed of the death. Identify patient's surrogate (next of kin or durable power of attorney [DPOA]).

3. Determine if patient's surrogate has been asked about organ and tissue donation and validate that donation request form has been signed. Notify organ request team per policy.

4. Provide family members and friends a private place to gather. Allow them time to ask questions (including those about medical care) or discuss grief.

5. Ask family members if they have requests for preparation or viewing of the body (e.g., washing the body, position of body, special clothing, shaving). Determine if they wish to be present or help with care of the body.

6. Contact support person (e.g., pastoral care, social work) to stay with family members not helping to prepare the body. Implement in timely manner a bereavement care plan after patient's death when family remains the focus of care (NCP, 2013).

7. Consult health care providers' orders for special care directives or specimens that are to be collected.

8. Perform hand hygiene; apply clean gloves, gown, or protective barriers.

9. Assess general condition of the body and note presence of dressings, tubes, and medical equipment. (If leaving room at this time, remove personal protective equipment and perform hand hygiene.)

Rationale column:

Certifies patient's death. Autopsy can determine cause of death and reveal more about a disease. Patient's legal representative and the health care provider or designated requester must sign an autopsy consent form.

Verifies that family has been notified of patient's death to avoid inappropriate communication of this sensitive information.

Federal guidelines require documentation that request has been made.

Creates safe environment for grieving family. Questions provide information about how they are coping with loss and their needs.

Respects individuality of patient and family and supports their right to having cultural or religious values and beliefs upheld. Provides closure for those who wish to help with body preparation (Hadders et al., 2014).

Provides family support during an emotional time.

Specimens may be used in determining cause of death.

Reduces transmission of microorganisms.

Validates if tissue damage was present before postmortem care.

NURSING DIAGNOSES

For patients:
- Risk for impaired skin integrity

For family members and significant others:
- Compromised family coping
- Deficient knowledge regarding organ donation
- Grieving
- Ineffective coping
- Powerlessness

Related factors/Risk factors are individualized based on the patient's, family's, and significant others' needs.

PLANNING

1. Expected outcomes following completion of procedure:
   - Body is free of new skin damage.

   - Significant others able to express grief.

Rationale column:

Careful handling of body prevents lacerations, bruises, or abrasions during postmortem care.

Significant others feel supported through their loss.

Clinical Decision Point *Immediately after death and before proceeding with other activities, place body in supine position and elevate head of bed 30 degrees to decrease livor mortis.*

2. Position patient supine in bed, arms at side, in a private room if possible. If patient has a roommate, explain and move him or her to another location temporarily.

Provides staff with larger area for postmortem care and for family members to gather in a private setting.

Clinical Decision Point *It is best practice to carry out "personal care after death" within 2 to 4 hours of death to preserve the deceased's appearance, condition, dignity, and ability to donate tissue (Henry and Wilson, 2012).*

STEP	RATIONALE
3. As soon as possible, a patient's death must be "pronounced" by someone in authority (e.g., physician in hospital or nursing facility or hospice nurse). This person completes forms certifying the cause, time, and place of death. The legal form is necessary for life insurance and financial and property issues. If hospice is helping, a plan for what happens after death is already in place (NIA, 2015)	These steps make it possible for an official death certificate to be prepared.
4. Direct NAP to gather needed equipment and arrange at bedside.	Because this is often an emotional time for family members, organized efficient care is important.

IMPLEMENTATION

STEP	RATIONALE
1. Help family members notify others of the death. Promptly notify the mortuary, as chosen by the family, and discuss plans for postmortem care.	Following a death, grieving persons have difficulty focusing on details and often need guidance. Being informed increases a sense of control.
2. If patient has made tissue donation, consult agency policy for care of the body guidelines.	Retrieval of tissues (e.g., eyes, bone, skin) may require special procedures.
3. Perform hand hygiene; apply clean gloves, gown, or protective barriers.	Reduces transmission of microorganisms.

Clinical Decision Point *Have family caregivers helping in postmortem care wear a gown and gloves to protect them from body fluids.*

STEP	RATIONALE
4. Identify patient using at least two identifiers (e.g., name and birthday or name and medical record number) according to agency policy. Tag the body and leave tag on the body as directed by agency policy.	Ensures correct patient. Complies with The Joint Commission standards and improves patient safety (TJC, 2016).
5. Remove indwelling devices (e.g., urinary catheter, endotracheal tube). Disconnect and cap off (no need to remove) intravenous lines. *Do not remove indwelling devices in cases of autopsy* (follow agency policy).	Creates normal appearance for family viewing of body. Removing intravenous catheters allows fluids to leak. Removal of tubes and lines is contraindicated if an autopsy is planned.
6. Clean the mouth and clean and replace dentures as soon as possible (Henry and Wilson, 2012). If dentures cannot be replaced, send them with body in clearly labeled denture cup and transport with body to mortuary. If culturally appropriate, close mouth with rolled-up towel under chin.	Gives face more natural appearance. If dentures are not replaced, it can be very difficult later for workers at funeral home to place dentures.
7. Place small pillow under head or position according to cultural preferences. Do not tie hands together on top of body. Check agency policy regarding need to secure hands and feet. Use only circular gauze bandaging on body.	Patient appears natural. Weight of limp arms causes skin damage and discoloration if hands are tied. Some agencies require securing appendages to prevent tissue damage when body is being moved.
8. Close eyes by applying light pressure for 30 seconds. Use saline-moistened gauze if corneal or eye donation is to take place (Henry and Wilson, 2012). Some cultures prefer that eyes remain open.	Closed eyes convey to some people a more peaceful and natural appearance. Gauze prevents corneal drying.
9. Groom and arrange hair into preferred style, if known. Remove any clips, hairpins, or rubber bands. Do not shave patient. Some faith groups prohibit shaving.	Hard objects damage or discolor face and scalp. Shaving too soon after death can cause bruising, so this is done by the funeral director. Explain this to the family if they request shaving (Henry and Wilson, 2012).
10. Wash soiled body parts. Some cultural practices require that family members clean the body (see Box 17.2).	Prepares body for viewing and reduces odors. Mortuary personnel provide complete bath.
11. Remove soiled dressings and replace with clean dressings, using paper tape or circular gauze bandaging.	Changing dressings controls odors and creates more acceptable appearance. Paper tape minimizes skin damage when tape is removed.

Clinical Decision Point *Turning a recently dead body to the side sometimes causes the flow of exhaled air. This is a normal event and not a sign of life.*

STEP	RATIONALE
12. Place absorbent pad under buttocks.	Relaxation of sphincter muscles at time of death causes release of urine or feces.

STEP	RATIONALE
13. Place clean gown on body. Some agencies require gown removal before placing body in shroud.	Provides privacy and prepares body for viewing.
14. Identify personal belongings that stay with body and those to be given to family.	Prevents loss of valuable or meaningful property.
15. If family requests viewing, respect individual cultural practices. Otherwise, place clean sheet over body up to chin with arms outside covers. Remove medical equipment from room. Provide soft lighting and chairs.	Maintains respect for patient and those viewing body. Prevents exposure of body parts. Removing medical equipment provides more peaceful, natural setting.
16. Allow family time alone with body and encourage them to say goodbye with religious rituals and in a culturally appropriate manner. Some families want time to sit quietly with the body, console each other, and share memories (NIA, 2015). Some cultural practices include maintaining silence at the time of death; whereas others express grief with intense emotional displays, loud wailing, or "falling out." Do not rush any grieving process.	Compassionate care provides family members with meaningful experience during early phase of grief. Ensure privacy and a safe environment. Provide chair at bedside for family member who might collapse.
17. After viewing, remove linens and gown per agency policy. Place body in shroud provided by the agency (see illustration).	Shroud protects injury to skin, avoids exposure of body, and provides barrier against potentially contaminated body fluids.

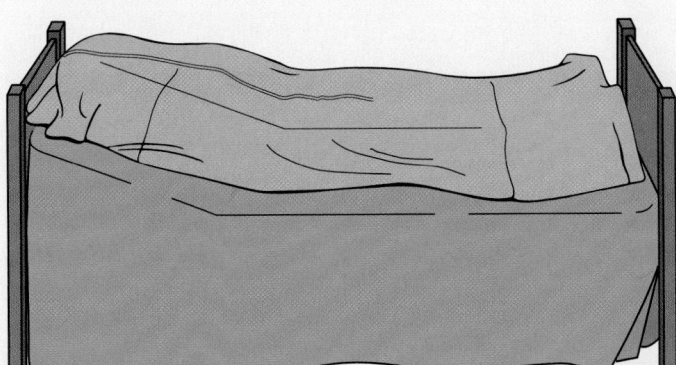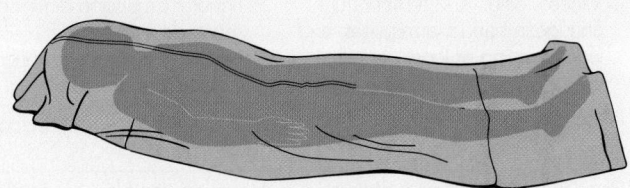

STEP 17 Body in shroud.

STEP	RATIONALE
18. Place identification label on outside of shroud if required by agency policy. Follow agency policy for marking a body that poses an infectious risk to others. Remove and dispose of personal protective equipment and perform hygiene.	Ensures proper identification of body. Reduces exposure of morgue and mortuary staff to contamination.
19. Arrange prompt transportation of body to the mortuary. If you anticipate a delay, transport body to the morgue.	Mortuary personnel get best results if embalming occurs before full rigor mortis (i.e., stiffening of body after death) occurs.

EVALUATION

1. Observe family members', friends', and significant others' response to the loss.	The need for referral or help is based on evaluation of person's unique response to loss.
2. Note appearance and condition of patient's skin during preparation of the body.	Provides information for postmortem care documentation.

Unexpected Outcomes
1. A family member becomes immobilized with grief and has difficulty functioning.
2. A grieving person becomes agitated and threatens or strikes out against others.

Related Interventions
- Enlist the help of a family member or trusted friend to provide direction and support.
- Call for assistance from a psychiatric nurse practitioner, spiritual care provider, or social worker who has a relationship with the family.
- Enlist help from security staff or crisis intervention professional if safety is a concern.

Recording and Reporting

- Record time of death in the nurses' notes in electronic health record (EHR) or chart, describe any resuscitative measures taken (if applicable), and note the name of the professional certifying the death.
- Record any special preparation of the body for autopsy or organ/tissue donation. Note whom you called and who made the request for organ/tissue donation.
- Record names of mortuary and names of family members consulted at the time of death and their relationship to the deceased.
- Record on appropriate form personal articles left on the body (e.g., teeth or glasses), jewelry taped to skin, or tubes and lines left in place. Note how valuables and personal belongings were handled and who received them. Secure signatures as required by agency policy.
- Record time the body was transported and its destination. Note the location of body identification tags.

Special Considerations
Pediatric

- Offer family members, especially parents, to be with the child throughout the dying process and help with body preparation.

- Parents frequently want to hold their child's body after death. Parents of deceased newborns often want a memento of their baby (e.g., picture, article of clothing, footprint, or lock of hair). Make every effort to honor parent requests.

Gerontological

- Some older adults have very small families and surviving circles of friends. Nurses and other care providers are sometimes the only human presence during death. Arrange for someone to be with the person when death is imminent.

Home Care

- Educate family members caring for a patient dying at home about what to expect at the time of death (Table 17.1).
- Consider the type of support that family members will need at the time of death and make arrangements.
- After death in the home, follow agency guidelines for body preparation and transfer and for disposal of durable medical equipment (e.g., tubing, needles, syringes), soiled dressings or linens, and medications. Instruct family members in safe and proper handling and disposal of medical waste.

TABLE 17.1

Physical Signs and Symptoms in the Final Stages of Dying

Physical Signs and Symptoms	Rationale	Intervention
Coolness, color, and temperature change in hands, arms, feet, and legs; mottling of legs; perspiration	Peripheral circulation diminished as blood shunts to vital organs Patient may feel cool to touch, but core temperature normal	Place socks on feet. Cover with light blanket. Do not use electric blanket because person is unable to report excess heat.
Increased sleeping	Decreased energy, psychological withdrawal, medications	Spend time with person; hold his or her hand. Speak to person, even if no response.
Disorientation, confusion of time, place, person	Metabolic changes, medications, changing sleep/wake cycles, decreased oxygenation	Identify self by name; reorient person to time and place. Decrease environmental stimuli.
Incontinence of urine and/or bowel	Decreased muscle tone and consciousness	Change bedding as appropriate. Use bed pads; try not to use indwelling catheters.
Upper airway secretions; noisy respirations	Decreased cough reflex, inability to expectorate secretions or clear throat, relaxation of glottis, decreased muscle tone	Elevate head with pillow or raise head of bed; turn head to side to drain secretions. Suction minimally.
Restlessness	Metabolic changes and decrease in oxygen to brain	Calm patient by speech and action; reduce light, rub back, stroke arms, or read aloud. Do not use restraints.
Decreased intake of food and fluids, nausea	Blood shunted away from gastrointestinal (GI) tract, causing decreased GI motility and anorexia; ketosis	Do not force patient to eat or drink; give ice chips or popsicles if desired. Provide mouth care.

Modified from Touhy TA, Jett KF: *Ebersole and Hess' gerontological nursing and healthy aging*, ed 4, St Louis, 2014, Elsevier.

♦ CLINICAL DEBRIEF

You are caring for a 79-year-old man hospitalized for abdominal pain, anorexia, weight loss, and weakness. He was treated 10 years earlier for prostate cancer. Test results now confirm that he has a large tumor in his abdomen and the cancer has spread to the lymph nodes. No medical interventions are available to cure his disease. When you enter the room, the patient tells you in an angry voice that he wants to transfer to a different hospital where people will help him fight his cancer.

1. Which approaches should you use in response to his statement?
2. The next day the patient reports mild abdominal pain and mentions that he has not had a bowel movement for 3 days. His wife reports to you that he has not had anything to eat or drink for 24 hours.
   a. What might be the cause of the patient not having a bowel movement?
   b. List three interventions to provide.

3. Four weeks later you take care of this patient again. His symptoms include weight loss, anorexia, worsening abdominal pain, depression, and anxiety. His wife tells you that the nurse practitioner told them about home hospice care. His wife says to you, "I'm still not sure if hospice would be best for us." Which key points would you include in a discussion with the patient and his wife about hospice care? Using SBAR, show how the nurse communicates her assessment with the other health care providers.

◆ REVIEW QUESTIONS

1. A patient with cancer is admitted into hospice care. What are the goals of hospice care? (Select all that apply.)
   1. Physical symptom management
   2. Provision of cultural and spiritual preferences
   3. Curative care
   4. Extending life as long as possible
   5. Providing a dignified death

2. A nurse suggests that a patient receive a palliative care consultation for symptom management related to anxiety and increasing pain. A family member asks the nurse if this means that the patient is dying and is now "in hospice." What should the nurse tell the patient and family about the care that she is receiving?
   1. Hospice (end-of-life care) and palliative care are the same thing.
   2. Palliative care is for any patient, any time with any chronic disease, in any setting.
   3. Palliative care strategies are primarily designed to treat the patient's illness.
   4. Palliative care interventions relieve the symptoms of illness and treatment.
   5. 1 and 3
   6. 2 and 4

3. A nurse has the responsibility of managing a deceased patient's postmortem care. Arrange the steps for postmortem care in the proper order.
   1. Bathe the deceased's body.
   2. Collect any needed specimens.
   3. Remove all drains and indwelling tubes.
   4. Position the body for family visit/viewing.
   5. Speak to the family members about their possible participation.
   6. Confirm that request for organ/tissue donation and/or autopsy has been made.
   7. Notify a support person (e.g., spiritual care provider, bereavement specialist) for the family.
   8. Accurately tag the body, indicating deceased's identity and safety issues regarding infection control.
   9. Elevate the head of the bed.

ⓔ *Visit the Evolve site for a complete list of Clinical Debrief and Review Questions answers.*

REFERENCES

Ache K, et al: Are advance directives associated with better hospice care? *J Am Geriatr Soc* 62:1091, 2014.

Albrecht TA, Taylor AG: Physical activity in patients with advanced-stage cancer: a systematic review of the literature, *Clin J Oncol Nurs* 16(3):293, 2012.

American Cancer Society (ACS): *Physical symptoms in the last 2 to 3 months of life*, ACS, 2014, http://www.cancer.org/treatment/nearingtheendoflife/nearing theendoflife/nearing-the-end-of-life-physical-symptoms. Accessed March 13, 2016.

Arbour R, Wiegand D: Self-described nursing roles experienced during care of dying patients and their families: a phenomenological study, *Intensive Crit Care Nurs* 30:211, 2014.

Arizmendi B, O'Connor M: What is "normal" in grief? *Aust Crit Care* 28:58, 2015.

Bailey FA, et al: Opioid pain medication orders and administration in the last days of life, *J Pain Symptom Manage* 44(5):681, 2012.

Bailey F, Harmon S: Palliative care: the last hours of day and life, *UpToDate*, 2016, http://www.uptodate.com/contents/palliative-care-the-last-hours-and-days-of-life. Accessed June 25, 2016.

Baker B, Ward-Smith P: Urinary incontinence: nursing considerations at the end of life, *Urol Nurs* 31(3):169, 2011.

Brazil K, et al: Family caregiver views on patient-centered care at the end of life, *Scand J Caring Sci* 26:513, 2012.

Brown M, Vaughan C: Care at the end of life: how policy and the law support practice, *Br J Nurs* 22(10):580, 2013.

Bullock K: The influence of culture on end-of-life decision making, *J Soc Work End Life Palliat Care* 7(1):83, 2011.

Burchum JR, Rosenthal LD: *Lehne's pharmacology for nursing care*, ed 9, St Louis, 2016, Elsevier.

Clabots S: Strategies to help initiate and maintain the end-of-life discussion with patients and family members, *Medsurg Nurs* 21(4):197, 2012.

Clark K, Currow D: Advancing research into symptoms of constipation at the end of life, *Int J Palliat Nurs* 20(8):370, 2014.

Curtis JR, et al: Randomized trial of communication facilitators to reduce family distress and intensity of end-of-life care, *Am J Respir Crit Care Med* 193(2):154, 2016.

Doherty M, Thompson H: Enhancing person-centered care through the development of a therapeutic relationship, *Br J Community Nurs* 19(10):502, 2014.

Dosser I, Kennedy C: Improving family carergivers' experiences of support at the end of life by enhancing communication: an action research study, *Int J Palliat Nurs* 20(12):608, 2014.

End-of-Life Nursing Education Consortium (ELNEC): *Peaceful death: recommended competencies and curricular guidelines for end-of-life nursing care*, American Association of Colleges of Nurses, 2015, http://www.aacn.nche.edu/elnec/publications/peaceful-death. Accessed March 13, 2016.

Findlater C, Thomson E: *Organ donation and management of the potential organ donor*, Anesthesia and Intensive Care Medicine, 2015, http://dx.doi.org/10.1016/j.mpaic.2015.04.013. Accessed March 13, 2016.

Fiorelli R, Jenkins W: Cultural competency in grief and loss, *Beginnings* 32(3):11, 2012.

Fowler MDM: *Guide to the code of ethics for nurses with interpretive statements: development, interpretation, and application*, ed 2, Silver Spring, MD, 2015, American Nurses Association.

Gillespie L, Raftery A: Nutrition in palliative and end-of-life care, *Br J Community Nurs* (Suppl):S15, 2014.

Guldin M: Complicated grief—a challenge in bereavement support in palliative care: an update of the field, *Prog Palliat Care* 22(3):136, 2014.

Hadders H, et al: Relatives' participation at the time of death: standardisation in pre and post-mortem care in a palliative medical unit, *Eur J Oncol Nurs* 18:159, 2014.

Hall A: An overview of end-of-life care in the community setting, *J Clin Nurs* 28(6):36, 2014.

Henry C, Wilson J: Personal care at the end of life and after death, *Nurs Times* 108(online issue):2012.

Hinderer K, Lee M: Assessing a nurse-led advance directive and advance care planning seminar, *Appl Nurs Res* 27:84, 2014.

Hockenberry MJ, Wilson D: *Wong's nursing care of infants and children*, ed 10, St Louis, 2015, Mosby.

Hodge D: Administering a two-stage spiritual assessment in healthcare settings: a necessary component of ethical and effective care, *J Nurs Manag* 23(1):27, 2015.

Hofmann SG, et al: The effect of mindfulness-based therapy on anxiety and depression: a meta-analytic review, *J Consult Clin Psychol* 78(2):169, 2010.

Hospice Foundation of America: 2015, http://www.hospicefoundation.org/. Accessed March 13, 2016.

Jeffers S: Nurse faculty perceptions of end-of-life education in the clinical setting: a phenomenological perspective, *Nurse Educ Pract* 14:455, 2014.

Keall R, et al: Therapeutic life review in palliative care: a systematic review of quantitative evaluations, *J Pain Symptom Manage* 49(4):747, 2015.

Kisvetrova H, et al: Spiritual support interventions in nursing care for patients suffering death anxiety in the final phase of life, *Int J Palliat Nurs* 19(12):599, 2013.

Koornstra R, et al: Management of fatigue in patients with cancer—a practical overview, *Cancer Treat Rev* 40:791, 2014.

Loggers E, et al: Predictors of intensive end-of-life and hospice care in Latino and white advanced cancer patients, *J Palliat Med* 16(10):1249, 2013.

Lowey SE, et al: Living with advanced heart failure or COPD: experiences and goals of individuals nearing the end of life, *Res Nurs Health* 36:349, 2013.

Luckett T, et al: Elements of effective palliative care models: a rapid review, *BMC Health Serv Res* 14:136, 2014.

Macauley R: The role of the principle of double effect in ethics education in US medical schools and its potential impact on pain management at the end of life, *J Med Ethics* 38(3):174, 2012.

Matzo M, Hill J: Peri-death nursing care. In Matzo M, Sherman D, editors: *Palliative care nursing: quality care at the end of life*, ed 4, New York, 2014, Springer.

McMahon M, Christopher K: Toward a mid-range theory of nursing presence, *Nurs Forum* 46(2):71, 2011.

Moir C, et al: Communicating with patients and their families about palliative and end-of-life care: comfort and educational needs of nurses, *Int J Palliat Nurs* 21(3):109, 2015.

Moyer D: Terminal delirium in geriatric patients with cancer at end of life, *Am J Hosp Palliat Care* 28(1):44, 2011.

National Consensus Project (NCP) for Quality Palliative Care: *Clinical practice guidelines for quality palliative care*, ed 3, 2013, http://www.nationalconsensusproject.org. Accessed March 13, 2016.

National Institute on Aging (NIA): *End of life: helping with comfort and care*, 2015, https://www.nia.nih.gov/health/publication/end-life-helping-comfort-and-care/things-do-after-someone-dies. Accessed March 13, 2016.

Nunn C: It's not just about pain: symptom management in palliative care, *Nurse Prescrib* 12(7):338, 2014.

Paice J: Pain at the end of life. In Ferrell B, et al, editors: *Textbook of palliative nursing*, ed 4, New York, 2015, Oxford University Press.

Quinn-Lee L, et al: Use of oxygen at the end of life: on what basis are decisions made?, *Int J Palliat Nurs* 18(8):369, 2012.

Regan A, et al: Improving end-of-life care for people with dementia, *Nurs Stand* 28(48):37, 2014.

Santucci G, Battista V: Methylnaltrexone for opioid-induced constipation in patients at the end of life, *Int J Palliat Nurs* 21(4):162, 2015.

Selman L, et al: Holistic models for end-of-life care: establishing place of culture, *Prog Palliat Care* 22(2):80, 2014.

Shaw C, Eldridge L: Nutritional considerations for the palliative care patient, *Int J Palliat Nurs* 21(1):7, 2015.

The Joint Commission (TJC): *2016 National Patient Safety Goals*, Oakbrook Terrace, IL, 2016, The Commission, http://www.jointcommission.org/standards_information/npsgs.aspx. Accessed March 13, 2016.

Touhy TA, Jett KF: *Ebersole and Hess' gerontological nursing and healthy aging*, ed 4, St Louis, 2014, Elsevier.

Ward L, et al: Relationships between bereavement and cognitive functioning in older adults, *Gerontology* 53(6):362, 2007.

Widera E, Block S: Managing grief and depression at the end of life, *Am Fam Physician* 86(3):259, 2012.

World Health Organization: *WHO definition of palliative care*, 2015, http://www.who.int/cancer/palliative/definition/en/. Accessed March 13, 2016.

Wynne L: Spiritual care at the end of life, *Nurs Stand* 28(2):41, 2013.

18 | Personal Hygiene and Bed Making

OBJECTIVES

Mastery of content in this chapter will enable the nurse to:
- Discuss clinical guidelines to use for providing personal hygiene to patients.
- Identify principles of aseptic technique applied while administering a bed bath.
- Administer a complete bed bath.
- Explain precautions to take when assisting patients with a tub bath or shower.
- Discuss precautions for minimizing transmission of infection during hygienic care.
- Identify clinical guidelines to follow when administering oral hygiene.
- Explain differences in providing oral hygiene to dependent versus unconscious patients.
- Identify clinical guidelines for administering hair, nail, and foot care.
- Comb, brush, and shampoo the hair of a bed-bound patient.
- Shave a male or female patient safely.
- Identify risk factors for foot and nail problems.
- Safely administer nail care.
- Change the linen on an unoccupied and occupied bed.

MEDIA RESOURCES

- evolve http://evolve.elsevier.com/Perry/skills
- Review Questions
- Case Studies
- ▶ Video Clips
- Audio Glossary
- Clinical Debrief and Review Questions Answers

PURPOSE

Hygiene is important for promoting and preserving physical and mental health. When you deliver hygiene to a patient, it is an excellent time to discuss health-related concerns, perform a physical assessment, and provide patient education. Providing personal hygiene is also necessary for an individual's comfort, safety, and sense of well-being.

STANDARDS OF CARE

- Agency for Healthcare Research and Quality (AHRQ), 2013—Bathing the Patient With Dementia
- Centers for Disease Control and Prevention (CDC), 2015—Oral Hygiene

- National Pressure Ulcer Advisory Panel (NPUAP): Prevention and Treatment of Pressure Ulcers: Clinical Practice Guideline, 2014—Bathing
- The Joint Commission (TJC), 2016—Patient Identification

PRINCIPLES FOR PRACTICE

- Regular bathing of all patients is essential to maintain skin integrity by promoting circulation and hydration.
- Bathing people with dementia is a complicated process of applying physical, emotional, and environmental factors to the care recipient's best advantage to promote a safe, acceptable, and comfortable bathing process for cleaning the person's skin (AHRQ, 2013a).

- When you provide patient hygiene, maintain a patient's privacy and comfort and encourage patients to participate in their hygienic care.

PATIENT-CENTERED CARE

- Always convey sensitivity and respect for a patient's personal cultural beliefs and habits in the way you provide hygiene.
- Skin problems cause changes that affect a patient's appearance and body image. Be sensitive to a patient's feelings while caring for skin problems.
- It is important to understand if a patient's ethnicity requires certain customs to be followed in the way personal hygiene is performed.
- Be sure to take each patient's preferences into consideration when providing hygiene. Simply asking patients about their preferences (e.g., products to use, best time to perform aspects of hygiene) can create a more trusting and nurturing environment.
- Depending on cultural considerations and the ability of a patient to help with care, it may be beneficial to involve a family member or significant other in the patient's hygiene so complete, culturally sensitive patient-centered care is provided.
- Preserve the dignity of patients with dementia by shifting the focus of care from tasks of bathing to needs and abilities of the person being bathed with emphasis on comfort, safety, autonomy, and self-esteem (AHRQ, 2013a).

EVIDENCED-BASED PRACTICE

Recent evidence supports the use of daily bathing with chlorhexidine gluconate (CHG) to reduce the rate of hospital-acquired infections.

- Multiple studies conducted in long-term acute care facilities and both medical and surgical intensive care units support that daily bathing with 2% CHG (cloths or in bath water) substantially reduces colonization and bloodstream health care–associated infections (HAIs), including methicillin-resistant *Staphylococcus aureus* (MRSA) and vancomycin-resistant *Enterococcus* (VRE) infections (Chen et al., 2013; Climo et al., 2013; Munoz-Price et al., 2012). A recent systematic review and meta-analysis confirmed that 2% CHG reduces central line–associated bloodstream infections (CLABSIs) (Shah et al., 2016). CHG-impregnated bathing cloths are more expensive than using CHG solution in bath water; however, both methods of bathing are effective. If using CHG solution in bath water, it is important to reserve a bath basin only for bathing and not for storage. Bathing should be provided daily. Use of CHG-impregnated bathing cloths is well tolerated by the skin and is effective against a wide spectrum of gram-positive and gram-negative bacteria, including MRSA.

SAFETY GUIDELINES

- Patients who are totally dependent on someone else require help with personal hygiene or must learn or adapt to new hygiene techniques. When providing personal hygiene, important safety principles to follow are prevention of infection and patient injury.
- Keep all personal-hygiene care items within a patient's reach. When the head of the bed is raised, the bedside stand is usually not within easy reach and must be moved forward. If a patient must leave the bed to go to the bathroom, be sure that there is a clear pathway to prevent falls.
- Use clean gloves when you anticipate contact with nonintact skin or mucous membranes or when there is or may likely be contact with drainage, secretions, excretions, or blood. Additional precautions requiring other personal protective equipment (PPE) may be necessary, depending on the patient's condition (see Chapter 9).
- To reduce the risk of infection, always perform hygiene measures moving from cleanest to less clean or dirty areas. This often requires you to change gloves and perform hand hygiene during care activities.
- When using water or solutions for hygiene care, be sure to test the solution temperature to prevent burn injury. This is especially important for patients with reduced sensation such as those with diabetes mellitus, peripheral neuropathy, or spinal cord injury. It is also important for patients unable to communicate.
- To avoid injury when performing hygiene care, use principles of body mechanics and safe patient handling (see Chapter 11).
- You are responsible and accountable for assessing and evaluating a patient before and after care to detect unexpected outcomes and give proper direction to nursing assistive personnel (NAP) when delegating hygiene care.
- Monitor laboratory findings such as coagulation studies before administering oral care to prevent bleeding.

THE SKIN

The skin is the largest organ in the human body; it protects the body from heat, light, injury, and infection. It serves to (1) help regulate body temperature; (2) store water, vitamin D, and fat; (3) help sense pain and other stimuli; and (4) prevent the entry of bacteria. Three primary layers make up the skin: the epidermis, dermis, and subcutaneous tissue. The skin covers the entire surface of the body and is continuous with mucous membranes of the mouth, eyes, ears, nose, vagina, and rectum. Thorough hygiene is essential for the integrity and function of each skin layer.

The epidermis, or outer skin layer, is the first line of defense against external injury and infection. Sebum, secreted from hair follicles from sebaceous glands, provides an acidic coating. This acidic coating protects the epidermis against penetration by chemicals and microorganisms. It also minimizes loss of water and plasma proteins.

Two types of sweat glands, the eccrine and apocrine glands, are distributed over the surface of the skin. Eccrine glands secrete a watery fluid (sweat) that helps control temperature through evaporation. The apocrine glands secrete sweat in the axillary and genital areas. Bacterial decomposition of sweat from the apocrine glands causes body odor.

The subcutaneous tissue layer contains blood vessels, nerves, lymph tissue, and loose connective tissue filled with fat cells. Fatty tissue insulates the body. Subcutaneous tissue also provides support for upper skin layers.

Bacteria reside on the outer surface of the skin. The resident bacteria are normal flora that do not cause disease but prevent disease-causing microorganisms from reproducing. Because a part of the skin is usually exposed to environmental irritants and is an active organ sensitive to physiological changes within the body, some skin problems commonly occur (Table 18.1).

TABLE 18.1

Common Skin Problems

Problem	Characteristics	Implications	Interventions
Dry skin 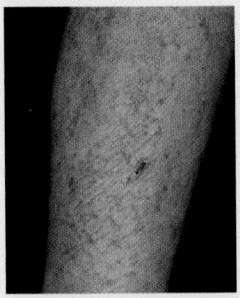	Flaky, rough texture caused by lack of moisture in outer stratum corneum, resulting in less pliable epidermis; most common on anterior surfaces of lower legs, knees, elbows, and backs of hands	Skin may crack, bleed, and become inflamed. As a result, redness, pruritus, and discomfort may develop.	Effective treatment of dry skin does not include limiting frequency of bathing but lies in bathing with warm, not hot, water and use of moisturizers (nonpetroleum). Use super-fatted soap (e.g., Dove) for cleaning. Rinse body of all soap well because residue left can cause irritation and breakdown. Add moisture to air through use of humidifier. Increase fluid intake when skin is dry.
Acne 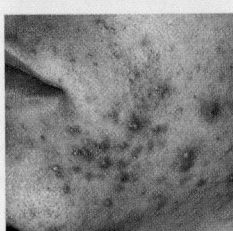 *(From James WD, et al: Andrew's diseases of the skin: clinical dermatology, ed 10, Philadelphia, 2007, Saunders.)*	Inflammatory, papulopustular skin eruption, usually involving bacterial breakdown of sebum; appears on face, neck, shoulders, and back	Infected material within pustule can spread if area is squeezed or picked. Permanent scarring can result.	Wash hair and skin each day with warm water and soap to remove oil. Use cosmetics sparingly because oily cosmetics or creams accumulate in pores and tend to make condition worse. Implement necessary dietary restrictions by eliminating foods found to aggravate condition. Use prescribed topical antibiotics for severe acne.
Hirsutism 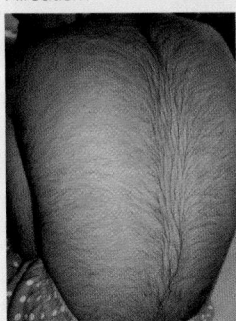 *(From Goyal D, et al: Coffin-Siris syndrome with Mayer-Rokitanksy-Küster-Hauser syndrome: a case report, J Med Case Report 4:354, 2010.)*	Excessive growth of body and facial hair, especially in women	May cause negative body image by giving female a male appearance.	Shaving is safest method to remove hair. Electrolysis and laser permanently remove hair. Tweezing and bleaching are temporary.
Skin rashes 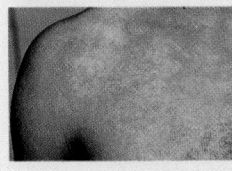	Skin eruption that results from overexposure to sun or moisture or from allergic reaction; may be flat or raised, localized or systemic, pruritic or nonpruritic	If skin is continually scratched, inflammation and infection may occur. Rashes also cause discomfort.	Wash area thoroughly and apply antiseptic spray or lotion to prevent further itching and aid healing process. Warm or cold soaks may relieve inflammation.
Contact dermatitis 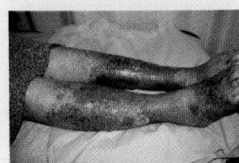 *(From Lewis SL, et al: Medical-surgical nursing: assessment and management of clinical problems, ed 8, St Louis, 2011, Mosby.)*	Acute or chronic eczematous rash characterized by abrupt onset with well-defined geometric margins of erythema, pruritus, pain, and appearance of scaly, oozing lesions; appears on head, neck, scalp, hands, legs, dorsum of feet, and trunk	Dermatitis is often difficult to eliminate because person is usually in continual contact with substance causing skin reaction. Substance may be hard to identify.	Identify and avoid contributing agents (e.g., cleaners, poison ivy or oak, cosmetics, latex, shoes/rubber). Treatment consists of removing contributing agent, if identified, and applying over-the-counter topical steroids or calamine lotion. In some cases prescription steroids may be ordered. Patients may also find comfort with tepid baths.

Continued

TABLE 18.1

Common Skin Problems—cont'd

Problem	Characteristics	Implications	Interventions
Abrasion	Scraping or rubbing away of epidermis may result in localized bleeding and later weeping of serous fluid	Infection occurs easily as result of loss of protective skin layer.	Nurses should always be careful not to scratch patients with their jewelry or fingernails. Wash abrasions with mild soap and water. Dressing or bandage could increase risk for infection because of retained moisture.

(From Cottran SR et al: From the teaching collection of the Department of Dermatology, *University of Texas, Southwestern Medical School, Dallas.)*

THE MOUTH

The oral cavity, which is lined with a normally moist and intact light pink mucous membrane, contains the teeth and gums. The membranous lining protects underlying organs; secretes mucus to keep the oral cavity lubricated; and absorbs water, salts, and other solutes. Saliva, a clear viscous fluid secreted by the mucous and salivary glands of the mouth, helps to prevent dental caries and plaque formation and lubricates the oral cavity. Lubrication of the oral cavity aids in chewing and swallowing. Saliva provides a means for removing cellular and bacterial debris that can cause infection, particularly fungal infection (Villa et al., 2015). Hyposalivation results in dry mouth, or xerostomia, and effects taste, swallowing, digestion, nutrition, and denture fit (Villa et al., 2015).

The teeth are organs of chewing, or mastication. Dentin, a hard, ivorylike substance that surrounds the pulp cavity, forms the major part of a tooth (Fig. 18.1). A layer of enamel, visible in the oral cavity, covers the upper part of the tooth, or crown. The periodontal membrane, just below the gum margins, surrounds the tooth root and holds it firmly in place. A tooth receives its blood, lymph, and nerve supply from the base of the tooth socket within the jaw. Healthy teeth are smooth, shiny, and properly aligned.

The gums, or gingivae, are mucous membranes with underlying supportive fibrous tissue. They encircle the necks of erupted teeth to hold them firmly in place. The gums normally are pink, moist, firm, and relatively inelastic.

THE HAIR

Hair grows from follicles located within the dermis of the skin (Fig. 18.2). Tiny blood vessels supply nourishment for each follicle for normal hair growth. Each hair has a shaft extending from the follicle. Sebaceous glands secrete the oily substance (i.e., sebum) into each follicle, which lubricates the hair and scalp. The hair shaft is normally shiny and pliant and is not excessively oily, dry, or brittle. The primary function of hair is to act as the first line of protection. For example, hair protects the scalp from injury. Eyebrows and eyelashes protect the eyes from foreign particles.

Special hair-care practices focus on care for scalp, axilla, and pubic areas. Hair growth, distribution, and pattern are indicators of a person's health status. Hormonal changes, emotional and physical stress, aging, intake of toxins (e.g., arsenic, cocaine), gender, race, nutrition, infection, and certain diseases affect hair characteristics. A person's appearance and sense of well-being often

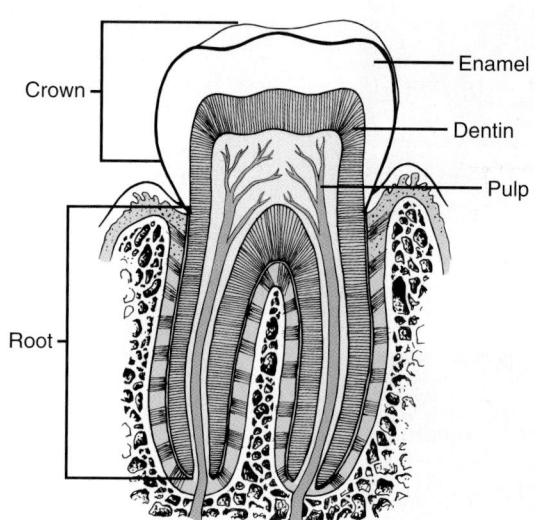

FIG 18.1 Normal tooth.

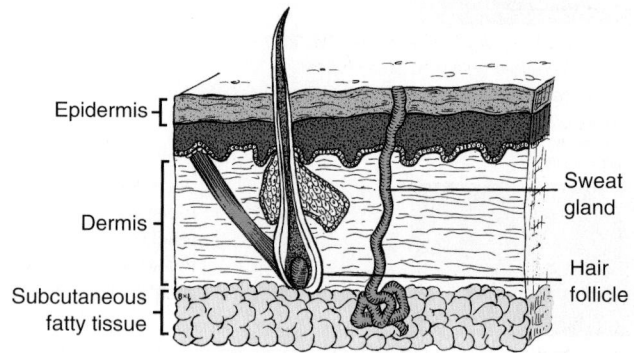

FIG 18.2 Cross section of hair follicle and supporting structures.

depend on the way the hair looks and feels. Illness or disability sometimes prevents patients from maintaining daily hair care.

THE NAILS

The nails are epithelial tissues that grow from the root of the nail bed, located in the skin at the nail groove. A normal, healthy nail is transparent, smooth, and convex, with a pink nail bed and translucent white tip. A normal color indicates adequate oxygenation to peripheral tissues. Pigment deposits or bands are common in nail beds of patients with dark skin. The feet and nails require

special care to prevent infection, odor, and injury. Problems typically result from abuse or poor care. Foot pain can often change a walking gait, causing strain on different muscle groups.

◆ SKILL 18.1 Complete or Partial Bed Bath

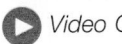 *Video Clip*

Bathing removes sweat, oil, dirt, and microorganisms from the skin. It also stimulates circulation and provides a refreshed and relaxed feeling. For some patients a bath is a time for socialization and pleasure, especially for those who are bedridden or seriously disabled.

The National Pressure Ulcer Advisory Panel and The European Pressure Ulcer Advisory Panel revised the stages of pressure injuries and redefined important points for skin care (NPUAP, 2014). Although these were intended for pressure injury prevention, they provide sound principles for good bathing techniques.

- Clean the skin at the time of soiling and at routine intervals. Individualize frequency of cleaning according to patient need and preference. Problems such as incontinence, wound drainage, or excessive diaphoresis often require bathing several times a day; whereas other patients such as the elderly and infants should be bathed only once or twice a week to prevent removal of protective skin oils.
- Avoid hot or excessively cold water and use a mild cleansing agent that minimizes irritation.
- Avoid use of force and friction on the skin when bathing patients. Do not massage reddened areas, especially over bony prominences, because this can promote pressure injury formation.
- Minimize environmental factors that lead to skin drying such as low humidity (less than 40%) and exposure to cold. Depending on a patient's age and physical condition, maintain room temperature between 20° and 23°C (68° and 74°F). Infants, older adults, and acutely ill patients may need a warmer temperature. However, certain critically ill patients require cooler room temperatures to lower the metabolic demands of the body. Controlling drafts and eliminating lingering odors from draining wounds, vomitus, bedpans, or urinals also improve a patient's comfort.
- Use bathing as a time to interact with and assess a patient. When giving a complete bath, perform a physical assessment of all body systems and discuss issues of concern for a patient.
- During bathing help patients through normal joint range-of-motion (ROM) exercises to promote circulation and joint integrity.
- For patients who tire easily, consider giving a partial versus complete bed bath.

There are two categories of baths: cleansing and therapeutic. Cleansing baths include the bed bath, tub bath, sponge bath at the sink, shower, and prepackaged disposable bed bath (Box 18.1). The type of cleansing bath to use depends on the assessment of a patient's physical capabilities and the degree of hygiene required. When a person is unable to perform personal care because of illness or disability, you are responsible for helping with bathing. You can also clean and groom hair, shave a patient, and clean the nails during or immediately after a bath.

Health care providers generally order therapeutic baths for a specific effect such as soothing the skin or promoting the healing process. Types of therapeutic baths include the following:

BOX 18.1

Types of Baths

- **Complete bed bath:** Bath administered to totally dependent patient in bed.
- **Partial bed bath:** Bed bath that consists of bathing only body parts that would cause discomfort if left unbathed such as the hands, face, axilla, and perineal area. Partial bath also includes washing back and providing back rub. Dependent patients in need of partial hygiene or self-sufficient bedridden patients who are unable to reach all body parts receive a partial bed bath.
- **Sponge bath at the sink:** Involves bathing from a bath basin or sink with patient sitting in a chair. Patient is able to perform part of the bath independently. Nurse helps with hard-to-reach areas.
- **Tub bath:** Involves immersion in a tub of water that allows more thorough washing and rinsing than a bed bath. Patients may require nurse's help. Some agencies have tubs equipped with lifting devices that facilitate positioning dependent patients in the tub.
- **Shower:** Patient sits or stands under a continuous stream of water. The shower provides more thorough cleaning than a bed bath but can be tiring.
- **Disposable bed bath/travel bath:** The bag bath contains several soft, nonwoven cotton cloths that are premoistened in a solution of no-rinse surfactant cleaner and emollient. The bag bath offers an alternative because of the ease of use, reduced time bathing, and patient comfort (Meiner, 2010).

- *Sitz bath:* Cleans and reduces pain and inflammation of perineal and anal areas. It is used for patients who have undergone rectal or perineal surgery or childbirth or who have local irritation from hemorrhoids or fissures. A patient sits in a special tub or basin (see Chapter 42).
- *Medicated bath (addition of over-the-counter, herbal, or health care provider–ordered ingredient to bath):* Relieves skin irritation and creates an antibacterial and drying effect.

Perineal care (see Procedural Guideline 18.1) involves thorough cleaning of a patient's external genitalia and surrounding skin. A patient routinely receives perineal care during a bath. However, patients at risk for acquiring an infection need more frequent perineal care such as those who have incontinence-associated dermatitis (IAD), indwelling Foley catheter, or who are postpartum or recovering from rectal or genital surgery.

Delegation and Collaboration

Assessment of the patient's skin, pain level, and ROM cannot be delegated to nursing assistive personnel (NAP). The skill of bathing can be delegated to NAP. The nurse instructs the NAP about:

- Not massaging reddened skin areas during bathing.
- Contraindications to soaking a patient's feet.
- Reporting any signs of impaired skin integrity to the nurse.

- Proper ways to position male and female patients with musculo-skeletal limitations or an indwelling Foley catheter or other equipment (e.g., intravenous [IV] tubing).

Equipment

- Washcloths and bath towels
- Bath blanket
- Bar or liquid soap, or 4-oz bottle of 4% chlorhexidine gluconate (CHG) (dispensed in a single bath-size bottle)

- Toiletry items (deodorant, lotion)
- Disposable wipes
- Warm water
- Clean hospital gown or patient's own pajamas or gown
- Laundry bag
- Clean gloves
- Washbasin
- Eye patch/shield and nonallergenic tape (for unconscious patient)

STEP	RATIONALE

ASSESSMENT

STEP	RATIONALE
1. Identify patient using at least two identifiers (e.g., name and birthday or name and medical record number) according to agency policy.	Ensures patient safety. Complies with The Joint Commission standards and improves patient safety (TJC, 2016).
2. Perform hand hygiene. Assess room environment for safety (e.g., check room for spills; make sure that equipment is working properly and that bed is in locked, low position).	Reduces transmission of microorganisms. Identifies safety hazards in patient environment that could cause or potentially lead to harm (QSEN, 2014).
3. Assess patient's fall risk status (if partial bathing out of bed or self-bath is to be performed) (see Chapter 14).	Allows you to anticipate needed precautions such as having patient sit on chair in front of basin.
4. Assess patient's tolerance for bathing: activity tolerance, comfort level, musculoskeletal function, and presence of shortness of breath.	Determines patient's ability to perform or tolerate bathing and type of bath to administer (e.g., tub bath, bed bath).
5. Assess patient's cognitive (Mini-Mental State Examination) and functional status (e.g., Barthel's index or the index of activities of daily living [ADLs] [AHRQ, 2013a] to measure self-care ability). For patients with suspected dementia, observe behavior especially after telling patient it is bath time; does he or she become agitated?	Every person entering a long-term care setting should be formally assessed for cognitive and functional status (AHRQ, 2013a). Functional status assesses a patient's capacity for self-bathing and how much supervision/help is needed to accomplish daily ADL tasks. Every attempt should be made to avoid bathing people against their will (AHRQ, 2013a)

Clinical Decision Point *Patients with dementia may become agitated. Observe for behaviors such as restlessness, yelling, and fighting with caregivers.*

STEP	RATIONALE
6. Assess patient's visual status, ability to sit without support, hand grasp, ROM of extremities (see Chapter 6).	Further determines degree of help needed for bathing.
7. Assess for presence and position of external medical device/equipment (e.g., IV line or oxygen tubing).	Affects how you will position patient and plan bathing activities.
8. Assess patient's bathing preferences (AHRQ, 2013a): How often does the person bathe? What time of day? Is there anything in the past that might affect frequency of bathing (such as growing up without indoor plumbing)? How does the person bathe now (tub, shower, at sink, only with prompting)? Does the person use any special products, robes, towels, or equipment during bathing (e.g., scented soaps, music, back brush, or sponge) to make the experience more enjoyable? Is the person especially modest?	Allows patient to participate in plan of care. Promotes patient's comfort and willingness to cooperate. Using a patient's established routine may reduce agitation in a patient with dementia.
9. Ask if patient has noticed any problems related to condition of skin and genitalia.	Provides information to direct physical assessment of skin and genitalia during bathing. Also influences selection of skin-care products.
10. Before or during bath, assess condition of patient's skin. Note presence of dryness, indicated by flaking, redness, scaling, and cracking or excessive moisture, inflammation, or pressure injuries (see Chapter 39).	Provides baseline for comparison of skin integrity over time.
11. Identify risks for skin impairment: older age, immobilization, reduced sensation, nutrition and hydration, excess skin moisture or drainage, shear or friction on skin, vascular insufficiencies, presence of external devices. *Option:* Use a pressure injury assessment tool (e.g., Braden Scale; see Chapter 39).	Risk factors increase the likelihood of injury to the skin because of pressure, impaired tissue synthesis, softening of or friction on tissues, and impaired circulation.

STEP	RATIONALE
12. Assess patient's comfort on a 0-to-10 pain scale.	Bath can soothe and comfort patient. Provides baseline measure.
13. Assess patient's knowledge and perceptions of the importance of skin hygiene, preventive measures to take, and common skin problems encountered (see Table 18.1).	Determines patient's willingness to learn and type of instruction required.
14. Review medical record for orders for specific precautions concerning patient's movement or positioning and whether there is an order for a therapeutic bath. Note and confirm with patient any allergies or sensitivities to bath products.	Prevents accidental injury to patient during bathing activities. Determines level of help that patient needs. Prevents allergic reactions to hygiene products during bathing.

NURSING DIAGNOSES

- Activity intolerance
- Bathing/self-care deficit
- Deficient knowledge regarding skin care
- Impaired physical mobility
- Impaired skin integrity
- Risk for impaired skin integrity
- Risk for infection

Related factors are individualized based on patient's condition or needs.

PLANNING

1. Expected outcomes following completion of procedure:	
• Skin is free of excretions, drainage, or odor.	Skin is clean.
• Skin shows decreased redness, cracking, flaking, and scaling.	Indicates reduction in skin dryness.
• Joint ROM remains same or improves from previous measurement.	Repeated ROM exercise during bathing helps prevent contractures and promotes joint movement.
• Patient expresses sense of comfort and relaxation.	Bath relaxes patient and removes sources of discomfort.
• Patient tolerates bath without fatigue or chilling.	Fatigue during bathing indicates worsening of chronic cardiopulmonary conditions.
• Patient describes benefits and techniques of proper hygiene and skin care.	Demonstrates learning with ability to repeat back to demonstrate understanding.
2. Explain procedure and ask patient for suggestions on how to prepare supplies. If partial bath, ask how much of bath patient wishes to complete.	Promotes patient's cooperation, participation, and promotion of self-care as appropriate.
3. Adjust room temperature and ventilation, close room doors and windows, and draw room divider curtain.	Warm room that is free of drafts prevents rapid loss of body heat during bathing. Privacy provides for patient's mental and physical comfort.
4. Prepare equipment and place supplies on bedside table. If it is necessary to leave room, be sure that call light is within patient's reach, bed is in low position, and wheels are locked.	Avoids interrupting procedure or leaving patient unattended to retrieve missing equipment. Provides for patient safety.

Clinical Decision Point *Never leave the bedside without ensuring that appropriate number of side rails have been raised (see agency policy). The number of side rails depends on the patient's fall risk assessment; however, having all side rails raised is considered a restraint.*

IMPLEMENTATION

1. Offer patient bedpan or urinal. Apply clean gloves to help patient as needed. Provide toilet tissue and dispose of any excrement properly. Dispose of gloves if applied and perform hand hygiene. Provide patient towel and moist washcloth.	Patient feels more comfortable after voiding. Prevents interruption of bath.
2. Perform hand hygiene. If patient has nonintact skin or skin is soiled with drainage, excretions, or body secretions, apply new pair of clean gloves before beginning bath.	Reduces transmission of microorganisms.
3. Raise bed to comfortable working height. Lower side rail closest to you and help patient assume comfortable supine position, maintaining body alignment. Bring patient toward side closest to you (staying supine).	Aids access to patient. Maintains patient's comfort throughout procedure. Uses proper body mechanics, thus minimizing strain on back muscles. If patient is overweight, use other caregiver or lift device for positioning (see Chapter 11).

STEP	RATIONALE

4. Place bath blanket over patient. Have patient hold top of bath blanket and remove top sheet from under bath blanket without exposing patient. Place soiled linen in laundry bag.

Blanket provides warmth and privacy.
Take care to avoid linen contacting uniform.

5. Remove patient's gown or pajamas.

Provides full exposure of body parts during bathing.

   a. If gown has snaps on sleeves, simply unsnap and remove gown without pulling IV tubing (if present).

   b. If gown has no snaps and if an extremity is *injured* or has reduced mobility, begin removal from *unaffected* side first.

Undressing unaffected side first allows easier manipulation of gown over body part with reduced ROM.

   c. If patient has an IV line and gown with no snaps, remove gown from arm *without* IV line first. Then remove gown from arm with IV line (see illustration). Pause IV fluid infusion by pressing appropriate sensor on IV pump. Remove IV tubing from pump; use regulator to slow IV infusion. Remove IV bag from pole (see illustration) and slide IV bag and tubing through arm of patient's gown (see illustration). Rehang IV bag (see illustration), reconnect tubing to pump, open regulator clamp, and restart IV fluid infusion by pressing appropriate sensor on IV pump. If IV fluids are infusing by gravity, check IV flow rate and regulate if necessary. *Do not disconnect IV tubing to remove gown.*

Manipulation of IV tubing and bag can disrupt IV infusion flow rate.

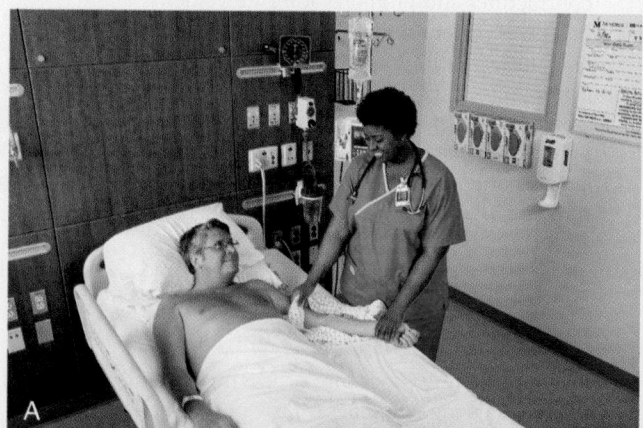
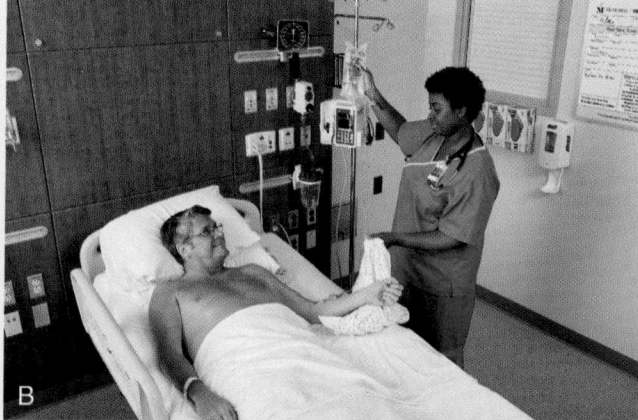
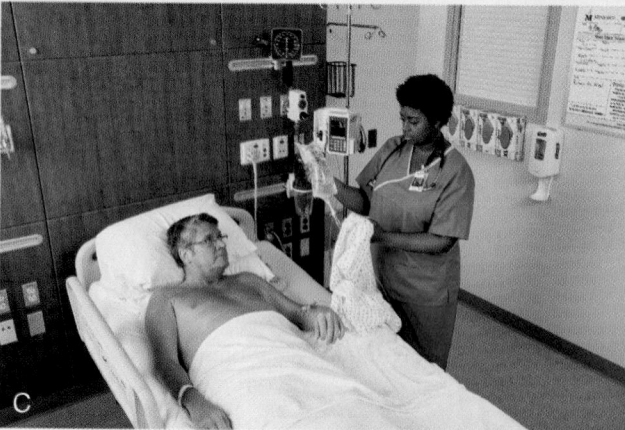
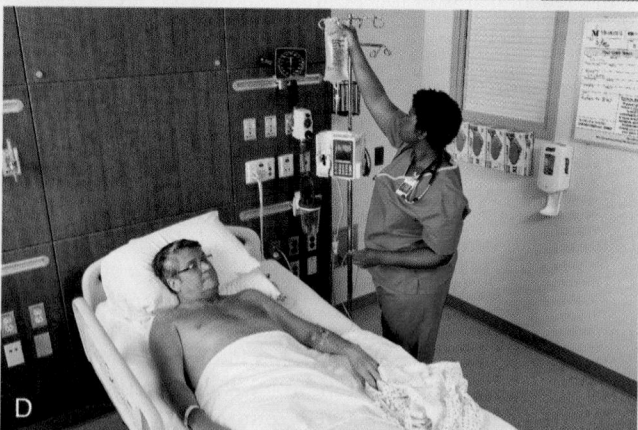

STEP 5c A, Remove patient's gown. **B,** Remove IV bag from pole. **C,** Slide IV tubing and bag through arm of patient's gown. **D,** Rehang IV bag.

STEP	RATIONALE

6. Raise side rail. Lower bed temporarily to lowest position and raise on return after you fill wash basin two-thirds full with warm water. Place basin along with supplies on over-bed table and position over patient's bed. Check water temperature and have patient place fingers in water.

Raising side rail and lowering bed maintains patient's safety. Warm water promotes comfort, relaxes muscles, and prevents unnecessary chilling. Use of over-bed table allows you to move to opposite side of bed without having to move equipment. Tests water temperature to prevent burns to skin.

7. Lower side rail. Remove pillow (if tolerated). Raise head of bed 30 to 45 degrees if allowed. Place bath towel under patient's head. Place second bath towel over patient's chest.

Removal of pillow makes it easier to wash patient's ears and neck. Placement of towels prevents soiling of bed linen and bath blanket.

8. Wash face.

Clinical Decision Point *Do not use bath water with 4% liquid CHG added or 2% CHG bathing cloths (see Procedural Guideline 18.2) on the eyes or face (AHRQ, 2013b).*

a. Inquire if patient is wearing contact lenses. You may choose to remove at this time.

Prevents accidental injury to eyes.

b. Form a mitt with washcloth (see illustration); immerse in water and wring thoroughly.

Mitt retains water and heat better than loosely held washcloth; keeps cold edges from brushing against patient and prevents splashing.

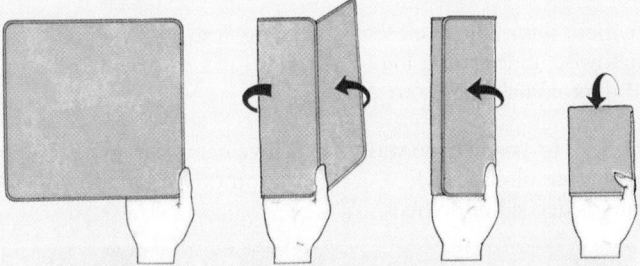

STEP 8b Steps for folding washcloth to form a mitt.

c. Wash patient's eyes with plain warm water, using a clean area of cloth for each eye and bathing from inner to outer canthus (see illustrations). Soak any crusts on eyelid for 2 to 3 minutes with warm, damp cloth before attempting removal. Dry around eyes thoroughly but gently.

Soap irritates eyes. Use of separate sections of mitt reduces infection transmission. Bathing eye gently from inner to outer canthus prevents secretions from entering nasolacrimal duct. Pressure causes internal injury.

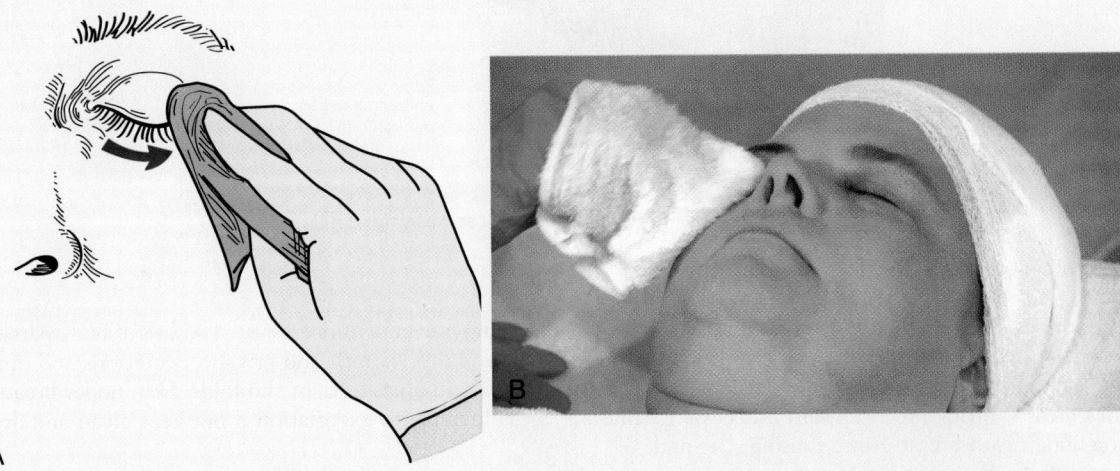

STEP 8c Wash eye from inner to outer canthus. **A,** Direction for cleaning eye. **B,** Washing eye from inner to outer canthus.

STEP	RATIONALE
d. Ask if patient prefers to use soap on face. Otherwise wash, rinse, and dry forehead, cheeks, nose, neck, and ears without using soap. Ask men if they want to be shaved (see Procedural Guideline 18.4).	Soap tends to dry face, which is exposed to air more than other body parts.
e. Provide eye care for unconscious patient.	Patients who are unconscious have lost the normal protective corneal reflex of blinking, increasing the risk for corneal drying, abrasions, and eye infection.
(1) Instill eyedrops or ointment per health care provider's order (see Chapter 19).	
(2) In the absence of blink reflex, keep eyelids closed. Close eye gently, using back of your fingertip, before placing eye patch or shield. Place tape over patch or shield. Do not tape eyelid.	When blink reflex is absent, patient loses a protective mechanism. Keeping eyelids closed maintains eye moisture and prevents injury.
9. Wash upper extremities and trunk. *Option:* Change bath water at this time. Obtain new 6-quart basin and mix contents of a 4-ounce bottle of 4% CHG with warm water (Petlin et al., 2014).	Evidence shows that CHG use in daily bathing can reduce incidence of hospital-acquired infections (Petlin et al., 2014; Shah et al., 2016). CHG reduces bacteria for up to 24 hours and prevents infection (AHRQ, 2013b).

Clinical Decision Point *When using CHG 4% in a bath basin of water, use one washcloth for washing each major body part. Then dispose of cloth and use a new cloth for the next body part (Petlin et al., 2014). Dipping cloth back into basin contaminates solution and makes CHG less effective. Do not rinse after bathing with CHG solution. Allow CHG to dry on the skin to achieve antimicrobial effects.*

STEP	RATIONALE
a. Remove bath blanket from patient's arm that is closest to you. Place bath towel lengthwise under arm using long, firm strokes from distal to proximal (fingers to axilla).	Long, firm strokes promote venous return.
b. Raise and support arm above head (if possible) to wash axilla, rinse, and dry thoroughly (see illustration). Apply deodorant to underarms as needed or desired.	Movement of arm exposes axilla and exercises normal ROM of joint. Deodorant controls body odor.

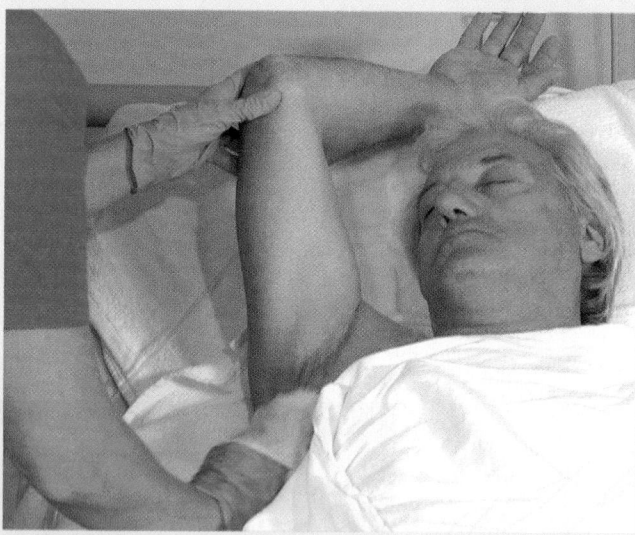

STEP 9b Position of patient's arm for washing axilla.

STEP	RATIONALE
c. Move to other side of bed and repeat steps with other arm.	
d. Cover patient's chest with bath towel and fold bath blanket down to umbilicus. Bathe chest with long, firm strokes. Take special care with skin under female patient's breasts, lifting breast upward if necessary while bathing underneath breast. Rinse if using soap and water and dry well.	Draping prevents unnecessary exposure of body parts. Towel maintains warmth and privacy. Secretions and dirt collect easily in areas of tight skinfolds. Skin under breasts is vulnerable to excoriation if not kept clean and dry.

STEP	RATIONALE

10. Wash hands and nails.

  a. Fold bath towel in half and lay it on bed beside patient. Place basin on towel. Immerse patient's hand in water. Allow hand to soak for 3 to 5 minutes before cleaning fingernails (see Skill 18.4). **NOTE:** Do not soak fingers of patient with diabetes mellitus. Remove basin and dry hand well. Repeat for other hand.

Soaking softens cuticles and calluses of hand, loosens debris beneath nails, and enhances feeling of cleanliness. Thorough drying removes moisture from between fingers. Soaking hands of patient with diabetes mellitus can lead to maceration and risk for infection.

11. Check temperature of bath water and change water if necessary; otherwise continue.

Warm water maintains patient's comfort.

Clinical Decision Point *If using CHG solution in bath water, do not discard water. One bottle of CHG soap is sufficient for a complete bath.*

12. Wash abdomen.

  a. Place bath towel lengthwise over chest and abdomen. (You may need two towels.) Fold bath blanket down to just above pubic region. Bathe, rinse, and dry abdomen with special attention to umbilicus and skinfolds of abdomen and groin. Keep abdomen covered between washing and rinsing. Dry well.

Keeping skinfolds clean and dry helps prevent odor and skin irritation. Moisture and sediment that collects in skinfolds predispose skin to maceration.

  b. Apply clean gown or pajama top by dressing affected side first. *Option:* You may omit this step until completion of bath.

Maintains patient's warmth and comfort. Allows easier manipulation of gown over body part with reduced ROM.

Clinical Decision Point *If one extremity is injured or immobilized, always dress affected side first.*

13. Wash lower extremities.

  a. Cover chest and abdomen with top of bath blanket. Expose near leg by folding blanket toward midline. Be sure that other leg and perineum remain draped. Place bath towel under leg as you support patient's knee and ankle.

Prevents overexposure. Method of placement supports patient's joint.

  b. Wash leg using long, firm strokes from ankle to knee and knee to thigh (see illustration). Assess condition of extremities.

Promotes circulation and venous return. Assessment is key to identifying signs and symptoms of venous thrombosis.

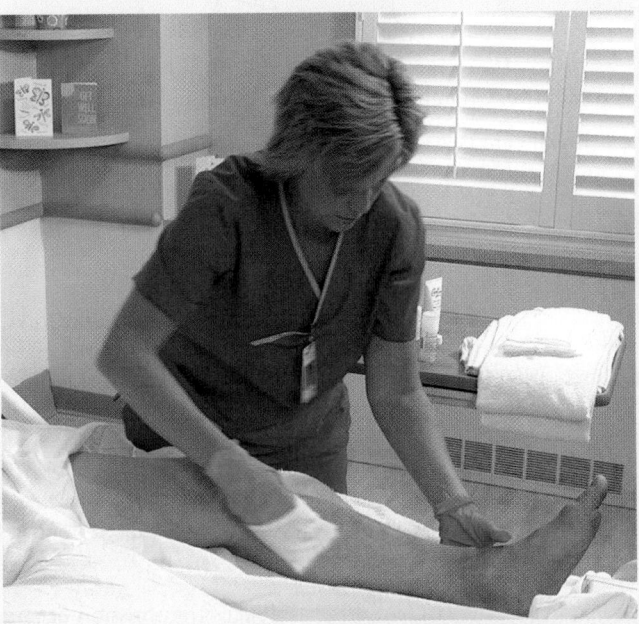

STEP 13b Washing patient's leg.

Clinical Decision Point *During the bath assess for signs of warmth, redness, swelling, tenderness, and pain in the lower extremities because these might be early signs of deep vein thrombosis (DVT).*

STEP	RATIONALE

   c. Clean foot, making sure to bathe between toes. Clean and file nails as needed (check agency policy) (see Skill 18.4). Dry toes and feet completely.

Secretions and moisture are often present between toes, predisposing patient to maceration and skin breakdown.

   d. Raise side rail; remove towel; move to opposite side of bed, lower side rail, place dry towel under second leg, and repeat steps 13b and c for other leg and foot. Apply light layer of moisturizing lotion to both feet. When finished, remove used towel.

Moisturizers are effective in reducing dry skin; however, in excess they can cause maceration.

   e. Cover patient with bath blanket, raise side rail, and change bath water (if using plain soap and water).

Decreased bath water temperature causes chilling. Clean water reduces microorganism transmission.

14. Wash back.

   a. Apply clean gloves (if not already applied). Lower side rail. Help patient assume prone or side-lying position, using safe patient-handling techniques (see Chapter 11) (as applicable). Place towel lengthwise along patient's side.

Exposes back and buttocks for bathing.

   b. If fecal material is present, enclose in fold of underpad or toilet tissue and remove with disposable wipes.

Skinfolds near buttocks and anus may contain fecal secretions and microorganisms.

   c. Keep patient draped by sliding bath blanket over shoulders and thighs during bathing. Wash, rinse, and dry back from neck to buttocks with long, firm strokes. Pay special attention to folds of buttocks and anus.

Maintains warmth and prevents unnecessary exposure.

   d. Clean buttocks and anus, washing front to back (see illustration). Clean, rinse, and dry area thoroughly. If needed, place clean, absorbent pad under patient's buttocks.

Cleaning buttocks after back prevents contamination of water.

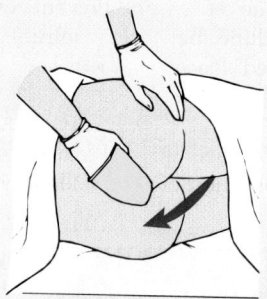

STEP 14d Clean buttocks and anus, washing front to back.

15. While patient is supine, provide perineal care (see Procedural Guideline 18.1).

Clinical Decision Point *At end of bath, if you have used 4% CHG solution, skin may feel sticky for a few minutes. Do NOT wipe off. Allow to air dry (AHRQ, 2013b).*

16. Massage back if patient desires.

Promotes patient relaxation.

17. Apply body lotion to skin and topical moisturizing agents to dry, flaky, reddened, or scaling areas. **NOTE:** If using CHG solution for bathing, only use a product compatible with CHG (AHRQ, 2013b).

Dry skin results in reduced pliability and cracking. Moisturizers help to prevent skin breakdown.

Clinical Decision Point *Massage is contraindicated in the presence of acute inflammation and where there is the possibility of damaged blood vessels or fragile skin (NPUAP, 2014). Massage of the legs is also contraindicated because of the possible presence of a blood clot, which could become dislodged.*

18. Remove and dispose of gloves and perform hand hygiene before helping patient complete grooming (e.g., combing hair, shaving).

Reduces transmission of microorganisms. Promotes patient's body image.

19. Check function and position of external devices (e.g., indwelling catheters, nasogastric tubes, IV tubes, braces).

Ensures that bathing activities did not disrupt systems.

STEP	RATIONALE
20. Replace top bed linen by pulling sheet and bedspread from foot of bed to cover patient before removing bath blanket. Apply gloves if linen is soiled. *Option:* Make occupied bed at this time (see Procedural Guideline 18.6).	Maintains patient warmth and privacy.
21. Place bed in low, locked position and raise appropriate number of side rails so they do not restrain patient from exiting bed safely. Make sure that patient is in comfortable position with call light and personal possessions in reach.	Maintains patient safety. Reaching for call light or personal items can lead to a fall.
22. Disinfect/rinse and dry bed basin according to agency policy. This is especially important if using CHG solution. DO NOT use basin for CHG as storage container for supplies (Petlin et al., 2014).	Reduces transmission of microorganisms. Evidence has shown that basins are frequently contaminated with microbes, and some has found that bacteria grew in up to 98% of the basins (Johnson et al., 2009).
23. Perform hand hygiene and leave room.	Reduces transmission of microorganisms.

EVALUATION

1. Observe skin; pay particular attention to areas that were previously soiled, reddened, flaking, scaling, or cracking or that showed early signs of breakdown. Inspect areas normally exposed to pressure.

   Bathing should leave skin clean and clear. If there are signs of skin irritation (e.g., redness, blistering), take steps to reduce pressure.

2. Observe ROM during bathing.

   Measures joint mobility.

3. Ask patient to rate level of comfort (on a scale of 0 to 10).

   Determines changes in level of comfort during bathing.

4. Ask if patient feels tired (on a scale of 0 to 10).

   Measures tolerance to bathing activity.

5. **Use Teach-Back:** "I want to be sure I explained the importance of keeping your skin clean, especially while in the hospital. Tell me why we want to bathe you daily." Revise your instruction now or develop a plan for revised patient or family caregiver teaching if patient or family caregiver is not able to teach back correctly.

   Determines patient's and family caregiver's level of understanding of instructional topic.

Unexpected Outcomes	Related Interventions
1. Areas of excessive dryness, rashes, irritation, or pressure injury appear on skin.	• Review agency skin-care policy regarding special cleansing and moisturizing products. • If using CHG soap, it may become necessary to reduce frequency of bathing. Sensitivity to CHG is rare. • Limit frequency of complete baths. • Complete pressure injury assessment (see Chapter 39). • Institute turning and positioning measures to keep patient off pressure injury. • Obtain special bed surface if patient is at risk for skin breakdown. • Notify health care provider and/or obtain wound consultation.
2. Patient becomes excessively tired and unable to cooperate or participate in bathing.	• Reschedule bathing to a time when patient is more rested. • Patients with cardiopulmonary conditions and breathing difficulties require pillow or elevated head of bed during bathing. • Notify health care provider about changes in patient's fatigue level. • Perform hygiene measures in stages between scheduled rest periods.
3. Patient seems unusually restless or complains of discomfort.	• Use less stressful method of bathing such as a disposable bath (see Procedural Guideline 18.2). • Consider analgesia before bathing. • Schedule rest periods before bathing.

Recording and Reporting

- Record procedure, observations (e.g., breaks in skin, inflammation, or areas of pressure injury), level of patient participation, and how the patient tolerated procedure in nurses' notes in electronic health record (EHR) or chart.
- Report evidence of alterations in skin integrity, break in suture line, or increased wound secretions to nurse in charge or health care provider. Patient may require special skin care.
- Document your evaluation of patient and family caregiver learning.

Special Considerations
Teaching

- Teach patients how to inspect surfaces between skinfolds and explain the signs of irritation or breakdown. Use simple language.
- Consider the need to include a family caregiver in learning the bathing process. Plan for a return demonstration.

Pediatric

- Some adolescents require and/or prefer more frequent bathing as a result of more active sebaceous glands.
- Young adolescent girls should learn basic perineal hygiene measures and know why they are predisposed to urinary tract infections.

Gerontological

- Older adults with incontinence need meticulous skin care to reduce incontinence-associated dermatitis (IAD) and the risk of infection. The use of barrier creams is sometimes recommended to keep the skin intact and free from infections.

- If patients have signs of dementia, caregiver behavior, especially 5 seconds before a bath, may be considered by the patient to be an assault. Behaviors that trigger agitation include confrontational communication; invalidation of the patient's feelings; absence of personal restraint; touching feet, axilla, or perineal area; non–bath-related communications; and failing to prepare the resident for the bath (AHRQ, 2013a).
- When giving a patient with dementia a bath, follow these guidelines (AHRQ, 2013a):
  - Do not rush and speak in a low pleasant voice, giving information before and all through the bathing process.
  - If agitation occurs, use distraction; bring up a pleasant topic; or use other distraction such as music, singing, holding an object, or eating.
  - Concentrate on the person's feelings and reactions. Pay attention and do not converse with others.

Home Care

- Type of bath chosen depends on assessment of the home, availability of running water, and condition of bathing facilities.
- In the home set up equipment according to patient's established routines.
- Patients at risk for falls may benefit from the following:
  - Installation of grab bars in shower
  - Adhesive strips applied to shower or tub floor
  - Addition of a shower chair or placement of a chair or stool

Long-Term Care

- Tubs in long-term care settings frequently come equipped with electronic thermometers to measure water temperature. The tubs also have hydraulic lifts to help residents into the tub.

PROCEDURAL GUIDELINE 18.1 *Perineal Care*

Perineal care involves thorough cleaning of the patient's external genitalia and surrounding skin. A patient routinely receives perineal care during a complete bed bath (see Skill 18.1). However, patients who have fecal or urinary incontinence, an indwelling Foley catheter, or rectal or genital surgery may need more frequent perineal care. This is especially important for patients with indwelling Foley catheters in the effort to reduce catheter-associated urinary tract infection (CAUTI). Wear clean gloves during perineal care because of the risk of contact with infectious organisms present in fecal, urinary, or vaginal secretions. To avoid embarrassment, always act in a professional and sensitive manner and provide patient privacy at all times.

Delegation and Collaboration

The skill of perineal care can be delegated to nursing assistive personnel (NAP). The nurse instructs the NAP to:

- Avoid any physical restriction that affects proper positioning of patient.
- Properly position a patient with an indwelling Foley catheter.
- Inform the nurse of any perineal drainage, excoriation, or rash observed.

Equipment

- Washcloths, bath towels, and bath blanket
- Cleaning product for bath (chlorhexidine gluconate [CHG] cloths can be used for perineal and catheter care; however,

some agencies do not use CHG because of concern over risk of mucosal irritation (see agency policy)
- Disposable wipes and wash basin
- Warm water
- Laundry bag
- Waterproof pad or bedpan
- Clean gloves
- Additional supplies when perineal care is provided other than during a bath: cotton balls or swabs, solution bottle or container filled with warm water or prescribed rinsing solution, waterproof bag

Procedural Steps

1. Identify patient using at least two identifiers (e.g., name and birthday or name and medical record number), according to agency policy (TJC, 2016).
2. Assess environment for safety (e.g., check room for spills, make sure that equipment is working properly and that bed is in locked, low position).
3. Assemble supplies. Provide privacy and explain procedure and importance in preventing infection.
4. Perform hand hygiene. Apply clean gloves. Place basin with warm water and cleansing solution on over-bed table.
5. **Perineal care for a female:**
   a. If patient is able to maneuver and handle washcloth, allow to clean perineum on own.

PROCEDURAL GUIDELINE 18.1 *Perineal Care—cont'd*

b. Help patient assume dorsal recumbent position. Note restrictions or a limitation in patient's positioning. Position waterproof pad under patient's buttocks.

c. Drape patient with bath blanket placed in shape of a diamond.

d. Fold both outer corners of bath blanket up around patient's legs onto abdomen and under hip (see illustration). Lift lower tip of bath blanket when you are ready to expose the perineum.

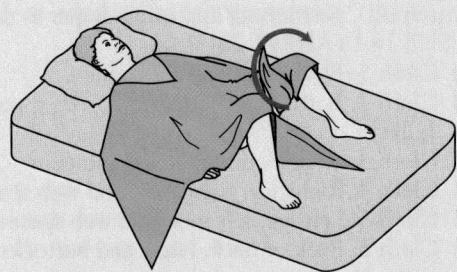

STEP 5d Drape patient for perineal care.

e. Wash and dry patient's upper thighs. (**NOTE:** If agency uses CHG solution for perineal care, do not rinse; allow to dry.)

f. Wash labia majora. Use nondominant hand to gently retract labia from thigh. Use dominant hand to wash carefully in skinfolds. Wipe in direction from perineum to rectum (front to back). Repeat on opposite side using separate section of washcloth or new washcloth. Rinse and dry area thoroughly.

g. Gently separate labia with nondominant hand to expose urethral meatus and vaginal orifice. With dominant hand wash downward from pubic area toward rectum in one smooth stroke (see illustration). Use separate section of cloth for each stroke. Clean thoroughly over labia minora, clitoris, and vaginal orifice. Avoid tension on indwelling catheter if present and clean area around it thoroughly.

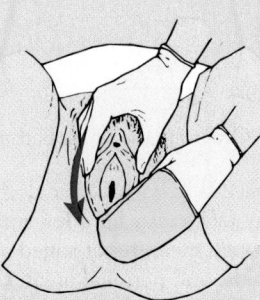

STEP 5g Clean from perineum to rectum (front to back).

h. Rinse and dry area thoroughly, using front-to-back method.

i. If patient uses bedpan, pour warm water over perineal area and dry thoroughly. (Exception: do not rinse if using CHG.)

j. Fold lower corner of bath blanket back between patient's legs and over perineum. Ask patient to lower legs and assume comfortable position.

6. Perineal care for a male:

a. If patient is able to maneuver and handle washcloth, allow him to clean perineum on his own.

b. Help patient to supine position. Note restriction in mobility.

c. Fold lower half of bath blanket up to expose upper thighs. Wash and dry thighs.

d. Cover thighs with bath towels. Raise bath blanket to expose genitalia. Gently raise penis and place bath towel underneath. Gently grasp shaft of penis. If patient is uncircumcised, retract foreskin. If patient has an erection, defer procedure until later.

e. Wash tip of penis at urethral meatus first. Using circular motion, clean from meatus outward (see illustration). Discard washcloth and repeat with clean cloth until penis is clean. Rinse and dry gently and thoroughly. (Exception: do not rinse if using CHG.)

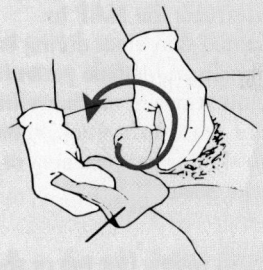

STEP 6e Use circular motion to clean tip of penis.

f. Return foreskin to its natural position.

Clinical Decision Point *After administering male perineal care for uncircumcised males, make sure that foreskin is in its natural position. This is extremely important in patients with decreased sensation in their lower extremities. Tightening foreskin around shaft of penis causes local edema; discomfort; and, if not corrected, may cause permanent urethral damage.*

g. Take a new washcloth and gently clean shaft of penis and scrotum by having patient abduct legs. Pay special attention to underlying surface of penis. Lift scrotum carefully and wash underlying skinfolds. Rinse and dry thoroughly. (Exception: do not rinse if using CHG.)

h. Fold bath blanket back over patient's perineum and help him to comfortable position.

7. For both female and male patient, avoid placing tension on an indwelling catheter, if present, and clean around it thoroughly during procedure.

8. Observe perineal area for any irritation, redness, or drainage that persists after perineal hygiene.

9. Dispose of gloves and used supplies in proper receptacles and perform hand hygiene.

10. Use Teach-Back: "We talked about how to wash your genital area to reduce the chance of infection. Describe for me how to wash your genital area." Revise your instruction now or develop a plan for revised patient or family caregiver teaching if patient or family caregiver is not able to teach back correctly.

PROCEDURAL GUIDELINE 18.2 *Use of Disposable Bed Bath, Tub, or Shower*

The use of disposable washcloths impregnated with an antiseptic solution such as chlorhexidine gluconate (CHG) is more common now in acute care hospitals, especially critical care settings. However, the cloths can be used in any setting. CHG cloths should be used for all bathing purposes, including once-a-day full-body bathing, incontinence care, or any other reasons for additional cleaning (AHRQ, 2013b). CHG replaces soap and water baths; thus the cloths should not be used as a "top coat" after bathing. Rather, CHG cloths clean and remove bacteria, and the antiseptic binds to the skin for persistent antibacterial activity lasting 24 hours (AHRQ, 2013b).

Although showers are available to patients in acute care, you will see tub and shower bathing more commonly in long-term care settings. When patients use a tub or shower, follow guidelines to maintain patient safety to prevent falls.

Delegation and Collaboration
The skill of bathing in a tub or shower or using disposable cloths for bathing can be delegated to nursing assistive personnel (NAP). The nurse instructs the NAP to:
- Not massage reddened skin areas during bathing.
- Properly position male and female patients with musculoskeletal limitations or an indwelling Foley catheter or other equipment (e.g., intravenous tubing).
- Report changes in skin or perineal area or signs of impaired skin integrity to the nurse.

Equipment
- Washcloths and bath towels (for tub or shower), bath blanket, cleaning product, toiletry items (deodorant, lotion), disposable wipes, clean hospital gown or patient's own pajamas or gown, laundry bag
- Prepackaged, disposable bathing cloths
- Clean gloves

Procedural Steps
1. Identify patient using at least two identifiers (e.g., name and birthday or name and medical record number) according to agency policy (TJC, 2016).
2. Assess environment for safety (e.g., check room for spills; make sure that equipment is working properly and that bed is in locked, low position) and provide privacy.
3. Assess degree of help patient will need for bathing, risk for falling (e.g., ability to stand, get into a tub), patient's risk for skin breakdown, and presence of allergy or sensitivity to bathing solution (e.g., CHG) (see Skill 18.1).
4. Perform hand hygiene and apply clean gloves.
5. Arrange supplies and toiletry items at bedside if using bathing cloths; otherwise prepare supplies and equipment in patient's bathroom or a shower room.
6. **Bathing cloths:** (This procedure follows the AHRQ [2013b] universal bathing protocol for decolonization, used commonly in critical care and acute care hospitals.)
   a. Adjust room temperature and ventilation, close room doors and windows, and draw room divider curtain.
   b. Position patient supine or in a position of comfort. Use a bath blanket to drape areas of body not being cleaned as bath proceeds (see Skill 18.1).
   c. Help patient remove old gown (see Skill 18.1).
   d. *Option:* Warm package of bathing cloths in a microwave, following package directions. Do not use a

microwave that is used for food preparation. The cleaning pack contains six premoistened cloths.

Clinical Decision Point *Check temperature of cloth after warming and have patient check as well to prevent burns to the skin.*

   e. Wash patient's face and eyes with plain warm water (see Skill 18.1).
   f. Use all six bathing cloths in the following order (see illustration), positioning and using drapes as described in Skill 18.1 (AHRQ, 2013b):
   (1) Cloth 1: Neck, shoulders, and chest
   (2) Cloth 2: Both arms, both hands, web spaces, and axilla
   (3) Cloth 3: Abdomen and groin/perineum
   (4) Cloth 4: Right leg, right foot, and web spaces
   (5) Cloth 5: Left leg, left foot, and web spaces
   (6) Cloth 6: Back of neck, back, and buttocks.

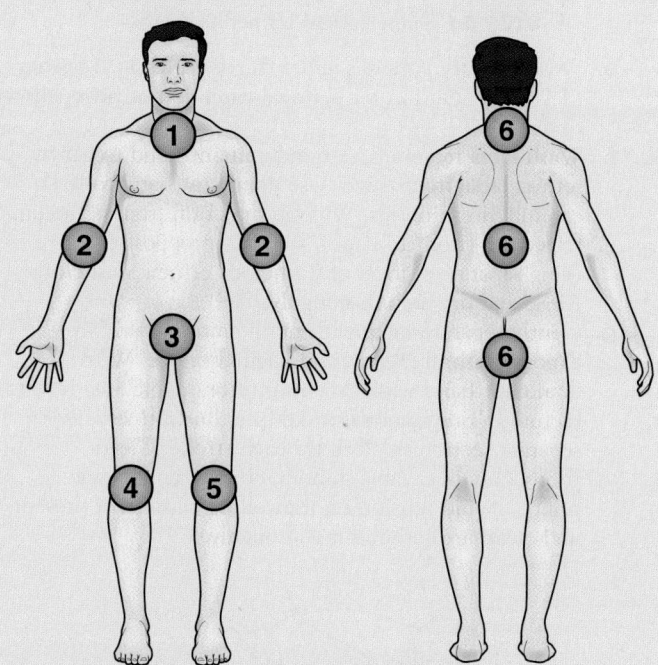

STEP 6f Order for use of six bathing cloths.

   g. Firmly massage skin with CHG cloth. Tell patient that the skin may feel sticky for a few minutes.
   h. Ensure thorough cleaning of soiled areas such as the neck, skinfolds, and perineal areas. CHG is safe to use on perineal areas, including external mucosa. It is also safe for superficial wounds, including stage 1 and stage 2 decubitus pressure injuries (AHRQ, 2013b).
   i. Do NOT rinse, wipe off, or dry with another cloth. Allow to air dry (AHRQ, 2013b).
   j. CHG cloths have built-in moisturizers. Skin may feel sticky for a few minutes.
   k. If additional moisturizer is needed, use only CHG-compatible products.
   l. Dispose of leftover cloths, help patient to comfortable position, and assist in applying clean gown.

PROCEDURAL GUIDELINE 18.2 *Use of Disposable Bed Bath, Tub, or Shower—cont'd*

7. Tub bath or shower:

  a. Assess patient's fall risk status; consider patient's physical ability to stand, get into tub, and review orders for precautions concerning his or her movement or positioning. A health care provider's order usually is needed for tub bath or shower.

  b. Schedule use of shower or tub.

  c. Check tub or shower for cleanliness. Use cleaning techniques outlined in agency policy. Place rubber mat on tub or shower bottom. Place skid-proof disposable bath mat or towel on floor in front of tub or shower.

  d. Place hygiene and toiletry items within easy reach of tub or shower.

  e. Help patient to bathroom if necessary. Have him or her wear robe and skid-proof slippers to bathroom.

  f. Demonstrate how to use call signal for help. Place "occupied" sign on bathroom door. Close door.

  g. Fill bathtub halfway with warm water. Check temperature of bath water, have patient test it, and adjust it if it is too warm or too cold. Explain which faucet controls hot water.

Clinical Decision Point *Do not use bath oil in tub water because this can cause slipping and resultant fall.*

  h. If patient is taking shower, turn shower on and adjust water temperature before he or she enters shower stall. Use shower seat or tub chair if available (see illustration).

  i. Tell patient that you will not allow him or her to remain in tub longer than 20 minutes. Check on patient every 5 minutes. Remove and dispose of gloves; perform hand hygiene.

  j. Apply clean gloves. Return to bathroom when patient signals and knock before entering.

  k. For patient who is unsteady, drain tub of water before he or she attempts to get out. Place bath towel over patient's shoulders. Help him or her get out of tub as needed and help with drying. If possible, have a shower chair available for patient to sit.

  l. Help patient as needed to don clean gown or pajamas, slippers, and robe. (In home, extended care, or rehabilitation setting, encourage patient to wear regular clothing.)

  m. Help patient to room and to comfortable position in bed or chair. Leave call light in reach.

  n. Clean tub or shower according to agency policy. Remove soiled linen and place in dirty laundry bag. Discard disposable equipment in proper receptacle. Place "unoccupied" sign on bathroom door. Return supplies to storage area.

  o. Remove and dispose of gloves. Perform hand hygiene.

8. Evaluate condition of patient's skin. Pay attention to areas that were previously soiled, reddened, flaking, scaling, or showing signs of breakdown.

9. Ask patient to rate level of fatigue and comfort

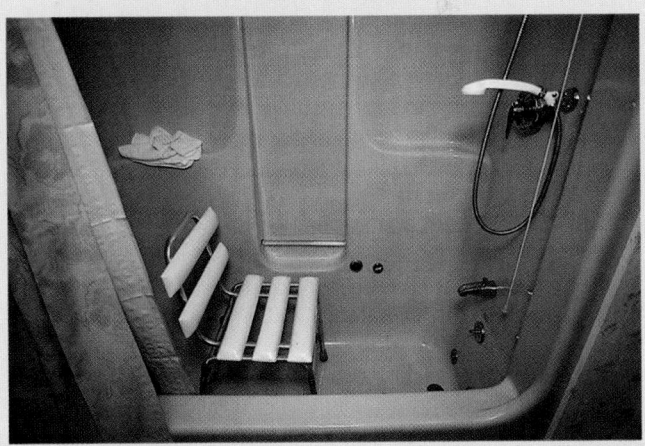

STEP 7h Shower seat for patient safety.

◆ SKILL 18.2   Oral Hygiene

Maintenance of daily oral hygiene, including brushing, flossing, and rinsing, is essential for the prevention and control of plaque-associated oral diseases. In addition to preventing inflammation and infection, oral hygiene in general promotes comfort, ease of swallowing for better food intake, and verbal communication. Brushing cleans the teeth of food particles, plaque (the cause of dental caries), and bacteria; massages the gums; and relieves discomfort from unpleasant odors and tastes. Flossing removes tartar that collects at the gum line. Rinsing removes dislodged food particles and excess toothpaste.

When a patient becomes ill, many factors influence the need for oral hygiene. Offer oral hygiene help as required, from preparing needed supplies to actually brushing a patient's teeth. Plan the frequency of care on the basis of a patient's clinical condition and the condition of his or her oral cavity. For example, a stroke patient who has difficulty swallowing may require care as often as every 4 hours; a patient on a ventilator will require special care to reduce the chances of developing ventilator-associated pneumonia (VAP) (see Skill 18.3).

In addition to recommendations for the general population, there are oral-care regimens designed to relieve discomfort and facilitate healing of chemotherapy- and radiation therapy–related mucositis, stomatitis, and xerostomia. These types of oral lesions are very painful and interfere with a patient's nutrition. Specific regimens are discussed later in this chapter.

Delegation and Collaboration

The skill of oral hygiene (including toothbrushing, flossing, and rinsing) can be delegated to nursing assistive personnel (NAP). However, the nurse is responsible for assessing the patient's gag reflex to determine if the patient is at risk for aspiration. The nurse instructs the NAP about:

- Types of changes in oral mucosa (e.g., presence of lesions or open areas) for which to observe and report to the nurse.

- Reporting patient's complaints of pain or occurrence of bleeding during oral care.
- Being aware of special precautions such as aspiration precautions, including:
  - Keeping head of bed (HOB) raised 30 to 45 degrees (not lower).
  - Explaining need to report excessive coughing or choking during procedure.
- Not flossing when a patient has a bleeding tendency.

Equipment

- Soft-bristled toothbrush (hard toothbrush damages enamel and gums)
- Nonabrasive fluoride toothpaste or dentifrice
- Dental floss
- Chlorhexidine gluconate (CHG) 0.12% (optional, see agency policy)
- Tongue depressor
- Penlight
- Water glass with cool water, straw
- Normal saline or an essential oil-antiseptic mouth rinse (optional)
- Emesis basin
- Bath towels to place over patient's chest; paper towels
- Clean gloves
- *Option:* Moisturizing lubricant for lips

STEP	RATIONALE

ASSESSMENT

STEP	RATIONALE
1. Identify patient using at least two identifiers (e.g., name and birthday or name and medical record number) according to agency policy.	Ensures patient safety. Complies with The Joint Commission standards and improves patient safety (TJC, 2016).
2. Assess environment for safety (e.g., check room for spills; make sure that equipment is working properly and that bed is in locked, low position.	Identifies safety hazards in patient environment that could cause or potentially lead to harm (QSEN, 2014).
3. Perform hand hygiene and apply clean gloves.	Reduces transmission of microorganisms in blood or saliva.
4. Instruct patient not to bite down during assessment of oral cavity. Using a penlight and tongue depressor, inspect integrity of lips, teeth, buccal mucosa, gums, palate, and tongue (see Chapter 6).	Determines status of patient's oral cavity and extent of need for oral hygiene. Provides baseline to determine change after hygiene.
5. Identify presence of common oral problems.	Helps determine type of hygiene and information that patient requires for self-care.
a. *Dental caries:* Chalky-white discoloration of tooth or presence of brown or black discoloration	
b. *Gingivitis:* Inflammation of gums	May indicate periodontal disease.
c. *Periodontitis:* Receding gum lines, inflammation, gaps between teeth	May indicate periodontal disease.
d. *Halitosis:* Bad breath	May indicate periodontal disease.
e. *Cheilosis:* Cracking lips	
f. *Stomatitis:* Inflammation of mouth tissues or structures	
g. *Mucositis:* Inflammation of oral mucous membrane	
h. Dry, cracked, coated tongue	
6. Remove gloves and perform hand hygiene.	Prevents transmission of microorganisms.
7. Review medical record and assess patient's risk for oral hygiene problems:	Certain conditions increase likelihood of impaired oral cavity integrity and need for preventive care.
a. Dehydration: Inability to take fluids or food by mouth; health care provider's order prohibiting food or fluids by mouth (NPO) for a procedure or because of patient's condition	Causes excess drying and fragility of mucous membranes and lips; increases accumulation of thick secretions on tongue and gums.
b. Presence of nasogastric or oxygen tubes; mouth breathers	Causes drying of mucosa.
c. Chemotherapeutic drugs	Drugs kill rapidly multiplying cells, including sloughing of normal cells lining oral cavity. Mucositis with ulcers and inflammation can develop.
d. Radiation therapy to head and neck	Reduces salivary flow and lowers pH of saliva; leads to stomatitis and tooth decay (NCI, 2016).
e. Presence of artificial airway (e.g., endotracheal tube)	Tube irritates gums and mucosa. Excess secretions accumulate on teeth and tongue.
f. Blood-clotting disorders (e.g., leukemia, aplastic anemia)	Predisposes to inflammation and bleeding of gums.
g. Oral surgery, trauma to mouth	Break in mucosa increases risk for infection. Vigorous brushing can disrupt suture lines.

STEP	RATIONALE
h. Aging	With advancing age mucosa becomes thin and less elastic.
i. Chemical injury	Results from irritants such as alcohol, tobacco, acidic foods, or side effects of medications (e.g., antibiotics, steroids, antidepressants).
j. Diabetes mellitus	Prone to dryness of mouth, gingivitis, periodontal disease, and loss of teeth.
8. Determine patient's oral hygiene practices.	Identifies errors in patient's technique, deficiencies in preventive oral hygiene, patient's level of knowledge regarding dental care.
a. Frequency of toothbrushing and flossing	American Dental Association (2016a) recommends brushing teeth at least twice a day with ADA-accepted fluoride toothpaste and once-a-day flossing.
b. Type of toothpaste, dentifrice, and mouth rinse used (assess if chlorhexidine is indicated for use)	Antimicrobial mouth rinses and toothpastes decrease bacteria and stop bacterial growth in dental plaque, which can cause an early, reversible form of gum disease called *gingivitis* (ADA, 2016a).
c. Last dental visit and frequency of visits	The ADA recommends regular dental visits; however, frequency of visits can vary for each patient and should be determined by his or her dentist (ADA, 2013).
9. Assess patient's ability to grasp and manipulate toothbrush.	Determines level of help required from nurse. Some older patients or people with musculoskeletal or nervous system alterations are unable to hold toothbrush with firm grip or manipulate brush. Large-handled toothbrushes or a toothbrush handle pushed through a small rubber ball may be of help.

NURSING DIAGNOSES

- Bathing/self-care deficit
- Deficient knowledge regarding oral hygiene care
- Impaired oral mucous membrane
- Risk for infection

Related factors are individualized based on patient's condition or needs.

PLANNING

1. Expected outcomes following completion of procedure:	
• Patient expresses feeling of mouth cleanliness.	Hygiene measures remove secretions and thickened mucosa.
• Oral cavity structures have normal characteristics:	Hygiene measures maintain integrity of teeth and healthy oral mucosa.
• Oral mucosa is moist, intact, and of normal color.	
• Gums are pink, firm, and adherent to neck of teeth.	
• Teeth are clean, smooth, and shiny.	
• Tongue is pink and without secretions or coating.	
• Patient describes correct oral hygiene techniques.	Demonstrates understanding of instruction.
• Patient makes choices regarding hygiene procedure and helps by flossing and brushing.	Patient is able to manage self-care.
2. Gather equipment and supplies at bedside.	Avoids interrupting procedure or leaving patient unattended to retrieve missing equipment.
3. Explain procedure to patient and discuss preferences regarding use of hygiene aids.	Some patients feel uncomfortable about having nurse care for their basic needs. Patient involvement with procedure minimizes anxiety.

IMPLEMENTATION

1. Perform hand hygiene. Close room doors and draw room divider curtain.	Reduces transmission of microorganisms. Privacy ensures patient's mental and physical comfort.
2. Arrange supplies on bedside table so within easy reach.	Creates organized workspace.

STEP	RATIONALE

3. Raise bed to comfortable working height. Raise HOB to at least semi-Fowler's position (unless contraindicated) and lower side rail. Move patient or help patient move close to side from which you choose to work. A side-lying position can be used.

Raising bed and positioning patient promote good body mechanics and prevent nurse from muscle strain. Semi-Fowler's position helps prevent patient from choking or aspirating. **NOTE:** If patient is overweight, use safe handling techniques (see Chapter 11).

4. Place towel over patient's chest.

Prevents soiling of patient's gown.

5. Perform hand hygiene. Apply clean gloves.

Prevents transmission of microorganisms in body fluids.

6. Apply toothpaste to brush bristles. Hold brush over emesis basin. Pour small amount of water over toothpaste.

Moisture aids in distribution of toothpaste over tooth surfaces.

7. Patient may help by brushing. Hold toothbrush bristles at 45-degree angle to gum line (see illustration). Be sure that tips of bristles rest against and penetrate under gum line. Brush inner and outer surfaces of upper and lower teeth by brushing from gum to crown of each tooth. Clean biting surfaces of teeth by holding top of bristles parallel with teeth and brushing gently back and forth (see illustration). Brush sides of teeth by moving bristles back and forth (see illustration).

Angle allows brush to reach all tooth surfaces and clean under gum line where plaque and tartar accumulate. Back-and-forth motion loosens food particles caught between teeth and along chewing surfaces.

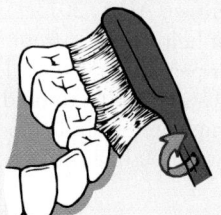 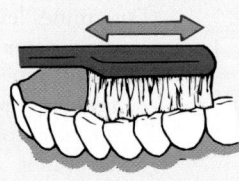 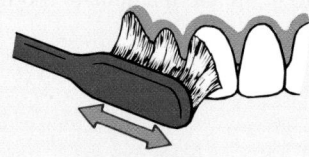

STEP 7 Directions of brush for toothbrushing.

8. Have patient hold brush at 45-degree angle and lightly brush over surface and sides of tongue (see illustration). Avoid initiating gag reflex.

Microorganisms collect and grow on surface of tongue and contribute to bad breath. Gagging may cause aspiration of toothpaste.

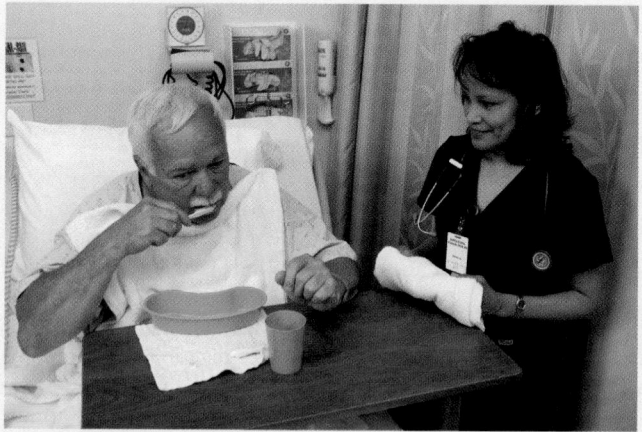

STEP 8 Nurse observe patient's toothbrushing technique, including brushing of tongue.

9. Allow patient to rinse mouth thoroughly with water by taking several sips of water (may use straw), swishing water across all tooth surfaces, and spitting into emesis basin. Use this time to observe patient's brushing technique and teach importance of brushing teeth twice a day.

Rinsing removes food particles.

STEP	RATIONALE

10. Have patient rinse teeth with antiseptic mouthwash for 30 seconds. Then have him or her spit rinse into emesis basin.

The ADA (2016b) recommends that an antiseptic mouthwash is effective in helping to prevent or control tooth decay, reduce plaque, prevent or reduce gingivitis, reduce the speed that tartar forms on the teeth, or produce a combination of these effects. Avoid using commercial brands of mouthwash that contain alcohol, which is drying to oral mucosa.

11. Help to wipe patient's mouth.

Promotes sense of comfort.

12. Allow patient to floss. Floss between all teeth. Hold floss against tooth while moving it up and down sides of teeth. Instruct patient in importance of daily flossing (see illustrations).

Flossing once daily removes plaque and decay-causing bacteria between teeth and under gum line, preventing gum disease.

Immunocompromised patients are sometimes on precautions that prohibit use of floss or Waterpiks because of dislodging bacteria and possible bleeding of gums.

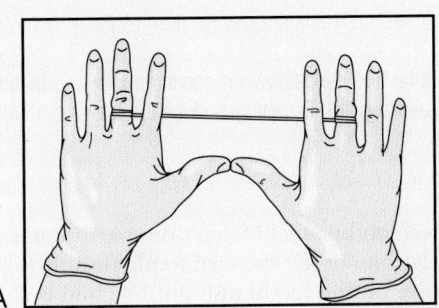 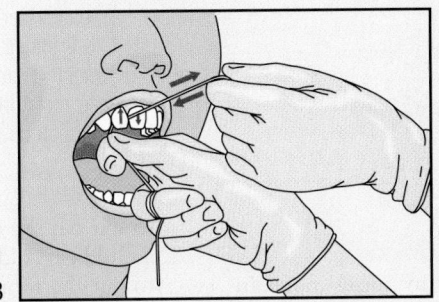 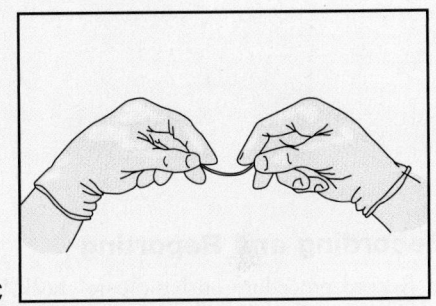

STEP 12 Flossing. **A,** Dental floss is held between middle fingers to floss upper teeth. **B,** Floss is moved in up-and-down motions between teeth. Floss is moved up and down from crown to gum line. **C,** Floss is held with index fingers to floss lower teeth.

13. Allow patient to rinse mouth thoroughly with cool water and spit into emesis basin. Help to wipe his or her mouth. Apply moisturizing lubricant to lips (if patient desires).

Rinsing removes plaque and tartar from oral cavity.

14. Help patient to comfortable position with call light in reach, remove emesis basin and over-bed table, raise side rail if appropriate, and lower bed to original position.

Provides for patient comfort and safety.

15. Wipe off bedside table, discard soiled linen in dirty laundry bag, remove soiled gloves, and return equipment to proper place.

Proper disposal of soiled equipment prevents spread of infection.

16. Perform hand hygiene.

Reduces transmission of microorganisms.

EVALUATION

1. Ask patient if any area of oral cavity feels uncomfortable or irritated.

Pain indicates need for further inspection for possible breaks in oral mucosa or identification of stomatitis or infection.

2. Apply clean gloves and inspect condition of oral cavity. Perform hand hygiene.

Determines effectiveness of hygiene and rinsing.

3. Observe patient brushing and flossing.

Evaluates patient's ability to demonstrate correct technique.

4. **Use Teach-Back:** "We discussed what is important for taking proper care of your teeth and gums. Tell me how often you should brush your teeth and what to use." Revise your instruction now or develop a plan for revised patient or family caregiver teaching if patient or family caregiver is not able to teach back correctly.

Determines patient's and family caregiver's level of understanding of instructional topic.

Unexpected Outcomes	Related Interventions
1. Mucosa is dry and inflamed. Tongue has thick coating.	• Increase patient's hydration. • Increase frequency of oral care, focusing on tongue brushing.
2. Cheilosis—Dry, cracked lips	• Apply moisturizing lubricant to patient's lips.

STEP	RATIONALE

3. Gum margins are retracted from teeth, with localized areas of inflammation. Bleeding occurs around gum margins.	• Report findings because patient may have an underlying bleeding tendency.
	• Switch to softer-bristled toothbrush or sponge toothette.
	• Avoid vigorous brushing and flossing.
	• Determine best-practice oral regimen for mucositis and stomatitis. Common regimens used to promote healing and comfort include:
	  • Use fluoride toothpaste.
	  • Use one of the following rinses made with salt and/or baking soda (NCI, 2016):
	    • 1 teaspoon salt in 4 cups of water
	    • 1 teaspoon baking soda in 1 cup (8 ounces) of water
	    • $\frac{1}{2}$ teaspoon salt and 2 tablespoons baking soda in 4 cups of water

4. Mucosa becomes inflamed from repeated chemotherapy administration, and a lesion from sloughing of tissue develops. These conditions can also be caused by radiation therapy used to treat head and neck cancers.	• An antibacterial rinse 2 to 4 times a day for gum disease; rinse for 1 to 2 minutes • If dry mouth (xerostomia) and hyposalivation occur, additional rinses to increase moisture may be used. Brushing and gentle flossing should be continued as well.

Recording and Reporting

- Record procedure on basic care check list in nurses' notes in electronic health record (EHR) or chart.
- Record condition of oral cavity in nurses' notes in EHR or chart.
- Document your evaluation of patient and family caregiver learning.
- Report bleeding, pain, or presence of lesions to nurse in charge or health care provider.

Special Considerations
Teaching

- Educate patients about methods to prevent tooth decay (e.g., reduce intake of carbohydrates, especially sweet, sticky snacks between meals; brush within 30 minutes of eating sweets; rinse mouth thoroughly with water or alcohol-free antiseptic mouth rinse; use fluoride toothpaste). Use simple language and available teaching materials at proper literacy level.
- Educate patients to visit a dentist regularly (based on dentist's recommendations) for professional cleaning and oral examination; frequency of visits varies for each patient and should be determined by his or her dentist (ADA, 2013).
- When teaching special oral-care regimens, include family caregiver.
- Avoid mints if conditions of the mouth are associated with ulcerations of the oral mucosa.

Pediatric

- Every infant should receive an oral-health risk assessment from his or her primary health care provider or qualified health care professional by 6 months of age (AAPD, 2014).
- Oral hygiene measures should be started no later than the time of eruption of the first primary tooth. Toothbrushing should be performed for children by a parent twice daily, using a soft toothbrush of age-appropriate size and the correct amount of fluoridated toothpaste (AAPD, 2014).
- As soon as a child has a tooth, use a smear (size of a grain of rice) of fluoride toothpaste. Clean the teeth right after breakfast and before bedtime. Once a child turns 3, use a pea-size amount of fluoride toothpaste. When a child is able, teach him or her

to spit out the excess toothpaste, but don't rinse with water. As a child gets older, let him or her use own toothbrush. It is best to put the toothpaste on the toothbrush until a child is about age 6. Until children are 7 or 8 years old, they will need help to brush their teeth. Try brushing their teeth first and letting them finish (AAP, 2014).
- Teach parents that infants should not be put to bed with a bottle; this causes tooth decay and ear infections. Limit snacks to three to four per day. Avoid sugary snacks and drinks and sticky candy.

Gerontological

- A number of normal age-related changes occur in the oral cavity. Thinning of the oral mucosa and decreased vascularity of the gingivae predispose older adults to injury and periodontal disease. Loss of tissue elasticity and decreased mass and strength of the muscles make chewing more difficult. Loss of the alveolar bone can loosen natural teeth.
- The number of taste buds declines with advancing age. In an attempt to enhance the taste of food, some older adults choose salty and sugary foods, which erode tooth enamel and expose dentin.
- It is recommended that an adult not smoke, chew tobacco, or use snuff. Smoking may impair blood flow to the gums, reducing the amount of oxygen and nutrients to the tissues and making them more vulnerable to infection. Chemicals in tobacco smoke cause inflammation and cell damage and can weaken the immune system. Nicotine is toxic to cells that make new connective tissue and also increases the production of an enzyme that breaks down tissue (National Institute of Dental and Craniofacial Research, 2015).
- Some older adults may find it difficult to maintain good oral hygiene with flossing and brushing because of decreased dexterity and decreasing eyesight.

Home Care

- During the initial admission, document the condition of a patient's mouth, teeth, and gums, thus providing a baseline for assessing the patient's ability to comply with special diets and fluid intake and carry out oral hygiene practices.

PROCEDURAL GUIDELINE 18.3 *Care of Dentures*

 Video Clip

Oral bacteria from multiple strains and *Candida* species are found on acrylic dentures (Villa et al., 2015). Encourage patients who wear dentures to continue to care for them and provide this care as frequently as with natural teeth. Loose dentures can cause discomfort and make it difficult for patients to chew food and speak clearly. Routine denture care reduces the risk for gingival infection. Offer dental care after every meal and before a patient goes to bed. Some patients are unable to care for their dentures, and nurses become responsible for providing denture and oral care. Dentures are a patient's personal property; thus be sure to handle them with care because they are easy to break. Reinsert them as soon as possible. Note that it is common for patients to choose to not wear their dentures during an acute illness.

Delegation and Collaboration
The skill of denture care can be delegated to nursing assistive personnel (NAP). The nurse instructs the NAP to:
- Not use hot or excessively cold water when caring for dentures.
- Inform the nurse if there are cracks in dentures.
- Inform the nurse if the patient has any oral discomfort.

Equipment
- Soft-bristled toothbrush or denture toothbrush
- Denture dentifrice or toothpaste, denture adhesive *(optional)*
- Glass of water
- Emesis basin or sink
- 4 × 4–inch gauze
- Washcloth
- Denture cup (for storage)
- Clean gloves

Procedural Steps
1. Identify patient using at least two identifiers (e.g., name and birthday or name and medical record number) according to agency policy (TJC, 2016).
2. Assess environment for safety (e.g., check room for spills; make sure that equipment is working properly and that bed is in locked, low position).
3. Perform hand hygiene.
4. Ask patient if dentures fit and if there is any gum or mucous membrane tenderness or irritation. Ask patient about denture care and product preferences.
5. Determine if patient has necessary dexterity to clean dentures independently or requires help.
6. Position patient comfortably sitting up in bed or help him or her walk from bed to chair placed in front of sink.
7. Fill emesis basin with tepid water. (If using sink, place washcloth in bottom of sink and fill sink with approximately 2.5 cm [1 inch] of water.)
8. Apply clean gloves.
9. Ask patient to remove dentures. If patient is unable to do this independently, grasp upper plate at front with thumb and index finger wrapped in gauze and pull downward. Gently lift lower denture from jaw and rotate one side downward to remove from patient's mouth. Place dentures in emesis basin or sink lined with washcloth and 2.5 cm (1 inch) of water.
10. Apply cleaning agent to brush and brush surfaces of dentures (see illustration). Hold dentures close to water. Hold brush horizontally and use back-and-forth motion to clean biting surfaces. Use short strokes from top of denture to biting surfaces to clean outer teeth surfaces. Hold brush vertically and use short strokes to clean inner teeth surfaces. Hold brush horizontally and use back-and-forth motion to clean undersurface of dentures (see Skill 18.2).

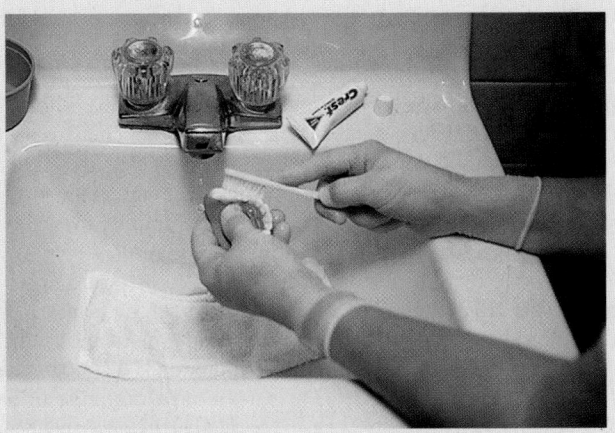

STEP 10 Brushing surface of dentures.

11. Rinse thoroughly in tepid water. If water is too cold, dentures can crack. If it is too hot, dentures can become warped and no longer fit.
12. Some patients use an adhesive to seal dentures in place. Apply a thin layer to undersurface before inserting.
13. If patient needs help with inserting dentures, moisten upper denture and press firmly to seal it in place. Insert moistened lower denture (if applicable). Ask if denture(s) feel comfortable.
14. Some patients prefer to store their dentures to give gums a rest and reduce risk for infection. Store in tepid water in enclosed, labeled denture cup. Keep denture cup in a secure place labeled with patient's name to prevent loss when not worn (e.g., at night, during surgery).
15. Dispose of supplies. Remove and discard gloves and perform hand hygiene.
16. Return patient to a comfortable position. Leave call light in reach.

◆ SKILL 18.3 Performing Mouth Care for an Unconscious or Debilitated Patient

Unconscious or debilitated patients pose challenges because of their risk for alterations of the oral cavity from drying of the mucous membrane, thickened secretions, and the inability to eat or drink. They are susceptible to infection because of the change in the normal flora of the oral cavity and at risk for infection because of increased plaque formation from the dryness of the mouth and decreased salivation. Dryness of the oral mucosa is also caused by mouth breathing and oxygen therapy. Respiratory secretions often are thick and place patients at risk for ineffective airway clearance, requiring oral suction (see Chapter 25). Debilitated patients are also at risk for aspiration. Although saliva production is decreased, saliva is present and can pool in the back of the oral cavity, which is a contributing factor for aspiration in patients with reduced gag reflexes. The secretions in the oral cavity change very rapidly to gram-negative pneumonia-producing bacteria if aspiration occurs.

The critically ill patient with an endotracheal tube who is on mechanical ventilation is at risk for ventilator-associated pneumonia (VAP). Once intubated, an endotracheal tube causes a bypass of normal airway defenses, which also causes a rapid change in the normal oral flora (CDC, 2015). Some patients require mouth care as often as every 1 to 2 hours until the mucosa returns to normal. Proper hygiene requires keeping the mucosa moist and removing secretions as they accumulate in the back of the throat. The Institute for Healthcare Improvement and the American Academy of Critical Care Nursing have recommended use of 0.12% chlorhexidine gluconate (CHG) as part of daily oral care (CDC, 2015; Wiech and Bayer, 2012) in critically ill patients. Many hospitals use an oral care bundle to reduce incidence of VAP, including toothbrushing every 12 hours before the application of CHG; CHG 0.12% rinse every 12 hours; and keeping the head of bed (HOB) elevated 30 to 45 degrees or more unless contraindicated to prevent aspiration of oral secretions. Recently, however, research has shown that routine oral care with CHG prevents nosocomial pneumonia in cardiac surgery patients but may not decrease VAP in noncardiac surgery patients (Klompas et al., 2014). Check agency policy regarding use of CHG in oral care.

Because many debilitated patients have either a reduced or absent gag reflex as a result of change in consciousness or a neurological injury, providing oral care requires protecting patients from choking and aspiration. The safest technique is to have two nurses provide care. You provide oral care while another nurse or nursing assistive personnel (NAP) suctions oral secretions as necessary with a Yankauer suction tip (see Chapter 25). You can also delegate oral care to two NAPs with instructions. Evaluate the level and frequency of oral care on a daily basis during assessment of the oral cavity. Routine suctioning of the mouth and pharynx is required to manage oral secretions to reduce the risk for aspiration.

Delegation and Collaboration

The skill of providing oral hygiene to an unconscious or debilitated patient can be delegated to NAP. The nurse is responsible for assessing a patient's gag reflex. The nurse instructs the NAP to:
- Have another NAP help and properly position patient for mouth care.
- Be aware of special precautions such as aspiration precautions.
- Use an oral suction catheter for clearing oral secretions (see Skill 25.1).
- Report signs of impaired integrity of oral mucosa to the nurse.
- Report any bleeding of mucosa or gum or excessive coughing or choking to the nurse.

Equipment

- Small pediatric, soft-bristled toothbrush, toothette sponges, or suction toothbrushes for patients for whom brushing is contraindicated
- Antibacterial solution per organization protocol (e.g., CHG)
- Fluoride toothpaste
- Water-based mouth moisturizer
- Tongue blade
- Penlight
- Oral suction equipment
- Oral airway (uncooperative patient or patient who shows bite reflex)
- Water-soluble lip lubricant
- Water glass with cool water
- Face and bath towel
- Emesis basin
- Clean gloves

STEP	RATIONALE

ASSESSMENT

1. Identify patient using at least two identifiers (e.g., name and birthday or name and medical record number) according to agency policy.	Ensures patient safety. Complies with The Joint Commission standards and improves patient safety (TJC, 2016).
2. Assess environment for safety (e.g., check room for spills; make sure that equipment is working properly and that bed is in locked, low position).	Identifies safety hazards in patient environment that could cause or potentially lead to harm (QSEN, 2014).
3. Perform hand hygiene and apply clean gloves.	Reduces transmission of microorganisms in blood or saliva.
4. Assess for presence of gag reflex by placing tongue blade on back half of tongue.	Helps in determining aspiration risk.

STEP	RATIONALE

Clinical Decision Point *Patients with impaired gag reflex still require oral care; however, they have a higher risk for aspiration. Keep suction equipment available when caring for patients who are at risk for aspiration.*

5. Inspect condition of oral cavity (see Chapter 6).	Determines condition of oral cavity and need for hygiene. Establishes baseline to show improvement following oral care.
6. Remove gloves. Perform hand hygiene.	Prevents transmission of infection.
7. Assess patient's risk for oral hygiene problems (see Skill 18.2).	Certain conditions increase likelihood of alterations in integrity of oral cavity mucosa and structures, necessitating more frequent care.
8. Assess patient's respirations or oxygen saturation.	Helps in early recognition of aspiration.

NURSING DIAGNOSES

- Impaired oral mucous membrane
- Risk for aspiration
- Risk for infection

Related factors are individualized based on patient's condition or needs.

PLANNING

1. Expected outcomes following completion of procedure:	
• Oral cavity structures have normal characteristics: buccal mucosa and tongue are pink, moist, and intact; gums are moist and intact; teeth are clean, smooth, and shiny; tongue is pink and without coating; lips are moist, smooth, and without cracks.	Degree of improvement in condition of oral cavity following oral hygiene depends on extent of secretions or changes that existed before care.
• Debilitated patient expresses feeling of mouth cleanliness.	Comfort achieved.
• Oropharynx remains clear of secretions.	Secretions removed, thus avoiding aspiration.
2. Gather equipment and supplies at bedside.	Avoids interrupting procedure or leaving patient unattended to retrieve missing equipment.
3. Explain procedure to patient or family caregiver if present.	Even debilitated or intubated patients are usually able to hear. Explanation can reduce anxiety.

IMPLEMENTATION

1. Pull curtain around bed or close room door.	Provides privacy.
2. Perform hand hygiene and apply clean gloves.	Reduces transfer of microorganisms.
3. Place towel on over-bed table and arrange equipment. If needed, turn on suction machine and connect tubing to suction catheter.	Prevents soiling of tabletop. Equipment prepared in advance ensures smooth, safe procedure. Supplies within reach create organized workspace.
4. Raise bed to appropriate working height; lower side rail. Unless contraindicated (e.g., head injury, neck trauma), position patient in Sims' or side-lying position. Turn patient's head toward mattress in dependent position with HOB elevated at least 30 degrees.	Use of good body mechanics with bed in high position prevents injury. Allows secretions to drain from mouth instead of collecting in back of pharynx. Prevents aspiration. If patient is overweight, follow safe handling techniques for positioning (see Chapter 11).
5. Place towel under patient's head and emesis basin under chin.	Prevents soiling of bed linen.
6. Remove dentures or partial plates if present.	Allows for thorough cleaning of prosthetics later. Provides clearer access to oral cavity.
7. If patient is uncooperative or having difficulty keeping mouth open, insert an oral airway. Insert upside down and turn airway sideways and over tongue to keep teeth apart. Insert when patient is relaxed if possible. Do not use force.	Prevents patient from biting down on nurse's fingers and provides access to oral cavity.

Clinical Decision Point *Never place fingers into the mouth of an unconscious or debilitated patient. This could occlude the airway. Also, the normal response is to bite down.*

STEP	RATIONALE
8. Clean mouth using brush moistened in water. Apply toothpaste or use antibacterial solution first to loosen crusts. Hold toothbrush bristles at 45-degree angle to gum line. Be sure that tips of bristles rest against and penetrate under gum line. Brush inner and outer surfaces of upper and lower teeth by brushing from gum to crown of each tooth; clean biting surfaces of teeth by holding top of bristles parallel with teeth and brushing gently back and forth (see Skill 18.2). Brush sides of teeth by moving bristles back and forth. Use toothette sponge if patient has bleeding tendency or use of toothbrush is contraindicated. Suction any accumulated secretions. Moisten brush with clear water or CHG solution to rinse. Clean lips and mucosa with toothette (see illustration). Use brush or toothette to clean roof of mouth, gums, and inside cheeks. Gently brush tongue but avoid stimulating gag reflex (if present). Repeat rinsing several times and use suction to remove secretions. Use towel to dry off lips.	Brushing action removes food particles between teeth and along chewing surfaces and crusts for mucosa. Do not use commercial swabs because they do not clean teeth. Repeated rinsing removes all debris and helps to moisten mucosa. Suction removes secretions and fluids that collect in posterior pharynx, thus reducing aspiration risk.
9. Apply thin layer of water-soluble moisturizer to lips (see illustration).	Lubricates lips to prevent drying and cracking.
10. Inform patient that procedure is completed. Return him or her to comfortable and safe position.	Provides meaningful stimulation to unconscious or less-responsive patient.
11. Raise side rails as appropriate and return bed to locked, low position. Leave call light in reach.	Reduces risk of falls from bed.
12. Clean equipment and return to its proper place. Place soiled linen in dirty laundry bag.	Proper disposal of soiled equipment prevents spread of infection.
13. Remove and dispose of gloves in proper receptacle and perform hand hygiene.	Reduces transmission of microorganisms.

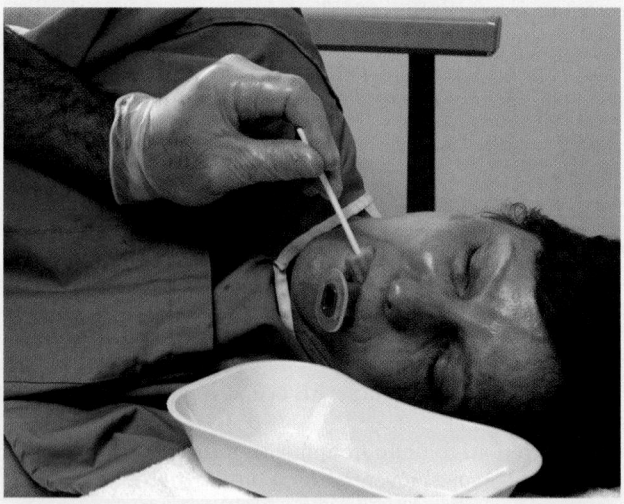

STEP 8 Cleaning lips and mucosa around oral airway with toothette.

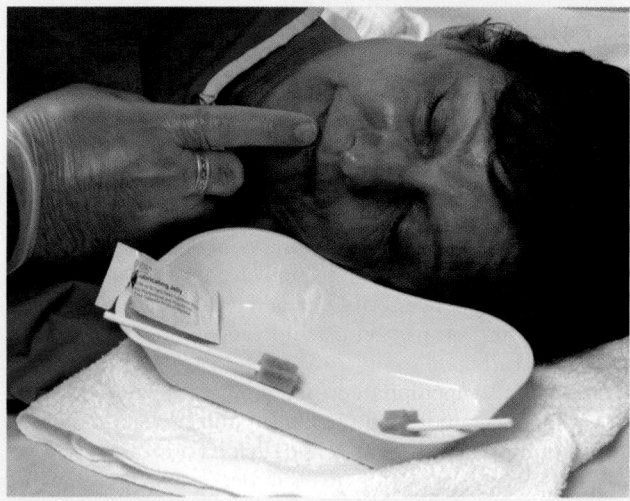

STEP 9 Application of water-soluble moisturizer to lips.

EVALUATION

1. Apply clean gloves and use tongue blade and penlight to inspect oral cavity.	Determines efficacy of cleaning. Once thick secretions are removed, underlying inflammation or lesions may be revealed.
2. Ask debilitated patient if mouth feels clean.	Evaluates level of comfort.
3. **Use Teach-Back:** "I explained what is needed to reduce your husband's risk of choking on secretions in his throat. Tell me the ways you will prevent him from choking when you give mouth care at home." Revise your instruction now or develop a plan for revised patient or family caregiver teaching if patient or family caregiver is not able to teach back correctly.	Determines patient's and family caregiver's level of understanding of instructional topic.

STEP	RATIONALE
Unexpected Outcomes 1. Secretions or crusts remain on mucosa, tongue, or gums. 2. Localized inflammation or bleeding of gums or mucosa is present. 3. Lips are cracked or inflamed. 4. Patient aspirates secretions.	**Related Interventions** • Provide more frequent oral hygiene. • Provide more frequent oral hygiene with toothette sponges. • Apply water-based mouth moisturizer to provide moisture and maintain integrity of oral mucosa. • Chemotherapy and radiation can cause mucositis (inflammation of mucous membranes in mouth) because of sloughing of epithelial tissue. Room temperature saline rinses, bicarbonate and sterile water rinses, and oral care with a soft-bristled toothbrush decrease severity and duration of mucositis. • Apply moisturizing gel or water-soluble lubricant to lips more often. • Suction oral airway as secretions accumulate to maintain airway patency (see Chapter 25). • Elevate patient's HOB to facilitate breathing. • If aspiration is suspected, notify health care provider. Prepare patient for chest x-ray film examination.

Recording and Reporting

- Record procedure, appearance of oral cavity, presence of gag reflex, and patient's response to procedure in medical record in nurses' notes in electronic health record (EHR) or chart.
- Document your evaluation of patient and family caregiver learning.
- Report any unusual findings (e.g., bleeding, ulceration, choking response) to nurse in charge or health care provider.

Special Considerations
Teaching

- Family members may care for debilitated patient in the home. Instruction in how to perform mouth care is necessary so family caregiver understands how to protect patient from aspirating

while thoroughly cleaning oral cavity. Use the teach-back technique by observing family caregiver perform mouth care procedure effectively or asking them to describe the procedure.

Home Care

- Irrigate oral cavity with bulb syringe; if unavailable, substitute gravy baster or large syringe. Caution family caregiver against instilling a large amount of water or rinsing agent in the oral cavity because of the risk of aspiration. Observe caregiver use baster.
- Encourage family caregiver to clean patient's mouth at least twice a day. If patient breathes through mouth, a soft-bristled toothbrush moistened and used every 1 to 2 hours will keep mouth moist and fresh.

PROCEDURAL GUIDELINE 18.4 *Hair Care—Combing and Shaving*

A person's comfort, appearance, and sense of well-being are influenced by how the hair looks and feels. Brushing, combing, and shaving are basic hygiene measures for all patients unable to provide self-care. Most long-term care facilities have beauty shops where patients can go for professional hair care. An immobilized patient's hair soon becomes tangled if not brushed or combed regularly. Dressings may leave sticky adhesive, blood, or antiseptic solutions on the hair. Diaphoresis leaves hair oily and unmanageable. Proper hair care is important to a person's body image.

Certain chemotherapy agents and radiation therapy cause loss of hair (alopecia). Many patients choose to wear a wig; however, some choose to wear hair scarves or turbans. Table 18.2 describes common hair and scalp conditions and nursing interventions.

Dependent patients with beards or mustaches need help keeping facial hair clean, especially after eating. Shaving facial hair is a task most men prefer to do for themselves daily. Because some religions and cultures forbid cutting or shaving any body hair, be certain to obtain consent from these patients. Make sure to be aware if patients are at risk for bleeding before shaving.

Delegation and Collaboration

The skills of combing and shaving can be delegated to nursing assistive personnel (NAP). The nurse instructs the NAP to:

- Properly position a patient with head or neck mobility restrictions.
- Report how the patient tolerated the procedure and any concerns (e.g., neck pain).
- Use an electric razor for any patient at risk for bleeding tendencies.

Equipment
Hair Care

- Wide-tooth comb and hairbrush

Shaving With Razor

- New disposable or electric razor
- Clean gloves
- Bath towel(s), mirror, washcloth, washbasin
- Shaving cream or soap, aftershave lotion (if patient desires and not contraindicated)

Continued

PROCEDURAL GUIDELINE 18.4 *Hair Care—Combing and Shaving—cont'd*

Mustache Care
- Scissors, brush or comb
- Bath towel
- Gooseneck lamp or overhead light

Procedural Steps
1. Identify patient using at least two identifiers (e.g., name and birthday or name and medical record number) according to agency policy (TJC, 2016).
2. Perform hand hygiene. Inspect condition of hair and scalp. Inspect for presence of any infestation (e.g., pediculosis). NOTE: Apply clean gloves and gown if infestation is suspected; discard gloves and perform hand hygiene after inspection.
3. Assess patient's hair-care and shaving product preferences (e.g., shampoo, aftershave lotion, skin conditioner).
4. Assess if patient has bleeding tendency. Review medical history, medications, and laboratory values (e.g., platelet count, anticoagulation studies).

Clinical Decision Point *Have any patient on anticoagulants or who has low platelets use an electric razor.*

5. Assess patient's ability to manipulate comb, brush, or razor.
6. Gather equipment and supplies at patient's bedside. Explain your intent to provide hair/beard care. Ask patient to explain during procedure steps that he or she uses to comb hair and/or shave. Ask patient to indicate if he or she becomes uncomfortable during procedure.
7. Position patient sitting in chair or up in bed with head elevated 45 to 90 degrees (as tolerated).
8. Provide privacy; close door or pull curtain. Arrange supplies at bedside table and adjust lighting.
9. Perform hand hygiene and apply clean gloves if necessary.
10. **Combing and brushing hair:**
    a. Part hair into two sections and then separate it into two more sections (see illustrations).
    b. Brush or comb from scalp toward hair ends.

TABLE 18.2

Hair and Scalp Problems

Characteristics	Implications	Interventions
Dandruff—Scaling of scalp accompanied by itching; in severe cases dandruff on eyebrows	Dandruff causes embarrassment; if it enters eyes, conjunctivitis may develop.	Shampoo regularly with medicated shampoo; in severe cases obtain health care provider's advice.
Ticks—Small gray-brown parasites that burrow into skin and suck blood	Ticks transmit several diseases, including Rocky Mountain spotted fever, Lyme disease, and tularemia.	Do not pull ticks from skin because sucking apparatus remains and may become infected; placing drop of oil on tick or covering it with petrolatum eases removal; oil suffocates tick.
Pediculosis capitis (head lice)—Tiny gray brown–white parasitic insects that attach to hair strands; about size of a sesame seed; nits or eggs look like oval particles attached at an angle to hair shaft; bites or pustules may be observed behind ears and at hairline	Head lice are difficult to remove and, if not treated, may spread to furniture and other people.	Check entire scalp. Use medicated shampoo for eliminating lice or permethrin (Nix), available as a crème rinse. *Caution against use of products containing lindane because the ingredient is toxic and known to cause adverse reactions* (National Pediculosis Association, 2016). Remove patient's clothing before treatment and apply new clothing following treatment. Repeat treatment according to product directions. Check hair for nits and comb with nit comb for 2 to 3 days until sure all lice and nits have been removed. Manual removal of lice is best option when treatment has failed. Vacuum infested areas of home. Wash linens in hot water and dry for at least 30 minutes.
Pediculosis corporis (body lice)—Tend to cling to clothing; thus may not be easily seen; suck blood and lay eggs on clothing and furniture	Patient itches constantly; scratches on skin may become infected; hemorrhagic spots may appear on skin where lice are sucking blood. It may spread to other people.	Patient should bathe or shower thoroughly; after skin is dried, apply lotion for eliminating lice; after 12 to 24 hours another bath or shower should be taken; bag infested clothing or linen until laundered. Vacuum items that cannot be washed.
Pediculosis pubis (crab lice)—Found in pubic hair; gray-white with red legs	Lice may spread through bed linen, clothing, furniture, or sexual contact.	Shave hair of affected area; clean as for body lice; if lice were sexually transmitted, partner must be notified.
Hair loss (alopecia)—Balding patches in periphery of hairline; hair becomes brittle and broken; caused by diseases, medication side effects, and improper use of hair-care products and hair-styling devices	Patches of uneven hair growth and loss alter patient's appearance.	Offer patients access to scarves, hairpieces, or wigs. Stop hair-care practices that damage hair.

PROCEDURAL GUIDELINE 18.4 *Hair Care—Combing and Shaving—cont'd*

  c. Moisten hair lightly with water, conditioner, or alcohol-free detangle product before combing.
  d. Move fingers through hair to loosen any larger tangles.
  e. Using a wide-tooth comb, start on either side of head and insert comb with teeth upward to hair near scalp. Comb through hair in circular motion by turning wrist while lifting up and out. Continue until all hair is combed through and comb into place to shape and style.

11. Shaving with disposable razor:
  a. Place bath towel over patient's chest and shoulders.
  b. Run warm water in washbasin. Check water temperature.
  c. Place washcloth in basin and wring out thoroughly. Apply cloth over patient's entire face for several seconds.
  d. Apply approximately ¼ inch shaving cream or soap to patient's face. Smooth cream evenly over sides of face, on chin, and under nose.
  e. Hold razor in dominant hand at 45-degree angle to patient's skin. Begin by shaving across one side of patient's face using short, firm strokes in direction that

hair grows (see illustration). Use nondominant hand to gently pull skin taut while shaving. Ask patient if he feels comfortable.
  f. Dip razor blade in water because shaving cream accumulates on edge of blade.
  g. After all facial hair is shaved, rinse face thoroughly with warm, moistened washcloth.
  h. Dry face thoroughly and apply aftershave lotion if desired. Remove towel.

12. Shaving with electric razor:
  a. Place bath towel over patient's chest and shoulders.
  b. Apply skin conditioner or preshave preparation.
  c. Turn razor on and begin by shaving across side of face. Gently hold skin taut while shaving over surface of skin. Use gentle downward stroke of razor in direction of hair growth.
  d. After completing shave, remove towel and apply aftershave lotion as desired unless contraindicated.

13. Mustache and beard care:
  a. Place bath towel over patient's chest and shoulders.
  b. If necessary, gently comb mustache or beard.
  c. Allow patient to use mirror and direct areas to trim with scissors.
  d. After completing, remove towel.

14. Help patient assume desired comfortable position. Leave call light in reach.

15. Return reusable equipment to proper place. Discard soiled linen in dirty laundry bag. Perform hand hygiene.

16. Ask patient how hair and scalp feel.

17. Inspect condition of shaved area and skin underneath beard or mustache. Look for areas of localized bleeding from cuts and areas of dryness.

18. Ask patient if face feels clean and comfortable.

19. Use Teach-Back: "I want to be sure I explained to you the risks of using a regular razor at home. Tell me what type of razor you should use and why this is important. Tell me the things to watch for with a bleeding tendency." Revise your instruction now or develop a plan for revised patient or family caregiver teaching if patient or family caregiver is not able to teach back correctly.

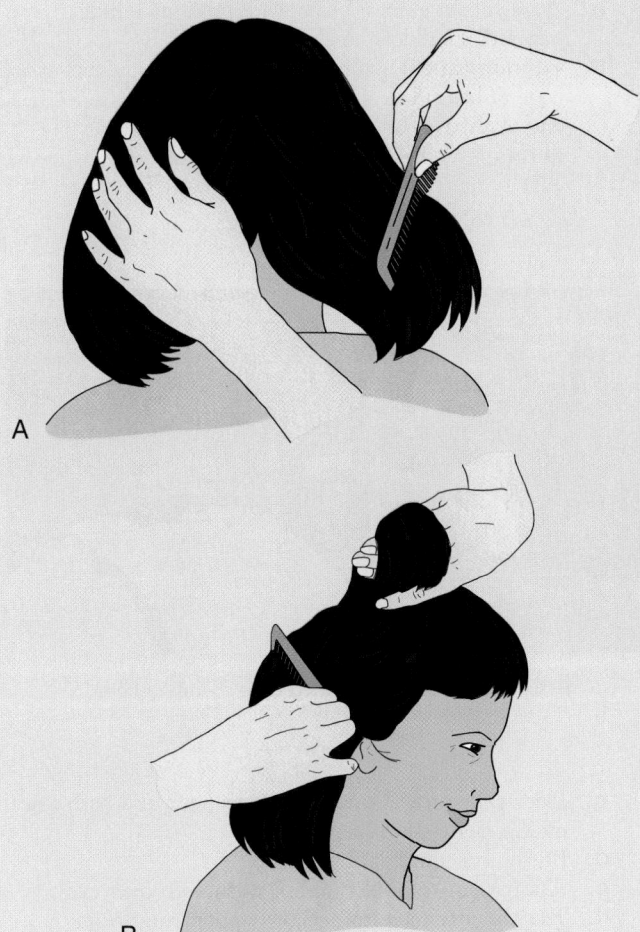

STEP 10a Parting hair. **A,** Part hair down the middle and divide it into two main sections. **B,** Part main section into two smaller sections.

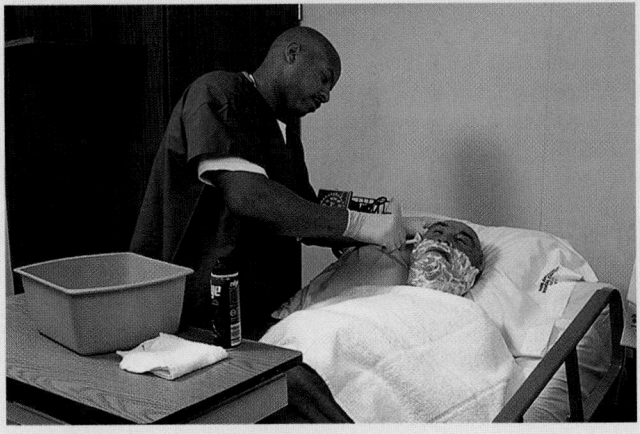

STEP 11e Shaving patient using short, firm strokes.

PROCEDURAL GUIDELINE 18.5 *Hair Care—Shampooing*

The frequency of shampooing depends on the condition of the hair and a person's daily routines and cultural preferences. Dry hair, which commonly results from aging and protein deficiency, requires less frequent shampooing than oily hair. In some health care agencies you need a health care provider's order to shampoo a patient who is dependent or has limited mobility because it is challenging to find ways to shampoo the hair without causing injury to a patient's neck.

Remind hospitalized patients that more frequent shampooing is necessary when they remain in bed for extended periods of time, have excessive perspiration, or undergo treatments that leave blood or solutions in the hair. Two types of shampooing are available for patients: (1) traditional shampoo and water, or (2) a disposable dry shampoo cap. You can shampoo patients who are allowed to sit in a chair in front of a sink. Make sure that a patient's condition does not contraindicate neck hyperextension. Caution is needed with patients who have suffered neck injuries because flexion and hyperextension of the neck could cause further injury. In addition, patients with positional vertigo are not able to tolerate neck hyperextension if it increases their dizziness. A folded towel placed under the neck on the edge of the sink provides added comfort.

If a patient cannot sit in a chair or be transferred to a stretcher, shampoo the hair with the patient in bed, using traditional shampoo and water or a disposable shampoo product.

Delegation and Collaboration

The skill of shampooing the hair of bed-bound patients and the use of a disposable shampoo product can be delegated to nursing assistive personnel (NAP). The nurse instructs the NAP about:

- Proper way to position a patient with a head or neck mobility restriction.
- Knowledge of care for lice, stressing steps to take to prevent transmission to other patients.

Equipment
- Bath towels
- Clean gloves; clean gown (*optional*) (if patient has known head lice)
- Clean comb and brush

Regular Shampoo
- Washcloth
- Shampoo, hair conditioner (*optional*), hydrogen peroxide (*optional*)
- Water pitcher with warm water
- Plastic shampoo board, wash basin
- Bath blanket, waterproof pad
- Hydrogen peroxide and saline (*optional*)

Disposable Shampoo
- Disposable shampoo cap product

Procedural Steps
1. Identify patient using at least two identifiers (e.g., name and birthday or name and medical record number) according to agency policy (TJC, 2016).
2. Inspect condition of hair and scalp before beginning shampoo. This determines if special shampoos or treatments are necessary (e.g., dandruff, lice, removal of blood). If draining head wounds are suspected, apply clean gloves. If lice are present, wear disposable gown in addition to gloves (National Pediculosis Association, 2016).
3. Review medical record to determine that there are no contraindications to procedure. Check agency policy for health care provider order as needed. Certain medical conditions such as head and neck injuries, spinal cord injuries, and arthritis place patient at risk for injury during shampooing because of positioning and manipulation of patient's head and neck.
4. Assess environment for safety (e.g., check room for spills; make sure that equipment is working properly and that bed is in locked, low position) (QSEN, 2014).
5. Explain procedure to patient, using simple language.
6. Perform hand hygiene. Assemble equipment at bedside, including pitcher with warm water.
7. Provide privacy by closing room door or curtain dividers. Raise bed to comfortable working height and lower side rail on side on which you will stand.
8. **Shampooing bed-bound patient with shampoo board:**
   a. Apply clean gloves. Place waterproof pad under patient's shoulders, neck, and head.
   b. Position patient supine with head and shoulders at top edge of bed. Place shampoo board under patient's head and washbasin under end of trough spout (see illustration). Be sure that trough spout extends beyond edge of mattress.

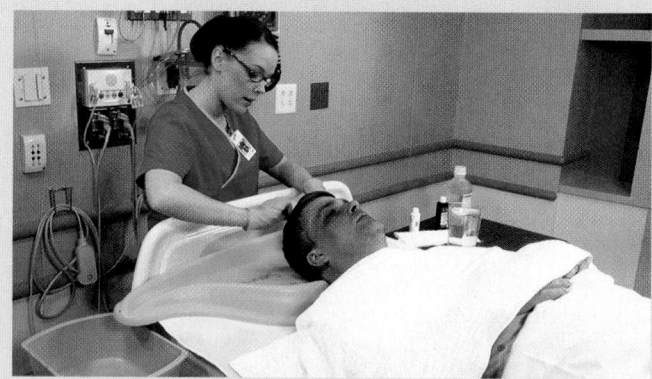

STEP 8b Patient positioned over shampoo board.

   c. Place rolled towel under patient's neck and bath towel over patient's shoulders.
   d. Brush and comb patient's hair.
   e. Ask patient to hold towel or washcloth over eyes.
   f. Test water temperature. Slowly pour water from pitcher over hair until it is completely wet (see illustration). If hair contains matted blood, apply hydrogen peroxide to dissolve clots and rinse with saline. Apply small amount of shampoo.

PROCEDURAL GUIDELINE 18.5 *Hair Care—Shampooing—cont'd*

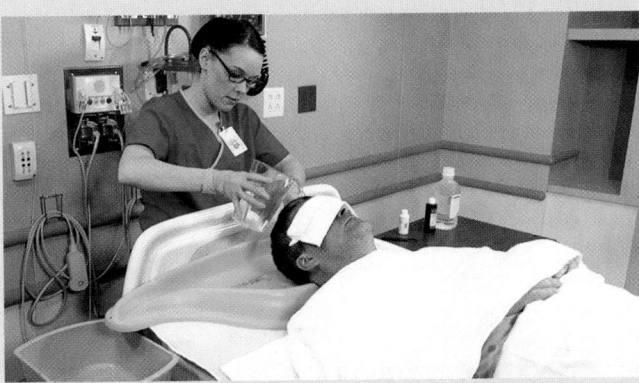

STEP 8f Nurse pouring water over patient's hair.

g. Work up lather with both hands. Start at hairline and work toward back of neck. Lift head slightly with one hand to wash back of head. Shampoo sides of head. Massage scalp by applying pressure with fingertips.

h. Rinse hair with water. Make sure that water drains into basin. Repeat rinsing until hair is free of soap. (If you need to refill pitcher, raise side rail when leaving bedside.)

i. Apply conditioner or crème rinse if requested and rinse hair thoroughly.

j. Wrap patient's head in bath towel. Dry face with cloth used to protect eyes. Dry off any moisture along neck or shoulders.

k. Dry patient's hair and scalp. Use second towel if first one becomes saturated.

l. Comb hair to remove tangles and dry with dryer if desired.

m. Apply oil preparation or conditioning product to hair if desired by patient.

n. Variation for patients with coarse, curly hair: Condition hair after washing. To untangle hair, use wide teeth of comb. Beginning at nape of neck, comb small subsections of hair, starting at hair ends. Continue to work through small sections until hair is free of tangles.

o. Help patient to comfortable position and complete styling of hair. Leave call light in reach.

p. Dispose of supplies. Store reusable supplies. Remove gloves and perform hand hygiene.

9. Shampooing with disposable shampoo product:

a. Patient can be sitting on chair or in bed. Apply clean gloves.

b. Comb hair to remove any tangles or debris.

c. Open package, apply cap, and secure all hair beneath cap (see illustration).

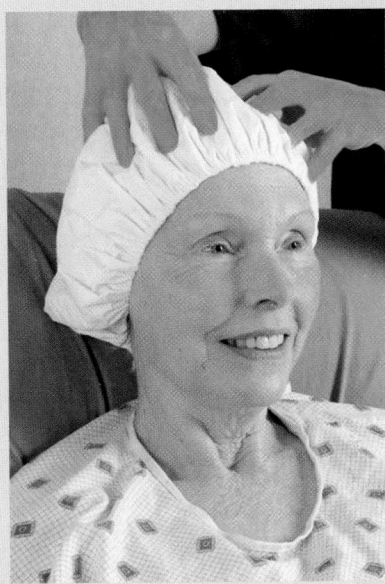

STEP 9c Patient wearing disposable shampoo cap.

d. Massage head through cap. Check fitting around head to maintain correct fit.

e. Massage 2 to 4 minutes according to directions on package; additional time may be required for longer hair or hair matted with blood.

f. Discard cap in trash; do not dispose of in toilet because it may clog plumbing.

g. If patient desires, towel dry hair. Brush or comb patient's hair.

h. Remove gloves. Perform hand hygiene.

i. Help patient to comfortable position with call light in reach.

10. Inspect condition of hair and scalp.

11. Use Teach-Back: "During the shampoo we discussed ways to reduce risk of getting exposed to lice in your home. Tell me three ways to reduce the chance of exposing yourself and others to lice." Revise your instruction now or develop a plan for revised patient or family caregiver teaching if patient or family caregiver is not able to teach back correctly.

◆ SKILL 18.4   Performing Nail and Foot Care

The best time to provide nail and foot care is during a patient's daily bath. Many agencies require a health care provider's order before you can trim nails. Feet and nails often require special care to prevent infection, odors, pain, and injury to soft tissues. Often people are unaware of foot or nail problems until discomfort or pain occurs. Common foot and nail problems are presented in Table 18.3. For proper foot and nail care, instruct patients to protect the feet from injury, keep them clean and dry, and wear appropriate footwear. Instruct patients how to properly inspect the feet for lesions, dryness, or signs of infection. To maintain and promote foot and nail health, patients should visit a podiatrist when necessary. This is especially important for patients with foot disorders, peripheral vascular diseases (PVDs), or diabetes mellitus; older adults; and patients who are immunocompromised.

TABLE 18.3

Common Foot and Nail Problems

Condition	Characteristics	Implications	Interventions
Callus	Thickened part of epidermis, consisting of mass of horny, keratotic cells; usually flat, painless, and found on undersurface of foot or palm of hand; caused by local friction or pressure	Foot calluses may cause discomfort when wearing tight-fitting shoes.	Refer patient to podiatrist; do not self-treat. Use of orthotic devices cushions and redistributes weight and pressure off calluses.
Corns	Keratosis caused by friction and pressure from shoes; mainly on toes, over bony prominence; usually cone-shaped, round, and raised; calluses with painful core	Conical shape compresses underlying dermis, making it thin and tender. Pain is aggravated by tight-fitting shoes. Patients may suffer alteration in gait because of pain.	Refer patient to podiatrist. Avoid use of oval corn pads, which increase pressure on toes. Use wider, softer shoes.
Plantar warts	Fungating lesions on sole of foot caused by papillomavirus	Warts may be contagious, are painful, and make walking difficult.	Refer patient to podiatrist.
Athlete's foot (tinea pedis)	Fungal infection of foot; scaliness and cracking of skin between toes and on soles of feet; small blisters containing fluid may appear, apparently induced by constricting footwear	Athlete's foot can spread to other body parts, especially hands. It is contagious and frequently recurs.	Feet should be well ventilated. Drying feet well after bathing and applying powder help prevent infection. Wearing clean socks or stockings reduces incidence. Health care provider orders application of griseofulvin, miconazole nitrate, or tolnaftate.
Ingrown nails	Toenail or fingernail growing inward into soft tissue around nail; results from improper nail trimming, poor shoe fit, or heredity	Ingrown nails can cause localized pain when pressure is applied.	Treatment is frequent warm soaks (exception: patient with diabetes mellitus) in antiseptic solution and removal of part of nail that has grown into skin. Teach patient proper nail-trimming techniques. Refer to podiatrist.
Paronychia	Inflammation of tissue surrounding nail after hangnail or other injury; occurs in people who frequently have their hands in water; common in patients with diabetes mellitus	Area can become infected.	Treatment is warm compresses or soaks (exception: patient with diabetes mellitus) and local application of antibiotic ointments. Paronychia can be prevented by careful manicuring.
Foot odors	Result of excess perspiration promoting microorganism growth and possibly faulty foot hygiene or improper footwear	Excess perspiration causes discomfort.	Frequent washing, use of foot deodorants and powders, and clean footwear prevent or reduce this problem.

Patients most at risk for developing serious foot problems are those with peripheral neuropathy and PVD. These two disorders, commonly found in patients with diabetes mellitus, cause a reduction in blood flow to the extremities and a loss of sensory, motor, and autonomic nerve function. As a result, a patient is unable to feel heat and cold, pain, pressure, and positioning of the foot or feet. The reduction in blood flow impairs healing and promotes risk for infection. The development of diabetic foot ulcers has three contributing factors: (1) peripheral neuropathy (changes in the function and efficiency of the nerves), (2) ischemia (decrease in the blood flow related to plaque formation in arteries), and (3) a pivotal event (trauma caused by banging the toe or stepping on a foreign object). If foot ulcers do not heal, they can become infected quickly and lead to gangrene and subsequent amputation.

Delegation and Collaboration

The skill of nail and foot care of patients *without diabetes mellitus* or *circulatory compromise* can be delegated to nursing assistive personnel (NAP). The nurse instructs the NAP about:

- Not trimming patient's nails (unless permitted by agency or health care provider).
- Special considerations for patient positioning.
- Reporting any breaks in skin, redness, numbness, swelling, or pain to the nurse.

Equipment

- Washbasin
- Emesis basin
- Washcloth and towel
- Nail clippers (check agency policy)
- Soft nail or cuticle brush
- Plastic applicator stick
- Emery board or nail file
- Body lotion
- Disposable bath mat
- Clean gloves

STEP	RATIONALE

ASSESSMENT

1. Identify patient using at least two identifiers (e.g., name and birthday or name and medical record number) according to agency policy.

   Ensures patient safety. Complies with The Joint Commission standards and improves patient safety (TJC, 2016).

2. Assess environment for safety (e.g., check room for spills; make sure that equipment is working properly and that bed is in locked, low position).

   Identifies safety hazards in patient environment that could cause or potentially lead to harm (QSEN, 2014).

3. Perform hand hygiene and apply clean gloves. Inspect all surfaces of fingers, toes, feet, and nails. **NOTE:** *This can be done during the bath.* Pay close attention to areas of dryness, inflammation, or cracking. Also inspect areas between toes and on heels and soles of feet. Inspect socks for stains.

   Integrity of feet and nails determines frequency and level of hygiene required. Heels, soles, and sides of feet are prone to irritation from ill-fitting shoes. Socks may become stained from bleeding or draining ulcer.

4. Assess circulation to extremities bilaterally: inspect color of skin; palpate temperature of toes, feet, and fingers and capillary refill of nails; palpate radial and ulnar pulse of each hand and dorsalis pedis pulse of foot; note character and symmetry of pulses (see Chapters 5 and 6). Remove gloves and perform hand hygiene.

   Extremities should always be assessed bilaterally to check for symmetry. Weak/absent pulses, pallor, decreased capillary refill and temperature are all signs of peripheral artery disease (PAD), which occurs when blood vessels in legs are narrowed or blocked by fatty deposits and blood flow to feet and legs decreases. Swelling, redness, and varicose veins indicate venous insufficiency (SVS, 2011).

5. Observe patient's walking gait (when appropriate). Have him or her walk down hall or walk straight line while wearing comfortable shoes or slippers (if able). Ask if patient has pain when walking (use pain scale).

   Alterations in bony structures of feet may cause pain, imbalance, and unsteady gait.

6. Ask if patient has history of leg pain on walking that is relieved with rest.

   Claudicating pain is related to ischemia with diabetic and neuropathic disorders.

7. Ask if patient uses nail polish and polish remover frequently.

   Chemicals in these products cause excessive dryness of nails.

8. Assess type of footwear patient wears: Does patient wear socks? Compression hose? Are shoes tight or ill fitting? Are garters or knee-high nylons worn? Is footwear clean?

   Some types of shoes and footwear predispose patient to foot and nail problems (e.g., infection, areas of friction, ulcerations).

9. Identify patient's risk for foot or nail problems.

   Certain conditions increase likelihood of foot or nail problems (e.g., diabetes mellitus, immunocompromised).

   a. Older adult

   Poor vision, lack of coordination, or inability to bend over contributes to difficulty in performing foot and nail care. Normal physiological changes of aging can result in brittle nails. Discolored, extremely thickened, and deformed nails can indicate infection, fungus, or disease (Anastasi et al., 2013).

   b. Diabetes mellitus

   Vascular changes reduce blood flow to peripheral tissues. Break in skin integrity places patient with diabetes mellitus at high risk for skin infection.

   c. Heart failure, renal disease

   Both conditions increase tissue edema, particularly in dependent areas (e.g., feet). Edema reduces blood flow to neighboring tissues.

   d. Cerebrovascular accident (stroke)

   Presence of residual foot or leg weakness or paralysis results in altered walking patterns. Altered gait pattern causes increased friction and pressure on feet.

STEP	RATIONALE
10. Assess for use of home remedies.	It is always a good idea to evaluate patient's self-care routine. Patient's personal care practices may overlap or clash with prescribed medical treatment. Collaborate with patient when possible to ensure best outcome possible.
a. Over-the-counter (OTC) liquid preparations to remove corns or warts	Patients with diabetes mellitus or circulatory insufficiency should seek professional treatment and avoid self-treating.
b. Cutting corns or calluses with razor blade or scissors	Carries risk for cutting skin, which can lead to infection.
c. Use of oval corn pads	May exert pressure on toes, thereby decreasing circulation to surrounding tissues. Seek professional treatment.
d. Application of adhesive tape	Skin of older adult is thin and delicate and prone to tearing when adhesive tape is removed.
11. Assess patient's ability to care for nails or feet: visual alterations, fatigue, and musculoskeletal weakness.	Extent of patient's ability to perform self-care determines degree of help required from nurse and need to educate family caregiver.

NURSING DIAGNOSES

- Bathing/self-care deficit
- Deficient knowledge regarding foot and nail care
- Impaired physical mobility
- Impaired skin integrity
- Ineffective tissue perfusion
- Risk for infection

Related factors are individualized based on patient's condition or needs.

PLANNING

1. Expected outcomes following completion of procedure:	
• Nails are smooth. Cuticles and tissues surrounding nail are clear and of normal color. Surfaces of feet are smooth.	Excess skin layers are removed. Nail integrity and cleanliness are maintained.
• Patient walks freely, without pain or unusual gait.	Foot care removes excess skin layers or shortens nails so patient can walk more comfortably.
• Patient explains or demonstrates nail care correctly.	Patient learns self-care skill.
2. Gather equipment and supplies at bedside on over-bed table.	Avoids interrupting procedure or leaving patient unattended to retrieve missing equipment.
3. Explain procedure to patient, including fact that proper soaking of nails on hands requires several minutes in warm water. Exception: Patients with diabetes mellitus do not soak hands or feet.	Patient must be willing to place fingers in basin up to 10 minutes. Patient may become anxious or tired.
4. Obtain health care provider's order for cutting nails (required by most agencies). Obtaining order for podiatry consultation should be initiated if patient has diabetes mellitus, PAD, or PVD.	Patient's skin may be cut accidentally. Certain patients are more at risk for infection, depending on their medical condition. A podiatrist should assess and develop a regular schedule for nail care for patients with vascular insufficiency or peripheral neuropathy.

IMPLEMENTATION

1. Perform hand hygiene and apply clean gloves.	Reduces transmission of infection. Easy access to equipment prevents delays.
2. Pull curtain around bed or close room door to provide privacy.	Maintaining patient's privacy reduces anxiety.
3. Help ambulatory patient sit in chair and place disposable bath mat on floor under patient's feet. Help bedfast patient to supine position with head of bed elevated 45 degrees and place waterproof pad on mattress (keep side rail up until ready to begin).	Sitting in chair facilitates immersing feet in basin. Bath mat protects feet from exposure to soil or debris.
4. Fill washbasin with warm water. Test water temperature. Place basin on floor or lower side rail and place basin on pad on mattress. Have patient immerse feet. If patient has diabetes mellitus, peripheral neuropathy, or PVD, go to Step 13 to begin foot care.	Prevents accidental burns to patient's skin.

STEP	RATIONALE

Clinical Decision Point *Patients who have diabetes mellitus, peripheral neuropathy, or PVD should not soak their hands and feet because of the increased risk of maceration that makes skin susceptible to infection.*

STEP	RATIONALE
5. Adjust over-bed table to low position and place it over patient's lap.	Easy access prevents accidental spills.
6. Fill emesis basin with warm water and place basin on towel on over-bed table. Test water temperature.	Warm water softens fingernails and thickened epidermal cells. Prevents accidental burns to patient's skin.
7. Instruct patient to place fingers in emesis basin and arms in comfortable position.	Prolonged positioning causes discomfort unless normal anatomical alignment is maintained.
8. Allow feet and fingernails to soak 5 to 10 minutes. If patient has diabetes mellitus, peripheral neuropathy, or PVD, skip this step and go straight to Step 9.	Goal is to soften debris beneath nails so it can be removed easily.
9. Clean gently under fingernails with end of plastic applicator stick while fingers are immersed (see illustration).	Removes debris under nails that harbors microorganisms.
10. Use soft cuticle brush or nailbrush to clean around cuticles to decrease overgrowth.	Nailbrush helps to prevent inflammation and injury to cuticles. The cuticle slowly grows over the nail and must be pushed back with a soft nail brush regularly.
11. Remove emesis basin and dry fingers thoroughly.	Thorough drying impedes fungal growth and prevents maceration of tissues.

Clinical Decision Point *Check agency policy for appropriate process for cleaning beneath nails. Do not use an orange stick or end of cotton swab; these splinter and can cause injury.*

STEP	RATIONALE
12. *Check agency policy on nail care regarding filing and trimming.* Trim nails straight across at level of finger or follow curve of finger, ensuring that you do not cut down into nail grooves (see illustration). Use disposable emery board and file nail to ensure that there are no sharp corners.	Trimming straight across avoids skin overgrowth at nail edges, which can lead to ingrown nails or infection. Filing nail straight across to eliminate sharp nail edges minimizes risk that nail can injure the adjacent finger (Anastasi et al., 2013).
13. Move over-bed table away from patient. Begin foot care by scrubbing callused areas of feet with washcloth.	Provides easier access to feet. Friction removes dead skin layers.
14. Clean between toes with washcloth.	
15. Dry feet thoroughly and trim or cut toenails (see Step 12).	Moisture can cause skin maceration.
16. Apply lotion to feet and hands. Rub in thoroughly. Do not leave excess lotion between toes.	Lotion lubricates dry skin by helping to retain moisture.
17. Help patient back to bed and into comfortable, safe position, leaving call light within reach.	
18. Sanitize equipment according to organizational policy and return equipment to proper place. Emery boards should be disposable. Dispose of soiled linen in dirty laundry bag. Remove gloves and perform hand hygiene.	Reduces transmission of infection.

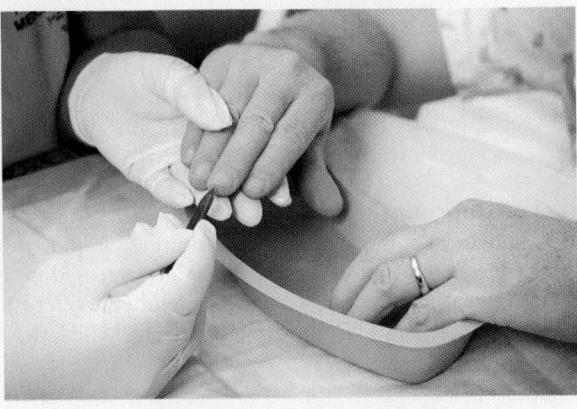

STEP 9 Clean under fingernails.

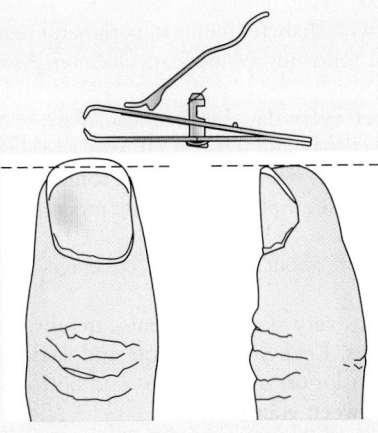

STEP 12 Trim nails straight across when using nail clipper.

STEP	RATIONALE

EVALUATION

1. Inspect nails, areas between fingers and toes, and surrounding skin surfaces.
2. If possible, have patient stand and walk and rate any pain.

3. Observe patient's walk after foot and nail care.
4. **Use Teach-Back:** "We discussed how to prevent infection in the skin around your nails. This is important because you have diabetes. Tell me the tips you should follow to protect your feet from infection." Revise your instruction now or develop a plan for revised patient or family caregiver teaching if patient or family caregiver is not able to teach back correctly.

Inspection enables you to evaluate condition of skin and nails and allows you to note any remaining rough nail edges.
Evaluates if nail care removed excess skin or uneven nail surfaces that can cause discomfort.
Evaluate level of comfort and mobility achieved.
Determines patient's and family caregiver's level of understanding of instructional topic.

Unexpected Outcomes
1. Cuticles and surrounding tissues are inflamed and tender to touch.

2. Localized areas of tenderness occur on feet with calluses or corns at point of friction.

3. Ulcerations involving toes or feet may remain.

Related Interventions
- Repeat nail care.
- Evaluate need for antifungal cream.
- Change in footwear or corrective foot surgery may be needed for permanent improvement in calluses or corns.
- Refer patient to podiatrist.
- Institute wound care policies (see Chapters 39 and 40).
- Consult with wound care specialist and/or podiatrist.
- Increase frequency of assessment and hygiene.

Recording and Reporting
- Record procedure and observations of condition of nails and skin around nails in medical record in nurses' notes in electronic health record (EHR) or chart.
- Report any areas of discomfort, breaks in skin, or ulcerations to nurse in charge or health care provider.
- Document your evaluation of patient and family caregiver learning.

Special Considerations
Teaching
- Use a variety of teaching formats regarding foot and nail care (e.g., brochures, videos, DVDs) that are consistent with patient's health literacy level. Instruct patient not to walk barefoot or use corn or callus products. Include family caregiver in foot and nail care education.
- Instruct a patient with diabetes mellitus, peripheral neuropathy, or PVD to do the following (American Diabetes Association, 2014):
  - Check your feet every day. Look at your bare feet for red spots, cuts, swelling, and blisters. If you cannot see the bottoms of your feet, use a mirror or ask someone for help.
  - Be more active. Plan a physical activity program with your health care team.
  - Ask your doctor about Medicare coverage for special shoes.
  - Wash your feet every day. Dry them carefully, especially between the toes. Keep your skin soft and smooth. Rub a thin coat of skin lotion over the tops and bottoms of your feet, but not between your toes.
  - If you can see and reach your toenails, trim them when needed.
  - Wear shoes and socks at all times. Never walk barefoot.
  - Wear comfortable shoes that fit well and protect your feet. Check inside your shoes before wearing them. Make sure that the lining is smooth and there are no objects inside.
  - Protect your feet from hot and cold. Wear shoes at the beach or on hot pavement.
  - Do not put your feet into hot water. Test water before putting your feet in it just as you would before bathing a baby. Never use hot water bottles, heating pads, or electric blankets. You can burn your feet without realizing it.
  - Put your feet up when sitting. Wiggle your toes and move your ankles up and down for 5 minutes 2 or 3 times a day. Do not cross your legs for long periods of time.
  - Do not smoke. See more at: http://www.diabetes.org/living-with-diabetes/complications/foot-complications/foot-care.html#sthash.Kzope5wg.dpuf.

Pediatric
- Teach a parent how to assess a child's nails and trim them to prevent the child from scratching the skin.
- Use appropriate-size clippers for infants and small children (check agency policy). *Do not use scissors.*

Gerontological
- Changes in aging skin include thinning of epidermis and subcutaneous fat and dryness because of decreased activity of oil and sweat glands. These changes are often evident in the feet. In addition, nails become discolored, thickened, deformed, and brittle.
- PVD, peripheral neuropathy, and long periods of limited exercise or bed rest impact balance, stability, and sensory impairment, resulting in impaired mobility.

- Older adults may lose the dexterity and coordination needed to trim nails regularly.

Home Care

- Assess the home for any areas where a person could accidentally injure the feet such as rugs, objects that block pathways, or uneven walks or flooring.

- Encourage patients to not go barefoot or wear open-toed shoes.
- *Alternative therapy:* Apply moleskin to friction areas of the foot or feet or wrap small pieces of lamb's wool around toes to reduce irritation from corns or bunions.
- Place contact information of podiatrist, health care provider, and home care nurse close by for easy access.

PROCEDURAL GUIDELINE 18.6 *Making an Occupied Bed*

The hospital bed is the piece of equipment a patient uses the most. It should be comfortable, safe, and adaptable to various positions. The typical hospital bed consists of a firm mattress on a metal frame that you can raise or lower horizontally. The frame is divided into three sections so the operator can raise and lower the head and foot of the bed separately and incline the entire bed with the head up or down. Table 18.4 shows common bed positions. Each bed sits on four casters that allow you to move it easily. Each caster has a brake to make sure the bed is stationary. Beds have side rails (adjustable metal frames) that you can raise or lower by pushing or pulling a knob located on both sides of the bed. Research shows that the risk for patient falls is greater when side rails on both sides of a bed are raised because patients try to climb over the rails to exit the bed. Raising only one rail (when there are only two) or three (when there are four rails) gives patients an exit to move independently.

At times it is necessary to make a bed that is occupied by a patient who cannot tolerate being out of bed. If a patient is confined to bed, you should make the bed in a way that conserves time and the patient's energy. A patient's weight, ability to move and turn, pain acuity, and restrictions related to clinical condition or treatment all affect the number of individuals who need to be

---

TABLE 18.4		
Common Bed Positions		
Position	**Description**	**Uses**
Fowler's 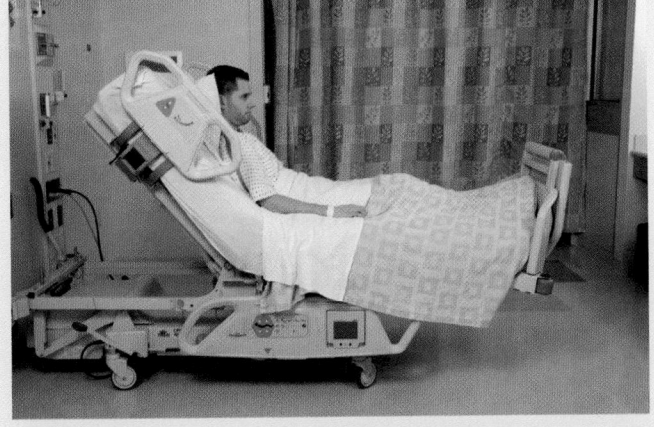	Head of bed raised to angle of 45 to 90 degrees; semisitting position; foot of bed may also raise at knee	Preferred while patient eats; used during nasogastric tube insertion and nasotracheal suction; promotes lung expansion
Semi-Fowler's 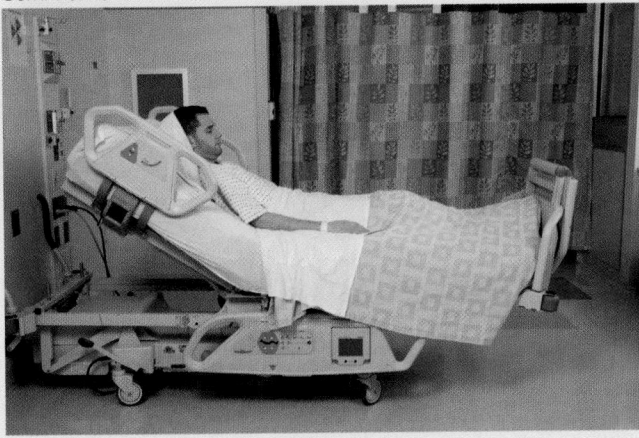	Head of bed raised approximately 30 to 45 degrees; incline less than Fowler's position; foot of bed may also raise at knee	Promotes lung expansion; relieves strain on abdominal muscles Used when patients receive gastric feedings to reduce risk for aspiration

Continued

PROCEDURAL GUIDELINE 18.6 *Making an Occupied Bed—cont'd*

TABLE 18.4

Common Bed Positions—cont'd

Position	Description	Uses
Trendelenburg's 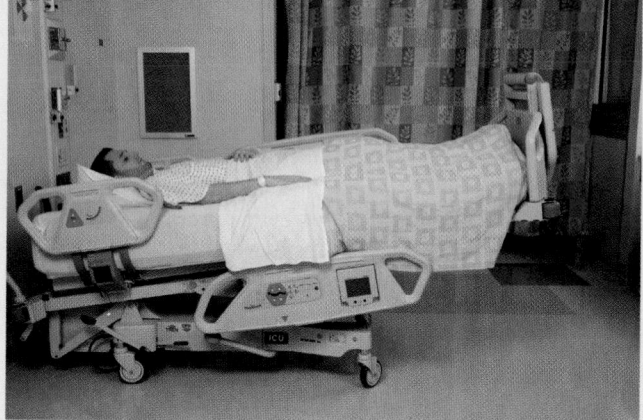	Entire bedframe tilted with head of bed down	For postural drainage; facilitates venous return in patients with poor peripheral perfusion
Reverse Trendelenburg's 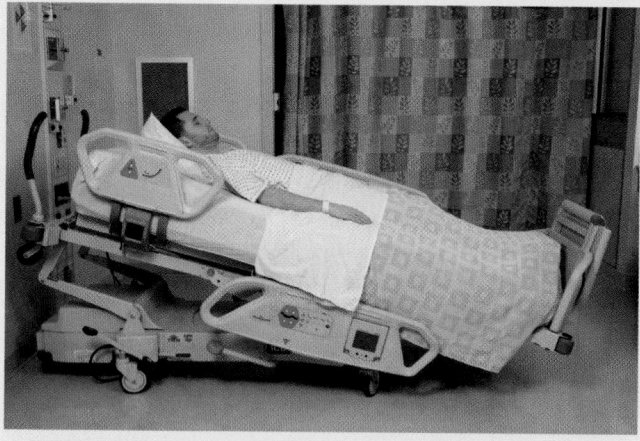	Entire bedframe tilted with foot of bed down	Used infrequently; promotes gastric emptying and prevents esophageal reflux
Supine or flat 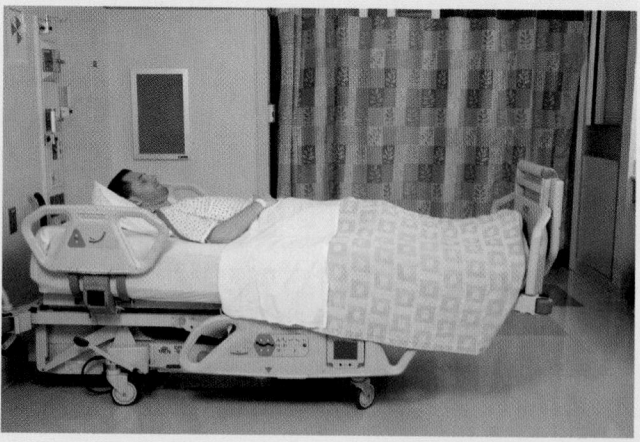	Entire bedframe horizontally parallel with floor	For patients with vertebral injuries and in cervical traction; position used for patients who are hypotensive and generally preferred by patients for sleeping

involved in making an occupied bed. Using safe patient-handling techniques when you turn and position a patient over bed linen is essential (see Chapter 11). In cases in which a patient experiences severe pain, an analgesic administered 30 to 60 minutes before making a bed can control pain and maintain comfort.

Even though a patient is unable to get out of bed, encourage self-help as much as possible. For example, if patients can turn, help in moving up in bed, or hold top sheets during application, have them do so. These activities help maintain a patient's strength and mobility and allow participation in hygiene care.

PROCEDURAL GUIDELINE 18.6 *Making an Occupied Bed—cont'd*

Delegation Considerations

The skill of making an occupied bed can be delegated to nursing assistive personnel (NAP). The nurse instructs the NAP about:

- Any position or activity restrictions that apply.
- Looking for wound drainage or loosened equipment that might be found in the bed linens.
- When to obtain help from other caregivers for positioning a patient during linen change and the importance of using good body mechanics and supporting patient alignment.
- Using special precautions (e.g., aspiration precautions [see Chapter 31] or positioning for tube-feeding infusion [see Chapter 32]) when positioning a patient during bed making.

Equipment

- Linen bags
- Mattress pad (change only when soiled)
- Bottom sheet (flat or fitted)
- Drawsheet (*optional*)
- Top sheet, blanket, bedspread, pillowcases
- Waterproof pads (*optional*)
- Clean gloves (if linen is soiled or there is risk of exposure to body fluids)
- Antiseptic cleanser
- Washcloth

Procedural Steps

1. Review medical record and assess restrictions in mobility/positioning of patient.
2. Organize supplies and close room door or divider curtain to provide privacy.
3. Assess environment for safety (e.g., check room for spills; make sure that equipment is working properly and that bed is in locked position and appropriate number of side rails are raised).
4. Perform hand hygiene. Apply clean gloves if patient has been incontinent or if drainage is present on linen.
5. Explain procedure to patient, noting that patient will be asked to turn over layers of linen.
6. Raise bed to a comfortable working height; lower head of bed (HOB) as tolerated, keeping patient comfortable. Remove call light.

Clinical Decision Point *If patient is on aspiration precautions or receiving tube feeding, keep HOB no lower than 30 degrees.*

7. Lower side rail on side where you are standing. Loosen all top linen. Remove bedspread and blanket separately, leaving patient covered with top sheet. If blanket or spread is soiled, place in linen bag. If to be reused, fold into square and place over back of chair.
8. Cover patient with clean bath blanket by unfolding it over top sheet. Have patient hold top edge of bath blanket or tuck blanket under shoulders. Grasp top sheet under bath blanket at patient's shoulders and bring sheet down to foot of bed. Remove sheet and discard in dirty laundry bag.
9. Position patient on far side of bed, turned onto side and facing away from you. **NOTE:** This is when another caregiver can help you by standing at bedside across from

you. Encourage patient to use side rail to turn. Adjust pillow under patient's head.

10. Assess to make sure that there is no tension on any external medical devices.
11. Loosen bottom linens, moving from head to foot. Fanfold or roll any cloth pads, drawsheet (if present), and bottom sheet (in that order) toward patient. Tuck edges of old linen just under patient's buttocks, back, and shoulders (see illustration). Do not fanfold mattress pad (if it is to be reused). Remove any disposable pads and discard in receptacle.

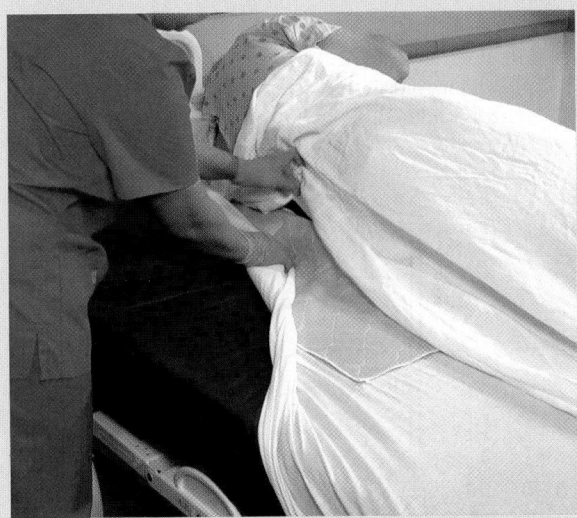

STEP 11 Tuck all soiled linen from one side of bed alongside patient's back.

12. Clean, disinfect, and dry mattress surface if it is soiled or has moisture (see agency policy).
13. Apply clean linens to the exposed half of bed in separate layers. When needed, start with a new mattress pad by placing it lengthwise with center crease in middle of bed. Fanfold pad to center of bed alongside patient. Repeat process with bottom sheet.
14. Pull new fitted sheet smoothly over mattress corner at top and bottom of bed. If using a flat sheet, allow edge of sheet to hang about 25 cm (10 inches) over mattress edge at head of bed. Be sure that lower hem of bottom flat sheet lies seam down and with bottom edge of mattress.
15. If bottom sheet is flat, miter top corner at HOB. Face HOB diagonally. Place hand away from HOB under top corner of mattress, lift, and with other hand tuck edge of bottom sheet smoothly under mattress so side edges of sheet above and below mattress meet when brought together.
16. If bottom sheet is flat, miter top corner at HOB.
    a. Face HOB diagonally. Place hand away from HOB under top corner of mattress, near mattress edge, and lift.
    b. With other hand, tuck top edge of bottom sheet smoothly under mattress so side edges of sheet above and below mattress meet when brought together.
    c. To miter a corner, pick up top edge of sheet at about 45 cm (18 inches) from top end of mattress (see illustration).

Continued

PROCEDURAL GUIDELINE 18.6 *Making an Occupied Bed—cont'd*

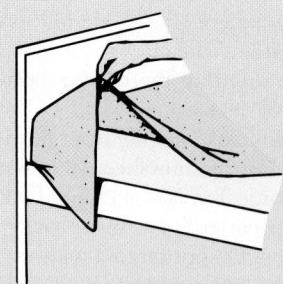

STEP 16c Top edge of sheet picked up.

d. Lift sheet and lay it on top of mattress to form a neat triangular fold with lower base of triangle even with mattress side edges (see illustration).

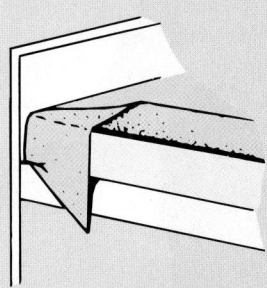

STEP 16d Sheet on top of mattress in a triangular fold.

e. Tuck lower edge of sheet, which is hanging free below the mattress, under the mattress. Tuck with palms down, without pulling triangular fold.

f. Hold part of sheet covering side of mattress in place with one hand (see illustrations). With other hand pick up top of triangular linen fold and bring it down over side of mattress. Tuck under mattress with palms down without pulling fold (see illustration).

17. Tuck remaining part of sheet under mattress, moving toward foot of bed. Keep linen smooth.

18. Place new drawsheet along middle of bed lengthwise. Fanfold or roll drawsheet on top of clean bottom sheet. Tuck under patient's buttocks and torso without touching old linen.

19. Add waterproof pad (absorbent side up) over drawsheet with seam side down. Fanfold toward patient. Continue to keep clean and soiled linen separate. Also keep linen under patient as flat as possible because patient will need to roll over old and new layers of linen when you are ready to make other side of bed.

20. Advise patient that he or she will be rolling over a thick layer of linens. Keeping patient covered; ask him or her to roll toward you slowly over layers of linen and to not raise the hips (see illustration). Stress the need to roll while staying aligned.

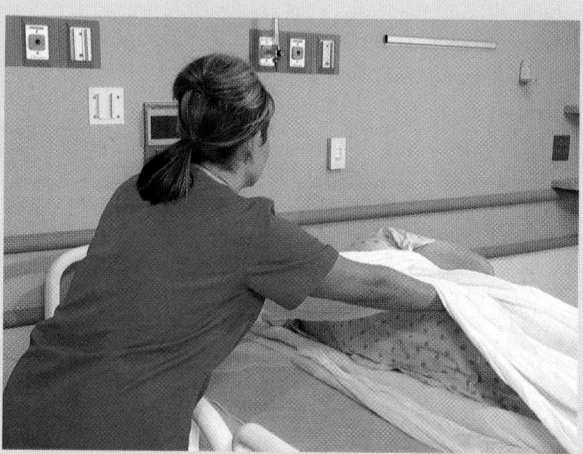

STEP 20 Patient begins rolling over layers of linen.

21. You will now raise side rail and move to opposite side of bed. *Option:* The caregiver helping you will help position patient. Have patient roll away from you toward other side of bed, over all of the folds of linen. Again have patient keep hips still.

22. Loosen edges of soiled linen from under mattress. Remove soiled linen by folding into a bundle or square.

23. Hold linen away from your body and place it in laundry bag.

24. Clean, disinfect, and dry other half of mattress as needed.

25. Pull clean, fanfolded or rolled mattress pad; sheet; drawsheet; and pad out from beneath patient toward you. Smooth all linen out over mattress from head to foot of bed. Help patient roll back to supine position and reposition pillow.

26. If bottom sheet is fitted, pull corners over mattress edges. If flat sheet is used, miter top corner of bottom flat sheet (see Steps 16a–f).

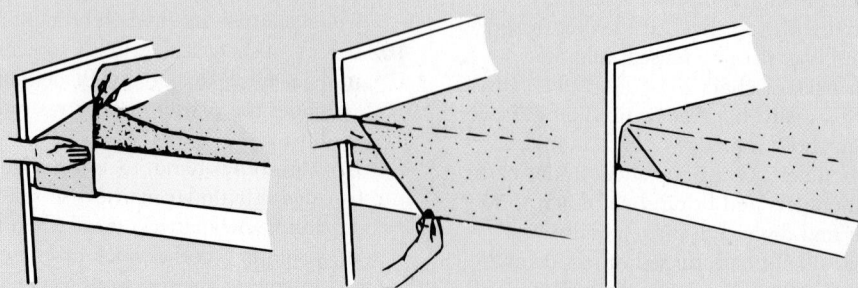

STEP 16f Triangular fold placed over side of mattress; sheet tucked under mattress.

PROCEDURAL GUIDELINE 18.6 *Making an Occupied Bed—cont'd*

27. Facing side of bed, grasp remaining edge of bottom flat sheet. Lean back slightly, keep back straight, and pull while tucking excess linen under mattress from HOB to foot of bed. Avoid lifting mattress during tucking.
28. Smooth fanfolded drawsheet over bottom sheet (tucking is optional). Smooth waterproof pads, making sure that bed surface is wrinkle free.
29. Place top sheet over patient with vertical centerfold lengthwise down middle of bed and with seam side of hem facing up. Open sheet out from head to foot and unfold over patient. Be sure that top edge of sheet is even with top edge of mattress.
30. Place clean or reused bed blanket on bed over patient. Make sure that top edge is parallel with top edge of sheet and 15 to 20 cm (6 to 8 inches) from edge of top sheet. Raise side rail.
31. Go to other side of bed. Lower side rail. Spread sheet and blanket out evenly.
32. Have patient hold onto sheet and blanket while you remove bath blanket; discard in linen bag.
33. Make cuff by turning edge of top sheet down over top edge of blanket.
34. Make horizontal toe pleat; stand at foot of bed and fanfold in sheet and blanket 5 to 10 cm (2 to 4 inches) across bed. Pull sheet and blanket up from bottom to make fold approximately 15 cm (6 inches) from bottom edge of mattress.
35. Standing at side of bed, tuck in remaining part of sheet and blanket under foot of mattress. Tuck top sheet and blanket together. Be sure that toe pleats are not pulled out.
36. Make modified mitered corner with top sheet and blanket. Follow Steps 16a–f). After making triangular fold, do not tuck tip of triangle (see illustration).
37. Go to other side of bed. Repeat Steps 35 and 36.
38. Change pillowcase. Have patient raise head. While supporting neck with one hand, remove pillow. Allow patient to lower head. Remove soiled case and place in linen bag. Grasp clean pillowcase at center of closed end. Gather case, turning it inside out over the hand holding it. With the same hand, pick up middle of one end of pillow. Pull pillowcase down over pillow with other hand. Do not hold pillow against your uniform. Be sure that pillow corners fit evenly into corners of case. Reposition pillow under patient's head.
39. Place call light within patient's reach on bedrail or pillow; return bed to locked, low position; and raise side rail (as needed).
40. Place all linen in dirty laundry bag. Remove and dispose of gloves.
41. Arrange and organize patient's room and perform hand hygiene.
42. During procedure inspect skin for areas of irritation. Observe patient for signs of fatigue, dyspnea, pain, or other sources of discomfort.

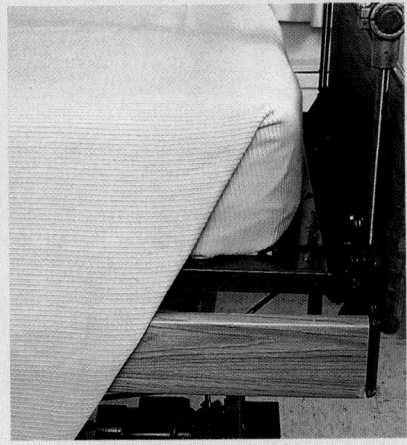

STEP 36 Modified mitered corner.

PROCEDURAL GUIDELINE 18.7 *Making an Unoccupied Bed*

A bed may be made with the patient out of the bed (unoccupied) or in the bed (occupied). In some settings bed linen is not changed every day; however, you always need to change any wet or soiled linen promptly. Moisture on bed linen can easily lead to skin breakdown. An unoccupied bed is one left open with the top sheets fanfolded down. A postoperative surgical bed is prepared for patients returning from the operating room (OR) or procedural area. The bed is left with the top sheets fanfolded lengthwise and not tucked in to facilitate a patient's transfer from a stretcher. A closed bed, which is made with the top sheets pulled up to the head of the bed, is made by the housekeeping department after a patient is discharged and the bed is cleaned.

Delegation and Collaboration
The skill of making an unoccupied bed can be delegated to nursing assistive personnel (NAP). The nurse instructs the NAP about:

- Position or activity restrictions that apply to patient's ability to get out of and back into bed.
- The type of special linen to use if patient is on an airflow mattress.

Equipment
- Linen/laundry bags
- Mattress pad (change only when soiled)
- Bottom sheet (flat or fitted)
- Drawsheet (*optional*)
- Waterproof pads (*optional*)
- Top sheet, blanket, spread, pillowcases
- Clean gloves (If linen is soiled or if there is risk of exposure to body fluids)
- Antiseptic cleanser
- Washcloth

Continued

PROCEDURAL GUIDELINE 18.7 *Making an Unoccupied Bed—cont'd*

Procedural Steps

1. Perform hand hygiene. Arrange supplies at beside.
2. Assess environment for safety (e.g., check room for spills; make sure that equipment is working properly and that bed is in locked, low position).
3. Pull room divider curtain or close room door to provide privacy. Follow steps for transferring patient to bedside chair or recliner (see Chapter 11).
4. Lower remaining side rails on bed and raise bed to comfortable working position.
5. Apply clean gloves if linen is soiled with body fluids. Remove all linen, hold away from uniform, and place in laundry bag. Avoid shaking or fanning linen.
6. Straighten mattress and wipe off any moisture with a washcloth moistened in antiseptic solution (consult agency housekeeping guidelines). Dry thoroughly.
7. Apply all bottom linen on one side of bed before moving to opposite side.
   a. For fitted sheet: Make sure that fitted sheet is placed smoothly over mattress and top and bottom mattress edge. Fit corners on one end and then the other.
   b. For flat sheet: Place sheet over mattress. Allow about 25 cm (10 inches) to hang over side mattress edge. Lower hem of sheet should lie seam down, even with bottom edge of mattress. Pull remaining top part of sheet over top edge of mattress. While standing at head of bed, miter top corner of bottom sheet (see Procedural Guideline 18.6, Step16a–f). Tuck remaining part of flat bottom sheet under mattress.
   c. *Optional:* Apply drawsheet and/or waterproof pad laying centerfold along middle of bed lengthwise. Smooth drawsheet/pad over mattress. Tuck excess edge of drawsheet under mattress, keeping palms down.
8. Move to opposite side of bed. Repeat Step 7.
9. Place top sheet over bed with vertical centerfold lengthwise down middle of bed. Open sheet out from head to foot, being sure that top edge of sheet is even with top edge of mattress. *Optional:* Spread a blanket or bedspread evenly over top sheet in same fashion.
10. Standing on one side at foot of bed, lift mattress corner slightly with one hand and with other hand tuck top sheet and blanket or spread under mattress.
11. Make modified mitered corner with top sheet, blanket, and spread. After making triangular fold, leave tip of triangle untucked (see Procedural Guideline 18.6, Step 36).
12. Make cuff by turning edge of top sheet down over top edge of blanket and spread.
13. Standing on one side at foot of bed, lift mattress corner slightly with one hand and with other hand tuck top sheet, blanket, and spread under mattress. Be sure that toe pleats are not pulled out.
14. Make modified mitered corner with top sheet, blanket, and spread. After making triangular fold, do not tuck tip of triangle (see Procedural Guideline 18.6, Step 36).
15. Go to other side of bed. Spread sheet, blanket, and spread out evenly. Make cuff with top sheet and blanket (closed bed). Make modified corner at foot of bed. Alternatively, fanfold sheet, blanket, and spread at foot of bed, with top layer ready to be pulled up (this leaves an open bed).
    Optional: Make horizontal toe pleat; stand at foot of bed and fanfold in sheet 5 to 10 cm (2 to 4 inches) across bed. Pull sheet up from bottom to make fold approximately 15 cm (6 inches) from bottom edge of mattress.
16. Apply clean pillowcase.
17. Place call light within patient's reach on bedrail or pillow and return bed to lowest position, allowing for patient transfer. Help patient to bed.
18. Place linen bag in dirty laundry bag. Remove and dispose of gloves.
19. Arrange and organize patient's room and perform hand hygiene.

◆ CLINICAL DEBRIEF

A 78-year-old male has a 3-year history of type 1 diabetes mellitus and hypertension. He was just discharged after 5 days of hospitalization with diagnoses of healing right-heel ulcer and controlled hypertension. His discharge summary notes that he requires help with daily dressing changes for the ulcer. He lives alone and is able to perform all routine activities of daily living (ADLs). During the initial home visit his vital signs were as follows: temp 37°C, pulse 86, BP 135/85, respiratory rate 30. The home health nurse noted a right-heal ulcer 2 cm × 2 cm; no drainage noted. A 4 × 4 dressing was applied, covered, and wrapped with gauze cling wrap. The nurse assessed that, although the patient understands the need for the daily dressing changes, he is not able to state which precautions are needed to prevent any recurrence.

1. List three actions that he should follow for maintaining good foot care.
2. A patient with diabetes mellitus has risk for oral problems for which of the following reasons?

1. Break in mucosa increases risk for infection. Vigorous brushing can disrupt suture lines.
2. Mucosa becomes thin and less elastic.
3. Irritation of oral mucosa.
4. Dryness of mouth with gingivitis.
3. Using SBAR show how would you communicate with the health care team about this patient's status.

◆ REVIEW QUESTIONS

1. A critically ill patient with an endotracheal tube and on mechanical ventilation is at risk for ventilator-associated pneumonia (VAP) for which of the following reasons? (Select all that apply.)
   1. The mucus inside the artificial airway grows gram-negative bacteria.

2. An endotracheal tube bypasses normal airway defenses, leading to a change in the normal oral flora.
3. A critically ill patient often has a reduced gag reflex.
4. Presence of an endotracheal tube makes it impossible to suction oral secretions.
5. Critically ill patients have an abnormal amount of mucosa released in oral cavity.

2. Which of the following actions are steps used when making an unoccupied bed? (Select all that apply.)
1. Raise bed to working height.
2. Wear clean gloves at all times.
3. Apply all bottom linen on one side of bed before moving to opposite side.
4. Remove soiled linen and place on the floor.
5. Tuck top sheet and blanket in at bottom of bed using a modified mitered corner.
6. Keep top blanket at head of bed when procedure is completed.
7. Make horizontal toe pleat with all top layers of linen.

3. Place the following steps for providing oral care to a debilitated patient in the correct order.
1. Remove dentures or partial plates if present.
2. Apply thin layer of water-soluble moisturizer to lips.
3. Perform hand hygiene and apply clean gloves.
4. Brush inner and outer surfaces of upper and lower teeth by brushing from gum to crown of each tooth; then clean biting surfaces of teeth.
5. If needed, turn on suction machine and connect tubing to suction catheter.
6. Position patient in side-lying position with head turned toward mattress in dependent position.
7. If patient is uncooperative or having difficulty keeping mouth open, insert an oral airway.

ⓔ *Visit the Evolve site for a complete list of Clinical Debrief and Review Questions answers.*

REFERENCES

Agency for Healthcare Research and Quality (AHRQ): *National guideline clearinghouse: bathing persons with dementia,* 2013a, https://www.guideline.gov/content.aspx?id=44984. Accessed April 2, 2016.

Agency for Healthcare Research and Quality (AHRQ): *Universal ICU decolonization: an enhanced protocol,* 2013b, http://www.ahrq.gov/professionals/systems/hospital/universal_icu_decolonization/universal-icu-ape4.html. Accessed April 2, 2016.

American Academy of Pediatric Dentistry (AAPD): *Guideline on infant oral health care,* 2014, http://www.aapd.org/media/policies_guidelines/g_infantoralhealthcare.pdf. Accessed April 2, 2016.

American Academy of Pediatrics (AAP): *Brushing up on oral health: never too late to start,* 2014, https://www.healthychildren.org/English/healthy-living/oral-health/Pages/Brushing-Up-on-Oral-Health-Never-Too-Early-to-Start.aspx. Accessed April 2, 2016.

American Dental Association (ADA): *American Dental Association statement on regular dental visits,* 2013, http://www.ada.org/en/press-room/news-releases/2013-archive/june/american-dental-association-statement-on-regular-dental-visits. Accessed April 2, 2016.

American Dental Association (ADA): *Mouth healthy,* 2016a, http://www.mouthhealthy.org/en/az-topics/b/brushing-your-teeth. Accessed April 2, 2016.

American Dental Association (ADA): *Learn more about mouth rinses,* 2016b, http://www.ada.org/en/science-research/ada-seal-of-acceptance/product-category-information/mouthrinses. Accessed April 2, 2016.

American Diabetes Association: *Foot care,* 2014, http://www.diabetes.org/living-with-diabetes/complications/foot-complications/foot-care.html. Accessed April 2, 2016.

Anastasi JK, et al: HIV peripheral neuropathy and foot care management: a review of assessment and relevant guidelines, *Am J Nurs* 113(12):4, 2013.

Centers for Disease Control and Prevention (CDC): *Oral and dental health,* 2015, http://www.cdc.gov/nchs/fastats/dental.htm. Accessed April 2, 2016.

Chen W, et al: Effects of daily bathing with chlorhexidine and acquired infection of methicillin-resistant *Staphylococcus aureus* and vancomycin-resistant *Enterococcus:* a meta-analysis, *J Thorac Dis* 5(4):518, 2013.

Climo MW, et al: Effect of daily chlorhexidine bathing on hospital-acquired infection, *N Engl J Med* 368:533, 2013.

Johnson D, et al: Patients' bath basins as potential sources of infection: a multi-center sampling study, *Am J Crit Care* 18(1):31, 2009.

Klompas M, et al: Reappraisal of routine oral care with chlorhexidine gluconate for patients receiving mechanical ventilation: systematic review and meta-analysis, *JAMA Intern Med* 174(5):751, 2014.

Meiner S: *Gerontologic nursing,* ed 4, St Louis, 2010, Mosby.

Munoz-Price LS, et al: Effectiveness of stepwise interventions targeted to decrease central catheter-associated bloodstream infections, *Crit Care Med* 40(5):1464, 2012.

National Cancer Institute (NCI): *Oral complications of chemotherapy and head/neck radiation (PDQ),* 2016, http://www.cancer.gov/cancertopics/pdq/supportivecare/oralcomplications/Patient. Accessed April 2, 2016.

National Institute of Dental and Craniofacial Research: *Older adults and oral health,* 2015, http://www.nidcr.nih.gov/oralhealth/OralHealthInformation/OlderAdults/. Accessed April 2, 2016.

National Pediculosis Association: *Welcome to HeadLice.org,* 2016, http://www.headlice.org/index.html. Accessed July 8, 2016.

National Pressure Ulcer Advisory Panel (NPUAP): *Prevention and treatment of pressure ulcers: clinical practice guideline,* 2014, http://www.npuap.org/wp-content/uploads/2014/08/Quick-Reference-Guide-DIGITAL-NPUAP-EPUAP-PPPIA-Jan2016.pdf. Accessed April 2, 2016.

Petlin A, et al: Chlorhexidine gluconate bathing to reduce methicillin-resistant *Staphylococcus aureus* acquisition, *Crit Care Nurse* 34(5):17, 2014.

Quality and Safety Education for Nurses (QSEN): *Pre-licensure KSAs,* 2014, http://qsen.org/competencies/pre-licensure-ksas/. Accessed April 2, 2016.

Shah HN, et al: Bathing with 2% chlorhexidine gluconate: evidence and costs associated with central line–associated bloodstream infections, *Crit Care Nurs Q* 39(1):42, 2016.

The Joint Commission (TJC): *2016 National Patient Safety Goals,* 2016, http://www.jointcommission.org/standards_information/npsgs.aspx. Accessed April 2, 2016.

The Society for Vascular Surgery (SVS): *Chronic venous insufficiency,* 2011, https://vascular.org/patient-resources/vascular-conditions/chronic-venous-insufficiency. Accessed April 2, 2016.

Villa A, et al: Diagnosis and management of xerostomia and hyposalivation, *Ther Clin Risk Manag* 5(11):45, 2015.

Wiech E, Bayer D: Simple interventions for ventilator-associated pneumonia, *Nursing2012 Crit Care* 7(3):19, 2012.

19 | Care of the Eye and Ear

OBJECTIVES

Mastery of content in this chapter will enable the nurse to:
- Explain safety guidelines used in the care of eye and ear prostheses.
- Identify patient-centered care guidelines used in caring for eye and ear prostheses.
- Correctly remove, store, clean, and insert a contact lens.
- Correctly perform eye and ear irrigations.
- Describe techniques that determine whether a hearing aid functions properly.
- Correctly remove, clean, and reinsert a hearing aid.

MEDIA RESOURCES

- evolve http://evolve.elsevier.com/Perry/skills
- Review Questions
- Audio Glossary
- Clinical Debrief and Review Questions Answers

PURPOSE

Vision and hearing are two special senses that help people carry out all daily and recreational activities. Risks to a patients' eye or ear structures or function can alter independence, safety, body image, and self-confidence. The skills in this chapter show how to help patients protect their vision and hearing and use artificial sensory devices correctly to replace or restore sensory function.

STANDARDS OF CARE

- American Academy of Audiology, 2015—Clinical Practice Guidelines: adult patients with severe-to profound unilateral sensorineural hearing loss
- The Joint Commission, 2016—National Patient Safety Goals, Patient Identification

PRINCIPLES FOR PRACTICE

- Meaningful sensory stimuli help people learn about their environment.
- Receiving and understanding environmental stimuli promote healthy functioning.
- Alteration in a patient's vision and hearing affects health literacy, independence, and adherence to medical and pharmacological therapies.
- Artificial sensory aids can restore some vision and hearing loss. However, these aids must fit and work properly for patients to function optimally in their environments.
- When caring for patients who use aids to help with visual or auditory loss, it is important that you and the health care team, along with the patient and his or her family, understand how to clean and care for these aids. Breakage or loss of an aid is expensive.

PATIENT-CENTERED CARE

- When a patient is without visual or hearing devices, communication is altered, and the patient is isolated socially and becomes more dependent (American Academy of Audiology, 2015; Ekberg et al., 2014).
- The noises within hospitals, rehabilitation centers, and skilled nursing facilities make hearing difficult. The hard flooring surfaces, medical equipment, televisions, and constant need to speak with other health care professionals all produce noise.
- Hearing-impaired patients need time to adjust to their hearing aid. For example, increased background noise makes hearing with an aid even more difficult. The noisy environments of hospitals and other health care facilities further contribute to adjustment to hearing aids (Dawes et al., 2014).
- When a patient has auditory impairments, the increased background noise in an unfamiliar environment often makes a patient more anxious and decreases his or her ability to adjust to new surroundings.
- At times you use touch to get the attention of a patient with severe visual loss or decreased hearing. Remember to ask patients if touch is permitted. In some cultures same-sex caregivers are required before touch can be used.

- Understand the cause of a person's sensory loss and then determine the patient's own perception of the reason for the loss.
- Identify a patient's usual practices in using and maintaining sensory assistive devices.

EVIDENCE-BASED PRACTICE

Dual sensory impairment (DSI), the concurrent losses in vision and hearing, has the potential to cause cognitive function decline or contribute to acute confusion or depression and increased mortality risk (Gopinath et al., 2013; Heine et al., 2015; Vreeken et al., 2014).

- DSI in rehabilitation or long-term care settings affects a patient's independence, socialization, and success in using assistive devices and rehabilitation services (Dawes et al., 2014; Tremblay, 2015).
- There is mounting evidence that there are central effects of biological aging and peripheral pathology that affect a person's neural detection of sound, which occurs as early as middle age (Tremblay, 2015). Older adults may not actually perceive their hearing loss because initially it is mild; however, as it progresses, they usually avoid or delay hearing evaluation (Chou et al., 2011; Mick et al., 2014).
- There are multiple definitions and classifications of levels of vision impairment and blindness, which adds to the complexity in understanding DSI (Gopinath et al., 2013). In addition, the psychosocial and functional impacts of DSI are not well understood when compared with those of a single sensory impairment (Roets-Merken et al., 2014).
- Identify patients at risk for hearing impairments: male over age 65, male or female over age 75, resident in nursing facility, existing visual impairment, chronic ear infection, prolonged exposure to loud noises, and use of ototoxic medication (Chou et al., 2011; Heine et al., 2015).

- Involving patients with DSI in volunteer work has been shown to result in fewer depressive symptoms compared to people without sensory loss who volunteer (White, 2015).
- Patients with DSI have unique communication needs that require a thorough assessment (Roets-Merken et al., 2014).

SAFETY GUIDELINES

- Whenever you care for patients with sensory alterations, safety is a priority. Anticipate how the sensory alteration places a patient at risk for injury (e.g., ability to maneuver through home, climb stairs, and respond to alarms).
- Select interventions on the basis of the type of sensory loss, patient preference, and patient safety.
- Orient patient to any new environment or changes within an existing environment to minimize safety hazards (e.g., visual loss affects a patient's ability to see the edge of the stairs). In addition, educate family caregivers about the best way to help the patient adapt to sensory loss.
- When patients have visual impairments, they may have difficulty with tasks requiring visual detail (e.g., reading prescriptions or syringe scales). This increases the risk of improper administration of medications in the home setting. In addition, certain eye conditions such as cataracts and macular degeneration cause a patient difficulty when adjusting to changes in contrast and brightness.
- Provide additional time for patients with hearing loss to ask repeated questions about their care or upcoming procedure.
- If a patient must sign a consent form for a procedure or surgery, be sure to have a method to verify that patient read, heard, and understood the procedure.

PROCEDURAL GUIDELINE 19.1 *Eye Care for Comatose Patients*

Comatose patients do not have the natural protective mechanisms of blinking and eye lubrication to protect the cornea. Critically ill patients often develop ocular surface disorders such as exposure keratopathy. Critically ill patients are often on mechanical ventilators and thus heavily sedated, which alters the normal blinking reflex (Jammal et al., 2012).

The blinking reflex flushes debris out of the eye. When patients are heavily sedated or in a coma, tear production is reduced, thus decreasing the normal lubrication of the corneal surface. Tears maintain a moist environment, lubricate the eyes, wash away foreign material and cell debris, prevent organisms from adhering to the ocular surface, and transport oxygen to the outer eye surface. When a patient's normal protective eye mechanisms are not effective, eye care is a must. Left unprotected, damage to the cornea can occur. This damage ranges from corneal scarring, infection, premature cataract formation, or vision changes. Simple eye hygiene measures such as moisture chambers, lubrication, and corneal surface protection are the best interventions to decrease the risk for or prevent damage to the cornea (Werli-Alvarenga et al., 2013).

Delegation and Collaboration

The skill of providing basic eye care for a comatose patient can be delegated to nursing assistive personnel (NAP). However, it is the nurse's responsibility to assess a patient's eyes and administer the sterile lubricant. The nurse instructs the NAP to:

- Adapt the skill for specific patients (e.g., using skin-sensitive tape to affix eye pads for patients with sensitive skin).
- Immediately report any eye drainage or irritation to the nurse for further assessment.

Equipment

- Clean gloves
- Warm water
- Normal saline solution
- Clean washcloth
- Cotton balls
- Eye pads or patches
- Paper tape
- Eyedropper bulb syringe
- Sterile lubricant or eye preparations as ordered
- *Option:* A moisture chamber (e.g., polyethylene covers or polyacrylamide hydrogel dressing that seals off the eye from the environment) may also be used; verify with agency policy.

Procedural Steps

1. Perform hand hygiene.
2. Observe patient's eyes for drainage, irritation, redness, and lesions. Apply clean gloves if drainage is present.

Continued

PROCEDURAL GUIDELINE 19.1 *Eye Care for Comatose Patients*—cont'd

3. Continually explain each step of the procedure. It is unknown how much a comatose patient can hear; thus it is important to continually orient a patient to any procedure.
4. Assess for blink reflex (see Chapter 6).
5. Examine the pupils; determine if pupils are equal and round and react to light and accommodation (PERRLA) (see Chapter 6).
6. Observe patient's eye movements, noting symmetry of movement.
7. Explain procedure to patient and family caregivers.
8. Position patient in supine position.
9. Use clean washcloth or cotton balls moistened with warm water or saline and gently wipe each eye from inner to outer canthus. Use a separate, clean cotton ball or corner of the washcloth for each eye.

Clinical Decision Point *Be sure water is warm and not hot to avoid damaging eye.*

10. Use an eyedropper to instill the prescribed lubricant (e.g., saline, methylcellulose, liquid tears) as ordered, wiping away any excess lubricant.

11. If the blink reflex is absent, gently close patient's eyes and apply eye patches or pads. Secure patch, being careful not to tape a patient's eyes.
12. Dispose of excess material, remove gloves, and perform hand hygiene.
13. Remove eye pads or patches every 4 hours or as ordered and observe condition of patient's eyes for drainage, irritation, redness, and lesions.
14. **Use Teach-Back:** "I want to be sure you understand what I explained about why I'm instilling these eye drops. Tell me why the eye drops are important." Revise your instruction now or develop plan for revised patient or family caregiver teaching if patient or family caregiver is not able to teach back correctly.
15. Document eye examination findings, administration of lubricant, and family caregiver learning on flow sheet or in nurses' notes in electronic health record (EHR) or chart.
16. Notify health care provider if signs of irritation or infection are present.

PROCEDURAL GUIDELINE 19.2 *Taking Care of Contact Lenses*

A contact lens is a thin, concave disk that fits directly over the cornea of the eye. It is transparent over at least the pupil and may be colorless or tinted. Contact lenses correct refractive errors of the eye or abnormalities in the shape of the cornea that distort vision. They are relatively easy to apply and remove.

Today rigid gas permeable (RGP) and soft contact lens are available. RGP lens are smaller than the soft lens, and initial awareness of the lens is present; but total comfort usually occurs within a couple of weeks. RGP lens are removed at the end of the day. Daily disposable soft contact lenses are made of a flexible hydrogel plastic and cover the entire cornea and a small rim of the sclera. Contact lenses must accommodate patient needs for comfort, vision correction, and convenience and must be prescribed by an eye care professional (American Optometric Association, 2015).

It is important to remember that all lenses must be removed periodically to prevent infection and corneal damage and that proper cleaning is necessary before reinserting a lens. As contact lenses are worn, secretions and foreign matter adhere to the lens surface (American Optometric Association, 2015). It is extremely important to determine whether patients wear contact lenses, particularly when they are admitted to hospitals or agencies in unresponsive or confused states. If a seriously ill patient is wearing contact lenses and this fact goes undetected, severe corneal injury can result.

Delegation and Collaboration
The skill of taking care of contact lenses can be delegated to nursing assistive personnel (NAP). However, it is the nurse's responsibility to assess a patient's eyes. The nurse directs the NAP to:
- Know a patient's specific type of contact lens, including cleaning solutions and routine, wear schedule, storage, and replacement schedule.

- Report immediately to the nurse any eye pain or discomfort, redness, swelling, tearing, or drainage.
- Carefully handle the lens to prevent damage and injury.

Equipment
- Bath towels or waterproof pads
- Sterile saline solution
- Sterile lens care solution(s) for cleaning, disinfecting, and rinsing
- Sterile wetting or conditioning solution (depends on care regimen)
- Sterile enzyme solution (depends on care regimen)
- Flashlight or penlight
- Clean lens storage container
- Suction cup (optional)
- Powder-free, clean gloves

Procedural Steps
1. Identify patient using at least two identifiers (e.g., name and birthday or name and medical record number) according to agency policy (TJC, 2016).
2. Inspect patient's eyes or ask patient if contact lens is in place.

Clinical Decision Point *If a patient is unconscious or confused, you must assess for presence of contact lenses, which are often difficult to detect if they are colorless (untinted).*

3. Determine if patient is able to manipulate and hold contact lenses and if glasses are available for periods when contacts are not in use. Determine patient's usual routine for wearing, cleaning, and storing lenses.
4. Assess patient for any unusual visual signs/symptoms (e.g., change in visual acuity, blurred vision, halos, photophobia).

PROCEDURAL GUIDELINE 19.2 *Taking Care of Contact Lenses—cont'd*

5. Review types of medication prescribed for patient: sedatives, hypnotics, muscle relaxants, antihistamines, or another medication that decreases blink reflex and subsequent lubrication of cornea.
6. Explain procedure to patient.
7. Perform hand hygiene.
8. Verify expiration date of all solutions and assemble equipment at bedside.
9. Be sure that your fingernails are short and smooth.
10. Position patient in supine or high-Fowler's position in bed.
11. Apply clean gloves. Place towel just below patient's face.
12. Removing lenses:
    a. Removal of soft lens: Follow Steps (1) through (6) for each eye.
       (1) If you are unable to visualize the lens, shine a penlight or flashlight sideways onto the eye to locate the position of the lens.
       (2) Add 2 or 3 drops of sterile saline solution to patient's eye.
       (3) If possible, ask patient to look straight ahead. Retract lower eyelid and expose lower edge of lens.
       (4) Use pad of index finger to slide lens off cornea down onto lower sclera (white of the eye).
       (5) Pull upper eyelid down gently with thumb of other hand and compress lens slightly between thumb and index finger.
       (6) Gently pinch lens and lift out without allowing edges to stick together. Place lens in storage case.

Clinical Decision Point *If lens edges stick together, place lens in palm and soak thoroughly with sterile saline solution. Gently roll lens with index finger in back-and-forth motion. If necessary, soak lens in storage solution, which may return lens to normal shape.*

    b. Removal of hard lenses: Follow Steps (1) through (6) for each eye.
       (1) Inspect the eye to be sure that lens is positioned directly over the cornea. If you are unable to visualize the lens, shine a penlight or flashlight sideways onto the eye to locate the position of the lens.

Clinical Decision Point *If lens is not positioned directly over the cornea, have patient close eyelid, place index and middle fingers of one hand on eyelid just beside the lens and beneath, and gently attempt to massage lens back into place. If lens cannot be repositioned, an immediate referral to an ophthalmologist is needed.*

       (2) Place index finger on outer corner of patient's eye and gently draw skin back toward ear.
       (3) Ask patient to blink. Do not release pressure until blink is completed.

Clinical Decision Point *For patients unable to open eye or blink on command, use a lens suction cup to remove lens from eye. Gently apply suction cup to lens surface and lift out.*

       (4) If lens does not dislodge, gently retract eyelid beyond edge of lens. Press lower eyelid gently against lower edge of lens to dislodge lens.
       (5) Allow both eyelids to close slightly and grasp lens as it rises from the eye. Cup lens in hand.
       (6) Inspect lens to be sure that it is intact. Place it in storage container.
    c. After lenses are removed, inspect eye for redness, pain, or swelling of eyelids or conjunctiva; discharge; or excess tearing.
13. Cleaning and storage: Typical cleaning and disinfecting of contact lenses (verify specific method for lenses):
    a. Apply 1 or 2 drops of cleaning solution to lens in palm of hand. Using index finger (soft lenses) or little finger (rigid lenses), rub lens gently but thoroughly on both sides for 20 to 30 seconds.
    b. Holding lens over emesis basin, rinse thoroughly with recommended rinsing solution.

Clinical Decision Point *Do not use tap water, bottled water, homemade saline, or distilled water for cleaning, rinsing, or storage (FDA, 2015). Tap water contains microbes and may be absorbed into the lenses, making them uncomfortable to wear. Tap and distilled water have been associated with Acanthamoeba keratitis, a corneal infection that is resistant to treatment and cure (FDA, 2015). Periodic cleaning with enzymatic cleaner and/or heat disinfecting may be part of the prescribed regimen. Follow prescriber's instructions and schedules.*

    c. Place lens in proper storage case compartment: "R" for right lens and "L" for left. Rigid lenses are placed inside up.
    d. Fill with recommended disinfectant or storage solution.
    e. Secure cover(s) over storage case. Label case with patient's name, identification number, and room number.
14. Inserting lenses:
    a. Inserting a soft lens: Follow Steps (1) through (5) for each eye.
       (1) Remove right lens from storage case and rinse with recommended rinsing solution; inspect lens for foreign materials, tears, and other damage.
       (2) Hold lens on tip of index finger of dominant hand with concave side up.
       (3) Inspect lens from side at eye level to ensure that it is not inverted (see illustration).

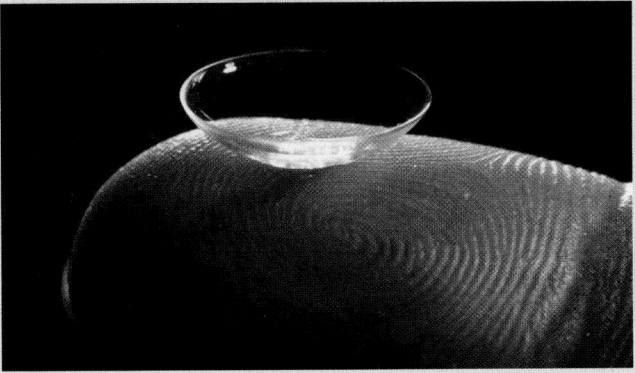

STEP 14a(3) Correct position of soft lens before insertion.

Continued

PROCEDURAL GUIDELINE 19.2 *Taking Care of Contact Lenses—cont'd*

(4) Using middle or index finger of opposite hand, retract upper lid until iris is exposed (see illustration). Using middle finger of hand holding the lens, pull down lower lid.

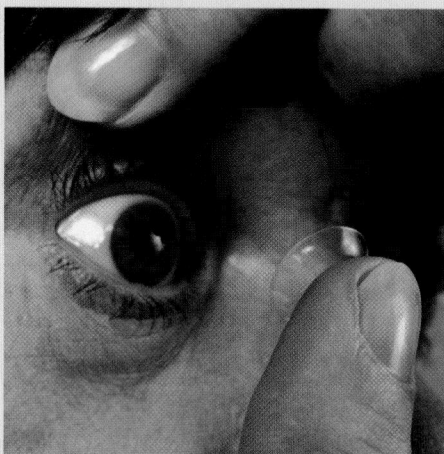

STEP 14a(4) Correct position of hands for soft lens insertion.

   (5) Instruct patient to look straight ahead and focus on an object in the distance. Gently place lens directly on cornea and release lids slowly, starting with lower lid.

  b. Inserting a rigid lens: Follow Steps (1) through (6) for each eye.

   (1) Remove right lens from storage case; attempt to lift lens straight up.

   (2) Hold lens on tip of index finger of dominant hand with concave side up.

   (3) Inspect the lens to ensure that it is moist, clean, clear, and free of chips or cracks.

   (4) Wet lens surfaces with a few drops of prescribed wetting solution.

   (5) Using middle finger of hand holding lens, pull down lower lid (see illustration).

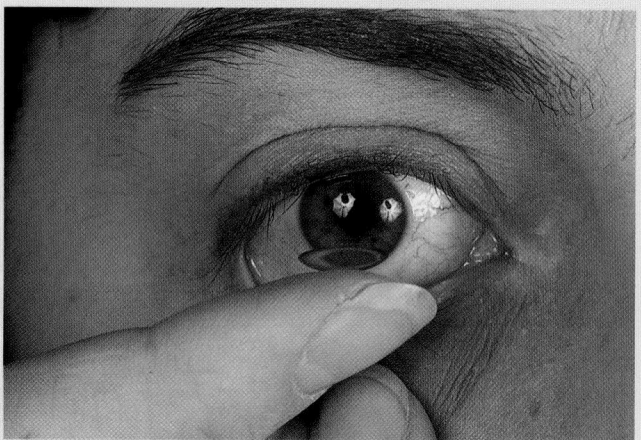

STEP 14b(5) Hand position for rigid lens insertion.

(6) Instruct patient to look straight ahead and focus on an object in the distance (see illustration). Gently place lens directly on cornea and release lids slowly, starting with lower lid.

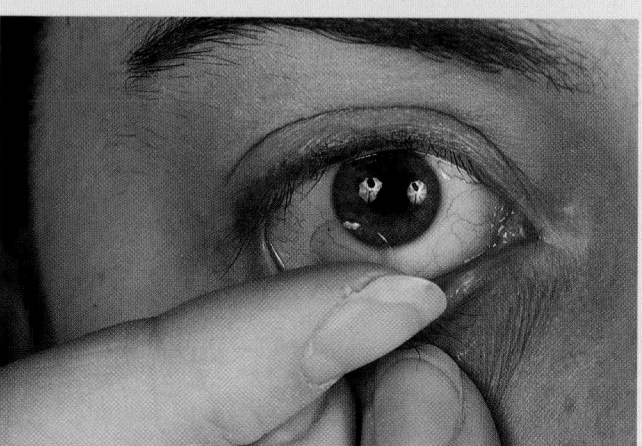

STEP 14b(6) Instruct patient to look straight ahead and focus on an object in the distance.

   (a) Ask patient to close eyes briefly and avoid blinking.

15. Inspect eye to ensure that lens is on cornea.

Clinical Decision Point *If lens is on sclera rather than cornea, ask patient to slowly close eye and look toward the lens. Gentle pressure on the eyelid may help to center the lens on the cornea. Ask patient to blink a few times.*

16. Ask patient to cover other eye with hand and report if vision is clear and lens is comfortable.
17. Repeat procedure to insert lens in other eye.
18. Discard solution from storage case and rinse case thoroughly with sterile lens storage solution. Sterilize or replace case as recommended by manufacturer. Allow case to air dry. Dispose of towel, remove gloves, and perform hand hygiene.
19. Ask patient if lens feels comfortable after removal and reinsertion of lenses.
20. Ask patient if there is blurred vision, pain, and foreign body sensation.
21. Observe eye for drainage or redness.
22. **Use Teach-Back:** "I want to be sure you understand how to clean your contact lenses. Describe for me the way to clean your lenses." Revise your instruction now or develop plan for revised patient or family caregiver teaching if patient or family caregiver is not able to teach back correctly.

◆ SKILL 19.1 Eye Irrigation

Chemical injuries to the eye are work related, caused by common household cleaning solutions or other fumes and aerosols. Acid burns such as bleach, toilet cleaners, and battery fluid cause a haze on the cornea, which often clears; and there is a good chance of recovery. Alkaline burns such as lye, ammonia, and dishwasher detergent often cause permanent injury to the eye. Alkaline burns cause very rapid, irreversible damage (Serrano et al., 2013). A chemical injury to the eye is an emergency and requires flushing the eye with copious amounts of irrigation fluid. Cool tap water is recommended because it is effective, is immediately available for first aid, and initially helps to dilute the concentration of the chemical. Tap water irrigation is also used in emergency situations when a foreign object has entered the eye. It is important to flush out the eye with clean water or saline while seeking medical care. Irrigate immediately with copious amounts of cool water or saline for at least 15 minutes to minimize corneal damage (Chau et al., 2012; Serrano et al., 2013). If the person wears a contact lens that did not wash out with the irrigation, have him or her try to remove the lens. The goal in treating ocular chemical injury is to prevent or reduce visual loss caused by the burn (Serrano et al., 2013).

Delegation and Collaboration

The skill of eye irrigation cannot be delegated to nursing assistive personnel (NAP). The nurse directs the NAP to:

- Report any patient complaint of discomfort or excess tearing following irrigation.

Equipment

- Emergency: Cool tap water
- Prescribed irrigating solution: volume usually 30 to 180 mL at 32° to 38° C (90° to 100° F) (For chemical flushing, use normal saline or lactated Ringer's solution in large volume to provide continuous irrigation over 15 minutes.)
- pH test strip
- Sterile basin or bag of solution
- Curved emesis basin
- Waterproof pad or towel
- 4 × 4–inch gauze pads
- Soft bulb syringe, eyedropper, or intravenous (IV) tubing
- Clean gloves
- Penlight
- Medication administration record (MAR)

STEP	RATIONALE

ASSESSMENT

1. In acute emergent situations: Use copious amounts of clear cool water (normal saline, or lactated Ringer's if quickly available) to flush eyes for at least 15 minutes. Sometimes irrigating volumes up to 20 L or more is required to change pH to physiological levels (pH testing should be done) (Singh et al., 2013).

Minimizes corneal damage (Chau et al., 2012).

2. If not an immediate emergency, identify patient using at least two identifiers (e.g., name and birthday or name and medical record number) according to agency policy.

Ensures correct patient. Complies with The Joint Commission standards and improves patient safety (TJC, 2016).

Clinical Decision Point When eye irrigation is an emergency treatment for a chemical burn follow agency protocol, (i.e., usually copious eye irrigation with cool water, normal saline, or lactated Ringer's solution). When possible, determine the chemical. However, do not stop to obtain a history or an eye examination. Irrigation is the immediate treatment; delays in irrigation by as little as 20 seconds have been associated with more severe injury in alkaline burns. Once the acute phase is over, an irrigation solution that buffers alkali or acid chemical is then selected, and further examination of the eye is possible (Serrano et al., 2013).

3. Review health care provider's medication order, including solution to be instilled and affected eye(s) (right, left, or both) to receive irrigation.

Ensures safe and correct administration of irrigant.

4. Obtain history of the injury to assess reason for eye irrigation (e.g., type of injury, when it occurred).

Determines amount and type of solution and immediacy of need for treatment.

5. Determine patient's ability to open affected eye.

Spasm of the eyelid or pain makes opening the eye difficult. Local anesthetics such as proparacaine or tetracaine cause topical numbness and are used before eye examination procedures.

6. If time permits, do a complete eye examination, including determining if pupils are equal and round and react to light and accommodation (PERRLA) (see Chapter 6). Have patient look in all directions to determine if there are any visible foreign bodies.

Provides baseline information and determines presence of any foreign bodies.

STEP	RATIONALE
7. Observe eye for redness, excessive tearing, discharge, and swelling. Ask patient about symptoms of itching, burning, pain, blurred vision, or photophobia.	Establishes baseline signs and symptoms.
8. Ask patient to rate level of pain. Use scale of 0 to 10.	Establishes baseline for level of pain. Adequate pain control is essential to more complete eye examination by an ophthalmologist (Serrano et al., 2013).
9. Assess patient's ability to cooperate.	Determines level of assistance needed.

NURSING DIAGNOSES

- Acute pain
- Risk for infection
- Risk for injury

Related factors/Risk factors are individualized based on patient's condition or needs.

PLANNING

1. Expected outcomes following completion of procedure:	
• Patient demonstrates minimal anxiety during and after irrigation.	Potential for anxiety and pain is high during emergency.
• Patient verbalizes reduced pain, burning, or itching and improved visual acuity after irrigation.	Reflects effectiveness of procedure in removing irritant.
• Patient maintains normal pupillary reaction and eye movement after irrigation.	Reflects effectiveness of procedure in minimizing exposure to irritant and preventing eye damage.
2. Discuss procedure with patient.	Decreases patient anxiety.
3. Check accuracy and completeness of each MAR with health care provider's written medication or procedure order. Check patient's name, irrigation solution name and concentration, route of administration, and time for administration. Compare MAR with label of eye irrigation solution.	The order sheet is the most reliable source and only legal record of drugs or procedure that patient is to receive. Ensures that patient receives correct medication.
4. Assemble supplies at bedside.	Provides easy access to supplies.
5. Help patient to side-lying position on side of affected eye. Turn head toward affected eye. If both eyes are affected, place patient supine for simultaneous irrigation of both eyes.	Position facilitates flow of solution from inner to outer canthus, preventing contamination of unaffected eye and nasolacrimal duct.

IMPLEMENTATION

1. Perform hand hygiene. Apply clean gloves.	Reduces transmission of microorganisms. Protects hands from chemical irritants.
2. Remove any contact lens if possible (see Procedural Guideline 19.2). Remove gloves after contact lens is removed. Reapply new gloves.	Prompt removal of lenses is needed to safely and completely irrigate foreign substances from patient's eyes. Removal of gloves following contact lens removal prevents reintroduction of chemical transferred from lens to glove.

Clinical Decision Point *In an emergency such as first aid for a chemical burn, do not delay by removing patient's contact lens before irrigation. Do not remove lens unless rapid swelling is occurring. Flush eye from the inner to outer canthus with cool tap water immediately (Chau et al., 2012; Serrano et al., 2013).*

3. Explain to patient that eye can be closed periodically and that no object will touch it.	Informing patients what to expect decreases anxiety and reassures them.
4. Place towel or waterproof pad under patient's face and curved emesis basin just below patient's cheek on side of affected eye.	Catches irrigation fluid.
5. Using gauze moistened with prescriber's solution (or normal saline), gently clean visible secretions or foreign material from eyelid margins and eyelashes, wiping from inner to outer canthus.	Minimizes transfer of material into eye during irrigation. Prevents secretions from entering nasolacrimal duct.

STEP	RATIONALE

6. Explain next steps to patient and encourage relaxation:

    a. With gloved finger gently retract upper and lower eyelids to expose conjunctival sacs.

Retraction minimizes blinking and allows irrigation of conjunctiva.

    b. To hold lids open, apply gentle pressure to lower bony orbit and bony prominence beneath eyebrow. Do not apply pressure over eye.

7. Hold irrigating syringe, dropper, or IV tubing approximately 2.5 cm (1 inch) from inner canthus.

Direct contact with irrigation equipment may injure eye.

8. Ask patient to look toward brow. Gently irrigate with steady stream toward lower conjunctival sac, moving from inner to outer canthus (see illustration).

Minimizes force of stream on patient's cornea. Flushes irritant out and away from the other eye and nasolacrimal duct.

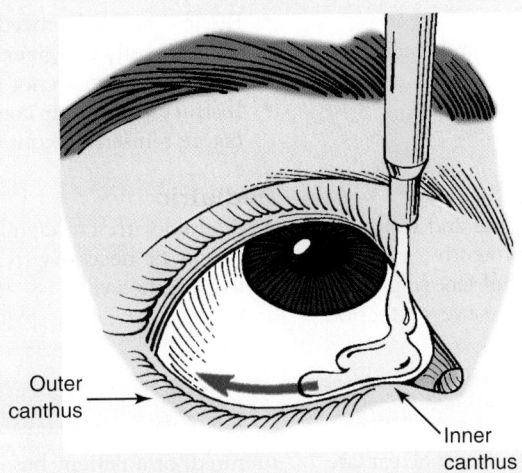

Outer canthus

Inner canthus

STEP 8 Irrigation of eye from inner to outer canthus.

9. Reinforce importance of procedure and encourage patient by using calm, confident, soft voice.

Reduces anxiety.

10. Allow patient to blink periodically.

Lid closure moves secretions from upper conjunctival sac.

11. Continue irrigation with prescribed solution volume or time or until secretions are cleared. (**NOTE:** In emergent situation: An irrigation of 15 minutes or more is needed to flush chemicals.)

Assessment of eye secretion pH may be necessary if eye was exposed to an acidic or basic solution during injury (Chau et al., 2012).

12. Blot excess moisture from eyelids and face with gauze or towel.

13. Dispose of soiled supplies, remove gloves, and perform hand hygiene.

Reduces transmission of microorganisms.

EVALUATION

1. Observe for verbal and nonverbal signs of anxiety during irrigation.

Verifies that patient is adequately comforted.

2. Assess patient's comfort level after irrigation.

Verifies effective removal of irritant.

3. Inspect eye for movement and to determine if pupils are equal, round, and react to light and accommodation (PERRLA).

Impaired reaction to light, accommodation, or movement may indicate injury.

4. Ask patient about improved visual acuity. Have patient read written material.

Corneal damage from irritant can result in altered visual acuity (e.g., blurred vision, cloudiness).

5. **Use Teach-Back:** "I want to be sure I explained why it is important to take your eye drops at home. Tell me the purpose of the drops and when you should use them." Revise your instruction now or develop a plan for revised patient or family caregiver teaching if patient and family caregiver are not able to teach back correctly.

Determines patient's and family caregiver's level of understanding of instructional topic.

STEP	RATIONALE

Unexpected Outcomes

1. Anxiety.

Related Interventions

- Reinforce rationale for irrigation.
- Allow patient to close eye periodically during irrigation.
- Instruct patient to take slow, deep breaths.

2. Patient complains of pain or foreign body sensation in eye following irrigation, excessive tearing, or photophobia.

- Advise patient to close eye and avoid eye movement.
- Immediately notify health care provider or eye care practitioner.

Recording and Reporting

- Record in nurses' notes in electronic health record (EHR) or chart the condition of eye and patient's report of pain and visual symptoms. Record amount and type of irrigation in patient's MAR.
- Document your evaluation of patient and family caregiver learning.
- Report continuing symptoms of pain or blurred vision.

Special Considerations
Teaching

- Help patient identify potential hazards at home and work and take steps to prevent accidents. Personal protective eyewear, such as goggles, face shields, safety glasses, or full-face respirators must be used when an eye hazard exists. The eye protection

chosen for specific work situations depends on the nature and extent of the hazard, the circumstances of exposure, other protective equipment used, and personal vision needs (CDC, 2013).

- Review first-aid procedures for eye emergencies with patient and/or family caregiver.
- Instruct patient to not press or rub an injured eye.
- Instruct patient to consult with personal eye care physician before reinserting contact lens.

Pediatric

- A child with a foreign body or chemical in the eye may panic. It may be necessary to restrain the child to safely and quickly irrigate the eye.

◆ SKILL 19.2 **Ear Irrigation**

The common indications for irrigation of the external ear are presence of foreign bodies, local inflammation, and buildup of cerumen (ear wax) in the ear canal. The procedure is not without potential hazards. Usually irrigations are performed with liquid warmed to body temperature to avoid vertigo or nausea in patients. Ear irrigations are effective when the use of commercial drops is unsuccessful in removing cerumen buildup (Harkin, 2015). The greatest danger during ear irrigation is trauma to the tympanic membrane by forcing irrigant into the ear canal under pressure. Damage to the external auditory meatus may occur by scratching the lining of the canal if a patient suddenly moves or if there is inadequate control of the irrigating syringe. Drying the ear improperly may lead to acute otitis externa (infection of the outer ear).

Ear emergencies can include the presence of foreign bodies, insect bites, or percussion injuries. In addition, a patient can also have damage from inside the ear, which includes blood and drainage. Sometimes the cause of bloody drainage may be the result of a head or neck injury. If a head or neck injury is suspected, immobilize the patient. Cover the outside of the ear with a sterile dressing (if available), get medical help immediately, and do not irrigate the ear. In addition, do not irrigate the ear if vegetable matter or an insect is present in the canal; the tympanic membrane is

ruptured; or a patient has otitis externa, myringotomy tubes, or a mastoid cavity (US National Library of Medicine, 2016).

Delegation and Collaboration

The skill of administering ear irrigation cannot be delegated to nursing assistive personnel (NAP). The nurse directs the NAP to:

- Immediately report any potential side effects of ear irrigation (e.g., pain, drainage, dizziness).
- Help a patient when ambulating because some light-headedness may be present, which increases a patient's risk for falling.

Equipment

- Clean gloves
- Otoscope (optional)
- Irrigation or bulb syringe
- Basin for irrigating solution (Use sterile basin if sterile irrigating solution is used [when tympanic membrane is ruptured].)
- Emesis basin for drainage or irrigating solution exiting the ear
- Towel
- Cotton balls or 4 × 4–inch gauze
- Prescribed irrigating solution warmed to body temperature or mineral oil, over-the-counter softener
- Medication administration record (MAR) (print or electronic)

STEP	RATIONALE

ASSESSMENT

1. Identify patient using at least two identifiers (e.g., name and birthday or name and medical record number) according to agency policy. Compare identifiers with information on patient's MAR or medical record.

Ensures correct patient. Complies with The Joint Commission Standards and improves patient safety (TJC, 2016).

STEP	RATIONALE
2. Review health care provider's medication order, including solution to be instilled and affected ear(s): right (AU), left (AS), or both (AD) to receive irrigation.	Ensures safe and correct administration of medication.
3. Review medical record for history of ruptured tympanic membrane, placement of myringotomy tubes, or surgery of the auditory canal.	These conditions contradict irrigation.
4. Inspect pinna and external auditory meatus for redness, swelling, drainage, abrasions, and presence of cerumen or foreign objects.	Findings provide baseline to monitor effects of medication or solution.
a. Always attempt to remove foreign objects in ear by first simply straightening ear canal.	This may cause object to fall out.

Clinical Decision Point *If vegetable matter such as a dried bean or pea is occluded in the canal, do not perform irrigation. The material can swell on contact with water and cause further damage to the canal (Harkin, 2015; Hockenberry and Wilson, 2015).*

STEP	RATIONALE
5. Use otoscope to inspect deeper parts of auditory canal and tympanic membrane. *Caution:* Do not push an object further into the ear canal.	Verifies if tympanic membrane is intact.
6. Ask if patient is experiencing discomfort, using a scale of 0 to 10.	Pain is symptomatic of external ear infection or inflammation.
7. Note patient's ability to hear clearly.	Occlusion of auditory canal by cerumen or foreign object can impair hearing.
8. Review patient's knowledge of purpose for irrigation and normal care of ears.	May indicate need for instruction regarding hygiene.

NURSING DIAGNOSES

- Deficient knowledge regarding purpose for irrigation
- Pain (acute or chronic)
- Risk for injury

Related factors/Risk factors are individualized based on patient's condition or needs.

PLANNING

STEP	RATIONALE
1. Expected outcomes following completion of procedure:	
• Patient denies pain during instillation.	Fluid is properly instilled.
• Patient demonstrates hearing conversation more clearly in affected ear.	Obstruction in ear canal is resolved.
• Patient is able to discuss purpose of irrigation and describe correct ear-care techniques.	Feedback reflects patient's learning.
• Patient's canal is clear of cerumen, foreign material, and discharge.	Inflammation, irritation, and occlusion of canal are relieved.
2. Check accuracy and completeness of each MAR with health care provider's written medication or procedure order. Check patient's name, drug name and dosage, route of administration, and time for administration. Compare MAR with label of ear irrigation solution.	The order sheet is the most reliable source and only legal record of drugs or procedure that patient is to receive. Ensures that patient receives correct medication.
3. If patient is found to have impacted cerumen, instill 1 or 2 drops of mineral oil or over-the-counter softener into ear twice a day for 2 to 3 days before irrigation.	Loosens cerumen and ensures easier removal during irrigation.
4. Explain procedure. Prepare patient that irrigation may cause sensation of dizziness, ear fullness, and warmth.	Prepares patient to anticipate effects of irrigation and promotes cooperation.

IMPLEMENTATION

STEP	RATIONALE
1. Perform hand hygiene and arrange supplies at bedside.	Reduces transfer of microorganisms; helps nurse perform procedure smoothly.
2. Close curtain or room door.	Maintains privacy.

STEP	RATIONALE
3. Help patient to sitting or lying position with head turned toward affected ear. Place towel under patient's head and shoulder and have patient, if able, hold emesis basin under affected ear.	Position minimizes leakage of fluids around neck and facial area. Solution will flow from ear canal to basin.
4. Pour prescribed irrigating solution into basin. Check temperature of solution by pouring small drop on your inner forearm. **NOTE:** If sterile irrigating solution is used, sterile basin is required.	
5. Apply clean gloves. Gently clean auricle and outer ear canal with gauze or cotton balls. Do *not* force drainage or cerumen into ear canal.	Prevents infected material from reentering ear canal. Forceful instillation of solution into occluded canal can cause injury to eardrum.
6. Fill irrigating syringe with solution (approximately 50 mL).	Enough fluid is needed to provide a steady irrigating stream.
7. For adults and children over 3 years old, gently pull pinna up and back. In children 3 years or younger, pinna should be pulled down and back (Hockenberry and Wilson, 2015). Adults can lie supine. Place tip of irrigating device just inside external meatus. Leave space around irrigating tip and canal.	Pulling pinna straightens external ear canal. Prevents obstruction of canal with device, which can lead to increased pressure on tympanic membrane.
8. Slowly instill irrigating solution by holding tip of syringe 1 cm (½ inch) above opening to ear canal. Direct fluid toward superior aspect of ear canal. Allow it to drain out into basin during instillation. Continue until canal is cleaned or solution is used (see illustration).	Slow instillation prevents buildup of pressure in ear canal and ensures contact of solution with all canal surfaces.

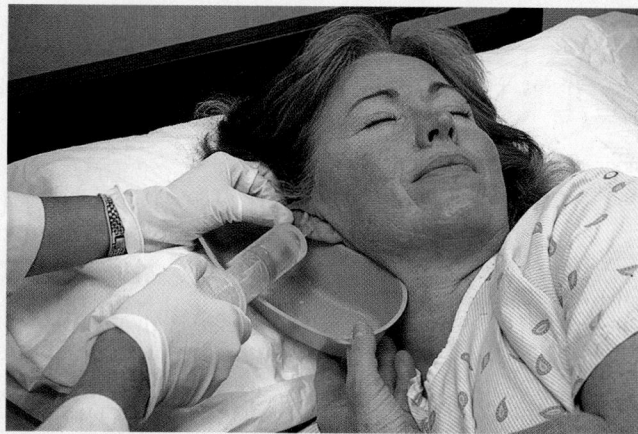

STEP 8 Tip of syringe does not occlude ear canal during irrigation.

9. Maintain flow of irrigation in steady stream until pieces of cerumen or exudate flow from canal.	Constant flow of fluid loosens cerumen.
10. Periodically ask if patient is experiencing pain, nausea, or vertigo.	Symptoms indicate that irrigating solution is too hot or too cold or instilled with too much pressure.
11. Drain excessive fluid from ear by having patient tilt head toward affected side.	Excess fluid may promote microorganism growth if not drained.
12. Dry outer ear canal gently with cotton ball. Leave cotton ball in place for 5 to 10 minutes.	Drying prevents buildup of moisture that can lead to otitis externa.
13. Help patient to sitting position.	Maintains comfort.
14. Remove gloves, dispose of supplies, and perform hand hygiene.	Reduces transmission of infection.

EVALUATION

1. Ask patient if discomfort is noted during instillation of solution.	Fluid instilled improperly under pressure causes discomfort.
2. Ask patient about sensations of light-headedness or dizziness.	Instillation of fluid into ear can cause some light-headedness or dizziness, which can put patient at risk for falling.

STEP	RATIONALE
3. Reinspect condition of meatus and canal.	Determines if solution relieves symptoms and removes foreign materials.
4. Assess patient's hearing acuity.	Determines if hearing is improved.
5. **Use Teach-Back:** "I want to be sure you understand how I showed you to insert the syringe for an ear irrigation. Show me how you would do this for your mother." Revise your instruction now or develop a plan for revised patient or family caregiver learning if patient or family caregiver is not able to teach back correctly.	Determines patient's and family caregiver's level of understanding of instructional topic.

Unexpected Outcomes	Related Interventions
1. Patient complains of increased ear pain during irrigation.	• Rupture of eardrum may have occurred. Stop irrigations and notify health care provider immediately.
2. Ear canal remains occluded with cerumen.	• Repeat irrigation.
3. Foreign body remains in ear canal.	• Refer patient to otolaryngologist if foreign object remains after irrigation.

Recording and Reporting

- Record the procedure, amount of solution instilled, time of administration, and ear receiving irrigation on flow sheet or in nurses' notes in electronic health record (EHR) or chart.
- Document your evaluation of patient and family caregiver learning.
- Record appearance of external ear and patient's hearing acuity on flow sheet or in nurses' notes in EHR or chart.
- Report adverse effects/patient response and/or withheld drugs to nurse in charge or health care provider.

Special Considerations
Teaching

- Instruct patient that cerumen has an antibacterial effect that maintains an acid pH in the auditory canal.

- Instruct patients to clean ears daily with a washcloth, soap, and warm water.
- Warn patients against placing objects (including cotton swabs) in ears.

Pediatric

- When cleaning the ear of a small child, be certain that child's head is immobilized to prevent puncturing eardrum. It may be necessary to have child's parent or staff participate (Hockenberry and Wilson, 2015).

Home Care

- Instruct patient to use a clean bulb syringe for irrigation. Mineral oil drops or over-the-counter otic preparations can help with removal of cerumen.

◆ SKILL 19.3 Care of Hearing Aids

Hearing is vital for normal communication and orientation to sounds in the environment. Hearing impairment is most common in older adults. Many patients do not seek professional help for this impairment, nor do they consistently wear aids (Ekberg et al., 2014). According to the National Institute on Deafness and other Communication Disorders (NIDCD, 2015), hearing loss affects 36 million people. In addition, 50% of residents in assisted-living and residential facilities are hearing impaired. People who do not wear a hearing aid often say that it is because of the quality of sound that the aid produces (Dawes et al., 2014).

Initially a person with hearing loss may deny the condition or think that there is a stigma attached to the actual hearing loss or the need for a hearing aid (Ross, 2015). Any hearing loss has social implications, and the person may not engage in social activities. In addition, in social situations people with a hearing aid often believe that, once their aid is observed, conversation occurs "around them" (Ekberg et al., 2014). There are also many safety considerations. Not only do people with hearing loss have difficulty hearing car horns and emergency sirens, they also have difficulty understanding patient education and, as a result, may not manage their symptoms or therapies safely.

When your patient has a hearing aid, your role is to understand how it functions and how to help the patient care for it. It is the role of a hearing professional to determine which type of aid the patient needs and how to establish the best auditory settings for individual patients (Mestayer, 2014). For people with hearing loss, a proper hearing aid improves the ability to hear and understand spoken words. Several styles of hearing aids are available to patients today (Table 19.1). Hearing aids amplify sound so it is heard at a more effective level. All hearing aids have four basic components:

1. A microphone, which receives and converts sound into electrical signals
2. An amplifier, which increases the strength of the electrical signal
3. A receiver, which converts the strengthened signal back into sound
4. A power source (batteries)

All hearing aids do not work the same. The two main types of electronic hearing aids are analog and digital. Analog technology converts sound waves into electrical waves, which are amplified. These are custom built to meet the needs of the user and programmed by the manufacturer according to the specifications of

TABLE 19.1

Types of Hearing Aids

Type	Advantages	Disadvantages	Cautions
In-the-ear (ITE) hearing aids fit completely in the outer ear and are used for mild-to-severe hearing loss. 	Design of the aid can improve sound transmission through telephone calls. Some ITEs have a *telecoil,* which is a magnetic circuit that allows users to receive sound through the circuitry of the hearing aid versus the microphone.	ITE aids are damaged by earwax and ear drainage, and their small size can cause adjustment problems and feedback.	Not usually worn by children because the casings need to be replaced as the ear grows
Behind-the-ear (BTE) hearing aids are worn behind the ear and are connected to a plastic ear mold that fits inside the outer ear. 	Sound travels through the ear mold into the ear. People of all ages wear BTE aids for mild-to-profound hearing loss.	Poorly fitting BTE ear molds can cause feedback, a whistling sound caused by the fit of the hearing aid.	May not be appropriate for children or adults who are active in sports because of potential for damage of the device
Completely-in-canal (CIC) aids are customized to fit the size and shape of the ear canal. 	Canal aids are used for mild to moderately severe hearing loss and are largely concealed in the ear canal.	Because of their small size, canal aids may be difficult for the user to adjust and remove and may not be able to hold additional devices such as a telecoil.	Expensive and not recommended for children Can also be damaged by earwax and ear drainage

Data from National Institute on Deafness and Other Communication Disorders (NIDCD): *Hearing aids,* 2013, http://www.nidcd.nih.gov/health/hearing/pages/hearingaid.aspx#hearingaid_01. Accessed January 2016.

the audiologist. Digital technology converts sound waves into numerical codes. The aid is programmed to amplify some frequencies more than others. Digital aids give the audiologist more flexibility in fine-tuning the aid to meet the patient's needs. These aids can be programmed to focus sounds coming from a specific direction (NIDCD, 2013).

It is a challenge to adjust one's communication style to accommodate a patient with a hearing impairment. Use the patient as a resource for identifying the communication techniques that are generally helpful. Be sure that a patient can see your face; speak slowly in a normal tone; and rephrase rather than repeat if he or she cannot understand you. Also remember that a patient is unable to hear alerts such as fire alarms or overhead announcements.

Delegation and Collaboration

This skill of caring for a hearing aid can be delegated to nursing assistive personnel (NAP). The nurse directs the NAP to:

- Report ear pain, inflammation, drainage, odor, or changes in hearing.
- Identify alternative ways to communicate with a patient while the aid is not in use.
- Learn how to carefully handle the aid to prevent damage or injury.

Equipment

- Soft towel and washcloth
- Facial tissues
- Brush or wax loop
- Storage case
- Warm water and soap
- Spare battery, size depends on aid (*optional*)
- Clean gloves (if drainage present)

STEP	RATIONALE

ASSESSMENT

1. Identify patient using at least two identifiers (e.g., name and birthday or name and medical record number) according to agency policy.

   Ensures correct patient. Complies with The Joint Commission Standards and improves patient safety (TJC, 2016).

2. Determine whether patient can hear clearly with hearing aid by talking slowly and clearly in normal tone of voice.

   Inability to hear may indicate a problem with the hearing aid or battery or that that particular model is no longer effective for patient.

3. Ask if patient is able to manipulate and hold hearing aid or, preferably, observe patient insert aid independently.

   Determines level of assistance required in care.

4. Assess if hearing aid is working by removing from patient's ear. Close battery case and turn volume slowly to high. Cup hand over hearing aid. If you hear a squealing sound (feedback), it is working. If no sound is heard, replace batteries and test again.

   May indicate malfunctioning of hearing aid.

5. Determine patient's usual hearing aid–care practices.

   Provides information as to how patient cares for device and identifies patient preferences.

6. Assess patient for any unusual physical or auditory signs/symptoms (pain, itching, redness, discharge, odor, tinnitus, decreased acuity). If hearing is reduced, ask: when did this start, is it present all the time, does the quality of hearing acuity change with male versus female voices, adult versus children's voices?

   May indicate injury, infection, or cerumen accumulation.

7. Inspect ear mold for cracked or rough edges.

   Poorly fitting hearing aids cause irritation and/or discomfort to external ear canal.

8. Inspect for accumulation of cerumen around aid and plugging of opening in aid.

   Cerumen can block sound reception (Harkin, 2015; White, 2015).

9. Assess patient's knowledge of and routines for cleaning and caring for hearing aid.

   Determines compliance with and knowledge of self-care.

NURSING DIAGNOSES

- Deficient knowledge regarding hearing aid care
- Impaired verbal communication
- Risk for injury
- Risk for situational low self-esteem

Related factors/Risk factors are individualized based on patient's condition or needs.

PLANNING

1. Expected outcomes following completion of procedure:
   - Patient verbalizes comfort after removal and reinsertion of hearing aid.

     Hearing aid is removed or inserted properly and positioned correctly.
   - Patient responds appropriately to normal conversation and environmental sounds.

     Hearing aid and batteries are operational. Aid is secure and unobstructed.
   - Patient demonstrates proper care of hearing aid.

     Learning is achieved.

2. Discuss procedure with patient. Explain all steps before removing aid.

   Patient can help in planning by explaining additional tips for care. Patient may be confused or anxious if verbal instructions are given after removal of hearing aid.

3. Assemble supplies at bedside. Place towel over work area.

   Provides easy access to supplies. Towel catches aid if accidentally dropped and avoids breakage.

4. Have patient assume supine, side-lying, or sitting position in bed or chair.

   Provides easy access for nurse. Promotes patient comfort.

IMPLEMENTATION

1. Perform hand hygiene and apply clean gloves if patient has ear drainage.

   Reduces transmission of microorganisms.

STEP	RATIONALE
2. Removing and cleaning hearing aid(s)	
a. Patient or nurse turns hearing aid(s) volume off, usually by turning volume control to left or toward patient's nose. Then grasp aid securely and gently remove device following natural ear contour.	Prevents feedback (whistling) during removal. Prevents dropping hearing aid. Prevents injury to ear.

Clinical Decision Point *Some hearing aids such as the completely-in-canal (CIC) device do not have a volume control but are turned off by opening the battery door. Other aids have the volume control located on the remote. Be sure that your patient knows the importance of having the volume turned off when the aid is not in use.*

STEP	RATIONALE
b. Hold aid over towel and wipe exterior with tissue to remove cerumen.	Prevents breakage or damage if aid is dropped. Cerumen may irritate canal and interfere with fit.
c. Inspect all openings in aid for accumulated cerumen. Carefully remove cerumen with wax loop or other device supplied with hearing aid.	Cerumen may block sound from receiver. It may also block pressure equalization channel and create feeling of ear pressure.

Clinical Decision Point *The pressure equalization channel is a tiny hole through the entire length of the ear mold and should be clear for the entire length. The receiver points into the ear through another opening. It is easily damaged. NEVER insert anything into the receiver port!*

STEP	RATIONALE
d. Inspect ear mold for rough edges or any frays in cords.	May irritate ear canal.
e. Open battery door, place hearing aid in labeled storage container, and allow it to air dry.	Allows drying of internal components. Protects against breakage and loss.
f. Assess ear for redness, tenderness, discharge, or odor.	Signs may indicate injury or infection.
g. Repeat procedure for other hearing aid if bilateral.	
h. Place towel beneath patient's ear(s). Wash ear canal(s) with washcloth moistened in soap and water. Rinse and dry.	Absorbs excess water. Removes cerumen from ear canal. Removes soap residue and water that may harbor microbes or damage aid.
i. Dispose of towels, remove gloves, and perform hand hygiene.	Reduces transmission of microorganisms.
j. If storing hearing aid(s), place each in dry storage case with desiccant material. Label case with patient's name and room number. If more than one aid, note right or left. Indicate in patient's medical record where aid is stored.	Protects hearing aid against damage, moisture, and breakage. Documents how and where hearing aid is stored.
3. Inserting hearing aid(s)	
a. Remove hearing aid(s) from storage case and check battery (see assessment). Check that volume is off.	
b. Identify hearing aid as either right (marked "R" or red color coded) or left (marked "L" or blue color coded).	Proper orientation prevents damage and injury.
c. When possible, allow patient to insert aid. Otherwise hold hearing aid with thumb and index finger of dominant hand so canal (long part with holes) is at bottom. Insert pointed end of ear mold into ear canal. Follow natural ear contours to guide aid into place.	Prevents dropping. Proper positioning prevents injury. Pulling on ear may distort canal and make insertion more difficult.
d. Anchor any separate pieces, as in case of behind-the-ear (BTE) aid or body aid.	Prevents pieces from falling and breaking.
e. Adjust or have patient adjust volume gradually to comfortable level for talking to patient in regular voice 3 to 4 feet away. Rotate volume control toward nose to increase volume and away from nose to decrease volume.	Gradual adjustment prevents discomfort and injury to ear.
f. Repeat insertion for other hearing aid, if bilateral	
g. Close and store case. Remove and dispose of gloves. Perform hand hygiene.	Preserves desiccant. Prevents loss. Reduces transmission of microorganisms.

EVALUATION

1. Ask patient to rate level of comfort after removal or insertion.	Verifies proper technique and positioning.

STEP	RATIONALE
2. Observe patient during normal conversation and in response to environmental sounds.	Verifies that aid is operational, correctly positioned, unobstructed, and effective.
3. **Use Teach-Back:** "I want to be sure you understand what I showed you to remove, clean, and reinsert your father's hearing aid. Let's take time now and show me how to do it." Revise your instruction now or develop a plan for revised patient or family caregiver teaching if patient or family caregiver is not able to teach back correctly.	Determines patient's and family caregiver's level of understanding of instructional topic.

Unexpected Outcomes	Related Interventions
1. Patient is unable to hear conversations or environmental sounds. Patient's verbal responses are inappropriate.	• Check function, type, and placement of battery and replace it if indicated. • Increase volume if adjustable. • Inspect aid and ear canal for cerumen blockage. • Refer to audiologist for reassessment.
2. Patient experiences discomfort or pain, inflammation, drainage, or odor from affected ear.	• Remove aid and inspect for sharp or rough edges. Refer to provider for repair. • Assess ear for signs of injury or infection. • Confirm correct R or L placement. Reposition hearing aid.

Recording and Reporting

- Record removal of hearing aid, storage location if not reinserted after cleaning, and patient's preferred communication techniques on flow sheet or in nurses' notes in electronic health record (EHR) or chart. If family takes aid home, be sure that this information is recorded.
- Document your evaluation of patient and family caregiver learning.
- Report any signs or symptoms of infection or injury or sudden decrease in hearing acuity.

Special Considerations
Teaching

- Instruct family that batteries are toxic if swallowed and keep them away from pets and children.
- Patients should insert the aid after their hair is dried and any hair spray applied. Heat from the hair dryer or perfumes and hair spray can damage the aid.
- Dogs in particular and cats are attracted to the smell of used hearing aids. Advise patient to protect the hearing aids and their pets by properly storing the aids out of reach.
- Encourage patients to identify helpful communication tips and teach them to others. Many patients find facial cues informative. Speakers must:
  1. Face patient, stay within 3 to 4 feet away, and keep hands away from mouth.
  2. Get patient's attention before speaking.
  3. Rephrase rather than repeat when a patient cannot understand.
  4. Reduce background noise or move to a quiet area.

Pediatric

- Children are more often fitted with BTE hearing aids because the ear canal is still growing.
- The aid is made less conspicuous with hair styling or becomes a statement of fashion and personality with a brightly colored or transparent case.
- Children need help to prevent acoustic feedback (whistling), which they are unable to hear. This is usually eliminated by removing and reinserting the device and making sure that no hair is caught between the ear mold and canal or lowering the volume of the device (Hockenberry and Wilson, 2015).

Gerontological

- Advise patient to protect the hearing aid from water, alcohol, hair spray or cologne, perspiration, rain, and snow and to avoid exposing it to extremes of temperature.
- Encourage patient to store hearing aids and batteries with desiccant or in an electronic dryer to prolong life, minimize repairs, and preserve batteries.
- The small size of some hearing aids may make them difficult to manipulate, particularly for individuals with decreased dexterity or visual acuity. Consult an audiologist to identify an aid that accommodates a patient's particular need.

Home Care

- Determine presence and willingness of family caregiver to perform necessary care of hearing aid.
- Assess patient's home and determine need for special precautions given patient's limited hearing.

◆ CLINICAL DEBRIEF

A 68-year-old married man and his wife have two grown children who are married with children. He has worn a bilateral in-the-ear (ITE) hearing aids for the last 10 years. He knows how to care for his aids. He is comfortable and satisfied with them. When the aids are working well, he notes that he hears his family and co-workers clearly, has minimal distortion in large gatherings, and is able to distinguish emergency sirens and car horns when he is driving. Three weeks ago he had a recent upper respiratory tract infection, and since that time both he and his wife have noticed changes in his hearing acuity. He is now visiting his primary care clinic to see what can be done with his hearing before he goes back to the audiologist.

1. He thinks that he has diminished hearing in the left ear and senses drainage from that ear. Which assessments should the nurse complete?

2. Their preschool- and school-age grandchildren visit frequently and are curious about the hearing aids. Neither the patient nor his wife remembers any patient education regarding hearing aid safety related to young children. What will you include in a teaching session regarding hearing aid safety?

3. During your assessment you identify that he has excessive wax and purulent drainage in his left ear. Using SBAR (Situation, Background, Assessment, and Recommendation), communicate this information to the health care team.

◆ REVIEW QUESTIONS

1. The nurse decides to check the functioning of the hearing aid. Place the following steps in appropriate order for cleaning the hearing aid.
   a. Wash ear canal.
   b. Place hearing aid in storage case.
   c. Perform hand hygiene and apply clean gloves.
   d. Grasp aid securely and remove from ear following natural ear contour.
   e. Use brush to clean holes in aid.
   f. Have patient turn hearing aid volume off.
      1. f, d, c, a, b, e
      2. c, f, d, e, a, b
      3. c, f, d, a, e, b
      4. f, d, c, e, a, b

2. Which important nursing responsibilities pertain to eye irrigations? (Select all that apply.)
   1. Irrigating the eye immediately in emergent situations
   2. Removing dried secretions with moistened gauze
   3. Gently securing the eyelids with paper tape
   4. Checking for the pupillary response
   5. Preventing injury to the patient's corneas

3. When caring for a patient who is hearing impaired, which approaches best facilitate communication? (Select all that apply.)
   1. Speaking slightly more loudly than usual
   2. Speaking slightly more slowly using a normal tone
   3. Standing so patient can see the nurse's face
   4. Rephrasing rather than repeating
   5. Using hand gestures to help explain what is being said

ⓔ *Visit the Evolve site for a complete list of Clinical Debrief and Review Questions answers.*

REFERENCES

American Academy of Audiology: *Clinical Practice Guidelines: adult patients with severe-to profound unilateral sensorineural hearing loss*, 2015, http://www.audiology.org/sites/default/files/PractGuidelineAdultsPatientsWithSNHL.pdf. Accessed May 18, 2016.

American Optometric Association: *Contact lens safety*, 2015, http://www.contactlenssafety.org/lenstypes.html. Accessed September, 2015.

Centers for Disease Control and Prevention (CDC): *Eye safety*, 2013, http://www.cdc.gov/niosh/topics/eye/. Accessed May 7, 2016.

Chau JPC, et al: A systematic review of methods of eye irrigation for adults and children with ocular chemical burns, *Worldviews Evid Based Nurs* 9(3):129, 2012.

Chou R, et al: *Screening for hearing loss in adults ages 50 years and older: a review of the evidence for the US Preventive Services Task Force*, Rockville, MD, 2011, Agency for Health Care Research and Quality.

Dawes P, et al: "Getting used to" hearing aids from the perspective of adult hearing-aid users, *Int J Audiol* 53:861, 2014.

Ekberg K, et al: Addressing patients' psychosocial concerns regarding hearing aids within audiology appointments for older adults, *Am J Audiol* 23:337, 2014.

Food and Drug Administration (FDA): *Contact lens risks*, US Food and Drug Administration, 2015, http://www.fda.gov/MedicalDevices/Productsand MedicalProcedures/HomeHealthandConsumer/ConsumerProducts/ContactLenses/ucm062589.htm. Accessed May 7, 2016.

Gopinath B, et al: Dual sensory impairment in older adults increases the risk of mortality: a population-based study, *PLoS ONE* 8(3):e55054, 2013.

Harkin H: Ear care and irrigation with water: an update, *Practice Nurse* 45(7):24, 2015.

Heine C, et al: The dual sensory loss in older adults: a systematic review, *Gerontologist* 55(5):913, 2015.

Hockenberry MJ, Wilson D: *Wong's nursing care of infants and children*, ed 10, St Louis, 2015, Mosby.

Jammal H, et al: Exposure keratopathy in sedated and ventilated patients, *J Crit Care* 27:537, 2012.

Mestayer K: Looking for hearing aids? Find the right professional first, *Hearing Health* Spring:34, 2014.

Mick P, et al: The association between hearing loss and social isolation in older adults, *Otolaryngol Head Neck Surg* 150(3):378, 2014.

National Institute on Deafness and Other Communication Disorders (NIDCD): *Hearing aids*, 2013, http://www.nidcd.nih.gov/health/hearing/pages/hearingaid.aspx#hearingaid_01. Accessed January, 2016.

National Institute on Deafness and Other Communication Disorders (NIDCD): *Quick statistics*, 2015, http://www.nidcd.nih.gov/health/statistics/Pages/quick.aspx. Accessed January, 2016.

Roets-Merken LM, et al: Screening for hearing, visual, and dual sensory impairment in older adults using behavioural cues: a validation study, *Int J Nurs Stud* 51:1434, 2014.

Ross M: The "stigma" of hearing loss and hearing aids, *Hearing Loss Magazine*, July/August:28, 2015.

Serrano F, et al: Traumatic eye injuries, *JEMS* 38(12):56, 2013.

Singh P, et al: Ocular chemical injuries and their management, *Oman J Ophthalmol* 6(2):83, 2013.

The Joint Commission (TJC): *National Patient Safety Goals*, Oakbrook Terrace, IL, 2016, The Commission. http://www.jointcommission.org/standards_information/npsgs.aspx. January 2016.

Tremblay KL: The ear-brain connection: older ears and older brains, *Am J Audiol* 24:117, 2015.

US National Library of Medicine: *Medline plus: ear emergencies*, 2016, https://www.nlm.nih.gov/medlineplus/ency/article/000052.htm, Accessed September 2016.

Vreeken HL, et al: Dual sensory loss: a major-age related increase of comorbid hearing loss and ownership in visually impaired adults, *Geriatr Gerontol Int* 14:570, 2014.

Werli-Alvarenga A, et al: Nursing interventions for adult intensive care patients with risk for corneal injury: a systematic review, *Int J Nurs Knowl* 24910:25, 2013.

White S: Practical implementation tips: dual sensory loss, *Guidel in Practice* 18(6):30, 2015.

20 | Safe Medication Preparation

OBJECTIVES

Mastery of content in this chapter will enable the nurse to:

- Discuss nursing roles and responsibilities in medication administration.
- Discuss National Patient Safety Goals for medication administration.
- Discuss factors that contribute to medication errors.
- Differentiate among different types of medication actions.
- List and discuss the six rights of medication administration.

- Identify the system of measurement for a given prescribed medication.
- Accurately calculate medication doses.
- Describe the safety features of medication delivery systems.
- Identify guidelines for safe administration of medications.
- Implement nursing actions to prevent medication errors.
- Discuss methods used to educate patients about prescribed medications.

MEDIA RESOURCES

- evolve http://evolve.elsevier.com/Perry/skills
- Review Questions
- Case Studies

- Audio Glossary
- **NSO** Nursing Skills Online
- Clinical Debrief and Review Questions Answers

PURPOSE

Safe and accurate medication administration is a challenging and important nursing responsibility. All professional nurses need to understand the implications involved in medication administration. Safe medication administration requires good judgment, critical thinking, and clinical decision-making skills. This includes thorough patient assessment and an understanding of pharmacotherapeutics, pharmacokinetics, growth and development, nutrition, and mathematics.

STANDARDS OF CARE

- Centers for Disease Control and Prevention (CDC), 2012—Medication Safety Basics
- Institute for Safe Medication Practices (ISMP), 2011—ISMP Acute Care Guidelines for Timely Administration of Scheduled Medications
- Institute for Safe Medication Practices (ISMP), 2013—ISMP's List of Error-Prone Abbreviations, Symbols, and Dose Designations

- The Joint Commission (TJC), 2016—National Patient Safety Goals

PRINCIPLES FOR PRACTICE

Pharmacological Concepts
Medication Names

NSO *Nursing Skills Online Safe Medication Administration Module / Lesson 1*

Some medications have as many as three different names. The chemical name describes the drug composition and molecular structure such as N-acetyl-para-aminophenol, commonly known as Tylenol. The chemical name provides an exact description of its composition and molecular structure. It is rarely used in clinical practice. A manufacturer who first develops a medication provides the generic name (e.g., acetaminophen is the generic name for Tylenol). The generic name is the name that is listed in official publications such as the *United States Pharmacopeia* (USP). A medication trade name or brand name is used to market the medication. The trade name has the symbol™ at the upper right of the name, indicating a manufacturer trademark of the name (e.g., Panadol™, Tempra™, Tylenol™).

Many companies choose brand and generic names that are easy to remember and can be very similar, which contributes to medication errors. The USP identifies several problematic medications with similar names and spelling such as Lamictal for epilepsy and Lamisil for fungal infections; Levoxine for hypothyroidism and Lanoxin for heart failure; Zebeta for hypertension and Diabeta for type 2 diabetes. The ISMP (2015a) and TJC (2015) both publish a list of medications that are frequently confused with one another. Another measure to help address the confusion around drugs having similar names includes the use of tall-man lettering (ISMP, 2013). This measure uses capital letters in specific parts of a word and helps distinguish dissimilarities in drug names; for example, TEGretol (for seizures) can be confused with TRENtal, which is prescribed for intermittent claudication; but the tall-man letters emphasize the difference in the drug name.

The physical appearances of some drugs with similar color, size, and shape have led to medication errors. For example, St. Joseph's aspirin and Crestor, a lipid-lowering agent, have a similar peach color, size, and circular shape. Generic drugs are often prescribed as a more cost-efficient substitution for brand-name medications. However, there may be dramatic differences in appearance of generic drugs, depending on the manufacturer (Greene et al., 2011). Patients may be confused as to why their medication has a different color or shape when the prescription is refilled. However, you find medications under a variety of different names and must be careful to obtain the exact name and spelling before administering a medication.

Classification

Medications with similar characteristics are categorized by their class. Medication classification indicates the effect of a medication on a body system, the symptoms the medication relieves, or the desired effect of the medication. For example, patients with type 2 diabetes often take oral hypoglycemic medications to control their blood glucose levels. The sulfonylureas are one classification of 11 medications used to treat hyperglycemia. Some medications are part of more than one class. For example, aspirin is an analgesic, antipyretic, and antiinflammatory medication.

Medication Forms

Medications are available in a variety of forms or preparations. The form of the medication determines its route of administration. The composition of a medication influences its absorption and metabolism. Many medications are made in several forms such as tablets, caplets, or suppositories. When administering a medication, be certain to use the proper form (Table 20.1).

Pharmacokinetics

A medication must enter a patient's body; be absorbed and distributed to cells, tissues, or a specific organ; and then alter physiological function to be therapeutic. Pharmacokinetics is the study of how medications enter the body, reach their site of action, are metabolized, and exit the body. Understanding pharmacokinetics allows you to properly time medication administration, select an administration route, and judge a patient's response to medications. Absorption is the passage of medication molecules into the blood from the site of administration. Factors that influence the rate of absorption include the administration route, ability of a medication to dissolve, blood flow to the administration site, body surface area, and lipid solubility of a medication (Table 20.2). After a medication is absorbed, it is distributed to tissues and organs and finally to the site of drug action. The rate and extent of distribution depends on circulation, cell membrane permeability, and protein binding. Poor perfusion (e.g., heart failure) alters medication distribution. A medication must pass through biological membranes to reach certain organs. Some membranes are barriers to the passage of medications. For example, the blood-brain barrier allows only fat-soluble medications to pass into the brain and cerebrospinal fluid. The degree to which medications bind to serum proteins such as albumin affects distribution. Most medications bind to albumin to some extent. When this happens, they are unable to exert pharmacological activity. Only the unbound, or "free," medication is active. Older adults and patients with liver disease or malnutrition have reduced albumin, which increases their risk for medication toxicity.

After a medication reaches its site of action, it is metabolized into a less active or inactive form. Biotransformation occurs under the influence of enzymes that detoxify, degrade (break down), and remove biologically active chemicals. Most biotransformation occurs in the liver; although the lungs, kidneys, blood, and intestines also play a role. Patients (e.g., older adults and those with chronic disease) are at risk for medication toxicity if their organs cannot metabolize medications effectively.

The final aspect of pharmacokinetics is excretion, the process by which medications exit the body through the lungs, exocrine glands, bowel, kidneys, and liver. The chemical makeup of a medication determines the organ of excretion. For example, gaseous and volatile compounds such as alcohol and nitrous oxide exit through the lungs. The site of excretion poses implications for nursing care. For example, when medications exit through sweat glands, you provide skin care to reduce irritation. You must know if a drug is excreted through the intestines because the administration of laxatives or enemas increases peristalsis, accelerates excretion, and thus lessens the time for drug effects. When patients have reduced renal function, they are at risk for medication toxicity since kidneys are the main organs for medication excretion.

Types of Medication Action

Medications vary in the way they act and their types of action. Patients do not always respond in the same way to each successive dose of a medication. Sometimes the same medication causes very different responses in different patients. Therefore it is

TABLE 20.1

Forms of Medication

Form	Description
Medication Forms Commonly Prepared for Administration by Oral Route	
Solid Forms	
Caplet	Shaped like a capsule and coated for ease of swallowing
Capsule	Medication encased in a gelatin shell
Tablet	Powdered medication compressed into a hard disk or cylinder; in addition to primary medication, contains binders (adhesive to allow powder to stick together), disintegrators (to promote table dissolution), lubricants (for ease of manufacturing), and fillers (for convenient tablet size)
Enteric coated	Coated tablet that does not dissolve in stomach; coating dissolves in intestine, where medication is absorbed
Liquid Forms	
Elixir	Clear fluid containing water and alcohol; often sweetened
Extract	Concentrated medication form made by removing the active part of the medication from its components. Extracts are prepared as a syrup or dried form of pharmacologically active medication, usually made by evaporating solution
Aqueous solution	Substance dissolved in water and syrups
Aqueous suspension	Finely dissolved drug particles in liquid medium must be shaken; when left standing, particles settle to bottom of container
Syrup	Medication dissolved in concentrated sugar solution
Tincture	Alcohol extract from plant or vegetable
Other Oral Forms and Terms Associated With Oral Preparations	
Troche (lozenge)	Flat, round tablet that dissolves in mouth to release medication; not meant for ingestion
Aerosol	Aqueous medication sprayed and absorbed in mouth and upper airway; not meant for ingestion
Sustained release	Tablet or capsule that contains small particles of a medication coated with material that requires a varying amount of time to dissolve
Medication Forms Commonly Prepared for Administration by Topical Route	
Ointment (salve or cream)	Semisolid, externally applied preparation, usually containing one or more medications
Liniment	Usually contains alcohol, oil, or soapy emollient applied to skin
Lotion	Semiliquid suspension that usually protects, cools, or cleans skin
Paste	Medication preparation that is thicker than ointment; absorbed through skin more slowly than ointment; often used for skin protection
Transdermal patch or disk	Medicated disk or patch embedded with medication that is applied to skin Drug absorbed through skin over a designated period of time (e.g., 24 hours)
Medication Forms Commonly Prepared for Administration by Parenteral Route	
Solution	Sterile preparation that contains water/normal saline with one or more dissolved compounds
Powder	Sterile particles of medication that are dissolved in a sterile liquid (e.g., water, normal saline) before administration
Medication Forms Commonly Prepared for Instillation Into Body Cavities	
Suppository	Solid dosage form mixed with gelatin and shaped in form of a pellet for insertion into body cavity (rectum or vagina) (Suppository melts when it reaches body temperature and is then absorbed.)
Intraocular disk	Small, flexible oval (similar to a contact lens) consisting of two soft outer layers and a middle layer containing medication; slowly releases medication when moistened by ocular fluid.

essential to understand all the effects that medications have on patients.

Therapeutic Effects

Each medication has a therapeutic effect (i.e., the intended or desired physiological response of a medication). For example, you administer morphine sulfate, an analgesic, to relieve a patient's pain. Sometimes a single medication has many therapeutic effects. For example, aspirin relieves pain and reduces fever and tissue inflammation. Knowing the desired therapeutic effect for each medication allows you to provide patient education and accurately evaluate its desired effect.

Adverse Effects

Adverse drug events or effects (ADEs) are unintended, undesirable, and often unpredictable. Although sometimes they are apparent immediately, unfortunately they often take weeks or months to develop. Early clinical recognition of ADEs is the important first step in identification. ADEs range from mild (e.g., rashes or photosensitivity to light) to potentially fatal (anaphylaxis). Prompt recognition and reporting of ADEs prevent serious injury to patients. Always assess patients who may be at high risk for an ADE such as pregnant women and patients with chronic disorders (e.g., hypertension, epilepsy, heart disease, psychoses) (Burchum and Rosenthal, 2016). Health care providers report

TABLE 20.2

Medication Absorption

Absorption Factor	Physiologic Effects
Route of administration	Topical applications on skin absorb slowly. Medications applied to mucous membranes and respiratory airways absorb quickly. Oral medications pass through the gastrointestinal tract and absorb slowly. The intravenous route produces the most rapid absorption because the medication is available immediately when it enters the systemic circulation.
Ability to dissolve	Solutions and liquid suspensions absorb more readily than tablets or capsules. Acidic medications pass through the gastric mucosa rapidly and absorb rapidly, whereas basic medications (pH greater than 7.0) do not absorb before reaching the small intestine.
Blood flow	When the administration site contains a rich blood supply, medications absorb rapidly.
Body surface area	A medication in contact with a large surface area (e.g., small intestine) absorbs faster than one in contact with smaller surface area (e.g., stomach).
Lipid solubility	Medications that are highly lipid soluble absorb more readily.

adverse events to the Food and Drug Administration (FDA) using the MedWatch program (USFDA, 2015).

Side Effects

Every medication has the potential for harm. No medication is totally safe and absolutely free of nontherapeutic effects. Side effects are predictable and often unavoidable secondary effects produced at a usual therapeutic drug dose. They are either harmless or cause injury. The intensity of side effects is often dose dependent. If the side effects are serious enough to outweigh the benefits of the therapeutic action of a medication, the health care provider will likely discontinue the medication. Patients commonly stop taking medications because of side effects such as anorexia, nausea, vomiting, dizziness, drowsiness, dry mouth, constipation, and diarrhea. Report any side effect to the health care provider to ensure that it is not incorrectly interpreted as a more serious adverse medication reaction.

Toxic Effects

Toxic effects develop after prolonged intake of a medication or when a medication accumulates in the blood because of impaired metabolism or excretion. Excess amounts of a medication within the body sometimes have lethal effects, depending on the action of the medication. For example, toxic levels of morphine, an opioid, cause severe respiratory depression and death. Antidotes are available to treat specific types of medication toxicity. For example, naloxone, an opioid antagonist, reverses the effects of opioid toxicity.

Idiosyncratic Reactions

An idiosyncratic reaction is an unpredictable effect in which a patient overreacts or underreacts to a medication or has a reaction different from normal. Predicting which patients will have an idiosyncratic response is impossible. For example, lorazepam is an antianxiety medication that may cause agitation and delirium when given to an older adult.

Allergic Reactions

Allergic reactions also are adverse unpredictable responses to a medication. Exposure to an initial dose of a medication causes a patient to become sensitized immunologically. The medication acts as an antigen, which causes antibodies to be produced. With repeated administration a patient develops an allergic response to the drug, its chemical preservatives, or a metabolite. An allergic reaction ranges from mild to severe, depending on the patient and the medication (Table 20.3). Among the different

TABLE 20.3

Mild Allergic Reactions

Symptom	Description
Urticaria (hives)	Raised, irregularly shaped skin eruptions with varying sizes and shapes; reddened margins and pale centers
Rash	Small, raised vesicles that are usually reddened; often distributed over the entire body
Pruritus	Itching of the skin; accompanies most rashes
Rhinitis	Inflammation of mucous membranes lining the nose, causing swelling and a clear watery discharge

classes of medications, antibiotics cause a high incidence of allergic reactions. Severe or anaphylactic reactions, which are life threatening, are characterized by sudden constriction of bronchiolar muscles, edema of the pharynx and larynx, severe wheezing, and shortness of breath. Some patients become severely hypotensive, necessitating emergency resuscitation measures.

It is common practice for hospitalized patients with known drug allergies to have their allergy information recorded in a clearly identifiable place. This allows all caregivers to be aware of each patient's allergies. In many agencies this information is recorded in a special section of the electronic health record (EHR), on the front of a patient's hard-copy medical record or chart, in the medication administration record (MAR), or on a specially designed label that is applied to the front of a patient's chart. Patients also receive color-coded allergy identification bands to wear around the wrist. *Always record a patient's allergies in the MAR.* Patients who are cared for in other settings (e.g., home or community clinics) and have a known history of an allergy to a medication or substance should wear an identification bracelet or medal, which alerts all health care providers to the allergies in case a patient is found unconscious or is unable to communicate (Fig. 20.1). It is often common that patients list having an allergy to a drug when it is not a true allergy but rather a severe side effect or an adverse drug effect (ADE). It is important for the nurse to be aware of the difference between a true allergy and a side effect. Ask the patient which type of reaction he or she experiences and offer him or her examples such as nausea versus hives.

Medication Tolerance and Dependence

Medication tolerance occurs over time. It is usually noted clinically when patients receive the same medication for long periods and

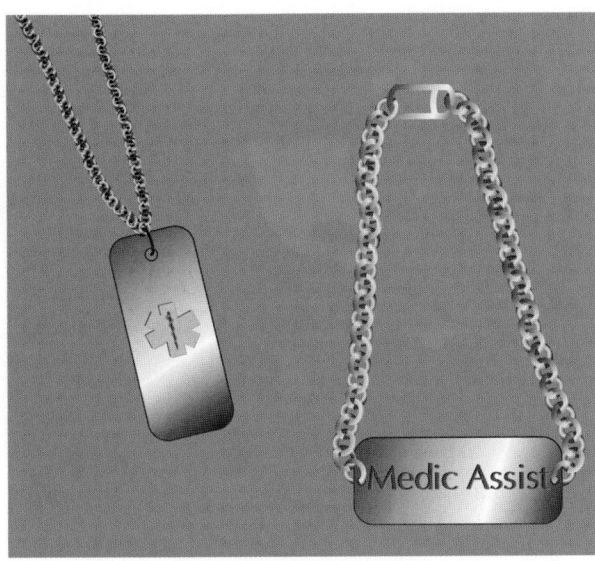

FIG 20.1 Identification bracelet and medal.

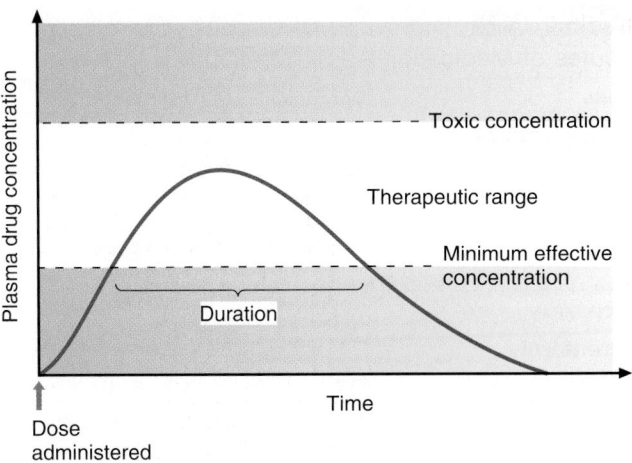

FIG 20.2 The therapeutic range of medication occurs between the minimum effective concentration and the toxic concentration. *(From Burchum J, Rosenthal L: Lehne's pharmacology for nursing care, ed 9, St Louis, 2016, Saunders.)*

require higher doses to produce the desired therapeutic effect. Medications known to produce tolerance include opium alkaloids (e.g., morphine), nitrates, and ethyl alcohol. Patients hospitalized for acute episodes of illness usually do not develop tolerance. It may take a month or longer for tolerance to occur.

Medication tolerance is not the same as medication dependence. Two types of medication dependence exist: psychological (or addiction) or physical. In psychological dependence a patient desires the medication for benefit other than the intended effect. Physical dependence is a physiological adaptation to a medication that manifests itself by intense physical disturbance when the medication is withdrawn. When patients receive medications for a short term such as for postoperative pain, dependence is rare. If a patient is dependent on alcohol, a higher-than-usual medication dose is necessary for the desired effect of the medication.

Medication Interactions

When one medication modifies the action of another medication, a medication interaction occurs. Medication interactions are common in individuals taking many medications. Some medications increase or diminish the action of other medications and alter the way in which another medication is absorbed, metabolized, or eliminated from the body. When two medications have a synergistic effect, their combined effect is greater than the effect of one drug given separately. For example, alcohol is a central nervous system depressant that has a synergistic effect with antihistamines, antidepressants, and narcotic analgesics. Sometimes a medication interaction is the desired effect. Health providers often combine medications to create an interaction that has a therapeutic effect. For example, a patient with hypertension may receive several medications such as diuretics and vasodilators, which act together to control the blood pressure when one medication alone is not effective.

Medication Dose Responses

A medication undergoes absorption, distribution, metabolism, and excretion after administration. Medications take time to enter the bloodstream, except when administered intravenously. When a medication is prescribed, the goal is a constant blood level within a safe therapeutic range. The minimum effective concentration (MEC) is the plasma level of the medication below which the effect of the medication does not occur. The toxic concentration is the

level at which toxic effects occur. The safe therapeutic range is between the MEC and the toxic concentration (Fig. 20.2). When a medication is administered repeatedly, its serum level fluctuates between doses. The highest level is called the *peak concentration*, and the lowest level is called the *trough concentration*. After peaking, the serum concentration falls progressively. With intravenous (IV) infusions, the peak concentration occurs quickly, but the serum level also begins to fall immediately. Some medication doses (e.g., vancomycin or gentamicin) are based on peak and trough serum levels. A patient's trough level is drawn as a blood sample 30 minutes before administering the drug, and the peak level is drawn whenever the drug is expected to reach its peak concentration. The results of the blood test reveal if the drug is reaching its therapeutic blood level.

All medications have a biological half-life, which is the time it takes for excretion processes to lower the serum medication concentration by half. To maintain a therapeutic plateau, a patient needs to receive regular fixed doses. For example, pain medications are most effective for some cancer patients when they are given around the clock (ATC) rather than when a patient intermittently complains of pain because the body maintains an almost constant level of pain medication (Burchum and Rosenthal, 2016). After an initial medication dose, the patient receives each successive dose when the previous dose reaches its half-life. The patient and nurse need to follow regular dosage schedules and administer prescribed doses at correct intervals. Know the following time intervals of medication action to anticipate the effect of a medication:

- *Onset of medication action:* Time it takes after a medication is administered for it to produce a response
- *Peak action:* Time it takes for a medication to reach its highest effective peak concentration
- *Trough:* Minimum blood serum concentration of medication reached just before the next scheduled dose
- *Duration of action:* Length of time during which a medication is present in a concentration great enough to produce a therapeutic effect
- *Plateau:* Blood serum concentration reached and maintained after repeated, fixed doses

Routes of Administration

The route prescribed for administering a medication (Table 20.4) depends on its properties and desired effect and on a patient's

TABLE 20.4

Routes of Medication Administration

Route	Description
Nonparenteral	
Oral, buccal	By mouth/mucous membrane
Sublingual	Under the tongue
Topical	On the skin (as a cream or patch) and eyedrops/eardrops
Suppository	Into the rectum or vagina
Parenteral	
Intramuscular (IM)	Into a muscle
Subcutaneous	Into the subcutaneous tissue of the skin
Intradermal (ID)	Into the dermis of the skin
Epidural	Into the epidural space
Intravenous (IV)	Into a vein

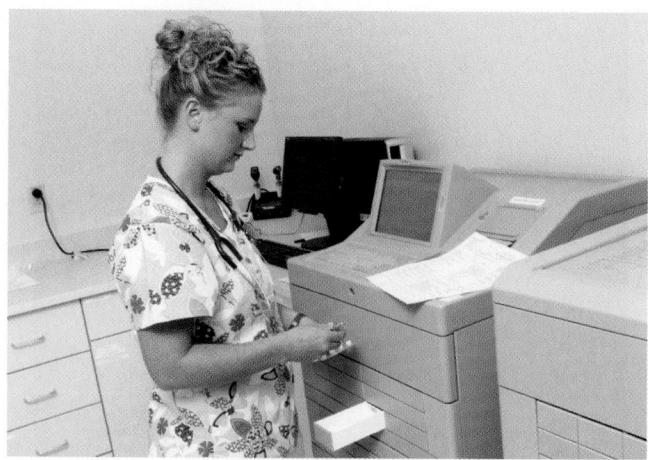

FIG 20.3 Automated medication dispensing system.

physical and mental condition. Because of what you know about each patient, you need to collaborate with a health care provider in determining the best route for a patient's medical condition. Table 20.5 summarizes the factors that influence the choice of administration routes.

Medication Distribution

Health care providers write medication orders, pharmacists dispense medications, and nurses verify and deliver medications to patients. Verification is the three-system check to ensure safe medication administration. The first check is the health care provider ordering the right drug for the right purpose. The pharmacist is the second check to ensure that the drug is appropriate and ordered correctly and then provided to the unit correctly. Finally, the nurse verifies the drug before administration with the three checks for accuracy to be sure that it is appropriate and ordered correctly.

A number of technologies for medication distribution have the potential for reducing medication errors and ADEs. The technologies include computerized provider order entry (CPOE), automated medication dispensing system (AMDS), and bar coding (Ghaemmaghami, 2014; Wittich et al., 2014).

Computerized Provider Order Entry

CPOE is a system that allows health care providers to enter orders for medications electronically, eliminating the need for written orders. CPOE increases the accuracy and legibility of medication orders, creates evidence-based order sets, and strengthens nursing documentation and coordination of care (Ghaemmaghami, 2014). Decision support software integrated into a CPOE system allows for automatic drug allergy checks, dosage indications, baseline laboratory result checks, and identification of potential drug interactions. When a health care provider enters an order through CPOE, the information about the order immediately transmits to the pharmacy and ultimately to the nurses' medication administration record (MAR) without the need for written transcription.

Distribution Systems

Systems for storing and distributing medications vary. Agencies providing nursing care have special areas for stocking and dispensing medications. Special medication rooms, portable locked carts, computerized medication cabinets, and individual storage units

next to patients' rooms are examples of storage areas used. Medication storage areas must be locked when unattended.

Unit Dose

The standard for medication distribution is the unit-dose system. The system uses an AMDS or carts containing a drawer with a 24-hour supply of medications for each patient. Each drawer has a label with the name of the patient and the designated room. The unit dose is the ordered dose of medication that the patient receives at one time. Each medication form is wrapped in a foil or paper container separately. Liquid doses come in prepackaged foil or plastic cups (e.g., for use in long-term care or the home setting). The cart also contains limited amounts of stock medication for special situations. At a designated time each day the pharmacist or a pharmacy technician refills the drawers in the cart with a fresh supply. Controlled substances are not in the individual patient drawer; they are in a larger locked drawer to keep them secure. A unit-dose system is designed to reduce the number of medication errors and saves steps in dispensing medications.

Automated Medication Dispensing System

AMDSs are variations of unit-dose and floor stock systems (Fig. 20.3). The systems within the health care agency are networked with one another and with other computer systems in the agency (e.g., computerized medical record). AMDSs control the dispensing of all medications, including opioid narcotics. Each nurse has a security code, which allows access to the system. If your agency uses a system that requires bioidentification, you have to place your finger on a screen to access the computer. Once logged onto the AMDS, you select a patient's name and medication profile. Then you select the medication, dosage, and route from a list displayed on the computer screen. The system opens the medication drawer or dispenses the medication to the nurse, records the event, and charges it to the patient. If the system is connected to the patient's medical record, information about the medication (e.g., name, dose, time) and the name of the nurse who retrieved it from the AMDS are recorded in the record. There is evidence of an increase in reported medication errors with use of the system and a reduction in dispensing errors through the use of alerts that are embedded within the clinical decision support system (Rochais et al., 2014).

The bar code medication administration (BCMA) system is often used to identify the patient, the medication, and the identification tag of the nurse administering the medication before recording this information in the patient's computerized medical

TABLE 20.5

Factors Influencing Choice of Administration Routes

Advantages	Disadvantages/Contraindications
Oral, Buccal, Sublingual Routes	
Routes are easy and comfortable to administer, convenient, economical; may produce local or systemic effects; and rarely cause anxiety for patient.	Routes are avoided when patient has alterations in GI function (e.g., nausea and vomiting), with reduced GI motility (after general anesthesia or bowel inflammation), and with surgical resection of part of GI tract. Gastric secretions destroy some medications. Oral administration is contraindicated in patients who are NPO and unable to swallow (e.g., patients with neuromuscular disorders, esophageal strictures, and mouth lesions). Do not give oral medications when patient has gastric suction or before certain diagnostic tests or surgery. An unconscious or confused patient is unable or unwilling to swallow or hold sublingual medication under tongue or buccal medication in cheek. Oral medications sometimes irritate lining of GI tract, discolor teeth, or have an unpleasant taste.
Subcutaneous, Intramuscular, Intravenous, Intradermal, Epidural Routes	
Routes provide means of administration when oral medications are contraindicated. More rapid absorption occurs than with topical or oral routes.	There are risks for introducing infection, and medications are expensive. Some patients experience pain from repeated needlesticks. Avoid subcutaneous, IM, and ID routes in patients with bleeding tendencies. There is risk for tissue damage with subcutaneous injections.
IV infusion provides medication delivery when patient is critically ill or long-term therapy is necessary. If peripheral perfusion is poor, IV route is preferred over injections. Epidural provides excellent pain control.	IV and IM routes have higher absorption rates, thus placing patients at higher risk for reactions. It limits mobility during administration, and there is risk for infection.
Skin	
Topical	
Topical skin applications provide primarily local effect. Route is usually painless. Limited side effects occur.	Extensive applications often require dressings that are bulky for a patient when maneuvering. Do not apply to skin if abrasions are present, unless that is the reason for order. Medications can be absorbed by person applying them if gloves are not worn.
Transdermal	
Transdermal applications provide prolonged systemic effects with limited side effects.	Application leaves oily or pasty substance on skin and may soil clothing. Some patients have sensitivity to adhesive.
Mucous Membranes (Includes Eyes, Ears, Nose, Vaginal, Rectal, Buccal, and Sublingual Routes)	
Therapeutic effects are provided by local application to involved sites. Aqueous solutions are readily absorbed and capable of causing systemic effects. Mucous membranes provide route of administration when oral medications are contraindicated.	Mucous membranes are highly sensitive to some medication concentrations. Insertion of rectal and vaginal medications often causes embarrassment. Rectal suppositories are contraindicated if patients have had rectal surgery or if active rectal bleeding is present. If eardrum is ruptured, otic medications are usually contraindicated.
Inhalation	
Inhalation provides rapid relief for local respiratory problems. An inhaled form of insulin is also available. Route provides easy access for introduction of general anesthetic gases.	Some local agents cause serious systemic effects. If patients are unable to administer inhaler correctly, medication is ineffective. Inhalation is difficult to learn for older adults and children.
Intraocular Disk	
Route is advantageous in that it does not require frequent administration (e.g., as for eyedrops). Patient can also wear disk when sleeping or swimming. Dry eyes do not affect medication delivery.	Local reactions such as tearing, itching, or redness of the eyes occur. Patient needs to know how to insert disk into and remove from eye. Medication is often expensive. Medication is contraindicated in patients with eye infections.

GI, Gastrointestinal; *ID,* intradermal; *IM,* intramuscular; *IV,* intravenous; *NPO,* nothing by mouth.

record. Agencies that implement AMDS with BCMA often reduce the incidence of medication errors.

Special Handling of Controlled Substances

As a nurse you are responsible for following legal regulations when administering controlled substances (medications with potential for abuse). Violations of the Controlled Substances Act may result in fines, imprisonment, and loss of license. Health care agencies have policies for the proper storage and distribution of controlled

substances, including opioids (Box 20.1). Many agencies use computerized systems for medication access and distribution.

Bar Coding

Bar-code labels are required on all medications, vaccines, and over-the-counter (OTC) drugs used in health care agencies (Wittich et al., 2014). EHR technology is used to improve patient care quality and coordination by providing health care providers easier access to patient information in a secure format. The use of

Guidelines for Safe Opioid Administration and Control

- All controlled substances are stored in a securely locked, substantially constructed cabinet (i.e., automated medication dispensing system [AMDS]) or a locked room.
- Authorized nurses carry a set of keys or an individual computer entry code for the AMDS.
- An inventory record is used each time a controlled substance is dispensed. Records are often kept electronically and provide an accurate ongoing account of the medications used, wasted, and remaining. If you find a discrepancy, correct and report it immediately.
- Use a special inventory record to document a patient's name, date, name of medication, dose, time of medication administration, and signature of nurse dispensing the medication.
- A second nurse witnesses disposal of the unused part if a nurse gives only part of a dose of a controlled substance. Computerized systems record the nurses' names electronically. If paper records are kept, both nurses sign their names on the form. Follow agency policy for appropriate waste of opioids. Do not place wasted part of medications in sharps containers.

TABLE 20.6

Equivalents of Measurement

Metric	Household
1 mL	15 drops (gtt)
5 mL	1 teaspoon (tsp)
15 mL	1 tablespoon (tbsp)
30 mL	2 tablespoon (tbsp)
240 mL	1 cup (c)
480 mL (approximately 500 mL)	1 pint (pt)
960 mL (approximately 1 L)	1 quart (qt)
3840 mL (approximately 4 L)	1 gallon (gal)

electronic bar codes on medication labels and packaging has the potential to improve patient safety in a number of ways. Bar codes electronically link with a hospital computer system. A patient's MAR entered into the computer database and encoded in the patient's wristband is accessible to a nurse through a handheld device. The device scans the patient's wristband and then displays the MAR. When administering a medication, the nurse scans the bar code on the drug and the patient's medical record number on the wristband. The computer processes the scanned information, charts it, and updates the patient's MAR record appropriately. The use of bar codes improves accuracy of patient identification, provides alert to potential medication error, and improves medical record keeping.

Systems of Medication Measurement

NSO *Nursing Skills Online Safe Medication Administration Module / Lesson 3*

The proper administration of medication depends on your ability to compute medication doses accurately and measure medications correctly. A careless mistake in placing a decimal point or adding a zero to a dosage can lead to fatal errors. The health care provider and patient depend on you to check doses before administering medications. Medication therapy uses metric, apothecary, and household systems of measurement. The apothecary system is used infrequently today. The most common medication measurement system is the metric system.

Metric System

As a decimal system the metric system is the most logically organized of the measurement systems. Metric units are easy to convert and compute through simple multiplication and division. Each basic unit of measure is organized into units of 10. Multiplying or dividing by 10 forms secondary units. In multiplication the decimal point moves to the right; in division the decimal moves to the left. For example:

$$10 \text{ mg} \times 10 = 100 \text{ mg}$$
$$10 \text{ mg} \div 10 = 1 \text{ mg}$$

The basic units of measure in the metric system are the meter (length), the liter (volume), and the gram (weight). For drug calculations you will primarily use volume and weight units. In the metric system lowercase or capital letters designate the basic units:

$$\text{Gram} = \text{g or Gm}$$
$$\text{Liter} = \text{l or L}$$

Use only lowercase letters for abbreviations for subdivisions of major units:

$$\text{Milligram} = \text{mg}$$
$$\text{Milliliter} = \text{mL}$$

When writing medication dosages in metric units, health care providers and nurses use either fractions or multiples of a unit. Convert fractions to decimals:

$$500 \text{ mg or } 0.5 \text{ g, not } \tfrac{1}{2} \text{ g}$$
$$10 \text{ mL or } 0.01 \text{ L, not } \tfrac{1}{100} \text{ L}$$

Many actual or potential medication errors happen with the use of fractions or decimal points. Use practice standards when medications are ordered in fractions to prevent errors. For example, never use a trailing zero (e.g., 1.0 mg) and always include a zero before a decimal point (e.g., 0.1 mL) (ISMP, 2013; TJC, 2015).

Household Measurement

Household measures are familiar to most people, but these are no longer recommended for medication administration because of the variability in the size of household utensils. Household measures include drops, teaspoons, tablespoons, and cups for volume and ounces and pounds for weight. A transition period may be necessary during which the household measure can be listed in parentheses immediately following the metric measure (e.g., 5 mL [one teaspoonful]). To calculate medications accurately, you need to know common equivalents of metric and household units (Table 20.6).

Solutions

Solutions of various concentrations are used for injections, irrigations, and infusions. A solution is a given mass of solid substance dissolved in a known volume of fluid or a given volume of liquid dissolved in a known volume of another fluid. Solutions are available in units of mass per units of volume (e.g., g/mL or g/L). You can also express the concentration of a solution as a percentage. A 10% solution is 10 g of solid dissolved in 100 mL of solution. A proportion also expresses concentrations. A 1/1000 solution represents a solution containing 1 g of solid in 1000 mL of liquid or 1 mL of liquid mixed with 1000 mL of another liquid.

PATIENT-CENTERED CARE

- A nurse's responsibility when administering medications safely must include effective communication with staff, pharmacy, patients, and family caregivers.
- Patients are an important resource for understanding the knowledge they have about their medications, their perceptions about the effects of medications, and their expectations for treatment.
- Consider factors that influence patient's abilities to communicate effectively such as anxiety, pain, hearing, or their cultural background. Therapeutic communication is essential to nursing practice and critical in safe medication administration.
- A new scientific field, pharmacogenetics, involves the study of the genetic influence on drug response that occurs from inherited metabolic defects or deficiencies. The most common mechanism of genetic influence on medications is the alteration in drug metabolism. The outcome is either a reduced benefit or increased toxicity of the medication (Burchum and Rosenthal, 2016). As a nurse you cannot detect a genetic abnormality. However, you can learn to become aware of cultural differences in drug responses to better monitor drug therapy.
- Culturally a patient's values and beliefs affect medication response.
- A patient's level of education, prior experience with medication therapy, and the family's influence on actions significantly influence medication adherence. For example, in some cultures it is not acceptable to complain about gastrointestinal problems; thus it is common for patients not to report nausea, vomiting, and bowel changes related to medication use.
- Use of herbal and homeopathic remedies in some cultures alters response to a medication.
- Ethnicity needs to be considered when medications are prescribed and administered.

Safe Medication Administration

Standards are actions that help ensure safe nursing practice. Standards for medication administration are set by health care agencies, nursing profession, and other organizations (Box 20.2). Most agencies have procedure manuals that contain policies about which medications nurses can and cannot deliver. The types and dosages that nurses may administer often vary from unit to unit within an agency. Professional standards such as *Nursing: Scope and Standards of Practice* (ANA, 2015) apply to the activity of safe medication administration. To prevent medication errors follow the six rights of medication administration consistently every time you administer medications. Many medication errors are linked in some way to an inconsistency in adhering to the six rights:

1. Right medication
2. Right dose
3. Right patient
4. Right route
5. Right time
6. Right documentation

BOX 20.2

The Joint Commission 2016 Hospital National Patient Safety Goals: Implications for Medication Administration

- Identify patient correctly. Use at least two patient identifiers (neither can be patient's room number) when providing care, treatment (e.g., medications), or services.
- Improve the effectiveness of communication among caregivers.
- Verbal or telephone orders require a verification "read-back" of the complete order or test result by the person receiving the order/test result.
- Standardize a list of abbreviations, acronyms, symbols, and dose designations that are *not* to be used throughout an organization.
- Improve the safety of using medications.
- Identify and at a minimum annually review a list of look-alike/sound-alike drugs used by the organization.
- Before a procedure, label all medications and medication containers (e.g., syringes) that are not labeled. Do this in areas where medicines and supplies are set up, such as on and off the sterile field in perioperative and other procedural settings. Labels include drug name, strength, amount, expiration date when not used within 24 hours, and expiration time when expiration occurs in less than 24 hours.
- Take extra care with patients who take anticoagulants. Use only oral unit-dose products and premixed infusions. When heparin is administered intravenously and continuously, use programmable infusion pumps.
- Maintain and communicate accurate patient medication information.
- Accurately and completely reconcile medications across the continuum of care.
- There is a process for comparing the patient's current medications with those ordered for the patient while under the care of the health care organization.
- Communicate a complete list of the patient's medications to the next provider of service when a patient is referred or transferred to another setting, service, or level of care. Also provide the complete list to the patient on discharge from the agency.
- Encourage patients' active involvement in their own care as a patient safety strategy.

Modified from The Joint Commission: *2016 National Patient Safety Goals*, Oakbrook Terrace, IL, 2016, The Commission, http://www.jointcommission.org/standards_information/npsgs.aspx. Accessed April 2, 2016.

Right Medication

At the time of admission, when transferring to a different unit, and when discharging patients from a hospital, assess their medication regimen, especially if they were admitted to the hospital because of a problem with medication self-administration. A strategy to reduce medication errors at transition points is the process of medication reconciliation. Patients often leave the hospital with a basic knowledge of their medications but are unable to safely self-administer them once they return home. When patients enter a health care agency, it is critical for health care providers to have an accurate list of the medications they are currently prescribed to take and any OTC medications being used.

A medication order is required for every medication that you administer to a patient. Some health care providers write orders by hand in a patient's chart. However, many agencies use CPOE, eliminating the need for handwritten orders and enhancing patient safety (Ghaemmaghami, 2014). Regardless of how an order is received, you compare the health care provider's orders with the

MAR or electronic MAR (eMAR) when the medication is ordered initially. Nurses verify medication information whenever new MARs are written or distributed or when patients transfer from one nursing unit or health care setting to another (TJC, 2015).

The ISMP (2013) and TJC published a list of error-prone and prohibited abbreviations that have been found to increase the incidence of errors in medication administration (Table 20.7). You are responsible for using correct abbreviations and verifying that the order was transcribed accurately.

Medication Orders. You must have a medication order before administering medications to a patient. Verbal and telephone orders are optional forms of orders when written or electronic communication between the health care provider and nurse is not possible. When you receive a verbal or telephone order, you write or enter the order on the health care provider's order sheet. You then read-back the order for verification and document the read-back. The name of the health care provider and your signature are included. The health care provider will countersign the order at a

---

TABLE 20.7

Institute for Safe Medication Practice List of Error-Prone Abbreviations

These abbreviations, symbols, and dose designations were reported to the Institute for Safe Medication add Practice (ISMP) through the USP-ISMP Medication Error Reporting Program for being frequently misinterpreted and involved in harmful medication errors. They should NEVER be used when communicating medical information. This includes internal communications, telephone/verbal prescriptions, computer-generated labels, labels for drug storage bins, medication administration records, and pharmacy and prescriber computer order entry screens. The Joint Commission (TJC) has established a National Patient Safety Goal that specifies that certain abbreviations must appear on the do-not-use list of an accredited organization; these items are highlighted with a double asterisk (**).

Abbreviations	Intended Meaning	Misinterpretation	Correction
μg	Microgram	Mistaken as "mg"	Use "mcg"
AD, AS, AU	Right ear, left ear, each ear	Mistaken as OD, OS, OU (right eye, left eye, each eye)	Use "right ear," "left ear," or "each ear"
OD, OS, OU	Right eye, left eye, each eye	Mistaken as AD, AS, AU (right ear, left ear, each ear)	Use "right eye," "left eye," or "each eye"
BT	Bedtime	Mistaken as "BID" (twice daily)	Use "bedtime"
Cc	Cubic centimeters	Mistaken as "u" (units)	Use "mL"
D/C	Discharge or discontinue	Premature discontinuation of medication if D/C (intended to mean "discharge") has been misinterpreted as "discontinued" when followed by a list of discharge medications	Use "discharge" and "discontinue"
IJ	Injection	Mistaken as "IV" or "intrajugular"	Use "injection"
IN	Intranasal	Mistaken as "IM" or "IV"	Use "intranasal" or "NAS"
HS	Half-strength	Mistaken as bedtime	Use "half-strength"
hs	At bedtime, hour of sleep	Mistaken as half-strength	Use "bedtime"
IU**	International unit	Mistaken as IV (intravenous) or 10 (ten)	Use "units"
o.d. or OD	Once daily	Mistaken as "right eye" (OD—*oculus dexter*), leading to oral liquid medications administered in the eye	Use "daily"
OJ	Orange juice	Mistaken as OD or OS (right or left eye); drugs meant to be diluted in orange juice may be given in the eye	Use "orange juice"
Per os	By mouth, orally	The "os" can be mistaken as "left eye" (OS—*oculus sinister*)	Use "PO," "by mouth," or "orally"
q.d. or QD**	Every day	Mistaken as q.i.d., especially if the period after the "q" or the tail of the "q" is misunderstood as an "i"	Use "daily"
qhs	Nightly at bedtime	Mistaken as "qhr" or every hour	Use "nightly"
qn	Nightly or at bedtime	Mistaken as "qhr" or every hour	Use "nightly" or "at bedtime"
q.o.d. or QOD**	Every other day	Mistaken as q.d. (daily) or q.i.d. (4 times daily) if the "o" is poorly written	Use "every other day"
q.d.	Daily	Mistaken as q.i.d. (4 times daily)	Use "daily"
q6PM, etc.	Every evening at 6 PM	Mistaken as every 6 hours	Use "6 PM nightly" or "6 PM daily"
SC, SQ, sub q	Subcutaneous	SC mistaken as SL (sublingual); SQ mistaken as "5 every"; the "q" in "sub q" has been mistaken for "every" (e.g., a heparin dose ordered "sub q 2 hours before surgery" misunderstood as every 2 hours before surgery)	Use "subcut" or "subcutaneously"

TABLE 20.7

Institute for Safe Medication Practice List of Error-Prone Abbreviations—cont'd

Abbreviations	Intended Meaning	Misinterpretation	Correction
ss	Sliding scale (insulin) or "½"; (apothecary)	Mistaken as "55"	Spell out "sliding scale"; use "one-half" or "½"
SSRI	Sliding scale regular insulin	Mistaken as selective-serotonin reuptake inhibitor	Spell out "sliding scale (insulin)"
SSI	Sliding scale insulin	Mistaken as Strong Solution of Iodine (Lugol's)	Spell out "sliding scale (insulin)"
i/d	One daily	Mistaken as "tid"	Use "1 daily"
TIW or tiw	3 times a week	Mistaken as "3 times a day" or "twice a week"	Use "3 times weekly"
U or u**	Unit	Mistaken as the number 0 or 4, causing a 10-fold overdose or greater (e.g., 4U seen as 40 or 4u seen as 44); mistaken as "cc" so dose given in volume instead of units (e.g., 4u seen as 4cc)	Use "unit"
UD	As directed ("ut dictum")	Mistaken as unit dose (e.g., diltiazem 125 mg IV infusion "UD" misinterpreted as meaning to give the entire infusion as a unit [bolus] dose)	Use "as directed"

Used with permission, Institute for Safe Medication Practices (ISMP): ISMP's list of error-prone abbreviations, symbols, and dose designations, 2013, https://www.ismp.org/tools/errorproneabbreviations.pdf. Accessed April 2, 2016.
**These abbreviations are included on The Joint Commission "minimum list" of dangerous abbreviations, acronyms, and symbols that must be included on the "Do Not Use" list of an organization, effective January 1, 2011.

BOX 20.3

Guidelines for Verbal and Telephone Orders

- Only authorized staff receive and record verbal or telephone orders. Agency identifies in writing the staff who are authorized.
- Clearly identify patient's name, room number, and diagnosis.
- **Read back** all orders to health care provider (TJC, 2015).
- Use clarification questions to avoid misunderstandings.
- Write "VO" (verbal order) or "TO" (telephone order), including date and time, name of patient, and complete order; sign the name of the health care provider and nurse.
- Follow agency policies; some agencies require documentation of the "read-back" or two nurses to review and sign telephone or verbal orders.
- Health care provider co-signs the order within the time frame required by the agency (usually 24 hours; verify agency policy).

later time, usually within 24 hours after making it (see agency policy). Box 20.3 provides guidelines for safely taking verbal or telephone orders for medications.

Five common types of orders based on frequency and/or urgency of medication administration orders are: standing; prn orders; and single (one-time) orders, which include stat orders and now orders. Each order needs to include the patient's name, the drug ordered, dosage, route of administration, and time(s) of administration.

You carry out a *standing order* until the health care provider cancels it by another order or until a prescribed number of days elapse. A standing order sometimes indicates a final day or number of doses. Many agencies have a policy for automatically discontinuing standing orders.

A medication can be ordered to be given only when a patient requires or requests it. This is a prn order. You must assess a patient thoroughly to determine whether he or she needs the medication. A prn order usually has a minimum interval set for the time of administration.

Single (one-time) orders are common for preoperative medications or medications given before diagnostic procedures. The medication is ordered to be given only once at a specified time. A stat order means that you give a single dose of medication immediately and only once. Stat orders are used for emergencies when a patient's condition changes suddenly. A now order is more specific than a one-time order and is used when a patient needs a medication quickly but not as soon as a stat order. When you receive a now order, you have up to 90 minutes to give the drug (see agency policy). The Joint Commission (2015) discourages the use of range orders; there continue to be concerns about providing enough guidance to nurses while still allowing them to address the individual needs of a patient. An example of a poorly written range order is "give morphine sulfate 2 to 6 mg IV push every 2 to 4 hours prn for pain." This order is not specific with regard to guidelines needed to give a correct dose. A range order must provide objective measures for nurses to use to determine the correct dose. An example of a clearly written range order is "give Lortab 1-2 tab every 4 hours prn pain. For pain 1-5, 1 tab; for pain 5-10, 2 tabs." A range order should include specific indications (e.g., pain-rating score, temperature level) especially for use of a medication indicated for more than one reason (e.g., ibuprofen, which could be indicated for pain or fever) (Rosier, 2012).

Once you determine that information on the patient's MAR is accurate, use the MAR to prepare and administer medications. When preparing medications from bottles or containers, *compare the label of the medication container with the MAR 3 times:* (1) before removing the container from the supply drawer or shelf, (2) as the amount of medication ordered is removed from the container, and (3) at the patient's bedside before administering the medication to the patient. Never prepare medications from unmarked containers or containers with illegible labels (TJC, 2016). With unit-dose prepackaged medications, check the label with the MAR when taking medications out of the medication dispensing system. Finally, verify all medications at the patient's bedside with the patient's MAR and use at least two identifiers before giving the patient any medications (TJC, 2015).

If a patient questions a medication, stop and recheck to be certain that there is no mistake. An alert patient or family caregiver will know whether a medication is different from those received before. In most cases the medication order has been changed, or the drug is manufactured by a different company than the patient has been using at home. However, attention to a patient's question is how errors are identified and prevented.

Right Dose

The unit-dose system is designed to minimize errors. When a medication is prepared from a larger volume or strength than needed or when the health care provider orders a system of measurement different from that which the pharmacist supplies, the chance of error increases. After calculating the doses of high-risk medications such as insulin or warfarin, compare the calculation with one done independently by a second nurse. This is especially important if it is an unusual calculation or involves a potentially toxic drug.

After calculating doses, prepare medications accurately. Use syringes and sealed droppers when it is necessary to measure medications accurately. For example, ISMP (2016) recommends the use of an oral syringe that measures in mL. If an oral solution is available only in a bulk size (such as a bottle) or if the patient-specific dose is less than the unit dose amount (e.g., dose is 3 mL when the unit dose product is 5 mL), the pharmacy should prepare the patient-specific dose in an oral syringe (or cup) and dispense it to the unit (ISMP, 2016). Nurses are no longer encouraged to pour medications into graduated cups because of the risk of medication errors. When preparing medication in an oral syringe, draw up the medication slowly to prevent air bubbles from entering the syringe. Air displaces the medication and leads to inaccurate doses. For the home, ISMP is now recommending that the patient or family caregiver be provided an oral syringe or dosing cup that accurately measures the medication.

Medication errors occur when pills need to be split. Studies show that the accuracy of split tablets is questionable, even if a tablet is scored (ISMP, 2015b). In addition, in the home setting patients may assume that tablets in containers have already been split when they have not or split them again when they have been split already (ISMP, 2015b).

To promote patient safety in some inpatient settings, pharmacists split medications, label and package them, and return them to the nurse for administration. Because pill splitting can be problematic in the home, determine if a patient has the manual dexterity or visual acuity to split tablets. If possible, determine if his or her pharmacy can split the pill or encourage the health care provider to order medications that do not require splitting.

Tablets are sometimes crushed and mixed with food. Be sure to clean the crushing device completely before crushing the tablet. Remnants of previously crushed medications increase concentration of the medication or result in a patient receiving part of an unprescribed medication. Mix crushed medications with very small amounts of food or liquid. Do not use a patient's favorite foods or liquids because medications alter their taste and decrease the patient's desire for them. This is especially a concern for pediatric patients. *Always check to determine whether a medication can be crushed* (see Chapter 21). Some medications (e.g., enteric-coated or slow-release) have special coatings to prevent them from being absorbed too quickly. These medications should not be crushed.

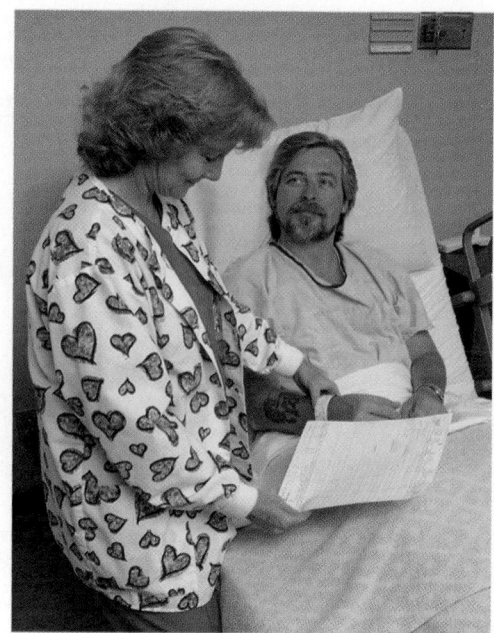

FIG 20.4 Before administering any medications, check patient's identification and allergy bracelets.

Refer to the "Do Not Crush List" (ISMP, 2015c) to ensure that a medication is safe to crush.

Right Patient

Medication errors often occur because one patient gets a drug intended for another patient. Therefore a key step in administering medications safely is being sure that you give the right medication to the right patient. It is difficult to remember every patient's name and face. Before giving a medication to a patient, always use at least two patient identifiers (TJC, 2016). Acceptable patient identifiers include the patient's name, an identification number assigned by a health care agency such as the medical record number, or date of birth. Do not use a patient's room number as an identifier. The required identification process mandates collecting patient identifiers reliably when a patient is first admitted to a health care agency. Once identifiers are assigned to a patient (e.g., putting identifiers on an armband and placing the armband on the patient), a nurse uses them to match the patient with the patient name on the MAR.

To identify a patient correctly in an acute care setting, at the patient's bedside compare the patient identifiers on the MAR with those on his or her identification bracelet (Fig. 20.4). Asking patients to state their full names and identification information provides a third way to verify that you are giving medications to the right patient. If an identification bracelet becomes smudged or illegible or is missing, get a new one for the patient. In health care settings that are nonacute care settings (e.g., long-term care agency), The Joint Commission does not require the use of armbands for identification. However, nurses must use a system to verify the patient's identification with at least two identifiers, such as resident picture, before administering medications (TJC, n.d.).

In addition to using two identifiers, some agencies use a wireless bar-code scanner to help identify the right patient (Fig. 20.5). This system requires the nurse to scan a personal bar code that is commonly placed on the nurse's name badge first. Then a bar code is

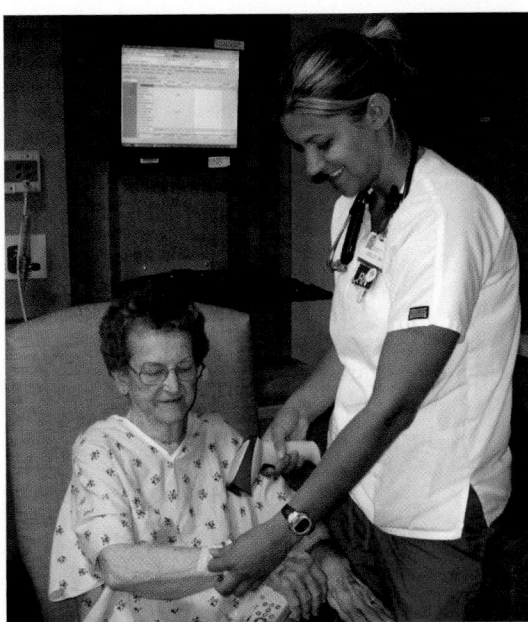

FIG 20.5 Nurse using bar-code scanner to identify patient during medication administration.

scanned from the single-dose medication package. Finally, the nurse scans the patient's armband. All of this information is stored in the computer for documentation purposes. The system helps prevent medication errors because it provides another step to ensure that the right patient receives the right medication.

Right Route

The health care provider's order must designate a route of administration. If the route of administration is missing or if the specified route is not the recommended route, consult the health care provider immediately. Recent evidence shows that medication errors involving the wrong route are common. For example, enteral and parenteral medications may become confused in the pediatric setting where liquid medications are frequently given orally. When oral medications are prepared in parenteral syringes, there is an increased risk of giving an oral medication through the parenteral route (ISMP, 2016). The injection of a liquid intended for oral use produces local complications such as sterile abscess or fatal systemic effects. Medication companies label parenteral medications "for injectable use only." Label the syringe after preparing a medication (TJC, 2016), include the location if appropriate (e.g., right eye), and always use different syringes for enteral and parenteral medication administration (ISMP, 2016).

Right Time

Safe medication administration involves adherence to prescribed doses and dosage schedules. Some agencies set schedules for medication administration. However, nurses are able to alter this schedule based on knowledge about a medication. For example, at some agencies medications that are taken once a day are given at 9:00 AM. However, if a medication works best when given at bedtime, the nurse administers it before the patient goes to sleep. In addition, acute care agencies use guidelines from the ISMP and Centers for Medicaid and Medicare Services (CMS, 2011; ISMP, 2011c) to determine safe, effective, and timely administration of scheduled medications. According to ISMP (2011a) and CMS (2011) guidelines, hospitals need to determine which medications are not eligible for scheduled dosing times and must be given at precise times (e.g., stat doses, first-time or loading doses, one-time doses). In addition, hospitals must determine which medications are time-critical scheduled and which are non–time-critical scheduled. With time-critical medications (e.g., antibiotics, anticoagulants, insulin, immunosuppressives), early or delayed administration of maintenance doses of more than 30 minutes before or after the scheduled dose will most likely cause harm or result in subtherapeutic responses in a patient. Non–time-critical medications include medications in which the timing of administration most likely will not affect the desired effect of the medication if the medication is given 1 to 2 hours before or after its scheduled time. Thus you administer time-critical–scheduled medications at a precise time or within 30 minutes before or after the scheduled time. You administer medications identified as non–time-critical within 1 to 2 hours of their scheduled time. Know your agency policies about the timing of medications to ensure that you administer medications at the right time (ISMP, 2011b).

Always know why a medication is ordered for a certain time of the day and whether you are able to alter the time schedule. For example, two medications are ordered, one q8h (every 8 hours) and the other 3 times per day. Both medications are scheduled 3 times a day over 24 hours. The health care provider intends for you to give the q8h medication ATC to maintain its therapeutic blood levels. In contrast, you need to give the other medication during the waking hours. Each agency has a recommended time schedule for medications ordered at frequent intervals. You can alter these recommended times if necessary or appropriate.

Give priority to medications that must act at certain times. For example, give insulin at a precise interval before a meal. Give antibiotics on time ATC to maintain therapeutic blood levels. Some medications require your clinical judgment to determine the proper time for administration. Administer a prn sleeping medication when the patient is ready for bed. You always document whenever there is a call to the patient's health care provider to obtain a change in a medication order.

When preparing patients for discharge, help them plan schedules based on preferred medication intervals, pharmacokinetics of the medication, and the patient's daily schedule. For patients who have difficulty remembering when to take medications, make a chart that lists the times when they should take each medication or prepare a special container to hold each timed dose.

Right Documentation

Accurate documentation allows nurses and other health care providers to communicate with one another and improves medication safety. Many medication errors result from inaccurate documentation. Therefore always document accurately at the time of administration and verify any inaccurate documentation before administering medications. To ensure the right documentation, first make sure that the information on your patient's MAR corresponds exactly with the health care provider's order and the label on the medication container. Written orders and medication forms must include the patient's name; the name of the ordered medication; and the medication dosage, route, and frequency. If there is any question about a medication order because it is incomplete, illegible, vague, or not understood, contact the health care provider before administering the medication.

Never document that you have administered a medication until you have actually given it. Document the name of the medication, the dose, the time of administration, and the route on the patient's MAR as soon as it is administered.

Also document the site of any injections and the patient's response to medications. You need to document response to drugs such as therapeutic or if ADE or side effects occur. For example, if pain medication is administered, you must reassess and document if the drug was effective in controlling pain. Your efforts to ensure proper documentation help provide safe care.

Medication Preparation

It is legally advisable to administer only the medications that you prepare. Administering a medication prepared by another nurse increases the opportunity for errors. You must perform several steps before actual administration of medications, including interpreting medication labels, converting measurement units within a system or between systems, and calculating medication doses. The importance of checking similar names and verifying the correct drug cannot be overemphasized.

Interpreting Medication Labels

Medication labels include several basic pieces of information: the trade name of the drug in large letters, the generic name in smaller letters, the form of the drug, the dosage, the expiration date, the lot number, and the name of the manufacturer (Fig. 20.6). The trade name given by the manufacturer suggests the action of the drug, and the generic name is the chemical name.

Clinical Calculation

To administer medications safely, use your mathematics skills to safely calculate dosages and mix solutions. This skill is important because medications are not always dispensed in the unit of measure in which they are ordered. Medication companies package and bottle medications in standard dosages. For example, a patient's health care provider orders 20 mg of a medication that is packaged in 40-mg vials. You are responsible for converting available units of volume and weight to the desired doses. Therefore be aware of approximate equivalents in all major measurement systems and make use of conversion tables. In addition to medication administration, nurses use volume and weight conversions in a variety of other nursing activities, including converting fluid ounces to milliliters to measure intake and output (I&O) or converting volume equivalents to calculate IV flow rates.

Conversions Within One System. Converting measurements within one system is relatively easy; simply divide or multiply in the metric system. For example, to change milligrams to grams, divide by 1000 or move the decimal three points to the left.

$$1000 \text{ mg} = 1 \text{ g}$$
$$350 \text{ mg} = 0.35 \text{ g}$$

To convert liters to milliliters, multiply by 1000 or move the decimal three points to the right.

$$1 \text{ L} = 1000 \text{ mL}$$
$$0.25 \text{ L} = 250 \text{ mL}$$

To convert units of measurement within the household system, consult an equivalency table. For example, when converting fluid ounces to quarts, you first need to know that 32 ounces is the equivalent of 1 quart. To convert 8 ounces to a quart measurement, divide 8 by 32 to get the equivalent, ¼ or 0.25 quart.

Conversion Between Systems. You will frequently determine the correct dose of a medication by converting weights or volumes from one system of measurement to another. To convert from one measurement system to another, use equivalent measurements. Tables of equivalent measurements are available in all health care agencies. The pharmacist is also a good resource.

Before making a conversion, compare the measurement system available with that ordered. For example, a health care provider orders Robitussin 30 mL, but the patient only has tablespoons at home. To properly instruct a patient, convert milliliters to tablespoons, which requires you to know the equivalency or refer to a table such as Table 20.6. ISMP (2011a; 2016) prefers the patient be provided with an oral syringe that measures in milliliters (mL) for measurement accuracy.

Dosage Calculations. Dosage calculations are necessary when the dose on the medication label differs from the dose ordered. There are several dose-calculation methods, including

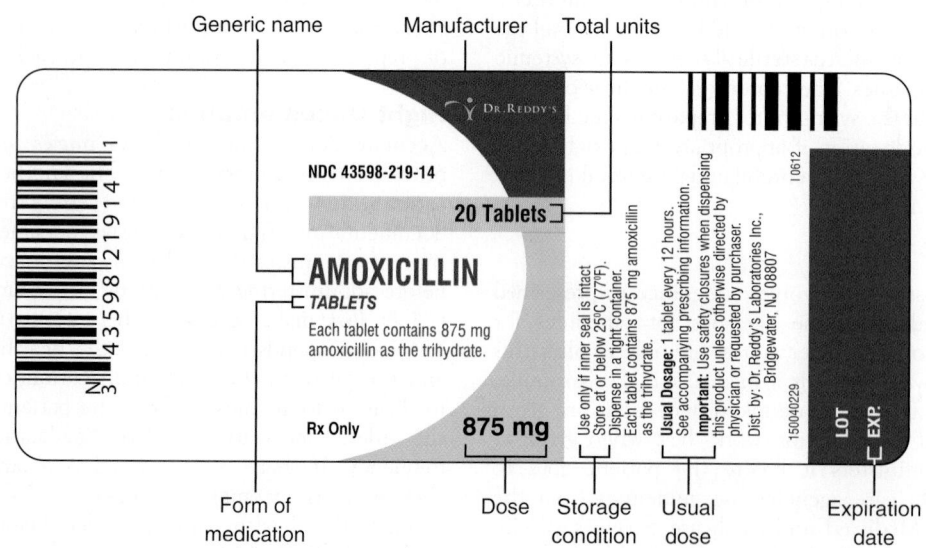

FIG 20.6 Interpreting medication label. (*Courtesy Dr. Reddy's Laboratories, Inc.*)

Formula Method

$$\frac{D}{H} = V = \text{Amount to give}$$

D is the desired dose or the dose ordered by the health care provider for the patient (e.g., 250 mg of penicillin PO 4 times daily).
H is the drug dose on hand or available for use. The dose is on the drug label (e.g., penicillin tablets 250 mg each).
V is the volume (liquid) or vehicle (number of tablets, capsules) that delivers the available dose.

NOTE: The desired dose (D) and the on-hand dose (H) must be in the same unit of measurement. If they are in different units, you must convert before completing the formula.

Dimensional Analysis

Use the following steps to solve medication problems using dimensional analysis:

1. Identify the unit of measure that you need to administer. For example, if you are giving a pill, you will usually be giving a tablet or a capsule; for parenteral or oral medications, the unit is milliliters.
2. Estimate the answer in your mind.
3. Place the name or appropriate abbreviation for *x* on the left side of the equation (e.g., *x* tab, *x* mL).
4. Place available information from the problem in a fraction format on the right side of the equation. Place the abbreviation or unit that matches what you are going to administer (determined in Step 1) in the numerator.
5. Look at the medication order and add other factors into the problem. Set up the numerator so it matches the unit in the previous denominator.
6. Cancel out like units of measurement on the right side of the equation. You should end up with only one unit left in the equation, and it should match the unit on the left side of the equation. Reduce to the lowest terms if possible and solve the problem or solve for *x*. Label your answer.
7. Reduce to the lowest terms if possible and solve the problem or solve for *x*. Label your answer.
8. Compare your estimate from Step 1 with your answer in Step 2.

formula (Box 20.4), dimensional analysis (Box 20.5) and ratio and proportion (Box 20.6). The most common methods are ratio-proportion or use of a formula.

The Formula Method

Dose ordered: Demerol 50 mg IM
Medication available: 100 mg in 1 mL

Step 1.

$$\frac{\text{Dose ordered}}{\text{Dose on hand}} \times \text{Amount on hand} = \text{Amount to administer}$$

Step 2. Calculate your answer:

$$\frac{50 \text{ mg}}{100 \text{ mg}} \times 1 \text{ mL} \times = 0.5 \text{ mL}$$

Dimensional Analysis Method. When the dose ordered has the same label as the dose available

The Ratio-and-Proportion Method

1. The numbers in a ratio are separated by a colon (:).
2. A proportion is an equation that has two ratios of equal value.
3. The first and last numbers are called the *extremes*. The second and third numbers are called the *means*.
4. Write a proportion in one of three ways:
   a. 1:2 = 5:10
   b. 1:2 :: 5:10
   c. ½ = ⁵⁄₁₀
5. Make sure that all the terms are in the same unit or system of measurement.
6. Label all the terms in the proportion.
7. Place the ratio you know (e.g., information on the drug label) first.
8. Put the terms of the ratio in the same sequence (e.g., mg:mL = mg:mL).
9. Cross-multiply the means and the extremes and then divide both sides by the number for the *x* to obtain the dosage.
10. Always label the answer.

Dose ordered: 0.5 g
Tablets available: 0.25 g per tablet

Step 1. The starting factor is 0.5 g.
The answer label is tablets (i.e., how many tablets should be given?)
Step 2. Formulate the conversion equation:
The equivalent needed is 1 tablet = 0.25 g.

$$\frac{0.5 \text{ g}}{1} \times \frac{1 \text{ tab}}{0.25 \text{ g}} = \text{tabs}$$

Cancel labels (g). **NOTE:** If properly written, all labels except the answer label will cancel.
Step 3. Solve the equation. Reduce the numerical values and multiply the numerators and denominators.

Ratio-and-Proportion Method. A ratio indicates the relationship between two numbers.

Dose ordered: Phenytoin solution 100 mg by mouth
Medication available: 125 mg/5 mL

Step 1. Set up the proportion:

$$\frac{125 \text{ mg}}{5} \times \frac{100 \text{ mg}}{x \text{ mL}}$$

Step 2. Cross multiply the equation:

$$125x = 100 \times 5$$
$$125x = 500$$

Step 3. Divide both sides by the number before *x*:

$$\frac{125x}{125} = \frac{500}{125}$$
$$x = \frac{500}{125}$$
$$x = 4 \text{ mL}$$

Pediatric Doses. Calculating children's medication doses requires caution (Hockenberry and Wilson, 2015). Evidence shows that children are at risk for experiencing an ADE as a result of their metabolic rate (Burchum and Rosenthal, 2016). Factors contributing to errors include workload, distractions, and lack of knowledge (Gann, 2015; Wittich et al., 2014). The child's age, weight, and maturity of body systems all affect the ability to metabolize and excrete medication. Other factors that influence medication dosages in children include the difficulty in evaluating the desired effect and the hydration status of the child. In most cases the health care provider will calculate the dose for a child before ordering the medication. However, it is your responsibility to be aware of the safe dosage range for any medication administered, and you should recheck/recalculate to confirm correct dose. Different formulas and methods are used to calculate drug doses in children. The two most common methods of calculating pediatric dosages are based on the child's weight or body surface area (BSA). Refer to a pediatric pharmacology resource, a pharmacist, or the health care provider if you have to calculate a medication based on BSA. Most of the time you calculate medications based on the child's weight.

Older Adult Dosages. Older adults also require special consideration during medication administration (Box 20.7). The changes of aging alter pharmacokinetics. In addition to physiological changes of aging, behavioral and social/economic issues influence the older adult's use of medications.

A common problem for older adults is polypharmacy. There is no consensus definition for polypharmacy, although the common definitions include five or more concurrent drugs or the mixing of nutritional or herbal supplements with medications (Burchum and Rosenthal, 2016; Touhy and Jett, 2014). Older adults experience polypharmacy when they seek relief from a variety of symptoms (e.g., constipation, insomnia, pain) and see multiple health care providers. When determining polypharmacy, review all older adults' prescribed medications and all other supplements and OTC medications. Polypharmacy increases the risk of adverse effects and interactions with other medications.

The nurse, health care provider, and pharmacist share the responsibility of reducing or eliminating the risk factors associated with medication regimens that older adults receive. Safety precautions include assessing a patient's health status, current medication regimen (including OTC drugs and herbal products), the reason for existing and proposed medications, and any environmental factors that influence accurate and safe medication administration by the patient and family caregiver(s).

EVIDENCE-BASED PRACTICE

Many medication errors occur when nurses become distracted or lose focus during medication administration or fail to follow best-practice protocols and procedures related to medication administration (Raban and Westbrook, 2014). Research reveals that $3.5 billion is spent every year as a result of 450,000 preventable medication errors (Williams et al., 2014). Nurses become interrupted while accessing dispensing systems, depositing medications into delivery containers, and confirming orders on computer screens. The majority of distractions have been identified as a result of interruptions by patients, family, friends of the patient, or other health care professionals (Raban and Westbrook, 2014; Williams et al., 2014; Yoder et al., 2015). Nurses need systems in place to avoid distractions to help prevent medication errors, including:

- Wearing a medication safety vest, sash or red apron.
- Using visible medication preparation signs.
- Medication administration checklists.
- Staff and patient education.
- Establishing no-interruption zones (NIZs) defined by a red tape outline around the medication AMDS.

NURSING PROCESS

Application of the nursing process ensures that critical thinking and clinical judgment are integrated into a patient's care. As a nurse your role extends beyond simply giving drugs to a patient. You are also responsible for understanding why your patient is receiving the drug therapy; monitoring patients' responses to medications; providing education to patients and family caregivers; and informing health care providers when medications are effective, ineffective, or no longer necessary.

Assessment

Before administering medications, perform a physical assessment, which will reveal physical findings for any indications or contraindications for medication therapy (e.g., inability to swallow because of mucositis). Be sure to also assess the patient's sensory, motor, and cognitive functions to determine if the patient can prepare and administer medications at home. Continue your assessment by determining if the patient has a history of medication allergies. When assessing for medication allergies, you must differentiate between actual allergic reactions, which can be life threatening, and drug sensitivities, which are uncomfortable side effects. In an acute care setting patients with allergies wear identification bands that list each medication allergy. All allergies and types of reactions are noted on the patient's admission notes, medication records, and history and physical examination. *Never give a patient a medication when there is a known allergy.*

Your assessment also involves identifying medications that a patient takes every day at home, including prescriptions, OTC preparations, and herbal supplements. Determine how long the patient has taken each medication, current dosage schedule, and whether he or she has had any adverse effects to any of the medications. The patient should know the name, purpose, dosage, route, and side effects of medications and supplements that are being taken. Often patients take many medications and carry a list that

---

BOX 20.7

Safe Medication Administration in Older Adults

- Consult with the health care provider to keep the medication plan as simple as possible (Burchum and Rosenthal, 2016).
- Keep instructions clear and simple and provide written materials in large print (Burchum and Rosenthal, 2016).
- Minimize distractions and make sure that older adult is comfortable (Touhy and Jett, 2014).
- Teach the complications and interactions of all over-the counter medications (Touhy and Jett, 2014).
- Teach the older adult to set up a daily or weekly schedule for medications using memory aids such as a calendar (Touhy and Jett, 2014). Have a family caregiver help with medication administration as needed.
- Monitor patient's response to medications to assess for overuse or underuse of the medication and anticipate possible dosage modifications (Touhy and Jett, 2014).
- Reduce the chance of errors by color coding or labeling medication bottles (Touhy and Jett, 2014).
- Include patient's family caregiver or key support person in any type of instruction.
- Evaluate teaching by having patient repeat back instructions.

includes this information. Patients have different levels of understanding. One patient may describe a diuretic as a "water pill," whereas another describes it as a drug to minimize swelling and lower blood pressure. By assessing the patient's level of knowledge, you determine the need for teaching. If a patient is unable to understand or remember pertinent information, it may be necessary to involve a family member.

Complete appropriate assessments, which may include vital signs, laboratory data, and the nature and severity of symptoms. If data contraindicate medication administration, hold the drug and notify the health care provider. When in doubt about medication information, check available medication references or the pharmacy.

Planning

During planning organize nursing activities to ensure the safe administration of medications. Current evidence shows that distractions or hurrying during preparation for medication administration increases the risk for medication errors (Yoder et al., 2015). The following are general goals of medication administration:

- Patient achieves therapeutic effect of the prescribed medication.
- There are no patient complications related to the prescribed medication.
- Patient and/or family caregiver understand medication therapy.
- Patient and family caregiver self-administer medication safely (when appropriate).

Implementation

Nursing interventions focus on safe and effective drug administration. This includes careful medication preparation, accurate and timely administration, and patient education.

Preadministration Activities

1. Identify the medication action, purpose, side effects, and nursing implications for administering and monitoring. Ensure that the medication order has not expired. Follow agency policy for medication order renewal.
2. Minimize distractions during medication preparation (e.g., discussion with staff, phone call, pager), close the door of the medication room or post "Do Not Disturb" signage, and do not perform other tasks while preparing a medication. Do not allow interruptions.
3. Make sure that the information on the medication computer sheet or MAR corresponds exactly with the health care provider's written order and with the medication container label. Do not interpret illegible handwriting; clarify with health care provider.
4. Read the label on the medication container and compare it with the MAR **at least 3 times:** before removing the container from the supply drawer, when placing the medication in an administration syringe, and just before administering the medication to the patient.
5. Double-check all calculations and other high-risk medication administration processes (e.g., insulin, patient-controlled analgesia) and verify with another nurse.
6. Review any preadministration assessments (e.g., vital signs, review of laboratory results).
7. Use good hand-hygiene technique. Avoid touching tablets and capsules. Use sterile technique for parenteral medications. Wear clean gloves when administering parenteral medications and certain topical medications.

8. Administer only those medications that you personally prepare. Do not ask another person to administer medications that you prepare. Keep medications secure.
9. When preparing medications, be sure that the label is clear and legible and that the drug is mixed properly; has not changed in color, clarity, or consistency; and has not expired.
10. Keep tablets and capsules in their wrappers and open them at the patient's bedside. This allows you to review each medication with the patient. If a patient refuses medication, there will be no question which one was withheld.
11. TJC (2016) has a standard for labeling syringes, including before a procedure labeling all medicines that are not labeled (e.g., medicines in syringes and basins). This should be done in the area where medicines and supplies are set up.

Medication Administration

1. Follow the *six rights* of medication administration.
2. Inform the patient of the name, purpose, action, and common side effects of each medication. Evaluate his or her knowledge of the medication and provide appropriate teaching using teach-back technique.
3. Stay with the patient until the medication is taken. Provide help as necessary. Do not leave medication at the bedside without a health care provider's order. For example, some patients may take their own vitamins while in the hospital.
4. Respect the patient's right to refuse a medication. If the medication wrapper remains intact, return the medication to the patient's unit-dose drawer. When medication is refused, determine the reason and take action accordingly.

Postadministration Activities

1. Record medications immediately after administration (see agency policy). Include the drug name, dose, route, time, and your signature.
2. Document preassessment as required (e.g., blood pressure measurement before antihypertensives).
3. Document postassessment data pertinent to patient's response. This is especially important when giving prn drugs.
4. If a patient refuses a medication, document that it was not given, the reason for refusal, and when you notified the health care provider.

Evaluation

After you administer a medication, consider how the medication is expected to affect the patient and evaluate his or her condition and response to it. Look for therapeutic and adverse effects. If adverse effects develop, you need to recognize the clinical signs and respond quickly:

1. Monitor for evidence of therapeutic effects, side effects, and adverse reactions. This includes monitoring physical response (e.g., heart rhythm, blood pressure, urine output, or laboratory results).
2. When a medication is given for relief of symptoms, ask the patient to report if symptoms have diminished or been relieved. In addition, reassess the patient after medication is administered (e.g., 30 minutes after medicating for pain).
3. Observe injection sites for bruises, inflammation, localized pain, numbness, or bleeding.
4. Evaluate that patient and family caregiver understand purpose of medication therapy, dose regimens, and ability to self-administer medication by using teach-back techniques.

REPORTING MEDICATION ERRORS

Medication errors often harm patients because of inappropriate medication use. Errors include inaccurate prescribing; administering the wrong medication, by the wrong route, and in the wrong time interval; and administering extra doses or failing to administer a medication. Medication errors are related to professional practice, health care product design, or procedures and systems such as product labeling and distribution. When an error occurs, the patient's safety and well-being become the top priority. A nurse assesses and examines the patient's condition and notifies the health care provider of the incident as soon as possible. Once the patient is stable, the nurse reports the incident to the appropriate person in the agency (e.g., manager or supervisor).

As a nurse you are responsible for preparing a written incident or occurrence report that must be filed usually within 24 hours of an incident (see agency policy) (see Chapter 4). The incident report is an internal audit tool and not a permanent part of the medical record. To legally protect the health care professional and agency, do not refer to an incident report in the nurses' notes in the EHR or chart. Agencies use incident reports to track incident patterns and initiate performance improvement programs as needed. Depending on the circumstances and the severity of the outcome, the nurse or agency may be responsible for reporting the incident to TJC, MedWatch (FDA Medical Products Reporting Program), or USP Medication Errors Reporting Program.

It is good risk management to report all medication errors, including mistakes that do not cause obvious or immediate harm or near misses. You should feel comfortable in reporting an error and not fear repercussions from managerial staff. Even when a patient suffers no harm from a medication error, the agency can still learn why the mistake occurred and what to do in the future to avoid similar errors. There are strategies that you can implement to prevent medication errors (Box 20.8).

PATIENT AND FAMILY TEACHING

A well-informed patient is more likely to take medications correctly. However, many patients have limited health literacy, meaning that they do not understand how to read medication labels and calculate doses. You will also care for patients who do not speak English. Thus any education requires a thorough assessment of a patient's learning needs and abilities. It is legally mandated by the National Standards for Culturally and Linguistically Appropriate Services (CLAS) in health care to provide easy-to-understand print and multimedia materials in the languages commonly used by the populations in a service area (USDHHSOMH, n.d.).

Provide an individualized approach to teaching, using visual aids, instructional booklets written in simple language or the patient's language, or even videotapes or DVDs. When teaching patients about their medications, include people identified as being significant to the patient's recovery (e.g., family caregivers or home care providers).

Begin instruction as soon as possible so you can have several teaching sessions. It is ideal to use instructional materials written no higher than a sixth-grade reading level. Provide instructions written in the patient's language if available. When providing instruction, have the patient or family caregiver repeat the name and use for each medication plus the dosing instructions. Current recommendations suggest the use of teach-back as a method to confirm patient learning and improve health care provider education (Nouri and Rudd, 2015). Have the patient explain for you the

---

BOX 20.8

Steps to Prevent Medication Errors

- Follow the six rights of medication administration.
- Only prepare medications for one patient at a time.
- Be sure to read labels at least 3 times (comparing MAR with label): When removing medication from storage, before taking to patient's room, before giving medication.
- Use at least two patient identifiers every time you administer medications (e.g., patient name, birthday, hospital number) whenever administering a medication.
- Do not allow any other activity to interrupt administration of medication to a patient (e.g., phone call, pager, discussion with other staff).
- Double-check all calculations and other high-risk medication administration processes (e.g., patient-controlled analgesia) and verify with another nurse.
- Do not interpret illegible handwriting; clarify with the health care provider.
- Question unusually large or small doses.
- Document all medications as soon as they are given.
- When you have made or discovered an error, reflect on what went wrong and ask how you could have prevented it. Complete an occurrence report per agency policy.
- Evaluate the context or situation in which a medication error occurred. This helps to determine if nurses have the necessary resources for safe medication administration.
- When repeated medication errors occur within a work area, identify and analyze the factors that may have caused the errors and take corrective action.
- Attend in-service programs on the medications you commonly administer.
- Ensure that you are well rested when caring for patients. Nurses make more errors when they are tired (Murphy and While, 2012).
- Involve and educate patients when administering medications. Address patients' concerns about medications before administering them (e.g., concerns about their appearance or side effects).
- Follow established agency policies and procedures when using technology to administer medications (e.g., automated medication dispensing system [AMDS] and bar-code scanning). Medication errors occur when nurses "work around" the technology (e.g., override alerts without thinking about them) (Voshall et al., 2013).

MAR, Medication administration record.

---

topic you taught him or her so you can confirm understanding. Have the patient demonstrate preparation of each medication. Provide time to discuss problem scenarios (e.g., side effects develop or a syringe becomes contaminated) to test the patient's knowledge of what to do should something go wrong. Determine if the patient requires a compliance aid or memory cue. This is especially important in older adults. If the patient speaks another language, have a professional interpreter available during instruction. Do not use a family member as an interpreter. Medication dose containers organized by the hours and days of the week are very useful. In the event that patients miss a dose of medication, they need to know how to adjust their medication schedule safely.

Evaluating the effectiveness of teaching ensures that a patient can administer medications in a safe manner. One method of evaluating patient understanding is to create medication cards with the generic and trade names of the medication on the front of the card and all pertinent medication information on the back of the card. Another method is to have patients read labels on prepared medications. Remember that medication bottles often have fine print and are difficult to read for the patient with impaired vision. Have the pharmacy prepare these types of patients with large-print labels. If the patient correctly identifies the name of the medication, ask him or her the following questions:

- Why are you taking this medication?
- How often do you take this medication and at what time of day?
- What side effects can occur with this medication?
- If this side effect occurs, what are you going to do about it?

Be sure to also assess the patient's sensory, motor, and cognitive functions (e.g., ability to open medication bottles). Impairments may affect the patient's ability to safely self-administer medications, and family caregivers or home health aides may need to help with medication administration. Many self-help devices are also available for purchase (e.g., pill boxes with times displayed and electronic dispensers).

✦ CLINICAL DEBRIEF

A 72-year-old male patient visits the medical clinic 1 month after a myocardial infarction (heart attack). He denies any chest pain since his angioplasty, which involved insertion of a stent into one of his coronary arteries to dilate the artery and improve blood flow to the heart. He is currently taking an antidepressant, a thyroid supplement, a stool softener, and a cardiac drug (beta-adrenergic blocker). In addition, he takes melatonin, an herbal preparation for sleep. The health care provider has recently revised the cardiac medication to metoprolol. He is now instructed to take 75 mg by mouth twice daily. The nurse notes that the drug is available in 150-mg tablets. The patient tells the clinic nurse that he has experienced some weakness and dizziness over the past week.

1. Which of the medications taken by the patient are likely to cause weakness and dizziness? Which nursing interventions should be included if he is experiencing these issues?
2. What might the health care provider who prescribed the medication do after receiving the nurse's report of the patient's weakness and dizziness? Use one of the methods provided to calculate the number of tablets of medication to administer.
3. As the nurse, which factors would be important for you to assess so the patient may take the 75-mg dose safely? Using SBAR, show how you would communicate with the health care team about this patient.

✦ REVIEW QUESTIONS

1. The health care provider has written the following orders. Which orders do you need to clarify before administering the medication? (Select all that apply and provide rationale for your answers. Rewrite the order so it follows the ISMP current medication order safety guidelines.)
   1. Timoptic .25% solution 1 drop OD BID
   2. Metoprolol 12.50 mg QD
   3. Insulin glargine 6 u SC twice a day
   4. Enalapril 2.5 mg. PO three times a day; hold for systolic blood pressure <100
2. An older adult states that she cannot see her medication bottles clearly to determine when to take her prescription. What should the nurse do? (Select all that apply.)
   1. Provide a pill-dispensing system that allows the patient or family caregiver to prepare medications for each day of the week
   2. Provide larger, easier-to-read labels on medication bottles
   3. Tell the patient what is in each container of medication
   4. Have a family caregiver administer the medication
   5. Use teach-back to ensure that patient knows what medication to take and when.

3. The nurse must take a verbal order during an emergency on the unit. Which of the following guidelines can be used for taking verbal or telephone orders? (Select all that apply.)
   1. Only authorized staff receive and record verbal or telephone orders. Agency identifies in writing the staff who are authorized.
   2. Clearly identify patient's name, room number, and diagnosis.
   3. Read back all orders to health care provider.
   4. Use clarification questions to avoid misunderstandings.
   5. Write "VO" (verbal order) or "TO" (telephone order), including date and time, name of patient, and complete order; sign the name of the health care provider and nurse.

ⓔ *Visit the Evolve site for a complete list of Clinical Debrief and Review Questions answers.*

REFERENCES

American Nurses Association (ANA): *Nursing scope and standards of practice*, ed 3, Silver Springs, MD, 2015, The Association.

Burchum J, Rosenthal L: *Lehne's pharmacology for nursing care*, ed 9, St Louis, 2016, Saunders.

Center for Disease Control and Prevention: *Medication Safety Program*, 2012, http://www.cdc.gov/medicationsafety/basics.html. Accessed July 7, 2016.

Centers for Medicare & Medicaid (CMS): *Medication administration guidance update*, 2011, CMS, https://www.cms.gov/Surveycertificationgeninfo/downloads/SCLetter12_05.pdf. Accessed June 23, 2015.

Gann M: How informatics nurses use bar-code technology to reduce medication errors, *Nursing* 45(3):60, 2015.

Ghaemmaghami V: Computerized provider order entry: advancing technology today, saving lives tomorrow, *AORN* 100(6):683, 2014.

Greene JA, et al: Why do the same drugs look different? Pills, trade dress, and public health, *N Engl J Med* 365(1):83, 2011.

Hockenberry MJ, Wilson D: *Wong's nursing care of infants and children*, ed 10, St Louis, 2015, Mosby.

Institute for Safe Medication Practices (ISMP): *Statement on use of metric measurements to prevent errors with oral liquids*, 2011a, https://www.ismp.org/pressroom/PR20110808.pdf. Accessed August 8, 2016.

Institute for Safe Medication Practices (ISMP): *Acute care guidelines for timely administration of scheduled medications*, 2011b, http://www.ismp.org/Tools/guidelines/acutecare/tasm.pdf. Accessed April 2, 2016.

Institute for Safe Medication Practices (ISMP): *Guidelines for timely medication administration: response to the CMS "30 minute" rule*, 2011c, http://www.ismp.org/Newsletters/acutecare/articles/20110113.asp. Accessed April 2, 2016.

Institute for Safe Medication Practices (ISMP): *ISMP's list of error-prone abbreviations, symbols, and dose designations*, 2013, ISMP, https://www.ismp.org/tools/errorproneabbreviations.pdf. Accessed April 2, 2016.

Institute for Safe Medication Practices: *Targeted medication safety best practices for hospitals: frequently asked questions*, 2014, https://www.ismp.org/tools/bestpractices/faq/FAQ-BP4.pdf. Accessed August 8, 2016.

Institute for Safe Medication Practices (ISMP): *ISMP's list of confused drug names*, 2015a, ISMP, https://www.ismp.org/tools/confuseddrugnames.pdf. Accessed April 2, 2016.

Institute for Safe Medication Practices (ISMP): *Tablet splitting: do it only if you "half" to, and then do it safely*, 2015b, https://www.ismp.org/newsletters/acutecare/articles/20060518.asp. Accessed April 2, 2016.

Institute for Safe Medication Practices (ISMP): *Oral dosage forms that should not be crushed*, 2015c, http://www.ismp.org/tools/donotcrush.pdf. Accessed April 2, 2016.

Institute for Safe Medication Practices (ISMP): *2016-2017 targeted medication safety best practices for hospitals*, 2016, http://www.ismp.org/tools/bestpractices/TMSBP-for-Hospitals.pdf. Accessed August 7, 2016.

Murphy M, While A: Medication administration practices among children's nurses: a survey, *Br J Nurs* 21(15):928, 2012.

Nouri S, Rudd R: Health literacy in the "oral exchange": an important element of patient provider communication, *Patient Educ Couns* 98(5):565, 2015.

Raban M, Westbrook J: Are interventions to reduce interruptions and errors during medication administration effective? A systematic review, *BJM Qual Saf* 23:414, 2014.

Rochais E, et al: Nursing perception of the impact of automated dispensing cabinets on patient safety and ergonomics in a teaching health center, *J Pharm Pract* 27(2):150, 2014.

Rosier P: Facing up to the challenge of range orders, *Nursing* 42(12):64, 2012.

The Joint Commission (TJC): *Comprehensive accreditation manual for hospitals*, Oakbrook Terrace, IL, 2015, The Commission.

The Joint Commission (TJC): *Standards FAQ details: two patient identifiers*, nd, https://www.jointcommission.org/standards_information/jcfaqdetails.aspx?StandardsFaqId=1054&ProgramId=46. Accessed July 7, 2016.

The Joint Commission (TJC): *2016 National Patient Safety Goals*, Oakbrook Terrace, IL, 2016, The Commission. http://www.jointcommission.org/standards_information/npsgs.aspx. Accessed April 2, 2016.

Touhy T, Jett K: *Ebersole and Hess' gerontological nursing & health aging*, ed 4, St Louis, 2014, Elsevier.

US Department of Health and Human Services Office of Minority Health (USDHHSOMH): *National standards for culturally and linguistically appropriate services (CLAS) in health and health care*, nd, https://www.thinkculturalhealth.hhs.gov/pdfs/enhancednationalclasstandards.pdf. Accessed April 2, 2016.

US Food and Drug Administration (USFDA): *MedWatch: the FDA safety information and adverse event reporting program*, 2015, http://www.fda.gov/safety/medwatch/default.htm. Accessed April 2, 2016.

Voshall B, et al: Barcode medication administration work-arounds, *J Nurs Adm* 43(10):530, 2013.

Williams T, et al: Implementing evidence-based medication safety interventions on a progressive care unit, *AJN* 114(11):53, 2014.

Wittich C, et al: Medication errors: an overview for clinicians, *Mayo Clin Proc* 89(8):1116, 2014.

Yoder M, et al: The effect of a safe zone on nurse interruptions, distractions, and medication administration errors, *J Infus Nurs* 38(2):140, 2015.

21 | Nonparenteral Medications

OBJECTIVES

Mastery of content in this chapter will enable the nurse to:
- Describe common principles to follow in the administration of medications.
- Discuss patient-centered practices to use to improve a patient's medication adherence.
- Safely and correctly administer a medication by oral, enteral, and topical routes.
- Identify guidelines for administering oral, enteral, and topical medications.
- Describe factors to assess before administering medications.

- Differentiate types of topical administrations that require sterile technique and those that require clean medical aseptic technique.
- Instruct patients in the proper use of a metered-dose inhaler (MDI), a dry powder inhaler (DPI), and small-volume nebulizer.
- Identify conditions contraindicating the administration of medications by various oral and topical routes.
- Prepare a teaching plan regarding medication use for a selected patient.

MEDIA RESOURCES

- evolve http://evolve.elsevier.com/Perry/skills
- Review Questions
- Audio Glossary

- ▶ Video Clips
- NSO Nursing Skills Online
- Clinical Debrief and Review Questions Answers

PURPOSE

Administration of nonparenteral medications includes those that are given orally, enterally, and topically. Nonparenteral medications exclude any medication administered via an injection or intravenous infusion. The nonparenteral route chosen depends on the properties and desired effects of the medication and the physical and mental condition of a patient. There are many reasons why it may be necessary to change from one route to another. When this occurs, you are responsible for consulting with a health care provider for an order or conferring with the pharmacist to safely meet a patient's needs.

STANDARDS OF CARE

- Food and Drug Administration (FDA), 2013—Best practices for tablet splitting
- Institute for Safe Medication Practices (ISMP), 2011—ISMP acute care guidelines for timely administration of scheduled medications
- Institute for Safe Medication Practices (ISMP), 2015—Oral dosage forms that should not be crushed
- Institute for Safe Medication Practices (ISMP), 2013—ISMP's list of error-prone abbreviations, symbols, and dose designations

Examples of Topical Medication Routes

1. *Sublingual:* Medication placed under the tongue; is dissolvable
2. *Buccal:* Medication placed between the upper or lower molar teeth and cheek area; is dissolvable
3. *Direct application to skin or mucosa:* Lotion, ointment, cream, powder, foam, spray, patch, and disk
4. *Direct application to mucous membrane:* Eyedrops, gargling, swabbing the throat; *Spraying:* Instillation into nose or throat
5. *Inhalation of medicated aerosol spray:* Distributes medication throughout the nasal passages and the tracheobronchial airway; two types of devices designed for this purpose: metered-dose inhalers (MDIs) and small-volume nebulizers
6. *Inhalation of dry powder medication:* Distributes medication in powder form throughout the tracheobronchial airway; device designed for this purpose: dry powder inhaler (DPI)
7. *Inserting drug into a body cavity:* Rectal or vaginal suppositories, vaginal creams, or foams

- Institute for Safe Medication Practices (ISMP), 2015—ISMP's list of confused drug names
- Institute for Safe Medication Practices (ISMP), 2016—2016-2017 targeted medication safety best practices for hospitals
- The Joint Commission (TJC), 2016—2016 National Patient Safety Goals

PRINCIPLES FOR PRACTICE

- The major principle of practice with nonparenteral medication administration is patient safety (see Safety Guidelines).
- The oral route (by mouth) is the easiest and most desirable way to administer medications.
- Topical administration of medications involves applying drugs directly to skin or mucous or tissue membranes. See Box 21.1 for examples of topical medication routes.
- You apply medications to the skin by spraying, painting, or spreading medication over a localized area. Transdermal patches (adhesive-backed medicated disks), which are applied to the skin, provide a continuous release of medication over several hours or days.
- Medications applied to membranes such as the cornea of the eye or the rectal mucosa are absorbed quickly because of the vascularity of the membrane and can also have systemic effects. In addition, you can experience systemic effects of a topical medication if you do not wear clean gloves.

PATIENT-CENTERED CARE

- An excellent time to provide patient education is during medication administration. You must assess the patient's and family caregiver's health literacy, health beliefs, and cultural practices.
- The goal of patient education is to improve patient adherence to medication regimens. Patients fail to adhere to medication regimens because of patient, medication, and provider issues. Patient issues include medication knowledge, health literacy, and financial limitations. Clear, concise, and at times one-on-one patient education does improve adherence to medication, which in turn improves patient outcomes (Ari, 2015; Berben et al., 2011).
- Print materials used for instruction should be written at an appropriate reading level (6th to 8th grade) and delivered in a manner that meets individual patient needs such as visual impairment or hearing or cognitive impairments. Involve family caregivers in the education sessions because they may be the ones administering medications.
- Cognitive impairment and depression interact with health literacy. Individualized patient education techniques that simplify tasks and patient roles may help to overcome cognitive load and suboptimal performance in self-medication administration (O'Conor et al., 2015).
- Medication issues include complex medication regimens and medication discrepancies. Provider issues include poor instruction, inappropriate prescriptions, and lack of provider knowledge about adherence. Patients need explanations about the purpose of medications, benefits, expected effects, and how to plan a daily schedule.
- Health beliefs vary by culture and influence how patients manage and respond to medication therapy. Differences in values, attitudes, and beliefs affect a patient's adherence to medication therapy. For example, herbal remedies and alternative therapies may be common practice in some cultures and interfere with prescribed medications. It is also important to consider cultural influences on drug response, metabolism, and side effects if a patient is not responding to drug therapy as expected. For example, certain cultural food preferences may have food-drug interactions.
- Vegetarian diets can affect warfarin or medications for glycemic control. A change in the medication may be necessary by the prescriber, or the patient may need counseling about how to change his or her dietary patterns.

EVIDENCE-BASED PRACTICE

- Medication competency is a skill that all nurses must possess to improve the quality and safety of medication administration. When nurses follow guidelines such as the "Six Rights of Medication Administration (see Chapter 20)" and the ISMP for timely administration, correct crushing and splitting of pills, avoiding confusing abbreviations, and double-checking for sound-alike drugs, medication errors are reduced (ISMP 2013, 2015b).
- Knowledge of technology and nurse competencies is essential to increase patient safety and promote best practices (Johansson-Pajala et al., 2014; Sulosaari et al., 2011).
- Bar code medication administration (BCMA) or automated dispensing medication cabinets enhance verification of the right patient, right drug, right dose, right route, and right time in the presence of medication administration technology and help to reduce medication errors (Bonkowski et al., 2013; Seibert et al., 2014).
- Evidence suggests that a quiet environment free of distractions and interruptions reduces errors when a nurse is preparing medications. Having a medication zone free of distractions, clutter, and interruptions helps to reduce the risk for medication errors (Tzeng et al., 2013; Yoder et al., 2015).
- Follow best practices for calculating medication doses, double-check the calculations, and *do not* administer if the dosage appears incorrect. Follow agency policy for drug calculations for the very young or high-risk medications (e.g., cardiotonics, insulin, and some opioid medications) (Kim and Bates, 2013).
- Best-practice guidelines for safe medication administration require critical thinking, clinical decision-making competency, and theoretical and clinical practice competency. Medication administration is not a routine nursing action. You must critically

think about the medications you are giving. Ask yourself: "Is the medication still appropriate for the patient's condition, or do I need to contact the health care provider?" "This pill looks different. I need to verify with pharmacy" (Teunissen et al., 2013).

SAFETY GUIDELINES

- Safe medication administration requires you to follow the six rights of medication administration for all nonparenteral medications: Right Medication, Right Patient, Right Dose, Right Route, Right Time, and Right Documentation. Also know the ISMP and TJC guidelines, drug actions and interactions, potential side effects and adverse effects, and how to safely administer medication through various nonparenteral routes.
- Assess a patient's sensory function, including sight, hearing, touch, and physical coordination and dexterity. Sensory function and coordination deficits impair a patient's ability to see medications, read labels at home, and discriminate one medication from another. Coordination and dexterity impairments impair a patient's ability to open prescription bottles and dispense the correct dosage.
- Patients often receive more than one oral medication at a time. Evaluate each medication for potential drug-drug or drug-food interactions. When unsure, consult with a pharmacist to clarify the risk of an interaction and determine the measure to reduce it.
- Always assess for drug allergies. If patient reports having an allergy, ask about the type of reaction that occurred.
- Evaluate if patient can take medication with food. In most cases the presence of food in the stomach delays drug absorption. However, some medications must be taken before meals, and others may need to be taken with meals. Some drugs irritate the stomach lining and need to be taken with food.
- For all medications administered, review the order for patient's name, drug, dosage, route, and time of administration.
- Use the correct equipment for administering all medications. For example, when delivering liquid medications, use only unit dose containers dispensed by the pharmacy (ISMP, 2016).
- For all medications administered, gather information pertinent to the drug(s) ordered: purpose, normal dosage and route, common side effects, time of onset and peak, contraindications, and nursing implications.
- Determine if medications require any specific nursing actions (e.g., obtaining vital signs, drug levels, or electrolytes) before administration.
- If patients are mentally and physically able, prepare them for discharge by instructing them in self-administration techniques. Include family caregivers if possible.
- Check the expiration date for all medications.

◆ SKILL 21.1 Administering Oral Medications

 Video Clip   NSO   Nursing Skills Online Administration of Nonparenteral Medications Module / Lesson 6

Patients are usually able to ingest or self-administer oral medications with few problems. If oral medications are contraindicated (e.g., inability to swallow, gastric suction), take precautions to protect patients from aspiration (see Skill 31.3). Nurses usually prepare medications in areas designed for medication preparation or at unit-dose carts.

The form or preparation of an oral medication affects how well it is absorbed after it is ingested. Liquids are absorbed faster than tablets or capsules and are usually absorbed in the stomach. Give an oral medication with a meal if its absorption is enhanced by food in the stomach. Some medications must be taken between meals, 2 to 3 hours later (Burchum and Rosenthal, 2016).

Other oral medications are absorbed in the intestinal tract. Enteric-coated preparations resist being dissolved by gastric juices. The enteric coating protects the stomach lining from irritation by the medication. These preparations are absorbed in the small intestine. Never crush or split an enteric-coated medication. Crushing or splitting these preparations causes the medication to be released too early; the medication may become inactive in the stomach or fail to reach the intended site of action (ISMP, 2015a).

Delegation and Collaboration

The skill of administering oral medications cannot be delegated to nursing assistive personnel (NAP). The nurse instructs the NAP about:

- Potential side effects of medications and to report their occurrence.
- Informing nurse if patient condition changes or worsens (e.g., pain, itching, or rash) after medication administration.

Equipment

- Automated, computer-controlled drug-dispensing system or unit-dose medication cart
- Oral syringes marked "oral use only"
- Glass of water, juice, or preferred liquid and drinking straw
- Device for crushing or splitting tablets (optional)
- Paper towels
- Medication administration record (MAR) (electronic or printed)
- Clean gloves (if handling an oral medication) NOTE: Gloves must be worn when administering an oral chemotherapy drug.

STEP	RATIONALE

ASSESSMENT

1. Check accuracy and completeness of each MAR with health care provider's medication order. Check patient's name and drug name, dosage, and route and time of administration. Clarify incomplete or unclear orders with health care provider before administration.

The health care provider's order is the most reliable source and only legal record of drugs that patient is to receive. Ensures that patient receives correct medication (Sulosaari et al., 2011). Handwritten MARs are a source of medication errors (Alassaad et al., 2013).

STEP	RATIONALE
2. Review pertinent information related to medication, including action, purpose, normal dose and route, side effects, time of onset and peak action, and nursing implications.	Allows you to anticipate effects of drug and observe patient's response.
3. Assess for any contraindications to patient receiving oral medication, including being on NPO status, inability to swallow, nausea/vomiting, bowel inflammation, reduced peristalsis, recent gastrointestinal (GI) surgery, gastric suction, and decreased level of consciousness (LOC). Notify health care provider if any contraindications are present.	Alterations in GI function can interfere with drug absorption, distribution, and excretion. Giving oral medications to patients with impaired swallowing or decreased LOC increases their risk for aspiration (Park et al., 2013). Patients with GI suction do not receive actions of oral medications because the medications are suctioned from the GI tract before they are absorbed.
4. Assess risk for aspiration using a dysphagia screening tool if available (see Skill 31.3). Protect patient from aspiration by assessing swallowing ability (Box 21.2).	Aspiration occurs when food, fluid, or medication intended for GI administration is inadvertently administered into the respiratory tract. Patients with altered ability to swallow are at higher risk for aspiration (Kelly et al., 2011; Park et al., 2013).
5. Assess patient's medical, medication and diet history, and history of allergies. List any drug allergies on each page of MAR and prominently display on patient's medical record. When allergies are present, patient should wear an allergy bracelet.	Information reflects patient's need for and potential responses to medication. Information reveals potential food and drug interactions. Communication of allergies is essential for safe, effective care.
6. Gather and review physical assessment findings and laboratory data that influence drug administration such as vital signs and results of renal and liver function studies.	Data may reveal need to contraindicate drug administration. Renal and liver function status affects metabolism and excretion of medications (Burchum and Rosenthal, 2016).
7. Assess patient's knowledge regarding health and medication use, medication schedule, and ability to prepare medications.	Determines patient's need for medication education and guidance needed to achieve drug adherence (e.g., involvement of family caregiver).
8. Assess patient's preference for fluids and determine if medications can be given with these fluids. Maintain fluid restrictions as prescribed.	Some fluids interfere with medication absorption (e.g., dairy products affect tetracycline). Offering fluids during drug administration is an excellent way to increase patient's fluid intake. Fluids ease swallowing and facilitate absorption from the GI tract. However, fluid restrictions exist; skillful planning of fluid intake must coordinate with medication times and type of medications (To et al., 2013).

NURSING DIAGNOSES

- Deficient knowledge regarding drugs and medication administration
- Impaired swallowing

- Noncompliance
- Readiness for enhanced self-health management

- Risk for aspiration

Related factors/Risk factors are individualized based on patient's condition or needs.

BOX 21.2

Protecting the Patient From Aspiration

- Assess patient's ability to swallow and cough and check for presence of gag reflex.
- Prepare oral medication in form that is easiest to swallow.
- Allow patient to self-administer medications if possible.
- If patient has unilateral (one-sided) weakness, place medication in stronger side of mouth.
- Administer pills one at a time, ensuring that each medication is properly swallowed before next one is introduced.
- Thicken regular liquids or offer fruit nectars if patient cannot tolerate thin liquids.

- Avoid straws because they decrease control patient has over volume intake, which increases risk of aspiration.
- Have patient hold and drink from a cup if possible.
- Time medications to coincide with meals or when patient is well rested and awake if possible.
- Administer medications using another route if risk of aspiration is severe.

STEP	RATIONALE

PLANNING

1. Expected outcomes following completion of procedure:

- Patient responds appropriately to desired medication effect.

Drug has exerted its therapeutic action.

- Patient denies any GI discomfort or symptoms of alterations.

Oral medications can irritate GI mucosa.

- Patient explains purpose of medication and drug dosage schedule.

Demonstrates understanding of drug therapy.

2. Explain procedure to patient. Be specific if patient wishes to self-administer medications.

Makes patient a participant in care, which minimizes anxiety. Begins patient teaching regarding medications. Prepares patient to self-administer drug, which increases feelings of independence.

3. Collect appropriate equipment and MAR.

Promotes time management and efficiency when preparing medications for all patients.

4. Plan preparation of medication to avoid interruptions and distractions. Do not take phone calls or talk with others. See agency policy.

Interruptions contribute to medication administration errors (Prakash et al., 2014; Yoder et al., 2015).

IMPLEMENTATION

1. Prepare medications.

a. Perform hand hygiene.

Reduces transfer of microorganisms.

b. Arrange medication tray and cups in medication preparation area or move medication cart to position outside patient's room.

Organization of equipment saves time and reduces error.

c. Log on to automated dispensing system (ADS) or unlock medicine drawer or cart.

Medications are safeguarded when locked in cabinet, cart, or ADS.

d. Prepare medications for *one patient at a time*. Follow the six rights of medication administration. Keep all pages of MARs or computer printouts for one patient together or look at only one patient's medication administration computer screen.

Prevents preparation errors.

e. Select correct medication from ADS, unit-dose drawer, or stock supply. Compare name of medication on label with MAR or computer printout (see illustration). Exit ADS after removing drug(s).

Reading label and comparing it against transcribed order reduces errors. Exiting ADS ensures that no one else can remove medications using your identity. *This is the first check for accuracy.*

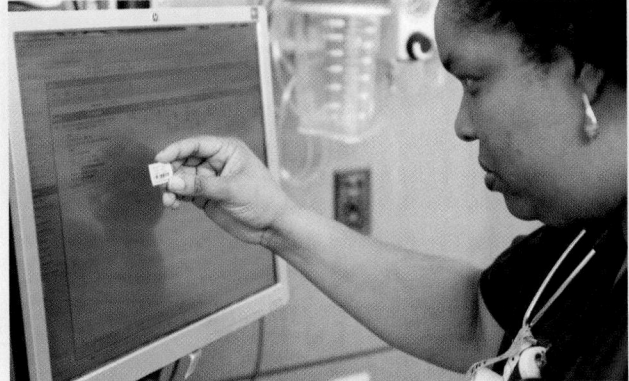

STEP 1e Nurse compares label of medication with transcribed medication order on computerized MAR.

f. Check or calculate medication dose as necessary. Double-check any calculation. Check expiration date on all medications and return outdated medication to pharmacy.

Double-checking pharmacy calculations reduces risk for error. Agency policy may require you to check calculations of certain medications such as insulin with another nurse (Kim and Bates, 2013). Expired medications may be inactive or harmful to patient.

STEP	RATIONALE

g. If preparing a controlled substance, check record for previous medication count and compare current count with available supply. Controlled drugs may be stored in computerized locked cart (see Chapter 20).

Controlled substance laws require nurses to carefully monitor and count dispensed narcotics.

h. Prepare solid forms of oral medications.

(1) To prepare unit-dose tablets or capsules, place packaged tablet or capsule directly into medication cup without removing wrapper. Administer medications only from containers with labels that are clearly marked.

Wrappers maintain cleanliness and identify drug name and dose, which can facilitate teaching.

(2) When using a blister pack, "pop" medications through foil or paper backing into a medication cup.

Packs provide a 1-month supply, with each "blister" usually containing a single dose.

(3) If it is necessary to give half the dose of medication, pharmacy should split, label, package, and send medication to unit.

In health care agencies, only pharmacy should split tablets to ensure patient safety (FDA, 2013). Reduces contamination of tablet.

(4) Place all tablets or capsules that patient will receive in one medicine cup, except for those requiring pre-administration assessments (e.g., pulse rate or blood pressure). Place those medications in separate additional cup with wrapper intact.

Keeping medications that require pre-administration assessments separate from others serves as reminder and makes it easier to withhold drugs as necessary.

(5) If patient has difficulty swallowing and liquid medications are not an option, use a pill-crushing device. Clean device before using. Place medicine between two cups, and grind and crush (see illustration). Mix ground tablet in small amount (teaspoon) of soft food (custard or applesauce).

Large tablets are often difficult to swallow. Ground tablet mixed with palatable soft food is usually easier to swallow.

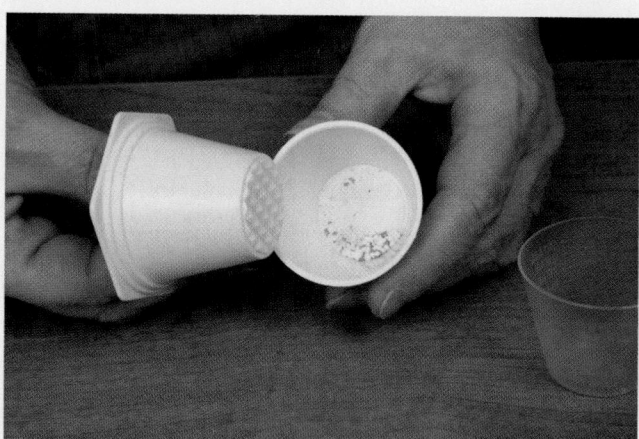

STEP 1h(5) Crushing tablet with pill-crushing device.

Clinical Decision Point *Not all medications can be crushed safely. Consult with a pharmacist or the ISMP Do Not Crush List (ISMP, 2015a).*

i. Prepare liquids.

(1) Use unit-dose container with correct amount of medication. Gently shake container. Administer medication packaged in a single-dose cup directly from the single-dose cup. Do not pour medicine into another cup.

Using unit-dose container with correct dosage of medication provides most accurate dose of medication (ISMP, 2016). Shaking container ensures that medication is mixed before administration.

STEP	RATIONALE

Clinical Decision Point *On the basis of current best practice (ISMP, 2016; Paparella, 2014), liquid medications that are not available or are not in correct dose in a unit-dose container should be dispensed by the pharmacy in special oral syringes marked "Oral Use Only." These syringes do not connect to any type of parenteral (e.g., intravenous [IV]) tubing. In addition, current evidence shows that liquid measuring devices on patient care units result in inaccurate dosing. Having oral medications prepared in the pharmacy ensures that you give the most accurate dose of a medication possible and prevents parenteral administration of oral medications.*

(2) Administer medications in only oral use syringes prepared by pharmacy (see illustration). *Do not* use hypodermic syringe or syringe with needle or syringe cap (see Chapter 20).	Only use syringes specifically designed for oral use when administering liquid medications. If using hypodermic syringes, the medication may be administered parenterally accidentally; or the syringe cap or needle, if not removed from the syringe before administration, may become dislodged and accidentally aspirated during administration of oral medications (ISMP, 2010; ISMP, 2016).
	Allows more accurate measurement of small amounts.

STEP 1i(2) Use special oral medication syringes to prepare small amounts of liquid medications.

j. Return stock containers or unused unit-dose medications to shelf or drawer. Label medication cups and poured medications with patient's name before leaving medication preparation area. Do not leave drugs unattended.	Ensures that correct medications are prepared for correct patient.
k. Before going to patient's room, compare patient's name and name of medication on label of prepared drugs with MAR.	Reading labels a second time reduces errors. *This is the second check for accuracy.*
2. Administer medications.	
a. Take medication(s) to patient at correct time (see agency policy). Medications that require exact timing include stat, first-time or loading doses, and one-time doses. Give time-critical scheduled medications (e.g., antibiotics, anticoagulants, insulin, anticonvulsants, immunosuppressive agents) at exact time ordered (no later than 30 minutes before or after scheduled dose). Give non–time-critical scheduled medications within a range of 1 or 2 hours of scheduled dose (ISMP, 2011). During administration, apply six rights of medication administration. Perform hand hygiene.	Hospitals must adopt medication administration policy and procedure for timing of medication administration that considers nature of the prescribed medication, specific clinical application, and patient needs (CMS, 2011; ISMP, 2011). Time-critical scheduled medications are those for which early or delayed administration of maintenance doses of greater than 30 minutes before or after the scheduled dose may cause harm or result in substantial suboptimal therapy or pharmacological effect. Non–time-critical medications are those for which early or delayed administration within a specified range of either 1 or 2 hours should not cause harm or result in substantial suboptimal therapy or pharmacological effect (CMS, 2011; ISMP, 2011).

STEP	RATIONALE

b. Identify patient using at least two identifiers (e.g., name and birthday or name and medical record number) according to agency policy. Compare identifiers with information on patient's MAR or medical record.

Ensures correct patient. Complies with The Joint Commission standards and improves patient safety (TJC, 2016).

c. At patient's bedside, again compare MAR or computer printout with names of medications on medication labels and patient name. Ask patient if he or she has allergies.

This is the third check for accuracy and ensures that patient receives correct medication.
Confirms patient's allergy history.

d. Explain the purpose of each medication, action, and most common possible adverse effects. Allow sufficient time for patient to ask questions.

Patient has the right to be informed, and patient understanding of each medication improves adherence with drug therapy.

e. Perform necessary pre-administration assessment (e.g., blood pressure, pulse) for specific medications. Ask patient if he or she has allergies.

Determines whether specific medications should be withheld at that time. Confirms patient's allergy history.

Clinical Decision Point *If patient expresses concern regarding accuracy of a medication, do not give the medication. Explore patient's concern and verify prescriber's order before administering. Listening to patient's concerns may prevent a medication error.*

f. Help patient to sitting or Fowler's position. Use side-lying position if he or she is unable to sit. Have patient stay in this position for 30 minutes after administration.

Decreases risk for aspiration during swallowing.

g. *For tablets:* Patient may wish to hold solid medications in hand or cup before placing in mouth. Offer water or preferred liquid to help patient swallow medications.

Patient can become familiar with medications by seeing each drug. Choice of fluid can improve fluid intake.

Clinical Decision Point *If administering an oral chemotherapy medication, you can administer it from the cup directly into the patient's mouth, or apply gloves before handling pill or tablet. Never use bare hands to touch a chemotherapy medication as residue can be absorbed through your skin (Dana Farber Cancer Institute, 2015).*

h. *For orally disintegrating formulations (tablets or strips):* Remove medication from packet just before use. Do not push tablet through foil. Place medication on top of patient's tongue. Caution against chewing it.

Orally disintegrating formulations begin to dissolve when placed on tongue. Water is not needed. Careful removal from packaging is necessary because tablets and strips are thin and fragile.

i. *For sublingually administered medications:* Have patient place medication under tongue and allow it to dissolve completely (see illustration). Caution patient against swallowing tablet.

Drug is absorbed through blood vessels of undersurface of tongue. If swallowed, it is destroyed by gastric juices or rapidly detoxified by liver, preventing therapeutic blood level.

j. *For buccal administered medications:* Have patient place medication in mouth against mucous membranes of cheek and gums until it dissolves (see illustration).

Buccal medications act locally or systemically as they are swallowed in saliva.

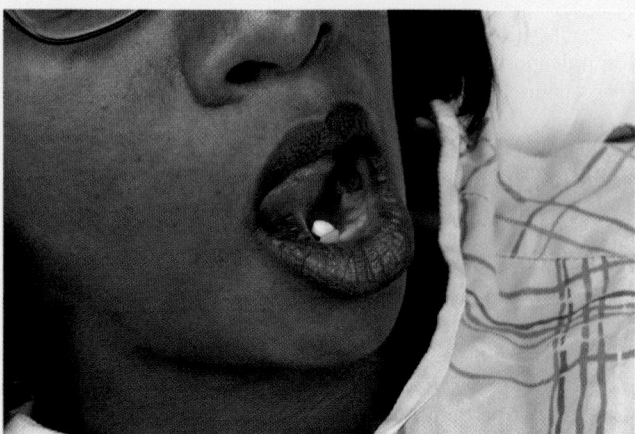

STEP 2i Proper placement of sublingual tablet in sublingual pocket.

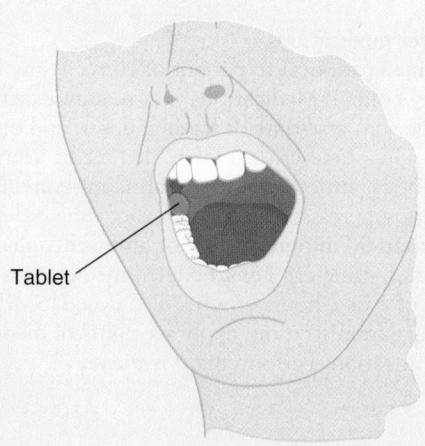

Tablet

STEP 2j Buccal administration of tablet.

STEP	RATIONALE

Clinical Decision Point *Avoid administering anything by mouth until orally disintegrating buccal or sublingual medication is completely dissolved.*

k. *For powdered medications:* Mix with liquids at bedside and give to patient to drink.	When prepared in advance, powdered drugs thicken; some even harden, making swallowing difficult.
l. *For crushed medications mixed with food:* Give each medication separately in teaspoon of food.	Ensures that patient swallows all of medicine.
m. *For lozenge:* Caution patient against chewing or swallowing lozenges.	Lozenges act through slow absorption through oral mucosa, not gastric mucosa.
n. *For effervescent medication:* Add tablet or powder to glass of water. Administer immediately after dissolving.	Effervescence improves unpleasant taste and often relieves GI problems.
o. If patient is unable to hold medications, place medication cup to lips and gently introduce each drug into mouth one at a time. A spoon can also be used to place pill in patient's mouth. Do not rush or force medications.	Administering a single tablet or capsule eases swallowing and decreases risk for aspiration.

Clinical Decision Point *If tablet or capsule falls to the floor, discard it and repeat preparation. Drug is contaminated.*

p. Stay until patient swallows each medication completely or takes it by the prescribed route. Ask patient to open mouth if uncertain whether medication has been swallowed.	Ensures that patient receives ordered dose. If left unattended, patient may not take dose or may save drugs, causing health risks.
q. For highly acidic medications (e.g., aspirin), offer patient a nonfat snack (e.g., crackers) if not contraindicated by his or her condition.	Reduces gastric irritation. Fat content of foods may delay drug absorption.
3. Help patient return to position of comfort.	Maintains patient's comfort.
4. Dispose of soiled supplies and perform hand hygiene. Return cart to medication room if used. Clean work area.	Reduces spread of microorganisms.

5. Replenish stock such as cups and straws, return cart to medication room, and clean work area.	Enhances efficiency and reduced transfer of microorganisms.

EVALUATION

1. Return to bedside to evaluate patient's response to medications at times that correlate with onset, peak, and duration of the medication.	Evaluates therapeutic benefit of medication and helps to detect onset of side effects or allergic reactions. Sublingual medications act in 15 minutes; most oral medications act in 30 to 60 minutes.
2. Ask patient or family caregiver to identify medication name and explain purpose, action, dose schedule, and potential side effects.	Determines level of knowledge gained by patient and family caregiver.
3. **Use Teach-Back:** "I want to be sure I showed you how to use your sublingual nitroglycerin. Show me where you will place the tablet in your mouth." Revise your instruction now or develop a plan for revised patient or family caregiver teaching if patient or family caregiver is not able to teach back correctly.	Determines patient's and family caregiver's level of understanding of instructional topic.

STEP	RATIONALE
Unexpected Outcomes 1. Patient exhibits adverse effects (e.g., side effect, toxic effect, allergic reaction). 2. Patient refuses medication. 3. Patient is unable to explain drug information.	**Related Interventions** • Notify health care provider and pharmacy. • Withhold further doses. • Assess vital signs. • Symptoms such as urticaria, rash, pruritus, rhinitis, and wheezing may indicate an allergic reaction and need for emergency medications. • Add allergy information to patient's medical record. • Assess why patient is refusing medication. • Provide further instruction • Do not force patient to take medications. • Notify health care provider. • Further assess patient's or family caregiver's knowledge of medications and guidelines for drug safety. • Further instruction or different approach to instruction is necessary.

Recording and Reporting

• Record drug, dose, route, and time administered on patient's MAR immediately after administration, not before. Include initials or signature.
• Record patient's response to medication, patient teaching, and validation of patient's understanding on flow sheet or in nurses' notes in electronic health record (EHR) or chart.
• If drug is withheld, record reason on flow sheet or in nurses' notes in EHR or chart and follow agency policy for noting withheld doses.
• Report adverse effects/patient response and/or withheld drugs to nurse in charge or health care provider. Depending on medication, immediate health care provider notification may be required.

Special Considerations
Teaching

• Instruct patient and family caregiver about specific information pertaining to drug regimen (purpose, action, dose, dosage intervals, side effects, foods to avoid or take with drugs). If patient is taking multiple medications, consider recommending a dose organizer.
• All patients should learn the basic guidelines for drug safety in the home (see Skill 43.3).

Pediatric

• Liquid forms of medication are safer to swallow to avoid aspiration of small pills.
• Children refuse bitter or distasteful oral preparations. Mix the drug with a small amount (about 1 tsp) of a sweet-tasting substance such as jam, applesauce, sherbet, ice cream, or fruit puree. Do not use honey for infants because of the risk of botulism. Offer the child juice or a flavored ice pop after medication administration. Do not place medication in an essential food item such as milk or formula; the child may refuse the food at a later time.
• Measure the liquid medications with a plastic calibrated oral dosing syringe or a spoon. Calibrated spoons have proven to be most accurate for the pediatric population (Beckett et al., 2012).

Gerontological

• Physiological changes of aging influence how oral medications are distributed, absorbed, and excreted. Common changes include loss of elasticity in oral mucosa; reduction in parotid gland secretion, causing dry mouth; delayed esophageal clearance; impaired swallowing; reduction in gastric acidity and stomach peristalsis; increased susceptibility to highly acidic drugs; reduced liver function, resulting in altered drug metabolism; and reduced renal function and colon motility, slowing drug excretion (Touhy and Jett, 2014). Both altered drug metabolism and excretion may lead to drug toxicity (Burchum and Rosenthal, 2016).
• Give medications with a full glass of water (unless restricted) to aid passage of the drug. Give patient time to swallow.
• Patients may have several health problems or chronic conditions requiring the use of multiple drugs, often prescribed by different health care providers. Polypharmacy creates a high risk for drug interactions and adverse reactions (Burchum and Rosenthal, 2016).

Home Care

• When measuring liquid medications at home, instruct patients and family caregivers how to accurately use a dosing cup to administer medications in the home (see Chapter 20).
• See Skills 43.3 and 44.6.

◆ SKILL 21.2 **Administering Medications Through a Feeding Tube**

NSO *Nursing Skills Online Administration of Nonparenteral Medications Module / Lesson 2*

Patients who have enteral feeding tubes are unable to receive food or medications by mouth. Nasogastric feeding tubes generally are small-bore tubes that are inserted into the stomach via one of the nares (see Chapter 32). For long-term enteral feedings, a percutaneous endoscopic gastrostomy (PEG) tube or a jejunostomy tube may be inserted surgically. *Do not administer medications into nasogastric tubes that are inserted for decompression.*

In addition to administering the correct medication, it is important that the enteral access connector be appropriate for the type of enteral tube (TJC, 2014). These devices are not compatible with Luer or needleless connectors. They are designed for specific enteral feeding tubes. The goal of these new access connectors is to reduce enteral tube misconnections and medication errors (Guenther, 2015; TJC, 2014).

Preferably medications administered by enteral tubes should be in liquid form. However, when the liquid form of the medication is not available, you need to prepare an oral medication tablet or capsule by crushing or dissolving it. Hospital pharmacies may be able to provide the prescribed medication in a liquid suspension, which does not affect its effectiveness (Salmon et al., 2013). However, *do not crush* sublingual, sustained-release, chewable, long-acting, or enteric-coated medications. Consult with the hospital pharmacist about whether you can crush or dissolve a medication. Always verify correct placement of a nasogastric tube before administering medications (see Skill 32.2).

Delegation and Collaboration

The skill of administering medications by enteral feeding tubes cannot be delegated to nursing assistive personnel (NAP). The nurse instructs the NAP to:

- Keep the head of the bed elevated a minimum of 30 degrees (preferably 45 degrees) for 1 hour after medication administration; follow agency policy.
- Report immediately to the nurse coughing, choking, gagging, or drooling of liquid or dissolved pills.
- Report to the nurse occurrence of possible medication side effects (specific to medication).

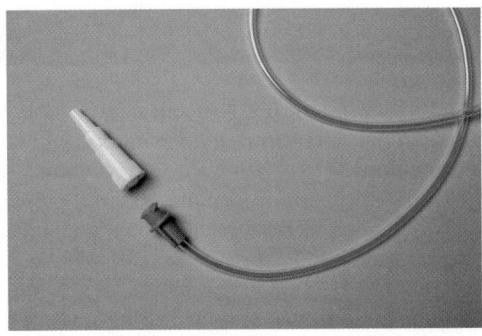

FIG 21.1 Enteral connector.

Equipment

- Medication administration record (MAR) (electronic or printed)
- Appropriate medication syringe or 60-mL Asepto syringe for large-bore tubes only
- Enteral-only connector (ENFit) designed to fit the specific enteral tube (TJC, 2014) (Fig. 21.1)
- Gastric pH test strip (scale of 1 to 11)
- Graduated container
- Medication to be administered
- Pill crusher if medication in tablet form
- Water or sterile water for immunocompromised patients
- Tongue blade or straw to stir dissolved medication
- Clean gloves
- Stethoscope and pulse oximeter (for evaluation)

STEP	RATIONALE

ASSESSMENT

1. Check accuracy and completeness of each MAR with health care provider's medication order. Check patient's name, drug name and dosage, route of administration, and time for administration. Clarify incomplete or unclear orders with health care provider before administration.

The health care provider's order is the most reliable source and only legal record of drugs that patient is to receive. Ensures that patient receives correct medication (Sulosaari et al., 2011). Handwritten MARs are a source of medication errors (Alassaad et al., 2013).

2. Review pertinent information related to medication, including action, purpose, normal dose and route, side effects, time of onset and peak action, and nursing implications.

Allows you to anticipate effects of drug and observe patient's response.

3. Assess for any contraindications to receiving enteral medications, including presence of bowel inflammation, reduced peristalsis, recent gastrointestinal (GI) surgery, and gastric suction that cannot be turned off.

Alterations in GI function can interfere with drug absorption, distribution, and excretion. Patients with GI suction do not benefit from medication because it may be suctioned from the GI track before it is absorbed.

4. Assess patient's medical, medication, and diet history and history of allergies. List patient's food and drug allergies on each page of the MAR and prominently display it on the patient's medical record per agency policy. When patient has allergy, provide allergy bracelet. If you identify contraindications, withhold medication and inform health care provider.

Information reflects patient's need for and potential responses to medications. Information also indicates potential food and drug interactions. Some drugs may require tube feeding to be stopped for an hour before and 2 hours after dose (Burchum and Rosenthal, 2016). Communication of allergies is essential for safe, effective care.

5. For postoperative patient review postoperative orders for type of enteral tube care.

Manipulation and irrigation of tube or instillation of medications may be contraindicated.

STEP	RATIONALE
6. Gather and review physical assessment data (e.g., bowel sounds, abdominal distention) and laboratory data (e.g., renal and liver function) that may influence drug administration.	Physical examination findings or laboratory data may contraindicate drug administration.
7. Check with pharmacy for availability of liquid preparation for patient's medications. Prescriber may need to change dosage form.	When possible, liquid formulation of the medication is the best option. The agency pharmacy may have the ability to provide a liquid preparation that is compatible with the enteral nutrition formula (Klang et al., 2013; Zhu and Zhou, 2013). Reduces risk for aspiration.
8. Before administration of enteral medications, verify placement of feeding tube (see Skill 32.2) and determine that tube is placed in the stomach or small intestine correctly.	Ensures that point of medication absorption is not bypassed by feeding tube. For example, some medications (e.g., antacids) are absorbed in the stomach. If the patient's tube is placed in the intestines, these medications are not absorbed because the stomach is bypassed by the tube (McIntyre and Monk, 2014).

NURSING DIAGNOSES

- Feeding self-care deficit
- Impaired swallowing
- Risk for aspiration

Related factors/Risk factors are individualized based on patient's condition or needs.

PLANNING

1. Expected outcomes following completion of procedure:	
• Patient experiences desired medication effect within period of onset of medication.	Drug has exerted its therapeutic action.
• Patient's feeding tube remains patent after administration of medication.	Patent enteral tube indicates passage of medication into stomach, ensuring proper absorption. If tube becomes blocked, administration of other medications and feedings are not possible.
• Patient does not aspirate during or after medication administration.	Patient safety in medication administration is maintained.
2. Collect appropriate equipment and MAR.	Ensures time management and efficiency.

IMPLEMENTATION

1. Perform hand hygiene. Prepare medications for instillation into feeding tube (see Skill 21.1). Check medication label against MAR 2 times. Fill graduated container with 50 to 100 mL of tepid water. Use sterile water for immunocompromised or critically ill patients (Allen, 2015; Malone, 2014).	*These are the first and second checks for accuracy.* Preparation process ensures that right patient receives right medication. Tepid water prevents abdominal cramping, which can occur with cold water.

Clinical Decision Point *Whenever possible, use liquid medications instead of crushed tablets. If you have to crush tablets, flush the tubing before and after the medication administration to prevent the drug from adhering to the inside of the tube. In addition, make sure that concentrated medications are thoroughly diluted. Never add crushed medications directly to a tube feeding (Guenther and Boullatta, 2013).*

a. *Tablets:* Crush each tablet into a fine powder, using pill-crushing device or two medication cups (see Skill 21.1). Dissolve each tablet in separate cup of 30 mL of warm water.	Fine powder dissolves more easily, reducing chance of occluding feeding tube.
b. *Capsules:* Ensure that contents of capsule (granules or gelatin) can be expressed from covering (consult with pharmacist). Apply gloves and open capsule or pierce gel cap with sterile needle and empty contents into 30 mL of warm water (or solution designated by drug company). Gel caps dissolve in warm water, but this may take 15 to 20 minutes.	Ensures that contents of capsules are in solution to prevent occlusion of tube.
c. Prepare liquid medication according to Skill 21.1.	

STEP	RATIONALE

2. Take medication(s) to patient at correct time (see agency policy). Medications that require exact timing include stat, first-time or loading doses, and 1-time doses. Give time-critical scheduled medications (e.g., antibiotics, anticoagulants, insulin, anticonvulsants, immunosuppressive agents) at exact time ordered (no later than 30 minutes before or after scheduled dose). Give non–time-critical scheduled medications within a range of 1 or 2 hours of scheduled dose (ISMP, 2011). During administration, apply six rights of medication administration. Perform hand hygiene.

Hospitals must adopt medication administration policy and procedure for timing of medication administration that considers nature of the prescribed medication, specific clinical application, and patient needs (CMS, 2011; ISMP, 2011). Time-critical scheduled medications are those for which early or delayed administration of maintenance doses of greater than 30 minutes before or after the scheduled dose may cause harm or result in substantial suboptimal therapy or pharmacological effect. Non–time-critical medications are those for which early or delayed administration within a specified range of either 1 or 2 hours should not cause harm or result in substantial suboptimal therapy or pharmacological effect (CMS, 2011; ISMP, 2011).

3. Identify patient using at least two identifiers (e.g., name and birthday or name and medical record number) according to agency policy. Compare identifiers with information on patient's MAR or medical record.

Ensures correct patient. Complies with The Joint Commission standards and improves patient safety (TJC, 2016).

4. At patient's bedside again compare MAR or computer printout with names of medications on medication labels and patient name. Ask patient if he or she has allergies.

This is the third check for accuracy and ensures that patient receives correct medication. Confirms patient's allergy history.

5. Explain procedure to patient and discuss purpose of each medication, action, and possible adverse effects. Allow patient to ask any questions about the drugs.

Helps patient be a participant in care, which minimizes anxiety. Patient has right to be informed, and patient's understanding of each medication improves adherence to drug therapy. Begins patient teaching regarding medications.

6. Assist patient to sitting position. Elevate head of bed to minimum of 30 degrees and preferably 45 degrees (unless contraindicated) or sit patient up in a chair (Malone, 2014).

Reduces risk for aspiration, keeping head above stomach.

7. If continuous enteral tube feeding is infusing, adjust infusion pump setting to hold tube feeding.

Feeding solution should not infuse while residuals are checked or medications are administered. The presence of a feeding solution may impede drug absorption (Klang et al., 2013).

8. Apply clean gloves. Check placement of feeding tube (see Skill 32.2) by observing gastric contents and checking pH of aspirate contents. *Gastric pH less than 5.0 is a good indicator that tip of tube is correctly placed in stomach* (Clifford et al., 2015).

Ensures proper tube placement and reduces risk of introducing fluids into respiratory tract.

9. Check for gastric residual volume (GRV). Draw up 10 to 30 mL of air into a 60-mL syringe and connect syringe to feeding tube. Flush tube with air and pull back slowly to aspirate gastric contents (see illustration). Determine GRV using either scale on syringe or a graduate container. Return aspirated contents to stomach unless a single GRV exceeds 250 mL (see agency policy). When GRV is excessive, hold medication and contact health care provider.

Large residuals indicate delayed gastric emptying and put patient at increased risk for aspiration (Malone, 2014).

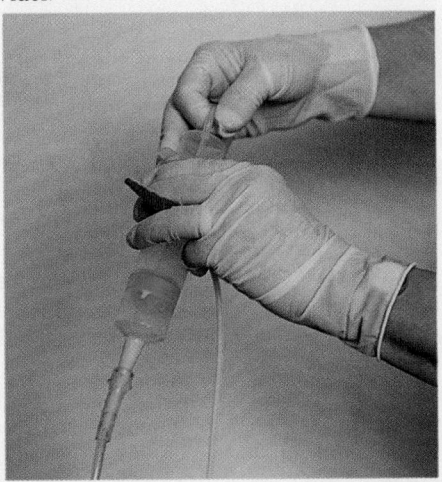

STEP 10 Aspirate stomach contents for residual volume.

STEP	RATIONALE

10. Irrigate the tubing.

   a. Pinch or clamp enteral tube and remove syringe. Draw up 30 mL of water into syringe. Reinsert tip of syringe into tube, release clamp, and flush tubing. Clamp tube again and remove syringe.

Pinching or clamping tubing prevents leakage or spillage of stomach contents. Flushing ensures that tube is patent.

   b. Using the appropriate enteral connector (see Fig. 21.1), attach to enteral tube.

Standardization of connector tubing improves patient safety. Tubing standards are designed to reduce tubing misconnections that result in patient injury (TJC, 2014).

Clinical Decision Point *Verify that the connector meets the ISO tubing connector standards (TJC, 2014). Do not attach the enteral tubing to a standardized Luer syringe or needleless device (Guenther, 2015; TJC, 2014).*

11. Remove bulb or plunger of syringe and reinsert syringe into tip of feeding tube.

Removal of bulb or plunger prepares syringe for delivery of medications.

12. Administer dose of first liquid or dissolved medication by pouring into syringe (see illustration). Allow to flow by gravity.

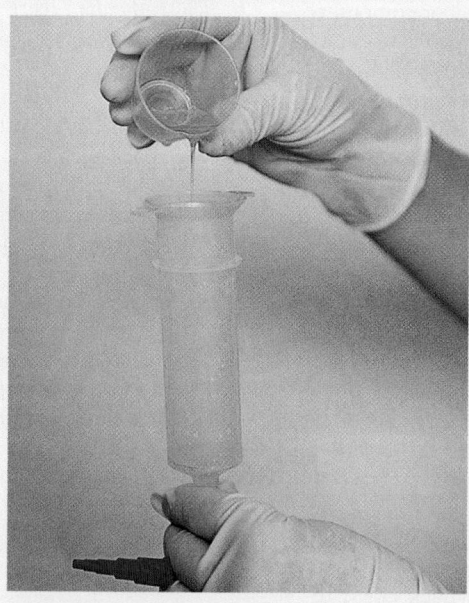

STEP 12 Pour liquid medication into syringe.

Clinical Decision Point *Sometimes it is necessary to transfer oral medications into a medication cup for enteral administration. If medication does not flow freely, raise the height of the syringe to increase the rate of flow or try having the patient change position slightly because the end of the feeding tube may be against the gastric mucosa. If these measures do not improve the flow, a gentle push with bulb of Asepto syringe or plunger of the syringe may facilitate flow of fluid.*

   a. If giving only one dose of medication, flush tubing with 30 to 60 mL of water after administration.

Maintains patency of enteral tube and ensures that medication passes through tube to stomach (Klang et al., 2013).

   b. To administer more than one medication, give each separately and flush between medications with 15 to 30 mL of water.

Allows for accurate identification of medication if dose is spilled. In addition, some medications may be incompatible, and giving medication separately followed by a flush solution decreases the risk for medication incompatibilities (Zhu and Zhou, 2013).

   c. Follow last dose of medication with 30 to 60 mL of water.

Maintains patency of enteral tube and ensures passage of medication into stomach (Blumenstein et al., 2014).

13. Clamp proximal end of feeding tube if tube feeding is not being administered and cap end of tube.

Prevents air from entering stomach between medication doses.

14. When continuous tube feeding is being administered by infusion pump, follow medication administration. If medications are not compatible with feeding solution, hold feeding for additional 30 to 60 minutes (Klang et al., 2013).

Allows for adequate absorption of medication and avoids potential drug-food interaction between medication and enteral feeding (Zhu and Zhou, 2013).

STEP	RATIONALE
15. Help patient to comfortable position and keep head of bed elevated for 1 hour (see agency policy).	Reduces risk of aspiration.
16. Dispose of soiled supplies, rinse graduated container and syringe with tap water, remove and dispose of gloves, and perform hand hygiene.	Reduces spread of microorganisms.

EVALUATION

1. Observe patient for signs of aspiration such as choking, gurgling, gurgling speech, breath sounds, and difficulty breathing.	Provides for prompt intervention if aspiration has occurred
2. Return within 30 minutes to evaluate patient's response to medications.	Monitoring patient's response evaluates therapeutic benefit of drug and helps detect onset of side effects or allergic reactions.
3. **Use Teach-Back:** "I want to be sure I explained clearly why your father must take his medications through his feeding tube. Tell me why he is receiving his medications through his feeding tube." Revise your instruction now or develop a plan for revised patient or family caregiver teaching if patient or family caregiver is not able to teach back correctly.	Determines patient's and family caregiver's level of understanding of instructional topic.

Unexpected Outcomes	Related Interventions
1. Patient exhibits signs of aspiration, including respiratory distress, changes in vital signs, or changes in oxygen saturation.	• Stop all medications/fluids through feeding tube. • Elevate head of bed and stay with patient. • Assess vital signs and breath sounds while another staff member notifies health care provider.
2. Patient does not receive medication because of blocked enteral tube.	• For newly inserted tube, notify health care provider and obtain x-ray film confirmation of placement. • Requires interventions to unclog tube to ensure drug delivery (Box 21.3).
3. Patient exhibits adverse effects (side effect, toxic effect, allergic reaction).	• Withhold further doses. • Always notify health care provider and pharmacy when patient exhibits adverse effects. • Symptoms such as urticaria, rash, pruritus, rhinitis, and wheezing indicate allergic reaction. • Enter patient allergy in medical record.

Recording and Reporting

- Record in nurses' notes in electronic health record (EHR) or chart the method used to check placement of enteral tube, GRV, and pH of stomach aspirate.
- Record actual time that each drug was administered on MAR immediately after administration, not before. Include initials or signature.

- Record patient's response to medication, patient teaching, and validation of patient understanding on flow sheet or in nurses' notes in EHR or chart.
- Record total amount of water used for medication administration on proper intake and output (I&O) form.
- Report adverse effects, patient response, and/or withheld drugs to nurse in charge or health care provider.

BOX 21.3

Unclogging a Blocked Feeding Tube

- Prevent tube from becoming blocked by flushing it with at least 15 to 30 mL of tepid water before and after administering each dose of medication, 30 to 60 mL after last dose of medication, before and after checking gastric residual volumes, and every 4 to 12 hours around the clock (refer to agency policies).
- Gently flush tube with large-bore syringe and warm water. Do not use small-bore syringe because this exerts too much pressure and may rupture tube.

- If irrigation with water is not effective, obtain an order for a pancrelipase tablet and follow manufacturer guidelines for tube irrigation. In addition, a declogging stylus may be used (see agency policy).
- The tube may have to be removed, and a new one inserted if the medication is urgent.

Modified from Blumenstein I, et al.: Gastroenteric tube feeding: techniques, problems and solutions, *World J Gastroenterol* 20(26):8505, 2014, http://doi.org/10.3748/wjg.v20.i26.8505.

Special Considerations
Teaching
- Teach patient or family caregiver how to store medications and tube-feeding supplements (see Chapter 32).
- Demonstrate to family caregiver how to prepare medications, including crushing them if appropriate.
- Demonstrate to patient or family caregiver how to verify correct placement of tube.

- Teach family caregiver the importance of consistent flushing of feeding tube before and after medication administration.

Pediatric
- Volumes for instillation of medications or for irrigation of enteral tubes should be small enough to clear tubing (Hockenberry and Wilson, 2015).

◆ SKILL 21.3 Applying Topical Medications to the Skin

▶ *Video Clip* **NSO** *Nursing Skills Online Administration of Nonparenteral Medications Module / Lesson 3*

Topical administration of medication involves applying drugs locally to the skin, mucous membranes, or tissues. Topical drugs such as lotions, patches, pastes, and ointments primarily produce local effects; but they can create systemic effects if absorbed through the skin. Systemic effects are more likely to occur if the skin is thin, drug concentration is high, contact with the skin is prolonged, or the drug is applied to skin that is not intact. In addition, skin hydration and environmental humidity affect percutaneous absorption of a medication. An increase in skin hydration increases absorption (Lawton, 2013). Apply topical drugs using gloves and applicators to protect from accidental exposure. Skin encrustations and dead tissue harbor microorganisms and block contact of medications with the affected tissue or membrane.

Never apply new medication over a previously applied medication because it will decrease the therapeutic benefit to a patient. Always clean the skin or wound thoroughly before applying a new dose of a topical medication. Apply each type of medication, whether an ointment, lotion, powder, or patch, in a specific way to ensure proper penetration and absorption (Lawton, 2013).

Delegation and Collaboration
The skill of administering most topical medications, including skin patches, cannot be delegated to nursing assistive personnel (NAP).

However, some facilities (e.g., long-term care) may allow NAP to apply some forms of topical agents (e.g., skin barriers) to irritated skin or for the protection of the perineum during morning or perineal care. Check agency policies. The nurse instructs the NAP to:
- Report immediately to the nurse any skin irritation, burning, blistering, or increased itching.
- Not apply any dressing over the topical medication unless instructed to do so.

Equipment
- Clean gloves (for intact skin) or sterile gloves (for nonintact skin)
- Cotton-tipped applicators or tongue blades *(optional)*
- Ordered medication (powder, cream, lotion, ointment, spray, patch)
- Basin of warm water, washcloth, towel, nondrying soap
- Sterile dressing, tape
- Felt-tip pen *(optional)*
- Medication administration record (MAR) (electronic or printed)
- Plastic wrap, transparent dressing (if ordered) *(optional)*

STEP	RATIONALE

ASSESSMENT

1. Check accuracy and completeness of each MAR with health care provider's medication order. Check patient's name, drug name and dosage, route of administration, and time for administration. Clarify incomplete or unclear orders with health care provider before administration.

The order sheet is the most reliable source and only legal record of medications that patient is to receive. Ensures that patient receives correct medications (Sulosaari et al., 2011). Handwritten MARs are a source of medication errors (Alassaad et al., 2013).

2. Review pertinent information related to medication, including action, purpose, normal dose and route, side effects, time of onset and peak action, and nursing implications.

Allows you to anticipate effects of drug and observe patient's response.

3. Assess condition of skin or membrane where medication is to be applied (see Chapter 6). If there is an open wound, perform hand hygiene and apply clean gloves. First wash site thoroughly with mild, nondrying soap and warm water, rinse, and dry. Be sure to remove any previously applied medication or debris. Also remove any blood, body fluids, secretions, or excretions. Assess for symptoms of skin irritation such as pruritus or burning. Remove gloves when finished. Perform hand hygiene.

Cleaning site thoroughly promotes proper assessment of skin surface. Assessment provides baseline to determine change in condition of skin after therapy. Application of certain topical agents can lessen or aggravate these symptoms.

Cleaning removes any residual medication from the previous dose, which reduces potential adverse medication reactions or skin irritation (Cohen, 2013).

STEP	RATIONALE
4. Assess patient's medical and medication history and history of allergies (including latex and topical agent). Ask if patient has had reaction to a cream or lotion applied to skin. List drug allergies on each page of the MAR and prominently display it on the patient's medical record per agency policy. When patient has allergy, provide allergy bracelet.	Information reflects patient's need for and potential responses to medications. Allergic contact dermatitis is relatively common and can worsen dermatological (skin) condition. In addition, some patients may be allergic to preservatives or fragrances in topical medications. Latex allergy requires use of nonlatex gloves. Communication of allergies is essential for safe and effective care.
5. Determine amount of topical agent required for application by assessing skin site, reviewing health care provider's order, and reading application directions carefully (a thin, even layer is usually adequate).	An excessive amount of topical agent can irritate skin chemically, negate effectiveness of drug, and/or cause adverse systemic effects such as decreased white blood cell (WBC) counts.
6. Assess patient's knowledge of action and purpose of medication being given, application schedule, and willingness to adhere to drug regimen.	Reveals patient's level of understanding and whether instruction is necessary.
7. Determine if patient or family caregiver is physically able to apply medication by assessing grasp, hand strength, reach, and coordination.	Necessary if patient is to self-administer drug at home.

NURSING DIAGNOSES

- Deficient knowledge regarding drug and medication application
- Impaired physical mobility
- Impaired skin integrity
- Pain (acute or chronic)
- Readiness for enhanced self-health management
- Risk for infection

Related factors/Risk factors are individualized based on patient's condition or needs.

PLANNING

1. Expected outcomes following completion of procedure:	
• Patient is able to identify drug and describe action, purpose, dose, side effects, and schedule of medication.	Demonstrates learning.
• Patient is able to apply medication without help on prescribed schedule.	Demonstrates learning and compliance.
• With repeated applications, skin becomes clear, without inflammation or drainage from lesions.	Existing lesions heal and/or disappear as result of therapeutic action of medication.
2. Collect appropriate equipment and MAR.	Ensures time management and efficiency.

IMPLEMENTATION

1. Perform hand hygiene. Prepare medications for application. Check label of medication against MAR 2 times (see Skill 21.1). Preparation usually involves taking bottle or tube of lotion, cream, ointment, or patch out of storage and to patient's room. Check expiration date on container.	Reduces transmission of infection. *These are the first and second checks for accuracy.* Process ensures that right patient receives right medication.
2. Take medication(s) to patient at correct time (see agency policy). Medications that require exact timing include stat, first-time or loading doses, and 1-time doses. Give time-critical scheduled medications (e.g., antibiotics, anticoagulants, insulin, anticonvulsants, immunosuppressive agents) at exact time ordered (no later than 30 minutes before or after scheduled dose). Give non–time-critical scheduled medications within a range of 1 or 2 hours of scheduled dose (ISMP, 2011). During administration, apply six rights of medication administration. Perform hand hygiene.	Hospitals must adopt medication administration policy and procedure for timing of medication administration that considers nature of the prescribed medication, specific clinical application, and patient needs (CMS, 2011; ISMP, 2011). Time-critical scheduled medications are those for which early or delayed administration of maintenance doses of greater than 30 minutes before or after the scheduled dose may cause harm or result in substantial suboptimal therapy or pharmacological effect. Non–time-critical medications are those for which early or delayed administration within a specified range of either 1 or 2 hours should not cause harm or result in substantial suboptimal therapy or pharmacological effect (CMS, 2011; ISMP, 2011).
3. Help patient to comfortable position. Arrange supplies at bedside.	Allows easy access to application site.

STEP	RATIONALE
4. Identify patient using at least two identifiers (e.g., name and birthday or name and medical record number) according to agency policy. Compare identifiers with information on patient's MAR or medical record.	Ensures correct patient. Complies with The Joint Commission standards and improves patient safety (TJC, 2016).
5. At patient's bedside again compare MAR or computer printout with names of medications on medication labels and patient name. Ask patient if he or she has allergies.	*This is the third check for accuracy* and ensures that patient receives correct medication. Confirms patient's allergy history.
6. Explain procedure to patient and discuss purpose of each medication, action, and possible adverse effects. Allow patient to ask any questions about the drugs.	Helps patient be a participant in care, which minimizes anxiety. Patient has the right to be informed, and his or her understanding of each medication improves adherence to drug therapy. Begins patient teaching regarding medications.
7. If skin is broken, apply sterile gloves. Otherwise apply clean gloves.	Reduces spread of microorganisms.
8. Apply topical creams, ointments, and oil-based lotions.	
a. Expose affected area while keeping unaffected areas covered.	Provides visualization for application and protects privacy.
b. Wash, rinse, and dry affected area before applying medication if not done earlier (see Assessment, Step 3).	Cleaning removes microorganisms from remaining debris and any surface medication (Cohen, 2013).
c. If skin is excessively dry and flaking, apply topical agent while skin is still damp.	Increased skin hydration and surface humidity enhance absorption of topical medication (Lawton, 2013).
d. After washing, remove gloves, perform hand hygiene, and apply new clean or sterile gloves.	Sterile gloves are used when applying agents to open, noninfectious skin lesions. Changing gloves prevents cross-contamination of infected or contagious lesions. Gloves also protect you from topical absorption of the medication and subsequent drug effects (Lawton, 2013).
e. Place required amount of medication in palm of gloved hand and soften by rubbing briskly between hands.	Softening topical agent makes it easier to spread on skin.
f. Tell patient that initial application of agent may feel cold. Once medication is softened, spread it evenly over skin surface, using long, even strokes that follow direction of hair growth. Do not vigorously rub skin. Apply to thickness specified by manufacturer instructions.	Ensures even distribution and sufficient dosage of medication. Technique prevents irritation of hair follicles.
g. Explain to patient that skin may feel greasy after application.	Ointments often contain oils.
9. Apply antianginal (nitroglycerin) ointment.	
a. Remove previous dose paper. Fold used paper containing any residual medication with used sides together and dispose of it in biohazard trash container. Wipe off residual medication with tissue.	Prevents overdose that can occur with multiple-dose papers left in place. Proper disposal protects you and others from accidental exposure to medication.
b. Write date, time, and your initials on new application paper.	Label provides reference to prevent missing doses.
c. Antianginal (nitroglycerin) ointments are usually ordered in inches and can be measured on small sheets of paper marked off in 1.25 cm (½-inch) markings. Unit-dose packages are available. Apply desired number of inches of ointment to paper-measuring guide (see illustration).	Ensures correct dose of medication.

Clinical Decision Point *Unit-dose packages are available.* **NOTE:** *One package equals 2.5 cm (1 inch); smaller amounts should not be measured from this package.*

d. Select new application site: Apply nitroglycerin to chest area, back, abdomen, or anterior thigh (Burchum and Rosenthal, 2016). Do not apply on nonintact skin or hairy surfaces or over scar tissue.	Application sites are rotated to reduce skin irritation. Application on nonintact skin may result in increased absorption of medication. Application on hairy surfaces or scar tissue may decrease absorption (Burchum and Rosenthal, 2016).

STEP	RATIONALE

e. Apply ointment to skin surface by holding edge or back of paper-measuring guide and placing ointment and wrapper directly on skin (see illustration). Do not rub or massage ointment into skin.

Minimizes chance of ointment covering gloves and later touching nurse's hands. Medication is designed to absorb slowly over several hours; massaging increases absorption rate.

f. Secure ointment and paper with transparent dressing or strip of tape. Apply dressing or plastic wrap only when instructed by pharmacy (Lawton, 2013).

Prevents staining of clothing or inadvertent removal of medication. Covering topical medications with dressing or plastic wrap increases heat and skin humidity and rate of absorption of medication (Cohen, 2013; Lawton, 2013).

10. Apply transdermal patches (e.g., analgesic, nicotine, nitroglycerin, estrogen).

a. If old patch is present, remove it and clean area. Be sure to check between skinfolds for patch.

Failure to remove old patch can result in overdose. Many patches are small, clear, or flesh colored and can be easily hidden between skinfolds. Cleaning removes residual medication traces of previous patch.

b. Dispose of old patch by folding in half with sticky sides together. Some facilities require patch to be cut before disposal (see agency policy). Dispose of it in biohazard trash bag.

Proper disposal prevents accidental exposure to medication.

c. Date and initial outer side of new patch before applying it and note time of administration. Use soft-tip or felt-tip pen.

Visual reminder prevents missing or extra doses. Ballpoint pen damages patch and alters medication delivery.

d. Choose a new site that is clean, intact, dry, and free of hair. Some patches have specific instructions for placement locations (e.g., Testoderm patches are placed on scrotum; a scopolamine patch is placed behind the ear; *never apply* an estrogen patch to breast tissue or waistline). Do not apply patch on skin that is oily, burned, cut, or irritated in any way.

Ensures complete medication absorption. Estrogen patches should never be placed on the breast, genitals, or other reproductive organs. There is a risk for systemic absorption of the hormone, which can increase patient's risk for breast, testicular, or ovarian cancers (Cohen, 2013).

e. Carefully remove patch from its protective covering by pulling off liner. Hold patch by edge without touching adhesive edges.

Touching only edges ensures that patch will adhere and that medication dose has not changed. Removing protective covering allows medication to be absorbed through skin.

f. Apply patch. Hold palm of one hand firmly over patch for 10 seconds. Make sure that it sticks well, especially around edges. Apply overlay if provided with patch.

Adequate adhesion prevents loss of patch, which results in decreased dose and effectiveness.

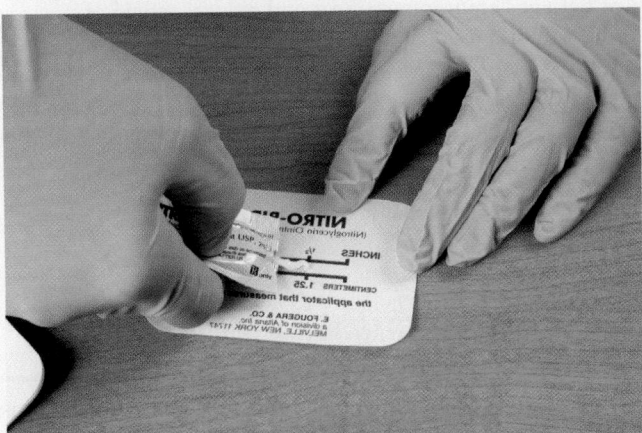

STEP 9c Ointment spread in inches over measuring guide.

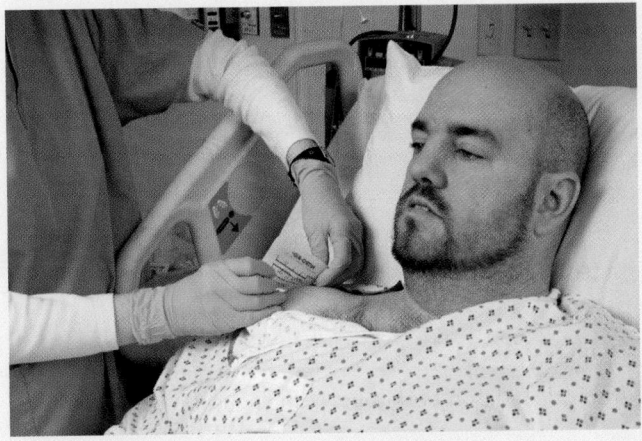

STEP 9e Nurse applies wrapper with medication to patient's skin.

STEP	RATIONALE

Clinical Decision Point *Never apply heat such as with a heating pad over a transdermal patch because this results in an increased rate of absorption with potentially serious adverse effects (Cohen, 2013; Lawton, 2013).*

g. Do not apply patch to previously used sites for at least 1 week.	Rotation of site reduces skin irritation from medication and adhesive (Lawton, 2013).
h. Instruct patient that transdermal patches are never to be cut in half; a change in dose would require prescription for new strength of transdermal medication.	Cutting transdermal patch in half would alter intended medication delivery of transdermal system, resulting in inadequate or altered drug levels.

Clinical Decision Point *It is recommended to have a daily "patch-free" interval of 10 to 12 hours because tolerance develops if patches are used 24 hours a day every day (Burchum and Rosenthal, 2016). Apply a new patch each morning, leave in place for 12 to 14 hours, and remove in the evening.*

i. Instruct patient to always remove old patch and clean skin before applying new one. Patients should not use alternative forms of medication when using patches. For example, patients should not apply nitroglycerin ointment in addition to patch unless specifically ordered to do so by their health care provider.	Use of patch with additional or alternative drug preparation can result in toxicity or other side effects.
11. Administer aerosol sprays (e.g., local anesthetic sprays).	
a. Shake container vigorously. Read container label for distance recommended to hold spray away from area, usually 15 to 30 cm (6 to 12 inches).	Mixing ensures delivery of fine, even spray. Proper distance ensures that fine spray hits skin surface. Holding container too close results in thin, watery distribution.
b. Ask patient to turn face away from spray or briefly cover face with towel while spraying neck or chest.	Prevents inhalation of spray.
c. Spray medication evenly over affected site (in some cases, time spray for a period of seconds).	Ensures that affected area of skin is covered with thin spray.
12. Apply suspension-based lotion.	
a. Shake container vigorously.	Mixes powder throughout liquid to form well-mixed suspension.
b. Apply small amount of lotion to small gauze dressing or pad and apply to skin by stroking evenly in direction of hair growth.	Method of application leaves protective film of powder on skin after water base of suspension dries. Technique prevents irritation to hair follicles.
c. Explain to patient that area will feel cool and dry.	Water evaporates to leave thin layer of powder.
13. Apply powder.	
a. Be sure that skin surface is thoroughly dry. With your nondominant hand, fully spread apart any skinfolds such as between toes or under axilla and dry with towel.	Minimizes caking and crusting of powder. Fully exposes skin surface for application.
b. If area of application is near face, ask patient to turn face away from powder or briefly cover face with towel.	Prevents inhalation of powder.
c. Dust skin site lightly with dispenser so area is covered with fine, thin layer of powder. *Option:* Cover skin area with dressing if ordered by health care provider.	Thin layer of powder has slight lubricating properties, which reduces friction and promotes drying (Burchum and Rosenthal, 2016).
14. Help patient to comfortable position, reapply gown, and cover with bed linen as desired.	Provides for patient's sense of well-being.
15. Dispose of soiled supplies in receptacle especially designated for such articles, remove and dispose of gloves, and perform hand hygiene.	Keeps patient's environment neat and reduces spread of infection and residual medication to others.

EVALUATION

1. Inspect condition of skin between applications.	Determines if skin condition is improving or verifies that skin is intact and not irritated.
2. Have patient keep diary of doses taken.	Confirms adherence to prescribed therapy.
3. Observe patient or family caregiver apply topical medication.	Return demonstration measures learning.

STEP	RATIONALE
4. Use Teach-Back: "I want to be sure I explained the action of the dose of medicine you are taking and the side effects of cortisone cream medication. In your own words, tell me how the drug works, your correct dose, and any side effects." Revise your instruction now or develop a plan for revised patient or family caregiver teaching if patient or family caregiver is not able to teach back correctly.	Determines patient's and family caregiver's level of understanding of instructional topic.

Unexpected Outcomes	Related Interventions
1. Skin site appears inflamed and edematous with blistering and oozing of fluid from lesions. These signs indicate subacute inflammation or eczema that can develop if skin lesions are getting worse.	• Hold medication. • Notify health care provider; alternative therapies may be needed.
2. Patient is unable to explain information about drug or does not administer as prescribed.	• Identify possible reasons for noncompliance and explore alternative approaches or options.

Recording and Reporting

- Record actual time that each drug was administered, type of agent applied, strength, and site of application in MAR immediately after administration, not before. Include initials or signature.
- Record patient's response to medication, patient teaching, and validation of patient's understanding on flow sheet or in nurses' notes in electronic health record (EHR) or chart.
- Describe condition of skin before each application on flow sheet or in nurses' notes in EHR or chart.
- Report adverse effects/patient response and/or withheld drugs to nurse in charge or health care provider. Depending on medication, immediate health care provider notification may be required.

Special Considerations
Teaching

- Instruct patient and family caregiver to (Cohen, 2013):
  - Not apply to irritated or damaged skin.
  - Not use heating pads, hot water bottle, or warm compresses over medication.
  - Only use a bandage or plastic wrap if instructed by a pharmacist.
  - Use medication exactly as prescribed.
  - Contact health care provider if medication comes in contact with eyes or other mucous membranes such as the mouth.
- Instruct patients to use only warm-water rinse without soap for cleaning inflamed skin.
- If a transdermal patch begins to peel off before the next dose is due, remove it, clean the skin, and apply a new patch to a different area rather than taping over the patch (ASHP, 2013a).

Gerontological

- Changes in the skin of an older-adult patient include increased fragility, wrinkling, dryness, flaking, and increased tendency to bruise. Be aware of these changes when applying topical medications to ensure proper application.

Home Care

- Instruct patient to wrap applicators, used patches, and similar materials and dispose of them into cardboard or plastic disposable containers. Careful disposal is necessary to ensure the safety of patient, other adults, pets, and children.

◆ **SKILL 21.4** **Administering Ophthalmic Medications**

▶ *Video Clip* **NSO** *Nursing Skills Online Administration of Nonparenteral Medications Module / Lesson 4*

Common eye (ophthalmic) medications are in the form of drops and ointments, including over-the-counter preparations such as artificial tears and vasoconstrictors. However, many patients receive prescribed ophthalmic drugs for eye conditions such as glaucoma and infection and following cataract extraction. In addition, there is a third type of delivery system, the intraocular disk. Medications delivered by disk resemble a contact lens; but the disk is placed in the conjunctival sac, not on the cornea, and it remains in place for up to 1 week.

The eye is the most sensitive organ to which you apply medications. The cornea is richly supplied with sensitive nerve fibers. Care must be taken to prevent instilling medication directly onto the cornea. The conjunctival sac is much less sensitive and thus a more appropriate site for medication instillation.

Any patient receiving topical eye medications should learn correct self-administration of the medication, especially patients with glaucoma, who must often undergo lifelong medication administration for control of their disease. You can easily instruct patients while administering medications. Family caregivers often administer eye medications when patients are unable to manipulate applicators (e.g., arthritis or neurological condition), immediately after eye surgery, and when a patient's vision is so impaired that it is difficult to assemble needed supplies and handle applicators correctly.

Delegation and Collaboration

The skill of administering ophthalmic medications cannot be delegated to nursing assistive personnel (NAP). The nurse instructs the NAP about:

- The specific potential side effects of medications and to report their occurrence.
- The potential for temporary burning or blurring of vision after administration of eye medications.

Equipment

- Appropriate medication (eyedrops with sterile eyedropper, ointment tube, medicated intraocular disk)

- Clean gloves
- Medication administration record (MAR) (electronic or printed)

Eyedrops/Ointment

- Cotton ball or tissue
- Wash basin filled with warm water and washcloth
- Eye patch and tape (*optional*)

STEP	RATIONALE

ASSESSMENT

1. Check accuracy and completeness of each MAR with health care provider's medication order. Check patient's name, drug name and dosage, route (one or both eyes), and time for administration. Clarify incomplete or unclear orders with health care provider before administration.

   The order sheet is the most reliable source and only legal record of medications that patient is to receive. Ensures that patient receives correct medications (Sulosaari et al., 2011). Handwritten MARs are a source of medication errors (Alassaad et al., 2013).

2. Review pertinent information related to medication, including action, purpose, normal dose and route, side effects, time of onset and peak action, and nursing implications.

   Allows you to anticipate effects of drug and observe patient's response.

3. Assess condition of external eye structures (see Chapter 6). This may be done just before drug instillation (if drainage is present, apply clean gloves).

   Provides baseline to determine if local response to medications occurs. Also indicates need to clean eye before drug application.

4. Determine whether patient has any symptoms of eye discomfort or visual impairment.

   Certain eye medications act to either lessen or increase these symptoms.

5. Assess patient's medical and medication history and history of allergies (including latex). List drug allergies on each page of the MAR and prominently display it on the patient's medical record per agency policy. When patient has allergy, provide allergy bracelet.

   Factors influence how certain drugs act. Reveals patient's need for and likely response to medication. Communication of allergies is essential for safe and effective care.

6. Assess patient's level of consciousness (LOC) and ability to follow directions.

   If patient becomes restless or combative during procedure, greater risk for accidental eye injury exists.

7. Assess patient's knowledge regarding drug therapy and desire to self-administer medication.

   Indicates need for health teaching. Motivation influences teaching approach.

8. Assess patient's ability to manipulate and hold dropper or ocular disk.

   Reflects patient's ability to learn to self-administer drug.

NURSING DIAGNOSES

- Deficient knowledge regarding drug and self-administration
- Impaired physical mobility

- Pain (acute or chronic)
- Readiness for enhanced self-health management

- Risk for injury

Related factors/Risk factors are individualized based on patient's condition or needs.

PLANNING

1. Expected outcomes following completion of procedure:
   - Patient experiences desired effect of medication.
   - Patient denies discomfort.
   - Patient experiences no side effects, and symptoms (e.g., irritation) are relieved.
   - Patient is able to discuss information about medication and technique correctly.
   - Patient demonstrates self-instillation of eyedrops.
2. Collect appropriate equipment and MAR.

Drug is administered correctly without injury to patient.
Drug is administered correctly without injury to patient.
Drug is distributed and absorbed properly.

Demonstrates learning.

Demonstrates learning.
Ensures time management and efficiency.

STEP	RATIONALE

IMPLEMENTATION

1. Perform hand hygiene and prepare medications for instillation. Check label of medication against MAR 2 times (see Skill 21.1). Preparation usually involves taking eyedrops out of refrigerator and rewarming to room temperature before administering to patient. Check expiration date on container.

Reduces transmission of infection. Warming eyedrops reduces eye irritation.

These are the first and second checks for accuracy. Process ensures that right patient receives right medication.

2. Take medication(s) to patient at correct time (see agency policy). Medications that require exact timing include stat, first-time or loading doses, and 1-time doses. Give time-critical scheduled medications (e.g., antibiotics, anticoagulants, insulin, anticonvulsants, immunosuppressive agents) at exact time ordered (no later than 30 minutes before or after scheduled dose). Give non–time-critical scheduled medications within a range of 1 or 2 hours of scheduled dose (ISMP, 2011). During administration, apply six rights of medication administration. Perform hand hygiene.

Hospitals must adopt medication administration policy and procedure for timing of medication administration that considers nature of the prescribed medication, specific clinical application, and patient needs (CMS, 2011; ISMP, 2011). Time-critical scheduled medications are those for which early or delayed administration of maintenance doses of greater than 30 minutes before or after the scheduled dose may cause harm or result in substantial suboptimal therapy or pharmacological effect. Non–time-critical medications are those for which early or delayed administration within a specified range of either 1 or 2 hours should not cause harm or result in substantial suboptimal therapy or pharmacological effect (CMS, 2011; ISMP, 2011).

3. Help patient to comfortable sitting position. Arrange supplies at bedside.

Ensures an organized procedure.

4. Identify patient using at least two identifiers (e.g., name and birthday or name and medical record number) according to agency policy. Compare identifiers with information on patient's MAR or medical record.

Ensures correct patient. Complies with The Joint Commission standards and improves patient safety (TJC, 2016).

5. At patient's bedside again compare MAR or computer printout with names of medications on medication labels and patient name. Ask patient if he or she has allergies.

This is the third check for accuracy and ensures that patient receives correct medication. Confirms patient's allergy history.

6. Explain procedure to patient and sensations to expect. Discuss purpose of each medication, action, and possible adverse effects. Allow patient to ask any questions about the drugs. Patients who self-instill medications may be allowed to give drops under nurse's supervision (check agency policy). Tell patients receiving eyedrops (mydriatics) that vision will be blurred temporarily and sensitivity to light may occur.

Helps patient be a participant in care, which minimizes anxiety. Patient has right to be informed, and patient's understanding of each medication improves adherence to drug therapy. Begins patient teaching regarding medications.

Clinical Decision Point *Instruct and reinforce that patient should not drive or operate machinery or perform any activity that requires clear vision until vision and sensitivity to light returns to normal.*

7. Instill eye medications.
   a. Apply clean gloves. Ask patient to lie supine or sit back in chair with head slightly hyperextended, looking up.

Position provides easy access to eye for medication instillation and minimizes drainage of medication into tear duct.

Clinical Decision Point *Do not hyperextend the neck of a patient with cervical spine injury.*

   b. If drainage or crusting is present along eyelid margins or inner canthus, gently wash away. Soak any dried crusts with warm, damp washcloth or cotton ball over eye for several minutes. Always wipe clean from inner to outer canthus (see illustration). Remove gloves and perform hand hygiene.

Soaking allows easy removal of crusts without applying pressure to eye. Cleaning from inner to outer canthus avoids entrance of microorganisms into lacrimal duct (Burchum and Rosenthal, 2016).

   c. Explain that there might be temporary burning sensation from drops.

Corneas are highly sensitive.

STEP	RATIONALE

d. Instill eyedrops.

(1) *Option:* Apply clean gloves if eye drainage present. Hold clean cotton ball or tissue in nondominant hand on patient's cheekbone just below lower eyelid.

Prevents transmission of infection. Cotton or tissue absorbs medication that escapes eye.

(2) With tissue or cotton ball resting below lower lid, gently press downward with thumb or forefinger against bony orbit, exposing conjunctival sac. Never press directly against patient's eyeball.

Prevents pressure and trauma to eyeball and prevents fingers from touching eye.

(3) Ask patient to look at ceiling. Rest dominant hand on patient's forehead; hold filled medication eyedropper approximately 1 to 2 cm (¼ to ½ inch) above conjunctival sac.

Action moves cornea up and away from conjunctival sac and reduces blink reflex. Prevents accidental contact of eyedropper with eye and reduces risk of injury and transfer of microorganisms to dropper (ophthalmic medications are sterile).

(4) Drop prescribed number of drops into conjunctival sac (see illustration).

Conjunctival sac normally holds 1 or 2 drops. Provides even distribution of medication across eye.

(5) If patient blinks or closes eye, causing drops to land on outer lid margins, repeat procedure.

Therapeutic effect of drug is obtained only when drops enter conjunctival sac.

(6) When administering drops that may cause systemic effects, apply gentle pressure to patient's nasolacrimal duct with clean tissue for 30 to 60 seconds over each eye, one at a time (see illustration). Avoid pressure directly against patient's eyeball.

Prevents overflow of medication into nasal and pharyngeal passages. Prevents absorption into systemic circulation (ASHP, 2013b).

(7) After instilling drops, ask patient to close eyes gently.

Helps distribute medication. Squinting or squeezing eyelids forces medication from conjunctival sac (ASHP, 2013b).

e. Instill ophthalmic ointment.

(1) *Option:* Apply clean gloves if eye drainage present. Holding applicator above lower lid margin, apply thin ribbon of ointment evenly along inner edge of lower eyelid on conjunctiva (see illustration) from inner to outer canthus.

Reduces transmission of infection. Distributes medication evenly across eye and lid margin.

(2) Have patient close eye and rub lid lightly in circular motion with cotton ball if not contraindicated. Avoid placing pressure directly against patient's eyeball.

Further distributes medication without traumatizing eye.

(3) If excess medication is on eyelid, gently wipe it from inner to outer canthus.

Promotes comfort and prevents trauma to eye.

(4) If patient needs an eye patch, apply clean one by placing it over affected eye so entire eye is covered. Tape securely without applying pressure to eye.

Clean eye patch reduces risk of infection.

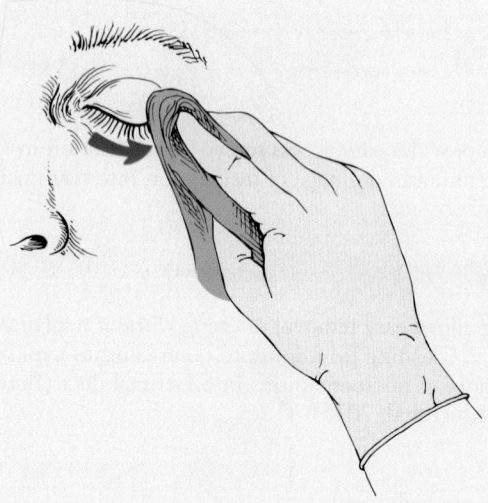

STEP 7b Clean eye, washing from inner to outer canthus before administering drops or ointment.

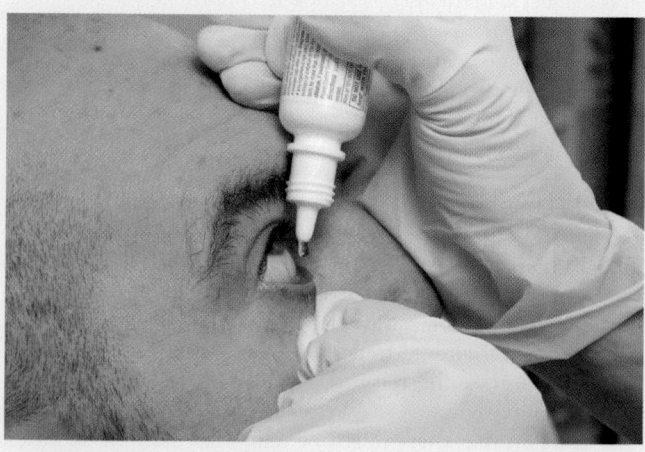

STEP 7d(4) Hold eyedropper over lower conjunctival sac.

STEP	RATIONALE

f. Insert intraocular disk.

   (1) Apply clean gloves. Open package containing disk. Gently press your fingertip against disk so it adheres to your finger. It may be necessary to moisten gloved finger with sterile saline. Position convex side of disk on your fingertip.

Allows you to inspect disk for damage or deformity.

   (2) With your other hand gently pull patient's lower eyelid away from eye. Ask patient to look up.

Prepares conjunctival sac for receiving medicated disk and moves sensitive cornea away.

   (3) Place disk in conjunctival sac so it floats on sclera between iris and lower eyelid (see illustration).

Ensures delivery of medication.

   (4) Pull patient's lower eyelid out and over disk (see illustration). You should not be able to see disk at this time. Repeat if you can see disk.

Ensures accurate medication delivery.

8. After administering eye medications, remove and dispose of gloves and soiled supplies; perform hand hygiene.

Reduces spread of microorganisms.

9. Remove intraocular disk.

  a. Perform hand hygiene and apply clean gloves. Gently pull downward on lower eyelid using your nondominant hand.

Exposes disk.

  b. Using forefinger and thumb of your dominant hand, pinch disk and lift it out of patient's eye (see illustration).

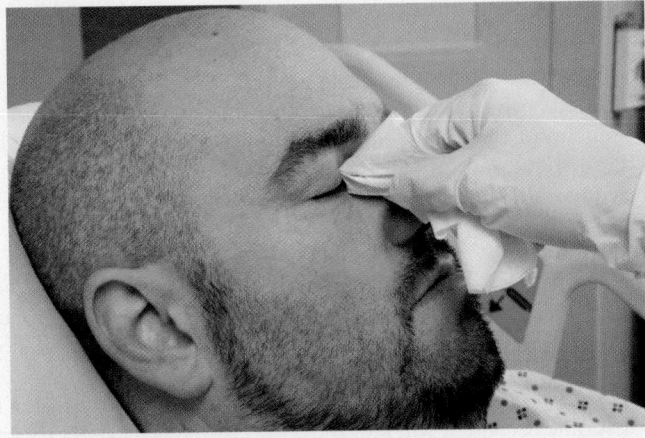

STEP 7d(6) Apply gentle pressure against nasolacrimal duct after giving eye medications.

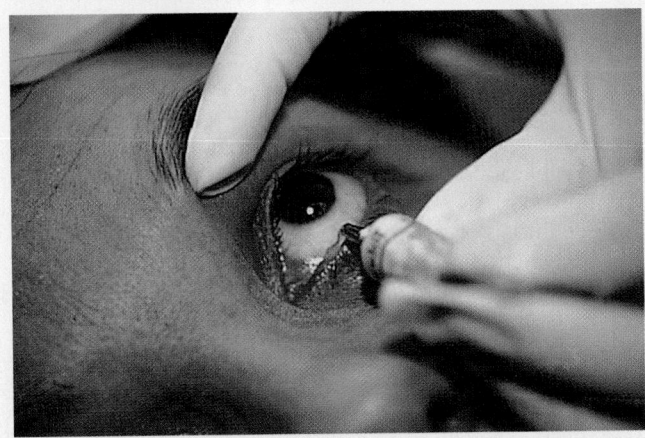

STEP 7e(1) Nurse applies ointment along inner edge of lower eyelid from inner to outer canthus.

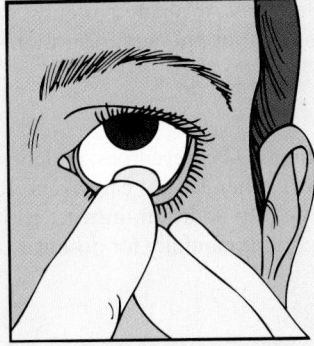

STEP 7f(3) Place intraocular disk in conjunctival sac between iris and lower eyelid.

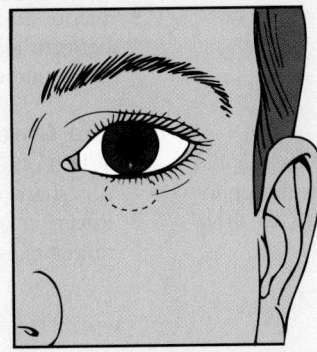

STEP 7f(4) Gently pull patient's lower eyelid over disk.

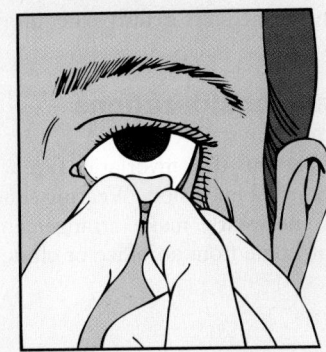

STEP 9b Carefully pinch disk to remove it from patient's eye.

STEP	RATIONALE

EVALUATION

1. Observe response to medication by assessing visual changes, asking if symptoms are relieved, and noting any side effects or discomfort felt.

2. Ask patient to discuss purpose of drug, action, side effects, and technique of administration.

3. **Use Teach-Back:** "I want to be sure I showed you how to insert the intraocular disk. Show me how to insert it into your left eye." Revise your instruction now or develop a plan for revised patient or family caregiver teaching if patient or family caregiver is not able to teach back correctly.

Evaluates effects of medication.

Determines patient's level of understanding.

Determines patient's and family caregiver's level of understanding of instructional topic.

Unexpected Outcomes	Related Interventions
1. Patient complains of burning or pain or experiences local side effects (e.g., headache, bloodshot eyes, local eye irritation). Drug concentration and patient's sensitivity both influence chances of side effects developing.	• Eyedrops may have been instilled onto cornea, or dropper touched surface of eye. • Notify health care provider for possible adjustment in medication type and dosage.
2. Patient experiences systemic effects from drops (e.g., increased heart rate and blood pressure from epinephrine, decreased heart rate and blood pressure from timolol).	• Notify health care provider immediately. • Remain with patient. Assess vital signs. • Withhold further doses.
3. Patient is unable to explain drug information or steps for taking eyedrops and/or has trouble manipulating dropper.	• Repeat instructions and include family caregiver as appropriate. Include return demonstration.

Recording and Reporting

• Record drug, concentration, dose or strength, number of drops, site of application (left, right, or both eyes), and time of administration on MAR immediately after administration, not before. Include initials or signature.

• Record patient teaching and validation of patient's understanding on flow sheet or in nurses' notes in electronic health record (EHR) or chart.

• Record objective data related to tissues involved (e.g., redness, drainage, irritation), any subjective data (e.g., pain, itching, altered vision), and patient's response to medications. Note any side effects experienced on flow sheet or in nurses' notes in EHR or chart.

• Report adverse effects/patient response and/or withheld drugs to nurse in charge or health care provider. Depending on medication, immediate health care provider notification may be required.

Special Considerations
Teaching

• Warn patients that mydriatics (agent used to dilate the pupils) temporarily blur vision. Wearing sunglasses reduces photophobia. If necessary, make arrangements for someone to drive patient home from an office or clinic visit.

• Patients who receive medications that paralyze the ciliary muscles of the eye (e.g., scopolamine, atropine, and cycloplegics) should not drive or attempt to perform any activity that requires acute vision after receiving medication.

Pediatric

• Infants often clench the eyes tightly to avoid eyedrops. Place the drops at the nasal corner where the lids meet with the infant supine. When the infant opens the eye, the medication will flow into it.

• If the eye ointment is to be given once a day, administer at bedtime because it will blur the child's vision (Hockenberry and Wilson, 2015).

Gerontological

• Before discharging an older adult, evaluate patient's ability to perform all the necessary steps for the administration of eyedrops and ointments.

Home Care

• When using over-the-counter (OTC) eyedrops, patients should not share medications with other family caregivers. Risk for infection transmission is high. In addition, instruct patients to follow manufacturer instructions carefully for dosing.

◆ SKILL 21.5 Administering Ear Medications

Ear (otic) medications are usually in a solution and instilled by drops. When administering ear medications, be aware of certain safety precautions. Internal ear structures are very sensitive to temperature extremes; administer eardrops at room temperature. Instilling cold drops can cause vertigo (severe dizziness) or nausea and debilitate a patient for several minutes. Although structures of the outer ear are not sterile, use sterile drops and solutions in case the eardrum is ruptured. A final safety precaution is to avoid forcing any solution into the ear. Do not occlude the ear canal with a medicine dropper because this can cause pressure within the canal during instillation and subsequent injury to the eardrum. If you follow these precautions, instillation of eardrops is a safe and effective therapy.

Equipment

- Medication administration record (MAR) (electronic or printed)
- Medication bottle with dropper
- Cotton-tipped applicator, cotton balls
- Clean gloves if drainage is present

Delegation and Collaboration

The skill of administering ear medications cannot be delegated to nursing assistive personnel (NAP). The nurse instructs the NAP about:

- Potential side effects of medications and to report their occurrence.
- The potential for dizziness or irritation after administration of ear medications.

STEP	RATIONALE

ASSESSMENT

1. Check accuracy and completeness of each MAR with health care provider's medication order. Check patient's name, drug name and dosage, route, and time for administration. Clarify incomplete or unclear orders with health care provider before administration.

   The order sheet is the most reliable source and only legal record of medications that patient is to receive. Ensures that patient receives correct medications (Sulosaari et al., 2011). Handwritten MARs are a source of medication errors (Alassaad et al., 2013).

2. Review pertinent information related to medication, including action, purpose, normal dose and route (one or both ears), side effects, time of onset and peak action, and nursing implications.

   Allows you to anticipate effects of drug and observe patient's response.

3. Assess condition of external ear structures (see Chapter 6). This may be done just before drug instillation (if drainage is present, apply clean gloves).

   Provides baseline to determine if local response to medications occurs. Also indicates need to clean ear before drug application.

4. Determine whether patient has any symptoms of ear discomfort or hearing impairment.

   Certain ear medications act to either lessen or increase these symptoms. Occlusion of external ear canal by swelling, drainage, or cerumen can impair hearing acuity and cause pain.

5. Assess patient's medical and medication history and history of allergies (including latex), and medication history. List drug allergies on each page of the MAR and prominently display it on the patient's medical record per agency policy. When patient has allergy, provide allergy bracelet.

   Factors influence how certain drugs act. Reveals patient's need for medication.
   Communication of allergies is essential for safe and effective care.

6. Assess patient's level of consciousness (LOC) and ability to follow directions.

   If patient becomes restless or combative during procedure, greater risk for accidental ear injury exists.

7. Assess patient's knowledge regarding drug therapy and desire to self-administer medication.

   Indicates need for health teaching. Motivation influences teaching approach.

8. Assess patient's ability to manipulate and hold ear dropper.

   Reflects patient's ability to learn to self-administer drug.

NURSING DIAGNOSES

- Deficient knowledge regarding drug and self-administration
- Impaired physical mobility
- Pain (acute or chronic)
- Readiness for enhanced self-health management
- Risk for injury

Related factors/Risk factors are individualized based on patient's condition or needs.

STEP	RATIONALE

PLANNING

1. Expected outcomes following completion of procedure:
   - Patient experiences desired effect of medication.
   - Patient denies discomfort.
   - Patient experiences no side effects, and symptoms (e.g., dizziness, ear irritation) are relieved.
   - Patient is able to discuss information about medication and technique correctly.
   - Patient demonstrates self-instillation of eardrops.
2. Collect appropriate equipment and MAR.

Drug is administered correctly without injury to patient.
Drug is administered correctly without injury to patient.
Drug is distributed and absorbed properly.

Demonstrates learning.

Demonstrates learning.
Ensures time management and efficiency.

IMPLEMENTATION

1. Perform hand hygiene and prepare medications for instillation. Check label of medication against MAR 2 times (see Skill 21.1). Preparation usually involves taking eardrops out of refrigerator and rewarming to room temperature before administering to patient. Check expiration date on container.

   Hand hygiene reduces transmission of infection. Ear structures are very sensitive to temperature extremes. Cold may cause vertigo and nausea.
   These are the first and second checks for accuracy. Process ensures that right patient receives right medication.

2. Take medication(s) to patient at correct time (see agency policy). Medications that require exact timing include stat, first-time or loading doses, and 1-time doses. Give time-critical scheduled medications (e.g., antibiotics, anticoagulants, insulin, anticonvulsants, immunosuppressive agents) at exact time ordered (no later than 30 minutes before or after scheduled dose). Give non–time-critical scheduled medications within a range of 1 or 2 hours of scheduled dose (ISMP, 2011). During administration apply six rights of medication administration. Perform hand hygiene.

   Hospitals must adopt medication administration policy and procedure for timing of medication administration that considers nature of the prescribed medication, specific clinical application, and patient needs (CMS, 2011; ISMP, 2011). Time-critical scheduled medications are those for which early or delayed administration of maintenance doses of greater than 30 minutes before or after the scheduled dose may cause harm or result in substantial suboptimal therapy or pharmacological effect. Non–time-critical medications are those for which early or delayed administration within a specified range of either 1 or 2 hours should not cause harm or result in substantial suboptimal therapy or pharmacological effect (CMS, 2011; ISMP, 2011).

3. Arrange supplies at bedside.
4. Identify patient using at least two identifiers (e.g., name and birthday or name and medical record number) according to agency policy. Compare identifiers with information on patient's MAR or medical record.

   Ensures correct patient. Complies with The Joint Commission standards and improves patient safety (TJC, 2016).

5. At patient's bedside again compare MAR or computer printout with names of medications on medication labels and patient name. Ask patient if he or she has allergies.

   This is the third check for accuracy and ensures that patient receives correct medication. Confirms patient's allergy history.

6. Explain procedure to patient and sensations to expect. Discuss purpose of each medication, action, and possible adverse effects. Allow patient to ask any questions about the drugs. Patients who self-instill medications may be allowed to give drops under nurse's supervision (check agency policy).

   Helps patient be a participant in care, which minimizes anxiety. Patient has right to be informed, and patient's understanding of each medication improves adherence to drug therapy. Begins patient teaching regarding medications.

7. Position patient on side (if not contraindicated) with ear to be treated facing up, or patient may sit in chair or at bedside. Stabilize patient's head with his or her own hand. *Option:* Apply clean gloves if ear drainage present.

   Facilitates distribution of medication into ear.

STEP	RATIONALE

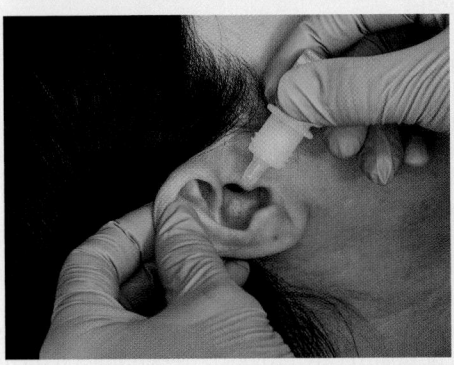
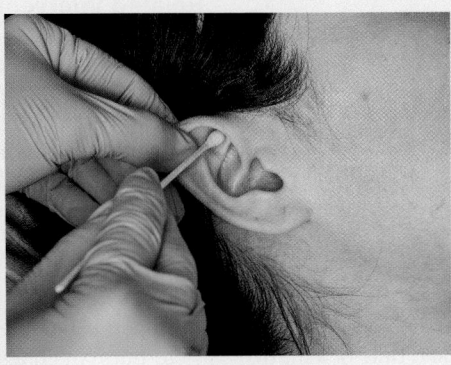
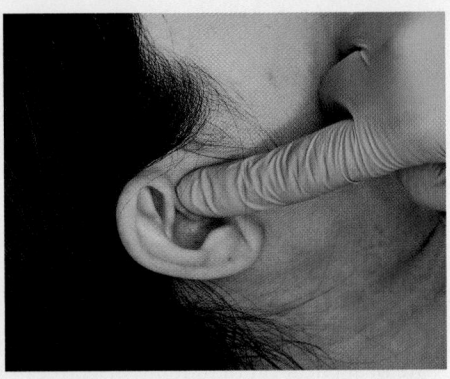

STEP 8 Pull pinna up and back for adults and children older than 3 years.

STEP 9 Always clean only outer canal. Do not push cerumen or secretions into ear.

STEP 11 Nurse applies gentle pressure to tragus of ear after instilling drops.

8. Straighten ear canal by pulling pinna up and back to 10 o'clock position (adult or child older than age 3) (see illustration) or down and back to 6 to 9 o'clock position (child under age 3).

   Straightening ear canal provides direct access to deeper ear structures. Anatomical differences in younger children and infants necessitate different methods of positioning canal (Hockenberry and Wilson, 2015).

9. If cerumen or drainage occludes outermost part of ear canal, wipe out gently with cotton-tipped applicator (see illustration). Take care not to force cerumen into canal.

   Cerumen and drainage harbor microorganisms and can block distribution of medication into canal. Occlusion blocks sound transmission.

10. Instill prescribed drops holding dropper 1 cm (½ inch) above ear canal.

    Avoiding contact with external ear canal prevents contamination of dropper, which could contaminate medication in container.

11. Ask patient to remain in side-lying position for a few minutes. Apply gentle massage or pressure to tragus of ear with finger (see illustration).

    Allows complete distribution of medication. Pressure and massage move medication inward.

12. If ordered, gently insert part of cotton ball into outermost part of canal. Do not press cotton into canal.

    Prevents escape of medication when patient sits or stands.

13. Remove cotton after 15 minutes. Help patient to comfortable position after drops are absorbed.

    Allows time for drug distribution and absorption.

14. Dispose of soiled supplies in proper receptacle, remove and dispose of gloves, and perform hand hygiene.

    Reduces spread of microorganisms.

EVALUATION

1. Observe response to medication by assessing hearing changes, asking if symptoms are relieved, and noting any side effects or discomfort felt.

   Evaluates effects of medication.

2. Ask patient to discuss purpose of drug, action, side effects, and technique of administration.

   Determines patient's level of understanding.

3. **Use Teach-Back:** "I want to be sure I clearly showed you how to administer eardrops. Let's take this time we have, show me how to place eardrops in your right ear." Revise your instruction now or develop a plan for revised patient or family caregiver teaching if patient or family caregiver is not able to teach back correctly.

   Determines patient's and family caregiver's level of understanding of instructional topic.

STEP	RATIONALE

Unexpected Outcomes

Ear canal remains inflamed, swollen, tender to palpation. Drainage is present.

Patient's hearing acuity does not improve.

Related Interventions

- Hold next dose.
- Notify health care provider for possible adjustment in medication type and dosage.
- Notify health care provider.
- Cerumen may be impacted, requiring ear irrigation.

Recording and Reporting

- Record drug, concentration, dose or strength, number of drops, site of application (left, right, or both ears), and time of administration on MAR immediately after administration, not before. Include initials or signature.
- Record patient teaching and validation of patient's understanding on flow sheet or in nurses' notes in electronic health record (EHR) or chart.
- Record objective data related to tissues involved (e.g., drainage, tenderness, irritation), any subjective data (e.g., ear pain, ringing in ears, change in hearing acuity), and patient's response

to medications. Note any side effects experienced in nurses' notes in EHR or chart.

- Report adverse effects/patient response and/or withheld drugs to nurse in charge or health care provider. Depending on medication, immediate health care provider notification may be required.

Pediatric

- Insert cotton pledgets loosely into ear canal to prevent medication from flowing out. To prevent cotton from absorbing medication, premoisten it with a few drops of medication (Hockenberry and Wilson, 2015).

◆ SKILL 21.6   Administering Nasal Instillations

Patients with nasal sinus problems may receive drugs by spray, drops, or tampons. The most commonly administered form of nasal instillation is a decongestant spray or drops used to relieve sinus congestion and cold symptoms. Many over-the-counter (OTC) nasal preparations contain sympathomimetic drugs (e.g., Neo-Synephrine). These drugs are relatively safe when administered nasally because only small doses are needed. However, the drugs can enter the systemic circulation by way of the nasal mucosa or by the gastrointestinal tract if an excess amount is swallowed, causing restlessness, nervousness, tremors, or insomnia in some patients. Long-term use of decongestant nasal spray can actually worsen nasal congestion because of a rebound effect. Nasal sprays are easy for a patient to self-administer. Health care providers treat severe nosebleeds by placing nasal packing or tampons, which are treated with epinephrine to slow bleeding.

Delegation and Collaboration

The skill of administering nasal instillations cannot be delegated to nursing assistive personnel (NAP). The nurse directs the NAP about:

- Potential side effects of medications and to report their occurrence to the nurse.
- Reporting any bloody nasal drainage to the nurse.

Equipment

- Prepared medication with clean dropper or spray container
- Facial tissue
- Small pillow (*optional*)
- Washcloth (*optional*)
- Clean gloves
- Medication administration record (MAR) (electronic or printed)

STEP	RATIONALE

ASSESSMENT

1. Check accuracy and completeness of each MAR with health care provider's medication order. Check patient's name, drug name and dosage, route (which sinus), and time for administration. Clarify incomplete or unclear orders with health care provider before administration.

2. Review pertinent information related to medication, including action, purpose, normal dose and route, side effects, time of onset and peak action, and nursing implications.

The order sheet is the most reliable source and only legal record of medications that patient is to receive. Ensures that patient receives the correct medications (Sulosaari et al., 2011). Handwritten MARs are a source of medication errors (Alassaad et al., 2013).

Allows you to anticipate effects of drug and observe patient's response.

STEP	RATIONALE
3. Assess patient's medical history (e.g., hypertension, heart disease, diabetes, and hyperthyroidism), medication history, and history of allergies. List drug allergies on each page of the MAR and prominently display it on the patient's medical record per agency policy. When patient has allergy, provide allergy bracelet.	These conditions contraindicate use of decongestants that stimulate central nervous system. Communication of allergies is essential for safe and effective care.
4. Perform hand hygiene. Use penlight and inspect condition of nose and sinuses (see Chapter 6). Palpate sinuses for pain or tenderness. Note type of drainage if present.	Provides baseline to monitor effects of medication. Presence of discharge interferes with drug absorption. Clear nasal discharge indicates sinus problem. Yellow or greenish discharge indicates infection.
5. Assess patient's knowledge regarding use of nasal instillations, technique for instillation, and willingness to learn self-administration.	Requires health teaching regarding use of drugs. Motivation influences teaching approach.

NURSING DIAGNOSES

- Deficient knowledge regarding drug action and purpose
- Pain (acute or chronic)
- Readiness for enhanced self-health management
- Risk for injury

Related factors/Risk factors are individualized based on patient's condition or needs.

PLANNING

1. Expected outcomes following completion of procedure:	
• Patient is able to breathe without difficulty through nose.	Nasal congestion has been relieved.
• Patient's nasal sinuses are clear, moist, pink, and without drainage after repeated instillations (applies to antiinfective medications).	Inflammation of mucosa has been relieved.
• Patient is able to explain purpose of medication and administers nasal instillations correctly.	Feedback reflects patient's learning.
2. Collect appropriate equipment and MAR.	Ensures time management and efficiency.

IMPLEMENTATION

1. Perform hand hygiene and prepare medications for instillation. Check label of medication against MAR 2 times (see Skill 21.1). Preparation usually involves taking nasal drops or sprays out of storage and into patient's room. Check expiration date on container.	*These are the first and second checks for accuracy.* Process ensures that right patient receives right medication.
2. Take medication(s) to patient at correct time (see agency policy). Medications that require exact timing include stat, first-time or loading doses, and 1-time doses. Give time-critical scheduled medications (e.g., antibiotics, anticoagulants, insulin, anticonvulsants, immunosuppressive agents) at exact time ordered (no later than 30 minutes before or after scheduled dose). Give non–time-critical scheduled medications within a range of 1 or 2 hours of scheduled dose (ISMP, 2011). During administration, apply six rights of medication administration. Perform hand hygiene.	Hospitals must adopt medication administration policy and procedure for timing of medication administration that considers nature of the prescribed medication, specific clinical application, and patient needs (CMS, 2011; ISMP, 2011). Time-critical scheduled medications are those for which early or delayed administration of maintenance doses of greater than 30 minutes before or after the scheduled dose may cause harm or result in substantial suboptimal therapy or pharmacological effect. Non–time-critical medications are those for which early or delayed administration within a specified range of either 1 or 2 hours should not cause harm or result in substantial suboptimal therapy or pharmacological effect (CMS, 2011; ISMP, 2011).
3. Identify patient using at least two identifiers (e.g., name and birthday or name and medical record number) according to agency policy. Compare identifiers with information on patient's MAR or medical record.	Ensures correct patient. Complies with The Joint Commission standards and improves patient safety (TJC, 2016).
4. At patient's bedside again compare MAR or computer printout with names of medications on medication labels and patient name. Ask patient if he or she has allergies.	*This is the third check for accuracy* and ensures that patient receives correct medication. Confirms patient's allergy history.

STEP	RATIONALE

5. Explain procedure to patient and sensations to expect. Discuss purpose of each medication, action, and possible adverse effects. Allow patient to ask any questions about drugs. Patients who self-instill medications may be allowed to give drops under nurse's supervision (check agency policy). Tell patients receiving nasal instillation that they may experience burning or stinging of mucosa or choking sensation as medication trickles into throat.

Helps patient be a participant in care, which minimizes anxiety. Patient has right to be informed, and patient's understanding of each medication improves adherence to drug therapy. Begins patient teaching regarding medications.

6. Arrange supplies and medications at bedside. Apply clean gloves (if drainage is present).

Reduces spread of microorganisms; ensures smooth, orderly procedure.

7. Gently roll or shake container. Instruct patient to clear or blow nose gently unless contraindicated (e.g., risk of increased intracranial pressure or nosebleed).

Ensures distribution of medication. Allows medication to reach sinuses.

8. Administer nose drops.
   a. Help patient to supine position and position head properly (ASHP, 2013c).

   Proper positioning provides access to specific nasal passages.

      (1) For access to posterior pharynx, tilt patient's head backward.
      (2) For access to ethmoid or sphenoid sinus, tilt head back over edge of bed or place small pillow under patient's shoulder and tilt head back (see illustration).
      (3) For access to frontal and maxillary sinus, tilt head back over edge of bed or pillow with head turned toward side to be treated (see illustration).

   Position allows medication to drain into affected sinus.

   b. Support patient's head with nondominant hand.

   Prevents straining neck muscles.

   c. Instruct patient to breathe through mouth.

   Mouth breathing reduces chance of aspirating nasal drops into trachea and lungs.

   d. Hold dropper 1 cm (½ inch) above nares and instill prescribed number of drops toward midline of ethmoid bone.

   Avoids contamination of dropper. Instilling toward ethmoid bone facilitates distribution of medication over nasal mucosa.

   e. Have patient remain in supine position 5 minutes.

   Prevents premature loss of medication through nares.

   f. Offer facial tissue to blot runny nose but caution patient against blowing nose for several minutes.

   Provides comfort but allows for absorption of medication.

9. Administer nasal spray.
   a. Help patient into upright position with head tilted slightly forward.

   Proper positioning permits medication spray to reach nasal passages.

   b. Instruct or assist patient to insert tip of nasal spray into appropriate nares and occlude other nostril with finger (see illustration). Point spray tip toward side and away from center of nose (ASHP, 2013d).

   Allows for proper administration of medication.

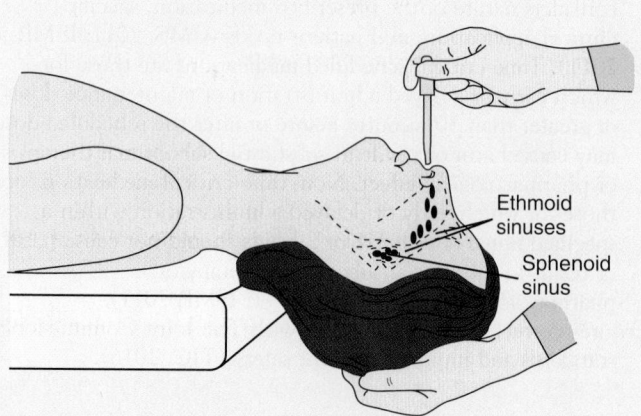

STEP 8a(2) Position for instilling nose drops into ethmoid or sphenoid sinus.

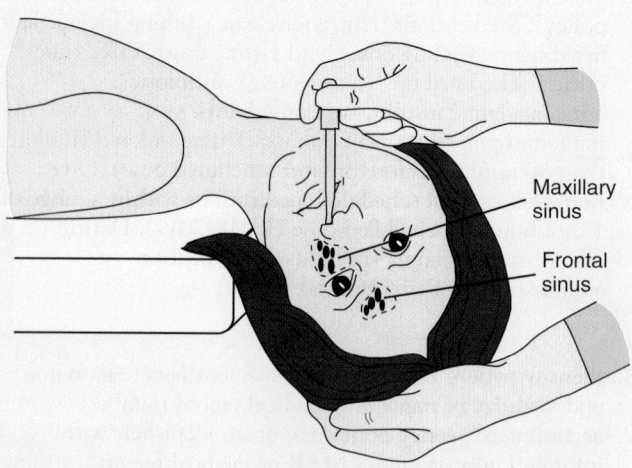

STEP 8a(3) Position for instilling nose drops into frontal and maxillary sinus.

STEP	RATIONALE

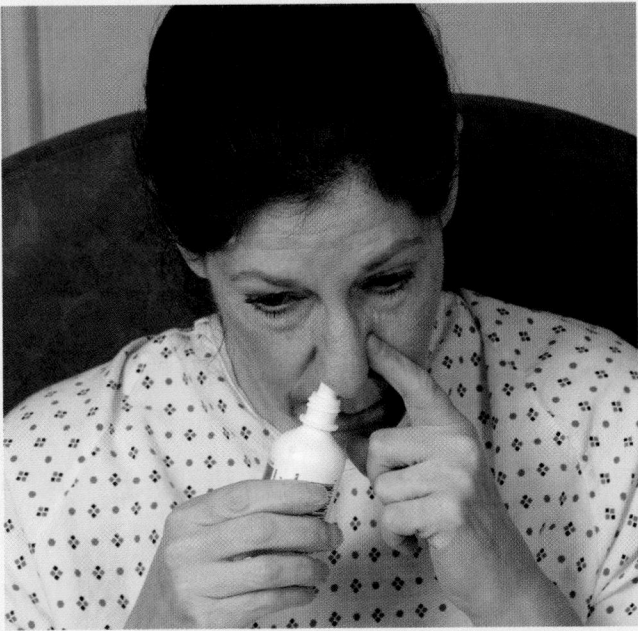

STEP 9b Occlude other nostril before self-administering nasal spray.

c. Have patient spray medication into nose while inhaling. Help him or her remove nozzle from nose and instruct to breathe out through mouth.

Allows for proper administration and distribution of nasal medication as high into nasal passages as possible.

d. Offer facial tissue to blot runny nose but caution patient against blowing nose for several minutes.

Provides comfort but allows for absorption of medication.

Clinical Decision Point *Some medications are designed for one spray per dose. Examples include calcitonin, desmopressin, and sumatriptan. It is essential to ensure that the patient understands the correct number of sprays to use per dose to prevent overdosing.*

10. Help patient to a comfortable position after medication is absorbed.

Restores comfort.

11. Dispose of soiled supplies, remove and dispose of gloves, and perform hand hygiene.

Reduces spread of microorganisms.

EVALUATION

1. Observe patient for onset of side effects 15 to 30 minutes after administration.

Drugs absorbed through mucosa can cause systemic reaction.

2. Ask if patient is able to breathe through nose after decongestant administration. May be necessary to have patient occlude one nostril at a time and breathe deeply.

Determines effectiveness of decongestant medication.

3. Reinspect condition of nasal passages between instillations.

Condition of mucosa reveals response to medication.

4. Ask patient to describe risks of overuse of decongestants and methods for administration.

Feedback ensures that patient can self-administer drugs properly.

5. Have patient demonstrate self-medication.

Feedback demonstrates learning.

6. **Use Teach-Back:** "I want to be sure I explained the importance to not overuse your nasal spray. Explain to me why it is important not to overuse nasal sprays." Revise your instruction now or develop a plan for revised patient or family caregiver teaching if patient or family caregiver is not able to teach back correctly.

Determines patient's and family caregiver's level of understanding of instructional topic.

STEP	RATIONALE

Unexpected Outcomes

1. Patient is unable to breathe easily through nasal passages. Mucosa appears swollen, and congestion is unrelieved, possibly because of rebound effect.
2. Nasal mucosa remains inflamed and tender, with discharge from nares.
3. Patient complains of sinus headache. Sinuses remain congested.

Related Interventions

- Stop medication use.
- Notify health care provider and consider alternative therapy.

- Consider alternative therapy.
- Consider alternative therapy.

Recording and Reporting

- Record drug name, concentration, number of drops, nares into which drug was instilled, and actual time of administration on MAR immediately after administration, not before. Include initials or signature.
- Record patient's response to medication, patient teaching, and validation of patient's understanding on flow sheet or in nurses' notes in electronic health record (EHR) or chart.
- Report any unusual systemic or adverse effects/patient response and/or withheld drugs to nurse in charge or health care provider.

Special Considerations
Teaching

- Instruct patients that each family caregiver should have a different dropper or spray applicator. Instruct patients to wash or rinse applicators after each use.

- Use OTC nasal sprays or nose drops for only one illness; bottles easily become contaminated with bacteria.
- Overuse of nasal sprays and drops can cause rebound sinus congestion, resulting in sinus pain and headache.

Pediatric

- Infants are nose breathers, and the possible congestion caused by nasal medications may inhibit their sucking. Administer nose drops if ordered 20 to 30 minutes before feedings (Hockenberry and Wilson, 2015).

◆ SKILL 21.7 Using Metered-Dose Inhalers (MDIs)

NSO *Nursing Skills Online Administration of Nonparenteral Medications Module / Lesson 6*

Medications administered with handheld inhalers are dispersed through an aerosol spray, mist, or powder that penetrates the airways. Pressurized metered-dose inhalers (pMDIs), breath-actuated metered-dose inhalers (BAIs), and dry powder inhalers (DPIs) deliver medications that produce local effects such as bronchodilation. Some of these medications are absorbed rapidly through the pulmonary circulation and create systemic side effects (e.g., albuterol may cause palpitations, tremors, and tachycardia). Patients who receive drugs by inhalation frequently suffer from asthma and chronic respiratory disease. Drugs administered by inhalation provide control of airway hyperactivity or bronchial constriction. Because patients depend on these medications for disease control, patient education is vital for correct use of inhalers and to ensure effectiveness of inhaled medications (Lareau and Hodder, 2012).

An MDI is a small, handheld device that disperses medication into the airways through an aerosol spray or mist by activation of a propellant. Dosing is usually achieved with 1 or 2 puffs. DPIs deliver inhaled medication in a fine powder formulation to the respiratory tract (see Procedural Guideline 21.1). The deeper passages of the respiratory tract provide a large surface area for drug absorption, and the alveolar-capillary network absorbs medication rapidly.

An MDI delivers a measured dose of the drug with each push of a canister. Approximately 5 to 10 lbs of pressure is needed to activate the aerosol. This is difficult for some older patients because hand strength diminishes with age. Because use of an MDI requires coordination during the breathing cycle, many patients spray only the back of their throats and fail to receive a full dose. The inhaler must be depressed to expel medication just as the patient inhales. This ensures that medication reaches the lower airways. A patient with poor coordination may need to use a spacer device or a BAI to administer the medication properly. A spacer device decreases the amount of medication deposited into the oropharyngeal mucosa. Some spacers have a one-way valve that activates on inhalation, thereby removing the need for good hand-breath coordination (Burchum and Rosenthal, 2016). Box 21.4 summarizes common problems that occur when using an inhaler.

Delegation and Collaboration

The skill of administering MDIs cannot be delegated to nursing assistive personnel (NAP). The nurse instructs the NAP about:

- Potential side effects of medications and to report their occurrence to the nurse.
- Reporting breathing difficulty (e.g., paroxysmal or sustained coughing, audible wheezing) to the nurse.

Equipment

- Inhaler device with medication canister (MDI or DPI) (Fig. 21.2A–C)
- Spacer device such as AeroChamber or InspirEase (*optional*)
- Facial tissues (*optional*)
- Stethoscope
- Medication administration record (MAR) (electronic or printed)
- Peak flowmeter (*optional*)

BOX 21.4

Common Problems in Using an Inhaler

- *Not taking the medication as prescribed:* Taking either too much or too little.
- *Incorrect activation:* This usually occurs through pressing the canister *before* taking a breath. These actions should be done simultaneously so the drug can be carried down to the lungs with the breath.
- *Forgetting to shake the inhaler:* The drug is in a suspension; therefore particles may settle. If the inhaler is not shaken, it may not deliver the correct dose of the drug.
- *Not waiting long enough between puffs:* A delay between puffs is needed before taking a second puff; otherwise an incorrect dose may be delivered, or the drug may not penetrate into the lungs.
- *Failure to clean the valve:* Particles may jam the valve in the mouthpiece unless it is cleaned occasionally. This is a frequent cause of failure to get 200 puffs from one inhaler.
- *Failure to observe whether the inhaler is actually releasing a spray:* If it is not, this should be checked with the pharmacist.
- *Failure to recognize when the canister is empty:* This occurs when the metered-dose inhaler has no built-in dose counter or instructions in dose counting.

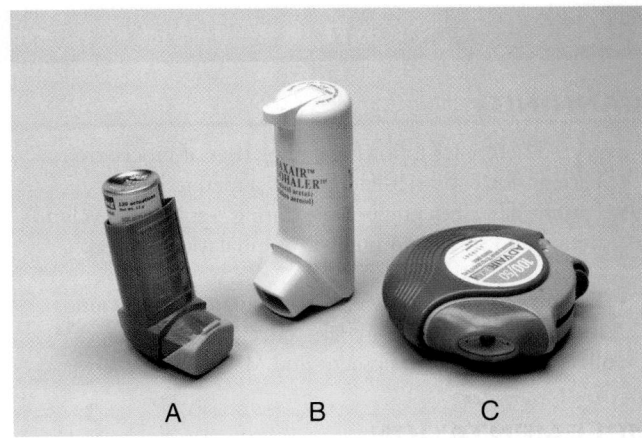

FIG 21.2 Types of inhalers. **A,** Metered-dose inhaler (MDI). **B,** Breath-actuated inhaler (BAI). **C,** Dry powder inhaler (DPI).

STEP	RATIONALE

ASSESSMENT

1. Check accuracy and completeness of each MAR with health care provider's medication order. Check patient's name, drug name and dosage, route, and time for administration. Clarify incomplete or unclear orders with health care provider before administration.	The order sheet is the most reliable source and only legal record of medications that patient is to receive. Ensures that patient receives correct medications (Sulosaari et al., 2011). Handwritten MARs are a source of medication errors (Alassaad et al., 2013).
2. Review pertinent information related to medication, including action, purpose, normal dose and route, side effects, time of onset and peak action, and nursing implications.	Allows you to anticipate effects of drug and observe patient's response.
3. Assess patient's medical and medication history and history of allergies. List drug allergies on each page of the MAR and prominently display it on the patient's medical record per agency policy. When patient has allergy, provide allergy bracelet.	Factors influence how certain drugs act. Reveals patient's need for medication. Communication of allergies is essential for safe and effective care.
4. Assess respiratory pattern and auscultate breath sounds (see Chapter 6). Also assess exercise tolerance; does patient develop shortness of breath easily?	Establishes baseline of airway status for comparison during and after treatment.
5. Assess patient's ability to hold, manipulate, and depress canister and inhaler.	Any impairment of grasp or presence of hand tremors interferes with patient's ability to depress canister within inhaler. Spacer device is often necessary.
6. If patient was previously instructed in self-administration, have him or her demonstrate how to use the device.	Often patients who have adequate understanding of how to use an inhaler forget the procedure. Ongoing assessment of inhaler technique identifies areas for further education and reinforcement (Ari, 2015).
7. Assess patient's readiness and ability to learn (e.g., asks questions about medication; is alert; participates in own care; is not fatigued, in pain, or in respiratory distress).	One-on-one patient assessment prepares patient for self-management and greater adherence to inhaler use (Ari, 2015). In some situations mental or physical limitations affect patient's ability to learn and methods used for instruction.
8. Assess patient's knowledge and understanding of disease and purpose and action of prescribed medications.	Knowledge of disease is essential for patient to realistically understand use of inhaler.

NURSING DIAGNOSES

- Activity intolerance
- Anxiety
- Deficient knowledge regarding use of MDI

- Impaired gas exchange
- Ineffective breathing pattern
- Readiness for enhanced self-health management

- Risk for injury

Related factors/Risk factors are individualized based on patient's condition or needs.

STEP	RATIONALE

PLANNING

1. Expected outcomes following completion of procedure:
  - Patient correctly self-administers a metered dose.
  - Patient describes proper time during respiratory cycle to inhale and spray and number of inhalations for each administration.
  - Patient's breathing pattern improves, and lung sounds indicate that airways are less restrictive.

2. Collect appropriate equipment and MAR.

Demonstrates learning.
Demonstrates learning and ensures correct administration of medication.

Demonstrates therapeutic effect of medication in improving gas exchange.
Ensures time management and efficiency.

IMPLEMENTATION

1. Perform hand hygiene and prepare medications for inhalation. Check label of medication against MAR 2 times (see Skill 21.1). Preparation usually involves taking inhaler device out of storage and into patient's room. Check expiration date on container.

These are the first and second checks for accuracy. Process ensures that right patient receives right medication.

2. Take medication(s) to patient at correct time (see agency policy). Medications that require exact timing include stat, first-time or loading doses, and 1-time doses. Give time-critical scheduled medications (e.g., antibiotics, anticoagulants, insulin, anticonvulsants, immunosuppressive agents) at exact time ordered (no later than 30 minutes before or after scheduled dose). Give non–time-critical scheduled medications within a range of 1 or 2 hours of scheduled dose (ISMP, 2011). During administration apply six rights of medication administration. Perform hand hygiene.

Hospitals must adopt medication administration policy and procedure for timing of medication administration that considers nature of the prescribed medication, specific clinical application, and patient needs (CMS, 2011; ISMP, 2011). Time-critical scheduled medications are those for which early or delayed administration of maintenance doses of greater than 30 minutes before or after the scheduled dose may cause harm or result in substantial suboptimal therapy or pharmacological effect. Non–time-critical medications are those for which early or delayed administration within a specified range of either 1 or 2 hours should not cause harm or result in substantial suboptimal therapy or pharmacological effect (CMS, 2011; ISMP, 2011).

3. Identify patient using at least two identifiers (e.g., name and birthday or name and medical record number) according to agency policy. Compare identifiers with information on patient's MAR or medical record.

Ensures correct patient. Complies with The Joint Commission standards and improves patient safety (TJC, 2016).

4. At patient's bedside again compare MAR or computer printout with names of medications on medication labels and patient name. Ask patient if he or she has allergies.

This is the third check for accuracy and ensures that patient receives correct medication. Confirms patient's allergy history.

5. Explain procedure to patient. Be specific if patient wishes to self-administer drug. Explain where and how to set up at home. Discuss purpose of each medication, action, and possible adverse effects. Allow patient to ask any questions about the drugs. Explain what a metered dose is and how to administer. Warn about overuse of inhaler and side effects.

Helps patient be a participant in care, which minimizes anxiety. Patient has right to be informed, and patient's understanding of each medication improves adherence to drug therapy. Begins patient teaching regarding medications.

6. Allow adequate time for patient to manipulate inhaler, canister, and spacer device (if provided). Explain and demonstrate how canister fits into inhaler.

Patient must be familiar with how to use equipment.

Clinical Decision Point *If using an MDI that is new or has not been used for several days, push a "test spray" into the air to prime the device before using. This ensures that the MDI is patent and the metal canister is positioned properly.*

7. Explain and demonstrate steps for administering MDI without spacer.

Simple one-on-one instruction and demonstration of step-by-step administration allows patient to ask questions at any point during procedure and increases patient adherence to inhaler use (Ari, 2015).

a. Remove mouthpiece cover from inhaler after inserting MDI canister into holder.

b. Shake inhaler well for 2 to 5 seconds (five or six shakes).

Ensures mixing of medication in canister.

STEP	RATIONALE
c. Hold inhaler in dominant hand.	
d. Have patient stand or sit and instruct him or her to position inhaler in one of two ways:	
(1) Have patient place the mouthpiece in the mouth between the teeth and over the tongue, aimed toward back of throat, with lips closed tightly around it. Do not block the mouthpiece with the teeth or tongue (see illustration).	Ensures proper fit to inhale medication.
(2) Position mouthpiece 2 to 4 cm (1 to 2 inches) in front of widely opened mouth (see illustration), with opening of inhaler toward back of throat. Lips should not touch inhaler.	Directs aerosol spray toward airway. This is best way to deliver medication without a spacer.
e. While holding the mouthpiece away from the mouth, have patient take deep breath and exhale completely.	Empties lung volume and prepares airway to receive medication.
f. With inhaler positioned, have patient hold it with thumb at mouthpiece and index and middle fingers at top. This is a three-point or bilateral hand position.	Hand position ensures proper activation of MDI and distribution of dosage (Burchum and Rosenthal, 2016).
g. Instruct patient to tilt head back slightly and inhale slowly and deeply through mouth for 3 to 5 seconds while depressing canister fully.	Medication is distributed to airways during inhalation.
h. Have patient hold breath for about 10 seconds.	Allows tiny drops of aerosol spray to reach deeper branches of airways.
i. Remove MDI from mouth before exhaling and exhale slowly through nose or pursed lips.	Keeps small airways open during exhalation.
8. Explain and demonstrate steps to administer MDI using spacer device.	Simple one-on-one instruction and demonstration of step-by-step administration allows patient to ask questions at any point during procedure and increases patient adherence to inhaler use (Ari, 2015).
a. Remove mouthpiece cover from MDI and mouthpiece of spacer device.	Inhaler fits into end of spacer device.
b. Shake inhaler well for 2 to 5 seconds (five or six shakes).	Ensures mixing of medication in canister.
c. Insert MDI into end of spacer device.	Spacer device traps medication released from MDI; patient then inhales drug from device. These devices improve delivery of correct dose of inhaled medication (Barrons et al., 2011).
d. Instruct patient to place spacer device mouthpiece in mouth and close lips. Do not insert beyond raised lip on mouthpiece. Avoid covering small exhalation slots with lips.	Medication should not escape through mouth.
e. Have patient breathe normally through spacer device mouthpiece (see illustration).	Allows patient to relax before delivering medication.

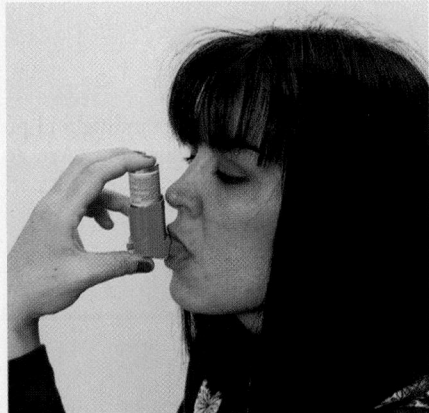

STEP 7d(1) Patient opens lips and places inhaler mouthpiece in mouth with opening toward back of throat.

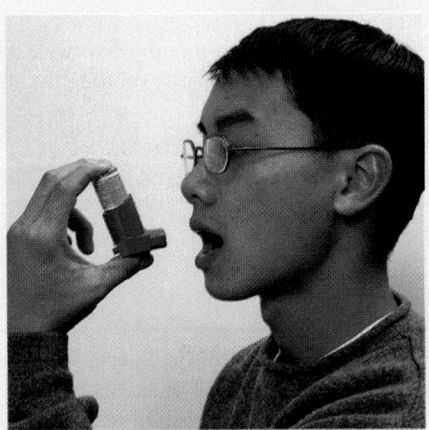

STEP 7d(2) Patient positions inhaler mouthpiece 2 to 4 cm (1 to 2 inches) from widely open mouth. This is considered the best way to deliver medication without a spacer.

STEP	RATIONALE

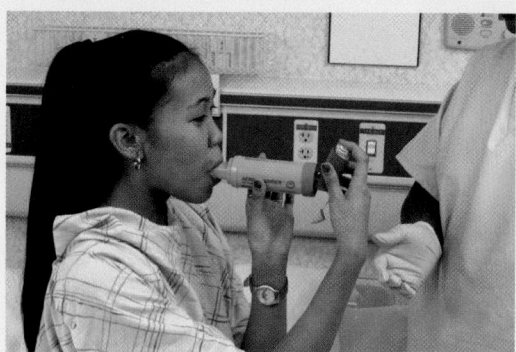

STEP 8e   Using spacer device with an MDI.

f. Instruct patient to depress medication canister, spraying one puff into spacer device.

Device contains fine spray and allows patient to inhale more medication. The spacer increases drug delivery and deposition of the medication on the oropharyngeal mucosa (Burchum and Rosenthal, 2016).

g. Patient breathes in slowly and fully (for 5 seconds).

Ensures that particles of medication are distributed to deeper airways.

h. Instruct patient to hold full breath for 10 seconds.

Ensures full drug distribution.

9. Instruct patient to wait 20 to 30 seconds between inhalations (if same medication) or 2 to 5 minutes between inhalations (if different medications).

Drugs must be inhaled sequentially. Always administer bronchodilators before steroids so dilators can open airway passages (Burchum and Rosenthal, 2016).

10. Instruct patient to not repeat inhalations before next scheduled.

Drugs are prescribed at intervals during day to provide constant drug levels and minimize side effects. Beta-adrenergic MDIs are used either on an "as needed" basis or regularly every 4 to 6 hours.

11. Warn patients that they may feel gagging sensation in throat caused by droplets of medication on pharynx or tongue.

This occurs when medication is sprayed and inhaled incorrectly.

12. About 2 minutes after last dose, instruct patient to rinse mouth with warm water and spit water out.

Steroids may alter normal flora of oral mucosa and lead to development of fungal infection. Rinsing out patient's mouth reduces risk of fungal infection (Ari, 2015).

13. Clean the MDI.

Removes residual medication and reduces spread of microorganisms.

a. For daily cleaning, instruct patient to remove medication canister, rinse inhaler and cap with warm running water, and be sure that inhaler is completely dry before reuse. Do not get valve mechanism of canister wet.

Water damages valve mechanism of canister.

b. Instruct patient to clean mouthpiece twice a week with a mild dishwashing soap, rinse thoroughly, and dry completely before storage.

14. Ask if patient has any questions.

Clarifies misconceptions or misunderstanding and provides opportunity for further patient education (Ari, 2015).

15. Help patient to comfortable position and perform hand hygiene.

Reduces spread of microorganisms and promotes patient comfort.

EVALUATION

1. Auscultate patient lungs, listen for abnormal breath sounds, and obtain peak flow measures if ordered.

Determines patient response to medication.

2. Have patient explain and demonstrate steps in use and cleaning of inhaler.

Return demonstration provides feedback for measuring patient's learning.

3. Ask patient to explain drug schedule and dose of medication.

Improves likelihood of adherence to therapy.

4. Ask patient to describe side effects of medication and criteria for calling health care provider.

Allows patient to recognize signs of overuse and need to seek medical support when drugs are ineffective.

STEP	RATIONALE
5. **Use Teach-Back:** "I want to be sure I clearly showed you how to use your inhaler. Let's take this time; show me how you will use the inhaler to take your medicine." Revise your instruction now or develop a plan for revised patient or family caregiver teaching if patient or family caregiver is not able to teach back correctly.	Determines patient's and family caregiver's level of understanding of instructional topic.

Unexpected Outcomes	Related Interventions
1. Patient's respirations are rapid and shallow; breath sounds indicate wheezing.	• Evaluate vital signs and respiratory status. • Notify health care provider. • Reassess type of medication and/or delivery method.
2. Patient needs bronchodilator more than every 4 hours (may indicate respiratory problem).	• Reassess type of medication and delivery methods needed. • Notify health care provider.
3. Patient experiences cardiac dysrhythmias (light-headedness, syncope), especially if receiving beta-adrenergic medications.	• Withhold all further doses of medication. • Evaluate cardiac and pulmonary status (see Chapter 6). • Notify health care provider for reassessment of type of medication and delivery method.

Recording and Reporting

- Record drug administered, dose or strength, route, number of inhalations, and actual time administered on MAR immediately after administration, not before. Include initials or signature.
- Record patient teaching and validation of patient's understanding on flow sheet or in nurses' notes in electronic health record (EHR) or chart.
- Record on flow sheet or in nurses' notes in EHR or chart patient's response to MDI (e.g., breath sounds), evidence of side effects (e.g., arrhythmia, feelings of anxiety), and ability to use MDI.
- Report adverse effects/patient response and/or withheld drugs to nurse in charge or health care provider.

Special Considerations
Teaching

- Allow for one-on-one supervised practice of the procedures. Patients may have difficulty timing an inhalation with activation of the medication canister without repeated instruction (Ari, 2015).
- Teach patient to keep track of the number of inhalations in the MDI (Box 21.5).
- Teach patients to use small, handheld peak flowmeters to monitor response to therapy when inhalers are prescribed (Barrons et al., 2011). A peak flowmeter measures the peak expiratory flow rate (PEFR), which is a person's maximum speed of expiration (Box 21.6).

Pediatric

- A spacer is of benefit to young children because they have difficulty coordinating inhaler activation and inhaling (Hockenberry and Wilson, 2015).
- Educate child and parent about the need to use the inhaler during school hours. Help family find resources within the school or day care facility. Many school systems do not permit self-administration of MDIs. Follow school policy regarding

---

BOX 21.5

Counting Doses in a Metered-Dose Inhaler

Most metered-dose inhalers (MDIs) currently do not have automatic dose counters. Patients need to keep careful track of the number of inhalations used in their MDIs. Failure to do so may result in patients using an empty inhaler during an acute exacerbation of a respiratory problem. To track doses:

- Note first day of use on a calendar.
- Note number of inhalations in the canister (e.g., 200 inhalations per MDI).
- Note number of inhalations used per day (e.g., 2 inhalations a day 3 times a day equals 6 inhalations per day).
- Divide the total number of inhalations in the canister by the number of inhalations needed per day to determine the number of days that the inhaler should last (e.g., 200 inhalations divided by 6 inhalations per day equals approximately 33 days of 3 times–a-day dosing).
- Mark on a calendar the date the inhaler will be empty and obtain a refill of the inhaler a few days before this target date.

BOX 21.6

How to Use a Peak Flowmeter

1. Move the marker to the bottom of the numbered scale, and connect the mouthpiece to the peak flowmeter.
2. Have patient stand up if able.
3. Have patient take a deep breath, filling the lungs completely.
4. Have the patient place the lips tightly around the mouthpiece of the flowmeter and then blow as hard and as fast as possible with a single breath.
5. Note the final position of the marker. This is the patient's peak flow rate.
6. Have the patient repeat the steps blowing into the peak flowmeter two more times. Record the highest reading of the three.

having the MDI available for use during school hours. A health care provider's order may be necessary.

Gerontological
- Older adults may be unable to depress medication canisters because of weakened grasp or inability to coordinate actuation

of the canister with inhalation. The use of a spacer device may be helpful.

Home Care
- Remind patients to carry prescribed inhalers to use as immediate treatment in case of an acute asthma attack.

PROCEDURAL GUIDELINE 21.1 *Using Dry Powder–Inhaled (DPI) Medications*

Dry powder inhalers (DPIs) hold dry powder medication and create an aerosol when the patient inhales through a reservoir that contains the medication. In contrast with the metered-dose inhaler (MDI), a DPI has no propellant. DPIs require less manual dexterity; and, because the device is breath activated, there is no need to coordinate puffs with inhalation. Compared with MDIs, DPIs deliver more medication to the lungs (Burchum and Rosenthal, 2016). A DPI does not require a spacer. Medication inside a DPI can clump if the patient lives in a humid climate. Some patients cannot inhale fast enough to administer the entire dose of medication.

Delegation and Collaboration
The skill of administering DPI medications cannot be delegated to nursing assistive personnel (NAP). The nurse directs the NAP about:
- Potential side effects of medications and to report their occurrence to the nurse.
- Reporting paroxysmal coughing, audible wheezing, and patient's report of breathlessness or difficulty breathing to the nurse.

Equipment
- DPI (see Fig. 21.2C)
- Stethoscope
- Wash basin or sink with warm water
- Medication administration record (MAR) (electronic or printed)
- Facial tissues *(optional)*

Procedural Steps
1. Check accuracy and completeness of each MAR with health care provider's medication order. Check patient's name, drug name and dosage, route (which sinus), and time for administration. Clarify incomplete or unclear orders with health care provider before administration.
2. Review pertinent information related to medication, including action, purpose, normal dose and route, side effects, time of onset and peak action, and nursing implications.
3. Assess patient's medical and medication history and history of allergies. List drug allergies on each page of the MAR and prominently display it on the patient's medical record per agency policy. When patient has allergy, provide allergy bracelet.
4. Assess respiratory pattern and auscultate breath sounds (see Chapter 6).
5. Assess patient's knowledge of medication and readiness to learn (e.g., asks questions about medication, requests education in use of DPI, is mentally alert, participates in own care).
6. Assess patient's ability to learn. Patient should not be fatigued, in pain, or in respiratory distress; assess level of understanding of technical vocabulary terms.

7. Determine patient's ability to hold, manipulate, and activate DPI.
8. If previously instructed in self-administration of DPI, assess patient's technique in using it.
9. Perform hand hygiene, prepare medication for inhalation, and check label on inhaler against MAR 2 times (see Skill 21.1). Preparation usually involves taking inhaler device out of storage and into patient's room. *These are the first and second checks for accuracy. Check expiration date on container.*
10. Take medication to patient at correct time (see agency policy). Give medications that require exact or precise timing when ordered, give time-critical medications at time ordered (no later than 30 minutes before or after), and give non–time-critical medications within 1 or 2 hours of scheduled dose (CMS, 2011; ISMP, 2011). During administration apply six rights of medication administration. Perform hand hygiene.
11. Identify patient using at least two identifiers (e.g., name and birthday or name and medical record number) according to agency policy. Compare identifiers with information on patient's MAR or medical record.
12. At patient's bedside again compare MAR or computer printout with names of medications on medication labels and patient name. *This is the third check for accuracy.* Ask patient if he or she has allergies.
13. Explain procedure and discuss purpose of each medication, action, and possible adverse effects. Allow patient to ask any questions about the drugs. Explain what a DPI is and how to administer. Warn about overuse of inhaler and side effects.
14. If DPI has an external counter, note number indicated to determine doses remaining. Otherwise use technique in Box 21.5 for counting doses.
15. Prepare DPI for administration. Perform hand hygiene. Some DPIs require loading medication before administration; some require rotation of a lever to load medication or insert a capsule; and some require insertion of a disk into inhaler device. Follow manufacturer specific instructions.

Clinical Decision Point *The patient's inhaled breath pulls the drug into the airway. DPIs may differ as to how fast the patient should inhale the medication; consult specific instructions of manufacturer. In addition, do not shake DPI because powdered medication may spill out of device.*

16. Have patient exhale fully and then place lips over mouthpiece of DPI and inhale quickly and as deeply as possible. Remove inhaler from mouth as soon as inhalation is complete.

PROCEDURAL GUIDELINE 21.1 *Using Dry Powder–Inhaled (DPI) Medications—cont'd*

17. Have patient hold breath for 10 seconds or as long as possible and then exhale. Do not exhale into DPI.

18. Instruct patients that, unlike with other inhaled medications, they may not taste or feel the dry powder or there may be a slight sweet taste.

19. After using DPI, have patient rinse mouth with warm water and spit it out to reduce throat irritation and prevent oral candidiasis.

20. Return DPI to closed position or remove loaded capsule or disk if necessary. If an external counter is present, note number, which should be one less than the number in Step 14.

21. Have patient demonstrate use of DPI at next scheduled dose. Ask him or her to discuss purpose, action, and side effects of medication.

22. Auscultate breath sounds, evaluate respiratory rate, and ask patient about his or her ease of breathing.

23. Record drug, dose or strength, route, number of inhalations, and time administered on MAR immediately after administration, not before. Include initials or signature.

24. Record patient teaching and validation of patient's understanding in nurses' notes in electronic health record (EHR) or chart.

25. **Use Teach-Back:** "I want to be sure I explained how often you need to use this DPI medication. Tell me when you will use this medication." Revise your instruction now or develop a plan for revised patient or family caregiver teaching if patient or family caregiver is not able to teach back correctly.

✦ SKILL 21.8 Using Small-Volume Nebulizers

Nebulization is a process of adding medications or moisture to inspired air by mixing particles of various sizes with air. Adding moisture to the respiratory system through nebulization improves clearance of pulmonary secretions. Medications such as bronchodilators, mucolytics, and corticosteroids are often administered by nebulization.

Small-volume nebulizers convert a drug solution into a mist that is then inhaled by a patient into his or her tracheobronchial tree. The droplets in the mist are much finer than those created by metered-dose inhalers (MDIs) or dry powder inhalers (DPIs). A face mask or a mouthpiece held between the teeth delivers a nebulized mist. A nebulized medication is designed to create a local effect, but it can be absorbed into the bloodstream through the alveoli. As a result, systemic effects from the medication may occur.

Delegation and Collaboration

In many health care agencies a respiratory therapist performs the skill of administering medications by nebulizer. The nurse must be aware of the type and actions of the inhaled medication that the patient is receiving. The skill of administering medications by nebulizer cannot be delegated to nursing assistive personnel (NAP). The nurse instructs the NAP about:

- Potential side effects of medications and to report their occurrence to the nurse.
- Reporting paroxysmal coughing, ineffective breathing patterns, and other respiratory difficulties to the nurse.

Equipment

- Medication ordered and diluent (if needed)
- Medicine dropper or syringe
- Nebulizer bottle and tubing assembly
- Small-volume nebulizer machine (often called *handheld nebulizer* or *nebulizer*)
- Pulse oximeter and peak flow device
- Stethoscope
- Medication administration record (MAR) (electronic or printed)
- *Option:* nose clip

STEP	RATIONALE

ASSESSMENT

1. Check accuracy and completeness of each MAR with health care provider's medication order. Check patient's name, drug name and dosage, route, and time for administration. Clarify incomplete or unclear orders with health care provider before administration.

The order sheet is the most reliable source and only legal record of medications that patient is to receive. Ensures that patient receives correct medications (Sulosaari et al., 2011). Handwritten MARs are a source of medication errors (Alassaad et al., 2013).

2. Review pertinent information related to medication, including action, purpose, normal dose and route, side effects, time of onset and peak action, and nursing implications.

Allows you to anticipate effects of drug and observe patient's response.

3. Assess patient's medical and medication history and history of allergies. List drug allergies on each page of the MAR and prominently display it on the patient's medical record per agency policy. When patient has allergy, provide allergy bracelet.

These factors influence how certain drugs act. Information also reflects patient's need for medications and risk for side effects. Communication of allergies is essential for safe and effective care.

STEP	RATIONALE
4. Assess patient's grasp and ability to assemble, hold, and manipulate nebulizer equipment.	Any impairment of cognition or grasp or the presence of hand tremors affects patient's ability to use equipment.
5. Assess pulse, respirations, breath sounds, pulse oximetry, and peak flow measurement (if ordered) before beginning treatment.	Establishes baseline for comparison during and after treatment.
6. Assess patient's knowledge of medication and readiness to learn (e.g., patient asks questions about medication, requests education in use of nebulizer, is mentally alert, participates in own care).	Determines level of instruction needed to assume self-administration.
7. Assess patient's ability to learn. Patient should not be fatigued, in pain, or in respiratory distress; assess level of understanding of technical vocabulary terms.	Determines best time to provide instruction and techniques to use.
8. Assess patient's ability to manipulate nebulizer mouthpiece and tubing.	Presence of mobility restrictions indicates need for assistance.

NURSING DIAGNOSES

- Activity intolerance
- Anxiety
- Deficient knowledge regarding use of nebulizers

- Impaired gas exchange
- Ineffective breathing pattern

- Readiness for enhanced self-health management
- Risk for injury

Related factors/Risk factors are individualized based on patient's condition or needs.

PLANNING

1. Expected outcomes following completion of procedure:	
• Patient's breathing pattern is effective.	Demonstrates therapeutic effect of medication.
• Patient's oxygen saturation level is adequate.	Demonstrates therapeutic effect of medication.
• Patient describes side effects of medication and criteria for calling health care provider (e.g., low peak flow rate).	Increases likelihood of adherence to therapeutic regimen.
• Patient demonstrates self-administration of nebulized dose of medication correctly.	Demonstrates proper administration of medication and documents learning.
2. Collect appropriate equipment and MAR.	Ensures time management and efficiency.

IMPLEMENTATION

1. Perform hand hygiene and prepare medications for inhalation. Check label of medication against MAR 2 times (see Skill 21.1). Preparation usually involves taking medication vial out of storage and taking to patient's room. Check expiration date on container.	*These are the first and second checks for accuracy.* Process ensures that right patient receives right medication.
2. Take medication(s) to patient at correct time (see agency policy). Medications that require exact timing include stat, first-time or loading doses, and 1-time doses. Give time-critical scheduled medications (e.g., antibiotics, anticoagulants, insulin, anticonvulsants, immunosuppressive agents) at exact time ordered (no later than 30 minutes before or after scheduled dose). Give non–time-critical scheduled medications within a range of 1 or 2 hours of scheduled dose (ISMP, 2011). During administration, apply six rights of medication administration. Perform hand hygiene.	Hospitals must adopt medication administration policy and procedure for timing of medication administration that considers nature of the prescribed medication, specific clinical application, and patient needs (CMS, 2011; ISMP, 2011). Time-critical scheduled medications are those for which early or delayed administration of maintenance doses of greater than 30 minutes before or after the scheduled dose may cause harm or result in substantial suboptimal therapy or pharmacological effect. Non–time-critical medications are those for which early or delayed administration within a specified range of either 1 or 2 hours should not cause harm or result in substantial suboptimal therapy or pharmacological effect (CMS, 2011; ISMP, 2011).
3. Identify patient using at least two identifiers (e.g., name and birthday or name and medical record number) according to agency policy. Compare identifiers with information on patient's MAR or medical record.	Ensures correct patient. Complies with The Joint Commission standards and improves patient safety (TJC, 2016).

STEP	RATIONALE

4. At patient's bedside again compare MAR or computer printout with names of medications on medication labels and patient name. Ask patient if he or she has allergies.

This is the third check for accuracy and ensures that patient receives correct medication. Confirms patient's allergy history.

5. Explain procedure to patient. Be specific if patient wishes to self-administer drug. Discuss purpose of each medication, action, and possible adverse effects. Allow patient to ask any questions about the drugs. Explain how to assemble nebulizer and proper use.

Helps patient be a participant in care, which minimizes anxiety. Patient has right to be informed, and patient's understanding of each medication improves adherence to drug therapy. Begins patient teaching regarding medications (Ari, 2015).

6. Assemble nebulizer equipment per manufacturer directions.

Assembly may vary slightly with different manufacturers. Proper assembly ensures safe delivery of medication.

7. Add prescribed medication by pouring medicine into nebulizer cup. (*Option:* You may use a medicine dropper or syringe to instill medication.)

Ensures proper dose and delivery of ordered medication.

8. Attach top to nebulizer cup and be sure that it is secure. Then connect cup to mouthpiece or face mask.

Prevents loss of medication.

9. Connect tubing to both aerosol compressor and nebulizer cup.

Ensures aerosol delivery to mouthpiece.

10. Have patient hold mouthpiece between lips with gentle pressure, but be sure lips are sealed (see illustration).

Prevents escape of nebulized medication.

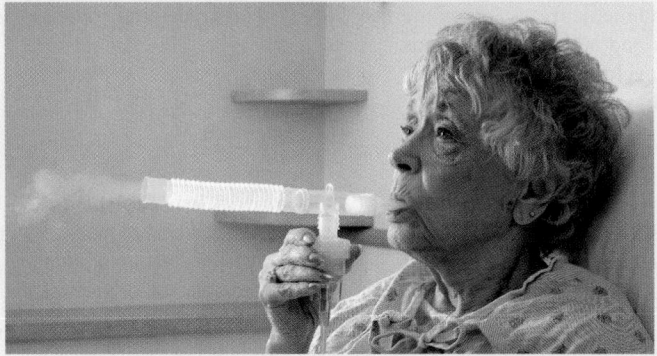

STEP 10 Nebulizer mouthpiece placed between patient's lips.

   a. If patient is an infant, child, or tired adult or unable to follow instructions, use face mask.

Use of face mask does not require patient to remember to hold mouthpiece correctly. Correct delivery ensures sufficient deposition of medication.

   b. Use special adapters for patients with tracheostomy.

Promotes greater deposition of medication in airways.

11. Turn on small-volume nebulizer machine and ensure that a sufficient mist begins to flow.

Verifies that equipment is working properly during delivery of medication.

12. Instruct patient take deep breath, slowly, to a volume slightly greater than normal. Encourage brief, end-inspiratory pause for about 2 to 3 seconds; then have patient exhale passively. *Option:* If needed, use a nose clip so patient breathes only through the mouth (Medline Plus, 2014).

Improves effectiveness of medication.

   a. If patient is dyspneic, encourage him or her to hold every fourth or fifth breath for 5 to 10 seconds.

Maximizes effectiveness of medication.

   b. Remind patient to repeat breathing pattern until drug is completely nebulized. This usually takes about 10 to 15 minutes (Medline Plus, 2014).

Maximizes effectiveness of medication.

     (1) Some health care providers set time limit as length of treatment rather than waiting for medication to completely nebulize.

   c. Tap nebulizer cup occasionally during and toward end of treatment.

Releases droplets that are clinging to side of cup, thus allowing for renebulization of solution.

   d. Monitor patient's pulse during procedure, especially if beta-adrenergic bronchodilators are used.

Enables you to observe for potential side effects of medications.

STEP	RATIONALE
13. When medication is completely nebulized, turn off machine. Rinse nebulizer cup per agency policy. Dry completely and store tubing assembly per agency policy.	Proper storage reduces transfer of microorganisms.
14. If steroids are nebulized, instruct patient to rinse mouth and gargle with warm water after nebulizer treatment. Have patient spit out solution.	Removes medication residue from oral cavity and helps to prevent oral candidiasis, a possible adverse effect of inhaled steroid therapy.
15. After nebulizer treatment is complete, have patient take several deep breaths and cough to expectorate mucus.	Nebulized medication is often ordered to open airways and promote expectoration of mucus.
16. Help patient to comfortable position and perform hand hygiene.	Reduces spread of microorganisms and promotes patient comfort.

EVALUATION

1. Assess patient's respirations, breath sounds, cough effort, sputum production, pulse oximetry, and peak flow measures if ordered.	Determines status of breathing pattern and adequacy of ventilation/gas exchange. Allows comparison with baseline data and evaluation of effectiveness of procedure.
2. Ask patient to explain drug schedule.	Improves likelihood of adherence to therapy.
3. Ask patient to describe side effects of medication and criteria for calling health care provider.	Allows patient to recognize signs of overuse and need to seek medical support when drugs are ineffective.
4. **Use Teach-Back:** "I want to be sure I was clear about how to put together the nebulizer and add medications. Show me the steps for assembling the nebulizer and adding medications." Revise your instruction now or develop a plan for revised patient or family caregiver teaching if patient or family caregiver is not able to teach back correctly.	Determines patient's and family caregiver's level of understanding of instructional topic.

Unexpected Outcomes	Related Interventions
1. Patient's breathing pattern is ineffective; respirations are rapid and shallow; breath sounds indicate wheezing.	• Reassess type of medication and/or delivery method. • Notify health care provider.
2. Patient experiences paroxysms of coughing. Aerosolized particles can irritate posterior pharynx.	• Reassess type of medication and/or delivery method. • Notify health care provider.
3. Patient experiences cardiac dysrhythmias (light-headedness, syncope), especially if receiving beta-adrenergics.	• Withhold all further doses of medication. Assess vital signs. • Notify health care provider for reassessment of type of medication and delivery method.

Recording and Reporting

- Record drug, dose and strength, route, length of treatment, and time administered on MAR immediately after administration, not before. Include initials or signature.
- Record patient teaching and validation of patient's understanding on flow sheet or in nurses' notes in electronic health record (EHR) or chart.
- Record patient's response to treatment on flow sheet or in nurses' notes in EHR or chart.
- Report adverse effects/patient response and/or withheld drugs to nurse in charge or health care provider.

Special Considerations
Teaching

- Teach patient not to store medication in nebulizer for later use.
- Advise patients taking long-acting beta-agonists about possible adverse effects, including nervousness, restlessness, tremor, headache, nausea, rapid or pounding heart rate, and dizziness.
- Teach patients how to use small, handheld peak flowmeters to monitor response to therapy when inhaled drugs are prescribed (Barrons et al., 2011) (see Box 21.6).

Pediatric

- Use a mask for the nebulizer treatment if child is too young to hold mouthpiece correctly for the duration of the treatment (Hockenberry and Wilson, 2015).
- Instruct child to breathe normally with mouth open to provide a direct route to the airways for the medication.
- Educate child and parent about the need to use the nebulizer during school or day care hours. Help family find resources within the school or day care facility. Follow school policy regarding having the nebulizer and medication available for use during school hours. A health care provider's order may be necessary.

Gerontological

- Older adults with a weak grasp, hand tremors, or coordination problems may not be able to manipulate or hold a nebulizer.

Home Care

- When at home, rinse nebulizer parts after each use with clear water and air dry (Roy et al., 2011; Medline Plus, 2014).

◆ SKILL 21.9 Administering Vaginal Instillations

NSO | *Nursing Skills Online Administration of Nonparenteral Medications Module / Lesson 7*

Female patients who develop vaginal infections often require topical application of antiinfective agents. Vaginal medications are available in foam, jelly, cream, or suppository form. Medicated irrigations or douches can also be given. However, their excessive use can lead to vaginal irritation.

Vaginal suppositories are oval shaped and come individually packaged in foil wrappers. They are larger and more oval than rectal suppositories (Fig. 21.3). Storage in a refrigerator prevents the solid suppositories from melting. You insert a suppository into the vagina with an applicator or a gloved hand. After insertion, body temperature causes the suppository to melt for effective medication distribution. You can insert foam, jellies, and creams with an inserter or applicator. Patients often prefer administering their own vaginal medications, and you should give them privacy to do so. Offer the patient a perineal pad to wear after drug instillation to collect excess drainage. Because vaginal medications are frequently given to treat infection, any discharge is often foul smelling. Follow good aseptic technique and offer a patient frequent opportunities for perineal hygiene (see Procedural Guideline 18.1).

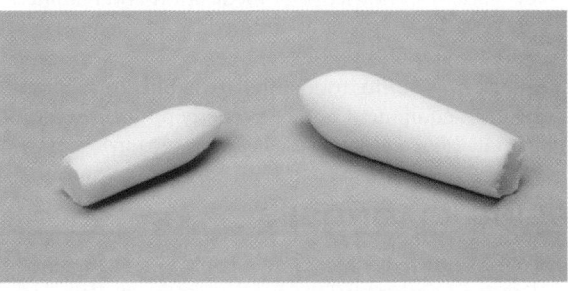

FIG 21.3 Vaginal suppositories *(right)* are larger and more oval than rectal suppositories *(left)*.

Delegation and Collaboration

The skill of administering vaginal medications cannot be delegated to nursing assistive personnel (NAP). The nurse instructs the NAP about:

- Potential side effects of medications and to report their occurrence to the nurse.
- Reporting any change in comfort level or new or increased vaginal discharge or bleeding to the nurse.

Equipment

- Vaginal cream, foam, jelly, tablet, suppository, or irrigating solution
- Applicators (Fig. 21.4) (if needed)
- Clean gloves
- Tissues
- Towels and/or washcloths

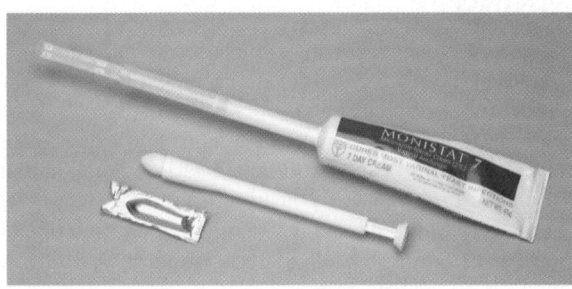

FIG 21.4 From top: Vaginal cream with applicator, applicator, and vaginal suppository. *(From Lilley LL et al: Pharmacology and the nursing process, ed 6, St Louis, 2011, Mosby.)*

- Perineal pad; drape or sheet
- Water-soluble lubricants
- Bedpan
- Irrigation or douche container (if needed)
- Medication administration record (MAR) (electronic or printed)
- *Option:* Gooseneck lamp

STEP	RATIONALE

ASSESSMENT

1. Check accuracy and completeness of each MAR with health care provider's medication order. Check patient's name, drug name and dosage, route, and time for administration. Clarify incomplete or unclear orders with health care provider before administration.

2. Review pertinent information related to medication, including action, purpose, normal dose and route, side effects, time of onset and peak action, and nursing implications.

3. Assess patient's medical and medication history and history of allergies. List drug allergies on each page of the MAR and prominently display it on the patient's medical record per agency policy. When patient has allergy, provide allergy bracelet.

4. Perform hand hygiene and apply clean gloves. During perineal care inspect condition of vaginal tissues; note if drainage is present. Remove gloves and perform hand hygiene.

5. Ask if patient is experiencing any symptoms of pruritus, burning, or discomfort.

The order sheet is the most reliable source and only legal record of medications that patient is to receive. Ensures that patient receives correct medications (Sulosaari et al., 2011). Handwritten MARs are a source of medication errors (Alassaad et al., 2013).

Allows you to anticipate effects of drug and observe patient's response.

These factors influence how certain drugs act. Information also reflects patient's need for medications and risk for side effects. Communication of allergies is essential for safe and effective care.

Prevents transmission of microorganisms. Identifies symptoms of vaginal irritation or infection.

Identifies symptoms of vaginal irritation or infection.

STEP	RATIONALE
6. Review patient's knowledge of medication and readiness to learn (e.g., asks questions about medication, requests education in use of suppository).	Indicates need for health teaching. Understanding influences adherence to therapy.
7. Assess patient's ability to manipulate applicator, suppository, or irrigation equipment and to properly position self to insert medication (may be done just before insertion).	Presence of mobility restrictions indicates need for help.

NURSING DIAGNOSES

- Deficient knowledge regarding vaginal medication administration
- Impaired physical mobility
- Pain (acute or chronic)
- Sexual dysfunction

Related factors/Risk factors are individualized based on patient's condition or needs.

PLANNING

1. Expected outcomes following completion of procedure:	
• Vaginal tissues are pink and smooth. Genitalia are clear and without discharge.	Tissues take on normal characteristics.
• Patient denies symptoms of discomfort and expresses relief from symptoms of infection/inflammation. Small amount of discharge the color of medication is present.	Inflammation or infection has resolved. When suppository or cream becomes distributed, small amount may escape from vaginal orifice.
• Patient is able to discuss information about prescribed drug.	Feedback reflects patient's learning.
• Patient demonstrates self-administration of suppository, medication, or irrigation.	Demonstrates learning.
2. Collect appropriate equipment and MAR.	Ensures time management and efficiency.

IMPLEMENTATION

1. Perform hand hygiene. Prepare suppository for administration. Check label of medication against MAR 2 times (see Skill 21.1). Preparation usually involves taking suppository out of refrigerator and taking to patient's room. Check expiration date on container.	*These are the first and second checks for accuracy.* Process ensures that right patient receives right medication.
2. Take medication(s) to patient at correct time (see agency policy). Medications that require exact timing include stat, first-time or loading doses, and 1-time doses. Give time-critical scheduled medications (e.g., antibiotics, anticoagulants, insulin, anticonvulsants, immunosuppressive agents) at exact time ordered (no later than 30 minutes before or after scheduled dose). Give non–time-critical scheduled medications within a range of 1 or 2 hours of scheduled dose (ISMP, 2011). During administration, apply six rights of medication administration. Perform hand hygiene.	Hospitals must adopt medication administration policy and procedure for timing of medication administration that considers nature of the prescribed medication, specific clinical application, and patient needs (CMS, 2011; ISMP, 2011). Time-critical scheduled medications are those for which early or delayed administration of maintenance doses of greater than 30 minutes before or after the scheduled dose may cause harm or result in substantial suboptimal therapy or pharmacological effect. Non–time-critical medications are those for which early or delayed administration within a specified range of either 1 or 2 hours should not cause harm or result in substantial suboptimal therapy or pharmacological effect (CMS, 2011; ISMP, 2011).
3. Identify patient using at least two identifiers (e.g., name and birthday or name and medical record number) according to agency policy. Compare identifiers with information on patient's MAR or medical record.	Ensures correct patient. Complies with The Joint Commission standards and improves patient safety (TJC, 2016).
4. At patient's bedside again compare MAR or computer printout with names of medications on medication labels and patient name. Ask patient if he or she has allergies.	*This is the third check for accuracy* and ensures that patient receives correct medication. Confirms patient's allergy history.
5. Explain procedure to patient. Be specific if patient plans to self-administer medication. Discuss purpose of each medication, action, and possible adverse effects. Allow patient to ask any questions about the drugs. Explain procedure if patient plans to self-administer medication.	Helps patient be a participant in care, which minimizes anxiety. Patient has right to be informed, and patient's understanding of each medication improves adherence to drug therapy. Begins patient teaching regarding medications.

STEP	**RATIONALE**

6. Arrange supplies at bedside, and apply clean gloves. Close door or pull curtain.

Reduces transfer of microorganisms.

7. Have patient void (using bathroom facilities or bedpan). Help her lie in dorsal recumbent position. Patients with restricted mobility in knees or hips may lie supine with legs abducted.

Voiding prevents passing of urine during insertion of suppository. Position provides easy access to and good exposure of vaginal canal. Dependent position also allows suppository to completely dissolve in vagina.

8. Keep abdomen and lower extremities draped.

Minimizes patient's embarrassment by limiting exposure.

9. Be sure that vaginal orifice is well illuminated by room light. Otherwise position portable gooseneck lamp.

Proper insertion requires visualization of external genitalia if not self-administered.

10. Insert vaginal suppository.

    a. Remove suppository from wrapper and apply liberal amount of water-soluble lubricant to smooth or rounded end (see illustration). Be sure that suppository is at room temperature. Lubricate gloved index finger of dominant hand.

Lubrication reduces friction against mucosal surfaces during insertion. Use of petroleum jelly may leave residue that harbors bacteria and yeast fungi.

    b. With nondominant gloved hand gently separate labial folds in front-to-back direction.

Exposes vaginal orifice.

    c. With dominant gloved hand insert rounded end of suppository along posterior wall of vaginal canal the entire length of finger (7.5 to 10 cm [3 to 4 inches]) (see illustration).

Proper placement of suppository ensures equal distribution of medication along walls of vaginal cavity.

    d. Withdraw finger and wipe away remaining lubricant from around orifice and labia with tissue or cloth.

Maintains comfort.

11. Apply cream or foam.

    a. Fill cream or foam applicator following package directions.

Dose is based on volume in applicator.

    b. With nondominant gloved hand gently separate labial folds.

Exposes vaginal orifice.

    c. With dominant gloved hand gently insert applicator approximately 5 to 7.5 cm (2 to 3 inches). Push applicator plunger to deposit medication into vagina (see illustration).

Allows equal distribution of medication along vaginal walls.

    d. Withdraw applicator and place on paper towel. Wipe off residual cream from labia or vaginal orifice with tissue or cloth.

Maintains patient comfort.

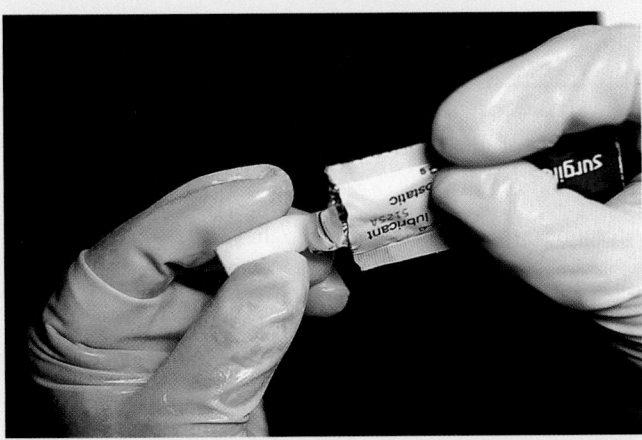

STEP 10a Lubricate tip of suppository.

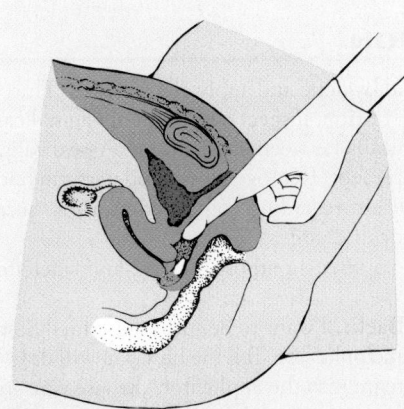

STEP 10c Angle of vaginal suppository insertion.

STEP	RATIONALE

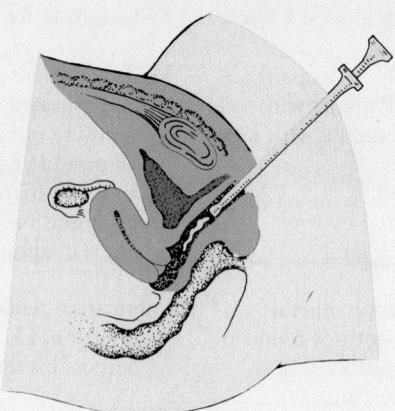

STEP 11c Applicator inserted into vaginal canal. Plunger pushed to instill medication.

12. Administer irrigation or douche.	
a. Place patient on bedpan with absorbent pad underneath.	Allows hips to be higher than shoulders and solution to reach posterior wall of vagina. Bedpan collects solution.
b. Be sure that irrigation or douche fluid is at body temperature. Run fluid through container nozzle (priming the tubing).	Body temperature promotes patient comfort. Priming tubing removes air and moistens nozzle tip.
c. Gently separate labial folds and direct nozzle toward sacrum, following floor of vagina.	Correct angle allows nozzle access into vagina.
d. Raise container approximately 30 to 50 cm (12 to 20 inches) above level of vagina. Insert nozzle 7 to 10 cm (3 to 4 inches). Allow solution to flow while rotating nozzle. Administer all irrigating solution.	Rotating nozzle allows irrigation of all areas in vagina.
e. Withdraw nozzle and help patient to comfortable sitting position.	Remaining solution drains by gravity.
f. Allow patient to remain on bedpan for a few minutes. Clean perineum with soap and water.	Ensures that all solution drains from vagina. Provides comfort for patient.
g. Help patient off bedpan. Dry perineal area.	Provides comfort.
13. Instruct patient who received suppository, cream, or tablet to remain on her back for at least 10 minutes.	Allows melting and spreading of medication throughout vaginal cavity and prevents loss through vaginal orifice.
14. If using an applicator, wash with soap and warm water, rinse, air dry, and then store for future use.	Vaginal cavity is not sterile. Soap and water help to remove bacteria and residual cream from applicator.
15. Offer perineal pad when patient resumes ambulation.	Provides patient comfort.
16. Discard gloves by turning them inside out and dispose of them and other soiled equipment in appropriate receptacle. Perform hand hygiene.	Reduces spread of microorganisms.

EVALUATION

1. Perform hand hygiene and apply clean gloves. Thirty minutes after administration, inspect condition of vaginal canal and external genitalia between applications. Assess vaginal discharge if present. Remove gloves and perform hand hygiene.	Determines whether vaginal medication effectively reduced irritation or inflammation of tissues.
2. Question patient regarding continued pruritus, burning, discomfort, or discharge.	Determines whether symptoms are relieved.
3. Ask patient to discuss purpose, action, and side effects of medication.	Reflects patient's understanding of drug therapy.
4. **Use Teach-Back:** "I want to be sure I explained how to use the vaginal cream applicator. Tell me how you will draw the correct amount of cream into the applicator." Revise your instruction now or develop a plan for revised patient or family caregiver teaching if patient or family caregiver is not able to teach back correctly.	Determines patient's and family caregiver's level of understanding of instructional topic.

STEP	RATIONALE
Unexpected Outcomes 1. Patient reports localized pruritus and burning. 2. Patient is unable to discuss drug therapy correctly. 3. Patient is unable to self-administer medications.	**Related Interventions** • Results of infection or inflammation, but may be possible side effects of some medications (e.g., miconazole). • Monitor symptoms; report to health care provider. • Repeat instructions or assess if patient is able to learn. • Include family caregiver when appropriate. • Reinstruction is necessary.

Recording and Reporting

• Record drug (or solution if vaginal instillation), dose, type of instillation, and time administered on MAR immediately after administration, not before. Include initials or signature.
• Record patient response to medication, patient teaching, and validation of understanding and ability to self-administer medication on flow sheet or in nurses' notes in electronic health record (EHR) or chart.
• Report to health care provider if patient states that symptoms do not disappear or symptoms get worse.
• Report adverse effects/patient response and/or withheld drugs to nurse in charge or health care provider.

Special Considerations
Teaching

• Encourage patient to take *all* of the medication as prescribed, for the prescribed amount of time, to ensure effectiveness of the treatment.

• Women taking antifungal medications for the treatment of vaginal infections should abstain from sexual intercourse until the treatment is completed and the infection is resolved. Women should be told to continue to take the medication even if actively menstruating. Patients should notify the health care provider if symptoms persist past the treatment time period (Burchum and Rosenthal, 2016).
• Many women prefer to self-administer vaginal irrigations and medications. These procedures may be self-administered while patient is sitting on the toilet. Ensure that patient is able to perform the procedure correctly.

Gerontological

• Older adults may have difficulty manipulating suppository, applicator, or irrigating equipment. If so, a family caregiver may need instruction on how to administer the medication.

◆ SKILL 21.10 Administering Rectal Suppositories

NSO *Nursing Skills Online Administration of Nonparenteral Medications Module / Lesson 7*

A rectal suppository is a form of medication that acts when it melts and is absorbed into the rectal mucosa. Rectal medications exert either local effects on gastrointestinal (GI) mucosa (e.g., promoting defecation) or systemic effects (e.g., relieving nausea or providing analgesia). The rectal route is not as reliable as oral or parenteral routes in terms of drug absorption and distribution. However, the medications are relatively safe because they rarely cause local irritation or side effects. Rectal medications are contraindicated in patients with recent surgery on the rectum, bowel, or prostate gland; rectal bleeding or prolapse; and very low platelet counts (Burchum and Rosenthal, 2016).

Rectal suppositories are thinner and more bullet shaped than vaginal suppositories (see Fig. 21.3). The rounded end prevents anal trauma during insertion. When you administer a rectal suppository, placing it past the internal anal sphincter and against the rectal mucosa is important. Improper placement can result in expulsion of the suppository before the medication dissolves and is absorbed into the mucosa. If a patient prefers to self-administer a suppository, give specific instructions so the medication is deposited correctly. Do not cut the suppository into sections to divide the dosage; the active drug may not be distributed evenly within the suppository, and the result may be an inaccurate dose (Burchum and Rosenthal, 2016)

Delegation and Collaboration

The skill of rectal medication administration cannot be delegated to nursing assistive personnel (NAP). The nurse instructs the NAP about:

• Reporting expected fecal discharge or bowel movement to the nurse.
• Potential side effects of medications and to report their occurrence to the nurse.
• Informing nurse of any rectal pain or bleeding.

Equipment

• Rectal suppository
• Water-soluble lubricating jelly
• Clean gloves
• Tissue
• Drape
• Medication administration record (MAR) (electronic or printed)

STEP	RATIONALE

ASSESSMENT

1. Check accuracy and completeness of each MAR with health care provider's medication order. Check patient's name, drug name and dosage, route, and time for administration. Clarify incomplete or unclear orders with health care provider before administration.

2. Review pertinent information related to medication, including action, purpose, normal dose and route, side effects, time of onset and peak action, and nursing implications.

3. Review patient's medical history for history of rectal surgery or bleeding, cardiac problems, history of allergies, and medication history. List drug allergies on each page of the MAR and prominently display it on the patient's medical record per agency policy. When patient has allergy, provide allergy bracelet.

4. Review any presenting signs and symptoms of GI alterations (e.g., constipation or diarrhea).

5. Assess patient's ability to hold suppository and position self to insert medication.

6. Review patient's knowledge of purpose of drug therapy and interest in self-administering suppository.

The order sheet is the most reliable source and only legal record of medications that patient is to receive. Ensures that patient receives correct medications (Sulosaari et al., 2011). Handwritten MARs are a source of medication errors (Alassaad et al., 2013).

Allows you to anticipate effects of drug and observe patient's response.

Conditions may contraindicate use of suppository. Communication of allergies is essential for safe and effective care.

Conditions indicate use of suppository.

Mobility restriction indicates need for nurse to help with drug administration.

Indicates need for health teaching. Level of motivation influences teaching approach.

NURSING DIAGNOSES

- Constipation
- Deficient knowledge regarding suppository administration
- Impaired physical mobility
- Pain (acute or chronic)
- Readiness for enhanced self-health management

Related factors/Risk factors are individualized based on patient's condition or needs.

PLANNING

1. Expected outcomes following completion of the procedure:
   - Patient reports relief or reduction in symptoms for which medication is prescribed.
   - Patient describes purpose of medication.
   - Patient demonstrates self-administration of rectal suppository.

2. Collect appropriate equipment and MAR.

Drug acts effectively.

Feedback reflects patient's learning.
Demonstrates learning.

Ensures time management and efficiency.

IMPLEMENTATION

1. Perform hand hygiene and prepare suppository for administration. Check label of medication against MAR 2 times (see Skill 21.1). Check expiration date on container.

2. Take medication(s) to patient at correct time (see agency policy). Medications that require exact timing include stat, first-time or loading doses, and 1-time doses. Give time-critical scheduled medications (e.g., antibiotics, anticoagulants, insulin, anticonvulsants, immunosuppressive agents) at exact time ordered (no later than 30 minutes before or after scheduled dose). Give non–time-critical scheduled medications within a range of 1 or 2 hours of scheduled dose (ISMP, 2011). During administration, apply six rights of medication administration. Perform hand hygiene.

These are the first and second checks for accuracy. Process ensures that right patient receives right medication.

Hospitals must adopt medication administration policy and procedure for timing of medication administration that considers nature of the prescribed medication, specific clinical application, and patient needs (CMS, 2011; ISMP, 2011). Time-critical scheduled medications are those for which early or delayed administration of maintenance doses of greater than 30 minutes before or after the scheduled dose may cause harm or result in substantial suboptimal therapy or pharmacological effect. Non–time-critical medications are those for which early or delayed administration within a specified range of either 1 or 2 hours should not cause harm or result in substantial suboptimal therapy or pharmacological effect (CMS, 2011; ISMP, 2011).

STEP	RATIONALE
3. Identify patient using at least two identifiers (e.g., name and birthday or name and medical record number) according to agency policy. Compare identifiers with information on patient's MAR or medical record.	Ensures correct patient. Complies with The Joint Commission standards and improves patient safety (TJC, 2016).
4. At patient's bedside again compare MAR or computer printout with names of medications on medication labels and patient name. Ask patient if he or she has allergies.	*This is the third check for accuracy* and ensures that patient receives correct medication. Confirms patient's allergy history.
5. Explain procedure to patient. Be specific if patient wishes to self-administer drug. Discuss purpose of each medication, action, and possible adverse effects. Allow patient to ask any questions about the drugs. Explain procedure if patient plans to self-administer medication.	Helps patient be a participant in care, which minimizes anxiety. Patient has right to be informed, and patient's understanding of each medication improves adherence to drug therapy. Begins patient teaching regarding medications.
6. Arrange supplies at bedside, and apply clean gloves. Close room curtain or door.	Reduces transfer of microorganisms. Maintains privacy and minimizes embarrassment.
7. Help patient assume left side-lying Sims' position with upper leg flexed upward.	Position exposes anus and relaxes external anal sphincter. Left side-lying Sims' position lessens likelihood of suppository or feces being expelled.
8. If patient has mobility impairment, help into lateral position. Obtain help to turn patient and use pillows under upper arm and leg.	Provides support during procedure and patient comfort.
9. Keep patient draped with only anal area exposed.	Maintains privacy and facilitates relaxation.
10. Examine condition of anus externally. *Option:* Palpate rectal walls as needed (e.g., if impaction is suspected) (see Chapter 6). If you palpate rectal walls, dispose of gloves by turning them inside out and placing them in proper receptacle if they become soiled. Otherwise keep gloves on your hands and proceed to Step 12.	Determines presence of active rectal bleeding. Palpation determines whether rectum is filled with feces, which interferes with suppository placement. Reduces spread of infection.

Clinical Decision Point *Do not palpate patient's rectum if there is a recent history of rectal surgery. A suppository is contraindicated in the presence of active bleeding and diarrhea (Burchum and Rosenthal, 2016).*

STEP	RATIONALE
11. Perform hand hygiene and apply new pair of clean gloves (if previous gloves were soiled and discarded).	Minimizes contact with fecal material to reduce transmission of infection.
12. Remove suppository from foil wrapper and lubricate rounded end with water-soluble lubricant. Lubricate gloved index finger of dominant hand. If patient has hemorrhoids, use liberal amount of lubricant and touch area gently.	Lubrication reduces friction as suppository enters rectal canal.
13. Ask patient to take slow, deep breaths through mouth and relax anal sphincter.	Forcing suppository through constricted sphincter causes pain.
14. Retract patient's buttocks with nondominant hand. With gloved index finger of dominant hand, insert suppository gently through anus, past internal sphincter, and against rectal wall, 10 cm (4 inches) in adults (see illustration) or 5 cm (2 inches) in infants and children. You should feel rectal sphincter close around your finger.	Suppository needs to be against rectal mucosa for eventual absorption and therapeutic action.

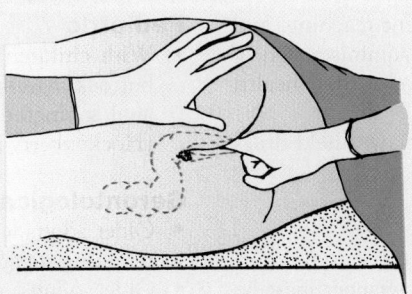

STEP 14 Insert rectal suppository past sphincter and against rectal wall.

STEP	RATIONALE

Clinical Decision Point *Do not insert suppository into a mass of fecal material; this will reduce effectiveness of medication.*

15. *Option:* A suppository may be given through a colostomy (not ileostomy) if ordered. Patient should lie supine. Use small amount of water-soluble lubricant for insertion.	
16. Withdraw finger and wipe patient's anal area.	Provides comfort.
17. Ask patient to remain flat or on side for 5 minutes.	Prevents expulsion of suppository.
18. Discard gloves by turning them inside out and dispose of them and used supplies in appropriate receptacle. Perform hand hygiene.	Reduces transfer of microorganisms.
19. If suppository contains laxative or fecal softener, place call light within reach so patient can obtain help to reach bedpan or toilet.	Ability to call for help provides patient with sense of control over elimination.
20. If suppository was given for constipation, remind patient *not* to flush commode after bowel movement.	Allows staff to evaluate results of suppository.

EVALUATION

1. Return to bedside within 5 minutes to determine if suppository was expelled.	Determines if drug is distributed properly. Reinsertion may be necessary.
2. Ask if patient experienced localized anal or rectal discomfort during insertion.	Determines whether insertion of suppository was irritating.
3. Evaluate patient at time of peak drug effect for relief of symptoms for which medication was prescribed.	Determines effectiveness of medication.
4. **Use Teach-Back:** "I want to be sure I explained clearly to you how to insert a rectal suppository. Describe the steps you take to insert the suppository." Revise your instruction now or develop a plan for revised patient or family caregiver teaching if patient or family caregiver is not able to teach back correctly.	Determines patient's and family caregiver's level of understanding of instructional topic.

Unexpected Outcomes	Related Interventions
1. Patient's symptoms are unrelieved.	• Explore alternative therapy.
2. Patient experiences decreased heart rate during rectal suppository insertion.	• Unintended vagal stimulation may occur, resulting in bradycardia in some patients.
	• Monitor heart rate of patient. Rectal route may not be suitable for certain cardiac conditions.
3. Patient reports rectal pain during insertion.	• Suppository may need more lubrication.
	• Rectal route may not be suitable; assess and notify health care provider.

Recording and Reporting

- Record the drug, dosage, route, and actual time and date of administration on MAR immediately after administration, not before. Include initials or signature.
- Record patient response to medication, patient teaching, and validation of patient understanding and self-administration of suppository on flow sheet or in nurses' notes in electronic health record (EHR) or chart.
- Report adverse effects/patient response and/or withheld drugs to nurse in charge or health care provider.

Special Considerations
Teaching

- Be certain that patient is aware that the foil wrapper must be removed before insertion and that the suppository is to be inserted rectally and not taken orally. If patient chooses to self-administer suppositories or if a family caregiver plans to administer, teach principles and techniques of infection control to prevent contact with and spread of fecal material.

Pediatric

- With children it is often necessary to gently hold or tape the buttocks together for 5 to 10 minutes to relieve pressure on the anal sphincter until the urge to expel the suppository is gone (Hockenberry and Wilson, 2015).

Gerontological

- Older adults with loss of sphincter control may have difficulty retaining suppository.
- Older adults may have difficulty manipulating suppository, applicator, or irrigating equipment. If so, a family caregiver may need instruction on how to insert the medication.

◆ CLINICAL DEBRIEF

A 75-year-old African-American homemaker is hospitalized for 3 days with a diagnosis of dehydration, following a week of gastroenteritis. She has a history of hypertension, asthma, angina (heart pain), and osteoarthritis in her hands. She also has an abscess on her right calf that was caused by an infected bug bite. Her medications include:

- Hydrochlorothiazide 25 mg every morning by mouth (PO) (diuretic)
- Diltiazem SR capsule, 60 mg twice a day PO (calcium channel blocker)
- Albuterol MDI 2 puffs 4 times a day (inhaled bronchodilator)
- Bacitracin topical ointment (500 units/g) applied topically to wound twice a day (antibiotic)
- Nitroglycerin transdermal patch, 0.2 mg/h, one each morning topically (nitrate)
- Nitroglycerin sublingual tablets, 400 mcg, as needed for chest pain (nitrate)

1. She is discharged and has a home nurse follow-up. On initial history she tells the nurse that she sometimes feels dizzy when she changes position. She also complains of a cough. The nurse decides to do a cardiopulmonary assessment first. While listening to her breath sounds, the nurse notes that she has three nitroglycerin transdermal patches on her chest. What should the nurse do first?

2. While inspecting her abscess, the nurse finds that there is a thick crust of old medication on the wound. She explains, "I don't like to waste the medication that is already there, so I just put the new medicine on top of it." How should the nurse intervene?

3. The nurse returns to the home 2 days later and notices that she is still not cleaning the wound and that the wound is larger (3 × 5 cm), is blistered, and has yellow, foul-smelling drainage. Using SBAR, show how to communicate with other home care nurses for this patient.

◆ REVIEW QUESTIONS

1. A patient is to receive medications through a small-bore nasogastric feeding. Which nursing actions are appropriate? (Select all that apply.)
   1. Verifying tube placement after medications are given
   2. Mixing all medications together and giving all at once
   3. Using an enteral tube syringe to administer medications
   4. Flushing tube with 30 to 60 mL of water after the last dose of medication
   5. Checking for gastric residual before giving the medications
   6. Keeping the head of the bed elevated 30 to 60 minutes after the medications are given

2. The nurse is caring for a patient who is receiving nitroglycerin ointment. Which nursing interventions are most appropriate to protect the nurse against accidental exposure? (Select all that apply.)
   1. Cleaning skin thoroughly before applying the next dose of medication
   2. Wearing gloves when applying the ointment
   3. Using the appropriate applicator to apply the medication
   4. Drawing blood to test for therapeutic drug values
   5. Wearing gloves to discard used ointment wrappers
   6. Performing hand hygiene immediately after mediation application

3. A nurse is administering a metered-dose inhaler (MDI) with a spacer to a patient with chronic obstructive pulmonary disease. Place the steps of the procedure in the correct order.
   1. Insert MDI into end of spacer.
   2. Perform a respiratory assessment.
   3. Remove mouthpiece from MDI and spacer device.
   4. Place spacer mouthpiece into patient's mouth and instruct patient to close lips around it.

5. Depress medication canister, spraying 1 puff into spacer device.
6. Shake inhaler for 2 to 5 seconds.
7. Instruct patient to hold breath for 10 seconds.
8. Instruct patient to breathe in slowly through mouth for 3 to 5 seconds.

ⓔ *Visit the Evolve site for a complete list of Clinical Debrief and Review Questions answers.*

REFERENCES

Alassaad A, et al: Prescription and transcription errors in multidose-dispensed medications on discharge from hospital: an observational and interventional study, *J Eval Clin Pract* 19:185, 2013.

Allen SM: As a flushing agent for enteral nutrition, does sterile water compared with tap water affect associated risk of infection in critically ill patients, *Ala Nurse* March-April-May:5, 2015.

American Society of Health-System Pharmacists (ASHP): *How to use a transdermal patch properly*, 2013a, http://www.safemedication.com/safemed/MedicationTips Tools/HowtoAdminister/How-to-Use-Transdermal-Patches. Accessed May 14, 2016.

American Society of Health-System Pharmacists (ASHP): *How to use eyedrops properly*, 2013b, http://www.safemedication.com/safemed/medicationtipsTools/ HowtoAdminister?howtouseEyedropsProperly. Accessed May 14, 2016.

American Society of Health-System Pharmacists (ASHP): *How to use nose drops properly*, 2013c, http://www.safemedication.com/safemed/MedicationTipsTools/ HowtoAdminister/HowtoUseNoseDropsProperly.aspx. Accessed May 14, 2016.

American Society of Health-System Pharmacists (ASHP): *How to use nasal spray properly*, 2013d, http://www.safemedication.com/safemed/MedicationTipsTools/ HowtoAdminister/HowtoUseNasalSpraysProperly.aspx. Accessed May 14, 2016.

Ari A: Patient education and adherence to aerosol therapy, *Respir Care* 60(6):941, 2015.

Barrons R, et al: Inhaler device selection: special considerations in elderly patients with chronic obstructive pulmonary disease, *Am J Health Syst Pharm* 68(13): 1221, 2011.

Beckett V, et al: Accurately administering oral medication to children isn't child's play, *Arch Dis Child* 97:838, 2012.

Berben L, et al: Which interventions are used by health care professionals to enhance medication adherence in cardiovascular patients? A survey of current clinical practice, *Eur J Cardiovasc Nurs* 10(1):14, 2011.

Blumenstein I, et al: Gastroenteric tube feeding: techniques, problems and solutions, *World J Gastroenterol* 20(26):8505, 2014.

Bonkowski J, et al: Effect of barcode-assisted medication administration on emergency department medication errors, *Acad Emerg Med* 20:801, 2013.

Burchum JR, Rosenthal LD: *Lehne's pharmacology for nursing care*, ed 8, Philadelphia, 2016, Saunders.

Centers for Medicare and Medicaid Services (CMS): *Updated guidance on medication administration*, 2011, http://www.ismp.org/download/files/updated_IGs_ Medication_Adminis_Nov-18-11.pdf. Accessed January 25, 2016.

Clifford P, et al: Following the evidence: enteral tube placement and verification in neonates and young children, *J Perinat Neonatal Nurs* 29(2):149, 2015.

Cohen H: Prevent adverse drug events from topical medications, *Nursing* 43(7):68, 2013.

Dana Farber Cancer Institute: *Five Things You Need to Know About Oral Chemotherapy* March 2, 2015, http://blog.dana-farber.org/insight/2015/03/ five-things-you-need-to-know-about-oral-chemotherapy/ Accessed May 14, 2016.

Food and Drug Administration (FDA): *Best practices for tablet splitting*, 2013, http:// www.fda.gov/Drugs/ResourcesForYou/Consumers/BuyingUsingMedicine Safely/EnsuringSafeUseofMedicine/ucm184666.htm. Accessed January 25, 2016.

Guenther P: New enteral connectors: raising awareness, *Nutr Clin Pract* 29:612, 2015.

Guenther P, Boullatta J: Drug administration by enteral feeding tube, *Nursing* 43(12):26, 2013.

Hockenberry M, Wilson D: *Wong's nursing care of infants and children*, ed 10, St Louis, 2015, Mosby.

Institute for Safe Medication Practices (ISMP): *Never use parenteral syringes for oral medications*, 2010, http://www.accessdata.fda.gov/psn/transcript.cfm?show=94 #9. Accessed January 25, 2016.

Institute for Safe Medication Practices (ISMP): *ISMP acute care guidelines for timely administration of scheduled medications,* 2011, http://www.ismp.org/Tools/guidelines/acutecare/tasm.pdf. Accessed May 9, 2016.

Institute for Safe Medication Practices (ISMP): *ISMP's list of error-prone abbreviations, symbols, and dose designations,* 2013, http://www.ismp.org/Tools/errorproneabbreviations.pdf. Accessed January 25, 2016.

Institute for Safe Medication Practices (ISMP): *Oral dosage forms that should not be crushed,* 2015a, http://www.ismp.org/tools/donotcrush.pdf. Accessed May 8, 2016.

Institute for Safe Medication Practices (ISMP): *ISMP's list of confused drug names,* 2015b, http://www.ismp.org/Tools/confuseddrugnames.pdf. Accessed January 25, 2016.

Institute for Safe Medication Practices (ISMP): *2016-2017 targeted medication safety best practices for hospitals,* 2016, http://ismp.org/tools/bestpractices/default.aspx. Accessed January 25, 2016.

Johansson-Pajala R, et al: Nurses' self-reported medication competence in relation to their pharmacovigilant activities in clinical practice, *J Eval Clin Pract* 21:145, 2014.

Kelly J, et al: An analysis of two incidents of medicine administration to a patient with dysphagia, *J Clin Nurs* 20(1–2):146, 2011.

Kim J, Bates DW: Medication administration errors by nurses: adherence to guidelines, *J Clin Nurs* 22:290, 2013.

Klang M, et al: Osmolality, pH, and compatibility of selected oral liquid medications with an enteral nutrition product, *JPEN J Parenter Enteral Nutr* 37:869, 2013.

Lareau S, Hodder R: Teaching inhaler use in chronic obstructive lung disease patients, *J Am Acad Nurse Pract* 24:113, 2012.

Lawton S: Safe and effective application of topical treatments to the skin, *Nurs Stand* 23(42):50, 2013.

Malone A: Clinical guidelines from the American Society for Parenteral and Enteral Nutrition: best practices recommendations for patient care, *J Infus Nurs* 37(3):179, 2014.

McIntyre CM, Monk HM: Medication absorption considerations in patient with postpyloric enteral feeding tubes, *Am J Health Syst Pharm* 71(7):549, 2014.

Medline Plus, US National Library of Medicine: *How to use a nebulizer,* 2014, https://www.nlm.nih.gov/medlineplus/ency/patientinstructions/000006.htm Accessed May 15, 2016.

National Alert Network (NAN): Move toward full use of metric dosing: eliminate dosage cups that measure liquid in fluid drams. Use cups that measure mL, *National Alert Network,* June 30, 2015, https://www.ismp.org/NAN/files/NAN-20150630.pdf. Accessed May 8, 2016.

O'Conor R, et al: Health literacy, cognitive function, proper use and adherence in inhaled asthma controller medications among older adults, *Chest* 147(5):1307, 2015.

Paparella S: Adopt the 2014-2015 targeted best practices for medication safety, *J Emerg Nurs* 40(3):263, 2014.

Park YH, et al: Prevalence and associated factors of dysphagia in nursing home residents, *Geriatr Nurs* 34(3):212, 2013.

Prakash V, et al: Mitigating errors caused by interruptions during medication verification and administration: interventions in a simulated ambulatory chemotherapy setting, *BMJ Qual Saf* 23(11):884, 2014.

Roy A, et al: Inhaler device administration, techniques, and adherence to inhaled corticosteroids in patients with asthma, *Prim Care Respir J* 20(20):148, 2011.

Salmon D, et al: Pharmaceutical and safety considerations of tablet crushing in patients undergoing enteral intubation, *Int J Pharm* 443:146, 2013.

Seibert HH, et al: Effect of barcode technology with electronic medication administration record on medication accuracy rates, *Am J Health Syst Pharm* 71:209, 2014.

Sulosaari V, et al: An integrative review of the literature on registered nurses' medication competence, *J Clin Nurs* 20(3–4):464, 2011.

Teunissen R, et al: Clinical relevance of risk factors associated with medication administration time errors, *Am J Health Syst Pharm* 70:1052, 2013.

The Joint Commission (TJC): *Sentinel alert event: managing risk during transition to new ISO connector standards,* 2014, http://www.jointcommission.org/assets/1/6/SEA_53_Connectors_8_19_14_final.pdf. Accessed January 25, 2016.

The Joint Commission (TJC): *National Patient Safety Goals,* Oakbrook Terrace, IL, 2016, The Commission, http://www.jointcommission.org/standards_information/npsgs.aspx. Accessed January 25, 2016.

To T, et al: Oral medication administration in patients with restrictions in oral intake: a snapshot survey, *J Res Pharm Pract* 43:177, 2013.

Touhy TA, Jett KF: *Ebersole and Hess' nursing & healthy aging,* ed 4, St Louis, 2014, Elsevier.

Tzeng H, et al: Medication error-related issues in nursing practice, *Medsurg Nurs* 22(1):13, 2013.

Yoder M, et al: The effect of a safe zone on nurse interruptions, distractions, and medication administration errors, *J Infus Nurs* 38(2):140, 2015.

Zhu L, Zhou Q: Therapeutic concerns when oral medications are administered nasogastrically, *J Clin Pharm Ther* 38:272, 2013.

SKILLS AND PROCEDURES

OBJECTIVES

Mastery of content in this chapter will enable the nurse to:

- Correctly prepare injectable medications from a vial and an ampule.
- Identify advantages, disadvantages, and risks of administering medications by each parenteral route.
- Evaluate the effectiveness and outcomes of administering medications by each parenteral route.
- Explain the importance of selecting the proper-size syringe and needle for an injection.
- Discuss factors to consider when selecting injection sites.
- Discuss ways to promote patient comfort while administering an injection.
- Correctly administer intradermal, subcutaneous, and intramuscular injections.
- Compare the risks of three different intravenous routes.
- Correctly administer an intravenous medication by intravenous piggyback, intermittent infusion, or bolus.
- Initiate, maintain, and discontinue a continuous subcutaneous infusion.

MEDIA RESOURCES

- evolve http://evolve.elsevier.com/Perry/skills
- Review Questions
- ▶ Video Clips
- Audio Glossary
- **NSO** Nursing Skills Online
- Clinical Debrief and Review Questions Answers

PURPOSE

Medications administered by the *parenteral* route enter body tissues and the circulatory system by injection. Injected medications are more quickly absorbed than oral medications. Parenteral routes are used when patients are vomiting or cannot swallow, when rapid onset of a medication is needed, and/or when patients are restricted from taking oral fluids. These medication administration procedures are invasive and thus pose greater risks than those associated with administering nonparenteral medications (see Chapter 21).

Each type of injection requires a certain set of skills to ensure that the medication reaches the proper location. There are four routes for parenteral administration:

1. *Subcutaneous injection:* Injection into tissues just under the dermis of the skin
2. *Intramuscular (IM) injection:* Injection into the body of a muscle
3. *Intradermal (ID) injection:* Injection into the dermis just under the epidermis
4. *Intravenous (IV) injection or infusion:* Injection into a vein

STANDARDS OF CARE

- Centers for Medicare & Medicaid Services (CMS), 2015—Preparation and Administration of Drugs
- Infusion Nurses Society, 2016—Infusion Nursing Standards of Practice
- Institute for Safe Medication Practices (ISMP), 2011; 2012; 2015—Safe Medication Preparation
- The Joint Commission, 2016—Patient Identification

PRINCIPLES FOR PRACTICE

- When managing a patient's medications, communicate clearly with the interprofessional team, assess and incorporate the patient's priorities of care and preferences, and use the best evidence when making decisions about patient care.
- Use technology (e.g., bar scanning, electronic medication administration record [MAR]) that is available in your agency when preparing and giving medications.

- Educate patients and family caregivers about each medication they take while you are administering medications. Patients often are able to identify inappropriate medications. Make sure that you answer all of their questions before administering medications. Educate family caregivers if appropriate.
- Minimize a patient's discomfort when giving an injection:
  - Use sharp, beveled needles in the shortest length and smallest gauge possible.
  - Change the needle if liquid medication coats the shaft of the needle.
  - Position and flex a patient's limbs to reduce muscular tension.
  - Divert the patient's attention away from the injection procedure.
  - Apply a vapocoolant spray (e.g., Flouri-Methane spray or ethyl chloride) or topical anesthetic (e.g., EMLA cream) to an injection site before giving a medication when possible, or place wrapped ice on the site for a minute before injection.

PATIENT-CENTERED CARE

- Research shows that ethnicity, genetics, and culture influence drug response, pharmacokinetics, and pharmacodynamics, and patient adherence and education (Burchum and Rosenthal, 2016; Giger, 2017; Tantisira et al., 2015).
- Knowledge about variations in therapeutic dose and adverse effects is essential in administering medications to different ethnic groups. Some patients experience a therapeutic response at a different dosage than recommended and require careful monitoring.
- You need skill in communicating with and educating diverse patient populations. For example, if a patient values patience and modesty, make your questions specific and take time when assessing his or her knowledge about adverse drug effects.
- Cultural assessment also yields information about dietary preferences, tobacco and alcohol use, and use of herbal remedies that affect drug action and response.
- Cultural context is essential in planning education for patients and families (Burchum and Rosenthal, 2016).

EVIDENCE-BASED PRACTICE

There is increasing evidence that addresses practice guidelines for administration of IM injections. IM injection technique has been modified over the past several years in response to evidence and research about best practices for patient assessment and site selection (Ogston-Tuck, 2014b). In the past site selection was not evidence based, and needle selection was based on nursing preference and ritualistic practice (Greenway, 2014). There is now enough consensual evidence to develop guidelines for administration of IM injections. On the basis of this evidence:

- Select needle size based on patient gender, weight and body mass index, condition, site, drug, and volume.
- Make the ventrogluteal site the first choice wherever possible for deep IM injections because there are reduced risks of nerve or muscle injury.
- Assess the skin and the patient's condition before and after an IM injection.
- Inject at 90 degrees, dartlike, to the hub of the needle and inject at 1 mL per second.
- Wait at least 10 seconds before withdrawing the needle.

SAFETY GUIDELINES

Patient safety in administering medication involves following the six rights of medication administration (see Chapter 20). Follow these guidelines to ensure safe medication administration:

- Be vigilant during medication administration. Avoid distractions while preparing an injection.
- Be sure that your patients receive the appropriate medications. Know why your patient is receiving each medication; know what you need to do before, during, and after medication administration; and evaluate the effectiveness of medications and any adverse effects after administration.
- Verify that the medications have not expired.
- Use at least two identifiers before administering medications and check against the MAR. Follow agency policy for patient identification (TJC, 2016).
- Clarify unclear medication orders and ask for help whenever you are uncertain about an order or calculation. Consult with your peers, pharmacists, and other health care providers and be sure that you have resolved all concerns related to medication administration before preparing and giving medications.
- Follow all policies related to use of the technology and do not use "work-arounds." A **work-around** bypasses a procedure, policy, or problem in a system. Nurses who use "work-arounds fail to follow agency protocols, policies, or procedures during medication administration in an attempt to get medications administered to patients in a more timely manner.
- Use strict aseptic technique during medication preparation and administration (Table 22.1).
- Most of the time you cannot delegate medication administration. Ensure that you follow standards set by the Nurse Practice Act in your state and guidelines established by your health care agency. Licensed practical nurses (LPNs) or licensed vocational nurses (LVNs) usually can administer medications via the oral (PO), subcutaneous, IM, and ID routes. Some states allow certified medication assistants (CMAs) to administer certain types of medications (e.g., oral medication) in long-term care facilities.
- No-interruption zones (NIZs) have been recommended by the Institute for Safe Medication Practices (2012). NIZs are created

TABLE 22.1	
Preventing Infection During an Injection	
Principle	**Technique**
Prevent contamination of solution	Ampules should not sit open, and medication should be removed quickly.
Prevent needle contamination	Avoid letting needle touch contaminated surface (e.g., outer edges of ampule or vial, outer surface of needle cap, your hands, countertop, or table surface). Avoid touching length of plunger or inner part of barrel. Keep tip of syringe covered with cap or needle.
Prepare skin	Wash skin soiled with dirt, drainage, or feces with soap and water. Use friction and a circular motion while cleaning with an antiseptic swab. Swab from center of site and move outward in a 5-cm (2-inch) radius.
Reduce transfer of microorganisms	Perform hand hygiene for a minimum of 15 seconds.

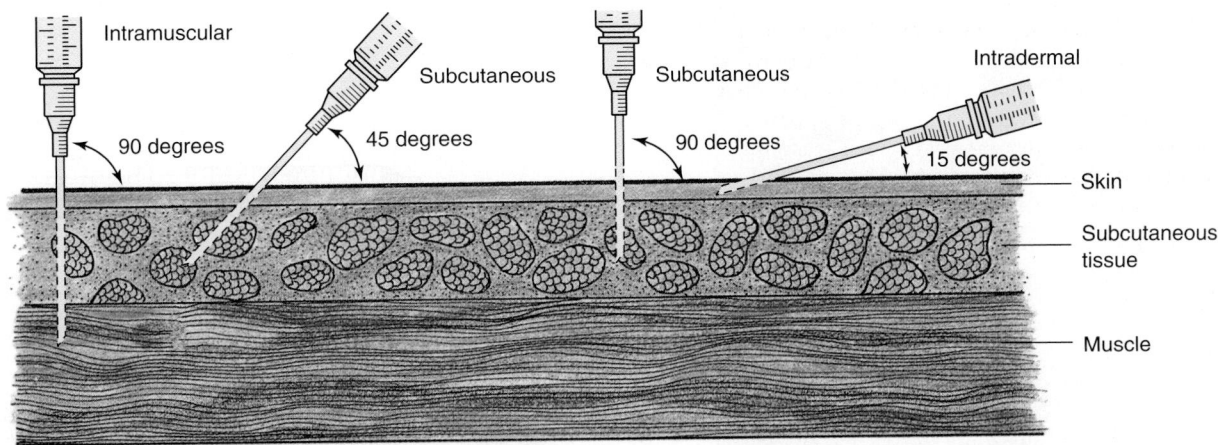

FIG 22.1 Comparison of angles of insertion of intramuscular (90 degrees), subcutaneous (45 or 90 degrees), and intradermal (15 degrees) injections.

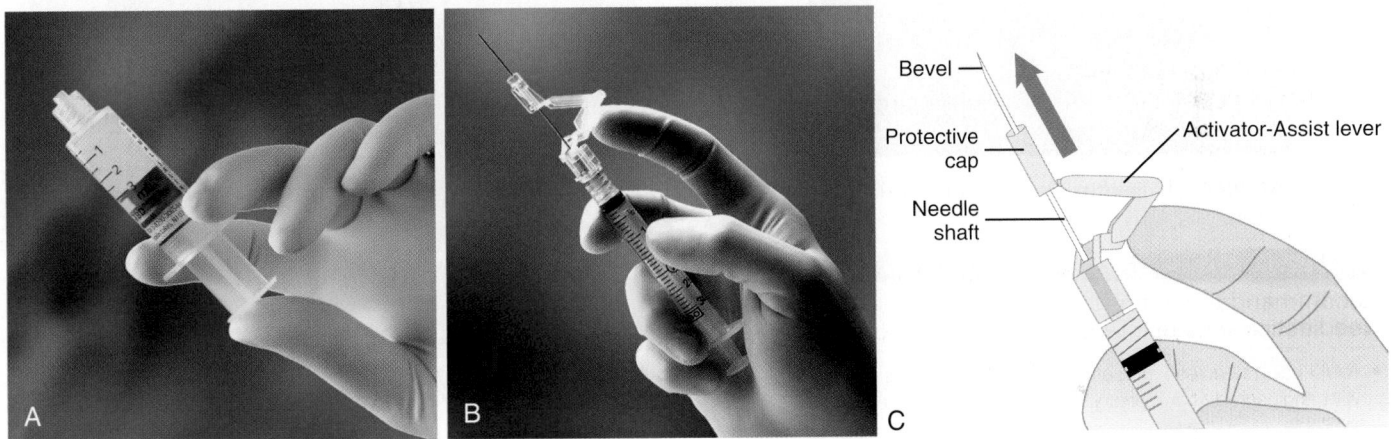

FIG 22.2 A, Needleless system. **B,** Safety needle system. **C,** Detail of safety needle system. (**A** *and* **B** *Courtesy and ©Becton, Dickinson and Company.*)

by placing red tape or tile borders on the floor around medication carts. Nurses standing in these zones are not to be interrupted.

- Insert the needle at the proper angle, smoothly, and quickly (Fig. 22.1). Do not hesitate and slowly push the needle into tissue.
- Inject the medication slowly but smoothly.
- Hold the syringe steady once the needle is in the tissue to prevent tissue damage.
- Withdraw the needle smoothly at the same angle used for insertion.
- Gently apply an antiseptic pad (e.g., alcohol) or dry, sterile gauze pad to the site.
- Apply gentle pressure at the injection site.
- Rotate injection sites to prevent the formation of indurations and abscesses.

Needlestick Prevention

The most frequent route of exposure to bloodborne disease for health care workers is from needlestick injuries (OSHA, n.d.). These injuries occur when health care workers recap needles, mishandle intravenous (IV) lines and needles, or leave needles at a patient's bedside. However, the implementation of safe needle

devices can prevent needlestick injuries (OSHA, n.d.). The Needlestick Safety and Prevention Act is a federal law that mandates health care agencies to use safe needle devices to reduce the frequency of needlestick injury (see Fig. 22.2C). Employers are required to maintain a current exposure control plan and seek employee input when considering changing medical devices (OSHA, n.d.).

A sharp (needle, lancet) with engineered sharps injury protection (SESIP) is a device that is effective in preventing needlesticks. One type of SESIP is a blunt-end cannula; another is a safety syringe equipped with a plastic guard or sheath that slips over the needle as it is withdrawn from the skin (Fig. 22.2A-C). The guard immediately covers the needle, eliminating the chance for a needlestick injury. A variety of other SESIP devices are found in needleless IV line connection systems (see Chapter 29). Box 22.1 lists recommendations for health care workers to reduce their risk of needlestick injuries.

Special puncture- and leak-proof containers are available in health care agencies for the disposal of sharps. Containers are made so only one hand needs to be used when disposing of an uncapped needle. In addition, containers must stand upright, not be allowed to overfill, and be colored red or labeled with a biohazard symbol (Fig. 22.3).

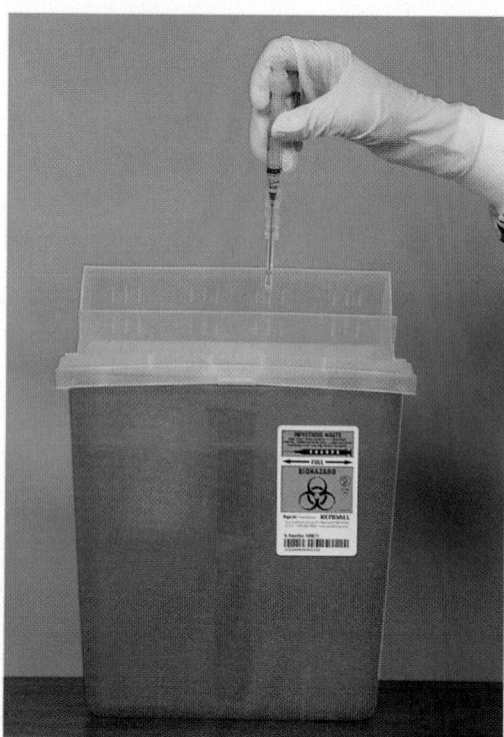

FIG 22.3 Sharps disposal using only one hand.

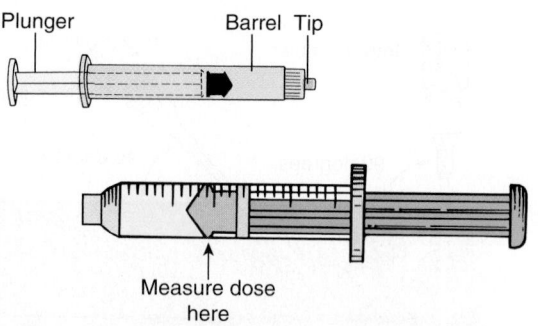

FIG 22.4 Parts of a syringe.

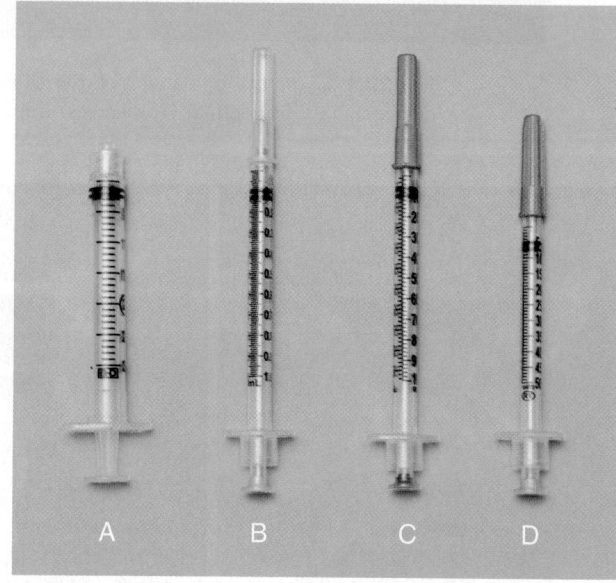

FIG 22.5 Examples of types of syringes. **A,** 5-mL syringe. **B,** 3-mL syringe. **C,** Tuberculin syringe marked in 0.01 (hundredths) for doses of less than 1 mL. **D,** Insulin syringe marked in units (50).

BOX 22.1

Recommendations for the Prevention of Needlestick Injuries

- Avoid using needles when effective needleless systems or sharps with engineered sharps injury protection (SESIP) safety devices are available.
- Do not recap any needle after medication administration.
- Plan safe handling and disposal of needles before beginning a procedure.
- Immediately dispose of needles, needleless systems, and SESIP into puncture-proof and leak-proof sharps disposal containers.
- Maintain a sharps injury log that reports the following: type and brand of device involved in the incident; location of the incident (e.g., department or work area); description of the incident; and privacy of the employees who have had sharps injuries.
- Attend education offerings on bloodborne pathogens and follow recommendations for infection prevention, including receiving the hepatitis B vaccine.
- Participate in the selection and evaluation of SESIP devices with safety features within your agency whenever possible.

Data from Occupational Safety and Health Administration (OSHA): *Bloodborne pathogens and needlestick injuries,* 77 FR 19934, 2012, https://www.osha.gov/FedReg_osha_pdf/FED20120403.pdf. Accessed April 3, 2016.

Equipment

Administer parenteral medication by using a needle and a syringe, available in a variety of sizes. Determine the appropriate size of syringe, length and gauge of needle, volume of solution, and medication route. These decisions are based on the quantity and type of medication prescribed and the body size of a patient. Most syringes come with needleless systems or safety needles that help prevent needlestick injuries. A variety of electronic infusion pumps deliver IV or continuous subcutaneous infusions. Infusion pumps ensure a constant and accurate delivery of medication.

Syringes

Syringes are single use, disposable, and either Luer-Lok or non–Luer-Lok. The design of the syringe tip influences the name. They are packaged separately in a paper wrapper or rigid plastic container. Syringes come with or without a sterile needle and with a needleless SESIP device. The parts of a syringe are shown in (Fig. 22.4). Non–Luer-Lok syringes use needles or needleless devices that slip onto the tip. Luer-Lok syringes (Fig. 22.5A) use standard needles or needleless devices that are twisted onto the tip and lock themselves in place. The Luer-Lok design prevents the accidental removal of a needle from the syringe.

Syringes come in a variety of sizes, ranging in capacity from 0.5 to 60 mL (Fig. 22.5). When you select a syringe, choose the smallest syringe size possible to improve accuracy of medication preparation. In addition, avoid injecting a large volume of fluid into tissues. A 1- to 3-mL syringe is usually adequate for a subcutaneous or IM injection. Larger volumes create pain and discomfort for a patient. Syringes are most commonly marked in a scale of tenths of a milliliter (see Fig. 22.5A). You use tuberculin (TB) syringes to prepare small amounts of medication for intradermal (ID) and subcutaneous injections (see Fig. 22.5B). Insulin syringes (see Fig. 22.5C-D) hold 0.3 mL to 1 mL, and low-dose insulin syringes (30 units per 0.3 mL or 50 units per 0.5 mL) hold 0.3 mL to 1 mL.

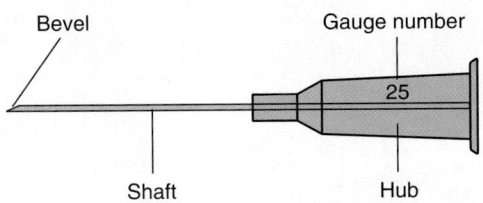

FIG 22.6 Parts of a needle.

Both come with preattached needles and are calibrated in units. Most insulin syringes are U-100s, designed for use with U-100–strength insulin. Each milliliter of solution contains 100 units of insulin.

Use a larger syringe to administer some IV medications and irrigate drainage tubes. Some syringes are packaged with their needle attached; and some syringes require you to change the needle based on the viscosity of the medication, route of administration, gender, and size of the patient. Before use carefully examine the syringe to determine the measurement scale and ensure that you use the correct syringe for preparing the ordered medication.

Needles

Some needles come attached to syringes. Others come packaged individually to allow flexibility in selecting the right needle for a patient. Needles are disposable, and most are made of stainless steel. A needle has three parts: the hub, which fits onto the tip of a syringe; the shaft, which connects to the hub; and the bevel, or slanted tip (Fig. 22.6). The needle hub, shaft, and bevel must remain sterile at all times. To prevent contamination, use gentle force to place the needle onto the syringe with the cap intact (Fig. 22.7A–B). Some needles come with filters for preparation of medications. Never use filters when administering a medication.

The tip of a needle, or the bevel, is always slanted. The bevel creates a narrow slit when injected into tissue that quickly closes after the needle is removed to prevent leakage of medication, blood, or serum. Longer beveled tips are sharper and narrower, which minimizes tissue discomfort during a subcutaneous or IM injection.

Most needles vary in length from ¼ to 3 inches (Fig. 22.8). Choose the needle length according to a patient's size and weight and the type of tissue into which the medication is to be injected. Current evidence suggests that needle length should be based on the patient's weight (Davidson and Rourke, 2013). There should be a 5-mm depth of muscle penetration to achieve an IM injection (Hibbard et al., 2015). A child or slender adult generally requires a shorter needle. Use longer needles (1 to 1½ inches) for IM injections and a shorter needle (⅜ to ⅝ inch) for subcutaneous injections. As the needle gauge becomes smaller, the needle diameter becomes larger. The selection of a gauge depends on the viscosity of fluid to be injected or infused; the greater the viscosity, the larger the gauge.

Disposable Injection Units

Single-dose, prefilled, disposable syringes are available for some medications. You do not need to prepare medication doses, except perhaps to expel unneeded parts of medication or air.

However, it is important to check the medication and concentration carefully because prefilled syringes appear very similar. Prefilled unit-dose systems such as Tubex and Carpuject injection systems include reusable plastic syringe holders and disposable, prefilled, sterile, glass cartridge units. To assemble a prefilled system,

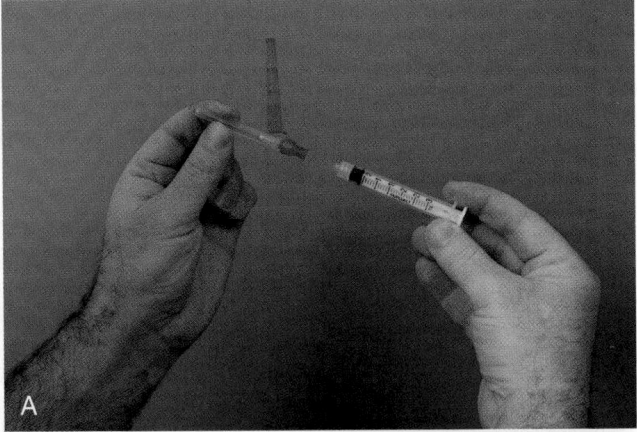

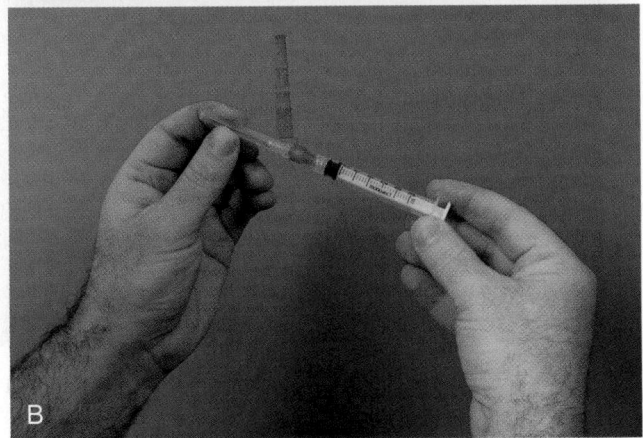

FIG 22.7 A, Capped needle placed on syringe tip. **B,** Needle secured.

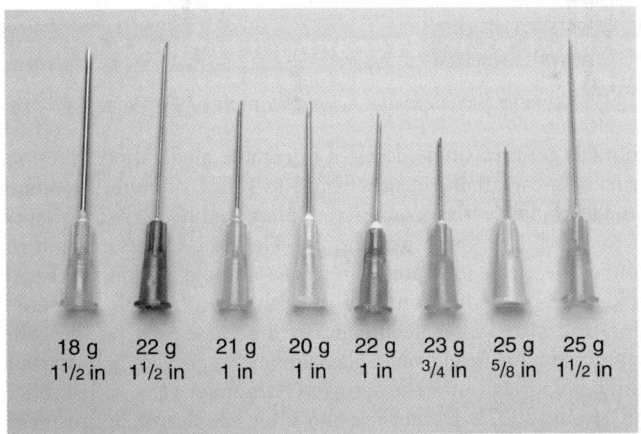

| 18 g | 22 g | 21 g | 20 g | 22 g | 23 g | 25 g | 25 g |
| 1½ in | 1½ in | 1 in | 1 in | 1 in | ¾ in | ⅝ in | 1½ in |

FIG 22.8 Needles come in a variety of gauges and lengths. Choose correct needle, gauge, and length for the injection ordered. (*Lilley LL, et al: Pharmacology for nurses and the nursing process, ed 7, St Louis, 2012, Mosby.*)

place the cartridge, barrel first, into the plastic syringe holder (Fig. 22.9A). Following manufacturer instructions, turn the plunger rod to the left (counterclockwise) (see Fig. 22.9B) and then lock to the right (clockwise) until it "clicks" (see Fig. 22.9C). Finally remove the needle guard and advance the plunger (see Fig. 22.9D) to expel air and any excess medication as with a regular syringe. The cartridge may be used with SESIP needles. After giving a medication, dispose of the glass cartridge safely in a puncture- and leak-proof container. This design reduces the risk for needlestick injury.

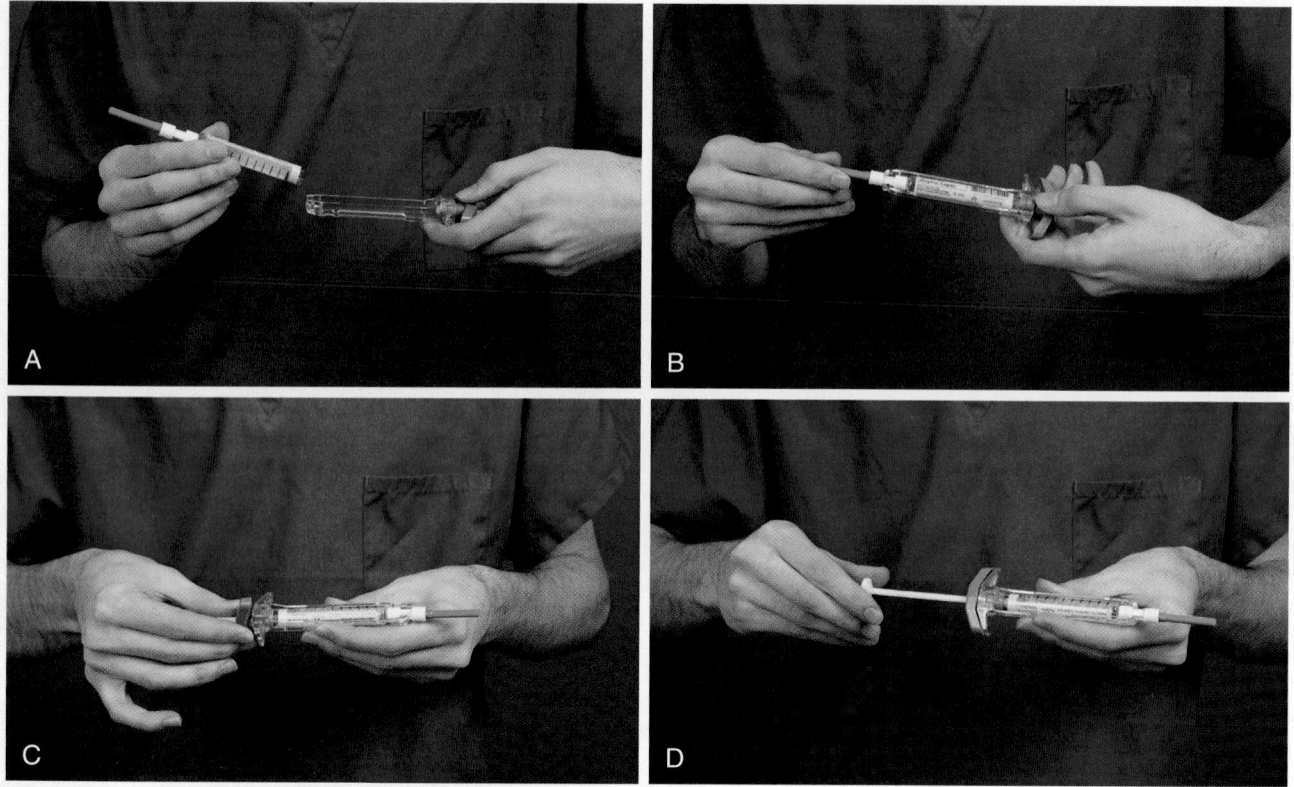

FIG 22.9 A, Carpuject syringe holder and prefilled sterile cartridge with needle. **B,** Assembling the Carpuject. **C,** Cartridge slides into syringe barrel, turns, and locks at needle end. **D,** Plunger screws into cartridge end.

◆ SKILL 22.1   Preparing Injections: Ampules and Vials

NSO *Nursing Skills Online Administration of Parenteral Medications: Injections Module / Lesson 2*

Ampules contain single doses of injectable medication in a liquid form and are available in sizes from 1 to 10 mL or more. An ampule is made of glass with a constricted, prescored neck that is snapped off to allow access to a medication (Fig. 22.10A). A colored ring around the neck indicates where the ampule is prescored to be broken easily. Medication is easily withdrawn from the ampule by aspirating with a filter needle and syringe. Use filter needles when preparing medication from a glass ampule to prevent glass particles from being drawn into the syringe (Alexander et al., 2014; Nicoll and Hesby, 2002). *Do not* use the filter needle to administer the medication. Place an appropriate-size needle on the syringe after withdrawing the medication.

A vial is a single- or multi-dose plastic or glass container with a rubber seal at the top (see Fig. 22.10B). After you open a single-dose vial discard it, regardless of the amount of medication used (Alexander et al., 2014). A multi-dose vial contains several doses of a medication and thus can be used several times, although only for a single patient. When using a multi-dose vial, write the date that the vial is opened on the vial label. Verify agency policy as to how long an opened multi-dose vial may be used. Properly discard a multi-dose vial when the allowed time for being open has expired.

A metal or plastic cap protects a rubber seal of the vial. Remove the cap when you first prepare the vial for use. Vials may contain liquid or dry forms of medications; medications that are unstable in solution are packaged in dry form. The vial label specifies the solvent or diluents used to dissolve the medication and the amount needed to prepare a desired medication concentration. Normal saline and sterile distilled water are the most common solutions.

Some vials have two chambers separated by a rubber stopper. One chamber contains the diluent solution; the other contains the dry medication. Before preparing the medication, push on the upper chamber to dislodge the rubber stopper and allow the powder and the diluent to mix. Unlike an ampule, a vial is a closed system. You must inject air into the vial to permit easy withdrawal of the solution. Some medications, even when in a vial, may need to be drawn up with a filter needle because of the nature of the medication. Agency policies and package inserts from the manufacturer indicate drugs that should be prepared with a filter needle.

Occasionally the health care provider orders an injectable medication that must be reconstituted because it comes in a powdered form. This frequently occurs with a time-sensitive injectable medication, which must be administered within a specific time period to guarantee full drug effectiveness.

Delegation and Collaboration

The skill of preparing injections from ampules and vials cannot be delegated to nursing assistive personnel (NAP).

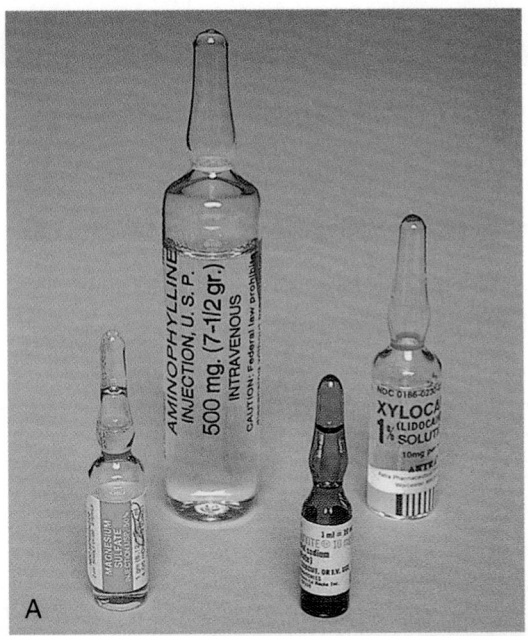

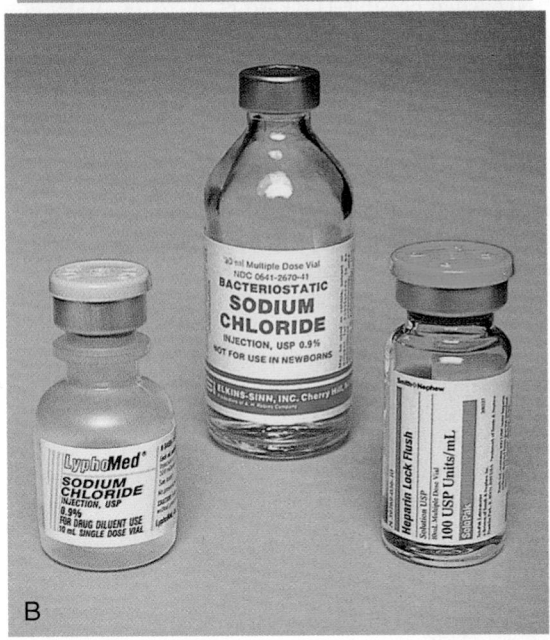

FIG 22.10 A, Medication in ampules. **B,** Medication in vials.

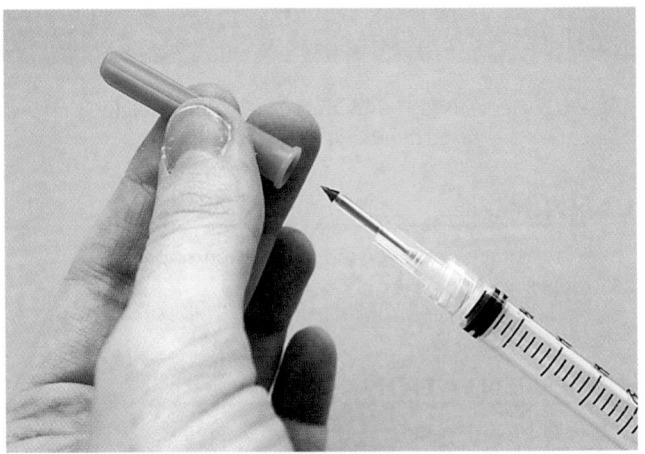

FIG. 22.11 Syringe with needleless vial access adapter.

Equipment

Medication in an Ampule
- Syringe, needle, and filter needle
- Small sterile gauze pad or unopened alcohol swab

Medication in a Vial
- Syringe and two needles
- Needles:
  - Needleless blunt-tip vial access cannula (Fig. 22.11) or needle (with safety sheath) for drawing up medication (if needed)
  - Filter needle if indicated
- Small, sterile gauze pad or alcohol swab
- Diluent (e.g., 0.9% sodium chloride or sterile water if indicated)

Both
- Medication administration record (MAR) or computer printout
- Sharps with engineered sharps injury protection (SESIP) safety needle for injection
- Medication in vial or ampule
- Puncture-proof container for disposal of syringes, needles, and glass

STEP	RATIONALE

ASSESSMENT

1. Check accuracy and completeness of each MAR or computer printout with health care provider's written medication order. Check patient's name, medication name and dosage, route of administration, and time of administration. Recopy or reprint any part of MAR that is difficult to read.

The order sheet is the most reliable source and only legal record of medications that patient is to receive. Ensures that patient receives the correct medications (Mandrack et al., 2012). Illegible MARs are a source of medication errors (Alassaad et al., 2013).

2. Assess patient's medical and medication history.

Determines need for medication or possible contraindications for medication administration.

3. Assess patient's history of allergies. Know type of allergies and normal allergic response.

Do not prepare medication if there is a known patient allergy.

4. Review medication reference information for action, purpose, side effects, and nursing implications.

Allows you to administer drug properly and monitor patient's response.

STEP	RATIONALE
5. Assess patient's body build, muscle size, and weight if giving subcutaneous or intramuscular (IM) medication.	Determines type and size of syringe and needle for injection.

PLANNING

1. Expected outcomes following completion of procedure: • Proper dose is prepared. • No air bubbles are in syringe barrel.	Ensures right dose. Air bubbles displace medication. Elimination of air ensures accuracy of medication dose.

IMPLEMENTATION

1. Perform hand hygiene and prepare supplies.	Reduces transmission of microorganisms.
2. Prepare medications.	
a. If using a medication cart, move it outside patient's room.	Organization of equipment saves time and reduces error.
b. Unlock medication drawer or cart or log onto computerized medication dispensing system.	Medications are safeguarded when locked in cabinet, cart, or computerized medication dispensing system.
c. Follow agency's no-interruption zone (NIZ) policy. Prepare medications for one patient at a time. Keep all pages of MARs or computer printouts for one patient together or look at only one patient's electronic MAR at a time.	Preventing distractions reduces medication preparation errors. Use NIZ when possible (Prakash et al., 2014; Yoder et al., 2015).
d. Select correct drug from stock supply or unit-dose drawer. Compare label of medication with MAR computer printout or computer screen.	Reading label and comparing it with transcribed order reduce errors. *This is the first check for accuracy.*
e. Check expiration date on each medication, one at a time.	Medications used past their expiration date are sometimes inactive, less effective, or harmful to patients.
f. Calculate drug dose as necessary. Double-check calculation. Ask another nurse to check calculations if needed.	Double-checking reduces error.
g. If preparing a controlled substance, check record for previous drug count and compare with supply available.	Controlled substance laws require careful monitoring of dispensed narcotics.
h. Do not leave drugs unattended.	Nurse is responsible for safekeeping of drugs.
3. Prepare ampule.	
a. Tap top of ampule lightly and quickly with finger until fluid moves from its neck (see illustration).	Dislodges any fluid that collects above neck of ampule. All solution moves into lower chamber.

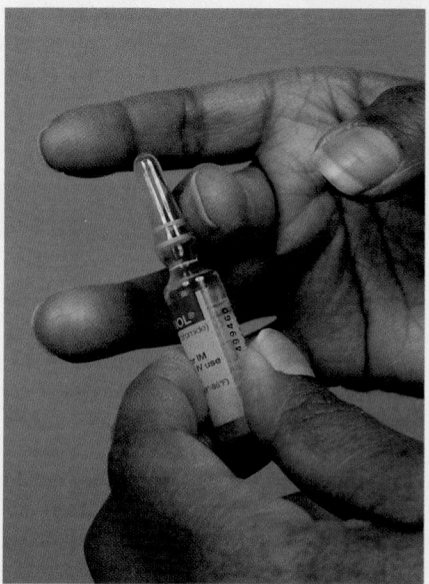

STEP 3a Tapping ampule moves fluid down neck.

STEP	RATIONALE
b. Place small gauze pad around neck of ampule (see illustration).	Protects fingers from trauma as glass tip is broken off. Do not use opened alcohol swab to wrap around top of ampule because alcohol may leak into ampule.
c. Snap neck of ampule quickly and firmly away from hands (see illustration).	Protects your fingers and face from shattering glass.
d. Draw up medication quickly, using filter needle long enough to reach bottom of ampule to access medication.	System is open to airborne contaminants. Filter needles filter out any fragments of glass (Alexander et al., 2014).
e. Hold ampule upside down or set it on flat surface. Insert filter needle into center of ampule opening. Do not allow needle tip or shaft to touch rim of ampule.	Broken rim of ampule is considered contaminated. When ampule is inverted, solution dribbles out if needle tip or shaft touches rim of ampule.
f. Aspirate medication into syringe by gently pulling back on plunger (see illustration).	Withdrawal of plunger creates negative pressure within syringe barrel, which pulls fluid into syringe.

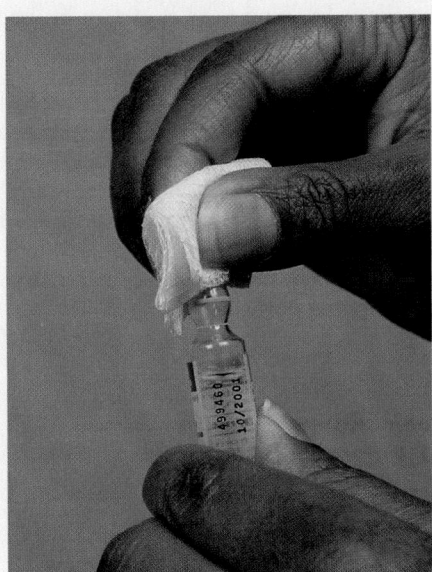

STEP 3b Gauze pad placed around neck of ampule.

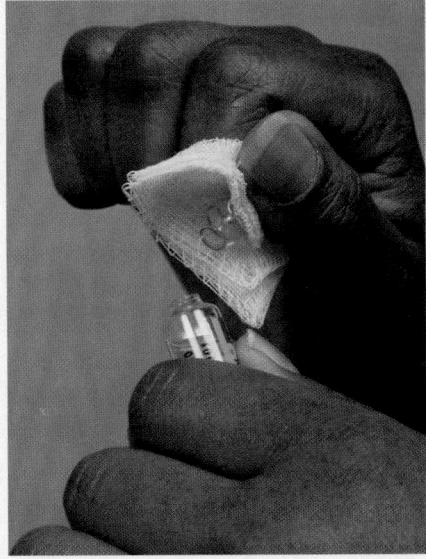

STEP 3c Neck snapped away from hands.

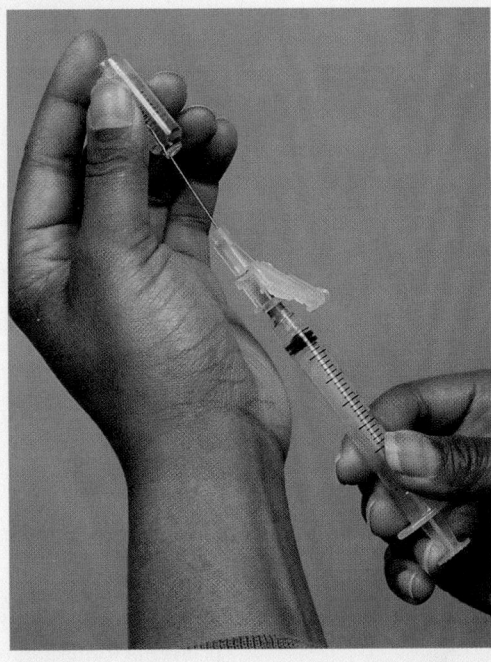

STEP 3f Medication aspirated with ampule inverted.

STEP	RATIONALE
g. Keep needle tip under surface of liquid. Tip ampule to bring all fluid within reach of needle.	Prevents aspiration of air bubbles.
h. If you aspirate air bubbles, do not expel air into ampule.	Air pressure forces fluid out of ampule, and medication will be lost.
i. To expel excess air bubbles, remove needle from ampule. Hold syringe vertically with needle pointing up. Tap side of syringe to cause bubbles to rise toward needle. Draw back slightly on plunger and push plunger upward to eject air. Do not eject fluid.	Withdrawing plunger too far removes it from barrel. Holding syringe vertically allows fluid to settle in bottom of barrel. Pulling back on plunger allows fluid within needle to enter barrel so fluid is not expelled. You then expel air at top of barrel and within needle.
j. If syringe contains excess fluid, use sink for disposal. Hold syringe vertically with needle tip up and slanted slightly toward sink. Slowly eject excess fluid into sink. Recheck fluid level in syringe by holding it vertically.	Safely disperses excess medication into sink. Position of needle allows you to expel medication without having it flow down needle shaft. Rechecking fluid level ensures proper dose.
k. Cover needle with its safety sheath or cap. Replace filter needle with regular SESIP needle.	Minimizes needlesticks. Filter needles cannot be used for injection.
4. Prepare vial containing a solution.	
a. Remove cap covering top of unused vial to expose sterile rubber seal. If a multi-dose vial has been used before, cap is already removed. Firmly and briskly wipe surface of rubber seal with alcohol swab and allow it to dry.	Vial comes packaged with cap that cannot be replaced after seal removal. Not all drug manufacturers guarantee that rubber seals of unused vials are sterile. Swabbing with alcohol reduces transmission of microorganisms. Allowing alcohol to dry prevents alcohol from coating needle and mixing with medication.
b. Pick up syringe and remove needle cap or cap covering needleless access device. Pull back on plunger to draw amount of air into syringe equivalent to volume of medication to be aspirated from vial.	Injecting air into vial prevents buildup of negative pressure in vial when aspirating medication.

Clinical Decision Point *Some medications and agencies require use of a filter needle when preparing medications from vials. Check agency policy or medication reference. If you use a filter needle to aspirate medication, you need to change it to a regular SESIP needle of the appropriate size to administer medication (Alexander et al., 2014).*

c. With vial on flat surface, insert tip of needle or needleless device through center of rubber seal (see illustration). Apply pressure to tip of needle during insertion.	Center of seal is thinner and easier to penetrate. Using firm pressure prevents dislodging rubber particles that could enter vial or needle.

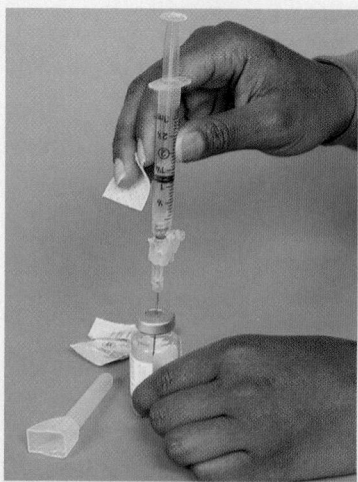

STEP 4c Insert safety needle through center of vial diaphragm (with vial flat on table).

d. Inject air into air space of vial, holding on to plunger. Hold plunger firmly; plunger is sometimes forced backward by air pressure within vial.	Injection of air creates vacuum needed to get medication to flow into syringe. Injecting into air space of vial pr events formation of bubbles and an inaccurate dose.

STEP	RATIONALE
e. Invert vial while keeping firm hold on syringe and plunger. Hold vial between thumb and middle fingers of nondominant hand (see illustration). Grasp end of syringe barrel and plunger with thumb and forefinger of dominant hand to counteract pressure in vial.	Inverting vial allows fluid to settle in lower half of container. Position of hands prevents forceful movement of plunger and permits easy manipulation of syringe.
f. Keep tip of needle or needleless device below fluid level.	Prevents aspiration of air.
g. Allow air pressure from vial to fill syringe gradually with medication. If necessary, pull back slightly on plunger to obtain correct amount of medication.	Positive pressure within vial forces fluid into syringe.
h. When you obtain desired volume, position needle or needleless device into air space of vial; tap side of syringe barrel gently to dislodge any air bubbles (see illustration). Eject any air remaining at top of syringe into vial.	Forcefully striking barrel while needle is inserted in vial may bend needle. Accumulation of air displaces medication and causes dose errors.
i. Remove needle or needleless access device from vial by pulling back on barrel of syringe.	Pulling plunger rather than barrel causes plunger to separate from barrel, resulting in loss of medication.
j. Hold syringe at eye level at 90-degree angle to ensure correct volume and absence of air bubbles. Remove any remaining air by tapping barrel to dislodge any air bubbles. Draw back slightly on plunger; then push it upward to eject air. Do not eject fluid. Recheck volume of medication.	Holding syringe vertically allows fluid to settle in bottom of barrel. Tapping dislodges air to top of barrel. Pulling back on plunger allows fluid within needle to enter barrel so you do not expel fluid. You then expel air at top of barrel and within needle.

Clinical Decision Point *When preparing medication from single-dose vial, do not assume that volume listed on label is total volume in vial. Some manufacturers provide small amount of extra liquid, expecting loss during preparation. Be sure to draw up only desired volume.*

k. If you need to inject medication into patient's tissue, change needle with regular SESIP to appropriate gauge and length according to route of medication administration.	Inserting needle through rubber stopper dulls beveled tip. New needle is sharper and, because no fluid is along shaft, does not track medication through tissues. Filter needles cannot be used for injection.
l. Cover needle with its safety sheath or cap.	Minimizes needlesticks.
m. For multi-dose vial, make label that includes date of opening, concentration of drug per milliliter, and your initials.	Ensures that nurses will prepare future doses correctly. You discard some drugs within a certain time frame after mixing.
5. Prepare vial containing powder (reconstituting medications).	
a. Remove cap covering vial of powdered medication and cap covering vial of proper diluent. Firmly swab both rubber seals with alcohol swab and allow alcohol to dry.	Allowing alcohol to dry prevents it from coating needle and mixing with medication.
b. Draw up manufacturer suggestion for volume and type of diluent into syringe following Steps 4b through 4j.	Prepares diluent for injection into vial containing powdered medication.

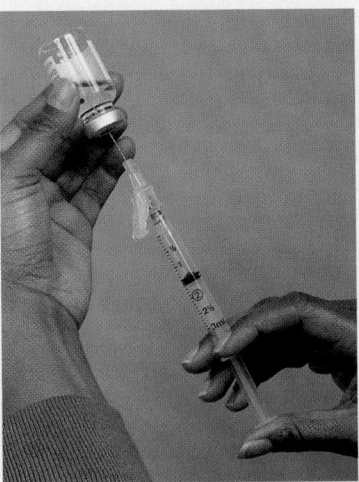

STEP 4e Withdraw fluid with vial inverted.

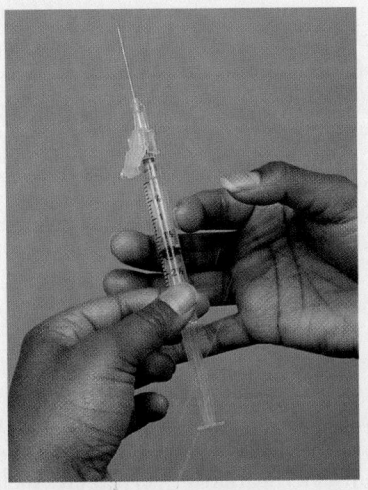

STEP 4h Hold syringe upright; tap barrel to dislodge air bubbles.

STEP	RATIONALE
c. Insert tip of needle or needleless device through center of rubber seal of vial of powdered medication. Inject diluent into vial. Remove needle.	Diluent begins to dissolve and reconstitute medication.
d. Mix medication thoroughly. Roll in palms. Do not shake.	Ensures proper dispersal of medication throughout solution and prevents formation of air bubbles.
e. Reconstituted medication in vial is ready to be drawn into new syringe. Read label carefully to determine dose after reconstitution.	Once you add diluent, concentration of medication (mg/mL) determines dose you give. Reading medication label carefully decreases medication errors.
f. Draw up reconstituted medication into syringe. Insert needleless device/needle into vial. Do not add air. Then follow Steps 4e through 4l.	Prepares medication for administration.

Clinical Decision Point *require that you verify dose of certain me Some agencies dications (e.g., insulin and heparin) for accuracy with another nurse. Check guidelines before administering medication.*

6. Compare label of medication with MAR, computer screen, or computer printout.	*This is the second check for accuracy.*
7. Dispose of soiled supplies. Place broken ampule and/or used vials and used needle or needleless device in puncture- and leak-proof container. Clean work area and perform hand hygiene.	Proper disposal of glass and needle prevents accidental injury to staff. Controls transmission of infection.

EVALUATION

1. Just before administering drug to patient, compare MAR with label of prepared drug and compare dose in syringe with desired dose.	Ensures that dose is accurate. *This is the third check for accuracy.*

Unexpected Outcomes	Related Interventions
1. Air bubbles remain in syringe.	• Expel air from syringe and add medication to it until you prepare correct dose.
2. Incorrect dose of medication is prepared.	• Discard prepared dose. • Prepare correct new dose.

PROCEDURAL GUIDELINE 22.1 *Mixing Parenteral Medications in One Syringe*

Some medications need to be mixed from two vials or from a vial and an ampule. Mixing compatible medications avoids the need to give a patient more than one injection. Most patient care units have medication compatibility charts. Compatibility charts are in drug reference guides, posted within patient care unit med rooms, or available electronically. If you are uncertain about medication compatibilities, consult a pharmacist. When mixing medications, you must correctly aspirate fluid from each type of container. When using multi-dose vials, do not contaminate the contents of the vial with medication from another vial or ampule.

When mixing medications from a vial and an ampule, prepare medications from the vial first. Then withdraw medication from the ampule using the same syringe and a filter needle. When mixing medications from two vials, do not contaminate one medication with another, ensure that the final dose is accurate, and maintain aseptic technique.

Give special consideration to the proper preparation of insulin, which comes in vials. Insulin is the hormone used to treat diabetes mellitus. It is classified by rate of action, including short, medium, and long duration. Often patients with diabetes mellitus receive a combination of different types of insulin to control their blood glucose levels. Before preparing insulin, gently roll all cloudy insulin preparations (Humulin-N) between the palms of your hands to resuspend the insulin (Burchum and Rosenthal, 2016).

If more than one type of insulin is required to manage a patient's diabetes, you can mix them into one syringe if they are compatible. Always prepare the short- or rapid-acting insulin first to prevent it from being contaminated with the longer-acting insulin (Burchum and Rosenthal, 2016). In some settings insulin is not mixed. Box 22.2 lists recommendations for mixing insulins.

Delegation and Collaboration
The skill of mixing medications in one syringe cannot be delegated to nursing assistive personnel (NAP). The nurse directs the NAP about:
• Potential side effects of medications and the need to immediately report their occurrence to the nurse.

Equipment
• Single- or multi-dose vials and ampules containing medication
• Syringe and two needles

PROCEDURAL GUIDELINE 22.1 *Mixing Parenteral Medications in One Syringe—cont'd*

- Needles:
  - Needleless blunt-tip vial access cannula or needle for drawing up medication
  - Filter needle if indicated
  - Sharps with engineered sharps injury protection (SESIP) needle for injection
- Alcohol swab
- Puncture-proof container for disposing of syringes, needles, and glass
- Medication administration record (MAR) or computer printout
- Medication in vial or ampule

Procedural Steps

1. Check accuracy and completeness of MAR or computer printout with health care provider's written medication order. Check patient's name, medication name and dosage, route of administration, and time of administration. Recopy or reprint any part of MAR that is difficult to read.
2. Review pertinent information related to medication, including action, purpose, side effects, and nursing implications.
3. Assess patient body build, muscle size, and weight if giving subcutaneous or intramuscular (IM) medication.
4. Consider compatibility of medications to be mixed and type of injection.

BOX 22.2

Recommendations for Mixing Insulins

- Patients whose blood glucose levels are well controlled on a mixed-insulin dose need to maintain their individual routine when preparing and administering their insulin.
- Do not mix insulin with any other medications or diluents unless approved by the health care provider.
- Never mix insulin glargine (Lantus) or insulin detemir (Levemir) with other types of insulin.
- Inject rapid-acting insulins mixed with NPH insulin within 15 minutes before a meal.
- Verify insulin doses with another nurse while you are preparing the injection.

---

5. Check expiration date of medication printed on vial or ampule.
6. Perform hand hygiene.
7. Prepare medication for one patient at a time following the six rights of medication administration (see Chapter 20). Select an ampule or vial from the unit-dose drawer or automated dispensing system. Compare the label of each medication with the MAR or computer printout. In the case of insulin, ensure that correct type(s) of insulin are prepared. *This is the first check for accuracy.*
8. Mixing medications from two vials (see illustration):
   a. Take syringe with needleless device or filter needle and aspirate volume of air equivalent to first medication dose (vial A).
   b. Inject air into vial A, making sure that needle or needleless device does not touch solution (see illustration A).
   c. Holding on to plunger, withdraw needle or needleless device and syringe from vial A. Aspirate air equivalent to second medication dose (vial B) into syringe.
   d. Insert needle or needleless device into vial B, inject volume of air into vial B, and withdraw medication from vial B into syringe (see illustration B).
   e. Withdraw needle or needleless device and syringe from vial B. Ensure that proper volume has been obtained.
   f. Determine on syringe scale what the combined volume of medications should measure.
   g. Insert needle or needleless device into vial A, being careful not to push plunger and expel medication within syringe into vial. Invert vial and carefully withdraw the desired amount of medication from vial A into syringe (see illustration C).
   h. Withdraw needle or needleless device and expel any excess air from syringe. Check fluid level in syringe for proper dose. Medications are now mixed.

Clinical Decision Point *If too much medication is withdrawn from second vial, discard syringe and start over. Do not push medication back into either vial.*

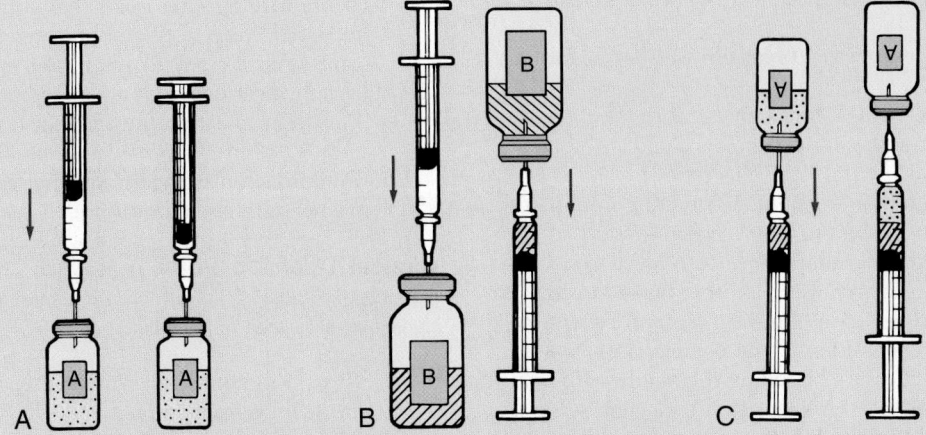

STEP 8 A, Inject air into vial A. **B,** Inject air into vial B and withdraw dose. **C,** Withdraw medication from vial A; medications are now mixed.

Continued

PROCEDURAL GUIDELINE 22.1 *Mixing Parenteral Medications in One Syringe—cont'd*

i. Change needle or needleless device for appropriate-size needle if medication is being injected. Keep needle or needleless device capped until administration time.

9. Mixing insulin:

    a. If patient takes insulin that is cloudy, roll bottle of insulin between hands to resuspend insulin preparation.

    b. Wipe off tops of both insulin vials with alcohol swab.

    c. Verify insulin dose against MAR.

Clinical Decision Point *If long-acting insulin glargine (Lantus) is ordered, note that this is a clear insulin and it should not be mixed with other insulin preparations.*

    d. If mixing rapid- or short-acting insulin with intermediate- or long-acting insulin, take insulin syringe and aspirate volume of air equivalent to dose to be withdrawn from intermediate- or long-acting insulin first (see illustration). If two intermediate- or long-acting insulins are mixed, it makes no difference which vial is prepared first.

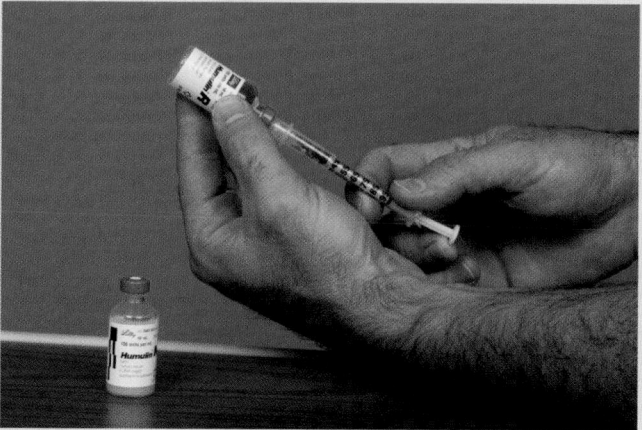

STEP 9g Withdraw short-acting insulin.

    k. Invert vial and carefully withdraw desired amount of insulin into syringe (see illustration).

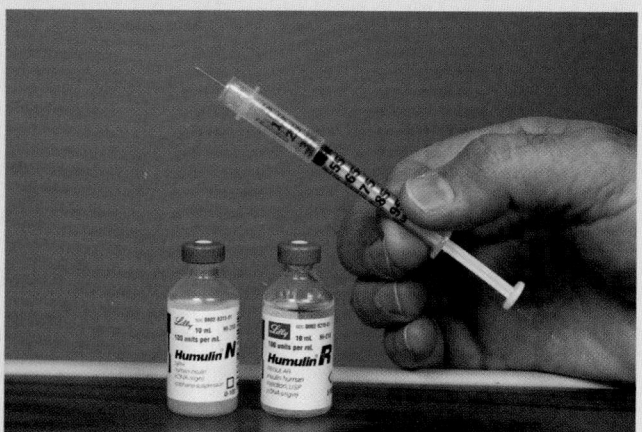

STEP 9d Aspirate air equivalent to dose to be withdrawn from intermediate insulin.

    e. Insert needle and inject air into vial of intermediate- or long-acting insulin. Do not let tip of needle touch solution.

    f. Remove syringe from vial of insulin without aspirating medication.

    g. With the same syringe, inject air equal to the dose of rapid- or short-acting insulin into vial and withdraw correct dose into syringe (see illustration).

    h. Remove syringe from rapid- or short-acting insulin and remove any air bubbles to ensure accurate dose.

    i. Verify short-acting insulin dosage with MAR and show insulin prepared in syringe to another nurse to verify that correct dosage of insulin was prepared. Determine which point on syringe scale the combined units of insulin should measure by adding the number of units of both insulins together (e.g., 4 units Regular + 10 units NPH = 14 units total). Verify combined dosage.

    j. Place needle of syringe back into vial of intermediate- or long-acting insulin. Be careful not to push plunger and inject insulin in syringe into vial.

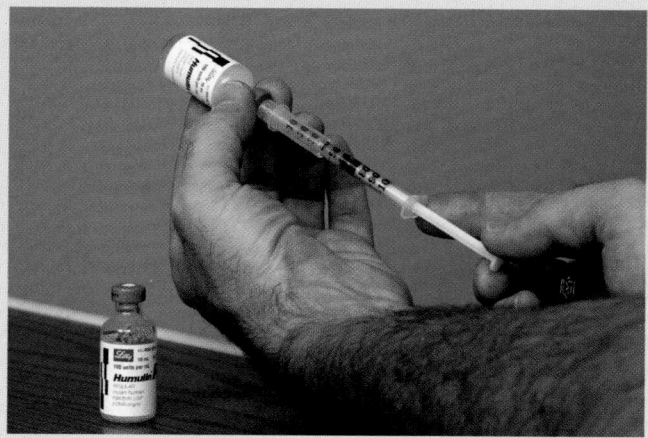

STEP 9k Withdraw intermediate insulin.

    l. Withdraw needle and check fluid level in syringe. Verify with another nurse that correct total dose was prepared. Keep needle of prepared syringe sheathed or capped until ready to administer medication.

10. Mixing medications from a vial and an ampule:

    a. Prepare medication from vial first, following Skill 22.1, Step 4.

    b. Determine on syringe scale what combined volume of medications should measure.

Clinical Decision Point *If needleless access device was used in preparing medication from vial, change needleless system to a filter needle to remove medication from ampule.*

    c. Next, using the same syringe, prepare second medication from ampule, following Step 3 in Skill 22.1.

    d. Withdraw filter needle from ampule and verify fluid level in syringe. Change filter needle to appropriate SESIP needle. Keep device or needle sheathed or capped until administering medication.

PROCEDURAL GUIDELINE 22.1 *Mixing Parenteral Medications in One Syringe—cont'd*

   e. Check syringe carefully for total combined dose of medications.

11. Compare MAR, computer screen, or computer printout with prepared medication and labels on vials/ampules. *This is the second check for accuracy.*

12. Dispose of soiled supplies. Place used ampules and/or vials and needle or needleless device in puncture- and leak-proof container.

13. Clean work area and perform hand hygiene.

14. Check syringe again carefully for total combined dose of medications.

15. *The third check for accuracy occurs at patient's bedside.*

◆ SKILL 22.2 Administering Intradermal Injections

▶ *Video Clip* **NSO** *Nursing Skills Online Administration of Parenteral Medications: Injections Module / Lesson 3*

Intradermal (ID) injections are used for skin testing (e.g., tuberculosis screening and allergy tests). Because such medications are potent, you inject them into the dermis, where blood supply is reduced and drug absorption occurs slowly. A patient may have an anaphylactic reaction if the medications enter the circulation too rapidly. For patients with a history of multiple allergies, the health care provider may perform skin testing. Skin testing often requires you to visually inspect the test site; therefore make sure that the ID sites are free of lesions and injuries and relatively hairless. The inner forearm and upper back are ideal locations.

Use a tuberculin (TB) or small syringe with a short ($\frac{1}{8}$- to $\frac{3}{8}$-inch), fine-gauge (25 to 27) needle to administer an ID injection. The angle of insertion for an ID injection is 5 to 15 degrees (see Fig. 22.1). Inject only small amounts of medication (0.01 to 0.1 mL) intradermally. If a bleb does not appear or if the site bleeds after needle withdrawal, the medication may have entered subcutaneous tissues. In this situation skin test results will not be valid.

Delegation and Collaboration

The skill of administering ID injections cannot be delegated to nursing assistive personnel (NAP). The nurse directs the NAP about:

- Potential medication side effects or allergic response signs and to report their occurrence to the nurse.
- Reporting any change in the patient's vital signs or condition to the nurse.

Equipment

- Syringe: 1-mL TB syringe with preattached 25- or 27-gauge needle, $\frac{1}{8}$- to $\frac{3}{8}$-inch
- Small gauze pad
- Alcohol swab
- Vial or ampule of medication
- Clean gloves
- Medication administration record (MAR) or computer printout
- Puncture-proof container

STEP	RATIONALE

ASSESSMENT

1. Check accuracy and completeness of MAR or computer printout with health care provider's original medication order. Check patient's name, medication name and dosage, route of administration, and time of administration. Recopy or reprint any part of MAR that is difficult to read.

   The order sheet is the most reliable source and only legal record of medications that patient is to receive. Ensures that patient receives the correct medications (Mandrack et al., 2012). Illegible MARs are a source of medication errors (Alassaad et al., 2013).

2. Review medication reference information about expected reaction/anticipated effects when testing skin with specific allergen or when giving medication and appropriate time to read site.

   Type of reaction depends on patient's ability to mount a cell-mediated immune response. Knowledge of expected and adverse reactions to skin testing helps you determine for which symptoms to monitor, how frequently, and when to reassess patient.

3. Assess patient's history of allergies: known type of allergens and normal allergic reaction.

   You do not administer any medication if there is known patient allergy. Medications are potent and can cause severe anaphylaxis.

4. Assess for contraindication to ID injections such as reduced local tissue perfusion. Assess for history of severe adverse reactions or necrosis that happened after previous ID injection.

   Decreased perfusion reduces absorption of medication. Prior history of severe reactions increases the risk for future severe reactions.

STEP	RATIONALE
5. Assess patient's knowledge of purpose and response to skin testing.	Patients need to know when to return for follow-up reading of skin test and when and how to report any reaction.
6. Check date of expiration for medication.	Dose potency increases or decreases when outdated.

NURSING DIAGNOSES

- Anxiety
- Fear
- Deficient knowledge regarding skin testing

Related factors are individualized based on patient's condition or needs.

PLANNING

1. Expected outcomes following completion of procedure:	
• Patient experiences very mild burning sensation during injection but no discomfort after injection.	Normal reaction to medication deposited in dermis.
• Small, light-colored bleb approximately 6 mm (¼ inch) in diameter forms at site and gradually disappears. Minimal bruising may be present.	Medication is in dermis and eventually absorbed. Bruising is result of minor bleeding from capillaries.
• Patient is able to identify signs of skin reaction and their significance.	Demonstrates learning.

IMPLEMENTATION

1. Prepare medications for one patient at a time using aseptic technique and avoiding distractions (see Skill 22.1). Check label of medication carefully with MAR or computer printout 2 times (see Skill 22.1 or Procedural Guideline 22.1) when preparing medication.	Ensures that medication is sterile. Preventing distractions reduces medication preparation errors. Use no-interruption zone (NIZ) when possible (Prakash et al., 2014; Yoder et al., 2015). *These are the first and second checks for accuracy* and ensure that correct medication is administered.
2. Take medication(s) to patient at correct time (see agency policy). Medications that require exact timing include stat, first-time or loading doses, and one-time doses. Give time-critical scheduled medications (e.g., antibiotics, anticoagulants, insulin, anticonvulsants, immunosuppressive agents) at exact time ordered (no later than 30 minutes before or after scheduled dose). Give non–time-critical scheduled medications within a range of 1 or 2 hours of scheduled dose (ISMP, 2011). During administration apply six rights of medication administration.	Hospitals must adopt medication administration policy and procedure for timing of medication administration that considers nature of the prescribed medication, specific clinical application, and patient needs (DHHS, 2011; ISMP, 2011). Time-critical scheduled medications are those for which early or delayed administration of maintenance doses of greater than 30 minutes before or after the scheduled dose may cause harm or result in substantial suboptimal therapy or pharmacological effect. Non–time-critical medications are those for which early or delayed administration within a specified range of either 1 or 2 hours should not cause harm or result in substantial suboptimal therapy or pharmacological effect (DHHS, 2011; ISMP, 2011).
3. Close room curtain or door.	Provides privacy.
4. Identify patient using at least two identifiers (e.g., name and birthday or name and medical record number) according to agency policy. Compare identifiers with information on patient's MAR or medical record.	Ensures correct patient. Complies with The Joint Commission standards and improves patient safety (TJC, 2016). Some agencies are now using a bar-code system to help with patient identification.
5. At patient's bedside again compare MAR or computer printout with names of medications on medication labels and patient name. Ask patient if he or she has allergies.	*This is the third check for accuracy* and ensures that patient receives correct medication. Confirms patient's allergy history.
6. Discuss purpose of each medication, action, and possible adverse effects. Allow patient to ask any questions. Tell him or her that injection will cause slight burning or sting.	Patient has right to be informed, and patient's understanding of each medication improves adherence to drug therapy. Helps minimize patient's anxiety.
7. Perform hand hygiene and apply clean gloves. Keep sheet or gown draped over body parts not requiring exposure.	Reduces transmission of infection.

STEP	RATIONALE
8. Select appropriate site. Note lesions or discolorations of skin. If possible, select site three to four finger widths below antecubital space and one hand width above wrist. If you cannot use forearm, inspect upper back. If necessary, use sites appropriate for subcutaneous injections.	An ID injection site is free of discoloration or hair so you can see results of skin test and interpret them correctly (WHO, 2015a).
9. Help patient to comfortable position. Have him or her extend elbow and support it and forearm on flat surface.	Stabilizes injection site for easy accessibility.
10. Clean site with antiseptic swab. Apply swab at center of site and rotate outward in circular direction for about 5 cm (2 inches). *Option:* Use vapocoolant spray (e.g., ethyl chloride) before injection.	Mechanical action of swab removes secretions containing microorganisms. Decreases pain at injection site.
11. Hold swab or gauze between third and fourth fingers of nondominant hand.	Gauze or swab remains readily accessible when withdrawing needle.
12. Remove needle cap from needle by pulling it straight off.	Preventing needle from touching sides of cap prevents contamination.
13. Hold syringe between thumb and forefinger of dominant hand with bevel of needle pointing up.	Smooth injection requires proper manipulation of syringe parts. With bevel up, you are less likely to deposit medication into tissues below dermis.
14. Administer injection.	
a. With nondominant hand stretch skin over site with forefinger or thumb.	Needle pierces tight skin more easily.
b. With needle almost against patient's skin, insert it slowly at 5- to 15-degree angle until resistance is felt. Advance needle through epidermis to approximately 3 mm (⅛ inch) below skin surface. You will see bulge of needle tip through skin (see illustration).	Ensures that needle tip is in dermis. You obtain inaccurate results if you do not inject needle at correct angle and depth (WHO, 2015a).
c. Inject medication slowly. Normally you feel resistance. If not, needle is too deep; remove and begin again.	Slow injection minimizes discomfort at site. Dermal layer is tight and does not expand easily when you inject solution.

Clinical Decision Point *It is not necessary to aspirate because dermis is relatively avascular.*

d. While injecting medication, note that small bleb (approximately 6 mm [¼ inch]) resembling mosquito bite appears on skin surface (see illustration).	Bleb indicates that you deposited medication in dermis.
e. After withdrawing needle, apply alcohol swab or gauze gently over site.	Do not massage site. Apply bandage if needed.
15. Help patient to comfortable position.	Gives patient sense of well-being.

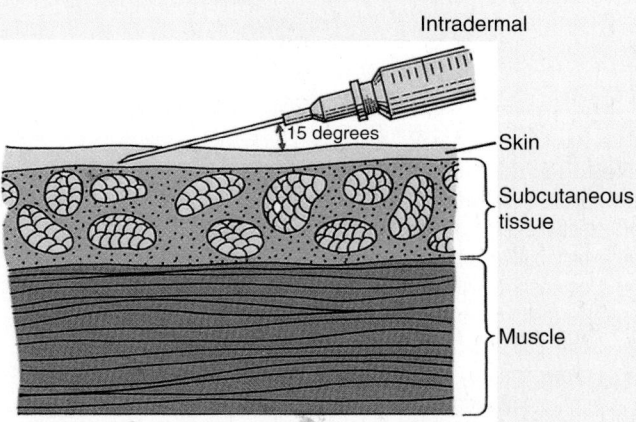

STEP 14b Intradermal needle tip inserted into dermis.

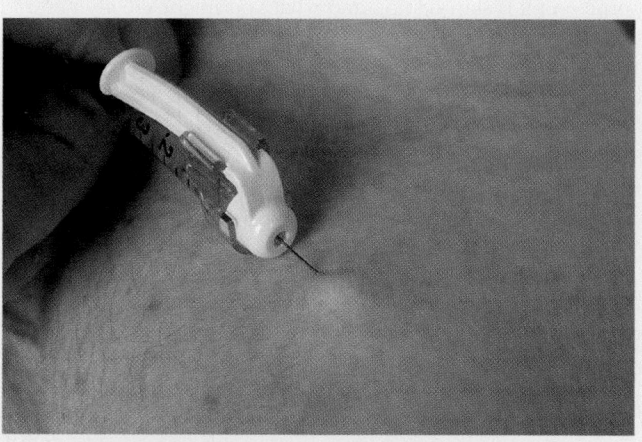

STEP 14d Injection creates small bleb.

STEP	RATIONALE
16. Discard uncapped needle or needle enclosed in safety shield and attached syringe in puncture- and leak-proof receptacle.	Prevents injury to patients and health care personnel. Recapping needles increases risk for a needlestick injury (OSHA, n.d.).
17. Remove gloves and perform hand hygiene.	Reduces transmission of microorganisms.
18. Stay with patient for several minutes and observe for any allergic reactions.	Dyspnea, wheezing, and circulatory collapse are signs of severe anaphylactic reaction and are likely to occur immediately after injection.

EVALUATION

1. Return to room in 15 to 30 minutes and ask if patient feels any acute pain, burning, numbness, or tingling at injection site.	Continued discomfort could indicate injury to underlying tissues.
2. Ask patient to discuss implications of skin testing and signs of hypersensitivity.	Patient's ability to recognize signs of skin testing helps to ensure timely reporting of results.
3. Inspect bleb. *Option:* Use skin pencil and draw circle around perimeter of injection site. Read TB test site at 48 to 72 hours; look for induration (hard, dense, raised area) of skin around injection site of:	Determines if reaction to antigen occurs; indication positive for tuberculosis or tested allergens. Site must be read at various intervals to determine test results. Pencil marks make site easy to find. You determine results of skin testing at various times, based on type of medication used or type of skin testing completed. Manufacturer directions determine when to read test results.
• 15 mm or more in patients with no known risk factors for tuberculosis.	Degree of reaction varies based on patient condition.
• 10 mm or more in patients who are recent immigrants; injection drug users; residents and employees of high-risk settings; patients with certain chronic illnesses; children less than 4 years of age; and infants, children, and adolescents exposed to high-risk adults.	
• 5 mm or more in patients who are human immunodeficiency virus (HIV) positive, have fibrotic changes on chest x-ray film consistent with previous tuberculosis infection, have had organ transplants, or are immunosuppressed.	
4. Use Teach-Back: "I want to be sure I explained to you the purpose of TB skin testing and what you might see after the test. Explain to me what the injection site might look like in 2 to 3 days." Revise your instruction now or develop a plan for revised patient or family caregiver teaching if patient or family caregiver is not able to teach back correctly.	Determines patient's and family caregiver's level of understanding of instructional topic.

Unexpected Outcomes	Related Interventions
1. Patient complains of localized pain or continued burning at injection site, indicating potential injury to nerve or vessels.	• Assess injection site. • Notify patient's health care provider.
2. Raised, reddened, or hard zone (induration) forms around ID test site.	• Notify patient's health care provider. • Document sensitivity to injected allergen or positive test if tuberculin skin testing was completed.
3. Patient has adverse reaction with signs of urticaria, pruritus, wheezing, and dyspnea.	• Notify patient's health care provider. • Follow agency policy for appropriate response to drug reactions (e.g., administration of antihistamine such as diphenhydramine or epinephrine). • Add allergy information to patient's record.

Recording and Reporting

- Record drug, dose, route, site, time, and date on MAR in nurses' notes in electronic health record (EHR) or chart immediately after administration, not before. Correctly sign MAR according to agency policy.
- Record area of ID injection and appearance of skin in nurses' notes in EHR or chart.
- Report any undesirable effects from medication to patient's health care provider and document adverse effects according to agency policy.
- Record patient teaching, validation of understanding, and patient's response to medication in nurses' notes in EHR or chart.

Special Considerations

Teaching

- Instruct patient not to squeeze medication out of injection site.
- Teach patient that negative skin tests may not rule out allergies, especially when low concentrations of medication are used.

- Patient should wear medical identification band listing all allergies.
- Caution patient not to wash off pencil markings around injection site.
- Explain to patient how to observe for skin reactions.

Pediatric

- Children who are exposed to people with confirmed or suspected infectious tuberculosis should be tested for it immediately following exposure (Hockenberry and Wilson, 2015).
- Children with ongoing exposure to high-risk individuals (e.g., HIV-infected, homeless, incarcerated) should be tested for tuberculosis every 2 to 3 years (Hockenberry and Wilson, 2015).

Gerontological

- The skin of the older adult is less elastic and must be held taut to ensure that ID injection is administered correctly.

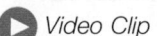 **SKILL 22.3** **Administering Subcutaneous Injections**

▶ *Video Clip* **NSO** *Nursing Skills Online Administration of Parenteral Medications: Injections Module / Lesson 4*

Subcutaneous injections involve depositing medication into the loose connective tissue underlying the dermis. Because subcutaneous tissue does not contain as many blood vessels as muscles, medications are absorbed more slowly than with intramuscular (IM) injections. Physical exercise or application of hot or cold compresses influences the rate of drug absorption by altering local blood flow to tissues. Any condition that impairs blood flow is a contraindication for subcutaneous injections.

Subcutaneous tissue is sensitive to irritating solutions and large volumes of medications. Thus you only administer small volumes (0.5 to 1.5 mL) of water-soluble medications subcutaneously to adults. In children, you give smaller volumes up to 0.5 mL (Hockenberry and Wilson, 2015). Examples of subcutaneous medications include epinephrine, insulin, allergy medications, opioids, and heparin. Because subcutaneous tissue contains pain receptors, the patient often experiences some discomfort.

The best subcutaneous injection sites include the outer aspect of the upper arms, the abdomen from below the costal margins to the iliac crests, and the anterior aspects of the thighs (Fig. 22.12). These areas are easily accessible and are large enough to allow rotating multiple injections within each anatomical location.

Choose an injection site that is free of skin lesions, bony prominences, and large underlying muscles or nerves. Site rotation prevents the formation of lipohypertrophy or lipoatrophy in the skin. A patient's body weight and adipose tissue indicate the depth of the subcutaneous layer. Therefore choose the needle length and angle of insertion on the basis of a patient's weight and an estimation of the amount of subcutaneous tissue (Ogston-Tuck, 2014a). Nurses typically use a 25-gauge, 16-mm (⅝-inch) needle inserted at a 45-degree angle or a 12-mm (½-inch) needle inserted at a 90-degree angle to administer subcutaneous medications to a normal-size adult patient. Some children require only a 12-mm (½-inch) needle. If the patient is obese, pinch the tissue and use a needle long enough to insert through fatty tissue at the base of the skinfold. Thin patients often do not have sufficient tissue for subcutaneous injections; the upper abdomen is usually the best site in this case. To ensure that a subcutaneous medication reaches the subcutaneous tissue, follow this rule: If you can grasp 5 cm (2 inches) of tissue, insert the needle at a 90-degree angle; if you can grasp only 2.5 cm (1 inch) of tissue, insert the needle at a 45-degree angle.

Research on insulin administration shows that insulin needles that are 8 mm (⁵⁄₁₆ inch) or longer often enter the muscles of men and people with a body mass index (BMI) of 25 or less. Shorter or 4- to 5-mm (³⁄₁₆-inch) needles were associated with less pain, adequate control of blood sugars, and minimal leakage of medication (Diggle, 2014; Hirsch et al., 2012). Thus, when administering insulin, needles of ³⁄₁₆ inch (4 to 5 mm) administered at a 90-degree angle should be used to reduce pain and achieve adequate control of blood sugars with minimal adverse effects for people of all BMIs, including children (AADE, 2013).

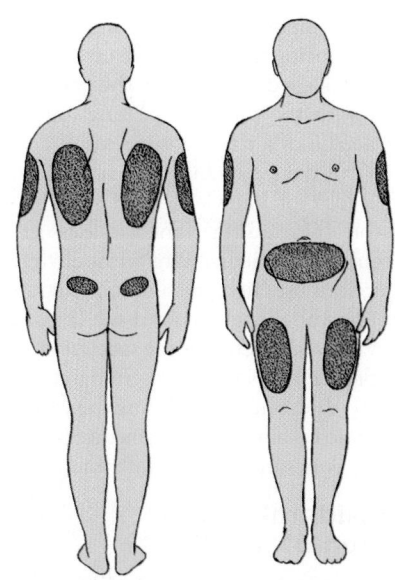

FIG 22.12 Common sites for subcutaneous injections.

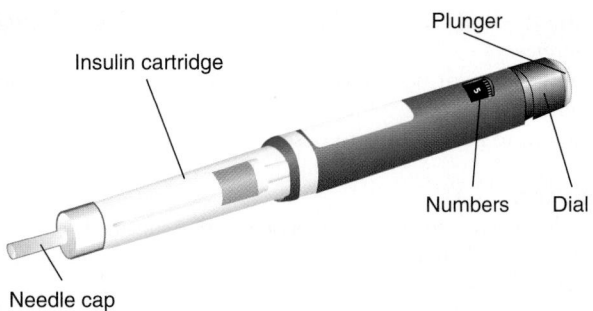

FIG 22.13 Insulin injection pen. *(From Lewis SL, et al: Medical-surgical nursing: assessment and management of clinical problems, ed 10, St Louis, 2017, Mosby.)*

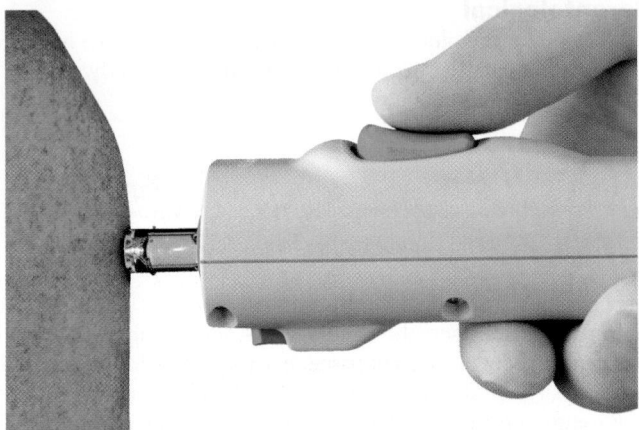

FIG 22.14 Jet injection system is held perpendicular to skin. *(Image courtesy Pharmajet. All rights reserved.)*

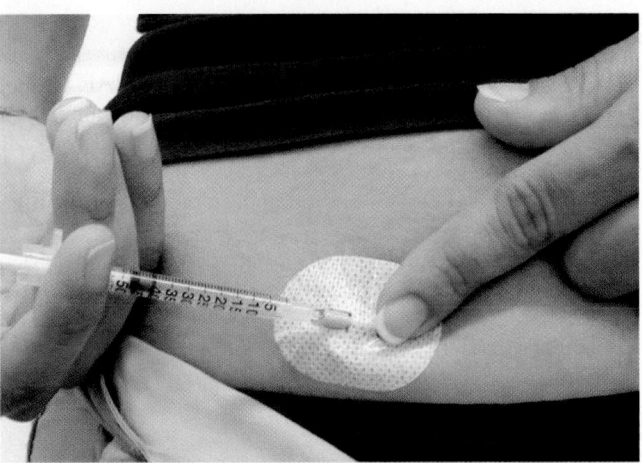

FIG 22.15 Subcutaneous device. *(Image courtesy IntraPump Infusion Systems. All rights reserved.)*

BOX 22.3

General Guidelines for Insulin Administration

- Store vials of insulin in the refrigerator, not the freezer. Keep vials currently being used at room temperature. Do not inject cold insulin.
- Inspect vials before each use for changes in appearance (e.g., clumping, frosting, precipitation, change in clarity or color), indicating lack of potency.
- Do not interchange insulin types unless approved by the patient's health care provider.
- Preferred injection sites include the abdomen, avoiding a 5-cm (2-inch) radius around the umbilicus and the outer aspect of the thighs.
- Have patient self-administer insulin whenever possible.
- Patients who take insulin need to self-monitor their blood glucose.
- All patients who take insulin should carry at least 15 g carbohydrate (e.g., 4 ounces of fruit juice, 4 ounces of regular soft drink, 8 ounces of skim milk, 6 to 10 hard candies) in the event of a hypoglycemic reaction.

Adapted from American Diabetes Association (ADA): Diabetes care in the hospital, nursing home, and skilled nursing facility, *Diabetes Care* 38(S1):S80, 2015.

Several different devices are available for administration of subcutaneous injections. *Injection pens* allow patients to self-administer medications (e.g., epinephrine, insulin, or interferon) subcutaneously (Fig. 22.13). They offer a convenient delivery method using prefilled, disposable cartridges. The patient pinches the skin, inserts the needle, and injects a predetermined medication dose. Teaching is essential to ensure that patients use the correct injection technique and deliver the correct dose of medication. Teach patients the importance of priming the pen before use. Priming involves pointing the pen needle up in the air, dialing one or two units (see package directions) on the pen, and then pressing the plunger fully with the thumb, repeating until a drop appears. This clears the needle of air and ensures a full dose is ready. The disadvantages of this device include increased risk for needlestick injury and user's lack of knowledge and skill in administration technique (Ogston-Tuck, 2014a). The *needleless jet injection system* administers subcutaneous medications without the use of needles. Needle-free injections use high pressure to penetrate the skin with the medication into the subcutaneous tissue (Fig. 22.14). Another option for subcutaneous injection is the *subcutaneous injection device* (e.g., insuflon) (Fig. 22.15), which is inserted into the subcutaneous tissue; the needle is then removed, leaving the cannula in the tissue to provide an avenue for administering medications for up to 3 days without having to puncture the skin with each injection.

Special Considerations for Administration of Insulin

Most patients manage type 1 diabetes mellitus with insulin injections. Anatomical injection site rotation is no longer necessary because newer human insulins carry a lower risk for skin hypertrophy. Patients choose one anatomical area (e.g., the abdomen) and systematically rotate sites within that region, which maintains consistent insulin absorption from day to day. Absorption rates of insulin vary on the basis of the injection site. Insulin is most quickly absorbed in the abdomen and most slowly in the thighs (Burchum and Rosenthal, 2016).

The timing of injections is critical to correct insulin administration. Health care providers plan insulin injection times based on blood glucose levels and when a patient will eat. Knowing the peak action and duration of the insulin is essential when developing an effective diabetes management plan. Table 22.2 compares a variety of insulin preparations. Box 22.3 provides general guidelines for insulin administration.

Special Considerations for Administration of Heparin

Heparin therapy provides therapeutic anticoagulation to reduce the risk for thrombus formation by suppressing clot formation. Therefore patients receiving heparin are at risk for bleeding, including bleeding gums, hematemesis, hematuria, or melena.

TABLE 22.2

Comparison of Insulin Preparations

Insulin Type*	Onset	Peak Effect (Hours)	Duration of Action (Hours)
Rapid-Acting			
Insulin lispro (Humalog)	15-30 min	$\frac{1}{2}$-1$\frac{1}{2}$	3-5
Insulin aspart (NovoLog)	10-20 min	1-3	3-5
Insulin glulisine (Apidra)	15-30 min	$\frac{1}{2}$-1$\frac{1}{2}$	3-4
Short-Acting			
Regular insulin† (e.g., Humulin R, Novolin R)	30-60 min	2$\frac{1}{2}$-5	Up to 7
Intermediate-Acting			
Isophane insulin suspension (NPH)	1$\frac{1}{2}$-4 h	4-12	Less than 24
Long-Acting			
Insulin glargine (Lantus)‡	1$\frac{1}{2}$ h	No peak identified	Greater than 24
Insulin detemir (Levemir)‡	0.8-2 h	Peak unknown	Up to 24

Data from Skidmore L: Mosby's 2015 nursing drug reference, ed 28, St Louis, 2015, Saunders.
*All insulins are available in 100-unit strengths.
†This is the only insulin approved for intravenous or intramuscular use.
‡Cannot be mixed with other insulins.

Results from coagulation blood tests (e.g., activated partial thromboplastin time [aPTT] and partial thromboplastin time [PTT]) allow you to monitor the desired therapeutic range for heparin therapy.

Before administering heparin, assess for preexisting conditions that contraindicate its use, including cerebral or aortic aneurysm, cerebrovascular hemorrhage, severe hypertension, and blood dyscrasias. In addition, assess for conditions in which increased risk for hemorrhage is present: recent childbirth; severe diabetes and renal disease; liver disease; severe trauma; and active ulcers or lesions of the gastrointestinal (GI), genitourinary (GU), or respiratory tract. Assess the patient's current medication regimen, including use of over-the-counter (OTC) and herbal medications (e.g., garlic, ginger, ginkgo, horse chestnut, or feverfew), for possible interaction with heparin. Other medications that interact with heparin include aspirin, nonsteroidal antiinflammatory drugs (NSAIDs), cephalosporins, antithyroid agents, probenecid, and thrombolytics.

You administer heparin subcutaneously or intravenously. Low-molecular-weight heparins (LMWHs) (e.g., enoxaparin) are more effective than heparin in some patients. The anticoagulant effects are more predictable (Burchum and Rosenthal, 2016). LMWHs have a longer half-life and require less laboratory monitoring but are expensive. To minimize the pain and bruising associated with LMWH, it is given subcutaneously on the right or left side of the abdomen, at least 5 cm (2 inches) away from the umbilicus (the patient's "love handles"). Administer LMWH in its prefilled syringe with the attached needle and do not expel the air bubble in the syringe before giving the medication. There is some new evidence to support a slower injection rate of 30 seconds to reduce bruising and pain (Akbari Sari et al., 2014; Sanofi-Aventis, 2014).

Delegation and Collaboration

The skill of administering subcutaneous injections cannot be delegated to nursing assistive personnel (NAP). The nurse directs the NAP about:

- Potential medication sides effects and to immediately report their occurrence to the nurse.

Equipment

- Proper size syringe and sharps with engineered sharps injury protection (SESIP) needle:
  - Subcutaneous: syringe (1- to 3-mL) and needle (25- to 27-gauge, $\frac{1}{8}$- to $\frac{5}{8}$-inch)
  - *Immunizations:* 23- to 25-gauge, $\frac{5}{8}$-inch needle (CDC, 2015)
  - Subcutaneous U-100 insulin: insulin syringe (1 mL) with preattached needle (28- to 31-gauge, $\frac{5}{16}$- to $\frac{5}{16}$-inch)
  - Subcutaneous U-500 insulin: 1 mL tuberculin (TB) syringe with needle (25- to 27-gauge, $\frac{1}{2}$- to $\frac{5}{8}$-inch)
- Small gauze pad (*optional*)
- Alcohol swab
- Medication vial or ampule
- Clean gloves
- Medication administration record (MAR) or computer printout
- Puncture-proof container

STEP	RATIONALE

ASSESSMENT

1. Check accuracy and completeness of each MAR or computer printout with health care provider's written medication order. Check patient's name, medication name and dosage, route of administration, and time of administration. Recopy or reprint any part of MAR that is difficult to read.

The order sheet is the most reliable source and only legal record of medications that patient is to receive. Ensures that patient receives the correct medications (Mandrack et al., 2012). Illegible MARs are a source of medication errors (Alassaad et al., 2013).

STEP	RATIONALE
2. Assess patient's medical and medication history.	Determines need for medication or possible contraindications for medication administration.
3. Assess patient's history of allergies: known type of allergies and normal allergic reaction.	Do not prepare medication if there is known patient allergy.
4. Review medication reference information for medication action, purpose, normal dose, side effects, time and peak of onset, and nursing implications.	Allows you to administer medication safely and monitor patient's response to therapy.
5. Check date of expiration for medication.	Dose potency increases or decreases when outdated.
6. Observe patient's previous verbal and nonverbal responses toward injection.	Anticipating patient's anxiety allows you to use distraction to reduce pain awareness.
7. Assess for contraindication to subcutaneous injections such as circulatory shock or reduced local tissue perfusion.	Reduced tissue perfusion interferes with drug absorption and distribution.
8. Assess patient's symptoms before initiating medication therapy.	Provides information to evaluate desired effect of medication.
9. Assess adequacy of patient's adipose tissue.	Adipose tissue influences methods for administering injections.
10. Assess relevant laboratory results (e.g., blood glucose, partial thromboplastin).	Provides baseline for measuring drug response.
11. Assess patient's knowledge of medication.	Poses implications for patient education.

NURSING DIAGNOSES

- Acute pain
- Anxiety

- Deficient knowledge regarding medication administration or drug therapy

- Fear
- Ineffective health maintenance

Related factors are individualized based on patient's condition or needs.

PLANNING

1. Expected outcomes following completion of procedure:	
• Patient experiences no pain or mild burning at injection site.	Medications may cause minor tissue irritation.
• Patient achieves desired effect of medication with no signs of allergies or undesired effects.	Medication administered without patient injury.
• Patient explains purpose, dosage, and effects of medication.	Demonstrates learning.

IMPLEMENTATION

1. Perform hand hygiene and prepare medication using aseptic technique. Check label of medication carefully with MAR or computer printout 2 times (see Skill 22.1 or Procedural Guideline 22.1) when preparing medication.	Ensures that medication is sterile. *These are the first and second checks for accuracy* and ensure that correct medication is administered.
2. Take medication(s) to patient at correct time (see agency policy). Medications that require exact timing include stat, first-time or loading doses, and one-time doses. Give time-critical scheduled medications (e.g., antibiotics, anticoagulants, insulin, anticonvulsants, immunosuppressive agents) at exact time ordered (no later than 30 minutes before or after scheduled dose). Give non–time-critical scheduled medications within a range of 1 or 2 hours of scheduled dose (ISMP, 2011). During administration apply six rights of medication administration.	Hospitals must adopt medication administration policy and procedure for timing of medication administration that considers nature of the prescribed medication, specific clinical application, and patient needs (DHHS, 2011; ISMP, 2011). Time-critical scheduled medications are those for which early or delayed administration of maintenance doses of greater than 30 minutes before or after the scheduled dose may cause harm or result in substantial suboptimal therapy or pharmacological effect. Non–time-critical medications are those for which early or delayed administration within a specified range of either 1 or 2 hours should not cause harm or result in substantial suboptimal therapy or pharmacological effect (DHHS, 2011; ISMP, 2011).
3. Close room curtain or door.	Provides privacy.
4. Identify patient using at least two identifiers (e.g., name and birthday or name and medical record number) according to agency policy. Compare identifiers with information on patient's MAR or medical record.	Ensures correct patient. Complies with The Joint Commission standards and improves patient safety (TJC, 2016). Some agencies are now using a bar-code system to help with patient identification.

STEP	RATIONALE
5. At patient's bedside again compare MAR or computer printout with names of medications on medication labels and patient name. Ask patient if he or she has allergies.	*This is the third check for accuracy* and ensures that patient receives correct medication. Confirms patient's allergy history.
6. Discuss purpose of each medication, action, and possible adverse effects. Allow patient to ask any questions. Tell patient that injection will cause slight burning or sting.	Patient has right to be informed, and patient's understanding of each medication improves adherence to drug therapy. Helps minimize patient's anxiety.
7. Perform hand hygiene and apply clean gloves. Keep sheet or gown draped over body parts not requiring exposure.	Reduces transmission of infection. Respects dignity of patient while exposing injection area.
8. Select appropriate injection site. Inspect skin surface over sites for bruises, inflammation, or edema. Do not use an area that is bruised or has signs associated with infection.	Injection sites are free of abnormalities that interfere with drug absorption. Sites used repeatedly become hardened from lipohypertrophy (increased growth in fatty tissue).

Clinical Decision Point *Applying ice to the injection site for 1 minute before the injection may decrease the patient's perception of pain (Hockenberry and Wilson, 2015).*

STEP	RATIONALE
9. Palpate sites and avoid those with masses or tenderness. Be sure that needle is correct size by grasping skinfold at site with thumb and forefinger. Measure fold from top to bottom. Make sure that needle is one-half length of fold.	You can mistakenly give subcutaneous injections in muscle, especially in abdomen and thigh sites. Appropriate size of needle ensures that you inject medication into subcutaneous tissue (Hirsch et al., 2012; Ogston-Tuck, 2014a).
a. When administering insulin or heparin, use abdominal injection sites first, followed by thigh injection site.	Risk for bruising is not affected by site.
b. When administering LMWH subcutaneously, choose site on right or left side of abdomen, at least 5 cm (2 inches) away from umbilicus.	Injecting LMWH on side of abdomen helps decrease pain and bruising at injection site (Sanofi-Aventis, 2014).
c. Rotate insulin site within an anatomical area (e.g., abdomen) and systematically rotate sites within that area.	Rotating injection sites within same anatomical site maintains consistency in day-to-day insulin absorption.
10. Help patient into comfortable position. Have him or her relax arm, leg, or abdomen, depending on site selection.	Relaxation of site minimizes discomfort.
11. Relocate site using anatomical landmarks.	Injection into correct anatomical site prevents injury to nerves, bone, and blood vessels.
12. Clean site with antiseptic swab. Apply swab at center of site and rotate outward in circular direction for about 5 cm (2 inches) (see illustration).	Mechanical action of swab removes secretions containing microorganisms.

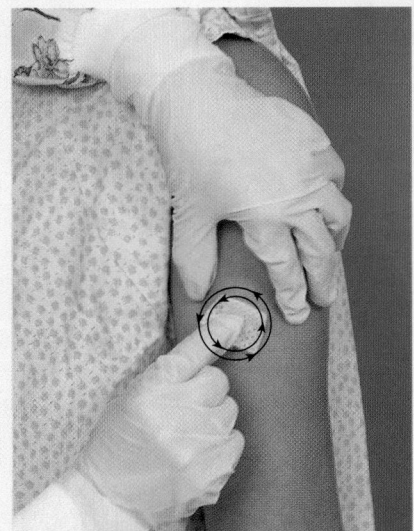

STEP 12 Clean site with circular motion.

STEP	RATIONALE
13. Hold swab or gauze between third and fourth fingers of nondominant hand.	Swab or gauze remains readily accessible for use when withdrawing needle after the injection.
14. Remove needle cap or protective sheath by pulling it straight off.	Preventing needle from touching sides of cap prevents contamination.

STEP	RATIONALE

15. Hold syringe between thumb and forefinger of dominant hand; hold as dart (see illustration).

Quick, smooth injection requires proper manipulation of syringe parts.

16. Administer injection:

   a. For average-size patient, hold skin across injection site or pinch skin with nondominant hand.

Needle penetrates tight skin more easily than loose skin. Pinching elevates subcutaneous tissue and desensitizes area.

   b. Inject needle quickly and firmly at 45- to 90-degree angle (see illustration). Release skin if pinched. *Option:* When using injection pen or giving heparin, continue to pinch skin while injecting medicine.

Quick, firm insertion minimizes discomfort. (Injecting medication into compressed tissue irritates nerve fibers.) Correct angle prevents accidental injection into muscle.

   c. For obese patient pinch skin at site and inject needle at 90-degree angle below tissue fold.

Obese patients have fatty layer of tissue above subcutaneous layer.

   d. After needle enters site, grasp lower end of syringe barrel with nondominant hand to stabilize it. Move dominant hand to end of plunger and slowly inject medication over several seconds (see illustration). When giving heparin, inject over 30 seconds (Akbari Sari et al., 2014; Sanofi-Aventis, 2014). Avoid moving syringe.

Movement of syringe may displace needle and cause discomfort. Slow injection of medication minimizes discomfort.

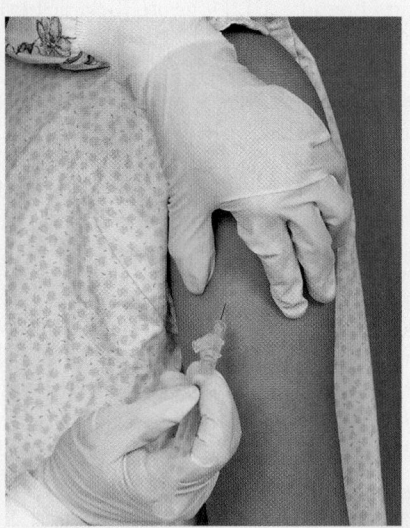

STEP 15 Hold syringe as if grasping a dart.

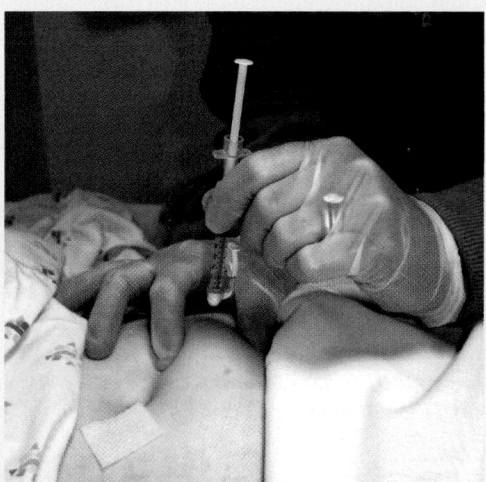

STEP 16b Subcutaneous injection. Angle and needle length depend on thickness of skinfold.

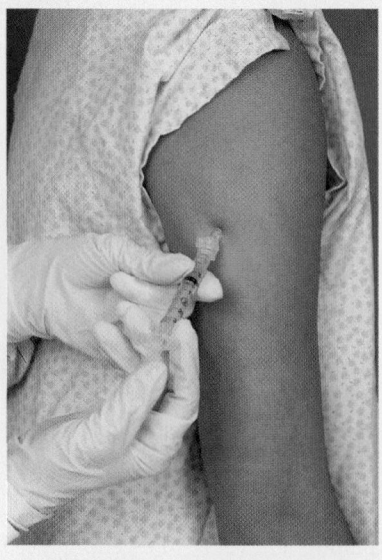

STEP 16d Inject medication slowly.

STEP	RATIONALE

Clinical Decision Point *Aspiration after injecting a subcutaneous medication is not necessary. Piercing a blood vessel in a subcutaneous injection is very rare. Aspiration after injecting heparin and insulin is not recommended (Lilley et al., 2012).*

    e. Withdraw needle quickly while placing antiseptic swab or gauze gently over site.

17. Apply gentle pressure to site. *Do not massage site.* (If heparin is given, hold alcohol swab or gauze to site for 30 to 60 seconds.)

18. Help patient to comfortable position.

19. Discard uncapped needle or needle enclosed in safety shield (see illustrations) and attached syringe into puncture- and leak-proof receptacle.

Supporting tissues around injection site minimizes discomfort during needle withdrawal. Dry gauze may minimize patient discomfort associated with alcohol on nonintact skin.

Aids absorption. Massage can damage underlying tissue. Time interval prevents bleeding at site.

Gives patient sense of well-being.

Prevents injury to patients and health care personnel. Recapping needles increases risk for needlestick injury (OSHA, n.d.).

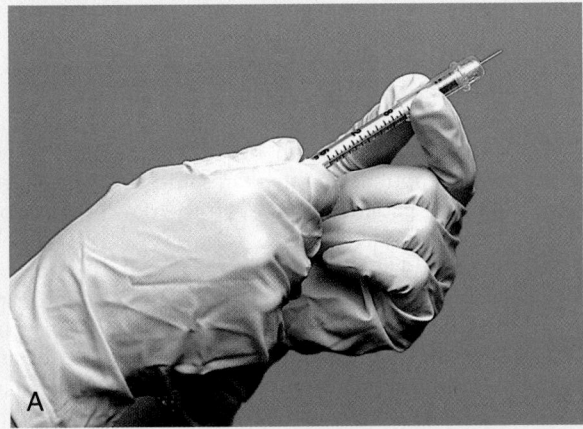 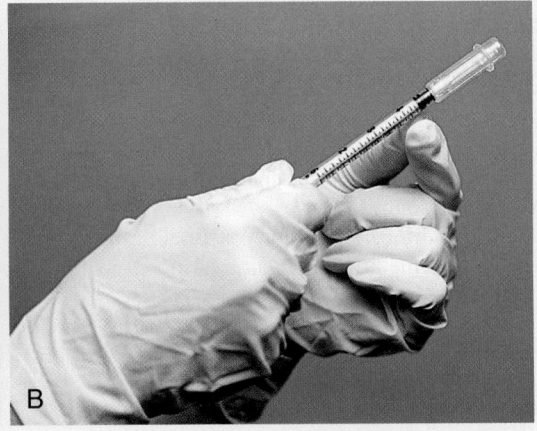

STEP 19 Needle with plastic guard to prevent needlesticks. **A,** Position of guard before injection. **B,** After injection guard locks in place, covering needle.

20. Remove gloves and perform hand hygiene.

21. Stay with patient for several minutes and observe for any allergic reactions.

Reduces transmission of microorganisms.

Dyspnea, wheezing, and circulatory collapse are signs of severe anaphylactic reaction.

EVALUATION

1. Return to room in 15 to 30 minutes and ask if patient feels any acute pain, burning, numbness, or tingling at injection site.

2. Inspect site, noting bruising or induration. Provide warm compress to site.

3. Observe patient's response to medication at times that correlate with onset, peak, and duration of medication. Review laboratory results as appropriate (e.g., blood glucose, partial thromboplastin).

4. Use Teach-Back: "I want to be sure I explained to you the reason for this subcutaneous injection. Tell me why you are receiving this injection." Revise your instruction now or develop a plan for revised patient or family caregiver teaching if patient or family caregiver is not able to teach back correctly.

Continued discomfort may indicate injury to underlying bones or nerves.

Bruising or induration indicates complication associated with injection.

Adverse effects of parenteral medications develop rapidly. Evaluate effect of medication on basis of onset, peak, and duration of action.

Determines patient's and family caregiver's level of understanding of instructional topic.

STEP	RATIONALE
Unexpected Outcomes 1. Patient complains of localized pain, numbness, tingling, or burning at injection site. 2. Patient displays adverse reaction with signs of urticaria, eczema, pruritus, wheezing, and dyspnea. 3. Hypertrophy of skin develops from repeated subcutaneous injection.	**Related Interventions** • Assess injection site; may indicate potential injury to nerve or tissues. • Notify patient's health care provider and do not reuse site. • Monitor patient's heart rate, respirations, blood pressure, and temperature. • Follow agency policy or guidelines for appropriate response to allergic reactions (e.g., administration of antihistamine such as diphenhydramine or epinephrine) and notify patient's health care provider immediately. • Add allergy information to patient's record. • Do not use site for future injections. • Instruct patient not to use site for 6 months.

Recording and Reporting

- Immediately after administration, record medication, dose, route, site, time, and date given on MAR in nurses' notes in electronic health record (EHR) or chart. Correctly sign MAR according to agency policy.
- Record patient teaching, validation of understanding, and patient's response to medication in nurses' notes in EHR or chart.
- Report any undesirable effects from medication to patient's health care provider and document adverse effects in record.

Special Considerations
Teaching

- Instruct patient to wear medical identification bracelet indicating important medical information, including bleeding tendencies, illnesses (e.g., diabetes), and allergies.
- Patients who require daily injections need to learn techniques of self-administration (see Skill 44.6). Teach injection techniques to a family caregiver.

Pediatric

- Administer only amounts up to 0.5 mL subcutaneously to small children (Hockenberry and Wilson, 2015).

Gerontological

- Aging patients have less elastic skin and reduced subcutaneous skinfold thickness. The upper abdominal site is the best site to use when the patient has little subcutaneous tissue.

Home Care

- Improper disposal of used needles and sharps in the home setting poses a health risk to the public and waste workers. Several options for safe sharps disposal at home exist, including allowing patients to transport their own sharps containers from home to collection sites (e.g., doctor's office, a hospital, or a pharmacy); mailing their used syringes to a collection site (mail-back programs); syringe exchange programs; or special devices that destroy the needle on the syringe, rendering it safe for disposal. If the patient cannot implement any of these options, have him or her dispose of needles and other sharps in a hard plastic or metal container with a tightly sealed lid (e.g., empty detergent bottle or coffee can). Pamphlets for safe home disposal of sharps are on the Environmental Protection Agency (EPA) website (EPA, 2014).
- Most insulin preparations have bacteriostatic properties that inhibit bacterial growth on the skin. Therefore patients with diabetes may reuse their syringes at home if they can recap the needles safely. Syringes should be discarded when the needles become dull or bent or contact any surface other than the skin. Wiping the needle off with alcohol is not recommended because the silicon coating on the needle is removed, making injections more painful. Immunocompromised patients and patients with poor personal hygiene, acute illness, or open hand wounds should not reuse syringes (American Diabetes Association, 2015).
- Teach injection techniques that minimize patient discomfort to patient and family caregiver.

◆ SKILL 22.4 Administering Intramuscular Injections

▶ Video Clip **NSO** *Nursing Skills Online Administration of Parenteral Medications: Injections Module / Lesson 5*

The intramuscular (IM) injection route deposits medication into deep muscle tissue, which has a rich blood supply, allowing medication to absorb faster than by the subcutaneous route. Any factor that interferes with local tissue blood flow affects the rate and extent of drug absorption. There is an increased risk for injecting drugs directly into blood vessels using the IM route.

The viscosity of the medication, injection site, patient's weight, and amount of adipose tissue influence needle size selection. Determine needle gauge by the medication to be administered. Therefore, whenever administering a medication by the IM route, first verify that the injection is justified (Nicoll and Hesby, 2002; WHO, 2015b). Some medications such as hepatitis B and tetanus, diphtheria, and pertussis (Tdap) immunizations are only given intramuscularly.

Use a longer and heavier-gauge needle to pass through subcutaneous tissue and penetrate deep muscle tissue (see Fig. 22.1). A patient's body mass index (BMI) and the amount of adipose tissue influence needle size selection. Many needles available in health care settings are not long enough to reach the muscle, especially in female patients and those who are obese (Bhalla et al., 2013; Dayananda et al., 2014; Palma and Strohfus, 2013). Because most agencies have needles that range in length from only ⅜ to 1½ inches, investigate different medication routes, especially when IM injections are ordered for patients who are obese females.

The angle of insertion for an IM injection is 90 degrees. Muscle is less sensitive to irritating and viscous medications. A normal, well-developed adult patient tolerates 2 to 5 mL of medication into a larger muscle without severe muscle discomfort (Hopkins and Arias, 2013: Nicoll and Hesby, 2002). However, larger volumes of medication (4 to 5 mL) are unlikely to be absorbed properly. Children, older adults, and thin patients tolerate only 2 mL of an IM injection. Do not give more than 1 mL to small children and older infants, and do not give more than 0.5 mL to smaller infants (Hockenberry and Wilson, 2015).

Rotate IM injection sites to decrease the risk for hypertrophy. Emaciated or atrophied muscles absorb medication poorly; thus avoid their use when possible. The **Z**-track method, a technique for pulling the skin during an injection, is recommended for IM injections (Nicoll and Hesby, 2002). It prevents leakage of medication into subcutaneous tissues, seals medication in the muscle, and minimizes irritation. To use the **Z**-track method, apply the appropriate-size needle to the syringe and clean and select an IM site, preferably in a large, deep muscle such as the ventrogluteal. Pull the overlying skin and subcutaneous tissues approximately 2.5 to 3.5 cm (1 to 1½ inches) laterally to the side with the ulnar side of the nondominant hand. Hold the skin in this position until you have administered the injection (Fig. 22.16A). Inject the needle deeply into the muscle. To reduce injection site discomfort, the CDC (2015) recommends there is no longer any need to aspirate after the needle is injected when *administering vaccines* (CDC, 2015). However, follow agency policy for aspirating vaccines after injecting an IM needle. Keep the needle inserted for 10 seconds to allow the medication to disperse evenly. Release the skin after withdrawing the needle. This leaves a zigzag path that seals the needle track wherever tissue planes slide across one another (see Fig. 22.16B). The medication is sealed in the muscle tissue.

Injection Sites

When selecting an IM site, determine that the site is free of pain, infection, necrosis, bruising, and abrasions. Also consider the location of underlying bones, nerves, and blood vessels and the volume of medication that you will administer. Because of the sciatic nerve location, the dorsogluteal muscle is not recommended as an injection site.

Ventrogluteal Site

The ventrogluteal muscle involves the gluteus medius; it is situated deep and away from major nerves and blood vessels. This site is the preferred and safest site for all adults, children, and infants, especially for medications that have larger volumes and are more viscous and irritating (Hockenberry and Wilson, 2015; Hopkins and Arias, 2013; Nicoll and Hesby, 2002). The ventrogluteal site is recommended for volumes greater than 2 mL (Hopkins and Arias, 2013; Nicoll and Hesby, 2002). Research shows that injuries such as fibrosis, nerve damage, abscess, tissue necrosis, muscle contraction, gangrene, and pain are associated with all the common IM sites *except* the ventrogluteal site (Hopkins and Arias, 2013).

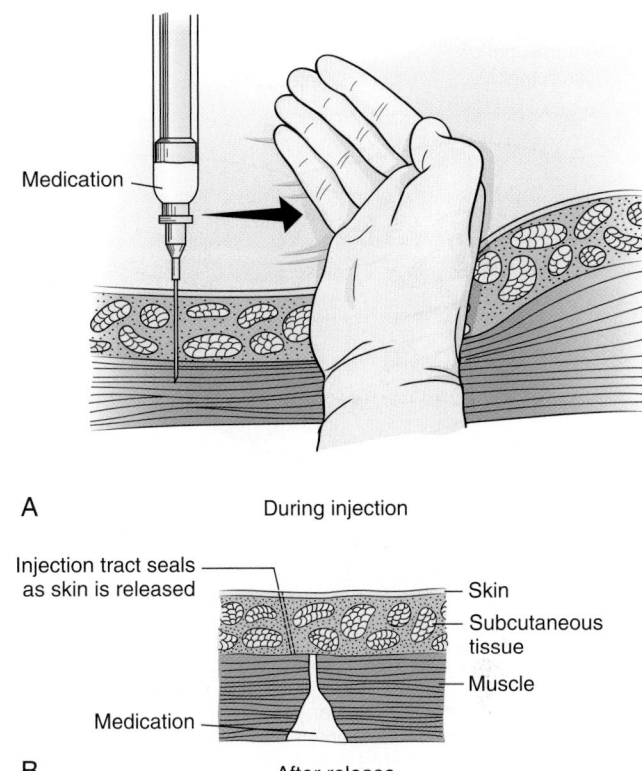

Medication

A   During injection

Injection tract seals as skin is released — Skin
— Subcutaneous tissue
Medication — — Muscle

B   After release

FIG 22.16 A, Pulling on overlying skin with dorsum of hand during IM injection moves tissue to prevent later tracking. **B,** Z-track left after injection prevents deposit of medication through sensitive tissue.

To locate the ventrogluteal muscle, have a patient lie in either the supine or lateral position; place the heel of your hand over the greater trochanter of the patient's hip with the wrist almost perpendicular to the femur. Use your right hand for the left hip and the left hand for the right hip. Point the thumb toward the patient's groin; point the index finger to the anterior superior iliac spine; and extend the middle finger back along the iliac crest toward the buttock. The index finger, the middle finger, and the iliac crest form a V-shaped triangle. The injection site is the center of the triangle (Fig. 22.17A) To relax this muscle, patients lie on their side or back, flexing the knee and hip (see Fig. 22.17B).

Vastus Lateralis Muscle

The vastus lateralis muscle is another injection site used in adults and is the preferred site for administration of biologics (e.g., immunizations) to infants, toddlers, and children (Hockenberry and Wilson, 2015). The muscle is thick and well developed; it is located on the anterior lateral aspect of the thigh. It extends in an adult from a hand breadth above the knee to a hand breadth below the greater trochanter of the femur (Fig. 22.18A). Use the middle third of the muscle for injection. The width of the muscle usually extends from the midline of the thigh to the midline of the outer side of the thigh. With young children or cachectic patients, it helps to grasp the body of the muscle during injection to be sure that the medication is deposited in muscle tissue. To help relax the muscle, ask the patient to lie flat with the knee slightly flexed and foot externally rotated or assume a sitting position (see Fig. 22.18B).

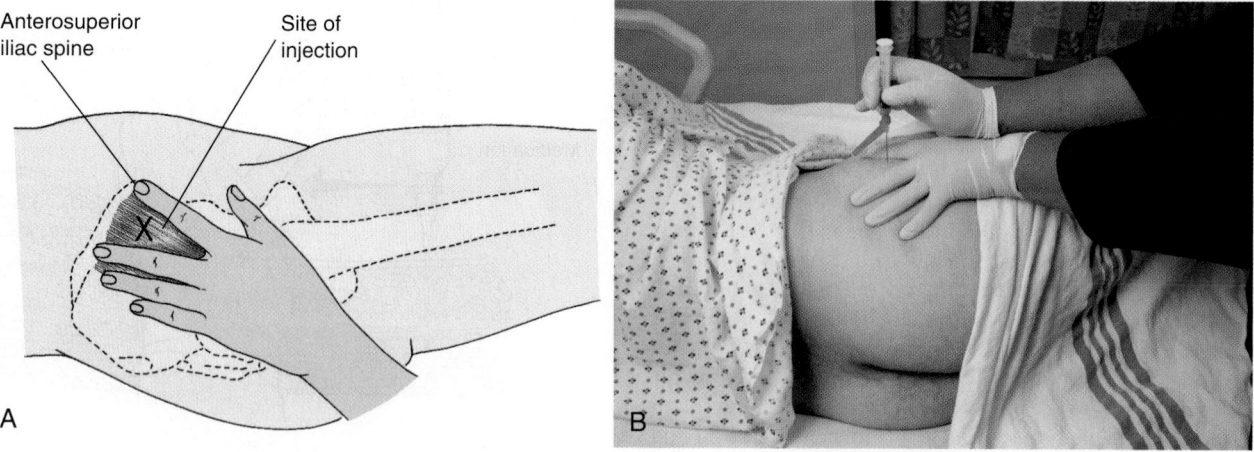

FIG 22.17 A, Anatomical view of ventrogluteal injection site. **B,** Injection at ventrogluteal site avoids major nerves and blood vessels.

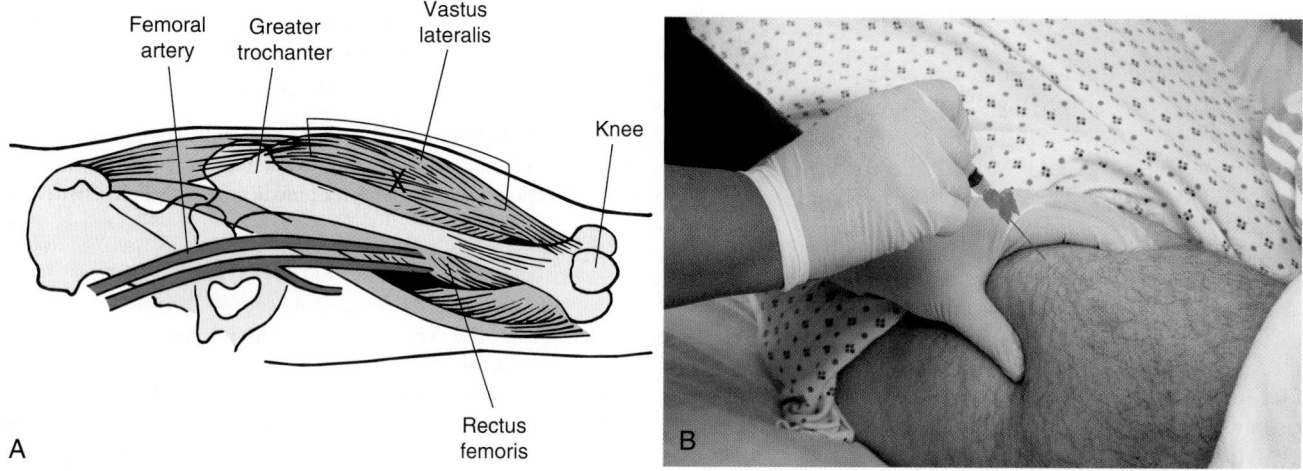

FIG 22.18 A, Landmarks for vastus lateralis site. **B,** Giving IM injection in vastus lateralis site.

Deltoid Muscle

Although the deltoid site is easily accessible, it is not well developed in many adults. There is potential for injury because the axillary, radial, brachial, and ulnar nerves and the brachial artery lie within the upper arm under the triceps and along the humerus. Use this site for small medication volumes (2 mL or less) (Hopkins and Arias, 2013; Nicoll and Hesby, 2002). *Carefully assess the condition of the deltoid muscle; consult medication references for suitability of medication; and carefully locate the injection site using anatomical landmarks.* Use this site for small medication volumes; for administration of routine immunizations in toddlers, older children, and adults; or when other sites are inaccessible because of dressings or casts.

Locate the deltoid muscle by fully exposing the patient's upper arm and shoulder and asking him or her to relax the arm at the side or by supporting the patient's arm and flexing the elbow. Do not roll up any tight-fitting sleeve. Allow the patient

to sit, stand, or lie down. Palpate the lower edge of the acromion process, which forms the base of a triangle in line with the midpoint of the lateral aspect of the upper arm. The injection site is in the center of the triangle, about 3 to 5 cm (1.2 to 2 inches) below the acromion process (Fig. 22.19A). You locate the apex of the triangle by placing four fingers across the deltoid muscle with the top finger along the acromion process. The injection site is three finger widths below the acromion process (see Fig. 22.19B).

Delegation and Collaboration

The skill of administering IM injections cannot be delegated to nursing assistive personnel (NAP). The nurse directs the NAP about:

- Potential medication side effects and to immediately report their occurrence to the nurse.
- Reporting any change in the patient's condition to the nurse.

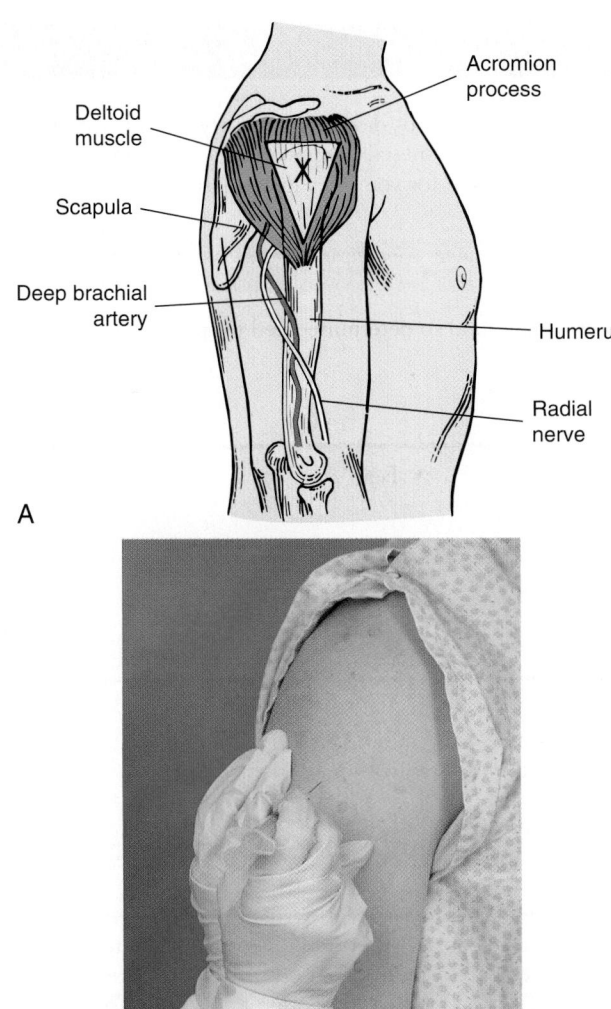

FIG 22.19 A, Landmarks for deltoid site. **B,** Giving IM injection in deltoid site.

Equipment

- Proper-size syringe and sharps with engineered sharps injury protection (SESIP) needle:
  - *IM:* Syringe 2 to 3 mL for adult, 0.5 to 1 mL for infants and small children
  - Needle length corresponding to site of injection, age, gender, and size of patient. Refer to following guidelines; length needed may vary outside of these guidelines for patients who are smaller or larger than average.

NEEDLE LENGTH FOR IMMUNIZATIONS
(BASED ON CDC 2015 GUIDELINES)

Site	Child	Adult
Ventrogluteal	$\frac{1}{2}$-1 inch	$1\frac{1}{2}$ inch
Vastus lateralis	$\frac{5}{8}$-1 inch	$\frac{5}{8}$-1 inch
Deltoid	$\frac{1}{2}$-1 inch	1-$1\frac{1}{2}$ inches

Gender-Male	Gender-Female	Needle Length
Less than 130 pounds	Less than 130 pounds	$\frac{5}{8}$-1 inch
130-152 pounds	130-152 pounds	1 inch
153-260 pounds	153-200 pounds	1-$1\frac{1}{2}$ inches
260+ pounds	200+ pounds	1-$1\frac{1}{2}$-inches

- Needle gauge often depends on length of needle; administer biologicals and medication in aqueous solution with a 20- to 25-gauge needle. Use 18- to 21-gauge needles for medications in oil-based solutions
- Alcohol swab
- Small gauze pad
- Vial or ampule of medication
- Clean gloves
- Medication administration record (MAR) or computer printout
- Puncture-proof container

STEP	RATIONALE

ASSESSMENT

1. Check accuracy and completeness of each MAR or computer printout with health care provider's written medication order. Check patient's name, medication name and dosage, route of administration, and time of administration. Recopy or reprint any part of MAR that is difficult to read.

   The order sheet is the most reliable source and only legal record of medications that patient is to receive. Ensures that patient receives the correct medications (Mandrack et al., 2012). Illegible MARs are a source of medication errors (Alassaad et al., 2013).

2. Assess patient's medical and medication history.

   Determines need for medication or possible contraindications for medication administration.

3. Assess patient's history of allergies: known type of allergies and normal allergic reaction.

   Do not prepare medication if there is a known patient allergy.

4. Review medication reference information for medication action, purpose, normal dose, side effects, time of peak onset, and nursing implications.

   Allows you to administer medication safely and monitor patient's response to therapy.

5. Check date of expiration for medication.

   Dose potency increases or decreases when outdated.

6. Observe patient's previous verbal and nonverbal responses toward injection.

   Anticipating patient's anxiety allows you to use distraction to reduce pain awareness.

STEP	RATIONALE
7. Assess for contraindication to IM injections such as muscle atrophy, reduced blood flow, or circulatory shock.	Atrophied muscle absorbs medication poorly. Factors interfering with blood flow to muscles impair drug absorption.
8. Assess patient's symptoms before initiating medication therapy.	Provides information for you to evaluate desired effects of medication.

Clinical Decision Point *Because of the documented adverse effects of IM injections, other routes of medication injection are preferred. Consider contacting health care provider for alternative route of medication administration.*

9. Assess patient's knowledge regarding medication to be received.	Provides background to determine need for patient education.

NURSING DIAGNOSES

- Acute pain
- Anxiety
- Deficient knowledge regarding medication administration or drug therapy
- Fear

Related factors are individualized based on patient's condition or needs.

PLANNING

1. Expected outcomes following completion of procedure:

• Patient experiences no pain or mild burning at injection site.	Medications may cause minor tissue irritation.
• Patient achieves desired effect of medication with no signs of allergies or undesired effects.	Medication administered without patient injury.
• Patient explains purpose, dosage, and effects of medication.	Demonstrates learning.

IMPLEMENTATION

1. Prepare medications for one patient at a time using aseptic technique. Keep all pages of MARs or computer printouts for one patient together or look at only one patient's electronic MAR at a time. Check label of medication carefully with MAR or computer printout 2 times (see Skill 22.1 and Procedural Guideline 22.1) when preparing medication.	Ensures that medication is sterile. Preventing distractions reduces medication preparation errors. Use no-interruption zone (NIZ) when possible (Prakash et al., 2014; Yoder et al., 2015). *These are the first and second checks for accuracy* and ensure that correct medication is administered.
2. Take medication(s) to patient at correct time (see agency policy). Medications that require exact timing include stat, first-time or loading doses, and one time doses. Give time-critical scheduled medications (e.g., antibiotics, anticoagulants, insulin, anticonvulsants, immunosuppressive agents) at exact time ordered (no later than 30 minutes before or after scheduled dose). Give non–time-critical scheduled medications within a range of 1 or 2 hours of scheduled dose (ISMP, 2011). During administration apply six rights of medication administration.	Hospitals must adopt medication administration policy and procedure for timing of medication administration that considers nature of prescribed medication, specific clinical application, and patient needs (DHHS, 2011; ISMP, 2011). Time-critical scheduled medications are those for which early or delayed administration of maintenance doses of greater than 30 minutes before or after scheduled dose may cause harm or result in substantial suboptimal therapy or pharmacological effect. Non–time-critical medications are those for which early or delayed administration within a specified range of either 1 or 2 hours should not cause harm or result in substantial suboptimal therapy or pharmacological effect (DHHS, 2011; ISMP, 2011).
3. Close room curtain or door.	Provides privacy.
4. Identify patient using at least two identifiers (e.g., name and birthday or name and medical record number) according to agency policy. Compare identifiers with information on patient's MAR or medical record.	Ensures correct patient. Complies with The Joint Commission standards and improves patient safety (TJC, 2016). Some agencies are now using a bar-code system to help with patient identification.
5. At patient's bedside again compare MAR or computer printout with names of medications on medication labels and patient name. Ask patient if he or she has allergies.	*This is the third check for accuracy* and ensures that patient receives correct medication. Confirms patient's allergy history.
6. Discuss purpose of each medication, action, and possible adverse effects. Allow patient to ask any questions. Tell patient that injection will cause a slight burning or sting.	Patient has right to be informed, and patient's understanding of each medication improves adherence to drug therapy. Helps minimize patient's anxiety.

STEP	RATIONALE
7. Perform hand hygiene and apply clean gloves. Keep sheet or gown draped over body parts not requiring exposure.	Reduces transmission of infection. Respects patient's dignity while exposing injection site.
8. Select appropriate site. Note integrity and size of muscle. Palpate for tenderness or hardness. Avoid these areas. If patient receives frequent injections, rotate sites. Use ventrogluteal if possible.	Ventrogluteal is preferred injection site for adults. It is also preferred site for children of all ages (Hockenberry and Wilson, 2015; Nicoll and Hesby, 2002; Ogston-Tuck, 2014b).
9. Help patient to comfortable position. Position patient depending on chosen site (e.g., sit, lie flat, on side, or prone).	Reduces strain on muscle and minimizes injection discomfort.

Clinical Decision Point *Ensure that medical condition (e.g., circulatory shock, orthopedic surgery) does not contraindicate patient's position for injection.*

10. Relocate site using anatomical landmarks.	Injection into correct anatomical site prevents injury to nerves, bone, and blood vessels.
11. Clean site with antiseptic swab. Apply swab at center of site and rotate outward in circular direction for about 5 cm (2 inches).	Mechanical action of swab removes secretions containing microorganisms.
a. *Option:* Apply EMLA cream on injection site at least 1 hour before IM injection or use vapocoolant spray (e.g., ethyl chloride) just before injection.	Decreases pain at injection site.
12. Hold swab or gauze between third and fourth fingers of nondominant hand.	Swab or gauze remains readily accessible for use when withdrawing needle after injection.
13. Remove needle cap or sheath by pulling it straight off.	Preventing needle from touching sides of cap prevents contamination.
14. Hold syringe between thumb and forefinger of dominant hand; hold as dart, palm down.	Quick, smooth injection requires proper manipulation of syringe parts.
15. Administer injection:	
a. Position ulnar side of nondominant hand just below site and pull skin laterally approximately 2.5 to 3.5 cm (1 to 1½ inches). Hold position until medication is injected. With dominant hand inject needle quickly at 90-degree angle into muscle (see Fig. 22.16A).	Z-track creates zigzag path through tissues that seals needle track to avoid tracking medication. A quick dartlike injection reduces discomfort. Use Z-track for all IM injections (Hopkins and Arias, 2013; Nicoll and Hesby, 2002; Ogston-Tuck, 2014b).
b. *Option:* If patient's muscle mass is small, grasp body of muscle between thumb and forefingers.	Ensures that medication reaches muscle mass (CDC, 2015; Hockenberry and Wilson, 2015).
c. After needle pierces skin, still pulling on skin with nondominant hand, grasp lower end of syringe barrel with fingers of nondominant hand to stabilize it. Move dominant hand to end of plunger. Avoid moving syringe.	Smooth manipulation of syringe reduces discomfort from needle movement. Skin remains pulled until after medication is injected to ensure Z-track administration.
d. Pull back on plunger 5 to 10 seconds. If no blood appears, inject medication slowly at rate of 10 sec/mL (Nicoll and Hesby, 2002).	Aspiration of blood into syringe indicates possible placement into a vein. Aspiration of blood into syringe indicates intravenous (IV) placement of needle. Slow injection rate reduces pain and tissue trauma and reduces chance of leakage of medication back through needle track (Hockenberry and Wilson, 2015; Nicoll and Hesby, 2002). The CDC (2015) no longer recommends aspiration when administering an immunization.

Clinical Decision Point *If blood appears in syringe, remove needle, dispose of medication and syringe properly, and prepare another dose of medication for injection to prevent injection of medication directly into the bloodstream.*

e. Once medication is injected, wait 10 seconds, then smoothly and steadily withdraw needle, release skin, and apply gauze gently over site (see Fig. 22.16B).	Allows time for medication to absorb into muscle before removing syringe. Dry gauze minimizes discomfort associated with alcohol on nonintact skin.
16. Apply gentle pressure to site. *Do not massage site.* Apply bandage if needed.	Massage damages underlying tissue.
17. Help patient to comfortable position.	Gives patient sense of well-being.

STEP	RATIONALE
18. Discard uncapped needle or needle enclosed in safety shield and attached syringe into puncture- and leak-proof receptacle.	Prevents injury to patients and health care personnel. Recapping needles increases risk for needlestick injury (OSHA, n.d.).
19. Remove gloves and perform hand hygiene.	Reduces transmission of microorganisms.
20. Stay with patient for several minutes and observe for any allergic reactions.	Dyspnea, wheezing, and circulatory collapse are signs of severe anaphylactic reaction.

EVALUATION

1. Return to room in 15 to 30 minutes and ask if patient feels any acute pain, burning, numbness, or tingling at injection site.	Continued discomfort may indicate injury to underlying bones or nerves.
2. Inspect site; note any bruising or induration. Apply warm compress to site.	Bruising or induration indicates complication associated with injection. Document findings and notify health care provider.
3. Observe patient's response to medication at times that correlate with onset, peak, and duration of medication.	IM medications are absorbed rapidly. Adverse effects of parenteral medications develop rapidly. Evaluate effect of medication based on onset, peak, and duration of actions of medication.
4. Use Teach-Back: "I want to be sure I explained to you the purpose of this IM injection. Explain to me why you are receiving the injection and what you might expect to feel during the injection." Revise your instruction now or develop a plan for revised patient or family caregiver teaching if patient or family caregiver is not able to teach back correctly.	Determines patient's and family caregiver's level of understanding of instructional topic.

Unexpected Outcomes	Related Interventions
1. Patient complains of localized pain or continued burning at injection site, indicating potential injury to nerve or vessels.	• Assess injection site. • Notify patient's health care provider.
2. During injection blood is aspirated.	• Immediately stop injection and remove needle. • Prepare new syringe of medication for administration.
3. Patient displays adverse reaction with signs of urticaria, eczema, pruritus, wheezing, and dyspnea.	• Follow agency policy or guidelines for appropriate response to allergic reactions (e.g., administration of antihistamine such as diphenhydramine or epinephrine). • Notify patient's health care provider immediately. • Add allergy information to patient's record.

Recording and Reporting

- Immediately after administration, record medication, dose, route, site, time, and date given on MAR in nurses' notes in electronic health record (EHR) or chart. Correctly sign MAR according to agency policy.
- Record patient teaching, validation of understanding, and patient's response to medication in nurse's notes in EHR or chart.
- Report any undesirable effects from medication to patient's health care provider and document adverse effects in record.

Special Considerations
Teaching

- Patients who require regular injections (e.g., vitamin B$_{12}$) need to learn techniques of self-administration. Teach a family caregiver injection techniques and the importance of rotating sites to decrease the risk for hypertrophy.
- Instruct patient and family caregiver to observe injection sites for complications and immediately report complications to the health care provider.
- Instruct patient and family caregiver to observe for effectiveness of medication and adverse reactions and report ineffectiveness

of medication and adverse reactions to the health care provider.
- Have patient perform several return demonstrations of medication preparation to validate that learning has taken place.

Pediatric
- Children can be very anxious or fearful of needles. Help with proper positioning and holding the child is sometimes necessary. Distraction such as blowing bubbles and pressure at the injection site before giving the injection can help alleviate anxiety (Hockenberry and Wilson, 2015).

Gerontological
- Older patients may have decreased muscle mass, which reduces drug absorption from IM injections. In addition, older adults

may have loss of muscle tone and strength that impairs mobility, placing them at high risk for falls from guarding an injection site.

Home Care
- Self-administration of an IM injection is difficult, especially in the ventrogluteal site. Teach a family caregiver to identify and administer injections in this site.
- Instruct adult patients who require frequent injections to apply EMLA cream to the injection site before administration.
- Instruct patients about the need for safe disposal of syringes and needles (see Skill 22.3, Home Care Considerations).
- See Skill 43.1 for information about modifying safety risks in the home.

◆ SKILL 22.5   Administering Medications by Intravenous Bolus

NSO *Nursing Skills Online Administration of Parenteral Medications: Intravenous Medications Module I Lesson 2*

In the past nurses often mixed medications into large volumes of intravenous (IV) fluids (500 to 1000 mL). However, today's safety standards and evidence-based practice no longer support this practice on a routine basis (INS, 2016; ISMP, 2011; TJC, 2016). Many patient safety risks such as incorrect calculation, poor aseptic technique, incorrect labeling, pump programming errors, lack of medication knowledge, and mix-up with another medication occur when nurses have to prepare medications in IV containers on patient care units. There are a number of current best practices for preparation and administration of IV medication (Box 22.4).

An IV bolus is one method of medication administration currently practiced on patient care units. It introduces a concentrated dose of a medication directly into a vein by way of an existing IV access. An IV bolus or "push" usually requires small volumes of fluid, which is an advantage for patients who are at risk for fluid overload. Administering medications by IV bolus is common in emergencies when you need to deliver a fast-acting medication quickly. Because these medications act quickly, it is essential that you monitor patients closely for adverse reactions. Agencies have policies and procedures that identify the medications that nurses are allowed to administer by IV push and other IV routes. These policies are based on the medication, compatibility and availability of staff, and type of monitoring equipment available. There are advantages and disadvantages to administering IV push medications (Box 22.5).

The IV bolus is a dangerous method to administer medications because it allows no time to correct errors. Administering an IV push medication too quickly can cause death. Therefore be very careful in calculating the correct amount of the medication to give and the rate of administration (see agency policy or manufacturer directions). In addition, a bolus may cause direct irritation to the lining of blood vessels; thus always confirm placement of the IV catheter or needle. Never give an IV bolus if the insertion site appears edematous or reddened or if the IV fluids do not flow at the ordered rate. Accidental injection of some medications into tissues surrounding a vein can cause pain, sloughing of tissues, and abscesses.

BOX 22.4

Best Practices for Administration of Intravenous Solutions and Medications

- Use standardized concentrations and dosages of medication.
- Use standardized procedures for ordering, preparing, and administering intravenous (IV) medications.
- Administer solutions and medications prepared and dispensed from the pharmacy or commercially prepared when possible.
- Never prepare high-alert medications (e.g., heparin, dopamine, dobutamine, nitroglycerin, potassium, antibiotics, or magnesium) on a patient care unit.
- Use standardized infusion concentrations of "high-alert" medications.
- Limit the use of add on devices to reduce risk of contamination and accidental disconnection.
- Standardize the storage of IV medications.
- Do not add medications to infusing containers of IV solutions.
- Use the mnemonic CATS PRRR to help remember safety checks for administering IV medications: C, compatibilities; A, allergies; T, tubing correct; S, site checked; P, pump safety checked; R, right rate; R, release clamps; R, return and reassess the patient.
- Use standardized label practices. Bold patient name, generic drug name, and patient-specific dose.
- Perform a medication reconciliation at each care transition (e.g., transfer, discharge) and when a new medication is ordered.
- Correctly use technology such as intelligent-infusion devices, bar code–assisted medication administration, and electronic medication administration record.

Adapted from Infusion Nurses Society: Infusion therapy standards of practice, *J Intraven Nurs* 39(1S), 2016; Institute for Safe Medication Practices (ISMP): Guidelines for standard order sets, 2010, http://www.ismp.org/tools/guidelines/StandardOrderSets.pdf. Accessed April 3, 2016; Institute for Safe Medication Practices (ISMP): *Principles of designing a medication label for intravenous piggyback medication for patient specific, inpatient use,* 2015, http://www.ismp.org/Tools/guidelines/labelFormats/Piggyback.asp. Accessed April 3, 2016; and The Joint Commission: *2016 National Patient Safety Goals,* 2016, http://www.jointcommission.org/standards_information/npsgs.aspx. Accessed April 3, 2016.

BOX 22.5

Advantages and Disadvantages of the Intravenous Push Method

Advantages	Disadvantages
• There is rapid onset of medication effects, which is useful in patients experiencing critical or emergent health problems.	• *Not all medications can be delivered by IV push.*
	• There is higher risk for infusion reactions; some are mild to severe because the medication action peaks quickly.
• Medications can be prepared quickly and given over a shorter time than by intravenous (IV) piggyback.	
• Doses of short-acting medications can be titrated on basis of a patient's needs and responses to the drug therapy. This is important for infants, children, and older patients.	• When giving medication quickly (e.g., less than 1 minute), there is very little opportunity to stop the injection if an adverse reaction occurs.
	• Risk for infiltration and phlebitis is increased, especially if a highly concentrated medication, a small peripheral vein, or a short venous access device is used.
• Method provides a more accurate dose of medication delivered because no medication is left in intravenously.	• Hypersensitivity reaction can cause an immediate or delayed systemic reaction to a medication, requiring supportive measures.

Verify the rate of administration of IV push medication using agency guidelines or a medication reference manual. The Institute for Safe Medication Practices (ISMP, 2015) has identified the following strategies to reduce harm from rapid IV push medications:

- Use commercially available or pharmacy prepared IV push medication whenever possible.
- Do not dilute IV push medications unless recommended by the manufacturer, agency policy, or reference literature.
- IV push medications should be administered at the rate recommended by the manufacturer, agency policy, or reference literature.
- Appropriately label of clinical prepared syringes.

Verify the rate of administration of IV push medication and compatibility using agency guidelines or a medication reference manual. Review the amount of medication that a patient will receive each minute, the recommended concentration, and rate of administration. For example, if a patient is to receive 6 mL of a medication over 3 minutes, give 2 mL of the IV bolus medication every minute. Understand the purpose of the medication and any potential adverse reactions related to the rate and route of administration. Some IV medications can only be given IV push safely when a patient is being monitored continuously for dysrhythmias, blood pressure changes, or other adverse effects. Therefore you can push some medications only in specific areas within a health care agency (e.g., critical care unit). Confirm agency guidelines regarding requirements for special monitoring.

IV push medications are given through either an existing continuous IV infusion or an intermittent venous access (commonly called a *saline lock*). A saline lock is an IV catheter with a small "well" or chamber covered by a rubber cap. An IV catheter can be converted into a lock by inserting a special rubber-seal injection cap into the end of the catheter (see Chapter 29). Use of a lock saves time by eliminating constant monitoring of an IV line. It also offers better mobility, safety, and comfort for patients by eliminating the need for a continuous IV line. After you administer an IV bolus through an intermittent venous access, flush with a normal saline solution to keep it patent.

Delegation and Collaboration

The skill of administering medications by IV bolus cannot be delegated to nursing assistive personnel (NAP). The nurse directs the NAP about:

- Potential medication actions and side effects of the medications and to immediately report their occurrence to the nurse.
- Reporting any patient complaints of moisture or discomfort around IV insertion site.
- Obtaining any required vital signs and reporting them to the nurse.

Equipment

- Watch with second hand
- Clean gloves
- Antiseptic swab
- Medication in vial or ampule
- Proper-size syringes for medication and saline flush with needleless device or sharps with engineered sharps injury protection (SESIP) needle (21- to 25-gauge)
- Intravenous lock: Vial of normal saline flush solution (saline recommended [Alexander et al., 2014]); if agency continues to use heparin flush, the most common concentration is 10 units/mL; check agency policy.
- Medication administration record (MAR) or computer printout
- Puncture-proof container

STEP	RATIONALE

ASSESSMENT

1. Check accuracy and completeness of each MAR or computer printout with health care provider's written medication order. Check patient's name, medication name and dosage, route of administration, and time of administration. Recopy or reprint any part of MAR that is difficult to read.

The order sheet is the most reliable source and only legal record of medications that patient is to receive. Ensures that patient receives the correct medications (Mandrack et al., 2012). Illegible MARs are a source of medication errors (Alassaad et al., 2013).

2. Assess patient's medical and medication history.

Identifies need for medication.

3. Review medication reference information for medication action, purpose, side effects, normal dose, time of peak onset, how slowly to give medication, and nursing implications such as need to dilute medication or administer it through a filter.

Knowledge of medication allows you to give it safely and monitor patient's response to therapy.

STEP	RATIONALE
4. If you give medication through an existing IV line, determine compatibility of medication with IV fluids and any additives within IV solution.	IV medication is not always compatible with IV solution and/or additives, and a new site may need to be initiated.
5. Perform hand hygiene. Assess condition of IV needle insertion site for signs of infiltration or phlebitis.	Do not administer medication if site is edematous or inflamed.
6. Assess patency of patient's existing IV infusion line or saline lock (see Chapter 29).	For medication to reach venous circulation effectively, IV line must be patent, and fluids must infuse easily.
7. Check patient's history of medication allergies: known allergens and normal allergic response.	IV bolus delivers medication rapidly. Allergic response is immediate.
8. Assess patient's symptoms before initiating medication therapy.	Provides information to evaluate desired effects of medication.
9. Assess patient's understanding of purpose of drug therapy.	Provides background to determine need for patient education.

NURSING DIAGNOSES

- Acute pain
- Deficient knowledge regarding medication administration or drug therapy

Related factors are individualized based on patient's condition or needs.

PLANNING

1. Expected outcomes following completion of procedure:	
• Patient experiences no medication side effects or adverse reactions.	Medication administered safely with desired therapeutic effect achieved.
• IV site remains intact, without signs of swelling or inflammation or symptoms of tenderness at site.	Medication infuses without complications to IV site and surrounding tissues.
• Patient explains purpose and side effects of medication.	Demonstrates learning.

IMPLEMENTATION

1. Prepare medications for one patient at a time using aseptic technique. Keep all pages of MARs or computer printouts for one patient together or look at only one patient's electronic MAR at a time. Check label of medication carefully with MAR or computer printout 2 times (see Skill 22.1 and Procedural Guideline 22.1) when preparing medication.	Ensures that medication is sterile. Preventing distractions reduces medication preparation errors. Use no-interruption zone (NIZ) when possible (Prakash et al., 2014; Yoder et al., 2015). *These are the first and second checks for accuracy* and ensure that correct medication is administered.

Clinical Decision Point *Some IV medications require dilution before administration. Verify with agency policy or pharmacy if dilution is permitted. If a small amount of medication is given (e.g., less than 1 mL), dilute medication in small amount (e.g., 5 mL) of normal saline or sterile water so it does not collect in the "dead spaces" (e.g., Y-site injection port, IV cap) of the IV delivery system.*

2. Take medication(s) to patient at correct time (see agency policy). Medications that require exact timing include stat, first-time or loading doses, and one time doses. Give time-critical scheduled medications (e.g., antibiotics, anticoagulants, insulin, anticonvulsants, immunosuppressive agents) at exact time ordered (no later than 30 minutes before or after scheduled dose). Give non–time-critical scheduled medications within a range of 1 or 2 hours of scheduled dose (ISMP, 2011). During administration apply six rights of medication administration.	Hospitals must adopt medication administration policy and procedure for timing of medication administration that considers nature of prescribed medication, specific clinical application, and patient needs (DHHS, 2011; ISMP, 2011). Time-critical scheduled medications are those for which early or delayed administration of maintenance doses of greater than 30 minutes before or after the scheduled dose may cause harm or result in substantial suboptimal therapy or pharmacological effect. Non–time-critical medications are those for which early or delayed administration within a specified range of either 1 or 2 hours should not cause harm or result in substantial suboptimal therapy or pharmacological effect (DHHS, 2011; ISMP, 2011).
3. Close room curtain or door.	Provides privacy.

STEP	RATIONALE
4. Identify patient using at least two identifiers (e.g., name and birthday or name and medical record number) according to agency policy. Compare identifiers with information on patient's MAR or medical record.	Ensures correct patient. Complies with The Joint Commission standards and improves patient safety (TJC, 2016). Some agencies are now using a bar-code system to help with patient identification.
5. At patient's bedside again compare MAR or computer printout with names of medications on medication labels and patient name. Ask patient if he or she has allergies.	*This is the third check for accuracy* and ensures that patient receives correct medication. Confirms patient's allergy history.
6. Discuss purpose of each medication, action, and possible adverse effects. Allow patient to ask any questions. Explain that you will give medication through existing IV line. Encourage patient to report symptoms of discomfort at IV site.	Keep patient informed of planned therapies, minimizing anxiety. Patients who verbalize pain at IV site help detect IV infiltrations early, lessening damage to surrounding tissues.
7. Perform hand hygiene and apply clean gloves.	Reduces transmission of infection.
8. IV push (existing IV line):	
a. Select injection port of IV tubing closest to patient. Use needleless injection port.	Follows provisions of Needle Safety and Prevention Act of 2001 (OSHA, n.d.).

Clinical Decision Point *Never administer IV medications through tubing that is infusing blood, blood products, or parenteral nutrition solutions.*

b. Clean injection port with antiseptic swab. Allow to dry.	Prevents transfer of microorganisms during blunt cannula insertion.
c. *Connect syringe to IV line:* Insert needleless tip of syringe containing drug through center of port (see illustration).	Prevents introduction of microorganisms. Prevents damage to port diaphragm and possible leakage from site.
d. Occlude IV line by pinching tubing just above injection port (see illustration). Pull back gently on plunger of syringe to aspirate for blood return.	Final check ensures that medication is being delivered into bloodstream.

Clinical Decision Point *In the case of smaller-gauge IV needles, blood return sometimes is not aspirated even if IV line is patent. If IV site does not show signs of infiltration and IV fluid is infusing without difficulty, give IV push.*

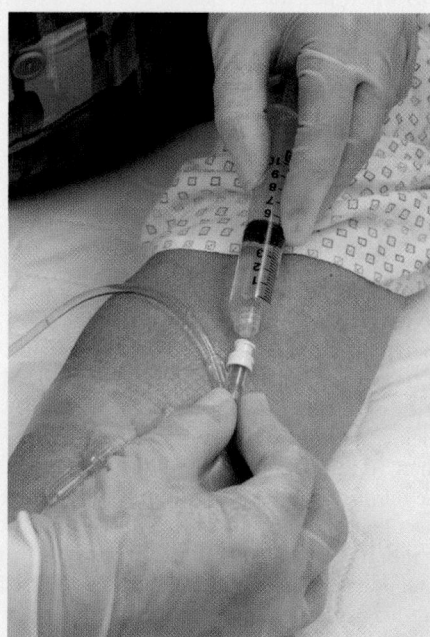

STEP 8c Connect syringe to IV line with needleless blunt cannula tip.

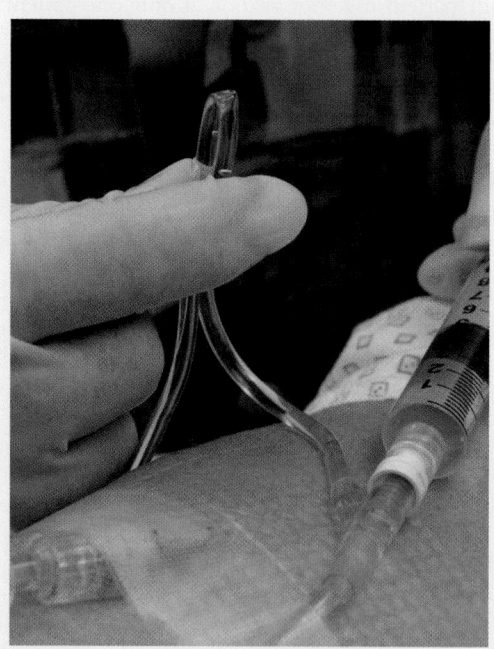

STEP 8d Occlude IV tubing above injection port.

STEP	RATIONALE

e. Release tubing and inject medication within amount of time recommended by agency policy, pharmacist, or medication reference manual. Use watch to time administrations (see illustration). You can pinch IV line while pushing medication and release it when not pushing medication. Allow IV fluids to infuse when not pushing medication.

Ensures safe medication infusion. Rapid injection of IV drug can be fatal. Allowing IV fluids to infuse while pushing IV drug enables medication to be delivered to patient at prescribed rate.

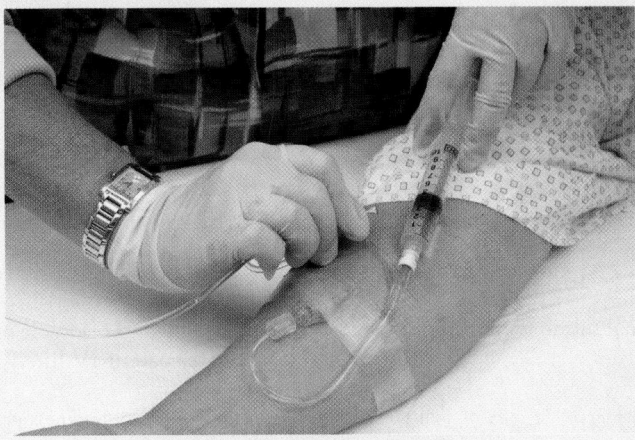

STEP 8e Use watch to time IV push medication.

f. After injecting medication, withdraw syringe and recheck IV fluid infusion rate.

g. If IV medication is incompatible with IV fluids, stop IV fluids, clamp IV line, and flush with 10 mL of normal saline or sterile water (see agency policy). Then give IV bolus over appropriate amount of time and flush with another 10 mL of normal saline or sterile water at *same rate* as medication was administered.

h. If IV line that currently is hanging is a medication, disconnect it and administer IV push medication as outlined in Step 9. Verify agency policy for stopping IV fluids or continuous IV medications. If unable to stop IV infusion, start new IV site (see Chapter 29) and administer medication using IV push (IV lock) method.

9. IV push (IV lock):

   a. Prepare flush solutions according to agency policy.

      (1) *Saline flush method (preferred method):* Prepare two syringes filled with 2 to 3 mL of normal saline (0.9%). Many agencies do not provide prefilled normal saline syringes for flushing IV lines.

      (2) Heparin flush method (refer to agency policy).

   b. Administer medication:

      (1) Clean injection port with antiseptic swab.

      (2) Insert needleless tip of syringe with normal saline 0.9% through center of injection port of IV lock (see illustrations).

Injection of bolus may alter rate of fluid infusion. Rapid fluid infusion can cause circulatory fluid overload.

Allows IV bolus to be administered without risks associated with IV incompatibilities. Ensure that agency guidelines permit flushing lines with incompatible medications. A new site may need to be initiated.

Avoids giving patient sudden bolus of medication in existing IV line.

Normal saline is effective in keeping IV locks patent and is compatible with wide range of medications (Patidar et al., 2014).

Prevents transfer of microorganisms during needle insertion.

STEP	RATIONALE

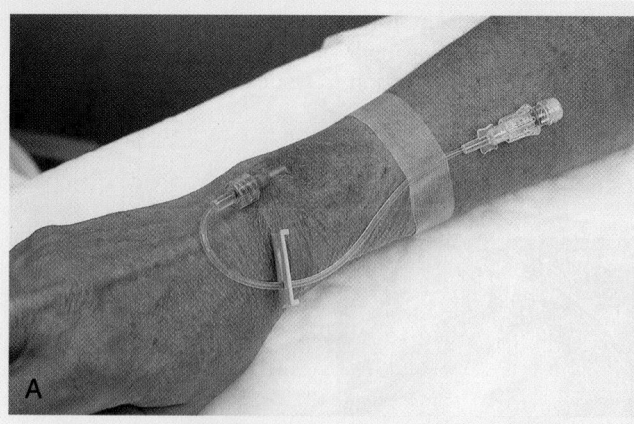 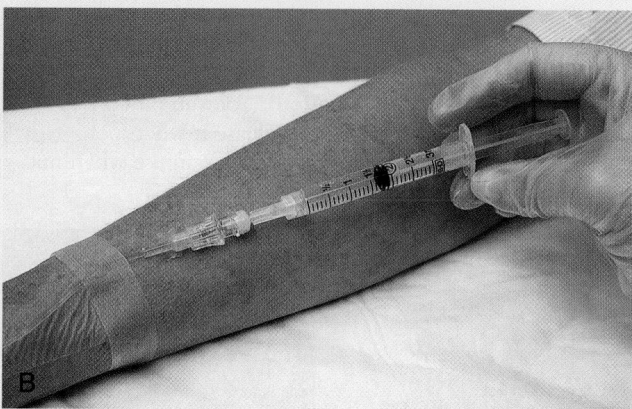

STEP 9b(2) A, IV catheter with saline lock adapter. **B,** Syringe inserted into injection port.

(3) Pull back gently on syringe plunger and check for blood return.	Indicates if needle or catheter is in vein.
(4) Flush IV site with normal saline by pushing slowly on plunger.	Clears needle and reservoir of blood. Flushing without difficulty indicates patent IV line.

Clinical Decision Point *Carefully observe the area of skin above the IV catheter. Note any puffiness or swelling as the IV site is flushed, which could indicate infiltration into the vein, requiring removal of catheter.*

(5) Remove saline-filled syringe.	
(6) Clean injection port with antiseptic swab.	Prevents transmission of microorganisms.
(7) Insert needleless tip of syringe containing prepared medication through injection port of IV lock.	Allows administration of medication.
(8) Inject medication within amount of time recommended by agency policy, pharmacist, or medication reference manual. Use watch to time administration.	Many medication errors are associated with IV pushes being administered too quickly. Following guidelines for IV push rates promotes patient safety.
(9) After administering bolus, withdraw syringe.	
(10) Clean injection port with antiseptic swab.	Prevents transmission of microorganisms.
(11) Flush injection port.	
(a) Attach syringe with normal saline and inject flush at same rate that medication was delivered.	Flushing IV line with saline prevents occlusion of IV access device and ensures that all medication is delivered. Flushing IV site at same rate as medication ensures that any medication remaining within IV needle is delivered at the correct rate.
10. Dispose of SESIP covered needles and syringes in puncture- and leak-proof container.	Prevents accidental needlestick injuries and follows CDC guidelines for disposal of sharps (OSHA, n.d.).
11. Stay with patient for several minutes and observe for any allergic reactions.	Dyspnea, wheezing, and circulatory collapse are signs of anaphylactic reaction.
12. Remove clean gloves and perform hand hygiene.	Reduces transmission of microorganisms.

EVALUATION

1. Observe patient closely for adverse reactions during administration and for several minutes thereafter.	IV medications act rapidly.
2. Observe IV site during injection for sudden swelling and for 48 hours after IV push.	Swelling indicates infiltration into tissues surrounding vein. Signs of infiltration may not occur for 48 hours.
3. Assess patient's status after giving medication to evaluate effectiveness of the medication.	Some IV bolus medications can cause rapid changes in patient's physiological status. Some medications require careful monitoring and assessment and possibly future laboratory testing (e.g., vasopressors and antiarrhythmics require blood pressure and heart rate monitoring, and heparin requires laboratory studies after administration to determine therapeutic levels).

STEP	RATIONALE
4. Use Teach-Back: "I want to be sure I explained to you why you are receiving this IV bolus medication. Can you explain to me what the medication is for and when to call the nurse?" Revise your instruction now or develop a plan for revised patient or family caregiver teaching if patient or family caregiver is not able to teach back correctly.	Determines patient's and family caregiver's level of understanding of instructional topic.

Unexpected Outcomes	Related Interventions
1. Patient develops adverse reaction to medication.	• Stop delivering medication immediately and follow agency policy or guidelines for appropriate response to allergic reaction (e.g., administration of antihistamine such as diphenhydramine or epinephrine) and reporting of adverse drug reactions. • Notify patient's health care provider of adverse effects immediately. • Add allergy information to patient's record.
2. IV medication is incompatible with IV fluids (e.g., IV fluid becomes cloudy in tubing) (see agency policy).	• Stop IV fluids and clamp IV line. • Flush IV line with 10 mL of 0.9% sodium chloride or sterile water. • Give IV bolus over appropriate amount of time. • Flush with another 10 mL of 0.9% sodium chloride or sterile water at same rate as medication was administered. • Restart IV fluids with new tubing at prescribed rate. • If unable to stop IV infusion, start new IV site (see Chapter 29) and administer medication using IV push (IV lock) method.
3. IV site shows symptoms of infiltration or phlebitis (see Chapter 29).	• Stop IV infusion immediately or discontinue access device and restart in another site. • Determine how much damage IV medication can produce in subcutaneous tissue. • Provide IV extravasation care (e.g., injecting phentolamine around IV infiltration site) as indicated by agency policy, use a medication reference, and consult pharmacist to determine appropriate follow-up care.

Recording and Reporting

- Immediately record medication administration, including drug, dose, route, time instilled, and date and time administered on MAR in nurses' notes in electronic health record (EHR) or chart. Include initials or signature.
- Record patient teaching, validation of understanding, and patient's response to medication in nurse's notes in EHR or chart.
- Report any adverse reactions to patient's health care provider. Patient's response sometimes indicates need for additional medical therapy.
- Record patient's medication response in nurses' notes in EHR or chart.

Special Considerations
Teaching

- Teach patient and/or family caregiver that effects of IV push medications occur rapidly. Explain reasons for giving medication slowly and teach signs of adverse effects.

Pediatric

- The therapeutic dosage of IV push medications for infants and children is often small and difficult to prepare accurately, even with a tuberculin syringe. You need to infuse these medications slowly and in small volumes because of the risk for fluid volume overload (Hockenberry and Wilson, 2015). To maintain pediatric patient safety, carefully follow agency policies when administering medications via IV bolus.

Gerontological

- The renal and metabolic systems do not function as efficiently because of the aging process. To reduce the risk for adverse effects of IV push medications, have good drug knowledge about adverse effects and drug interactions. Older patients may tolerate IV push medications if they are given over longer periods of time.

Home Care

- IV push medications are frequently given in the home. Nurses, pharmacists, and health care providers need to collaborate closely in the care of these patients. Patients and family caregivers who are independently responsible for managing IV medications need to understand all aspects of administration safety. Adequate eyesight and manual dexterity are necessary to manipulate the syringe. Patients need to understand their venous access device, rate to give medications, and how to flush their access device. Patients need to store their medications safely and dispose of their IV supplies, and they should know whom to contact in case of an emergency.

NSO *Nursing Skills Online Administration of Parenteral Medications: Intravenous Medications Module / Lesson 3*

One method of administering intravenous (IV) medications uses small volumes (25 to 250 mL) of compatible IV fluids infused over a desired period of time. This method reduces the risk for rapid dose infusion and provides independence for patients. Patients must have an established IV line that is kept patent by either a continuous infusion or intermittent flushes of normal saline. You can administer intermittent infusion of medication with any of the following methods.

- *Piggyback.* A piggyback is a small (25- to 250-mL) IV bag or bottle connected to a short tubing line that connects to the *upper* Y-port of a primary infusion line or to an intermittent venous access such as a saline lock. The IV container that holds the medication is labeled following the IV piggyback medication format of the Institute for Safe Medication Practices (ISMP, 2015). The piggyback tubing is a microdrip or macrodrip system (see Chapter 29). The set is called a *piggyback* because the small bag or bottle is set *higher* than the primary infusion bag or bottle. In the piggyback setup the main line does not infuse when a compatible piggybacked medication is infusing. The port of the primary IV line contains a back-check valve that automatically stops the flow of the primary infusion once the piggyback infusion flows. After the piggyback solution infuses and the solution within the tubing falls below the level of the primary infusion drip chamber, the back-check valve opens, and the primary infusion starts to flow again.
- *Volume-Control Administration.* Volume-control administration sets (e.g., Volutrol, Buretrol, Pediatrol) are small (50- to 150-mL) containers that attach just below the primary infusion bag or bottle. The set is attached and filled in a manner similar to that used with a regular IV infusion. However, the priming filling of the set is different, depending on the type of filter (floating valve or membrane) within the set. Follow package directions for priming sets.
- *Mini-Infusion Pump.* The mini-infusion pump is battery operated and delivers medication in very small amounts of fluid (5 to 60 mL) within controlled infusion times using standard syringes (Fig. 22.20).

Needle Safety

The Needle Safety and Prevention Act of 2001 mandates that health care agencies use safe needle devices and manufactured needleless systems to reduce needlestick injury. Systems with catheter ports or Y-connector sites are designed to contain a needle housed in a protective covering. Needleless infusion lines allow a direct connection with the IV line via a recessed connection port, a blunt-ended cannula, or shielded-needle device, eliminating the risk for exposure to an IV needle (OSHA, n.d.).

Delegation and Collaboration

The skill of administering IV medications by piggyback, intermittent infusion sets, and mini-infusion pumps cannot be delegated to nursing assistive personnel (NAP). The nurse directs the NAP about:

- Potential medication actions and side effects and to immediately report their occurrence to the nurse.
- Reporting any patient complaints of moisture or discomfort around IV insertion site.
- Reporting any change in patient's condition or vital signs to the nurse.

Equipment

- Adhesive tape (*optional*)
- Antiseptic swab
- Clean gloves
- IV pole
- Medication administration record (MAR) or computer printout
- Puncture-proof container

Piggyback or Mini-Infusion Pump
- Medication prepared in 50- to 250-mL labeled infusion bag or syringe
- Prefilled syringe of normal saline flush solution (for saline lock only)
- Short microdrip, macrodrip, or mini-infusion IV tubing set with blunt-end (needleless) cannula attachment
- Needleless device
- Mini-infusion pump if indicated

Volume-Control Administration Set
- Volutrol or Buretrol
- Infusion tubing with needleless system attachment
- Syringe (1 to 20 mL)
- Vial or ampule of ordered medication

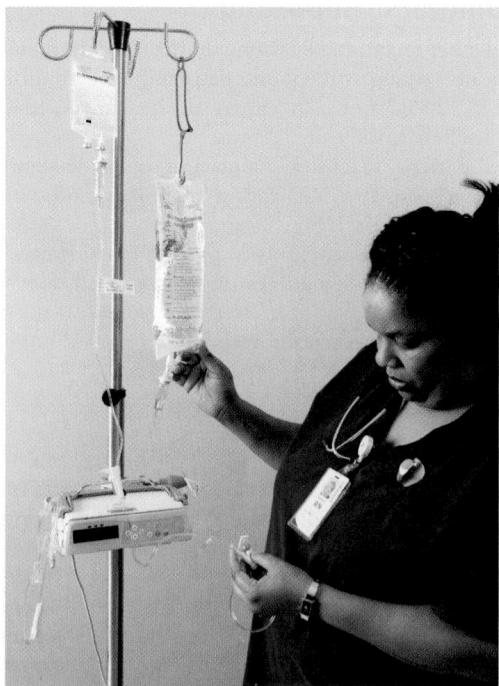

FIG 22.20 Mini-infusion pump.

STEP	RATIONALE

ASSESSMENT

1. Check accuracy and completeness of each MAR or computer printout with health care provider's written medication order. Check patient's name, medication name and dosage, route of administration, and time of administration. Recopy or reprint any part of MAR that is difficult to read.

The order sheet is the most reliable source and only legal record of medications that patient is to receive. Ensures that patient receives the correct medications (Mandrack et al., 2012). Illegible MARs are a source of medication errors (Alassaad et al., 2013).

2. Assess patient's medical and medication history.

Determines need for medication or possible contraindications for medication administration.

3. Assess patient's history of allergies: known type of allergens and normal allergic reaction.

IV administration of medication may cause rapid response. Allergic response is immediate.

4. Review medication reference information for medication action, purpose, normal dose, side effects, time and peak of onset, how slowly to give medication, and nursing implications (e.g., need to dilute medication, administer through filter).

Allows you to administer medication safely and monitor patient's response to therapy.

5. If you give medication through existing IV line, determine compatibility of medication with IV fluids and any additional additives within IV solution.

IV medication is sometimes not compatible with IV solution and/or additives.

Clinical Decision Point *Never administer IV medications through tubing that is infusing blood, blood products, or parenteral nutrition solutions.*

6. Assess patency and placement of patient's existing IV infusion line or saline lock (see Chapter 29).

Do not administer medication if site is edematous or inflamed.

Clinical Decision Point *If patient's IV site is saline locked, clean the port with alcohol and assess the patency of the IV line by flushing it with 2 to 3 mL of sterile sodium chloride.*

7. Assess patient's symptoms before initiating medication therapy.

Provides information to evaluate desired effects of medication.

8. Assess patient's knowledge of medication.

Provides background to determine need for patient education.

NURSING DIAGNOSES

- Deficient knowledge regarding medication administration or drug therapy
- Risk for imbalanced fluid volume
- Risk for ineffective health maintenance

Related factors/Risk factors are individualized based on patient's condition or needs.

PLANNING

1. Expected outcomes following completion of procedure:
   - Patient experiences no adverse reactions.
   - Medication infuses within desired time frame.
   - IV site remains intact without signs of swelling, inflammation, or symptoms of tenderness at site.
   - Patient explains medication purposes, action, side effects, and dosage.

Medication was administered safely with desired therapeutic effect.
IV line remains patent.
Fluid infuses into vein, not tissues.
Demonstrates learning.

IMPLEMENTATION

1. Prepare medications for one patient at a time using aseptic technique. Check label of medication carefully with MAR or computer printout 2 times (see Skill 22.1 and Procedural Guideline 22.1) when preparing medication. Pharmacy prepares piggyback and prefilled syringes. You prepare medication for Volutrol.

Ensures that medication is sterile. Preventing distractions reduces medication preparation errors. Use no-interruption zone (NIZ) when possible (Prakash et al., 2014; Yoder et al., 2015).
These are the first and second checks for accuracy and ensure that correct medication is administered.

STEP	RATIONALE

2. Take medication(s) to patient at correct time (see agency policy). Medications that require exact timing include stat, first-time or loading doses, and one time doses. Give time-critical scheduled medications (e.g., antibiotics, anticoagulants, insulin, anticonvulsants, immunosuppressive agents) at exact time ordered (no later than 30 minutes before or after scheduled dose). Give non–time-critical scheduled medications within a range of 1 or 2 hours of scheduled dose (ISMP, 2011). During administration apply six rights of medication administration.

Hospitals must adopt medication administration policy and procedure for timing of medication administration that considers nature of the prescribed medication, specific clinical application, and patient needs (DHHS, 2011; ISMP, 2011). Time-critical scheduled medications are those for which early or delayed administration of maintenance doses of greater than 30 minutes before or after the scheduled dose may cause harm or result in substantial suboptimal therapy or pharmacological effect. Non–time-critical medications are those for which early or delayed administration within a specified range of either 1 or 2 hours should not cause harm or result in substantial suboptimal therapy or pharmacological effect (DHHS, 2011; ISMP, 2011).

3. Close room curtain or door. Perform hand hygiene and apply clean gloves.

Provides privacy. Reduces infection transmission.

4. Identify patient using at least two identifiers (e.g., name and birthday or name and medical record number) according to agency policy. Compare identifiers with information on patient's MAR or medical record.

Ensures correct patient. Complies with The Joint Commission standards and improves patient safety (TJC, 2016).

Some agencies are now using a bar-code system to help with patient identification.

5. At patient's bedside again compare MAR or computer printout with names of medications on medication labels and patient name. Ask patient if he or she has allergies.

This is the third check for accuracy and ensures that patient receives correct medication. Confirms patient's allergy history.

6. Discuss purpose of each medication, action, and possible adverse effects. Allow patient to ask any questions. Explain that you will give medication through existing IV line. Encourage patient to report symptoms of discomfort at site.

Keep patient informed of planned therapies, minimizing anxiety. Patients who verbalize pain at IV site help detect IV infiltrations early, lessening damage to surrounding tissues.

7. Administer infusion.

   a. Piggyback infusion:

     (1) Connect infusion tubing to medication bag (see Chapter 29). Fill tubing by opening regulator flow clamp. Once tubing is full, close clamp and cap end of tubing.

Filling infusion tubing with solution and freeing air bubbles prevent air embolus.

     (2) Hang piggyback (see illustration) medication bag above level of primary fluid bag. (Use hook to lower main bag.)

Height of fluid bag affects rate of flow to patient.

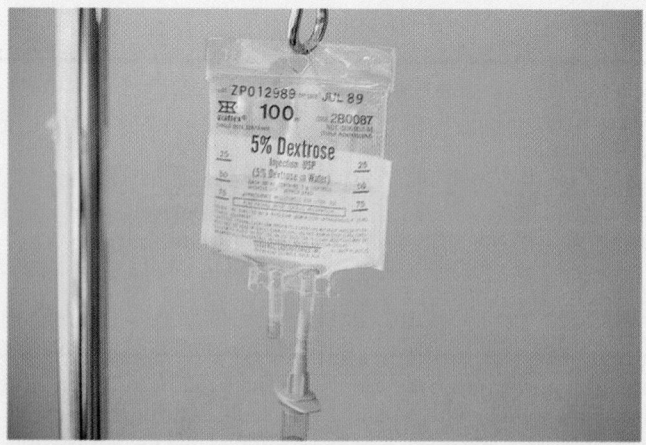

STEP 7a(2) Small-volume minibag for piggyback infusion.

     (3) Connect tubing of piggyback infusion to appropriate connector on upper Y-port of primary infusion line:

Connection allows IV medication to enter main IV line.

STEP	RATIONALE

(a) *Needleless system:* Wipe off needleless port of main IV line with alcohol swab, allow to dry, and insert cannula tip of piggyback infusion tubing (see illustrations).

Use needleless connections to prevent accidental needlestick injuries (INS, 2016; OSHA, n.d.).

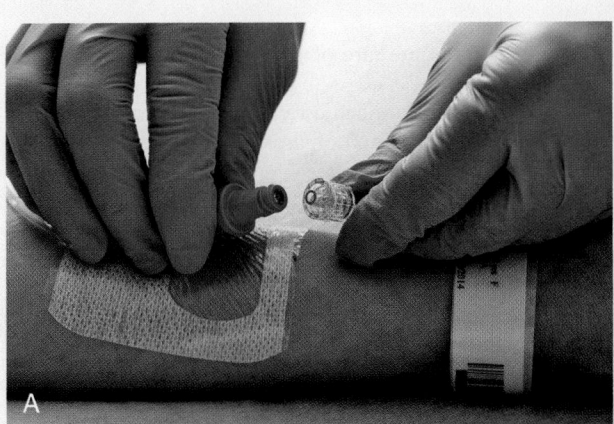 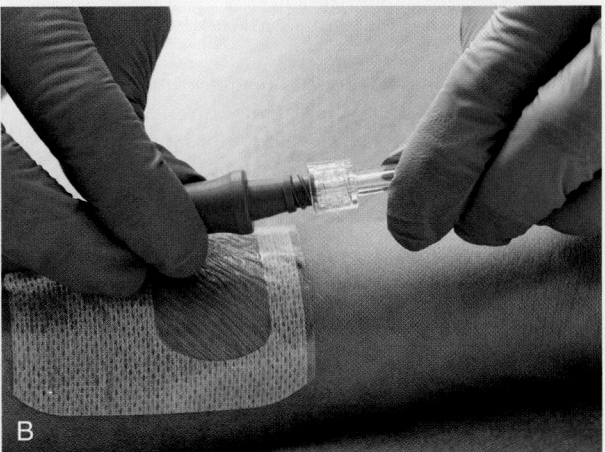

STEP 7a(3)(a) A, Needleless lock cannula system. **B,** Blunt-ended cannula inserts into port and locks.

(4) *Option:* Normal saline lock: Follow Steps 9a(1) through 9b(6) in Skill 22.5 to flush and prepare lock. Wipe off port with alcohol swab, let dry, and insert tip of piggyback infusion tubing via needleless access.

Flushing of lock ensures patency.

(5) Regulate flow rate of medication solution by adjusting regulator clamp or IV pump infusion rate. Infusion times vary. Refer to medication reference or agency policy for safe flow rate.

Provides slow, safe, intermittent infusion of medication and maintains therapeutic blood levels.

(6) Once medication has infused:

  (a) Continuous infusion: Check flow rate of primary infusion. Primary infusion automatically begins after piggyback solution is empty.

Back-check valve on piggyback prevents flow of primary infusion until medication infuses. Checking flow rate ensures proper administration of IV fluids.

  (b) Normal saline lock: Disconnect tubing, clean port with alcohol, and flush IV line with 2 to 3 mL of sterile 0.9% sodium chloride. Maintain sterility of IV tubing between intermittent infusions.

(7) Regulate continuous main infusion line to ordered rate.

Infusion of piggyback sometimes interferes with main line infusion rate.

(8) Leave IV piggyback and tubing in place for future drug administration (see agency policy) or discard in puncture- and leak-proof container.

Establishing secondary line produces route for microorganisms to enter main line. Repeated changes in tubing increase risk for infection transmission.

b. Volume-control administration set (e.g., Volutrol):

  (1) Fill Volutrol with desired amount of IV fluid (50 to 100 mL) by opening clamp between Volutrol and main IV bag (see illustration).

Small volume of fluid dilutes IV medication and reduces risk of fluid infusing too rapidly.

  (2) Close clamp and check to be sure that clamp on air vent Volutrol chamber is open.

Prevents additional leakage of fluid into Volutrol. Air vent allows fluid in Volutrol to exit at regulated rate.

  (3) Clean injection port on top of Volutrol with antiseptic swab.

Prevents introduction of microorganisms during needle insertion.

  (4) Remove needle cap or sheath and insert needleless syringe or syringe needle through port and inject medication (see illustration). Gently rotate Volutrol between hands.

Rotating mixes medication with solution to ensure equal distribution in Volutrol.

STEP	RATIONALE
(5) Regulate IV infusion rate to allow medication to infuse in time recommended by agency policy, pharmacist, or medication reference manual.	For optimal therapeutic effect, medication should infuse in prescribed time interval.
(6) Label Volutrol with name of medication; dosage, total volume, including diluent; and time of administration following ISMP (2015) safe-medication label format.	Alerts nurses to medication being infused. Prevents other medications from being added to Volutrol.
(7) If patient is receiving continuous IV infusion, check infusion rate after Volutrol infusion is complete.	Ensures appropriate rate of administration.
(8) Dispose of uncapped needle or needle enclosed in safety shield and syringe in puncture- and leak-proof container. Discard supplies in appropriate container. Perform hand hygiene.	Prevents accidental needlesticks (OSHA, n.d.). Reduces transmission of microorganisms.
c. Mini-infusion administration:	
(1) Connect prefilled syringe to mini-infusion tubing; remove end cap of tubing.	Special tubing designed to fit syringe delivers medication to main IV line.
(2) Carefully apply pressure to syringe plunger, allowing tubing to fill with medication.	Ensures that tubing is free of air bubbles to prevent air embolus.
(3) Place syringe into mini-infusion pump (follow product directions) and hang on IV pole. Be sure that syringe is secured (see illustration).	Secure placement is needed for proper infusion.

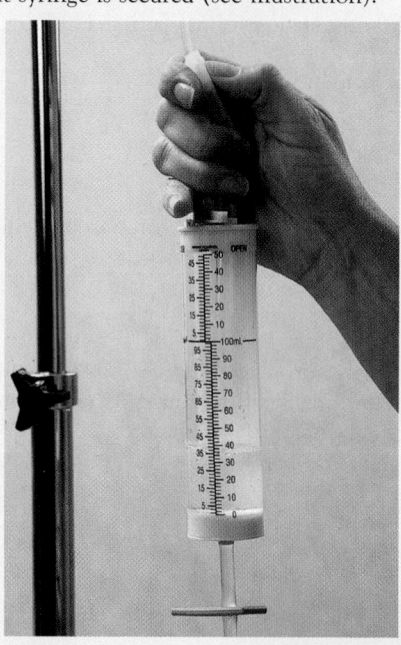

STEP 7b(1) Fill volume-control administration device.

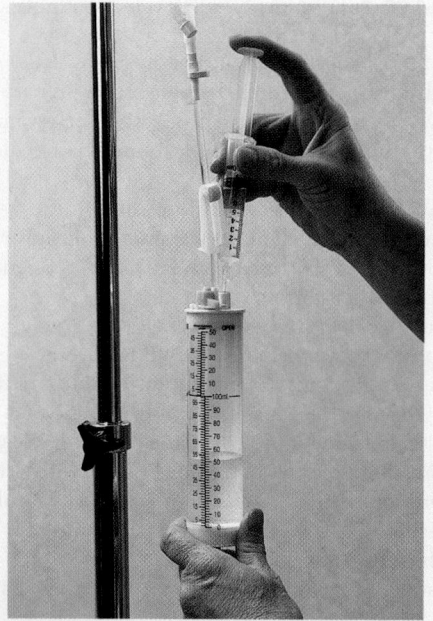

STEP 7b(4) Medication injected into device.

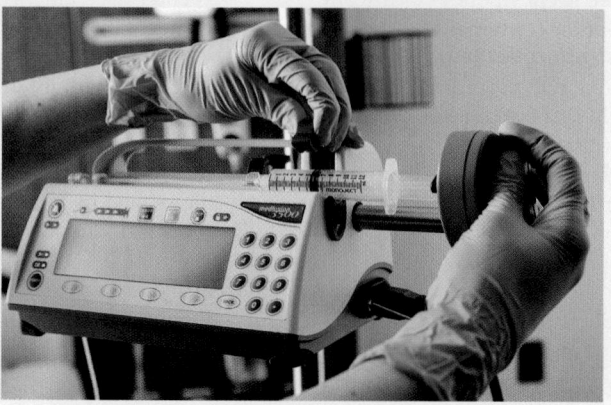

STEP 7c(3) Ensure that syringe is secure after placing it into mini-infusion pump.

STEP	RATIONALE
(4) Connect end of mini-infusion tubing to main IV line or saline lock:	Establishes route for IV medication to enter main IV line.
(a) *Existing IV line:* Wipe off needleless port on main IV line with alcohol swab, allow to dry, and insert tip of mini-infusion tubing through center of port.	Needleless connections reduce risk for accidental needlestick injuries (OSHA, n.d.).
(b) *Normal saline lock:* Follow Steps 9a(1) through 9b(6) in Skill 22.5 to flush and prepare lock. Wipe off port with alcohol swab, allow to dry, and insert tip of mini-infusion tubing.	
(5) Set pump to deliver medication within time recommended by agency policy, pharmacist, or medication reference manual. Press button on pump to begin infusion.	Pump automatically delivers medication at safe, constant rate based on volume in syringe.
(6) Once medication has infused:	
(a) *Main IV infusion:* Check flow rate. Infusion automatically begins to flow once pump stops. Regulate infusion to desired rate as needed.	Maintains patent primary IV fluids.
(b) *Normal saline lock:* Disconnect tubing, clean port with alcohol, and flush IV line with 2 to 3 mL of sterile 0.9% sodium chloride. Maintain sterility of IV tubing between intermittent infusions.	
8. Dispose of supplies in puncture- and leak-proof container.	Prevents accidental needlesticks (OSHA, n.d.).
9. Remove gloves and perform hand hygiene.	Reduces transmission of microorganisms.
10. Stay with patient for several minutes and observe for any allergic reactions.	Dyspnea, wheezing, and circulatory collapse are signs of severe anaphylactic reaction.

EVALUATION

1. Observe patient for signs or symptoms of adverse reaction.	IV medications act rapidly.
2. During infusion periodically check infusion rate and condition of IV site.	IV must remain patent for proper drug administration. Infiltration of IV site requires discontinuing infusion.
3. Ask patient to explain purpose and side effects of medication.	Evaluates patient's understanding of instruction.
4. Use Teach-Back: "I want to be sure I explained to you the reason for this IV medication. Can you explain to me why you are receiving the medication and what to report to the nurse?" Revise your instruction now or develop a plan for revised patient or family caregiver teaching if patient or family caregiver is not able to teach back correctly.	Determines patient's and family caregiver's level of understanding of instructional topic.

Unexpected Outcomes	Related Interventions
1. Patient develops adverse or allergic reaction to medication.	• Stop medication infusion immediately.
	• Follow agency policy or guidelines for appropriate response to allergic reaction (e.g., administration of antihistamine such as diphenhydramine or epinephrine) and reporting of adverse medication reactions.
	• Notify patient's health care provider of adverse effects immediately.
	• Add allergy information to patient record per agency policy.
2. Medication does not infuse over established time frame.	• Determine reason (e.g., improper calculation of flow rate, poor positioning of IV needle at insertion site, infiltration).
	• Take corrective action as indicated.
3. IV site shows signs of infiltration or phlebitis (see Chapter 29).	• Stop IV infusion and discontinue access device.
	• Treat IV site as indicated by agency policy.
	• Insert new IV catheter if therapy continues.
	• For infiltration determine how harmful IV medication is to subcutaneous tissue. Provide IV extravasation care (e.g., injecting phentolamine around IV infiltration site) as indicated by agency policy or consult pharmacist to determine appropriate follow-up care.

Recording and Reporting

- Immediately record medication, dose, route, infusion rate, and date and time administered on MAR in nurses' notes in electronic health record (EHR) or chart. Include initials or signature.
- Record volume of fluid in medication bag or Volutrol on intake and output (I&O) form.
- Record patient teaching, validation of understanding, and patient's response to medication in nurse's notes in EHR or chart.
- Report any adverse reactions to patient's health care provider.

Special Considerations
Teaching

- Review all IV medications with patient and family caregivers, including why patient is receiving the medication and potential adverse effects, including allergic responses.
- Teach patient and/or family caregivers not to alter the ordered rate of infusion without consulting the health care provider. IV medications need to be infused at a specified rate to achieve their desired effect and avoid adverse effects.
- Teach patient and/or family caregiver to report any adverse effects immediately.

Pediatric

- Infants and young children are more vulnerable to alterations in fluid balance and do not adjust quickly to changes in it. Therefore, to assess fluid balance, monitor I&O carefully when infusing IV medications (Hockenberry and Wilson, 2015).

Gerontological

- Altered pharmacokinetics of medications and the effects of polypharmacy place older adults at risk for medication toxicity. Carefully monitor the response of older adults to IV medications (Touhy and Jett, 2014).
- Older adults are at risk for developing fluid volume overload and require careful assessment for signs of overload and heart failure.

Home Care

- Patients or family caregivers who administer IV medications at home require education about the steps of medication administration. The patient or family caregiver needs to perform several return demonstrations of IV medication administration before performing this skill independently. In addition, patients and family caregivers need to know signs of IV medication administration complications such as phlebitis and infiltration and what to do for any problems.

◆ SKILL 22.7   Administering Continuous Subcutaneous Medications

NSO   *Nursing Skills Online Administration of Parenteral Medications: Intravenous Medications Module / Lesson 4*

The continuous subcutaneous infusion (CSQI or CSCI) route of medication administration is used for selected medications (e.g., opioids, insulin). The route is also effective with medications to stop preterm labor (e.g., terbutaline) and to treat pulmonary hypertension (e.g., treprostinil sodium). One factor that determines the infusion rate of CSQI is the rate of medication absorption. Most patients can absorb 1 to 2 mL/hour of medication, but the rate of absorption is more dependent on osmotic pressure than rate of administration (Alexander et al., 2014; Arthur, 2015).

With CSQI patients are able to manage their illness and/or pain without the risks and expenses involved with intravenous (IV) medication administration (Bartz et al., 2014). The route is relatively easy for patients and families to learn and understand in the home setting. CSQI improves oncological and postoperative pain control in infants, children, and adults (Arthur, 2015; Oldenmenger et al., 2012). Box 22.6 summarizes benefits associated with the use of CSQI for pain management.

Patients with diabetes mellitus using CSQI for management of blood glucose levels receive intense diabetes self-management education from qualified diabetes educators and insulin pump trainers. The newest system, Medtronic MiniMed (2015), integrates an insulin pump with real-time continuous glucose monitoring (Fig. 22.21). Patients with diabetes mellitus using insulin pumps generally require less insulin because it is absorbed and used more efficiently (Buchko, 2012; Heinemann et al., 2015). Box 22.7 lists criteria for selecting insulin pumps for patient use.

The procedure to initiate and discontinue CSQI therapy is similar, regardless of the type of medication being delivered.

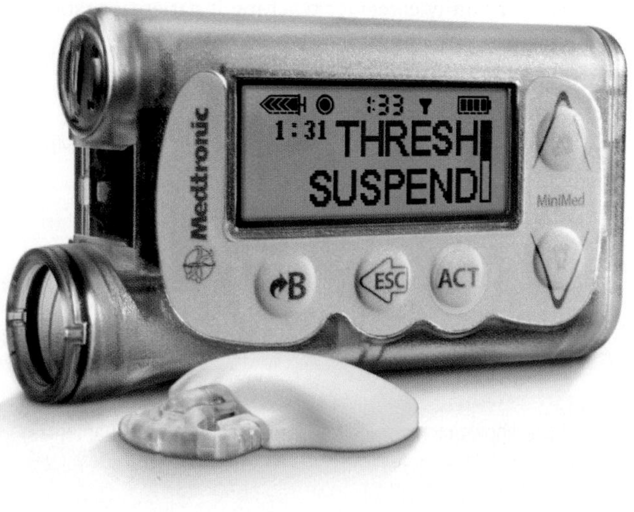

BOX 22.6

Pain Management Benefits With Use of Continuous Subcutaneous Infusion

- Benefits patients with poor venous access
- Provides pain relief to patients who are unable to tolerate oral pain medications
- Allows patients greater mobility
- Onset of action about 20 minutes
- Better pain control than intramuscular injections
- Lower rates of infection

Modified from Arthur A: Innovations in subcutaneous infusions, *J Infus Nurs* 38(3):179, 2015; Bartz L, et al: Subcutaneous administration of drugs in palliative care: result of a systematic observational study, *J Pain Symptom Manag* 48(4):540, 2014.

FIG 22.21 Mini-Med Paradigm REAL-Time Insulin CSQI Pump and Continuous Glucose Monitoring System. (*Courtesy Medtronic, Inc., Northridge, CA.*)

Patient Selection Criteria for Use of Insulin Pumps

- Possesses strong motivation and commitment to use diabetes management skills
- Requires or desires improved control of blood glucose levels
- Requires greater flexibility than allowed by traditional insulin injection schedules
- Is willing to participate in a formal diabetes education program
- Possesses strong critical thinking and problem-solving skills
- Accepts responsibilities associated with the self-management of diabetes
- Is able to perform self-blood glucose monitoring and operate the insulin pump
- Displays evidence of effective coping patterns
- Has family support systems available
- Secures financial resources to cover costs associated with CSQI

Data from Heinemann L, et al: Insulin pump risks and benefits: a clinical appraisal of pump safety, standards, adverse event reporting, and research needs, *Diabetes Care* 38(4):716, 2015.
CSQI, Continuous subcutaneous infusion.

However, nursing assessment and interventions vary, depending on the type of medication administered. For example, if the medication is for diabetes glucose management, you evaluate the patient's blood glucose levels and monitor episodes of hypoglycemia or hyperglycemia (Carchidi et al., 2011).

Use a small-gauge (25 to 27) winged butterfly IV needle or special commercially prepared Teflon cannula to deliver medications. Although Teflon cannulas generally are more expensive, they are more comfortable for the patient and have lower rates of complications than winged IV needles. The cannulas are associated with fewer needlestick injuries. Base the choice of needle type on agency guidelines or patient preference. Use the needle with the shortest length and the smallest gauge necessary to establish and maintain the infusion.

Use the same anatomical sites for subcutaneous injections and the upper chest. Site selection depends on a patient's activity level and the type of medication delivered. For example, pain medications given to ambulatory patients are best delivered in the upper chest, which allows a patient to move freely. Insulin is absorbed most consistently in the abdomen; thus choose a site in the abdomen away from the waistline. Always avoid sites where the tubing of the pump could be disturbed. Rotate sites used for medication administration at least every 2 to 7 days or whenever complications such as leaking occur (Alexander et al., 2014; Arthur, 2015; INS, 2016).

The CSQI route requires a computerized pump with safety features, including lockout intervals and warning alarms. Ideally medication pumps are individualized on the basis of the medication being delivered and a patient's needs. You also need to consider the availability and cost of the pump and its supplies. When possible, have patients select the pump that fits their individual and home needs and is easiest to use.

Delegation and Collaboration

The skill of administering CSQI medications cannot be delegated to nursing assistive personnel (NAP). The nurse directs the NAP about:

- Potential medication side effects or reactions and to immediately report their occurrence to the nurse.
- Reporting complications (e.g., leaking, redness, discomfort) at the CSQI needle insertion site to the nurse.
- Obtaining any required vital signs and reporting them to the nurse.

Equipment

Initiation of CSQI
- Clean gloves
- Alcohol swab
- Antibacterial skin preparation such as chlorhexidine
- Small (25- to 27-gauge) winged IV catheter with attached tubing or CSQI-designed catheter (e.g., Sof-Set)
- Infusion pump
- Occlusive, transparent dressing
- Tape
- Medication in appropriate syringe or container
- Medication administration record (MAR) or computer printout

Discontinuing CSQI
- Clean gloves
- Small, sterile gauze dressing
- Tape or adhesive bandage
- Alcohol swab and chlorhexidine (*optional*)
- Puncture-proof container

STEP	RATIONALE

ASSESSMENT

1. Check accuracy and completeness of each MAR or computer printout with health care provider's written medication order. Check patient's name, medication name and dosage, route of administration, and time of administration. Recopy or reprint any part of MAR that is difficult to read.

The order sheet is the most reliable source and only legal record of medications that patient is to receive. Ensures that patient receives the correct medications (Mandrack et al., 2012). Illegible MARs are a source of medication errors (Alassaad et al., 2013).

2. Assess patient's medical and medication history.

Determines need for medication or possible contraindications for medication administration.

3. Assess patient's history of allergies: known type of allergens and normal allergic reaction.

CSQI administration of medications may cause rapid response. Allergic response is immediate.

4. Collect drug reference information necessary to administer drug safely, including action, purpose, side effects, normal dose, time of peak onset, how slowly to give medication, and nursing implications.

Knowledge of medication allows you to give medication safely and monitor patient's response to therapy.

STEP	RATIONALE
5. Assess patient's previous verbal and nonverbal response to needle insertion.	Anticipating patient's anxiety allows you to use distraction to reduce pain awareness.
6. If an analgesic is being administered, assess patient's pain severity using a scale from 0 to 10; 0 being no pain and 10 being the worst pain ever experienced.	Provides an objective measure of pain severity.
7. Assess for contraindications to CSQI (e.g., thrombocytopenia or reduced local tissue perfusion).	Any existing coagulation disorder contraindicates heparin infusion. Reduced tissue perfusion interferes with medication absorption and distribution.
8. Assess adequacy of patient's adipose tissue to determine appropriate infusion site.	Physiological changes of aging or patient illness influence amount of subcutaneous tissue, which affects choice of catheter insertion site.
9. Assess patient's knowledge regarding medication to be received and use of medication pump.	Provides background to determine need for patient education.
10. Assess patient's symptoms before initiating medication therapy. Determine severity of pain (if using analgesia) or measure blood glucose level (if using insulin).	Provides information to evaluate desired effects of CSQI medication.

NURSING DIAGNOSES

- Anxiety
- Deficient knowledge regarding CSQI therapy
- Fear
- Ineffective health maintenance
- Pain (acute, chronic)
- Risk for infection
- Risk for injury

Related factors/Risk factors are individualized based on patient's condition or needs.

PLANNING

1. Expected outcomes following completion of procedure: • Needle insertion site remains free from infection. • Patient achieves desired effect of medication with no signs of adverse reactions. • Patient explains purpose, dosage, and effects of medication and verbalizes understanding of CSQI therapy.	Risk for infection at needle insertion site is potential complication of CSQI therapy. Medication is delivered safely with desired therapeutic effect achieved. Demonstrates learning.

IMPLEMENTATION

1. Review manufacturer directions for pump.	Ensures proper use of equipment.
2. Perform hand hygiene. Prepare medication using aseptic technique or check dose on prefilled syringe. Connect syringe and prime tubing with medication, being careful not to lose any medication. Compare label of medication with MAR or computer printout 2 times.	Ensures that medication is sterile. Checking label of medication with transcribed order reduces error. *This is the first check for accuracy* and ensures that correct medication is administered.
3. Obtain and program medication administration pump. Place syringe in pump.	Ensures that medication dose administered is accurate.
4. Read label on prefilled syringe and compare with MAR or computer printout.	*This is the second check for accuracy.*
5. Identify patient using at least two identifiers (e.g., name and birthday or name and medical record number) according to agency policy. Compare identifiers with information on patient's MAR or medical record.	Ensures correct patient. Complies with The Joint Commission standards and improves patient safety (TJC, 2016). Some agencies are now using a bar-code system to help with patient identification.
6. At patient's bedside again compare MAR or computer printout with names of medications on medication labels and patient name. Ask patient if he or she has allergies.	*This is the third check for accuracy* and ensures that patient receives correct medication. Confirms patient's allergy history.
7. Discuss purpose of each medication, action, and possible adverse effects. Allow patient to ask any questions. Tell patient that needle insertion will cause slight burning or stinging.	Patient has right to be informed, and patient's understanding of each medication improves adherence to drug therapy.
8. Position patient supine, drape, and provide for privacy.	Respects patient's dignity.

STEP	RATIONALE

9. Initiate CSQI:

a. Be sure that patient is comfortable, sitting or lying down.

Eases pain associated with insertion of needle.

b. Select appropriate injection site free of irritation and away from bony prominences and waistline. Most common sites used are subclavicular and abdomen.

Ensures proper medication absorption.

c. Perform hand hygiene and apply clean gloves. Clean injection site with alcohol using circular motion, followed by antiseptic, using straight cleaning strokes. Allow both agents to dry.

Reduces risk for infection at insertion site.

d. Hold needle in dominant hand and remove needle guard.

Prepares needle for insertion.

e. Gently pinch or lift up skin with nondominant hand.

Ensures that needle will enter subcutaneous tissue.

f. Gently and firmly insert needle at 45- to 90-degree angle (see illustration). Some shorter prepackaged needles (e.g., Sof-Set, Subcutaneous-Set) are inserted at a 90-degree angle. Refer to manufacturer directions.

Decreases pain related to insertion of needle.

g. Release skinfold and apply tape over "wings" of needle.

Secures needle.

Clinical Decision Point *Some cannulas have a sharp needle covered with a plastic catheter. In this case remove the needle and leave the plastic catheter in the skin.*

h. Place occlusive, transparent dressing over insertion site (see illustration).

Protects site from infection and allows you to assess site during medication infusion.

i. Attach tubing from needle to tubing from infusion pump and turn pump on.

Allows you to administer medication.

j. Dispose of any sharps in appropriate leak- and puncture-proof container. Discard used supplies, remove gloves, and perform hand hygiene.

Prevents accidental needlestick injuries and follows CDC guidelines for disposal of sharps (OSHA, n.d.).

k. Inspect site before leaving patient and instruct patient to inform you if site becomes red or begins to leak.

Initiate new site with new needle whenever erythema or leaking occurs. If site is free from complications, rotate needle every 2 to 7 days (Alexander et al., 2014; Arthur, 2015; INS, 2016).

l. Stay with patient for several minutes and observe for any allergic reactions.

Dyspnea, wheezing, and circulatory collapse are signs of severe anaphylactic reaction.

10. Discontinue CSQI:

a. Verify order and establish alternative method for medication administration if applicable.

If medication will be required after discontinuing CSQI, a different medication and/or route is often necessary to continue to manage patient's illness or pain.

b. Stop infusion pump.

Prevents medication from spilling.

c. Perform hand hygiene and apply clean gloves.

Follows CDC recommendations to prevent accidental exposure to blood and body fluids (OSHA, n.d.).

d. Remove dressing without dislodging or removing needle. Discard properly.

Exposes needle.

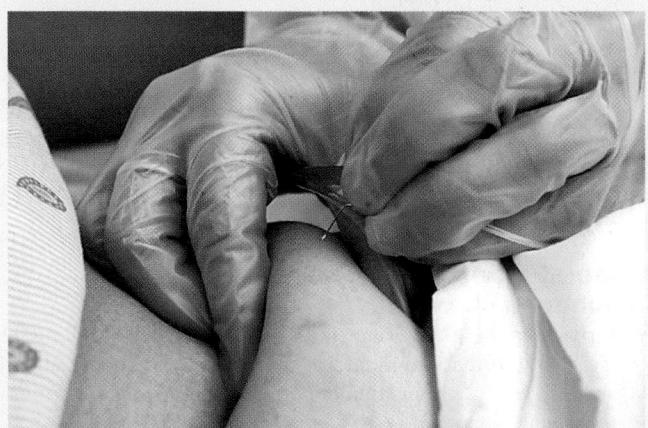

STEP 9f Insert butterfly needle into subcutaneous tissue of abdomen.

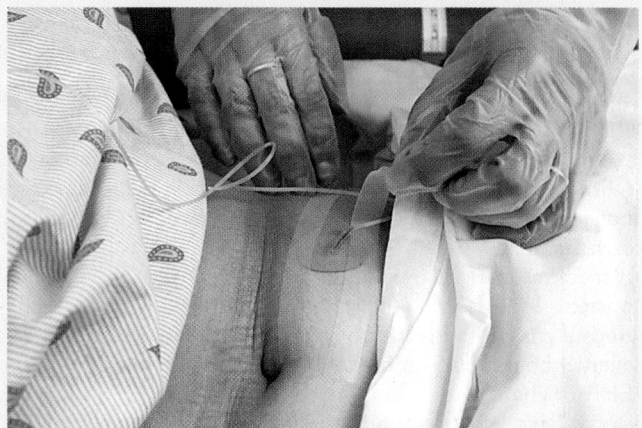

STEP 9h Place transparent dressing over insertion site.

STEP	RATIONALE

Clinical Decision Point *If site is infected, clean it with alcohol and antiseptic. Apply triple antibiotic cream to site if it is excoriated (abraded).*

e. Remove tape from wings of needle and pull needle out at same angle at which it was inserted.	Minimizes patient discomfort.
f. Apply gentle pressure at site until no fluid leaks out of skin.	Dressing adheres to site if skin remains dry.
g. Apply small sterile gauze dressing or adhesive bandage to site.	Prevents bacterial entry into puncture site.
11. Dispose of uncapped needles and syringes in puncture- and leak-proof container.	Prevents accidental needlestick injuries and follows CDC guidelines for disposal of sharps (OSHA, n.d.).
12. Remove and dispose of gloves and perform hand hygiene.	Reduces transmission of microorganisms.

EVALUATION

1. Evaluate patient's response to medication.	Determines effect of therapy. Decreased or absent response to medication may indicate that patient is not receiving medication into subcutaneous tissue (e.g., pump malfunction, medication leaking at site).
2. Assess site at least every 4 hours for redness, pain, drainage, or swelling.	Indicates infection at insertion site.
3. Use Teach-Back: "I want to be sure you understand your continuous infusion into your skin and the medication you are receiving. Tell me in your own words why you have a continuous infusion to receive your medication." Revise your instruction now or develop a plan for revised patient or family caregiver teaching if patient or family caregiver is not able to teach back correctly.	Determines patient's and family caregiver's level of understanding of instructional topic.

Unexpected Outcomes	**Related Interventions**
1. Patient complains of localized pain or burning at insertion site; or site appears red or swollen or is leaking, indicating potential infection or needle dislodgement.	• Remove needle and place new needle in different site. • Continue to monitor original site for signs of infection and notify health care provider if you suspect infection.
2. Patient displays signs of allergic reaction to medication.	• Stop delivering medication immediately and follow agency policy or guidelines for appropriate response to allergic reaction (e.g., administration of antihistamine such as diphenhydramine or epinephrine) and reporting of adverse drug reactions. • Notify patient's health care provider of adverse effects immediately. • Add allergy information to medical record.
3. CSQI becomes dislodged.	• Stop infusion, apply pressure at site until no fluid leaks out of skin, cover site with gauze dressing or adhesive bandage, and initiate new site. • Assess patient to determine effects of not receiving medication (e.g., assess patient's pain level using age-appropriate pain scale, obtain blood glucose level).

Recording and Reporting

- After initiating CSQI, immediately chart medication, dose, route, site, time, date, and type of medication pump in nurses' notes in electronic health record (EHR) or chart. Use initials or signature.
- If medication is an opioid, follow agency policy to document waste.
- Record patient's response to medication and appearance of site every 4 hours or according to agency policy in nurses' notes in EHR or chart.
- Record patient teaching, validation of understanding, and patient's response to medication in nurse's notes in EHR or chart.

- Report any adverse effects from medication or infection at insertion site to patient's health care provider and document according to agency policy. Patient's condition often indicates need for additional medical therapy.

Special Considerations
Teaching

- Instruct patient to wear medical alert bracelet along with medical information, including disease (e.g., diabetes), allergies, and a contact phone number for the pump manufacturer for technical support.
- Instruct patients to carry back-up batteries and extra medication if they are going to be away from home.

BOX 22.8

Education Topics for Patients Receiving Insulin With Continuous Subcutaneous Infusion

- Blood glucose monitoring
- Meal planning and food choices
- Incorporating exercise into daily routine
- How to program and use the insulin pump
- Illness guidelines and management
- Management of hypoglycemia
- Prevention and management of hyperglycemia
- Prevention of infection, especially at CSQI infusion site
- Problem-solving and decision-making skills when pump malfunctions
- Special considerations and precautions (e.g., what to do with pump when showering and sleeping)

Modified from American Diabetes Association (ADA): Standards of medical care in diabetes—2014, *Diabetes Care* 37(1):S14, 2014; Heinemann L, et al: Insulin pump risks and benefits: a clinical appraisal of pump safety, standards, adverse event reporting and research needs, *Diabetes Care* 38(4):716, 2015. *CSQI,* Continuous subcutaneous infusion.

- Patients receiving insulin require intensive diabetes management education (Box 22.8).
- Never immerse pumps in water or expose them to x-ray films or magnetic resonance imaging.

Pediatric

- CSQI improves glycemic control in children and adolescents. There is a decreased rate of severe hypoglycemia, catheter-site infection, and weight gain (Hockenberry and Wilson, 2015).
- Insulin pumps offer more flexibility for adolescents, placing the responsibility of diabetes management on the child. Extensive child and family education is needed in using CSQI (Hockenberry and Wilson, 2015).
- Clean and change CSQI sites in children every 48 to 72 hours or at the first signs of inflammation (Hockenberry and Wilson, 2015).

Gerontological

- CSQI delivers isotonic IV solutions to dehydrated older adults, known as *hypodermoclysis therapy*. This method of providing hydration avoids the need to transfer a patient from home or long-term care facility to an acute care hospital. A health care provider may order use of hyaluronidase to facilitate dispersion and absorption of 1000 mL or more of hydration solutions (INS, 2016). Infuse fluids slowly (e.g., 30 mL/hour) during the first hour of therapy. If the patient remains comfortable, you can increase the rate of infusion. Usually infusion rates do not exceed 60 mL/hour. The rate and volume should not exceed those used for intravenous infusion (INS, 2016). Hypodermoclysis is an easy-to-use, safe, and cost-effective alternative to IV hydration for older adults (Scales, 2011).

Home Care

- Patients in the home using CSQI need a responsible family caregiver if available. Educate the patient and family caregiver about the desired effect of the medication, side effects and adverse effects of the medication, operation of the pump, how to evaluate the effectiveness of the medication, when and how to assess and rotate injection sites, and when to call a health care provider for problems. Patients need to know where and how to obtain and dispose of all required supplies.
- Patients managing CSQI at home may use an antibacterial soap (e.g., Hibiclens, pHisoHex) instead of alcohol and chlorhexidine to clean insertion site.

◆ CLINICAL DEBRIEF

The nurse is developing a plan of care for an alert and oriented patient with thrombophlebitis of the left leg who received heparin 5000 units subcutaneously on admission to the unit and every 8 hours; this is the fourth day after admission. The heparin comes prepared from the pharmacy in a single-dose vial.

1. Which information does the nurse need to know about the medication and the vial before administration?
2. Which information does the nurse need to know about the patient before administration of the heparin?
3. Which aspects of the patient's care related to the administration of heparin can the nurse delegate to the nursing assistive personnel (NAP)?
4. The male patient weighs 100 kg (220 lbs). The drug calculation has determined that 1 mL of heparin needs to be administered. Which size syringe and needle will be used to administer the injection?
5. The patient is complaining of soreness and tenderness at the heparin injection site. Using SBAR, show how you would communicate with the health care team about this patient.

◆ REVIEW QUESTIONS

1. Place the steps of administering an intradermal injection in the correct order.
   1. Inject medication slowly.
   2. Note the presence of a bleb.
   3. Advance needle through epidermis to 3 mm.
   4. Using nondominant hand, stretch skin over site with forefinger.
   5. Insert needle at a 5- to 15-degree angle into skin until resistance is felt.
   6. Clean site with antiseptic swab.
2. A patient with diabetes is receiving insulin using a continuous subcutaneous infusion pump. Place the steps of discontinuing the insulin pump in the correct order.
   1. Perform hand hygiene and apply clean gloves.
   2. Stop infusion pump.
   3. Remove dressing and discard properly.
   4. Apply gentle pressure to site until no fluid is leaking from skin.
   5. Verify order and establish an alternate route for medication if applicable.
   6. Apply small sterile gauze dressing to site.
   7. Remove tape from wings of needle and pull needle out.

3. You are administering an intravenous (IV) push medication to a patient who has a compatible IV fluid running through IV tubing. Place the following steps in the appropriate order.

1. Release tubing and inject medication within amount of time recommended by agency policy, pharmacist, or medication reference manual. Use watch to time administration.

2. Select injection port of IV tubing closest to patient. Whenever possible, injection port should accept a needleless syringe. Use IV filter if required by medication reference or agency policy.

3. After injecting medication, release tubing, withdraw syringe, and recheck fluid infusion rate.

4. Connect syringe to port of IV line. Insert needleless tip or small-gauge needle of syringe containing prepared drug through center of injection port.

5. Clean injection port with antiseptic swab. Allow to dry.

6. Occlude IV line by pinching tubing just above injection port. Pull back gently on syringe plunger to aspirate blood return.

ⓔ *Visit the Evolve site for a complete list of Clinical Debrief and Review Questions answers.*

REFERENCES

Akbari Sari A, et al: Slow versus fast subcutaneous heparin injections for preventing bruising and site-pain intensity, *Cochrane Database Syst Rev* (7):CD008077, 2014. doi: 10.1002/14651858.CD008077.pub3.

Alassaad A, et al: Prescription and transcription errors in multidose-dispensed medication on discharge from hospital: an observational and interventional study, *J Eval Clin Pract* 19(1):185, 2013.

Alexander M, et al: *Core curriculum for infusion nursing*, ed 4, Philadelphia, 2014, Williams & Wilkins.

American Association of Diabetes Educators (AADE): *Teaching injection technique to people with diabetes*, 2013, http://www.diabeteseducator.org/export/sites/aade/_resources/pdf/research/InjectionEducationPracticeGuide.pdf. Accessed July 4, 2015.

American Diabetes Association (ADA): Diabetes care in the hospital, nursing home, and skilled nursing facility, *Diabetes Care* 38(S1):S80, 2015.

Arthur A: Innovations in subcutaneous infusions, *J Infus Nurs* 38(3):179, 2015.

Bartz L, et al: Subcutaneous administration of drugs in palliative care: result of a systematic observational study, *J Pain Symptom Manag* 48(4):540, 2014.

Bhalla MC, et al: Predictors of epinephrine autoinjector needle length inadequacy, *Am J Emerg Med* 31(12):1671, 2013.

Buchko B, et al: Improving care of patients with insulin pumps during hospitalization: translating the evidence, *J Nurs Care Qual* 27(4):333, 2012.

Burchum J, Rosenthal L: *Lehne's pharmacology for nursing care*, ed 9, St Louis, 2016, Saunders.

Carchidi C, et al: Clinical effectiveness and cost-effectiveness of continuous subcutaneous insulin infusion for diabetes: systematic review and economic evaluation, *Am J Matern Child Nurs* 36(1):32, 2011.

Centers for Disease Control and Prevention (CDC): *CMS hospital conditions participation: medication administration and safe opioid use*, 2015, http://www.themha.org/education/2015-CMS-Hospital-Conditions-of-Participation/CMS-2015-MEDICATION-ADM-SAFE-OPIOID-USE.aspx. Accessed July 7, 2016.

Centers for Disease Control and Prevention (CDC): *Vaccine administration: epidemiology and prevention of vaccine-preventable diseases*, 2015, http://www.cdc.gov/vaccines/pubs/pinkbook/vac-admin.html. Accessed April 3, 2016.

Davidson K, Rourke L: Teaching best evidence: deltoid intramuscular injection technique, *J Nurs Educ Pract* 3(7):122, 2013.

Dayananda L, et al: Intended intramuscular gluteal injections: are they truly intramuscular?, *J Postgrad Med* 60(2):175, 2014.

Department of Health and Human Services, Centers for Medicare & Medicaid (DHHS): *Updated guidance on medication administration*, Hospital Appendix A of State Operations Manual, Baltimore, 2011, Department of Health and Human Services.

Diggle D: Are you FIT for purpose? The importance of getting injection technique right, *J Diabetes Nurs* 18:50, 2014.

Environmental Protection Agency (EPA): *Disposal of medical sharps*, 2014, http://www.epa.gov/osw/nonhaz/industrial/medical/disposal.htm. Accessed April 3, 2016.

Giger JN: *Transcultural nursing: assessment and intervention*, ed 7, St Louis, 2017, Mosby.

Greenway K: Rituals in nursing: intramuscular technique, *J Clin Nurs* 23(23):3583, 2014.

Heinemann L, et al: Insulin pump risks and benefits: a clinical appraisal of pump safety, standards, adverse event reporting, and research needs, *Diabetes Care* 38(4):716, 2015.

Hibbard P, et al: Approach to immunizations in healthy adults, *UpToDate*, 2015, http://www.uptodate.com/contents/approach-to-immunizations-in-healthy-adults. Accessed April 3, 2016.

Hirsch LJ, et al: Glycemic control, reported pain and leakage with a 4 mm (32 G pen needle in obese and nonobese adults with diabetes: a post hoc analysis, *Curr Med Res Opin* 28(8):1305, 2012.

Hockenberry MJ, Wilson D: *Wong's nursing care of infants and children*, ed 10, St Louis, 2015, Mosby.

Hopkins U, Arias C: Large-volume IM injections: a review of best practices, *Oncol Nurse Advisor* 32:2013. http://www.oncologynurseadvisor.com/chemotherapy/large-volume-im-injections-a-review-of-best-practices/article/281208/. Accessed April 3, 2016.

Infusion Nurses Society: Infusion therapy standards of practice, *J Intraven Nurs* 39(Suppl 1):1S, 2016.

Institute for Safe Medication Practices (ISMP): *Acute care guidelines for timely administration of scheduled medications*, 2011, http://www.ismp.org/Tools/guidelines/acutecare/tasm.pdf. Accessed April 3, 2016.

Institute for Safe Medication Practices (ISMP): *Side tracks on the safety express. Interruptions lead to errors and unfinished. Wait, what was I doing?*, 2012, http://www.ismp.org/newsletters/acutecare/showarticle.aspx?id=37. Accessed April 3, 2016.

Institute for Safe Medication Practices (ISMP): *Principles of designing a medication label for intravenous piggyback medication for patient-specific inpatient use*, 2015, http://www.ismp.org/Tools/guidelines/labelFormats/Piggyback.asp. Accessed April 3, 2016.

Lilley LL, et al: *Pharmacology and the nursing process*, ed 7, St Louis, 2012, Mosby.

Mandrack M, et al: Nursing best practices using automated dispensing cabinets: nurses' key role in improving medication safety, *Medsurg Nurs* 21(3):134, 2012.

Medtronic MiniMed: *MiniMed Paradigm REAL-Time insulin pump and continuous glucose monitoring system*, 2015, http://www.medtronic.eu/your-health/diabetes/device/insulin-pumps/paradigm-real-time-system/index.htm. Accessed April 6, 2016.

Nicoll L, Hesby A: Intramuscular injection: an integrative research review and guideline for evidence-based practice, *Appl Nurs Res* 16(2):159, 2002.

Occupational Safety and Health Administration (OSHA): *Bloodborne pathogens and needlestick prevention*, nd, https://www.osha.gov/SLTC/bloodbornepathogens/index.html. Accessed April 3, 2016.

Ogston-Tuck S: Subcutaneous injection technique: an evidence based approach, *Nurs Stand* 29(3):53, 2014a.

Ogston-Tuck S: Intramuscular injection technique: an evidence based approach, *Nurs Stand* 29(4):55, 2014b.

Oldenmenger W, et al: Efficacy of opioid rotation to continuous parenteral hydromorphone in advanced cancer patients failing on other opioids, *Support Care Cancer* 20(8):1639, 2012.

Palma S, Strohfus P: Are IM injections IM in obese and overweight females? A study in injection technique, *Appl Nurs Res* 26(4):e1, 2013.

Patidar A, et al: Comparative efficacy of heparin saline and normal saline flush for maintaining patency of peripheral intravenous lines: a randomized control trial, *Int J Health Sci Res* 4(3):159, 2014.

Prakash V, et al: Mitigating errors caused by interruptions during medication verification and administration: interventions in a simulated ambulatory chemotherapy setting, *BMJ Qual Saf* 23(11):884, 2014.

Sanofi-Aventis: *Lovenox subcutaneous injection*, 2014, http://www.lovenox.com/hcp_default.aspx, Accessed July 5, 2015.

Scales K: Use of hypodermoclysis to manage dehydration, *Nurs Older People* 23(5):16, 2011.

Tantisira K, et al: Overview of pharmacogenomics, *UpToDate*, 2015, http://www.uptodate.com/contents/overview-of-pharmacogenomics. Accessed April 3, 2016.

The Joint Commission (TJC): *2016 National Patient Safety Goals*, 2016, http://www.jointcommission.org/standards_information/npsgs.aspx. Accessed April 3, 2016.

Touhy TA, Jett KF: *Ebersole and Hess' gerontological nursing & healthy aging*, ed 4, St Louis, 2014, Elsevier.

World Health Organization (WHO): *Tuberculosis*, 2015a, http://www.who.int/mediacentre/factsheets/fs104/en/. Accessed April 3, 2016.

World Health Organization (WHO): *Injection safety*, 2015b, http://www.who.int/injection_safety/en/. Accessed April 3, 2016.

Yoder M, et al: The effect of a safe zone on nurse interruptions, distractions, and medication administration errors, *J Infus Nurs* 38(2):140, 2015.

23 | Oxygen Therapy

OBJECTIVES

Mastery of content in this chapter will enable the nurse to:
- Discuss indications for oxygen therapy.
- Describe methods for administering oxygen therapy.
- Demonstrate applying an oxygen-delivery device.
- Demonstrate administering oxygen therapy to a patient with an artificial airway.
- Demonstrate obtaining peak expiratory flow rate (PEFR) measurements.
- Demonstrate proper use of incentive spirometry.
- Demonstrate use of noninvasive positive-pressure ventilation (NPPV) using continuous positive airway pressure (CPAP) or bi-level positive airway pressure (BiPAP).
- Demonstrate care of a patient receiving mechanical ventilation.

MEDIA RESOURCES

- evolve http://evolve.elsevier.com/Perry/skills
- Review Questions
- Audio Glossary
- Case Studies
- ▶ Video Clips
- Clinical Debrief and Review Questions Answers

PURPOSE

Oxygen therapy is the administration of supplemental oxygen (O_2) to a patient to prevent or treat hypoxemia. Routes of administration include, but are not limited to, nasal cannula, face masks, noninvasive ventilation, and positive-pressure ventilators. Special care is required for each of the separate delivery devices.

STANDARDS OF CARE

- AARC Clinical Practice Guideline, 2012—Humidification During Invasive and Noninvasive Mechanical Ventilation
- AARC Clinical Practice Guideline, 2011—Incentive Spirometry
- American Thoracic Society (ATS), 2015—Long-Term Oxygen Therapy
- Institute for Healthcare Improvement (IHI), 2012—Care Bundle for Ventilator-Associated Pneumonia (VAP)
- The Joint Commission (TJC), 2016—Patient Safety Goals

PRINCIPLES FOR PRACTICE

- Oxygen therapy is used in a variety of conditions to treat hypoxia, which is a condition in which there is insufficient oxygen to meet the metabolic demands of the tissues and cells (Box 23.1).

- Hemoglobin is the carrier of respiratory gases, oxygen, and carbon dioxide (CO_2). It combines with a gas to carry it to and from the cells. Decreased hemoglobin levels reduce the amount of oxygen transported to the cells and carbon dioxide transported away from the cells.
- Hemoglobin levels and acid-base status directly affect oxygenation. Acidemia increases the ability of hemoglobin to release oxygen to the tissues. Alkalemia decreases the ability of hemoglobin to release oxygen to the tissues.
- Pain and anxiety affect patient oxygenation. Therefore assess patient's pain, pulse oximetry (SpO_2) values, level of consciousness, developmental level, and observed behaviors (Hockenberry and Wilson, 2015; Lewis et al., 2017).
- Treat oxygen therapy as a medication. As with any drug, continuously monitor the dosage or concentration of oxygen and routinely check the health care provider's orders to verify that the patient is receiving the prescribed oxygen concentration. Follow the six rights of medication administration when administering oxygen (see Chapter 20).
- Contraindications to oxygen therapies include those that increase the patient's risk for respiratory failure. For example, patients with certain types of congenital heart defects and chronic pulmonary diseases should receive oxygen sparingly. In patients with congenital heart defects, oxygen affects blood flow through the heart and lungs. In patients with chronic

Signs and Symptoms Associated With Acute Hypoxia

- Apprehension, anxiety, behavioral changes
- Decreased level of consciousness, confusion, drowsiness, altered concentration
- Increased pulse rate
- Increased rate and depth of respiration or irregular respiratory patterns
- Decreased lung sounds, adventitious lung sounds (e.g., crackles, wheezes)
- Elevated blood pressure evolving to decreased blood pressure
- Pulse oximetry (SpO$_2$) less than 90%
- Dyspnea
- Use of accessory muscles of respiration, rib retractions
- Cardiac dysrhythmias
- Pallor, cyanosis
- Increased fatigue
- Dizziness

Care Bundle for Ventilator-Associated Pneumonia

- Good hand hygiene
- Internal endotracheal cuff pressure at 25 to 30 cm H$_2$O every 2 hours
- Head of bed at 30 to 45 degrees
- Prophylaxis for deep vein thrombosis and peptic ulcer disease
- Daily interruptions of sedation to assess accurately for readiness to extubate
- Oral care with chlorhexidine 0.12% every 12 hours and general oral care every 2 hours secondary to microbial colonization within the mouth
- Complete subglottal suctioning to decrease risk of oral fluid aspiration
- Accurate and timely documentation
- Timely ventilator circuit changes and removal of condensation
- Provide for mobility through turning and repositioning every 2 hours

Data from Institute for Healthcare Improvement (IHI): *How-to guide: prevent ventilator-associated pneumonia*, 2012, available at www.ihi.org. Accessed November 2015; Lamb KD: Year in review 2014: mechanical ventilation, *Respir Care* 60(4):606, 2015; Urden L et al: *Priorities in critical care nursing*, ed 7, St Louis, 2016, Mosby.

pulmonary diseases, oxygen therapy increases the patient's risk for elevated carbon dioxide in the blood (hypercarbia).

PATIENT-CENTERED CARE

- Take time to explain to the patient and family caregiver the oxygen setup and necessary safety precautions needed when oxygen is in use.
- Patients and visitors with limited English proficiency may not be able to understand signs posted in the room and need help.
- Safely accommodate valued practices of cultural groups when using oxygen. For example, some cultures burn incense, which does not have a flame, to promote healing of ill members. When oxygen is used in the home, designate areas where patients can safely burn incense and encourage family members to bring the ashes to the bedside. Some cultures light candles to celebrate or honor holidays and may accept the use of battery-operated candles while in the hospital (Spector, 2013). Collaborate with family members and religious leaders about how to accommodate these practices during illness and recovery.

EVIDENCE-BASED PRACTICE

- Recent research suggests that high-flow nasal cannula (HFNC) may be used in place of noninvasive positive-pressure ventilation (NPPV) in certain patients with acute respiratory failure (Gaunt et al., 2015). It may also be used instead of bag-valve-mask ventilation when preoxygenating patients immediately before intubation (Messika et al., 2015).
- Early studies indicate that the use of ventilator-associated pneumonia (VAP) prevention bundles have decreased the rates of VAP (Chahoud et al., 2015). The Institute for Healthcare Improvement (IHI, 2012) created the five-step "Ventilator Bundle" (Box 23.2).
- There are significant issues regarding defining VAP and ventilator-associated events (VAEs) (Munaco et al, 2014). The Centers for Disease Control and Prevention (CDC) developed a lengthy algorithm for clinicians to use to accurately diagnose these complications. This algorithm can be viewed at http://www.cdc.gov/nhsn/PDFs/pscManual/10-VAE_FINAL.pdf. The key points in the definition of VAE are the "deterioration in respiratory status after a period of stability or improvement on the ventilator, evidence of infection or inflammation, and laboratory evidence of respiratory infection …. Patients must be mechanically ventilated for more than 2 calendar days to be eligible for VAE" (CDC, 2016, p. 10-3).
- Adult patients who have received mechanical ventilation reported several feelings during their experience, including:
  - Fear caused by dependence on ventilator and loss of control of their life
  - Disconnection from reality
  - Impaired sense of body image
  - Development of adaptation patterns, including maintaining a strong belief and developing communication methods
  - Feeling concern and caring from others, including health care professionals, who helped patients' sense of security (Tsay et al., 2013).
- NPPV does not have a significant effect on gas exchange, exercise tolerance, lung function, respiratory muscle strength, or sleep efficiency in patients with chronic obstructive pulmonary disease (COPD) (Striuk et al., 2013).
- There is no evidence to support that incentive spirometer (IS) alone prevents pulmonary complications in patients who have undergone upper abdominal surgery (do Nascimento et al., 2014; Tyson et al., 2015).

SAFETY GUIDELINES

- Know a patient's normal range of vital signs and pulse oximetry (SpO$_2$) values.
- Be aware of environmental conditions. Patients with chronic respiratory diseases have difficulty maintaining optimal oxygen levels in polluted environments.
- If a patient is to receive home oxygen therapy, complete an environmental assessment to determine respiratory hazards in the home such as the use of gas stoves or kerosene space heaters or the presence of smokers in the home (see Chapter 43).
- Document a patient's smoking history. Smoking damages the mucociliary clearance mechanism of the lungs and paralyzes the ciliary action, resulting in a decreased ability to clear mucus from the airways. Chronic bronchitis is caused primarily by

smoking and results in pooling of mucus in the airways, creating an environment for the development of infections. Long-term chronic bronchitis ultimately results in hypoxia.

- Know a patient's most recent hemoglobin values and past and current arterial blood gas (ABG) values.
- Oxygen is a medication. Increasing the oxygen liter flow rate for shortness of breath is similar to doubling heart, asthma, or other medications.
- Provide education to patient and family about home oxygen therapy so they understand proper use of the equipment. Safety measures for oxygen use are very important (see Chapter 43) (Box 23.3).
- Have suction equipment available to help clear airway secretions, particularly in patients with artificial airways such as an endotracheal tube or tracheostomy.
- Most agencies require that a self-inflating resuscitation bag and appropriate-size mask should be available in patient rooms, particularly in patients requiring mechanical ventilation.

◆ SKILL 23.1   Applying an Oxygen-Delivery Device

 Video Clip

Various diseases (e.g., pneumonia, chronic obstructive pulmonary disease [COPD]) require the use of oxygen therapy. Pneumonia results in impaired gas exchange because of fluid and secretions in the lung, which decrease the diffusion of oxygen from the lungs to the arterial blood supply. Some patients with COPD require the use of oxygen, particularly at home. These patients may require oxygen 24 hours a day; therefore care is taken to plan administration around patient needs (Grindrod, 2015).

Oxygen-Delivery Devices

Oxygen therapy is inexpensive, widely available, and used in a variety of settings. Patients with decreased tissue oxygenation benefit from controlled oxygen administration. Long-term oxygen treatment can improve survival in COPD (Grindrod, 2015).

Selection of the type of oxygen delivery system is made on the basis of the level of oxygen support that the patient needs, the severity of the hypoxia, and the disease process. Consider other factors such as the patient's age and developmental level, level of health and orientation, presence of an artificial airway, whether the setting is in the hospital or the home, type of home environment, and type of support and care given after discharge.

Oxygen-delivery devices fall into one of two categories, high flow or low flow, depending on their ability to provide enough flow to match the patient's spontaneous minute volume. Matching a patient's spontaneous minute volume is imperative for patient comfort and adequate oxygen delivery. High-flow devices discourage entraining room air, which dilutes the inspired oxygen concentration (FiO$_2$). High-flow devices include Venturi mask (Fig. 23.1), large-volume nebulizer, and blender masks. A newer type of high-flow device is the high-flow nasal cannula (Fig. 23.2). Low-flow devices include nasal cannula (Fig. 23.3) and simple face mask (Fig. 23.4), nonrebreather, and partial rebreather masks (Fig. 23.5). These devices deliver set percentages of oxygen, and each one has advantages and disadvantages. You can estimate approximate FiO$_2$ by the flow rate (Table 23.1)

An oxygen flowmeter regulates the flow rate in liters per minute (Fig. 23.6). Oxygen cylinders used in hospital and institutional care

settings include large H cylinders and smaller E cylinders (Fig. 23.7). In addition, still smaller, easily transported cylinders are available for use in the home. Patients using home oxygen commonly use concentrators, some of which are portable.

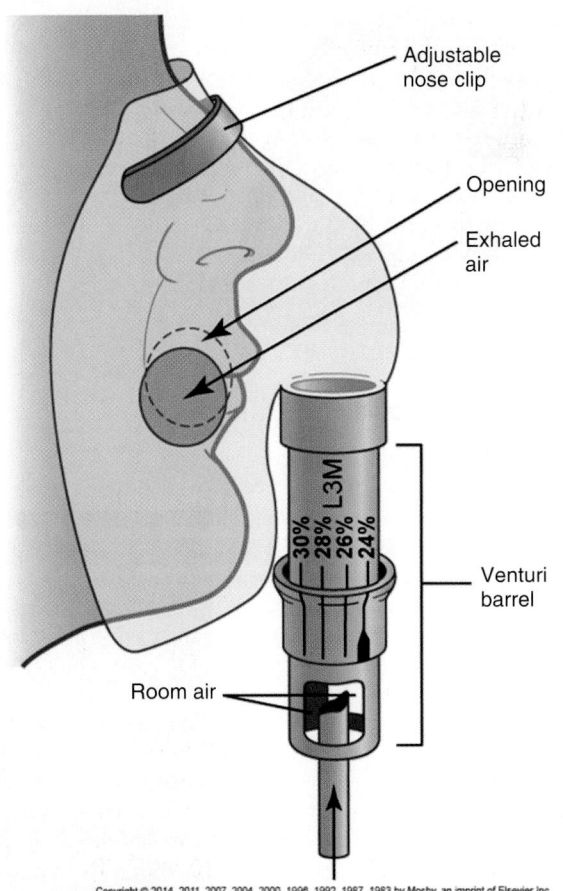

Copyright © 2014, 2011, 2007, 2004, 2000, 1996, 1992, 1987, 1983 by Mosby, an imprint of Elsevier Inc.

FIG 23.1 Venturi mask.

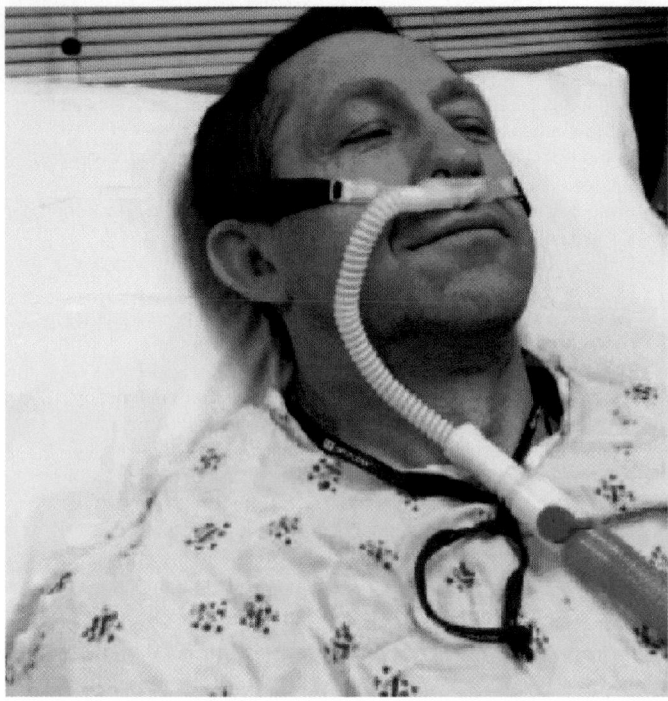

FIG 23.2 High-flow nasal cannula. (*Courtesy Fisher & Paykel Healthcare.*)

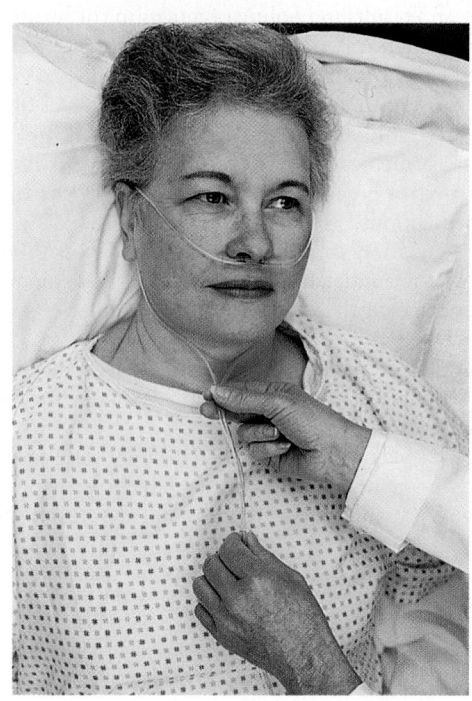

FIG 23.3 Nasal cannula adjusted for proper fit.

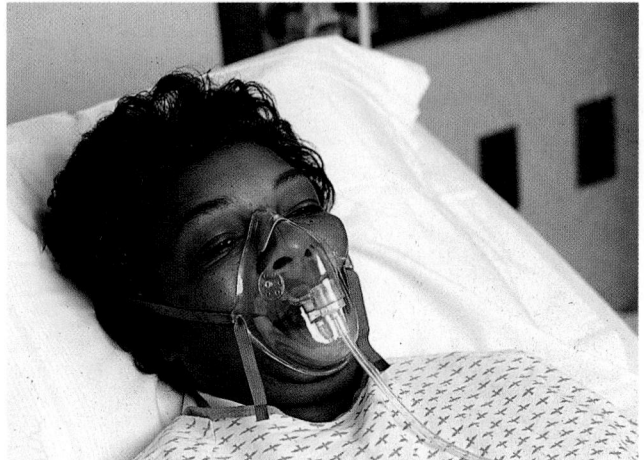

FIG 23.4 Simple face mask.

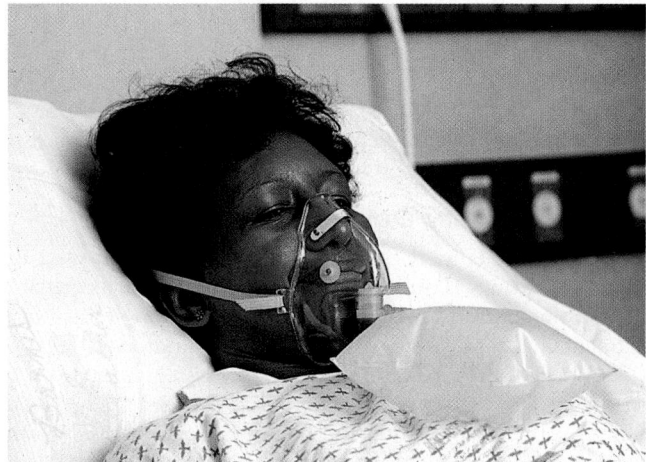

FIG 23.5 Plastic face mask with reservoir bag.

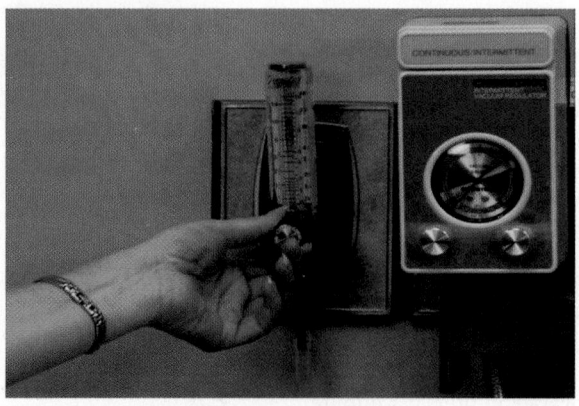

FIG 23.6 Oxygen flowmeter.

TABLE 23.1

Oxygen Delivery Systems

Delivery System	FiO₂ Delivered	Advantages	Disadvantages
Low-flow delivery devices Nasal cannula	1-6 L/min: 24%-44%	Safe and simple Easily tolerated Effective for low concentrations Does not impede eating or talking Inexpensive, disposable	Unable to use with nasal obstruction Drying of mucous membranes Can dislodge easily May cause skin irritation or breakdown Patient's breathing pattern affects exact FiO₂
Oxygen-conserving cannula (Oxymizer)	8 L/min: up to 30%-60%	Indicated for long-term O₂ use in the home Allows increased O₂ concentration and lower flow	Cannula cannot be cleaned More expensive than standard cannula
Simple face mask	6-12 L/min: 35%-50%	Useful for short periods of time such as patient transportation	Contraindicated for patients who retain CO₂ May induce feelings of claustrophobia Therapy interrupted with eating or drinking Increased risk for aspiration
Partial nonrebreather (Bag should always remain partially inflated. Therefore flow rate must be high enough to prevent collapse of bag.)	10-15 L/min; 60%-90%	Useful for short periods Delivers increased FiO₂ Easily humidifies O₂ Does not dry mucous membranes	Hot and confining May cause skin irritation Interferes with eating, drinking, and talking Bag may twist and deflate
High-flow delivery devices Venturi mask	24%-50%	Provides specific amount of O₂ with humidity added Administers low, constant O₂	Mask and humidity may irritate skin Interferes with eating, drinking, and talking
High-flow nasal cannula	Adjustable FiO₂ (0.21-1.0) with a modifiable flow (up to 60 L/min)	Wide range of FiO₂; can use on adults, children, and infants	FiO₂ dependent on patient respiratory pattern and input flow; risk for infection (Messika et al., 2015; Urden et al., 2016)

FiO₂, Fraction of inspired oxygen concentration.

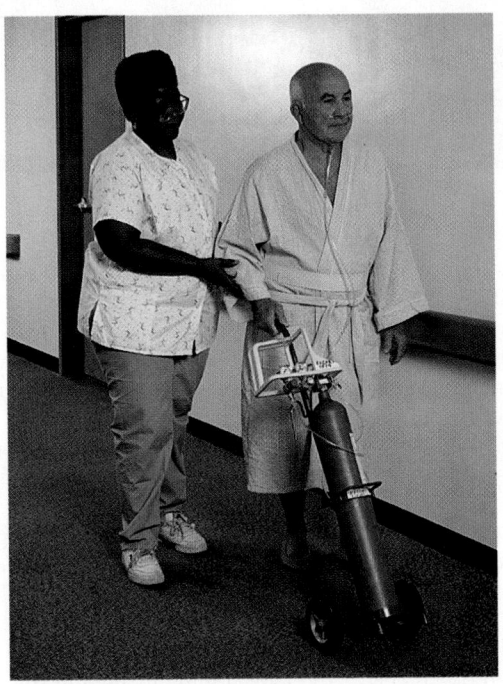

FIG 23.7 Smaller E tank for portability.

Nasal Cannula

Several types of oxygen cannula are used to deliver oxygen to the patient (see Table 23.1). A nasal cannula is a simple, effective, and comfortable device for delivering oxygen to a patient (see Fig. 23.3). It allows a patient to breathe through the mouth or nose, is available for all age-groups, and is adequate for short- or long-term use. The two tips of the cannula, about 1.5 cm (½ inch) long, protrude from the center of a disposable tube and are inserted into the nostrils. Oxygen is delivered via the cannula. At flow rates greater than 4 L/min, humidification helps prevent drying of nasal and oral mucous membranes.

A high-flow nasal cannula (HFNC) consists of an air-oxygen blender that has an adjustable FiO₂ (Fig. 23.8). It is used in patients prone to severe oxygen desaturation and is currently recommended for use in critical care settings. This system can deliver heated and humidified air/oxygen mixture at high flows, up to 60 L/min (Spoletini et al., 2015). The oxygen gas is then delivered to the patient via wide-bore nasal prongs (Messika et al., 2015). HFNC has been used in the neonatal population, and there is increasing evidence to support its use in adults with acute respiratory failure (Gaunt et al., 2015; Roca and Masclans, 2015).

An oxygen-conserving cannula is indicated for patients who require higher oxygen concentrations than what can be provided via traditional nasal cannula. The cannula possesses a built-in reservoir that allows for increasing oxygen concentration at a lower flow rate, which can increase patient comfort (Fig. 23.9).

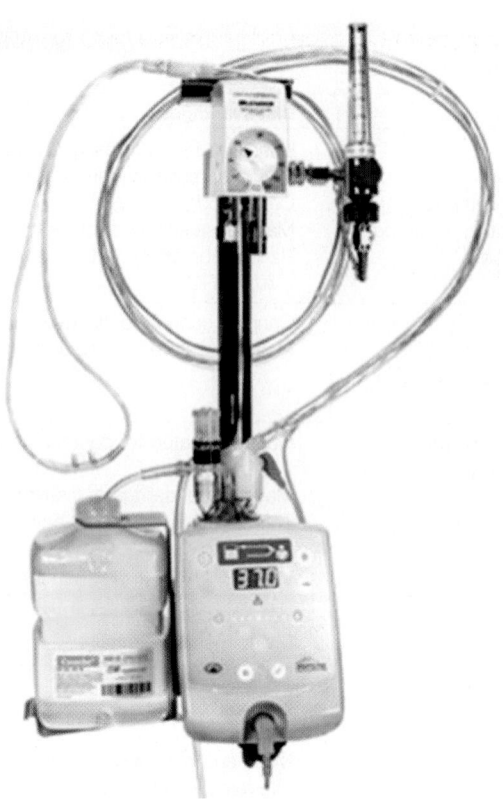

FIG 23.8 High-flow nasal cannula blender. (*Comfort Flo® Humidification System courtesy Teleflex Medical.*)

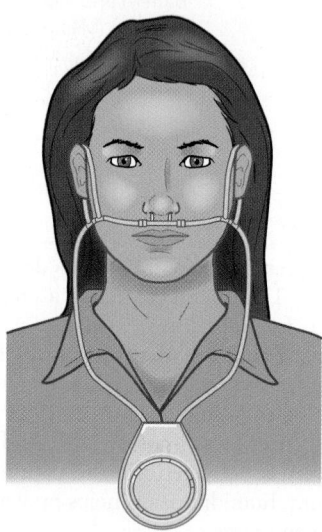

FIG 23.9 Oxygen-reserving cannula. (*From Lewis S, et al: Medical-surgical nursing: assessment and management of clinical problems, ed 9, St Louis, 2014, Mosby.*)

Oxygen Mask

Oxygen masks are used to administer oxygen therapy (see Table 23.1). The simple face mask (see Fig. 23.4) is for short-term oxygen therapy. It fits loosely and delivers oxygen concentrations from 35% to 50% or 60%.

A plastic face mask with a reservoir bag (see Fig. 23.5) and a Venturi mask (see Fig. 23.1) deliver higher concentrations of oxygen. When used as a nonrebreather, the plastic face mask with a reservoir bag delivers 60% to 90% oxygen at appropriate flow rate. This oxygen mask maintains a high-concentration oxygen supply in the reservoir bag. Frequently inspect the bag to make sure

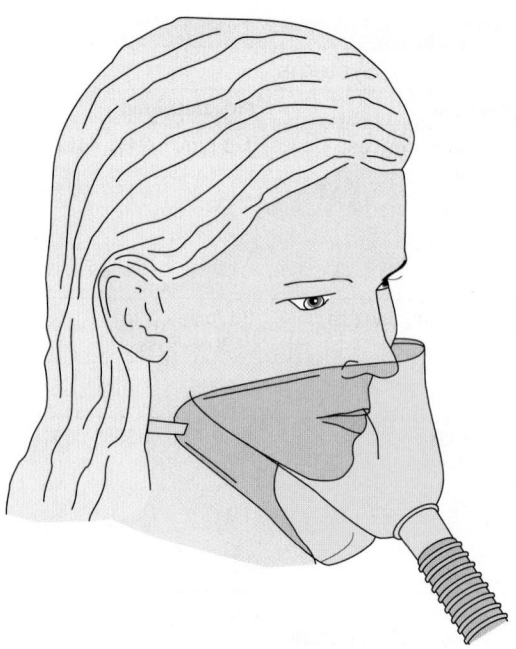

FIG 23.10 Face tent for oxygen delivery. (*From Hockenberry MJ, Wilson D: Wong's nursing care of infants and children, ed 10, St Louis, 2015, Mosby.*)

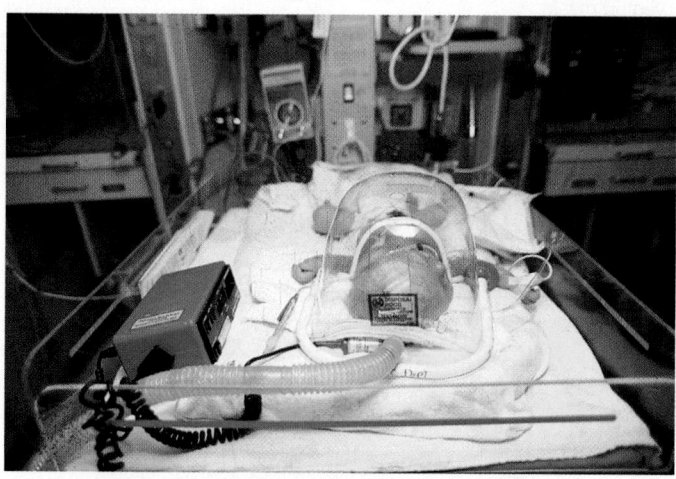

FIG 23.11 Oxygen tent.

that it is fully inflated. If it is *not fully inflated*, the patient may breathe in large amounts of exhaled carbon dioxide.

A Venturi mask is a cone-shaped high-flow device with entrainment ports of various sizes at the base of the mask, which delivers a more precise concentration of oxygen to a patient (see Fig. 23.1). The concentration of oxygen delivered ranges from 24% to 50% and is based on the flow of the gas. The nurse or respiratory therapist adjusts the ports on the mask to permit regulation of FiO_2.

The face tent is a shield-like device that fits under a patient's chin and sweeps around the face (Fig. 23.10). It is used primarily for humidification and for oxygen only when a patient cannot or will not tolerate a tight-fitting mask. Because it is so close to a patient's face, there is no way to estimate how much oxygen is delivered to him or her.

Oxygen hoods (Fig. 23.11) are commonly used in the pediatric setting. These devices are able to provide high concentrations of humidified oxygen. This is particularly useful in the child with airway inflammation, croup, or other respiratory tract infections.

Delegation and Collaboration

The skill of applying a nasal cannula or oxygen mask can be delegated to nursing assistive personnel (NAP). The nurse is responsible for assessing patient's respiratory system, response to oxygen therapy, and setup of oxygen therapy, including adjustment of oxygen flow rate. The nurse directs the NAP by:

- Informing how to safely adjust the device (e.g., loosening the strap on the oxygen cannula or mask) and clarifying its correct placement and positioning.
- Instructing to inform the nurse immediately about any changes in vital signs; changes in pulse oximetry (SpO_2); changes in level of consciousness (LOC); skin irritation from the cannula, mask, or straps; or patient complaints of pain or breathlessness.
- Instructing personnel to provide extra skin care around patient's ears and nose.

Equipment

- Oxygen-delivery device as ordered by health care provider
- Oxygen tubing (consider extension tubing)
- Humidifier, if indicated
- Sterile water for humidifier
- Face shield as needed for risk of splash
- Clean gloves, if secretions are present
- Oxygen source
- Oxygen flowmeter
- Appropriate "Oxygen in use" signs
- Pulse oximeter
- Stethoscope

STEP	RATIONALE

ASSESSMENT

STEP	RATIONALE
1. Identify patient using at least two identifiers (e.g., name and birthday or name and medical record number) according to agency policy.	Ensures correct patient. Complies with The Joint Commission standards and improves patient safety (TJC, 2016).
2. Perform hand hygiene. Perform respiratory assessment, including symmetry of chest wall expansion, chest wall abnormalities (e.g., kyphosis), temporary conditions (e.g., pregnancy, trauma) affecting ventilation, respiratory rate and depth, sputum production, and lung sounds (see Chapter 6) and for signs and symptoms associated with hypoxia (see Box 23.1).	Reduces transmission of microorganisms. Changes in ventilation and gas exchange resulting in hypoxia require oxygen therapy.
3. Observe for behavioral changes (e.g., apprehension, anxiety, confusion, decreased ability to concentrate, decreased LOC, fatigue, and dizziness).	Decreased levels of oxygen (hypoxia) or increased levels of carbon dioxide (hypercapnia) affect a person's cognitive abilities, interpersonal interactions, and mood (Lewis et al., 2017).

Clinical Decision Point *Patients with sudden changes in their vital signs, LOC, or behavior may be experiencing profound hypoxia. Patients who demonstrate subtle changes over time may have worsening of a chronic or existing condition or a new medical condition (Lewis et al., 2017).*

STEP	RATIONALE
4. Assess airway patency and remove airway secretions by having patient cough and expectorate mucus or by suctioning (see Chapter 25). **Note:** Apply clean gloves if there is risk of contacting mucus.	Secretions plug the airway, decreasing amount of oxygen that is available for gas exchange in lungs.
5. Inspect condition of skin around nose and ears.	Provides baseline for monitoring development of skin breakdown from medical device irritation.

Clinical Decision Point *Excessive amounts of secretions, signs of respiratory distress (increased work of breathing, increased respiratory rate), presence of rhonchi on auscultation, excessive coughing, or decrease in patient pulse oximeter can indicate need for suctioning.*

STEP	RATIONALE
6. If available, note patient's most recent arterial blood gas (ABG) results or SpO_2 value. Remove and discard gloves if worn; perform hand hygiene.	Objectively documents patient's pH, arterial oxygen, arterial carbon dioxide, or arterial oxygen saturation.
7. Review patient's medical record for medical order for oxygen, noting delivery method, flow rate, duration of oxygen therapy, and parameters for titration of oxygen settings.	Ensures safe and accurate oxygen administration. Safe oxygen delivery includes the six rights of medication administration (see Chapter 20).
8. Assess patient's and family caregiver's level of understanding about oxygen therapy.	Determines level of instruction required.

NURSING DIAGNOSES

- Anxiety
- Deficient knowledge regarding purpose of oxygen therapy
- Fatigue
- Impaired gas exchange
- Ineffective airway clearance
- Ineffective breathing pattern
- Risk for impaired skin integrity

Related factors/Risk factors are individualized based on patient's condition or needs.

STEP	RATIONALE

PLANNING

1. Expected outcomes following completion of procedure:
   - Patient's SpO_2 and/or ABGs return to or remain within normal limits or baseline levels.

   Objective determinants of stable or improved oxygenation.

   - Patient's vital signs remain stable or return to baseline.

   When there is no underlying cardiovascular disease, patients adapt to decreased oxygen levels by increasing pulse and blood pressure. This is a short-term adaptive response. Once signs of hypoxia are reduced or controlled, patient's vital signs usually return to normal.

   - Patient's work of breathing decreases.

   Pulmonary conditions such as pneumonia or asthma cause varying degrees of airway narrowing. With improved oxygenation, patient's airways are open, and work of breathing decreases.

   - Patient experiences increased lung expansion.

   Improved oxygenation helps to resolve collapsed and constricted airways, improves work of breathing, and thus improves lung expansion.

   - Patient's level of consciousness (LOC) returns to baseline.

   Improvement in oxygenation relieves hypoxia and improves patient's mental status.

   - Patient verbalizes improved levels of comfort; and subjective sensations of anxiety, fatigue, and breathlessness decrease.

   Increased oxygen levels in the blood reduce patient's anxiety, fatigue, and breathlessness.

   - Patient's ears, nares, and nasal mucosa remain intact.

   Intact skin indicates no device-related pressure to underlying skin and mucous membrane (Pittman et al., 2015; Schallom et al., 2015).

2. Explain procedure to patient and family caregiver.

   Explanation decreases patient's anxiety and reduces oxygen consumption. Increases adherence and cooperation of patient and family caregiver.

3. Gather equipment/supplies and complete necessary charges according to agency policy.

   Provides organized implementation of the oxygen-delivery device.

IMPLEMENTATION

1. Perform hand hygiene. Apply face shield if risk of exposure to splashing mucus exists. Apply gloves if patient has oral or nasal secretions.

   Reduces transmission of microorganisms.

2. Adjust bed to appropriate height and lower side rail on side nearest you. Check locks on bed wheel.

   Minimizes caregiver's muscle strain and prevents injury. Prevents bed from moving.

3. Attach oxygen-delivery device (e.g., cannula, mask) to oxygen tubing and attach end of tubing to humidified oxygen source adjusted to prescribed flow rate (see Fig. 23.6).

   Humidity prevents drying of nasal and oral mucous membranes and airway secretions. Flowmeters with smaller calibrations may be required for patients requiring low-dose oxygen such as pediatric patients or patients with chronic obstructive pulmonary disease (COPD) (Hockenberry and Wilson, 2015; Restrepo and Walsh, 2012).

4. Apply oxygen device:
   a. Place tips of the cannula into patient's nares. If tips are curved, they should point downward inside nostrils. Then loop cannula tubing up and over patient's ears. Adjust lanyard so cannula fits snugly but not too tight without pressure to patient nares and ears (see Fig. 23.3).

   Tips of cannula direct flow of oxygen into patient's upper respiratory tract.

   b. Apply a mask by placing it over patient's mouth and nose. Then bring straps over patient's head and adjust to form a comfortable but tight seal (see Fig. 23.4).

   A properly fitting device that does not create pressure on nares or ears is comfortable, and patient is more likely to keep it in place; reduces risk for skin breakdown (Schallom et al., 2015).

5. Maintain sufficient slack on oxygen tubing and secure to patient's clothes.

   Allows patient to turn head without causing mask to shift position or dislodge nasal cannula.

6. Observe for proper function of oxygen-delivery device:

   Ensures patency of delivery device and accuracy of prescribed oxygen flow rate (see Table 23.1).

   a. *Nasal cannula:* Cannula is positioned properly in nares; oxygen flows through tips.

   Provides prescribed oxygen rate and reduces pressure on tips of nares.

STEP	RATIONALE
b. *Partial* or *nonrebreather mask* (see Fig. 23.5): Mask seals tightly around mouth. Reservoir fills on exhalation and almost collapses on inspiration. Reservoir should not collapse completely.	Easily humidifies oxygen and does not dry mucous membranes (Restrepo and Walsh, 2012). Useful for short-term therapy of 24 hours or less.
c. *Oxygen-conserving cannula (Oxymizer):* Fit as for nasal cannula. Reservoir is located under patient's nose or worn as a pendant.	Delivers higher flow of oxygen with nasal cannula. Delivers 2:1 ratio (e.g., 6 L/min nasal cannula is approximately equivalent to 3.5 L/min with Oxymizer device).
d. *Nonrebreather mask:* Apply as regular mask. Contains one-way valves with reservoir; exhaled air does not enter reservoir bag. Can be combined with nasal cannula to provide higher inspired oxygen concentration (FiO_2).	Device of choice for short-term high FiO_2 delivery. Valves on mask side ports permit exhalation but close during inhalation to prevent inhaling room air.
e. *Simple face mask:* Select appropriate flow rate (see Fig. 23.4)	Used for short-term oxygen therapy.
f. *Venturi mask* (see Fig. 23.1): Apply as regular mask. Select appropriate flow rate (see Table 23.1).	Used when high-flow device is desired.
g. *Face tent* (see Fig. 23.10): Apply tent under patient's chin and over mouth and nose. It will be loose, and a mist is always present.	Excellent source of humidification; however, you cannot control oxygen concentrations, and patient who requires high oxygen cannot use this device.
h. *High-flow nasal cannula* (see Fig. 23.8): Fit as for nasal cannula.	Used when high oxygen delivery is required.
7. Verify setting on flowmeter and oxygen source for proper setup and prescribed flow rate.	Ensures delivery of prescribed oxygen therapy in conjunction with specific cannula/mask.
8. Check cannula/mask every 8 hours or as agency policy indicates. Keep humidification container filled at all times.	Ensures patency of cannula and oxygen flow. Oxygen is a dry gas; when it is administered via nasal cannula of 4 L/min or more, you must add humidification so patient inhales humidified oxygen (ATS, 2015a).
9. Post "Oxygen in use" signs on wall behind bed and at entrance to room.	Alerts visitors and care providers that oxygen is in use (ATS, 2015a).
10. Properly dispose of gloves (if used) and perform hand hygiene.	Reduces transmission of microorganisms.

EVALUATION

1. Monitor patient's response to changes in oxygen flow rate with SpO_2. **NOTE:** Monitor ABGs when ordered; however, obtaining ABG measurement is an invasive procedure, and ABGs are not measured frequently.	Continual monitoring with SpO_2 is required for patients on oxygen therapy. Base changes in supplemental oxygen on individual patient's oxygen saturation levels.
2. Perform physical assessment, listening to lung sounds; palpating chest excursion; inspecting color and condition of skin; and observing for decreased anxiety, improved LOC and cognitive abilities, decreased fatigue, and absence of dizziness. Measure vital signs.	Evaluates patient's response to supplemental oxygen. As patient's oxygen level improves, physical signs and symptoms improve.
3. Assess adequacy of oxygen flow each shift or as agency policy dictates.	Ensures patency of oxygen delivery device.
4. Observe patient's external ears, bridge of nose, nares, and nasal mucous membranes for evidence of skin breakdown.	Oxygen therapy sometimes causes drying of nasal mucosa. The delivery device can cause skin breakdown where device comes in contact with face, neck, and ears (Schallom et al., 2015).
5. Use Teach-Back: "I want to be sure I explained how oxygen will help you. Explain to me why oxygen is beneficial for you to use right now." Revise your instruction now or develop a plan for revised patient or family caregiver teaching if patient or family caregiver is not able to teach back correctly.	Determines patient's and family caregiver's level of understanding of instructional topic.

STEP	RATIONALE
Unexpected Outcomes	**Related Interventions**
1. Patient experiences skin irritation or breakdown (e.g., at ears, bridge of nose, nares, other pressure areas), sinus pain, or epistaxis.	• Increase humidification to oxygen-delivery system. • Provide appropriate skin care. Do not use petroleum-based gel around oxygen because it is flammable (American Lung Association, 2016).
2. Patient experiences continued hypoxia.	• Notify health care provider. • Obtain health care provider's orders for follow-up SpO_2 monitoring or ABG determinations. • Consider measures to improve airway patency, including but not limited to coughing techniques and oropharyngeal or orotracheal suctioning.
3. Patient experiences nasal and upper airway mucosa drying.	• If oxygen flow rate is greater than 4 L/min, use humidification (Restrepo and Walsh, 2012). At rates greater than 5 L/min, nasal mucous membranes dry, and pain in frontal sinuses may develop (Lewis et al., 2017). • Assess patient's fluid status and increase fluids if appropriate. • Provide frequent oral care.

Recording and Reporting

• Record the respiratory assessment findings, method of oxygen delivery, oxygen flow rate, patient's response to intervention, any adverse reactions or side effects, or change on flow sheet in nurses' notes in electronic health record (EHR) or chart.

• Document your evaluation of patient and family caregiver learning.

• Report any unexpected outcome to health care provider or nurse in charge.

Special Considerations
Teaching

• If oxygen therapy continues after discharge, teach patient and family caregiver the importance of and rationale for it, how to use the oxygen-delivery device, how to contact the supplier of medical equipment, and when to contact the health care provider (see Chapter 44).

• Discuss safety precautions for oxygen use (see Box 23.3) with patient and family caregiver.

• Discuss signs of carbon dioxide retention (e.g., confusion, headache, decreased LOC, somnolence, carbon dioxide narcosis, respiratory arrest) that patient or family caregiver needs to report to the health care provider.

Pediatric

• Some infants and small children are able to tolerate a nasal cannula. Secure the prongs of the cannula with transparent tape or strips of transparent dressing over the child's cheek.

• Sometimes infants receive oxygen therapy via an oxygen hood. Place the hood over the patient's head (see Fig. 23.10).

• Inspect toys placed in the tent for safety and suitability. Any source of sparks (e.g., from mechanical or electrical toys) is a potential fire hazard (Hockenberry and Wilson, 2015).

• Provide comfort and reassurance to the child. Make sure that he or she is able to see someone nearby. Children may still be held by their parents while receiving oxygen via nasal cannula or face mask (Hockenberry and Wilson, 2015).

Gerontological

• Because of the fragility of older adults' skin and mucous membranes, offer oral hygiene and skin care more frequently. Water-based gels such as Aquagel are useful but also dry quickly and need more frequent application.

Home Care

• Obtain appropriate referrals to determine if patient meets the standards for third-party reimbursement (e.g., PaO_2 55 mm Hg or less or SaO_2 less than 88%). Exceptions apply when patients have pulmonary hypertension, cor pulmonale, erythrocytosis, edema, or impaired mental status; they are eligible with a PaO_2 of 56 to 59 mm Hg (ATS, 2015b).

• Oxygen tubing in the home setting is available in lengths of 15 m (50 feet).

• Provide information about a reliable oxygen-therapy equipment vendor within the community to determine if patient and family are able to use a home-fill system with an oxygen concentrator, which provides patient opportunity to fill portable canister as needed (Aguiar et al., 2015).

• Consider using oxygen-conserving devices (e.g., Oxymizer) that administer oxygen in a pulse-dosed flow during inhalation only. These reduce the use and cost of long-term oxygen therapy.

◆ **SKILL 23.2**   **Administering Oxygen Therapy to a Patient With an Artificial Airway**

Patients with an artificial airway require constant humidification to the airway (see Chapter 25). An artificial airway bypasses the normal filtering and humidification process of the nose and mouth. The two devices that supply humidified gas to an artificial airway are a T tube and a tracheostomy collar.

The T tube, also called a *Briggs adaptor*, is a T-shaped device with a 15-mm ($\frac{1}{3}$-inch) connection that connects an oxygen source to an artificial airway such as an endotracheal (ET) tube or

tracheostomy (Fig. 23.12). A tracheostomy mask is a curved device with an adjustable strap that fits around a patient's neck (Fig. 23.13).

Delegation and Collaboration

The skill of administering oxygen therapy to a patient with an artificial airway cannot be delegated to nursing assistive personnel (NAP). The nurse collaborates with the respiratory therapist when caring for this patient. The nurse directs the NAP about:

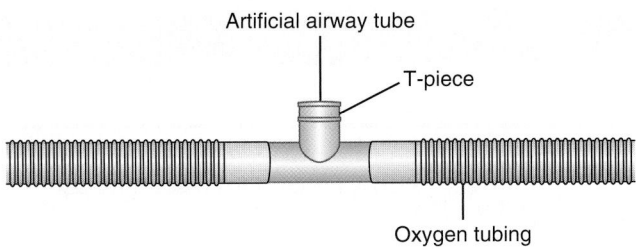

Artificial airway tube

T-piece

Oxygen tubing

FIG 23.12 T tube.

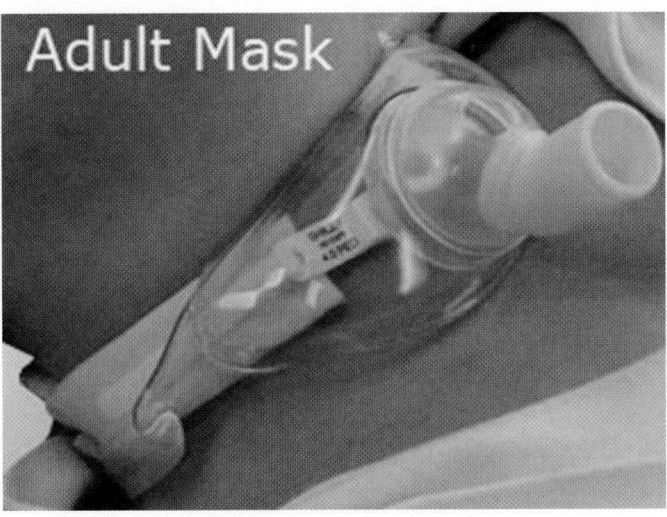

FIG 23.13 Tracheostomy mask. (*Courtesy Marcpac Company.*)

- Patient-specific variations for application or adjustment of the T tube or tracheostomy collar (e.g., methods to avoid device-related pressure areas or pulling on the artificial airway, methods for handling accumulated secretions in devices).
- Immediately reporting to the nurse increase in anxiety, changes in vital signs, and increase in airway secretions.

Equipment

- T tube or tracheostomy collar
- Large-bore oxygen tubing
- Nebulizer
- Sterile water for nebulizer
- Oxygen or gas source
- Clean gloves
- Mask and/or barrier gown (if patient isolation orders dictate)
- Goggles (if splash risk exists)

- Flowmeter
- Yankauer or tonsillar tip suction catheter
- Connecting tubing (at least 6 feet)
- Suction machine or wall suction device
- Pulse oximeter
- Stethoscope

STEP	RATIONALE

ASSESSMENT

STEP	RATIONALE
1. Identify patient using at least two identifiers (e.g., name and birthday or name and medical record number) according to agency policy.	Ensures correct patient. Complies with The Joint Commission standards and improves patient safety (TJC, 2016).
2. Perform hand hygiene. Assess patient's respiratory status, including symmetry of chest wall expansion, respiratory rate and depth, sputum production, and lung sounds (see Chapter 6); assess for signs and symptoms associated with hypoxia (see Box 23.1). Assess condition of lips around endotracheal tube or of tracheal stoma. **Note:** Apply clean gloves if there is risk of contacting mucus. Apply mask if there is risk of mucus splash.	Changes in ventilation and gas exchange resulting in hypoxia require oxygen therapy. Provides baseline for monitoring of tissue breakdown from irritation of medical device. Reduces transmission of microorganisms.
3. Observe for patent airway and remove airway secretions by having patient cough and by suctioning (see Chapter 25).	Secretions plug airway, decreasing amount of oxygen available for gas exchange in lung. Secretions also occlude T tube or tracheostomy collar, impeding oxygen delivery to patient.
4. Observe for behavioral changes (e.g., apprehension, anxiety, confusion, decreased ability to concentrate, decreased LOC, fatigue, and dizziness).	Decreased levels of oxygen (hypoxia) or increased levels of carbon dioxide (hypercapnia) affect a person's cognitive abilities, interpersonal interactions, and mood (Lewis et al., 2017).

Clinical Decision Point *Patients with artificial airways who develop sudden changes in their vital signs, level of consciousness (LOC), or behavior may be experiencing hypoxia secondary to airway obstruction. The airway must be determined to be patent before oxygen is administered. If patients continue with signs of hypoxia once obstruction is removed or ruled out, oxygen should be applied.*

STEP	RATIONALE
5. Monitor pulse oximetry (SpO$_2$) and, if available, note patient's most recent arterial blood gas (ABG) results. Remove gloves and other PPE, perform hand hygiene.	Objectively documents patient's pH, arterial oxygen, arterial carbon dioxide, or arterial oxygen saturation.
6. Review patient's medical record for medical order for oxygen, noting delivery method, flow rate, and duration of oxygen therapy.	Ensures safe and accurate oxygen administration. Safe oxygen delivery includes the six rights of medication administration (see Chapter 20).
7. Assess patient's and family caregiver's level of understanding of purpose of oxygen therapy.	Determines level of instruction or support needed.

STEP	RATIONALE

NURSING DIAGNOSES

- Anxiety
- Deficient knowledge regarding purpose of therapy
- Fatigue
- Impaired gas exchange
- Ineffective airway clearance
- Ineffective breathing pattern
- Risk for impaired tissue integrity

Related factors are individualized based on patient's condition or needs.

PLANNING

STEP	RATIONALE
1. Expected outcomes following completion of procedure: • Patient's signs of hypoxia are reduced or eliminated. • Patient's vital signs remain stable or return to baseline.	Patient demonstrates improved oxygenation. When there is no underlying cardiovascular disease, patient adapts to decreased oxygen levels by increasing pulse and blood pressure. This is a short-term adaptive response. Once signs of hypoxia are reduced or controlled, patient's vital signs usually return to normal.
• Patient's work of breathing decreases.	With improved oxygenation, tissue oxygen demand is met, and work of breathing decreases.
• Patient experiences increased lung expansion.	Improved oxygenation helps to resolve collapsed and constricted airways, improve work of breathing, and thus improve lung expansion.
• Patient's LOC returns to baseline.	Improvement in oxygenation relieves hypoxia and improves patient's mental status.
• ABG values or SpO$_2$ saturation returns to normal or baseline.	Documents physiological response to oxygen therapy.
• Tracheal stoma remains intact without irritation or peristomal skin breakdown.	Tension on tracheal stoma from oxygen therapy equipment has potential to cause pressure on stoma and surrounding skin (Pittman et al., 2015).
2. Explain purpose of **T** tube or tracheostomy collar to patient and family caregiver.	Explanation decreases patient's anxiety and reduces oxygen consumption. Education increases adherence to treatment plan and cooperation of patient and family caregiver.

IMPLEMENTATION

STEP	RATIONALE
1. Gather equipment/supplies and complete necessary charges according to agency policy.	Ensure that you have the necessary equipment to apply oxygen-delivery device appropriately.
2. Perform hand hygiene, apply clean gloves and goggles; consider use of barrier gown and mask.	Reduces transmission of microorganisms by preventing contact with pulmonary secretions. Patients with excessive secretions or forceful productive coughs place caregiver at risk for splash contact.
3. Attach **T** tube or tracheostomy mask to large-bore oxygen tubing and to humidified room air or oxygen source as indicated.	Provides supplemental humidification to avoid drying of airway. This is necessary because of loss of oral and nasal passages that naturally humidify air.
4. If health care provider orders oxygen, adjust flow rate to 10 L/min or as ordered. Adjust nebulizer to proper oxygen concentration (FiO$_2$) setting. Attach **T** tube to artificial airway. Place tracheostomy collar over tracheostomy tube and adjust straps so it fits snugly.	Flow rate ensures humidification; nebulizer regulates FiO$_2$.
5. Observe that **T** tube does not pull on artificial airway or cause pressure on adjacent skin and tissue. Observe for secretions within **T** tube or tracheostomy collar and suction as necessary (see Chapter 25).	Pulling effect on tube increases patient's discomfort and causes pressure to side of patient's mouth or tracheal stoma, which increases risk for device-related pressure injuries (Pittman et al., 2015; Schallom et al., 2015).
6. Observe oxygen tubing frequently for accumulation of fluid caused by condensation. If fluid is present, drain tube away from patient, disconnect from collar or **T** tube, and discard fluid in proper receptacle.	Excess water is medium for bacterial growth. Draining contaminated water into proper receptacle prevents contamination of entire humidifying unit.
7. Set up suction equipment at patient's bedside.	Humidification increases airway secretions.
8. Remove personal protective equipment (gloves, goggles, mask, and/or gown); perform hand hygiene.	Reduces transmission of microorganisms.

STEP	RATIONALE

EVALUATION

1. Monitor patient's vital signs and SpO_2.

Continuous monitoring of vital signs and SpO_2 allows for continual noninvasive, cost-effective trending of patient's vital signs and oxygen saturation.

2. Perform respiratory assessment and observe for any behavioral changes indicative of hypoxia.

Monitors changes in patient's respiratory assessment and cognitive status in response to supplemental oxygen.

3. Observe position of oxygen-delivery device and condition of adjacent tissues to ensure that there is no pulling on artificial airway or pressure areas.

Pulling on artificial airway or pressure on adjacent tissues results in damage to oral cavity or stoma.

4. Use Teach-Back: "I want to be sure I explained how oxygen will help your mother. Explain to me why oxygen is attached to your mother's tracheostomy tube." Revise your instruction now or develop a plan for revised patient or family caregiver teaching if patient or family caregiver is not able to teach back correctly.

Determines patient's and family caregiver's level of understanding of instructional topic.

Unexpected Outcomes

1. Patient experiences tracheal stoma or lip irritation; thick, tenacious secretions; pressure areas on neck or near stoma site.

2. Patient experiences continued hypoxia.

Related Interventions

- Implement measures to protect patient from medical device pressure injuries (MDPIs) (see Chapter 39).
- Increase frequency of suctioning and airway care (see Chapter 25).
- Determine if cause of continued hypoxia is oxygen-delivery device, plugging of airway, oxygen flow rate, or a new clinical problem.
- Notify health care provider of continued or worsening hypoxia.

Recording and Reporting

- Record the respiratory assessment findings; method of oxygen delivery, flow rate, condition of tracheal stoma or lips, patient's response; any adverse reactions on the flow sheet in nurses' notes in electronic health record (EHR) or chart.
- Document your evaluation of patient and family caregiver learning.
- Report any unexpected outcome to health care provider or nurse in charge.

Special Considerations
Teaching
- See teaching considerations for Skill 23.1.

Home Care

- Some patients who are at home have both a permanent tracheostomy and a **T** tube or a tracheostomy collar. The patient or caregiver needs to be physically able to perform tracheostomy care and suctioning techniques and must understand how to manage oxygen (see Chapters 25 and 44).

◆ SKILL 23.3 Using Incentive Spirometry

Incentive spirometry helps a patient deep breathe. It works by providing visual feedback that helps encourage the patient to take long, deep, slow breaths (Smetana, 2016). The use of an incentive spirometer (IS) alone is not recommended to prevent postoperative pulmonary complications. It should be used in combination with other pulmonary maneuvers such as deep breathing and coughing, early mobilization of the patient, and directed coughing (do Nascimento et al., 2014; Smetana, 2016).

The two types of ISs are flow oriented and volume oriented. Flow-oriented ISs have one or more plastic chambers with freely movable colored balls. The advantage of a flow-oriented IS is the slow, steady expansion of the lung. As a patient inhales slowly, the balls elevate to a premarked area (Fig. 23.14). A patient's goal is to keep the balls elevated for as long as possible to ensure maximal sustained inhalation. Even if a very slow inspiration does not elevate the balls, this pattern helps a patient improve lung expansion.

Volume-oriented devices use a bellows that a patient must raise to a predetermined volume by inhaling slowly (Fig. 23.15). The

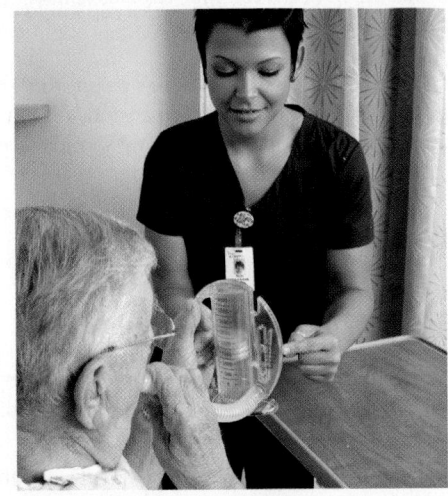

FIG 23.14 Flow-oriented incentive spirometer.

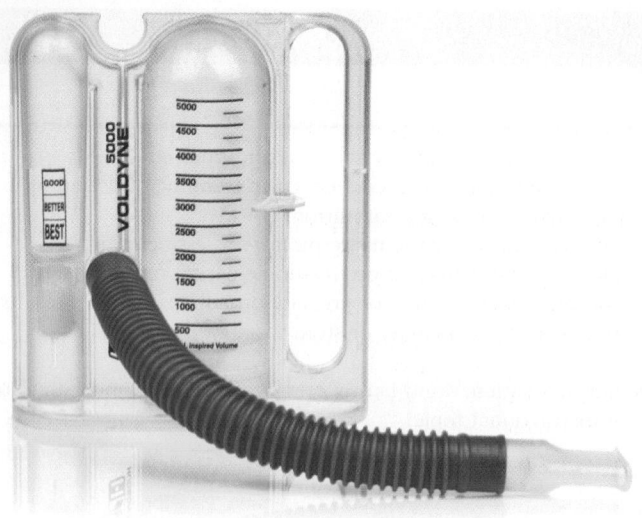

FIG 23.15 Volume-oriented incentive spirometer.

advantage of the volume-oriented IS is that a patient can achieve a known inspiratory volume and measure it with each breath.

Delegation and Collaboration

The skill of helping a patient to use incentive spirometry can be delegated to nursing assistive personnel (NAP). The nurse is responsible for assessing and monitoring the patient, evaluating the patient response, educating the patient about the proper use of the IS, and evaluating that education. The nurse directs the NAP by:

- Informing about the patient's target goal for incentive spirometry.
- Informing to immediately notify the nurse about any unexpected outcomes such as chest pain, excessive sputum production, and fever.

Equipment

- Flow- or volume-oriented IS
- Stethoscope
- Pulse oximeter monitor

STEP	RATIONALE

ASSESSMENT

1. Identify patient using at least two identifiers (e.g., name and birthday or name and medical record number) according to agency policy.	Ensures correct patient. Complies with The Joint Commission standards and improves patient safety (TJC, 2016).
2. Review medical record to identify patients who will benefit from the use of an IS (e.g., existing pulmonary disease, obesity, debilitating chronic illness, heavy smokers, patients with a neuromuscular disease, or patients with sickle cell disease with acute chest syndrome (Smetana, 2016). In addition, identify selected postoperative patients who would benefit from combining IS with other airway clearance measures (Tyson et al., 2015).	Alerts health care personnel to patients at risk for respiratory complications during illness or after surgery.
3. Assess patient for confusion, cognitive impairment, ability to follow directions, age, developmental level, level of consciousness, and decreased necessary motor skills (Smetana, 2016).	Determines risks for difficulty performing incentive spirometry.

Clinical Decision Point *Patients who are unable to follow directions or who are not developmentally or physically able to perform the actions associated with this skill are not candidates for this intervention. This assessment allows the nurse ability to identify whether to use the flow-oriented versus volume-oriented IS.*

4. Perform hand hygiene. Assess patient's respiratory status, including symmetry of chest wall expansion, respiratory rate and depth, sputum production, and lung sounds (see Chapter 6). Also obtain a pulse oximeter reading.	Reduces transmission of microorganisms. Decreased chest wall movement, crackles or decreased lung sounds, increased respiratory rate, or increased sputum production can indicate a need for incentive spirometry to improve lung expansion.
5. Assess level of pain at rest and during activity (e.g., coughing) using a 0-to-10 scale.	Pain decreases effective incentive spirometry by restricting chest expansion.
6. Review health care provider's order for incentive spirometry.	Health care agencies often require a medical order for incentive spirometry to receive third-party reimbursement.

NURSING DIAGNOSES

- Acute pain
- Impaired breathing pattern
- Impaired gas exchange
- Ineffective airway clearance

Related factors are individualized based on patient's condition or needs.

STEP	RATIONALE

PLANNING

1. Expected outcomes following completion of procedure:
- Patient demonstrates correct use of IS.

Demonstrates learning.

- Patient achieves target volume and number of repetitions per hour.

Demonstrates increased lung expansion.

- Patient has improved breath sounds and increased pulse oximeter reading.

Incentive spirometry helps patient deep breathe and manage airway secretions.

2. Explain procedure to patient and family caregiver.

Understanding purpose of incentive spirometry and its proper use improves compliance with use.

3. Indicate to patient where target volume is on IS. **NOTE:** If possible, demonstrate use of IS.

Encourages patients to "do better" with each breath and meet or exceed target volume. When patients have a visual target, they can gauge their improvement.

IMPLEMENTATION

1. Gather equipment/supplies and complete necessary charges according to agency policy.

Ensures that you have the necessary equipment.

2. Perform hand hygiene.

Reduces transmission of microorganisms.

3. Position patient in most erect position (e.g., high-Fowler's if tolerated) in bed or chair.

Promotes optimal lung expansion during respiratory maneuver.

4. Instruct patient to hold IS upright, exhale normally and completely through mouth, and place lips tightly around mouthpiece (Fig. 23.16).

Allows for proper function of IS (Smetana, 2016). Showing patient how to correctly place mouthpiece is reliable technique for teaching psychomotor skill and enables patient to ask questions.

5. Instruct patient to take a slow, deep breath and maintain constant flow, like pulling through a straw. If flow-oriented IS, inhalation should raise the ball. If volume-oriented IS, inhalation should raise the piston. Remove mouthpiece at point of maximal inhalation; then have patient hold his or her breath for 3 seconds and exhale normally.

Maintains maximal inspiration; reduces risk for progressive collapse of individual alveoli.

Clinical Decision Point *Some patients are unable to hold their breath for 3 seconds. Encourage them to do their best and try to extend the duration of breath holding. Allow patients to rest between IS breaths to prevent hyperventilation and fatigue.*

6. Have patient repeat maneuver, encouraging him or her to reach prescribed goal.

Ensures correct use of IS and patient's understanding of use.

7. Encourage patient to independently use IS at prescribed frequency. Frequently prescribed timing schedules of IS use are up to 30 deep breaths with 30- to 60-second rests between sets of 10 (Smetana, 2016).

Repeated use of IS improves lung expansion and promotes clearing of airways. Encouraging patients to perform independently gives them a sense of control over their care.

8. Perform hand hygiene.

Reduces transmission of microorganisms.

EVALUATION

1. Observe patient's ability to use incentive spirometry by return demonstration.

Determines patient's ability to perform breathing exercise correctly.

2. Assess if patient is able to achieve target volume or frequency.

Measures adherence to therapy and lung expansion.

3. Auscultate chest during respiratory cycle and obtain pulse oximeter reading (Smetana, 2016).

Documents lung expansion, identifies any abnormal lung sounds, and determines if airways are clear. Identifies improvement in pulse oximeter readings.

4. Use Teach-Back: "I want to be sure I explained how and when to use the IS. Show me how to use your IS, and tell me how frequently you should use it." Revise your instruction now or develop a plan for revised patient teaching if patient is not able to teach back correctly.

Determines patient's level of understanding of instructional topic.

STEP	RATIONALE

Unexpected Outcomes

1. Patient is unable to achieve incentive spirometry target volume.

Related Interventions

- Encourage patient to attempt incentive spirometry more frequently, followed by rest periods.
- Teach cough-control exercises.
- Teach patient how to splint and protect incision sites during deep breathing.
- Administer ordered analgesic if acute pain is inhibiting use of IS.

2. Patient has decreased lung expansion and/or abnormal breath sounds or decreased pulse oximeter readings.

- Teach patient cough-control exercises.
- Provide help with suctioning if patient cannot cough up secretions effectively.

3. Patient develops hyperventilation.

- Encourage longer rest periods between breaths.

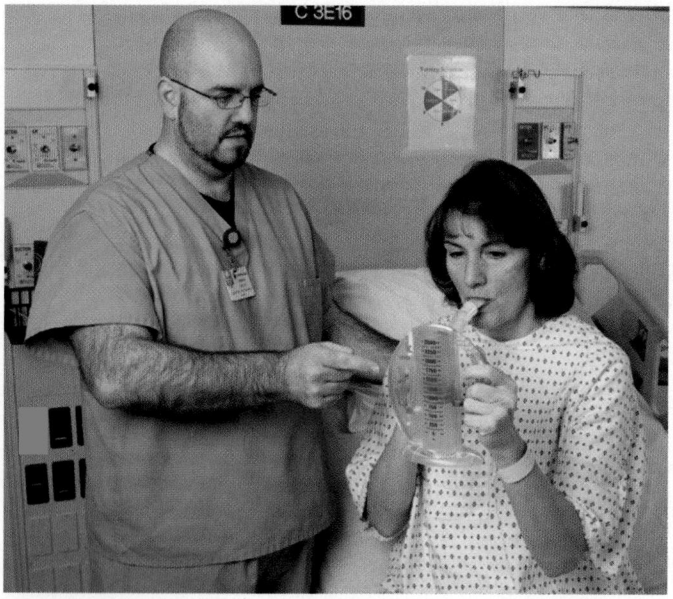

FIG 23.16 Proper placement of lips around incentive spirometer.

Recording and Reporting

- Record lung sounds, respiratory rate, and pulse oximeter readings before and after incentive spirometry; frequency of use; volumes achieved; and any adverse effects on flow sheet in nurses' notes in electronic health record (EHR) or chart.
- Document your evaluation of patient learning.

Special Considerations
Teaching

- Teach patient to examine sputum for consistency, amount, and color changes. Sputum should become clearer over time and decrease in volume.

Pediatric

- Incentive spirometry is not typically used in pediatrics except for school-age children; a pediatric patient needs the fine-motor skills and ability to follow instructions to use an IS effectively (Hockenberry and Wilson, 2015).
- Allowing a child to play with and try out the IS helps to decrease his or her anxiety and encourages participation in care.
- Use games or bubbles and pinwheels to encourage small children to take deep breaths. These activities help achieve the same goals as incentive spirometry in some children.

Gerontological

- Older adults with chronic illnesses or arthritis have difficulty coordinating the use of the IS. They require additional time to demonstrate the procedure (Touhy and Jett, 2014).
- Weakened respiratory muscles and decreased elastic recoil properties of the lungs affect a patient's ability to cough and deep breathe. Therefore it takes an older adult longer to achieve the target volume (Touhy and Jett, 2014).
- An older adult may be more able to use the volume-oriented IS versus the flow-oriented IS (Lunardi et al., 2014).

> **SKILL 23.4   Care of a Patient Receiving Noninvasive Positive-Pressure Ventilation**

Noninvasive positive-pressure ventilation (NIPPV or NPPV), or noninvasive ventilation (NIV), maintains positive airway pressure and improves alveolar ventilation without the need for an artificial airway. There are two types of NIPPV: continuous positive airway pressure (CPAP) and bi-level positive airway pressure (BiPAP). BiPAP and CPAP are usually applied via a mask covering the nose or both the mouth and nose (Fig. 23.17), but those who require home CPAP may wear nasal prongs instead (Cross, 2012; Hill and Kramer, 2016; Pooboni et al., 2013; Preston, 2013).

NIPPV is used both in acute care settings and increasingly more in home care settings to treat a variety of conditions, including obstructive sleep apnea (OSA), chronic obstructive pulmonary disease (COPD), cardiogenic pulmonary edema, respiratory failure, and neuromuscular disorders. It is commonly used in these conditions to avoid the complications of invasive ventilation strategies, including pneumonia and aspiration (Gale et al., 2015; Hill and Kramer, 2016; Pooboni et al., 2013). It should not be used in patients who cannot protect their airway or in patients with an

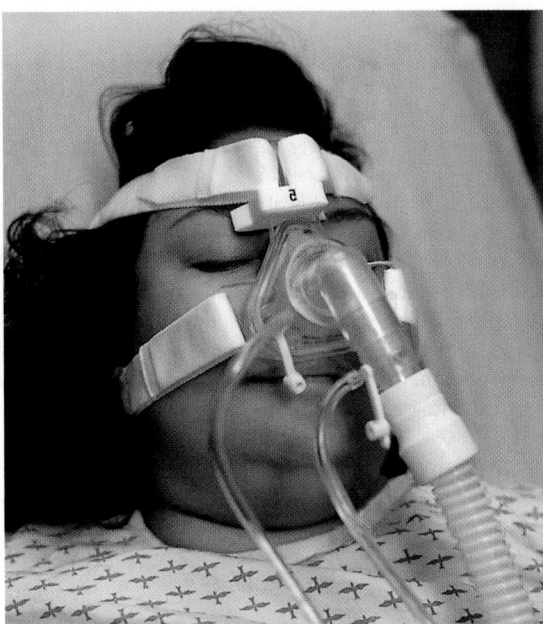

FIG 23.17 CPAP mask.

TABLE 23.2

Problems Associated With Continuous Positive Airway Pressure and Bi-Level Positive Airway Pressure

Problem	Cause
Discomfort	Mask that fits over patient's nose is tight fitting. Oxygen flow rate causes dry mucous membranes.
Psychosocial	Relationship with sleep partner is difficult. There are possible sensations of claustrophobia.
Risks to skin integrity	Tight fit of mask causes diaphoresis, pressure, and increased risk for skin breakdown. Patients need to remove mask to relieve pressure.
Hypercapnia	Although CPAP improves alveolar function, which increases carbon dioxide clearance from the blood, it also causes air trapping. In some patients this causes a rise in carbon dioxide levels. Initially you need to monitor patient's ABG levels.
Gastric distention	CPAP/BiPAP force more air into the stomach, which causes distention and discomfort.
Noise	Some patients find the older machines very noisy, interfering with sleep and leisure activities such as watching television or listening to music.

Data from Pooboni et al: *Noninvasive ventilation procedures,* 2013, http://emedicine.medscape.com/article/1417959-overview, November 2015.
ABG, Arterial blood gas; *BiPAP,* bi-level positive airway pressure; *CPAP,* continuous positive airway pressure.

inadequate respiratory drive or apnea and should be used with caution in patients with facial injuries, uncooperative patients, or hemodynamically unstable patients (Cross, 2012).

The advantages of this type of ventilation versus invasive ventilation include an increased ability to communicate with caregivers and family, better ability to cough and clear secretions, and allowance for eating and drinking. There are disadvantages, problems, and concerns to this type of ventilation (Table 23.2). The mask must fit tight and have a good seal to prevent air from leaking. This pressure can cause feelings of claustrophobia and intolerance in patients, which can lead to issues with adherence to therapy. The tight-fitting mask can also lead to skin breakdown, particularly on the bridge of the nose (Cross, 2012; Schallom et al., 2015).

Delegation and Collaboration

The skill of caring for a patient receiving noninvasive ventilation cannot be delegated to nursing assistive personnel (NAP). The nurse collaborates with the respiratory therapist when providing care for the patient. However, the skills of patient positioning, therapeutic coughing, and CPAP/BiPAP mask application can be delegated to NAP. The nurse directs the NAP by:
- Informing about the need to immediately report to the nurse any changes in patient's vital signs; oxygen saturation; mental status; skin color; or skin abrasions, bruising, or blistering around mask area.
- Informing about the need to immediately report to the nurse any ventilator or CPAP/BiPAP machine alarms or patient monitor alarms.

- Instructing on how to modify care such as for how long the mask can be removed, oral care, or any special skin care needs.
- Informing about the prescribed settings on the NIPPV equipment and instructing personnel to immediately notify the nurse of any change in settings or patient comfort.

Equipment

(**NOTE:** When device is used in the home, the home care equipment vendor provides the equipment.)
- Nasal mask/full face mask (with quick-release straps), or nasal pillows
- Oxygen source and tubing
- CPAP/BiPAP health care provider order
- Humidification source
- BiPAP and/or CPAP ventilator
- Delivery tubing
- Pulse oximetry
- Clean gloves
- Personal protective equipment as appropriate
- Stethoscope
- Suction equipment
- Self-inflating manual-resuscitation bag-valve-mask device

STEP	RATIONALE

ASSESSMENT

1. Identify patient using at least two identifiers (e.g., name and birthday or name and medical record number) according to agency policy.

Ensures correct patient. Complies with The Joint Commission standards and improves patient safety (TJC, 2016).

STEP	RATIONALE
2. Assess patient's respiratory status, including symmetry of chest wall expansion, respiratory rate and depth, oxygen saturation, sputum production, and lung sounds (see Chapter 6). When possible, ask patient about dyspnea and observe for signs and symptoms associated with hypoxia (see Box 23.1).	Decreased chest wall movement, crackles or decreased lung sounds, increased respiratory rate, increased sputum production, or signs of worsening hypoxia may make patient a candidate for noninvasive positive-pressure ventilation or changes in NIPPV settings.
3. Observe patient's skin over bridge of nose, around external ears, back of head.	The mask can place pressure on skin and increase risk for skin breakdown (Schallom et al., 2015).
4. Observe patient's ability to clear and remove airway secretions by coughing.	Secretions plug the airway, decreasing amount of oxygen that is available for gas exchange in the lung.
5. Perform hand hygiene. Assess patient's vital signs, pulse oximetry; when available, note patient's most recent arterial blood gas (ABG) results.	Objectively documents patient's pH, arterial oxygen, arterial carbon dioxide, or arterial oxygen saturation. Identifies need for NIPPV.
6. Assess patient's level of consciousness, behaviors, and ability to maintain and protect airway.	Patients who cannot maintain their own airway or who are uncooperative are not candidates for NIPPV.

Clinical Decision Point *NIPPV is contraindicated in patients in cardiac or respiratory arrest or with facial deformities, hemodynamic instability, inability to protect airway, severe agitation, excessive secretions, or high inspired oxygen concentration (FiO_2) requirements (Wiegand, 2011). Its use in palliative care and end-of-life care is still being investigated (Gale et al., 2015).*

STEP	RATIONALE
7. Review patient's medical record for medical order for CPAP/BiPAP and appropriate settings.	Health care provider's order is necessary for this therapy.
8. Assess patient's and family caregiver's understanding of purpose of CPAP and ongoing maintenance.	Determines level of instruction required.

NURSING DIAGNOSES

- Activity intolerance
- Deficient knowledge regarding purpose of CPAP
- Impaired comfort
- Impaired gas exchange
- Risk for aspiration
- Risk for impaired skin integrity
- Sleep deprivation

Related factors/Risk factors are individualized based on patient's condition or needs.

PLANNING

1. Expected outcomes following completion of procedure:	
• Patient has increased lung expansion.	Patient experiences improved gas exchange when lungs are expanded.
• Patient maintains ABG levels and/or pulse oximetry (SpO_2) readings improve or remain normal.	NIPPV delivered appropriately based on patient assessment data.

Clinical Decision Point *When first initiating CPAP/BiPAP, it is important to monitor gas exchange, especially in patients with COPD, cardiogenic pulmonary edema, or acute respiratory failure. You do this to observe for carbon dioxide retention. If patient has "do not resuscitate" orders or is receiving palliative care services, careful consideration is given before starting noninvasive ventilation (Preston, 2013).*

• Patient experiences reduction in feelings of dyspnea and work of breathing.	In patients with acute conditions dyspnea usually improves. Patients with chronic pulmonary diseases often require nocturnal CPAP/BiPAP indefinitely to achieve long-term benefits.
• Patient's vital signs and respiratory assessment parameters improve.	Reduced pulse and respiratory rate, improved mental status, improved skin color, and decreased use of accessory and abdominal muscles occur because patient's work of breathing decreases as level of oxygenation improves.
• Patient's skin around bridge of nose, ears, and back of head remains clear without breakdown.	Mask applied properly and monitored for pressure occurrence.
• Patient able to describe how to use CPAP in the home setting.	Demonstrates learning.
2. Explain to patient and family the purpose and reasons for CPAP/BiPAP.	Helps reduce sense of claustrophobia from mask. In addition, information reduces anxiety and increases cooperation and adherence to therapy.

STEP	RATIONALE

IMPLEMENTATION

1. Collaborate with the respiratory therapist to gather equipment/supplies and complete necessary charges according to agency policy.

Ensures that you have necessary equipment to apply the NIPPV system.

2. Perform hand hygiene; apply clean gloves. Apply mask, gown, and goggles if secretions are projectile or if patient is in isolation.

Reduces transmission of microorganisms and exposure to pulmonary secretions.

3. Adjust bed to appropriate height and lower side rail on side nearest you. Check locks on bed wheel.

Minimizes caregiver's muscle strain and prevents injury. Prevents bed from moving.

4. Determine correct mask size. Use masking chart to determine correct size (S, M, L, XL). **NOTE:** *It is imperative that mask have quick-release straps.*

Mask should fit snugly over patient's nose (CPAP) or nose and/or mouth (BiPAP) to create a tight seal for delivering positive pressure. In case of emergency (e.g., vomiting, respiratory arrest), quick-release straps allow mask to be removed quickly. This system also allows patient to remove mask quickly as needed (Urden et al., 2016).

Clinical Decision Point *A patient receiving NIPPV via a full face mask should **never** be restrained. The patient must be able to remove the mask if he or she begins to vomit, needs to remove excess secretions, or reposition a mask that has moved. A displaced mask can force the patient's jaw inward, which can obstruct the patient's airway (Urden et al., 2016).*

5. Connect CPAP/BiPAP device-delivery tubing to pressure generator.

Ensures that patient is receiving proper NIPPV as ordered.

6. Connect patient to pulse oximetry.

It is important to continually monitor patient's level of oxygenation when initiating NIPPV.

7. Set CPAP/BiPAP initial settings per physician order:

These settings allow health care team to determine initial patient response.

   a. CPAP: 5 to 15 cm H_2O is the typically prescribed pressure range (Pooboni et al., 2013)

CPAP provides single positive pressure throughout breathing cycle, which helps to keep alveoli open at end-expiration.

   b. BiPAP: Inspiratory pressure is usually set at 10 to 12 cm H_2O initially and can be titrated up to 15-20 cm H_2O as patient condition dictates; expiratory pressure is usually set at 5-7 cm H_2O initially and can be titrated up as patient condition warrants (Pooboni et al., 2013).

BiPAP supplies pressure at both inhalation and exhalation. The inhalation pressure is set according to health care provider's order and helps prevent airway closure. Expiratory pressure is set according to health care provider's order and keeps alveoli open at end-expiration (Cross, 2012; Preston, 2013).

8. Select FiO_2 level as indicated and per prescriber order.

Patients on NIPPV may also need supplemental oxygen to decrease signs and symptoms of hypoxia (Hill and Kramer, 2016).

9. Ensure that humidification and heating appliances are connected and on.

Humidification of gas is thought to improve comfort in patients receiving NIPPV (Restrepo and Walsh, 2012).

10. Ensure that mask is tight fitting, no air leak is present, and there are no excessive pressure points.

An ill-fitting mask leads to loss of pressure getting into airways or dyssynchrony with ventilator. It also can lead to air blowing into eyes, which can cause patient discomfort (Wiegand, 2011). Pressure points around mask area can cause device-related pressure injuries (Schallom et al., 2015).

11. If patient is to use CPAP at home, have patient or family caregiver demonstrate mask placement and adjustment of settings.

Return demonstration indicates learning.

12. Dispose of supplies as appropriate, remove gloves and other personal protective equipment, and perform hand hygiene.

Reduces transmission of microorganisms.

13. Continuous care of patient

   a. Ensure that all alarms are on and active and that ventilator circuit is intact and properly functioning.

Ensures patient safety.

   b. Ensure that emergency resuscitation equipment is at bedside.

Allows for quick resuscitation in case of worsening patient condition (Wiegand, 2011).

   c. Investigate any and all alarms that come with ventilator/CPAP machine and/or patient monitor.

Alarms can alert health care team to problems with patient or with circuit that adversely affects patient status.

   d. Change patient's position every 2 hours or encourage patient to change position every 2 hours.

Reduces incidence of atelectasis or pneumonia secondary to stasis of secretions.

STEP	RATIONALE

EVALUATION

1. Observe for decreased anxiety, improved level of consciousness and cognitive abilities, decreased fatigue, and absence of dizziness.

2. Measure vital signs, perform respiratory assessment and observe skin color, and ask patient to describe sense of dyspnea.

3. Monitor pulse oximetry.

4. Observe skin integrity over bridge of patient's nose every 2 hours. Ask patient about level of comfort (Hill and Kramer, 2016).

5. If NIPPV is planned for use in home, observe and monitor patient's and family's ability to manipulate CPAP or BiPAP machine/ventilator and face mask.

6. **Use Teach-Back:** "I want to be sure I explained how NIPPV works and why you are receiving this therapy. Explain to me why this therapy is necessary." Revise your instruction now or develop a plan for revised patient or family caregiver teaching if patient or family caregiver is not able to teach back correctly.

Determines patient's response to NIPPV. As hypoxia and hypercapnia are reduced or corrected, patient's behavioral assessment parameters improve.

Physical assessment parameters reveal oxygenation status.

Documents patient's level of oxygenation. When first initiating NIPPV, it is important to obtain ABG levels in patients in whom abnormal gas exchange is suspected, after the first hour, and per agency protocol.

Mask that is too tight causes skin breakdown, and frequent skin assessment is necessary (Pittman et al., 2015; Schallom et al., 2015).

Determines patient's ability to perform self-care and adhere to CPAP/BiPAP plan. Success of noninvasive ventilation depends largely on patient acceptance and adherence (Gale et al., 2015).

Determines patient's and family caregiver's level of understanding of instructional topic.

Unexpected Outcomes	Related Interventions
1. Patient experiences hypoxia, hypercapnia, or other signs of worsening respiratory function.	• Notify health care provider. • Reassess patient. • Determine correct settings and integrity of NIPPV.
2. Patient develops skin breakdown at mask sites or sites where mask straps are located such as bridge of nose, nasal septum, or ears.	• Notify health care provider. • Place protective synthetic coverings on nasal bridge or areas of irritation/possible irritation to protect skin. • Fit mask so it is tight enough to not cause air leak but loose enough to not cause skin breakdown. • Reassess patient (Pooboni et al., 2013).
3. Patient states sense of smothering or claustrophobia.	• Explain system to patient again. • Demonstrate use of quick-release straps. • Have patient demonstrate use of quick-release straps.
4. Stomach distention secondary to positive-pressure air being forced into esophagus and trachea (Pooboni et al., 2013).	• Notify health care provider. • Be prepared for possible insertion of nasogastric tube (see Chapter 35).

Recording and Reporting

• Record respiratory assessment findings, CPAP/BiPAP settings, vital signs and pulse oximetry, patient response, patient teaching outcomes, and skin assessment on flow sheet in nurses' notes in electronic health record (EHR) or chart.

• Document your evaluation of patient and family caregiver learning.

• Report to charge nurse or health care provider sudden change in patient's behavior or respiratory status and any decline in ABG levels or pulse oximetry values.

Special Considerations
Teaching

• Teach patient and family caregiver the prescribed hours to use the machine. If not in use for 24 hours/day, work with the family caregiver to identify the ideal time for use (e.g., bedtime, watching television).

• Teach patient and family caregiver how to apply the mask, connect it to the machine, and add oxygen if ordered.

• Instruct family caregiver to bring the machine, along with a list of correct settings, to the hospital any time patient is admitted.

Home Care

• The durable medical equipment provider, the home care nurse, and the primary care nurse develop a teaching plan to ensure that patient and family have working knowledge of the system before discharge.

• When patients require home NIPPV, instruct in complete care of the CPAP/BiPAP system. Skills include assembling the system, cleaning it, and maintaining the equipment daily.

• Teach patient and family caregiver what to do in case of respiratory distress or power failure.

• Notify appropriate power company so, in the event of a power outage, the home is on priority for restoring power.

• Follow the safety precautions for oxygen use (see Box 23.3).

PROCEDURAL GUIDELINE 23.1 *Use of a Peak Flowmeter*

For patients who have measurable changes in the flow of their airways such as patients with asthma or reactive airway disease, peak expiratory flow rate (PEFR) measurements are useful. The PEFR is the maximum flow that a patient forces out during one quick, forced expiration and is measured in liters per minute. Use these measurements as an objective indicator of a patient's current status or the effectiveness of treatment. Decreased PEFR may indicate the need for further interventions such as increased doses of bronchodilators, antiinflammatory medications, or even seeking emergency medical attention. Normal PEFR values vary according to a person's age, gender, and size.

Patients with asthma perform PEFR measures in the home to monitor the status of their airways. Health care providers usually recommend that patients measure and record their PEFR during the following times: same time every day (values are lowest in the morning and typically highest between noon and 5 PM), before taking asthma medicines, during asthma symptoms or an asthma attack, after taking medicine for an asthma attack, and other times recommended by their health care provider (NHLBI, 2013).

Delegation and Collaboration
Initial assessment of the patient's condition is a nursing responsibility and cannot be delegated. The skills of follow-up PEFR measurements in a stable patient can be delegated to nursing assistive personnel (NAP). The nurse instructs the NAP to:
- Report immediately to the nurse patient's difficulty breathing or decrease in PEFR measurement.

Equipment
- Peak flowmeter (Fig. 23.18)
- Patient diary/action plan (if appropriate)

Procedural Steps
1. Review medical record for patient's baseline PEFR (if available).
2. Assess previous PEFR readings and the target set by patient's health care provider.
3. Help patient to stand or to high-Fowler's position or any other position that promotes optimum lung expansion.
4. Assess patient's baseline knowledge of when and how to use PEFR and correct response to results.
5. Slide clean mouthpiece into base of the numbered scale.
6. Instruct patient to take a deep breath through nose and slowly blow out through mouth. Take second deep breath.
7. Have patient place meter mouthpiece in mouth and close lips, making a firm seal.
8. Have patient blow out as hard and fast as possible through mouth only.
9. Monitor PEFR results and assess if patient is in expected range.
10. Inform patient of his or her individualized acceptable range and mark on meter.
11. If patient is to record PEFR at home, have him or her demonstrate how to record it accurately on chart using "traffic light" pattern. A system of asthma zones—green, yellow, and red—is commonly used. Green indicates that the PEFR is 80% to 100% of patient's personal best value

and means that he or she should continue with the currently prescribed treatment regimen. Yellow indicates that the PEFR is 50% to 90% of the personal best and that the person should add the prescribed quick-relief medication to the treatment regimen and continue with his or her daily long-term control medications. Red indicates that the PEFR is less than 50% of the patient's personal best and that the person should take the prescribed quick-relief medication and seek medical attention (NHLBI, 2013) (Fig. 23.19).

12. **Use Teach-Back:** "I want to make sure that I showed you how to correctly measure your PEFR. Show me how you would use this PEFR device." Revise your instruction now or develop a plan for revised patient or family caregiver teaching if patient or family caregiver is not able to teach back correctly.
13. Compare patient's PEFR with his or her personal best.
14. Record PEFR measurement before and after therapy and patient's ability and effort to perform PEFR in electronic health record (EHR) or chart.
15. Instruct patient to clean unit weekly following manufacturer instructions.

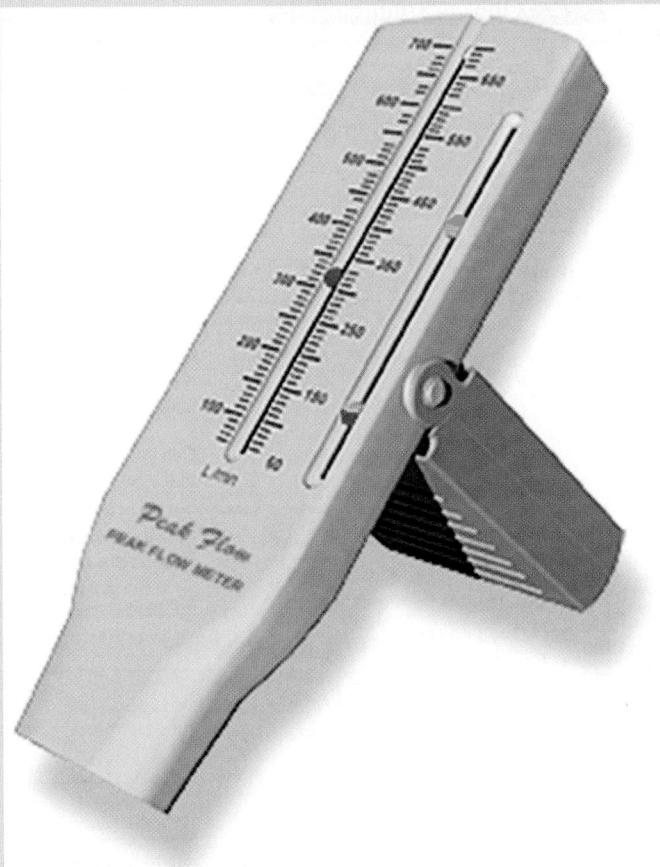

FIG 23.18 Peak flowmeter. (*Courtesy Philips Respironics.*)

Continued

PROCEDURAL GUIDELINE 23.1 *Use of a Peak Flowmeter—cont'd*

Asthma Action Plan

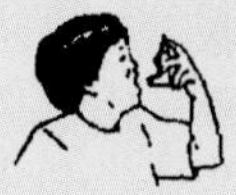

You can use the colors of a traffic light to help learn about your asthma medicines.

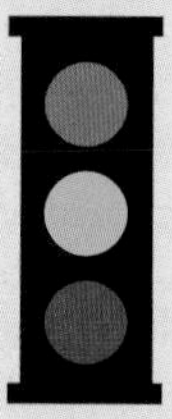

1. **Green** means **Go.**
   Use preventive medicine.
2. **Yellow** means **Caution.**
   Use quick-relief medicine.
3. **Red** means **Stop.**
   Get help from a doctor.

Name:_____

Doctor:_____ Date:_____

Phone for doctor or clinic:_____

Emergency contact phone and name:_____

1. Green — Go

- Breathing is good
- No cough or wheeze
- Can work and play

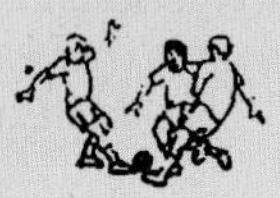

Peak flow number

_____ to _____

Personal best peak flow _____

Use preventive medicine.

Medicine	How much to take	When to take it
_____	_____	_____
_____	_____	_____

5 to 60 minutes before exercise, use this medicine:

_____

2. Yellow — Caution

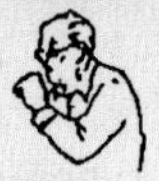

Cough 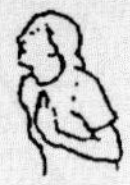   Wheeze 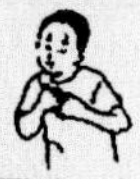   Tight chest

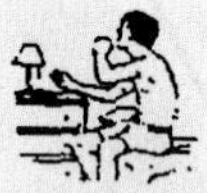

Wake up at night

Peak flow number

_____ to _____

(50% to 80% of my best peak flow)

Take quick-relief medicine to keep an asthma attack from getting bad

Medicine	How much to take	When to take it
_____	_____	_____
(short-acting beta$_2$ agonist)		
_____	_____	_____
_____	_____	_____

If symptoms return to Green Zone after 1 hour of taking above quick-relief medication, take_____ (medicine) and _____ (medicine).

If symptoms **do not** return to Green Zone after 1 hour of taking the quick-relief medication, take_____ (medicine) and add _____(medicine).
  (short-acting beta$_2$ agonist)   (oral steroid)

Call your doctor if symptoms do not improve within_____ hours after taking the oral steroid or if your symptoms are in the Red Zone.

3. Red — Stop — Danger

- Medicine is not helping
- Breathing is hard and fast
- Nose opens wide
- Can't walk
- Ribs show
- Can't talk well

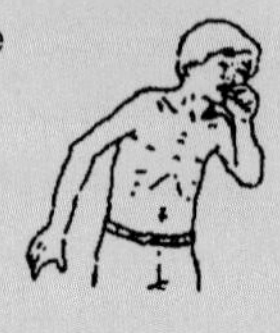

Peak flow number

_____ to _____

(50% or less of personal best)

Get help from a doctor now!
Take these medicines until you talk with the doctor.

Medicine	How much to take	When to take it
_____	_____	_____
(short-acting beta$_2$ agonist)		
_____	_____	_____
(oral steroid)		
_____	_____	_____

Go to the emergency department immediately or call the ambulance if you cannot reach your doctor and you are still in the Red Zone after 15 minutes.

These signs signal **DANGER:**
- Difficulty walking or breathing
- Mental confusion
- Fingernails or lips are blue

Call the ambulance.

FIG 23.19 Asthma action plan. (*From Hockenberry MJ, Wilson D: Wong's nursing care of infants and children, ed 10, St Louis, 2015, Mosby.*)

◆ **SKILL 23.5** Care of a Patient on a Mechanical Ventilator

Mechanical ventilation is a life-saving therapy used for patients who have an inability to protect their airway or who have an illness that leads to respiratory failure. It can be used for a short period of time or as a long-term means of support for those who cannot support their own respiratory effort such as those with neuromuscular disorders (Lewis et al., 2017). Patients receiving mechanical ventilation are most often in an intensive care unit but may be seen in skilled nursing facilities or home settings. The nurse must collaborate with the respiratory therapist when caring for patients receiving mechanical ventilation. At many institutions the respiratory therapist is charged with caring for and monitoring the ventilator.

There are two types of mechanical ventilation: positive pressure and negative pressure. Positive-pressure ventilation is the usual method of ventilation that delivers a positive pressure to inflate the lungs. An artificial airway such as an endotracheal (ET) tube or tracheostomy tube is necessary for positive-pressure mechanical ventilation (see Chapter 25). Multiple complications are associated with positive-pressure ventilation, including decreased cardiac output, aspiration, barotrauma, and ventilator-associated events (VAEs) such as ventilator-associated pneumonia (VAP) (see Chapter 25). Be alert for these side effects.

Negative-pressure ventilation is a noninvasive, negative-pressure ventilation technique that mimics normal physiological ventilation. It is used for the chronic management of patients with primary neuromuscular illnesses that interfere with normal respiratory muscle function such as multiple sclerosis and muscular dystrophy. It generally is not used during times of acute illness. The nurse or respiratory therapist fits a patient with a poncho or shell that is connected to the ventilator. Air is removed from between the patient's chest wall and the interior wall of the poncho or shell, causing the negative pressure that allows the chest to pull outward, causing the patient to inhale. Exhalation is passive. A patient using negative-pressure ventilation does not need an artificial airway (Lewis et al., 2017).

The skill described in this chapter focuses on positive-pressure mechanical ventilation frequently used in acute, subacute, and some selective home care settings. Many types of positive-pressure mechanical ventilators are available for acute care use (Fig. 23.20).

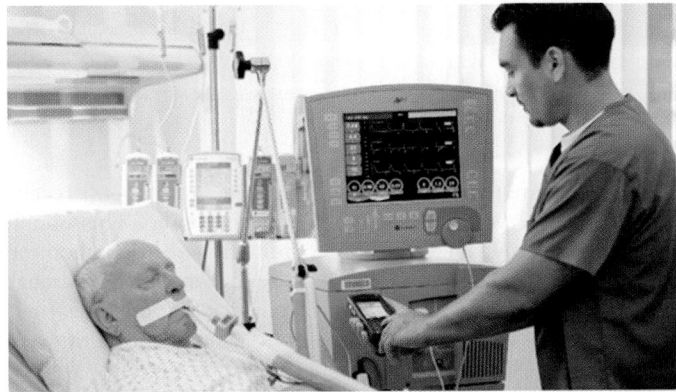

FIG 23.20 Positive-pressure ventilator. (*Courtesy and © Becton, Dickinson and Company.*)

Modes of Positive-Pressure Mechanical Ventilation

There are many different modes of mechanical ventilation to support different conditions and physiological processes. Mechanical ventilation controls or helps a patient's respirations when he or she is unable to maintain adequate gas exchange because of respiratory or ventilatory failure (Table 23.3). The ventilator takes over the physical work of moving air into and out of the lungs, but it does not replace or alter the physiological function of the lung. Mechanical ventilation maintains or improves ventilation, oxygenation, and breathing pattern. Patients with impaired ventilation have low oxygen level (hypoxemia), retained carbon dioxide (hypercapnia), and difficulty breathing.

It is important that patients remain on mechanical ventilation only as long as necessary because there is an increased mortality risk associated with positive-pressure ventilation. In addition, as the length of time needed for mechanical ventilation increases, there is an increased risk of failure to wean from the ventilator (Urden et al., 2016). Caring for a patient on mechanical ventilation and weaning from it require interprofessional collaboration.

Alarms and Settings

The mechanical ventilator has a number of settings to adjust the amount of oxygen delivered, the number of breaths per minute, the amount of tidal volume, the time for inspiration and expiration, and the pressure at which each breath is delivered. The goal of providing oxygenation is to maintain a PaO_2 of >60 mm Hg using an FiO_2 of 40% or less. Table 23.4 lists the ventilator parameters with which you need to become familiar to care for a patient on positive-pressure mechanical ventilation.

There are several alarms on the ventilator to ensure patient safety. Each ventilator is a little different; however, the basic alarms are similar. Alarms common to all ventilators include high-pressure, low-pressure, low-exhaled volume, and oxygen alarms (Table 23.5). You need to know how to respond to the ventilator alarms and which nursing actions are required to preserve the patient's respiratory status. The two most frequent alarms are the high-pressure and low-pressure alarms. The high-pressure alarm is usually set at 10 to 20 cm greater than the peak inspiratory pressure (Lewis et al., 2017). When this alarm sounds, it indicates that the ventilator has met resistance to delivering the tidal volume and requires more pressure to inflate the lungs. The low-pressure alarm sounds when the ventilator has no resistance to inflating the lung. All ventilator alarms require immediate nursing intervention to prevent patient harm.

Ventilator-Associated Events

VAP, a type of VAE, is the leading cause of death among all health care–associated infections (HAIs). VAP has a 20% to 50% mortality rate in patients receiving mechanical ventilation and adds approximately $40,000 to the costs of a patient's hospital stay. The Centers for Disease Control and Prevention (CDC) assembled several organizations, including the American Association of Critical Care Nurses (AACN), the American Thoracic Society (ATS), the American College of Chest Physicians, and the American Association for Respiratory Care (AARC) in an attempt to develop a clear definition of VAP and a valid reporting system for this complication (CDC, 2016). The simplified way to identify VAP includes observing deterioration in the patient's respiratory status

TABLE 23.3

Modes of Mechanical Ventilation

Types	Description	Nursing Considerations
Continuous positive airway pressure (CPAP)	Applies positive pressure during entire respiratory cycle. Used to help open alveoli at end expiration, thereby improving oxygenation.	Used for patients who breathe spontaneously but have hypoxemic respiratory failure; useful during weaning. Patients with COPD may tire after long hours of CPAP and require increased pressure support. Is used in both invasive and noninvasive ventilation modes.
Pressure support ventilation (PSV)	Preset amount of positive pressure used to help augment patient's spontaneous inspiratory efforts. Patient determines rate and tidal volume.	Spontaneous breathing mode. Helps overcome resistance of airway and ventilator tubing. Reduces patient work of breathing and improves ventilator-patient synchrony.
Assist-control (AC) or continuous mandatory ventilation (CMV)	Patient initiates breathing, but backup control delivers preset number of breaths at set volume.	Volume-controlled CMV used in patients with weak respiratory muscles that are spontaneously breathing. Watch for volutrauma. Pressure-controlled CMV used in patients with increased airway resistance or decreased lung compliance. Watch for hypercapnia. Sedation may be needed to control respiratory rate.
Synchronized intermittent mandatory ventilation (SIMV)	Ventilator delivers set number of breaths at specified volume. Some patients breathe spontaneously between SIMV breaths at volumes differing from those set on the machine.	Volume-controlled IMV is primary method of ventilation in many settings. Requires frequent monitoring during weaning from mechanical ventilation. May increase patient's work of breathing.
Pressure-regulated volume-control ventilation (PRVCV or PRVC)	Variation of CMV combining the feature of both volume- and pressure-control settings. The ventilator delivers a preset tidal volume at the lowest possible airway pressure. That pressure will not exceed preset maximum pressure limit.	Used in patient with changing pulmonary mechanics and dynamics. Potential complications are limited when compared with AC or pressure controlled–intermittent mandatory ventilation (PC-IMV) modes.
Airway pressure release ventilation (APRV)	Inspiratory and expiratory levels of CPAP are applied for predetermined periods of time. Spontaneous breathing can occur at both levels.	Spontaneous breathing mode that recruits alveoli with decreased risk of high peak pressures, decreasing risk of barotrauma. Patient should be monitored for hypercapnia.
High-Frequency		
High-frequency jet ventilation (HFJV)	Delivers gas rapidly under low pressure via special injector cannula. Delivers 100-600 cycles/min with lower-than-normal tidal volumes.	Patient on any mode of high-frequency ventilation requires continuous sedation and neuromuscular blocking agent administration. Not commonly used in adults; more commonly used in neonates. Requires intensive monitoring and care.
High-frequency oscillatory ventilation (HFOV)	Delivers 900-3000 cycles/min with very small tidal volumes. Airway pressure controlled.	Most common of high-frequency types: maintains alveolar ventilation with low airway pressure; useful for treating esophageal or bronchopleural fistulas; helps avert barotraumas in high-risk patients if used early in treatment. Not commonly used in adults; more commonly used in infants and children. Requires use of continuous sedation and neuromuscular blocking agent. Requires intensive monitoring and care.

Data from Urden L, et al: *Priorities in critical care nursing,* ed 7, St Louis, 2016, Mosby.
COPD, Chronic obstructive pulmonary disease.

after a period of stability while on the ventilator, objective evidence of inflammation or infection, and laboratory evidence of respiratory infection. A patient can be considered for VAP only after he or she has received mechanical ventilation for more than 2 calendar days (CDC, 2016).

In an attempt to decrease the incidence of VAEs, practice bundles have been developed and implemented at health care facilities across the country. The Institute for Healthcare Improvement (IHI) has developed a widely used Ventilator Bundle (IHI, 2012) (see Box 23.2).

Another care practice that is implemented for patients receiving mechanical ventilation is the ABCDE bundle. This bundle includes *a*wakening and *b*reathing *c*oordination, *d*elirium monitoring and management, and early *e*xercise and mobility. Although this care bundle has not been used in practice for very long, there is some evidence of a decreased amount of time spent on the ventilator, decreased amount of delirium, and lower mortality when it is used (Lamb, 2015; Urden et al., 2016).

Other interventions exist, although they are not listed specifically within the care bundles that are being used to decrease the

TABLE 23.4

Ventilator Parameters

Parameter	Definition	Ventilator Setting
Tidal volume (V_t)	Amount of air inspired and expired with each breath; can be set by ventilator or can measure patient's own spontaneous breaths	6-12 mL/kg of ideal body weight. Use lower volumes in patients with ARDS.
Respiratory rate (R or RR)	Number of breaths delivered by ventilator per minute	Usual rate is 10-16 breaths/min. However, the rate can be set 4-20 breaths/min, with lower rates used during ventilator weaning.
Fraction of inspired oxygen (FiO_2)	Amount of oxygen that patient receives	Ideally less than 40% to maintain PaO_2 >60 mm Hg and SpO_2 >90%.
Positive end-expiratory pressure (PEEP)	Positive pressure applied at end-expiration of ventilator breaths to open alveoli and improve oxygenation	5 cm H_2O may be used to approximate physiological PEEP. May require higher levels (10-20 cm H_2O) in respiratory failure (e.g., refractory hypoxemia). If patient has a PEEP greater than 10 cm H_2O, the circuit should not be interrupted.
Sensitivity	Determines patient's inspiratory effort required to trigger the ventilator	A breath can be triggered by a change in either flow or pressure. Pressure trigger is usually 0.5-1.5 cm below baseline. Flow trigger is usually 1-3 L/min below baseline.
I:E ratio	Comparison of inspiratory (I) to expiratory (E) time	Example: Inspiration 0.5 seconds, expiration 1 second, then I:E = 1:2. Usually set at 1:2 to 1:1.5 because expiration is typically longer than inspiration. Can use inverse ratios for certain disease states such as ARDS in attempt to open alveoli.
Exhaled minute ventilation (V_E)	Measures exhaled minute ventilations in liters	Alarm set at 15% greater than patient's average V_E.

Data from Urden L, et al: *Priorities in critical care nursing,* ed 7, St Louis, 2016, Mosby; and Wiegand D: *AACN procedure manual for critical care,* ed 6, St Louis, 2011, Mosby.
ARDS, Acute respiratory distress syndrome; *PEEP,* Positive end-expiratory pressure.

TABLE 23.5

Troubleshooting Mechanical Ventilation

Ventilator Alarm	Possible Causes	Nursing Interventions
Sudden increase in peak airway pressure (high-pressure alarm)	Coughing Airway plugging/excess secretions Changes in patient position Pneumothorax Incorrect ET tube position Kinked ventilator circuit Excessive water in ventilator circuit Patient biting tube Patient not in synchrony with ventilator Ventilator malfunction	Clear secretions by suctioning. Reposition patient. Assess breath sounds and chest wall movement. Verify placement of ET tube. Verify centimeter level of ET tube. Check circuit; unkink tubing. Drain ventilator tubing. Insert bite block. Sedate patient. Notify health care provider if interventions do not fix the cause.
Gradual increase in peak airway pressure	Decreasing lung compliance Exacerbation of acute process	Evaluate breath sounds; suction. Check for reversible causes: airway plugging, bronchospasm. Notify health care provider if interventions don't fix the alarm.
d=Decrease in peak airway pressure (low-pressure alarm)	Patient disconnected from ventilator Leak in ventilator circuit ET tube displaced into pharynx Cuff not inflated properly Improved lung compliance Decrease in amount of secretions	Check for disconnection. Evaluate circuit connections; tighten loose connections. Assess cuff for appropriate pressure (see Skill 25.5).
Change in minute ventilation or tidal volume	Leak in ET cuff Patient stops spontaneously breathing Other conditions that trigger low- or high-pressure alarms	Check cuff seal (see Skill 25.5). Evaluate patient.
Increase in respiratory rate	Patient anxiety Increased metabolic demand Hypoxia	Reassure patient. Evaluate body temperature, heart rate, and rhythm. Monitor pulse oximetry.

Continued

TABLE 23.5

Troubleshooting Mechanical Ventilation—cont'd

Ventilator Alarm	Possible Causes	Nursing Interventions
Apnea	Respiratory arrest Oversedation Incidental extubation	Reverse/discontinue sedating medications. Provide breaths via self-inflating resuscitation bag. Prepare for reintubation if tube dislodged and patient requires it.
Ventilator inoperative or low battery	Equipment malfunction Machine not plugged in	Plug in machine. Notify respiratory therapist. Provide breaths via self-inflating resuscitation bag if necessary.

Data from Urden L, et al: *Priorities in critical care nursing*, ed 7, St Louis, 2016, Mosby; and Wiegand D: *AACN procedure manual for critical care*, ed 6, St Louis, 2011, Elsevier.
ET, endotracheal.

risk of VAEs. One of these interventions is to maintain the ET tube cuff pressure at least 20 cm H_2O pressure to decrease the risk of microaspiration of oral secretions or gastric contents (Bouadma et al., 2012). Refer to Skill 25.5 for directions for this procedure. Other interventions include specially coated ET tubes, using ET tubes that allow for drainage of subglottic secretions (Bouadma et al., 2012; Urden et al., 2016), and turning and repositioning the patient every 2 hours.

Delegation and Collaboration

The skill of caring for a patient on a mechanical ventilator cannot be delegated to nursing assistive personnel (NAP). The nurse will collaborate with a respiratory therapist when caring for this patient. The nurse directs the NAP about:
- Reporting immediately to the nurse any change in the patient's respiratory status, vital signs, or oxygen saturation and if patient indicates breathlessness.
- Informing the nurse immediately if any of the ventilator alarms sound.
- Helping in daily care such as bathing and repositioning the patient.

Equipment

- Artificial airway
- Appropriate mechanical ventilator
- Heater and humidifier for circuit
- Oxygen source
- Pulse oximetry (SpO_2) probe and monitor
- Electrocardiogram (ECG) monitoring (if in intensive care unit or by institution policy)
- Capnography ($EtCO_2$) window and monitor (if available)
- Stethoscope
- 5- or 10-mL syringe
- Oral airway/bite block, as needed
- Manual self-inflating resuscitation bag (bag-valve-mask) with oxygen connecting tubing and flowmeter
- Appropriately sized resuscitation face mask
- Cuff pressure monitoring device
- Sedation monitoring scale (e.g., Richmond Agitation Sedation Scale) if patient receiving sedation
- Clean gloves
- Goggles (if splash risk exists); mask and gown if patient's isolation orders indicate
- Suction equipment at bedside (in-line/individual catheters)
- Suction equipment for subglottic and oral suctioning
- Chlorhexidine solution (0.12%), oral swab, and toothbrush for oral care
- Method for patient communication (e.g., letter/picture board, common word lists)
- Ventilator flow sheet to document ventilator changes and settings (may be a paper flow sheet part of the electronic health record (EHR)

STEP	RATIONALE

ASSESSMENT

1. Identify patient using at least two identifiers (e.g., name and birthday or name and account number, according to agency policy).

Ensures correct patient. Complies with The Joint Commission standards and improves patient safety (TJC, 2016).

2. Assess patient's level of consciousness (LOC) and ability to cooperate with mechanical ventilation and tolerate need for special positioning such as HOB at 30 degrees.

Determines patient's ability to cooperate and understand aspects of care. Anxious and combative patients may require sedation to tolerate mechanical ventilation.

3. Assess patient's need for sedation (check agency policy).

Sedation is often used in mechanically ventilated patients to reduce respiratory efforts, decrease oxygen demand, ensure patient synchrony with the ventilator, and improve arterial blood gas (ABG) and oxygen saturation levels (Lillie, 2012).

Clinical Decision Point *When patients on mechanical ventilation become excessively anxious or combative or try to override the ventilator, sedation is often used. Be aware that heavy sedation is associated with increased length of time on the ventilator, increased risk of delirium, and increased mortality (Lillie, 2012). Follow agency policy for the specific indications for sedation and the specific protocol for administering and monitoring sedation levels for these patients.*

STEP	RATIONALE
4. Perform hand hygiene. Assess patient's respiratory status, including symmetry of chest wall expansion, respiratory rate and depth, sputum production, and lung sounds (see Chapter 6), and assess for signs and symptoms associated with hypoxia (see Box 23.1).	Reduces transmission of microorganisms. Decreased chest wall movement; crackles, decreased, or absent lung sounds; increased respiratory rate; increased sputum production; or signs of worsening hypoxia indicate need for mechanical ventilation or changes in current ventilator settings to improve oxygenation and ventilation.
5. Assess patient's cardiovascular condition, including blood pressure, heart rate, regularity of heart rate, and quality of peripheral pulses (see Chapter 6).	Positive-pressure mechanical ventilation can increase patient's intrathoracic pressure. This can cause a decrease in cardiac output and cardiovascular function (Wiegand, 2011).
6. Assess for signs and symptoms of inadvertent extubation (able to vocalize, low-pressure ventilator alarms, decreased or absent breath sounds, gastric distention, changes in ET tube depth according to markings, changes in $EtCO_2$ waveform and values, patient holding tube with hand).	Inadvertent extubation can lead to decrease in patient oxygenation and cardiopulmonary status.

Clinical Decision Point *Sometimes patients tolerate inadvertent extubation. The nurse needs to carefully assess the patient and be prepared to apply a different type of oxygen-delivery device (nasal cannula, face mask, or NIPPV) or to reintubate the patient (Hill and Kramer, 2016). The nurse may need to perform bag-valve-mask ventilation until a provider who can reintubate the patient arrives in the room.*

STEP	RATIONALE
7. Check ventilator, $EtCO_2$ (if available), SpO_2, and ventilator and cardiac alarms at beginning of each shift and periodically throughout care and compare with health care provider's orders.	Verifies that ventilator settings are as ordered by health care provider. Ensures patient safety.
8. Apply clean gloves and verify placement of artificial airway through auscultation of lung sounds, verification of distal tip marking on ET tube and/or $EtCO_2$ value. Determine that tube is secure and stable (see Chapter 25).	Prevents migration of tube into right or left bronchus and accidental extubation.

Clinical Decision Point *When patients have periodic chest x-ray film examinations, verify placement of the artificial airway.*

STEP	RATIONALE
a. Auscultate over trachea for presence of air leak. When air leak is present, you hear movement of air over trachea. Assess and compare inhaled and exhaled tidal volumes as measured by ventilator.	Cuff of artificial airway needs to be inflated to create a seal for positive-pressure ventilation to occur.
b. Use cuff pressure monitoring device.	Cuff pressure of ET tube should be between 20 and 30 cm H_2O (Bouadma et al., 2012). Use 10-mL syringe to inflate or deflate cuff to achieve desired pressure.

Clinical Decision Point *ET tube cuff pressures need to be monitored carefully. Pressures that are too low lead to microaspiration of oral and subglottic secretions, which increase the patient's risk of developing VAP. If the cuff pressures are too high, the patient is at risk of developing tracheal mucosa damage (Branson et al., 2014). Hypopharyngeal suctioning should be performed before a cuff is deflated to decrease risk of aspiration of secretions (Bauman and Hyzy, 2016).*

STEP	RATIONALE
9. Ensure that suctioning system is functioning properly.	It is important to know that the emergency equipment is functioning before needing it (Schreiber, 2015).
10. Observe for patent airway and, if necessary, remove airway secretions by suctioning (see Chapter 25). Remove and dispose of gloves and perform hand hygiene.	Secretions plug airway, decreasing amount of oxygen that is available for gas exchange in lung. Secretions also occlude T tube or tracheostomy collar, impeding oxygen delivery to patient.

Clinical Decision Point *Routine suctioning of the patient should be avoided. Indications for suctioning include the presence of a saw-tooth pattern in the pressure and flow curves on the ventilator, increased peak inspiratory pressures or decreased tidal volumes, decrease in patient's SpO_2, visible secretions in the airway, inability of patient to cough effectively, or suspected aspiration (AARC, 2010; Branson et al., 2014).*

STEP	RATIONALE
11. Assess integrity of patient's oral mucous membrane and skin around tube stabilization device (Pittman et al., 2015).	Provides baseline for health care provider to recognize signs of oral mucous membrane or skin breakdown.
12. If available, note patient's most recent ABG results or SpO_2. Determine if any factors have changed during mechanical ventilation.	Objectively documents patient's pH, arterial oxygen, arterial carbon dioxide, or arterial oxygen saturation.

STEP	RATIONALE
13. Determine method for communication with patient. If possible, review previous communication techniques with patient and family.	Patients with an artificial airway and mechanical ventilation cannot communicate verbally. In addition, some of these patients are too weak to use a note pad to communicate their needs. Therefore assessing for and determining communication needs before instituting mechanical ventilation is ideal (Grossbach et al., 2011). However, each time patient has a new caregiver, assess communication preferences.
14. Review patient's medical record for medical order for mechanical ventilation, noting mode of ventilation, respiratory rate, oxygen setting, pressure support, positive end-expiratory pressures (PEEP), and tidal volume.	Mechanical ventilation and changes in ventilator settings require health care provider's order. Knowing mode of ventilation should key nurse on priority values to monitor.

NURSING DIAGNOSES

- Dysfunctional ventilatory weaning response
- Impaired gas exchange
- Impaired verbal communication

- Impaired spontaneous ventilation
- Ineffective airway clearance
- Ineffective breathing pattern

- Risk for infection
- Risk for impaired oral mucous membrane

Related factors/Risk factors are individualized based on patient's condition or needs.

PLANNING

1. Expected outcomes following completion of procedure:

- Patient has improved lung expansion.

- Patient maintains or has improving PaO$_2$, PaCO$_2$, and pH levels and oxygen saturation within normal range or at patient baseline.
- Patient's vital signs and respiratory assessment parameters improve.

- Patient experiences reduction in feelings of dyspnea and work of breathing. **Note:** Dyspnea scales are available to provide more objective data.
- Patient uses communication board, paper and pencil, or computer to state needs.

As patient's lungs and lung mechanics improve, lung expansion increases.

Verifies that ventilator settings are effective in improving or maintaining patient's level of oxygenation and ventilation.

Reduced pulse and respiratory rate, improved mental status, improved skin color, and decreased use of accessory and abdominal muscles occur because patient's work of breathing decreases as level of oxygenation improves.

Indicates effectiveness of therapy.

Appropriate communication system matches patient's abilities. Helps to express patient's needs and wishes (Grossbach et al., 2011).

2. Explain ventilator system to patient and family caregiver and be sure to include purpose of and reasons for initiation of mechanical ventilation.

Reinforces need for ventilation to improve patient condition.

3. Position patient with HOB elevated 30 to 45 degrees (unless contraindicated).

Positioning patients with HOB elevated 30 to 45 degrees or higher significantly reduces gastric reflux, thereby decreasing risk for aspiration and VAP (AACN, 2010; IHI, 2012; Munro and Ruggiero, 2014).

IMPLEMENTATION

1. Perform hand hygiene; apply clean gloves. Apply mask, gown, and goggles if secretions are projectile or if isolation precautions secondary to infectious status indicate.	Reduces transmission of microorganisms and exposure to pulmonary secretions.
2. Attach mechanical ventilator to ET or tracheostomy tube if not already attached or connected to patient. Observe for proper functioning of mechanical ventilator.	Connects artificial airway to ventilator and ensures closed system, which enables ventilator to exert appropriate pressure or volume to meet patient's oxygen and ventilation demands.

Clinical Decision Point *The mechanical ventilator requires programming of accurate settings before attaching to the patient. This is most often the responsibility of the respiratory therapist as prescribed by the health care provider; however, it is usually a collaborative responsibility of the nurse.*

STEP	RATIONALE
3. Verify that ET or tracheostomy tube is properly positioned during an inspiratory and expiratory cycle by listening to both lungs and assessing chest wall symmetry. Capnography can also be used to verify proper placement (Bauman and Hyzy, 2016). When chest x-ray film is available, observe tube placement.	Properly placed artificial airway ensures that both lungs are ventilated equally. Improper airway placement leads to unilateral lung ventilation or inadequate oxygenation.
4. Observe patient for synchronization with mechanical ventilation and response to therapy.	Ensures that patient is comfortable using ventilator and has not experienced any adverse hemodynamic effects.
5. Monitor heart rate, blood pressure, respiratory rate, temperature, and cardiac rhythm routinely (see agency policy).	Implementation of mechanical ventilation results in decreased venous return and associated hemodynamic changes. The patient is also at increased risk for developing an infection; thus temperature needs to be monitored (Wiegand, 2011).
6. Reassess and mark level of ET tube at lips or nares (see Chapter 25). Ensure that ET tube is secured.	Provides measure to compare with baseline for depth of tube placement. ET tube must be placed through vocal cords into trachea. Helps to ensure that tube is not too close to carina or in right main-stem bronchus. ET tube may be secured with use of tape or commercial tube holder.
7. Ensure that suction equipment is set up and functioning, including oral suctioning (see Chapter 25).	Need to provide airway care and suctioning of ET or tracheostomy tube as needed to prevent plugging of airway and reduce risk for infection.
8. Reposition patient regularly (minimum of every 2 hours), maintaining an HOB elevation of 30 to 35 degrees. In some instances patient may even be placed in prone position. Monitor SpO$_2$ levels during and after positioning.	Elevated HOB positioning improves oxygenation and ventilation. It reduces stasis of secretions, which can lead to atelectasis or pneumonia. In addition HOB elevation reduces risk for aspiration of stomach content secretions into patient's airway (AACN, 2011). SpO$_2$ drops during position change and recovers once patient is completely positioned. In other patients a change in position results in a sustained drop in SpO$_2$, thus indicating that patient is unable to tolerate that particular position at that time. Regular turning reduces risk of pressure injury development involving the skin.
	Prone positioning is reserved for critically ill patients with severe illness and requires assistance of four or five staff members or a specialty bed (Wiegand, 2011). **NOTE:** A recent systematic review shows no clear evidence on the effectiveness of routine lateral repositioning or the effects of a single turn for critically ill patients (Hewitt et al., 2016).

Clinical Decision Point *The oral cavity should be suctioned before repositioning. Cuff pressures should be checked after repositioning (Branson et al., 2014).*

STEP	RATIONALE
9. Collaborate with health care provider frequently about status of patient, response to therapy, and ongoing monitoring.	Assesses oxygenation status and continued need for mechanical ventilation.
a. Monitor SpO$_2$ continuously.	Provides ability to continually assess oxygenation levels.
b. Monitor EtCO$_2$ continually (if available and indicated) and serial ABG levels to detect possible overventilation or inadequate alveolar ventilation.	Allows you to continuously monitor integrity of ventilator circuit and quickly evaluate response to therapy or changes to ventilator settings (Walsh et al., 2011). Overventilation causes respiratory alkalosis from decreased carbon dioxide. Inadequate alveolar ventilation causes respiratory acidosis from increased carbon dioxide retention.
c. Obtain ABG levels with changes in patient's condition or ventilator changes per provider order.	Provides more accurate measure of oxygen saturation and partial pressures of oxygen and carbon dioxide.
10. Perform hourly safety checks on patient and ventilator system:	
a. Make sure that patient can reach call light.	Provides mechanism for patient to contact health care personnel.
b. Check security of all ventilator connections; make sure that alarms are all turned on, including both high- and low-pressure alarms and volume alarms.	Ensures continuous safe and proper functioning of ventilator system. Enables you to identify and correct problems in a timely manner.

STEP	RATIONALE
c. Verify that all ventilator settings are correct and correspond to health care provider's orders.	Maintains integrity of system and ensures that all settings are consistent with health care provider's orders.
d. Check and refill humidifier as needed. Check corrugated tubing for condensation; drain away from patient but not into humidifier and appropriately discard liquid.	Ensures continuous humidification. Condensation that returns to humidifier can cause possible bacterial contamination. Condensation that drains into patient can cause pneumonia or severe coughing episode that can lead to increased patient distress (Restrepo and Walsh, 2012).
e. When present, observe temperature gauges on panel of mechanical ventilator, making sure that gas is delivered at correct temperature. Desired temperature of inspired gas is 35° to 37° C (95° to 98.6° F).	The temperature of inspired gas artificially alters patient's body temperature.
11. Perform mouth care at least 4 times per 24 hours (see Chapter 18). Use chlorhexidine to brush teeth, gums, and tongue with soft toothbrush at least twice a day. Water-based moisturizer should be applied every 2 to 4 hours.	VAP is common, and it is associated with microaspiration of oropharyngeal secretions. Frequent mouth care reduces patient's risk for VAP. Oral care helps reduce risk for pneumonias (Hess, 2016).
12. Insert bite block if patient bites ET tube.	Prevents patient from occluding airway. Oral mucous membranes and tongue need to be monitored for any signs of breakdown.
13. Administer sedating drugs as indicated.	Sedating medications help to keep patient comfortable and breathe in synchrony with ventilator (Lillie, 2012).
14. Perform daily interruption in sedation; assess readiness to extubate.	This step is part of the IHI Ventilator Bundle. Sometimes patients need to be sedated to keep them comfortable or to increase synchrony with ventilator (Lillie, 2012). Providing daily interruptions of sedation decreases length of mechanical ventilation (IHI, 2012).
15. Administer medications (H_2 antagonists, sucralfate, or PPIs) as ordered for peptic ulcer disease (PUD) prophylaxis.	PUD prophylaxis is standard of care in most intensive care settings to prevent stress ulcer formation. It is also part of the IHI Ventilator Bundle (IHI, 2012).

Clinical Decision Point *There is some concern regarding the increased risk of developing a Clostridium difficile infection while taking these medications. Some research indicates that their use leads to an increased growth of gram-negative bacteria in the gastrointestinal system, which leads to an increased incidence of gram-negative aspiration pneumonia in ventilated patients (Munro and Ruggiero, 2014). Collaborate with the physician to determine the appropriate treatment regimen for the patient.*

STEP	RATIONALE
16. Institute deep vein thrombosis (DVT) prophylaxis as ordered per physician. This includes use of anticoagulants (if no contraindications such as bleeding are present) and sequential compression devices.	DVT prevention protocols reduce patient's risk of DVT (IHI, 2012).
17. Perform nursing activities to prevent hazards of immobility (e.g., help patient change position, perform range-of-joint motion exercise, and encourage independence and early mobility as tolerated) (see Chapter 12).	Maintaining activity and promoting early mobility avoids complications associated with decreased mobility such as pressure injuries, pneumonia, DVT, and activity intolerance. Patients receiving mechanical ventilation need help with activity but can ambulate.
18. Ensure that communication method is in place for patient. This includes letter/picture boards, common word and phrase lists, writing utensil and paper, or a computer/tablet.	Patients report feeling frightened, anxious, and disconnected during their time of short-term mechanical ventilation (Tsay et al., 2013). Communication strategies, including lip reading and patient gestures, help patient communicate his or her needs and feelings, which helps to decrease anxiety and fear (Grossbach et al., 2011).
19. Keep patient and family informed about progress and plan for weaning from mechanical ventilator.	Apprehension and anxiety occur when patient and family are not properly informed about progress, changes in care, or changes in ventilator setting. Patients and families need information and emotional support to successfully tolerate and wean from mechanical ventilation (Grossbach et al., 2011).
20. Remove and dispose of personal protective equipment; perform hand hygiene.	Reduces transmission of microorganisms and exposure to pulmonary secretions.

STEP	RATIONALE

EVALUATION

1. Monitor and evaluate patient's response to mechanical ventilation every 1 to 4 hours.

   a. *Neurological assessment:* LOC, orientation, sleepiness, changes in anxiety, sedation levels

   b. *Pulmonary assessment:* Lung sounds, airway clearance, work of breathing, breathing pattern, rate of respirations, SpO_2, $EtCO_2$.

   c. *Cardiovascular assessment:* Vital signs, heart rhythm, heart sounds, lower-extremity edema, pulse quality

2. Observe SpO_2 and $EtCO_2$ and monitor gas exchange.

3. Observe integrity of patient ventilator system.

4. Observe and evaluate effectiveness of communication methods:

   a. Ask patient if needs and concerns are addressed.

   b. Observe for signs of frustration (e.g., patient shaking head in irritation, crying, withdrawal).

   c. Observe patient/family and health care personnel use communication methods.

5. Use Teach-Back: "I want to be sure I explained how the ventilator works and why we are using it to treat your husband. Explain to me why mechanical ventilation is necessary." Revise your instruction now or develop a plan for revised patient or family caregiver teaching if patient or family caregiver is not able to teach back correctly.

Rationale column:

Patients requiring mechanical ventilation have unstable physiological status. It is important to perform key focused evaluation measures frequently as patient's condition warrants.

Documents patient's level of oxygenation and ventilation. Ensures adequate delivery of mechanical ventilation.

Communication, or lack of it, increases patient's frustration, sense of powerlessness, anxiety, and confusion during mechanical ventilation and weaning process (Grossbach et al., 2011).

Determines patient's and family caregiver's level of understanding of instructional topic.

Unexpected Outcomes

1. Patient experiences a VAE such as VAP.

2. Patient experiences no improvement in or worsening of respiratory status.

3. Patient experiences self-extubation.

4. Patient experiences barotrauma such as tension pneumothorax (an emergency situation).

5. Patient develops hemodynamic instability.

Related Interventions

- Notify health care provider.
- Remain with patient.
- Conduct complete cardiac and pulmonary assessment.
- Be prepared for initiation of antibiotic therapy.
- Notify health care provider.
- Reassess patient.
- Assess integrity of ventilator system.
- Expect ventilator change (increased PEEP levels, increase in respiratory rate or tidal volume).
- Maintain patent airway by suctioning and inserting oral airway.
- Provide oxygen.
- Assess patient's respiratory status and level of oxygenation and ventilation.
- Notify health care provider.
- Patient may need sedation and/or use of restraints to prevent this complication from occurring in the future (see Chapter 14).
- Remain with patient, remove patient from ventilator, and ventilate with bag-valve-mask (see Chapter 28).
- Notify health care provider.
- Ask NAP to obtain chest tube insertion kit.
- Ask additional personnel to obtain patient's vital signs.
- Notify health care provider.
- Stay with patient.
- Be prepared to change ventilator settings or initiate intravenous inotropes or vasopressors.

Recording and Reporting

- Record the following on the appropriate flow sheet in nurses' notes in electronic health record (EHR) or chart: respiratory assessment findings, mode of mechanical ventilation, oxygen level, actual patient tidal volume, actual patient respiratory rate, peak inspiratory pressure, vital signs, size and level of the ET tube, ABG results (if performed as a point of care test), patient level of comfort, sedation level scores (if sedation is used), and degree of bed elevation.

- Record on flow sheet or nurses' notes in EHR or chart any nursing interventions that are performed, including oral care, repositioning, range-of-motion exercises, medications that were administered, and suctioning.

- Document your evaluation of patient and family caregiver learning.
- Report to nurse in charge or health care provider sudden change in patient's respiratory status, ventilator-associated problems, or adverse reactions or side effects.

Special Considerations
Teaching

- Teach patient and family caregiver about the rationale for mechanical ventilation and the alarms and what they mean.
- Teach patient and family caregiver alternative communication techniques to reduce frustration and fear.
- Teach patient about rationale for all interventions, including oral care and frequent repositioning.

Pediatric

- Increasing numbers of children are on home mechanical ventilation. For this reason it is important to include the parent in the child's care as appropriate. Parents also need to be prepared that, when a readmission to a hospital occurs, because of the chronic nature of the illness the child may not be readmitted to an intensive care unit but rather may remain on the general medical or surgical area (Hockenberry and Wilson, 2015).
- Once the child is stable on the mechanical ventilator, promote normal or near-normal activities as the child's condition warrants (e.g., promote play, resume school activities, and encourage mobility).

Gerontological

- Presence of underlying chronic illnesses increase patient's risk for longer intensive care, hospital stays.

- Older adults are usually not able to tolerate the usual sedative or antianxiety medications ordered. The prescribed dose is based on patient's baseline kidney and liver functions (Touhy and Jett, 2014).

Home Care

- Planning for home ventilation is performed by a multidisciplinary team, including representatives of nursing, respiratory, dietary service, and social services; the home care nurse; the home care durable medical equipment company; and the patient's insurance company/health care payer (Garber and Guertin, 2012).
- Patients requiring home mechanical ventilation need to be assessed for acceptance of ventilator dependence and the ability to understand and demonstrate daily care of the artificial airway, ventilator, and ventilator circuit.
- Patients requiring home mechanical ventilation need their home environment, personal and monetary resources, and availability of home care nurses or staff assessed. Availability of community resources should also be assessed. The home electricity may need to be updated to support the equipment required to care for them (Garber and Guertin, 2012).
- Evaluate the following areas during each visit: oxygen flow, alarm system, inspiratory pressure, high-pressure alarm, tidal volume setting, humidifier, respiratory rate, tubing, temperature, resuscitation bag, tracheostomy care, breath sounds, suctioning, and tubing changes.
- Teach patient and family caregiver what to do in case of respiratory distress or power failure. Check to determine availability of emergency batteries.
- Instruct family caregiver in use of the bag-valve-mask (see Chapter 28).

◆ CLINICAL DEBRIEF

A 59-year-old man with a history of well-controlled chronic obstructive pulmonary disease (COPD) developed an upper respiratory tract infection 2 weeks ago and was treated with antibiotics. He completed his full course of antibiotics, but his symptoms continued. He has a 4-day history of fever greater than 39.4° C (102.8° F), fatigue, productive cough with yellow sputum, worsening dyspnea, and decreased activity tolerance. His health care provider does a complete examination, orders a chest x-ray film examination, and obtains a sputum specimen. Preliminary chest x-ray film results indicate right lower lobe pneumonia. He is admitted to a general medicine floor for treatment with intravenous (IV) antibiotics, supplemental oxygen at 2 L/min via nasal cannula, and pulmonary hygiene measures.

1. The nurse observes the patient and notices that he is fatigued, has difficulty speaking, and in general looks very uncomfortable. The nurse decides to do a focused assessment. Which systems will the nurse assess, and what information does the nurse expect to find?

2. The patient's condition continues to worsen, and the nurse notifies the physician. The provider, who is in the room, tells the nursing assistive personnel (NAP) to place the patient on a simple face mask at 50% FiO$_2$ with a flow rate of 10 L/min and to encourage the patient to use an incentive spirometer. Why should the nurse question this order?

3. The patient is placed on a Venturi mask at 45% FiO$_2$, the first dose of IV antibiotic is administered, and the patient continues to be in

distress. SpO$_2$ now is 85%, with a respiratory rate of 32 breaths/min, heart rate of 110 beats/min, BP 144/76, and temperature of 38.7° C (101.8° F). Crackles persist in the right lower lobe and are clear but diminished in all other lobes. Patient is using accessory muscles to breathe, and cough is no longer productive. Patient states in short two-word sentences that he can't breathe and that he thinks he is going to die. The nurse recognizes that the provider needs to be notified.

Using SBAR format, how should the nurse communicate the patient's status to the provider?

◆ REVIEW QUESTIONS

1. The nurse is caring for a patient receiving BiPAP ventilation via face mask for treatment of respiratory distress. Which interventions can be delegated to nursing assistant personnel (NAP)? (Select all that apply.)
   a. Educating the patient and family about the use of BiPAP
   b. Repositioning patient in bed or chair
   c. Titrating patient's FiO$_2$
   d. Adjusting mask if it becomes displaced
   e. Recording patient's SpO$_2$ level
   f. Assessing patient's respiratory status

2. The nurse is assessing a patient who is experiencing respiratory distress. Which findings would best indicate the need for supplemental oxygen therapy? (Select all that apply.)
   a. Shortness of breath
   b. PaO_2 58 mm Hg
   c. SpO_2 89%
   d. Diminished breath sounds in all lobes
   e. Cyanosis of oral mucous membranes

3. The nurse is teaching the patient how to use the peak flowmeter. The nurse asks the patient to demonstrate the procedure. Place the steps of using a peak flowmeter in the correct order.
   a. Have patient take deep breath and hold it.
   b. Place marker of meter at bottom of scale.
   c. Have patient place mouthpiece in his or her mouth.
   d. Have patient blow out as hard and fast as possible.
   e. Have patient stand up, if able.
   f. Record the value.

ⓔ *Visit the Evolve site for a complete list of Clinical Debrief and Review Questions answers.*

REFERENCES

Aguiar C, et al: Tubing length for long-term oxygen therapy, *Respir Care* 60(2):179, 2015.

American Association of Critical Care Nurses (AACN): *Practice alert: oral care for patients at risk for ventilator-associated pneumonia*, 2010. http://www.aacn.org/wd/practice/docs/practicealerts/oral-care-patients-at-risk-vap.pdf?menu=aboutus. Accessed February, 2016.

American Association of Critical Care Nurses (AACN): *Practice alert: prevention of aspiration*, 2011. http://www.aacn.org/wd/practice/docs/practicealerts/prevention-aspiration-practice-alert.pdf?menu=aboutus. Accessed February 24, 2016.

American Association for Respiratory Care (AARC): Endotracheal suctioning of mechanically ventilated patients with artificial airways 2010, *Respir Care* 55(6):758, 2010.

American Lung Association: *Supplemental oxygen*, 2016. http://www.lung.org/lung-health-and-diseases/lung-disease-lookup/copd/diagnosing-and-treating/supplemental-oxygen.html. Accessed January 31, 2016.

American Thoracic Society (ATS): *Inpatient oxygen therapy*, 2015a. http://www.thoracic.org/copd-guidelines/for-health-professionals/exacerbation/inpatient-oxygen-therapy/index.php. Accessed November, 2015.

American Thoracic Society (ATS): *Long-term oxygen therapy*, 2015b. http://www.thoracic.org/copd-guidelines/for-health-professionals/management-of-stable-copd/long-term-oxygen-therapy/home-oxygen-therapy.php. Accessed January, 2016.

Bauman K, Hyzy R: *Endotracheal tube management and complications*, UpToDate, 2016. http://www.uptodate.com/contents/endotracheal-tube-management-and-complications. Accessed May 19, 2016.

Bouadma L, et al: Ventilator-associated pneumonia and its prevention, *Curr Opin Infect Dis* 25:395, 2012.

Branson R, et al: Management of the artificial airway, *Respir Care* 59(6):974, 2014.

Centers for Disease Control and Prevention (CDC): *Ventilator-associated event*, 2016. http://www.cdc.gov/nhsn/PDFs/pscManual/10-VAE_FINAL.pdf. Accessed January, 2016.

Chahoud J, et al: Ventilator-associated events prevention, learning lessons from the past: a systematic review, *Heart Lung* 44:251, 2015.

Cross A: Non-invasive ventilation in critical care, *Intern Med J* 42(Suppl 5):35, 2012.

do Nascimento P, et al: Incentive spirometry for prevention of postoperative pulmonary complication in upper abdominal surgery, *Cochrane Database Syst Rev* (2):CD006058, 2014.

Gale N, et al: Adapting to domiciliary non-invasive ventilation in chronic obstructive pulmonary disease: a qualitative interview study, *Palliat Med* 29(3):268, 2015.

Garber K, Guertin M: Home mechanical ventilation, RT, *J Respir Care Practitioners* 25(8):14, 2012.

Gaunt KA, et al: High-flow nasal cannula in mixed adult ICU, *Respir Care* 60(10):1383, 2015.

Grindrod K: Management of stable chronic obstructive pulmonary disease, *Br J Community Nurs* 20(2):58, 2015.

Grossbach I, et al: Promoting effective communication for patients receiving mechanical ventilation, *Crit Care Nurse* 31(3):46, 2011.

Hess D: *The ventilator circuit and ventilator-associated pneumonia*, UpToDate, 2016. http://www.uptodate.com/contents/the-ventilator-circuit-and-ventilator-associated-pneumonia. Accessed May 19, 2016.

Hewitt N, et al: *Lateral positioning for critically ill adult patients*, Cochrane Database for Systematic Reviews, May 12, 2016. http://onlinelibrary.wiley.com/doi/10.1002/14651858.CD007205.pub2/abstract;jsessionid=9F9AF8BEE55142635440D69ECD18468B.f04t01. Accessed October 15, 2016.

Hill N, Kramer N: *Troubleshooting problems with noninvasive positive pressure ventilation*, UpToDate, 2016. http://www.uptodate.com/contents/troubleshooting-problems-with-noninvasive-positive-pressure-ventilation. Accessed May 19, 2016.

Hockenberry MJ, Wilson D: *Wong's nursing care of infants and children*, ed 10, St Louis, 2015, Mosby.

Institute for Healthcare Improvement (IHI): *How-to guide: prevent ventilator-associated pneumonia*, 2012. www.ihi.org. Accessed November, 2015.

Lamb KD: Year in review 2014: mechanical ventilation, *Respir Care* 60(4):606, 2015.

Lewis S, et al: *Medical-surgical nursing: assessment and management of clinical problems*, ed 10, St Louis, 2017, Elsevier.

Lillie B: Friend or foe? Sedation during mechanical ventilation, RT, *J Respir Care Practitioners* 25(7):14, 2012.

Lunardi A, et al: Effect of volume-oriented versus flow-oriented incentive spirometry on chest wall volumes, inspiratory muscle activity, and thoracoabdominal synchrony in the elderly, *Respir Care* 59(3):420, 2014.

Messika J, et al: Use of high-flow nasal cannula oxygen therapy in subjects with ARDS: A 1-year observational study, *Respir Care* 60(2):162, 2015.

Munaco SS, et al: Preventing ventilator-associated events: complying with evidence-based practice, *Crit Care Nurs Q* 37(4):384, 2014.

Munro N, Ruggiero M: Ventilator-associated pneumonia bundle: reconstruction for best care, *AACN Adv Crit Care* 25(2):163, 2014.

National Heart, Lung, and Blood Institute (NHLBI): *How to use a peak flowmeter*, 2013. http://www.nhlbi.nih.gov/files/docs/public/lung/asthma_tipsheets.pdf. Accessed November, 2015.

Pittman J, et al: Medical device related hospital-acquired pressure ulcers, *JWOCN* 42(2):151, 2015.

Pooboni S, et al: *Noninvasive ventilation procedures*, 2013. http://emedicine.medscape.com/article/1417959-overview. Accessed November, 2015.

Preston W: The increasing use of non-invasive ventilation, *Practice Nurs* 24(3):114, 2013.

Restrepo R, Walsh B: Humidification during invasive and noninvasive mechanical ventilation, *Respir Care* 57(5):782, 2012.

Roca O, Masclans J: High-flow nasal cannula oxygen therapy: innovative strategies for traditional procedures, *Crit Care Med* 43(3):707, 2015.

Schallom M, et al: Pressure ulcer incidence in patients wearing nasal-oral versus full-face noninvasive ventilation masks, *Am J Crit Care* 24(4):349, 2015.

Schreiber M: Tracheostomy: site care, suctioning, and readiness, *Medsurg Nurs* 24(2):121, 2015.

Smetana G: *Strategies to reduce postoperative complications*, UpToDate, 2016. http://www.uptodate.com/contents/strategies-to-reduce-postoperative-pulmonary-complications. Accessed May 19, 2016.

Spector R: *Cultural diversity in health and illness*, ed 8, Upper Saddle River, NJ, 2013, Pearson Prentice Hall.

Spoletini G, et al: Heated humidified high-flow nasal oxygen in adults: mechanism of action and clinical implications, *Chest* 148(1):253, 2015.

Struik FM, et al: Nocturnal non-invasive positive pressure ventilation for stable chronic obstructive pulmonary disease (review), *Cochrane Database Syst Rev* (6):CD002878, 2013.

The Joint Commission (TJC): *National Patient Safety Goals 2016*, 2016. http://www.jointcommission.org/standards_information/npsgs.aspx. Accessed January, 2016.

Touhy T, Jett K: *Ebersole and Hess' gerontological nursing & healthy aging*, ed 4, St Louis, 2014, Mosby.

Tsay S, et al: The experiences of adult ventilator-dependent patients: a meta-synthesis review, *Nurs Health Sci* 15:525, 2013.

Tyson A, et al: The effect of incentive spirometry on postoperative pulmonary function following laparotomy: a randomized clinical trial, *JAMA Surg* 150(3):229, 2015.

Urden L, et al: *Priorities in critical care nursing*, ed 7, St Louis, 2016, Mosby.

Walsh B, et al: Capnography/capnometry during mechanical ventilation, *Respir Care* 56(4):503, 2011.

Wiegand D: *AACN procedure manual for critical care*, ed 6, St Louis, 2011, Mosby.

24 | Performing Chest Physiotherapy

SKILLS AND PROCEDURES

OBJECTIVES

Mastery of content in this chapter will enable the nurse to:

- Assess for the need to perform chest physiotherapy (CPT) maneuvers.
- Determine the need to modify or discontinue CPT maneuvers.
- Explain how to prepare a patient and family caregiver for the performance of each CPT maneuver.
- Perform the outlined CPT maneuvers, including standard and modified versions.
- Describe the use of an Acapella device and vest airway clearance system.
- Describe expected and unexpected outcomes of each CPT maneuver.
- Describe discharge teaching and planning related to the use of each CPT maneuver in the home setting.

MEDIA RESOURCES

- evolve http://evolve.elsevier.com/Perry/skills
- Review Questions
- Audio Glossary
- Clinical Debrief and Review Questions Answers

PURPOSE

Chest physiotherapy (CPT) is external chest wall manipulation, which includes one of a combination of or all of percussion, vibration, and postural drainage (PD) therapy to loosen and remove secretions from patients' airways (Strickland et al., 2013). CPT is usually followed by productive coughing or suctioning to remove secretions. Traditional CPT does not help children with pneumonia, bronchiolitis, or asthma; and it does not prevent atelectasis after extubation (Makic et al., 2015). In addition, routine use of CPT does not improve mortality rates of adults with pneumonia (Yang et al., 2013).

CPT is beneficial and an essential therapy in patients with cystic fibrosis (CF). For these patients a vest airway clearance system increases patient adherence to CPT. A vest airway clearance system is a method for delivering CPT that uses high-frequency chest wall compressions created by bursts of air for external chest wall compression. The Acapella device uses positive airway pressure to increase airway pressure, which helps a patient's ability to cough. Each of these therapies is broadly classified as an airway clearance therapy (ACT) by the American Association of Respiratory Care (AARC) (Strickland et al., 2013).

Careful patient assessment is a prerequisite for administering any ACTs. The auscultation of all the lung fields is essential to determine which regions would benefit from CPT. CPT maneuvers move secretions into the large central airways; then these secretions are removed through coughing or suctioning. PD requires specific positioning of a patient to position the targeted lung segment so gravity helps to remove secretions.

The Acapella device and the vest airway clearance system are very effective in helping with airway clearance. They are also used for patients with chronic lung diseases such as CF (Morrison and Agnew, 2014). The devices are used in hospital settings, but they also make it possible for patients to continue ACTs in the home and school environments as necessary.

STANDARDS OF CARE

- AARC Clinical Practice Guideline, 2013—Effectiveness of nonpharmacologic airway clearance therapies in hospitalized patients
- The Joint Commission, 2016—Patient identification

PRINCIPLES FOR PRACTICE

- Careful patient assessment is a prerequisite for administering any CPT and PD maneuver because the therapy is usually targeted to the affected areas as opposed to all the lung fields (Strickland et al., 2013).
- CPT and PD aim to remove secretions that accumulate in the airways of patients with CF.
- Surgical patients in the postoperative period and critically ill patients have excess secretions as a result of the effects of anesthesia, ineffective coughing because of incision pain or muscle weakness, and reduced mobility (Ambrosino and Makhabah, 2014). Mucus plugs, atelectasis, and lobular collapse occur when secretions accumulate in the airways. Early mobility and ambulation are more successful in promoting airway clearance than routine CPT (Strickland et al., 2013; Yang et al., 2013).

- CPT and PD are often used in combination with other therapies, including antibiotics, bronchodilators, mucolytic agents, and inhaled and nebulized medications in CF patients (Strickland et al., 2015). These other therapies reduce mucus production and promote airway clearance. The goals of these therapies are (1) to clear the airways of excessive secretions to reduce the work of breathing, and (2) to improve a patient's ability to cough up secretions (Morrison and Agnew, 2014).
- In the normal lung the mucociliary transport system clears the airways of excessive mucus and inhaled particles. Airways normally remain clear, and mucus is constantly being cleared almost as fast as it is made. Normal mucus remains thin, white, and watery.
- In various disease states mucus clearance slows down, or the cilia are overwhelmed by production of large quantities of mucus. The lungs no longer clear the mucus as fast as it is produced. Secretions stagnate in the airways, change color, and become thick and sticky (Volsko, 2013).

PATIENT-CENTERED CARE

- When patients' physiological capacities are weakened, they are often anxious because of their illness or surgery, and they may be in pain. It is important to complete a pain assessment and administer prescribed analgesics 20 to 30 minutes before initiating any CPT maneuvers. This ensures that the patient is comfortable and as pain free as possible.
- Assess your patient's activity tolerance. Patients with cardiopulmonary disease, severe arthritis, and certain musculoskeletal diseases often have diminished activity tolerance and cannot tolerate a complete CPT session. Plan CPT during short periods interspersed with rest periods, at a time when the patient is rested, and not immediately after a meal.
- Encourage mobility and ambulation to reduce postoperative pulmonary complications and promote airway clearance (Strickland et al., 2013)
- The patient with chronic pulmonary illnesses such as CF poses different challenges. Often these patients must devote several hours of their day to activities to assist in airway clearance. It is important that CPT and other airway clearance techniques do not impact a patient's quality of life (QOL). To maintain this QOL try to integrate CPT and airway techniques into his or her routine, personal goals, and social activities (Cross et al., 2012).
- When dealing with patients who have CF, devices such as the Acapella, the vest airway clearance system, and other airway clearance devices help these patients maintain their CPT schedule (dos Santos et al., 2013; Mesquinta et al., 2014).
- CPT skills include a great deal of patient touching. Some cultures consider it very poor taste to touch in public. In addition, the skills of physical therapy sometimes involve a gentle percussion or vibration of a patient's rib cage. Patients and families from cultures where violence is an everyday occurrence need detailed information about the procedure so they do not misunderstand the intent and objective of CPT. Always explain which type of touching is involved and what a patient may feel during the treatment. Provide an opportunity for a patient to temporarily stop and rest during the procedure (Giger, 2016).

EVIDENCE-BASED PRACTICE

- ACTs such as CPT and PD maneuvers are effective only in selected patients such as those with CF, bronchiectasis, other chronic pulmonary diseases, and some surgeries (Strickland et al., 2013). When disease processes alter the normal mechanisms of the body to clear the airway, therapies must be instituted to ensure that the airways remain free of secretions so the risk for pulmonary infection is reduced and the oxygen demands of the body are met. When secretions are stagnant, they obstruct airways, are conduits for bacterial colonization and infections, stimulate an inflammatory response, and contribute to airway and tissue damage (Volsko, 2013).
- Recent systematic review noted that CPT is not recommended routinely as additional treatment for pneumonia in adults (Makic et al., 2015). Careful assessment of medical history for smoking, pulmonary infections, and other conditions may indicate the need for CPT in selected adults at risk for complicated pneumonia (Yang et al., 2013).
- ACT is not recommended as routine in patients with chronic obstructive pulmonary disease (COPD) unless secretion retention is present (Strickland et al., 2013)
- In selected intubated patients in the intensive care unit (ICU), early and routine CPT benefits patients and improves airway patency, secretion clearance, and oxygen delivery to the tissues. In addition, early CPT reduces some ICU complications such as health care–acquired infections (Kohan et al., 2014).
- High-frequency chest wall oscillators such as the vest airway clearance system (see Procedural Guideline 24.2) are effective in aiding sputum clearance for a variety of adult and pediatric lung diseases (Sisson, 2013).
- The use of the Acapella device (see Procedure Guideline 24.1) improves patient satisfaction and adherence to airway clearance therapies (Sisson, 2013).

SAFETY GUIDELINES

- Know a patient's normal range of vital signs. Conditions such as CF and complicated pneumonia requiring CPT can affect a patient's vital signs. The degree of change is related to the level of hypoxia, overall cardiopulmonary status, and tolerance to the procedure.
- Know a patient's current medications. Some medications, particularly diuretics and antihypertensives, cause fluid and hemodynamic changes. These changes affect a patient's tolerance of the positional changes. Steroid medications, age, and malnutrition increase a patient's risk for pathological rib fractures and often contraindicate rib vibration.
- Know a patient's medical and surgical history. Certain conditions such as increased intracranial pressure, spinal cord injuries, abdominal aneurysm resection, bone metastases, or severe osteoporosis contraindicate the positional changes of postural drainage (Box 24.1). Thoracic trauma contraindicates percussion and vibration.
- Know a patient's level of cognitive function. Alteration in mental status often makes it difficult or impossible for a patient to understand the procedure and participate in coughing and expectorating secretions.
- Have suction machine equipment available to help clear airway secretions (see Chapter 25).
- Patients who receive long-term steroid therapy are at risk for pathological fractures. Physical maneuvers such as chest percussion and vibration may be contraindicated because of the risk for rib fractures. These patients benefit from individualized airway clearance measures such as the Acapella device (dos Santos et al., 2013; Strickland et al., 2013).

BOX 24.1

Contraindications for Postural Drainage

- Increased intracranial pressure
- Head and neck injury until stabilized
- Active hemorrhage with hemodynamic instability
- Recent spinal surgery (e.g., laminectomy) or acute spinal injury
- Active hemoptysis
- Empyema
- Bronchopleural fistula
- Pulmonary edema associated with heart failure
- Large pleural effusions
- Pulmonary embolism

- Aged, confused, or anxious patients who are unable to tolerate position change
- Rib fracture, with or without flail chest
- Surgical wound or healing tissue

Trendelenburg's position is contraindicated for the following:

- Uncontrolled hypertension
- Distended abdomen
- Esophageal surgery
- Recent gross hemoptysis
- Uncontrolled airway at risk for aspiration

Modified from White G: *Basic clinical lab competencies for respiratory care: an integrated approach*, ed 5, Clifton Park, NY, 2013, Cengage Learning.

✦ SKILL 24.1   Performing Postural Drainage

Postural drainage (PD) is the use of positioning techniques to drain secretions from specific segments of the lungs and bronchi into the trachea (Fig. 24.1). Each position drains a specific corresponding section of the tracheobronchial tree from the upper, middle, or lower lung field into the trachea (Table 24.1). Additional coughing or airway suctioning helps remove secretions from the trachea.

Use physical assessment findings and a review of chest x-ray films to determine which lung segments require PD. Patients needing PD usually have chronic conditions, which impact their activity tolerance. Knowing which lung segments require PD promotes patient cooperation, adherence to therapy, and prevention of excessive fatigue. In addition, use knowledge of a patient's condition and disease process and the extent of the pathological condition to individualize the PD therapy.

Delegation and Collaboration

The skill of PD can be delegated to nursing assistive personnel (NAP). It is the nurse's responsibility to assess the patient, review laboratory and x-ray film examination results, and determine that the patient is stable and able to tolerate the procedure. The nurse instructs the NAP to:

- Immediately report to the nurse changes in patient's comfort level, changes in breathing pattern, and tolerance of the procedure.
- Use specific patient precautions related to disease, mobility status, position restrictions, or treatment.

Equipment

- Stethoscope
- Pulse oximeter
- Trendelenburg's hospital bed or tilt table (more common in pediatric agencies)
- Water in pitcher and glass
- Tissues and paper bag
- Chair (for draining upper lobes)
- Extra pillows
- Clear graduated screw-top container for sputum collection (optional)
- Oral hygiene care products
- Suction equipment (if patient unable to cough and clear own secretions)
- Clean gloves (*when there is risk of exposure to patient's respiratory secretions*)
- Patient education materials

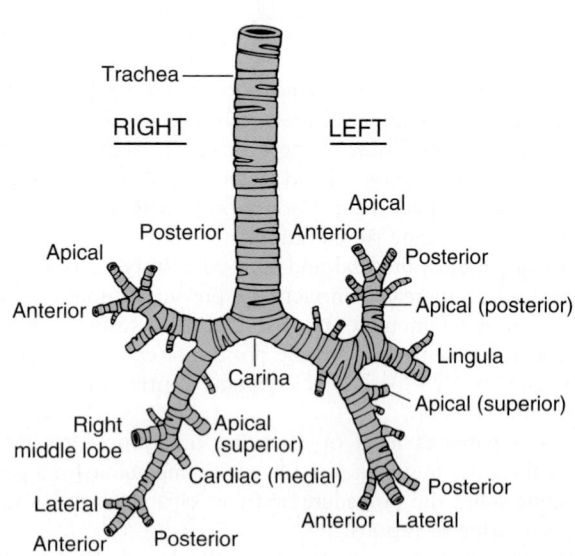

FIG 24.1 Tracheobronchial tree. (*Modified from Frownfelter DL, Dean E: Principles and practice of cardiopulmonary therapy, ed 43, St Louis, 2006, Mosby.*)

TABLE 24.1

Positions and Procedures for Drainage, Percussion, and Vibration

Area and Procedure	Anatomical Area	Position of Patient

Left and Right Upper Lobe Anterior Apical Bronchi

Position patient in chair, or high-Fowler's, leaning back. Percuss and vibrate with heel of hands at shoulders and fingers over collarbones (clavicles) in front; do both sides at same time. Note body posture and arm position of nurse. Nurse's back is kept straight, and elbows and knees are slightly flexed.

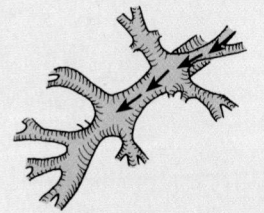 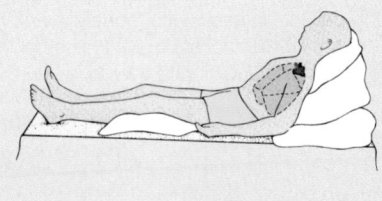

Direction of mucus flow through upper lobe anterior apical bronchi.

Anterior apical segments
Position hands for chest physiotherapy over left and right upper anterior apical bronchi.

Left and Right Upper Lobe Posterior Apical Bronchi

Position patient in chair, leaning forward on pillow or table. Percuss and vibrate with hands on either side of upper spine. Do both sides at same time.

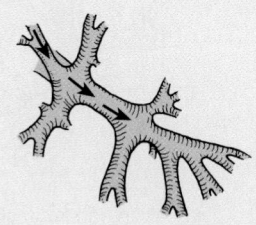 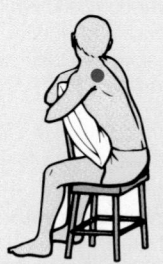

Direction of mucus flow through upper lobe posterior apical bronchi.

Posterior apical segments
Position hands for chest physiotherapy over left and right upper lobe posterior apical bronchi.

Left and Right Anterior Upper Lobe Bronchi

Position patient flat on back with small pillow under knees. Percuss and vibrate just below clavicle on either side of sternum.

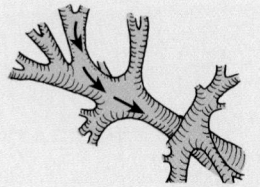 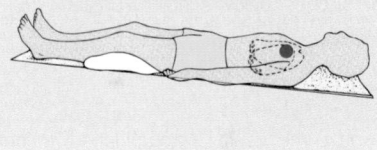

Direction of mucus flow through anterior upper bronchi.

Left and right anterior upper lobe segments
Position hands for chest physiotherapy over right and left anterior upper lobe bronchi.

Left Upper Lobe Lingular Bronchus

Position patient on right side with arm overhead in Trendelenburg's position, with foot of bed raised 30 cm (12 inches), as tolerated.* Place pillow behind back, and roll patient one-quarter turn onto pillow. Percuss and vibrate lateral to left nipple below axilla.

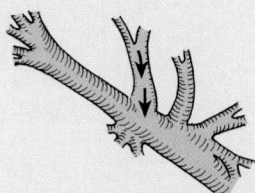 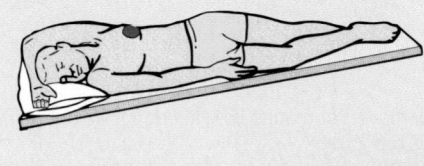

Direction of mucus flow through left upper lobe lingular bronchus.

Left upper lobe lingular segment
Position hands for chest physiotherapy over left upper lobe lingular bronchus.

Right Middle Lobe Bronchus

Position patient on left side or abdomen. Place pillow behind back, and roll patient one-quarter turn onto pillow. Percuss and vibrate to right nipple below axilla.

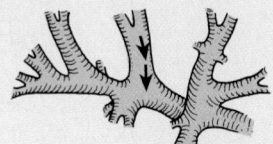 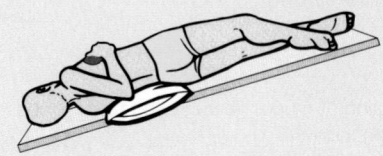

Direction of mucus flow through right middle lobe bronchus.

Right middle lobe segment
Position hands for chest physiotherapy over right middle lobe bronchus.

Continued

TABLE 24.1

Positions and Procedures for Drainage, Percussion, and Vibration—cont'd

Area and Procedure	Anatomical Area	Position of Patient
Left and Right Anterior Lower Lobe Bronchi Position patient on back, with foot of bed elevated to 45-50 cm (18-20 inches). Have knees bent on pillow. Percuss and vibrate over lower anterior ribs on both sides. Direction of mucus flow through anterior lower lobe bronchi.	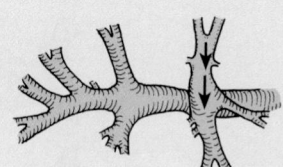	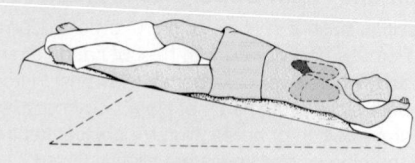 Left and right anterior lower lobe segments Position hands for chest physiotherapy over left and right anterior lower lobe bronchi.
Right Lower Lobe Lateral Bronchus Position patient on abdomen in Trendelenburg's position with foot of bed raised 45-50 cm (18-20 inches), as tolerated. Percuss and vibrate on left and right sides of chest below shoulder blades (scapulas) posterior to midaxillary line. Direction of mucus flow through right lower lobe lateral bronchus.	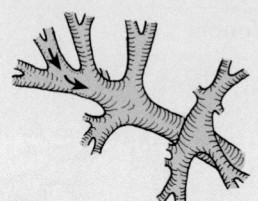	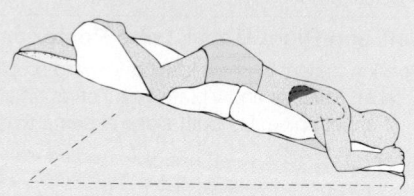 Right lower lateral lobe segment Position hands for chest physiotherapy over right lower lobe lateral bronchus.
Left Lower Lobe Lateral Bronchus Position patient on right side in Trendelenburg's position with foot of bed raised 45-50 cm (18-20 inches), as tolerated. Percuss and vibrate on left side of chest below scapulas posterior to midaxillary line. Direction of mucus flow through left lower lobe lateral bronchus.	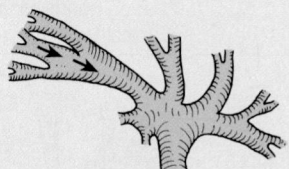	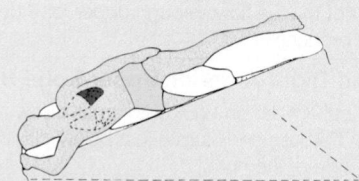 Left lower lobe lateral segment Position hands for chest physiotherapy over left lower lobe lateral bronchus.
Right and Left Lower Lobe Superior Bronchi Position patient flat on stomach with pillow under stomach. Percuss and vibrate below scapula on either side of spine. Direction of mucus flow through lower lobe superior bronchi.	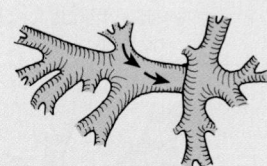	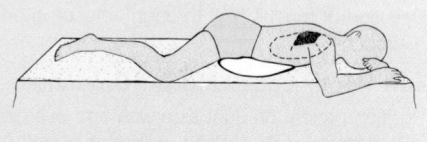 Right and left lower lobe superior segments Position hands for chest physiotherapy over right and left lower lobe superior bronchi.
Right and Left Posterior Basal Bronchi Position patient on stomach in Trendelenburg's position with foot of bed raised 45-50 cm (18–20 inches), as tolerated. Percuss and vibrate over low posterior ribs on either side of spine. Direction of mucus flow through posterior basal bronchi.	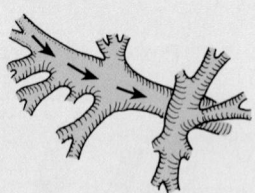	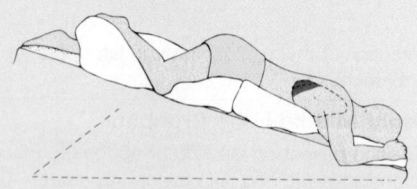 Right and left posterior segments Position hands for chest physiotherapy over right and left posterior lower lobe bronchi.

*In adult settings, Trendelenburg's position is not used as frequently. Verify use with agency policy and health care provider's order.

STEP	RATIONALE

ASSESSMENT

1. Identify patient using at least two identifiers (e.g., name and birthday or name and medical record number) according to agency policy.

Ensures correct patient. Complies with The Joint Commission standards and improves patient safety (TJC, 2016).

2. Assess patient for history of decreased level of consciousness, decreased activity tolerance, and muscle weakness or chronic disease processes such as complicated pneumonia and chronic obstructive pulmonary disease (COPD) (see Box 24.1).

Conditions that pose risk for impaired airway clearance require PD.

Clinical Decision Point *If the use of Trendelenburg's position or other postures causes severe hypertension, severe hypoxemia, or severe shortness of breath, therapy is contraindicated (see Box 24.1). In addition, when patients have a risk for or a history of gastroesophageal reflux disease (GERD), which is regurgitation of stomach contents into the esophagus, the head-down positions should not be used.*

3. Review medical record and assess patient for signs and symptoms, including x-ray film changes consistent with atelectasis, lobar collapse pneumonia, or bronchiectasis; ineffective coughing; thick, sticky, tenacious, and discolored secretions that are difficult to cough up.

Indicates need to perform postural drainage. X-ray film data and signs and symptoms indicate accumulation of pulmonary secretions and ineffective airway clearance. Chest physical therapy (CPT) is an additional therapy to improve removal of airway secretions (Ambrosino and Makhabah, 2014).

4. Auscultate all lung fields for decreased breath sounds and adventitious lung sounds.

Findings identify specific lung segments needing drainage.

5. Obtain vital signs and pulse oximetry (SpO_2) before PD treatment.

Provides baseline to evaluate patient's response and tolerance to therapy.

6. Determine patient's and family caregiver's understanding of and ability to perform home postural drainage.

Identifies potential areas for instruction for discharge planning. Home PD is essential for airway secretion management in patients with cystic fibrosis (CF) (Morrison and Agnew, 2014).

7. Use a 0-to-10 pain scale to determine patient's level of comfort.

Determines patient's level of pain and if preprocedure analgesia is needed.

NURSING DIAGNOSES

- Acute pain
- Deficient knowledge regarding postural drainage and airway clearance
- Impaired gas exchange
- Ineffective airway clearance
- Ineffective breathing pattern

Related factors are individualized based on patient's condition or needs.

PLANNING

1. Expected outcomes following completion of procedure:
   - Lung sounds improve or become clear to auscultation.
   - Sputum is more easily expectorated or suctioned out.

   - Secretions appear more normal in color and consistency.

   - SpO_2 levels increase and dyspnea decreases.

   - Chest x-ray film shows improvements: lobar collapse and atelectasis are decreased or eliminated.

Clearing of airways confirms effectiveness of procedure.

PD maneuvers loosen airway secretions, facilitating secretion removal.

When infection is present, returning to normal indicates resolving infection.

As secretions are removed, patient exchange of respiratory gases improves, and dyspnea gradually declines.

PD drains secretions into major airways, facilitating removal during coughing and CPT. As a result, there is visual improvement on chest x-ray film.

2. Prepare patient for procedure:
   a. If patient has an increased pain rating on assessment, administer analgesia 20 minutes before CPT maneuvers.
   b. Explain purpose and rationale for procedure. Explain positioning, sensations, how long it will take, and any discomforts or side effects.
   c. Unless contraindicated, encourage high fluid intake (minimum of 1500 mL) daily. Maintain record of fluid intake and output.

Pain control is essential for patient to actively participate in PD maneuvers and cough forcefully to clear airways.

Helps promote cooperation. Well-prepared patient is usually more relaxed and comfortable, which is essential for effective drainage.

Fluids may thin secretions and make them easier to cough up. Patients need close monitoring and encouragement when first starting high fluid intake program.

STEP	RATIONALE
d. Plan treatments so they do not overlap with meals or tube feeding. Avoid PD 1 to 2 hours before or 1 to 2 hours after meals or bolus tube feedings. Stop all continuous gastric tube feedings for 30 to 45 minutes before PD. Check for residual feeding in patient's stomach; if greater than 100 mL, hold treatment.	Performing PD when patient's stomach is empty helps avoid gastric reflux or vomiting and aspiration of stomach contents.
e. Schedule treatments at appropriate times during day.	Scheduling of PD avoids conflict with other interventions and/or diagnostic testing.

Clinical Decision Point *If patient is receiving inhaled bronchodilator, nebulizers, or aerosol treatment, provide PD 20 minutes after such therapy. PD following bronchodilator therapy enhances patient oxygenation during procedure (Strickland et al., 2015).*

STEP	RATIONALE
f. Have patient remove any tight or restrictive clothing.	Helps patient relax and promotes deep breathing.

IMPLEMENTATION

STEP	RATIONALE
1. Close room door or pull curtains around patient's bed. Perform hand hygiene and apply clean gloves as indicated.	Maintains privacy. Reduces transmission of microorganisms.
2. Use findings from physical assessment and chest x-ray film to select congested areas for draining. Consult with primary health care provider as needed.	Individualized treatment helps relieve specific areas of congestion identified during patient assessment.
3. Help patient to desired position to drain congested areas (see Table 24.1). Place pillows for support and comfort. Drape patient appropriately.	Proper patient positioning assists gravity in helping movement of secretions from peripheral airways to larger bronchi, where they can be cleared (Volsko, 2013).
4. Have patient maintain position for 10 to 15 minutes.	In adults draining each area takes time.
5. After 10 to 15 minutes of drainage in selected postures, perform chest percussion and vibration (see Procedural Guideline 24.2) over affected lung region. Table 24.1 shows all postures and hand placement for percussion and vibration.	Provides mechanical forces to help move airway secretions.
6. After 10 to 15 minutes of drainage in first posture, have patient sit up and cough. If indicated, save expectorated secretions in clear container. If patient cannot cough, suctioning is necessary (see Chapter 25).	Any secretions moved to central airways are removed by cough or suctioning before placing patient into next drainage position. Coughing is most effective when patient is sitting up and leaning forward.

Clinical Decision Point *Sometimes patients experience transient dyspnea and fatigue because of airway irritation and bronchospasm from the secretions. These patients often benefit from an oscillating or vibrating device such as an Acapella device (see Procedural Guideline 24.1).*

STEP	RATIONALE
7. Have patient rest briefly if necessary between positions. Note pulse oximeter readings.	Short rest periods between postures prevent fatigue and increase tolerance. SpO$_2$ values may fall slightly.
8. Have patient take sips of water.	Keeping mouth moist aids in expectoration of secretions.
9. Repeat Steps 3 to 8 until all affected areas selected are drained. Make sure that each treatment does not exceed 30 to 60 minutes.	Drainage is used only to drain areas involved and is based on individual assessment.
10. Offer to help patient with oral hygiene.	Promotes comfort and reduces bad breath.
11. Remove gloves and perform hand hygiene.	Reduces transmission of microorganisms.

EVALUATION

STEP	RATIONALE
1. Auscultate lung fields.	Clearance of secretions usually relieves gurgling, early inspiratory crackles, and palpable crepitus.
2. Inspect character and amount of sputum.	Determines if more secretions are coughed up and if they are thinned adequately.
3. Review diagnostic reports, including sputum collections/cultures, chest x-ray films, and arterial blood gas (ABG) levels.	Provides objective data on improvements in lung function.
4. Obtain vital signs, pulse oximetry.	Procedure can result in dysrhythmias and decreases in oxygen saturation, below 90%, in some patients.

STEP	RATIONALE
5. Use Teach-Back: "I want to be sure I explained why you need to position yourself over the back of a chair with a pillow supporting your chest. Tell me why this position is important." Revise your instruction now or develop a plan for revised patient or family caregiver teaching if patient or family caregiver is not able to teach back correctly.	Determines patient's and family caregiver's level of understanding of instructional topic.

Unexpected Outcomes	Related Interventions
1. Patient experiences severe dyspnea, bronchospasm, hypoxemia, or hypercarbia and/or is unable to tolerate treatment.	• Discontinue, modify, or shorten treatments. • Administer bronchodilator or nebulizer therapy 20 minutes before CPT. • Suction and ventilate with bag-valve-mask to improve patient oxygenation. Closely monitor ABG levels, oxygen saturation, and vital signs (Kohan et al., 2014).
2. No improvement in chest assessment or chest x-ray film examination results.	• Initially increase treatments and encourage and teach coughing exercises. • Increase hydration (if medically appropriate). • Notify health care provider because patient may need sputum culture, change in antibiotics, mucolytics, or a bronchoscopy to remove thick mucus plugs.
3. Hemoptysis occurs; or patient develops acute hypotension, severe chest pain, vomiting, aspiration, and/or dysrhythmias.	• Stop therapy, place patient in high-Fowler's position, and obtain vital signs. • Call for help and notify health care provider. • Remain with patient; keep patient comfortable, calm, warm, and quiet. • If patient vomits or aspirates, suction airway and place him or her on his or her side. • Reapply patient's oxygen device if ordered.

Recording and Reporting

• Record pretherapy and posttherapy assessment findings, SpO₂ readings, and chest x-ray film results; frequency and duration of treatment; postures used and bronchial segments drained; cough effectiveness; need for suctioning; color, amount, and consistency of sputum; hemoptysis or other unexpected outcomes; and patient's tolerance and reactions in the nurses' notes in electronic health record (EHR) or chart.

• Document your evaluation of patient and family caregiver learning.

Special Considerations
Teaching

• Instruct patient and family caregiver that the best times for treatments are (1) in the morning before breakfast, when patient can clear secretions that accumulate overnight; and (2) about 1 hour before bedtime, so lungs are clear before sleeping and patient has time after treatment to cough up any mobilized secretions. Frequency depends on need and patient's tolerance and varies from once daily to every 2 to 4 hours in an acute situation.

• Instruct family caregiver how to recognize when patient's respiratory status requires breathing exercises or PD.

Pediatric

• In a child with CF, PD is a cornerstone therapy and is usually performed at least twice daily, on rising in the morning and in the evening (Hockenberry and Wilson, 2015).

• Many CF patients benefit from the use of the vest airway clearance system (see Procedural Guideline 24.2) (Hockenberry and Wilson, 2015; Morrison and Agnew, 2014).

• CPT is not beneficial in the treatment of bronchiolitis in children younger than 2 years of age (Roqué i Figuls et al., 2012).

• Children with pneumonia, bronchiolitis, and asthma have limited benefits with the administration of CPT (Makic et al., 2015).

Gerontological

• Take extra care and thoroughly assess when using PD in older adults. Certain medications such as antihypertensive and cardiac drugs may increase the risk for dizziness when positions are changed rapidly. Therefore change positions more slowly and closely assess for any changes in oxygen saturation or vital signs with position changes (Touhy and Jett, 2014).

• Older adults with chronic cardiac and pulmonary conditions do not always tolerate a supine or side-lying position for PD. If a patient experiences a decrease in oxygen saturation (decreased SpO₂) or increased breathlessness in these positions, reposition him or her to a semi-Fowler's position and perform CPT.

Home Care

• Teach patient and family caregiver how to assume PD positions at home. Some positions need modification to meet patient needs. For example, if the patient is very short of breath, place him or her in a supine, side-lying semi-Fowler's or side-lying Trendelenburg's position to drain lateral lower lobes.

• Obtain foam wedge or multiple pillows for correct positioning.

• If eligible, refer patient to a pulmonary rehabilitation program.

PROCEDURAL GUIDELINE 24.1 *Using an Acapella Device*

The Acapella device is a handheld airway clearance device (Fig. 24.2). It includes two types, which are designed to match patient's expiratory flow rates and work of breathing. The blue device is for patients who cannot maintain their expiratory flow above 15 L/min for greater than 3 seconds. The green device is for patients who can maintain expiratory flow above or equal to 15 L/min for at least 3 seconds (dos Santos et al., 2013). The device has a control that can adjust the frequency of oscillations and resistance to expiratory flow. Positive expiratory pressure stabilizes airways and improves aeration of the distal lung areas. During exhalation, pressure from the airways is transmitted to the Acapella device, which helps mucus dislodge from the airway walls and as a result prevents airway collapse, accelerates expiratory flow, and moves mucus toward the trachea (Strickland et al., 2013). Some patients with cystic fibrosis may benefit more from this device than from standard chest physiotherapy (Volsko, 2013). However cystic fibrosis patients must receive some type of routine airway clearance therapy daily.

Delegation and Collaboration

The skill of using an Acapella device can be delegated to nursing assistive personnel (NAP). The nurse is responsible for performing respiratory assessment, determining that the procedure is appropriate and that a patient is able to tolerate it, and evaluating a patient's response to it. The nurse instructs the NAP to:

- Be alert for patient's tolerance of procedure such as comfort level and changes in breathing pattern and immediately report changes to the nurse.
- Use specific patient precautions such as positioning restrictions related to disease or treatment.

Equipment

- Stethoscope
- Pulse oximeter
- Water and glass
- Chair
- Tissues and paper bag
- Clear graduated screw-top container
- Suction equipment (if patient unable to cough and clear own secretions)
- Acapella device (see Fig. 24.2)
- Clean gloves (if there is a risk of exposure to patient's respiratory secretions)
- Patient education materials

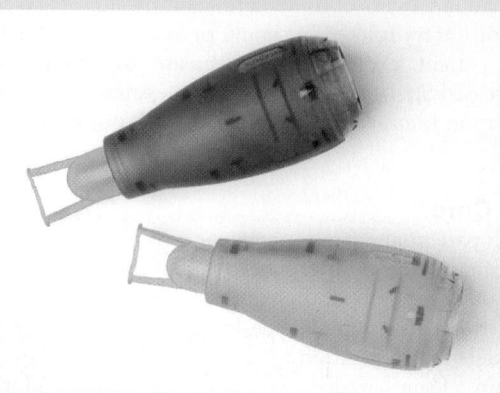

FIG 24.2 Acapella device. (*Used with permission, Smithsmedical.com.*)

Procedural Steps

1. Identify patient using at least two identifiers (e.g., name and birthday or name and medical record number) according to agency policy (TJC, 2016).
2. Verify the need for a health care provider's order per agency policy.
3. Perform respiratory assessment to determine lung segments requiring percussion and/or vibration (Volsko, 2013).
4. Assess patient's and family's understanding of the device and procedure and explain and clarify procedure as needed.
5. Prepare prescribed Acapella device:

Clinical Decision Point *Verify that the correct device is used to match patient's expiratory flow rate. Blue: patients who cannot maintain their expiratory flow above 15 L/min for greater than 3 seconds. Green: patients who can maintain expiratory flow above or equal to 15 L/min for at least 3 seconds.*

    a. Initial setting: turn Acapella frequency adjustment dial counterclockwise to lowest resistance setting.
    b. As patient improves or is more proficient, adjust the proper resistance level upward by turning the dial clockwise. This initial setting helps patient adjust to the device.

Clinical Decision Point *Determine if aerosol drug therapy is ordered. If so, attach a nebulizer to the end of the Acapella valve.*

6. Instruct patient to:
    a. Sit comfortably.
    b. Take in a breath that is larger than normal but not to fill lungs completely. Instruct patient to inhale to about 75% of inspiratory capacity.
    c. Place mouthpiece into mouth, maintaining a tight seal.
    d. Hold breath for 2 to 3 seconds.
    e. Try not to cough and to exhale slowly for 3 to 4 seconds through the device while it vibrates.

Clinical Decision Point *If patient cannot maintain an exhalation for this length of time, adjust the dial clockwise. Clockwise adjustment increases the resistance of the vibrating opening, which allows the patient to exhale at a lower flow rate. Or it may be necessary to change from the blue to green device.*

    f. Repeat cycle for 5 to 10 breaths as tolerated.
    g. Remove mouthpiece and perform one or two forceful exhalations and "huff" coughs.
    h. Repeat Steps a to g as ordered.
7. Auscultate lung fields.
8. Obtain vital signs, SpO_2.
9. Inspect color, character, and amount of sputum.
10. Help patient with oral hygiene.
11. **Use Teach-Back:** "I want to be sure I effectively showed you how to use this device. Show me how you use the Acapella device during this airway treatment." Revise your instruction now or develop a plan for revised patient or family caregiver teaching if patient or family caregiver is not able to teach back correctly.
12. Review Unexpected Outcomes for Skill 24.1.
13. Document procedure and patient's tolerance. Document your evaluation of patient learning.

PROCEDURAL GUIDELINE 24.2 *Performing Percussion and Vibration*

During postural drainage a nurse, respiratory therapist, or trained family caregiver sometimes uses physical maneuvers such as percussion and vibration on the rib cage over lung tissue. The clinician uses techniques on specific parts of the rib cage over each affected lung region. Normally the mucociliary escalator and cough transport of the body can clear airway secretions effectively. However, when a patient's ability to clear the airways is reduced, the techniques of percussion and vibration are combined with postural drainage (see Skill 24.1).

Percussion is the manual external clapping of a patient's chest wall with cupped hands or with a mechanical device in a rhythmic fashion to loosen secretions from the bronchial walls. You apply vibration to a patient's external chest wall by placing both hands (one over the other) over the areas to be vibrated. Then you tense and contract the shoulder and arm muscles to create a vibration while the patient exhales to mobilize secretions (Strickland et al., 2013). Vibration augments the natural movement of the rib cage during exhalation and helps with secretion clearance. Never use the clavicles, breast tissue, sternum, spine, waist, and abdomen for percussion and vibration; only perform these maneuvers over the ribs.

High-Frequency Chest Wall Compression

High-frequency chest wall compression (HFCWC) consists of an inflatable vest linked to an air-pulse generator. One HFCWC device is the vest airway clearance system, which helps to loosen and remove secretions from the airways (Fig. 24.3). HFCWC systems deliver high-frequency, small-volume expiratory pulses to a patient's external chest wall. This mechanical action helps to loosen and mobilize airway secretions (Volsko, 2013). It is beneficial for selected patients with neuromuscular diseases, cystic fibrosis, and ineffective coughing and airway clearance. In addition, patients with sputum production of 25 to 30 mL/day also benefit from this device because HFCWC decreases the viscosity of mucus, making it easier to cough productively (Volsko, 2013).

Delegation and Collaboration

The skill of performing percussion and vibration can be delegated to trained nursing assistive personnel (NAP) (see agency policy).

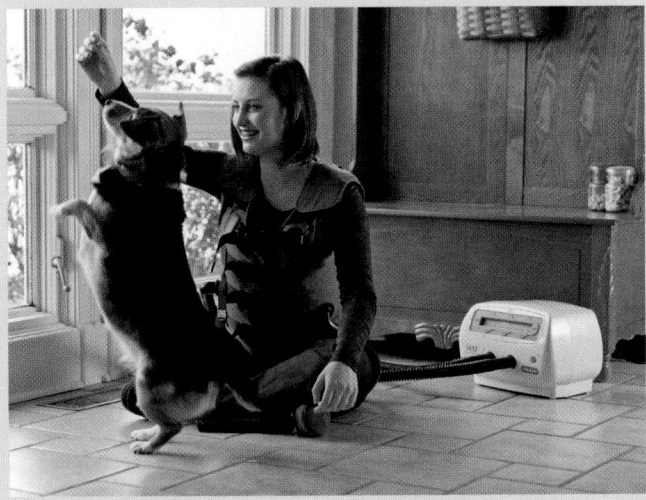

FIG 24.3 High-frequency chest wall oscillation vest for home use. (*Copyright ©2012 Hill-Rom Services, Inc. Reprinted with permission. All rights reserved.*)

The nurse is responsible for the respiratory assessment and review of the patient's chest x-ray film (with a physician) to determine patient stability, which areas of the lungs are affected, and specific positions for the patient to assume. The nurse instructs the NAP about:

- Any patient precautions related to disease or treatment.
- Reporting to the nurse any problems with tolerance of the procedure, pain, dyspnea, or changes in vital signs.

Equipment

- Stethoscope
- Hospital bed (tilt table placed in Trendelenburg's position, optional; check agency policy)
- Chair (for upper lobes)
- One-to-four pillows
- Water pitcher and glass
- Tissues and paper bag
- Clear graduated screw-top container
- Mechanical vibrator or percussor (*optional*)
- HFCWC device such as the vest airway clearance system
- Single layer of clothing
- Clean gloves (if there is a risk for exposure to patient's respiratory secretions)
- Oral hygiene care: toothbrush, toothpaste, mouthwash, or chlorhexidine oral rinse if ordered
- Suction equipment (*optional*)
- Stethoscope, pulse oximeter

Procedural Steps

1. Identify patient using at least two identifiers (e.g., name and birthday or name and medical record number) according to agency policy (TJC, 2016).
2. Assess patient and review medical record for signs, symptoms, and conditions that indicate need to perform percussion and vibration (see Skill 24.1, Assessment).
3. Perform respiratory assessment (including vital signs, pulse oximetry, inspection, and palpation) to assess breathing pattern, including muscles used for breathing, respiratory rate and depth, extent of excursion, chest wall movement, and oxygen saturation.
4. Auscultate lung sounds over lung segments drained during postural drainage (see Skill 24.1).

Clinical Decision Point *Percussion and/or vibration are contraindicated with rib fracture, fracture of other rib cage structures such as clavicle or sternum, pain, severe dyspnea, and severe osteoporosis. Thin, frail patients with osteoporosis are most susceptible to injury and are taught other secretion control measures (e.g., forceful coughing, humidification).*

5. Inspect and gently palpate rib cage over affected bronchial segment(s) for pain, tenderness, abnormal configuration, abnormal excursion or chest wall movement during breathing, and muscle tension. Percussion or vibration is contraindicated if one of these assessment findings is present because the treatment has the potential to cause further injury and impair chest wall motion.
6. Determine patient's understanding and assess ability to cooperate with therapy, both in hospital and at home.
7. Explain procedure in detail: patient's positioning, sensations, how it will be done, how long it will take, use of vest (if applicable), and any discomforts or side effects.

Continued

PROCEDURAL GUIDELINE 24.2 *Performing Percussion and Vibration—cont'd*

8. Help patient relax and deep breathe during procedure. Have him or her practice exhaling slowly through pursed lips while relaxing chest wall muscles and blow out using abdominal muscles, not rib cage muscles.

9. Perform hand hygiene and apply clean gloves as appropriate.

10. Elevate bed to comfortable working height and stand close to bed with arms directly in front and knees slightly bent.

11. Use findings from physical assessment and chest x-ray film to select congested areas of lung. Position patient in appropriate drainage position (see Table 24.1) and place pillows for support and comfort.

12. Perform percussion and vibration.
    a. Percussion and vibration with hands
       (1) Perform percussion for 3 to 5 minutes in each position as tolerated. Begin on appropriate part of chest wall over draining area (see Table 24.1). Always ask if patient is experiencing any discomfort such as undue pressure or stinging of the skin.
       (2) Place hands side by side on chest wall over area to be drained. Cup hands with fingers and thumbs held tightly together. Make sure that entire outer part of hand makes contact with chest wall to avoid air leaks (see illustration).

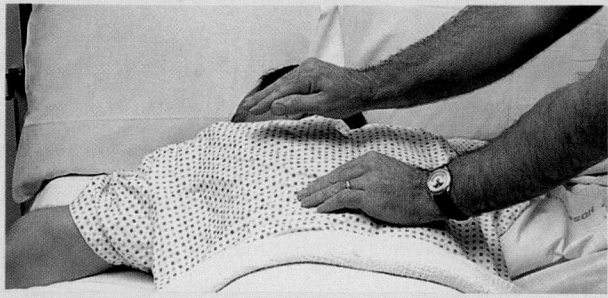

STEP 12a(2) Chest wall percussion, alternating hand clapping against patient's chest wall.

       (3) When clapping, most arm movement comes from the elbow and wrist joints. Clapping is often done for 5 minutes without stopping or for 2 to 3 minutes, alternating with vibration.
       (4) Alternately clap chest with cupped hands to create rhythmic popping sound resembling galloping horse. Perform clapping at moderate or fast speed, whichever is most comfortable and effective.
       (5) Perform chest wall vibration over each affected area (see Table 24.1). Perform vibrations in sets of three followed by coughing so any loosened secretions are expectorated.
          (a) Place flat part of hand over area and have patient take slow, deep breath through nose.
          (b) Gently resist chest wall as it rises during inhalation.
          (c) Have patient hold breath for 2 to 3 seconds and exhale through pursed lips, while contracting abdominal muscles and relaxing chest wall muscles. Chest wall relaxes and falls.
          (d) While patient is exhaling, gently push down and vibrate chest wall with flat part of hand (Volsko, 2013).

       (e) Repeat vibration 3 times and have patient cascade cough by taking deep breath and doing series of small coughs until end of breath. Instruct patient not to inhale between coughs. Vibrate chest wall as patient coughs. When applying pressure to ribs, always follow natural movement of rib cage. Allow patient to sit up and cough as needed.

Clinical Decision Point *When a patient has excessive pulmonary secretions, which occur with cystic fibrosis, a mechanical vibrator instead of manual vibration is more effective in removing them.*

       (f) Monitor patient's tolerance of vibration and ability to relax chest wall and breathe properly as instructed.
       (g) Perform a total of three or four sets of three vibrations with vibration followed by coughing over each lung segment as tolerated. Strength and frequency of vibration will vary.
    b. HFCWC device:
       (1) Place vest on patient and assess for proper fit.
          (a) With vest deflated, adjust closures so it fits comfortably.
          (b) Vest should rest on shoulder and extend to top of hip bone.
       (2) Assess chest wall motion. Breathing should not be restricted when vest is deflated.
       (3) Connect tubing to the generator and ports of the vest. Turn on power.
       (4) Adjust pressure control as ordered; usually pressure is between 5 and 6.
       (5) Adjust frequency; usually set between 10 and 15 Hz.
       (6) Administer any aerosol therapy as prescribed.
       (7) Depress and maintain pressure on the hand/foot control to initiate vest therapy.
       (8) After 5 to 10 minutes, release hand/foot control.

13. Instruct patient to cough or suction if he or she is unable to cough up mucus (see Chapter 25).

14. Continue with treatment; usually 15 to 30 minutes.

15. Help patient with oral hygiene.

16. Remove gloves and perform hand hygiene.

17. If long-term therapy is needed, teach patient and significant others the procedure for home use for Acapella or HFCWC devices. If they cannot learn or use, refer for outpatient or home care follow-up.

18. Auscultate lung fields.

19. Obtain vital signs, pulse oximetry.

20. Inspect color, character, and amount of sputum.

21. **Use Teach-Back:** "We discussed the importance of using this vest to manage your respiratory secretions. Tell me why it is important to keep your airways clear of secretions." Revise your instruction now or develop a plan for revised patient or family caregiver teaching if patient or family caregiver is not able to teach back correctly.

22. Document procedure and patient's response. Document your evaluation of patient learning.

◆ CLINICAL DEBRIEF

A 29-year-old college student has a history of cystic fibrosis (CF). He is on the lung transplant list and adheres to his chest physical therapy (CPT) and medication regimen. One week ago he developed a cold, which continued to worsen, and his respiratory secretions were difficult to clear with his usual treatments. He was admitted to the hospital 3 days ago for complicated pneumonia, with a respiratory rate of 30 breaths/min and 90% saturation (SaO_2) on 2 L/min of oxygen via nasal cannula. He has a fever of 38.8°C (101.8°F). Chest x-ray film showed bilateral lower lobe pneumonia and lobar collapse of his right middle lobe.

1. On the basis of the chest x-ray film findings, what would you expect to find on physical examination of the chest, and which additional signs and symptoms would you expect to see?
2. Chest physiotherapy (CPT) was ordered. Which positions would you use for postural drainage (PD)?
3. After 24 hours of aggressive CPT and PD, a chest x-ray film examination was repeated. It showed no improvement. Using SBAR, show how would you communicate with the health care team about this patient?

◆ REVIEW QUESTIONS

1. Your patient is to have postural drainage 3 times a day. Which of the following are necessary to prepare the patient for postural drainage? (Select all that apply.)
   1. Encourage adequate fluid intake.
   2. Provide a light meal 30 minutes before.
   3. Explain the procedure and positioning techniques.
   4. Review any chest x-ray films and auscultate all lung fields.
   5. Coordinate treatments with other respiratory or medical therapies.
   6. Plan on performing chest physiotherapy (CPT) on all lung regions.
2. Your patient is scheduled for postural drainage (PD). Place the following steps in correct order.
   1. Obtain vital signs and pulse oximetry.
   2. Position patient in proper position to drain selected lung segment.
   3. Maintain position for 10 to 15 minutes.
   4. Perform chest physiotherapy maneuvers.
   5. Perform respiratory assessment.
   6. Provide rest period between positions.
3. Your patient experiences severe dyspnea and hemoptysis during a session of percussion and vibration. After stopping the treatment, what is the priority nursing intervention?
   1. Notify the health care provider.
   2. Administer a bronchodilator to ease the dyspnea.
   3. Assess the patient.
   4. Elevate the head of the patient's bed.

ⓔ *Visit the Evolve site for a complete list of Clinical Debrief and Review Questions answers.*

REFERENCES

Ambrosino N, Makhabah D: *Physiotherapy in the ICU*, July 2014, http://www.rtmagazine.com/2014/07/physiotherapy-icu/. Accessed January 26, 2016.

Cross JL, et al: Evaluation of the effectiveness of physiotherapy techniques on quality of life at six months' postexacerbation of COPD (MATREX): a randomized controlled equivalence trial, *BMC Pulm Med* 12:33, 2012.

dos Santos AP, et al: Mechanical behaviors of Flutter VRP1, Shaker, and Acapella devices, *Respir Care* 58(2):298, 2013.

Giger JN: *Transcultural nursing*, ed 7, St Louis, 2016, Mosby.

Hockenberry MJ, Wilson D: *Wong's nursing care of infants and children*, ed 10, St Louis, 2015, Mosby.

Kohan M, et al: Effects of expiratory ribcage compression before endotracheal suctioning on arterial blood gases in patients receiving mechanical ventilation, *Nurs Crit Care* 19(5):255, 2014.

Makic MBF, et al: Continuing to challenge practice to be evidence based, *Crit Care Nurse* 35(2):39, 2015.

Mesquinta FOS, et al: Scintigraphic assessment of radio-aerosol pulmonary disposition with the Acapella positive-pressure device and various nebulizer configurations, *Respir Care* 59(3):328, 2014.

Morrison L, Agnew J: *Oscillating devices for airway clearance in people with cystic fibrosis*, 2014, http://onlinelibrary.wiley.com/doi/10.1002/14651858.CD006842.pub3/abstract.

Roqué i Figuls M, et al: Chest physiotherapy for acute bronchiolitis in paediatric patients between 0 and 24 months old, *Cochrane Database Syst Rev* (2):CD004873, 2012.

Sisson JH, et al: Vest chest physiotherapy airway clearance is associated with nitric oxide metabolism, *Pulm Med* 23: article ID 291375, 2013.

Strickland SL, et al: AARC Clinical Practice Guideline: effectiveness of nonpharmacologic airway clearance therapies in hospitalized patients, *Respir Care* 58(12):2187, 2013.

Strickland SL, et al: AARC Clinical Practice Guideline: effectiveness of pharmacologic airway clearance therapies in hospitalized patients, *Respir Care* 60(7):1071, 2015.

The Joint Commission (TJC): *National Patient Safety Goals*, 2016, Oakbrook Terrace, IL, 2016, The Commission, http://www.jointcommission.org/standards_information/npsgs.aspx. Accessed January 25, 2016.

Touhy TA, Jett KF: *Ebersole and Hess' Gerontological nursing and healthy aging*, ed 4, St Louis, 2014, Mosby.

Volsko TA: Airway clearance therapy: finding the evidence, *Respir Care* 58(10):1669, 2013.

Yang M, et al: Chest physiotherapy for pneumonia in adults, *Cochrane Database Syst Rev* (2):CD006338, 2013.

25 | Airway Management

OBJECTIVES

Mastery of content in this chapter will enable the nurse to:
- Identify safety guidelines for managing a patient's airway.
- Discuss patient-centered approaches to airway management.
- Describe the nursing interventions for airway management.
- Discuss the indications for airway suctioning.
- Discuss the indications for tracheostomy care.

- Correctly perform oropharyngeal, nasopharyngeal and nasotracheal, and tracheal suctioning; endotracheal care; and tracheostomy tube care.
- Correctly inflate a cuff on an endotracheal or tracheostomy tube.
- Change a tracheostomy tube or inner cannula.

MEDIA RESOURCES

- evolve http://evolve.elsevier.com/Perry/skills
- Review Questions
- ▶ Video Clips
- Audio Glossary

- **NSO** Nursing Skills Online
- Clinical Debrief and Review Questions Answers
- Animations

PURPOSE

Airway management involves nursing interventions to maintain the patency of a patient's nose, mouth, upper airway, trachea, and lower airway of the respiratory system. The primary goal of airway management is to protect the airway, which will help promote and maintain adequate tissue oxygenation.

STANDARDS OF CARE

- AARC Clinical Practice Guideline, 2004—Nasotracheal Suctioning
- AARC Clinical Practice Guideline, 2010—Endotracheal Suctioning of Mechanically Ventilated Patients With Artificial Airways
- AARC Clinical Practice Guideline, 2012—Humidification During Invasive and Noninvasive Mechanical Ventilation
- Institute for Healthcare Improvement (IHI), 2012—How-to Guide: Prevent Ventilator-Associated Pneumonia
- The Joint Commission (TJC), 2016—Patient Safety Goals – Patient Identification
- AARC Clinical Practice Guidelines, 2011—Capnography/capnometry

PRINCIPLES FOR PRACTICE

- Various techniques for airway management are available to promote an open or patent airway, which has the potential to become obstructed by mucus, mechanical obstruction (i.e., soft tissue in upper airway), or a foreign body.
- Hydration, positioning, nutrition, chest physiotherapy techniques, deep breathing, coughing, humidity, incentive spirometry, and aerosol therapy are noninvasive techniques that are helpful in maintaining a patent airway.
- When patients are unable to protect their own airway or clear airway secretions with coughing, chest physiotherapy, or other noninvasive techniques, more invasive measures such as suctioning or inserting an artificial airway are needed.
- An artificial airway is a plastic or rubber device (such as a tracheostomy or endotracheal tube) that is inserted into the upper or lower respiratory tract to facilitate ventilation or the removal of secretions.

PATIENT-CENTERED CARE

- Artificial airways alter patients' ability to communicate, possibly causing feelings of fear, frustration, anxiety, and vulnerability.

- Recommendations to improve communication for patients with an altered airway include developing alternate means of and establishing an environment that promotes effective communication among the patient, the family, and the members of the health care team (Grossbach et al., 2011; Tsay et al., 2013).
- Assess for anger and frustration when patients with artificial airways try to communicate, and consider the need for individualized and creative communication methods (Grossbach et al., 2011; Tsay et al., 2013).
- Nurses need to thoroughly educate patients and their families using plain language that is culturally appropriate and verify that they understand any procedures or tests.
- Collaboration with families is essential when providing alternative means of communication for patients. Once communication is established, a patient and family will have more trust in the care provided, which will promote cooperation and rapport (Grossbach et al., 2011).
- Patients and families who have English as their second language or do not speak English require additional attention from nurses and other health care providers to prevent misunderstanding treatment options.
- Obtain professional translators or other communication aids so patients and families understand the need for an artificial airway and the subsequent treatments.
- Assess the functional skills of the patient. Ensure that functioning hearing aids are in place and working so communication with a hearing impaired patient is possible. Allow patients to wear their glasses and use communication devices such as picture or letter boards. Assess patient's dominant hand and muscle strength if writing boards are to be used (Grossbach et al., 2011).

EVIDENCE-BASED PRACTICE

- There are significant concerns regarding defining ventilator-associated pneumonia (VAP) and ventilator-associated events (VAEs). The Centers for Disease Control and Prevention (CDC, 2016) developed a lengthy algorithm for clinicians to use to accurately diagnose these complications.
  - The key points in the definition of VAE are "deterioration in respiratory status after a period of stability or improvement on the ventilator, evidence of infection or inflammation, and laboratory evidence of respiratory infection.
  - Patient must be mechanically ventilated for more than 2 calendar days to be eligible for VAE (CDC, 2016).
- VAP/VAE bundles are available to help guide nursing practice (see also Skill 23.5). Key interventions included in these bundles are the following:
  - Elevation of the head of bed (HOB) between 30 and 45 degrees
  - Daily interruption of sedation and daily assessment of patient's readiness to extubate
  - Peptic ulcer disease prophylaxis
  - Deep venous thrombosis prophylaxis (unless contraindicated)
  - Daily oral care with chlorhexidine
  - Delirium monitoring and management
  - Early exercise and mobility (IHI, 2012; Lamb, 2015)
- Closed endotracheal suctioning techniques are preferred over open endotracheal suctioning techniques in patients who have undergone open heart surgery. Closed suctioning has fewer traumatic effects on mean arterial blood pressure and pulse oximetry than open suctioning (Özden and Görgülü, 2014).

- Closed-circuit suctioning has more advantages than disadvantages when compared with open circuit suctioning such as avoiding loss of positive end-expiratory pressure (PEEP), which decreases amount of hypoxemia, costs, and caregiver exposure to pulmonary secretions (Branson et al., 2014).
- New products are being developed to decrease the risk of biofilm formation on endotracheal tubes (ET). Biofilm is associated with increased risks of developing VAP.
  - These new products include systems that scrape the inside of the ET to remove the secretions.
  - Silver-coated, gardine-coated, and gendine-coated ETs are also being investigated for their effectiveness in preventing biofilm formation (Branson et al., 2014).
- Automated cuff pressure-control devices used to measure cuff pressures on artificial airways are more consistent and possibly lead to better airway care (Branson et al., 2014).

SAFETY GUIDELINES

- Know a patient's baseline range of vital signs and oxygen saturation levels. Baseline physiological measures serve as a means to identify individual abnormalities and recognize the worsening of an illness.
- Know a patient's medical history. Smoking alters normal mucociliary clearance. Certain disorders such as chronic obstructive pulmonary disease (COPD), asthma, cystic fibrosis, pneumonia, thoracic surgery, chest trauma, and abdominal surgery place patients at increased risk for an obstructed airway.
- Identify conditions that increase a patient's risk for aspiration of gastric contents into the lung, resulting in airway obstruction. These include the presence of enteral feeding tubes or nasal and oral gastric tubes, a decreased level of consciousness, and a decreased swallowing ability.
- Use caution when suctioning patients with head injuries. The suction procedure causes an elevation in intracranial pressure (ICP) (Galbiati and Paola, 2015). Reduce this risk by presuctioning hyperventilation, which results in hypocarbia. This in turn induces vasoconstriction, thereby reducing the risk of elevated ICP.
- Determine if a patient has a history of nasal problems such as nasal trauma, nasal polyps, deviated nasal septum, or chronic sinusitis. Allergy problems may cause mucosal swelling that narrows nasal passages, which affects the ability to easily pass a suction catheter.
- Review a patient's respiratory assessments from the past 12 or 24 hours. These are relative baseline measurements that help to distinguish between gradual and acute changes in a patient's status.
- Perform a systematic pulmonary assessment of upper and lower airways, including identifying respiratory rate, respiratory pattern, accessory muscle use, breath sounds, ability to cough effectively, integrity of the rib cage, and the characteristics of sputum production.
- Identify and become familiar with the use of equipment available at the agency. Many types of artificial airways, suction catheters, and suction machines are available. Knowing how to operate the equipment before use promotes positive outcomes.
- Test all equipment before use. Have adequate supplies on hand at the bedside. Equipment must work properly to provide safe nursing care. Determine that the suction machine is generating adequate negative suction pressure and that suction catheters and appropriate equipment are available at the bedside.

- Know the side effects of medications and other therapies. Some medications such as beta-adrenergic blockers have the side effect of bronchospasm. An adverse effect of opioids and sedatives is respiratory depression. Similarly, too much oxygen reduces the drive to breathe in patients with chronic hypercapnia (elevated arterial carbon dioxide tension). Some position changes affect a patient adversely. For example, in patients with

impaired spinal cord innervations of the respiratory muscles, supine positions place the diaphragm at a mechanical disadvantage and increase the risk for aspiration.
- The instillation of normal saline when performing endotracheal suctioning is no longer encouraged and is not a supported practice (Branson et al., 2014).

◆ SKILL 25.1   Performing Oropharyngeal Suctioning

 Video Clip   **NSO** *Nursing Skills Online Airway Management Module / Lesson 2*

A Yankauer, or tonsillar tip, suction device is used for oropharyngeal suctioning (i.e., the removal of pharyngeal secretions through the mouth) (Fig. 25.1). A Yankauer suction catheter is made of rigid, minimally flexible plastic. The tip of this suction catheter usually has one large and several small openings through which the mucus enters with application of negative pressure. The Yankauer suction catheter is angled to facilitate removal of secretions through a patient's mouth. Oropharyngeal suctioning only removes secretions from the back of the throat. Perform oral suctioning when a patient is able to cough effectively but is unable to clear secretions such as for a patient with a neuromuscular injury who cannot manage his or her own oral secretions. Patients with artificial airways and impaired swallowing require use of the Yankauer suction device to provide oral hygiene.

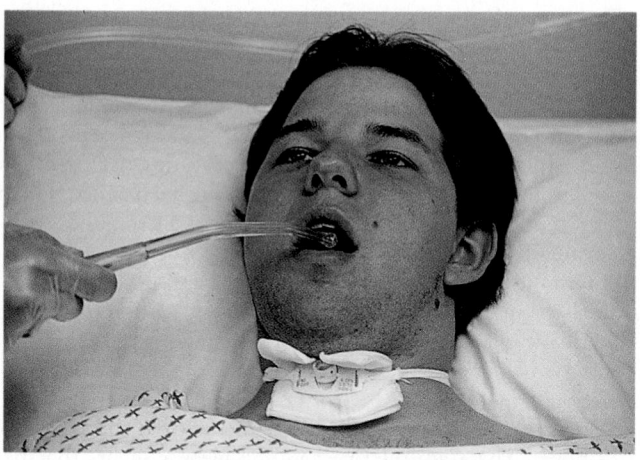

FIG 25.1 Oropharyngeal suctioning.

Delegation and Collaboration

The skill of performing oropharyngeal suctioning can be delegated to nursing assistive personnel (NAP). Do not delegate this skill for patients with oral or neck surgery in the immediate postoperative period. The nurse is responsible for assessing the patient's respiratory status. The nurse directs the NAP about:

- Appropriate suction limits for oropharyngeal suctioning for a particular patient (e.g., the appropriate suction pressure, expected frequency of suctioning, and expected color and volume of secretions).
- The risks of applying excessive or inadequate suction pressure.
- Avoiding mouth sutures, applying suction against sensitive tissues, and dislodging tubes in the patient's nose or mouth.
- Avoiding stimulation of the gag reflex.
- Immediately reporting to the nurse any change in vital signs, pulse oximetry (SpO_2), sputum (i.e., bloody), difficulty breathing, or discomfort during or after the procedure.

Equipment

- Yankauer or tonsillar tip suction catheter
- Clean gloves
- Towel, cloth, or disposable paper drape
- Mask, goggles, or face shield; isolation gown if indicated
- Disposable cup or nonsterile basin
- Tap water or normal saline (about 100 mL)
- Suction machine or wall suction device with regulator
- Connecting tubing (6 feet)
- Oral airway (if indicated)
- Washcloth (if indicated)
- Pulse oximeter, stethoscope
- Manual self-inflating resuscitation bag (bag-valve-mask) with oxygen connecting tubing

---

STEP	RATIONALE

ASSESSMENT

1. Identify patient using at least two identifiers (e.g., name and birthday or name and medical record number) according to agency policy.

Ensures correct patient. Complies with The Joint Commission standards and improves patient safety (TJC, 2016).

2. Identify risk factors for airway obstruction: impaired cough or gag reflex, weakened respiratory muscles, impaired swallowing, and decreased level of consciousness.

Risk factors prevent patient from protecting airway from aspiration or clearing secretions safely.

3. Assess for signs and symptoms of hypoxia: anxiety, change in level of consciousness, change in vital signs, decreased SpO_2, adventitious sounds (see also Box 23.1).

Suctioning of oropharyngeal airway is indicated with alterations in oxygenation associated with secretion accumulation.

STEP	RATIONALE
4. Obtain patient's oxygen saturation level via SpO$_2$ (see Chapter 5). Keep pulse oximeter in place.	Provides an objective baseline measure of oxygen saturation and an early indication of changes in oxygenation status. Aids in assessment of patient during and after oropharyngeal suctioning.
5. Determine patient's ability to hold or manipulate catheter and his or her knowledge about use of suction catheter and procedure.	Encourages cooperation; minimizes risks and anxiety. Identifies teaching needs. Physical factors such as impaired mobility of upper extremities prevent patient from using catheter to help control oral secretions.
6. Assess for signs and symptoms of upper airway obstruction: gurgling on inspiration or expiration, restlessness, obvious excessive oral secretions, drooling, gastric secretions or vomitus in mouth, or coughing without clearing secretions from upper airway.	Secretions pool in upper airway, which can cause total airway obstruction and hypoxia. The risk for aspiration of gastric contents and airway obstruction is increased in patients with vomiting; delayed gastric emptying; impairment in esophageal sphincter control, cough, swallowing, or gag reflex; or those receiving enteral feedings.
7. Auscultate for presence of adventitious sounds (see Chapter 6 and Skill 25.2).	Determines if lower airway secretions are present and establishes baseline.

NURSING DIAGNOSES

- Deficient knowledge regarding use of suction
- Impaired gas exchange

- Impaired swallowing
- Ineffective airway clearance
- Ineffective breathing pattern

- Risk for aspiration
- Risk for infection

Related factors/Risk factors are individualized based on patient's condition or needs.

PLANNING

1. Expected outcomes following completion of procedure:	
• No gurgling sounds are heard in patient's pharynx on inspiration and expiration.	Suctioning is effective. Secretions are removed from large upper airway.
• Drooling is diminished or absent.	Excessive drooling indicates that patient is unable to handle oral secretions.
• Vomitus or gastric secretions are absent from mouth.	Gastric secretions retained in oral cavity increase patient's risk for aspiration pneumonia.
• SpO$_2$ improves or remains at patient's normal baseline.	Removal of secretions helps to improve oxygen saturation level.

Clinical Decision Point *In patients with chronic pulmonary disease, the SpO$_2$ value may remain the same after oropharyngeal suctioning. This baseline value may be lower than the typical normal values of greater than 95% (Grindrod, 2015).*

2. Perform hand hygiene. Gather equipment/supplies. Close room door or curtain.	Ensures well organized procedure. Provides patient privacy.
3. Explain to patient how procedure helps clear airway secretions and relieves some breathing problems. Explain that coughing, gagging, or (less commonly) sneezing is normal and lasts only a few seconds. Encourage patient to cough out secretions and show how to splint painful areas during procedure. Practice coughing if able.	Gagging or coughing occurs when posterior pharynx is suctioned or as a result of excess secretions. Coughing secretions out of lower airway or posterior pharynx decreases amount of suctioning required. Splinting reduces abdominal incision discomfort during coughing or gagging.
4. Position patient in semi-Fowler's or sitting position. Place towel, cloth, or paper drape across patient's neck and chest.	Promotes patient comfort and removal of airway secretions. Towel protects gown and bed linen from contamination by secretions.

IMPLEMENTATION

1. Apply clean gloves. Apply mask or face shield if splashing is likely. Wear gown if isolation precautions are indicated.	Reduces transmission of microorganisms.
2. Fill cup or basin with approximately 100 mL of water or normal saline.	Helps to clean catheter after suctioning and assesses that equipment functions.
3. Connect one end of connecting tubing to suction machine and other to Yankauer suction catheter. Turn on suction machine; set vacuum regulator to appropriate setting (infants 80–100 mm Hg; children 100–120 mm Hg; adults 100–150 mm Hg) (AARC, 2004).	Prepares suction apparatus. Pressures should not exceed 150 mm Hg because elevated pressure settings increase risk for trauma to oral mucosa (AARC, 2004).

STEP	RATIONALE
4. Check that suction machine is functioning properly by placing tip of catheter in water or normal saline and suctioning small amount from cup or basin.	Ensures that equipment functions and lubricates catheter.
5. Remove patient's oxygen mask if present. Nasal cannula may remain in place. Keep oxygen mask near patient's face.	Allows access to mouth. Reduces chance of hypoxia.

Clinical Decision Point *Be prepared to quickly reapply supplemental oxygen if SpO$_2$ value falls below 90% or respiratory distress develops during or at the end of oropharyngeal suctioning. Be prepared to use the bag-valve-mask if patient has serious acute respiratory distress or decline in SpO$_2$.*

STEP	RATIONALE
6. Insert catheter into mouth along gum line to pharynx. Move catheter around mouth until secretions have cleared. Encourage patient to cough. Replace oxygen mask.	Movement of catheter prevents suction tip from invaginating oral mucosal surfaces and causing trauma. Coughing moves secretions from lower airway into mouth and upper airway.

Clinical Decision Point *Be careful when using a Yankauer tip suction catheter with a patient who had recent oral or head/neck surgery. Aggressive suctioning and excessive coughing should not be used or encouraged in patients who have undergone throat surgery such as a tonsillectomy. These acts can aggravate the operative site, increasing the risk of infection or bleeding (Hockenberry and Wilson, 2015).*

STEP	RATIONALE
7. Rinse catheter with water or normal saline in cup or basin until connecting tubing is cleared of secretions. Turn off suction. Place catheter in clean, dry area.	Rinses catheter and reduces probability of transmission of microorganisms. Clean suction tubing enhances delivery of set suction pressure.
8. Wash face if secretions are present on patient's skin.	Prevents skin breakdown.
9. Observe respiratory status. Repeat procedure if indicated. May need to use standard suction catheter to reach into trachea if respiratory status not improved (see Skill 25.2).	Directs nurse to continue, cease intervention, or choose another intervention.
10. Remove towel, cloth, or disposable drape and place in trash or in laundry if soiled. Reposition patient; Sims' or side-lying position encourages drainage and should be used if patient has decreased level of consciousness.	Reduces transmission of microorganisms. Facilitates drainage of oral secretions.
11. Discard remainder of water or normal saline into appropriate receptacle. Rinse basin in warm soapy water and dry with paper towels (check agency policy). Discard disposable cup into appropriate receptacle.	Reduces transmission of microorganisms and maintains medical asepsis. Moist environment encourages microorganism growth.

Clinical Decision Point *Keep catheter in nonairtight container such as brown paper or plastic bag attached to bedrail or in suction canister area. Do not store the catheter where it will come in contact with secretions or excretions, which promote bacterial growth.*

STEP	RATIONALE
12. Remove gloves, mask, or face shield and dispose of in appropriate receptacle. Perform hand hygiene.	Reduces transmission of microorganisms to other patients and equipment.
13. Position patient and provide oral hygiene as needed.	Promotes patient's comfort.

EVALUATION

1. Compare assessment findings before and after procedure. — Identifies physiological response to suction procedure.
2. Auscultate chest and airways for adventitious sounds. — Presence of lower airway adventitious sounds suggests need for lower airway suctioning.

3. Inspect mouth for any vomitus or remaining secretions. — Clear oral airway is necessary to prevent aspiration.
4. Obtain and record postsuction SpO$_2$ value. Compare with presuction level. — Provides objective measure of effectiveness of suction procedure (AARC, 2004).
5. **Use Teach-Back:** "I want to be sure I explained how to suction your mouth and why it should be performed. Show me how you will use this suction catheter." Revise your instruction now or develop a plan for revised patient or family caregiver teaching if patient or family caregiver is not able to teach back correctly. — Determines patient's and family caregiver's level of understanding of instructional topic.

STEP	RATIONALE
Unexpected Outcomes 1. Patient's respiratory distress increases. 2. Bloody secretions are suctioned.	**Related Interventions** • Suction further or implement nasal or tracheal suctioning (Skill 25.2). • Evaluate need for other means to protect airway (e.g., oral intubation, oral airway, positioning). • Provide supplemental oxygen. • Notify health care provider. • Assess oral cavity for trauma or lesions. • Reduce amount of suction pressure used. • Observe catheter tip for nicks, which cause mucosal trauma. • Increase frequency of oral hygiene.

Recording and Reporting

• Record the amount, consistency, color, and odor of secretions; number of times suctioned; patient's response to suctioning; and presuction and postsuction cardiopulmonary assessment findings on flow sheet or nurses' notes in electronic health record (EHR) or chart.
• Record patient's and family caregiver's understanding through teach-back for safe oral suctioning.
• Report any unresolved outcomes such as worsening respiratory distress to the health care provider.

Special Considerations

Teaching

• Instruct patient and family caregiver not to allow catheter to fall to the floor. If this occurs, teach patient and family caregiver how to clean or obtain a clean catheter (see Home Care considerations).
• Provide information regarding signs and symptoms of worsening respiratory status.

Pediatric

• Airways of infants and children are smaller than those of an adult; even small amounts of mucus cause airway obstruction. Smaller suction catheters may need to be used (Hockenberry and Wilson, 2015).
• Bulb syringes may be used to suction the oral cavity in newborns and infants. To properly use a bulb syringe, compress the bulb before inserting into mouth to decrease the risk of forcing the secretions into lower airways. If the bulb syringe cannot remove the secretions, use appropriate-size mechanical suction equipment (Hockenberry and Wilson, 2015).
• Use lower suction pressures with infants and children than with adults (Hockenberry and Wilson, 2015).
• Position infants with breathing problems or excessive vomitus in side-lying position to decrease risk of aspiration (Hockenberry and Wilson, 2015).

• Suctioning, particularly for young infants, should be completed for only 5 seconds because of risk of deoxygenation. Allow 30 to 60 seconds for patient to reoxygenate (Hockenberry and Wilson, 2015).
• Complete oral suctioning first and then nasal suctioning to decrease the risk of aspiration, particularly for newborn infants (Hockenberry and Wilson, 2015).

Gerontological

• Patients with dysphagia may benefit from oral suctioning before, during, and after meals.
• Oral mucosa in older adults is fragile (Touhy and Jett, 2014). Use a lower suction pressure if bleeding starts to occur.
• Older adults are prone to aspiration of oral secretions because of decreased cough and gag reflexes and increased incidence of dysphagia (Touhy and Jett, 2014).

Home Care

• Make sure that patient and family caregiver know how to clean and disinfect or change the secretion collection container every 24 hours according to home care protocol. Many agencies seal and dispose of the entire disposable secretion collection canister as biohazardous material.
• Assess knowledge level of patient and family caregiver to determine amount of instruction required and frequency of home health visits necessary to reach goals.
• Assess home for the presence of respiratory irritants, including cigarette smoke, dust, pollen, animal dander, mold, and chemicals.

Long-Term Care

• As many as 60% of patients who live in nursing homes have evidence of dysphagia, which makes them prone to aspiration. Ensure that dysphagia screens are performed for all patients and that properly functioning equipment is available in the agency (Touhy and Jett, 2014).

◆ SKILL 25.2   Airway Suctioning

NSO *Nursing Skills Online Airway Management Module / Lessons 1, 3, and 4*

Suctioning is necessary when patients are unable to clear respiratory secretions. If the secretions are only in the nose and mouth, only the pharynx requires suctioning. However, in most instances you will suction both the pharynx and the trachea. Suction secretions from the pharynx as often as necessary using oropharyngeal suctioning (see Skill 25.1). Secretions that are not removed are more likely to be aspirated into the lungs, increasing the risk for infection, ventilator-associated pneumonia, and respiratory failure. Retained lower airway secretions require the use of tracheal suction to remove.

Tracheal airway suctioning is a sterile procedure. It extends into the lower airway and is indicated to remove respiratory secretions and maintain optimum ventilation and oxygenation in patients who are unable to remove these secretions independently. This skill can be performed in people with or without an artificial airway.

Tracheal suctioning has many complications, including hypoxemia, cardiac dysrhythmias, changes in blood pressure (can be either hypertensive or hypotensive), laryngeal or bronchospasm, pain, infection, or bradycardia. Bradycardia is associated with stimulation of the vagus nerve. Respiratory or cardiac arrest can even occur as a result of tracheal suctioning. Nasal trauma and bleeding can develop from a suction catheter being introduced through the nares (Urden et al., 2016).

Patient assessment, not routine suctioning, guides the frequency of airway suctioning (Branson et al., 2014; Urden et al., 2016). Patient assessment factors indicating the need for suctioning include oxygen saturation below 90%; visible secretions in the airway; patient's inability to produce an effective, productive cough; auscultation of coarse crackles over the trachea; and acute respiratory distress. If the patient has an artificial airway in place and/or is mechanically ventilated, other indications for suctioning include the presence of a saw-tooth pattern on the flow-volume loop on the ventilator monitor, increased peak inspiratory pressure or decreased tidal volumes noted on the ventilator monitor, abnormal capnography waveforms, or suspected aspiration (AARC, 2010; Özden and Görgülü, 2012; Walsh et al., 2011; Wiegand, 2011).

Artificial Airway Suctioning

Endotracheal tubes (ETs) and tracheostomy tubes (TTs) are artificial airways inserted to maintain respiratory flow and prevent airway obstruction, provide a route for mechanical ventilation, permit easy access for secretion removal, and protect the airway from gross aspiration in patients with impaired cough or gag reflexes.

Endotracheal Tubes

NSO *Nursing Skills Online Airway Management Module / Lesson 4*

ET intubation is a procedure performed by a health care provider or other specially trained personnel (e.g., certified registered nurse anesthesiologist, respiratory therapist, or rescue personnel). An ET is inserted through the nares (nasotracheal tube) or most commonly through the mouth (oral ET) past the epiglottis and vocal cords into the trachea (Fig. 25.2A–B). Oral ETs are usually made of plastic or rubber. Adult (and some pediatric) sizes of ETs have a cuff molded onto the tube. When the cuff is inflated, it seals the airway around the tube to prevent the aspiration of oral secretions or gastric contents into the lung and/or to obstruct the escape of air from mechanical ventilator breaths through the upper airway. Some newer ETs also contain a port that can be connected for continuous subglottal suctioning.

The length of time that an ET should remain in place is controversial. Complications from long-term intubation include laryngeal and tracheal stenosis or a cricoid abscess (Urden et al., 2016). Sources differ on when a patient should be changed from an ET to a TT. The range of recommended length of time to be intubated is 7 to 10 days to as long as 21 days (Durbin, 2010; Morris et al., 2013; Urden et al., 2016). It is appropriate for you to consult with a health care provider if patients begin to show signs of complications from the airways themselves, such as erosion of the oral mucosa. Known benefits of having a TT versus an ET include less need for deeper sedation, shorter ventilator weaning time (time it takes to get a patient off a ventilator), and shorter ICU and hospital stay (Durbin, 2010).

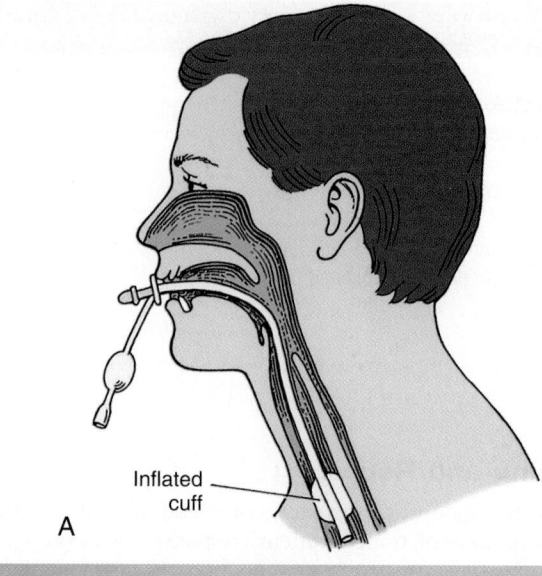

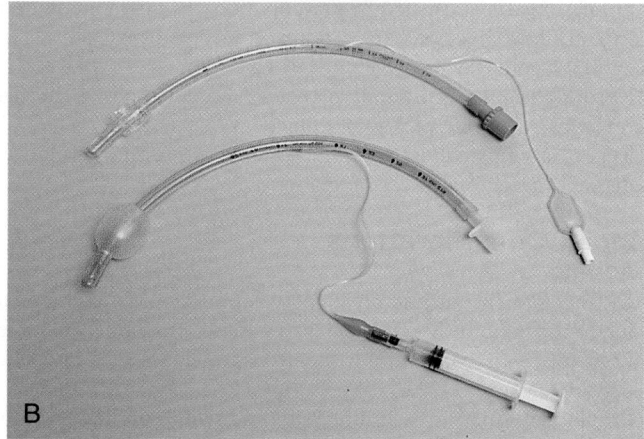

FIG 25.2 A, Endotracheal (ET) tube with inflated cuff. **B,** ET tubes with uninflated and inflated cuffs and syringe for inflation.

Tracheostomy Tubes

A TT can be temporary or permanent, depending on a patient's condition. It is inserted either surgically or percutaneously directly into the trachea through a small incision made in a patient's neck. Reasons for a TT include the need for prolonged mechanical ventilation, upper airway obstruction secondary to trauma or tumor, or difficulties with airway clearance that occurs in conditions such as spinal cord injury or neuromuscular disease (Myatt, 2015; Urden et al., 2016). TTs are made of several different materials, including polyvinyl chloride or silicone-based plastics and stainless steel or metallic compounds. Metal TTs are thermal sensitive and must be protected from extreme heat and cold to prevent tissue injury in a patient. Most metal and plastic TTs contain an inner cannula that is withdrawn temporarily for cleaning airway-occluding mucus without removing the entire TT (see Skill 25.4) (Myatt, 2015; Urden et al., 2016).

The use of closed-system suction catheters for suctioning artificial airways has increased in recent years. Use of a closed-system catheter (in-line) allows quicker lower airway suctioning without applying sterile gloves or a mask and does not interrupt ventilation and oxygenation in critically ill patients (see Procedural Guideline 25.1). With a closed-system method, the patient's artificial airway is not disconnected from the mechanical ventilator; therefore there is no loss of positive end-expiratory pressure (PEEP) (Branson et al., 2014). Other advantages of this system include a quicker, more efficient performance of the suctioning procedure (Özden and Görgülü, 2014). When comparing closed-versus-open suctioning, the incidence of ventilator-associated pneumonia (VAP) is unchanged (Branson et al., 2014). However, there is a decreased risk of infection for a health care provider from exposure to patient secretions with a closed system (Urden et al., 2016).

Delegation and Collaboration

The skill of artificial airway suctioning of newly inserted artificial airways cannot be delegated to nursing assistive personnel (NAP). At some agencies the NAP may suction a patient with a well-established tracheostomy that the nurse has determined to be stable. The nurse directs the NAP about:

- Any modifications of the skill such as the need for supplemental oxygen or the use of a clean-versus-sterile suction technique.
- Appropriate suction limits for suctioning ETs and TTs and risks of applying excessive or inadequate suction pressure.
- Reporting any changes in patient's respiratory status, level of consciousness, restlessness, secretion color and amount, and unresolved coughing or gagging.
- Reporting any change in patient's color, vital signs, or complaints of pain.

Equipment

- Stethoscope
- Pulse oximeter
- Portable or wall suction machine
- Connecting tubing (6 feet)
- Bedside table
- Mask, goggles, or face shield; gown if isolation procedures dictate

Endotracheal or Tracheostomy Suctioning

- Appropriate-size suction catheter, usually 12-16 Fr, (smallest diameter that will remove secretions effectively, preferably one that is no more than half of the internal diameter of the artificial airway to minimize decrease in PaO_2) (AARC, 2010; Branson et al., 2014)
- Two sterile gloves or one sterile and one clean glove
- Clean towel or paper drape
- Small Y-adapter (if catheter does not have a suction control port)
- Sterile basin or solution container
- Sterile normal saline solution or water, about 100 mL
- Pulse oximeter, stethoscope, and end-tidal CO_2 detector
- Manual self-inflating manual resuscitation bag-valve device with appropriate-size mask
- PEEP valve for resuscitation bag

STEP	RATIONALE

ASSESSMENT

1. Identify patient using at least two identifiers (e.g., name and birthday or name and medical record number) according to agency policy.

Ensures correct patient. Complies with The Joint Commission standards and improves patient safety (TJC, 2016).

2. Perform hand hygiene and apply gloves if risk of exposing self to secretions. Assess for signs and symptoms of upper and lower airway obstruction requiring suctioning: abnormal respiratory rate, adventitious lung sounds, nasal secretions, gurgling, drooling, restlessness, gastric secretions or vomitus in mouth, and coughing without clearing airway secretions and/or improving adventitious lung sounds.

Physical signs and symptoms result from secretions in upper and lower airways and decreased oxygen to the tissues. Presuction assessment provides baseline data to identify need for suctioning and measures the effectiveness of suction procedures (Branson et al., 2014).

3. Assess vital signs and signs and symptoms associated with hypoxia and hypercapnia: decreased pulse oximetry (SpO_2), increased pulse and blood pressure, apprehension, anxiety, lack of concentration, lethargy, decreased level of consciousness, confusion, dizziness, behavioral changes (e.g., irritability), irregular heart pulse, pallor, and cyanosis (a very late sign of hypoxia). Keep pulse oximeter on patient.

Physical signs and symptoms resulting from decreased tissue oxygenation. Provides presuction baseline to measure patient tolerance to suctioning and effectiveness of suctioning on SpO_2 levels.

4. Assess for risk factors for upper and lower airway obstruction, including chronic obstructive pulmonary disease, impaired mobility, decreased level of consciousness, nasal feeding tube, decreased cough or gag reflex, and decreased swallowing ability.

Risk factors can impair patient's ability to clear secretions from airway, increase risk for retaining secretions, and necessitate nasopharyngeal or nasotracheal suctioning (Urden et al., 2016).

5. Identify patients with an increased risk for ineffective airway clearance (e.g., patients with decreased level of consciousness, neuromuscular or neurological impairment, or anatomical factors that influence upper or lower airway function such as recent surgery head chest or neck tumors.

Changes in neurological status and neuromuscular impairment increase likelihood that patient is unable to clear respiratory secretions. Abnormal anatomy or head and neck surgery/ trauma and tumors in and around lower airway impair normal secretion clearance. Accumulating pulmonary secretions impede patient's ability to effectively clear airway through cough mechanism (Urden et al., 2016).

STEP	RATIONALE
6. Assess for excessive amounts of secretions or secretions visible in the artificial airway, signs of respiratory distress (increased work of breathing, increased respiratory rate), presence of rhonchi on auscultation, excessive coughing, increased peak inspiratory pressures (if on mechanical ventilator), saw-tooth pattern on ventilator monitor, or changes in capnography waveform (if patient on mechanical ventilator) or decrease in patient pulse oximeter (Branson et al., 2014).	Suctioning should only be performed as patient condition indicates and not in a scheduled fashion such as hourly (Lewis et al., 2017, Myatt, 2015).
7. Assess patency of ET with capnography/end-tidal carbon dioxide (CO_2) detector.	ET may become displaced or blocked by secretions. CO_2 detector is pH sensitive and can identify changes in CO_2 levels caused by retained secretions (Walsh et al., 2011).
8. Assess factors that may affect volume and consistency of secretions.	Thickened or copious secretions increase risk for airway obstruction.
a. Fluid balance	Fluid overload increases amount of secretions. Dehydration promotes thicker secretions.
b. Lack of humidity	Environment influences secretion formation and gas exchange. Airway suctioning is needed when patient cannot clear secretions effectively.
c. Infection (e.g., pneumonia)	Patients with respiratory infections are prone to increased secretions that are thicker and sometimes more difficult to expectorate.
9. For endotracheal suctioning assess patient's peak inspiratory pressure when on volume-controlled ventilation or tidal volume during pressure-controlled ventilation.	Increased peak inspiratory pressure or decreased tidal volume may indicate airway obstruction (Urden et al., 2016).

Clinical Decision Point *The patient's vital signs, pulse oximetry, end-tidal CO_2, and respiratory status will be assessed before and continuously throughout the procedure (Wiegand, 2011).*

STEP	RATIONALE
10. Identify contraindications to nasotracheal suctioning (AARC, 2004): occluded nasal passages; nasal bleeding; epiglottis or croup; acute head, facial, or neck injury or surgery; coagulopathy or bleeding disorder; irritable airway; laryngospasm or bronchospasm; gastric surgery with high anastomosis; myocardial infarction.	These conditions are contraindicated because passage of suction catheter through nasal route causes trauma to existing facial trauma/surgery, increases nasal bleeding, or causes severe bleeding in presence of coagulopathy or bleeding disorders. In presence of epiglottis or croup, laryngospasm, or irritable airway, passage of suction catheter through nose causes intractable coughing, hypoxemia, and severe bronchospasm, necessitating emergency intubation or tracheostomy. Hypoxemia could worsen cardiac damage in myocardial infarction (AARC, 2004).
11. Review sputum microbiology data in laboratory report.	Certain bacteria are easier to transmit or require isolation because of virulence or antibiotic resistance.
12. Determine presence of apprehension, anxiety, decreased ability to concentrate, lethargy, decreased level of consciousness (especially acute), increased fatigue, dizziness, behavioral changes (especially irritability), pallor, cyanosis, dyspnea, or use of accessory muscles.	These are signs and symptoms of hypoxia and/or hypercapnia, which can indicate need for suction. These signs can also help to identify patient's ability to cooperate with procedure.
13 Assess for patient's understanding of procedure and presence of any apprehension.	Reveals need for instruction or psychosocial support.

NURSING DIAGNOSES

- Anxiety
- Deficient knowledge regarding suctioning
- Fatigue

- Impaired comfort
- Impaired gas exchange
- Impaired spontaneous ventilation
- Impaired swallowing

- Ineffective airway clearance
- Ineffective breathing pattern
- Risk for aspiration
- Risk for infection

Related factors/Risk factors are individualized based on patient's condition or needs.

STEP	RATIONALE

PLANNING

1. Expected outcomes following completion of procedure:
   - Upper and lower airways demonstrate absent or diminished gurgles, crackles, rhonchi, and wheezes on inspiration and expiration.

     Absent or diminished adventitious sounds indicates that airways are cleared of secretions and are patent.

   - Heart rate, blood pressure, respiratory rate, and effort are within normal range for patient.

     When airway secretions are removed and oxygenation improves, patient's vital signs and respiratory assessment findings improve.

   - Patient's SpO_2 is at or above baseline whereas end-tidal carbon dioxide concentration (E_TCO_2), if being monitored, is at or below baseline.

     Demonstrates improvement in gas exchange (Branson et al., 2014; Wiegand, 2011).

Clinical Decision Point *While normal E_TCO_2 ranges from 35 to 45 mm Hg, it is important to ensure that the patient's value is below the normal baseline. Persons with pulmonary diseases often have abnormal CO_2 values.*

   - Patient's peak inspiratory pressure decreases back to baseline, and exhaled tidal volume increases back to baseline.

     Demonstrates removal of secretions (Wiegand, 2011).

2. Help patient to comfortable position, typically semi-Fowler's or high Fowler's.

   Reduces stimulation of gag reflex, promotes patient comfort and secretion drainage, and prevents aspiration.

3. If not already present, place pulse oximeter on patient's finger. Take reading and leave oximeter in place.

   Provides continuous SpO_2 value to determine patient's response to suctioning.

4. Explain to patient how procedure will help clear airway and relieve breathing difficulty. Explain that temporary coughing, sneezing, gagging, or shortness of breath is normal during procedure.

   Encourages cooperation and minimizes risks, anxiety, and pain of procedure.

IMPLEMENTATION

1. Perform hand hygiene and apply appropriate personal protective equipment (clean gloves and mask with face shield or goggles; gown if necessary).

   Reduces transmission of microorganisms.

2. Adjust bed to appropriate height (if not already done) and lower side rail on side nearest you. Check locks on bed wheel.

   Minimizes caregiver's muscle strain and prevents injury. Prevents bed from moving.

3. Connect one end of connecting tubing to suction device and place other end in convenient location near patient. Turn suction device on and set suction pressure to as low a level as possible and yet able to effectively clear secretions. This value is typically between 100 and 150 mm Hg in adults (between 60 and 100 mm Hg in neonates) (AARC, 2010). Suction pressure should not exceed 180 mm Hg (Branson et al., 2014). Occlude end of suction tubing to check pressure.

   Ensures equipment function. Excessive negative pressure damages tracheal mucosa and induces greater hypoxia (Wiegand, 2011).

4. Prepare suction catheter for all types of open suctioning.
   a. Using aseptic technique, open suction kit or catheter package. If sterile drape is available, place it across patient's chest or on bedside table. Do not allow suction catheter to touch any nonsterile surfaces.

      Prepares catheter, maintains asepsis, and reduces transmission of microorganisms. Provides sterile surface on which to lay catheter between passes.

   b. Unwrap or open sterile basin and place on bedside table. Be careful not to touch inside of basin. Fill with about 100 mL sterile normal saline solution or water (see illustration).

      Saline or water is used to clean tubing after each suction pass.

   c. If performing nasotracheal suctioning, open packet of water-soluble lubricant and apply small amount to catheter. **NOTE:** *Lubricant is not necessary for artificial airway suctioning.*

      Water-soluble lubricant helps avoid lipid aspiration pneumonia. Excessive amount of lubricant occludes catheter.

5. Apply sterile gloves to each hand or nonsterile glove to nondominant hand and sterile glove to dominant hand.

   Reduces transmission of microorganisms and maintains sterility of suction catheter.

STEP	RATIONALE
6. Pick up suction catheter with dominant hand without touching nonsterile surfaces. Pick up connecting tubing with nondominant hand. Secure catheter to tubing (see illustration).	Maintains catheter sterility. Connects catheter to suction.
7. Place tip of catheter into sterile basin and suction small amount of normal saline solution from basin by occluding suction vent.	Ensures equipment function. Lubricates internal catheter and tubing.
8. Suction airway.	
a. Nasopharyngeal and nasotracheal suctioning:	
(1) Have patient take deep breaths, if able, or increase oxygen flow rate with delivery device through cannula or mask (if ordered).	May help to decrease risks of hypoxemia.
(2) Lightly coat distal 6–8 cm (2–3 inches) of catheter with water-soluble lubricant.	Lubricates catheter for easier insertion.
(3) Remove oxygen-delivery device, if applicable, with nondominant hand.	Allows access to nares and catheter.

Clinical Decision Point *Be sure to insert catheter during patient inhalation, especially if inserting it into trachea, because epiglottis is open. Do not insert during swallowing or catheter will most likely enter esophagus.* **Never apply suction during insertion.** *Patient should cough. If patient gags or becomes nauseated, catheter is most likely in esophagus, and you need to remove it.*

(a) *Nasopharyngeal (without applying suction):* As patient takes deep breath, insert catheter following natural course of naris; slightly slant catheter downward and advance to back of pharynx. Do not force through naris. In adults insert catheter approximately 16 cm (6.5 inches); in older children, 8–12 cm (3 to 5 inches); in infants and young children, 4–7.5 cm (1.5–3 inches). Rule of thumb is to insert catheter distance from tip of nose (or mouth) to angle of mandible.	Ensure that catheter tip reaches pharynx for suctioning.

Clinical Decision Point *If resistance is met during insertion, you may need to try the other naris. Do not force the catheter up the nares because this will cause mucosal damage.*

(i) Apply intermittent suction for no more than 10–15 seconds by placing and releasing nondominant thumb over catheter vent. Slowly withdraw catheter while rotating it back and forth between thumb and forefinger.	Intermittent suction up to 10–15 seconds safely removes pharyngeal secretions. Suction time greater than 10 to 15 seconds increases risk for suction-induced hypoxemia (AARC, 2010; Branson et al., 2014).

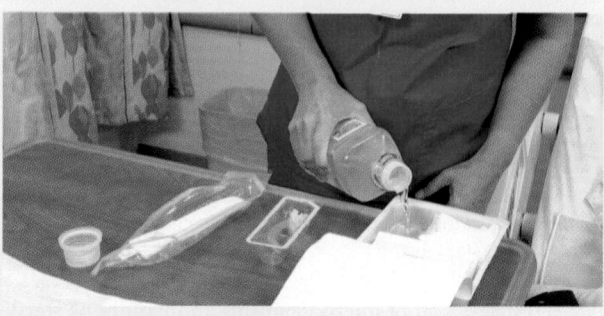

STEP 4b Pouring sterile saline into tray.

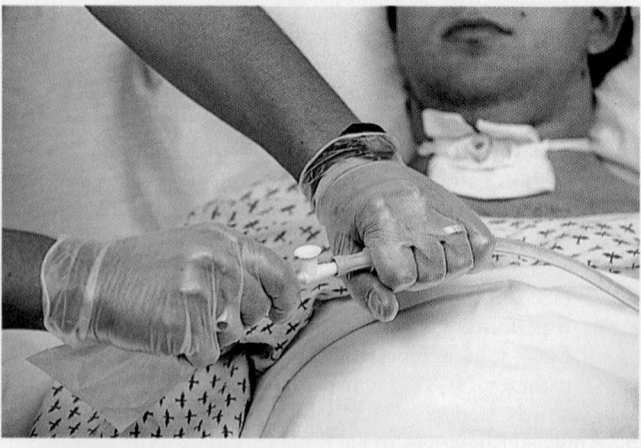

STEP 6 Attaching suction catheter to suction tubing.

STEP	RATIONALE

(b) *Nasotracheal* (without applying suction): As patient takes deep breath, advance catheter following natural course of naris. Advance catheter slightly slanted and downward to just above entrance into larynx and then trachea. While patient takes deep breath, quickly insert catheter: for adults insert approximately 16–20 cm (6–8 inches) into trachea (see illustration). Patient will begin to cough; then pull back catheter 1–2 cm (½ inch) before applying suction. **NOTE:** In older children, 16–20 cm (6–8 inches); in infants and young children, 8–14 cm (3–5½ inches).

Ensure that catheter tip reaches trachea for suctioning

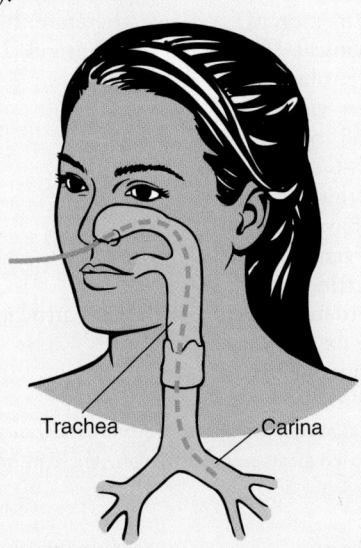

Trachea   Carina

STEP 8a(3)b Distance of insertion of nasotracheal catheter.

Clinical Decision Point *When using the nasal approach, perform tracheal suctioning before pharyngeal suctioning whenever possible. The mouth and pharynx contain more bacteria than the trachea. If copious oral secretions are present before beginning the procedure, suction mouth with oral suction device first.*

Clinical Decision Point *When there is difficulty passing the catheter, ask patient to cough or say "ahh" or try to advance the catheter during inspiration. Both measures help to open the glottis to permit passage of the catheter into the trachea.*

(i) *Positioning option:* In some instances turning patient's head helps you suction more effectively. If you feel resistance after insertion of catheter, use caution; it has probably hit the carina. Pull catheter back 1–2 cm (0.4–0.8 inches) before applying suction (AARC, 2004).

Turning patient's head to side elevates bronchial passage on opposite side. Turning head to right helps with suctioning of left main-stem bronchus; turning head to left helps you suction right main-stem bronchus. Suctioning too deep may cause tracheal mucosa trauma.

(ii) Apply intermittent suction for no more than 10–15 seconds by placing and releasing nondominant thumb over catheter vent. Slowly withdraw catheter while rotating it back and forth between thumb and forefinger.

Suction time greater than 15 seconds increases risk for suction-induced hypoxemia (AARC, 2010; Branson et al., 2014). Intermittent suction and rotation of catheter prevents injury to tracheal mucosa. If catheter "grabs" mucosa, remove thumb to release suction.

Clinical Decision Point *Monitor patient's vital signs and oxygen saturation throughout suctioning process. Stop suctioning if there is a 20 beats/min change (increase or decrease) in pulse rate or if SpO_2 falls below 90% or 5% from baseline.*

(4) Reapply oxygen-delivery device and encourage patient to take some deep breaths, if able.

Helps to decrease risk of hypoxia. Increases patient comfort.

STEP	RATIONALE

(5) Rinse catheter and connecting tubing with normal saline or water until cleared.

Secretions that remain in suction catheter or connecting tubing decrease suctioning efficiency.

(6) Assess for need to repeat suctioning. Do not perform more than two passes with catheter. Allow patient to rest at least 1 minute (AARC, 2010). Ask patient to deep breathe and cough.

Observe for alterations in cardiopulmonary status. Suctioning induces hypoxemia, irregular pulse, laryngospasm, and bronchospasm (AARC, 2010). Hyperoxygenation is recommended before, during, and after open suctioning to reduce suction-induced hypoxemia (Galbiati and Paola, 2015).

b. Artificial airway:

(1) When patient has an artificial airway, hyperoxygenate him or her with 100% oxygen for at least 30 to 60 seconds before suctioning by (1) pressing suction hyperoxygenation button on ventilator OR (2) increasing baseline fraction of inspired oxygen (FiO_2) level on mechanical ventilator OR; or (3) disconnecting ventilator, attaching self-inflating resuscitation bag-valve device to tube with nondominant hand (or have assistant do this), and administering 5–6 breaths over 30 seconds (or have assistant do this). **NOTE:** Some mechanical ventilators have a button that, when pushed, delivers 100% oxygen for a few minutes and then resets to previous setting.

Preoxygenation decreases risk of decreased arterial oxygen levels while ventilation or oxygenation is interrupted and volume is lost during suctioning (AARC, 2010). Some models of resuscitation bags do not deliver 100% oxygen; therefore this is not the best way to oxygenate patient (Wiegand, 2011).

(2) If patient is receiving mechanical ventilation, open swivel adapter or, if necessary, remove oxygen- or humidity-delivery device with nondominant hand.

Exposes artificial airway.

Clinical Decision Point *Suctioning can cause elevations in intracranial pressure (ICP) in patients with head injuries. Reduce this risk by presuction hyperoxygenation, which results in hypocarbia, which in turn induces vasoconstriction. Vasoconstriction reduces the potential for an increase in ICP (Urden et al., 2016).*

(3) Advise patient that you are about to begin suctioning. Without applying suction, gently but quickly insert catheter into artificial airway using dominant thumb and forefinger (it is best to try to time catheter insertion into artificial airway with inspiration) (see illustration). Advance catheter until you meet resistance or patient coughs; then pull back 1 cm (0.4 inch) (Wiegand, 2011).

Application of suction pressure while introducing catheter into trachea increases risk for damage to tracheal mucosa and increased hypoxia. Pulling back stimulates cough and removes catheter from mucosal wall so catheter is not resting against tracheal mucosa during suctioning. Shallow suctioning is recommended to prevent tracheal mucosa trauma (AARC, 2010; Wiegand, 2011).

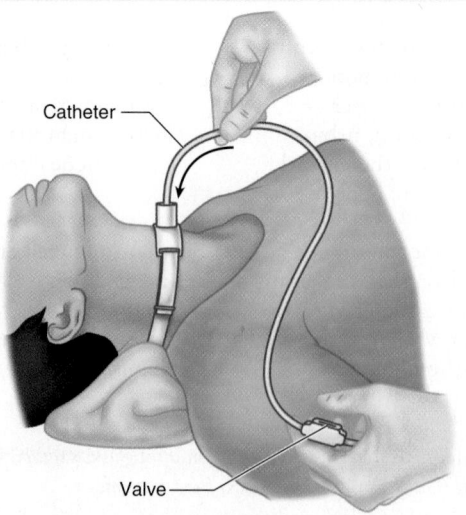

STEP 8b(3) Suctioning tracheostomy.

STEP	RATIONALE

Clinical Decision Point *If unable to insert catheter past the end of the ET, the catheter is probably caught in the Murphy eye (i.e., side hole at the distal end of the ET that allows for collateral airflow in the event of tracheal main-stem intubation). If this happens, rotate the catheter to reposition it away from the Murphy eye or withdraw it slightly and reinsert with the next inhalation. Usually the catheter meets resistance at the carina. One indication that the catheter is at the carina is acute onset of coughing because the carina contains many cough receptors. Pull the catheter back 1 cm (½ inch).*

(4) Apply intermittent suction for 10–15 seconds (AARC, 2010; Branson et al., 2014). Apply intermittent suction by placing and releasing nondominant thumb over vent of catheter; slowly withdraw catheter while rotating it back and forth between dominant thumb and forefinger. Do not use suction for greater than 15 seconds. Encourage patient to cough. Watch for respiratory distress.	Suction time greater than 15 seconds increases risk for suction-induced hypoxemia (AARC, 2010; Branson et al., 2014). Intermittent suction and rotation of catheter prevent injury to tracheal mucosa. If catheter "grabs" mucosa, remove thumb to release suction.

Clinical Decision Point *If patient develops respiratory distress during the suction procedure, immediately withdraw catheter and supply additional oxygen and breaths as needed. In an emergency administer oxygen directly through the catheter. Disconnect suction and attach oxygen at prescribed flow rate through the catheter. If the patient does not tolerate the suctioning procedure, you may need to consider switching to closed (in-line) suctioning or allowing longer recovery times. Notify health care provider if patient develops significant cardiopulmonary compromise during suctioning (Urden et al., 2016; Wiegand, 2011).*

(5) If patient is receiving mechanical ventilation, close swivel adapter or replace oxygen-delivery device. Hyperoxygenate patient for 30–60 seconds.	Reestablishes artificial airway. Helps to decrease risks of hypoxia.
(6) Rinse catheter and connecting tubing with normal saline until clear. Use continuous suction.	Removes catheter secretions. Secretions left in tubing decrease suctioning efficiency and provide environment for microorganism growth.
(7) Assess patient's vital signs, cardiopulmonary status, and ventilator measures for secretion clearance. Repeat Steps (1) through (6) once or twice more to clear secretions. Allow adequate time (at least 1 full minute) between suction passes.	Suctioning can induce dysrhythmias, hypoxia, and bronchospasm and impair cerebral circulation or adversely affect hemodynamic stability (Wiegand, 2011).

Clinical Decision Point *The number of suction passes should be based on patient assessment and presence of secretions. If secretions persist after two passes, allow patient more time to rest and recover from these procedures (Wiegand, 2011).*

(8) When pharynx and trachea are sufficiently cleared of secretions, perform oropharyngeal suctioning (Skill 25.1) to clear mouth of secretions. Do not suction nose again after suctioning mouth.	Removes upper airway secretions. More microorganisms generally are present in mouth. Upper airway is considered "clean," and lower airway is considered "sterile." You can use same catheter to suction from sterile to clean areas (e.g., tracheal suctioning to oropharyngeal suctioning) but not from clean to sterile areas.
9. When suctioning is complete, disconnect catheter from connecting tubing. Roll catheter around fingers of dominant hand. Pull glove off inside out so catheter remains coiled in glove. Pull off other glove over first glove in same way. Discard in appropriate receptacle. Turn off suction device.	Seals contaminants in gloves. Reduces transmission of microorganisms (Wiegand, 2011).
10. Remove towel, place in laundry or appropriate receptacle, and reposition patient. (Apply clean gloves to continue personal care.)	Reduces transmission of microorganisms. Promotes comfort.
11. If oxygen level was changed during procedure, readjust oxygen to original ordered level because patient's blood oxygen level should have returned to baseline.	Prevents absorption atelectasis (i.e., tendency for airways to collapse if proximally obstructed by secretions). Prevents oxygen toxicity while allowing patient time to reoxygenate blood.
12. Discard remainder of normal saline into appropriate receptacle. If basin is disposable, discard into appropriate receptacle. If basin is reusable, rinse it out and place it in soiled utility room.	Reduces transmission of microorganisms.
13. Remove personal protective equipment and discard into appropriate receptacle. Perform hand hygiene.	Reduces transmission of microorganisms.
14. Place unopened suction kit on suction machine table or at head of bed.	Provides immediate access to suction catheter for next procedure.
15. Help patient to comfortable position and provide oral hygiene as needed.	

STEP	RATIONALE

EVALUATION

1. Compare patient's vital signs, cardiopulmonary assessments, E_TCO_2 and SpO_2 values before and after suctioning. If on ventilator, compare FiO_2 and tidal volumes and peak inspiratory pressures.

Identifies physiological effects of suction procedure to restore airway patency.

2. Ask patient if breathing is easier and if congestion is decreased.

Provides subjective confirmation that suctioning procedure has relieved airway.

3. Auscultate lungs and compare patient's respiratory assessment before and after suctioning.

Provides objective information about any change in lung sounds.

4. Observe character of airway secretions.

Provides data to document presence or absence of respiratory tract infection or thickened secretions.

5. **Use Teach-Back**: "I need to suction your father and I want to be sure that I explained the suctioning procedure and when I need to do it. Please tell me in your own words why I'm suctioning him." Revise your instruction now or develop a plan for revised patient or family caregiver teaching if patient or family caregiver is not able to teach back correctly.

Determines patient's and family caregiver's level of understanding of instructional topic.

Unexpected Outcomes

1. Patient has decrease in overall cardiopulmonary status as evidenced by decreased SpO_2, increased E_TCO_2, continued tachypnea, continued increased work of breathing, and cardiac dysrhythmias.

2. Bloody secretions are returned after suctioning.

3. Patient has paroxysms of coughing or bronchospasm.

4. Inability to obtain secretions during suction procedure.

Related Interventions

- Limit length of suctioning.
- Determine need for more frequent suctioning, possibly of shorter duration.
- Determine need for supplemental or increase in supplemental oxygen. Supply oxygen between suctioning passes.
- Notify health care provider.
- Determine amount of suction pressure used. May need to be decreased.
- Ensure that suction is completed correctly using intermittent suction and catheter rotation. Do not apply suction until after catheter has been pulled back 1 cm (0.4 inches) to prevent applying suction while catheter is touching carina.
- Evaluate suctioning frequency.
- Provide more frequent oral hygiene.
- Administer supplemental oxygen.
- Allow patient to rest between passes of suction catheter.
- Consult with health care provider regarding need for inhaled bronchodilators or topical anesthetics.
- Evaluate patient's fluid status and adequacy of humidification on oxygen-delivery device.
- Assess for signs of infection.
- Determine need for chest physiotherapy (see Chapter 24).

Recording and Reporting

- Record the amount, consistency, color, and odor of secretions; size of catheter; route of suctioning; and patient's response to suctioning on flow sheet in nurses' notes in electronic health record (EHR) or chart.
- Record need for hyperoxygenation, type of hyperoxygenation, and % oxygenation used.
- Record patient's and family caregiver's understanding through teach-back.
- Document patient's presuctioning and postsuctioning vital signs, cardiopulmonary status, and ventilation measures on flow sheet in nurses' notes in EHR or chart.
- Report patient's intolerance to procedure or unexpected physiological changes to health care provider.

Special Considerations
Teaching

- Instruct patient that coughing increases and that there will be some discomfort during the procedure.
- Explain why supplemental oxygen is given before and after suctioning if indicated.

Pediatric

- The size of the suction catheter should occlude less than 70% of the artificial airway in infants and less than 50% of the artificial airway in children (AARC, 2010).
- Hyperoxygenate with 100% oxygen in pediatric patients and 10% increase of baseline in neonates before suctioning (Hockenberry and Wilson, 2015).

- Perform ET suctioning only when clinically indicated in infants and neonates. Clinical signs are notable changes in respiratory rate and breath sounds, increased secretions, bradycardia, or restlessness (Hockenberry and Wilson, 2015).
- Thick secretions are more difficult to remove because of small diameter of suction catheter. Normal saline should not be instilled in the airway in an attempt to thin the secretions (AARC, 2010).
- Make sure that distance suctioned is not greater than 0.5 cm (0.2 inches) beyond the tip of the artificial airway. To determine distance, place catheter near a sample artificial airway (Hockenberry and Wilson, 2015).
- Infant airways have less cartilage and may collapse easily, especially in premature infants or those with reactive airways.
- Suctioning should not last beyond 5 seconds, and negative pressure should not exceed 100 mm Hg (Hockenberry and Wilson, 2015).

Gerontological
- Older adults lose some properties of elastic recoil and gas exchange.
- Capillaries of older adults are often fragile, predisposing patient to bleeding problems.
- Patients with coronary artery disease are at greater risk for cardiopulmonary compromise.

Home Care
- Most patients with airway clearance problems at home have a tracheostomy,
- Instruct patient and family caregiver to clean and disinfect or change the secretion collection container every 24 hours according to home care or agency protocol.
- In the home setting stress the importance of brief intervals of applying suction pressure. Instruct those performing suctioning to hold their breath during the application of negative suction pressure to help them remember to not suction too long.

PROCEDURAL GUIDELINE 25.1 *Closed (In-Line) Suction*

NSO *Nursing Skills Online Airway Management Module / Lesson 4*

Closed suctioning (or in-line suctioning) is another method of suctioning an artificial airway. It involves the use of a multiuse suction catheter that is housed within a plastic sleeve and is attached to a patient's artificial airway (Fig. 25.3A–B). This method of suctioning is associated with decreased risk of hypoxia and cardiovascular complications when compared to open suctioning. It is also the recommended method of suctioning for patients who cannot tolerate loss of positive end-expiratory pressure (PEEP) such as those with severe respiratory disorders who require high amounts of PEEP or oxygen requirements (Wiegand, 2011).

Delegation and Collaboration
The skill of airway suction with a closed (in-line) suction catheter cannot be delegated to nursing assistive personnel (NAP). In special situations such as suctioning a well-established permanent tracheostomy, this procedure may be delegated to the NAP. The nurse is responsible for cardiopulmonary assessment and evaluation of patient. The nurse often collaborates with a respiratory therapist when assessing the patient and performing the suction procedure. The nurse directs the NAP about:
- Any individualized aspects of patient care that pertain to suctioning (e.g., position, duration of suction, pressure settings).
- Expected quality, quantity, and color of secretions and to inform the nurse immediately if there are changes.
- Patient's anticipated response to suction and to immediately report to the nurse changes in vital signs, complaints of pain, shortness of breath, confusion, or increased restlessness.

Equipment
- Closed-system or in-line suction catheter
- Sterile saline solution lavage containers (5 to 10 mL)
- Suction machine/source with regulator
- Connecting tubing (6 feet)
- Two clean gloves
- Oral suction kit/supplies for oropharyngeal suctioning
- Mask, goggles, or face shield; gown if isolation precautions indicate

- Pulse oximeter and stethoscope
- Manual self-inflating resuscitation bag (bag-valve-mask) with appropriate-size mask, while not necessary for the procedure, is safe to have on hand

Procedural Steps
1. Perform assessment as in Skill 25.2.
2. Perform hand hygiene. Gather equipment/supplies and close room door or curtain.
3. Identify patient using at least two identifiers (e.g., name and birthday or name and medical record number) according to agency policy (TJC, 2016).
4. Explain procedure to patient and the importance of coughing during the suctioning procedure. Even if patients cannot speak, they deserve to have information regarding the procedure.
5. Adjust the bed to appropriate height and lower side rail on the side nearest you. Check locks on the bed.
6. Help patient assume a position of comfort for both patient and nurse, usually semi- or high-Fowler's position. Place towel across patient's chest.
7. Apply clean gloves and face shield and attach suction:
   a. In many agencies a respiratory therapist attaches the catheter to the mechanical ventilator circuit. If catheter is not already in place, open suction catheter package using aseptic technique and attach closed suction catheter to ventilator circuit by removing swivel adapter and placing closed suction catheter apparatus on endotracheal tube (ET) or tracheostomy tube (TT). Connect Y on mechanical ventilator circuit to closed suction catheter with flex tubing (see Fig. 25.3A).
   b. Connect one end of connecting tubing to suction machine; connect other end to the end of a closed-system or in-line suction catheter. Turn suction device on, set vacuum regulator to appropriate negative pressure, and check pressure. Many closed-system suction catheters require slightly higher suction pressures (consult manufacturer guidelines).

Continued

PROCEDURAL GUIDELINE 25.1 *Closed (In-Line) Suction—cont'd*

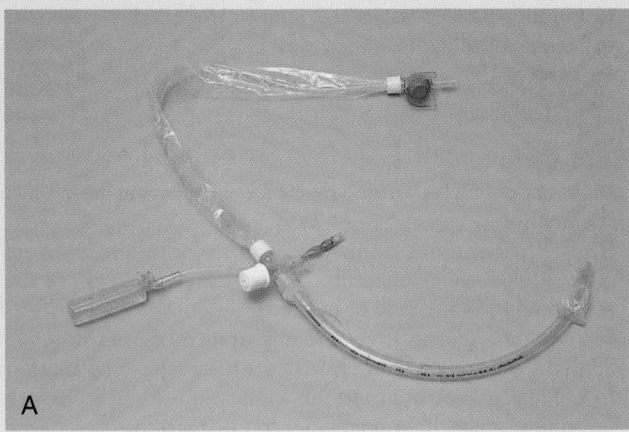

A

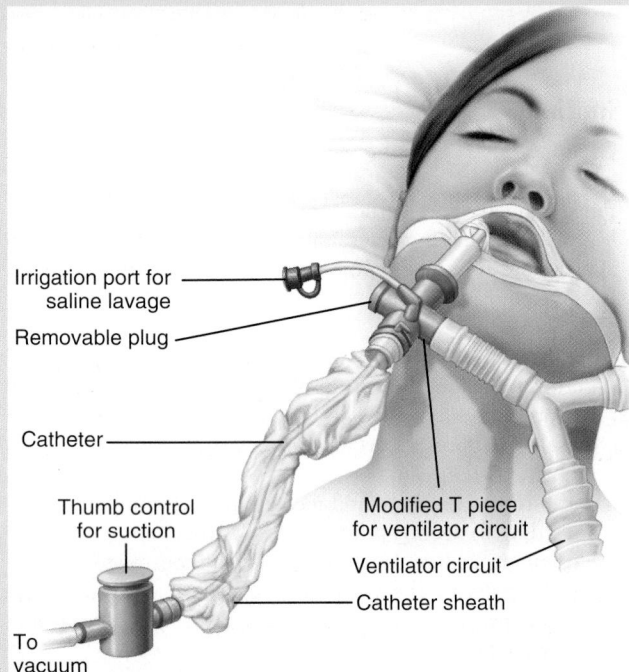

Irrigation port for
saline lavage

Removable plug

Catheter

Thumb control
for suction

Modified T piece
for ventilator circuit

Ventilator circuit

Catheter sheath

To
vacuum
B source

FIG 25.3 A, Closed-system suction catheter attached to endotracheal tube. **B,** Closed suction system attached to an endotracheal tube. (**B** *from Blanchard B: Thoracic surgery. In Rothrock JC, McEwen DR, eds. Alexander's care of the patient in surgery, ed 14, St Louis, 2011, Mosby.)*

8. Hyperoxygenate patient (usually 100% oxygen) by adjusting the fraction of inspired oxygen (FiO₂) setting on the ventilator or by using a temporary oxygen-enrichment program available on microprocessor ventilators according to agency policy or protocol. (Manual ventilation is not recommended.)
9. Unlock suction control mechanism if required by manufacturer. Open saline port and attach saline syringe or vial.
10. Pickup suction catheter enclosed in plastic sleeve with dominant hand.

11. Wait until patient inhales to insert catheter. Then insert catheter using a repeating maneuver of pushing catheter and sliding (or pulling) plastic sleeve back between thumb and forefinger until resistance is felt or patient coughs. Pull back 1 cm (0.4 inches) before applying suction to avoid tissue damage to tracheal carina.
12. Encourage patient to cough and apply suction by squeezing on suction control mechanism while withdrawing catheter. **NOTE:** It is difficult to apply intermittent pulses of suction and nearly impossible to rotate the catheter compared to standard catheter. Apply continuous suction for 10 to 15 seconds but no longer than 15 seconds as you remove the suction catheter (AARC, 2010; Branson et al., 2014). Be sure to withdraw catheter completely into plastic sheath and past the tip of the airway so it does not obstruct airflow.
13. Reassess cardiopulmonary status, including pulse oximetry (SpO₂) and ventilator measures, to determine need for subsequent suctioning or complications. Repeat Steps 8 to 12 one more time to clear secretions if patient condition indicates. Allow adequate time (at least 1 full minute) between suction passes for ventilation and reoxygenation.
14. When airway is clear, withdraw catheter completely into sheath. Be sure that colored indicator line on catheter is visible in the sheath. Attach sterile solution lavage container or sterile saline or water syringe to side port of suction catheter. Squeeze vial or push syringe while applying suction to rinse inner lumen of catheter. Use at least 5 to 10 mL of saline to rinse the catheter until it is clear of retained secretions, which can cause bacterial growth and increase the risk for infection (AARC, 2004). Lock suction mechanism if applicable and turn off suction.
15. Hyperoxygenate for at least 1 minute by following the same technique used to preoxygenate (Wiegand, 2011).
16. If patient requires oral or nasal suctioning, perform Skill 25.1 or 25.2 with separate standard suction catheter.
17. Place the Yankauer catheter on a clean, dry area for reuse with suction turned off or within patient's reach with suction on if patient is capable of suctioning his or her own mouth.
18. Reposition patient. Remove gloves, face shield, and other personal protective equipment; discard into appropriate receptacle; and perform hand hygiene.
19. Compare patient's vital signs and SpO₂ before and after suctioning.
20. Auscultate lung fields and compare with baseline.
21. Observe airway secretions.
22. Ask patient if breathing is easier and congestion is decreased.
23. **Use Teach-Back:** "I want to be sure I explained this suctioning procedure correctly. Please squeeze my hand if you understand these steps. Each time I suction you I will explain these steps again." Revise your instruction now or develop a plan for revised patient or family caregiver teaching if patient or family caregiver is not able to teach back correctly.

NSO *Nursing Skills Online Airway Management Module / Lesson 4*

Endotracheal tubes (ETs) are flexible, plastic tubes placed in the mouth or through the nose and advanced down into the trachea to establish short-term artificial airways to administer mechanical ventilation, relieve upper airway obstruction, protect against aspiration, and clear secretions (see Fig. 25.2). Routine care maintains correct position of the tube and good hygiene.

After insertion of an ET, the cuff is inflated, and the tube is secured with tape or a commercially available device. A cuff on an ET prevents the escape of air between the tube and the walls of the trachea and reduces the risk of aspiration when a patient is receiving mechanical ventilation (Box 25.1). The amount of air or water inserted in a cuff is based on two factors (i.e., the size of the patient's trachea and the external diameter of the artificial airway). If the cuff pressures are too high, permanent damage to the tracheal mucosa occurs, leading to complications such as tracheomalacia; tracheoesophageal fistula; or erosion of the innominate artery, which is rare but almost always fatal (Morris et al., 2013). If the cuff pressure is too low, the mechanical ventilation will not be effective; and the patient has an increased risk of aspiration, which increases the risk of developing ventilator-associated pneumonia (VAP) (Myatt, 2015).

Preventing tube-related complications is a critical component of care and depends on securing the tube and inflating the cuff properly. In many agencies these functions are the responsibility of respiratory therapy. However, the nurse is responsible for assessing the patient's respiratory status, ventilator settings and functioning, and integrity of the airway cuff.

Properly securing an ET prevents inadvertent extubation from coughing, gagging, or accidental pulling on the tube. Additional risks of movement of an artificial airway are tracheal stenosis; tracheomalacia; barotrauma; erosion of the innominate artery; and tracheoesophageal fistula, particularly when the cuff is overinflated (Branson et al., 2014). In addition, the risk for device-related pressure injuries increases because of pressure from the artificial airway on adjacent tissues (e.g., lips, oral mucosa) (Pittman et al., 2015).

Once a tube is inserted, confirmation of placement is achieved using a chest x-ray film and a disposable end-tidal CO_2 detector (Fig. 25.4) (Wiegand, 2011). Capnography, the noninvasive measurement of the partial pressure of carbon dioxide (CO_2) in exhaled breath expressed as the CO_2 concentration over time, is used to continuously monitor CO_2 once the patient is placed on mechanical ventilation. It is recommended as a reliable way to validate the correct placement of an ET (AARC, 2011). The CO_2 monitor measures CO_2 directly from the airway, with the sensor located on the airway adapter at the hub of the ET.

After a tube is inserted and secured and the cuff is inflated, your chief concern is to maintain patency of the ET and prevent a ventilator-associated event (VAE). Please refer to Chapter 23 for more information regarding VAE. In patients who cannot clear their secretions, periodic suctioning of the artificial airway achieves airway patency.

Delegation and Collaboration

This skill of performing ET care cannot be delegated to nursing assistive personnel (NAP). NAP may assist the nurse with ET care. Often the nurse collaborates with a respiratory therapist in performing this care. The nurse directs the NAP to:

- Immediately report any signs of respiratory problems or increased airway secretions.
- Immediately report if the ET appears to have moved or become obstructed or dislodged.
- Immediately report changes in patient's mood, level of consciousness, irritability, vital signs, decreased pulse oximetry value, or changes in end-tidal CO_2 values.

Equipment

- Towel
- ET and oropharyngeal suction equipment
- 1- or ½-inch-wide adhesive or waterproof tape (do not use paper or silk tape) or commercial ET holder and mouth guard (follow manufacturer instructions for securing)
- Oral airway and bite block (bite block is optional and only used is patient is biting ET)
- Suction equipment
- Clean gloves
- Adhesive remover swab or acetone on cotton ball
- Oral hygiene supplies: pediatric toothbrush (or suction toothbrush), toothette for edentulous patients

BOX 25.1

Indications for Cuff Inflation

Mechanical Ventilation	Risk of Aspirating Gastric Contents
• Continuous positive airway pressure	• Feeding tube, especially large-bore, in stomach
• Positive end-expiratory pressure (PEEP)	• Gastroesophageal reflux disease
• Inability to meet ventilatory requirements with cuff down	• Hiatal hernia
• Inability to meet oxygen requirements with cuff down	• During and after meals
	• Impaired gastric emptying
	• Decreased gag reflex
	• Impaired swallowing

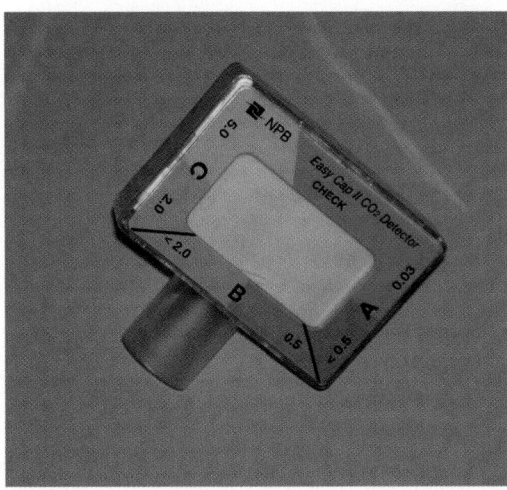

FIG 25.4 End-tidal CO_2 detector. (*Used by permission from Nellcor Puritan Bennett LLC, Boulder, Colo, doing business as Covidien.*)

- Cleaning solution: 0.12% to 0.20% chlorhexidine mouthwash, rinse, or gel
- Face cleaner (e.g., wet washcloth, towel, soap, shaving supplies
- Clean 2 × 2 gauze
- Tincture of benzoin, liquid adhesive, or skin preparation pads
- Tongue blade (optional)

- Mask, goggles, face shield (if indicated); gown if isolation procedures indicate
- Stethoscope
- Pulse oximeter, end-tidal CO_2 detector
- Another health care team member (need two people to perform some of the steps)
- Communication device (letter or picture board, tablet, paper and pen)

STEP	RATIONALE

ASSESSMENT

1. Identify patient using at least two identifiers (e.g., name and birthday or name and medical record number) according to agency policy.

2. Auscultate lungs and observe respiratory rate and depth.

3. Perform hand hygiene and apply gloves. Observe condition of tissues surrounding ET for impaired skin integrity (e.g., blistering, abrasions, pressure injuries) on nares, lips, cheeks, or corner of mouth; excess nasal or oral secretions; patient moving tube with tongue, biting tube or tongue, and foul-smelling mouth.

4. Observe patency of airway: excess intratracheal or endotracheal secretions, diminished airflow, and sign and symptoms of airway obstruction.

5. Observe for signs and symptoms of gurgling on expiration, decreased exhaled tidal volume (mechanically ventilated patient), signs and symptoms of inadequate ventilation (rising end-tidal carbon dioxide concentration [E_TCO_2], patient-ventilator dyssynchrony, or dyspnea), spasmodic coughing, tense test balloon on tube, flaccid test balloon on tube, and ability to speak or vocalize.

6. Observe for factors that increase risk for complications from ET: type and size of tube, movement of tube up and down trachea (in and out), duration of tube placement, presence of facial trauma, malnutrition, and neck or thoracic radiation.

7. Assess for patient's ability to verbalize around ET or for presence of audible air leak.

Ensures correct patient. Complies with The Joint Commission standards and improves patient safety (TJC, 2016).

Provides baseline measure of ventilation.
Presence of ET impairs ability of patient to swallow oral secretions. Patient is at increased risk for developing pressure areas from impaired circulation as tube is pulled or pressed against mucosal tissues (Pittman et al., 2015).

Buildup of secretions in ET impairs oxygen delivery and subsequent tissue oxygenation.

Cuff underinflation increases risk for aspiration, allows secretions to enter the trachea, and permits vocalization.
Cuff overinflation may cause ischemia or necrosis of tracheal tissue from obstruction of capillary bed, resulting in tracheomalacia or tracheoesophageal fistula (Myatt, 2015).

Tube rotating from side to side can cause medical device–related pressure injuries. Tube can become dislodged from lower airway (incidental extubation), or it can enter right main-stem bronchus. Longer duration of intubation is associated with increased risk for lower airway complications such as ventilator-associated event (VAE)/ventilator-associated pneumonia (VAP) (Bouadma et al., 2012).
Underinflated cuff allows passage of air through patient's vocal cords and increases patient's risk for aspiration (Morris et al., 2013).

Clinical Decision Point *When assessment indicates possible overinflation or underinflation of ET cuff, notify respiratory therapy and follow agency policy for correcting cuff pressures. Most sources agree that 20 cm H_2O is the lowest accepted pressure, but some sources recommend that the highest pressure to maintain the cuff is 25 cm H_2O (AACN, 2016; Dawson, 2014b; Myatt, 2015; Wiegand, 2011).*

8. Determine proper ET depth as noted by centimeters at lip or gum line. This line is marked on tube and recorded in patient's record at time of intubation and every shift.

9. Assess patient's knowledge of procedure.

Ensures that tube is at proper depth to adequately ventilate both lungs and that it is not too high, which causes vocal cord damage, or too low, which results in right main-stem intubation, in which only the right lung is ventilated.
Encourages cooperation, minimizes risks and anxiety. Identifies teaching needs.

NURSING DIAGNOSES

- Fatigue
- Impaired gas exchange
- Impaired skin integrity (or risk for)
- Impaired verbal communication

- Ineffective airway clearance
- Ineffective breathing pattern
- Risk for aspiration

- Risk for impaired oral mucous membrane
- Risk for infection

Related factors/Risk factors are individualized based on patient's condition or needs.

STEP	RATIONALE

PLANNING

1. Expected outcomes following completion of procedure:
   - ET remains in correct position in patient's trachea, evidenced by depth of tube same as when started or as ordered (same centimeter marking at gums or lips); bilateral breath sounds are equal; E_TCO_2 values remain at patient baseline.

   Maintaining ET position promotes adequate ventilation of lungs. Complications of lower airway and vocal cord trauma prevented.

   - Patient's skin around mouth and oral mucous membranes remains intact without evidence of pressure or other injury from biting or from ET itself.

   ET does not place undue pressure against corners of mouth, causing pressure area. Patient is not able to bite inner cheeks or tongue.

2. Perform hand hygiene. Gather equipment/supplies and arrange at bedside. Close room curtain or door.

   Ensures that nurse has the necessary equipment to implement all interventions that should be completed for patient. Ensures patient privacy.

3. Obtain assistance from available staff for this procedure.

   Reduces risk for accidental extubation of ET.

4. Assist patient in assuming comfortable position for both patient and you. Elevate patient's head of bed at least 30 degrees, unless patient is at risk for pressure injury.

   Provides access to site and facilitates completion of procedure. Prepares patient for oropharyngeal suctioning. Evidence favoring head-of-bed elevation to help prevent VAP is not apparent (Munro and Ruggiero, 2014). Position may decrease risk of aspiration (IHI, 2012).

5. Explain procedure and patient's need to participate, including not biting or moving ET with tongue, trying not to cough when tape is off ET, keeping hands down, and not pulling on tubing.

   Reduces anxiety, encourages cooperation, and reduces risk of accidental extubation.

IMPLEMENTATION

1. Perform hand hygiene. Apply clean gloves and mask, goggles, or face shield if indicated. Have assistant do so as well.

   Reduces transmission of microorganisms.

2. Place clean towel across patient's chest.

   Reduces soiling of bed clothes and linen.

3. Perform endotracheal or oropharyngeal suction if indicated (see Skills 25.1 and 25.2 and Procedural Guideline 25.1).

   Removes secretions. Diminishes patient's need to cough during procedure.

4. Connect Yankauer suction catheter to suction source and have it ready to use. Ensure that suction source/machine for oral suctioning is on and functioning properly.

   Need to have functioning equipment to perform oral care appropriately. Prepares suction apparatus.

5. Remove oral airway or bite block, if present, and place on towel.

   Provides access to and complete observation of patient's oral cavity.

Clinical Decision Point *If patient is biting the tube, do not remove bite block until absolutely necessary. This prevents obstruction of the ET and occlusion of the airway.*

6. Brush teeth with soft toothbrush, using solution or toothpaste that helps to break down plaque buildup on teeth. Suction oropharyngeal secretions as necessary.

   There may be need for pediatric toothbrush, depending on size of patient's oral cavity. It is recommended to brush teeth at least twice a day (AACN, 2010).

7. Use chlorhexidine solution and oral swabs to clean mouth. Suction oropharyngeal secretions as necessary. Apply mouth moisturizer to oral mucosa and lips after each cleaning.

   This step should be completed every 2 to 4 hours (AACN, 2010). The swabs, solution, and moisturizer may come in a prepackaged kit from manufacturer. The use of chlorhexidine mouthwash or gel is effective in reducing VAP (Munro and Ruggiero, 2014).

Clinical Decision Point *It may be useful to have the assistant constantly suction the oral cavity during the procedure. This helps to prevent the pooling and aspiration of oral secretions. Use continuous subglottic suctioning if available at your agency (Wiegand, 2011).*

STEP	RATIONALE
8. Prepare ET securement options: a. *Tape method:* Prepare tape by cutting piece of tape long enough to go completely around patient's head from naris to naris plus 15 cm (6 inches). This is typically 30–60 cm (12–24 inches) in total length. Lay tape adhesive-side up on bedside table. Cut and lay 8–15 cm (3–6 inches) of second piece of tape, adhesive sides together, in center of the long strip to prevent tape from sticking to hair. Smaller strip of tape should cover area between ears around back of head.	Preparing tape ahead decreases amount of time one has to manually hold ET throughout procedure, therefore decreasing risk of tube dislodgement. Adhesive tape needs to encircle head below ears with sufficient tape left to wrap around tube.
b. *Commercially available ET holder:* Open package per manufacturer instructions. Set device aside with head guard in place and Velcro strips open.	Commercial devices are latex free, fast, convenient, and disposable.

Clinical Decision Point *It is a nursing decision whether to use tape or a commercially available ET holder. There are advantages and disadvantages to both (Branson et al., 2014).*

STEP	RATIONALE
9. Remove old tape or device. a. *Tape:* While one person is holding and stabilizing ET, the other person should remove tape from patient, using adhesive tape remover. The tape will also need to be removed from ET itself.	Provides access to skin under tape for assessment and hygiene. Adhesive tape remover ensures easier, less traumatic removal of the tape.

Clinical Decision Point *Clean ET tube with soap and water as needed. Do not apply adhesive tape remover to the ET itself. This action will make it nearly impossible for the new tape to appropriately stick to the ET, which increases risk of tube dislodgement. Do not allow assistant to hold the tube away from the lips or nares. Doing so allows too much movement in the tube and increases the risk for tube movement and accidental extubation. Never let go of the ET because it could become dislodged.*

STEP	RATIONALE
b. *Commercially available device:* Remove Velcro strips from ET and remove ET holder from patient.	Velcro adhesive strips hold ET in place and provide marker to measure distance to patient's lips or gums. These devices all permit access to patient's mouth and lips for ease in oropharyngeal suctioning and oral hygiene.

Clinical Decision Point *Do not allow assistant to hold the tube away from the lips or nares. Doing so allows too much movement in the tube and increases the risk for tube movement and accidental extubation. Never let go of the ET because it could become dislodged.*

STEP	RATIONALE
10. Remove excess secretions or adhesive from patient's face. Clean facial skin with mild soap and water and dry thoroughly. Apply tape adherence product such as tincture of benzoin to face.	Application of tape adherence product is necessary for new tape or device to stay on patient's face (Wiegand, 2011).

Clinical Decision Point *Do not remove oral airway of bite block if patient is actively biting. Wait until the new tape or commercial device is partially or completely secured to ET.*

STEP	RATIONALE
11. Note level of ET by looking at mark or noting centimeter value on tube itself. Move oral ET to other side of mouth and ensure that tube marking at lip is unchanged. Perform oral care as needed on side where tube was initially positioned. Clean oral airway or bite block with warm soapy water and rinse well. Reinsert as necessary.	Changing sides of ET removes pressure and decreases risk of breakdown at corners of mouth and oral mucosa (Pittman et al., 2015; Wiegand, 2011).

Clinical Decision Point *The patient may cough excessively when the tube is being moved. The person who is holding the tube in place should be prepared for this and take extra caution while holding. In some instances the ET may need to be secured with the tape before the rest of the oral care is performed. In some cases the patient may need to be administered a dose of an antianxiety or sedating medication.*

The cuff of the ET may need to be deflated before changing its position. If this step needs to be performed, deep oral suctioning should be completed before deflation of the cuff, and oral care should not be performed until the cuff is properly reinflated (Wiegand, 2011).

STEP	RATIONALE

12. Secure tube (assistant continues to hold ET).
   a. Tape method:
   (1) Slip tape under patient's head and neck, adhesive side up. Take care not to twist tape or catch hair. Do not allow tape to stick to itself. It helps to gently stick end of tape to tongue blade, which serves as guide. Then slide tongue blade under patient's neck. Center tape so double-faced tape extends around back of neck from ear to ear.

Positions tape to secure ET in proper position. Don't allow tape to go over earlobe.

   (2) On one side of face secure tape from ear to naris (nasal ET) or over lip to ET (oral ET). Tear remaining tape in half lengthwise, forming two pieces that are 1–1.5 cm (0.4–0.6 inch) wide. Secure bottom half of tape across upper lip (oral ET) or across top of nose (nasal ET) to opposite ear (see illustration A). Wrap top half of tape around tube and up from bottom (see illustration B). Tape should encircle tube at least 2 times for security.

Secures tape to face. Using top tape to wrap prevents downward drag on ET.

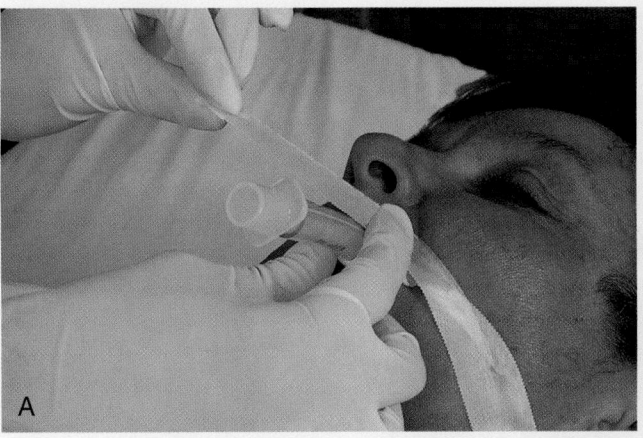 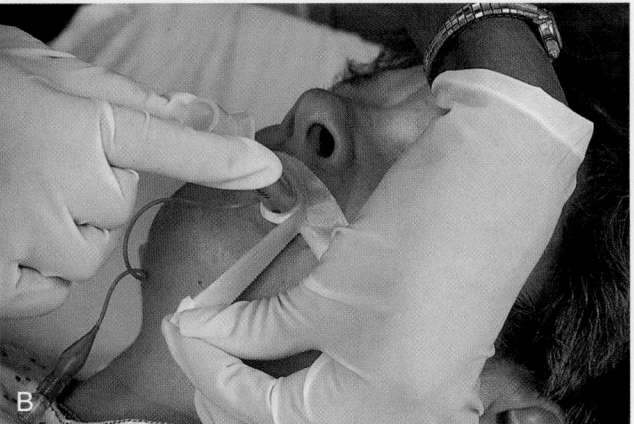

STEP 12a(2) A, Securing bottom half of tape across patient's upper lip. **B,** Securing top half of tape around tube.

   (3) Gently pull other side of tape firmly to pick up slack and secure to opposite side of face and ET same as first piece (see illustration).
   NOTE: ET is secured. Assistant can release hold. Check depth mark at lips or gum line.

Secures tape to face and tube. ET should be at same depth at lips or gum line. Check earlier assessment for verification of tube depth in centimeters.

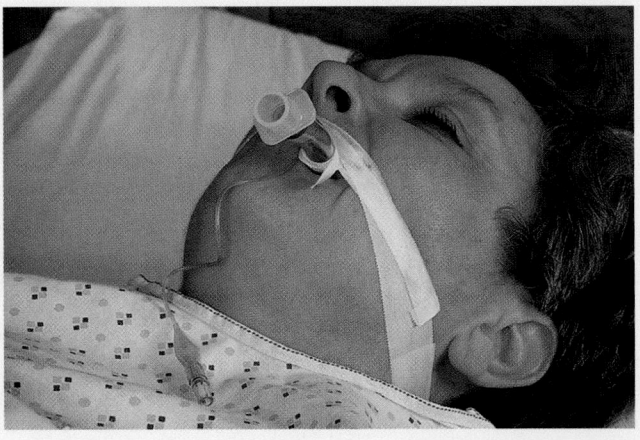

STEP 12a(3) Tape securing endotracheal tube.

STEP	RATIONALE

b. Commercially available ET tube securement device:

Clinical Decision Point *This step will only need to be completed if the device is visibly soiled and cannot be cleaned or if it is no longer adhering to the face and keeping the ET secure.*

STEP	RATIONALE
(1) Thread ET through opening designed to secure it. Be sure that pilot balloon is accessible.	Commercially available holders have a slit in front of holder designed to secure ET.
(2) Place strips of ET holder under patient at occipital region of head.	
(3) Verify that ET is at established depth using lip or gum line marker as guide.	Ensures that ET remains at correct depth as determined during assessment.
(4) Attach Velcro strips at base of patient's head. Leave 1 cm (0.4 inch) slack in strips.	
(5) Verify that tube is secure, it does not move forward from patient's mouth or backward down into patient's throat, and there are no pressure areas on oral mucosa or occipital region of head (see illustration).	Tube must be secure so it remains at correct depth. It can be secured without being tight and causing pressure.

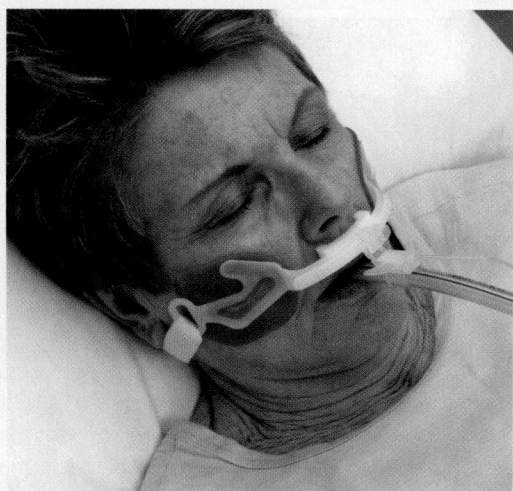

STEP 12b(5) Commercial endotracheal tube holder. *(Modified from Sills JR. Entry-level respiratory therapist exam guide, St Louis, 2000, Mosby.)*

STEP	RATIONALE
13. For unconscious patient reinsert oral airway without pushing tongue into oropharynx and secure with tape.	Prevents patient from biting ET and allows access for oropharyngeal suctioning. An oral airway is not used in a conscious, cooperative patient because it causes excessive gagging and pressure areas to mouth and tongue.
14. Clean rest of face and neck with soapy washcloth, rinse, and dry. Shave male patient as necessary.	Moisture and beard growth prevent adhesive tape adherence.

Clinical Decision Point *When shaving patients, take great care to keep the cuff inflation port away from the razor. The razor can inadvertently cut or nick the tubing, causing air loss from the cuff and the possible need for reintubation.*

Clinical Decision Point *If a nasotracheal tube is in place, all of the preceding steps will be completed, except that the tube will not be moved or its position changed. It is out of the scope of nurse practice to move the ET from one naris to another and could cause great harm to the patient.*

STEP	RATIONALE
15. Discard soiled items in appropriate receptacle. Remove towel and place in laundry.	Reduces transmission of microorganisms.
16. Reposition patient and ask him or her what else he or she needs.	Promotes comfort; gives patients opportunity to communicate their needs.
17. Remove gloves and mask, goggles, or face shield or gown; discard in receptacle; and perform hand hygiene. (Assistant performs same steps.) Place clean items (e.g., tincture of benzoin, oral care solution, excess swabs) in place of storage.	Reduces transmission of microorganisms. Ensures that contaminated gloves and hands do not touch clean items.

STEP	RATIONALE

EVALUATION

1. Compare respiratory assessments before and after ET care.	Identifies any physiological changes, including presence and quality of breath sounds after procedure.
2. Observe depth and position of ET according to health care provider recommendation.	Position of ET should not be altered.
3. Assess security of tape by *gently* tugging at tube.	Tape should remain attached to face. Patient may cough during tugging.
4. Assess skin around mouth and oral mucous membranes for intactness and pressure sores.	Tape should not tear skin. Pressure areas should be absent.
5. Compare E_TCO_2 values from before and after ET care.	Changes in E_TCO_2 can help identify displacement or dislodgement of ET.
6. Observe for excessive phonation, presence of gastric secretions in airway secretions, or tracheoesophageal fistula.	Occurs with inadequate or excessive cuff inflation.

Unexpected Outcomes	Related Interventions
1. Patient is extubated accidentally.	• Remain with patient while calling for help. • Ventilate with bag-valve-mask as needed. • Assess patient for airway patency, spontaneous breathing, and vital signs. • Prepare for reintubation.
2. ET moves in airway and becomes malpositioned.	• Call for help and repeat taping or securing procedure. Be prepared for chest x-ray film to confirm placement. • In very active patients without facial injury who are at risk for self-extubation, consider applying second piece of tape around back of head.
3. Patient has pressure injury in mouth or on lips and nares.	• Increase frequency of ET care. • Apply antimicrobial ointment per agency protocol. • Align oxygen and humidity supply tubing so they do not pull ET, creating pressure sores. • Monitor for infection. If skin tear is present on cheeks or over nose or upper lip, apply protective barrier such as stoma adhesive patch or hydrocolloid dressing and apply tape to it.
4. Cuff leak develops.	• Verify position of tube, notify respiratory therapy, and follow agency policy.

Recording and Reporting

- Document respiratory assessments before and after care, patient's tolerance of procedure, ordered and actual depth of ET, frequency of ET care, integrity of oral and nasal mucosa, pressure sore care (if performed), and frequency and extent of ET care on flow sheet in nurses' notes in electronic health record (EHR) or chart.
- Record repositioning of ET, side on which it is placed, and the securement technique used.
- Report unequal breath sounds, accidental extubation, cuff leak, or respiratory distress to the health care provider.

Special Considerations
Teaching

- Instruct patient and family caregivers not to manipulate the ET, tape, or ET holder. If patient is complaining or appears uncomfortable, instruct family caregiver to ask for the nurse.
- Instruct patient and family caregiver to inform the nurse if the tube causes gagging. Repositioning of the tube and/or sedation are options for reducing gagging.

Pediatric

- Neonatal and pediatric procedures for securing ETs and suctioning airways vary. Refer to agency protocols for specific procedures (Hockenberry and Wilson, 2015).
- Infant skin is more prone to tearing when removing tape (Hockenberry and Wilson, 2015).
- Because of infants' delicate skin, you will not always use adhesive tape remover to remove the tape or skin preparation before securing ET. ET holders are best used in this population as long as appropriate-size holders are available for the child.

Gerontological

- Older adult skin is more prone to tearing when removing tape.
- Older adults with tendency toward inadequate nutrition are more prone to complications (e.g., infection, breakdown of oral mucosa).

A tracheostomy is a surgical or percutaneous creation of a stoma through the neck and into the trachea that allows for the insertion of an artificial airway called a *tracheostomy tube (TT)*. TTs are placed in patients who require long-term airway management because of airway obstruction, airway clearance needs, and/or long-term need for mechanical ventilation (Hess and Altobelli, 2014; Myatt, 2015). A TT offers advantages over long-term endotracheal tube (ET) placement such as decreased risk of laryngeal and tracheal injury, less sedation, shorter ventilator weaning time (time it takes to get a patient off a ventilator) (Durbin, 2010), and improved comfort for the patient. Some TTs even allow more patient freedom in the performance of activities of daily living such as feeding, speaking, and mobility (Morris et al., 2013).

TTs are comprised of several components (Fig. 25.5). The shaft is the main component of the TT and is what sits inside the trachea, keeping the airway open. Flanges rest against the patient's neck and prevent the TT from migrating into the trachea. The 15-mm connector is located on the shaft or the inner cannula and is where the ventilator tubing or resuscitation bag attaches to the TT. The obturator is placed inside the TT and used during the TT insertion process and is replaced with an inner cannula (if necessary) once inserted. The inner cannula is located inside the shaft of the TT and is a safety feature because it can be quickly removed and replaced if obstructed (Dawson and Farrington, 2014a; Dawson, 2014b). TTs are curved and are commonly made of a synthetic material such as polyvinyl chloride (PVC), silicone, or polyurethane. The curved nature of the TT improves the ability of the tube to fit within the trachea (Hess and Altobelli, 2014; Wiegand,

2011). Metal tubes are rarely used because of their increased costs, their rigidity, and their lack of a cuff.

A TT is cuffed or uncuffed. A cuff on a TT serves the same purpose as the cuff on an ET. Cuffs are made of a balloonlike inflatable plastic typically inflated with air, although there are brands that are inflated with liquid such as water or saline. Uncuffed tubes allow patients the ability to clear the airway, but they provide no protection from aspiration. It is also more difficult to use positive-pressure ventilation in patients with these types of TTs (Hess and Altobelli, 2014, Myatt, 2015).

Some TTs allow a patient to speak. This ability to verbalize needs and wants provides psychological benefits to the patient. The openings in fenestrated tubes allow air to flow from the lungs over the vocal cords. However, these tubes must be used with caution; only patients who can swallow without aspiration should use them. There are speaking valves that can be used with TTs. The patient must have a cuffless TT in place or be able to tolerate the cuff being deflated without risk of respiratory distress or aspiration. Patients may not tolerate the speaking valves when first placed; therefore they will need to be carefully monitored for signs of intolerance or respiratory distress. It is possible to administer oxygen with a tracheotomy mask or via nasal cannula if the TT is small (Hess and Altobelli, 2014).

Nurses also need to monitor for emergency events such as tube obstruction or dislodgement. Box 25.2 is a list of equipment that should be kept in the room or at the bedside of any patient who has a tracheostomy. Table 25.1 describes the signs of tracheal tube obstruction or dislodgement and the interventions that should be performed.

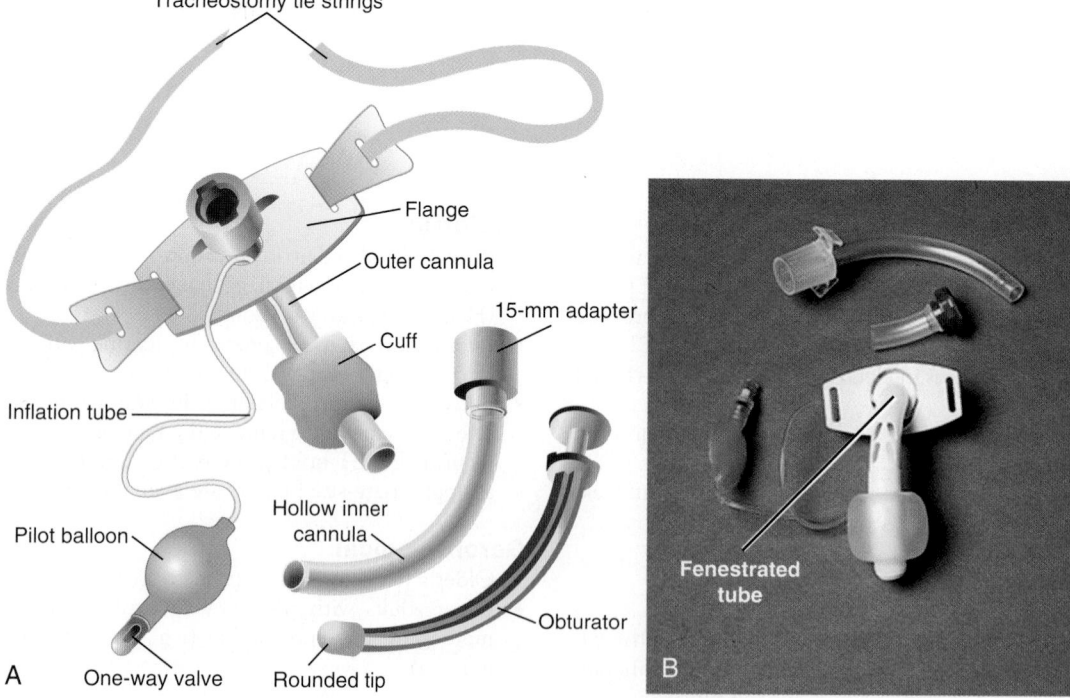

FIG 25.5 A, Parts of tracheostomy tube. **B,** Fenestrated tracheostomy tube with cuff, inner cannula, decannulation plug, and pilot balloon. (*From Lewis S, et al: Medical-surgical nursing: assessment and management of clinical problems, ed 9, St Louis, 2014, Mosby.*)

TABLE 25.1

Tracheostomy Emergencies

Emergency Type	Signs and Symptoms	Interventions

Tube dislodgement/ decannulation	• Inability to pass suction catheter past the length of the tube
	• Presence of subcutaneous emphysema near incision or stoma
	• Signs of respiratory distress
	• High-pressure alarm on ventilator
	• Flange of TT not flush with neck
	• Decreased SpO_2
	• Patient able to speak around the TT
		• Call for help
		• If stoma is less than 1 week old
		  • Notify surgeon
		  • Bag-mask ventilation
		  • Prepare for intubation or surgical reinsertion of new TT
		• If stoma is well established (typically greater than 1 week old)
		  • Replace with a new TT, inserting at a 90-degree angle into the trachea, then angling downward another 90 degrees

Tube obstruction	• Respiratory distress
	• Inability to pass suction catheter
	• Resistance felt when using the self-inflating resuscitation bag
		• Call for help
		• Remove and inspect the inner cannula (if one present); clean or replace with a new one
		• Mature site
		  • Replace the TT (if changing inner cannula did not relieve the obstruction)
		  • Patient may need more invasive intervention such as bronchoscopy
		• Immature site
		  • Ensure TT in correct position
		  • Prepare for more invasive intervention such as oral endotracheal intubation, tracheostomy revision, or placement of a longer TT

Hemorrhage	• More than minimal bleeding at stoma site	• Notify health care provider • Provide oxygen, if not already in place

Data from Dawson D: Essential principles: tracheostomy care in the adult patient, *Nurs Crit Care* 19(2):63-72, 2014; and Morris LL, et al: Tracheostomy care and complications in the intensive care unit, *Crit Care Nurse* 33(5):18, 2013.
TT, Tracheostomy tube.

BOX 25.2

Bedside Equipment for a Tracheostomy Patient

• Suction machine/equipment
• Suction tubing
• Suction catheters (Yankauer and tracheal)
• Sterile saline
• Additional tracheostomy tubes, one the same size as the current tube and another that is one size smaller
• Obturator
• Manual self-inflating resuscitation bag with appropriate-size mask
• 10-ml syringe

Delegation and Collaboration

The skill of performing tracheostomy care is not routinely delegated to nursing assistive personnel (NAP). In some settings patients who have well-established TTs may have the care delegated to NAP. The nurse is responsible for assessing a patient and evaluating for proper artificial airway care, often in collaboration with a respiratory therapist. The nurse is also responsible for educating the patient and family caregivers regarding care of an established tracheostomy in the home. The nurse directs the NAP to:

• Immediately report any changes in patient's respiratory status, level of consciousness, confusion, restlessness or irritability, or level of comfort.
• Immediately report any dislodgement or excessive movement of the TT.
• Immediately report abnormal color of the tracheal stoma and drainage.

Equipment

• Bedside table
• Person to help change the tracheostomy tie/holder
• Towel
• Artificial airway suction supplies (see Skill 25.2)
• Oropharyngeal suction supplies (see Skill 25.1)
• Sterile tracheostomy care kit, if available (be sure to collect supplies listed that are not available in kit), or two sterile 4 × 4–inch gauze pads
• Sterile cotton-tipped applicators
• Sterile tracheostomy dressing (precut and sewn surgical dressing)
• Sterile basin
• Sterile normal saline or water
• Small sterile brush (pipe cleaner) (or disposable inner cannula)
• Roll of twill tape, tracheostomy ties, or commercial tracheostomy holder
• Scissors
• Inner cannula that fits the patient's TT
• Pulse oximeter, end-tidal CO_2 detector
• Clean gloves (two pair)
• Personal protective equipment; goggles if concern regarding contact with secretions
• Self-inflating manual resuscitation bag-valve device and appropriate-size mask
• Extra sterile tracheostomy kit

STEP	RATIONALE

ASSESSMENT

1. Identify patient using at least two identifiers (e.g., name and birthday or name and medical record number) according to agency policy.

Ensures correct patient. Complies with The Joint Commission standards and improves patient safety (TJC, 2016).

2. Perform hand hygiene and apply clean gloves. Observe for signs and symptoms of gurgling on expiration, decreased exhaled tidal volume (mechanically ventilated patient), signs and symptoms of inadequate ventilation (rising end-tidal carbon dioxide concentration [$E_T CO_2$], patient-ventilator dyssynchrony, or dyspnea), spasmodic coughing, tense test balloon on tube, flaccid test balloon on tube, and ability to speak or vocalize (see Box 25.1).

Reduces contact with infectious microorganisms. Cuff underinflation increases risk for aspiration and allows secretions to enter trachea and permits vocalization. Cuff overinflation may cause ischemia or necrosis of tracheal tissue from obstruction of capillary bed, resulting in tracheomalacia or tracheoesophageal fistula (Myatt, 2015).

3. Observe for excess peristomal secretions, excess intratracheal secretions, soiled or damp tracheostomy ties, soiled or damp tracheostomy dressing, diminished airflow through tracheostomy tube, or signs and symptoms of airway obstruction requiring suctioning (see Skill 25.2).

Indicate need for tracheostomy care caused by presence of secretions at stoma site or within tracheostomy tube. Irritation of mucosa caused by tube itself can also cause increase in secretions (Wiegand, 2011).

4. Observe skin around tracheal stoma, under TT, and under tracheal ties for skin breakdown: blistering, erythema, drainage, or other discoloration.

Pressure areas related to TT increase patient's risk for medical device–related pressure injury (MDPI) formation (Pittman et al., 2015).

5. Assess patient's hydration status, humidity delivered to airway, status of any existing infection, patient's nutritional status, and ability to cough.

Determines factors that affect amount and consistency of secretions in tracheostomy and patient's ability to clear airway.

6. Assess patient's cardiopulmonary status, including pulse oximetry (SpO_2), $E_T CO_2$, vital signs, respiratory effort, lung sounds, and level of consciousness. Keep pulse oximeter in place.

Provides baseline to determine patient response to and tolerance of therapy.

7. Assess patient's or family caregiver's understanding of and ability to perform own tracheostomy care.

Allows you to identify potential need for instruction.

8. Check when tracheostomy care was last performed.

Tracheostomy care is provided at least every 4 to 8 hours and more often if indicated (e.g., increased airway or stoma secretions, infection [airway or stoma]) (Wiegand, 2011).

NURSING DIAGNOSES

- Deficient knowledge regarding tracheostomy care
- Impaired comfort
- Impaired gas exchange
- Impaired verbal communication
- Ineffective airway clearance
- Ineffective breathing pattern
- Risk for aspiration
- Risk for infection

Related factors/Risk factors are individualized based on patient's condition or needs.

PLANNING

1. Expected outcomes following completion of procedure:
   - Inner and outer cannulas of TT are free of secretions; ties are clean, secured snugly, and tied in double square knot.

   TT is patent and secure, optimizing amount of oxygen delivered to patient and limiting risk of infection from retained secretions.

   - Stoma site is pink; does not bleed; and is free of secretions, signs of infection, skin breakdown and pressure areas, and signs of granuloma formation.

   Indicates absence of infection at stoma site. Dry, intact tracheostomy stoma reduces risk for subsequent systemic infection.

   - No evidence of skin breakdown under tracheostomy ties or commercial tube holder.

   Patients with excessive secretions or diaphoresis are at risk for skin breakdown under TT stabilizer.

2. Have another nurse, NAP, or respiratory therapist help in this procedure (Wiegand, 2011).

   Prevents accidental extubation of TT.

3. Perform hand hygiene. Gather supplies and arrange at bedside. Close room door or curtain.

   Ensures a well-organized procedure. Ensures patient privacy.

4. Assist patient to comfortable position, raise head of bed to level of comfort.

5. Explain procedure and patient's participation.

   Encourages cooperation, minimizes risks, and reduces anxiety.

STEP	RATIONALE

Clinical Decision Point *At some agencies it is standard practice to have an extra TT that is the same size as the patient's current TT and a TT one size smaller at the bedside at all times in case there is an emergent need to replace the TT because of obstruction or dislodgement (Wiegand, 2011).*

IMPLEMENTATION

1. Apply personal protective equipment as necessary or ordered.

Reduces transmission of microorganisms.

2. Adjust bed to appropriate height and lower side rail on side nearest you. Check locks on bed wheel.

Minimizes caregiver's muscle strain and prevents injury. Prevents bed from moving.

3. Preoxygenate patient for 30 seconds or ask patient to take 5 to 6 deep breaths. Then suction tracheostomy (see Skill 25.2). Before removing gloves, remove soiled tracheostomy dressing and discard in glove with coiled catheter.

Removes secretions to avoid occluding outer cannula while inner cannula is removed. Reduces need for patient to cough.

4. Perform hand hygiene. Prepare equipment on bedside table.

Prepares equipment and allows for smooth, organized completion of tracheostomy care.

Tracheostomy cares should be performed every 4 to 8 hours or per agency protocol (Wiegand, 2011).

a. Open sterile tracheostomy kit. Open two 4 × 4–inch gauze packages using aseptic technique and pour normal saline on one package. Leave second package dry. Open two cotton-tipped swab packages and pour normal saline on one package. Do not recap normal saline.

b. Open sterile tracheostomy dressing package.

c. Unwrap sterile basin and pour about 0.5–2 cm (0.2–1 inch) of normal saline into it.

d. Open small sterile brush package and place aseptically into sterile basin.

e. Prepare TT fixation device.

(1) If using twill tape: Prepare length of twill tape long enough to go around patient's neck 2 times, about 60–75 cm (24–30 inches) for an adult. Cut ends on diagonal. Lay aside in dry area.

Cutting ends of tie on diagonal aids in inserting tie through eyelet.

(2) If using commercially available TT holder, open package according to manufacturer directions.

f. Open inner cannula package (if new one is to be inserted such as with disposable inner cannulas or if patient does not tolerate being disconnected from oxygen source while cleaning reusable inner cannula).

5. Apply sterile gloves. Keep dominant hand sterile throughout procedure.

Reduces transmission of microorganisms.

6. Remove oxygen source if present.

Clinical Decision Point *It is important to stabilize TT at all times during tracheostomy care to prevent injury, unnecessary discomfort, or accidental extubation. Have an assistant such as a NAP help during the procedure. Instruct assistant to apply clean gloves.*

7. Care of tracheostomy with reusable inner cannula:
a. While touching only outer aspect of tube, unlock and remove inner cannula with nondominant hand following line of tracheostomy. Drop inner cannula into normal saline basin.

Removes inner cannula for cleaning. Normal saline loosens secretions from inner cannula.

Clinical Decision Point *If patient is receiving mechanical ventilation, you may want the person assisting you to hold the TT stable and remove the ventilator tube from the connection while you remove the inner cannula. This action helps to ensure that the TT itself is not removed accidentally if difficulties removing the ventilator from the TT or removing the inner cannula from the TT occur.*

b. Place tracheostomy collar, T tube, or ventilator oxygen source over outer cannula. (**NOTE:** May not be able to attach T tube and ventilator oxygen devices to all outer cannulas when inner cannula is removed.)

Maintains supply of oxygen to patient as needed.

STEP	RATIONALE

Clinical Decision Point *If patient is unable to tolerate being disconnected from the ventilator, replace the inner cannula with a clean new one and reattach the ventilator to the tracheostomy. Then proceed with cleaning the original inner cannula as described in the next steps and store it in a sterile container until the next inner cannula change (Wiegand, 2011).*

c. To prevent oxygen desaturation in affected patients, quickly pick up inner cannula and use small brush to remove secretions inside and outside inner cannula (see illustration).	Tracheostomy brush provides mechanical force to remove thick or dried secretions.
d. Hold inner cannula over basin and rinse with sterile normal saline, using nondominant (clean) hand to pour normal saline.	Removes secretions and normal saline from inner cannula.
e. Remove oxygen source, replace inner cannula (see illustration), and secure "locking" mechanism. Reapply ventilator, tracheostomy collar, or T tube. Hyperoxygenate patient if needed.	Secures inner cannula and reestablishes oxygen supply.
8. Tracheostomy with disposable inner cannula:	
a. Remove new cannula from manufacturer packaging.	Prepares you for change of inner cannula.
b. While touching only outer aspect of tube, withdraw inner cannula and replace with new cannula. Lock into position.	Provides clean, sterile inner cannula for patient.

Clinical Decision Point *If patient is receiving mechanical ventilation, you may want the person assisting you to hold the TT stable and remove the ventilator tube from the connection while you remove the inner cannula. This action helps to ensure that the TT itself is not accidentally removed if difficulties removing the ventilator or the inner cannula from the TT occur.*

c. Dispose of contaminated cannula in appropriate receptacle and reconnect to ventilator or oxygen supply.	Prevents transmission of infection. Restores oxygen delivery.
9. Using normal saline-saturated cotton-tipped swabs and 4 × 4–inch gauze, clean exposed outer cannula surfaces and stoma under faceplate extending 5–10 cm (2–4 inches) in all directions from stoma (see illustration). Clean in circular motion from stoma site outward with dominant hand to handle sterile supplies. Do not go over previously cleaned area.	Aseptically removes secretions from stoma site. Moving in outward circle pulls mucus and other contaminants from stoma to periphery.
10. Using dry 4 × 4–inch gauze, pat lightly at skin and exposed outer cannula surfaces.	Dry surfaces prohibit formation of moist environment for microorganism growth and skin excoriation (Wiegand, 2011).
11. Secure tracheostomy.	

Clinical Decision Point *Some agencies do not recommend changing the securement device for the first 72 hours after insertion of the TT because of risk of stoma closure if the tube were to become dislodged accidentally (Wiegand, 2011).*

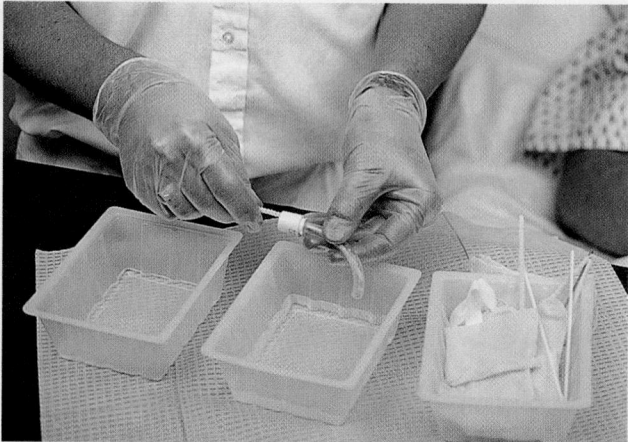

STEP 7c Cleaning tracheostomy inner cannula.

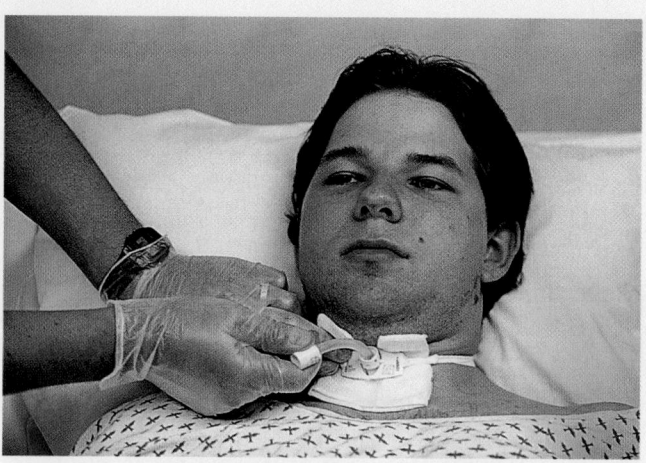

STEP 7e Reinserting inner cannula.

STEP	RATIONALE

a. Tracheostomy tie method:

(1) Instruct assistant, if available, to apply clean gloves and securely hold TT in place. With assistant holding TT, cut old ties. Ensure to not cut pilot balloon of cuff.

Prevents transmission of infection. Secures TT to prevent incidental dislodgement. If pilot balloon is cut, there is no ability to inflate cuff (Wiegand, 2011).

Clinical Decision Point *Assistant must not release hold on TT until new ties are firmly tied. If working without an assistant, do not cut old ties until new ties are in place and securely tied (Lewis et al., 2017). When ties are off, this is a good time to clean the back of the patient's neck and assess patient's skin under TT flange and under the ties or tube holder, making sure that skin is intact, free of pressure, and dry before applying securement device.*

(2) Take prepared twill tape, insert one end of tie through faceplate eyelet, and pull ends even (see illustration).

Diagonal cuts ensure ease of threading end of tie through holes of eyelet (Wiegand, 2011).

(3) Slide both ends of tie behind head and around neck to other eyelet and insert one tie through second eyelet.

(4) Pull snugly.

Secures TT.

(5) Tie ends securely in double square knot, allowing space for insertion of only one loose or two snug finger widths between tie and neck (see illustration).

One finger width of slack prevents ties from being too tight when tracheostomy dressing is in place and also prevents movement of tracheostomy tube into lower airway (Wiegand, 2011).

(6) Insert fresh 4 × 4–inch tracheostomy dressing under clean ties and faceplate (see illustration).

Absorbs drainage. Dressing prevents pressure on clavicle heads (Wiegand, 2011).

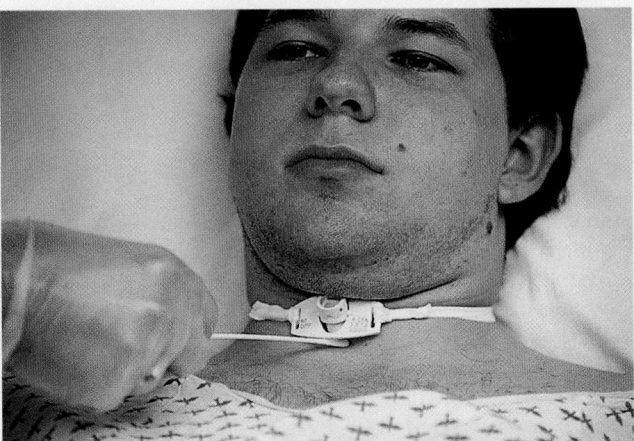

STEP 9 Cleaning around stoma.

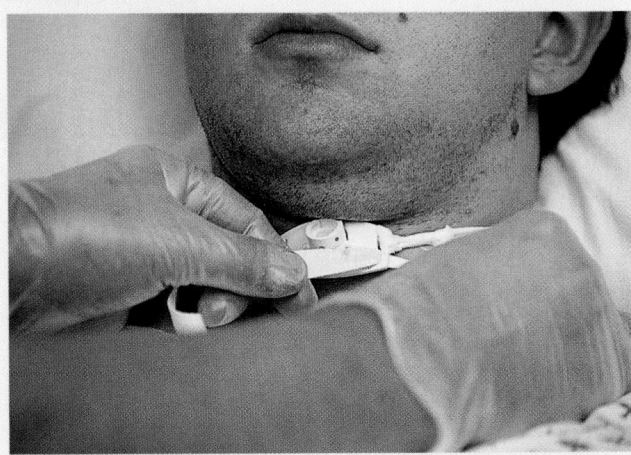

STEP 11a(2) Replacing tracheostomy ties. Do not remove old tracheostomy ties until new ones are secure.

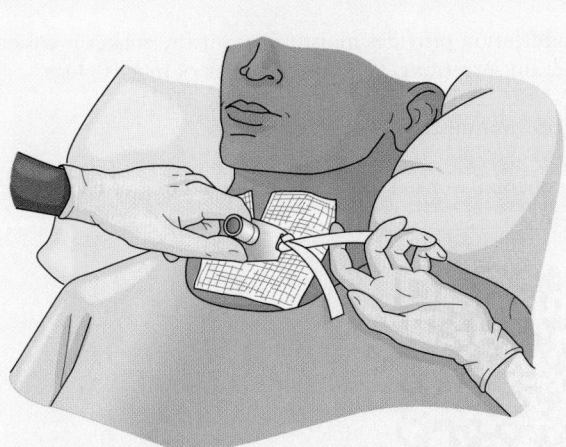

STEP 11a(5) Tracheostomy ties properly placed. (*From Sorrentino SA: Mosby's textbook for nursing assistants, ed 8, St Louis, 2013, Mosby.*)

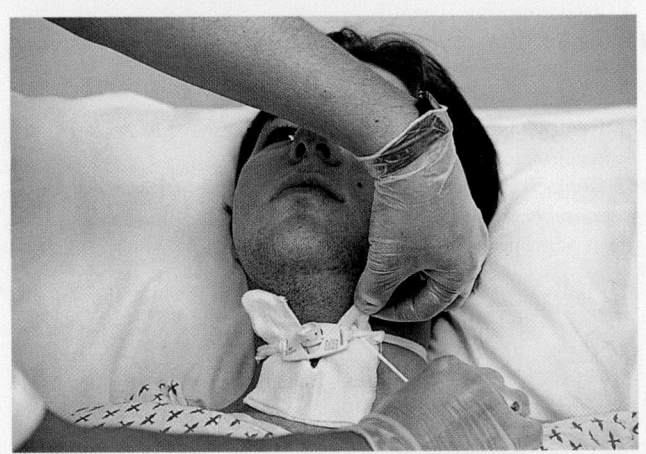

STEP 11a(6) Applying tracheostomy dressing.

STEP	RATIONALE

b. Tracheostomy tube holder method:

(1) Instruct assistant, if available, to apply clean gloves and securely hold TT in place. When an assistant is not available, leave old TT holder in place until new device is secure.

Prevents incidental dislodgement of tube.
Ensures that tracheostomy stays in correct position.

(2) Align strap under patient's neck. Be sure that Velcro attachments are on either side of TT.

(3) Place narrow end of ties under and through faceplate eyelets. Pull ends even and secure with Velcro closures (see illustration).

Ensures proper securement of TT.

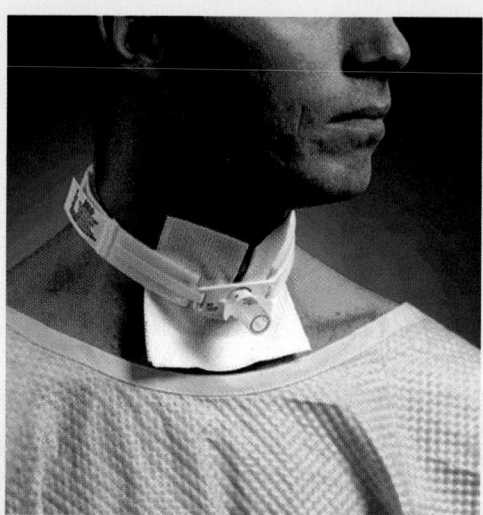

STEP 11b(3) Tracheostomy tube holder in place. (*Courtesy Dale Medical Products, Plainesville, MA.*)

(4) Verify that there is space for only one loose or two snug finger widths to be inserted under neck strap.

Ensures proper securement of TT without securement device being too tight.

Clinical Decision Point *Never cut a gauze pad to fit around TT. The cut fibers from the gauze pad may shed fibers that could be inhaled by patient and lead to pulmonary damage or infection. Use a manufactured pad for this purpose (Wiegand, 2011).*

12. Perform oral care with toothbrush or oral swabs and chlorhexidine rinse.

Use of chlorhexidine may decrease patient risk of developing a ventilator-associated event (VAE)/ventilator-associated pneumonia (VAP) and promotes patient comfort.

13. Reposition patient comfortably, with head of bed elevated at least 30 degrees (unless at risk for pressure injury) and assess respiratory status.

Promotes comfort. Some patients require posttracheostomy care suctioning.

14. Be sure that oxygen- or humidification-delivery sources are in place and set at correct levels.

Humidification provides moisture for airway, makes it easier to suction secretions, and decreases risk of mucus plugs (AARC, 2012: Restrepo and Walsh, 2012).

15. Remove gloves and face shield and discard in appropriate receptacle. Perform hand hygiene.

Reduces transmission of microorganisms.

16. Replace cap on reusable normal saline bottles. Store reusable liquids, date container, and store unused supplies in appropriate place.

Once opened, normal saline is considered free of bacteria for 24 hours.

STEP	RATIONALE

EVALUATION

1. Compare assessments before and after tracheostomy care.

2. Assess fit of new tracheostomy ties and ask patient if tube feels comfortable. Palpate tube for pulsation for air under the skin.

3. Inspect inner and outer cannulas for secretions.

4. Assess stoma, surrounding skin, and skin under ties for inflammation, edema, bleeding or discolored secretions.

5. Observe for excessive phonation, presence of gastric secretions in airway secretions, or tracheoesophageal fistula.

6. **Use Teach-Back:** "I want to be sure I explained how to clean your tracheostomy tube and place new ties. "Let's take time now and show me how to clean the tubing and place new ties." Revise your instruction now or develop a plan for revised patient or family caregiver teaching if patient or family caregiver is not able to teach back correctly.

Rationale:

Determines effectiveness of tracheostomy care and patient's tolerance of procedure.

Tracheostomy ties are uncomfortable and place patient at risk for tissue injury when they are too loose or too tight. A pulsating feeling in TT can indicate early signs of innominate artery erosion. Air under skin suggests presence of subcutaneous emphysema.

Presence of secretions on cannulas indicates need for more frequent tracheostomy care.

Broken skin places patient at risk for infection.
Stoma infection requires change in tracheostomy skin care plan.
Stomas located below second and third cartilage rings are at risk of causing innominate artery erosion (Wiegand, 2011).

Occurs with inadequate or excessive cuff inflation.

Determines patient's and family caregiver's level of understanding of instructional topic.

Unexpected Outcomes

1. Excessively loose or tight tracheostomy ties/tracheostomy holder.
2. Cuff leak develops.

3. Inflammation of tracheostomy stoma or pressure area around TT.

4. Accidental decannulation/dislodgement

5. Respiratory distress from mucus plugs in cannula.

Related Interventions

- Adjust ties or apply new ties/tracheostomy holder.
- Verify position of tube, notify respiratory therapy, and follow agency policy.
- Increase frequency of tracheostomy care.
- Apply topical antibacterial solution; apply bacterial barrier if ordered.
- Apply hydrocolloid or transparent dressing just under stoma to protect skin from breakdown.
- Consult with skin care specialist.
- Call for help.
- Replace old TT with new tube. Some experienced nurses or respiratory therapists may be able to reinsert TT quickly.
- Same-size ET can be inserted in stoma in an emergency.
- Insert suction catheter to confirm that new tube is in trachea.
- Be prepared to manually ventilate patients in whom respiratory distress develops with self-inflating resuscitation bag until tracheostomy is replaced.
- Notify health care provider.
- Remove inner cannula if applicable for cleaning or suction cannula.
- Notify health care provider if TT requires replacement.

Recording and Reporting

- Record respiratory assessments before and after care; type and size of tracheostomy tube and inner cannula; frequency and extent of care, including inner cannula, dressing and securement device changes; type, color, and amount of secretions; patient tolerance and understanding of procedure; and special care in event of unexpected outcomes in nurses' notes in electronic health record (EHR) or chart.
- Record condition of stoma and skin around stoma site and under dressing.
- Record any interventions that were performed to address patient complications.
- Record patient's and family caregiver's understanding through teach-back.

- Report accidental decannulation or respiratory distress to the health care provider.

Special Considerations
Teaching

- Different types of TTs have different faceplates. Some are rigid; others are not. Instruct caregivers not to lift up rigid faceplates or they will dislodge tube.
- Some commercial TT holders require removal of excess tie material to fit properly.
- If you anticipate long-term placement of tracheostomy, plan to teach patient and family caregiver tracheostomy care.
- Patients with new tracheostomy frequently have bloody secretions for 2 or 3 days after tubing change (Wiegand, 2011).

Pediatric

- Children generally have shorter necks, making the stoma more difficult to clean.
- Pediatric TTs (smaller than size 4) do not contain an inner cannula.
- Nurses perform routine TT changes weekly after a tract has formed, generally 5 days (Hockenberry and Wilson, 2015).

Gerontological

- Some older adults may have more fragile skin and are more prone to skin breakdown from secretions or pressure (Touhy and Jett, 2014).
- Some older adults with impaired nutrition do not heal well.

Home Care

- Coordinate with patient, family caregivers, and home care agencies to ensure ability to secure appropriate supplies for use at home.
- Coordinate with home care services to ensure that home has appropriate electricity to support the equipment, particularly if patient is receiving mechanical ventilation or requires suctioning
- See Skill 23.5, Home Care.

◆ CLINICAL DEBRIEF

A 65-year-old patient suffered a severe stroke 2 days and at this time cannot communicate verbally. The health care team is monitoring him for the ability to control his secretions and maintain an airway. The nurse walks into his room and notices cyanotic oral mucous membranes, pulse oximeter reading of 78%, and a large amount of oral secretions. The patient is gasping for air and tachypneic.

1. What should the nurse do first?

2. The nurse attempted to clear the patient's airway, but the patient continues to gasp for air; and the pulse oximeter improved only to 82%, even with the addition of 10 L oxygen via nonrebreather face mask. Rhonchi are noted on auscultation of breath sounds and trachea. The patient also continues to present with a large amount of oral secretions. The nurse recognizes that the provider needs to be notified. Using SBAR format, how should the nurse communicate the patient's status to the provider?

3. The patient was intubated; however, because of an inability to control secretions and maintain an airway, he was unable to be weaned off the ventilator. The decision was made to perform a tracheostomy. The nurse is teaching his wife about how the nurses will manage her husband's tracheostomy tube. What should be included in the teaching plan, and why are these interventions performed?

◆ REVIEW QUESTIONS

1. The nurse is assessing a patient with an endotracheal tube (ET) and receiving positive-pressure mechanical ventilation. Which assessment findings would alert the nurse for the need to perform endotracheal suctioning? (Select all that apply.)
1. Increased exhaled tidal volume above patient baseline
2. Auscultation of rhonchi in the lungs
3. Elevated exhaled carbon dioxide levels
4. Decreased peak inspiratory pressures noted on the ventilator
5. Presence of yellow fluid within the ET
6. Patient speaking around the ET tube

2. A patient who is receiving mechanical ventilation via tracheostomy tube (TT) is preparing for discharge home. Which statements, made by the patient's primary family caregiver, indicate an understanding of the care of this patient? (Select all that apply.)
1. "We should suction the tracheostomy tube every 4 hours during the day."
2. "We will need to rinse the nondisposable inner cannula with sterile saline to clean it."
3. "We should make sure that the tracheostomy holder is tight against the skin."
4. "We should check the pressure in the cuff at least 3 times a day."
5. "We will need to clean the stoma site at least every 8 hours and more frequently if there are secretions or signs of infection."

3. Put the steps of tracheal suctioning in order.
1. Hyperoxygenate the patient.
2. Assess for the need for suctioning.
3. Perform oropharyngeal suctioning.
4. Withdraw catheter while applying suction.
5. Insert catheter into endotracheal or tracheostomy tube.

ⓔ *Visit the Evolve site for a complete list of Clinical Debrief and Review Questions answers.*

REFERENCES

American Association of Critical Care Nurses (AACN): *AACN practice alert: Oral care for patients at risk for ventilator-associated pneumonia,* 2010, http://www.aacn.org/wd/practice/docs/practicealerts/oral-care-patients-at-risk-vap.pdf?menu=aboutus. Accessed April 14, 2016.

American Association of Critical Care Nurses (AACN): *AACN practice alert: Prevention of aspiration,* 2016, http://www.aacn.org/wd/practice/content/practicealerts/aspiration-practice-alert.pcms?menu=practice. Accessed April 14, 2016.

American Association of Respiratory Care (AARC): *AARC clinical practice guideline: nasotracheal suctioning—2004 revision & update,* 2004, http://www.rcjournal.com/cpgs/pdf/09.04.1080.pdf. Accessed April 14, 2016.

American Association of Respiratory Care (AARC): AARC clinical practice guidelines: endotracheal suctioning of mechanically ventilated patients with artificial airways, *Respir Care* 55(6):758, 2010.

American Association of Respiratory Care (AARC): AARC clinical practice guidelines: capnography/capnometry during mechanical ventilation, *Respir Care* 56(4):503, 2011.

American Association of Respiratory Care (AARC): Humidification during invasive and noninvasive mechanical ventilation, *Respir Care* 57(5):782, 2012.

Bouadma L, et al: Ventilator-associated pneumonia and its prevention, *Curr Opin Infect Dis* 25(4):395, 2012.

Branson RD, et al: Management of the artificial airway, *Respir Care* 59(6):974, 2014.

Centers for Disease Control and Prevention (CDC): *Ventilator-associated event (VAE),* 2016, http://www.cdc.gov/nhsn/PDFs/pscManual/10-VAE_FINAL.pdf. Accessed July 10, 2016.

Dawson C, Farrington M: Tracheostomy care: putting statements into action!, *ORL Head Neck Nurs* 32(1):14, 2014a.

Dawson D: Essential principles: tracheostomy care in the adult patient, *Nurs Crit Care* 19(2):63, 2014b.

Durbin CG: Tracheostomy: Why, When and How? *Respir Care* 55(8):1056–1068, 2010.

Galbiati G, Paola C: Effects of open and closed endotracheal suctioning on intracranial pressure and cerebral perfusion pressure in adult patients with severe brain injury: a literature review, *J Neurosci Nurs* 47(4):239, 2015.

Grindrod K: Management of stable chronic obstructive pulmonary disease, *Br J Community Nurs* 20(2):58, 2015.

Grossbach I, et al: Promoting effective communication for patients receiving mechanical ventilation, *Crit Care Nurse* 31(3):46, 2011.

Hess DR, Altobelli NP: Tracheostomy tubes, *Respir Care* 59(6):956, 2014.

Hockenberry MJ, Wilson D: *Wong's nursing care of infants and children,* ed 10, St Louis, 2015, Mosby.

Institute for Healthcare Improvement (IHI): *How-to guide: prevent ventilator-associated pneumonia*, 2012, www.ihi.org. Accessed April 14, 2016.

Lamb KD: Year in review 2014: mechanical ventilation, *Respir Care* 60(4):606, 2015.

Lewis S, et al: *Medical-surgical nursing: assessment and management of clinical problems*, ed 10, St Louis, 2017, Elsevier.

Morris LL, et al: Tracheostomy care and complications in the intensive care unit, *Crit Care Nurse* 33(5):18, 2013.

Munro N, Ruggiero M: Ventilator-associated pneumonia bundle reconstruction for best care, *AACN Adv Crit Care* 25(2):163, 2014.

Myatt R: Nursing care of patients with a temporary tracheostomy, *Nurs Stand* 29(26):42, 2015.

Özden D, Görgülü RS: Development of standard practice guidelines for open and closed system suctioning, *J Clin Nurs* 21:1327, 2012.

Özden D, Görgülü RS: Effects of open and closed suction systems on the haemodynamic parameters in cardiac surgery patients, *Nurs Crit Care* 20(3):118, 2014.

Pittman J, et al: Medical device–related hospital-acquired pressure ulcers, *J Wound Ostomy Continence Nurs* 42(2):151, 2015.

Restrepo RD, Walsh BK: Humidification during invasive and noninvasive mechanical ventilation, *Respir Care* 57(5):782, 2012.

The Joint Commission (TJC): *2016 national patient safety goals*, Oakbrook Terrace, IL, 2016, The Commission. http://www.jointcommission.org/standards_information/npsgs.aspx. Accessed July 10, 2016.

Touhy T, Jett K: *Ebersole and Hess' gerontological nursing & healthy aging*, ed 4, St Louis, 2014, Mosby.

Tsay S, et al: The experiences of adult ventilator-dependent patients: a meta-synthesis review, *Nurs Health Sci* 15:525–533, 2013.

Urden L, et al: *Priorities in critical care nursing*, ed 7, St Louis, 2016, Mosby.

Walsh BK, et al: Capnography/capnometry during mechanical ventilation, *Respir Care* 56(4):503, 2011.

Wiegand D: *AACN procedure manual for critical care*, ed 6, St Louis, 2011, Mosby.

26 | Cardiac Care

OBJECTIVES

Mastery of content in this chapter will enable the nurse to:
- Identify the indications to perform a 12-lead electrocardiogram (ECG) and cardiac monitor application.
- Determine correct electrode placement to obtain an accurate ECG tracing.
- Describe measures to reduce false alarms.

MEDIA RESOURCES

- evolve http://evolve.elsevier.com/Perry/skills
- Review Questions
- Audio Glossary
- **NSO** Nursing Skills Online
- Clinical Debrief and Review Questions Answers
- Animations

PURPOSE

The ECG is the graphic representation of the electrical activities, or conduction system, of the heart used for diagnostic and treatment purposes. Accuracy of these waveforms depends on the correct placement and clean application of electrodes to the skin.

STANDARDS OF CARE

- American College of Cardiology Foundation (ACCF)/American Heart Association (AHA) STEMI Guidelines, 2013—12-Lead ECG
- AHA: Practice Guidelines for Electrocardiographic Monitoring in Hospital Settings, 2004—Cardiac Monitoring
- AACN Practice Alert, 2013—Alarm Management
- The Joint Commission, 2016—Patient Identification

PRINCIPLES FOR PRACTICE

- 12-lead ECG provides a snapshot of the electrical activity of the heart from multiple views. It is a diagnostic tool to determine emergency treatment of patients with acute coronary syndrome or acute onset of potential life-threatening dysrhythmias. Accuracy and timeliness are the key principles of acquisition (O'Gara et al., 2013).
- Cardiac monitoring provides continuous ECG observation of the acutely ill patient. Proper placement of the ECG electrodes is essential to ensure real-time detection of arrhythmias (Drew et al., 2004; Sendelbach and Jepsen, 2013) (Table 26.1).

PATIENT-CENTERED CARE

- Placement of the electrodes requires exposure of a patient's chest. Measures to maintain the patient's modesty are essential.
- Women require special consideration with the placement of electrodes as close to the chest wall as possible, avoiding breast tissue.
- Patients and families, especially those with a cultural need for modesty, may need detailed information about the procedure so they do not misunderstand the intent and objective of cardiac monitoring.
- Always explain which type of physical interaction is involved to avoid misinterpretation of interventions.

EVIDENCE-BASED PRACTICE

The clinical indications for the acquisition of continuous cardiac monitoring and 12-lead ECG have been well established over the last several years. A recent research review by the American College of Cardiology and American Heart Association has provided an update of 12-lead ECG indications (O'Gara et al, 2013). Patient selection for ECG monitoring is the first step toward establishing appropriate alarms and response expectations. Indications and contraindications for 12-lead ECG acquisitions follow.

Indications

- Suspected acute coronary syndrome, including myocardial infarction
- Evaluation of implanted defibrillators and pacemakers
- Disorders of the cardiac rhythm
- Evaluation of syncope
- Evaluation of metabolic disorders
- Effects and side effects of pharmacotherapy
- Evaluation of primary and secondary cardiomyopathic processes

Contraindications

- No absolute contraindications to performing an ECG other than patient refusal exist.
- Some patients may have allergies or, more commonly, sensitivities to the adhesive used to affix the leads; in these cases hypoallergenic alternatives are available from various manufacturers.

TABLE 26.1

Common Basic Cardiac Rhythms

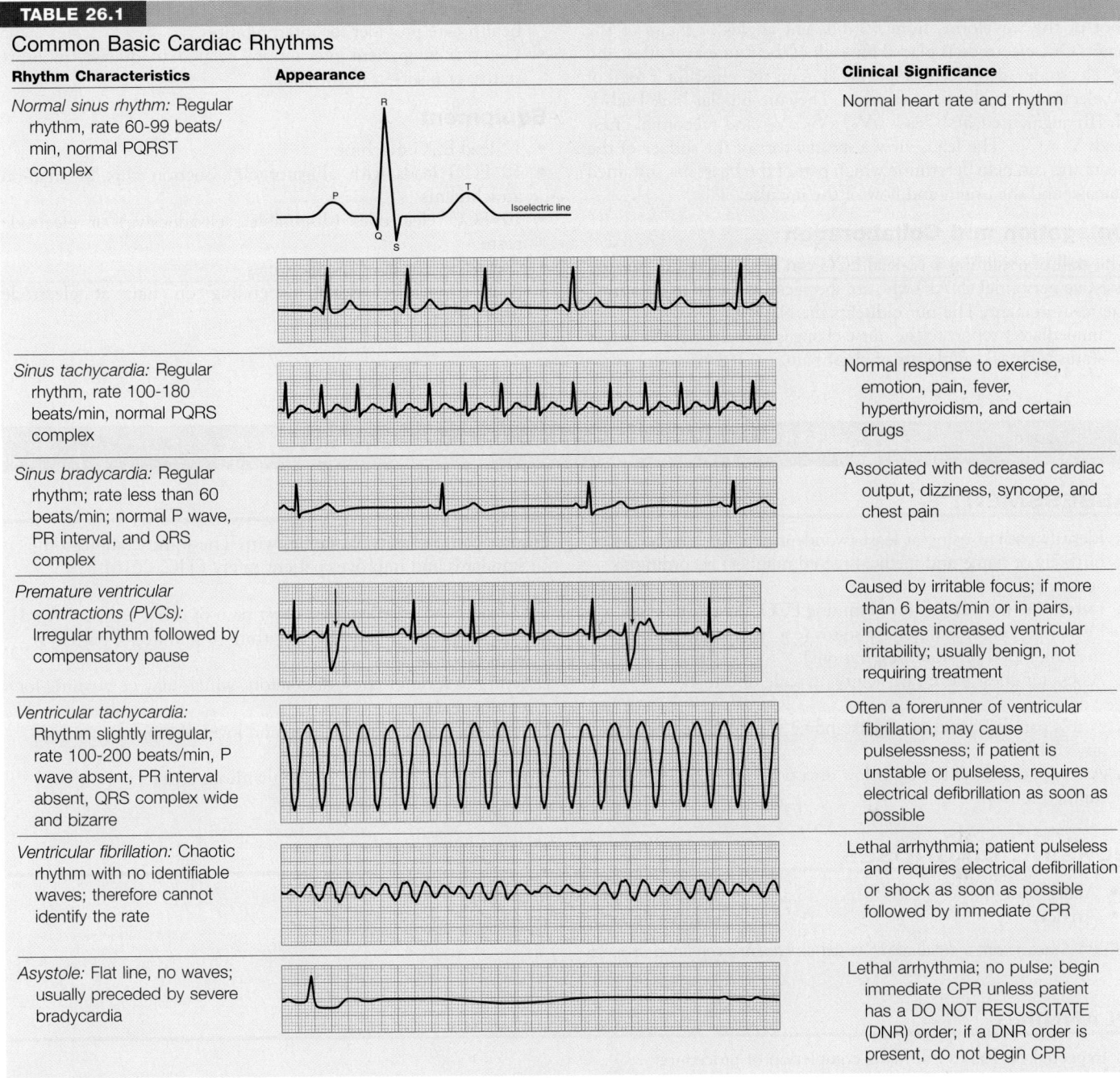

Rhythm Characteristics	Appearance	Clinical Significance
Normal sinus rhythm: Regular rhythm, rate 60-99 beats/min, normal PQRST complex		Normal heart rate and rhythm
Sinus tachycardia: Regular rhythm, rate 100-180 beats/min, normal PQRS complex		Normal response to exercise, emotion, pain, fever, hyperthyroidism, and certain drugs
Sinus bradycardia: Regular rhythm; rate less than 60 beats/min; normal P wave, PR interval, and QRS complex		Associated with decreased cardiac output, dizziness, syncope, and chest pain
Premature ventricular contractions (PVCs): Irregular rhythm followed by compensatory pause		Caused by irritable focus; if more than 6 beats/min or in pairs, indicates increased ventricular irritability; usually benign, not requiring treatment
Ventricular tachycardia: Rhythm slightly irregular, rate 100-200 beats/min, P wave absent, PR interval absent, QRS complex wide and bizarre		Often a forerunner of ventricular fibrillation; may cause pulselessness; if patient is unstable or pulseless, requires electrical defibrillation as soon as possible
Ventricular fibrillation: Chaotic rhythm with no identifiable waves; therefore cannot identify the rate		Lethal arrhythmia; patient pulseless and requires electrical defibrillation or shock as soon as possible followed by immediate CPR
Asystole: Flat line, no waves; usually preceded by severe bradycardia		Lethal arrhythmia; no pulse; begin immediate CPR unless patient has a DO NOT RESUSCITATE (DNR) order; if a DNR order is present, do not begin CPR

Martin, NK: *ECG strips from Barnes-Jewish Hospital Cardiac Care Unit,* St Louis, 2015, Elsevier.
CPR, Cardiopulmonary resuscitation.

SAFETY GUIDELINES

- Know the indications for the ordered 12-lead ECG. Patients suffering from chest pain need to have their 12-lead ECG within 10 minutes of the assessment and onset of pain. A 12-lead ECG will determine the next step in their treatment plan.
- Know a patient's current medications. Some medications, particularly beta blockers; some calcium channel blockers; and other antiarrhythmics can cause dysrhythmias.

◆ **SKILL 26.1** **Obtaining a 12-Lead Electrocardiogram**

NSO *Nursing Skills Online Cardiac Care Module / Lesson 2*

Electrical impulses of the heart are conducted to the surface of the body and are detected by electrodes placed on the skin of the limbs and torso. The electrodes carry these impulses to either a continuous monitor or a 12-lead electrocardiogram (ECG) machine. The appearance of the ECG pattern or wave form helps to diagnose whether there are any abnormalities in the electrical conduction through the heart. The 12-lead ECG provides a snap-shot of the waveforms from 12 different angles or views of the heart. One electrode is placed on each of the four extremities, and six electrodes are placed at specific sites on the chest for a total of 10 electrodes on the patient's skin. They are bipolar limb leads I, II, III; augmented limb leads aV_R, aV_L, aV_F; and precordial chest leads V_1 to V_6. The leads view a specific part of the surface of the heart and can help determine which part of the heart has sustained damage and the origin and flow of the impulse.

Delegation and Collaboration

The skill of obtaining a 12-lead ECG can be delegated to nursing assistive personnel (NAP) who are specifically trained in obtaining the measurement. The nurse directs the NAP to:

- Immediately report to the nurse changes in the patient's cardiac status such as complaints of chest pain.

- Immediately deliver the completed 12-lead ECG recording to a health care provider for interpretation.
- Use specific patient precautions related to disease, mobility status, or position restrictions.

Equipment

- 12-lead ECG machine
- 10 ECG leads with alligator clip, suction cup, or snap-on attachments
- 10 ECG electrodes (disposable, self-adhesive) or electrode paste
- Clean, dry towel or sponge wipes
- Hair clippers (optional depending on hair at electrode sites)

STEP	RATIONALE

ASSESSMENT

1. Identify patient using at least two identifiers (e.g., name and birthday or name and medical record number) according to agency policy.	Ensures patient safety. Complies with The Joint Commission standards and improves patient safety (TJC, 2016).
2. Determine indications for obtaining ECG. Assess patient's history and cardiopulmonary status (e.g., heart rate and rhythm, blood pressure, respirations).	If 12-lead ECG is ordered for chest pain or other ischemic signs and symptoms, obtain ECG within 10 minutes of patient's pain report.
3. Assess for chest pain; rate acuity on scale of 0 to 10.	Determines level of chest discomfort, which may be warning for cardiac ischemia.
4. Assess patient's level of understanding of procedure, including any concerns.	Determine extent of instruction and level of support required.
5. Assess patient's ability to follow directions and remain still in supine position.	Provides clear, accurate recording without artifact.

NURSING DIAGNOSES

- Acute pain
- Anxiety
- Deficient knowledge regarding purpose and steps of procedure
- Fear

Related factors are individualized based on patient's condition or needs.

PLANNING

1. Expected outcomes following completion of procedure: • Patient tolerates procedure without anxiety or discomfort. • Clear, accurate recording of ECG waveform is obtained.	Appropriate preparation and education decrease anxiety.
2. Close room door or bedside curtains.	Provides privacy.

IMPLEMENTATION

1. Prepare patient for procedure: a. Remove or reposition patient's clothing to expose only patient's chest and arms. Keep abdomen and thighs covered.	Facilitates correct placement of cardiac leads and maintains patient's modesty. Improper lead placement produces artifact, which necessitates repeating test or interpretation errors.
b. Place patient in supine position with head of bed no higher than 30 degrees.	Electrodes must be placed on anterior chest for standard 12-lead ECG (O'Gara et al., 2013).
c. Instruct patient to lie still without talking and do not cross legs.	Body movement or talking produces artifact, which may necessitate repeating test.
2. Turn on machine; enter required demographic information.	Turning machine on first helps you identify electrode and lead issues on application.
3. Perform hand hygiene.	Reduces transmission of microorganisms.

STEP	RATIONALE

4. Clean and prepare skin for isolated electrode placement with soap and water. Wipe area with rough washcloth or gauze or use edge of electrode to gently scrape skin. Clip excessive hair from electrode area.

Proper skin preparation before ECG electrodes are placed decreases skin impedance and signal noise, thereby producing clean, accurate recording. Do not use alcohol to clean area. It will dry out skin. Clipping hair in electrode area is preferred. Shaving leaves nicks that predispose to risk for infection.

5. Apply electrodes in correct positions. If using leads with suction cups, apply electrode paste to areas before attaching leads.
   a. Chest (precordial) leads (Fig. 26.1)
      - V1—Fourth intercostal space (ICS) at right sternal angle
      - V2—Fourth ICS at left sternal border
      - V3—Midway between V2 and V4
      - V4—Fifth ICS at midclavicular line
      - V5—Left anterior axillary line at level of V4 horizontally
      - V6—Left midaxillary line at level of V4 horizontally
   b. Extremities: One lead on each extremity (Fig. 26.2); right wrist, left wrist, left ankle, right ankle

Proper placement of leads is very important for accurate interpretation of 12-lead ECG. Ensure that correct lead is in correct location. If any leads are misplaced, ECG reading will be inaccurate (O'Gara et al., 2013).

6. Check 12-lead machine for messages to correct electrode or lead issues. If no messages occur, press button to obtain 12-lead ECG.

7. If you obtain ECG tracing without artifact, disconnect leads and wipe off excess electrode paste from chest.

Promotes comfort and hygiene.

8. If STAT, immediately deliver ECG tracing (if not computerized) to appropriate health care provider for interpretation.

If non-STAT 12-lead ECG, place in patient's chart or designated area.

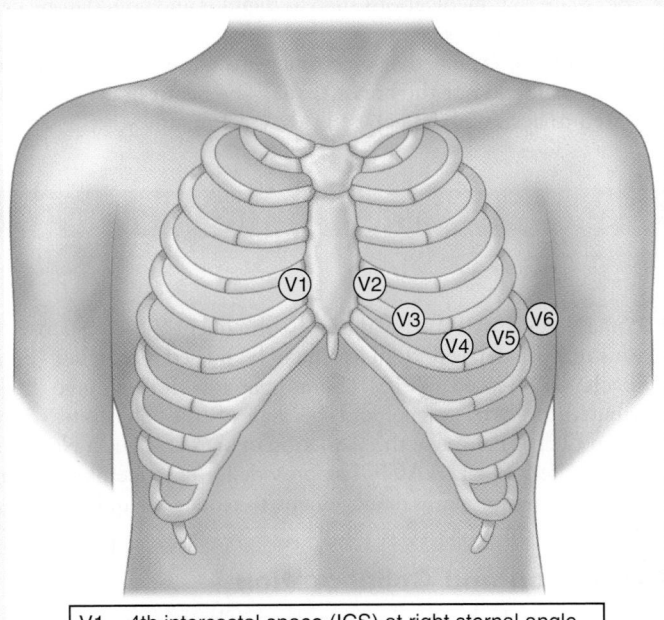

V1 – 4th intercostal space (ICS) at right sternal angle
V2 – 4th ICS at left sternal border
V3 – Midway between V2 and V4
V4 – Fifth ICS at midclavicular line
V5 – Left anterior axillary line at level of V4 horizontally
V6 – Left midaxillary line at level of V4 horizontally

FIG 26.1 Precordial (chest) lead placement for a standard 12-lead ECG.

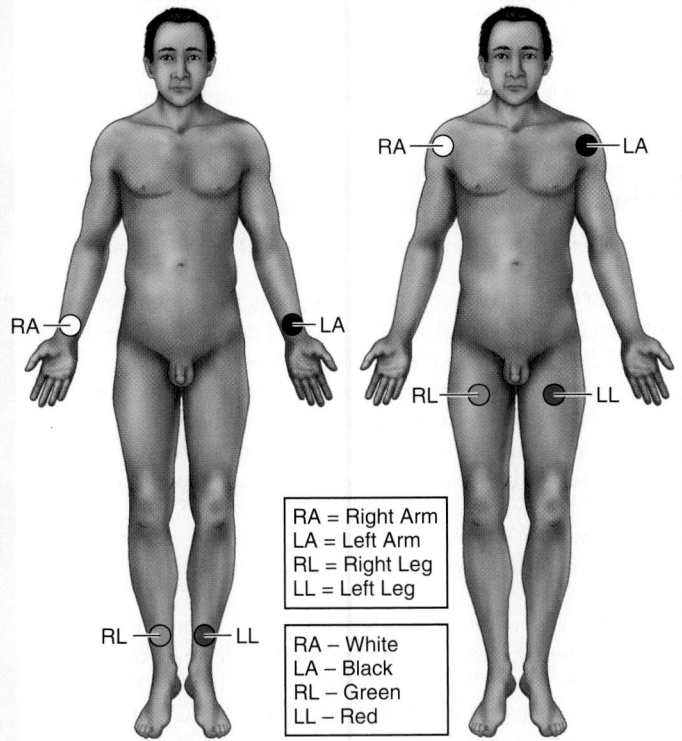

RA = Right Arm
LA = Left Arm
RL = Right Leg
LL = Left Leg

RA – White
LA – Black
RL – Green
LL – Red

FIG 26.2 Limb lead placement for a standard 12-lead ECG.

STEP	RATIONALE

EVALUATION

1. Note and document if patient is experiencing any chest discomfort during procedure.

2. Discuss findings and results of 12-lead ECG with health care provider to determine next steps in patient's treatment plan.

3. Use Teach-Back: "I want to be sure I explained why you need this ECG. Why are you receiving an ECG?" Revise your instruction now or develop a plan for revised patient teaching if patient is not able to teach back correctly.

Helps correlate ECG changes to symptoms of chest pain.

If myocardial infarction is identified, immediate steps will need to be taken to get patient to cardiac catheterization laboratory or consider use of thrombolytic medications.

Determines patient's level of understanding of instructional topic.

Unexpected Outcomes	Related Interventions

1. ECG cannot be interpreted:
  • Absence of tracing on one or more leads
  • Presence of artifact in ECG tracings
	• Inspect electrodes for secure placement.
	• Reposition any wires that move as a result of patient breathing or movement or vibrations in environment. Do not reposition electrodes if in correct position.
	• Remind patient who is moving that lying still is necessary to obtain good tracing.
	• If artifact looks like 60-cycle interference (very thick-lined waveform), unplug battery-operated equipment in room one item at a time to see if interference disappears. **NOTE:** 60-cycle interference is rare.
	• Repeat tracing.

2. Patient has chest pain or anxiety.	• Continue to monitor patient. • Reassess factors contributing to anxiety or distress. • Follow specific orders related to findings. • Notify health care provider.

Recording and Reporting

• Record date and time ECG was obtained, reason for obtaining ECG, and to whom ECG was given for interpretation in nurses' notes in electronic health record (EHR) or chart.
• Report any unexpected outcomes immediately.
• Document your evaluation of patient learning.

Special Considerations

• Be aware that medications such as digitalis and amiodarone can affect ECG results.
• For women, ensure that electrodes are placed directly on the chest wall and not the breast tissue. The breast may need to be lifted to accommodate chest leads V4, V5, V6.

◆ SKILL 26.2   Applying a Cardiac Monitor

NSO *Nursing Skills Online Cardiac Care Module / Lesson 3*

The use of continuous cardiac monitors is very common inside hospitals, clinics, and outpatient settings. The cardiac monitor can be a bedside, hard-wired monitor or a wireless transmitter used with telemetry systems. A continuous electrocardiogram (ECG) rhythm is obtained using 3 or 5 electrodes and leads on the patient. Cardiac monitors are attached to patients for immediate dysrhythmia detection; some dysrhythmias can be life threatening. They can also monitor a decrease or increase in heart rate. Most cardiac monitor systems have dysrhythmia detection software and provide alarms when dysrhythmias appear or heart rate limits are exceeded.

It is important to monitor only patients with clinical indications for cardiac monitoring. This can significantly decrease the number of false alarms (Sendelbach and Jepsen, 2013). In 2004 the American Heart Association developed guidelines for ECG monitoring in hospitalized patients (Drew et al., 2004) (Box 26.1).

Alarm fatigue develops when a person is exposed to an excessive number of alarms (Sendelbach and Jepsen, 2013). This situation can result in sensory overload, which may cause the person to

become desensitized to the alarms. Consequently the response to alarms may be delayed, or alarms may be missed altogether (Sendelbach and Jepsen, 2013). Some patient deaths have been attributed to alarm fatigue; and, because of this, The Joint Commission (2016) has made the reduction of alarm fatigue a National Patient Safety Goal. AACN has provided a practice alert listing some strategies for alarm management to reduce alarm fatigue and improve patient safety (Box 26.2).

Delegation and Collaboration

The skill of applying a cardiac monitor can be delegated to nursing assistive personnel (NAP) who are specifically trained. In some agencies the responsible party for monitoring ECG rhythms and alarms may also be that of a specifically trained NAP such as a telemetry technician. The nurse directs the NAP to:

• Immediately report to the nurse alarms or patient complaints of pain, shortness of breath, or hypotension.
• Ensure that the parameters for alarms and heart rate are set per the health care provider's orders.

BOX 26.1

Class I Indications for Continuous Cardiac Monitoring

- Postresuscitation patients
- Early phase of acute coronary syndromes
- Emergency percutaneous coronary interventions (PCI) or nonurgent PCI with complications
- Adults and children undergoing cardiac surgery
- New implantable defibrillation and/or pacemaker placement
- Temporary or transcutaneous pacemaker
- Atrioventricular block
- Suspected or known accessory pathway conduction
- Long QT syndrome
- Heart failure/pulmonary edema
- Indication for intensive care admission
- Procedures requiring conscious sedation or anesthesia
- Diagnosis of dysrhythmia in children

Modified from Drew BJ, et al: Practice standards for electrocardiographic monitoring in hospital settings: an American Heart Association scientific statement from the Councils on Cardiovascular Nursing, Clinical Cardiology, and Cardiovascular Disease in the Young: endorsed by the International Society of Computerized Electrocardiology and the American Association of Critical-Care Nurses, *Circulation* 26:110(17):2721, 2004.

BOX 26.2

Expected Practice and Nursing Actions for the Reduction of Alarm Fatigue

- Provide proper skin preparation for ECG electrodes.
- Change ECG electrodes daily.
- Customize alarm parameters and levels of ECG monitors.
- Customize delay and threshold settings on oxygen saturation via pulse oximetry (SpO_2) monitors.
- Provide initial and ongoing education about devices with alarms.
- Establish interprofessional teams to address issues related to alarms such as the development of policies and procedures.
- Monitor only patients with clinical indications for monitoring.

Adapted from Sendelbach S, Jepsen S: *AACN practice alert: alarm management,* 2013, http://www.aacn.org/wd/practice/docs/practicealerts/alarm-management-practice-alert.pdf. Accessed March 27, 2016.
ECG, Electrocardiogram.

Equipment

- Bedside cardiac monitor or telemetry transmitter
- Three or five ECG electrodes (disposable, self-adhesive)
- Three or five ECG leads with snap-on attachments
- Clean, dry towel, washcloth, or gauze
- Hair clippers (optional depending on hair at electrode sites)

STEP	RATIONALE

ASSESSMENT

1. Identify patient using at least two identifiers (e.g., name and birthday or name and medical record number) according to agency policy.

Ensures patient safety. Complies with The Joint Commission standards and improves patient safety (TJC, 2016).

2. Determine reason for continuous cardiac monitoring. Assess patient's history and cardiopulmonary status.

Knowing reason for monitoring allows for focused, improved response to an alarm.

3. Assess patient's level of understanding of procedure, including any concerns. Also assess for chest pain.

Determine extent of instruction and level of support required.

4. Check skin for excess oil or moisture. If present, wipe chest or limbs with clean, dry towel.

Provides clear, accurate recording without artifact.

NURSING DIAGNOSES

- Acute pain
- Anxiety
- Deficient knowledge regarding purpose and steps of procedure
- Fear

Related factors are individualized based on patient's condition or needs.

PLANNING

1. Expected outcomes following completion of procedure:
   - Patient tolerates procedure without anxiety or discomfort.
   - Clear, accurate ongoing recording of ECG rhythm is obtained.

Appropriate preparation decreases anxiety.

2. Close room door or bedside curtains.

Provides privacy.

IMPLEMENTATION

1. Prepare patient for procedure:
   a. Remove or reposition patient's gown to expose only patient's chest. Keep abdomen and thighs covered.

Facilitates correct placement of cardiac leads and maintains patient's modesty.

   b. Place patient in supine position.

Electrodes must be placed on anterior chest.

2. Perform hand hygiene.

Reduces transmission of microorganisms.

STEP	RATIONALE
3. Clean and prepare chest area for electrode placement with soap and water. Wipe area with rough washcloth or gauze or use edge of electrode to gently scrape area. Clip excessive hair from electrode area rather than shaving. Clipping reduces risk for infection.	Proper skin preparation before ECG electrodes are placed decreases skin impedance and signal noise, thereby producing a clean, accurate recording. Do not use alcohol to clean area. It will dry skin. Roughening skin helps remove epidermis outer layer to allow electrical signals to travel (Sendelbach and Jepsen, 2013).
4. Apply electrodes in correct positions for either a three- or five-electrode system (Fig. 26.3).	Proper placement of leads is very important for accurate dysrhythmia interpretation.
5. Attach monitor leads to electrodes. Colors of leads represent their polarity. White is negative. Black is positive. Red is ground or neutral. Two additional leads on five-lead system would include a green lead (positive or negative) and a brown lead (positive), which can be placed at a V lead locations on precordial chest.	Coloring system allows for consistent application of leads.
6. Check bedside monitor or telemetry station for any messages indicating electrode or lead issues. Troubleshoot as needed.	Monitoring system itself may detect bad electrode contact with skin or loose connection.
7. Check that the ECG rhythm can be visualized on bedside monitor, central station, or remote viewing station.	If staff is watching monitor remotely, communicate with them before you leave the room so you can correct any issues while on the phone with viewers. This call can also serve as notification that monitoring has started.
8. Change ECG electrodes daily or more often if electrode contact to skin is loose.	Changing ECG electrodes decreases the number of false alarms.
9. Customize alarm limits within 1 hour of assuming care of patient and on condition changes. Changes made should be in accordance with agency policies and health care provider's orders.	Customize alarms to individual patient needs to reduce false alarms and focus true alarms on reasons for monitoring (Sendelbach and Jepsen, 2013).

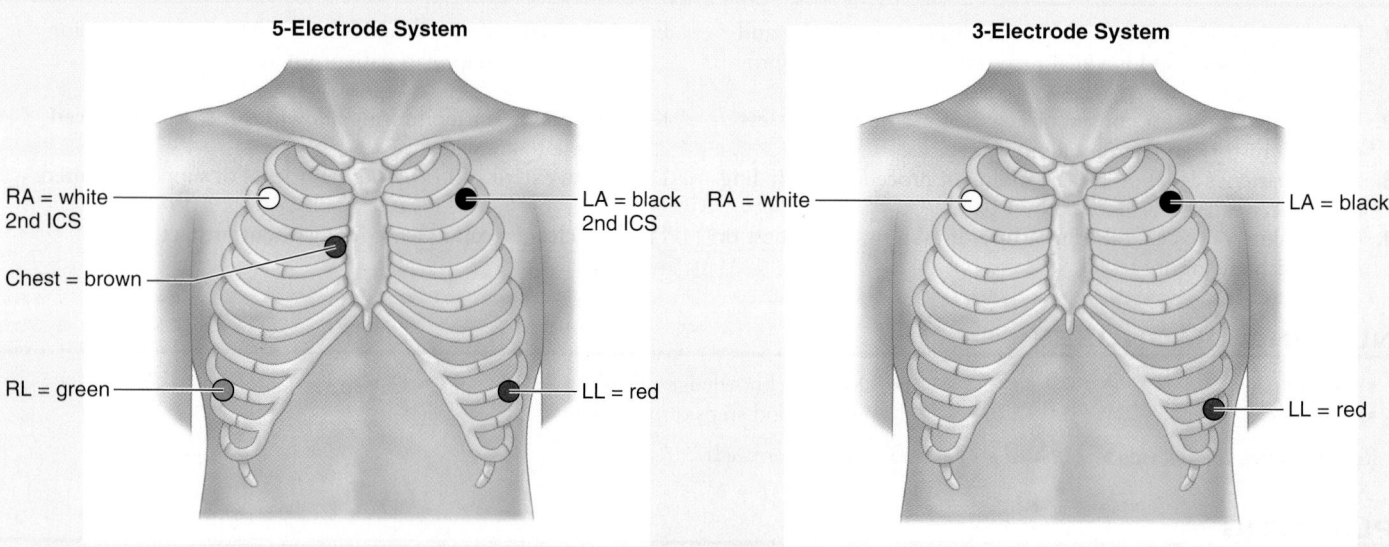

FIG 26.3 Cardiac monitor lead placement: three- or five-electrode systems. *ICS,* Intercostal space; *LA,* left arm; *LL,* left leg; *RA,* right arm; *RL,* right leg.

EVALUATION

1. Although procedure is painless, it is important to note and document if patient experienced any distress.	
2. Ensure that all appropriate alarms are ON.	Ensures accurate monitoring. Refer to agency policies.
3. **Use Teach-Back:** "I want to be sure I explained why you needed this monitoring. Why is this monitoring important?" Revise your instruction now or develop a plan for revised patient or family caregiver teaching if patient or family caregiver is not able to teach back correctly.	Determines patient's and family caregiver's level of understanding of instructional topic.

STEP	RATIONALE

Unexpected Outcomes

1. Monitor tracing cannot be interpreted:
   - Absence of tracing on one or more leads
   - Presence of artifact in ECG tracings

Related Interventions

- Inspect electrodes for secure placement. Replace as needed and provide new skin preparation.
- Reposition any wires that move as result of patient breathing or movement or vibrations in environment. Do not reposition electrodes if in correct position.
- If artifact looks like 60-cycle interference (very thick-lined waveform), unplug battery-operated equipment in room one item at a time to see if interference disappears. **NOTE:** 60-cycle interference is rare.

Recording and Reporting

- Review alarm trends and waveforms at least once a shift and on report of an alarm.
- Record at least one rhythm strip per shift per agency policy, either on paper or save to electronic health record (EHR).
- Document your evaluation of patient and family caregiver learning.
- Report any unexpected outcomes immediately to the health care provider.

Special Considerations
Pediatric

- In general, the mechanisms of dysrhythmias are the same in children as they are in adults; however, the appearance of the dysrhythmias on the ECG may differ because of developmental issues such as heart size, baseline heart rate, sinus and AV node function, and autonomic innervation.
- Be aware that medications such as digitalis and antiarrhythmics can affect ECG rhythms.
- The position of the brown lead can be changed to mirror one of the precordial (chest) lead positions, V1 to V6. The standard placement is for V1 at fourth ICS, right sternal border.

CLINICAL DEBRIEF

A 76-year-old female patient is postoperative day 2 following a partial colectomy for colon cancer. She has a history of myocardial infarction (MI) in 2008 with two stents. Your patient has turned on her call light and is complaining of nausea and chest pain. You immediately go to the patient's room. She states that she has been feeling this way for about 30 minutes. Vital signs are BP 96/50 (previous BP 128/70); pulse 120 (previous pulse 95), irregular; respiratory rate 28/minute, pulse oximetry (SpO$_2$) 90%, temp 37.5C. Lungs have crackles in the bases bilaterally. Apical pulse is very irregular. You decide to call the health care provider.

1. Based on the patient's complaint, what would you assess and which additional signs and symptoms would you expect to find?
2. Based on the patient's signs and symptoms, which orders can you anticipate? What could you delegate to the nursing assistive personnel (NAP)?
3. Using SBAR, show how you would communicate with the health care provider about this patient.

REVIEW QUESTIONS

1. Cardiac monitoring via telemetry has begun, and the telemetry technician keeps calling to report artifact on the patient's electrocardiogram (ECG) rhythm. How would you troubleshoot this artifact problem? (Select all that apply.)
   1. Moving electrodes to different locations on the chest
   2. Wiping electrode skin areas with alcohol
   3. Preparing skin by washing with soap and water and drying with a washcloth
   4. Not changing electrodes for 2 days
   5. Inspecting electrodes for secure placement
2. Indications for a 12-lead electrocardiogram (ECG) include: (Select all that apply.)
   1. Suspected acute coronary syndromes, including myocardial infarction
   2. Evaluation of implanted defibrillators and pacemakers
   3. Disorders of the cardiac rhythm
   4. Evaluation of syncope
   5. Evaluation of metabolic disorders
   6. Effects and side effects of pharmacotherapy
3. When preparing a patient for a 12-lead electrocardiogram (ECG), it is necessary to apply six precordial chest leads. Match the lead with the correct anatomical position on the patient's chest.
   1. V1   a. Fifth intercostal space (ICS) at midclavicular line
   2. V2   b. Left midaxillary line at level of V4 horizontally
   3. V3   c. Left anterior axillary line at level of V4 horizontally
   4. V4   d. Fourth ICS at right sternal border
   5. V5   e. Midway between V2 and V4
   6. V6   f. Fourth ICS at left sternal border

ⓔ *Visit the Evolve site for a complete list of Clinical Debrief and Review Questions answers.*

REFERENCES

Drew BJ, et al: Practice standards for electrocardiographic monitoring in hospital settings, *Circulation* 110:2721, 2004.
O'Gara PT, et al: 2013 ACCF/AHA guideline for the management of ST-elevation myocardial infarction: a report of the American College of Cardiology Foundation/American Heart Association Task Force on Practice Guidelines, *Circulation* 127(4):e362, 2013.
Sendelbach S, Jepsen S: AACN *practice alert: alarm management*, 2013, http://www.aacn.org/wd/practice/docs/practicealerts/alarm-management-practice-alert.pdf. Accessed March 27, 2016.
The Joint Commission (TJC): 2016 *National Patient Safety Goals*, Oakbrook Terrace, IL, 2016, The Commission, http://www.jointcommission.org/standards_information/npsgs.aspx. Accessed March 27, 2016.

27 | Closed Chest Drainage Systems

OBJECTIVES

Mastery of content in this chapter will enable the nurse to:
- Explain the physiology of normal respiration.
- List three common sites for chest tube placement.
- List three conditions requiring chest tube insertion.
- Describe closed chest drainage systems: water-seal and waterless systems.
- Describe principles and mechanisms of chest tube suction.

- Discuss measures to maintain patient safety during chest tube insertion, maintenance, and removal.
- Describe methods of troubleshooting chest tube systems.
- Discuss the nursing principles in caring for patients with chest tubes.
- Describe autotransfusion.

MEDIA RESOURCES

- evolve http://evolve.elsevier.com/Perry/skills
- Review Questions
- Audio Glossary

- **NSO** Nursing Skills Online
- Clinical Debrief and Review Questions Answers

PURPOSE

The purpose of a closed chest drainage system, with or without suction, is to promote drainage of air and fluid from the pleural space. Lung reexpansion occurs as the fluid or air is removed and the patient's oxygenation improves (Kane et al., 2013; Myatt, 2014). When air enters the pleural space, a pneumothorax occurs. When blood enters the pleural space, a hemothorax occurs. Pleural effusions occur when fluid enters the pleural space in response to infection, inflammation, or cancer.

STANDARDS OF CARE

- Scott et al., 2011—AACN Procedure Manual for Critical Care, Chest tube placement (assist)
- Atrium, 2015a—Evidence-based care of patients with chest tubes
- The Joint Commission, 2016—Patient identification

PRINCIPLES FOR PRACTICE

- The chest cavity is a closed structure bound by muscle, bone, connective tissue, vascular structures, and the diaphragm. This cavity has three distinct sections, each sealed from the others: one section for each lung and a third section for the mediastinum, which surrounds structures such as the heart, esophagus, trachea, and great vessels. The lungs are covered with a membrane called the *visceral pleura*. The interior chest wall is lined with a membrane called the *parietal pleura* (Fig. 27.1). The space between the visceral and parietal pleura is called the *pleural space* and is filled with approximately 7 to 20 mL of lubricating fluid to help the pleura slide during respiration (Kane et al., 2013; Widmaier et al., 2014).
- Trauma, disease, or surgery can result in air, blood, pus, or lymph fluid leaking into the intrapleural space, creating a positive pressure that collapses lung tissue (Shlamovitz, 2014). Small leaks (24% or less) are sometimes absorbed spontaneously and may not require a chest tube.
- A number of clinical conditions such as cancer, infection, pancreatitis, connective tissue disease, autoimmune diseases, asbestos exposure, certain drugs, or collagen vascular diseases increase pleural fluid entry or decrease fluid exit from the lung. This is called a *pleural effusion;* and, when present, a patient usually needs a diagnostic thoracentesis and pleural fluid analysis to determine the cause of the exudate (see Chapter 8) (Myatt, 2014).
- A pneumothorax is collapse of the lung caused by a collection of air in the pleural space. The loss of negative intrapleural pressure causes the lung to collapse. A traumatic pneumothorax develops as a result of penetrating chest trauma such as a

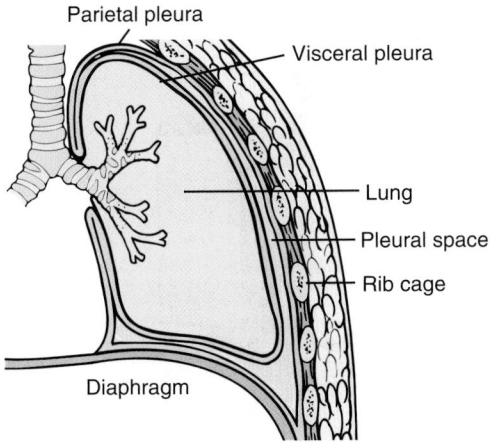

FIG 27.1 Partial structures of lungs.

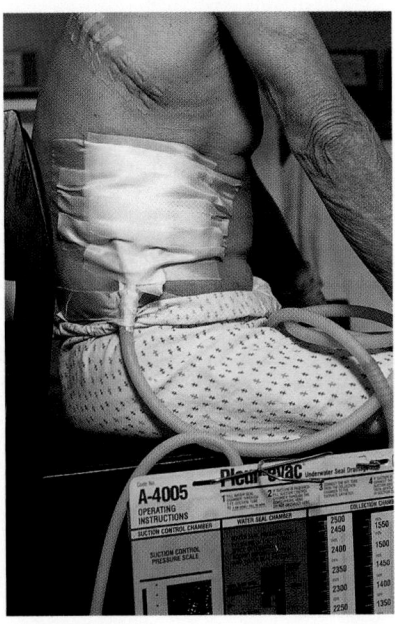

FIG 27.2 Pleural chest tube in place following thoracic surgery.

stabbing (open) or the chest striking the steering wheel in an automobile accident (closed). A spontaneous or primary pneumothorax sometimes occurs from the rupture of a small bleb (blister) on the surface of the lung or an invasive procedure such as insertion of a subclavian intravenous (IV) line. Secondary pneumothorax occurs because of underlying disease such as emphysema. A patient with a pneumothorax usually feels sharp chest pain that worsens on inspiration or coughing because atmospheric air irritates the parietal pleura.

- A tension pneumothorax, a life-threatening situation, occurs from rupture in the pleura when air accumulates in the pleural space more rapidly than it is removed. If left untreated, the lung on the affected side collapses; and the mediastinum shifts to the opposite (unaffected side), leading to tracheal deviation, reduced venous return, and subsequent decrease in cardiac output. Tracheal deviation is a late sign and may be absent in some cases (Zarogoulidis et al., 2014). Sudden chest pain, a fall in blood pressure, tachycardia, acute pleuritic pain, diaphoresis, dry cough, and cardiopulmonary arrest can occur.
- If emergent treatment is required, a needle decompression is achieved with a large-gauge needle (14 or 16 gauge) inserted into the second intercostal space, midclavicular line. A "hissing" sound is noted, followed by a rapid stabilization of the patient's vital signs and respiratory status (Bascom et al., 2014).
- A hemothorax is collapse of the lung caused by an accumulation of blood and fluid in the pleural cavity between the chest wall and the lung, usually as a result of trauma. It produces a counter pressure and prevents the full expansion of the lung. A hemothorax is also caused by rupture of small blood vessels from inflammatory processes such as pneumonia or tuberculosis. In addition to pain and dyspnea, signs and symptoms of shock can develop if blood loss is severe (US National Library of Medicine, 2014).
- Chest tube insertion is the treatment for most types of effusions, pneumothorax, hemothorax, and postoperative chest surgery or trauma. A chest tube is a large catheter inserted through the thorax to remove fluid (effusions), blood (hemothorax), and/or air (pneumothorax).
- A pleural chest tube (Fig. 27.2) is inserted when air or fluid enters the pleural space, compromising oxygenation or ventilation.
- The location of the chest tube indicates the type of drainage expected. Apical (second or third intercostal space) and

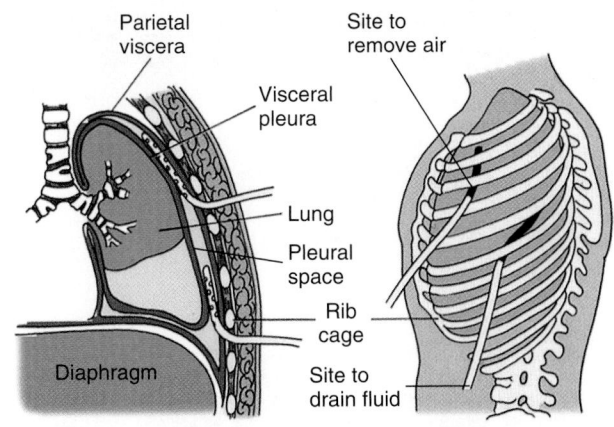

FIG 27.3 Diagram of sites for chest tube placement.

anterior chest tube placement promotes removal of air. Because air rises, these chest tubes are placed high, allowing evacuation of air from the intrapleural space and lung reexpansion (Fig. 27.3). The air is discharged into the atmosphere, and there is little or no drainage in the collection chamber.

- Chest tubes placed low (usually in the fifth or sixth intercostal space) and posterior or lateral drain fluid (see Fig. 27.3). Fluid in the intrapleural space is affected by gravity and localizes in the lower part of the lung cavity. Tubes placed in these positions drain blood and fluid. Fluid drainage is expected after open-chest surgery and with some chest trauma.
- A mediastinal chest tube is placed in the mediastinum, just below the sternum (Fig. 27.4), and is connected to a drainage system. This tube drains blood or fluid, preventing its accumulation around the heart. A mediastinal tube is commonly used after open-heart surgery.

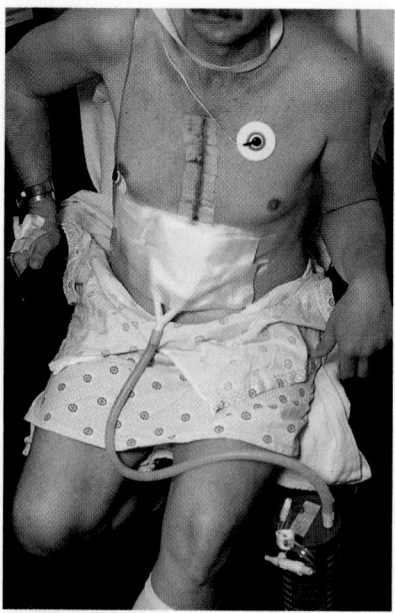

FIG 27.4 Mediastinal chest tube.

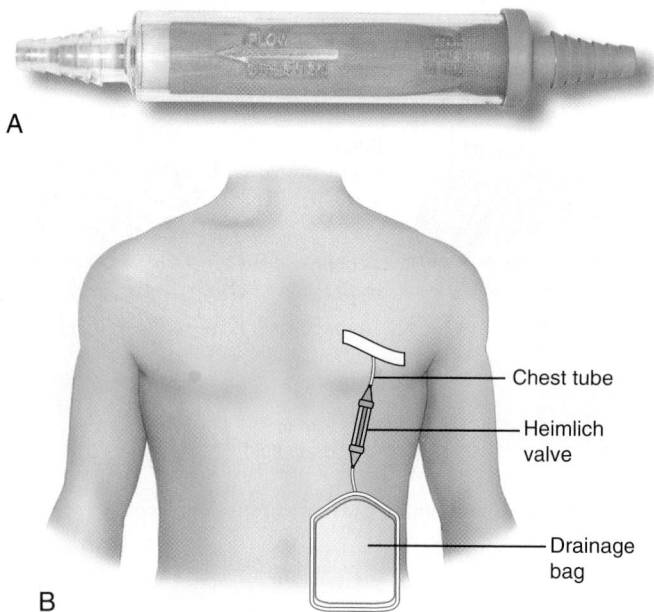

A

B

FIG 27.5 A, Heimlich chest drain valve is a specially designed flutter valve that is used in place of a chest drainage unit for small uncomplicated pneumothorax with little or no drainage and no need for suction. The valve allows for escape of air but prevents reentry of air into the pleural space. (*Image courtesy Becton, Dickenson and Company, Franklin Lakes, New Jersey. All rights reserved.*) **B,** Placement of valve between chest tube and drainage bag, which can be worn under clothing.

- In emergent situations a small pneumothorax catheter is inserted through the chest wall, and a rubber flutter one-way valve (e.g., a Heimlich valve) is attached to the catheter (Fig. 27.5A–B). As a patient exhales, the positive pressure generated by the air leaving the chest enters the tubing, causing the valve to open so air is released. During inspiration the tube

Chest tube

Heimlich valve

Drainage bag

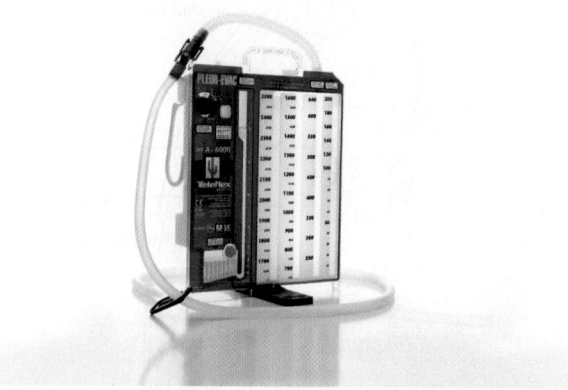

FIG 27.6 Disposable chest drainage systems. (*Multi-chamber Pleur-Evac image courtesy Teleflex Medical, Research Triangle Park, NC.*)

collapses on itself, preventing air from reentering the chest. This type of valve is not used when patients need fluid drained such as from a hemothorax or a pleural effusion (Lewis et al., 2017).

- Smaller "pigtail catheters" are also used and are less traumatic than the large-bore tubes. Ambulatory management with pigtail catheters is reasonable first-line treatment for spontaneous pneumothoraxes (Voisin et al., 2014).

- Mobile chest drains are devices that are lighter and self-contained; they allow patients to move with less restriction and cause less discomfort. These mobile systems rely on gravity or dry suction for drainage. They are ideal for home use for patients with persistent drainage or air leaks requiring prolonged need for a chest tube (Voisin et al., 2014).

- The disposable systems such as an Atrium or Pleur-Evac chest drainage system are one-piece molded plastic units that provide for a single- or multiple-chamber closed drainage system (Fig. 27.6). A single-chamber system allows air from a pneumothorax to bubble out of the water seal and escape through the air outlet while preventing it from reentering the intrapleural space. The drawback of a single-chamber system is that any chest drainage present collects in the same chamber that provides the water seal. If the single-chamber system fills with chest fluid, the water-seal level would rise, making it more difficult for the patient to expel any air. Thus single-chamber systems are not recommended for the evacuation of fluid. An increased height of fluid in the water seal increases the resistance to drainage on expiration and eventually stops the drainage entirely.

- A two- or three-chamber system drains both a hemothorax and a pneumothorax effectively. The two-chamber system permits liquid to flow into the collection chamber, and air flows into the water-seal chamber. A three-chamber system promotes the drainage of fluid and air with controlled suction. In both systems the first chamber provides a compartment for fluid or blood drainage and a second compartment for either a water seal or a one-way valve. In the three-chamber system the third compartment is for suction control, which may or may not be used. The disposable units appear to be the system of choice because they are cost-effective and some facilitate autotransfusion; they are occasionally used in open-heart surgeries.

PATIENT-CENTERED CARE

- Health care–acquired infections (HAIs) occur at the rate of 13 per 1000 patient days in U.S. intensive care units (ICUs). As patient advocates, nurses need to know the factors leading to HAIs, the related increased length of stay and financial burden of these infections (Zimlichman et al., 2013), and the burden patients and families experience because of higher mortality rates and prolonged hospitalizations. Invasive procedures such as mechanical ventilation, central venous catheters, and chest tubes can all increase the risk for HAIs.
- Infections occur rarely with chest tubes. They can range from skin infections at the insertion site to empyema and even necrotizing infections (Kwiatt et al., 2014; Mao et al., 2015; Rajan, 2013).
- Nurses must be vigilant for patient assessment findings that indicate the need for a chest tube and encourage deep-breathing exercises and early mobility, use of appropriate analgesia to promote activity, and patient education regarding these practices (Kane et al., 2013).

EVIDENCE-BASED PRACTICE

- Small chest tubes often become blocked by blood clots and fibrin. Large-bore catheters (such as 28F) safely remove secretions (Zardo et al., 2015).
- Milking and stripping a chest tube to clear the clots are controversial and when done on a routine basis do more harm than good (Makic et al., 2015). Stripping causes a dangerous increase in intrathoracic pressure, which damages the lung tissue (Atrium, 2014; Kane et al., 2013). Chest drainage stripping or milking demonstrates no safety or efficacy benefits, slightly increases intrathoracic pressure, and risks tissue damage (Atrium, 2014, 2015a; Makic et al., 2015).
- Careful management of chest tube drainage prevents chest tube occlusion:
  - Avoid dependent loops of the drainage tube; or, when these loops cannot be avoided (such as when the patient is sitting), lift and clear the tube every 15 to 30 minutes.
  - Keep the chest drainage tubing and the collection system below the level of the patient's chest. Keep the tubing above the collection system to allow drainage by gravity.
  - Tailor the length of the drainage tube to a patient. The tubing must be long enough to allow a patient to move but not so long that dependent loops hang down the side of the bed. If the tubing is coiled, looped, or clotted, the drainage is impeded and can result in a tension pneumothorax (Kane et al., 2013).

SAFETY GUIDELINES

- Document patient's baseline vital signs, oxygen saturation, lung sounds, and respiratory status. Changes in vital signs or respiratory status often indicate a malfunction of a chest drainage system.
- Observe the water seal for intermittent bubbling or a rise and fall of fluid that is synchronous with respirations (Kane et al., 2013). For example, in a spontaneously breathing patient the fluid level rises during inspiration and falls during expiration. When a patient is on a mechanical ventilator, the opposite occurs.
- Constant bubbling in the water seal or a sudden, unexpected stoppage of water-seal activity is considered abnormal and requires immediate attention (Kane et al., 2013).
- Unexpected stoppage of chest tube activity may indicate a blockage or lung reexpansion. In these situations immediate attention and correction are indicated. After 2 or 3 days, tidaling or bubbling on expiration is expected to stop, indicating that the lung has reexpanded (Kuhajda et al., 2014).
- In a waterless system look for a rise and fall of fluid in the diagnostic air-leak indicator synchronous with respirations. Constant left-to-right bubbling (when facing the indicator) or violent rocking is considered abnormal and indicates an air leak.
- Note the expected amount of chest tube drainage and monitor drainage on a regular basis (e.g., every hour initially and then every 4 hours). At the end of the shift, make a mark to indicate the fluid level with the date and time on the side of the drainage collection chamber. Note the drainage amount as output.
  - A sudden decrease in the amount of chest tube drainage can indicate a possible clot or obstruction in the chest tube (Kuhajda et al., 2014).
  - Notify a health care provider when there is a sudden increase of more than 250 mL of drainage over 1 hour, which can indicate fresh bleeding from the thorax (Kane et al., 2013; Mao et al., 2015).
  - Drainage from a pneumothorax is generally limited (Kane et al., 2013). Any fluid buildup is caused by chest tube insertion trauma. The chest tubes promote the removal of air from the intrapleural space.
- Know the expected color of the drainage. Drainage from recent open-chest surgery initially is bright red and gradually becomes serous as the postoperative course continues. Blood-tinged fluid usually indicates malignancy, pulmonary infarction, or severe inflammation. Frank blood indicates a hemothorax. Pus indicates an empyema, which is a collection of pus in the pleural cavity (Kane et al., 2013).
- In the water-seal system observe for constant, gentle bubbling in the suction-control chamber when it is connected to suction. In the waterless system a designated amount of suction is maintained by setting the suction source and dialing the prescribed suction level in the float ball column.
- Assess both types of systems for air leaks. If an air leak exists, determine whether it is in the patient (patient-centered air leak) or the chest tube system (system-centered air leak). To rule out an air leak as patient-centered, you assess the patient's respiratory status. Document and report any changes in lung sounds, pulse oximetry, respiratory rate, or mentation. Remember that continuous bubbling in the water-seal chamber with an absence of bubbles in the suction-control chamber indicates that there is a leak in the system (Kane et al., 2013). Ensure that all tubing connections are tight.
- Be sure that the drainage system is stable. Most chest drainage units have attached adjustable hangers that allow the device to hang on the side or end of the patient's bed. Many have a swing-out floor stand to reduce the chance of accidentally knocking over the chest drainage system if it is placed on the floor. Some manufacturers make a reusable drain caddy that allows the chest drainage system to be connected to an IV pole to facilitate patient movement and eliminate a chance of knocking over the system.

✦ SKILL 27.1 Managing Closed Chest Drainage Systems

NSO *Nursing Skills Online Closed Chest Drainage System Module / Lessons 1 and 3*

There are two types of commercial drainage systems: the water-seal and the waterless systems (Table 27.1). This skill reviews the nursing responsibilities and interventions related to the safe management of chest tubes. Review the roles and responsibilities of the health care provider for chest tube placement (Table 27.2).

Water-Seal Systems

NSO *Nursing Skills Online Closed Chest Drainage System Module / Lesson 2*

Two-Chamber Water-Seal System

On expiration fluid or air is forced out of the intrapleural space. Suction pulls air or fluid through the chest tube into the drainage collection chamber. On entering the drainage collection chamber, this fluid or air displaces the air present in the chamber by pushing it through the water-seal and out of the system into the atmosphere. The water-seal chamber is left open to air to drain. If the tubing is clamped, there is no mechanism for air to vent. To maintain the water-seal system, the chest tube system must remain upright. When it is tipped or overturned, the water-seal is disrupted.

Three-Chamber Water-Seal System

If suction is used, the three-chamber water-seal system (Fig. 27.7) is set up with the suction-control chamber added. A prescribed amount of sterile fluid (e.g., 20 cm of water) is poured into the suction-control chamber, which is then attached to a suction source by tubing. The amount of sterile water added depends on manufacturer recommendations. The chamber is filled to the set volume for the prescribed amount of suction. It is the height of the water in the suction-control chamber that determines the amount of suction. Sterile water is added several times a day because of evaporation. As the fluid level decreases, the amount of suction also declines.

If the suction source delivers more negative pressure than the suction-control chamber water level allows, the extra air pulled into the chamber causes vigorous bubbling. If this occurs, lower the suction source setting to reduce noise and evaporation of the fluid. The absence of bubbling indicates that no suction is being exerted into the system. Raise the suction setting to restore gentle bubbling.

The middle chamber is the water seal. The water seal allows air to exit from the pleural space on exhalation and prevents it from entering the pleural cavity or mediastinum on inhalation. When the appropriate amount of sterile water is added, a 2-cm water seal is established. To maintain effective water seal the chest drainage unit must remain upright, and you must monitor the water level in the water-seal chamber to check for evaporation. Bubbling in the water-seal chamber indicates an air leak.

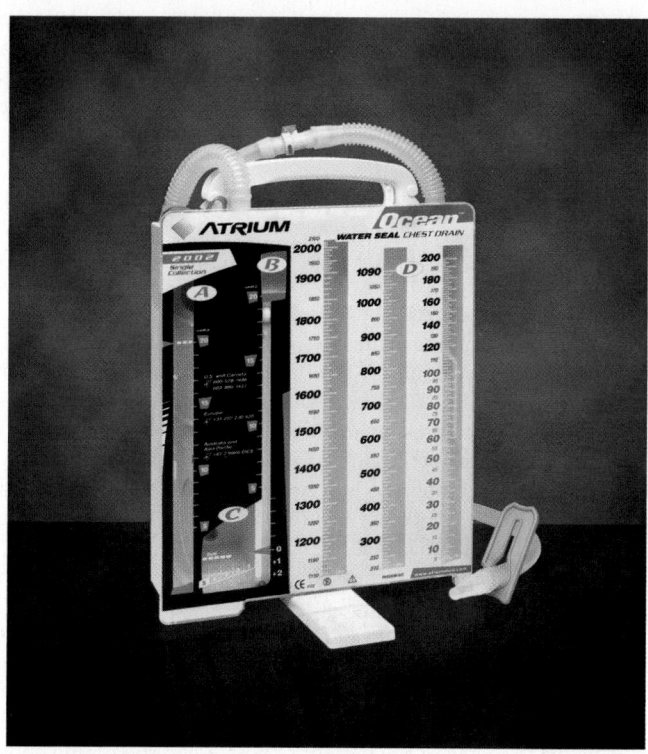

FIG 27.7 Disposable water-seal chest drainage system with suction. (*Used with permission, Atrium Medical Corp.*)

TABLE 27.1

Comparison of Chest Tube Drainage Systems

Drainage System Type	Function	Advantage	Disadvantage
Water-seal system (see Fig. 27.7)	Two-chamber provides one-way valve for chest drainage. Water seal prevents reentry of air into lung. Three-chamber adds a chamber to aid evacuation of chest drainage.	Easy setup and use Cost-effective	System must be kept upright to maintain seal. Drainage chamber may fill up quickly if patient has large amount of drainage. Sterile water must be added several times a day to maintain suction and water seal because of evaporation.
Waterless system (see Fig. 27.8)	Also provides three chambers, but no water is required to establish a seal.	Seal is maintained by a one-way valve Accidental tipping of system does not compromise patient's condition More space provided for drainage	Water must be added to an air-leak indicator if patient requires evaluation of an air leak.
Dry suction system (see Fig. 27.9)	Also provides three chambers, but suction is controlled by an integrated valve.	Easy setup Quiet operation Can be used when higher levels of suction are required	Sterile water must be added to system to provide a water seal.

Waterless Systems

Two-Chamber Waterless System

The principles of the waterless system are similar to those of the water-seal system except that fluid is not required for setup. Because water is not used, accidentally tipping the system does not compromise the patient's condition.

The water seal is replaced by a one-way valve (Fig. 27.8) located near the top of the system. Most of the container serves as the drainage chamber. The suction chamber does not depend on water. Instead it contains a float ball, which is set by a suction-control dial after the suction source is turned on.

A diagnostic air-leak indicator is located on the face of the unit. It requires the addition of 15 mL of fluid for visualization. The function of the indicator is to identify one of the following:

1. The lung is expanding normally. This is indicated by a gentle tidaling of the fluid in the diagnostic indicator.
2. The lung is probably reexpanded if after 2 or 3 days the tidaling has stopped.
3. There is an air leak in the system if, when facing the system, the observer sees the fluid bubbling left to right. Locate and correct the source of the air leak.

TABLE 27.2

Process for Insertion of Chest Tubes

Role	Purpose
Explain purpose, procedure, and possible complications to patient and have patient sign consent form.	Provides informed consent.
Have pain medication available to administer before or immediately after chest tube insertion as appropriate according to patient's condition.	Analgesia improves patient comfort throughout procedure and helps patient take appropriate deep breaths to promote lung expansion and drainage of fluid in pleural space.
Unless an emergent situation exists, perform "time out" before initiating procedure.	Verifies correct patient and procedure.
Perform hand hygiene. Clean chest wall with antiseptic.	Reduces transmission of microorganisms.
Apply mask and gloves.	Maintains surgical asepsis.
Drape area of chest tube insertion with sterile towels. Health care provider injects local anesthetic and allow time to take effect.	Maintains surgical asepsis. Decreases pain during procedure.
Health care provider makes a small incision over the rib space where tube is to be inserted. Thread a clamped chest tube through the incision. Health care provider clamps chest tube until system is connected to water seal.	Inserts chest tube into intrapleural space. Clamping prevents entry of atmospheric air into chest and worsening of pneumothorax.
Health care provider sutures chest tube in place if suturing is policy or health care provider preference.	Secures chest tube in place.
Cover chest tube insertion site with sterile 4 × 4–inch gauze and large dressing to form an occlusive dressing. Sterile petrolatum gauze is used around the tube.	Holds chest tube in place and occludes site around it. Helps stabilize chest tube and holds dressing tightly in place. Sterile petrolatum gauze helps prevent air leak.
Water-Seal System	
Remove connector cover from patient's end of chest drainage tubing with sterile technique. Secure drainage tubing to chest tube and drainage system.	Health care provider is responsible for making certain that system is set up properly, proper amount of water is in the water seal, dressing is secure, and chest tube is connected to drainage system securely.
Water-Seal Suction	
Connect system to suction or supervise a nurse connecting it to suction if suction is to be used.	Health care provider is responsible for determining and checking amount of fluid that is to be added to suction-control chamber and prescribing suction setting.
Waterless System	
Remove connector cover from patient's end of chest drainage tubing with sterile technique. Secure drainage tubing to chest tube and drainage system.	Health care provider is responsible for making certain that system is set up properly and chest tube is securely connected to drainage system.
Waterless Suction	
Turn on suction source. Set suction indicator (float ball or bellows) to prescribed setting.	Health care provider is responsible for prescribing level suction.
Health care provider or nurse adds sterile water or normal saline to diagnostic indicator on waterless system.	Allows quick assurance that system is functioning properly. Connects chest tube to drainage.
Unclamp chest tube.	Verifies correct chest tube placement.
In each system health care provider orders and reviews chest x-ray film studies.	

Three-Chamber Waterless System

When suction is ordered, attach the suction chamber port to the suction source by tubing, turn the suction on, and set the suction indicator (float ball or bellows) to the prescribed setting. If the suction indicator does not move to the prescribed level, increase the suction source setting until it does. The system is now functioning with suction.

There are usually two suction settings: one at either the suction-control chamber or the indicator setting and the other at the suction source. The settings are safety factors to reduce the possibility that the intrapleural tissues receive too much suction, causing injury.

Dry Suction System

Dry suction-control systems provide many advantages (Fig. 27.9), including higher suction pressure levels if needed, easy setup, no water in the suction-control chamber, and the absence of continuous bubbling, which provides for quiet operation. A self-compensating regulator controls dry suction units. A dial is set to the prescribed suction-control setting. These units are preset to −20 cm of water pressure, but they are adjustable from −10 to −40 cm. However, the dry suction-control systems require or have presealed sterile water to use in the water-seal chamber (Atrium, 2015b).

Delegation and Collaboration

The skill of chest tube management cannot be delegated to nursing assistive personnel (NAP). The nurse directs the NAP about:

- Proper positioning of the patient with chest tubes to facilitate chest tube drainage and optimal functioning of the system.
- Ambulating and transferring patient with chest drainage.
- Reporting changes in vital signs, complaints of chest pain or sudden shortness of breath, or excessive bubbling in water-seal chamber to the nurse immediately.
- Danger of any disconnection of drainage system, change in type and amount of drainage, sudden bleeding, or sudden cessation of bubbling.

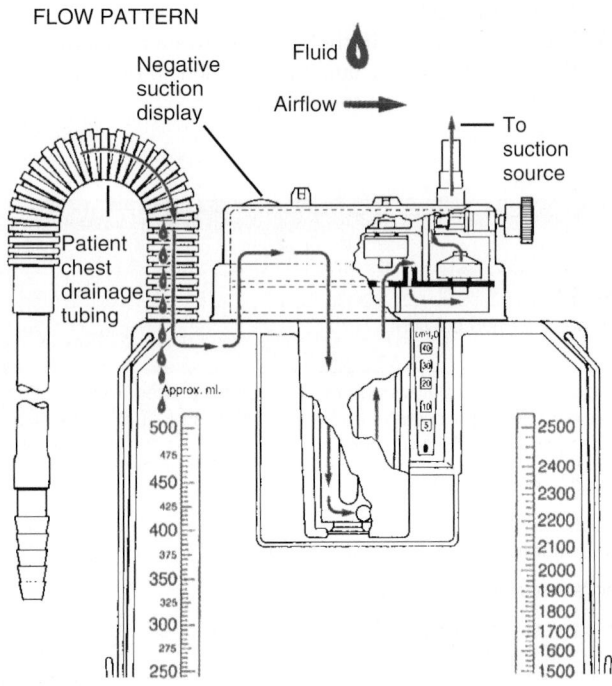

FIG 27.8 Disposable waterless chest drainage system with suction.

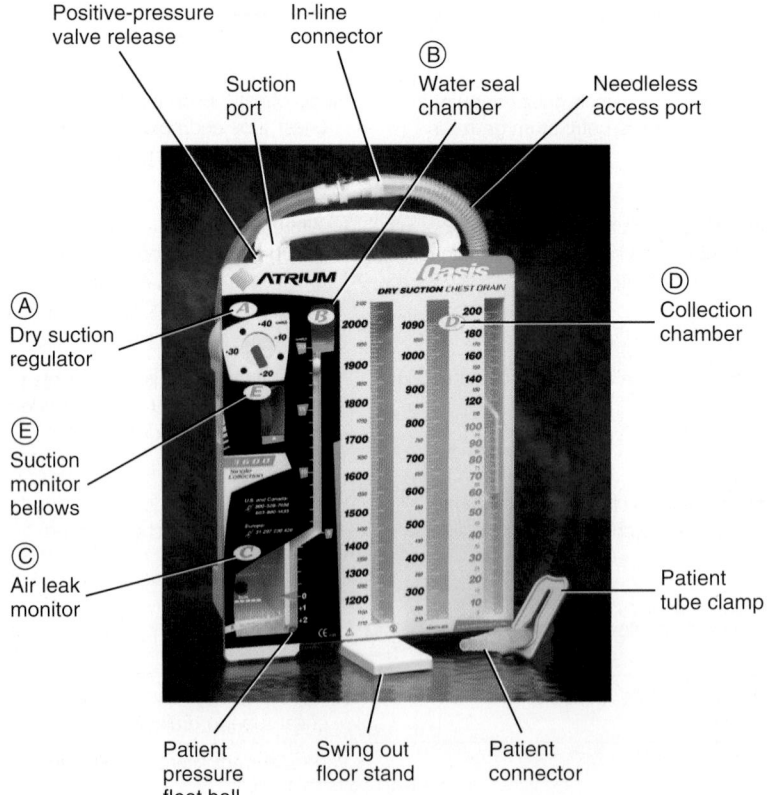

FIG 27.9 Dry suction chest drainage system. (*Used with permission, Atrium Medical Corp.*)

Equipment

- Prescribed chest drainage system
- Suction source and setup (wall canister or portable)
  - *Water-seal system:* Add sterile water or normal saline (NS) solution to cover the lower 2 cm of the water-seal chamber. Pour sterile water or NS into the suction-control chamber if suction is to be used (see manufacturer directions)
  - *Waterless system:* Add vial of 30- to 45-mL sterile sodium chloride or water (for diagnostic air-leak indicator), 20-mL syringe, 21-gauge needle, and antiseptic swab
  - Dry suction system
- Clean gloves
- Sterile gauze sponges
- Local anesthetic, if not an emergent procedure
- Chest tube tray (all items are sterile): Knife handle (1), knife blade No. 10 or disposable safety scalpel No. 10, chest tube clamp, small sponge forceps, needle holder, size 3-0 silk sutures, tray liner (sterile field), curved 8-inch Kelly clamps (2), 4 × 4–inch sponges (10), suture scissors, hand towels (3), sterile gloves
- Dressings: Petrolatum or Xeroform gauze, split chest-tube dressings, several 4 × 4–inch gauze dressings, large gauze dressings (2), and 4-inch tape
- Head cover
- Face mask/face shield
- Sterile gloves
- Two rubber-tipped hemostats (shodded) for each chest tube
- 2.5-cm (1-inch) waterproof adhesive tape or plastic zip ties for securing connections
- Stethoscope, sphygmomanometer, and pulse oximeter

STEP	RATIONALE

ASSESSMENT

STEP	RATIONALE
1. Identify patient using at least two identifiers (e.g., name and birthday or name and medical record number) according to agency policy.	Ensures correct patient. Complies with The Joint Commission standards and improves patient safety (TJC, 2016).
2. Perform a complete respiratory assessment, baseline vital signs, and pulse oximetry (SpO$_2$).	Baseline assessment and vital signs are essential for any invasive procedure. Chest tube insertion often causes respiratory distress.
a. Signs and symptoms of increased respiratory distress and hypoxia (e.g., decreased breath sounds over affected and unaffected lungs, marked cyanosis, asymmetrical chest movements, displaced trachea, shortness of breath, and confusion).	Signs and symptoms associated with respiratory distress are related to type and size of pneumothorax, hemothorax, or preexisting illness. Signs of hypoxia are related to inadequate oxygen to tissues.
b. Assess for sharp, stabbing chest pain or chest pain on inspiration, hypotension, and tachycardia. If possible, ask patient to rate level of comfort on a scale of 0 to 10.	Sharp stabbing chest pain with or without decreased blood pressure and increased heart rate may indicate tension pneumothorax. Presence of pneumothorax or hemothorax is painful, frequently causing sharp inspiratory pain. In addition, discomfort is associated with presence of a chest tube, not just with its insertion. As a result, patients tend to not cough or change position in an effort to minimize this pain (Kane et al., 2013).
3. Assess patient for known allergies. Ask patient if he or she has had a problem with medications, latex, or anything applied to skin.	Povidone-iodine or chlorhexidine are antiseptic solutions used to clean skin before tube insertion (Kuhajda et al., 2014). Lidocaine is a local anesthetic administered to reduce pain. The chest tube will be held in place with tape and sutures.
4. Review patient's medication record for anticoagulant therapy, including aspirin, warfarin, heparin, or platelet aggregation inhibitors such as ticlopidine or dipyridamole.	Anticoagulation therapy can increase procedure-related blood loss.
5. Review patient's hemoglobin and hematocrit levels.	Parameters reflect if blood loss is occurring, which may affect oxygenation.
6. For patients who have chest tubes, observe:	
a. Chest tube dressing and site surrounding tube insertion.	Ensures that dressing is intact and occlusive seal remains without air or fluid leaks and that area surrounding insertion site is free of drainage or skin irritation.
b. Tubing for kinks, dependent loops, or clots.	Maintains a patent, freely draining system, preventing fluid accumulation in chest cavity. When tubing is coiled, looped, or clotted, drainage is impeded, and there is an increased risk for tension pneumothorax or surgical emphysema (Kane et al., 2013; Rajan, 2013).
c. Chest drainage system should remain upright and below level of tube insertion.	An upright drainage system facilitates drainage and maintains water seal.
7. Determine patient's knowledge of procedure.	Encourages cooperation, minimizes risks and anxiety. Identifies teaching needs.

STEP	RATIONALE

NURSING DIAGNOSES

- Anxiety
- Acute pain
- Impaired gas exchange
- Risk for infection

Related factors/Risk factors are individualized based on patient's condition or needs.

PLANNING

1. Expected outcomes following completion of procedure:
- Patient is oriented and less anxious.
- Vital signs are stable.
- Patient reports no chest pain.
- Breath sounds are auscultated in all lobes. Lung expansion is symmetrical, SpO_2 is stable or improved, and respirations are unlabored.
- Chest tube remains in place, and chest drainage system remains airtight.
- Gentle tidaling (fluctuations or rocking) is evident in water-seal or diagnostic indicator.

Hypoxia is relieved.
Decreased hypoxia improves vital sign measures.
Reexpansion of lung reduces chest pain.
Reexpansion of lung promotes normal respirations.

Indicates correct placement and patency of chest tube drainage system.
Indicates that system is functioning normally. Reflects changes in intrapleural pressure.

IMPLEMENTATION

1. Check agency policy and determine whether informed consent is needed. Complete "Time Out" procedure.

Invasive medical procedures typically require informed consent. "Time Out" is completed to determine right patient, procedure, and location of insertion or incision site (Kane et al., 2013).

2. Review health care provider's order for chest tube placement.

Insertion of chest tube requires health care provider order.

3. Perform hand hygiene.

4. Set up water-seal system (or dry system with suction); see manufacturer guidelines.

a. Obtain chest drainage system. Remove wrappers and prepare to set up two- or three-chamber system.

Maintains sterility of system for use under sterile operating room conditions.

b. While maintaining sterility of drainage tubing, stand system upright and add sterile water or normal saline (NS) to appropriate compartments.

Reduces possibility of contamination.

(1) *Two-chamber system (without suction):* Add sterile solution to water-seal chamber (second chamber), bringing fluid to required level as indicated.

Water-seal chamber acts as one-way valve so air cannot enter pleural space (Kane et al., 2013).

(2) *Three-chamber system (with suction):* Add sterile solution to water-seal chamber (second chamber). Add amount of sterile solution prescribed by health care provider to suction-control chamber (third chamber), usually 20 cm H_2O pressure. Connect tubing from suction-control chamber to suction source. Tailor length of drainage tube to patient. **NOTE:** Suction control chamber vent must not be occluded when using suction (see illustration).

Depth of fluid level dictates highest amount of negative pressure that can be present within system. For example, 20 cm of water is approximately 20 cm of water pressure. Any additional negative pressure applied to the system is vented into the atmosphere through suction-control vent. This safety device prevents damage to pleural tissues from unexpected surge of negative pressure from suction source.
After chest tube is inserted, turn up the wall or portable suction device until water in suction-control bottle exhibits continuous, gentle bubbling.

Clinical Decision Point *When increasing suction, remember that increased bubbling does not result in more suction to the chest cavity, but only serves to evaporate the water more quickly.*

(3) *Dry suction system:* Fill water-seal chamber with sterile solution. Adjust suction-control dial to prescribed level of suction; suction ranges from −10 to −40 cm of water pressure. Suction-control chamber vent is never occluded when suction is used. **NOTE:** On dry suction system, *DO NOT* obstruct positive-pressure relief valve. This allows air to escape.

Automatic control valve on dry suction-control device adjusts to changes in patient air leaks and fluctuation in suction source and vacuum to deliver prescribed amount of suction.

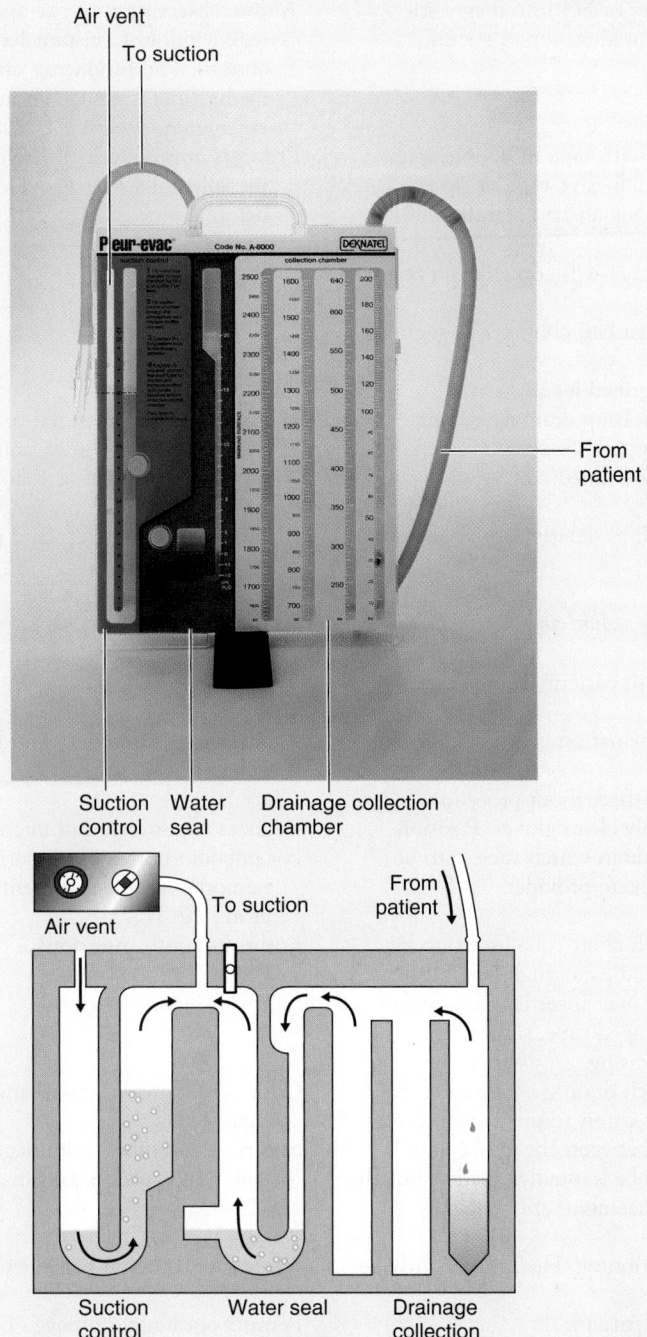

STEP 4b(2) *Top,* Pleur-Evac drainage system, a commercial three-chamber chest drainage device. *Bottom,* Schematic of drainage device.

STEP	RATIONALE
5. Set up waterless system (see manufacturer guidelines).	
a. Remove sterile wrappers and prepare to set up.	Maintains sterility of system for use under sterile operating room conditions.
b. For two-chamber system (without suction), nothing is added or needs to be done to system.	Waterless two-chamber system is ready for connecting to patient's chest tube after opening wrappers.
c. For three-chamber system (with suction), connect tubing from suction-control chamber to suction source.	Suction source provides additional negative pressure to system.

STEP	RATIONALE
d. Instill 15 mL of sterile water or NS into diagnostic indicator injection port located on top of system.	Allows observation of rise and fall of water in diagnostic air leak window. Constant left-to-right bubbling or rocking is abnormal and indicates air leak. This is not necessary for mediastinal drainage because there is no tidaling. In an emergency, system *does not* require water for setup.
6. Secure all tubing connections with tape in double-spiral fashion using 2.5-cm (1-inch) adhesive tape or zip ties (nylon cable) with a clamp (Bauman and Handley, 2011). Check system for patency by: **a.** Clamping drainage tubing that will connect to patient's chest tube. **b.** Connecting tubing from float ball chamber to suction source. **c.** Turning on suction to prescribed level.	Prevents atmospheric air from leaking into system and patient's intrapleural space. Provides chance to ensure airtight system before connection to patient.
7. Turn off suction source and unclamp drainage tubing before connecting patient to system. Suction source is turned on again after patient is connected.	Having patient connected to suction when it is initiated could damage pleural tissues from sudden increase in negative pressure. Tubing that is coiled or looped may become clotted and cause tension pneumothorax (Kane et al., 2013).
8. Administer premedication such as sedatives or analgesics as ordered.	Reduces patient anxiety and pain during procedure.

Clinical Decision Point *During procedure carefully monitor patient for changes in level of sedation.*

STEP	RATIONALE
9. Provide psychological support to patient (Kane et al., 2013). **a.** Reinforce preprocedure explanation. **b.** Coach and support patient throughout procedure.	Reduces patient anxiety and helps complete procedure efficiently.
10. Perform hand hygiene and apply clean gloves. Position patient for tube insertion so side in which tube is to be inserted is accessible to health care provider.	Reduces transmission of microorganisms. For pneumothorax, place patient in lateral supine position. For hemothorax, place patient in semi-Fowler's position (Kane et al., 2013).
11. Assist health care provider with chest tube insertion by providing needed equipment and local analgesic. Health care provider anesthetizes skin over insertion site, makes small skin incision, inserts clamped tube, sutures it in place, and applies occlusive dressing.	Ensures smooth insertion.
12. Help health care provider attach drainage tube to chest tube; remove clamp. Turn on suction to prescribed level.	Connects drainage system and suction (if ordered) to chest tube.
13. Tape or zip-tie all connections between chest tube and drainage tube. (**NOTE:** Chest tube is usually taped by health care provider at time of tube placement; check agency policy).	Secures chest tube to drainage system and reduces risk for air leak that causes breaks in airtight system (Shlamovitz, 2014).
14. Check systems for proper functioning. Health care provider orders chest x-ray film.	Verifies intrapleural placement of tube.
15. After tube placement position patient: **a.** Use semi-Fowler's or high-Fowler's position to evacuate air (pneumothorax) (Rajan, 2013). **b.** Use high-Fowler's position to drain fluid (hemothorax) (Rajan, 2013).	Permits optimum drainage of fluid and/or air.
16. Check patency of air vents in system. **a.** Water-seal vent must have no occlusion. **b.** Suction-control chamber vent is not occluded when suction is used. **c.** Waterless systems have relief valves without caps.	Permits displaced air to pass into atmosphere. Provides safety factor of releasing excess negative pressure into atmosphere. Provides safety factor of releasing excess negative pressure.
17. Position excess tubing horizontally on mattress next to patient. Secure with clamp provided so it does not obstruct tubing.	Prevents excess tubing from hanging over edge of mattress in dependent loop. Drainage collected in loop can occlude drainage system, which predisposes patient to tension pneumothorax (Kane et al., 2013).

STEP	RATIONALE
18. Adjust tubing to hang in straight line from chest tube to drainage chamber.	Promotes drainage and prevents fluid or blood from accumulating in pleural cavity.

Clinical Decision Point *Frequent gentle lifting of the drain allows gravity to help blood and other viscous material to move to the drainage bottle. Patients with recent chest surgery or trauma need to have the chest drain lifted on the basis of assessment of the amount of drainage; some patients might need chest tube drains lifted every 5 to 10 minutes until drainage volume decreases. However, when coiled or dependent looping of tubing is unavoidable, lift the tubing every 15 minutes at a minimum to promote drainage (Kane et al., 2013).*

STEP	RATIONALE
19. Place two rubber-tipped hemostats (for each chest tube) in easily accessible position (e.g., taped to top of patient's headboard). These should remain with patient when ambulating.	Chest tubes are double clamped under specific circumstances: (1) to assess for air leak (Table 27.3), (2) to empty or quickly change disposable systems, or (3) to assess if patient is ready to have tube removed.

Clinical Decision Point *In the event of a chest tube disconnection and risk of contamination, submerge the tube 2 to 4 cm (1 to 2 inches) below the surface of a 250-mL bottle of sterile water or NS until a new chest tube unit can be set up (Bauman and Handley, 2011).*

STEP	RATIONALE
20. Dispose of sharps in proper container, dispose of used supplies, and perform hand hygiene.	Reduces transmission of microorganisms.
21. Care of patient after chest tube insertion:	
a. Perform hand hygiene and apply clean gloves. Assess vital signs, oxygen saturation; skin color; breath sounds; rate, depth, and ease of respirations; and insertion site every 15 minutes for first 2 hours, and then at least every shift (see agency policy).	Provides immediate information about procedure-related complications such as respiratory distress and leakage.
b. Monitor color, consistency, and amount of chest tube drainage every 15 minutes for first 2 hours. Indicate level of drainage fluid, date, and time on write-on surface of chamber.	Provides baseline for continuous assessment of type and quantity of drainage. Ensures early detection of complications.

TABLE 27.3

Problem Solving With Chest Tubes

Assessment	Intervention
Air leak can occur at insertion site, at connection between tube and drainage device, or within drainage device itself. Determine when air leak occurs during respiratory cycle (e.g., inspiration or expiration). Continuous bubbling is noted in water-seal chamber that is attached to suction (Kane et al., 2013).	Check all connections between chest tube and drainage system to make sure they are tight. When in doubt, remove tape without disconnecting the tube to inspect connections. Inspect the chest drainage unit for cracks or breaks that can allow air into the system. Leaks are corrected when constant bubbling stops. If present on a chest drainage system such as the Sahara S 1100a Pleur-Evac, observe the air-leak meter to determine the size of the leak.
Assess for location of leak by squeezing the chest drainage tubing between your hands. If the bubbling stops, air leak is inside patient's thorax or at chest insertion site.	Release the pressure on the drainage tube, reinforce chest dressing, and notify health care provider immediately. Leaving chest tube clamped can cause collapse of lung, mediastinal shift, and eventual collapse of other lung from buildup of air pressure within the pleural cavity.
If bubbling still continues, it indicates that leak is in the drainage system.	Change the drainage system.
Assess for tension pneumothorax: • Severe respiratory distress • Low oxygen saturation • Chest pain • Absence of breath sounds on affected side • Tracheal shift to unaffected side • Hypotension and signs of shock • Tachycardia	Make sure that chest tubes are patent: remove clamps, eliminate kinks, or eliminate occlusion. Notify health care provider immediately and prepare for another chest tube insertion. A one-way flutter (Heimlich) valve or large-gauge needle may be used for short-term emergency release of pressure in the intrapleural space. Have emergency equipment, oxygen, and code cart available because condition is life threatening.
Water-seal tube is no longer submerged in sterile fluid because of evaporation.	Add sterile water to water-seal chamber until distal tip is 2 cm under surface level. Most chest drainage units are marked at the 2 cm level to indicate the fill line.

STEP	RATIONALE
(1) From mediastinal tube, expect less than 100 mL/hr immediately after surgery and no more than 500 mL in first 24 hours.	Sudden gush of drainage may result from coughing or changing patient's position (i.e., releasing pooled/collected blood rather than indicating active bleeding).
(2) From posterior chest tube, expect between 100 and 300 mL first 3 hours after insertion, with total of 500 to 1000 mL expected in first 24 hours. Drainage is grossly bloody during first several hours after surgery and changes to serous (Kane et al., 2013).	Acute bleeding indicates hemorrhage. Health care provider should be notified if there is more than 250 mL of bloody drainage in an hour (Kane et al., 2013).
(3) Expect little or no output from anterior chest tube that is inserted for a pneumothorax (Kane et al., 2013).	
c. Observe chest dressing for drainage.	Drainage around tube may indicate blockage.
d. Apply clean gloves. Palpate around tube for swelling and crepitus (subcutaneous emphysema) as noted by crackling.	Indicates presence of air trapping in subcutaneous tissues. Small amounts are commonly absorbed. Large amounts are potentially dangerous. Most occurrences of crepitus are minor (Mao et al., 2015).

Clinical Decision Point *Some patients may develop subcutaneous emphysema (i.e., a collection of air under the skin after chest tube placement), which can occur if tubing is blocked or kinked. When this occurs, a crepitus (a crackling sensation) is heard on auscultation.*

STEP	RATIONALE
e. Check tubing to ensure that it is free of kinks and dependent loops.	Promotes drainage.
f. Observe for fluctuation of drainage in tubing and water-seal chamber during inspiration and expiration. Observe for clots or debris in tubing.	If fluctuation or tidaling stops, it means that either the lung is fully expanded or system is obstructed (Bauman and Handley, 2011). In spontaneously breathing patient, fluid rises in water-seal or diagnostic indicator (waterless system) with inspiration and falls with expiration. The opposite occurs in patient who is mechanically ventilated. This indicates that system is functioning properly (Atrium, 2015b; Kane et al., 2013).
g. Keep drainage system upright and below level of patient's chest.	Promotes gravity drainage and prevents backflow of fluid and air into pleural space.
h. Check for air leaks by monitoring bubbling in water-seal chamber: Intermittent bubbling is normal during expiration when air is being evacuated from pleural cavity, but continuous bubbling during both inspiration and expiration indicates leak in system.	Absence of bubbling may indicate that lung is fully expanded in patient with pneumothorax. Check all connections and locate sources of air leak as described in Table 27.3.
i. Remove gloves and dispose of used soiled equipment in appropriate biohazard container. Perform hand hygiene.	Prevents accidents involving contaminated equipment.

EVALUATION

1. Evaluate patient for decreased respiratory distress and chest pain. Auscultate patient's lungs and observe chest expansion.	Determines status of lung expansion.
2. Monitor vital signs and SpO$_2$.	Determines if level of oxygenation has improved.
3. Reassess patient's level of comfort on scale of 0 to 10, comparing level with comfort before chest tube insertion.	Indicates need for analgesia. Patient with chest tube discomfort hesitates to take deep breaths and as a result is at risk for pneumonia and atelectasis.
4. Evaluate patient's ability to use deep-breathing exercises while maintaining comfort.	Indicates patient's ability to promote lung expansion and prevent complications.
5. Monitor continued functioning of system as indicated by reduction in amount of drainage, resolution of air leak, and complete reexpansion of the lung.	Detects early signs of system complications or indicates possible removal of chest tube.
6. Use Teach-Back: "I want to be sure I explained why you have a chest tube. Tell me the reason why you have it." Revise your instruction now or develop a plan for revised patient or family caregiver teaching if patient or family caregiver is not able to teach back correctly.	Determines patient's and family caregiver's level of understanding of instructional topic.

STEP	RATIONALE

Unexpected Outcomes

1. Patient develops respiratory distress. Chest pain, decrease in breath sounds over affected and unaffected lungs, marked cyanosis, asymmetrical chest movements, presence of subcutaneous emphysema around tube insertion site or neck, hypotension, tachycardia, and/or mediastinal shift are critical and indicate severe change in patient status such as excessive blood loss or tension pneumothorax.

2. Air leak is unrelated to patient's respirations.

3. There is no chest tube drainage.

4. Chest tube is dislodged.

5. Substantial increase in bright red drainage is observed.

Related Interventions

- Notify health care provider immediately.
- Collect set of vital signs and SpO_2.
- Prepare for chest x-ray film.
- Provide oxygen as ordered.

- See Table 27.3 for determining source of an air leak and problem solving.
- Notify health care provider.
- Observe for kink in chest drainage system.
- Observe for possible clot in chest drainage system.
- Observe for mediastinal shift or respiratory distress (medical emergency).
- Notify health care provider.
- Immediately apply pressure over chest tube insertion site.
- Have assistant obtain sterile petroleum gauze dressing. Apply as patient exhales. Secure dressing with tight seal. Dressing with tape over three of four sides may allow for escape of air if there is residual pneumothorax.
- Notify health care provider.
- Obtain vital signs.
- Monitor drainage.
- Assess patient's cardiopulmonary status.
- Notify health care provider.

Recording and Reporting

- Record respiratory assessment, type of drainage device, amount of suction if used, amount of drainage in chamber, and presence or absence of an air leak in nurses' notes in electronic health record (EHR) or chart. Document the integrity of the dressing and color and type of drainage for comparison between shifts.
- Record patient teaching and validation of understanding on flow sheet or nurses' notes in electronic health record (EHR) or chart.
- Record level of patient comfort and baseline vital signs, including oxygen saturation. If postoperative patient, record vital signs and oxygen saturation every 15 minutes for at least 2 hours after surgery on flow sheet or nurses' notes in EHR or chart.
- Report any unexpected outcomes immediately to nurse in charge or health care provider.

Special Considerations

Teaching

- Instruct patient and family caregivers regarding proper functioning of chest tube and drainage system.
- Inform patient to remain in bed if chest tube is attached to suction (Maliakal, 2011).
- Instruct patient to not lie on the tubing or allow it to get kinked to promote drainage (Maliakal, 2011).
- Instruct patient to immediately report any changes in chest comfort.
- Instruct patient to call immediately for help if the chest tube becomes dislodged.

Pediatric

- If possible, using pictures and special dolls, familiarize child and family with equipment before inserting chest drainage system (Hockenberry and Wilson, 2015).

- Chest tube drainage greater than 3 mL/kg/hr for more than 3 consecutive hours is excessive and may indicate postoperative hemorrhage. Notify the health care provider immediately (Hockenberry and Wilson, 2015).

Gerontological

- Fragility of the older adult's skin requires special care and planning for management of chest tube dressing. Frequently assess surrounding skin for signs of skin breakdown.

Home Care

- Patients with chronic conditions (e.g., uncomplicated pneumothorax, effusions, empyema) that require long-term chest tube may be discharged with smaller mobile drains (Voisin et al., 2014).
- Teach patient how to ambulate and remain active with a mobile chest tube drainage system.
- Instruct patient and family caregivers about when to contact health care provider regarding changes in the drainage system (e.g., chest pain, breathlessness, change in color or amount of drainage, leakage on the dressing around the chest tube).
- Provide patient and family caregiver information specific to the type of drain; when possible have patient demonstrate proper maintenance of the mobile drainage system. Most of these systems do not have a suction-control chamber and use a mechanical one-way valve instead of a water-seal chamber (Voisin et al., 2014).

◆ **SKILL 27.2**   **Assisting With Removal of Chest Tubes**

NSO *Nursing Skills Online Closed Chest Drainage System Module / Lesson 3*

Actual removal of a chest tube is most often the function of a physician or health care provider such as a physician's assistant or nurse practitioner (verify agency policy). Prepare a patient for chest tube removal by assessing the need for preremoval analgesia, obtaining the required medication orders, and instructing the patient about the process and what will be requested of him or her. There has been debate about the optimal timing of chest tube removal in relation to the respiratory cycle. Removal at full inspiration maximally expands the lungs and minimizes the potential space between the pleurae. Another recommendation is for chest tube removal at end expiration when the pressure difference between the chest cavity and the atmosphere is the lowest (Kwiatt et al., 2014). Cerfolio et al (2013) studied chest tube removal in patients after pulmonary resections. Half had their chest tube removed at full inspiration; half at full expiration. All patients performed the Valsalva maneuver during the tube removal. Of the patients who had their chest tubes removed at full inspiration, 32% had a larger or new pneumothorax compared with 19% in the exhalation group. The postremoval pneumothorax was only clinically significant in 2% of patients. Contrary to previous thinking, instruct the patient to exhale during chest tube removal while bearing down (Valsalva maneuver). An occlusive dressing is applied immediately after tube removal to maintain a tight seal.

Delegation and Collaboration

The skill of assisting with removal of chest tubes cannot be delegated to nursing assistive personnel (NAP). The nurse directs the NAP to:
- Immediately report to the nurse any patient sensations of shortness of breath, increased chest pain, dizziness, or increased anxiety.
- Report to the nurse any drainage on the dressing placed over the chest tube site.

Equipment

- Suture set
- Sterile scissors
- Sterile forceps
- Clean gloves
- Sterile gloves
- Face mask/face shield
- Prepared sterile dressing: petrolatum-impregnated gauze, 4 × 4–inch gauze dressings, and large dressings
- 4-inch adhesive tape or elastic bandage (Elastoplast) cut into strips
- Stethoscope, sphygmomanometer, pulse oximeter
- Disposable bed pad

STEP	RATIONALE

ASSESSMENT

1. Identify patient using at least two identifiers (e.g., name and birthday or name and medical record number) according to agency policy.	Ensures correct patient. Complies with The Joint Commission standards and improves patient safety (TJC, 2016).
2. Perform respiratory assessment and assess for lung reexpansion.	
a. Provide health care provider with results of chest x-ray film.	Reveals position of lung tissue in chest cavity and whether sufficient lung reexpansion has occurred (Kane et al., 2013).
b. Note trend in water-seal fluctuation over last 24 hours. Determine if bubbling is present.	Pleura of expanded lung seals holes on internal tip of chest tube, halting fluctuation in water seal. Halt in fluctuation for 24 hours indicates that lung is expanded. When bubbling is present, it usually indicates that lung has not fully expanded (Kane et al., 2013).
c. Confirm that drainage has decreased to less than 100-to-150 mL/day (Kirkwood, 2011).	Pleural drainage was removed, allowing lung to reexpand.
d. Percuss lung for resonance (see Chapter 6).	Normal resonance occurs with reexpansion.
e. Auscultate lung sounds.	Normal breath sounds are heard bilaterally with reexpansion.
3. Assess patient's level of comfort using a scale of 0 to 10 and determine when last analgesic medication was given.	Chest tube removal is often painful; additional analgesia or breathing exercises are often necessary (Kane et al., 2013).
4. Determine patient's understanding of chest tube removal procedure.	Encourages cooperation and minimizes risks and anxiety. Identifies teaching needs.
5. Do not clamp chest tube before removal. Assess for changes in vital signs, oxygen saturation, chest pain, apprehension, and symptoms of tension pneumothorax.	Clamping chest tube before removal to assess patient's tolerance is no longer recommended because there is no benefit to the practice. If a chest tube that was continuing to bubble is clamped, tension pneumothorax may occur (Briggs, 2010; Mao et al., 2015).

NURSING DIAGNOSES

- Acute pain
- Anxiety
- Risk for impaired gas exchange

Related factors/Risk factors are individualized based on patient's condition or needs.

STEP	RATIONALE

PLANNING

1. Expected outcomes following completion of procedure:
- Lung reexpansion is maintained.
- Patient does not experience discomfort.
- Spontaneous healing of chest tube insertion site occurs after removal of tube without infection or other complications.

2. Explain procedure to patient.

Source of air or fluid loss is sealed or has healed.

Pain management is achieved.

Large, nonporous occlusive dressing at puncture site promotes uncomplicated healing.

Reduces anxiety and promotes patient cooperation.

IMPLEMENTATION

1. Administer prescribed medication for pain relief about 30 minutes before procedure.

Reduces discomfort and relaxes patient. Medication reaches peak effect at time of tube removal. Patients report sensations ranging from pain to pulling when chest tube is removed (Kane et al., 2013).

2. Perform "Time Out" procedure with health care provider to verify patient identification, planned procedure, correct tube(s), and that chest tube is visible and patient position is correct.

The "Time Out" step is intended to reliably identify patient as individual for whom procedure is intended and to match procedure to patient (TJC, 2016).

3. Perform hand hygiene and apply clean gloves and face shield if needed.

Reduces transmission of microorganisms.

4. Help patient to sitting position on edge of bed, lying supine or on side without chest tubes. Place pad under chest tube site.

Health care provider prescribes patient's position to facilitate tube removal. Pad absorbs any drainage associated with tube removal.

5. Health care provider prepares an occlusive dressing of petrolatum-impregnated gauze on pressure dressing, sets it aside on sterile field, and applies sterile gloves.

Essential to prepare in advance for quick application to wound on tube withdrawal.

6. Support patient physically and emotionally while health care provider removes dressing and clips sutures.

Patients state that, when they know that the tube is being pulled, they can mentally prepare themselves for the procedure. Support from health care team reduces anxiety and promotes cooperation.

7. Health care provider asks patient to exhale completely and hold it while bearing down (Valsalva maneuver).

Prevents air from being sucked into chest as tube is removed (Cerfolio et al., 2013). A complication associated with removal of chest tubes is recurrent pneumothorax, which results from atmospheric air reentering pleural cavity. This occurs when patient inhales during tube removal.

8. Health care provider quickly pulls out chest tube and tightens and ties purse-string suture if present, after which patient is instructed to breathe normally.

This forms an airtight seal and prevents entry of air through chest wound. Sutures aid in skin closure (Kane et al., 2013; Rajan, 2013).

9. Health care provider applies sterile occlusive dressing over wound and firmly secures it in position with wide tape.

Keeps wound aseptic. Prevents entry of air into chest. Wound closure occurs spontaneously.

10. Health care provider inspects end of chest tube(s) before disposal to ensure entire removal.

On rare occasions chest tube is damaged by instruments, surgical wires, or manipulation that can lead to its breakage during removal (Mao et al., 2015). Inspection of end of chest tube helps to verify that all of tube was removed (Kirkwood, 2011).

11. Help patient to upright position supported by pillows.

Restores patient's comfort. Patients report that proper positioning following chest tube removal helps to relieve procedure-related sensations of pain and pulling (Rajan, 2013).

12. Remove used equipment from bedside. Dispose in appropriate receptacle.

Prevents spread of microorganisms.

13. Remove gloves and perform hand hygiene.

Reduces transmission of microorganisms.

STEP	RATIONALE

EVALUATION

1. Auscultate lung sounds.	Helps to confirm lung remains expanded.
2. Palpate skin over area where tube was inserted for subcutaneous emphysema.	Subcutaneous emphysema results from entrance of air into subcutaneous space. It is painful, and as a result patients may not take full lung expansion (Kane et al., 2013).
3. Evaluate for signs of respiratory distress immediately after tube removal and during first few hours after removal.	Provides for early notification of health care provider if adverse symptoms occur. Chest tubes may need reinsertion.

Critical Decision Point *If air is heard escaping from the chest tube site, reinforce the occlusive dressing and immediately notify health care provider.*

4. Evaluate patient's vital signs, oxygen saturation, pulmonary status, and psychological status.	Detects early signs and symptoms of complications.
5. Review chest x-ray film, if ordered.	Evidence does not support routine postremoval x-rays films in either adults or pediatric/neonatal patients (Reeb et al., 2013; Sepehripour et al., 2012). If complications are noted, bedside ultrasound imaging or computed tomography (CT) scan, which is better at identifying the chest cavity, may be ordered.
6. Ask about patient's level of pain or comfort. Observe for nonverbal cues of pain and assess level of discomfort on scale of 0 to 10.	Indicates that wound did not close well. Determines patient's tolerance of procedure.
7. Check chest dressing for drainage and patency. When changing dressing, note wound for signs of healing.	Ensures occlusion and proper healing of chest wound.
8. **Use Teach-Back:** "I want to be sure I explained about removing your chest tube. Tell me what you know about what we did." Revise your instruction now or develop a plan for revised patient or family caregiver teaching if the patient or family caregiver is not able to teach back correctly.	Determines patient's and family caregiver's level of understanding of instructional topic.

Unexpected Outcomes	**Related Interventions**
1. Dyspnea and labored respirations noted after chest tube removal; potential recurrence of pneumothorax, hemothorax, or effusion.	• Notify health care provider. • Obtain vital signs and oxygen saturation. • Stay with patient. • Prepare for possible chest tube reinsertion.
2. Infection is noted at insertion site.	• Assess patient's vital signs for elevated temperature, tachypnea, and tachycardia. Assess wound for drainage, odor, erythema, or increased pain.

Recording and Reporting

- Record removal of tube, amount and appearance of drainage in the collection bottle, appearance of wound and dressing, and patient's response and understanding of the procedure on flow sheet or in nurses' notes in electronic health record (EHR) or chart.
- Record vital signs and respiratory assessment on flow sheet or nurses' notes in EHR or chart.
- Report unexpected outcomes to nurse in charge or health care provider.

Special Considerations

Teaching

- Instruct patient and family caregiver to immediately report signs of chest pain, shortness of breath, or sensations of chest discomfort.

Pediatric

- Pediatric patients usually require analgesia (e.g., morphine sulfate 0.1 mg/kg in combination with midazolam before chest tube removal (Hockenberry and Wilson, 2015).
- EMLA (locally applied lidocaine/prilocaine anesthetic patch) placed under the occlusive dressing at the chest tube insertion site 1 hour before tube removal reduces pain of procedure. However, child may still feel the "pulling" sensation (Hockenberry and Wilson, 2015).

◆ SKILL 27.3 Autotransfusion of Chest Tube Drainage

NSO *Nursing Skills Online Closed Chest Drainage System Module / Lesson 4*

In autotransfusion blood lost from trauma, injury, or surgery is infused back into a patient's circulatory system. When reinfusion is linked with chest drainage, it is a relatively risk-free, inexpensive, and easy method of replacing blood. Benefits of autotransfusion include an immediate blood supply, no risk of transfusion reaction, and more oxygen supplied to vital organs (Bauman and Handley, 2011). Patients must also have a patent intravenous (IV) line in place (see Chapter 29). Autotransfusion is contraindicated in patients with coagulation disorders, infections, cancer, and preexisting liver or kidney dysfunction (Atrium, 2015c; Bauman and Handley, 2011).

Delegation and Collaboration

The skill of autotransfusion of chest tube drainage cannot be delegated to nursing assistive personnel (NAP). The nurse directs the NAP to:

- Immediately inform nurse of changes in patient's vital signs or pulse oximetry (SpO_2) levels.
- Immediately inform nurse about increased or decreased drainage from chest tube.

Equipment

- Adult/pediatric single-use chest drainage and autotransfusion unit (Fig. 27.10)
- *Optional:* Continuous autotransfusion system (ATS) with a blood-compatible infusion pump (check agency policy)
- Microaggregate blood filter (40-μm filter, see manufacturer instructions)
- Nonvented blood-compatible IV administration set
- Antiseptic swab
- Infusion pump (see manufacturer instructions)
- Replacement bag
- Gown, clean gloves, and mask as needed

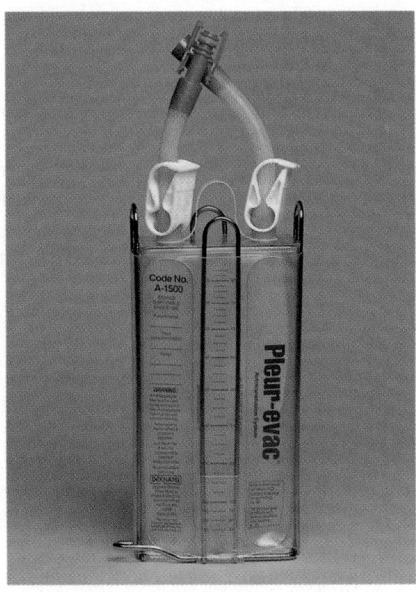

FIG 27.10 Example of autotransfusion unit.

STEP	RATIONALE

ASSESSMENT

1. Identify patient using at least two identifiers (e.g., name and birthday or name and medical record number) according to agency policy. Compare identifiers with information on patient's MAR or medical record.	Ensures correct patient. Complies with The Joint Commission standards and improves patient safety (TJC, 2016).
2. See Assessment for Skill 27.1.	
3. Determine presence of active bleeding (at least 50-to-100 mL/hr), through chest tube.	Indicates need for possible reinfusion of chest tube drainage.

Clinical Decision Point *Collected blood never remains in the chest drain or ATS blood bag for more than 6 hours before autotransfusion. Immediate use is preferred (Atrium, 2015c; Bauman and Handley, 2011).*

4. Assess IV site (see Chapter 29); note size of IV catheter. 18-gauge angiocatheter preferred.	Determines presence of adequate and patent IV site for administration of blood products.
5. Obtain baseline laboratory data (e.g., hemoglobin and hematocrit).	Provides data to measure effectiveness of reinfusion of chest drainage on patient's circulating blood volume.

NURSING DIAGNOSES

- Decreased cardiac output
- Ineffective peripheral tissue perfusion
- Risk for infection

Related factors/Risk factors are individualized based on patient's condition or needs.

STEP	RATIONALE

PLANNING

1. Expected outcomes following completion of procedure:

- Vital signs, hematocrit, and hemoglobin stabilize.

- Drainage system functions correctly and lung reexpands in 48 to 72 hours.
- IV line remains patent.

2. Explain procedure to patient.

Reinfusion reduces significant blood loss associated with closed chest drainage.

Negative pressure is reestablished in intrapleural space.

Patent IV is necessary for reinfusion of cleansed mediastinal tube drainage.

Reduces anxiety and promotes patient cooperation.

IMPLEMENTATION

1. System setup:

a. Set up ATS according to technique that maintains sterility of unit and following three steps printed on front of unit.

b. Make certain that all connections are tight and all clamps are open.

c. A 200-μm double-sided mesh filter is located in ATS bag to filter drainage.

d. ATS collection bag has capacity of 1000 mL marked in increments of 25 mL and an area for marking times and amounts.

Contamination of unit provides ready source of infection to patient.

Tight connections ensure airtight system and open clamps allow chest drainage to enter ATS bag.

Filtering drainage removes extraneous materials and microemboli.

Dark-red drainage is expected only during immediate postoperative period. This drainage turns serous over time.

Clinical Decision Point *Continuous ATS may be prescribed following cardiac surgery. This is a closed system with a specific infusion pump and IV circuit. This system requires specific education and is used in selected situations (Atrium, 2015c). Check agency policy.*

2. Perform hand hygiene and apply clean gloves.

3. Prepare chest drainage for reinfusion.

a. Following manufacturer directions, open replacement bag, and close two white clamps.

b. Use high-negativity relief valve to reduce excessive negativity.

c. *Bag transfer:*

   (1) Close clamp on chest drainage tubing.

   (2) Close clamps on top of initial ATS collection bag.

   (3) Connect chest drainage tube to new ATS bag.

   (4) Make certain that all connections are tight.

   (5) Open all clamps on chest drainage tube and replacement bag.

d. Connect connectors on top of initial collection bag and remove bag by lifting it from side hook and then from foot hook.

e. Secure replacement bag by connecting foot hook, replacing metal frame into side hook of chest drainage unit, and pushing down to secure frame onto hook.

f. Place thumbs on top of metal frame and push up with fingers to slide bag out; remove replacement bag.

4. Reinfuse chest drainage.

a. Use new microaggregate filter to reinfuse each autotransfusion bag.

b. Access bag by inverting it, wiping off port with antiseptic swab, and spiking through port with microaggregate filter and twisting.

c. With bag upside down, gently squeeze it to remove air and prime filter with blood.

Reduces transmission of microorganisms.

Contamination of unit provides ready source of contamination to patient. Closed clamps maintain closed system during replacement.

This eases removal of initial collection bag from metal support stand.

Prevents air from entering chest cavity through tube and collapsing lung.

Maintains closed system for reinfusion, preventing contamination of blood.

Establishes new ATS.

Ensures airtight system.

Reestablishes ATS.

Maintains closed system within bag and removes it for use in autotransfusion.

Provides safe attachment of replacement bag to chest drainage unit.

Prevents infusion of microemboli and provides maximal filtration for each bag.

Connects autotransfusion bag to transfusion tubing.

Gentle pressure is used to prevent hemolysis.

STEP	RATIONALE
d. Hang bag on IV pole and continue to prime tubing until all air is gone. Clamp tubing, attach it to patient's IV access, and adjust clamp to deliver reinfusion at appropriate rate.	Removes all air from transfusion tubing. Reinfusion is delivered by gravity, application of a blood cuff (not to exceed 150 mm Hg pressure), or blood-compatible IV pump (see Chapter 29).
e. If ordered, anticoagulants (Anticoagulant Citrate Dextrose Solution-A or Citrate Phosphate Dextrose Solution, USP) are added to reinfusion through self-sealing port in autotransfusion connector.	Prevents clotting in autotransfusion. Reversing heparin with protamine to preoperative levels or collection of nonheparinized blood following emergency chest trauma may require a citrate anticoagulant (Atrium, 2015c).
f. Monitor patient's vital signs and SpO$_2$ according to patient condition and agency policy. For some patients this may be as frequently as every 15 minutes; for other patients it may be every hour.	Patients who require autotransfusion usually have complex physiological needs, and their vital signs change quite rapidly. Consistent, frequent monitoring allows for timely identification of changes and initiation of appropriate interventions to restore physiological stability.
5. Discontinue autotransfusion.	
a. Clamp chest drainage tube only briefly and only if ordered by health care provider and connect it directly to chest drainage unit with red and blue connectors.	Clamping chest tube for any length of time can cause tension pneumothorax (Kane et al., 2013).
b. Open chest drainage tube clamp.	All drainage will be collected directly in drainage unit and discarded appropriately.
6. Discard used supplies and perform hand hygiene.	Reduces transmission of microorganisms.

EVALUATION

1. Monitor vital signs, hematocrit, and hemoglobin.	Helps determine effects of treatment.
2. Monitor chest drainage system and patient's lung sounds.	Helps determine proper functioning of system and its effectiveness.
3. Evaluate IV infusion site for infiltration and phlebitis.	Patent IV infusion site is maintained.
4. Use Teach Back: "I want to be sure I explained why you needed this procedure. Tell me why this was important." Revise your instruction now or develop a plan for revised patient or family caregiver teaching if patient or family caregiver is not able to teach back correctly.	Determines patient's and family caregiver's level of understanding of instructional topic.

Unexpected Outcomes	Related Interventions
1. Chest tube is dislodged.	• Immediately apply pressure over chest tube insertion site.
	• Have assistant apply sterile petrolatum-impregnated occlusive dressing.
	• Notify health care provider.
2. Patient has dyspnea, chest pain, and labored respirations.	• Verify that chest tube is patent and draining.
	• Obtain vital signs.
	• Notify health care provider.
3. Patient has signs of infection, fever, and chills.	• Obtain wound cultures as ordered.
	• Obtain vital signs.

Recording and Reporting

- Record drainage and reinfusion with times and amounts of each; include patient's response to reinfusion in nurses' notes in electronic health record (EHR) or chart. Describe condition of IV infusion site.
- Record patient teaching and validation of understanding on flow sheet or in nurses' notes in EHR or chart.

Special Considerations
Teaching

- Prepare patient and family caregivers for the procedure so they will understand when the patient's blood is reinfused. Patients and their families may have had this instruction before surgery but need reinforcement.

◆ CLINICAL DEBRIEF

A patient is in the intensive care unit following open heart surgery. He has a right pleural and mediastinal chest tube to drainage. His last vital signs were blood pressure (BP) 110/64 mm Hg; pulse 126 beats/min; respirations on mechanical ventilator 16 breaths/min; SpO_2 90%; temperature 37.2°C (99°F rectally). The last hourly chest tube drainage was 75 mL from the pleural tube and 100 mL from the mediastinal tube.

1. Why is it important to check vital signs, check for air leaks, and note the amount of chest drainage every 15 to 30 minutes for at least 2 hours after patient returns from surgery?

2. It is now 12 hours after surgery, and the patient is transferred from bed to chair. Immediately following this transfer you note drainage of 50 mL of dark red fluid. What are your actions?

3. Using SBAR, how would you document this episode with the patient's chest drainage as noted in question 2?

◆ REVIEW QUESTIONS

1. Patients with chest tubes that remove bloody drainage from the chest cavity usually are at risk for respiratory problems. These patients have many care priorities. What are two important priorities related to management of the chest tube system?
   1. Monitoring chest tube drainage
   2. Promoting activity
   3. Promoting airway clearance
   4. Maintaining chest tube patency
   5. Observing dressing

2. When caring for a patient with a chest tube, which activities can a nurse delegate to nursing assistive personnel (NAP)? (Select all that apply.)
   1. Proper positioning of the patient to facilitate chest tube drainage
   2. Helping to remove a chest tube
   3. How to ambulate and transfer a patient with chest drainage
   4. Reporting any abnormal vital signs, complaints of chest pain or shortness of breath
   5. Reinfusion of chest tube drainage
   6. Reporting any change in the amount of drainage or sudden bleeding

3. Correctly organize the following steps to autoinfuse chest tube drainage.
   a. Hang the bag on an intravenous (IV) pole and continue to prime the tubing until all air is gone.
   b. Access the bag by inverting it and spiking it through the spike port with the microaggregate filter and twisting.
   c. Use a new microaggregate filter to reinfuse each autotransfusion bag.
   d. If ordered, add anticoagulants to the reinfusion through the self-sealing port in the autotransfusion connector.
   e. With the bag upside down, gently squeeze it to remove the air and prime the filter with blood.
   f. Monitor patient's vital signs and SpO_2 according to patient condition and agency policy.

ⓔ *Visit the Evolve site for a complete list of Clinical Debrief and Review Questions answers.*

REFERENCES

Atrium: *Suggested readings regarding chest tube stripping*, 2014, Atrium Medical, http://www.atriummed.com/EN/chest_drainage/Documents/Chest_Tube_Stripping.pdf. Accessed January 29, 2016.

Atrium: *Evidence-based care of patients with chest tubes*, Hudson, NH, 2015a, http://www.atriummed.com/EN/chest_drainage/Documents/NTI2015Evidence-BasedCareofPatientswithChestTubes.pdf. Accessed January 29, 2016.

Atrium: *Managing chest drainage–autotransfusion*, Hudson, NH, 2015b, http://www.atriummed.com/pdf/ats%20ifu.pdf. Accessed January 29, 2016.

Atrium: *Oasis™ dry suction water seal drain*, Hudson, NH, 2015c, http://www.atriummed.com/en/chest_drainage/Documents/Oasis-GreenHandbook-010139.pdf. Accessed January 29, 2016.

Bascom R, et al: *Restoring an air-free pleural space in pneumothorax*, 2014, http://emedicine.medscape.com/article/1959416-overview#a2. Accessed January 30, 2016.

Bauman A, Handley C: Chest-tube care: the more you know the easier it gets, *Am Nurse Today* 6(9):27, 2011.

Briggs D: Nursing care and management of patients with interpleural drains, *Nurs Stand* 24(21):47, 2010.

Cerfolio RJ, et al: Optimal technique for the removal of chest tubes after pulmonary resection, *J Thorac Cardiovasc Surg* 145(6):1535, 2013.

Hockenberry MJ, Wilson D: *Nursing care of infants and children*, ed 10, St Louis, 2015, Mosby.

Kane C, et al: Chest tubes in the critically ill patient, *Dimens Crit Care Nurs* 32(3):112, 2013.

Kirkwood P: Chest tube removal (perform). In Weigand D, editor: *AACN Procedure Manual for Critical Care*, ed 6, St Louis, 2011, Elsevier.

Kuhajda I, et al: Tube thoracostomy; chest tube implantation and follow up, *J Thorac Dis* 6(S4):S470, 2014.

Kwiatt M, et al: Thoracostomy tubes: a comprehensive review of complications and related topics, *Int J Crit Illn Inj Sci* 4(2):143, 2014.

Lewis ML, et al: *Medical-surgical nursing: assessment and management of clinical problems*, ed 10, St Louis, 2017, Elsevier.

Makic MBF, et al: Continuing to challenge practice to be evidence based, *Crit Care Nurse* 35(2):39, 2015.

Maliakal M: Chest tubes, *Nursing* 7:33, 2011.

Mao M, et al: Complications of chest tubes: a focused clinical synopsis, *Curr Opin Pulm Med* 21:376, 2015.

Myatt R: Diagnosis and management of patients with pleural effusions, *Nurs Stand* 41:51, 2014.

Rajan C: *Tube thoracostomy management*, 2013, http://emedicine.medscape.com/article/1503275-overview#a5. Accessed January 4, 2016.

Reeb J, et al: Are daily routine chest radiographs necessary after pulmonary surgery in adult patients?, *Interact Cardiovasc Thorac Surg* 17(6):995, 2013.

Scott SS, et al: Chest tube placement (assist). In Weigand D, editor: *AACN Procedure Manual for Critical Care*, ed 6, St Louis, 2011, Elsevier.

Sepehripour AH, et al: Is routine chest radiography indicated following chest drain removal after cardiothoracic surgery?, *Interact Cardiovasc Thorac Surg* 14(6):834, 2012.

Shlamovitz GA: *Tube thoracostomy*, 2014, http://emedicine.medscape.com/article/80678-overview#a1. Accessed January 30, 2016.

The Joint Commission (TJC): *National Patient Safety Goals*, Oakbrook Terrace, IL, 2016, The Commission. http://www.jointcommission.org/standards_information/npsgs.aspx. Accessed January 30, 2016.

US National Library of Medicine: *MedlinePlus: Hemothorax*, 2014, https://www.nlm.nih.gov/medlineplus/ency/article/000126.htm. Accessed May 17, 2016.

Voisin F, et al: Ambulatory management of large spontaneous pneumothorax with pigtail catheters, *Ann Emerg Med* 64:222, 2014.

Widmaier EP, et al: *Vander's human physiology: the mechanisms of body function*, ed 13, Boston, 2014, McGraw-Hill.

Zardo P, et al: Chest tube management: state of the art, *Curr Opin Anesthesiol* 28:45, 2015.

Zarogoulidis P, et al: Pneumothorax: from definition to diagnosis and treatment, *J Thorac Dis* 6(S4):S372, 2014.

Zimlichman E, et al: Health-care associated infections: a meta-analysis of costs and financial impact on the US health care system, *JAMA Intern Med* 173(22):2039, 2013.

28 | Emergency Measures for Life Support

SKILLS AND PROCEDURES

OBJECTIVES

- Discuss indications for oral airway insertion.
- Identify need for automated external defibrillator (AED) application and indications for use.
- State indications for cardiopulmonary resuscitation (CPR).
- Discuss code management.

MEDIA RESOURCES

- evolve http://evolve.elsevier.com/Perry/skills
- Review Questions
- Audio Glossary
- Clinical Debrief and Review Questions Answers

PURPOSE

This chapter addresses the basic aspects of cardiopulmonary resuscitation (CPR) skills and concepts of critical thinking to apply during a cardiac arrest. Cardiopulmonary arrests are emergency situations that you must be prepared to handle at any time. You are expected to follow current resuscitation guidelines in a systematic and organized manner. The goal is to provide resuscitation in a timely manner to restore cardiopulmonary function and avoid poor neurological outcomes. All nurses and nursing students are required to be certified and maintain certification in basic life support (BLS).

STANDARDS OF CARE

- American Heart Association, 2015—Resuscitation Guidelines

PRINCIPLES OF PRACTICE

- In some cardiac arrests the cessation of circulating blood flow is caused by irregular heart rhythms known as dysrhythmias. The causes of dysrhythmias may include electrolyte disturbances, acute coronary syndrome, and certain prescribed or recreational medications. Lethal dysrhythmias include ventricular tachycardia (VT) and ventricular fibrillation (VF) and require a medically delivered electrical shock for treatment.
- Early defibrillation or shock may quickly return the heart to normal without further deterioration of a patient's status.
- Before most arrests, signs and symptoms of impending deterioration include tachycardia, hypotension, tachypnea, decreasing oxygen saturation below 90% despite provision of supplemental oxygen, and a decreasing urine output of less than 50 mL in 4 hours and are reasons for activating a rapid response team (AHRQ, 2014).
- Each agency has a specific code or signal to summon immediate assistance in the event of a cardiac and/or respiratory arrest; the arrest situation may be referred to as a "code" (e.g., "code blue," "code 7").

PATIENT-CENTERED CARE

- Whenever a patient requires resuscitation, his or her family is also a prime nursing concern. When caring for patients from diverse cultures and religions, consider an individual's meaning and interpretation of life support and resuscitation.
- Although individuals may be part of a specific cultural or religious group, an individual may not follow all aspects of that culture or religion. Therefore it is essential that you consider each individual's interpretation and wishes to ensure the right of self-determination.
- When necessary, use a professional language interpreter to explain the patient's status to him or her. In addition, use cultural and religious support personnel to facilitate understanding of the events.
- Be prepared to handle large numbers of visitors who may remain at the bedside to provide support for the family and/or pray for the patient. Collaborate with the family decision maker and leader to plan rotating visits at the bedside.
- Advance directives offer valuable information concerning a patient's resuscitation status and individual patient decisions regarding resuscitation efforts. Although advance directives are often addressed before or during a patient's hospitalization, you play an important role in encouraging patients to complete the document.

EVIDENCE-BASED PRACTICE

The Committee on Emergency Cardiac Care (Kleinman et al., 2015) reviews and conducts research on cardiac arrest treatment and outcomes and has created evidence-based guidelines for both initial care (BLS) and ongoing measures (advanced cardiovascular life support [ACLS]). The 2015 American Heart Association (AHA) resuscitation guidelines emphasize the importance of high-quality cardiopulmonary resuscitation (CPR), which includes continuous chest compression for bystanders, updated ACLS algorithms and pulseless dysrhythmias, and aggressive postresuscitation care (AHA, 2014). Methods to improve survival after cardiopulmonary arrest include (Kleinman et al., 2015):

- Immediate recognition and activation of emergency medical response.
- Early CPR that emphasizes chest compressions.
- Rapid defibrillation if indicated.
- Effective advanced cardiac life support

More data are available showing that high-quality CPR improves survival from cardiac arrest, including:

- Ensuring chest compressions of adequate rate.
- Ensuring chest compressions of adequate depth.
- Allowing full chest recoil between compressions.
- Minimizing interruptions in chest compressions.
- Avoiding excessive ventilation.
- Postcardiac care such as cooling to preserve neurological function (Callaway et al., 2015). Many hospitals have developed protocols for using external cooling techniques and intravascular cooling devices.
- Evaluation of allowing family members to remain in a patient's room during resuscitative efforts and invasive procedures confirms a remarkable level of approval and gratitude by participating family members (AACN, 2016). Survey of family members noted a significant reduction in posttraumatic stress and self-reports of a greater sense of resolution and fulfillment among witnesses of resuscitative efforts compared with nonwitnesses.

SAFETY GUIDELINES

- Know a patient's baseline vital signs, noting any irregularities in cardiac rhythm. Dysrhythmias can precipitate a cardiopulmonary arrest. Conditions that place a patient at risk for dysrhythmias include coronary artery disease, myocardial infarction, open-heart surgeries, acid-base imbalances, and toxicities.
- Know a patient's most recent serum electrolyte values. Electrolyte imbalances (e.g., potassium, magnesium, and calcium) can precipitate cardiopulmonary arrest.
- When a patient has been exposed to a chemical or drug, attempt to determine the type and amount of the substance involved. Certain chemicals (e.g., ethanol, tranquilizers, opiates) depress the respiratory center and can result in a respiratory arrest. Oversedation involving the use of patient-controlled analgesia (PCA) pumps or epidural administration can also contribute to respiratory depression. Overdoses of some drugs can cause ventricular dysrhythmias and cardiopulmonary arrest.
- The AHA *Get With the Guidelines—Resuscitation Registry* (2014) has set the goal for hospitals to deliver the first electrical shock to patients in VF in less than 2 minutes and 59 seconds. When electrical energy is used during an emergency, good skin contact between the pad and patient's chest is essential to avoid the release of live electricity into the environment.
- Clear communication to all others in the room is essential at the time of defibrillation so everyone is aware and does not touch the patient or the bed at the time of the shock.
- Know agency policy for activating the Rapid Response Team, which is composed of a critical care nurse, a physician or advanced practice nurse, and respiratory therapists who are present in many hospitals (AHRQ, 2014).

◆ SKILL 28.1 | Inserting an Oropharyngeal Airway

An oropharyngeal airway is a semicircular, minimally flexible, curved piece of hard plastic (Fig. 28.1). When inserted, it extends from just outside the lips, over the tongue, and to the pharynx (Fig. 28.2). Oral airways allow you to suction through a central core or along the side of the airway and maintain airway patency in an unconscious patient. Choose correct size of an oral airway on the basis of a patient's age and the width and length of his or her mouth. Size is correct if, when the flange is held parallel to the front teeth with the airway against the patient's cheek, the end of the curve reaches the angle of the jaw (Table 28.1).

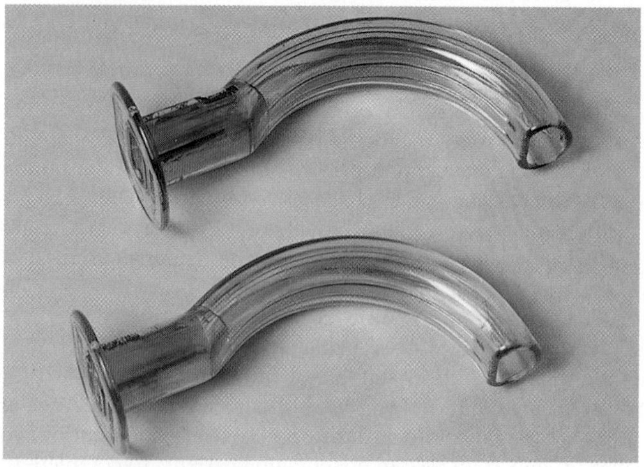

Delegation and Collaboration

The skill of inserting an oropharyngeal airway cannot be delegated to nursing assistive personnel (NAP). Respiratory therapists have the training to insert an oral airway. The nurse directs the NAP to:

FIG 28.1 Oral airways.

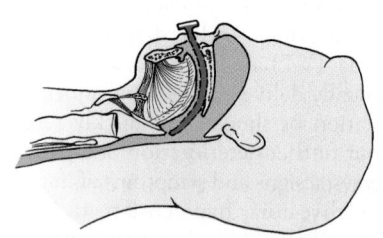

FIG 28.2 Placement of oral airway.

(see Table 28.1)

TABLE 28.1

Oral Airway Guidelines for Size* by Age

Size	Age
30 mm or size 000	Premature neonates
45 mm or size 00	Newborn
55 mm or size 0	Newborn to 1 year
60 mm or size 1	1–2 years
70 mm or size 2	2–6 years
80 mm or size 3	6–18 years
90 mm or size 4	Adult medium
100 mm or size 5	Adult large
110 mm or size 6	Adult extra large

*Measure from the corner of the mouth to the angle of the jaw just below the ear for size estimation.

- Immediately report to the nurse any signs of airway distress, vomiting, or change in level of consciousness.

Equipment

- Appropriate-size oral airway (see Table 28.1)
- Clean gloves
- Gown if indicated
- Tissues or washcloths
- Suction equipment if indicated
- Nonallergenic tape (optional)
- Face shield if indicated
- Tongue blade
- Stethoscope

STEP	RATIONALE

ASSESSMENT

1. Identify need to insert an oral airway. Signs and symptoms include upper airway gurgling with breathing, absent cough or gag reflex, increased oral secretions, excessive drooling, grinding teeth, clenched teeth, biting endotracheal or gastric tubes, and labored respirations.

   These conditions place patient at risk for obstruction of the upper airway. Use oral airways only in unconscious patients. They may stimulate vomiting or laryngospasm if inserted in a semiconscious or conscious patient.

2. Determine factors that may contribute to upper airway obstruction such as age (children have a proportionally larger tongue) or presence of a nasal or oral airway and drainage tubes (swallowing is more difficult with tubes in place).

   Allows you to accurately assess need for oral airway placement. Patients at greater risk for upper airway obstruction are infants; children; and adults with upper airway congestion, loss of consciousness, seizure disorders, neuromuscular diseases, or increased oral secretions.

3. Ensure that patient does not have dentures in place before attempting an oral airway insertion.

   Oral airway insertion can dislodge dentures and cause worsening airway obstruction.

Clinical Decision Point *Never insert an oral airway in a conscious patient or a patient with recent oral/facial trauma, oral surgery, or loose teeth. Never force an airway into place.*

4. Assess family caregiver's knowledge of procedure.

   Identifies learning needs of family. Patient will be unconscious.

NURSING DIAGNOSES

- Ineffective airway clearance
- Risk for aspiration

Related factors/Risk factors are individualized based on patient's condition or needs.

PLANNING

1. Expected outcomes following completion of procedure:
   - Patient's respiratory status improves, as evidenced by respirations with normal rate, easier removal of secretions, and lack of gurgling noise in throat with respirations.

     Airway is clear of secretions.

   - Patient is not able to grind teeth or bite tubes.

     Oral airway prevents tooth contact with other teeth or with tubes.

   - Patient's tongue does not obstruct airway.

     Oral airway keeps tongue in correct position to maintain patent airway.

2. Family caregiver can verbalize understanding of need for oropharyngeal airway.

   Teaching was successful.

STEP	RATIONALE

IMPLEMENTATION

1. Position unconscious patient in semi-Fowler's position if possible.

Provides easy access to oral cavity.

2. Perform hand hygiene and apply clean gloves and face shield (when possible).

Reduces transmission of microorganisms.

3. Whenever possible, use padded tongue blade to open patient's mouth; if necessary, use thumb and forefinger of nondominant hand to open jaws and teeth.

Provides access to oral cavity. To avoid a bite, do not insert your fingers into patient's mouth. Use extreme caution if manually opening patient's jaw and teeth.

4. Insert oral airway.

When inserting airway, take care not to push patient's tongue into pharynx.

   a. Hold oral airway with curved end up and insert distal end until airway reaches back of throat; then turn airway over 180 degrees and follow natural curve of tongue. *Option:* Hold airway sideways, insert halfway, and rotate 90 degrees while gliding it over natural curvature of tongue. Make sure that outer flange is just outside patient's lips.

Proper insertion of airway prevents displacement of patient's tongue into posterior oropharynx. Secure oral airway with tape on upper and lower flange.

Clinical Decision Point In a *pediatric patient,* **DO NOT rotate** the oral airway on insertion because the airway tip will damage the soft palate.

5. Suction secretions as needed.

Removes secretions; maintains patent airway.

6. Reassess patient's respiratory status; auscultate lungs.

Verifies respiratory status and patent airway.

7. Clean patient's face with soft tissue or washcloth.

Promotes hygiene.

8. Discard tissue into appropriate receptacle, place washcloth in dirty or soiled linen bag, remove gloves and face shield and discard in appropriate receptacle; perform hand hygiene.

Reduces transmission of microorganisms.

9. Administer mouth care frequently.

Increases patient comfort and removes debris. It also provides moisture to oral mucosal tissues.

Clinical Decision Point Oral airway will need to be removed, cleaned or discarded, and replaced in patients with excessive oral secretions. Frequent suctioning of the oral cavity may be required. Oral airways are not a long-term solution. They can create pressure on underlying tissue and cause significant lip and tongue erosion, which can result in a medical device–related pressure injury (MDPI) (Pittman et al., 2015).

EVALUATION

1. Observe patient's respiratory status and compare respiratory assessments before and after insertion of oral airway.

Identifies patient's response to insertion of airway.

2. Evaluate that airway is patent and that patient's tongue does not obstruct it.

Ensures route for oxygen delivery to patient.

3. Observe adjacent and underlying tissue for signs of redness, abrasion, or bruising.

Identifies early signs of MDPI.

4. Observe for patient pushing airway out with tongue or coughing.

Patient's ability to clear his or her own airway may have returned. Indicates reassessment of need for oral airway.

5. **Use Teach-Back:** "I want to be sure I explained why your loved one needs this oral airway. Tell me why it is important." Revise your instruction now or develop a plan for revised patient or family caregiver teaching if patient or family caregiver is not able to teach back correctly.

Determines patient's and family caregiver's level of instructional topic.

Unexpected Outcomes	Related Interventions
1. Patient continually coughs and gags when airway is inserted.	• Do not continue inserting airway if patient begins to gag. Stimulation of gag reflex can cause vomiting and aspiration. • Remove oral airway and position patient on side. • Reassess need for artificial airway prn.
2. Airway obstruction not relieved.	• Obtain immediate assistance. • Reinsert airway or determine from health care provider if another form of airway is needed. • Assess for other causes of obstruction.
3. Patient pushes airway out of place or out of mouth.	• Reassess patient's need for oral airway.
4. Unable to insert oral airway; patient is combative or you are unable to open his or her mouth.	• Get help. • Reassess patient's need for oral airway. • Provide sedation as ordered.

Recording and Reporting

- Record assessment findings while inserting oral airway; size of oral airway; other interventions performed at same time, especially positioning and suctioning; and patient's response to procedure on flow sheet or in nurses' notes in electronic health record (EHR) or chart.
- Document your evaluation of patient and family caregiver learning.

Special Considerations
Pediatric

- Oral airways are seldom used in treatment of airway obstruction in infants and children. Because the airway is narrow, they are often more occlusive than beneficial (Hockenberry and Wilson, 2015).

◆ SKILL 28.2   Using an Automated External Defibrillator

Defibrillation is the electrical attempt to stop a lethal cardiac arrhythmia such as ventricular fibrillation (VF). An automated external defibrillator (AED) allows for individuals trained only in basic life support to defibrillate. AEDs eliminate the need for training in rhythm interpretation and make early defibrillation practical and achievable. The AED is a defibrillator that incorporates a rhythm analysis system. The device attaches to a patient by two adhesive pads and connecting cables. Most AEDs are stand-alone boxes with a very simple three-step function (Fig. 28.3) and verbal prompts to guide the responder. All AEDs offer automated rhythm analysis, whereby the rhythm is compared to thousands of other rhythms stored in the AED computer software. On rhythm identification, some AEDs automatically provide the electrical shock after a verbal warning (fully automated). Other AEDs recommend a shock, if needed, and then prompt the responder to press the shock button.

Delegation and Collaboration

Basic life support certification provides hands-on training with an AED for laypeople, nursing assistive personnel (NAP), and licensed health care professionals. Most agencies using AEDs have given the authority to use it for all cardiopulmonary resuscitation (CPR)–

certified personnel, including NAP. Refer to specific agency policies for use of the AED.

Equipment

- AED
- Pair of AED adhesive pads

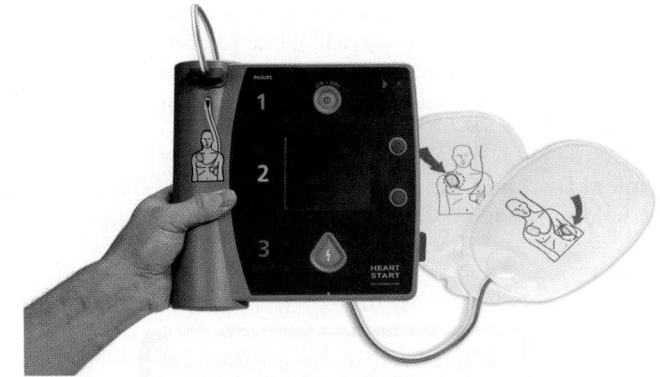

FIG 28.3 Automated external defibrillator device. (*Courtesy Philips Medical Systems.*)

STEP	RATIONALE

ASSESSMENT

1. Establish person's unresponsiveness and call for help. (In community settings have someone call 9-1-1.)

This information helps to determine if individual is unresponsive rather than asleep, intoxicated, hearing impaired, or postictal. Rapid response by qualified professionals ensures ongoing resuscitation support.

2. Establish absence of respirations and lack of circulation within 10 seconds: no pulse, no respirations, no movement.

Indicates need for emergency measures, including AED.

Clinical Decision Point *An AED should be applied only to a patient who is unconscious, not breathing, and pulseless. For children younger than 8 years old, AED pads designed for children should be used. When child pads are not available, use adult AED pads (Atkins et al., 2015).*

NURSING DIAGNOSES

- Decreased cardiac output
- Impaired spontaneous ventilation
- Ineffective breathing pattern
- Ineffective tissue perfusion

Related factors are individualized based on patient's condition or needs.

PLANNING

1. Expected outcomes following completion of procedure:
- Patient's cardiac rhythm is converted back to stable rhythm.
- Patient regains pulse and respirations.

Defibrillation provides electrical shock to convert a lethal dysrhythmia.
CPR and defibrillation were successful.

STEP	RATIONALE

IMPLEMENTATION

1. Assess patient for unresponsiveness, not breathing and pulselessness, and no movement within 10 seconds.

   These are indicators of cardiopulmonary arrest.

2. Activate code team in accordance with agency policy and procedure.

   First available person brings resuscitation cart and AED.

3. Start chest compressions and continue until AED is attached to patient and verbal prompt of device advises you, "Do not touch the patient."

   To minimize interruption time of chest compressions, continue CPR while AED is being applied and turned on.

4. Place AED next to patient near chest or head.

   Ensures easy access to device.

Clinical Decision Point *If the AED is immediately available, attach it to patient as soon as possible. The faster defibrillation is delivered, the better the survival rate (Kleinman et al., 2015).*

5. Turn on power (see illustration).

   Turning on power begins verbal prompts to guide you through the next steps.

6. Attach device. Place first AED pad on upper right sternal border directly below clavicle. Place second AED pad lateral to left nipple with top of pad a few inches below axilla (see illustration). Ensure that cables are connected to AED.

   Alternative pad placement of AED pads is not recommended. AEDs analyze most heart rhythms using lead II.

Clinical Decision Point *Do not attach pads to a wet surface, over a medication patch, or over a pacemaker or implanted defibrillator. Wet surfaces, implanted defibrillators, and medication patches reduce the effectiveness of the defibrillation attempt and result in complications.*

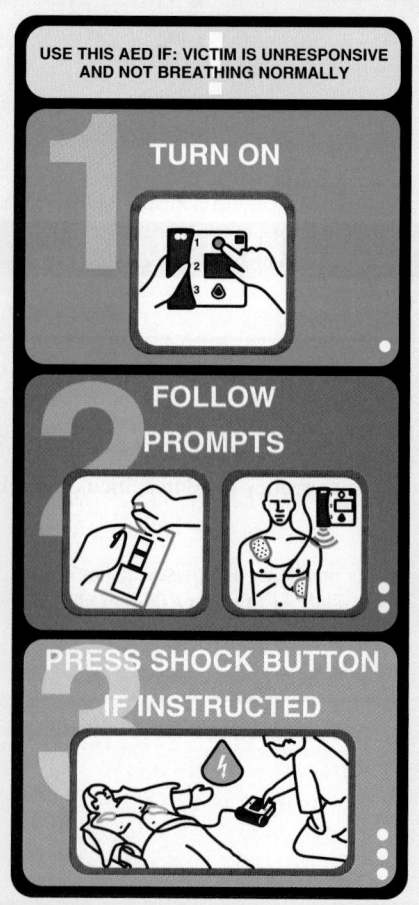

STEP 5 Power panel with AED prompts. *(Courtesy Philips Medical Systems.)*

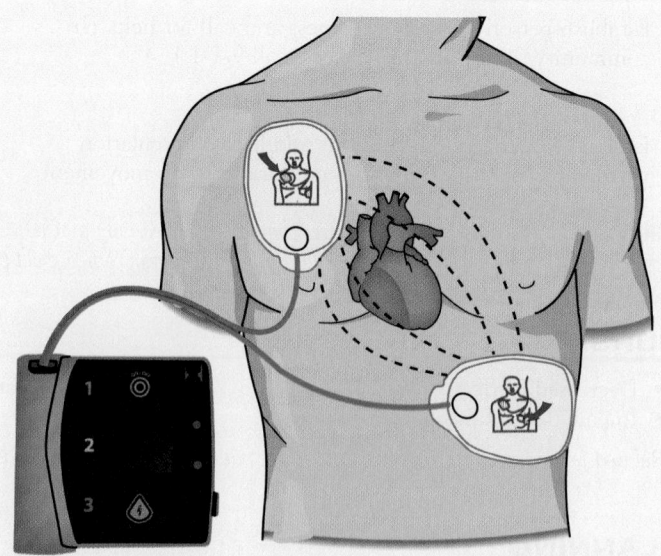

STEP 6 Placement of AED pads with device next to patient.

STEP	RATIONALE
7. Do NOT touch patient when AED prompts you. Direct rescuers and bystanders to avoid touching patient by announcing "Clear!" Allow AED to analyze the rhythm. Some devices require that an analysis button be pressed. The AED takes approximately 5 to 15 seconds to analyze the rhythm.	Each brand of AED is different; thus familiarity with the specific model that you are using is important. Not touching patient when directed prevents artifact errors, avoids all movement during analysis (Kleinman et al., 2015), and prevents shock from being delivered to bystanders.
8. Before pressing the shock button, announce loudly to clear the victim and perform a visual check to ensure that no one is in contact with him or her.	Clearing patient ensures safety for those involved in rescue efforts.
9. Immediately begin chest compression after the shock and continue for 2 minutes with a ratio of 30:2 (30 compressions and 2 breaths). Do NOT remove pads.	Continues cardiac perfusion.
10. Deliver two breaths using mouth-to-mouth with barrier device or mouth-to-mask device or bag-valve mask device. Watch for chest rise and fall. If second rescuer available, deliver 10 to 12 breaths/min or 1 breath every 5 to 6 seconds while continuing chest compressions.	In a hospital setting where protected methods of artificial ventilation are available, mouth-to-mouth without a barrier device is not recommended because of risk for microbial contamination.
11. After 2 minutes of CPR, AED will prompt you not to touch patient and will resume analysis of patient's rhythm. This cycle will continue until patient regains a pulse or health care provider determines death.	Determines patient status.

EVALUATION

1. Inspect pad adhesion to chest wall. If pads are not in good contact with chest wall, remove them and apply a new set. Attach new set of pads to AED.	Poor pad-skin contact reduces effectiveness of the shock, causes skin burns, or increases chance of shocking those involved in the rescue efforts. Always apply a new set of pads. Do NOT reuse.
2. Check for palpable pulse. Continue resuscitative efforts until patient regains pulse or health care provider determines death.	Evaluates circulatory status.
3. Provide updates to family on patient's status.	Use resources to keep family informed, including providers, chaplain, social workers. Screen family for possible family presence in the room.

Unexpected Outcomes	Related Interventions
1. Patient's heart rhythm does not convert into stable rhythm with pulse after defibrillation.	• Assess pad contact on patient's chest wall. • Do not touch patient during AED rhythm analysis. • Avoid placing AED pads over medication patches, pacemaker, or implantable defibrillator generators.
2. Patient's skin has burns under AED pads.	• Assess AED pad contact on chest. • Ensure that chest is dry before applying pads to chest. • Apply skin care as indicated if patient is resuscitated successfully.

Recording and Reporting

- Immediately report arrest via the agency-wide communication system, indicating exact location of victim.
- Cardiopulmonary arrest requires precise documentation. Most hospitals use a form designed specifically for in-hospital arrests.
- Record in nurses' notes in electronic health record (EHR) or chart or on designated CPR worksheet: onset of arrest, time and number of AED shocks (you will not know the exact energy level used by the AED), time and energy level of manual defibrillations, medications given, procedures performed, cardiac rhythm, use of CPR, and patient's response.

Special Considerations
Teaching

- If patient is at risk for cardiopulmonary arrest, instruct the family or caregivers in CPR or encourage them to obtain certification through an instructor from the hospital, American Red Cross, or American Heart Association.
- It is extremely helpful if family has a list of medications that patient is presently taking and a description of purpose of medications.

Pediatric

- Most AEDs are specifically designed for adult use only and are therefore not recommended for use in children younger than 8 years old or less than 25 kg (55 pounds) body weight (Atkins et al., 2015). Adult pads can be used if child pads are not available; be sure not to overlap pads. Manual defibrillation performed by health care personnel using lower energy settings (2 to 4 joules/kg) is the most common method of pediatric defibrillation (Atkins et al., 2015).

Home Care

- Patient and family should keep emergency numbers taped to the phone or consider programming them into a speed dial function on both home and mobile phones. Stress the use of 9-1-1.
- AEDs are available for use in the community and home setting

---

◆ SKILL 28.3   Code Management

All who respond to cardiopulmonary arrests should follow a simple, standardized, easy-to-remember approach. Initially a code is managed by the first responder performing the basic skills of cardiopulmonary resuscitation (CPR), which includes the primary survey of C (circulation), A (airway), B (breathing), and D (early defibrillation). These interventions continue until the code team arrives. The initial process also includes notification of the hospital resuscitation or code team. Most of the code team members have been trained in the advanced cardiac life support (ACLS) guidelines and the performance of the secondary survey: C (rhythm analysis of cardiac rhythm), A (airway intubation), B (confirmation of airway and ventilation), and D (differential diagnosis of the cause). Both surveys must be reassessed continually and managed as appropriate throughout the code situation.

The agency response team usually includes a physician, intensive care nurse, respiratory therapy personnel, anesthesiology personnel, and possibly radiology and laboratory technologists. A pastoral care representative is often available to be with the family.

The ability of a non-ACLS–certified nurse to initiate resuscitative efforts can prevent lethal dysrhythmias such as ventricular fibrillation from deteriorating to asystole (absence of cardiac electrical activity) and provide a chance for the heart to return to its normal rhythm. As soon as possible determine the patient's cardiac rhythm and, if appropriate, defibrillate the patient (see Skill 28.2). Table 28.2 summarizes basic cardiac arrhythmias. Early CPR and defibrillation delivered within the primary survey optimizes heart and brain function, leading to improved survivability. Equipment may be readily available at the bedside or in a designated area of

---

TABLE 28.2

Common Cardiac Dysrhythmias*

Rhythm Characteristics and Etiology	Clinical Significance and Management
Sinus Tachycardia	
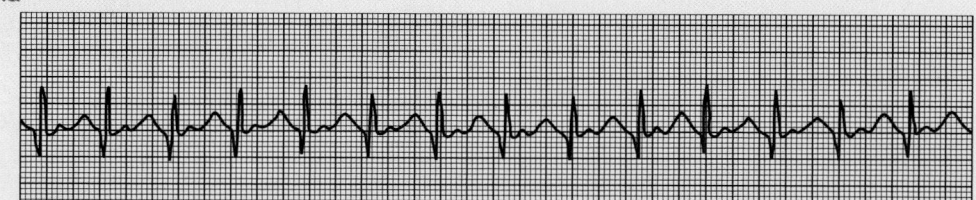	
Regular rhythm, rate 100–180 beats/min (higher in infants), normal P wave, normal QRS complex.	Some patients with heart disease are unable to increase their heart rate to meet increased oxygen demands.
Rate increase is often a normal response to exercise; emotion; or stressors such as pain, fever, pump failure, hyperthyroidism, and certain drugs (e.g., caffeine, nitrates, epinephrine, nicotine).	Correct underlying factors; discontinue drugs producing the side effect.
Sinus Bradycardia	
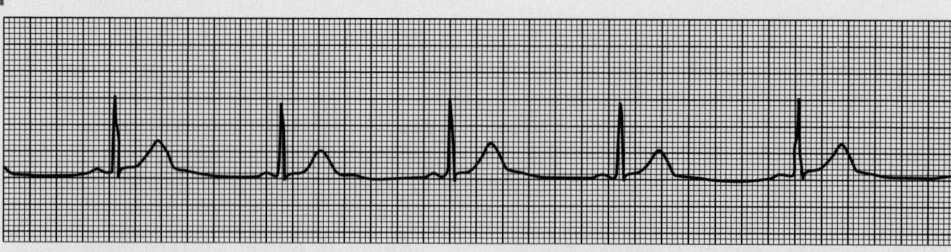	
Regular rhythm, rate less than 60 beats/min, normal P wave, normal PR interval, normal QRS complex.	No clinical significance unless associated with signs and symptoms of reduced cardiac output such as dizziness or syncope or presence of chest pain.
Rate decrease is a normal response to sleep or in well-conditioned athlete; diminished blood flow to SA node, vagal stimulation, hypothyroidism, increased intracranial pressure, or pharmacological agents (e.g., digoxin, propranolol, quinidine, procainamide) sometimes cause abnormal drops in rate.	Bradycardia with hypotension and decreased cardiac output is treated with atropine; pacemaker is sometimes necessary.

TABLE 28.2

Common Cardiac Dysrhythmias*—cont'd

| **Rhythm Characteristics and Etiology** | **Clinical Significance and Management** |

Atrial Fibrillation (A-fib)

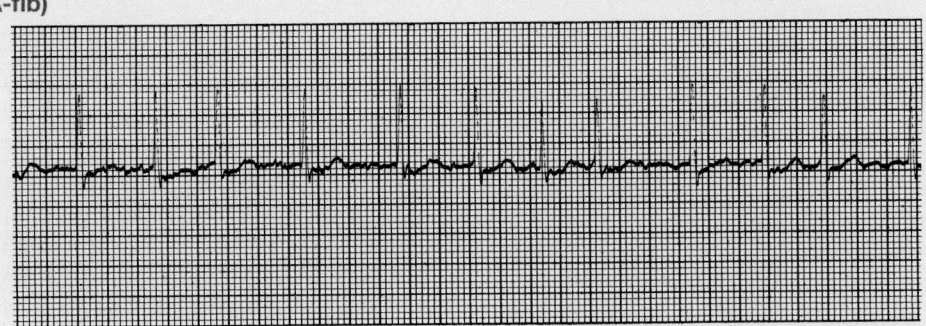

Chaotic, irregular atrial activity resulting in an irregular ventricular response. No identifiable P waves. Irregular ventricular response resulting in an irregular cardiac rate and rhythm. The conduction of the multiple atrial impulses across the atrioventricular (AV) node determines the rate.

Caused by aging, calcification of the sinoatrial (SA) node, or changes in myocardial blood supply.

There is loss of the atrial kick (part of the cardiac output squeezed in the ventricles with a coordinated atrial contraction), pooling of blood in the atria, and development of microemboli. The patient often complains of fatigue, a fluttering in the chest, or shortness of breath if the ventricular response is rapid. Dysrhythmia occurs commonly in the aging and older adult.

Ventricular Tachycardia

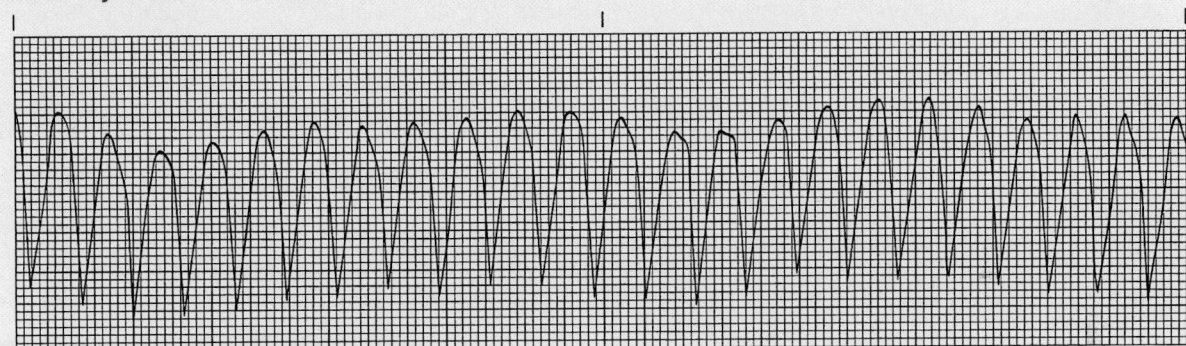

Rhythm slightly irregular, rate 100–200 beats/min, P wave absent, PR interval absent, QRS complex wide and bizarre, >0.12 second.

Results in decreased cardiac output caused by decreased ventricular filling time; often leads to severe hypotension and loss of pulse and consciousness.

Caused by changes in the normal pacemaker of the heart such as decrease in blood flow, ischemia, or embolus.

Acute loss of pulse and respiration. Immediate chest compressions and defibrillation are required.

Ventricular Fibrillation

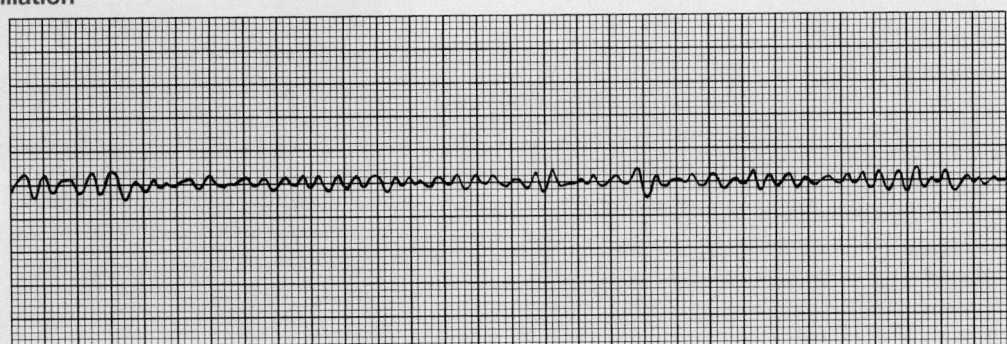

Uncoordinated electrical activity. No identifiable P, QRS, or T wave. Causes include sudden cardiac death, electrical shock, acute myocardial infarction, drowning, or trauma.

Acute loss of pulse and respiration. Immediate chest compressions and defibrillation are required. Availability of automated external defibrillator (AED) is recommended in public and/or private places where large numbers of people gather or where people who are at high risk for heart attack live.

Modified from Kleinman ME, et al: 2015 American Heart Association Guidelines for cardiopulmonary resuscitation and emergency cardiovascular care. Part 5: Adult basic life support and cardiopulmonary resuscitation quality, *Circulation* 132(suppl 2):S414, 2015.
*Refer to Table 26.1, Chapter 26 Cardiac Care.

TABLE 28.3

Adult, Child, and Infant Cardiopulmonary Resuscitation Techniques (Health Care Providers)

Technique	Adult	Child (1–8 Years Old)	Infant (Under 1 Year) Does Not Include Newborns
Chest compressions: Push hard and fast to allow complete recoil	Begin compressions if no pulse Lower half of sternum, between nipples Heel of one hand, other hand on top 5–6 cm (2–2.4 inches) One to two rescuers: 100–120/min at a rate of 30 compressions to 2 breaths (30:2) Continue until AED is available and ready to analyze rhythm	Begin compressions if no pulse or pulse <60/min Lower half of sternum, between nipples Heel of one hand or as for adults At least ⅓ depth of chest One rescuer: 30 compressions, 2 breaths (30:2) Two rescuers: 15 compressions, 2 breaths (15:2)	Begin compressions if no pulse or pulse <60/min Just below nipple line (lower half of sternum) Two fingers, two thumbs (encircling hands) One rescuer: 30 compressions, 2 breaths (30:2) Two rescuers: 15 compressions, 2 breaths (15:2)
Defibrillation using AED	Use adult pads AED should be applied as soon as available, and shock as soon as advised Resume compressions immediately after shock	Use child pads whenever possible If none, use adult pads but do not overlap them Apply AED as soon as available, and shock as soon as advised	If there is a shockable rhythm, manual defibrillation is used.
Airway	Head tilt–chin lift (HCP: Suspected trauma, use jaw thrust)	Head tilt–chin lift (HCP: Suspected trauma, use jaw thrust)	Head tilt–chin lift (HCP: Suspected trauma, use jaw thrust)
HCP: Rescue breathing mouth-to-mask or bag-valve mask without chest compressions	10–12 breaths/min (approximately 1 breath every 5–6 seconds)	12–20 breaths/min (approximately 1 breath every 3 seconds)	12–20 breaths/min (approximately 1 breath every 3 seconds)
HCP: Rescue breaths for CPR with advanced airway (endotracheal tube/tracheotomy)	8–10 breaths/min (approximately 1 breath every 6–8 seconds)	8–10 breaths/min (approximately 1 breath every 6–8 seconds)	8–10 breaths/min (approximately 1 breath every 6–8 seconds)

Data from Kleinman ME, et al: American Heart Association Guidelines for cardiopulmonary resuscitation and emergency cardiovascular care. Part 5: Adult basic life support, *Circulation* 132(suppl 2):S414, 2015; and Atkins DL, et al, American Heart Association Guidelines for cardiopulmonary resuscitation and emergency cardiovascular care. Part 11: Pediatric basic life support and cardiopulmonary resuscitation quality, *Circulation* 132(suppl 2):S519, 2015.
AED, Automated external defibrillator; *CPR,* cardiopulmonary resuscitation; *HCP,* health care provider.

the hospital unit. It is the nurse's responsibility to know how to use this equipment and to know its location and the contents of the resuscitation or crash cart.

CPR certification is a requirement of nurses and nursing students. Therefore CPR will not be covered in detail within this chapter. Table 28.3 summarizes some points regarding CPR skills, including differences in adult, child, and infant techniques.

Delegation and Collaboration

The skill of code management cannot be delegated to nursing assistive personnel (NAP). However, NAP who are certified in basic life support (BLS) techniques can perform the basic skills of CPR. Most NAP are certified in BLS and can use an automated external defibrillator (AED). Most agencies reserve the skill of manual defibrillation for licensed personnel who are ACLS certified or have received competency validation to perform manual defibrillation. All other skills in the code situation are directed by the code team leader and performed by nurses, respiratory therapists, and other health care professionals.

Equipment

- Crash cart (Fig. 28.4)—Most adult carts have the following equipment:
- Clean and sterile gloves, gown, protective eyewear
- Oxygen source
- Bag-valve mask device or resuscitation bag
- Oral airways
- Laryngoscope, handle, and laryngoscope straight and curved blades

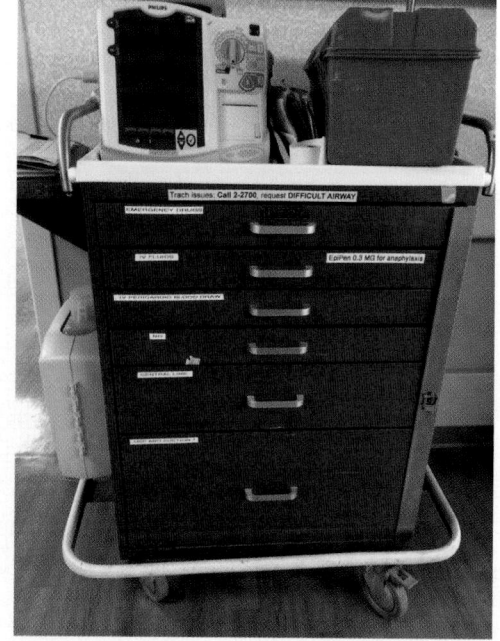

FIG 28.4 Emergency resuscitation cart.

- Endotracheal (ET) tubes, various sizes (5 to 9 mm for adults; 0 to 4 mm for pediatrics)
- Carbon dioxide detector to confirm ET tube placement
- Tape or commercial ET tube holder
- Backboard

- AED and/or manual defibrillator with AED/defibrillator pads
- Intravenous (IV) needles (sizes for adults and pediatrics)
- Central vascular access kit
- IV tubing and fluids (normal saline [NS] and 5% dextrose in water [D₅W])
- Syringes

- Laboratory specimen tubes
- Arterial blood gas kit
- Emergency medications
- ACLS guidelines or algorithms
- Suction source and suction equipment if not with crash cart

STEP	RATIONALE

ASSESSMENT

1. Determine if patient is unconscious by shaking him or her and shouting, "Are you OK?" Assess patient unresponsiveness.

Confirms that patient is unresponsive rather than intoxicated, sleeping, or hearing impaired. Substance abuse, hypoglycemia, toxicities, seizures, trauma, ketoacidosis, and shock also can cause unconsciousness.

Clinical Decision Point *If an unresponsive person has adequate respirations and pulse, remain until further help is present. Place victim in a modified lateral recovery position (see illustration). Continue to assess for the presence of respirations and pulse because a recurrent arrest may develop.*

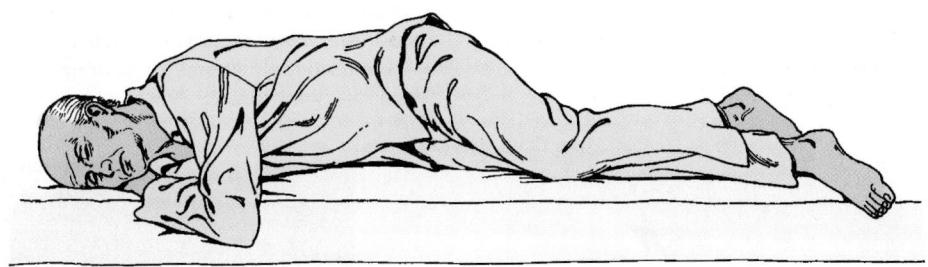

STEP 1 Recovery position.

NURSING DIAGNOSES

- Decreased cardiac output
- Impaired gas exchange
- Impaired spontaneous ventilation
- Ineffective breathing pattern

Related factors are individualized based on patient's condition or needs.

PLANNING

1. Expected outcomes following completion of procedure:
- Patient regains pulse and respirations.
- Patient receives postresuscitation care.
- Patient transported to intensive care unit (ICU) for ongoing care.

2. Immediately activate the agency code team or emergency medical services (EMS). Tell co-workers to bring AED (if available) and crash cart to bedside.

CPR was successful.
Ongoing treatment and support needed.
Resuscitation was successful.

Ensures timely application of defibrillation, CPR, and ACLS to arrest victim.

IMPLEMENTATION

Primary Survey: C (Circulation)

1. Check carotid pulse on adult or child; use brachial or femoral pulse in infant. Palpate for no more than 10 seconds (Kleinman et al., 2015).

2. Place victim on hard surface such as floor, ground, or backboard. Victim must be flat. Logroll victim to flat, supine position using spine precautions if trauma is suspected.

Carotid pulse is the easiest to locate in adults and children. Femoral pulse may also be palpated in child or infant.

External compression of heart is facilitated. Heart is compressed between sternum and spinal vertebrae, which must be on hard and firm surface. Do NOT delay the start of CPR. Positioning patient on hard surface may take more than one or two rescuers. You may need to wait to safely move him or her. Place on backboard or position patient as soon as appropriate help is present.

STEP	RATIONALE

Primary Survey: *A* (Airway)

3. Apply clean gloves and face shield.

   Reduces transmission of microorganisms.

4. Open airway.

   a. Head tilt–chin lift (no trauma) (see illustration) *or*

   Tongue is most common cause of blocked airway in unresponsive patient.

   b. Jaw thrust (cervical trauma is suspected) (see illustration)

   Suspect spinal cord injury in patients with trauma. Jaw-thrust maneuver prevents head extension and neck movement and further paralysis or spinal cord injury. Apply rigid cervical collar and immobilize patient as soon as possible to reduce cervical spine motion.

5. Determine if patient has spontaneous respirations.

   Determines level of resuscitation required.

Primary Survey: *B* (Breathing)

6. Attempt to ventilate patient with slow breaths using one of these methods.

   Slow breaths deliver air at low pressure to reduce risk of gastric distention.

   a. Mouth-to-mouth using barrier device.

   Forms airtight seal to prevent air from escaping through nose.

   b. Mouth-to-mask using pocket mask (see illustration).

   Provides secure seal and permits use of supplemental oxygen.

   c. Bag-valve mask device (see illustrations).

   Gives breaths with enough force to make chest rise.

7. If available, insert oral airway (see Skill 28.1).

   Maintains tongue on anterior floor of mouth and prevents obstruction of posterior airway by tongue.

8. Suction secretions if necessary or turn victim's head to one side unless trauma is suspected.

   Suctioning prevents airway obstruction. Turning patient's head to one side allows gravity to drain any secretions, decreasing risk of aspiration.

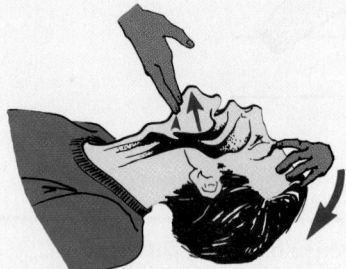

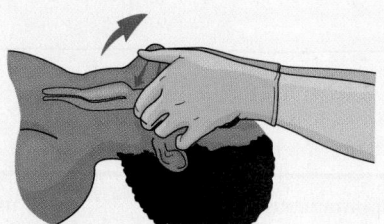

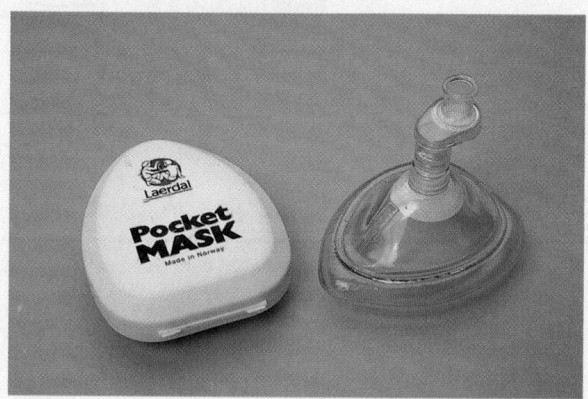

STEP 4a Head tilt–chin lift. *(From Sorrentino S: Mosby's textbook for nursing assistants, ed 7, St Louis, 2008, Mosby.)*

STEP 4b Jaw thrust without head tilt.

STEP 6b Pocket mask.

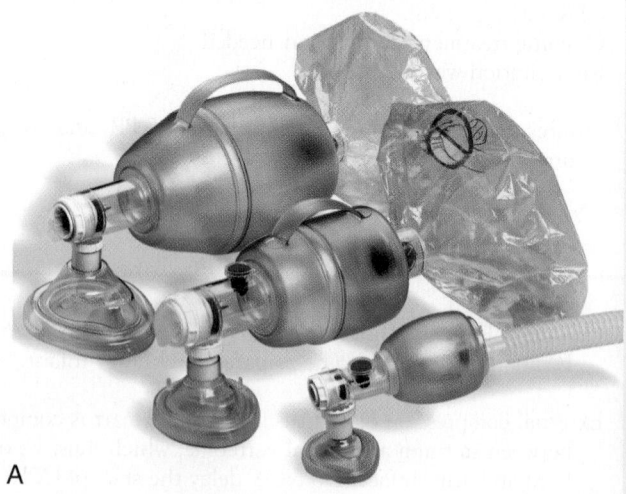

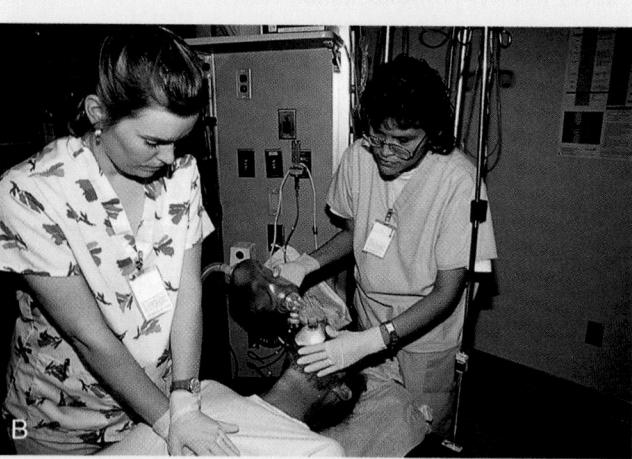

STEP 6c A, Bag-valve mask device. **B,** Two-rescuer breathing with bag-valve mask device. *(Courtesy Ambu USA.)*

STEP	RATIONALE

Primary Survey: *D* (Defibrillation)

9. If pulse is absent and AED is available, apply AED immediately as appropriate.

   Most successful defibrillation rates occur when AED is applied and used within 5 minutes following collapse. Survival rates decline when defibrillation is delayed.

   a. After one shock, resume CPR for 5 cycles (30:2, adult compressions:breath ratio) and begin rhythm analysis and shock sequence again (see Table 28.3).

   One shock followed by chest compressions for 5 cycles of 30:2 ratio provides sufficient blood flow and perfusion before another set of shocks is delivered (Kleinman et al., 2015).

10. If pulse is absent and an AED is unavailable, immediately initiate chest compressions.

    a. Assume correct hand position and compression ratio for patient (30:2 adult) (see Table 28.3; see illustrations).

    Specific hand position, compression depth, and ratio are different for adults, children, and infants to avoid injury to heart, lung, or liver (see Table 28.3).

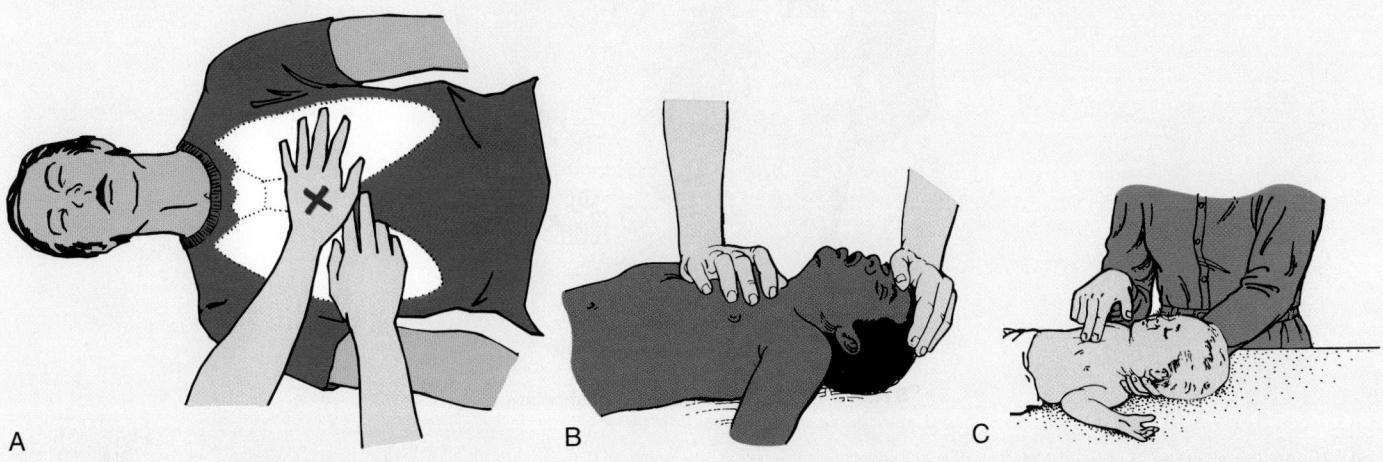

STEP 10a A, Proper hand position—adult. **B,** Proper hand position—child. **C,** Proper hand position—infant.

Clinical Decision Point *Ensure that fingers are off the ribs and lowermost part of the xiphoid process. This minimizes the chance of rib fracture that could result in punctured lung or liver laceration, which further compromises cardiopulmonary status. Continue chest compressions, ventilation, and AED use.*

Secondary Survey: Implementation

1. Give code leader brief verbal report on events performed before code team's arrival (i.e., code, vital signs, medical diagnosis, and code intervention).

   This information is critical in selection of appropriate treatment for patient.

2. On arrival of sufficient personnel, delegate tasks as appropriate while core group continues with resuscitation efforts.

   Delegation of duties is essential to meet critical needs of patient and his or her family in timely matter.

   a. Help victim's roommate and visitors away from code scene. Assign pastoral care or other nurses to communicate with patient's family. Consider allowing family to witness resuscitation (see agency policy).

   Family members who were allowed to witness resuscitation efforts have been found to have a significant reduction in posttraumatic stress and self-reports of a greater sense of resolution and fulfillment (AACN, 2016).

   b. Delegate someone to remove excess furniture or equipment from room.

   Provides room for emergency equipment and responders.

   c. Have someone bring patient's chart to bedside or have access to patient's electronic health record (EHR).

   Clarifies patient's medical condition, code status, and presence of any allergies.

   d. Assign nurse as recorder to record/document events of code.

   Ensures accurate documentation of events of code, medications, and treatments administered.

   e. Assign another nurse to get medications and supplies from crash cart to hand off to code team members. Bedside nurse is involved in tasks such as medication administration, vital signs, and helping with procedures.

   Provides code personnel with appropriate medication and equipment in timely fashion.

STEP	RATIONALE

Secondary Survey: C (Analysis of Cardiac Rhythm)

3. Attach manual defibrillator/monitor to patient using electrocardiogram (ECG) electrodes, quick-look paddles with gel pads, or "hands-off" defibrillation electrode to visualize cardiac rhythm (see illustration).

Cardiac rhythm monitor devices provide immediate rhythm display for analysis without disruption of rescue breathing and chest compression.

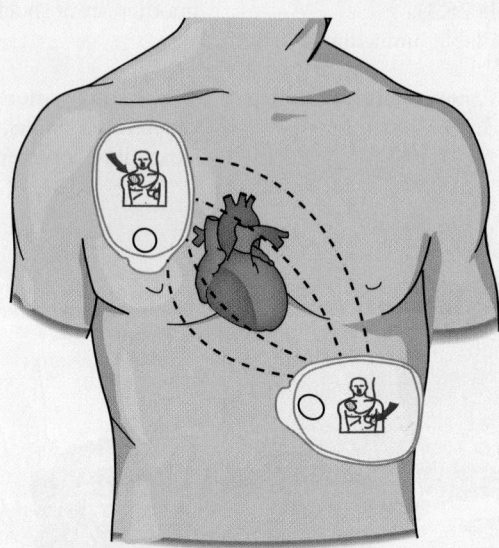

STEP 3 Paddle placement for defibrillation.

4. If cardiac rhythm is "shockable," continue CPR and help code team with manual defibrillation.

Manual defibrillation is performed by ACLS-certified personnel.

    a. Turn on defibrillator and select proper energy level following agency policy and equipment directions.

Energy is delivered in prescribed doses. Manual biphasic devices deliver shocks at a lower level (200 joules); monophasic waveforms use 360 joules.

    b. Apply conductive gel or gel pads to patient's chest where defibrillator paddles will be placed. Some defibrillators use "hands-off pads" that are applied to patient's chest and directly connect to manual defibrillator.

Good skin-to-paddle/pad contact ensures appropriate discharge of current and decreases chance of skin burns (Link et al., 2015).

    c. Place paddles or pads on patient's chest wall.

Ensures appropriate discharge of current.

    d. Verify that no one is in physical contact with patient, bed, or any item contacting patient during defibrillation. A warning must be called out before initiating charge.

Prevents accidental delivery of shock or injury to personnel.

5. Establish IV access (see Chapter 29) with large-bore IV needle (14– to 22–gauge) and begin infusion of 0.9% NS.

Provides a route for rapid drug administration and access for blood samples and fluid administration. Physiological saline is isotonic. Rapid fluid infusion facilitates dispersal of medication throughout cardiovascular system.

    a. If you cannot obtain peripheral IV access, health care provider may pursue central venous or intraosseous (IO) access.

Administration of emergency medications is dependent on vascular or IO access.

6. Help with procedures as needed.

Most equipment needed for special procedures during code is on the crash cart. Knowledge of crash cart contents is very helpful in the code to provide personnel with appropriate equipment.

7. Continue CPR until relieved (i.e., until victim regains spontaneous pulse and respiration, rescuer is exhausted and unable to perform CPR effectively, or physician discontinues CPR).

Interruptions in CPR are planned and organized. They usually occur during change of CPR personnel, defibrillation, and intubation. An interruption should not exceed 10 seconds (Kleinman et al., 2015).

STEP	RATIONALE

Secondary Survey: *A* (Intubate Airway)

8. If respirations are absent, help code team with ET intubation.

Intubation provides a patent airway and facilitates pulmonary ventilation. Laryngeal mask airway or esophageal-tracheal Combitube can also be used to provide advanced airway support.

   a. Have available laryngoscope handle, laryngoscope blades, curved and straight blades, ET tubes, stylet, suction, and tape or ET tube holder. Ensure that light source on laryngoscope is functional.

Light is necessary on laryngoscope to visualize vocal cords and intubate trachea. Batteries may need to be changed.

Secondary Survey: *B* (Confirmation of Airway and Ventilation)

9. Help in confirmation of ET tube placement or advanced airway support by auscultating lungs for bilateral breath sounds and monitoring the carbon dioxide (CO_2) detector to confirm correct airway placement (Link et al., 2015).

Auscultation of lungs and monitoring of exhaled CO_2 or esophageal detector device further verify correct airway placement and adequacy of ventilation and gas exchange.

Chest x-ray film is usually obtained after patient has been stabilized to confirm placement of ET tube and central venous catheters.

10. Ventilate using bag device on intubation. **Avoid hyperventilation.**

Increased intrathoracic pressure caused by incomplete exhalation results in reduced cardiac output (Link et al., 2015).

Secondary Survey: *D* (Differential Diagnosis)

11. Obtain ordered laboratory and diagnostic studies.

Aids in determination of cause of arrest.

EVALUATION

1. Reassess primary and secondary surveys throughout code event.
2. Palpate carotid pulse at 5 cycles or 2 minutes of CPR.
3. Observe for spontaneous return of respirations or heart rate every 2 minutes.

4. Ensure that interruptions in CPR are minimized.

5. **Use Teach-Back:** "I want to be sure I clearly explained what has happened to your loved one and why we performed cardiopulmonary resuscitation, known as CPR. In your own words, tell me why we had to perform CPR." Revise your instruction now or develop a plan for revised patient or family caregiver teaching if patient or family caregiver is not able to teach back correctly.

Keeps process organized and addresses immediate needs of patient.

Documents adequacy of external cardiac compressions.

Assessment of pulse, respiration, heart rate, and cardiac rhythm can occur after chest compressions and ventilation have been interrupted briefly every 2 minutes.

Interruptions are associated with reduced coronary artery perfusion pressure and lower mean coronary perfusion pressure (Link et al., 2015).

Determines patient's and family caregiver's level of understanding of instructional topic.

Unexpected Outcomes

1. Patient develops skeletal injury such as fractured ribs or sternum or internal organ injury such as lacerated lung or liver as result of chest compressions.

2. Patient's CPR is unsuccessful.

3. Rescuer is unassisted, tires, and is unable to continue.

Related Interventions

- Obtain appropriate diagnostic tests to document injuries.
- Assess patient's postarrest breathing for symmetry and pain.
- Assess for intrathoracic or intraabdominal bleeding (hematomas, increasing abdominal girth).
- Contact chaplain services.
- Contact social worker.
- Complete postmortem care on patient (see Chapter 17).
- Notify coroner and organ procurement agency in accordance with local hospital or state law.
- Provide for privacy for patient's family to grieve and mourn loss of loved one.
- Get help.

Recording and Reporting

- Immediately report arrest, indicating exact location of victim. In agency setting follow agency policy. In community setting activate the emergency response system.
- Record in nurses' notes in electronic health record (EHR) or chart or on designated CPR worksheet: onset of arrest, time and number of AED shocks (you will not know the exact energy level used by the AED), time and energy level of manual defibrillations, medications given, procedures performed, cardiac rhythm, use of CPR, patient's response and education and interventions provided to family.

Special Considerations
Teaching
- See Skill 28.2 for teaching considerations.

Pediatric
- All people involved in administering CPR must understand different breathing/compression ratios, hand (fingers) placement, and depth of compression in children and infants compared with adults.
- Infants and children experience respiratory arrest much more frequently than full cardiopulmonary arrest.

- Quick reference, color-coded guides are frequently used in pediatric codes to quickly determine appropriate drug doses and equipment sizes.

Gerontological
- In older adults compressions often result in rib or cartilage fractures.
- Remove loose-fitting dentures to avoid obstructing the airway. If dentures fit securely, leave them in to provide a tight seal when providing ventilations.

Home Care
- In the community and long-term care settings, patients may have implanted cardioverter defibrillators (ICDs) and/or pacemakers. For these patients, families need to know how to administer CPR and the specific capabilities of the patient's ICD/pacemaker. Placement of defibrillator or AED pads/paddles may need to be altered to avoid placement directly on top of an ICD or pacemaker generator. Remove medication patches from chest.
- Soft surfaces such as a mattress or car seat decrease efficiency of external cardiac compressions.

◆ CLINICAL DEBRIEF

You are the charge nurse for night shift on a general medical floor. Your next patient is 85 years old and admitted with heart failure. On your rounds you find your patient lying on the floor of the bathroom. You shake her and call her name. She is unresponsive. An automated external defibrillator (AED) is available down the hall.

1. What should you do first? Explain your choice.
   1. Apply the AED
   2. Call for help
   3. Check for a pulse
   4. Open airway and provide two breaths
2. Your co-worker arrives to the room with the AED. You've started chest compressions already. What is your next step? Explain your choice.
   1. Check for a pulse
   2. Call for help
   3. Tell your co-worker to apply the AED
   4. Continue with 8 to 10 breaths/min
3. The code team has arrived to continue resuscitation attempts on Mrs. Waters. Using an SBAR technique, how would you communicate to the arriving code team?

▶ REVIEW QUESTIONS

1. Which of the following techniques ensures the highest-quality chest compressions? (Select all that apply.)
   1. Minimizing interruption in chest compressions
   2. Avoiding full chest recoil
   3. Providing excessive ventilations
   4. Adequate depth and rate of compression
   5. Ensure AED is in place.
2. Place the following interventions in the correct sequence for beginning CPR.
   a. Check responsiveness.
   b. Begin 30 chest compressions.
   c. Provide 2 breaths.
   d. Attach the AED.
   e. Check for a pulse.

3. Review the following steps and place in correct order for using an automatic external defibrillator (AED).
   a. Start chest compressions.
   b. Apply AED pads to the patient.
   c. Perform a visual check to ensure that no one is in contact with the patient.
   d. Turn on the power.
   e. Assess for unresponsiveness, pulselessness, and breathlessness.
   f. Announce "Clear."
   g. Resume chest compressions.
   h. Press the shock button.

ⓔ *Visit the Evolve site for a complete list of Clinical Debrief and Review Questions answers.*

REFERENCES

AACN: Practice Alert: Family presence during resuscitation and invasive procedures, *Crit Care Nurse* 36(1):e11, 2016.

Agency for Healthcare Research and Quality (AHRQ): *Patient safety primer: rapid response systems,* psnet.ahrq.gov/primers/primer/4/rapid-response-systems, December 2014. Accessed May 21, 2016.

American Heart Association (AHA): *Resuscitation Fact Sheet,* April 2014, http://www.heart.org/idc/groups/heart-public/@private/@wcm/@hcm/@gwtg/documents/downloadable/ucm_434082.pdf. Accessed February 2016.

Atkins DL, et al: American Heart Association Guidelines for cardiopulmonary resuscitation and emergency cardiovascular care. Part 11: Pediatric basic life support and cardiopulmonary resuscitation quality, *Circulation* 132(Suppl 2):S519b, 2015.

Callaway CW, et al: Part 8: Post–cardiac arrest care: American Heart Association guidelines update for cardiopulmonary resuscitation and emergency cardiovascular care, *Circulation* 132(Suppl 1):S465, 2015.

Hockenberry MJ, Wilson D: *Wong's nursing care of infants and children,* ed 10, St Louis, 2015, Mosby.

Kleinman ME, et al: American Heart Association Guidelines for cardiopulmonary resuscitation and emergency cardiovascular care. Part 5: Adult basic life support and cardiopulmonary resuscitation quality, *Circulation* 132(Suppl 2):S414a, 2015.

Link MS, et al: Part 7: Adult advanced cardiovascular life support: American Heart Association Guidelines for cardiopulmonary resuscitation and emergency cardiovascular care, *Circulation* 132(Suppl 2):S444, 2015.

Pittman J, et al: Medical device related hospital-acquired pressure ulcers, *JWOCN* 42(2):151, 2015.

29 | Intravenous and Vascular Access Therapy

OBJECTIVES

Mastery of content in this chapter will enable the nurse to:

- Discuss current evidence-based practices for intravenous therapy.
- Discuss patient conditions requiring intravenous (IV) therapy.
- Identify safety guidelines for IV fluid administration.
- Explain how to prepare a patient and family caregiver for IV therapy.
- Discuss complications of IV therapy.
- Identify individualized outcomes for patients requiring IV therapy.
- Identify the educational needs of patients receiving IV therapy.
- Explain techniques for preventing transmission of infection for a patient receiving IV therapy.
- Demonstrate initiating IV therapy, regulating IV flow rate, changing IV solutions, changing IV tubing, changing IV dressings, and discontinuing a short-peripheral IV device.
- Identify common types of central vascular access devices (CVADs) and describe their care and maintenance.
- Identify the educational needs of patients with CVADs.

MEDIA RESOURCES

- evolve http://evolve.elsevier.com/Perry/skills
- Review Questions
- ▶ Video Clips
- Audio Glossary
- **NSO** Nursing Skills Online
- Clinical Debrief and Review Questions Answers

PURPOSE

Intravenous (IV) therapy is used to provide parenteral nutrition, transfuse blood products, provide a route for hemodynamic monitoring and a route for diagnostic testing, and to administer fluids and medications with the ability to rapidly/accurately change blood concentration levels by either continuous, intermittent, or IV push method. Each of these purposes poses risks to patients. The use of IV therapy for a patient is common in nursing practice and thus requires skill competency.

STANDARDS OF CARE

- Infusion Nurses Society (INS), 2016—Infusion Therapy Standards of Practice

- Occupational Safety and Health Administration (OSHA), 2012—Occupational Safe Exposure to Bloodborne Pathogens
- The Joint Commission (TJC), 2016—Patient Identification

PRINCIPLES FOR PRACTICE

- Evidence-based practices guide the safe, efficient, quality of care necessary to provide IV therapy.
- Successful IV therapy depends on patient preparation, site selection, catheter selection, and catheter insertion.
- Indications and protocols for vascular access device (VAD) selection and placement; management; prevention, assessment, and management of complications; and infusion therapy administration are established in organizational policies, procedures,

and/or practice guidelines and according to manufacturer directions for use (INS, 2016a).

- Assessments of a patient's anatomy and physiology of the circulatory system, fluid and electrolyte balance, disease pathophysiology, type and duration of prescribed therapy, allergies, and patient's response to illness play a key role in decision making to ensure safe delivery of infusion solutions or medications.
- For the skills in this chapter, follow the rights of medication administration for administrating parenteral solutions or medications: *Right* patient, *Right* drug/solution, *Right* dose/concentration, *Right* route, and *Right* date/time, and *Right* documentation (INS, 2016a; Phillips and Gorski, 2014). This includes knowledge of the solution or medication, how to initiate and regulate an infusion, how to operate and maintain the infusion equipment, and how to identify and correct any infusion-related complications and discontinue an infusion.

Intravenous Catheters

- To administer IV solutions and medications, a VAD is inserted into a vein. VADs can be peripheral devices (i.e., short-peripheral, midline) or central vascular access devices (CVADs) (i.e., tunneled, nontunneled, peripherally inserted central catheter [PICC], implanted port), depending on where the tip of the device resides. The choice of VADs can be overwhelming because sizes, number of lumens, and materials used to manufacture the devices vary.
- When selecting the appropriate VAD, consider a patient's prescribed therapy; length of treatment; duration the device remains in place; vascular characteristics; and patient's age, co-morbidities, history of infusion therapy, preference for VAD location, and resources available to care for the device (INS, 2016a).
- When continuous infusion of solutions or medications is not necessary, a short-peripheral IV line can be locked with preservative-free 0.9% sodium chloride (normal saline [NS]) in adults (INS, 2016a). Use commercially available prefilled syringes to reduce the risk of catheter-related bloodstream infection (CR-BSI). Use a minimum volume equal to twice the internal volume of the catheter system (INS, 2016a)
- In the case of CVADs, lock with either heparin 10 units per mL or preservative-free 0.9% NS according to the directions for use of the VAD (INS, 2016a).

Intravenous Solutions

- Many prepared IV solutions are available for use (Table 29.1).
- IV solutions fall into several categories: isotonic, hypotonic, and hypertonic. Isotonic solutions have the same osmolality as body fluids.
- Administer IV solutions carefully; isotonic solutions can cause increased risk for fluid overload in patients with renal or cardiac disease; hypotonic solutions can exacerbate a hypotensive state; and hypertonic solutions are irritating to the vein and can cause increased risk of heart failure and pulmonary edema.
- To prevent infusion-related complications, solutions and medications with an osmolarity greater than 900 mOsm/L are infused through a CVAD. Short-peripheral catheters should not be used for vesicant therapy, parenteral nutrition, or infusates with an osmolarity greater than 900 mOsm/L (INS, 2016a). In addition, solutions or medications with low or high pH have the potential to cause infusion-related complications such as phlebitis when administered with a short-peripheral or midline catheter (Alexander et al., 2014).

TABLE 29.1

Intravenous Solutions

Solution	Concentration	Other Names
Dextrose in Water Solutions		
Dextrose 5% in water*	Isotonic	D₅W
Dextrose 10% in water	Hypertonic	D₁₀W
Dextrose 50% in water	Hypertonic	D₅₀W
Saline Solutions		
0.45% sodium chloride (half NS)	Hypotonic	½ NS 0.45% NS
0.33% sodium chloride (one-third NS)	Hypotonic	⅓ NS
0.9% sodium chloride† (NS)	Isotonic	NS 0.9% NS 0.9% NaCl
3%–5% sodium chloride	Hypertonic	3%-5% NS 3%-5% NaCl
Dextrose in Saline Solutions		
Dextrose 5% in 0.9% sodium chloride	Hypertonic	D₅0.9% NaCl D₅0.9% NS D₅ NS
Dextrose 5% in 0.45% NaCl sodium chloride	Hypertonic	D₅0.45% NaCl D₅0.45% NS D₅ ½ NS
Multiple Electrolyte Solutions		
Lactated Ringer's‡	Isotonic	LR
Dextrose 5% in Lactated Ringer's	Hypertonic	D₅LR

LR, Lactated Ringer's; *NS*, normal saline.
*Dextrose is quickly metabolized, leaving free water to be distributed evenly in all fluid compartments (Alexander et al., 2014).
†Although it is isotonic because the total concentration of electrolytes equals plasma concentration, it contains 154 mEq of both sodium and chloride, which is a higher concentration of these electrolytes than is found in the plasma, which can cause fluid volume excess (Alexander et al., 2014).
‡Contains sodium, potassium, calcium, chloride, and lactate.

- Premixed solutions contain medications or electrolytes added by the manufacturer. These solutions have increased stability and allow for selecting the correct medication and diluents. However, the risk for medication errors increases because they come in varying dosages.
- A patient's specific fluid and electrolyte imbalance and serum electrolyte values guide selection of the appropriate IV fluid (Alexander et al., 2014).

PATIENT-CENTERED CARE

- Communication, comfort, and education are essential components of patient-centered care when delivering IV therapy. Successfully educating patients and family caregivers about the prescribed IV therapy and goals and expected outcomes of therapy may be difficult unless you give attention to patients' cultural and linguistic needs. Your ability to recognize diversity in patients, whether it is cultural, linguistic, or religious or caused by past experiences, will prepare you to be confident in providing IV therapy to them.

- Have patients participate in creating the plan of care, including their preferences regarding the degree of active involvement they choose. Although the skills in this chapter are performed by the nurse, engaging the patient in the decision-making process can give him or her a sense of control.
- Patient education includes clear and concise terms for all aspects of IV therapy and individualized training that includes self-care practices (Alexander et al., 2014).
- Patient teaching should also include care of the VAD, infection prevention, and potential VAD complications and signs and symptoms to report (INS, 2016a).
- Reduce anxiety and fear during the insertion of a VAD by preparing patients before insertion of a short-peripheral IV catheter. Place patients in a comfortable position, speak directly to them, and answer questions as honestly as possible. Ask patients if they have had IV therapy in the past. Know their concerns and expectations.
- When preparing for insertion, use techniques that minimize discomfort. Consider using local anesthetic agents (see agency policy) based on patient condition, needs, risks, benefits, and anticipated discomfort of the procedure (INS, 2016a).
- Some of the skills in this chapter include hands-on patient care, which may pose a problem in certain cultures where touching is not acceptable. Always explain what touching is involved and what the patient may experience.
- Allow the patient to have a family caregiver present and provide privacy during the procedure; if possible, assign same-sex caregivers to avoid opposite-sex touching.
- Pain is also expressed differently in different cultures, and you may see some cultures that encourage expressiveness and others that encourage stoicism; this is important to keep in mind when performing skills that may elicit a response to the pain of inserting or removing the tape and dressing from a VAD (Galanti, 2015).
- Consider patients' religious beliefs, especially when locking VADs with heparin. Heparin is derived from animal products (e.g., porcine, bovine) and may be in conflict with some religious beliefs (INS, 2016a).

EVIDENCE-BASED PRACTICE

It is expected that the nurse providing infusion therapy understands and implements evidence-based practice (INS, 2016a; Phillips and Gorski, 2014).

- Quality improvement includes surveillance and analysis of infection rates, infection prevention practices. and infusion-related patient quality indicators, such as occurrence of central line–associated bloodstream infection (CLABSI) and number of attempts for VAD insertion. Implementation of quality indicators and benchmarks develops a culture of accountability (INS, 2016a).
- Remove VADs on unresolved complication, discontinuation of infusion therapy, or when no longer necessary for the plan of care (INS, 2016a).
- Disinfection caps that contain a sponge saturated with 70% alcohol placed on the end of the needleless connector between

intermittent infusions protect the end and require less disinfection time or do not require disinfection before access (Phillips and Gorski, 2014). These caps have been shown to reduce intraluminal contamination and CLABSI rates (INS, 2016a).
- Primary and secondary continuous administration sets used to administer solutions other than lipid, blood, or blood products should be changed no more often than every 96 hours or according to agency policy (INS, 2016a).
- Randomized controlled trials have shown equivalent outcomes with heparin and sodium chloride lock solutions for multiple-lumen nontunneled CVADs, peripherally inserted central catheters, and implanted ports while accessed and when the access needle is removed. There is insufficient evidence to recommend one solution over the other (INS, 2016a).

SAFETY GUIDELINES

- Clinician competence is required for the use, placement, and management of VADs; the ability to recognize signs and symptoms of VAD-related complications; the use of infusion equipment; and knowledge of all aspects of administering infusion therapy (INS, 2016a). This includes knowledge of the solution or medication, how to initiate and regulate an infusion and operate and maintain the infusion equipment, and how to identify and correct any infusion-related complications and discontinue an infusion.
- Conduct a complete history and physical assessment, including vital signs, and review laboratory findings before initiating any solutions or medications. Consider prolonged environmental conditions that affect a patient's fluid status (e.g., exposure to hot, humid weather), leading to fluid and electrolyte imbalances, particularly in the infant, older adult, and chronically ill.
- Know the indications for prescribed therapy before initiating IV therapy. Obtain and review the health care practitioner's order to ensure appropriateness of the prescribed solution or medication for patient's age, health status, medical diagnosis, allergy status, acuity, VAD type and tip location, dose, frequency, and route of administration (INS, 2016b).
- Before initiating IV therapy, assess the patency and functioning of the VAD for aspiration of a blood return, absence of resistance, patient complaints of pain or discomfort when flushing, and all VAD complications (INS, 2016a, 2016b).
- Reduce risk for administration set misconnections by tracing path between IV container and patient, labeling administration sets near patient connection and solution container, routing tubings with different purposes in different directions, and providing education for patient, family caregivers, and nursing assistive personnel (NAP) to seek help with connecting or disconnecting devices or infusions.
- Maintain sterility of a patent IV system using Infusion Nurses Society (INS) standards (Box 29.1).
- Know and implement the standard precautions for infection control and the Occupational Safety and Health Administration (OSHA) standards for occupational exposure to bloodborne pathogens (Box 29.2).

BOX 29.1

INS Standards to Decrease Intravascular Infection Related to Intravenous Therapy

- Assess the VAD catheter-skin junction site and surrounding area for redness, tenderness, swelling, and drainage by visual inspection and palpation through the intact dressing. Assess short-peripheral catheters minimally at least every 4 hours or more if clinically indicated and daily for outpatient or home care patients. CVADs should be assessed at least daily.
- Change the dressing immediately to assess, clean, and disinfect the site in the event of drainage, tenderness, other signs of infection or if dressing becomes loose or dislodged.
- Perform hand hygiene before placing and providing any VAD-associated interventions.
- Perform dressing changes at a frequency based on the type of catheter and dressing. Short-peripheral catheter dressings are changed if the dressing becomes damp, loosened, and/or visibly soiled; if there is blood or drainage under the dressing; and at least every 5–7 days. Change CVAD dressings at least every 5–7 days for TSM dressings and at least every 2 days for gauze dressings that cover a catheter site or are under a TSM.
- Use approved antiseptic agents before venipuncture and when performing skin antisepsis. The preferred skin antiseptic is >0.5%

chlorhexidine gluconate (CHG) in alcohol solution. Tincture of iodine, an iodophor (povidone-iodine), or 70% alcohol may be used if CHG solution is contraindicated.
- Allow skin antiseptic to dry fully before dressing placement; alcoholic chlorhexidine solutions, for at least 30 seconds; iodophors, for at least 1.5–2 minutes.
- Use catheter stabilization device that allows visual inspection of access site.
- Use vigorous mechanical scrubbing methods when disinfecting needleless connectors before each access using 70% isopropyl alcohol, iodophors, or >0.5% chlorhexidine alcoholic solution. Disinfect before each access when multiple accesses are required.
- Change needleless connectors using aseptic no-touch technique no more frequently than 96-hour intervals.
- Use passive disinfection caps (e.g., isopropyl alcohol).
- Change administration sets based on solution administered and frequency of the infusion and immediately on suspected contamination or when integrity has been compromised.

Modified from Infusion Nurses Society: Infusion therapy standards of practice, *J Intraven Nurs* 39(suppl 1):1S, 2016.
CVAD, Central vascular access device; *INS*, Infusion Nurses Society; *TSM*, transparent semipermeable membrane; *VAD*, vascular access device.

BOX 29.2

Standards for Reducing Occupational Exposure to Bloodborne Pathogens

1. Gloves are necessary when there is a reasonable expectation that the employee may contact blood (e.g., during vascular access procedures or while changing intravenous (IV) administration sets).
2. Immediately place contaminated needles, needleless devices, and other sharps in puncture-resistant, leak-proof containers properly labeled as a biohazard; when the containers are full, seal and dispose of them properly.
3. Do not bend, shear, recap, or remove contaminated needles from the syringe after use.
4. Occupational Safety and Health Administration (OSHA) requires reports of needlestick injuries, and the health care agency must provide medical evaluation and follow-up.

5. Hepatitis B vaccinations should be made available to all employees who have occupational exposure.
6. Training and education about exposure prevention and use of protective equipment must be offered to high-risk workers who initiate IV therapy.
7. Each agency must have an infection control plan, including methods to reduce health care worker's exposure to biohazardous wastes.
8. Agencies must have engineering and work practice controls to eliminate or minimize employee exposure. Controls may include sharps disposal containers and self-sheathing needles.

Modified from Occupational Safety and Health Administration (OSHA): Occupational exposure to bloodborne pathogens, needlestick, and other sharps injuries: final rule, CFR 29, part 1910, *Fed Reg* 66:5317, 2001, updated April 2011, http://www.osha.gov/pls/oshaweb/owadisp.show_document?p_table=FEDERAL_REGISTER&p_id=16265. Accessed March 20, 2016.

◆ **SKILL 29.1**   **Insertion of a Short-Peripheral Intravenous Device**

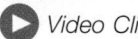 *Video Clip*   **NSO** *Nursing Skills Online Intravenous Fluid Therapy Module / Lessons 1 and 2*

An intravenous (IV) device provides access to the venous system to deliver solutions and medications or blood and blood products. Reliable venous access for infusion therapy administration is essential. Several vascular access devices (VADs) are available for use in peripheral veins (Fig. 29.1). Table 29.2 outlines the VAD options for peripheral administration. The commonly used over-the-needle catheters (ONCs) include (1) a metal stylet to pierce the skin; and (2) a catheter made of silicone, polyurethane, polyvinyl chloride, or polytetrafluoroethylene (Teflon) that threads into a vein and remains there for the infusion of fluid. Table 29.3 indicates appropriate uses for the more common short-peripheral catheter sizes.

Delegation and Collaboration

The skill of inserting a short-peripheral IV access device cannot be delegated to nursing assistive personnel (NAP). Delegation to licensed practical nurses (LPNs) varies by State Nurse Practice Act. The nurse instructs the NAP to:

- Notify the nurse if the patient complains of any IV site–related complications such as redness, pain, tenderness, swelling, bleeding, drainage, or leaking from under dressing.
- Notify the nurse if the patient's IV dressing becomes wet.
- Notify the nurse if the level of fluid in the IV bag is low or the electronic infusion device (EID) is alarming.

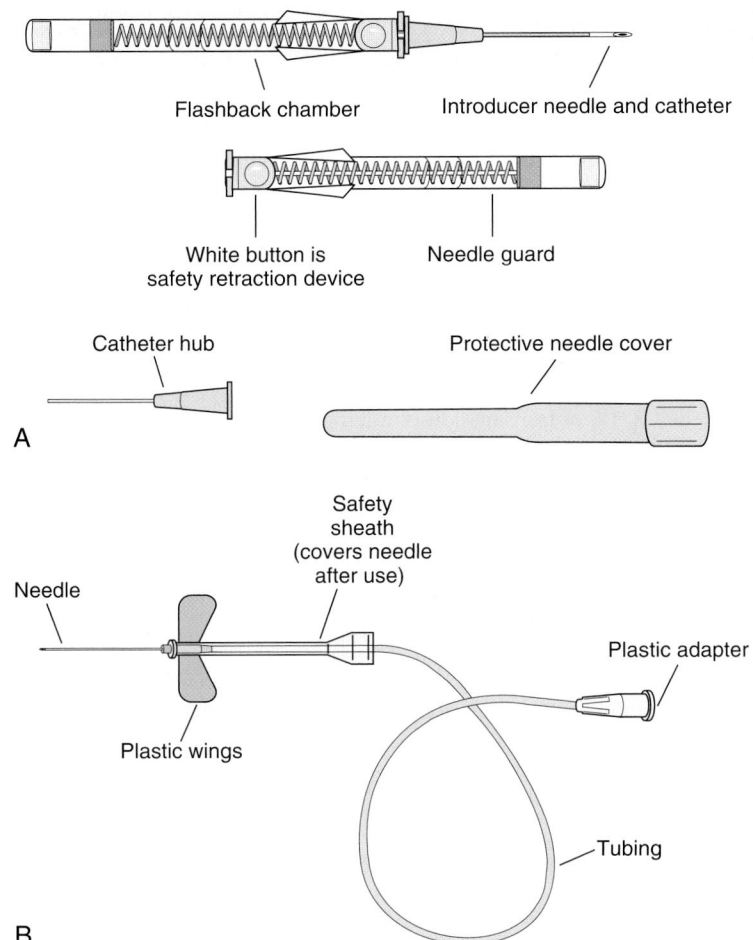

FIG 29.1 Intravenous access device options. **A,** Over-the-needle catheter (ONC) device. **B,** Steel butterfly needle.

TABLE 29.2

Peripheral Vascular Access Device Options

Type	Use	Types of Infusions
Steel needle winged butterfly	One-time infusion, IV push administration, venipuncture for phlebotomy (INS, 2016a)	Solutions or medications with an osmolarity less than 900 mOsm/L (INS, 2016a)
Short, over-the-needle catheter (ONC) (7.5 cm [less than 3 inches]); may be winged or nonwinged	Continuous infusion, intermittent infusion, short-term duration (INS, 2016a)	Solutions or medications with an osmolarity less than 900 mOsm/L (INS, 2016a)
Midline peripheral catheters (7.5 to 20 cm [3 to 8 inches])	Continuous infusion and intermittent infusion (1 to 4 weeks) (INS, 2016a)	Solutions or medications with an osmolarity less than 900 mOsm/L (INS, 2016a)

IV, Intravenous.

TABLE 29.3

Recommendations for Short-Peripheral Catheter Selection

Catheter Size (Gauge)	Clinical Indication
14, 16, 18	Trauma, surgery, rapid blood transfusions, and rapid fluid replacement
20	Continuous or intermittent infusions in adults; administration of blood transfusions in adults
22	Continuous or intermittent infusions in adults, pediatrics, neonates and the elderly; administration of blood or blood product in adults, pediatrics, neonates, and the elderly
24	Continuous or intermittent infusions in adults, pediatrics, neonates and the elderly; administration of blood or blood product in adults, pediatrics, neonates, and the elderly

Modified from Infusion Nurses Society (INS): *Policy and procedures for infusion therapy,* ed 5, Norwood, MA, 2016, INS.

Equipment

- Short-peripheral IV start kit supplies (available in some agencies): single-use tourniquet, tape, transparent semipermeable membrane (TSM) dressing or sterile gauze and sterile tape, antiseptic wipes (chlorhexidine gluconate [CHG]) solution preferred, povidone-iodine, or 70% alcohol), 2 × 2–inch gauze pads, and label.
- If kit is not available, gather all items separately.
- Appropriate short-peripheral IV catheter with safety mechanism for venipuncture (see Table 29.3) (INS, 2016a)
- Clean gloves (latex free for patients with latex allergy); sterile gloves are needed if palpating the site after skin antisepsis (INS, 2016a)
- Single-use hair clippers or scissors for hair removal if indicated
- Short extension tubing with fused needleless connector or separate needleless connector (also called *injection cap, saline lock, heparin lock, IV plug, buff cap, buffalo cap, or PRN adapter*)
- 5-mL prefilled syringe with preservative-free 0.9% sodium chloride (normal saline [NS]) (INS, 2016a)
- Antiseptic swabs
- Manufactured catheter stabilization device (if available) and skin protectant swab
- Prescribed IV solution or medication (see Chapter 22).

- IV infusion set (IV tubing), either macrodrip or microdrip, depending on prescribed rate; if using EID, appropriate administration set
- 0.2-micron filter for nonlipid (fat emulsions) solutions (may be incorporated into the infusion set)
- Protective equipment: Goggles and mask (optional based on agency policy)
- Electronic infusion device (EID) and IV pole
- Vein visualization device (optional based on agency policy)
- Stethoscope
- Watch with second hand to calculate drip rate
- Special patient gown with snaps at shoulder seams if available (makes removal with IV tubing easier)
- Needle disposal container (*sharps container* or *biohazard container*)

STEP	RATIONALE

ASSESSMENT

1. Review accuracy of health care provider's order: date and time, IV solution, route of administration, volume, rate, duration, and signature of ordering health care practitioner (Phillips and Gorski, 2014). Follow rights of medication administration (see Chapter 20).

Before IV therapy, an order from a health care provider is needed (INS, 2016a).
Verification that order is complete prevents medication errors.

   a. Check approved online database, drug reference book, or pharmacist about IV solution composition, purpose, potential incompatibilities, adverse reactions, and side effects.

Ensures safe and correct administration of IV therapy and appropriate selection of VAD.

2. Perform hand hygiene.

Reduces risk of transmission of microorganisms.

3. Assess patient's knowledge of procedure, reason for prescribed therapy, and arm placement preference.

Provides patient-centered care by determining level of emotional support and instruction needed.

4. Assess for clinical factors/conditions that will respond to or be affected by administration of IV solutions.

Provides baseline to determine effectiveness of prescribed therapy. A systems approach is recommended to assess for fluid and electrolyte imbalances (Phillips and Gorski, 2014).

   a. Body weight

Changes in body weight can be an indication of fluid loss or gain (Alexander et al., 2014).

   b. Clinical markers of vascular volume:
     (1) Urine output (decreased, dark yellow)

Kidneys respond to extracellular volume (ECV) deficit by reducing urine production and concentrating urine. Kidney disease can also cause oliguria.

     (2) Vital signs: blood pressure, respirations, pulse, temperature

Changes in blood pressure may be associated with fluid volume status (fluid volume deficit [FVD]) seen in postural hypotension.
Respirations can be altered in presence of acid-base imbalances.
Temperature elevations increase need for fluid requirements (temperature of 38.3°C [101°F] to 39.4°C [103°F] require at least 500 mL of fluid replacement within a 24-h period) (Weinstein and Hagle, 2014).

     (3) Distended neck veins (Normally veins are full when person is supine and flat when person is upright.)

Indicator of fluid volume status: flat or collapsing with inhalation when supine with ECV deficit; full when upright or semi-upright with ECV excess.

     (4) Auscultation of lungs

Crackles or rhonchi in dependent parts of lung may signal fluid buildup caused by ECV excess.

     (5) Capillary refill

Indirect measure of tissue perfusion (sluggish with ECV deficit).

   c. Clinical markers of interstitial volume
     (1) Skin turgor (Pinch skin over sternum or inside of forearm.)

Failure of skin to return to normal position after several seconds indicates FVD (Alexander et al., 2014).

     (2) Dependent edema (pitting or nonpitting) (see Chapter 6).

Edema is not usually apparent until 4.4–8.8 lbs (2–4 kg) of fluid is retained. A weight gain of 2.2 lbs (1 kg) is equivalent to the retention of 1 L of body water (Phillips and Gorski, 2014).

     (3) Oral mucous membrane between cheek and gum (see Chapter 6).

More reliable indicator than dry lips or skin. Dry between cheek and gums indicates ECV deficit.

   d. Thirst

Occurs with hypernatremia and severe ECV deficit. Not a reliable indicator for older adults (Phillips and Gorski, 2014).

   e. Behavior and level of consciousness:
     (1) Restlessness and mild confusion

Occurs with FVD or acid-base imbalance

     (2) Decreased level of consciousness (lethargy, confusion, coma)

Occurs with severe ECV deficit.
May occur with osmolality, fluid and electrolyte, and acid-base imbalances.

4. Determine if patient is to undergo any planned surgeries or procedures.

Allows anticipation and placement of appropriate VAD for infusion and avoids placement in an area that will interfere with medical procedures (INS, 2016a).

5. Assess available laboratory data (e.g., hematocrit, serum electrolytes, arterial blood gases, and kidney functions [blood urea nitrogen, urine specific gravity, and urine osmolality]).

Helps determine priority assessments and establishes baseline for determining if therapy is effective. Laboratory values are an assessment of hydration status (Alexander et al., 2014).

STEP	RATIONALE
6. Assess patient's history of allergies, especially to iodine, adhesive, or latex.	Equipment used during VAD insertion may contain substances to which patient is allergic. Will require use of latex-free gloves.

NURSING DIAGNOSES

- Anxiety
- Deficient knowledge regarding IV therapy

- Risk for electrolyte imbalance

- Risk for injury

Related factors/Risk factors are individualized based on patient's condition or needs.

PLANNING

1. Expected outcomes following completion of procedure:	
• Patient's VAD remains patent, and site is free from signs and symptoms of IV-related complications.	Ensures that patient receives prescribed infusion therapy and VAD is without complications (INS, 2016a).
• Vital signs are stable and within normal limits for patient.	Demonstrates response of body systems to fluid and electrolyte replacement (Alexander et al., 2014).
• Fluid and electrolyte balance returns to normal.	Proper solution is infused at proper rate and monitored, resolving fluid and electrolyte imbalance (Alexander et al., 2014).
• Patient is able to explain purpose and risks of IV therapy.	Demonstrates learning (INS, 2016a).
2. Collect appropriate equipment. Be sure you have the correct infusion set for the EID that is to be used.	Ensures patient safety.

IMPLEMENTATION

1. Identify patient using at least two identifiers (e.g., name and birthday or name and medical record number) according to agency policy. Compare identifiers with information on patient's MAR or medical record.	Ensures correct patient. Complies with The Joint Commission standards and improves patient safety (TJC, 2016).
2. Instruct patient about rationale for infusion, including solution and medications ordered, procedure for initiating an IV line, and signs and symptoms of complications (e.g., redness, pain, tenderness, swelling, bleeding, drainage, or leaking from under dressing).	Provides patient with information about procedure and promotes compliance (INS, 2016a). Informing patient may minimize anxiety.
3. Help patient to comfortable sitting or supine position. Provide adequate lighting.	Promotes comfort and relaxation of patient. Aids in successful vein location.
4. Perform hand hygiene. Collect and organize equipment on clean, clutter-free bedside stand or overbed table.	Reduces transmission of infection and contamination of equipment (INS, 2016a). Easy access to equipment improves efficiency.
5. Change patient's gown to more easily removed gown with snaps at shoulder if available.	Use of this gown decreases risk of inadvertently dislodging VAD or administration set when changing gown.
6. Select appropriate-size catheter; open and prepare sterile packages using sterile aseptic technique (see Chapter 10).	Use smallest-gauge peripheral catheter that will accommodate prescribed therapy and patient need (INS, 2016a).
7. Prepare short extension tubing with fused needleless connector or separate needleless connector (injection cap) to attach to catheter hub.	Needleless connectors protect health care workers by eliminating needles and potential for needlestick injuries when accessing VAD (INS, 2016a).
a. Remove protective cap from needleless connector and attach syringe with 1 to 3 mL 0.9% sodium chloride (normal saline), maintaining sterility. Slowly inject enough saline to prime (fill) short extension tubing and connector, removing all air. Leave syringe attached to tubing.	Replaces air with normal saline, preventing air from entering patient's vein later during VAD insertion.
b. Maintain sterility of end of connector by reapplying end caps, and set aside for attaching to catheter hub after successful venipuncture.	Prevents touch contamination, which allows microorganisms to enter infusion equipment and bloodstream.

Clinical Decision Point *Short extension sets may be used on short-peripheral catheters. Reduces catheter manipulation. For patient safety, all connections should be of Luer-Lok type (INS, 2016a). Many agencies use short extension tubing for continuous infusions and stand-alone saline locks (capped catheters).*

STEP	RATIONALE

8. Prepare IV tubing and solution for continuous infusion.

a. Check IV solution using six rights of medication administration (see Chapter 20) and review label for name and concentration of solution, type and concentration of any additives, volume, beyond-use and expiration dates, and sterility state. If using bar code, scan code on patient's wristband and then on IV fluid container. Be sure that prescribed additives such as potassium and vitamins have been added. Check solution for color and clarity. Check bag for leaks.

Reviewing label for accuracy reduces risk for medication errors (INS, 2016a).
Bar-code system reduces human error (INS, 2016a).
Risk for medication errors can be reduced with safe medication practices, including (INS, 2016a):
- Do not add medications to infusing containers of IV solutions (INS, 2016a).
- Do not use IV solutions that are discolored, contain precipitates, or are expired.
- Risk for transmission of infection can be reduced by not using leaking bags because integrity has been compromised.

b. Open IV infusion set, maintaining sterility. **NOTE:** EIDs sometimes have a dedicated administration set; follow manufacturer's instructions.

Prevents touch contamination, which allows microorganisms to enter infusion equipment and bloodstream.

c. Place roller clamp (see illustration A) about 2 to 5 cm (1 to 2 inches) below drip chamber and move roller clamp to "off" position (see illustration B).

Close proximity of roller clamp to drip chamber allows more accurate regulation of flow rate. Moving clamp to "off" prevents accidental spillage of IV solution during priming.

d. Remove protective sheath over IV tubing port on plastic IV solution bag (see illustration) or top of IV solution bottle while maintaining sterility.

Provides access for insertion of IV tubing spike into solution using sterile technique.

e. Remove protective cover from IV tubing spike while maintaining sterility of spike. Insert spike into port of IV bag using a twisting motion (see illustration). If solution container is glass bottle, clean rubber stopper on glass-bottled solution with antiseptic swab and insert spike into rubber stopper of IV bottle. Bottles require vented tubing.

Flat surface on top of bottled solution may contain contaminants, whereas opening to plastic bag is recessed. Prevents contamination of bottled solution during insertion of spike. If sterility of spike is compromised, discard IV tubing and obtain new one.

f. Compress drip chamber and release, allowing it to fill one-third to one-half full (see illustration).

Creates suction effect; fluid enters drip chamber to prevent air from entering tubing.

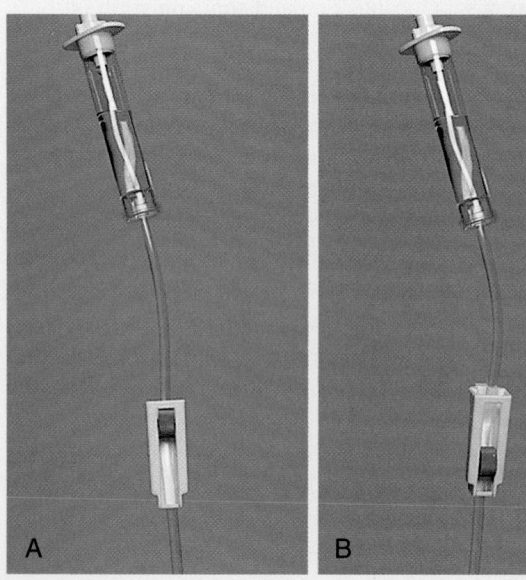

STEP 8c A, Roller clamp in open position. **B,** Roller clamp in closed position.

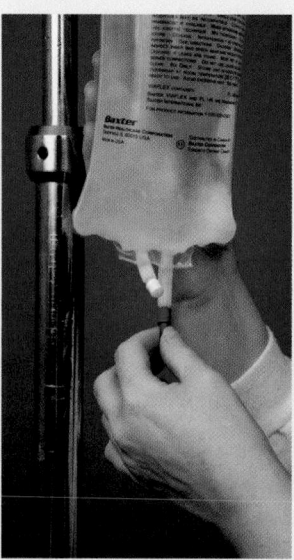

STEP 8d Removing protective sheath from IV tubing port.

STEP	RATIONALE
g. Prime air out of IV tubing by filling with IV solution: Remove protective cover on end of IV tubing (some tubing can be primed without removing protective cover) and slowly open roller clamp to allow fluid to flow from drip chamber to distal end of IV tubing. If tubing has a Y connector, invert Y connector when fluid reaches it to displace air. Return roller clamp to "off" position after priming tubing (filled with IV fluid). Replace protective cover on distal end of tubing. Label IV tubing with date according to agency policy and procedure.	Priming ensures that IV tubing is clear of air and filled with IV solution before connecting to VAD. Slowly filling tubing decreases turbulence and chance of bubble formation. Closing clamp prevents accidental loss of fluid. Maintains sterility. Labeling IV tubing allows for recognition of length of time that tubing has in use and when to change it.
h. Be certain that IV tubing is clear of air and air bubbles. To remove small air bubbles, firmly tap tubing where they are located. Check entire length of tubing to ensure that all air bubbles are removed (see illustration).	Large air bubbles may act as emboli (Cook, 2013).
i. If using optional long extension tubing (not short tubing in Step 7), remove protective cover and attach it to distal end of IV tubing, maintaining sterility. Then prime long extension tubing. Insert tubing into EID with power off.	Priming removes air from long extension tubing so it does not enter patient's vascular system. Facilitates starting infusion as soon as IV site is ready.
9. Perform hand hygiene.	Decreases potential risk of microbial contamination and cross-contamination (INS, 2016a).

Clinical Decision Point *Gloves are not necessary to locate vein but must be applied for VAD insertion using a no-touch technique where the site is not palpated after skin antisepsis (INS, 2016a, 2016b).*

STEP	RATIONALE
10. Apply tourniquet around upper arm about 10 to 15 cm (4 to 6 inches) above proposed insertion site (see illustration). Do not apply tourniquet too tightly. Check for presence of pulse distal to tourniquet. (*Option A:* Apply tourniquet on top of thin layer of clothing such as gown sleeve to protect fragile or hairy skin.) (*Option B:* Blood pressure cuff may be used in place of tourniquet: activate cuff and hold at approximately 50 mm Hg.)	Tourniquet should be tight enough to impede venous flow while maintaining arterial circulation (INS, 2016a, 2016b). If patient has fragile veins or bruises easily, tourniquet should be applied loosely or not at all to prevent damage to veins and bruising (INS, 2016a). Reduces trauma to skin.

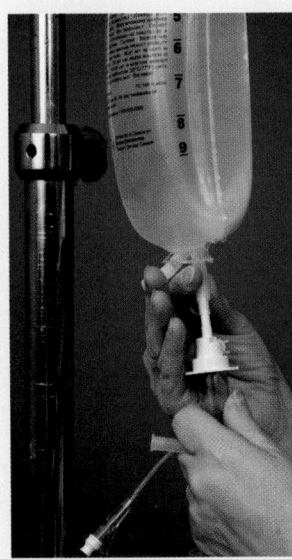

STEP 8e Inserting spike into IV bag.

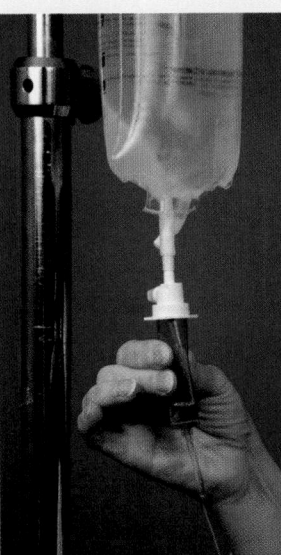

STEP 8f Squeezing drip chamber to fill with fluid.

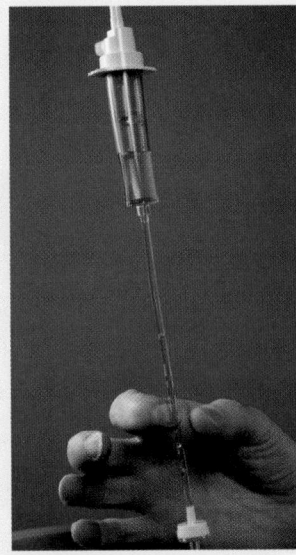

STEP 8h Removing air bubbles from tubing.

STEP	RATIONALE
11. Select vein for VAD insertion (see illustration). Veins on dorsal and ventral surfaces of arms (e.g., metacarpal, cephalic, basilic, or median) are preferred in adults.	Ensures adequate vein that is easy to puncture and less likely to rupture.
a. Use most distal site in nondominant arm if possible.	Patients with VAD placement in their dominant hand have decreased ability to perform self-care.
b. With your fingertip, palpate vein at intended insertion site by pressing downward. Note resilient, soft, bouncy feeling while releasing pressure (see illustration).	Fingertip is more sensitive and better for assessing vein location and condition.
c. Select well-dilated vein. Methods to improve vascular distention:	Increased volume of blood in vein at venipuncture site makes vein more visible.
(1) Position extremity lower than heart, have patient open and close fist slowly, and lightly stroke vein downward.	Use of gravity promotes vascular distention (INS, 2016a).
(2) Apply dry heat to extremity for several minutes.	Dry heat has been found to increase successful peripheral catheter insertion (INS, 2016a).

Clinical Decision Point *Vigorous friction, slapping or hard tapping of a vein, especially in older adults, can cause venous constriction and/or bruising and hematoma (Weinstein and Hagle, 2014).*

12. When selecting a vein: **a.** Avoid vein selection in:	
(1) Areas with pain on palpation, compromised areas, sites distal to compromised areas (e.g., open wounds, bruising, infection, infiltration, or extravasation) (INS, 2016a).	It would be difficult to assess for any signs or symptoms of complications if an IV device were inserted in an area already compromised.
(2) Upper extremity on side of breast surgery with axillary node dissection or lymphedema or after radiation, arteriovenous (AV) fistulas/grafts; or affected extremity from cerebrovascular accident (CVA) (INS, 2016a).	Increases risk for complications such as infection, lymphedema, or vessel damage.
(3) Site distal to previous venipuncture site, sclerosed or hardened veins, previous infiltrations or extravasations, areas of venous valves, or phlebitic vessels.	Such sites cause infiltration around newly placed VAD site and vessel damage.
(4) Fragile dorsal hand veins in older adults. Veins of lower extremities should not be used for routine IV therapy in adults because of risk of tissue damage and thrombophlebitis (INS, 2016a).	Veins have increased risk for infiltration.

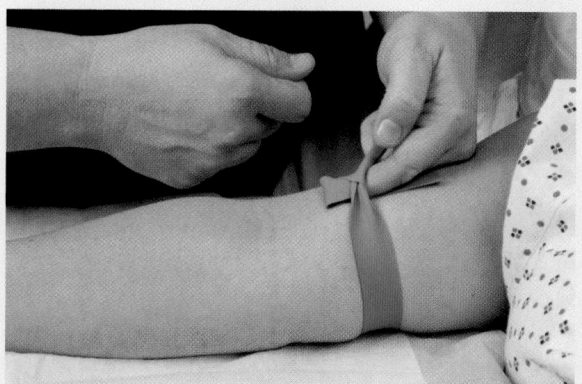

STEP 10 Tourniquet placed on arm for initial vein selection.

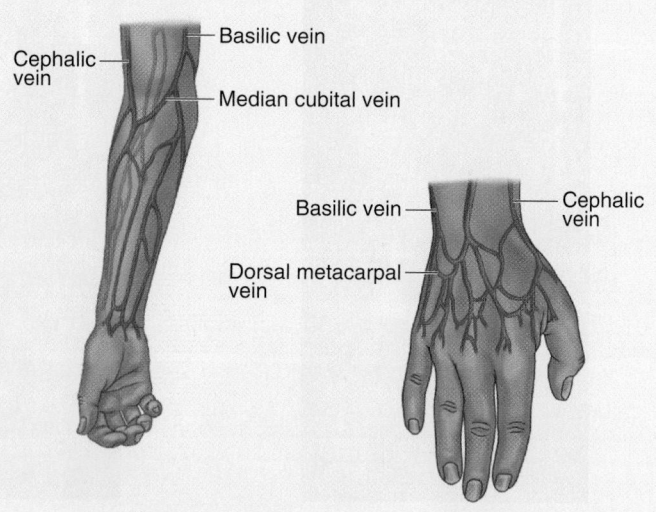

STEP 11 Cephalic, basilic, and median cubital veins are best for IV placement in adults.

STEP	RATIONALE
(5) Areas of flexion such as wrist or antecubital area (INS, 2016a).	Veins have increased risk for infiltration, phlebitis, or dislodgement.
(6) Ventral surface of wrist (10–12.5 cm [4–5 inches])	Venipuncture in ventral surface of wrist is painful and has potential for nerve damage (INS, 2016a).
b. Choose site that will not interfere with patient's activities of daily living (ADLs), use of assist devices, or planned procedures.	Keeps patient as mobile as possible.
13. Release tourniquet temporarily.	Restores blood flow and prevents venospasm when preparing for venipuncture.

Clinical Decision Point *If hair removal is needed, do not shave area with a razor. Shaving may increase risk of infection (INS, 2016a). Clip hair with scissors or hair clippers to prepare area for application of TSM dressing if necessary (explain to patient).*

Clinical Decision Point *Local anesthetic reduces discomfort associated with placement of a VAD. Both topical and injectable drugs can be used to reduce pain and require a health care provider's order. You may apply topical local anesthetic to intended IV site 30 minutes before procedure. Follow manufacturer recommendations and monitor for allergic reaction (Alexander et al., 2014; INS, 2016a).*

STEP	RATIONALE
14. Perform hand hygiene and apply clean gloves. Wear eye protection and mask (see agency policy) if splash or spray of blood is possible.	Decreases potential risk of microbial contamination and cross-contamination (INS, 2016a).
15. Place adapter end of short extension set (prepared in Step 7) or needless connector (injection cap) for saline lock nearby in sterile package.	Permits smooth, quick connection of infusion to short-peripheral catheter once vein is accessed.
16. If area of insertion is visibly soiled, clean site with antiseptic soap and water first and dry. Perform skin antisepsis with CHG solution using friction in back-and-forth motion (see illustration) for 30 seconds and allow to dry completely. If using alcohol or povidone-iodine, clean in concentric circle, moving from insertion site outward with swab. Allow drying time between agents if agents are used in combination (alcohol and povidone-iodine).	Mechanical friction in this pattern allows penetration of antiseptic solution to epidermal layer of skin (Alexander et al., 2014). Reduces incidence of catheter-related infections (Alexander et al., 2014). Allow any skin antiseptic agent to fully dry for complete antisepsis; alcoholic CHG solutions for at least 30 seconds; iodophors for at least 1.5 to 2 minutes (INS, 2016a).

Clinical Decision Point *If vein palpation is necessary after performing skin antisepsis, use sterile gloves for palpation or perform skin antisepsis again because touching cleaned area introduces microorganisms from your finger to site (INS, 2016a, 2016b).*

STEP	RATIONALE
17. Reapply tourniquet 10 to 15 cm (4 to 6 inches) above anticipated insertion site. Check for presence of pulse distal to tourniquet.	Pressure of tourniquet promotes vein distention. Diminished arterial flow prevents venous filling.
18. Perform venipuncture. Anchor vein below anticipated insertion site by placing thumb over vein 4 to 5 cm (1½ to 2 inches) distal to site (see illustration) and gently stretching skin against direction of insertion. Instruct patient to relax hand.	Stabilizes vein for needle insertion; prevents vein from rolling; and stretches skin taut, decreasing drag during insertion. Some devices require loosening needle (stylet) from catheter before venipuncture. Follow manufacturer directions for use.
a. Warn patient of a sharp stick. Hold VAD with needle bevel up. Align catheter on top of vein at 10- to 30-degree angle. Puncture skin and anterior vein wall (see illustration).	Accessing vein at an angle reduces risk of puncturing posterior vein wall. Superficial veins require smaller angle. Deeper veins require greater angle.

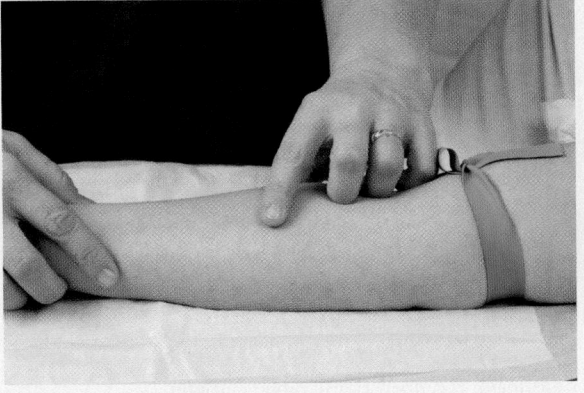

STEP 11b Palpate vein.

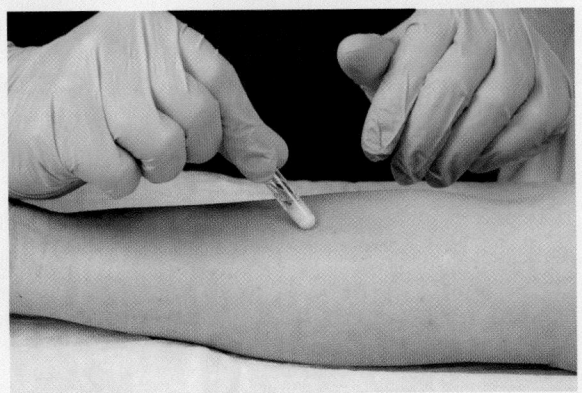

STEP 16 Clean site with >0.5% chlorhexidine alcoholic solution.

STEP	RATIONALE

Clinical Decision Point *Use each VAD only once for each insertion attempt.*

19. Observe for blood return in catheter or flashback chamber of catheter, indicating that bevel of needle has entered vein (see illustration A). Advance VAD approximately ¼ inch (0.6 cm) into vein and loosen stylet (needle) of ONC. Continue to hold skin taut while stabilizing VAD and, with index finger on push-off tab of VAD, advance catheter off needle into vein until hub rests at venipuncture site (see illustration B). *Do not reinsert stylet into catheter once catheter has been advanced into vein.* Advance catheter while safety device automatically retracts stylet (techniques for retracting stylet vary with different VADs). Place stylet directly into sharps container.

Increased venous pressure from tourniquet causes backflow of blood into catheter and/or flashback chamber. Some VADs have a notch in the stylet, allowing flash of blood into catheter. Stabilizing VAD allows for placement of catheter into vein and advancement of catheter off stylet.

Advancing entire stylet into vein may penetrate wall of vein, resulting in hematoma.

Advancing catheter with finger on open hub causes contamination (INS, 2016a).

Reinsertion of stylet can cause catheter to shear off and embolize into vein. Proper sharps disposal prevents needlestick injury (OSHA, 2012).

Clinical Decision Point *A single clinician should not make more than two attempts at initiating IV access and limit total attempts to no more than 4 (INS, 2016a).*

20. Stabilize VAD with nondominant hand and release tourniquet or blood pressure cuff with other. Apply gentle but firm pressure with middle finger of nondominant hand 3 cm (1¼ inches) above insertion site. Keep catheter stable with index finger.

Permits venous flow and reduces backflow of blood.

Digital pressure minimizes blood loss and allows attachment of extension set or needleless connector (INS, 2016b).

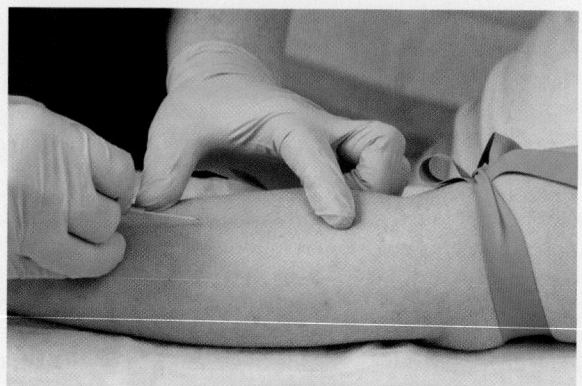

STEP 18 Stabilize vein below insertion site.

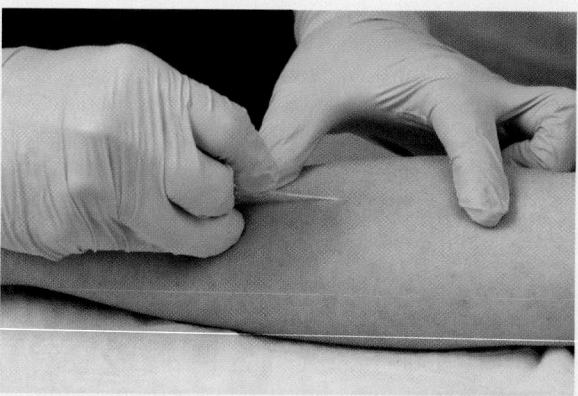

STEP 18a Puncture skin with catheter at 10- to 15-degree angle.

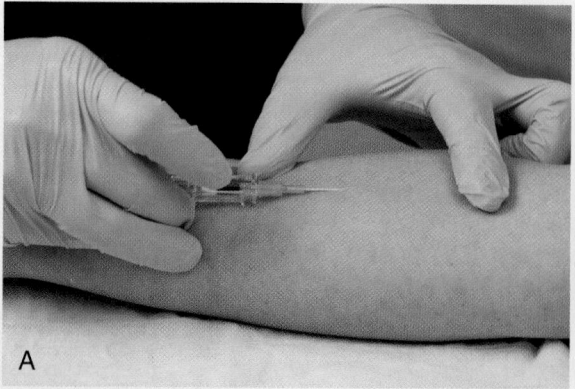

A

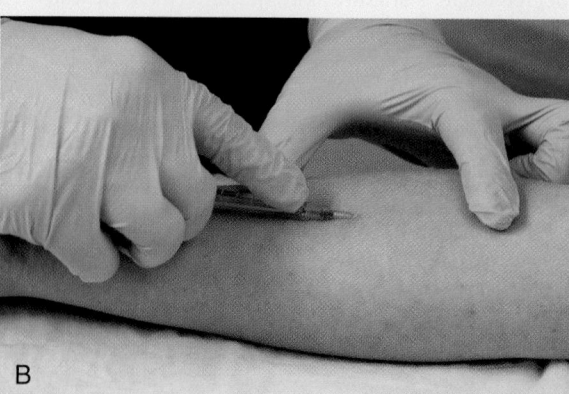

B

STEP 19 A, Observe for blood return in catheter and/or flashback chamber. **B,** Advance catheter into vein until hub rests at venipuncture site.

STEP	RATIONALE
21. Quickly connect Luer-Lok end of short extension tubing with needleless connector to end of catheter hub. Secure connection. Avoid touching sterile connection ends. *Option:* IV tubing can be attached directly to catheter hub in place of short extension tubing or needleless connector.	Prompt connection maintains patency of vein, minimizes blood loss, and prevents risk of exposure to blood. Maintains sterility.
22. Attach prefilled flush syringe of 0.9% sodium chloride to short extension set and aspirate to remove air and assess blood return. Slowly inject NS from prefilled syringe into VAD (see illustration A). Remove syringe and discard.	Aspirating air prevents air embolism. Blood return that is color and consistency of whole blood confirms placement of catheter in vein (INS, 2016a). Flushing prevents reflux of blood into catheter and occlusion (INS, 2016b). Initiates flow of fluid through IV catheter, preventing clotting of device. Swelling indicates infiltration, and catheter would need to be removed.
Option: To begin primary infusion, swab needleless connector with antiseptic swab and attach Luer-Lok end of IV tubing to needleless connector (see illustration B). Open roller clamp of IV tubing, turn on EID, and program it. Begin infusion at correct rate. If using gravity flow instead of EID, begin infusion by slowly opening roller clamp to regulate rate.	Initiates flow of fluid through IV catheter, preventing clotting of VAD.

Clinical Decision Point *Needleless connectors protect health care workers and decrease risk for needlestick injuries. They have different internal mechanisms for fluid displacement and vary in the flush-clamp-disconnect sequence to prevent reflux of blood into catheter on disconnection (INS, 2016a). The sequence depends on the type of internal mechanism (Phillips and Gorski, 2014):*

- Neutral displacement devices do not have a specified flush/clamp/disconnect sequence.
- For negative-pressure displacement devices, flush, clamp catheter, then disconnect syringe.
- For positive-pressure displacement, flush, disconnect syringe, then clamp catheter.

STEP	RATIONALE
23. Observe insertion site for swelling.	Swelling indicates infiltration, which requires immediate catheter removal.

24. Apply sterile dressing over site.
  a. **TSM dressing:**
    (1) Continue to secure catheter with nondominant hand. Remove adherent backing. Apply one edge of dressing and gently smooth remaining dressing over IV insertion site, leaving Luer-Lok connection between tubing and catheter hub uncovered. Gently press dressing to adhere to skin. Remove outer covering and smooth dressing gently over site (see illustration).
	Protects catheter insertion site and minimizes risk for infection (Phillips and Gorski, 2014). Allows visualization of insertion site and surrounding area for complications (INS, 2016a). Access to Luer-Lok connection between tubing and catheter hub facilitates changing tubing if necessary.

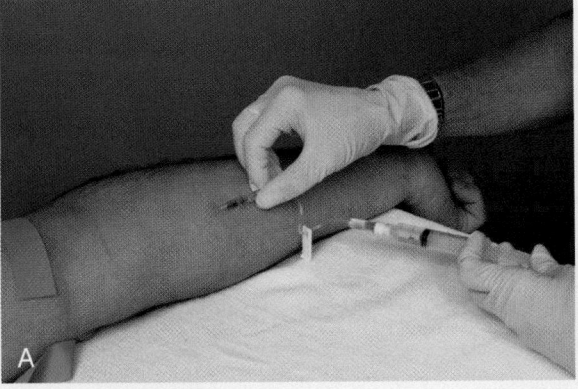
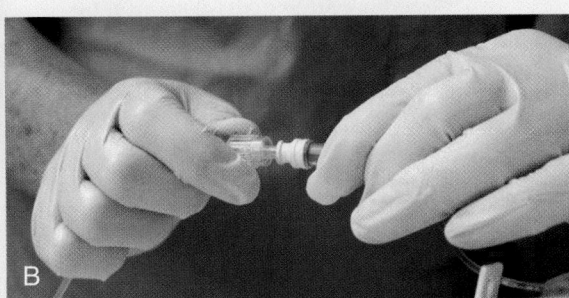

STEP 22 A, Flush short extension set after aspirating air and assessing blood return. **B,** Connect IV tubing to the short extension set that is attached to the catheter.

STEP	RATIONALE

(2) Place 2.5 cm (2-inch) piece of tape over Luer-Lok connection (see illustration). **Do not apply tape on top of TSM dressing.**

Removal of tape from TSM dressing can tear dressing and cause catheter dislodgement.

Tape on top of TSM dressing prevents moisture from being carried away from skin.

b. Sterile gauze dressing:

(1) Place 5-cm (2-inch) piece of sterile tape over catheter hub (see illustration).

Stabilizes catheter under gauze dressing.

(2) Place 2 × 2–inch gauze pad over insertion site and edge of catheter hub. Secure all edges with tape. Do not place tape over insertion site. Do not cover connection between IV tubing and catheter hub (see illustration).

Use gauze dressings for site drainage, excessive perspiration, or sensitivity/allergic reactions to TSM dressings (INS, 2016a; Phillips and Gorski, 2014).

(3) Fold 2 × 2–inch gauze in half and cover with 10-cm (4-inch) or 1 inch–wide tape so about an inch extends on each side. Place under Luer-Lok connection (see illustration). Secure Luer-Lok connection and tubing to tape on folded gauze with 2.5-cm (1-inch) piece of tape. Avoid applying tape or gauze around arm. Do not use rolled bandages with or without elastic to secure VAD. Taping Luer-Lok connection can be eliminated if engineered stabilization device is to be used.

Tape on top of gauze makes it easier to access hub/tubing junction. Gauze pad elevates hub off skin to prevent pressure area.

Prevents back-and-forth motion of catheter.

Rolled bandages do not secure VAD adequately, can impair circulation or flow of infusion, and obscure visualization for complications (INS, 2016a).

25. *Option:* Secure IV catheter using engineered stabilization device (follow manufacturer directions and agency policy).

Use of engineered stabilization devices that allow visual inspection of insertion site can reduce risk of VAD complications (i.e., phlebitis, infection, migration) and unintentional loss of access (INS, 2016a).

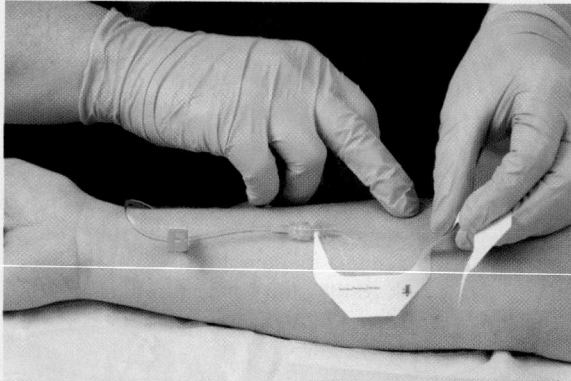

STEP 24a(1) Apply transparent semipermeable membrane (TSM) dressing.

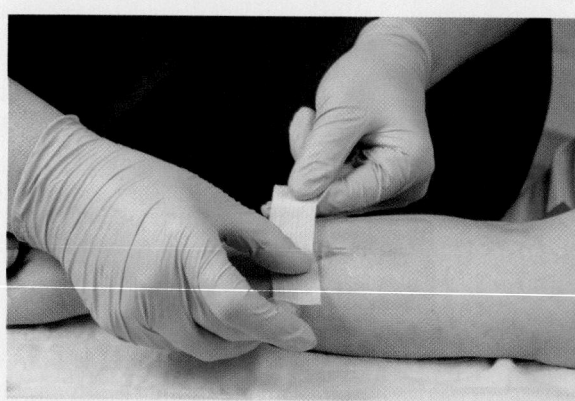

STEP 24a(2) Place tape over administration set tubing.

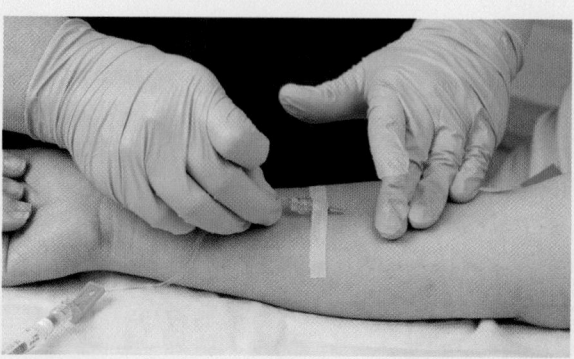

STEP 24b(1) Place sterile tape over catheter hub.

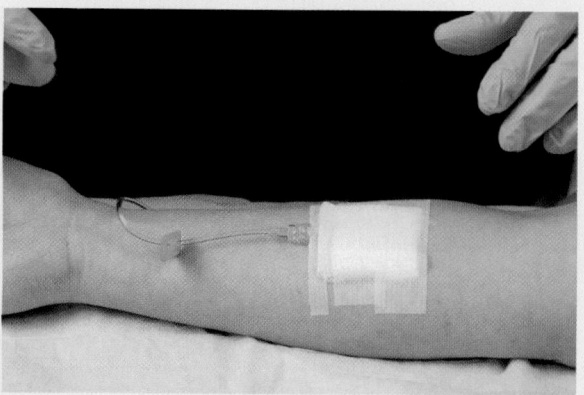

STEP 24b(2) Place 2 × 2–inch gauze over insertion site and catheter hub.

STEP	RATIONALE

a. Apply skin protectant to area of skin around IV site and allow to dry completely.

Risk for medical adhesive–related skin injury (MARSI) is increased as result of age, joint movement, and edema; use of skin protectant can decrease risk (INS, 2016a).

(2) Align anchoring pads with directional arrow pointing to insertion site. Press device retainer over top of Luer-Lok connection while supporting underneath connection.

(3) Stabilize catheter and peel off one side of liner and press to adhere to skin. Repeat on other side (see illustration).

(4) Monitor for medical adhesive–related skin injury (MARSI).

26. Loop extension or IV tubing alongside dressing on arm and secure with second piece of tape directly over tubing (see illustration).

Securing tubing reduces risk for dislodging catheter if IV tubing is pulled (i.e., loop comes apart before catheter dislodges).

27. Label dressing per agency policy. Include date and time of IV insertion, VAD gauge size and length, and your initials (see illustration).

Allows for recognition of type of device and length of time that device has been in place.

28. Dispose of any remaining sharps in appropriate sharps container. Discard supplies. Remove gloves and perform hand hygiene.

Reduces transmission of microorganisms; prevents accidental needlestick injuries (OSHA, 2012).

29. Instruct patient in how to move or turn without dislodging VAD.

Prevents accidental dislodgement of catheter.

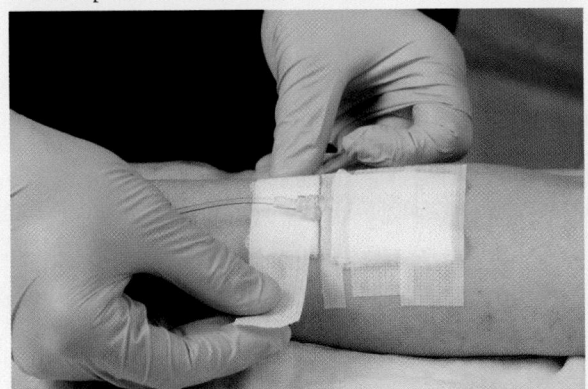

STEP 24b(3) Apply 2 × 2–inch gauze dressing under tubing junction.

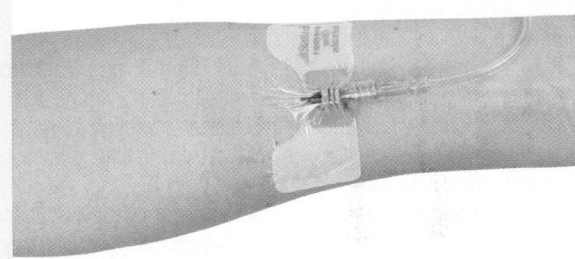

STEP 25a(3) Catheter stabilization device in place. (*Image Courtesy C.R. Bard, Inc., All rights reserved.*)

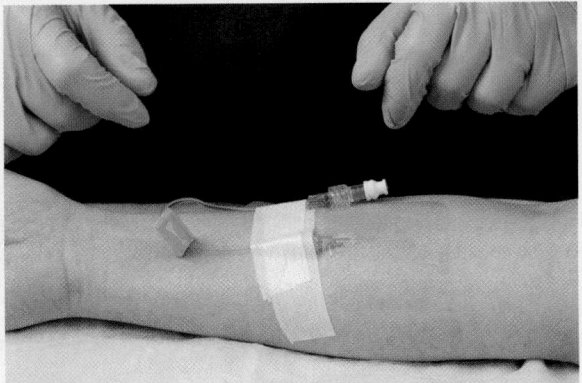

STEP 26 Loop and secure tubing.

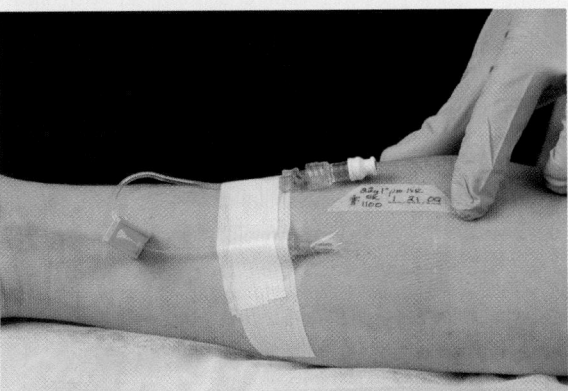

STEP 27 Label IV dressing.

STEP	RATIONALE

EVALUATION

1. Observe patient every 1 to 2 hours or at established intervals per agency policy and procedure for function, intactness, and patency of IV system and for correct infusion rate and accurate type/amount of IV solution infused by observing level in IV container.

Ensures delivery of prescribed volume over prescribed time and decreases risk for fluid and electrolyte imbalance.

2. Evaluate patient to determine response to therapy (e.g., laboratory values, input and output [I&O], weights, vital signs, postprocedure assessments).

Early recognition of complications leads to prompt treatment.

3. Evaluate patient at established intervals per agency policy and procedure for signs and symptoms of IV-related complications by inspecting and gently palpating skin around and above IV site over the dressing.

Identifies complications that compromise integrity of VAD or cause inaccurate IV solution flow rate.

Clinical Decision Point *If IV is positional, fluid will run slowly or stop, depending on position of patient's arm; if this continues, you may have to restart IV line.*

4. **Use Teach-Back:** "I want to make sure that I explained the problems that can happen with your IV. Tell me the signs or symptoms that you should tell me or the other nurses about." Revise your instruction now or develop a plan for revised patient or family caregiver teaching if patient or family caregiver is not able to teach back correctly.

Determines patient's and family caregiver's level of understanding of instructional topic.

Unexpected Outcomes

1. Fluid and electrolyte imbalances:
   a. Fluid volume deficit (FVD): decreased urine output, dry mucous membranes, decreased capillary refill, disparity in central and peripheral pulses, tachycardia, hypotension, shock.
   b. Fluid volume excess (FVE): dyspnea, crackles in lung, edema, and/or increased urine output.
   c. Electrolyte imbalances: abnormal serum electrolyte levels, changes in mental status, alterations in neuromuscular function, cardiac arrhythmias, and changes in vital signs.

2. IV-related complications
   a. Infiltration: pain, swelling, coolness to touch, or presence of blanching (white, shiny appearance at or above IV site) or redness (INS, 2016b).

   b. Catheter occlusion can occur from bent catheter, positional catheter (catheter resting against catheter wall), kink or knot in infusion tubing, clot formation, or precipitate formation from administration of incompatible medications or solutions (Alexander et al., 2014).

   c. Phlebitis (i.e., vein inflammation): pain, redness, warmth, swelling, induration, or presence of palpable cord along course of vein (INS, 2016a). Rate of infusion may be altered.

Related Interventions

- Notify health care provider.
- Requires readjusting infusion rate.
- Requires adjusting additives in IV line or type of IV fluid ordered.

- Stop infusion and remove IV catheter at first sign of infiltration (see Procedural Guideline 29.1).
- Elevate affected extremity.
- Avoid applying pressure, which can force solution into contact with more tissue, causing tissue damage.
- Use standard scale for assessing and documenting infiltration (INS, 2016a).
- Determine cause and consider catheter removal.
- Positional catheters can be repositioned to improve IV flow.
- Remove occluded IV catheter. Occluded catheters should not be flushed because an embolus can result from dislodging a clot (Alexander et al., 2014).
- Notify health care provider.
- Determine cause (i.e., chemical, mechanical, bacterial) and consider removal or replacement of VAD.
- *Chemical phlebitis:* Apply heat, elevate limb, consider slowing infusion rate, and determine if catheter removal is necessary (INS, 2016a).
- *Mechanical phlebitis:* Apply heat, elevate limb, monitor for 24–48 hours, consider catheter removal if signs and symptoms persist (INS, 2016a).
- *Bacterial phlebitis:* Remove IV catheter (INS, 2016a).
- Document phlebitis using a standardized scale, including nursing interventions per agency policy and procedure (Tables 29.4 and 29.5).

STEP	RATIONALE
d. Catheter-related infection can present as redness, swelling around or above IV site, pain, purulent drainage at insertion site, and body temperature elevations (INS, 2016a).	• Notify health care provider. Obtain order to culture drainage (INS, 2016a). • Remove IV catheter and culture purulent drainage from around IV site (see Chapter 7) (INS, 2016a).
e. Hematoma is bleeding under skin caused by trauma to vessel wall. It can occur during short-peripheral IV insertion if needle punctures either adjacent vessels or posterior vein wall or can be seen with multiple venipuncture attempts (Alexander et al., 2014).	• Remove IV catheter immediately and apply pressure and dry, sterile. • Monitor for additional bleeding. • Elevate extremity and monitor for circulatory, neurological, or motor dysfunction (Alexander et al., 2014).
f. Nerve injuries during short-peripheral IV insertion can occur. Be alert for patient complaints of paresthesias, including shocklike pain, tingling or pins and needles, burning, or numbness on insertion.	• Notify health care provider of any signs and symptoms of nerve injury (INS, 2016b). • Immediately stop VAD insertion and remove device if patient complains of symptoms of paresthesias (INS, 2016a). • Continue to monitor neurovascular status (INS, 2016b)

TABLE 29.4

Phlebitis Scale

Grade	Clinical Criteria
0	No symptoms
1	Erythema at access site with or without pain
2	Pain at access site with erythema and/or edema
3	Pain at access site with erythema and/or edema Streak formation Palpable venous cord
4	Pain at access site with erythema and/or edema Streak formation Palpable venous cord >2.5 cm (1 inch) in length Purulent drainage

Modified from Infusion Nurses Society (INS): *Policy and procedures for infusion therapy*, ed 5, Norwood, MA, 2016, INS.

TABLE 29.5

Visual Infusion Phlebitis Scale

Score	Observation
0	IV site appears healthy
1	One of the following signs is evident: Slight pain near IV site *or* slight redness near IV site
2	Two of the following signs are evident: • Pain at IV site • Erythema • Swelling
3	All of the following signs are evident: • Pain along the path of cannula • Induration
4	All of the following signs are evident and extensive: • Pain along the path of cannula • Erythema • Induration • Palpable venous cord
5	All of the following signs are evident and extensive: • Pain along the path of cannula • Erythema • Induration • Palpable venous cord • Pyrexia

Modified from Infusion Nurses Society (INS): *Policy and procedures for infusion therapy*, ed 5, Norwood, MA, 2016, INS.
IV, Intravenous.

Recording and Reporting

• Record in nurses' notes in electronic health record (EHR) or chart the number of attempts (successful and unsuccessful) and sites of insertion; precise description of insertion site (e.g., cephalic vein on dorsal surface of right lower arm, 2.5 cm [1 inch] above wrist); flow rate; method of infusion (gravity or EID); size and type, length, and brand of catheter; and time infusion started and patient's response to insertion. Use an infusion therapy flow sheet when available.

• If using an EID, document type and rate of infusion and device identification number.

• Record patient's status, IV fluid, amount infused, integrity and patency of system according to agency policy.

• Record patient's and family caregiver's level of understanding following instruction in nurses' notes in EHR or chart.

• Report to oncoming nursing staff: type of fluid, flow rate, status of VAD, amount of fluid remaining in present solution, expected time to hang subsequent IV container, and patient condition.

• Report to health care provider any signs and symptoms of IV-related complications.

• Record signs and symptoms of IV-related complications, including interventions and patient response to treatments.

Special Considerations
Teaching

• Instruct patient to notify nurse or NAP if any signs or symptoms of IV complications are noted (e.g., redness, pain, tenderness, swelling, bleeding, drainage, or leaking under dressing), if flow rate slows or stops, or if patient sees blood in the IV tubing or on the dressing

• Teach patient how to ambulate with IV pole; to protect IV when performing hygiene activities.

Pediatric

• Perform venipuncture in a neutral space to allow the child's room to be a safe place.

- In addition to the usual venipuncture sites, the four scalp veins are used in infants and toddlers and, if not walking, the dorsum of the foot.
- Needle selection is based on age: 26- to 24-gauge for neonates, 24- to 22-gauge for children (Hockenberry and Wilson, 2015).
- Use local anesthetics and distraction strategies to minimize distress associated with venipuncture (Alexander et al., 2014).
- Apply latex-free tubing or use a blood pressure cuff inflated to just below diastolic blood pressure.
- Allow older children to select IV site to increase cooperation so they believe that they have some control over their treatment.
- To maintain safety in positioning, have extra help when starting an IV line on a child. Use therapeutic hugging, usually in a sitting position, to provide close contact (Hockenberry and Wilson, 2015). NAP can help with positioning.
- Choose age-appropriate activities compatible with the maintenance of the IV infusion to maintain normal growth and development.

Gerontological

- Veins of the older population are very fragile; they have less subcutaneous support tissue, and their skin is thinning (Alexander et al., 2014). Avoid sites that are easily moved or bumped. Use a commercial protective device to protect the site and reduce manipulation (Fig. 29.2).
- In older patients the use of a 22- or 24-gauge catheter is appropriate for most therapies. Smaller-gauge catheters are less traumatizing to the vein but still allow blood flow to provide increased hemodilution of the IV solutions or medications (Alexander et al., 2014).
- If possible, avoid the back of the older adult's hand or the dominant arm for venipuncture because use of these sites interferes with their independence.
- As older adults lose subcutaneous tissue, the veins lose stability and roll away from the needle. To stabilize the vein, pull the skin taut and toward you with your nondominant hand and anchor the vein with your thumb.

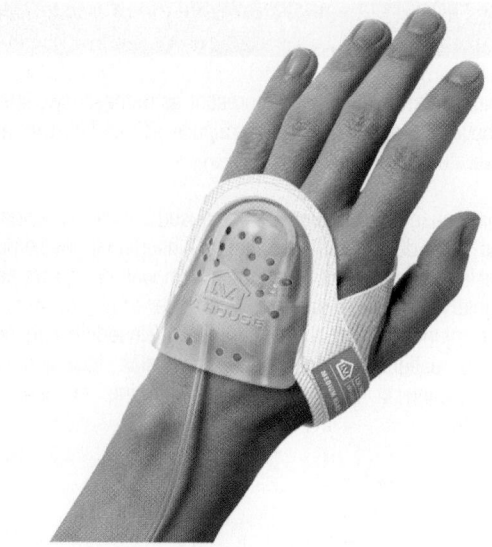

FIG 29.2 I.V. House Protective Device. (*Courtesy I.V. House.*)

Home Care

- Ensure that a patient is able and willing to self-administer IV therapy or that there is a reliable family caregiver to provide IV therapy care at home.
- Ensure that all sharps and equipment contaminated by blood are disposed of appropriately based on their community's standards. Some suppliers provide sharps containers for needle disposal. Teach patient and family caregiver appropriate sharps disposal.
- Instruct patient and family caregiver about procedures of IV therapy, including hand hygiene and aseptic technique while handling and proper disposal of syringes and other supplies. Observe patient and family caregiver performing tasks.
- Ensure availability of 24-hour assistance with provider of home infusion therapy pharmaceuticals, and equipment.
- Teach patient about activity restrictions (e.g., avoiding strenuous exercise of the arm with the IV line, protecting site while bathing/showering).

 SKILL 29.2 **Regulating Intravenous Flow Rates**

▶ *Video Clip* **NSO** *Nursing Skills Online Maintenance of Intravenous Fluid Therapy Module / Lesson 2*

Accurate infusion rates in intravenous (IV) therapy are essential in the safe delivery of solutions and medications (see Chapter 22). Appropriate regulation of infusion rates reduces complications (e.g., phlebitis, infiltration, fluid overload, or clotting of the vascular access device [VAD]) associated with IV therapy (INS, 2016b). Infusion rates can be affected by changes in patient position, flexion of the IV site extremity, occlusion of the IV device, venospasm, venous trauma, or manipulation of the VAD (Alexander et al., 2014). A patient achieves therapeutic outcomes and fewer complications when an IV system and flow rates are assessed systematically (Alexander et al., 2014).

There are a variety of methods for regulating infusion rates. Electronic infusion devices (EIDs) maintain correct flow rates and catheter patency and prevent an unexpected bolus of IV infusion for patient safety (INS, 2016a). Many EIDs provide a record of the volume of fluid infused over a period of time. An EID delivers a measured amount of fluid over a period of time (e.g., 100 mL/h) using positive pressure. An electronic sensor signals an alarm if the pressure in the system changes and the desired flow rate alters. The use of an EID does not absolve a nurse from checking to ensure that the pump is functioning and infusing at the prescribed rate or to detect infiltration or extravasation (INS, 2016a).

Manual flow-control devices include flow regulators (i.e., dial or barrel-shaped) and mechanical infusion devices without a power source (i.e., elastomeric devices, piston-driven pumps). These may be used when flow rate is not critical (Alexander et al., 2014; Phillips and Gorski, 2014). They are not recommended for use in infants and children because accuracy cannot be guaranteed (Alexander et al., 2014).

Flow regulators such as volume-control devices deliver small volumes with the aid of gravity. Patient and mechanical factors (e.g., height of the IV container, IV tubing size, or fluid viscosity) affect an IV gravity controller. One example of a volume-control device is a calibrated chamber placed between the IV container and the insertion spike and drip chamber of an administration set (see Chapter 22). A small volume of IV solution is placed in the chamber and regulated for administration. The advantage of this system is that, if the rate of the IV is inadvertently increased, only a limited amount of solution will infuse. With either type of device, a consistent monitoring is necessary to verify the accurate infusion of the IV solution and detect and prevent complications.

The capabilities of EID have increased over the years, allowing for enhanced patient safety (Weinstein and Hagle, 2014). Multifunctional EIDs or "smart pumps" have an embedded computer system with a drug library and are associated with reduced risk for infusion-related medication errors (Phillips and Gorski, 2014). The built-in software is programmed from health care pharmacy databases with unit-specific profiles (Fig. 29.3). The pump has an audible and visual alert when its setting does not match the pre-selected dose or volume limits, helping to prevent infusion errors. The use of "smart pump" with the potential reduction in serious medication errors and improved patient outcomes is becoming the standard of care across all settings (Phillips and Gorski, 2014). Know and follow your agency and manufacturer recommendations for selection and use of EIDs, alarm settings, pump controls, and features. Diligence is necessary on your part to assess and monitor patients because use of any EID or controller is not without risk of malfunction, placing a patient at risk for harm or injury.

Patients in alternative care settings (e.g., home care, long-term care) can receive infusion therapy with ambulatory pumps, which promote independence and improved quality of life. Most pumps weigh less than 2.7 kg (6 lbs) and range from palm size to fitting in a backpack. Programming capabilities range from rate adjustments, remote site adjustments, and therapy-specific settings.

Delegation and Collaboration

The skill of regulating IV flow rates cannot be delegated to nursing assistive personnel (NAP). Delegation to licensed practical nurses

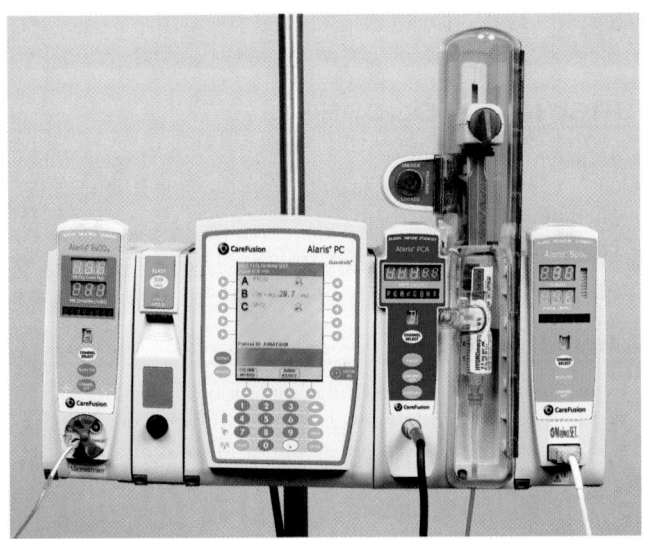

FIG 29.3 Smart pump. (*Photo courtesy Cardinal Health, Dublin, Ohio.*)

(LPNs) varies by state Nurse Practice Act. The nurse instructs the NAP to:
- Inform the nurse when the EID alarm signals.
- Inform the nurse when the fluid container is empty.
- Report any patient complaints of discomfort related to infusion such as pain, burning, bleeding, or swelling.

Equipment
- Watch with second hand
- Calculator, paper, and pencil
- Tape
- Label
- IV solution bag and appropriate administration set
- IV administration set: EID (*optional*)
- Clean gloves

STEP	RATIONALE

ASSESSMENT

1. Review accuracy and completeness of health care provider order in patient's medical record for patient name and correct solution: type, volume, additives, infusion rate, and duration of IV therapy. Follow six rights of drug administration (see Chapter 20).

   Ensures delivery of correct IV solution and prescribed volume over prescribed time.

2. Perform hand hygiene.

   Reduces transmission of microorganisms.

3. Apply clean gloves; inspect and gently palpate skin around and above IV site over dressing. Ask patient how IV site feels. Assess VAD for patency and signs and symptoms of IV-related complications (e.g., infiltration, occlusion of VAD, phlebitis, infection, patient complaints of pain, or leaking under dressing). Dispose of gloves; perform hand hygiene.

   Identifies complications that compromise integrity of VAD and may necessitate replacement of VAD. Reduces transmission of infection.

4. Assess IV system for patency from IV container to insertion site.

   Ensures delivery of prescribed volume over prescribed time.

5. Identify patient risk for fluid and electrolyte imbalance given type of IV solution (e.g., neonate, history of cardiac or renal disease).

   Helps prioritize assessments. Volume control needs to be strict. Guides choice of infusion device.

6. Assess patient's knowledge of how positioning of IV site affects flow rate.

   Fosters patient participation in maintaining most effective position of arm with IV equipment.

STEP	RATIONALE

NURSING DIAGNOSES

- Deficient fluid volume
- Deficient knowledge regarding IV therapy
- Excess fluid volume
- Risk for infection
- Risk for injury

Related factors/Risk factors are individualized based on patient's condition or needs.

PLANNING

1. Expected outcomes following completion of procedure:
   - Fluid and electrolyte levels remain within normal limits.
   - Patient receives prescribed volume of solution over prescribed time interval.
   - Patient's VAD remains patent, and site is free from signs and symptoms of IV-related complications.
   - Patient is able to explain how positioning of IV site affects rate and describe complications related to inaccurate flow rate.
2. Have paper and pencil or calculator to calculate flow rate.
3. Prepare patient and family caregiver by explaining procedure, its purpose, and what is expected of patient.
4. Check order to see how long each liter of fluid should infuse. If hourly rate (mL/h) is not provided in order, calculate it by dividing volume by hours. For example:

$$\text{mL/hr} = \frac{\text{Total infusion (mL)}}{\text{Hours of infusion}}$$

$$1000 \text{ mL/8 h} = 125 \text{ mL/h}$$

or if 3 L is ordered for 24 hours:

$$3000 \text{ mL/24 h} = 125 \text{ mL/h}$$

IV solution helps to maintain fluid and electrolyte levels. Patient achieves therapeutic outcomes.

Ensures that patient receives prescribed infusion therapy and that VAD is without complications (INS, 2016a).
Demonstrates learning (INS, 2016a).

Use mathematical calculations to obtain correct rate.
Decreases anxiety and promotes cooperation and compliance with therapy.
Basis of calculation to ensure infusion of solution over prescribed hourly rate.

Clinical Decision Point It is common for health care providers to write an abbreviated IV order such as "D$_5$W with 20 mEq KCl 125 mL/h continuous." This order implies that the IV should be maintained at this rate until an order has been written for the IV to be discontinued or changed to another order.

5. If keep vein open (KVO) rate is ordered, check agency policy regarding flow rate of KVO.

Prevents catheter clotting, thus preserving venous access while infusing a minimal amount of fluid. An order for KVO rate must specify an infusion rate as required by the rights of medication administration. Rates may vary from 0.5 mL/h to 30 mL/h based on type of VAD, patient specific therapy, and method of infusion (gravity or EID).

6. Use hourly rate to program electronic infusion device (EID) or, if gravity-flow infusion, use to calculate minute flow rate (gtt/mL),

EID automatically delivers correct minute flow rate. Gravity infusion requires calculation of gtt/mL.

7. Know calibration (drop factor), in drops per milliliter (gtt/mL), of infusion set used by agency:
   a. Microdrip: 60 gtt/mL: Used to deliver rates less than 100 mL/h.
   b. Macrodrip: 10 to 15 gtt/mL (depending on manufacturer). Used to deliver rates greater than 100 mL/h.

Microdrip tubing universally delivers 60 gtt/mL. Used when small or very precise volumes are to be infused.
There are different commercial parenteral administration sets for macrodrip tubing. Used when large volumes or fast rates are necessary. Know drip factor for tubing being used.

8. Select one of the following formulas to calculate minute flow rate (drops per minute) based on drop factor of infusion set:

Once you determine hourly rate, these formulas compute the correct flow rate.

    a. mL/h/60 min = mL/min

    Drop factor × mL/min = Drops/min

          or

    b. mL/h × Drop factor/60 min = Drops/min

STEP	RATIONALE

Calculate minute flow rate for a bag 1000 mL with 20 mEq KCl at 125 mL/h.

Microdrip:

$$125 \text{ mL/h} \times 60 \text{ gtt/mL} = 7500 \text{ gtt/h}$$

$$7500 \text{ gtt} \div 60 \text{ min} = 125 \text{ gtt/min}$$

When using microdrip, milliliters per hour (mL/h) always equals drops per minute (gtt/min).

Macrodrip:

$$125 \text{ mL/h} \times 15 \text{ gtt/mL} = 1875 \text{ gtt/h}$$

$$1875 \text{ gtt} \div 60 \text{ min} = 31 - 32 \text{ gtt/min}$$

Multiply volume by drop factor and divide product by time (in minutes).

IMPLEMENTATION

1. Identify patient using at least two identifiers (e.g., name and birthday or name and medical record number) according to agency policy. Compare identifiers with information on patient's MAR or medical record.

   Ensures correct patient. Complies with The Joint Commission standards and improves patient safety (TJC, 2016).

2. **Regulate gravity infusion.**

   a. Ensure that IV container is at least 76.2 cm (30 inches) above IV site for adults and increase height for more viscous fluids (Alexander et al., 2014).

   Pressure caused by gravity is necessary to overcome venous pressure and resistance from tubing and catheter.

   b. Slowly open roller clamp on tubing until you can see drops in drip chamber. Hold a watch with second hand at same level as drip chamber and count drip rate for 1 minute (see illustration). Adjust roller clamp to increase or decrease rate of infusion.

   Regulates flow to prescribed rate.

   c. Monitor drip rate at least hourly.

   Many factors influence drip rate; frequent monitoring ensures IV fluid administration as prescribed.

3. **Regulate EID (infusion pump or smart pump):** Follow manufacturer guidelines for setup of EID. Be sure you are using infusion tubing compatible with EID.

   Smart pumps with medication safety software are designed for administration of IV fluids that contain medications.

   a. Close roller clamp on primed IV infusion tubing.

   Prevents fluid leakage.

   b. Insert infusion tubing into chamber of control mechanism (see manufacturer directions) (see illustration). Roller clamp on IV tubing goes between EID and patient.

   Most EIDs use positive pressure to infuse. Infusion pumps propel fluid through tubing by compressing and milking IV tubing.

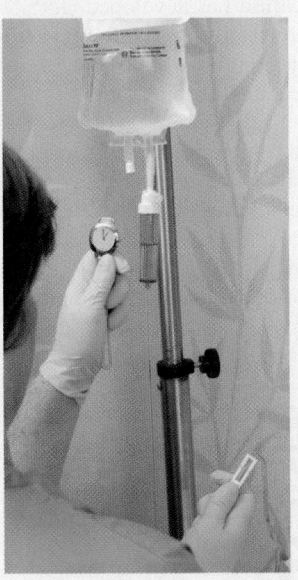

STEP 2b Nurse counting drip rate on gravity infusion.

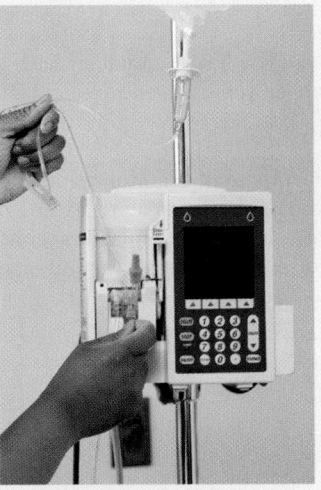

STEP 3b Insert IV tubing into chamber of control mechanism.

STEP	RATIONALE

c. Secure part of IV tubing through "air in line" alarm system. Close door (see illustration A) and turn on power button, select required drops per minute or volume per hour, close door to control chamber, and press start button (see illustration B). If infusing medication, access the EID library of medications and set appropriate rate and dose limits. If smart pump alarms immediately and shuts down, your settings were outside unit parameters.

Ensures safe administration of ordered flow rate or medication dose. Smart pumps require additional information such as patient unit and medication. Computer matches pump setting against a drug database (Harding, 2013).

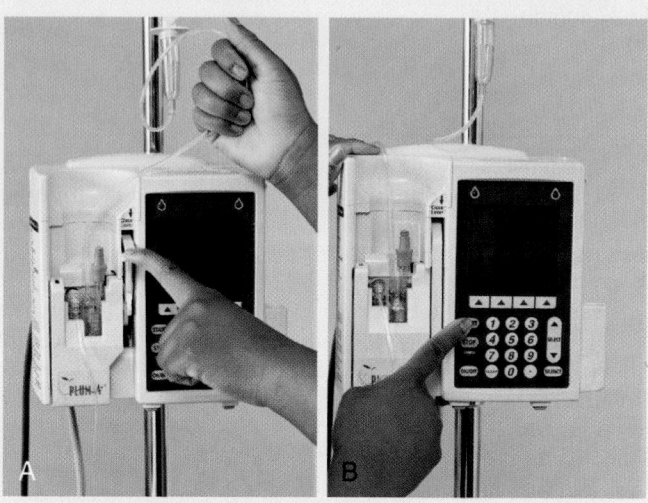

STEP 3c A, Close door of control mechanism. **B,** Select rate and volume to be infused and press start button.

Clinical Decision Point *An anti–free flow safeguard (preventing bolus infusion in the event of machine malfunction or when tubing is removed from machine) is an important element of an EID and is required. Always check and follow manufacturer recommendations for specific device features.*

d. Open infusion tubing drip regulator completely while EID is in use.

Ensures that pump freely regulates infusion rate.

e. Monitor infusion rate and IV site for complications according to agency policy. Use watch to verify rate of infusion, even when using EID.

Flow controllers and pumps do not replace frequent, accurate nursing evaluation. EIDs can continue to infuse IV solutions after a complication has developed (INS, 2016a).

f. Assess IV system from container to VAD insertion site when alarm signals.

Alarm indicates situation that requires attention. Empty solution container, tubing kinks, closed clamp, infiltration, clotted catheter, air in tubing, and/or low battery can trigger EID alarm.

4. Attach label to IV solution container with date and time container changed (check agency policy).

Provides reference to determine next time for container change, especially with keep vein open (KVO) rate that contains a specific infusion rate as ordered by health care provider.

5. Teach patient purpose of EID if infusion therapy is delivered by EID, purpose of alarms, to avoid raising hand or arm that affects flow rate, and to avoid touching control clamp.

Information allows patient to protect IV site and informs him or her about rationale for not altering control rate.

6. Remove and dispose of any used supplies; perform hand hygiene.

Prevents transmission of infection.

STEP	RATIONALE

EVALUATION

1. Observe patient every 1 to 2 hours (see agency policy), noting volume of IV fluid infused and rate of infusion.
2. Evaluate patient's response to therapy (e.g., laboratory values, input and output [I&O], weights, vital signs, postprocedure assessments).
3. Evaluate patient at established intervals per agency policy and procedure for signs and symptoms of IV-related complications.
4. **Use Teach-Back:** "I want to be sure that I explained the importance of your IV fluids running on time at the rate ordered. Tell me what you think may cause the pump to alarm and what you would do." Revise your instruction now or develop a plan for revised patient or family caregiver teaching if patient or family caregiver is not able to teach back correctly.

Ensures delivery of prescribed volume over prescribed time and decreases risk for fluid and electrolyte imbalance.

Provides ongoing evaluation of patient's fluid status, including monitoring for FVE or FVD. Early recognition of complications leads to prompt treatment.

Prevents complications that compromise integrity of VAD or cause inaccurate IV solution flow rate.

Determines patient's and family caregiver's level of understanding of instructional topic.

Unexpected Outcomes

1. Solution does not infuse at prescribed rate
   a. Sudden infusion of large volume of solution occurs; patient develops dyspnea, crackles in lung, dependent edema (edema in legs), and increased urine output, indicating FVE.

   b. IV solution runs slower than ordered.

2. IV patency is lost subsequent to IV solution container running empty.

Related Interventions

- Slow infusion rate: KVO rates must have specific rate ordered by health care provider.
- Notify health care provider immediately.
- Place patient in high-Fowler's position.
- Anticipate new IV orders.
- Anticipate administration of oxygen per order.
- Administer diuretics if ordered.
- Check for positional change that affects rate, height of IV container, kinking of tubing, or obstruction.
- Check VAD site for complications.
- Consult health care provider for new order to provide necessary fluid volume.
- Discontinue present IV infusion and restart new short-peripheral catheter in new site.

Recording and Reporting

- Record IV solution, rate of infusion in drops per minute (gtt/min) or milliliters per hour (mL/h), and integrity and patency of system in nurses' notes in electronic health record (EHR) or chart and on infusion therapy flow sheet according to agency policy.
- Record use of any EID or control device and identification number on that device.
- Record patient response (e.g., laboratory values, I&O, weights, vital signs, postprocedure assessments) to therapy and unexpected outcomes (e.g., signs and symptoms of FVE, FVD, or IV-related complications).
- Record patient's and family caregiver's level of understanding following instruction in nurses' notes in EHR or chart.
- At change of shift or when leaving on break, report rate of and volume left in infusion to nurse in charge or next nurse assigned to care for patient.

Special Considerations
Teaching

- Instruct patient to notify nurse if any signs or symptoms of IV complications are noted (e.g., redness, pain, tenderness, swelling, bleeding, drainage, or leaking from under dressing).
- Patient using an EID should know the significance of alarms and when to notify nursing.

- Teach patient about factors affecting flow rate, to protect IV site, and importance of not altering rate control.

Pediatric

- Do not use containers exceeding 150 mL in children younger than 2 years of age, exceeding 250 mL in children younger than 5 years of age, or exceeding 500 mL in children younger than 10 years of age. Always use tamper-resistant volume-controlled EIDs to ensure accurate fluid delivery (Alexander et al., 2014; Hockenberry and Wilson, 2015).

Gerontological

- Use an EID and microdrip tubing to administer IV solutions. Monitor vital signs, electrolyte levels, blood urea nitrogen (BUN), creatinine, urine output, and body weight (Alexander et al., 2014).

Home Care

- Ensure that patient is able and willing to operate an EID and administer IV therapy. If patient is unable to provide self-care, be sure that a reliable family caregiver is available in the home.
- Discuss proper EID function with patient. Consider use of an ambulatory-type device. Observe patient operating infusion EID and administering IV therapy.

- Teach patient and family caregiver what EID alarms mean, methods to troubleshoot them, and how to disconnect the IV tubing from the EID pump in the event of a pump failure.

- Ensure that patient's electrical outlets are properly grounded.
- Provide patient with a contact phone number to access 24 hours a day for problems.

◆ SKILL 29.3 **Changing Intravenous Solutions**

NSO *Nursing Skills Online Maintenance of Intravenous Fluid Therapy Module / Lesson 3*

Patients receiving intravenous (IV) therapy periodically require changes of IV solutions. IV containers include plastic bags and glass bottles. You change a container when there is an order for a new solution or when it becomes time to add a sequential container to avoid exceeding hang time (Alexander et al., 2014). It becomes clinically appropriate to change the type of solution, depending on a patient's fluid and electrolyte balance, response to therapy (e.g., therapeutic drug monitoring), and goals of therapy. The maximum hang time for routine replacement of IV containers is established by agency policy and procedure (INS, 2016a). Maximum hang time is based on factors such as the use of strict aseptic technique, whether the system remains closed without injection ports or add-on tubing, stability of the solution or medication being infused, and how long the solution in the IV container will last (Alexander et al., 2014). Organizational skills are necessary to manage changing IV containers or solutions in a manner that decreases the risk

of infusion-related complications such as an infusion container becoming empty or clotting of a vascular access device (VAD).

Delegation and Collaboration

The skill of changing an IV solution cannot be delegated to nursing assistive personnel (NAP). Delegation to licensed practical nurses (LPNs) varies by state Nurse Practice Act. The nurse instructs the NAP to:

- Inform the nurse when an IV container is near completion.
- Report any cloudiness or precipitate in the IV solution.
- Report alarm sounding on electronic infusion device (EID).
- Report any patient complaints of discomfort related to infusion such as pain, burning, bleeding, or swelling.

Equipment

- IV solution as ordered by health care provider

STEP	RATIONALE

ASSESSMENT

1. Review accuracy and completeness of health care provider's order in patient's medical record for patient name and correct solution: type, volume, additives, rate, and duration of IV therapy. Follow rights of drug administration (see Chapter 20).

Ensures delivery of correct IV solution and prescribed volume over prescribed time (INS, 2016a).

2. Note date and time when IV tubing and solution were last changed.

Ensures correct timing of tubing changes.

3. Determine patient understanding of need for continued IV therapy.

Indicates need for any patient education.

4. Perform hand hygiene and apply clean gloves; inspect and gently palpate skin around and above IV site over dressing. Assess VAD for patency and signs and symptoms of IV-related complications (e.g., infiltration, occlusion of VAD, phlebitis, infection, patient complaints of pain, or leaking under dressing).

Identifies complications that compromise integrity of VAD and necessitate replacement of VAD.

5. Check infusion system from solution container down to VAD insertion site for integrity, including but not limited to discoloration, cloudiness, leakage, expiration date. Determine compatibility of all IV solutions and additives by consulting approved online database, drug reference, or pharmacist. Discard gloves and perform hand hygiene.

If there has been a break in integrity of solution container, a new bag is needed (Alexander et al., 2014).
May indicate need for IV tubing change.
Incompatibilities cause physical, chemical, and therapeutic changes with adverse patient outcomes (Alexander et al., 2014). Reduces transmission of microorganisms.

6. Check pertinent laboratory data such as potassium level.

Compare data with baseline to determine ongoing response to IV solution administration.

NURSING DIAGNOSES

- Deficient fluid volume
- Deficient knowledge regarding IV infusion

- Risk for infection

- Risk for injury

Related factors/Risk factors are individualized based on patient's condition or needs.

STEP	RATIONALE

PLANNING

1. Expected outcomes following completion of procedure:
- IV solution is correct.
- Fluid and electrolyte levels return to normal.
- Patient's VAD remains patent, and site is free from signs and symptoms of IV-related complications.
- Patient and family caregiver can explain purpose of IV solution change.

Patient receives solution ordered for treatment of diagnosis.
IV solution helps to maintain fluid and electrolyte levels.
Ensures IV access for delivery of prescribed IV therapy (INS, 2016a).
Demonstrates learning (INS, 2016a).

2. Perform hand hygiene. Collect equipment. Have next solution prepared at least 1 hour before needed. If solution is prepared in pharmacy, ensure that it has been delivered to patient care unit. Allow solution to warm to room temperature if it has been refrigerated. Check that solution is correct and properly labeled. Check solution expiration date. Ensure that any light sensitivity restrictions are followed.

Reduces transmission of infection and contamination of equipment (INS, 2016a). Proper handling of solutions prevents IV-related complications such as occlusion. Checking that solution is correct prevents medication error.

3. Prepare patient and family caregiver by explaining procedure, its purpose, and what is expected of patient.

Decreases anxiety and promotes cooperation and compliance with therapy.

IMPLEMENTATION

1. Identify patient using at least two identifiers (e.g., name and birthday or name and medical record number) according to agency policy. Compare identifiers with information on patient's MAR or medical record.

Ensures correct patient. Complies with The Joint Commission standards and improves patient safety (TJC, 2016).

2. Change solution when fluid remains only in neck of container (about 50 mL) or when new type of solution has been ordered.

Prevents waste of solution.

3. Perform hand hygiene.

Reduces transmission of microorganisms.

4. Prepare new solution for changing. If using plastic bag, hang on IV pole and remove protective cover from IV tubing port. If using glass bottle, remove metal cap and metal and rubber disks.

Permits quick, smooth, organized change from old to new container.

5. Close roller clamp on existing solution to stop flow rate. Remove IV tubing from EID (if used). Then remove old IV solution container from IV pole. Hold container with tubing port pointing upward.

Prevents solution remaining in drip chamber from emptying while changing solutions. Prevents solution in bag from spilling.

6. Quickly remove spike from old solution container and, without touching tip, insert spike into new container (see illustrations).

Reduces risk for solution in drip chamber becoming empty and maintains sterility.

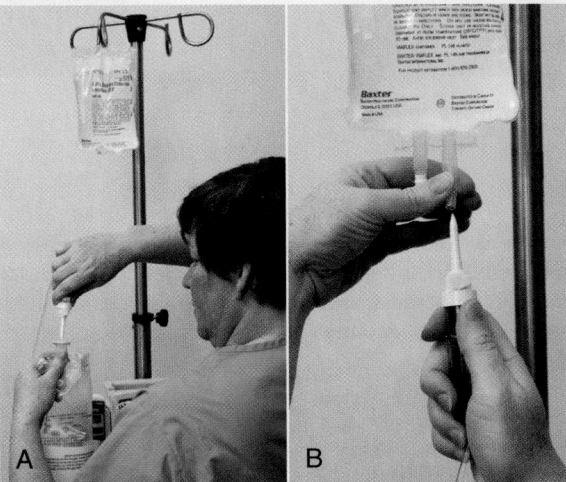

STEP 6 A, Quickly remove spike from old solution container. **B,** Without touching tip, insert spike into new container.

Clinical Decision Point *If spike becomes contaminated by touching an unsterile object, you will need a new IV tubing set.*

STEP	RATIONALE
7. Hang new container of solution on IV pole.	Gravity helps with delivery of fluid into drip chamber.
8. Check for air in IV tubing. If air bubbles have formed, remove them by closing roller clamp, stretching tubing downward, and tapping tubing with finger (bubbles rise in fluid to drip chamber) (see illustration).	Reduces risk of air entering tubing. Use of an air-eliminating filter also reduces risk.
9. Make sure that drip chamber is one-third to one-half full. If drip chamber is too full, level can be decreased by removing bag from IV pole, pinching off IV tubing below drip chamber, inverting container, squeezing drip chamber (see illustration), releasing and turning solution container upright, and releasing pinch on tubing.	Reduces risk for air entering IV tubing. If chamber is completely filled, you cannot observe or regulate drip rate.
10. Regulate flow to ordered rate by opening and adjusting roller clamp on IV tubing or by opening roller clamp and programming and turning on EID.	Maintains measures to restore fluid balance and deliver IV solution as ordered.
11. Place time label on side of container and label with time hung, time of completion, and appropriate intervals. If using plastic bags, mark only on label and not container.	Provides visual comparison of volume infused compared with prescribed rate of infusion.
12. Instruct patient on purpose of new IV solution, additives, flow rate, potential side effects, how to avoiding occluding tubing, and what to report.	Information informs patient about purpose for continued IV therapy and what to report and protects VAD patency.

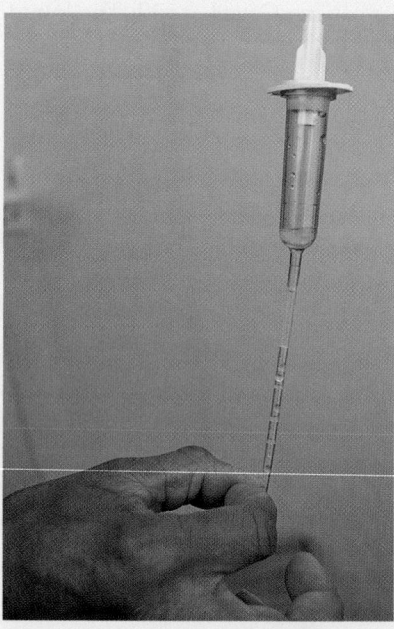

STEP 8 Tap tubing to cause air bubbles to rise up to drip chamber.

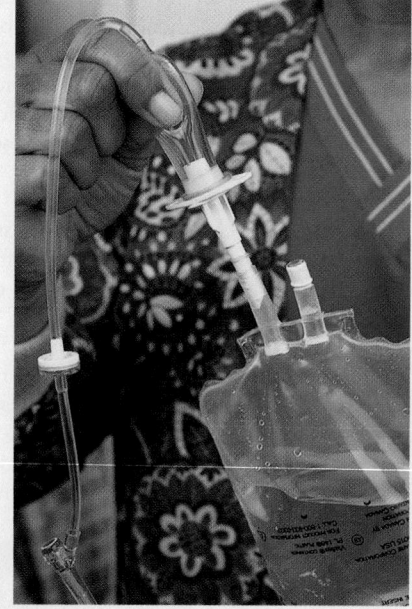

STEP 9 Squeeze drip chamber to fill with fluid. Be sure to leave chamber one-third to one-half full.

EVALUATION

1. Observe patient every 1 to 2 hours or at established intervals per agency policy and procedure for function, intactness, and patency of IV system; correct infusion rate; and type/amount of IV solution infused.	Ensures delivery of prescribed volume over prescribed time and decreases risk for fluid and electrolyte imbalance.
2. Evaluate patient to determine response to therapy (e.g., laboratory values, input and output [I&O], weights, vital signs, postprocedure assessments).	Provides ongoing evaluation of patient's fluid status.
3. Monitor patient for signs of fluid volume excess (FVE), fluid volume deficit (FVD), or signs and symptoms of electrolyte imbalances.	Early recognition of complications leads to prompt treatment.
4. Evaluate patient at established intervals per agency policy and procedure for signs and symptoms of IV-related complications.	Prevents complications that compromise integrity of VAD or cause inaccurate IV solution flow rate.

STEP	RATIONALE
5. **Use Teach-Back:** "We talked about the importance of your IV solutions running continuously. I want to be sure I explained this clearly. Tell me in your own words what you should do if you notice that the IV is not dripping." Revise your instruction now or develop a plan for revised patient or family caregiver teaching if patient or family caregiver is not able to teach back correctly.	Determines patient's and family caregiver's level of understanding of instructional topic.

Unexpected Outcomes	Related Interventions
1. Flow rate is incorrect; patient receives too little or too much solution.	• Notify health care provider if patient's anticipated infusion is 100 to 200 mL less than or greater than anticipated (per agency policy and procedure). • Evaluate patient for signs and symptoms of adverse effects of infusion (e.g., FVD or FVE). • Determine and correct cause of incorrect flow rate (e.g., change in position, tubing kink, loss of IV patency or intactness). • Use EID when accurate flow rate is critical.
2. Fluid and/or electrolyte imbalances	• Notify health care provider. • Anticipate orders for changes in IV solution or additives.

Recording and Reporting

- Record in nurse's notes or on appropriate flow sheet in electronic health record (EHR) or chart the IV solution, rate of infusion, and integrity and patency of system.
- Record use of any EID or control device and identification number on that device.
- Record in nurses' notes in EHR or chart what IV problems the patient and family caregiver know to report.
- Record patient response to therapy and unexpected outcomes (e.g., causes of flow rate inaccuracy).
- At change of shift or when leaving on break, report rate of and volume left in infusion to nurse in charge or next nurse assigned to care for patient.

Special Considerations
Teaching

- Inform patient of new solution, additives, and potential side effects, including those to report to the nurse.
- Instruct patient to notify nurse or NAP if flow rate slows or IV container is empty.

Home Care

- Ensure that patient and family caregiver are willing and able to perform an IV solution change.
- Teach patient and family caregiver how to perform an IV solution change. Observe them performing procedure.

◆ SKILL 29.4 Changing Infusion Tubing

NSO *Nursing Skills Online Maintenance of Intravenous Fluid Therapy Module / Lesson 3*

An important component of patient care is maintaining the integrity of the intravenous (IV) system through the conscientious use of infection-prevention principles. Administration sets are the primary method of delivering IV solutions to patients. In addition, patients may have add-on devices (e.g., filters, extension sets), which you connect to the primary administration set as indicated by the prescribed therapy. Secondary sets may be used as a method to administer medications in conjunction with the primary infusion (e.g., antibiotics). Depending on the solution or medication being infused and the method for administration (i.e., primary set with or without add-on device, secondary sets), adherence to infection-prevention principles must be followed to ensure positive patient outcomes. Luer-Lok connections should be used to prevent accidental tubing disconnection (INS, 2016a). When a short peripheral IV site is rotated to a different site or a central vascular access device (CVAD) is placed, the administration set should be changed (INS, 2016a). Follow agency policy and procedures for specific requirements (Table 29.6).

Administration sets used for parenteral nutrition (see Chapter 33) and blood or blood products (see Chapter 30) have specific criteria with which you need to be familiar when administering these advanced therapies (see agency policy). Whenever possible, schedule IV tubing changes when it is time to hang a new IV container (see Skill 29.3). To prevent entry of bacteria into the bloodstream, maintain sterility during tubing and solution changes. If the tubing and/or IV bag becomes damaged, is leaking, or becomes contaminated, it must be changed, regardless of the tubing change schedule.

Delegation and Collaboration

The skill of changing IV tubing cannot be delegated to nursing assistive personnel (NAP). Delegation to licensed practical nurses (LPNs) varies by state Nurse Practice Act. The nurse instructs the NAP to:

- Report to the nurse any leakage from or around the IV tubing.
- Report if tubing has become contaminated (lying on the floor).

Equipment

- Clean gloves
- Antiseptic swabs (chlorhexidine gluconate [CHG] solution preferred, povidone-iodine, or 70% alcohol)
- Label

Continuous IV Infusion
- Microdrip or macrodrip administration set of IV tubing as appropriate
- Add-on device as necessary (e.g., filters, extension set, needleless connector)
- Tubing label

Intermittent Extension Set
- 3- to 5-mL syringe filled with preservative-free 0.9% sodium chloride (normal saline [NS])
- Short extension tubing (if necessary), injection cap

STEP	RATIONALE

ASSESSMENT

1. Note date and time when IV tubing was last changed (see Table 29.6 for recommendations on administration set changes).	Decreases risk of infection.
2. Perform hand hygiene. Assess IV tubing for puncture, contamination, or occlusion that requires immediate change.	Compromised tubing results in fluid leakage and bacterial contamination.
3. Determine patient understanding of need for continued IV therapy.	Reinforces need for further instruction.

NURSING DIAGNOSES

- Deficient knowledge regarding IV therapy
- Risk for infection

Related factors/Risk factors are individualized based on patient's condition or needs.

PLANNING

1. Expected outcomes following completion of procedure:	
• Patient experiences no leakage of solution from or around IV tubing.	Intact system decreases risk for microbial contamination.
• Patient's IV tubing is patent, and patient receives prescribed IV therapy as ordered.	Brief interruption of IV infusion does not result in occlusion of vascular access device (VAD).
• Patient's VAD remains patent, and site is free from signs and symptoms of IV-related complications.	Adherence to administration set changes decreases risk of complications.
• Patient and family caregiver can explain purpose of tubing change and how patient can avoid occluding tubing.	Demonstrates learning.
2. Prepare patient by explaining procedure, its purpose, and what is expected of him or her.	Decreases anxiety, promotes cooperation, and prevents sudden movement of extremity, which could dislodge IV catheter.
3. Coordinate IV tubing changes with solution changes when possible.	Decreases number of times system is open.
4. Collect equipment.	Provides easy access to equipment for efficient procedure.

TABLE 29.6		
Intravenous Administration Set Changes		
Primary and Secondary Continuous Infusions	**Primary Intermittent Infusions**	**Use of Add-on Devices**
• Change no more frequently than every 96 hours for solutions *other* than lipid, blood, or blood products.	• Should be changed every 24 hours because of increased risk of infection with repeatedly disconnecting and reconnecting administration set.	• Should be minimized because each is a potential source of contamination and disconnection.
• In addition to routine changes, change the administration set whenever the short-peripheral IV site is changed or a new CVAD is placed.	• Aseptically attach a new, sterile covering device to the Luer end of the administration set after each intermittent use. *Avoid* attaching the exposed end of the administration set to port on the same set (e.g., looping).	• Use of administration sets with devices as part of the set is preferred.
• If the secondary set is removed from the primary set, the secondary set is now an intermittent set and should be changed every 24 hours.		• Aseptically change with insertion of new VAD or with each administration set replacement.
		• Change if the integrity of the product is compromised or suspected of being compromised.

CVAD, Central vascular access device; *IV,* intravenous; *VAD,* vascular access device.
Modified from Infusion Nurses Society (INS): *Policy and procedures for infusion therapy,* ed 5, Norwood, MA, 2016, INS.

STEP	RATIONALE

IMPLEMENTATION

1. Identify patient using at least two identifiers (e.g., name and birthday or name and medical record number) according to agency policy. Compare identifiers with information on patient's MAR or medical record.

   Ensures correct patient. Complies with The Joint Commission standards and improves patient safety (TJC, 2016).

2. Perform hand hygiene. Open new infusion set and connect add-on pieces (e.g., filters, extension tubing) using aseptic technique. Keep protective coverings over infusion spike and distal adapter. Place roller clamp about 2–2.5 cm (1–2 inches) below drip chamber and move roller clamp to "off" position. Secure all connections.

   Close proximity of roller clamp to drip chamber allows more accurate regulation of flow rate. Securing connections reduces risk later of air emboli and infection. Protective covers reduce entrance of microorganisms. All connections should be of Luer-Lok type (INS, 2016a).

3. Apply clean gloves. If patient's IV cannula hub is not visible, remove IV dressing (see Skill 29.5). Do not remove tape securing cannula to skin.

   Cannula hub must be visible to provide smooth transition when removing old and inserting new tubing.

4. Prepare IV tubing with new IV container. (See Skill 29.1, Step 8.)

5. Prepare IV tubing with existing continuous IV infusion bag.
   a. Move roller clamp on new IV tubing to "off" position.

      Prevents fluid spillage.

   b. Slow rate of infusion through old tubing to keep vein open (KVO) rate using EID or roller clamp.

      Prevents occlusion of VAD.

   c. Compress and fill drip chamber of old tubing.

      Ensures that drip chamber remains full until new tubing is changed.

   d. Invert container and remove old tubing. Keep spike sterile and upright.

      Solution in drip chamber will continue to run and maintain catheter patency.

   e. Insert spike of new infusion tubing into solution container. Hang solution bag on IV pole, compress drip chamber on new tubing, and release, allowing it to fill one-third to one-half full.

      Permits drip chamber to fill and promotes rapid, smooth flow of solution through tubing.

   f. Prime air out of IV tubing by filling with IV solution: Remove protective cover on end of tubing and slowly open roller clamp to allow solution to flow from drip chamber to distal end of IV tubing. If tubing has Y connector, invert Y connector when solution reaches it to displace air. Return roller clamp to "off" position after priming tubing (filled with IV solution). Replace protective cover on end of IV tubing. Place end of adapter near patient's IV site.

      Priming ensures that IV tubing is clear of air before connection with VAD and filled with IV solution. Slow fill of tubing decreases turbulence and chance of bubble formation. Closing clamp prevents accidental loss of fluid.
      Maintains sterility. Equipment is positioned for quick connection of new tubing.

   g. Stop EID or turn roller clamp on old tubing to "off" position.

      Prevents fluid spillage.

6. Prepare tubing with extension set or saline lock.
   a. If short extension tubing is needed, use sterile technique to connect new injection cap to new extension set or IV tubing.

      Prepares extension set for connecting with IV.

   b. Scrub injection cap with antiseptic swab for at least 15 seconds and allow to dry completely. Attach syringe with 3 to 5 mL of NS flush solution and inject through injection cap into extension set.

      Ensures effective disinfection (Phillips and Gorski, 2014). Maintains patency of catheter.

7. Reestablish infusion.
   a. Gently disconnect old tubing from extension tubing (or from IV catheter hub) and quickly insert Luer-Lok end of new tubing or saline lock into extension tubing connection (or IV catheter hub) (see illustrations for example of connecting tubing to short extension set).

      Allows smooth transition from old to new tubing, minimizing time system is open.

   b. For continuous infusion, open roller clamp on new tubing and regulate drip rate using roller clamp or insert tubing into EID, program to desired rate, and push on.

      Ensures catheter patency and prevents occlusion.

   c. Attach piece of tape or preprinted label with date and time of IV tubing change onto tubing below drip chamber.

      Provides reference to determine next time for tubing change.

   d. Form loop of tubing and secure it to patient's arm with strip of tape.

      Avoids accidental pulling against site and stabilizes catheter.

STEP	RATIONALE

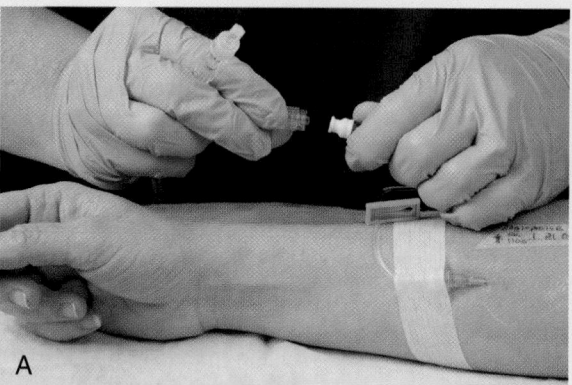

STEP 7a A, Disconnect old tubing. **B,** Insert adapter of new tubing.

8. Remove and discard old IV tubing. If necessary, apply new dressing (see Skill 29.5). Remove and dispose of gloves. Perform hand hygiene.	Reduces transmission of microorganisms.
9. Teach patient how to move and turn properly with IV tubing.	Prevents accidental occlusion or disconnection and contamination of IV tubing.

EVALUATION

1. Observe patient every 1 to 2 hours or at established intervals per agency policy and procedure for function, intactness, and patency of IV system and leaking at connection sites.	Ensures that IV system is functioning appropriately and minimizes risk of infection caused by breach in system integrity.
2. Evaluate patient at established intervals per agency policy and procedure for signs and symptoms of IV-related complications.	Prevents complications that compromise integrity of VAD or cause inaccurate IV solution flow rate.
3. **Use Teach-Back:** "Let's go over what we talked about earlier regarding the problems that can occur with your IV line. Tell me how you can prevent the tubing from being pinched off and which signs and symptoms you would report to me or another nurse." Revise your instruction now or develop a plan for revised patient or family caregiver teaching if patient or family caregiver is not able to teach back correctly.	Determines patient's and family caregiver's level of understanding of instructional topic.

Unexpected Outcomes
1. IV solution infuses more slowly than ordered.

Related Interventions
- Check for positional change that affects rate, height of IV container, kinking of tubing, or obstruction.
- Check for patency by opening roller clamp.
- Check VAD site for complications.
- Consult health care provider for new order to provide necessary fluid volume.

Recording and Reporting

- Record tubing change, type of solution, volume, and rate of infusion in nurses' notes in electronic health record (EHR) or chart. Use a special IV therapy flow sheet for parenteral solutions per agency policy.
- Record in nurses' notes in EHR or chart what IV problems the patient and family caregiver know to report.

Special Considerations
Teaching

- Instruct patient to notify nurse if fluid leaks from or around IV site or tubing or if tubing separates from catheter.

Home Care

- Ensure that patient is able and willing to perform IV tubing change and maintain IV access site or that there is a reliable person at home to provide this IV therapy care.
- Instruct patient or family caregiver in procedure for performing a sterile tubing change. Observe them performing procedure.

✦ SKILL 29.5 Changing a Short-Peripheral Intravenous Dressing

NSO *Nursing Skills Online Maintenance of Intravenous Fluid Therapy Module / Lesson 4*

Administration of solutions via the parenteral route is not without complications, which can be either systemic or local (Alexander et al., 2014). Systemic complications occur within the vascular system and are usually remote to the infusion site (e.g., septicemia, circulatory overload, and embolism). Local complications result from trauma to the inner layer of the vein (tunica intima) as a direct result of many factors such as poor insertion technique, inappropriate size of short-peripheral device (see Table 29.3), inadequate catheter stabilization, infusing a solution or medication with a pH or osmolarity not within suggested ranges (see Table 29.2), and poor assessment and incorrect technique for short-peripheral dressing changes (Alexander et al., 2014).

Short-peripheral intravenous (IV) catheters require strict adherence to infection-prevention measures to avoid complications associated with these devices. The skin insertion site is the most common source of colonization and catheter-related infections (Alexander et al., 2014). Short peripheral catheter transparent semipermeable membrane (TSM) dressing changes should be performed every 5 to 7 days, and gauze dressings every 2 days (INS, 2016a). If a gauze dressing is underneath a TSM, it should be changed every 2 days (INS, 2016a). Apply IV catheter dressings securely and change dressings immediately when wet, soiled, or loosened or if the integrity is compromised (INS, 2016b). Stabilization of short-peripheral catheters decreases risk of catheter-related complications and premature loss of access. Preferred options for stabilization include an adhesive engineered stabilization device used with a standard short-peripheral IV catheter or an integrated feature on the IV catheter with use of a bordered polyurethane dressing (INS, 2016a). Although sterile tape or surgical strips can be used, they are not as effective as an engineered stabilization device (Alexander et al., 2014; INS, 2016a).

Delegation and Collaboration

The skill of changing a short-peripheral IV dressing cannot be delegated to nursing assistive personnel (NAP). The nurse instructs the NAP to:

- Report to the nurse if a patient complains of moistness or loosening of an IV dressing.
- Protect the IV dressing during hygiene and activities of daily living (ADLs).

Equipment

- Antiseptic swabs (chlorhexidine gluconate [CHG]) solution preferred, povidone-iodine, or 70% alcohol)
- Adhesive remover (*optional*)
- Skin protectant swab
- Clean gloves
- Engineered stabilization device or precut strips sterile tape
- Commercially available IV site protection device (*optional*) (see Fig. 29.2)
- Sterile transparent semipermeable membrane (TSM) dressing

or

- Sterile 2 × 2– or 4 × 4–inch gauze pad

STEP	RATIONALE

ASSESSMENT

1. Determine when dressing was last changed. Dressing should be labeled to include date and time applied, size and type of vascular access device (VAD) insertion date.

2. Perform hand hygiene and apply clean gloves. Observe present dressing for moisture and intactness. Determine if moisture is from site leakage or external source.

3. Inspect and gently palpate skin around and above IV site over dressing. Assess VAD for patency and signs and symptoms of IV-related complications (e.g., infiltration, occlusion of VAD, phlebitis, infection, patient complaints of pain, or leaking under dressing). Remove and discard gloves.

4. Assess patient's understanding of need for continued IV infusion.

Rationale column:

Provides information regarding length of time that present dressing has been in place and allows planning for dressing change.

Nonadhering dressing increases risk for insertion site infection or dislodgement of VAD.

Identifies complications that compromise integrity of VAD and may necessitate its replacement.

Reveals need for patient instruction.

NURSING DIAGNOSES

- Acute pain
- Deficient knowledge regarding IV therapy
- Risk for infection

Related factors/Risk factors are individualized based on patient's condition or needs.

PLANNING

1. Expected outcomes following completion of procedure:
   - Patient's VAD remains patent, and site is free from signs and symptoms of IV-related complications.
   - Patient and family caregiver can explain procedure and purpose of VAD dressing change.

Rationale column:

Proper care maintains IV site.

Demonstrates learning.

STEP	RATIONALE

2. Explain procedure and purpose to patient and family caregiver. Explain that patient will need to hold affected extremity still. Explain how long procedure will take.

Decreases anxiety, promotes cooperation, and gives patient time frame around which to plan personal activities.

3. Perform hand hygiene. Collect equipment and organize on clean, clutter-free bedside stand or overbed table. Apply clean gloves.

Reduces transmission of infection and contamination of equipment (INS, 2016a).

IMPLEMENTATION

1. Identify patient using at least two identifiers (e.g., name and birthday or name and medical record number) according to agency policy. Compare identifiers with information on patient's MAR or medical record.

Ensures correct patient. Complies with The Joint Commission standards and improves patient safety (TJC, 2016).

2. Remove existing dressing:

Technique minimizes discomfort during removal. Use alcohol swab on TSM dressing next to patient's skin to loosen dressing.

   a. *For TSM dressing:* Stabilize catheter with nondominant hand (see illustration). Remove dressing by pulling up one corner and gently pulling straight out and parallel to skin. Repeat on all sides until dressing has been removed.

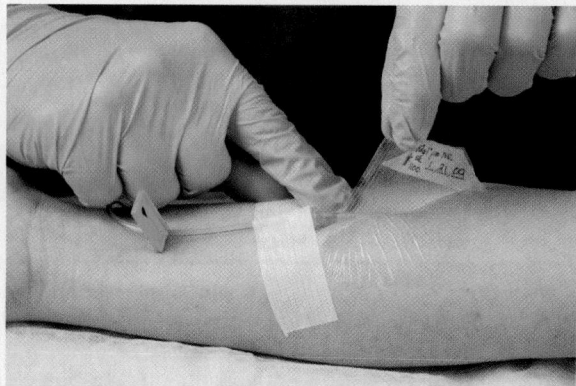

STEP 2a Remove transparent semipermeable membrane (TSM) dressing by pulling side laterally.

   b. *For gauze dressing:* Stabilize catheter hub while loosening tape and removing old dressing one layer at a time by pulling toward insertion site. Be cautious if tubing becomes tangled between two layers of dressing.

3. Assess VAD insertion site for signs and symptoms of IV-related complications. If complication exists, determine if VAD requires removal. Remove catheter if ordered by health care provider (see Procedural Guideline 29.1).

Presence of complication may necessitate VAD removal.

4. If catheter is to remain in place, assess integrity of engineered stabilization device. Continue to stabilize catheter and remove as recommended by manufacturer directions for use. Inspect for signs of adhesive-related skin injury from adhesive-based engineered stabilization devices.

Removing stabilization device allows for appropriate skin antisepsis before applying dressing and new stabilization device (INS, 2016a).

Stabilization prevents accidental dislodgement of VAD.

   NOTE: Some stabilization devices are designed to remain in place for length of time VAD is in as long as adequate stabilization is evident.

STEP	RATIONALE

Clinical Decision Point *Keep one finger over catheter at all times until dressing secures catheter hub. If patient is restless or uncooperative, it is helpful to have another staff member help with procedure.*

STEP	RATIONALE
5. While stabilizing IV line, perform skin antisepsis to insertion site with CHG solution using friction in back-and-forth motion for 30 seconds and allow to dry completely. If using alcohol or povidone-iodine, clean in concentric circle, moving from insertion site outward with the swab. Allow antiseptic solution to dry completely.	Reduces incidence of catheter-related infections (Alexander, et al., 2014). Allow any skin antiseptic agent to fully dry for complete antisepsis (INS, 2016a).
6. *Optional:* Apply skin protectant to area where you will apply tape, dressing, or engineered stabilization device. Allow to dry.	Coats skin with protective solution to maintain skin integrity, prevents irritation from adhesive, and promotes adhesion of dressing.
7. While stabilizing catheter, apply sterile dressing over site (procedures differ; follow agency policy).	
a. *TSM dressing:* Apply TSM dressing as directed in Skill 29.1, Step 24a.	Protects catheter insertion site and minimizes risk for infection (Phillips and Gorski, 2014). TSM dressing allows visualization of insertion site and surrounding area for complications (INS, 2016a).
b. *Sterile gauze dressing:* Apply sterile gauze dressing as directed in Skill 29.1, Step 24b.	Only use sterile tape under sterile dressing to prevent site contamination.
	Gauze dressing obscures observation of insertion site and is changed every 2 days (INS, 2016a).
8. **Option.** *Secure with new engineered catheter stabilization device:* Apply device as directed in Skill 29.1, Step 25.	Use of engineered stabilization devices can reduce risk for VAD complications (i.e., phlebitis, infection, migration) and unintentional loss of access (INS, 2016a).

Clinical Decision Point *Because Band-Aids are not occlusive and nonsterile tape increases the risk for insertion site infection, do not use either over catheter insertion points.*

STEP	RATIONALE
9. Remove and discard gloves and used equipment. Perform hand hygiene.	Prevents transmission of microorganisms.
10. *Optional:* Apply site protection device (e.g., I.V. House Ultra Protective Dressing®).	Reduces risk of VAD dislodgement (INS, 2016a).
11. Anchor extension tubing or IV tubing alongside dressing on arm and secure with tape directly over tubing. When using TSM dressing, avoid placing tape over dressing.	Prevents accidental dislodgement of VAD tubing.
12. Label dressing per agency policy. Information on label includes date and time of IV insertion, VAD gauge size and length, and your initials.	Communicates type of device and time interval for dressing change and site rotation.
13. Perform hand hygiene.	Reduces transmission of microorganisms.

EVALUATION

1. Evaluate function, patency of IV system, and flow rate after changing dressing.	Validates that IV line is patent and functioning correctly. Manipulation of catheter and tubing will affect rate of infusion.
2. Evaluate patient at established intervals per agency policy and procedure for signs and symptoms of IV line–related complications.	Identifies complications that compromise integrity of VAD or cause inaccurate IV solution flow rate.
3. **Use Teach-Back:** "I want to be sure that I explained reasons for why we change the IV dressing. Tell me in your own words the problems that you would report that would require us to change the dressing." Revise your instruction now or develop a plan for revised patient or family caregiver teaching if patient or family caregiver is not able to teach back correctly.	Determines patient's and family caregiver's level of understanding of instructional topic.

STEP	RATIONALE

Unexpected Outcomes

1. IV catheter is removed or dislodged accidentally.

2. IV solution is not infusing or runs more slowly than ordered.

Related Interventions

- Restart new short-peripheral IV line in other extremity or above previous insertion site if continued therapy is necessary.
- Check IV catheter for bending, kinking, or dislodgement because catheter may require replacement.
- Check for positional IV site and reposition catheter, applying new dressing if necessary.
- Check and adjust height of IV container and for kinking or obstruction of IV tubing.

Recording and Reporting

- Record in nurse's notes in electronic health record (EHR) or chart the time short-peripheral dressing was changed, reason for change, type of dressing material used, patency of system, and description of VAD site.
- Record in nurses' notes in EHR or chart what IV problems the patient and family caregiver know to report.
- Report to nurse in charge or oncoming nursing shift that dressing was changed and any significant information about integrity of system.
- Report to health care provider and document any complications, interventions, and response to treatment.

Special Considerations
Teaching

- Instruct patient to notify nurse if the dressing is wet, soiled, or loosened.

Pediatric

- Pediatric patients are not always able to understand explanations fully. Presence of parent or security toy during procedure helps to decrease fear and increase cooperation. Perform procedure on patient's toy or doll first.
- Help is necessary to keep patient still and protect IV catheter from dislodgement.
- Use commercially available IV site protectors to cover and protect the IV site in young active children.

- Use CHG with care in premature infants and those under 2 months of age due to the risks of skin irritation and chemical burns (INS, 2016a).
- Dried povidone-iodine should be removed with sodium chloride or sterile water for neonates with compromised skin integrity (INS, 2016b).

Gerontological

- Some older adults have fragile skin; therefore prevent skin tears by minimizing the use of tape or an engineered stabilization device directly on the skin and applying skin protectant before applying tape.
- Infiltration may go unnoticed because of the decreased elasticity of skin and loose skinfolds. Because of decreased tactile sensation, a large amount of fluid may infiltrate before pain occurs.

Home Care

- Instruct patient and family caregiver about the signs and symptoms of IV-related complications.
- Have patient or family caregiver demonstrate hand hygiene.
- Teach patient to protect IV site during bath or shower by wrapping in plastic bag and taping occlusively to keep dry.
- Teach patient and family caregiver what to do if dressing becomes compromised or if catheter comes out. If catheter comes out, apply gauze pressure dressing at site and notify home health agency nurse.

PROCEDURAL GUIDELINE 29.1 *Discontinuing a Short-Peripheral Intravenous Device*

NSO *Nursing Skills Online Intravenous Fluid Therapy Module / Lesson 4*

A short-peripheral intravenous (IV) catheter is discontinued when the prescribed length of therapy is completed or a complication occurs (e.g., phlebitis, infiltration, or catheter occlusion). The technique for discontinuing a short-peripheral IV catheter follows infection-prevention guidelines to minimize the chance of the patient acquiring an infection. Care must also be taken because the risk of catheter emboli may occur if the catheter breaks off during removal.

Delegation and Collaboration

The skill of discontinuing a short-peripheral intravenous line cannot be delegated to nursing assistive personnel (NAP). Delegation to licensed practical nurses (LPNs) varies by state Nurse Practice Act. The nurse instructs the NAP to:

- Report to the nurse any bleeding at the site after catheter has been removed.

- Report any complaints of pain or observation of redness at the site by the patient.

Equipment

- Clean gloves
- Sterile 2 × 2–inch or 4 × 4–inch gauze sponge
- Antiseptic swabs (chlorhexidine gluconate [CHG] solution preferred, povidone-iodine, or 70% alcohol)
- Tape

Procedural Steps

1. Review accuracy and completeness of health care provider's order for discontinuation of vascular access device (VAD).
2. Perform hand hygiene and collect equipment.

PROCEDURAL GUIDELINE 29.1 *Discontinuing a Short-Peripheral Intravenous Device—cont'd*

3. Identify patient using at least two identifiers (e.g., name and birthday or name and medical record number) according to agency policy. Compare identifiers with information on patient's MAR or medical record.
4. Apply clean gloves. Observe existing IV site for signs and symptoms of IV-related complications (redness, pain, tenderness, swelling, bleeding, drainage, or leaking from under dressing). Palpate catheter site through intact dressing.
5. Assess if patient is receiving an anticoagulant or has a history of a coagulopathy.
6. Assess patient's understanding of the reason for IV infusion to be discontinued.
7. Explain procedure to patient before you remove catheter. Explain that patient needs to hold affected extremity still.
8. Turn IV tubing roller clamp to "off" position or turn electronic infusion device (EID) off and roller clamp to "off" position.
9. Carefully remove VAD dressing and engineered stabilization device.
10. Stabilize IV catheter hub with middle finger of nondominant hand.

Clinical Decision Point *Never use scissors to remove the tape or dressing because you may accidentally cut the catheter.*

11. Place clean sterile gauze above insertion site and, using dominant hand, withdraw catheter using a slow, steady

motion and keeping the hub parallel to skin (see illustration).

Clinical Decision Point *Do not raise or lift catheter before it is completely out of the vein to avoid trauma or hematoma formation.*

12. Apply pressure to site for a minimum of 30 seconds until bleeding has stopped.
    NOTE: Apply pressure for at least 5 to 10 minutes if patient is on anticoagulants.
13. Inspect catheter for intactness after removal; note tip integrity and length.
14. Observe IV site for evidence of any complications such as redness, pain, tenderness, swelling, bleeding, or drainage. Monitor for 24 to 48 hours after removal for postinfusion phlebitis.
15. Apply clean, folded gauze dressing over insertion site and secure with tape.
16. Discard used supplies, remove gloves, and perform hand hygiene.
17. Document procedure in patient's medical record in EHR or chart.
18. **Use Teach-Back:** "I want to be sure that I explained to you why we are taking your IV out. In your own words tell me why we are removing the IV." Revise your instruction now or develop a plan for revised patient teaching if patient is not able to teach back correctly.

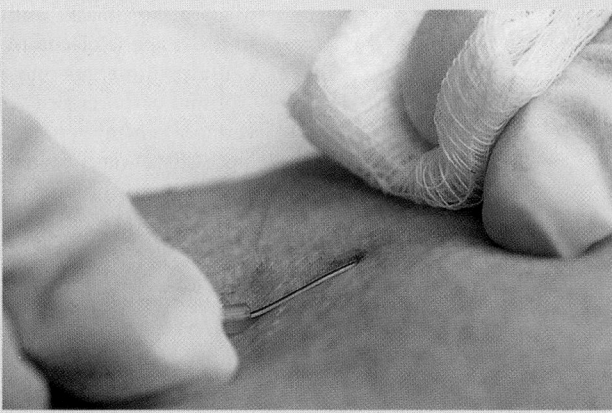

STEP 11 IV catheter is removed slowly, keeping catheter parallel to vein.

◆ SKILL 29.6   Managing Central Vascular Access Devices

The need for safe and convenient intravenous (IV) therapy has led to the development of vascular access devices (VADs) designed for long-term access to the venous or arterial systems. Physicians or competently trained nurses place these devices into the central vascular system. A central vascular access device (CVAD) differs from short-peripheral or midline catheters in that the farthest tip of the catheter ends in a larger blood vessel. The tip of a CVAD should be placed in the upper body in the lower segment of the superior or inferior vena cava at or near the cavoatrial junction (Fig. 29.4). Those placed in the lower body should end in the

inferior vena cava above the level of the diaphragm (INS, 2016a). CVADs placed in the femoral region are not recommended in adults (Ciocson et al., 2014).

Factors considered when determining placement of a CVAD include type and duration of infusion therapy (greater than 7 days), vascular characteristics, patient's age, co-morbidities, history of infusion therapy, and preference for VAD location (INS, 2016a). Also considered are the pH and osmolarity of the solution or medication to be administered. Your role is to anticipate a patient's need for a CVAD, assist the health care provider in placing a

CVAD, care for and maintain the device, administer solutions or medications, and assess for signs and symptoms of IV-related complications (Alexander et al., 2014).

Try to remain aware of the similarities and differences of each device (Table 29.7). Characteristics of the devices and the type of patient education affect care and maintenance of each CVAD. These devices are composed of silicone or polyurethane and can be coated with antibiotics, silver, minocycline/rifampin, or chlorhexidine (Phillips and Gorski, 2014).

Catheter tip configuration can be either open-ended or valve ended. Open-ended devices (e.g., Hickman, Broviac) have a catheter tip that is open like a "straw." Valve-ended catheters (e.g., Groshong) have a rounded catheter tip with a three-way pressure-activated valve that prevents reflux of blood into the catheter to reduce the risk of hemorrhage, air embolism, and occlusion. This technology can also be located in the catheter hub (e.g., PASV, SOLO2). Manufacturers of valved catheters state that heparin is not needed to maintain patency and recommend flushing with only 0.9% sodium chloride (normal saline [NS]) (Phillips and Gorski, 2014).

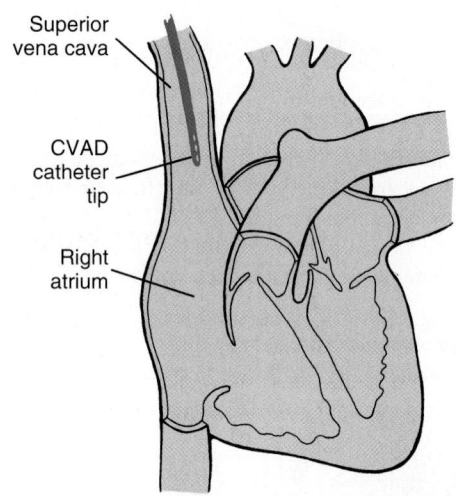

FIG 29.4 Catheter tip from CVAD lies in superior vena cava. *CVAD,* Central vascular access device.

CVADs have single or multiple lumens. The choice of the number of lumens depends on a patient's condition and prescribed therapy. Patients requiring numerous infusions and blood samplings may have a device placed with more than one lumen, allowing simultaneous administration of solutions and medications. In addition, multiple lumens allow for administration of incompatible solutions or medications at the same time. You access a CVAD through the hub of the device located on the end of each external lumen.

An implanted venous port is a CVAD that has a reservoir placed in a pocket under the skin with the catheter inserted into a major vessel (e.g., subclavian). The CVAD has no external lumen or hub. Instead you access an implanted venous port by inserting a special 90-degree angle noncoring needle through the skin into the self-sealing injection port in the septum of the reservoir. A port may not be used for extended periods (i.e., weeks) between infusions, and it is not necessary that the port remain accessed during these periods. To maintain the patency of a port, it is necessary to flush monthly with heparin solution or 0.9% sodium chloride in accordance with agency policies and procedures and manufacturer directions for use (INS, 2016a).

Complications associated with CVADs can include local or systemic infection. A local infection can develop around the catheter insertion site. A more serious infection of the bloodstream may be caused by contamination of the catheter from the skin of the patient or poor infection-prevention practices during insertion, care, and maintenance (Alexander et al., 2014). The implementation of the Institute for Healthcare Improvement (IHI) Central Line Bundle prevents infection. The key components of the IHI Central Line Bundle are:

- Hand hygiene before catheter insertion.
- Maximal sterile barrier precautions with insertion. (Inserter wears a cap, mask, and sterile gloves and gown; and a large sterile drape is placed over patient during insertion.)
- Chlorhexidine gluconate (CHG) skin antisepsis.
- Optimal catheter site selection, with avoidance of the femoral vein for central venous access in adult patients.
- Necessity of daily review of the condition of the line and insertion site with prompt removal of unnecessary lines.

Care of CVADs requires knowledge of the purpose and function of the devices and prevention of complications. Patients with

TABLE 29.7	
Central Vascular Access Devices	
Short-Term Devices	**Long-Term Devices**
Nontunneled Percutaneous	**External Tunneled (Hickman, Broviac, Groshong)**
• Length of dwell: Days to several weeks	• Length of dwell: Considered permanent
• Insertion sites: Subclavian, external/internal jugular, and femoral veins	• Insertion sites: Chest region through subclavian or jugular vein
• Insertion technique: Not surgically placed; can be done at bedside; direct puncture into intended vein without passing through subcutaneous tissue	• Insertion technique: Surgery required; tunneling of proximal end subcutaneously from insertion site and bringing it out through skin at an exit site (Fig. 29.6)
• Held in place with sutures or engineered securement device	• Held in place by a Dacron cuff coated in antimicrobial solution; in approximately 2–3 weeks scar tissue forms around cuff, fixing catheter in place
Peripherally Inserted Central Catheters (PICCs) (Fig. 29.5)	**Implanted Venous Ports**
• Length of dwell: As long as they function properly with no evidence of intravenous (IV)-related complications	• Length of dwell: Considered permanent
• Insertion sites: Antecubital fossa or upper arm (basilic or cephalic vein) and advanced until catheter tip reaches superior vena cava (SVC)	• Insertion sites: Chest, abdomen, or inner aspect of forearm
• Insertion technique: Not surgically placed; can be done at bedside, in home setting, or in radiology setting	• Insertion techniques: Requires surgery; catheter placed via subclavian or jugular vein and attached to reservoir located within a surgically created subcutaneous pocket (Fig. 29.7)
• Held in place with sutures or engineered securement device	• Sutured in place within surgically created pocket and accessed using a noncoring needle through the skin (Fig. 29.8)

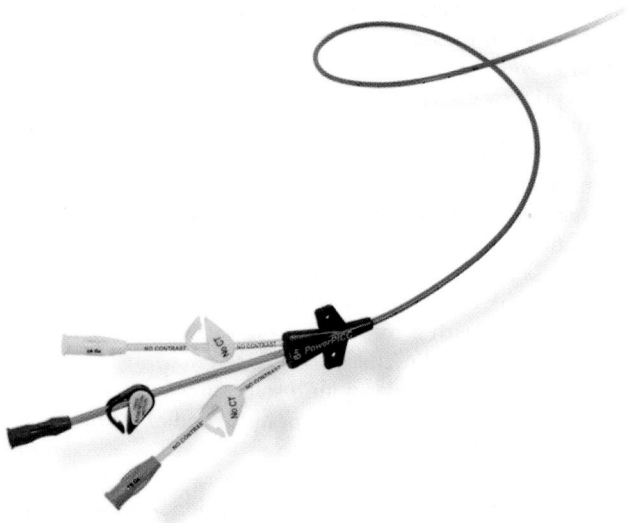

FIG 29.5 Peripherally inserted central catheter (PICC). (*Courtesy and copyright ©Bard Access Systems.*)

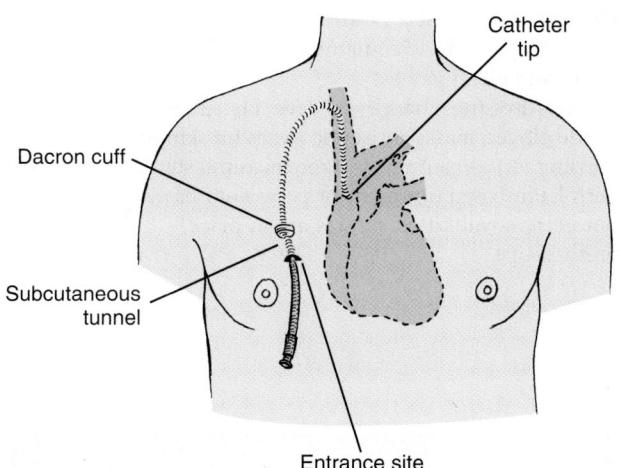

FIG 29.6 Tunneled catheter is in place, threaded into superior vena cava.

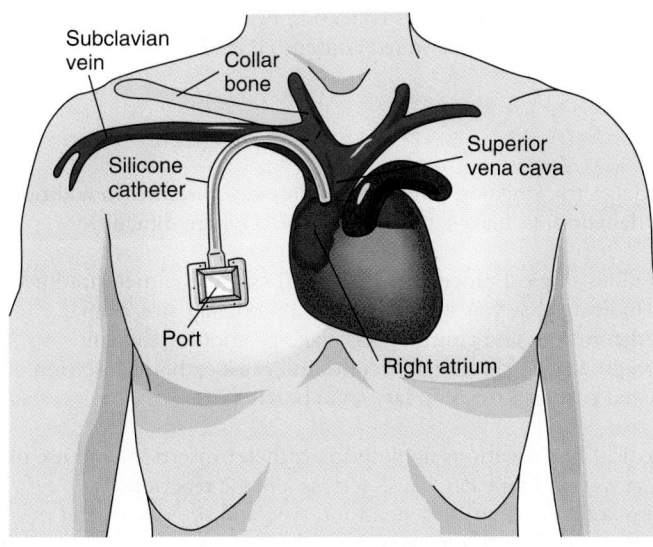

FIG 29.7 Implanted port and catheter.

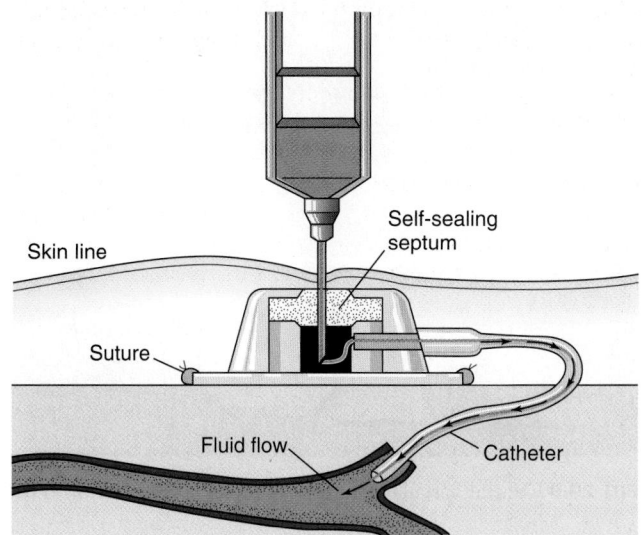

FIG 29.8 Cross-section of implanted port showing access of port with noncoring needle.

CVADs require health education and teaching about infection-prevention practices and skin care.

Delegation and Collaboration

The skill of managing a CVAD cannot be delegated to nursing assistive personnel (NAP). The nurse instructs the NAP to:

- Report the following to the nurse immediately: bleeding or swelling around CVAD insertion site; shortness of breath; loosened or soiled dressing; or if the patient has a fever or complains of pain at the site or catheter becomes dislodged.
- Inform nurse if the electronic infusion device (EID) alarm signals or if the fluid level in container is low or empty.
- Help with positioning patient during insertion and care.

Equipment

Insertion and Dressing Care

- Hair clippers
- CVAD insertion tray to include appropriate length catheter and introducer needle, sterile gauze, sterile drapes, disposable tape measure
- Maximum barrier supplies to include head covering, sterile gowns, masks, sterile gloves (powder free), antiseptic solution (alcoholic chlorhexidine solution is preferred; 70% isopropyl alcohol and povidone-iodine for chlorhexidine sensitivities), large full-body sterile drape with fenestration
- Protective eyewear
- Nonsterile gloves
- Gauze pads
- Surgical towels
- 1% lidocaine for use as local anesthetic as ordered by health care provider
- 3-mL syringe and small gauge needle for anesthetic administration
- 10-mL syringe
- Transparent semipermeable membrane (TSM) or 4 × 4 gauze dressing for catheter insertion site
- Engineered stabilization device
- Needleless connector for each lumen
- Skin protectant swab (*optional*)
- Sterile tape

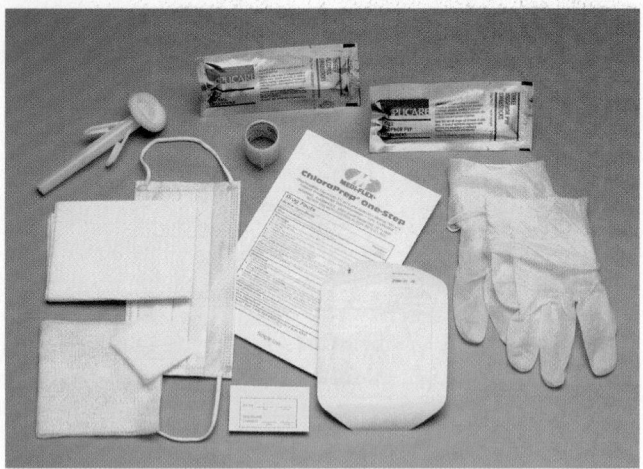

FIG 29.9 Central vascular access device (CVAD) insertion tray.

- Electronic infusion device
- Ultrasound (if available) with sterile wand cover and sterile transducer gel
  Site Care and Dressing Change
- CVAD dressing change kit (Fig. 29.9), which includes: sterile gloves, mask, antiseptic swabs for skin disinfection (chlorhexidine solution preferred, povidone-iodine, or 70% alcohol), transparent semipermeable membrane dressing (TSM), 4 × 4 gauze pads, tape measure, sterile tape, label
- Engineered stabilization device (if not sutured) for peripherally inserted central catheter (PICC) or nontunneled catheters
- Skin protectant swab
- Clean gloves

- Needleless injection cap(s) for each lumen(s)
  Blood Sampling
- Clean gloves
- Antiseptic swabs (CHG solution, povidone-iodine, or 70% alcohol)
- 5-mL Luer-Lok syringes
- 10-mL Luer-Lok syringes
- Vacuum system or blood transfer device (see agency policy)
- Blood tubes, including waste tubes, labels
- Needleless injection cap
- Syringe (5 mL or 10 mL; see agency policy) for discarded blood
- 10-mL syringe with 5 to 10 mL preservative-free 0.9% sodium chloride (normal saline [NS])
- 10-mL syringe with heparin flush solution
- Sterile cap to maintain sterility of distal end of IV tubing
  Changing the Injection Cap
- Clean gloves
- Antiseptic swabs (CHG solution, povidone-iodine, or 70% alcohol)
- Needleless injection cap(s)
- 10-mL syringe with 10 mL preservative-free 0.9% sodium chloride (NS)
- 10-mL syringe with heparin flush solution
  Discontinuation of a Nontunneled Catheter
- Personal protective equipment as indicated (goggles, gown, mask, and clean gloves)
- CVAD dressing change kit (see Fig. 29.9), which includes: sterile gloves, mask, antiseptic swabs for skin disinfection, TSM dressing, 4 × 4 gauze pads, tape measure, sterile tape, label
- Petroleum-based ointment or petroleum-based gauze, sterile
- Suture removal kit (if sutures are in place)
- Stethoscope

STEP	RATIONALE

ASSESSMENT

1. Review accuracy and completeness of health care provider's order for insertion of CVAD for size and type. Assess treatment schedule: times for administration of IV solutions, medications, and blood sampling. Follow rights of medication administration (see Chapter 20). Confirm that informed consent has been obtained and witnessed by health care provider who will perform procedure.

   Identifies patient's need for vascular access, evaluates response to therapy, and determines education needs. Insertion of central catheter requires informed consent (INS, 2016a).

2. Perform hand hygiene. Assess patient's hydration status: skin turgor, dryness of mouth, skin texture, and fluid intake and output.

   Reduces transmission of infection. Provides baseline. In addition, dehydration makes insertion of CVAD more difficult.

3. Assess patient for any surgical procedures of upper chest or anatomical irregularities of proposed insertion site.

   Previous surgical procedures or central vascular catheterizations indicate that you should not use a particular site. Spinal deformities and contractions make positioning difficult.

4. Assess CVAD placement site for skin integrity (open lesions) and signs of infection (i.e., redness, pain, tenderness, swelling, bleeding, or drainage). Apply gloves if drainage is present.

   Compromised skin integrity contraindicates catheter insertion and can lead to secondary complications.

5. Assess patient for allergy to iodine, lidocaine, latex, or CHG.

   Medications, solutions used during catheter insertion, and use of gloves and tape can cause serious allergic reactions.

6. Assess type of CVAD intended for placement. Review manufacturer directions concerning catheter and maintenance.

   Care and management depends on type and size of catheter or port, number of lumens, purpose of therapy.

STEP	RATIONALE
7. Assess for proper function of existing CVAD before therapy: integrity of catheter, ability to flush or infuse solution, ability to aspirate blood. Remove and discard gloves (if worn). Perform hand hygiene.	Blood return should be obtained and patency confirmed before infusion of solutions or medications (INS, 2016a).
8. Assess if any catheter lumens require flushing or if CVAD site needs dressing change by referring to medical record, nurses' notes, agency policies, and manufacturer-recommended guidelines for use.	Provides guidelines for maintaining catheter patency and preventing infection.
9. Assess patient's understanding of CVAD and knowledge of purpose, care, and maintenance. For long-term use ask patient or family caregiver to discuss steps in care and perform procedure (e.g., catheter site cleaning or dressing change).	Determines patient's and family caregiver's level of understanding and need for further patient education.

NURSING DIAGNOSES

- Deficient fluid volume
- Deficient knowledge regarding care of CVAD
- Excess fluid volume
- Impaired skin integrity
- Risk for infection
- Risk for injury

Related factors/Risk factors are individualized based on patient's condition or needs.

PLANNING

1. Expected outcomes following completion of procedure:	
• Insertion occurs without complication.	Placement of nontunneled CVAD carries risks such as pneumothorax, hematoma, air embolism, thrombosis, and infection.
• Catheter tip placement is appropriate at or near the cavoatrial junction as confirmed by x-ray.	Appropriate tip placement decreases risk of thrombotic complications or arrhythmias. Confirmation of tip location is required before use of CVAD (INS, 2016a).
• CVAD site is intact, with no evidence of signs or symptoms of postinsertion complications (e.g., catheter migration, redness, swelling, aching or pain).	Catheter is patent, properly placed, and without evidence of complications.
• Prescribed solutions and medications infuse without difficulty.	Catheter remains patent.
• Patient's CVAD is maintained routinely and remains patent; site is free from signs and symptoms of IV-related complications.	Care and maintenance of CVAD includes assessment, site care, dressing changes, injection cap changes, and flushing with aseptic technique (Alexander et al., 2014).
• Blood specimens are obtained, and CVAD patency is maintained.	Catheter remains patent after blood draws.
• Patient and family caregiver are able to explain purpose of CVAD and IV line therapy, care, and maintenance.	Demonstrates that patient and family caregiver have understanding and competency in caring for CVAD.
2. Explain procedure and purpose to patient and family caregiver. Explain to patient that he or she must not move during procedure. Offer opportunity at this time to toilet and offer pain medication (if needed).	Decreases anxiety, promotes cooperation, and prevents sudden movement during sterile procedure.
3. Perform hand hygiene. Collect and organize equipment on clean, clutter-free bedside stand or overbed table.	Reduces transmission of infection and contamination of equipment (INS, 2016a).

IMPLEMENTATION

1. Identify patient using at least two identifiers (e.g., name and birthday or name and medical record number) according to agency policy. Compare identifiers with information on MAR or medical record.	Ensures correct patient. Complies with The Joint Commission standards and improves patient safety (TJC, 2016).
2. **Catheter insertion: nontunneled device**	Ultrasound-guided venous access is recommended when internal jugular vein is going to be used and equipment and clinical expertise are available. Ultrasound is also used to place PICCs using brachial or basilic vein in children and adults (Heffner et al., 2015; Mitchell et al., 2015).

STEP	RATIONALE
a. Physician, with help from nurse, positions patient in Trendelenburg's or supine position for placement in vessels above heart, unless contraindicated.	Opens angle between clavicle and first rib; dilates veins to facilitate eventual catheter insertion.

Clinical Decision Point *Trendelenburg's position is contraindicated in patients with head injuries, increased intracranial pressure, certain respiratory conditions, and spinal cord injuries.*

STEP	RATIONALE
(1) Nurse places rolled towel or bath blanket between patient's shoulder blades, rotating them slightly to 10-degree angle. Turn patient's head away from intended insertion site.	Head down, below heart, promotes maximum filling and distention with increase in diameter of subclavicular vein (Phillips and Gorski, 2014); 10-degree tilt effectively achieves increase in diameter of vein.
b. Perform hand hygiene using antiseptic soap for 60 seconds.	Handwashing technique removes transient and resident bacteria from skin.
c. If necessary, use scissors or electric clippers to remove any hair around insertion site. Explain rationale to patient.	Transient microorganisms reside in body hair. Shaving can cause increased risk for infection (INS, 2016a).
d. Physician and nurse apply cap, mask, eyewear, surgical gown, and powder-free sterile gloves.	Maximum barrier precautions needed when inserting central vascular catheter (INS, 2016a).
e. Physician opens central vascular access kit. May have nurse add needed sterile equipment to kit for use during insertion (see Chapter 10).	Maintains sterile field.
f. Site preparation.	Reduces incidence of catheter-related infections (Alexander et al., 2014; CDC, 2011).
(1) Perform skin antisepsis with CHG solution using friction in back-and-forth motion for 30 seconds and allow to dry completely.	Allow any skin antiseptic agent to fully dry for complete antisepsis (INS, 2016a).
g. After cleaning site, physician and nurse remove gloves. Physician changes into second pair of sterile gloves, and nurse performs hand hygiene. (Check agency policy because some agencies require strict precautions.)	Gloves become contaminated from surface bacteria picked up in solution. Nurse functions as nonsterile circulator whose primary function is to ensure sterility of insertion field.
h. Physician uses large sterile drape and sterile towels to create sterile field. Physician finds anatomical landmarks and places sterile fenestrated drape appropriately over proposed insertion site.	Provides sterile work space for catheter insertion (INS, 2016a).
i. Physician arranges equipment in kit in preparation for catheter insertion.	Ensures smooth, orderly procedure.
j. Nurse sets up IV bag, primes and fills tubing, and covers end of tubing with sterile cap (see Skill 29.1).	IV tubing is ready to be connected to IV catheter.
k. Nurse scrubs top of 1% lidocaine bottle with antiseptic swab, allowing to dry completely, and holds bottle upside down if not in insertion kit. *Optional:* Topical local anesthetic agents can be applied before insertion with health care provider's order.	Removes surface bacteria; allows physician to withdraw lidocaine while maintaining asepsis. Lidocaine has potential for creating allergic reaction and tissue damage.
l. Physician injects needle into bottle and withdraws approximately 3 to 4 mL lidocaine. He or she injects needle into site for internal jugular puncture and anesthetizes venipuncture site, waiting 1 to 2 minutes for effect to take place.	Minimizes discomfort patient feels during venipuncture. Site has been documented to be safer for bedside insertion and ability to use ultrasound-guided insertion (Heffner et al., 2015; Mitchell et al., 2015).

Clinical Decision Point *Just before time of catheter insertion, ask patient to hold breath and strain. This is a Valsalva maneuver, which increases central venous pressure to prevent entry of air into the catheter. The Valsalva maneuver is the preferred method, although breath holding and humming may be a necessary option in uncooperative patients. In addition, if patient is unable to perform maneuvers, compress patient's abdomen gently.*

STEP	RATIONALE
m. Physician inserts IV catheter into internal jugular vein via ultrasound-guided access or using knowledge of vein anatomy. Usually this is done by locating vein with large-bore cannula, removing needle from cannula, threading wire into cannula and vein, removing cannula over wire, and threading central vein catheter over wire to appropriate location (Seldinger technique) (Alexander et al., 2014; Heffner et al., 2015).	Large vein is selected because it will be less irritated by hypertonic solutions or medications.

STEP	RATIONALE
n. Physician determines patency of line by withdrawing blood with 5-mL syringe, flushing with 0.9% sodium chloride, and placing needleless connectors on hub of each lumen. *Option:* VAD may be flushed with heparin based on type of catheter and agency policy and procedure.	Determines patency of device. Use of heparin, flush volume, and concentration vary by agency and type of catheter. Valved catheters are flushed with 0.9% sodium chloride only and do not require heparin.
o. Physician applies catheter securement device (e.g., engineered stabilization device, sutures, sterile tape, or surgical Steri-Strips) to secure central vascular catheter in place. Cover with TSM dressing.	Suturing catheter to skin at insertion site increases risk for infection. Catheter securement devices are noninvasive and preferred for preventing catheter dislodgement (INS, 2016a).
p. Physician removes sterile drapes and completes procedure. External catheter length is measured.	Measurement allows for comparison if dislodgement of CVAD is suspected (INS, 2016a).
q. Nurse initiates and regulates IV infusion to prescribed rate and connects to electronic infusion pump after receiving a chest x-ray confirmation of appropriate tip placement. Although chest x-ray is still the gold standard for determining tip placement, the use of transesophageal echocardiography, fluoroscopy, and C-arm can detect a catheter tip more readily and accurately compared with chest x-ray (Venugopal et al., 2013).	Maintains patency of VAD. Confirmation of tip placement prevents complications.

3. Insertion site care and dressing change

STEP	RATIONALE
a. Position patient in comfortable position with head slightly elevated. Have arm extended for PICC or midline device.	Provides access to patient.
b. Prepare dressing materials. *TSM dressing:* change at least every 5–7 days *Gauze dressing:* change at least every 2 days *Gauze under TSM:* change at least every 2 days	TSM dressings have advantage of allowing visualization of IV site. Gauze dressings and TSM are associated with a lower rate of catheter tip infection (Band et al., 2015, INS 2016a).
c. Perform hand hygiene and apply mask. Instruct patient to turn head away from site during dressing change or provide mask for patient.	Reduces transfer of microorganisms; prevents spread of airborne microorganisms over CVAD insertion site.
d. Apply clean gloves. Remove old TSM dressing by stabilizing catheter with nondominant hand. Remove dressing by pulling up one corner and gently pulling straight out and parallel to skin. Repeat on all sides until dressing has been removed.	Prevents unintentional catheter removal.
e. Remove catheter stabilization device if used and requires changing. Must use alcohol to remove adhesive stabilization devices.	Allows visualization of insertion site and allows for appropriate skin antisepsis (INS, 2016a). Use of alcohol minimizes risk for medical adhesive–related skin injury (MARSI) (INS, 2016a).

Clinical Decision Point *If sutures are used for initial catheter stabilization and become loosened or are no longer intact, alternative stabilization measures should be used. Use of an engineered stabilization device is recommended because sutures are associated with increased risk of infection (Alexander et al., 2014; INS, 2016a).*

STEP	RATIONALE
f. Inspect catheter, insertion site, and surrounding skin. Measure external CVAD length and compare to measurement from insertion if dislodgement is suspected. For PICC and midlines, measure upper-arm circumference 10 cm above antecubital fossa if clinically indicated and compare to baseline.	Insertion sites require regular inspection for early detection of signs and symptoms of IV-related complications (INS, 2016a). Measurement of external catheter length provides comparison to determine dislodgement; arm measurement with a 3-cm increase can indicate thrombosis (INS, 2016a).
g. Remove and discard clean gloves; perform hand hygiene. Open CVAD dressing kit using sterile technique and *apply sterile gloves* (Chapter 10). Area to be cleaned should be same size as dressing.	Sterile technique is required to apply new dressing.
h. Clean site:	Reduces incidence of catheter related infections (Alexander, et al., 2014; CDC, 2011).
(1) Perform skin antisepsis with CHG solution using friction in back-and-forth motion for 30 seconds and allow to dry completely.	Allow any skin antiseptic agent to dry fully for complete antisepsis (INS, 2016a).

STEP	RATIONALE

(2) Povidone-iodine and alcohol may be used in some settings or if patient is sensitive to CHG (see agency policy). If using alcohol or povidone-iodine, clean in concentric circle, moving from insertion site outward with swab. Allow to dry completely.

i. Apply skin protectant to area and allow to dry completely so skin is not tacky. Skin protectant must be used if adhesive stabilization device will be used.

Protects irritated or fragile skin from dressing and stabilization device, if used, and minimizes risk for MARSI.

j. *Option:* Use CHG-impregnated dressing for short-term CVADs.

CHG-impregnated dressings can reduce risk of infection (INS, 2016a). Use with caution in premature neonates and patients with fragile skin and/or complicated skin pathologies (INS, 2016a).

k. Apply sterile TSM dressing or gauze dressing over insertion site (see Skill 29.1, Step 24).

Protects catheter insertion site and minimizes risk for infection (Phillips and Gorski, 2014). Allows for clear visualization of catheter site between dressing changes (INS, 2016b).

l. Apply new catheter stabilization device according to manufacturer directions for use if catheter is not sutured in place (see Skill 29.1, Step 25).

Use of engineered stabilization devices that allow visual inspection of insertion site can reduce risk for VAD complications (i.e., phlebitis, infection, migration) and unintentional loss of access (INS, 2016a).

m. Apply label to dressing with date, time, and your initials.

Provides information about next dressing change.

n. Dispose of soiled supplies and used equipment. Remove gloves and perform hand hygiene.

Reduces transmission of microorganisms.

4. Blood sampling

a. Apply clean gloves.

Reduces transmission of microorganisms.
Prevents transfer of body fluids.

b. Turn off all infusions for at least 1 to 5 minutes before drawing blood. **NOTE:** If you cannot stop infusion, draw blood from peripheral vein.

Prevents dilution of sample. Prevents interruption of critical IV therapy.

c. When drawing through staggered multilumen catheters, draw from distal lumen (or one recommended by manufacturer).

Distal lumen typically is largest-gauge lumen (Phillips and Gorski, 2014).

d. Syringe method:
NOTE: Check agency policy for use of vacuum tube method with CVADs.

(1) Remove distal end of IV tubing or injection cap from catheter hub. Cover end of IV tubing with sterile cap to keep end of tubing sterile.

Maintains sterility of end of IV tubing. Drawing from needleless connector minimizes risk of blood exposure.

(2) Scrub catheter hub with antiseptic swab for at least 15 seconds and allow to dry completely.

Reduces risk of infection.

(3) Attach empty 5-mL syringe, unclamp catheter (if necessary), and withdraw 4 to 5 mL of blood for discard sample.

Discard sample reduces risk of drug concentrations or diluted specimen (Alexander et al., 2014). Drawing specimens for international normalized ratio (INR) studies from heparinized lines is not recommended (INS, 2016b).

(4) Clamp catheter (if necessary); remove syringe with blood and discard in appropriate biohazard container.

Valved catheters do not require clamping because clamp opens valve and allows reflux of blood into catheter.

(5) Scrub catheter hub with another antiseptic swab for 15 seconds and allow to dry completely.

(6) Attach second syringe(s) to obtain required volume of blood needed for specimen ordered.

Multiple syringes may be required, depending on specimens required and number of blood tubes needed.

(7) Unclamp catheter (if necessary) to withdraw blood.

(8) Once specimens are obtained, clamp catheter (if necessary) and remove syringe.

(9) Scrub catheter hub with antiseptic swab for 15 seconds and allow to dry completely.

STEP	RATIONALE

(10) Attach prefilled syringe with 10-mL 0.9% sodium chloride (NS) and flush catheter using the appropriate flush/clamp/disconnect sequence based on the type of needleless connector (e.g., neutral, negative or positive pressure displacement). Ensure that clamp is engaged (if available).

Flush with minimum volume of twice the internal volume of catheter with 0.9% sodium chloride (NS) (INS, 2016a). Refer to agency policy and procedure for flush volume requirements. Reduces risk for catheter clotting after procedure.

(11) Remove syringe and discard into appropriate biohazard container.

Reduces transmission of microorganisms.

f. Transfer blood using transfer vacuum device (see illustration).

Reduces risk of blood exposure.

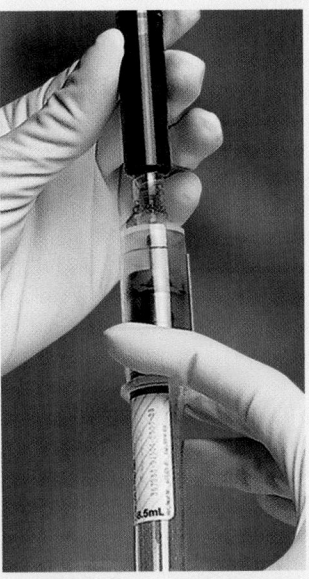

STEP 4f Blood specimen transfer device. *(Courtesy ©Becton Dickinson & Co.)*

g. Flush catheter with heparin flush based on type of catheter and agency policy and procedure using appropriate flush/clamp/disconnect sequence. Ensure that clamp is engaged (if available).

Prevents clot formation. Heparin flush volume and concentration vary by agency and type of catheter. Valved catheters are flushed with 0.9% sodium chloride (NS) only and do not require heparin.

Clinical Decision Point *Always use a 10-mL syringe or syringe designed to generate lower injection pressure (i.e., 10 mL–diameter syringe barrel) on central lines in adults to minimize pressure during injection (INS, 2016a).*

h. Remove syringe. Scrub exposed hub with antiseptic swab for 15 seconds and allow to dry. Attach new sterile injection cap or IV tubing to hub of catheter. Resume infusion as ordered or clamp catheter (if necessary).

Decreases risk of contamination.

i. Dispose of soiled equipment and used supplies. Remove gloves and perform hand hygiene.

Reduces transmission of microorganisms.

5. Changing injection cap

a. Determine if injection caps should be changed.

Injection caps should be changed no more frequently than 9-hour intervals, with primary administration set changed for continuous infusions if it is removed for any reason, if there is residual blood or debris in it, if it becomes contaminated, or according to agency policies and procedures (INS, 2016a).

b. Prepare new injection cap(s):

Understanding of types of injection caps ensures appropriate flush/clamp/disconnect sequence based on type of device (e.g., positive, negative, or neutral displacement valves) (INS, 2016a).

(1) Perform hand hygiene. Apply clean gloves. Remove cap from package. Do not contaminate sterile injection port.

Reduces transfer of microorganisms. Maintains sterility.

STEP	RATIONALE
(2) Keep protective cover on tip of injection cap.	Maintains sterility.
(3) Prime injection cap by attaching prefilled syringe and flushing with preservative-free 0.9% sodium chloride (NS) through cap until fluid is seen in protective cover. Keep syringe attached.	Removes air from system, preventing it from being introduced into vein (Alexander et al., 2014).
c. Based on catheter type, clamp catheter lumens one at a time by using slide or squeeze clamp, if necessary. If catheter is not clamped, ask patient to perform Valsalva maneuver as new cap is applied.	Prevents air from entering system when opened. Valsalva maneuver prevents air embolus (Phillips and Gorski, 2014).
d. Scrub catheter hub and injection cap with antiseptic swab for 15 seconds and allow to dry completely. Remove and dispose of old injection cap using aseptic technique.	Reduces transmission of microorganisms.
e. Scrub exposed catheter hub with antiseptic swab for 15 seconds and allow to dry completely. Connect new injection cap(s) on catheter hub.	Drying allows time for maximum antimicrobial activity of agents.
f. Flush catheter with 10-mL 0.9% sodium chloride (NS), followed by heparin flush based on type of catheter and agency policy and procedure using appropriate sequence to clamp/flush/disconnect based on type of needleless connector (e.g., neutral, negative, or positive pressure displacement). Ensure that clamp is engaged (if available).	Prevents clot formation. Heparin flush volume and concentration vary by agency and type of catheter. Valved catheters are flushed with 0.9% sodium chloride (NS) only and do not require heparin. Engaging clamp minimizes risk if injection cap loosens or comes off, which can cause infection, air embolism, and bleeding.
g. Dispose of all soiled supplies and used equipment. Remove gloves and perform hand hygiene.	Reduces transmission of microorganisms.
6. Discontinuing nontunneled catheters	
a. Verify health care provider's order to discontinue line. Check agency policy because most require health care providers to discontinue CVAD. In some settings advanced practice nurses or specially credentialed nurses can remove devices.	Verifies appropriateness of procedure. Only specially trained health care professional can remove CVAD.
b. If IV solutions or medications are to continue, arrange placement of a short-peripheral or midline before CVAD discontinuation. **NOTE:** Be aware of pH and osmolarity of solution or medication for appropriateness of conversion to short-peripheral or midline catheter.	Prevents interruption of IV therapy.
c. Position patient in supine flat or 10-degree Trendelenburg's position unless contraindicated.	Position promotes venous filling and prevents air embolus during catheter removal.
d. Perform hand hygiene.	Prevents transmission of microorganisms.
e. Turn off IV solutions infusing through central line and convert to alternate VAD.	Prevents fluid loss during CVAD removal.
f. Place moisture-proof pad under site.	Minimizes soiling of bed linen. Provides clean environment.
g. Apply gown, clean gloves, mask, and goggles.	Prevents transmission of microorganisms and exposure to bloodborne pathogens.
h. Gently remove CVAD dressing by stabilizing catheter with nondominant hand, pulling up one corner and gently pulling straight out and parallel to skin. Repeat on all sides until dressing has been removed.	Prevents skin tears. Allows inspection of CVAD insertion site before removal.
i. If catheter securement device is present, carefully remove catheter from device and remove device with alcohol.	Alcohol aids in removal of securement device without causing skin tear.
k. Remove gloves and perform hand hygiene; open CVAD dressing change kit and suture removal kit (if CVAD is sutured in place). Add items to sterile field. Apply sterile gloves.	Prevents transfer of organisms on soiled dressing to catheter insertion site.
l. Perform skin antisepsis of insertion site with CHG solution using friction in back-and-forth motion for 30 seconds and allow to dry completely. *Option:* If CVAD is sutured in place, remove sutures (see Skill 40.2).	Reduces risk of migration of microbes into catheter tract. Allows CVAD removal.

STEP	RATIONALE

Clinical Decision Point *All CVADs require measurements of total length and external catheter on insertion. PICC lines also require measurement of upper-arm circumference.*

m. Using nondominant hand, apply sterile 4 × 4–inch gauze to site. Instruct patient to take deep breath and perform Valsalva maneuver as catheter is withdrawn.

Valsalva maneuver reduces risk for air embolus by decreasing negative pressure in respiratory system.

n. With dominant hand slowly remove catheter in smooth, continuous motion an inch at a time. Keeping fingers near insertion site, immediately apply pressure to site and continue until bleeding stops. Stop removal procedure if resistance is met while removing catheter (INS, 2016b).

Gentle removal of catheter prevents stretching and breaking it. Damaged catheter may break off and leave piece in patient's arm.

Direct pressure reduces risk for bleeding and hematoma formation.

Clinical Decision Point *It is often necessary to apply pressure longer if patient is receiving anticoagulation therapy or has prolonged clotting times.*

o. Apply petroleum-based ointment or gauze to exit site. Apply sterile occlusive dressing such as TSM dressing or sterile gauze to site. Change dressing every 24 hours until healed.

Reduces chance of air embolism and seals skin-to-vein tract (Alexander et al., 2014). Allows for inspection of site for bleeding and infection until it is healed.

p. Label dressing with date, time, and your initials.

Identifies date of catheter removal and need for dressing change.

q. Inspect catheter integrity for intactness, especially along tip, and that length is appropriate for device. Discard in appropriate biohazard container.
NOTE: Catheter cultures should be performed when catheter is removed for suspected catheter-related bloodstream infection (CRBSI). Catheter cultures should not be obtained routinely (INS, 2016a).

If catheter tip is broken or compromised, place in container and label for possible follow-up and notify health care provider

r. Position patient in a supine position for 30 minutes after nontunneled CVAD removal (INS, 2016a). Be sure that short-peripheral IV line or midline is infusing at correct rate.

Reduces chance of air embolism.
Maintains prescribed IV solution therapy.

s. Dispose of soiled supplies; remove gloves and personal protective equipment. Perform hand hygiene.

Reduces transmission of microorganisms.

EVALUATION

1. Consult x-ray film (or echocardiography, fluoroscopy) examination reports for catheter placement.

A routine chest x-ray film examination is still gold standard to confirm position of catheter tip and presence of pneumothorax. However, other technologies are proving reliable.

2. Determine daily, in consultation with health care provider, the continued need for the CVAD.

Daily review of line necessity with prompt removal of unnecessary lines is practice recommended in the IHI central line–associated bloodstream infection (CLABSI) bundle (IHI, 2012).

3. Evaluate for postinsertion complications to include:

Complications after insertion can include pneumothorax, cardiac arrhythmias, and nerve injury (Phillips and Gorski, 2014). Prompt identification can allow for treatment, repositioning of catheter, or removal if necessary.

a. Auscultate breath sounds and evaluate for shortness of breath, chest pain, absent breath sounds.

Signs and symptoms of pneumothorax develop if CVAD pierces intrathoracic space.

b. Monitor vital signs, including heart rate and rhythm.

Evaluates for signs of cardiac arrhythmias.

c. Monitor patient complaints of pain, numbness, tingling, or weakness.

Signs of nerve injury from catheter insertion.

4. Evaluate patient to determine response to infusion therapy (e.g., laboratory values, input and output [I&O], weights, vital signs, postprocedure assessments).

IV solutions and additives maintain or restore fluid and electrolyte balance. Early recognition of complications leads to prompt treatment.

STEP	RATIONALE

5. Evaluate patient at established intervals for signs and symptoms of CVAD-related complications (Table 29.8) according to agency policy and procedure.

Prevents complications that compromise integrity of CVAD or cause inaccurate IV solution flow rate and allows for prompt intervention.

6. Observe all connection points, being sure that they are secure as directed by agency policy and procedure.

An intact system prevents accidental blood loss or entrance of air or microbes into the vasculature.

7. **Use Teach-Back:** "I want to be sure that I explained the purpose and care of your intravenous catheter. This catheter is placed in a large vein in your body and the problems we talked about can occur. Tell me in your own words the problems that might develop with your catheter and the signs and symptoms you would report to me or another nurse." Revise your instruction now or develop a plan for revised patient or family caregiver teaching if patient or family caregiver is not able to teach back correctly.

Determines patient's and family caregiver's level of understanding of instructional topic.

Unexpected Outcomes
1. For catheter complications, see Table 29.8.
2. Patient or family caregiver is unable to explain or perform CVAD care.

Related Interventions
- See Table 29.8.
- Indicates need for home care referral or additional instruction.

TABLE 29.8

Complications of Vascular Access Devices

Complication	Assessment	Prevention	Intervention
Catheter damage, breakage	Every shift observe for pinholes, leaks, tears. Assess for drainage from site after flushing.	Follow proper clamping procedure. Avoid sharp objects near catheter. Use needleless system device. A 10-mL syringe is preferred for flushing CVADs to avoid excessive pressure and potential catheter damage. Never flush against resistance.	Clamp catheter near insertion site and place sterile gauze over break or hole until repaired. Use only repair kit that is recommended by manufacturer. Remove catheter with order.
Occlusion: thrombus, fibrin sheath, fibrin tail, precipitation, malposition	Assess insertion site and sutures. Assess for blood return. Assess for ability to infuse fluid. Assess equipment. If port is in place, reassess and verify noncoring needle placement. Assess with syringe directly on catheter. Assess for discomfort or pain in shoulder, neck, ear, or arm at insertion site. Assess for neck or shoulder edema.	Follow routine flushing with positive pressure and/or use positive-pressure valve injection cap. Secure with catheter stabilization device to prevent tension on CVAD. A 10-mL syringe is preferred for flushing CVADs to avoid excessive pressure and potential catheter damage. Do not flush against resistance. Flush between medications. Flush vigorously after viscous solutions. Avoid mixing incompatible drugs. Avoid kinking catheter.	Reposition patient. Have patient cough and deep breathe. Raise patient's arm overhead. Obtain venogram if ordered. Administer thrombolytics if ordered. Remove catheter (CVAD requires order). Obtain x-ray film as ordered. Do not use a 1-mL syringe to instill saline because pressure exceeds 200 psi.
Infection and sepsis: catheter skin junction, tunnel, thrombus, port pocket, CLABSI	Assess catheter skin junction for redness, drainage, edema, or tenderness. Assess for signs of systemic infection. Monitor laboratory findings.	Use aseptic technique. Prevent contamination of catheter hub. Adhere to dressing change technique. Apply TSM dressing over catheter skin junction.	Obtain blood cultures from peripheral and CVAD if ordered. Remove catheter (CVAD requires order). Replace catheter.
Dislodgement	Assess length of catheter daily. Inform patient of possible catheter dislodgement. Identify edema at catheter skin junction or drainage. Palpate catheter skin junction and tunnel for coiling (catheter can feel cordlike underneath the skin). Assess for distended neck veins.	Loop and tape catheter securely. Use catheter stabilization device and TSM dressing. Avoid pulling on CVAD. Avoid manipulating catheter by hand.	Insert new catheter. Secure with catheter stabilization device. Teach patient not to manipulate catheter.

TABLE 29.8

Complications of Vascular Access Devices—cont'd

Complication	Assessment	Prevention	Intervention
Catheter migration (e.g., length of catheter moved from original position), pinch-off syndrome (e.g., compression of catheter between clavicle and first rib), port separation or catheter fracture (e.g., internal fracture or separation of catheter)	Assess for patient complaints of gurgling sounds. Assess for change in patency of catheter by evaluating change in flow rate, local irritation, swelling, occlusion, tenderness, pain, inability to aspirate fluid and/or blood. Pain at site when flushed or symptoms of embolus. Obtain x-ray film examination. Assess edema of arm and hand on side of insertion. Assess for distended neck veins. Assess for inability to infuse solutions. Assess length of catheter daily.	Avoid trauma. Avoid placement near site of local infection, scarring, or skin disorder.	Reposition under fluoroscopy as ordered. Remove catheter as ordered. Stop all fluid administration.
Skin erosion (e.g., mechanical loss of skin tissue), hematomas (e.g., local collection of blood), cuff extrusion (e.g., tissue at edges of insertion site separate), scar tissue formation over port	Assess for loss of viable tissue over septum site. Assess for separation of exit site edges. Assess for drainage at catheter skin junction. Assess for redness. Assess for edema, contusions. Note if tunneled catheter is exposed (Dacron cuff is visible.)	Maintain nutritional status. Avoid pressure or trauma. Rotate with each port access. Do not reinsert a noncoring needle in the same "hole" of a previous insertion. This creates a permanent hole in the septum. Do not use standard needle to access port.	Remove CVAD as ordered. Improve nutrition. Provide appropriate skin care.
Infiltration, extravasation	Assess for erythema. Assess for edema. Assess for spongy feeling. Assess for swelling around IV site and at termination of catheter tip. Assess for labored breathing. Assess for aspiration of fluid and/or blood. Assess for complaints of pain with infusion of solutions or medications (e.g., burning). Assess for no free-flow IV drip.	Immediately stop vesicant administration. Administer antidote or therapeutic medications to maintain tissue integrity according to protocol.	Apply cold/warm compresses according to specific vesicant protocol. Provide emotional support. Obtain x-ray film if ordered. Use antidotes per protocol. Discontinue IV solutions.
Pneumothorax, hemothorax, air emboli, hydrothorax	Assess for subcutaneous emphysema by inspecting and palpating skin around insertion site and along arm. Inspection may reveal edema where air is located, and air may travel if skin is loose. Palpation reveals a crackling sensation such as popping plastic bubble wrap. Assess for chest pain. Assess for dyspnea, apnea, hypoxia, tachycardia, hypotension, nausea, confusion.	Use injection cap on distal end when not in use. Do not leave catheter hub open to air. If appropriate for device, be sure that clamps are engaged.	Administer oxygen as ordered. Elevate feet. Aspirate air, fluid. If air emboli suspected, place patient on left side with head down. Remove catheter as ordered. Help with insertion of chest tubes as ordered.
Incorrect placement	Assess for cardiac dysrhythmias. Assess for hypotension. Assess for neck distention. Assess for narrow pulse pressure. Assess for inadequate blood withdrawal. Assess for retrograde flow of blood (flow of blood back into tubing usually caused by decreased pressure gradient between venous system and access device unit [e.g., IV infusion, heparin lock]).	Obtain x-ray film examination after placement. Reposition catheter as warranted.	Stop all fluid administration until placement is confirmed. Discontinue catheter (requires order). Obtain x-ray film and electrocardiogram (for PICC and CVAD). Administer support medications as ordered.

CLABSI, Central line–associated bloodstream infection; *CVAD*, central vascular access device; *CVC*, central venous catheter; *IV*, intravenous; *PICC*, peripherally inserted central catheter.

Recording and Reporting

- Immediately notify health care provider of signs and symptoms of any complications.
- Document catheter site care in nurses' notes in electronic health record (EHR) or chart, including catheter location; size of catheter; number of lumens; condition of catheter insertion site or port site, including skin integrity, external catheter length, mid-arm circumference for PICC; condition and type of securement device; date and time of dressing change; change of injection caps; flushes used; patency of catheter, including presence or absence of blood return; and patient's tolerance of the procedure.
- Document patient's and family caregiver's ability to explain instructions in EHR or chart.
- Document in nurses' notes in EHR catheter removal: patient position, appearance of site, length of catheter removed, integrity of catheter after removal, dressing applied, patient's tolerance of procedure, presence/absence of bleeding from site every 15 minutes for 1 hour, and any problems with removal.
- Document in nurses' notes in EHR blood draw: date, time, sample drawn, waste volume, and flushes used.
- Document in nurses' notes in EHR unexpected outcomes and CVAD complications, health care provider notification, interventions, and patient response to treatment.

Special Considerations

Teaching

- Instruct patient to report discomfort around the site; discomfort in arms, shoulders, or side of the neck; or any shortness of breath.
- Discuss and provide written emergency measures and telephone numbers of health care personnel to be used in case of catheter damage, dislodgement, swelling, redness, or leakage at insertion site; occlusion of catheter; temperature above 38°C (100.4°F) (see agency policy); and shaking chills.
- Provide written instruction for dressing changes, inspection of insertion site, flushing, and tubing changes.
- Arrange for instruction and return demonstration of skills by patient or family caregiver.
- Have patient or family caregiver maintain a list of caregivers and telephone numbers (e.g., health care provider, nurse, social worker, pharmacist, dietitian).

Pediatric

- Central vein catheters that are of a smaller diameter and shorter length are available for children and infants.
- Take care to secure infant catheters in a manner that does not allow them to twist. Small-diameter catheters are fragile, and twisting them causes them to tear.
- Amount and dosage of flush solution (heparin/sodium chloride) vary with age, size, and catheter diameter and length.
- Record volume of blood draws on I&O record.

Gerontological

- Some older adults have difficulty lying flat in bed, and a modification of the totally supine position during CVAD insertion is often necessary.
- PICC insertion may provide an alternative route of administration and reduce the risk of complications associated with subclavian or jugular insertion.

Home Care

- Initiate early referral for discharge planning to social service, counselor, or home care coordinator for assessment of resources.
- Provide patient with written list of providers for supplies and equipment.
- Provide patient with Kelly clamp *without* teeth (bulldog clamp) that can be used in the event of catheter rupture to prevent air embolism and instruct patient on use.
- Instruct patient or family caregiver in flushing technique, site care, and dressing change and observe them performing procedures.
- Instruct patient and family caregiver in adaptations of hospital procedures that they can make at home (e.g., good hand hygiene instead of sterile gloves).
- Provide education to the patient and family caregiver about how to recognize signs and symptoms of IV-related complications, actions to take, how to report, and methods for preservation of CVADs.
- Assess home environment and determine suitable area for dressing changes, avoiding areas where contaminants are potential hazards.
- Provide appropriate information about home disposal of soiled dressings and equipment (see Chapter 44).

◆ CLINICAL DEBRIEF

An 88-year-old female with a history of heart failure and gastric cancer was admitted to the hospital 24 hours ago for dehydration with mild confusion, decreased urine output, postural hypotension, and poor oral intake after receiving chemotherapy. She has been receiving D_5LR at 100 mL/h by gravity through a short-peripheral intravenous (IV) line since admission. Today her daughter tells you that her mother is having difficulty breathing and is asking for another pillow for her bed.

1. On the basis of her daughter's information, which clinical markers would you assess, and which additional signs and symptoms would you expect to find?
2. At morning rounds the health care team sees the patient and writes changes to the IV solution orders. In addition, orders are received to administer furosemide 10 mg slow IV push daily for 3 days. Based on the patient's signs and symptoms, which orders can you anticipate? How would you calculate the minute flow rate of an infusion set with a drop factor of 15 gtt/mL, and how would you ensure an accurate flow rate?
3. The following morning the patient complains of tenderness at her IV site. However, she no longer has dyspnea or other signs of fluid volume excess. Her past 24-hour intake was 1600 mL, and her output was 1700 mL. Serum electrolyte levels drawn this morning were within normal limits. She reported that she put some tape on her IV dressing last night because it was falling off. There is marked redness and swelling around the IV site with purulent drainage. Her temperature is 38.2°C (100.8°F). Using SBAR, show how you would communicate with the health care team about this patient.

◆ REVIEW QUESTIONS

1. Your patient has a tunneled central vascular access device (CVAD) placed, and you will be performing catheter care to include insertion site care, dressing change, injection cap change, and flush. Place the following steps in correct order:
   1. Connect injection cap on catheter hub, flush with 0.9% normal saline (NS), remove gloves, perform hand hygiene.
   2. Apply new stabilization device, transparent semipermeable membrane (TSM) dressing, label dressing.
   3. Perform hand hygiene, apply clean gloves and mask, remove old dressing.
   4. Perform skin antisepsis with chlorhexidine solution and allow to dry completely.
   5. Remove injection cap, scrub exposed catheter hub with antiseptic swab, let dry completely.
   6. Remove and discard clean gloves, perform hand hygiene, apply sterile gloves.

2. Which of the following steps are necessary when inserting a short-peripheral IV line? (Select all that apply.)
   1. Apply tourniquet to arm 10 to 15 cm (4 to 6 inches) above the intended insertion site.
   2. Clean skin using an approved antiseptic agent such as 70% isopropyl alcohol and allow to dry thoroughly.
   3. Stabilize the vein by placing the thumb proximal to the insertion site, stretching the skin in the direction of insertion.
   4. Use the smallest-gauge, shortest catheter available and insert with the bevel up at a 10- to 15-degree angle.
   5. Observe for blood in the flashback chamber of the catheter and advance the catheter off the needle into the vein.
   6. Release the tourniquet once the catheter has been secured and the dressing has been applied.

3. Identify the veins of the forearm as indicated on the diagram.

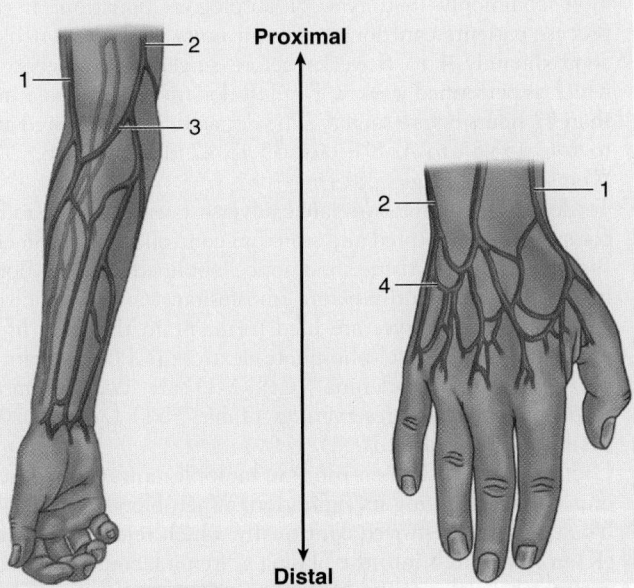

Proximal

Distal

ⓔ *Visit the Evolve site for a complete list of Clinical Debrief and Review Questions answers.*

REFERENCES

Alexander M, et al: *Core curriculum for infusion nursing,* ed 4, St Louis, 2014, Lippincott, Williams & Wilkins.

Band J, et al: Prevention of intravascular catheter-related infections, *UpToDate,* 2015, http://www.uptodate.com/contents/prevention-of-intravascular-catheter-related-infections. Accessed March 20, 2016.

Centers for Disease Control and Prevention (CDC): *Guidelines for the prevention of intravascular catheter-related infections,* Atlanta, GA, 2011, http://www.cdc.gov/hicpac/pdf/guidelines/bsi-guidelines-2011.pdf. Accessed March 20, 2016.

Ciocson M, et al: Central vascular access device: an adapted evidence-based clinical practice guideline, *J Vasc Access* 19(4):221, 2013.

Cook LS: Infusion-related air embolism, *J Infus Nurs* 36(1):26, 2013.

Galanti GA: *Caring for patients from different cultures,* ed 5, Philadelphia, 2015, University of Pennsylvania Press.

Harding AD: Intravenous smart pumps, *J Infus Nurs* 36(3):191, 2013.

Heffner A, et al: Overview of central line care, *UpToDate,* 2015, http://www.uptodate.com/contents/overview-of-central-venous-access?source=search_result&search=central+line&selectedTitle=1%7E150. Accessed July 20, 2016.

Hockenberry M, Wilson D: *Wong's nursing care of infants and children,* ed 10, St Louis, 2015, Elsevier.

Infusion Nurses Society (INS): Infusion therapy standards of practice, *J Intraven Nurs* 39(1S):2016a.

Infusion Nurses Society (INS): *Policy and procedures for infusion therapy,* ed 5, Norwood, MA, 2016b, INS.

Institute for Healthcare Improvement (IHI): *How-to guide: prevent central line–associated bloodstream infections,* Cambridge, MA, 2012, IHI. http://www.ihi.org/resources/Pages/Tools/HowtoGuidePreventCentralLineAssociatedBloodstreamInfection.aspx. Accessed March 20, 2016.

Mitchell E, et al: Principles of ultrasound-guided venous access, *UpToDate,* 2015, http://www.uptodate.com/contents/principles-of-ultrasound-guided-venous-access. Accessed July 20, 2016.

Occupational Safety and Health Administration (OSHA): *Bloodborne pathogens standard,* United States Department of Labor, last amended April 3, 2012, https://www.osha.gov/pls/oshaweb/owadisp.show_document?p_table=STANDARDS&p_id=10051. Accessed July 19, 2016.

Phillips LD, Gorski L: *Manual of IV therapeutics: evidenced-based practice for infusion therapy,* ed 6, Philadelphia, 2014, FA Davis.

The Joint Commission (TJC): *2016 National Patient Safety Goals,* Oakbrook Terrace, IL, 2016, TJ, http://www.jointcommission.org/standards_information/npsgs.aspx. Accessed March 20, 2016.

Venugopal AN, et al: Role of chest x-ray in citing central venous catheter tip: A few case reports with a brief review of the literature, *J Anaesthesiol Clin Pharmacol* 29(3):397–400, 2013.

Weinstein S, Hagle M: *Plumer's principles and practice of infusion therapy,* Philadelphia, 2014, Lippincott, Williams & Wilkins.

30 | Blood Transfusions

OBJECTIVES

Mastery of content in this chapter will enable the nurse to:
- Discuss indications for blood therapy.
- Demonstrate the following skills on selected patients: initiating blood therapy, implementing autotransfusion, and monitoring for adverse reactions to transfusion.
- Describe various transfusion reactions.
- Explain techniques for managing symptoms of adverse transfusion reactions.

MEDIA RESOURCES

- evolve http://evolve.elsevier.com/Perry/skills
- Review Questions
- ▶ Video Clips
- Audio Glossary

- **NSO** Nursing Skills Online
- Clinical Debrief and Review Questions Answers
- Animations

PURPOSE

The transfusion of blood and blood components restores and maintains quality of life for patients with hematological disorders, cancer, injury, or surgical intervention. A competent nurse must know not only the complexities of the ABO and Rh system, but also the numerous components of blood that can be transfused and the serious negative outcomes that can occur.

STANDARDS OF CARE

- American Association of Blood Banks (AABB), 2014—Technical Manual for Transfusing Blood and Blood Products
- Infusion Nurses Society (INS), 2016—Evidence-Based Practice Guidelines for Infusions
- Occupational Safety and Health Administration (OSHA), 2015—Occupational Safe Exposure to Bloodborne Pathogens
- The Joint Commission (TJC), 2016—Patient Identification

PRINCIPLES FOR PRACTICE

- Transfusion therapy or blood replacement is the intravenous (IV) administration of whole blood (Fig. 30.1), its components (Fig. 30.2A-B), or a plasma-derived product (Fig. 30.3) for therapeutic purposes (Alexander et al., 2014). Transfusions restore intravascular volume with whole blood or albumin, restore the oxygen-carrying capacity of blood with red blood cells, and provide clotting factors and/or platelets.
- The most common method of blood transfusion is allogeneic blood (blood donated from someone else).
- Autologous transfusion or autotransfusion is a method in which a patient's own blood is collected and reinfused for the purpose of intravascular volume replacement (AABB, 2014; Alexander et al., 2014). Patients who have a concern about

transfusion-related reactions or transmission of disease find positive advantages to autologous transfusion. It is ideal for preoperative blood donation, intraoperative cell salvage, and postoperative blood salvage. Preoperative blood donation is the most commonly used type of autologous donation. In this process patients can donate several units of their own blood approximately 4 to 6 weeks before surgery via phlebotomy, which is performed weekly. The last donation must occur more than 72 hours before surgery. The donated blood is stored at 1° to 6°C (33.8° to 42.8°F) for 35 to 42 days (AABB, 2014; Weinstein and Hagle, 2014).
- To decrease transfusion-related adverse events, blood and its components are treated and stored in controlled environments. Blood is a living tissue; and, once obtained via the donor, it must remain healthy before transfusion. Various anticoagulants and preservatives are used to maintain the shelf life of donated blood. Citrate-phosphate-dextrose (CPD) and citrate-phosphate-dextrose-adenine (CPDA-1) are two commonly used anticoagulant preservatives (Table 30.1) (AABB, 2014; Weinstein and Hagle, 2014).
- Caution is needed when infusing multiple units of blood or a unit of blood nearing its expiration. When blood is stored, red blood cells are destroyed continually, which releases potassium (K) from the cells into the plasma. Often a laboratory test of a patient's K level is ordered before administering a unit of blood.
- As a nurse your role during a blood transfusion is to carry out the health care provider's order by safely administering the blood/blood products and assessing a patient before, during, and after the transfusion and by promptly identifying and reporting any transfusion reactions.

ABO System

- There are three blood-typing systems: ABO, Rh, and human leukocyte antigen (HLA). These systems ensure a close match

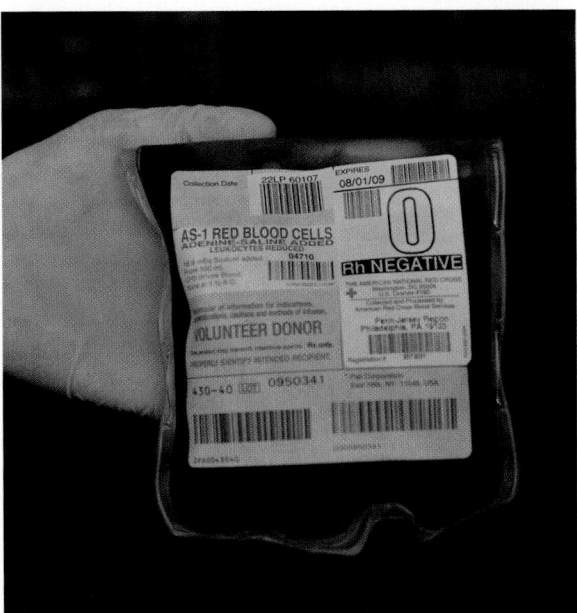

FIG 30.1 Unit of blood. (*Image courtesy American Red Cross.*)

TABLE 30.1

Types of Blood Preservatives

Anticoagulant Preservative	Composition	Shelf Life Provided (Days)
CPD	Citrate, phosphate, and dextrose	21
CPDA-1	CPD plus adenine	35
CPDA-1 additive system	CPD plus various preservative combinations	35–42

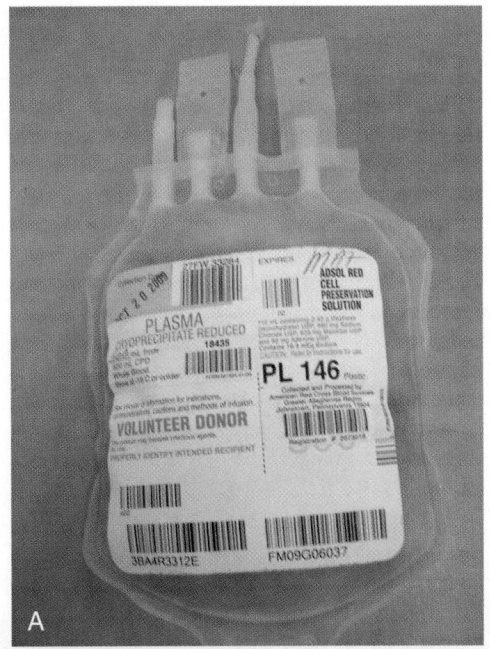

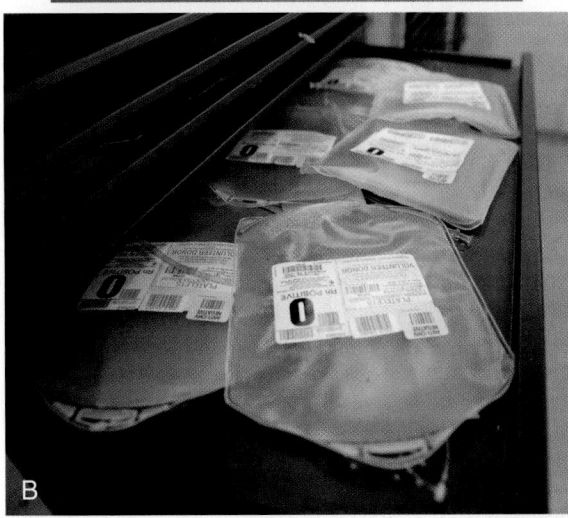

FIG 30.2 A, Bag of cryoprecipitate (Cryo). **B,** Bag of platelets. (*Images courtesy American Red Cross.*)

between transfused products and a recipient's blood. The ABO system uses the presence or absence of specific antigens on the surface of red blood cells to identify blood groups. When the type A antigen is present, the blood group is type A. When the type B antigen is present, the blood group is type B. When both A and B antigens are present, the blood group is type AB; and when neither A nor B antigens are present, the blood group is type O (AABB, 2014; Alexander et al., 2014) (Table 30.2).

- Antibodies that react against the A and B antigens are naturally present in the plasma of people whose red blood cells do not carry the antigen. These antibodies (agglutinins) react against the foreign antigens (agglutinogens). Incompatible red blood cells agglutinate (clump together) and result in a life-threatening hemolytic transfusion reaction. People with type A blood have anti-B antibodies; people with type B blood have anti-A antibodies. People with type AB blood have neither antibody and can receive all blood types. People with type O blood have both A and B antibodies and can receive only type O blood (AABB, 2014; Alexander et al., 2014).

Rh System

- The Rh factor is considered when matching blood components for transfusion. The Rh factor is another antigen in red blood cell membranes. Although nearly 50 types of Rh antigen may be present on the surface of red blood cells, the type D antigen is widely prevalent and is most likely to elicit an immune response. It is the presence or absence of the D antigen that

determines a person's Rh type. A person with the D antigen is Rh positive, and a person without the D antigen is Rh negative (AABB, 2014; Alexander et al., 2014). Unlike the ABO antigens, naturally occurring antibodies to the Rh(D) antigen do not occur. A person with Rh-negative blood must first be exposed to Rh-positive blood before any Rh antibodies are formed. A person with Rh-negative blood who is exposed to a large volume (200 mL or more) of Rh-positive blood will develop enough antibodies to cause a severe transfusion reaction with repeat exposure. These antibodies take up to 2 weeks to form (AABB, 2014).

- An Rh-negative mother previously exposed to Rh antigen can transfer Rh antibodies across the placenta to an Rh-positive fetus. This can result in severe fetal hemolysis (i.e., the breakdown of red blood cells, with resultant anemia and jaundice) and is often fatal to the infant. To prevent current or future fetal hemolysis, Rh(D) immunoglobulin (RhoGam) is given by intramuscular injection to the mother. RhoGam can suppress or destroy the fetal Rh-positive blood cells that have passed from the fetal to the maternal circulation.

TABLE 30.2

ABO System

Patient Blood Type (Rh Factor)	Red Blood Cell Antigen	Transfuse With Type A	Transfuse With Type B	Transfuse With Type AB	Transfuse With Type O	Transfusion Options
A (+)	A	Yes	No	No	Yes	A+, A– O+, O–
A (–)	A	Yes	No	No	Yes	A–, O–
B (+)	B	No	Yes	No	Yes	B+, B– O+, O–
B (–)	B	No	Yes	No	Yes	B–, O–
AB (+)	AB	Yes	Yes	Yes	Yes	A+, A– B+, B– O+, O– Universal recipient
AB (–)	AB	Yes	Yes	Yes	Yes	A– B– O–
O (+)	None	No	No	No	Yes	O+, O–
O (–)	None	No	No	No	Yes	O– Universal donor

Data from Alexander M et al: *Core curriculum for infusion nursing,* ed 4, Philadelphia, 2014, Lippincott, Williams & Wilkins.

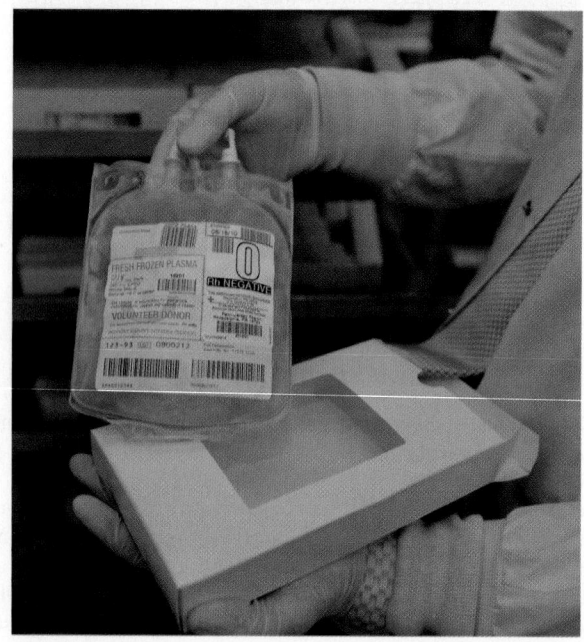

FIG 30.3 Bag of plasma. (*Image courtesy American Red Cross.*)

Human Leukocyte Antigen System

- Although most commonly linked to transplant rejection, HLAs are highly immunogenic antigens that can cause serious transfusion complications. HLA antibodies are located on the cell surface of leukocytes but can be found on all cells of the body (AABB, 2014; Phillips and Gorski, 2014). HLA complications most commonly seen are as follows:
  - Febrile nonhemolytic reaction (FNH)
  - Immune-mediated platelet refractoriness
  - Transfusion-related acute lung injury (TRALI)
  - Transfusion-associated graft-versus-host disease (TA-GVHD)

PATIENT-CENTERED CARE

- When administering blood products, you need to consider a patient's values and cultural and religious beliefs about blood therapy. A person's perception of his or her disease or health condition affects how receptive he or she is to receiving blood. Blood transfusion is often equated to severity of illness.
- Allay patient anxieties when possible and acknowledge their beliefs. A certain religion does not allow blood transfusions or organ donation if it involves blood exchange or the blood has not been removed from the organ (Galanti, 2015).
- When possible, it is helpful to consult a religious leader when caring for patients in need of blood therapy. Be familiar with agency policies and procedures to follow when patients refuse blood transfusions and inform the health care provider of a patient's decision.
- By law parents have the primary obligation to care for and make decisions about their minor children. However, the legal principle of *parens patriae* says that the state has an overriding interest in the health and welfare of its citizens. The parents' refusal can be interpreted as neglect. The nurse's role is to advocate for the patient and family, and he or she may need to identify new, alternative methods of transfusion. If necessary, the nurse coordinates with officials to petition juvenile or family court for temporary guardianship of the child.
- Another aspect of patient-centered care is safety, specifically the prevention of transfusion-related complications. Transfusion-related reactions occur most commonly from human error. To ensure safe patient outcomes, the National Quality Forum (NQF) endorses a list of serious reportable events (SREs), which outlines 28 events that are preventable. Regarding transfusion therapy, any "patient death or serious disability associated with a hemolytic reaction due to the administration of ABO/HLA–incompatible blood or blood products" is considered a Care Management Event and must be reported (NQF, 2011).

EVIDENCE-BASED PRACTICE

Compliance with standards and policies and ongoing education are essential to maintain patient safety and reduce potential errors. Safety and risk management are key factors in transfusion therapy. ABO incompatibilities are one of the most serious errors associated with transfusions and can have fatal outcomes (AABB, 2014; Phillips and Gorski, 2014). A human error most often involves misidentification of the patient or the unit of blood or mislabeling the pretransfusion blood sample. Advances in technology help to decrease transfusion-related errors:

- Bar-code technology helps prevent errors in the identification process between a patient and the compatible blood unit.
- Radiofrequency transponder microchips are used to standardize and document key steps in the blood collection and confirm the recipient–blood unit matching at a patient's bedside.
- Advanced technological laboratory screening procedures also help to ensure safe transfusions with regard to bloodborne pathogens.
- Screening identifies and thereby reduces pathogen transmission.
- Better assessment of blood and plasma cell integrity is available to avoid loss of blood component function.

- Blood alternative therapies with pharmacological developments such as colloids, crystalloids, erythropoietin, antifibrinolytics, and hematinics reduce the risks associated with transfusing human blood.

SAFETY GUIDELINES

- Administration of blood and blood components requires meticulous attention to detail (e.g., preparation, administration, and monitoring) to prevent life-threatening transfusion reactions (Table 30.3).
- Ensure that each blood unit is correctly labeled; check against patient's identification.
- Review agency policy and procedure regarding administration of blood or blood products.
- Two nurses should verify correct unit and correct patient before administration.
- Despite precautions, transfusion therapy carries risks. Compatibility of the patient and donor is essential. Human-related errors (e.g., improper labeling, poor hand-off between nurses and the person transporting blood, or the method used to complete a blood requisition) that may lead to the administration of incompatible transfusions can occur in every step of the

TABLE 30.3

Transfusion Reactions

Reaction	Mechanism	Onset	Signs and Symptoms	Prevention	Nursing Intervention
Febrile, nonhemolytic	Most common type of transfusion reaction; caused by WBC antigen-antibody reaction	May begin early in transfusion or as long as several hours after completion	Temperature increase of 1°C (2°F) or more above baseline, chills, rigors, general malaise	Premedicate as ordered with antipyretics if prior history of reaction. Use leukocyte-reduced blood products	**Stop transfusion.** Change administration set and administer 0.9% sodium chloride at rate to maintain patent IV access. Institute transfusion reaction protocol. Administer antipyretics as ordered to treat fever. Document clinical symptoms, when transfusion was stopped, notification of health care provider and blood bank, nursing interventions and response to interventions, and patient teaching.
Acute hemolytic transfusion reaction	Caused by ABO, Rh incompatibility; donor red cells incompatible with recipient's plasma that can be potentially fatal with as little as 10–15 mL of incompatible blood; usually caused by administration of blood with wrong ABO blood group as a result of misidentification or improper labeling	Within minutes of transfusion initiation	Fever with or without chills, tachycardia, hypotension, lumbar/flank pain, hemoglobinemia, hemoglobinuria, dyspnea, shock, oliguria or anuria, abnormal bleeding	Proper patient identification; proper labeling of blood sample; meticulous verification of ABO/Rh compatibility between donor and recipient before administration	**Stop transfusion.** Change administration set and administer 0.9% sodium chloride at rate to maintain patent IV access. Notify health care provider and blood bank. Monitor vital signs at least every 15 min. Administer ordered therapy to correct arterial blood pressure and coagulopathy. Insert Foley catheter. Monitor intake and output hourly. Assess for shock. Dialysis may be required. Obtain blood and urine samples and send to laboratory with unused part of unit of blood. Document reaction according to agency policy.

Continued

TABLE 30.3

Transfusion Reactions—cont'd

Reaction	Mechanism	Onset	Signs and Symptoms	Prevention	Nursing Intervention
Delayed hemolytic transfusion reaction (extravascular)	ABO, Rh incompatibility. Caused by donor plasma incompatible with recipient's red cells, usually the result of improperly identified blood sample, blood unit, or patient	Several hours after transfusion	Unexplained fever, unexplained decrease in Hgb/Hct, increased bilirubin levels, jaundice	Proper patient identification; proper labeling of blood sample	**Stop transfusion if in progress.** Change administration set and administer 0.9% sodium chloride at rate to maintain patent IV access. Notify health care provider and blood bank immediately. Monitor laboratory values for anemia. (Recognition is important because subsequent transfusions may cause an acute hemolytic reaction.) Most delayed hemolytic reactions require no treatment.
Allergic reaction (mild-to-moderate)	Thought to be caused by sensitivity reaction to foreign plasma protein in transfused product	Within minutes of transfusion initiation	Local erythema; hives; and urticaria, itching, or pruritus	May administer antihistamines before transfusion if prescribed	**Stop transfusion.** Change administration set and administer 0.9% sodium chloride at rate to maintain patent IV access. Notify health care provider and blood bank. Administer antihistamines as ordered. Monitor and document vital signs every 15 min. Transfusion may be restarted if fever, dyspnea, and wheezing are not present.
Allergic reaction (severe)	Caused by recipient allergy to a donor antigen (usually IgA) Agglutination of RBCs obstructing capillaries and blocking blood flow, causing symptoms to all major organ systems	Within minutes of transfusion initiation	Coughing, nausea, vomiting, respiratory distress, wheezing, hypotension, loss of consciousness, possible cardiac arrest	Transfusion of saline-washed or leukocyte-depleted RBCs	**Stop transfusion.** This is a life-threatening reaction. Change administration set and administer 0.9% sodium chloride at rate to maintain patent IV access. Notify health care provider and blood bank. Administer antihistamines, corticosteroids, epinephrine, and antipyretics as ordered. Monitor and document vital signs until stable. Initiate cardiopulmonary resuscitation if necessary.
Graft-versus-host disease	Donor lymphocytes destroyed by recipient's immune system In immunocompromised patients the donor lymphocytes are identified as foreign; however, patient's immune system is not capable of destroying, and in turn patient's lymphocytes are destroyed.	8 to 10 days after transfusion	Skin rash, diarrhea, fever, jaundice caused by liver dysfunction, bone marrow suppression	Administration of irradiated blood and leukocyte-depleted RBC products as prescribed	Administer methotrexate and corticosteroids as ordered for treatment of symptoms.

TABLE 30.3

Transfusion Reactions—cont'd

Reaction	Mechanism	Onset	Signs and Symptoms	Prevention	Nursing Intervention
Circulatory overload	Occurs with transfusion of excessive volume or excessively rapid rate; can lead to pulmonary edema	Anytime during or within 1–2 h after transfusion	Dyspnea, cough, crackles at lung bases, tachypnea, headache, hypertension, tachycardia, increased central venous pressure, distended neck veins	Administration of blood or component at prescribed rate, usually no greater than 2–4 mL/kg/h; particular attention paid to rate and volume in older adults, young children, and patients with cardiac and renal disorders. Administration of PRBCs instead of whole blood. Minimizing amount of saline infused with transfusion	**Slow or stop transfusion** as ordered. Elevate patient's head. Notify health care provider. Administer oxygen and diuretics as ordered. Monitor and document vital signs, including a cardiac and respiratory assessment.
Infectious disease transmission	Microorganism contamination of infused product	During transfusion to 2 h after transfusion. Complete transfusion within 4 h	High fever, chills, abdominal cramping, vomiting, diarrhea, profound hypotension, flushed skin, back pain	Proper care of blood or blood product from time of procurement through end of administration	**Stop transfusion.** Change administration set and maintain patent IV access. Notify health care provider and blood bank. Monitor and document vital signs. Obtain samples for blood culture and Gram stain from recipient. Administer IV fluids, broad-spectrum antimicrobials, vasopressors, and steroids as ordered.
Iron overload	Iron from donated blood binds to protein and is not eliminated	May occur with multiple transfusions or chronic transfusion therapy	Cardiac dysfunction, SOB, arrhythmias, HF, increased serum transferrin, increased liver enzymes, jaundice	Chelation, phlebotomy, monitoring of serum iron levels	Monitor patient for heart failure, cardiac disorder, liver disorder, serum transferrin.

Data modified from Alexander M, et al: *Core curriculum for infusion nursing*, ed 4, St Louis, 2014; American Association of Blood Banks (AABB): *Technical Manual of the American Association of Blood Banks,* ed 18, Bethesda, MD, 2014, American Association of Blood Banks.; and Phillips LD, Gorski L: *Manual of IV therapeutics: evidence-based practice for infusion therapy*, ed 6, Philadelphia, 2014, FA Davis.
Hct, Hematocrit; *HF*, heart failure; *Hgb*, hemoglobin; *IV*, intravenous; *PRBCs*, packed red blood cells; *RBC*, red blood cell; *SOB*, shortness of breath.

process. In addition, disease transmission is also a possibility (Alexander et al., 2014). Comprehensive screening and testing reduce these occurrences considerably; however, the administration of blood and blood products cannot be taken lightly because these complications result from human error during transfusion (Alexander et al., 2014). Complications resulting from immunological response to blood or blood products can be reduced by modifications such as washed or irradiated red blood cells or leukocyte-reduced blood.

◆ SKILL 30.1 Initiating Blood Therapy

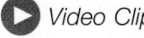 *Video Clip*   **NSO** *Nursing Skills Online Blood Therapy Module / Lessons 1 and 2*

Blood is administered for different clinical indications (Table 30.4). A patient's medical condition determines which blood component is indicated. A health care provider's order is required for the administration of a blood product. A nurse is responsible for understanding which components are appropriate in various situations. In addition, a nurse must ensure that a blood sample has been collected and sent to the laboratory within 72 hours for typing and compatibility screening. The blood sample collector must be meticulous when labeling the blood tube and ensure that it includes the patient's name and identification information based on agency policy (Alexander et al., 2014).

Blood is stored in a refrigerated environment. The refrigeration unit is regulated by the blood bank; blood should not be stored in refrigerators on the unit. In emergency situations rapid transfusion

TABLE 30.4

Blood and Blood Component Products*

Blood Product and Source	Volume and Infusion Time	Able to Transmit HIV/HBV	ABO/RH Testing Needed	Actions/Uses
Whole blood—Single donor: allogeneic or autologous	300–550 mL Within 4 h	Yes	Yes—Must be ABO identical; Rh–Yes	Replaces red cell mass and plasma volume; expected to raise Hgb 1 g/100 mL and Hct by 3% in nonhemorrhaging adult.
Packed RBCs—Single donor: allogeneic or autologous	250–350 mL Within 4 h	Yes	Yes/Yes	Preferred method of replacing RBC mass; expected to raise Hgb/Hct level same as whole blood.
Leukocyte-poor RBCs—Single donor: allogeneic or directed	200–250 mL Within 4 h	Yes	Yes/Yes	Replaces RBCs while preventing febrile, nonhemolytic transfusion reactions; reduces risk for CMV transmission.
Irradiated RBCs—Single donor: allogeneic or directed	250–350 mL Within 4 h	Yes	Yes/Yes	Replaces RBCs while preventing transfusion-associated graft-versus-host disease; used in immunodeficient patients (any blood component can be irradiated).
Fresh frozen plasma—Single donor	200–250 mL Infuse within 24 h of thawing Within 4 h	Yes	Yes/No	Replaces plasma without RBCs or platelets; contains most coagulation factors and complement; used in control of bleeding when replacement of coagulation factors is needed (e.g., DIC, TTP).
Cryoprecipitate—Multiple donors, pooled	5–20 mL/unit; 1 unit/10 kg body weight 1–2 mL/min Infuse within 6 h of thawing or 4 h of pooling	Yes	No/No	Replaces factors VIII, XIII, von Willebrand's factor, and fibrinogen.
Platelets—Multiple/random donor, pooled	40–70 mL/unit; 1 unit/10 kg body weight Within 6 h of pooling	Yes	Yes/Yes	Used in patients with thrombocytopenia. Certain microaggregate filters are not to be used with platelets—check manufacturer instructions.
Platelets—Single donor	200–500 mL Within 4 h	Yes	Yes/Yes	Single-donor platelets are most useful in immunologically refractory patients when given as HLA matched with recipient. Each unit expected to raise platelet count by 5,000–10,000/mL in a 70-kg patient.
Colloid components—Albumin 5% pooled	250–500 mL 1–10 mL/min	No	No/No	Oncotically equivalent to plasma; used to treat hypoproteinemia in burns and hypoalbuminemia in shock and ARDs; used to support blood pressure in dialysis and acute liver failure.
Colloid components—Albumin 25% pooled	50–100 mL 0.2–0.4 mL/min	No	No/No	Increases circulating blood volume by increasing intravascular oncotic pressure.

Data modified from Alexander M, et al: *Core curriculum for infusion nursing,* ed 4, St Louis, 2014; American Association of Blood Banks (AABB): *Technical Manual of the American Association of Blood Banks,* ed 18, Bethesda, Md, 2014, American Association of Blood Banks; and Phillips LD, Gorski L: *Manual of IV therapeutics: evidence-based practice for infusion therapy,* ed 6, Philadelphia, 2014, FA Davis.
ARD, Acute respiratory disease; *CMV,* cytomegalovirus; *DIC,* disseminated intravascular coagulation; *HBV,* hepatitis B virus; *Hct,* hematocrit; *Hgb,* hemoglobin; *HIV,* human immunodeficiency virus; *HLA,* human leukocyte antigen; *RBC,* red blood cell; *TTP,* thrombotic thrombocytopenic purpura.
*Other less commonly used blood components include factors VIII and IX concentrates, granulocytes, immunoglobulin, and saline-washed RBCs.

of cold blood may lead to dysrhythmias and a reduction of core temperature. Sometimes a blood-warmer machine is used for large transfusions of greater than 50 mL/kg/h or patients with cold agglutinins (Fig. 30.4). Do not heat blood products in a microwave or with hot water because this is dangerous and may destroy blood cells and result in hemolysis and severe reactions (Phillips and Gorski, 2014).

Delegation and Collaboration

The skill of initiating transfusion therapy cannot be delegated to nursing assistive personnel (NAP). The skill of initiating transfusion therapy by a licensed practical nurse (LPN) varies by State Practice Acts. After the transfusion has been started and the patient is stable, monitoring a patient by NAP does not relieve a registered nurse (RN) of the responsibility to continue to assess the patient during the transfusion. The nurse instructs the NAP about:

- Frequency of vital sign monitoring needed.
- What to observe such as complaints of shortness of breath, hives, and/or chills and reporting this information to the nurse.
- Obtaining blood components from the blood bank (check agency policy).

Equipment

- Y-type blood administration set (in-line filter) (**NOTE:** Depending on blood product, special tubing and filter are necessary.)
- Prescribed blood product
- 250-mL bag 0.9% sodium chloride (normal saline [NS]) intravenously
- 5- to 10-mL prefilled syringe with preservative-free 0.9% sodium chloride (NS)
- Antiseptic swabs (chlorhexidine solution preferred, povidone-iodine, or 70% alcohol)
- Clean gloves
- Tape
- Vital sign equipment: thermometer, blood pressure cuff, stethoscope, and pulse oximeter
- Signed transfusion consent form

Optional Equipment

- Rapid infusion pump
- Electronic infusion device (EID) (Verify that pump can be used to deliver blood and blood products.)
- *Option:* Leukocyte-depleting filter (**NOTE:** Agency may irradiate blood products within the blood bank.)
- Blood warmer (used mainly when large-volume or rapid transfusion is needed)
- Pressure bag
- Cardiac monitor for emergencies

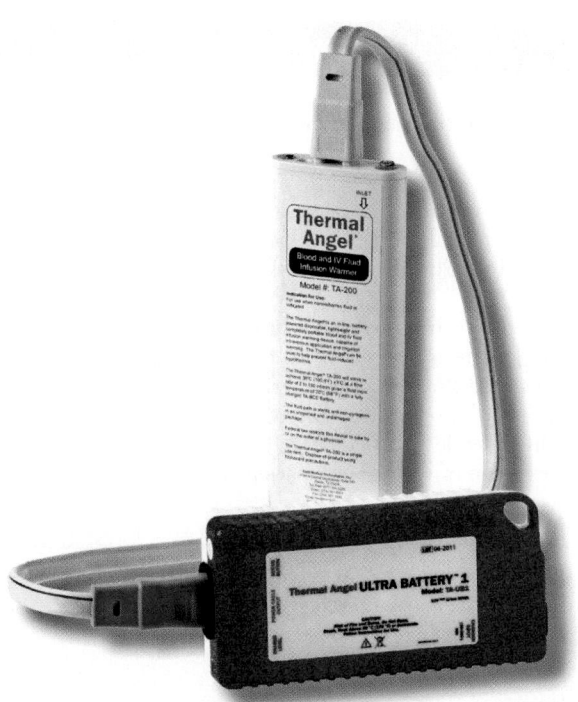

FIG 30.4 Blood-warming system. (*Used with permission of Estill Medical Technologies, Inc. All rights reserved.*)

STEP	RATIONALE

ASSESSMENT

1. Verify health care provider's order for specific blood or blood product with appropriate date, time to begin transfusion, special instructions (i.e., irradiated, leukocyte depleted), duration, and any pretransfusion or posttransfusion medications to administer.

A health care provider's order must be present before transfusing a blood product. Verifying order helps to ensure that appropriate blood component will be administered (AABB, 2014; Alexander et al., 2014; INS, 2016a). Premedications such as an antihistamine or antipyretic may be ordered, especially if patient demonstrated previous transfusion sensitivity.

2. Obtain patient's transfusion history and note known allergies and previous transfusion reactions. Verify that type and cross-match have been completed within 72 hours of transfusion.

Identifies patient's prior response(s) to transfusion of blood components. If patient has experienced reaction in the past, anticipate similar reaction and be prepared to rapidly intervene.

3. Verify that intravenous (IV) cannula is patent and without complications such as infiltration or phlebitis.

Patent IV ensures that transfusion will be infused within established time guidelines.

   a. Administer blood or blood components to an adult through a 14- to 24-gauge short-peripheral catheter with a 18- to 20-gauge appropriate for the general population, and a 14- to 18-gauge when rapid infusion is required (INS, 2016a; Phillips and Gorski, 2014).

The gauge of the IV cannula should be appropriate for accommodating the infusion of blood and/or blood components (INS, 2016a). Large-gauge cannulas promote rapid flow of blood components.

   b. Transfuse a neonate, pediatric, and older adult patient with a 22- to 24-gauge device (INS, 2016a).

Use of smaller cannula gauges such as 24 gauge often requires blood bank to divide the unit so each half can be infused within allotted time or with pressure-assisted devices.

   c. Appropriate-gauge central vascular access device (CVAD) may also be used.

Use of CVAD for administration of blood depends on catheter gauge and manufacturer recommendations for use (Phillips and Gorski, 2014).

4. Assess laboratory values such as hematocrit, coagulation values, platelet count, potassium.

Provides baseline for later evaluation of patient response to transfusion (INS, 2016a).

5. Check that patient has completed and signed transfusion consent properly before retrieving blood.

Informed consent is required before transfusion. The consent form should include risks, benefits, and treatment alternatives; right to accept or refuse transfusion; and opportunity to ask questions (AABB, 2014; INS, 2016a). Administration of albumin does not require informed consent.

STEP	RATIONALE
6. Know indications or reasons for transfusion (e.g., packed red blood cells [PRBCs] for patient with low hematocrit level from gastrointestinal bleeding or surgery blood loss).	Allows you to anticipate patient's response to therapy.
7. Obtain and record pretransfusion baseline vital signs (temperature, pulse, respirations, and blood pressure). If patient is febrile (temperature greater than 37.8°C [100°F]), notify health care provider before initiating transfusion.	Change from baseline vital signs during infusion alerts nurse to potential transfusion reaction or adverse effect of therapy (INS, 2016b; Phillips and Gorski, 2014).
8. Assess patient's need for IV fluids or medications while transfusion is infusing.	If IV medications need to be administered during transfusion, second IV site is necessary. No other infusions are to be administered through same IV site as blood transfusion. Administer blood or blood components only with 0.9% sodium chloride (NS) (INS, 2016a).
9. Assess patient's understanding of procedure and rationale.	Alleviates some of the anxiety patient may have.

NURSING DIAGNOSES

- Activity intolerance
- Altered health protection, risk for infection
- Decreased cardiac output

- Deficient fluid volume
- Deficient knowledge regarding transfusion

- Excess fluid volume
- Ineffective peripheral tissue perfusion

Related factors/Risk factors are individualized based on patient's condition or needs.

PLANNING

1. Expected outcomes following completion of the procedure:	
• Patient verbalizes understanding of rationale for therapy.	Indicates patient's understanding and ability to make informed decision for consent.
• Patient experiences improved activity tolerance.	Oxygenation is improved.
• Mucous membranes are pink, and patient has brisk capillary refill.	Tissue perfusion is improved.
• Patient's cardiac output returns to baseline.	Intravascular volume is restored.
• Patient's systolic blood pressure improves, and urine output is 0.5 to 1 mL/kg/h.	Parameters reflect optimal fluid status and adequate renal blood flow.
• Patient's laboratory values improve in targeted areas (e.g., hematocrit, coagulation values, platelet count).	Indicates that patient responds appropriately to blood or blood component infusion.

IMPLEMENTATION

1. Preadministration protocol:	
a. Obtain blood component from blood bank following agency protocol (see illustration).	Timely acquisition ensures that product is safe to administer. Agency protocol usually encompasses safeguards to ensure quality control throughout transfusion process.

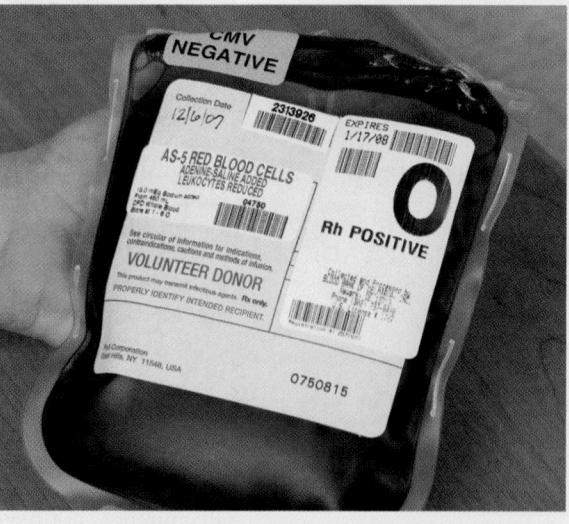

STEP 1a Unit of blood with label.

STEP	RATIONALE

b. Check blood bag for any signs of contamination (i.e., clumping/clots, gas bubbles, purplish color) and presence of leaks.

Blood should not be infused if integrity is compromised. Air bubbles, clumping, clots, and discoloration can be an indication of bacterial contamination or inadequate anticoagulation of stored component and are contraindications for transfusion of that product (Weinstein and Hagle, 2014).

Blood serves as medium for bacterial growth.

c. Verbally compare and correctly verify patient, blood product, and type with another person considered qualified by your agency (e.g., RN or LPN) before initiating transfusion. Check the following:

Strict adherence to verification procedures before administration of blood or blood components reduces risk for administering wrong blood to patient. Misidentification of patient is one of most important factors in transfusion errors (Weinstein and Hagle, 2014).

(1) Identify patient using at least two identifiers (e.g., name and birthday or name and medical record number) according to agency policy. Compare identifiers with information on patient's medication administration record (MAR) or medical record.

Ensures correct patient. Complies with The Joint Commission standards and improves patient safety (TJC, 2016).

(2) Transfusion record number and patient's identification number match.

Prevents accidental administration of wrong component.

Clinical Decision Point *If you notice a discrepancy during verification procedure, do not administer the product. Notify blood bank and appropriate personnel as indicated by agency policy. The product should be returned to the blood bank until the discrepancy is resolved (INS, 2016a; Phillips and Gorski, 2014).*

(3) Patient's name is correct on all documents. Check patient identification number and date of birth on identification band and patient record.

(4) Check unit number on blood bag with blood bank form to ensure that they are the same. Check expiration date and time.

(5) Blood type matches on transfusion record and blood bag. Verify that component received from blood bank is same component that health care provider ordered (e.g., packed red cells, platelets) (see illustration).

Ensures that patient receives correct therapy. Misidentification and improper labeling result in transfusing wrong ABO group (Alexander et al., 2014).

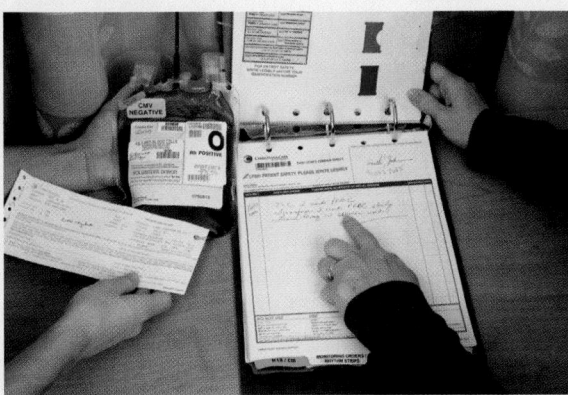

STEP 1c(5) Two clinicians verifying blood type with health care provider order.

(6) Check that patient's blood type and Rh type are compatible with donor blood type and Rh type (e.g., Patient A+: Donor A+ or 0+).

Verifies accurate donor blood type and compatibility.

(7) Check expiration date and time on unit of blood.

Never use expired blood because cell components deteriorate and may contain excess citrate ions. There is also a higher rate of infection with expired blood (AABB, 2014; Weinstein and Hagle, 2014).

STEP	RATIONALE
(8) Just before initiating transfusion, check patient identification information with blood unit label information (see illustration). Do not administer blood to patient without identification bracelet or blood identification bracelet (see agency policy).	Serves as last point of patient and blood confirmation (Phillips and Gorski, 2014).
(9) Both individuals verify patient and unit identification record process as directed by agency policy.	Documentation is legal medical record.
d. Review purpose of transfusion and ask patient to report any changes that he or she may feel during the transfusion.	Signs and symptoms of transfusion reactions include chills, low back pain, shortness of breath, rash, hives, or itching (Alexander et al., 2014). Prompt notification aids in early intervention.
e. Have patient void or apply clean gloves and empty urine drainage collection container.	If transfusion reaction occurs, urine specimen containing urine produced after initiation of transfusion will be sent to laboratory (Weinstein and Hagle, 2014).

Clinical Decision Point *Blood transfusion should be initiated within 30 minutes from time of release from blood bank. If this cannot be completed because of factors such as an elevated temperature, immediately return the blood to the blood bank and retrieve it when you can administer it (Weinstein and Hagle, 2014). It is important that the blood bag not be spiked until you ensure that no factors exist preventing transfusion.*

2. Administration:

a. Perform hand hygiene. Apply clean gloves. Reinspect blood product for signs of leakage or unusual appearance.	Using standard precautions reduces risk for transmission of microorganisms. Provides ongoing verification of blood product.
b. Open Y-tubing blood administration set for single unit. Use multiset if multiple units are to be transfused.	Y-tubing facilitates maintenance of IV line access with NS in case patient will need more than 1 unit of blood.
c. Set all clamp(s) to "off" position.	Setting clamps to "off" position prevents accidentally spilling and wasting product.
d. Use aseptic technique and spike bag of 0.9% sodium chloride (NS) IV bag with one of Y-tubing spikes. Hang bag on IV pole and prime tubing. Open upper clamp on normal saline side of tubing and squeeze drip chamber until fluid covers filter and one third to one half of drip chamber (see illustration).	Primes tubing with fluid to eliminate air in Y-tubing. Closing clamp prevents spillage and waste of fluid.

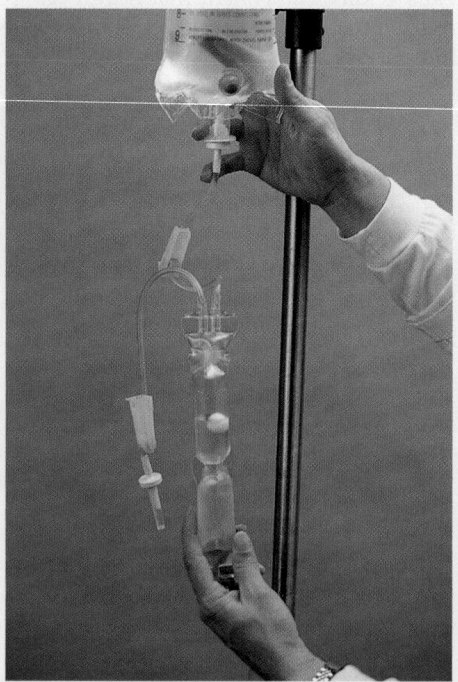

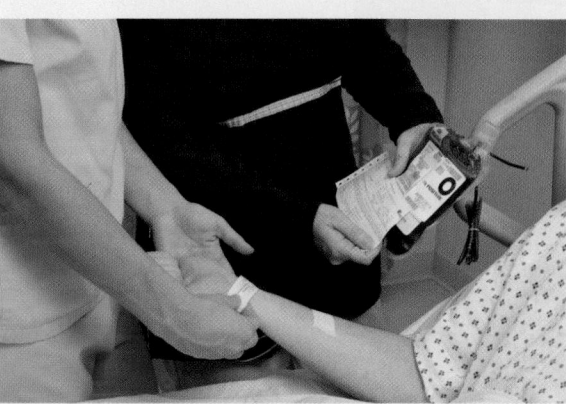

STEP 1c(8) Two clinicians verifying identification of patient and blood product.

STEP 2d Blood administration set primed with normal saline.

STEP	RATIONALE

e. Maintain clamp on blood product side of Y-tubing in "off" position. Open common tubing clamp to finish priming tubing to distal end of tubing connector. Close tubing clamp when tubing is filled with saline. All three tubing clamps should be closed. Maintain protective sterile cap on tubing connector.

This will completely prime tubing with saline, and IV line is ready to be connected to patient's vascular access device (VAD).

f. Prepare blood component for administration. Gently invert bag two or three times, turning back and forth. Remove protective covering from access port. Spike blood component unit with other Y-connection. Close normal saline clamp above filter, open clamp above filter to blood unit, and prime tubing with blood. Blood will flow into drip chamber (see illustration). Tap filter chamber to ensure that residual air is removed.

Gentle agitation suspends red blood cells in anticoagulant. Protective barrier drape may be used to catch any potential blood spillage. Tubing is primed with blood unit and ready for transfusion into patient.

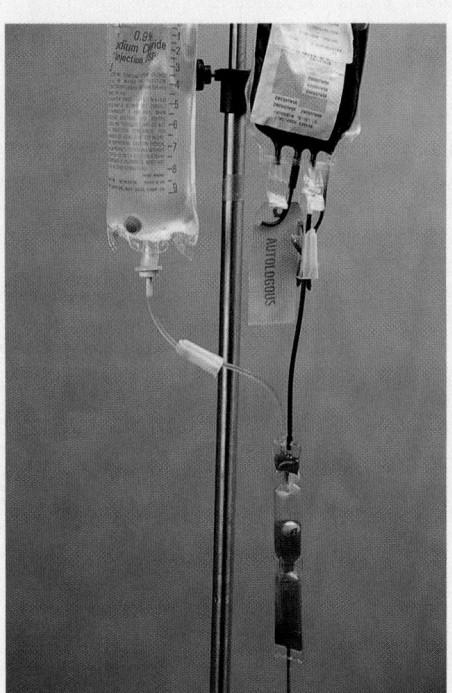

STEP 2f Unit of blood connected to Y-tubing setup.

Clinical Decision Point *NS is compatible with blood products, unlike solutions that contain dextrose, which cause coagulation of blood. Only use 0.9% sodium chloride (NS) to administer blood. No other solutions are to be administered with blood (piggybacked) (AABB, 2014; INS, 2016a).*

g. Maintaining asepsis, attach primed tubing to patient's VAD by first cleansing the catheter hub with an antiseptic swab. Then quickly connect NS-primed blood administration tubing directly to patient's VAD.

Reduces transmission of microorganisms from catheter hub. This initiates infusion of blood product into patient's vein.

h. Open common tubing clamp and regulate blood infusion to allow only 2 mL/min to infuse in initial 15 minutes. Remain with patient during first 15 minutes of transfusion. Initial flow rate during this time should be 1–2 mL/min or 10–20 gtt/min (using macrodrip of 10 gtt/mL).

Many transfusion reactions occur within first 15 minutes of transfusion (Phillips and Gorski, 2014). Infusing small amount of blood component initially minimizes volume of blood to which patient is exposed, thereby minimizing severity of reaction (Phillips and Gorski, 2014).

Clinical Decision Point *If signs of a transfusion reaction occur, **stop the transfusion,** start 0.9% sodium chloride (NS) with a new primed tubing attached directly to the VAD hub, and notify the health care provider immediately (see Skill 30.2). Do not discard the blood product or tubing because they need to be returned to the blood bank. Do not infuse saline through existing tubing because it will cause blood in tubing to enter patient.*

STEP	RATIONALE
i. Monitor patient's vital signs within 5 to 15 minutes of initiating transfusion and at completion of transfusion (AABB, 2014; Phillips and Gorski, 2014) or according to agency policy.	Frequently monitoring patient helps to quickly alert you to transfusion reaction (Weinstein and Hagle, 2014).
j. If there is no transfusion reaction, regulate rate of transfusion according to health care provider's orders based on drop factor for blood administration tubing (see Chapter 29).	Maintaining prescribed rate of flow decreases risk for fluid volume excess while restoring vascular volume. Drop factor for most blood tubing is 10 gtt/mL.

Clinical Decision Point *Do not let a unit of blood hang for more than 4 hours because of danger of bacterial growth. When a longer transfusion time is indicated clinically, the unit may be divided by the blood bank, and the part not being transfused can be properly refrigerated (Phillips and Gorski, 2014). Administration sets should be changed at the completion of each unit or every 4 hours to reduce bacterial contamination (INS, 2016a). Blood should only be stored in a refrigerator specific for blood or blood products to maintain appropriate temperature controls.*

Clinical Decision Point *Medications and solutions should not be infused into the same IV line with a blood component because of the possibility of incompatibility unless the drug or solution has been approved by the Food and Drug Administration (FDA) for use with blood administration. Maintain a separate IV access if patient requires IV solutions or medications (Phillips and Gorski, 2014).*

STEP	RATIONALE
k. After blood has infused, clear IV line with 0.9% sodium chloride (NS) and discard blood bag according to agency policy. When consecutive units are ordered, line patency with 0.9% sodium chloride (NS) at keep vein open (KVO) rate as ordered by health care provider and retrieve subsequent unit for administration.	Infusing IV NS allows remainder of blood in IV tubing to infuse and keeps IV line patent for supportive measures in case of transfusion reaction (Phillips and Gorski, 2014). KVO rate must specify infusion rate as required by rights of medication administration.
l. Appropriately dispose of all supplies. Remove gloves and perform hand hygiene.	Standard precautions during transfusion reduce transmission of microorganisms.

EVALUATION

1. Observe IV site and status of infusion each time vital signs are taken.	Detects presence of IV-related complications (e.g., infiltration, occlusion, phlebitis) and verifies continuous and safe infusion of blood product.
2. Observe for any signs of transfusion reactions such as chills, flushing, itching, dyspnea, or rash.	Compare presenting signs and symptoms to baseline assessment of patient before transfusion. These are early signs of transfusion reaction (see Table 30.3).
3. Observe patient and assess laboratory values to determine response to administration of blood component.	Aids in determining whether goals of therapy have been reached or if further blood component therapy will be required. Laboratory results may not reflect transfusion reaction for several hours.
4. Use Teach-Back: "I want to be sure that I explained the reason for your blood transfusion, including the risks and benefits? How can this transfusion help you?" Revise your instruction now or develop a plan for revised patient or family caregiver teaching if patient or family caregiver is not able to teach back correctly.	Determines patient's and family caregiver's level of understanding of instructional topic.

STEP	RATIONALE
Unexpected Outcomes	**Related Interventions**
1. Patient displays signs and symptoms of transfusion reaction such as chills, flushing, itching, dyspnea, or rash.	• Stop transfusion immediately. • Disconnect blood tubing at VAD hub and cap distal end with sterile connector to maintain sterile system. • Connect new normal saline solution and primed tubing directly to VAD hub to prevent any subsequent blood from infusing into patient from tubing. • Keep vein open with slow infusion of normal saline at 1–2 mL/min to ensure venous patency and maintain venous access for medication or to resume transfusion. • Notify health care provider. • See Table 30.3 for interventions.
2. Patient develops infiltration or phlebitis at venipuncture site.	• Transfusion should be stopped at first sign of infiltration, and IV line removed (see Procedural Guideline 29.1). • Insert new VAD in area above previous location or opposite arm. • Restart product if remainder can be infused within 4 hours of initiation of transfusion. • Institute nursing measures to reduce discomfort at infiltrated or phlebitic area.
3. Fluid volume overload occurs, and/or patient exhibits difficulty breathing or has crackles on auscultation of lungs.	• Slow or stop transfusion, elevate head of bed, and inform health care provider of physical findings. • Administer diuretics, morphine, and/or oxygen as ordered by health care provider. • Continue frequent assessments and closely monitor vital signs and intake and output.

Recording and Reporting

• Before transfusion record pretransfusion medications, vital signs, location and condition of IV site, and patient education in nurses' notes in electronic health record (EHR) or chart.
• Record the type and volume of blood component, blood unit/donor/recipient identification, compatibility, and expiration date according to agency policy, along with patient's response to therapy. Document on the transfusion record in nurses' notes in EHR or chart, medication administration record, flow sheet, and/or intake and output sheet, depending on agency policy.
• Record volume of NS and blood component infused.
• Record amount of blood received by autotransfusion and patient's response to therapy.
• Record vital signs before, shortly after initiation, and after transfusion.
• Document your evaluation of patient and family caregiver learning.
• Report signs and symptoms of a transfusion reaction immediately to the health care provider.
• Report to health care provider any intratransfusion/posttransfusion deterioration in cardiac, pulmonary, and/or renal status.

Special Considerations
Teaching

• Instruct patient and family caregiver regarding rationale for transfusion and anticipated amount of time for completion of transfusion.
• Discuss with patient and family caregiver the rationale for patient monitoring throughout transfusion.
• Instruct patient and family caregiver to notify nurse if patient experiences itching, swelling, dizziness, dyspnea, low back pain,

and/or chest pain because these may indicate a transfusion reaction.
• Instruct patient to inform nurse if redness, pain, tenderness, swelling, bleeding, drainage, or leaking from under dressing occurs at IV site.

Pediatric

• Infuse the first 50 mL or 20% of volume (whichever is smaller) of a blood transfusion very slowly in a pediatric patient. Nurse should stay with the child during this time frame (Hockenberry and Wilson, 2015).
• Smaller portions of blood are often available for use with pediatric patients (AABB, 2014).
• A 22- or 24-gauge cannula can be used to infuse PRBCs in small veins that do not need rapid flow rates (Alexander et al., 2014).
• Umbilical catheters or catheters placed in the small saphenous veins may be used in infants and/or pediatric patients (Alexander et al., 2014).

Gerontological

• Some older adults have decreased cardiac function, thus requiring a slower infusion time. Half units may be obtained if a patient is unable to tolerate the volume in a whole unit of blood or blood component.
• In older adults at risk for circulatory overload, regulate flow rate at 1 mL/kg/h.

Home Care

• Patients who have had prior transfusion reactions, acute angina, or heart failure are not good candidates for home transfusion.
• Nursing personnel must be present during the entire transfusion process and for 30 to 60 minutes after transfusion.

- Blood and blood products must be transported in a container with appropriate coolant. Verify and record the temperature at time of delivery.
- Initiate the transfusion as soon as possible after component is obtained from blood bank.
- When blood sample is obtained for blood typing and cross-matching, attach identification band to patient with full name and identification number used by laboratory. This provides clear identification of patient when blood component transfusion is initiated.

- Instruct patient and family caregiver regarding signs and symptoms of a delayed hemolytic transfusion reaction (i.e., unexplained fever, decrease in hemoglobin and hematocrit levels 2 to 14 days after transfusion) so they can report them and receive treatment if necessary.
- Return the container, empty bags, and tubing to the home care agency after completion of the transfusion.

◆ SKILL 30.2   Monitoring for Adverse Transfusion Reactions

NSO | *Nursing Skills Online Blood Therapy Module / Lesson 3*

Adverse transfusion reactions may occur any time during a transfusion of blood products. Life-threatening reactions usually occur within the first 15 minutes of transfusion. Remain with a patient during this time to monitor physiological responses.

Several types of adverse reactions may result from a blood transfusion (see Table 30.3). A hemolytic reaction is a systemic response to the administration of a blood product that is incompatible with that of the recipient. The product contains allergens to which the recipient is sensitive or allergic, or it is contaminated with pathogens. Some patients who have a history of frequent transfusion may receive premedication with diphenhydramine to combat acquired sensitivities.

Before a transfusion each blood unit undergoes extensive serological testing to reduce the risk for patients acquiring a bloodborne disease. Symptoms that indicate an adverse reaction range from fever, chills, and skin rash to hypotension and cardiac arrest. Some patients also experience a delayed transfusion reaction, which sometimes does not occur for days or weeks after the transfusion (AABB, 2014; Alexander et al., 2014). Other possible adverse outcomes that result from transfusion therapy include transmission

of diseases, circulatory overload, and transfusion-related acute lung injury (TRALI), characterized by noncardiogenic pulmonary edema with an onset within 6 hours of transfusion (Alexander et al., 2014; Phillips and Gorski, 2014). The most fatal risk for transfusion-associated death is the erroneous transfusion of ABO-incompatible allogeneic units (Phillips and Gorski, 2014). Agencies must report fatalities that occur as the result of a transfusion reaction to the Food and Drug Administration (NQF, 2011).

Delegation and Collaboration

The skill of monitoring for adverse blood transfusion reactions by a licensed practical nurse (LPN) varies by state Nurse Practice acts. After the transfusion has been started and the patient is stable, monitoring a patient by nursing assistive personnel (NAP) does not relieve a registered nurse (RN) of the responsibility to continue to assess the patient during the transfusion. The nurse instructs the NAP about:

- Frequency of vital sign monitoring needed.
- The signs and symptoms of a transfusion reaction that patient may exhibit and to immediately report these to the nurse.

STEP	RATIONALE
ASSESSMENT	
1. Identify patient using at least two identifiers (e.g., name and birthday or name and medical record number) according to agency policy.	Ensures correct patient. Complies with The Joint Commission standards and improves patient safety (TJC, 2016).
2. With initiation of a transfusion, observe patient for fever with or without chills.	Fever indicates onset of acute hemolytic reaction, febrile nonhemolytic reaction, or bacterial sepsis.
3. Assess patient for tachycardia and/or tachypnea and dyspnea.	Indicates acute hemolytic reaction or circulatory overload. In case of circulatory overload, cough may accompany these symptoms.
4. Observe patient for drop in blood pressure.	Hypotension indicates infectious disease transmission, an acute hemolytic reaction, and anaphylaxis.
5. Observe patient for hives or skin rash, including assessment of trunk and back.	These are early indications of an allergic reaction, anaphylaxis, or graft-versus-host disease, which occurs after transfusion.
6. Observe patient for flushing.	Early indication of acute hemolytic reaction or febrile nonhemolytic reaction. Sometimes localized flushing presents with an allergic reaction.
7. Observe patient for gastrointestinal symptoms.	Nausea and vomiting are present in acute hemolytic transfusion reactions, anaphylactic reactions, or infectious disease transmission.
8. Observe patient for wheezing, chest pain, and possible cardiac arrest.	These are all indications of anaphylactic reaction.
9. Be alert to patient complaints of headache or muscle pain in presence of fever.	Both indicate febrile nonhemolytic reaction.

STEP	RATIONALE
10. Monitor patient for disseminated intravascular coagulation (DIC), renal failure, anemia, and hemoglobinemia/hemoglobinuria by reviewing laboratory test results (complete blood count [CBC] with differential, hemoglobin [Hgb], hematocrit [Hct]).	All are late signs of an acute hemolytic reaction.
11. Auscultate patient's lungs before and during transfusion and monitor central venous pressure (CVP) if possible.	Crackles in bases of lungs and rising CVP are indications of circulatory overload.
12. Observe patient for jaundice and increased liver enzyme levels, indicating liver damage; and decreased red blood cells (RBCs), white blood cells (WBCs), and platelets, indicating bone marrow suppression.	These indicate graft-versus-host disease and would occur following transfusion.
13. In patients receiving massive transfusions, observe for mild hypothermia, cardiac dysrhythmias, hypotension, hypocalcemia, and hemochromatosis (iron overload).	Cold blood products affect cardiac conduction system, resulting in ventricular dysrhythmias. Other cardiac dysrhythmias, hypotension, and tingling indicate hypocalcemia, which occurs when citrate (used as a preservative for some blood products) combines with patient's calcium. Iron overload may occur after 10 transfusions (see Table 30.3). It usually occurs in patients who require chronic transfusions.

NURSING DIAGNOSES

- Acute pain
- Anxiety
- Decreased cardiac output
- Excess fluid volume
- Hyperthermia
- Hypothermia
- Impaired gas exchange
- Risk for infection

Related factors/Risk factors are individualized based on patient's condition or needs.

PLANNING

1. Expected outcomes following completion of procedure:	
• Patient's cardiac parameters (heart rate, blood pressure, CVP) return to baseline.	Intravascular volume is restored, reaction reversed.
• Patient maintains core body temperature of 36° to 37.2°C (97° to 99°F).	Helps to confirm absence of transfusion reaction, infection, and sepsis.
• Patient has urine output of 0.5 to 1 mL/kg/h.	Reflects optimal fluid status.
• Patient maintains oxygen saturation greater than 95%.	Improved tissue perfusion.
• Patient is comfortable.	Absence of transfusion reaction. Appropriate nursing measures keeps patient at ease.
2. Patient is able to explain signs and symptoms of a transfusion reaction.	Calms anxiety and helps patient/family caregiver anticipate nurse's actions.

IMPLEMENTATION

1. If you suspect transfusion reaction:	
a. **Immediately stop transfusion.**	Severity of reaction is related to amount of blood component infused and cause of reaction. It is critical to prevent any more blood from infusing into patient.
b. Remove blood component and tubing containing blood product. Replace them with new bag of 0.9% sodium chloride (normal saline [NS]) and tubing (see Chapter 29). Connect tubing directly to hub of vascular access device (VAD). *Exception:* If patient symptoms suggest mild allergic reaction, stop transfusion, administer antihistamine, and restart or discontinue transfusion per health care provider's order.	Prevents additional blood in tubing from being infused.
c. Maintain patent VAD using 0.9% sodium chloride (NS) at rate prescribed by health care provider.	NS keeps patent IV and provides route for emergency medications and fluids.
d. Obtain vital signs. Remain with patient for continuous monitoring and assessment. Do not leave patient alone.	Vital signs are objective measure of patient's condition, which can deteriorate rapidly.

STEP	RATIONALE
e. Notify health care provider.	Transfusion reactions require immediate medical intervention. Follow protocol for emergency interventions for anaphylactic reactions.
f. Notify blood bank.	Blood bank has procedure to follow when notified of transfusion reaction.
g. Obtain blood samples (if needed) from extremity opposite extremity receiving transfusion. Check agency policy regarding number and type of tubes to be used.	Typically one tube of blood will be cross-matched to pretransfusion sample to ensure that correct blood was given to recipient. Blood will be checked for antibodies to determine type of reaction. Second sample will be checked for free hemoglobin in serum, indicating hemolysis, and bilirubin level should be obtained.
h. Return remainder of blood component and attached blood tubing to blood bank according to agency policy.	Sample of this blood will be cross-matched to patient's pretransfusion and posttransfusion samples to determine if error in cross-matching occurred.
i. Monitor patient's vital signs every 15 minutes or per agency policy.	Maintains ongoing assessment of patient's cardiopulmonary status and response to treatment.
j. Administer prescribed medications according to type and severity of transfusion reaction.	Follow medical protocol or health care provider's orders.
(1) Epinephrine	Stimulates sympathetic nervous system to relieve respiratory distress and combat vasodilation in anaphylaxis.
(2) Antihistamine	Diminishes some aspects of allergic response by blocking histamine receptors.
(3) Antibiotics	Administered when bacterial contamination/sepsis is suspected.
(4) Antipyretics/analgesics	Administered to relieve fever and discomfort in acute hemolytic reactions, febrile nonhemolytic reactions, graft-versus-host disease, and bacterial sepsis.
(5) Diuretics/morphine	Treats circulatory overload by reducing intravascular volume (diuresis) and decreasing vascular tone (opioid effect).
(6) Corticosteroids	Stabilizes cell membranes, decreasing histamine release. Administered in severe allergic reactions.
(7) Intravenous (IV) fluids	Rapid administration of IV fluids counteracts some symptoms of anaphylactic shock.
k. In event of cardiac arrest, initiate cardiopulmonary resuscitation (see Chapter 28).	Anaphylaxis can quickly lead to cardiopulmonary arrest. Prompt resuscitation may prevent further complications.
l. Obtain first voided urine sample and send to laboratory. You may need to insert Foley catheter to obtain urine (see Chapter 34).	Hemoglobinuria occurs with acute hemolytic reactions. Degree of damage to kidneys is influenced by pH of urine and rate of urinary excretion. Attempts will be made to initiate diuresis and alkalinize urine. If kidney damage is severe, dialysis may be required.

EVALUATION

1. Continue monitoring patient for signs and symptoms of transfusion reactions.	Continued monitoring of patient's cardiopulmonary status and physiological response will indicate if reaction has been reversed.
2. **Use Teach-Back:** "I want to be sure that I explained the reactions that can occur when you are getting a blood transfusion. What signs and symptoms you would report?" Revise your instruction now or develop a plan for revised patient and family caregiver teaching if patient or family caregiver is not able to teach back correctly.	Determines patient's and family caregiver's level of understanding of instructional topic.

Unexpected Outcomes	**Related Interventions**
1. Patient's physiological status worsens.	• Appropriate interventions depend on type of transfusion reaction. Table 30.3 provides general guidelines.

Recording and Reporting

- Document the exact time transfusion reaction was first noted, all vital signs and other physiological assessments, treatments instituted, and patient response in nurses' notes in electronic health record (EHR) or chart. Complete transfusion reaction report (see agency policy).
- Document your evaluation of patient and family caregiver learning.
- Immediately report presence of transfusion reaction and patient's physical assessment findings to nurse in charge and health care provider.

Special Considerations
Teaching

- Teach patient and family caregiver signs and symptoms of transfusion reactions and steps to take if they occur.

Pediatric

- Irradiated RBCs and platelets are preferable in children under 6 years of age because of their immature immune systems and to avoid graft-versus-host disease.

Gerontological

- Administer blood components cautiously to older adults, considering both rate and amount of infusion, because they are at risk for developing circulatory overload.

Home Care

- Certain adverse outcomes (development of hepatitis) or transfusion reactions (delayed hemolysis) occur days to weeks after patient has received transfusion and may become evident in the home setting. It is important that patient, family caregiver, and home care workers be aware of signs and symptoms of adverse occurrences and steps to be taken should they occur.

◆ CLINICAL DEBRIEF

A 72-year-old man is admitted for a hip replacement and has donated 1 unit of autologous blood in the event that he needed transfusion therapy after surgery. Three weeks earlier his surgery was postponed because he had a case of pneumonia that required treatment with antibiotics. While he was awaiting hip surgery, he developed bleeding hemorrhoids that were surgically repaired yesterday. Today he tells you that he is very tired, and he passed a great deal of blood with several bowel movements during the night and earlier this morning. His coloring is pale, and skin is cool to the touch. Blood pressure has dropped since admission from 130/80 mm Hg to 100/66 mm Hg. His health care provider told him that he may need a blood transfusion. He had blood drawn this morning, and his hematocrit has dropped from 32% to 27%. The patient states that he is very concerned about being transfused, and he thinks that the blood he donated will not be good since it was over a month ago.

1. Based on his concerns, which items would be assessed in preparation for a blood transfusion?
2. After you obtain the unit of packed red blood cells (PRBCs) from the blood bank, the patient is taken for a procedure to stop the rectal bleeding that will last 1 to 2 hours before starting the blood transfusion. Which actions would you take while waiting for him to return?
3. About 30 minutes after initiating the first unit of packed red blood cells (PRBCs), he reports that he is itchy all over his body and presents with a rash and hives. Using SBAR, show how you would communicate with the health care team about this patient.

◆ REVIEW QUESTIONS

1. Which of the following steps are necessary for initiating a transfusion of packed red blood cells (PRBCs)? (Select all that apply.)
   1. Infuse blood component with 5% dextrose (D₅W).
   2. Follow agency policy to verify correct patient and blood product.

   3. Check appearance of blood for leaks, bubbles, clots, or purplish color.
   4. Infuse blood component over 4–6 hours to prevent fluid volume overload.
   5. Obtain vital signs before, after 5 to 15 minutes of initiating infusion, and at completion.
   6. Clear IV line with 0.9% saline after transfusion.
2. Your patient is experiencing an acute hemolytic transfusion reaction while receiving packed red blood cells (PRBCs). Place the following steps in the correct order:
   1. Obtain vital signs and remain with the patient.
   2. Stop the infusion.
   3. Obtain blood and urine samples.
   4. Replace the blood component and tubing with a new bag of 0.9% sodium chloride (normal saline [NS]) and new tubing.
   5. Notify the blood bank.
   6. Notify the health care provider.
3. Which of the following items must be verified to ensure that the correct blood component is transfused to the correct patient? (Select all that apply.)
   1. Verbally compare and correctly identify the patient's identity using two patient identifiers.
   2. Verify that the transfusion record number matches the patient's identification number.
   3. Check that the expiration date is not passed.
   4. Confirm that blood collection date is within 72 hours of the transfusion.
   5. Have two qualified individuals perform verifications before initiation of transfusion.
   6. Verify that the blood component and type to be infused match the patient's.

ⓔ *Visit the Evolve site for a complete list of Clinical Debrief and Review Questions answers.*

REFERENCES

Alexander M, et al: *Core curriculum for infusion nursing*, ed 4, Philadelphia, 2014, Lippincott, Williams & Wilkins.

American Association of Blood Banks (AABB): *Technical Manual of the American Association of Blood Banks*, ed 18, Bethesda, MD, 2014, American Association of Blood Banks.

Galanti GA: *Caring for patients from different cultures*, ed 5, Philadelphia, 2015.

Hockenberry MJ, Wilson D: *Wong's nursing care of infants and children*, ed 10, St Louis, 2015.

Infusion Nurses Society: Infusion therapy standards of practice, *J Intraven Nurs* 39(Suppl 1):1S, 2016a.

Infusion Nurses Society (INS): *Policy and procedures for infusion therapy*, ed 5, Norwood, MA, 2016b, INS.

National Quality Forum (NQF): *National voluntary consensus standards for patient safety: a consensus report*, Washington, DC, 2011, http://www.qualityforum.org/Publications/2011/02/Pt_safety_reporting_full.aspx. Accessed April 3, 2016.

Phillips LD, Gorski L: *Manual of IV therapeutics: evidence-based practice for infusion therapy*, ed 6, Philadelphia, 2014, FA Davis.

The Joint Commission (TJC): *2016 National Patient Safety Goals*, Oakbrook Terrace, IL, 2016, http://www.jointcommission.org/standards_information/npsgs.aspx. Accessed April 3, 2016.

Weinstein S, Hagle M: *Plumer's principles and practice of infusion therapy*, Philadelphia, 2014, Lippincott, Williams & Wilkins.

31 | Oral Nutrition

OBJECTIVES

Mastery of content in this chapter will enable the nurse to:
- Perform an accurate nutritional screening.
- Identify the need and collaborate with registered dietitian for a patient's nutritional assessment.
- Assess a patient's ability to swallow.
- Identify risk factors for aspiration.
- Evaluate a patient's tolerance of oral nutrition.
- Identify appropriate techniques to use to prevent a patient from aspirating.
- Demonstrate how to properly feed a patient who cannot self-feed.

MEDIA RESOURCES

- evolve http://evolve.elsevier.com/Perry/skills
- Review Questions
- ▶ Video Clips
- Audio Glossary
- Clinical Debrief and Review Questions Answers

PURPOSE

Nutrition is a basic component of health that affects a patient's rate of recovery from short-term and chronic illness, surgery, and injury. Malnutrition develops as a result of deficiency in dietary intake, increased requirements associated with a disease state, complications of an underlying illness such as poor absorption and excessive nutrient losses, or a combination of all of these factors (Barker et al., 2011).

Malnutrition is a major concern for older adults and patients with limited financial resources is malnutrition. In addition, it is a debilitating and highly prevalent condition for patients in acute hospital settings (Barker et al., 2011). The function and recovery of every organ system is affected by malnutrition. Complications from malnutrition include alterations in muscle, cardiorespiratory and gastrointestinal function, immune function, wound healing, and psychosocial effects. The Joint Commission (TJC, 2015) requires routine identification of malnutrition with screening of patients in health care settings. As a nurse you will provide nutritional screening and collaborate with registered dietitians and health care providers to determine the safest and best approaches for supporting patients' nutritional health.

STANDARDS OF CARE

- Academy of Nutrition and Dietetics, 2012— Nutrition for Older Adults
- *Healthy People 2020*, 2014—Nutrition and Weight Status
- The Joint Commission (TJC), 2015, 2016—Nutritional Screening, Patient Identification
- US Department of Agriculture (USDA) and US Department of Health and Human Services (USDHHS), 2015—Dietary Guidelines for Americans
- US Department of Agriculture (USDA): ChooseMyPlate, 2015—MyPlate Guidelines

PRINCIPLES FOR PRACTICE

- For hospitalized patients nutritional screening must be completed within 24 hours of a patient's admission to a hospital, within 14 days of admission to a long-term care facility, or within an agency-defined period of time in ambulatory and home care settings (TJC, 2015).
- When performing a nutritional screening, an aim is to identify common risk factors for nutritional problems (Box 31.1).
- Nutrition assessment is suggested for all patients who are identified to be at nutrition risk by nutrition screening (ASPEN, 2011). A thorough assessment is performed by a registered dietitian. Recommendations for improving nutritional status such as change in diet, alternative feeding methods, or further medical assessment and intervention stem from nutritional assessments.
- In an acute care setting quality nutritional care requires you to document weight and appetite loss and collaborate with health care providers to make dietary referrals.
- Patients who are malnourished have an increased length of hospital stay, and they are prone to experiencing more complications (e.g., infection rates, mortality) during their period of hospitalization than patients who are in a well-nourished state.

BOX 31.1

Risk Factors for Potential Nutritional Problems

- Clear- or full-liquid diets for more than 3 days without nutrient supplementation or with inappropriate or insufficient nutrient supplementation
- Intravenous feeding (dextrose and saline or saline) or NPO for more than 3 days without nutrient supplementation
- Low intake of prescribed diet or tube feedings
- Weight 20% above or 10% below desirable body weight (accounting for edema)
- Pregnancy weight gain deviating from normal patterns
- Diagnoses that increase nutritional needs or decrease nutrient intake (or both): cancer, malabsorption, diarrhea, hyperthyroidism, excessive inflammation, postoperative status, hemorrhage, infected or draining wounds, burns, infection, major trauma
- Chronic use of drugs, especially alcohol, which affects nutritional intake
- Alterations in chewing, swallowing, appetite, taste, and smell
- Body temperature consistently above 37° C (98.6° F) for more than 2 days
- Hematocrit: less than 43% in men, less than 37% in women; hemoglobin less than 14 g/dL in men, less than 12 g/dL in women
- Absolute decrease in lymphocyte count (less than 1500 cells/mm³)
- Elevated (greater than 250 mg/dL) or decreased (less than 130 mg/dL) total plasma cholesterol
- Serum albumin less than 3 g/dL in patients without renal or liver disease, generalized dermatitis, overhydration
- Remaining *NPO* (nothing by mouth)

Modified from Grodner M, et al: *Foundations and clinical applications of nutrition: a nursing approach,* ed 5, St Louis, 2012, Mosby.

- As a nurse you are responsible for preparing patients who are on oral diets by offering the type of assistance needed to help them successfully eat an adequate amount of food at a safe and comfortable pace.
- *Dietary Guidelines for Americans* was released in February 2015 and targets individuals 2 years and older (USDA and USDHHS, 2015). Dietary guidelines are reviewed regularly and modified based on the most current evidence related to nutrition, physical activity, and health. The intent is to promote health, reduce the risk of chronic diseases, and provide the basis for federal food and nutrition policy and education initiatives. The 2015 guidelines focus on foods and beverages that help achieve and maintain a healthy weight, promote health, and prevent disease.

PATIENT-CENTERED CARE

- An understanding of your patients' values, beliefs, and attitudes about food and how these values affect food purchase, preparation, and intake will allow you to help your patients make healthy food choices.
- Most Americans need to improve some aspect of their diet. A number of social factors influence diet. As a nurse, collaborate with a registered dietitian in considering a patient's: knowledge and attitudes about food and health, skills in being able to feed self and properly store and prepare food, social support, access and use of food assistance programs, and the economic price system affecting a patient (*Healthy People 2020,* 2014a).
- Individuals follow special patterns of food intake based on religion, cultural background, ethics, health beliefs, or concern about the environment. Such special diets (e.g., vegetarian, ovolactovegetarian) do not necessarily provide more or less

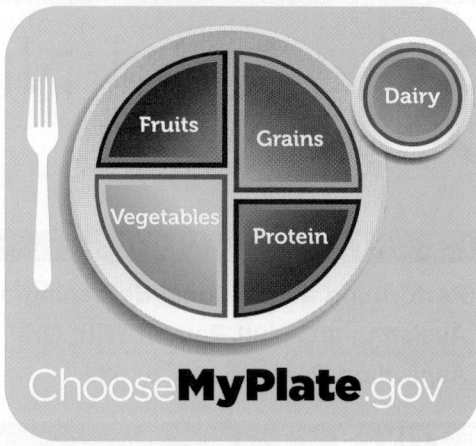

FIG 31.1 MyPlate showing the five essential food groups. *(From US Department of Agriculture [USDA] MyPlate.gov: ChooseMyPlate, 2010, http://www.choosemyplate.gov/. Accessed April 5, 2016.)*

nutritional benefit than diets based on ChooseMyPlate or other nutritional guidelines (USDA, 2015).
- Some cultures believe in the hot-and-cold theory of health and illness. Foods are classified as cold or hot based on their characteristics, independent of the temperature at which they are served. There is no universal agreement across cultures about which foods are hot and which foods are cold.
- The ChooseMyPlate program was developed by the US Department of Agriculture (USDA, 2015) (Fig. 31.1). ChooseMyPlate aims to help the American population choose healthier food and confront the obesity epidemic by providing a basic, visual guide for making food choices for a healthy lifestyle. A nurse's role is to match patient food preferences with healthier food choices when possible.

EVIDENCE-BASED PRACTICE

Safe nutritional support of hospitalized adult patients with obesity is an important priority of care. Following an extensive review of the literature, the Association of Parenteral and Enteral Nutrition (ASPEN) released clinical guidelines for the nutritional support of hospitalized adult patients with obesity (Choban et al., 2013):
- Critically ill patients with obesity experience more complications than patients with optimal body mass index.
- A nutritional support plan is recommended within 48 hours of admission to an intensive care unit.
- All hospitalized patients, regardless of body mass index, should be screened for nutritional risk, using nutritional assessment.

The Agency for Healthcare Research and Quality (AHRQ, 2013) has recently updated a geriatric nursing protocol for strategies to improve oral intake of older adults in nursing home/center environments. Strategies include the following:
- Conduct mealtime rounds to determine how much food is consumed and whether help is needed.
- Limit staff breaks to before or after patient mealtimes to ensure that adequate staff is available to help residents with meals.
- Help patient with mouth care and placement of dentures before food is served.
- Encourage family members to visit at meals.

- Ask family to bring favorite foods from home when appropriate. Ask about patient food preferences and honor them.
- Suggest small, frequent meals with adequate nutrients to help patients regain or maintain weight.
- Provide nutritious snacks.

SAFETY GUIDELINES

- Improper handling, preparation, and storage practices in the home environment may result in cases of foodborne illness (*Healthy People 2020*, 2014b). Children younger than 5, pregnant women, adults over 65, and people with weak immune systems are more likely to become ill from contaminated food; and, if they do become ill, the effects may be more serious (CDC, 2015). There are four principles for patients to follow in the home: cook to the right temperature, wash hands and surfaces (cutting boards, utensils, countertops) often, refrigerate promptly (summer—1 hour, winter—2 hours), and separate raw meats from other foods to prevent contamination (Box 31.2).
- Identify patients at risk for dysphagia and collaborate with other members, especially a speech-language pathologist of the health care team, to minimize complications such as aspiration pneumonia (NQF, 2010). The role of speech-language pathologists is to evaluate the stages of the swallow and make recommendations to physicians, nurses, dietitians, and family members (Tanner, 2014).

BOX 31.2

Food Safety Tips

- Wash hands, food-preparation surfaces, and utensils with warm soapy water before touching food.
- Cook meat, poultry, fish, and eggs until well done (180°F).
- Wash all fresh fruits and vegetables thoroughly.
- Do not eat raw meats or drink unpasteurized milk or juices.
- Do not use food past the expiration date on a package.
- Keep foods refrigerated at 40°F within 2 hours of cooking.
- Place leftover foods in refrigerator after cooking.
- Thaw frozen foods in the refrigerator.
- Discard food that you suspect spoiled. Place a date on time that food was first refrigerated.
- Do not use wooden cutting board; instead use plastic laminate or solid surface boards that can be disinfected.
- Clean the inside of the refrigerator and microwave regularly with bleach or soap.

Modified from Nix S: *Williams' basic nutrition and diet therapy,* ed 14, St Louis, 2013, Mosby.

- Ensure that patients receive the correct therapeutic diets. The Joint Commission and Centers for Medicare and Medicaid report that common dietary errors include wrong diet, meals meant for other patients, and meals delivered to patient when NPO.
- Assess a patient's level of consciousness before attempting any oral feeding.

◆ SKILL 31.1   Performing a Nutritional Screening and Physical Examination

Nurses screen for patients' actual and potential nutritional alterations by focusing on the effects of an illness, disease, or lifestyle on a patient's nutritional status such as recent weight loss and decreased oral intake. A nutrition risk screening refers to a rapid and simple set of usually two or three questions that have been validated to predict if a patient is malnourished or a malnutrition risk, helping to determine if a detailed nutritional assessment is indicated (Barker et al., 2011; Hammond and Litchford, 2012). Several common nutritional assessment tools are used in various health care agencies (Box 31.3).

Part of nutritional screening is application of physical examination findings (including height and weight). A nurse conducts a complete or focused physical examination at the time of a patient's admission to a health care agency. The extent of an examination is determined by a patient's condition. During an examination learn to recognize the physical signs that indicate a nutritional alteration (Table 31.1) and review laboratory results that further support a patient's nutritional status. Common biochemical markers that reflect nutritional status include albumin and prealbumin, complete blood count (CBC) with differential, ferritin, folate, total iron binding capacity with iron, reticulocyte count, vitamin B_{12}, and folate levels, which confirm a nutritional anemia diagnosis (NHLBI, 2014).

A nurse also collects a patient history at the time of admission. Dietary information from the history provides helpful information that will allow you to identify the adequacy of a patient's current diet, appetite changes, type of assistance a patient will need to eat, and food preferences. Findings from a nutritional screening determine if there is a need for consultation with a registered dietitian (RD) to complete a more in-depth assessment of a patient's nutritional status. In addition, assessment findings can lead to a medical referral for a speech-language pathologist (SLP) if the patient has

swallowing difficulties. However, SLPs are in short supply in many agencies (Donovan et al., 2013).

The Center for Medicare and Medicaid believes that RDs are best qualified to assess patients' nutritional treatment plans and design and implement nutritional treatment plans in consultation with the care team (Calloway, 2015). When you make referrals to RDs, it is important to know their role. Dietitians use a problem-solving method, the nutrition care process (NCP), to think critically and make decisions regarding nutrition therapy (Charney and Escott-Stump, 2012). The process is similar to the nursing process. The NCP has four interrelated steps: nutrition assessment, nutrition diagnosis, nutrition intervention, and nutrition monitoring and evaluation (ACEND, 2016; Charney and Escott-Stump, 2012). The RD first performs a comprehensive assessment of a patient's nutritional status, including medical, social, nutritional, and medication history; physical examination; anthropometric measurements; and laboratory data. The goal of the assessment is to develop an effective nutritional plan of care that addresses patients' nutritional problems. The RD then makes a nutritional diagnosis that describes alterations in a patient's nutritional status that a dietitian can treat independently (ACEND, 2016). The nutritional intervention is a purposely planned activity with the intent to resolve the nutrition diagnosis (i.e., to change a nutrition-related alteration). Nutrition monitoring and evaluation identifies patient progress, including patient understanding and adherence.

Delegation and Collaboration

The skill of performing and interpreting a nutritional screening and physical examination cannot be delegated to nursing assistive personnel (NAP). However, measurement of a patient's height and weight can be delegated. The nurse directs the NAP to:

BOX 31.3

Examples of Nutritional Screening Tools

- The Malnutrition Screening Tool (MST) is a simple; three-question tool assessing recent weight and appetite loss validated for use in general medical, surgical, and oncology patients. It was designed for use by non-nutrition–trained staff and uses a scoring system to identify patients at high nutrition risk, which can then provide a basis for dietetic referrals and intervention.
- The Malnutrition Universal Screening Tool (MUST) was designed to detect both undernutrition and obesity in adults. It can be used in multiple settings, including hospitals and nursing homes. Body mass index (BMI), unplanned weight loss, and the presence or absence of serious disease allows a score to be derived to indicate whether nutrition intervention is necessary. Not valid for children or renal failure patients.
- The Mini Nutritional Assessment (MNA) was developed for elderly patients (greater than or equal to 65 years of age) in hospitals, nursing homes, and the community. The original form considers anthropometrical, medical, lifestyle, dietary, and psychosocial factors in an 18-item assessment, using a points-based scoring system to determine if a patient is at risk of, or suffering from, malnutrition. The short-form MNA (MNA-SF) is a simple two-step nutrition screen, with the full MNA completed only for patients deemed at nutritional risk.
- Nutritional Risk Screening (NRS-2002) uses recent weight loss, decreased BMI, and reduced dietary intake, combined with a subjective assessment of disease severity (based on increased nutrition requirements and/or metabolic stress), to generate a nutrition risk score. The NRS tool has been recommended for use in hospitalized patients by ASPEN and may be useful for prompting the initiation of nutrition support.
- Subjective Global Assessment (SGA) is one of the most commonly used nutrition assessment tools. It requires completion of a questionnaire, which includes data on weight change, dietary intake change, gastrointestinal symptoms, changes in functional capacity in relation to malnutrition, and assessment of fat and muscle stores and the presence of edema and ascites. This tool allows for malnutrition diagnosis and classifies patients as either: A, well-nourished; B, mildly/moderately malnourished; or C, severely malnourished.

Adapted from Barker LA, et al: Hospital malnutrition: prevalence, identification and impact on patients and the healthcare system, *Int J Environ Res Public Health* 8(2):514, 2011.

- Measure patient's weight after voiding, at the same time of day and wearing same clothing.
- Use the internal bed scale according to agency guidelines (if applicable).
- Report inability to measure height if patient is nonambulatory.

TABLE 31.1

Physical Signs of Nutritional Status Alteration

Body Area	Indicators of Malnutrition
General appearance	Listless, apathetic, cachectic
Posture	Sagging shoulders, sunken chest, humped back
Hair	Stringy, dull, brittle, dry, thin and sparse, depigmented, easily plucked
Face and neck	Greasy, discolored, scaly, swollen, dark skin over cheeks and under eyes, lumpiness or flakiness of skin around nose and mouth
Skin	Rough, dry, scaly, pale, pigmented, irritated; bruises and petechiae
Lips	Dry, scaly, swollen, redness and swelling (cheilosis), angular lesions at corner of mouth or fissures or scars.
Mouth, oral mucous membranes	Swollen, deep red or magenta mucous membranes, oral lesions
Gums	Spongy, bleed easily, marginal redness, inflamed, receding
Tongue	Swelling, scarlet and raw, magenta color, beefy (glossitis), hyperemic and hypertrophic or atrophic papillae
Teeth	Missing, broken teeth
Eyes	Conjunctiva pale, redness of conjunctiva, dryness or infection, redness and fissuring of eyelid corners (angular palpebritis), Bitot's spots
Neck (glands)	Thyroid or lymph nodes enlarged
Nails	Spoon shaped (koilonychias), brittle, ridged
Legs and feet	Edema, tender calf, tingling, weakness, lesions
Muscles	Flaccid, poor tone, undeveloped, tender, impaired ability to walk
Nerve conduction and mental status	Inattentive, irritable, confused, burning and tingling of hands and feet, loss of position and vibratory sense

Modified from Nix S: *Williams' basic nutrition and diet therapy,* ed 14, St Louis, 2013, Mosby.

Equipment

- Scale (beam, electronic, bed with scale, wheelchair/chair)
- Nutritional screening form (data sheet and pen or computerized assessment form)
- Tongue blade, clean gloves, pen light for physical examination

STEP	RATIONALE

ASSESSMENT

1. Identify patient using at least two identifiers (e.g., name and birthday or name and medical record number), according to agency policy).

   Ensures correct patient. Complies with The Joint Commission standards and improves patient's safety (TJC, 2016).

2. Ask patient to report usual body weight (UBW), noting recent changes in weight. Ask if weight loss was intentional or unintentional.

   In adults weight is usually stable. A weight loss of more than 5% within 1 month is an indicator for further assessment, especially in an adult older than 65 years (Table 31.2).

STEP	RATIONALE

3. Perform hand hygiene. Measure actual body weight (ABW).

Women tend to underestimate their weight more than men, and for both sexes extent of underreporting increases as actual weight increases (Grodner et al., 2012).
Improves accuracy of ABW for comparison over time.

  a. Have patient void. Be sure that he or she is wearing underwear or hospital gown. Make sure that patient is weighed either barefoot or with same shoes. Weigh at same time of day.

  b. Make sure that beam scale has been calibrated. If ambulatory, help patient stand still on scale with weight evenly distributed on both feet.

Accurate measurement requires regularly calibrated and maintained scales. Standing still with equal weight distribution helps to obtain accurate weight (Grodner et al., 2012).

  c. If patient is unable to stand, use wheelchair or bed scale.

Decreases risk of falling.

  d. Record weight to nearest 0.1 kg (0.25 lb).

Provides precise measurement of weight.

4. Measure actual height.

On average, when asked, people report being slightly taller than they actually are (Grodner et al., 2012).
Ensures accurate height (Grodner et al., 2012).

  a. Help patient to standing position; have him or her stand erect with weight equally distributed on both feet.

  b. Instruct patient to let arms hang free at sides with palms facing thighs.

Prevents movement of shoulders, which will result in inaccurate measurement.

  c. Have patient look straight ahead, take a deep breath, and hold position while you bring horizontal bar firmly on top of head. Measure to nearest 0.1 cm ($\frac{1}{8}$ inch). Make sure that your eyes are level with bar to read measurement.

Steady position ensures accurate measurement. Provides precise measurement of height.

5. Calculate ideal body weight (IBW).

  a. Calculate via standard height and weight chart. IBW range for normal is 10% above and 10% below IBW.

Use IBW to compare with patient's actual weight to determine if he or she is at risk for nutritional alteration.

  b. Use the following formulas:
  Male: 48.1 kg (106 lbs) for first 5 feet; add 2.7 kg (6 lbs) per additional 2.5 cm (inch).
  Female: 45.4 kg (100 lbs) for first 5 feet; add 2.25 kg (5 lbs) per additional 2.5 cm (inch).

6. Calculate BMI (see illustration):

Body mass index (BMI) is a measure of body fat based on height and weight that applies to adult men and women (NHLBI, n.d.). Use this link for an automatic calculation:
http://www.nhlbi.nih.gov/health/educational/lose_wt/BMI/bmicalc.htm (NHLBI, n.d.)

$$BMI = \frac{Actual\ Body\ Weight\ (kg)}{Height^2(m^2)}$$

  a. Divide ABW in pounds by 2.2.

Converts pounds into kilograms.

  b. Convert height to inches. Multiply inches by 2.54.

Converts height in inches to centimeters.

  c. Divide height in centimeters by 100.

Converts height to meters.

  d. Divide weight in kilograms by the square of height in meters (m^2).

Computes BMI (Box 31.4).

  e. Optional formula for BMI
  weight (lbs)/ [height (in)]^2 × 703

TABLE 31.2		
Weight Change as an Indicator of Nutritional Status		
Weight Change (%)	**Time Period**	**Nutritional Status**
1–2	1 week	Moderate weight loss
Greater than 2	1 week	Severe weight loss
5	1 month	Moderate weight loss
Greater than 5	1 month	Severe weight loss

From Grodner M, et al: *Foundations and clinical applications of nutrition: a nursing approach*, ed 4, St Louis, 2012, Mosby.

BOX 31.4	
Classification of BMI in Adults	
Degree of Adiposity	**Body Mass Index**
Underweight	Less than 18.5 kg/m²
Normal weight	18.5–24.9 kg/m²
Overweight	25–29.9 kg/m²
Obesity (class 1)	30–34.9 kg/m²
Obesity (class 2)	35–39.9 kg/m²
Extreme obesity (class 3)	Greater than or equal to 40 kg/m²

From Expert Panel on the Identification, Evaluation, and Treatment of Overweight and Obesity in Adults: *The practical guide: identification, evaluation, and treatment of overweight and obesity in adults*, Bethesda, MD, 2000, National Institutes of Health.

| STEP | | | | | | | | | | | | | | | | RATIONALE |

To use the table, find the appropriate height in the left-hand column labeled Height. Move across to a given weight (in pounds). The number at the top of the column is the BMI at that height and weight. Pounds have been rounded off.

BMI	19	20	21	22	23	24	25	26	27	28	29	30	31	32	33	34	35
Height (inches)								Body Weight (pounds)									
58	91	96	100	105	110	115	119	124	129	134	138	143	148	153	158	162	167
59	94	99	104	109	114	119	124	128	133	138	143	148	153	158	163	168	173
60	97	102	107	112	118	123	128	133	138	143	148	153	158	163	168	174	179
61	100	106	111	116	122	127	132	137	143	148	153	158	164	169	174	180	185
62	104	109	115	120	126	131	136	142	147	153	158	164	169	175	180	186	191
63	107	113	118	124	130	135	141	146	152	158	163	169	175	180	186	191	197
64	110	116	122	128	134	140	145	151	157	163	169	174	180	186	192	197	204
65	114	120	126	132	138	144	150	156	162	168	174	180	186	192	198	204	210
66	118	124	130	136	142	148	155	161	167	173	179	186	192	198	204	210	216
67	121	127	134	140	146	153	159	166	172	178	185	191	198	204	211	217	223
68	125	131	138	144	151	158	164	171	177	184	190	197	203	210	216	223	230
69	128	135	142	149	155	162	169	176	182	189	196	203	209	216	223	230	236
70	132	139	146	153	160	167	174	181	188	195	202	209	216	222	229	236	243
71	136	143	150	157	165	172	179	186	193	200	208	215	222	229	236	243	250
72	140	147	154	162	169	177	184	191	199	206	213	221	228	235	242	250	258
73	144	151	159	166	174	182	189	197	204	212	219	227	235	242	250	257	265
74	148	155	163	171	179	186	194	202	210	218	225	233	241	249	256	264	272
75	152	160	168	176	184	192	200	208	216	224	232	240	248	256	264	272	279
76	156	164	172	180	189	197	205	213	221	230	238	246	254	263	271	279	287

Key

Obese (30+)
Overweight (25-29)
Normal (19-24)

STEP 6 Body mass index for BMI 35 and under. (*Data from National Heart, Lung, and Blood Institute: Body mass index table 1, https://www.nhlbi.nih.gov/health/educational/lose_wt/BMI/bmi_tbl.htm. Accessed November 29, 2016.*)

7. Obtain dietary information as you complete nursing history (see Chapter 6):
   a. Assess patient's diet history, including current diet, food choices/preferences, appetite, food allergies, and food intolerances. **NOTE:** In outpatient settings have patient bring 7-day food diary report.

   b. Assess for any cultural and religious preferences and/or restrictions in diet. Ask patient if family caregiver believes in "hot" versus "cold" foods for times when health changes occur.

   c. Determine medications and other dietary/herbal supplements that patient is taking (over-the-counter and prescribed). Be aware of common drug-drug and drug-nutrient interactions (consult pharmacist).

8. Perform physical assessment (see Chapter 6) (see Table 31.1), noting any physical changes reflecting nutritional deficiencies, patient's level of consciousness, responsiveness, and ability to swallow.
9. Review results of relevant laboratory tests (e.g., albumin, prealbumin, CBC).
10. During first meal determine patient's ability to manipulate eating utensils and self-feed.
11. Complete a nutritional screening tool if required by agency (see Box 31.3).

Assesses factors affecting diet adequacy and appetite (Tanner, 2014).

Knowing patient preferences will improve ability to plan diet that patient will accept. As a resource, the Food and Agriculture Organization (FAO) of the United Nations provides advice on food, food groups, and dietary patterns for different cultures (FAO, 2015).
Certain medications inhibit or increase action of other medications. Some nutrients interact with medications. For example, vitamin K–rich foods (green leafy vegetables) interfere with action of warfarin (anticoagulant).
Medications such as mineral oil laxatives impair nutrient use.
The most obvious signs of malnutrition on physical examination are apparent in the skin, mouth, muscles, and central nervous system. Difficulty swallowing predisposes patient to aspiration when eating.

Test data provide clues about nutritional status.

Difficulty in self-feeding creates significant risk for malnutrition (Meiner, 2015).
Valid tools include key elements for detecting patient's nutritional risk.

STEP	RATIONALE
12. Explain to patient that nutritional assessment is complete and how you intend to apply information in patient care.	Allows time for patient to ask questions about assessment and clarify information.

NURSING DIAGNOSES

- Deficient knowledge regarding nutritional needs/ recommendations
- Imbalanced nutrition less than body requirements
- Impaired swallowing
- Obesity
- Overweight
- Risk for overweight

Related factors/Risk factors are individualized based on patient's condition or needs.

IMPLEMENTATION

1. Provide patient help with feeding based on assessment findings (see Skill 31.2).	Level of assistance required depends on patient's motor skills, ability to attend, and ability to swallow and chew normally.
2. Institute aspiration precautions (see Skill 31.3) if needed.	Precautions lessen chance of patient aspirating food or liquid into tracheobronchial tree.

EVALUATION

1. Review history and physical findings. Note abnormal findings or areas of concern.	Permits prompt identification of risk for malnutrition and need for nutritional interventions.
2. Compare patient's actual weight for height with IBW. Compare BMI with recommended BMI for height/weight.	Determines nutritional risk factors and health-related conditions (NHLBI, 2012).
3. Compare normal laboratory test levels with patient's levels.	When considered with other nutritional parameters, abnormal values can indicate malnutrition (Grodner et al., 2012; Litchford, 2012).
4. Compute any score on nutritional screening tool.	Valid tools use scoring system to identify patients at high nutrition risk.
5. **Use Teach-Back:** "I want to be sure I explained why we need to do a nutritional screening for you. Tell me what the screening tells us? How we will use that information" Revise your instruction now or develop a plan for revised patient or family caregiver teaching if patient or family caregiver is not able to teach back correctly.	Determines patient's and family caregiver's level of understanding of instructional topic.

Unexpected Outcomes	Related Interventions
1. Patient is overweight if BMI greater than 25 kg/m^2 in an adult. Patient is obese if BMI is greater than 30 kg/m^2.	• Ensure that patient is receiving correct caloric diet. • Check that patient is being weighed on same scale, with same type of clothing/shoes, and at same time of day. • Consult with RD or health care provider so RD can conduct a nutritional assessment and calculate patient's caloric and protein intake and route of nutrition (enteral versus parenteral) (see Chapters 32 and 33).
2. Patient is underweight taking in insufficient intake.	• Consult with RD to determine needed calorie and protein intake and proper route of nutrition. • Implement measures to improve patient's appetite: appearance of served food, comfort of room, providing comfort measures before meal. • Include patient and family caregiver in developing a meal plan.
3. Nutritional screening tool score reflects high nutrition risk.	• Refer patient to RD.

Recording and Reporting

- Document assessment results on nurses' notes, flow sheet, and nutritional screening form in electronic health record (EHR) or chart.
- Document your evaluation of patient and family caregiver learning.
- Notify health care provider of abnormal findings.
- Make referral to the RD.

Special Considerations
Teaching

- To increase the awareness of healthy nutrition, educate patient and family caregiver about a case-specific nutritional diet.
- Provide patient and family caregiver resources to promote healthy eating (e.g., MyPlate Food Guidance System) (USDA, 2015) (Box 31.5).

Building a Healthy Eating Style

Following the USDA (2015) ChooseMyPlate guidelines will result in a healthier eating style:

- When selecting food and beverages, focus on variety, amount, and nutrition. Include all five food groups: fruits, vegetables, grains, protein foods, and dairy.
- Eat the right amount of calories for you based on your age, sex, height, weight, and physical activity level.
- A healthier eating style will help you avoid overweight and obesity and reduce your risk of diseases such as heart disease, diabetes, and cancer.
- Choose an eating style low in saturated fat, sodium, and added sugars.
- Read nutrition fact labels and ingredient lists carefully for the amounts of saturated fat, sodium, and added sugars in the foods and beverages you choose. Make food choices that follow these same guidelines.
- Eating foods with less sodium can reduce your risk of high blood pressure.
- Make small changes to create a healthier eating style. Think of each change as a personal "win" on your path to living healthier. Start with a few of these small changes.
  - Make half your plate fruits and vegetables.
  - Focus on whole fruits.
  - Vary your veggies.
  - Make half your grains whole grains.
  - Move to low-fat and fat-free dairy.
  - Vary your protein routine.
- Eat and drink the right amount for you. Support healthy eating for everyone.
- Create settings where healthy choices are available and affordable to you and others in your community.
- Professionals, policymakers, partners, industry, families, and individuals can help others in their journey to make healthy eating a part of their lives.
- See more at: http://www.choosemyplate.gov/MyPlate#sthash.qyz0YKJi.dpuf.

- Introduce technology nutrition tools such as nutrition smartphone applications and websites to encourage patient engagement with diet plan.

Gerontological

- Nutrition is one of the major determinants of successful aging. Food is not only critical to one's physiological well-being but also contributes to social, cultural, and psychological quality of life. Primarily nutrition helps promote health and functionality (Academy of Nutrition and Dietetics, 2012).
- Food insecurity occurs whenever the availability of nutritionally adequate and safe food or the ability to acquire food in socially accepted ways is inadequate or uncertain. Food insecurity is more prevalent in older adults with incomes below the poverty line who rent their homes, are less educated, are disabled, have a grandchild living in the house, and are participants in the Supplemental Nutrition Assistance Program (SNAP) (Academy of Nutrition and Dietetics, 2012).

Pediatric

- Anthropometric data include measurement of length, weight, and head circumference in children. Compare these measurements with standard growth charts to determine percentiles. The most commonly used growth charts are from the National Center for Health Statistics (Hockenberry and Wilson, 2015). These charts now include BMI for age and weight for stature percentiles.

Home Care

- Instruct patient and family caregiver about strategies for safe handling, preparation, and storage of food.
- Assess home environment to determine if patient or family caregiver can prepare a meal safely.

◆ SKILL 31.2 Assisting an Adult Patient With Oral Nutrition

Some patients are unable to feed themselves adequately because of the severity of their illness, which may cause musculoskeletal weakness, fatigue, pain, or debilitation. For example, a patient who loses fine-motor skills will have difficulty getting food from the plate into the mouth. Helping adults with feeding requires time, patience, knowledge of a patient's physical limitations and nutritional needs, and understanding a patient's preferences for foods and how to eat a meal. You can improve a patient's nutritional intake by helping with feedings directly or teaching family caregivers how to do so safely. It is important to maintain a patient's dignity during feeding and to actively involve him or her in eating. Encourage patients to make decisions about food choices and times for eating and help them use assistive devices correctly (when needed).

Hospitalized patients receive a number of different therapeutic oral diets that require a health care provider's order. A therapeutic diet treats many illness and disease states (Table 31.3). Refer to an agency dietary manual or confer with a registered dietitian (RD) for specific information about therapeutic diets. There are two ways to modify a regular diet: quantitatively or qualitatively (Grodner et al., 2012). Quantitative diets include modifications in number or size of meals served or amounts of specific nutrients such as six small feedings or kcalorie diets. Qualitative diets include

modifications in consistency, texture, or nutrients such as clear or full liquid. You can supplement any diet with oral nutrition supplements. In a health care setting you will often receive an order for a calorie count, which requires you to record the percentage of each food that a patient eats next to the food choice directly on the meal menu. The RD collects the menus to calculate caloric intake and determine the need for nutrition supplements or dietary change. For example, liquid supplements with or between meals can significantly increase protein and calorie intake but do not replace scheduled meals (Gaddey and Holder, 2014).

Altered dentition, improperly fitted dentures, oral lesions or infections, or diseases causing impaired digestion limit the types and consistencies of foods tolerated. Hemiplegia, fractured arm, quadriplegia, debilitating illness, or generalized weakness limits self-feeding ability and appetite. The presence of intravenous (IV) catheters or tubing, dressings, and bandages also limits mobility needed for self-feeding. Collaborate with an occupational therapist (OT) who can assess a patient's ability to self-feed and make recommendations for adaptive equipment and supplies for self-feeding. An adult who needs help to eat needs compassion and understanding. Use common sense when feeding an adult and provide a socially meaningful mealtime experience.

TABLE 31.3	

Progressive and Therapeutic Diets

Diet	Description
Clear-liquid	Foods that are clear and liquid at room or body temperature (e.g., water, apple or cranberry juice, gelatin, Popsicles), that leave little residue, and are easily absorbed; commonly ordered for short-term use (24 to 48 hours) after surgery, before diagnostic tests, and after episodes of diarrhea and vomiting
Full-liquid	Includes foods on clear-liquid diet plus addition of smooth-textured dairy products (e.g., milk and ice cream), strained soups and custard, refined cooked cereals, vegetable juice, and pureed vegetables; commonly ordered before or after surgery for patients who are acutely ill from infection or for patients who cannot chew or tolerate solid foods; must verify that patients are able to tolerate lactose before providing dairy products
Pureed	Includes foods on clear- and full-liquid diet plus easily swallowed foods that do not require chewing (e.g., scrambled eggs, pureed meats, vegetables, fruits, mashed potatoes). Ordered for patients with head and neck abnormalities or who have had oral surgery. Can be modified for low sodium, fat, or calorie count
Mechanical or dental-soft	Consists of all previous diets plus addition of lightly seasoned ground or finely diced meats, flaked fish, cottage cheese, cheese, rice, potatoes, pancakes, light breads, cooked vegetables, cooked or canned fruit, bananas, and peanut butter; avoid tough meats, nuts, bacon, and fruits with tough skins or membranes; ordered for patients who have chewing problems or mild GI problems; used as a transition diet from liquids to regular
Soft/low-residue	Addition of low-fiber, easily digested foods such as pastas, casseroles, moist tender meats, and canned cooked fruits and vegetables; includes foods that are easy to chew and simply cooked; does not permit fatty, rich, and fried foods; sometimes referred to as *low fiber*
High-fiber	Addition of fresh uncooked fruits, steamed vegetables, bran, oatmeal, and dried fruits; includes sufficient amounts of indigestible carbohydrates to relieve constipation, increase GI motility, and increase stool weight
Regular or diet as tolerated	No restrictions; permits patient preferences and allows for postoperative diet progression
Sample Therapeutic Diets	
Restricted fluids	Required in severe heart failure or kidney failure
Sodium-restricted	Low levels of sodium: may include a 4-g (no added salt), 2-g (moderate), 1-g (strict), or 500-mg (very strict) diet; may be ordered for patients with heart failure, renal failure, cirrhosis, or hypertension
Fat-modified	Low total and saturated fat and low cholesterol intake limited to less than 300 mg daily, and fat intake 30% to 35%; eliminates or reduces fatty foods for hypercholesterolemia, malabsorption disorders, and diarrhea
Diabetic	Essential treatment for patients with diabetes mellitus; provide patient with a diet recommended by the American Diabetes Association, which allows for patients to select set amount of food from basic food groups.

Adapted from Grodner M, et al: *Foundations and clinical applications of nutrition: a nursing approach*, ed 4, St Louis, 2012, Mosby.
GI, Gastrointestinal.

Delegation and Collaboration

The skill of assisting a patient with oral nutrition can be delegated to nursing assistive personnel (NAP). However, the nurse is responsible to determine if a patient is able to receive oral nutrition, including swallowing ability and dietary restrictions. The nurse directs the NAP by:

- Explaining any specific swallowing strategies/techniques unique to the patient.
- Reviewing when to stop feeding and report immediately to the nurse incidences of coughing, gagging, pocketing of food in the mouth, or difficulty swallowing.
- Cautioning to not rush the patient during eating.

Equipment

- Stethoscope
- Washcloths and towels
- Tongue blade
- Adaptive utensils as needed for self-feeding
- Straw
- Oral hygiene supplies; *Option:* solution for stomatitis care
- Clean gloves

STEP	RATIONALE

ASSESSMENT

1. Identify patient using at least two identifiers (e.g., name and birthday or name and medical record number), according to agency policy).

Ensures correct patient. Complies with The Joint Commission standards and improves patient's safety (TJC, 2016).

2. Review health care provider's diet order for type of diet and supplements.

Helps to ensure that patient will receive proper diet.

3. Assess presence and condition of teeth. (Apply clean gloves if there is risk of exposure to saliva.) Determine if dentures are poorly fitted. If patient has mouth discomfort, measure pain severity on a scale of 0 to 10 on a pain scale.

Absence of teeth and ill-fitting dentures inhibit normal chewing and influence preparation of food for safe swallowing (Kyle, 2011) (see Skill 31.3). Pain can reduce patient's appetite and ability to chew or swallow. These factors increase risk for dysphagia.

STEP	RATIONALE
4. Have patient speak and swallow. Watch for laryngeal movement. Ask patient to say "Ah" while using tongue blade and penlight. Check for midline uvula and symmetrical rise of uvula and soft palate. Use tongue blade to elicit gag reflex (see Chapter 6).	Patients with chronic neurological disease may experience cranial nerve damage (Remig and Weeden, 2012). Patient may experience impaired swallowing (cranial nerve IX) or loss of gag reflex, hoarseness, and nasal voice (cranial nerve X).
5. Determine to what extent patient is able to self-feed. Assess physical motor skills (e.g., ability to grasp utensils, hold cup and move utensil to mouth). Assess level of consciousness or ability to attend to feeding, visual acuity, and peripheral vision.	Patients with any level of independence should be encouraged to feed self as much as possible. Thorough understanding of patient's physical and cognitive limitations alerts you to type of help patient needs. Visual impairments make it difficult to see food and utensils (Chang and Roberts, 2011).
6. Assess patient's appetite, recent food and fluid intake, cultural and religious preferences for participating in mealtime, and food likes and dislikes.	Determines type of foods and size of meals that can potentially improve oral intake.
7. Assess for presence of generalized fatigue, pain, or shortness of breath.	Symptoms affect appetite and ability to participate in feeding. Patients eat better when rested.
8. Ask if patient feels nauseated. Also assess recent bowel pattern. Is patient passing flatus? Auscultate for bowel sounds.	Determines baseline assessment of gastrointestinal function.
9. Assess need for toileting, handwashing, and oral care (including dentures) before feeding.	Reduces interruptions and improves patient's appetite.
10. Review nursing history (see Skill 31.1) for patient's most recent weight and laboratory values.	Provides ongoing monitoring of patient's nutritional status.

NURSING DIAGNOSIS

- Activity intolerance
- Acute pain
- Feeding self-care deficit
- Impaired swallowing
- Risk for aspiration
- Risk for deficient fluid volume
- Risk for imbalanced nutrition: less than body requirements

Related factors/Risk factors are individualized based on patient's condition or needs.

PLANNING

1. Expected outcomes following completion of procedure:	
• Patient's weight is maintained or trends toward desired level.	Nutritional intake meets daily needs.
• Patient's nutrition-related laboratory values trend toward normal.	Biochemical markers along with nutritional assessment indicate nutritional status.
• Patient demonstrates increased ability to self-feed or open items on tray as appropriate.	Indicates increased strength, improved mental status, and increased well-being.
• Patient coughs appropriately with no indication of respiratory compromise.	Ineffective cough and respiratory compromise are indicators of dysphagia and aspiration.
• Patient completes meal.	Indicates normal vital signs and skin color during activity.
• Patient able to describe foods allowed within prescribed diet.	Demonstrates learning.
2. After assessment allow patient to rest 30 minutes before mealtime.	Assessment activities can be tiring. Short rest improves patient's energy level and ability to participate in feeding.
3. Administer ordered analgesic 30 minutes before meal if patient has discomfort.	Analgesic receives peak level during meal, improving patient's ability to self-feed.
4. Explain to patient how you plan to set up and help with meal. Allow time for questions.	Minimizes any anxiety and engages patient in mealtime.

IMPLEMENTATION

1. Prepare patient's room for mealtime.	
a. Perform hand hygiene. Clear over-bed table and arrange any needed supplies.	Reduces transmission of microorganisms and prepares room for food tray.
b. Help patient to comfortable sitting position in chair or place bed in high-Fowler's position. If patient is unable to sit, turn him or her on side with head of bed elevated and chin in down position.	Upright position facilitates swallowing, reducing aspiration risk. Conditions such as pressure injury, traction, or spinal surgery prevent positioning with head elevated.

STEP	RATIONALE

2. Prepare patient for meal.

   a. Help patient with elimination needs and to perform hand hygiene.

Increases patient's comfort and enjoyment of meal, which helps increase patient's nutritional intake.

   b. Apply clean gloves and offer oral hygiene. If patient has dentures, remove and rinse thoroughly and reinsert. Remove gloves and perform hand hygiene.

Moist, clean oral mucosa and teeth improve taste and appetite.

   c. Patients with oral mucositis (inflammation of mucous membranes) benefit from rinsing with solutions such as saline, saline-sodium bicarbonate mouthwash, sodium bicarbonate solution, topical anesthetics or from using mucosal coating agents (NCI, 2014). Consult with health care provider to determine best therapy.

Pain of stomatitis causes patients to avoid eating.

   d. Help patient put on eyeglasses or insert contact lenses if used.

Enhances patient's ability to self-feed and makes meal more visually appealing.

3. Check environment for distractions. Reduce noise level if possible. *Option:* If patient enjoys music, play a soothing, low-volume selection.

Pleasant environment enhances mealtime experience.

4. Obtain special assistive devices as needed and instruct on use. For example:

Devices facilitate self-feeding by improving ability to grasp, picking up foods with utensils, and drinking liquids.

   • Two-handled cup with spout in lid makes it easier to drink and hold and lift a cup. Avoids spills. Cup has wide base that prevents tipping over.

   • Plate with plate guard (see illustration) and nonskid bottom helps person with limited flexibility of hands or poor motor coordination or who uses only one hand.

   • Knife, fork, and spoon with large handles or attached splints help patient with limited hand function or a weak grip.

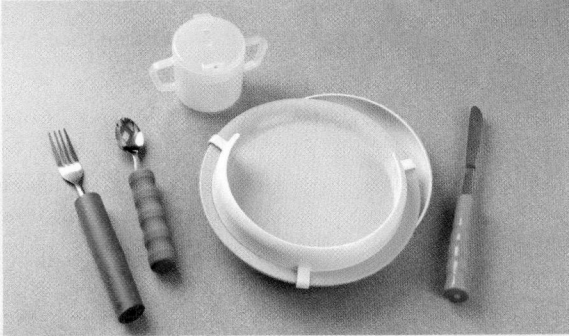

STEP 4 Mealtime adaptive equipment. *Clockwise from upper left:* Two-handled cup with lid, plate with plate guard, utensils with splints, and utensils with enlarged handles.

5. Assess meal tray for completeness and correct diet. Use this time (and during actual feeding) to instruct patient about diet, rationale for diet, food options, and dysphagia risks.

Prevents intake of incomplete or incorrect diet. Instruction more meaningful when applied during real time activity.

6. Ask in which order patient would like to eat his or her meal. Help to set up meal tray if patient unable to do so: open packages, cut up food, apply seasonings or condiments, place napkin.

Allows patient more independence and control. Small pieces are easier to chew and minimize risk for aspiration.

7. Watch patient successfully swallow first bites of food and drink. If patient is able to eat independently, stop here. Return after 15 or 20 minutes or stay at side for communication and additional teaching.

Aim is to make patient as self-sufficient as possible.

Clinical Decision Point *If patient is at risk for aspiration, stay at his or her side during feeding.*

STEP	RATIONALE

8. Help patient who cannot eat independently.

    a. Assume comfortable position.

Being comfortable prevents you from rushing patient through meal.

    b. If patient is visually impaired, identify food location on plate as if it were a clock (e.g., vegetables at 9 o'clock, meat at 3 o'clock) (see illustration).

Helps patient locate food items; may be able to feed self if given adequate information about food placement on tray.

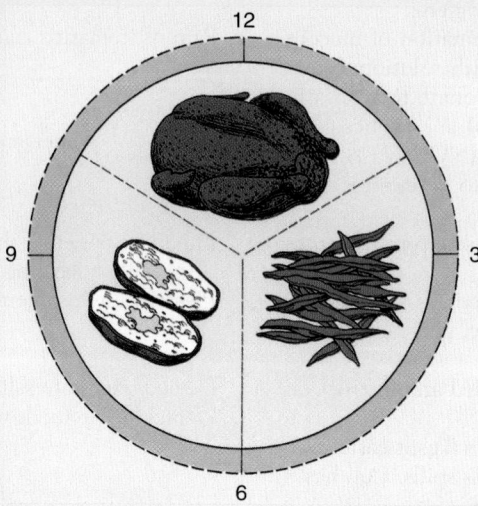

STEP 8b Clock setup to prepare food on a plate for the visually impaired patient.

    c. Ask patient in which order he or she would like to eat and cut food into bite-size pieces.

Gives patient more independence and control. Small bites reduce risk of aspiration (see Skill 31.3).

    d. Provide fluids as requested. Discourage patient from drinking all fluids at beginning of meal.

Promotes swallowing. Prevents patient from filling up on fluids.

    e. Pace feeding to avoid patient fatigue. Interact with patient during mealtime. Verbally encourage self-feeding attempts.

Social interaction may improve appetite.

    f. Use meal as opportunity to communicate with and educate patient about nutrition topics and discharge plan.

Offers extended time for teaching.

    g. Feed patient in manner that facilitates chewing and swallowing. Position patient's chin down and place food in stronger side of the mouth.

Chin-down position may help to reduce aspiration risk (see Skill 31.3).

9. Use appropriate feeding techniques for patients with special needs:

Decreased saliva production in older adults impairs swallowing. Aspiration results from decreased or absent gag reflex.

    a. *Older adult:* Feed small amounts at a time, observing biting, chewing, ability to manipulate tongue to form bolus of food, swallowing, and fatigue between bites. Be sure that patient has swallowed food. Offer variety of foods and frequent rest periods.

Clinical Decision Point *If you suspect that patient is aspirating, stop feeding immediately and suction airway (see Skill 31.3).*

    b. *Neurologically impaired patient:* Feed small amounts at a time and observe ability to chew, manipulate tongue to form bolus, and swallow. Have patient open mouth and check for food left inside cheeks (pocketing). Give small amount of thin liquid between bites.

Some patients with limited tongue strength and control are unable to move food to back of mouth for swallowing. Checking for "pocketed" food in mouth prevents aspiration (Remig and Weeden, 2012).

    c. *Patients with cancer:* Check for food aversions before and during meal. Monitor for fatigue.

Strong, abnormal sense of taste and smell are side effects of chemotherapy. Cancer patients can tire easily.

10. Help patient with hand hygiene and performing mouth care after meal is completed. (Apply gloves as needed.)

Maintains comfort.

11. Help patient to resting position, leave head elevated at least 45 degrees for 30–60 minutes after meal.

Reduces risk of aspiration from regurgitation.

12. Return patient's tray to appropriate place, remove and discard gloves, and perform hand hygiene.

Reduces transmission of microorganisms.

STEP	RATIONALE

EVALUATION

1. Monitor body weight daily or weekly.
2. Monitor laboratory values as indicated.

3. Monitor intake and output (I&O) (see Chapter 6) and complete intake measurement (e.g., observed intake, calorie count).
4. Observe patient's ability to self-feed, including ability to feed certain items, part, or all of meal.
5. Observe patient for choking, coughing, gagging, or food left in mouth during eating.
6. **Use Teach-Back:** "We discussed ways you can help feed your husband that make it easier for him to swallow. Tell me two ways to help feed him and why it is important." Revise your instruction now or develop a plan for revised family caregiver teaching if family caregiver is not able to teach back correctly.

Determines ongoing nutritional status.
Biochemical markers such as albumin and prealbumin help to identify changes in nutritional status.

Helps to determine what help patient needs with feeding.

Indicates dysphagia and possible aspiration.

Determines family caregiver's level of understanding of instructional topic.

Unexpected Outcomes
1. Patient is unable to eat entire meal or refuses to eat.

2. Patient chokes on food.

Related Interventions
- Determine if patient has other food preferences and cultural factors or religious restrictions.
- Ask patient what is affecting his or her ability to eat.
- Determine if patient's ability or desire to eat is better at other times of the day.
- Determine if patient is in pain or nauseated or if he or she has constipation. Implement appropriate interventions (e.g., administering analgesic, antiemetic, or cathartic; offering food or liquid at temperature patient prefers; offering small frequent meals).
- Provide more frequent oral care.
- If inability to eat meal is a repeated problem, collaborate with health care provider and RD.
- Stop feeding immediately; place on side with head forward and pointing down; suction food and secretions from mouth and airway.
- Contact health care provider if choking occurs repeatedly.
- Suggest appropriate referrals (e.g., speech-language pathologist, RD) (see Skill 31.3).

Recording and Reporting

- Record in nurses' notes in electronic health record (EHR) or chart the patient's type of diet, amount of feeding assistance needed, tolerance of diet, amount or percentage of the meal eaten (e.g., 25% of food consumed at breakfast), and calorie count (if ordered).
- If evaluating I&O, record fluid intake on appropriate form (see Chapter 6).
- If patient is receiving oral nutritional supplements (e.g., Ensure, Boost), record the amount taken and patient's tolerance (likes or dislikes, supplements to fill or replace meals) to the health care team.
- Report any swallowing difficulties, food dislikes, refusal to eat to health care provider and RD.
- Document your evaluation of family caregiver learning.

Special Considerations
Teaching
- See Teaching Considerations, Skill 31.1.

Pediatric

- Human milk is the most desirable complete diet for infants during the first 6 months. Infants who are breastfed or bottle-fed do not require additional fluids, especially water or juice, during the first 4 months of life. Excessive intake of water causes water intoxication, failure to thrive, and hyponatremia.
- Typically infants do not consume solid foods until 6 months of age. Iron-fortified infant cereal is usually the first solid food to offer. A common sequence for introducing solid food is one new food every 5 to 7 days; strained fruits followed by vegetables and finally meats are recommended (Hockenberry and Wilson, 2015).
- Do not mix solid foods in a bottle and feed through a nipple with a larger hole (Hockenberry and Wilson, 2015).

Gerontological

- Some older adults have diminished appetite because of loss of taste and smell and decreased number of taste buds (Chang and Roberts, 2011).
- Interactions between nutrients and medications affect taste of foods or metabolism, absorption, digestion, or excretion of drugs.

Home Care

- Assess financial resources of patient and family caregiver to determine if they are able to purchase nutritionally complete foods for patient.
- Help patient and family caregiver identify ways to make meals in the home pleasant and enjoyable experiences.

✦ SKILL 31.3   Aspiration Precautions

 Video Clip

Aspiration is the misdirection of oropharyngeal secretions or gastric contents into the larynx and lower respiratory tract (Metheny, 2012). It often occurs when secretions in the oral pharynx enter the trachea, or it may occur as a result of reflux of gastric content that enters the throat and then goes down the trachea. Patients at risk for aspiration include those with dysphagia (difficulty swallowing). The ability to swallow effectively and safely is necessary for safe transport of food and fluid through the mouth, pharynx, and esophagus to the stomach. It requires a complex and fine coordination of cranial nerves and the muscles of the tongue, pharynx, larynx, and jaw. Any alteration or delay in the swallowing process causes dysphagia.

Some of the conditions that increase the risk for dysphagia include severity of illness (e.g., sepsis, acute stroke, head and neck cancer, head trauma, dementia, and Parkinson's disease) and medical interventions that compromise the gag reflex (Kaspar and Ekberg, 2012). Medical interventions include sedation, mechanical ventilation, nasotracheal suctioning, and lying flat. Structural obstructions and medication side effects also cause difficulty swallowing (Sura et al., 2012) (Box 31.6). Symptoms of dysphagia vary, depending on the swallowing alteration. You should suspect dysphagia if a patient has frequent drooling, loss of food from the mouth during eating, pocketing food (holding food in the cheek), and spitting pieces of food out. In addition, a patient might experience choking or coughing when swallowing, a gurgling or wet-sounding voice quality (e.g., hoarseness), and having the sensation of food getting stuck in the throat after multiple attempts to swallow (Kyle, 2011; Mayo Clinic, 2014).

Inability to coordinate the complex, sequential swallowing mechanism slows eating, results in food being left in the mouth, and may lead to aspiration (Steele and Cichero, 2014). Gastric material and secretions in the mouth and pharynx and pathogenic bacteria enter the trachea and lungs (Eisenstadt, 2010). Aspiration pneumonia can be a fatal complication of dysphagia, especially in older adults. However, aspiration pneumonia will develop only if the material aspirated is pathogenic to the lungs and the patient's natural resistance to the material is compromised (Ebihara et al., 2016; Walker et al., 2009). Tachypnea (respirations above 26) is an early clue of aspiration (Eisenstadt, 2010). Other signs include cough; dyspnea (trouble breathing); decreased breath sounds; and abnormal breath sounds such as wheezing, rales, and rhonchi (see Chapter 6).

Silent or asymptomatic aspiration refers to passage of food or liquid into the trachea and lungs without producing a productive cough or other signs consistent with aspiration (Garon et al., 2009). As patients with dysphagia age, their perception of the urge to cough decreases, which further increases the risk for silent aspiration. The condition often results from sensory damage to the pharynx and muscle weakness in the throat and mouth that produces a lack of a protective cough reflex (Ebihara et al., 2016; Garon et al., 2009). Lack of outward signs such as coughing reduces awareness by the patient, family, and health team members that aspiration is occurring. This can result in longer periods of ingestion of food and liquid into the lungs and places the patient in a higher-risk group for the development of pneumonia (Garon et al., 2009). The more subtle signs associated with silent aspiration are easy to miss and include lack of speech, depressed alertness, wet quality to voice, drooling, difficulty controlling secretions, and absence of gag reflex.

Dysphagia Evaluation

As a nurse you work closely with patients and are in a key position to identify swallowing difficulties and make referrals to appropriate health care professionals. When your assessment shows that a patient is at risk for dysphagia and aspiration, referral for a more comprehensive examination is necessary (Box 31.7). The single most important measure to prevent aspiration is to place the patient on NPO until a dysphagia evaluation by a certified speech-language pathologist (SLP) can be performed; then a safe diet can resume. Early screening and intervention are crucial to preventing aspiration and pneumonia. Conduct your initial nutritional screening (see Skill 31.1) to determine the potential for both aspiration and safe oral intake. When you detect risk factors, consult the SLP for dysphagia screening. Dysphagia screening is a minimally invasive procedure that initially documents the likelihood that dysphagia is present, the need for further swallowing assessment, and the safety of patient intake. A functional oral assessment by an SLP includes acceptance of liquid and food, bolus formation, lip seal, mastication, dentition, salivation, pocketing,

---

BOX 31.6

Causes of Dysphagia

Neurogenic
- Stroke
- Cerebral palsy
- Guillain-Barré syndrome
- Multiple sclerosis
- Amyotrophic lateral sclerosis (Lou Gehrig's disease)
- Diabetic neuropathy
- Parkinson's disease

Myogenic
- Myasthenia gravis
- Aging
- Muscular dystrophy
- Polymyositis

Obstructive
- Benign peptic stricture
- Lower esophageal ring
- Candidiasis
- Head and neck cancer
- Inflammatory masses
- Trauma/surgical resection
- Anterior mediastinal masses
- Cervical spondylosis

Other
- Gastrointestinal or esophageal resection
- Rheumatological disorders
- Connective tissue disorders
- Vagotomy

tongue mobility, mandibular movements, propulsion of bolus along palatal vault, and impulsivity (Tanner, 2014). If the SLP finds serious abnormalities, the gold standard for dysphagia diagnosis is use of videofluoroscopy.

Dysphagia Management

Dysphagia management includes dietary modification by altering the consistency of food and liquids and is most effective when implemented using an interprofessional approach recommended by the SLP (Tanner, 2014). The SLP and registered dietitian (RD) are central to dysphagia management. An SLP specializes in swallowing disorders and makes treatment recommendations to a health care provider that may include texture modifications for food and liquids. The RD ensures that recommendations are balanced with the nutritional and caloric needs of patients. Appropriate food choices and consistency of liquids are individualized and based on which phase of swallowing is dysfunctional (Sura et al., 2012).

BOX 31.7

Criteria for Dysphagia Referral

Before Referral:

If the answer is yes to either of the following two questions, referral at this time is **not appropriate.**

- Is patient unconscious or drowsy?
- Is patient unable to sit in an upright position for a reasonable length of time?

Also Consider the Next Two Questions Before Making a Referral:

- Is the patient near the end of life?
- Does the patient have an esophageal problem that will require surgical intervention?

When Observing a Patient or Giving Mouth Care, Look for the Following:

- Open mouth (weak lip closure)
- Drooling liquids or solids
- Facial or tongue weakness
- Difficulty moving or swallowing secretions in the mouth
- Slurred, indistinct speech
- Hoarseness
- Poor posture or head control
- Weak involuntary cough
- Delayed cough (up to 2 minutes after swallow)
- General frailty, confusion, or dementia
- No spontaneous swallowing movements

If any of the above is present, the patient may have swallowing problems and need referral to a speech-language pathologist.

In October 2002 the American Dietetic Association published the National Dysphagia Diet Task Force (NDDTF) national dysphagia diet. The diet standards provide guidelines and standard terminology for food and texture modifications. The diet comprises four levels: dysphagia puree, dysphagia mechanically altered, dysphagia advanced, and regular (Table 31.4). There are also four levels of liquid: thin liquids (low viscosity) such as water, coffee, tea; nectarlike liquids (medium viscosity); honeylike liquids (viscosity of honey), and spoon-thick liquids (viscosity of pudding) (Academy of Nutrition and Dietetics, 2012; NDDTF, 2002).

Thickened liquids are commonly prescribed to prevent aspiration pneumonia (Frey and Ramsberger, 2011). A thickening agent alters flavor and texture qualities. There are often complaints about their taste and thickness, which increase nonadherence (Frey and Ramsberger, 2011). It is important to remember that the desired thickness of a liquid depends on a patient's swallowing deficit. Always read the label directions when modifying liquids to prepare the desired thickness correctly.

Consequences of Dysphagia

Physiological consequences of dysphagia include decreased appetite, weight loss, dehydration, malnutrition, pneumonia, and poststroke pneumonia (Sura et al., 2012). Dietary intake may be affected for long periods of time; and the malnutrition that occurs is secondary to insufficient protein, calorie, and micronutrient intake (Meiner, 2015). Dysphagia may affect a patient's quality of life. Understand the emotional impact of losing the ability to eat and drink safely. A patient's normal nutritional intake is altered because he or she either is unable to consume oral nutrition or has to make diet modifications to swallow without risk of aspiration. Emotional responses may include altered body image, embarrassment, social isolation, and depression. In addition, a patient may feel as though he or she is a burden to family caregivers.

Delegation and Collaboration

The skill of following aspiration precautions while feeding a patient can be delegated to nursing assistive personnel (NAP). However, the nurse is responsible for the ongoing assessment of a patient's risk for aspiration and determination of positioning and any special feeding techniques. The nurse directs the NAP to:

- Position patient upright (45 to 90 degrees preferred) or according to medical restrictions during and after feeding.
- Use aspiration precautions while feeding patients who need help and explain feeding techniques that are successful for specific patients.
- Immediately report any onset coughing, gagging, or a wet voice or pocketing of food to the nurse.

TABLE 31.4

National Dysphagia Diet Levels

Level	Description	Examples
NDD 1: Dysphagia pureed	Uniform, pureed, cohesive, pudding-like texture	Smooth hot cereals cooked to a "pudding" consistency; mashed potatoes; pureed meat and vegetables; pureed pasta on rice; yogurt
NDD 2: Dysphagia mechanically altered	Moist, soft textured. Easily forms a bolus	Cooked cereals; dry cereals moistened with milk; canned fruit (except pineapple); moist ground meat; well-cooked noodles in sauce/gravy; well cooked, diced vegetables
NDD 3: Dysphagia advanced	Regular foods (except very hard, sticky, or crunchy foods)	Moist breads (e.g., butter, jelly); well-moistened cereals, peeled soft fruits (peach, plum, kiwi); tender, thin-sliced meats; baked potato (without skin); tender, cooked vegetables
Regular	All foods	No restrictions

Modified from National Dysphagia Diet Task Force (NDDTF): *National dysphagia diet: standardization for optimal care*, Chicago, 2002, American Dietetic Association.
NDD, National Dysphasia Diet.

Equipment

- Chair or bed that allows patient to sit upright
- Thickening agents as designated by SLP (rice, cereal, yogurt, gelatin, commercial thickener)
- Tongue blade
- Penlight
- Oral hygiene supplies (see Chapter 18)
- Suction equipment (see Chapter 25)
- Clean gloves
- *Option:* Pulse oximeter

STEP	RATIONALE

ASSESSMENT

1. Review results of nutritional screening in medical record (see Skill 31.1).	Reveals risk patterns (e.g., patients with dysphagia often alter their eating patterns or choose foods that do not provide adequate nutrition).
2. Identify patient using at least two identifiers (e.g., name and birthday or name and medical record number), according to agency policy.	Ensures correct patient. Complies with The Joint Commission standards and improves patient safety (TJC, 2016).
3. Ask patient or family caregiver if patient has difficulties with chewing or swallowing various food textures.	Patients likely to aspirate certain foods more than others.
4. Assess for conditions that cause dysphagia and thus present risk for aspiration (see Box 31.6). Also assess signs and symptoms of dysphagia (e.g., drooling, hoarseness, food pocketing). Use dysphagia screening tool if available.	Patients with neurological or neuromuscular disease and those with trauma to or surgery of oral cavity or throat are at risk.
5. Assess mental status, including alertness, orientation, and ability to follow simple commands (e.g., open your mouth; stick out your tongue).	Disorientation and inability to follow commands present higher risk for dysphagia.
6. Assess patient's oral cavity, level of dental hygiene, missing teeth, or poorly fitting dentures. (Apply clean gloves if needed.)	Poor oral hygiene can result in decayed teeth, plaque, and periodontal disease and cause growth of bacteria in mouth, which can be aspirated (Eisenstadt, 2010).
7. Observe patient during previous mealtime for signs of dysphagia such as coughing, dyspnea, or drooling. Observe patient attempt to feed self; note type of food consistencies and liquids able to swallow. Note during and at end of meal if patient tires.	Detects abnormal eating patterns such as frequent clearing of throat or prolonged eating time. Chewing and sitting up for feeding bring on onset of fatigue (Meiner, 2015).
8. *Option:* Obtain baseline assessment oxygen saturation.	Research findings differ as to whether oximetry can reliably detect aspiration (ASHA, 2016; Lancaster, 2015).
9. Indicate on patient's electronic medical record (EMR), chart, or Kardex that dysphagia/aspiration risk is present. *Option:* Some agencies use different-colored meal trays to signify patients at risk for aspiration.	Identifying patient as dysphagic reduces risk that he or she will receive improperly prepared oral nutrition without supervision.

NURSING DIAGNOSES

- Impaired swallowing
- Risk for aspiration

Related factors/Risk factors are individualized based on patient's condition or needs.

PLANNING

1. Expected outcomes following completion of procedure:	
• Patient does not exhibit signs or symptoms of aspiration.	Interventions for preventing aspiration are successful.
• Patient maintains stable weight.	Patient is able to maintain adequate oral nutrition.
2. Provide patient 30 minutes of rest.	Fatigue increases risk of aspiration.
3. Explain to patient why you are observing him or her while he or she eats.	Signs or symptoms associated with aspiration indicate need for further swallowing evaluation such as fluoroscopic examination.
4. Explain to patient and family caregiver what you are going to do and why.	Increases patient cooperation and prepares family caregiver for being able to help.

IMPLEMENTATION

1. Perform hand hygiene and have patient or family caregiver (if going to help with feeding) perform hand hygiene.	Prevents transmission of microorganisms. Educates patient and family caregiver about need to maintain infection control practices.

STEP	RATIONALE
2. Apply clean gloves. Provide thorough oral hygiene, including brushing tongue, before meal.	Risk for aspiration pneumonia has been associated with poor oral hygiene (Eisenstadt, 2010).
3. Position patient upright (90 degrees) in chair or elevate head of patient's bed to a 45– to 90–degree angle or highest position allowed by medical condition during meal or position in chair.	Position facilitates safe swallowing and enhances esophageal motility (Metheny and Franz, 2013; Grodner et al., 2012; Ney et al., 2009). Side-lying position is an option if patient cannot have head elevated.
4. *Option:* Apply pulse oximeter to patient's finger; monitor during feeding.	Pulse oximetry may be reliable method of diagnosis of aspiration in most dysphagic stroke patients (Lancaster, 2015).
5. Using penlight and tongue blade, gently inspect mouth for pockets of food.	Pockets of food found inside cheeks occur when patient has difficulty moving food from mouth into pharynx; may lead to aspiration (Remig and Weeden, 2012). Patient is usually unaware of pocketing (Chang and Roberts, 2011).
6. Add thickener to thin liquids to create desired consistency per SLP assessment. Encourage patient to feed self.	Thin liquids are difficult to control in mouth and pharynx and are more easily aspirated (Garcia et al., 2010).
7. Have patient assume chin-tuck position. Remind patient to not tilt head backward when eating or while drinking.	Chin-tuck or chin-down position has traditionally been used to help reduce aspiration (Eisenstadt, 2010). However, a study of 47 patients with videofluoroscopic diagnosis of aspiration found that only 55% avoided aspiration during the chin-down posture (Terre and Mearin, 2012). More research is needed. Hyperextension of neck makes it easier for food to enter airway.
8. If patient unable to feed self, place ½ to 1 teaspoon of food on unaffected side of mouth, allowing utensil to touch mouth or tongue.	Small bites help patient swallow (Grodner et al., 2012). Provides tactile cue to food being eaten; avoids pocketing of food on weaker side.
9. Provide verbal coaching: remind patient to chew and think about swallowing. "Open your mouth. Feel the food in your mouth. Chew and taste the food. Raise your tongue to the roof of your mouth. Think about swallowing Close your mouth and swallow. Swallow again. Cough to clear your airway."	Verbal cueing keeps patient focused on normal swallowing (Metheny, 2012). Positive reinforcement enhances patient's confidence in ability to swallow. Double- or repeat-swallowing requires patient to use additional swallows to help clear any remaining food from unprotected airway (Garcia and Chambers, 2010).
10. Avoid mixing food of different textures in same mouthful. Alternate liquids and bites of food. Refer to RD for next meal if patient has difficulty with particular consistency.	Gradual increase in types and textures combined with constant monitoring ensures that patient is able to eat safely. Single textures are easier to swallow than multiple textures. Alternating solids with liquids removes food residue in mouth (Ney et al., 2009).
11. Monitor swallowing and observe for any respiratory difficulty. Observe for throat clearing, coughing, choking, gagging and drooling of food; suction airway as needed (see Chapter 25).	These are indications that suggest dysphagia and risk for aspiration (National Stroke Association, n.d.; DeFabrizio and Rajappa, 2010).
12. Minimize distractions, do not talk, and do not rush patient. Allow time for adequate chewing and swallowing. Provide rest period as needed during meal.	Environmental distractions and conversations during mealtime increase risk for aspiration (Chang and Roberts, 2011). Avoiding fatigue reduces aspiration risk.
13. Use sauces, condiments, and gravies to facilitate cohesive food bolus formation.	Cohesive food bolus helps to prevent pocketing or small food particles from entering the airway (Ney et al., 2009).
14. Ask patient to remain sitting upright for at least 30 to 60 minutes after meal.	Remaining upright after meals or snack reduces chance of aspiration by allowing food particles remaining in pharynx to clear (Frey and Ramsberger, 2011).
15. Provide thorough oral hygiene after meal (see Chapter 18).	Oral hygiene reduces plaque and secretions containing bacteria that can cause pneumonia, especially in patients with decreased immunity (Eisenstadt, 2010; Frey and Ramsberger, 2011).

STEP	RATIONALE
16. Remove gloves if worn. Return patient's tray to appropriate place and perform hand hygiene.	Reduces spread of microorganisms.

EVALUATION

1. Throughout meal observe patient's ability to swallow food and fluids of various textures and thickness without choking.

Indicates if there is ease with swallowing and absence of signs related to aspiration (DeFabrizio and Rajappa, 2010). Ability to swallow can improve or deteriorate (Nazarko, 2009).

2. Monitor pulse oximetry readings for high-risk patients during eating.

Deteriorating oxygen saturation levels indicate aspiration.

3. Monitor patient's intake and output (I&O), calorie count, and food intake.

Helps to detect malnutrition and dehydration resulting from dysphagia.

4. Weigh patient daily or weekly.

Determines if weight is stable and reflects nutritional status.

5. Observe patient's oral cavity after meal.

Determines presence of food pockets after meal that has included foods of various textures.

6. Use Teach-Back: "We talked about why your husband is at risk to aspirate his food. Tell me the things to observe for that will tell you if he is having trouble swallowing? What should you do if these things happen during a meal?" Revise your instruction now or develop a plan for revised family caregiver teaching if family caregiver is not able to teach back correctly.

Determines family caregiver's level of understanding of instructional topic.

Unexpected Outcomes	Related Interventions
1. Patient coughs, gags, complains of food "stuck in throat," and has wet quality to voice when eating.	• Stop feeding immediately and place patient on NPO. • Notify health care provider and suction as needed. • Anticipate consultation with SLP for swallowing exercises and techniques to improve swallowing.
2. Patient experiences weight loss over next several days/weeks.	• Discuss findings with health care provider and RD. Determine if increasing frequency or quality of foods is needed. • Nutritional supplements may be needed.

Recording and Reporting

- Record in nurses' notes in electronic health record (EHR) or chart the assessment findings, patient's tolerance of liquid and food textures, amount of help required, position during meal, absence or presence of any symptoms of dysphagia during feeding fluid intake, and amount eaten.
- Report any coughing, gagging, choking, or other swallowing difficulties to health care provider.
- Communicate with other health care staff that patient has dysphagia during hand-off communication.
- Document your evaluation of family caregiver learning.

Special Considerations
Pediatric

- Long-term effects for a child diagnosed with pediatric dysphagia include poor weight gain velocity and/or undernutrition (failure to thrive), aspiration pneumonia and/or compromised pulmonary status, food aversion, oral aversion, dehydration, and ongoing need for enteral or parenteral nutrition (ASHA, 2016).

- The primary goals of feeding and swallowing interventions for children are to safely support adequate nutrition and hydration, determine the optimum feeding methods/technique to maximize swallowing safety and feeding efficiency, collaborate with family caregiver to incorporate dietary preferences, attain age-appropriate eating skills in the most normal setting and manner possible, minimize the risk of pulmonary complications, and maximize the quality of life (ASHA, 2016).

Gerontological

- Hospital patients with dementia are at high risk for eating and feeding difficulties and inadequate food and fluid intake. Depending on the severity of their cognitive impairment, they may forget to eat, forget they have eaten, fail to recognize food, or eat things that are not food.
- Eating difficulties may have existed before hospitalization, but they are likely to worsen in the hospital because people with dementia often become more confused in an unfamiliar place. Different mealtime routines and foods add to the problem.

- Patients with dementia may not be able tell anyone that they are hungry or that they need help eating or more time to chew and swallow.
- Minimize the use of sedatives and hypnotics because these agents may impair the cough reflex and swallowing (Metheny, 2012).

Home Care
- Educate patient and family caregiver about aspiration precautions, particularly the techniques most effective for the patient, to prevent pneumonia (Tanner, 2014).

- Warn family caregiver that older adults with pneumonia often complain of significantly fewer symptoms than their younger counterparts; for this reason aspiration pneumonia is underdiagnosed in this group. Delirium may be the only manifestation of pneumonia in elderly people.
- Dysphagia in home care is best managed with a multidisciplinary approach that includes patient, family caregiver, health care provider, nurse occupational therapist, and SLP (Tanner, 2014).

◆ CLINICAL DEBRIEF

A 73-year-old patient with Alzheimer's disease is receiving medication that leaves him with a dry mouth. Results of a nutritional screening indicate difficulty swallowing. Symptoms include frequent coughing during a meal. The patient's respiratory rate is 18/min, heart rate 90. The speech-language pathologist (SLP) recommended a dysphagia mechanically altered diet with liquids thickened to medium viscosity. He currently weighs 138 lbs (62.7 kg) and is 182.88 cm (6 feet) tall. His daughter visits frequently at the assisted-living facility. Although he can feed himself, she usually feeds him during scheduled mealtimes in the busy dining room. She frequently gives him sips of her coffee and bites of his favorite oatmeal cookies. The daughter encourages him to bend his head backward to make sure that he drinks all of the liquid in a cup or glass.

1. Determine the patient's body mass index (BMI) and rate his nutritional status.
2. Identify three ways you should teach the daughter to help him swallow and decrease his aspiration risk. Include rationales for your actions.
3. The patient is in the dining area where a nurse assistant is feeding him. The nurse assistant gives the patient some moist ground meat and then cooked fruit. The nurse walks up to the patient's table and notices the patient coughing and beginning to gag. The nurse instructs the nurse assistant to stop feeding. The patient has a respiratory rate of 30 per minute and shows effort needed to breathe. Write an SBAR for this situation.

◆ REVIEW QUESTIONS

1. The nurse may delegate the following care to the nursing assistive personnel (NAP). (Select all that apply.)
   1. Nutritional screening
   2. Aspiration precautions
   3. Feeding a patient
   4. Interpreting pulse oximetry readings
   5. Measuring a patient's weight
2. A patient is unable to eat more than 25% of any meal because of pain and nausea. Which of the following interventions would be most important for the nurse to perform? (Select all that apply.)
   1. Encourage the patient to eat small amounts several times during the day.
   2. Ask the patient which foods and beverages cause the least amount of nausea.
   3. Record a chronology of what the patient has been eating for the past 2 days.
   4. Provide an analgesic 30 minutes before a meal.

3. A nurse is examining a patient just admitted to an acute medicine unit in the hospital.
   List three assessment findings of the skin that would indicate a possible nutritional problem:
   a.
   b.
   c.

ⓔ *Visit the Evolve site for a complete list of Clinical Debrief and Review Questions answers.*

REFERENCES

Academy of Nutrition and Dietetics: Position of the Academy of Nutrition and Dietetics: food and nutrition for older adults: promoting health and wellness, *J Acad Nutr Diet* 112:1255, 2012.

Accreditation Council of Education in Nutrition and Dietetics (ACEND): *ACEND Accreditation Standards for Nutrition and Dietetics Coordinated Programs (P)*, Chicago, 2016, The Association.

Agency for Healthcare Research and Quality (AHRQ): *National Guidelines Clearinghouse— Nutrition in aging.* In *Evidence-based geriatric nursing protocols for best practice*, 2013, http://www.guideline.gov/content.aspx?id=43931. Accessed April 4, 2016.

American Speech, Language, Hearing Association (ASHA): *Pediatric dysphagia: causes*, 2016, http://www.asha.org/PRPSpecificTopic.aspx?folderid=8589934965&section=Causes. Accessed April 4, 2016.

Association of Parenteral and Enteral Nutrition (ASPEN): Clinical guidelines: nutrition, assessment, and interventions in adults, *J Parenter Enter Nutr* 35(1):16, 2011.

Barker LA, Gout BS, et al: Hospital malnutrition: prevalence, identification and impact on patients and the healthcare system, *Int J Environ Res Public Health* 8(2):514, 2011.

Calloway SD: *The CMS and Joint Commission Dietary Standards 2015: what hospitals need to know*, 2015, http://www.kyha.com/docs/Presentations/DietaryStandards.pdf. Accessed April 4, 2016.

Centers for Disease Control and Prevention (CDC): *Challenges in food safety*, 2015, http://www.cdc.gov/foodsafety/challenges/index.html. Accessed April 4, 2016.

Chang C, Roberts B: Strategies for feeding patients with dementia, *Am J Nurs* 111(4):36, 2011.

Charney P, Escott-Stump S: Overview of nutrition diagnosis and intervention. In Mahan LK, Escott-Stump S, et al, editors: *Krause's food nutrition and the nutrition care process*, ed 13, Philadelphia, 2012, Saunders.

Choban P, et al: ASPEN Clinical guidelines: Nutrition support of hospitalized adult patients with obesity, *JPEN J Parenter Enteral Nutr* 37(6):714, 2013.

DeFabrizio M, Rajappa A: Contemporary approach to dysphagia management, *J Nurse Pract* 6(9):625, 2010.

Donovan NJ, et al: American Heart Association Council on Cardiovascular Nursing and Stroke Council. Dysphagia screening: state of the art: invitational conference proceeding from the State-of-the-Art Nursing Symposium, International Stroke Conference 2012, *Stroke* 44:e24, 2013.

Ebihara S, et al: Dysphagia, dystussia and aspiration pneumonia in elderly people, *J Thorac Disease* 8(3):632, 2016.

Eisenstadt E: Dysphagia and aspiration pneumonia in older adults, *J Acad Nurse Pract* 22:17, 2010.

Food and Agriculture Organization of the United Nations (FAO): *Food-based dietary guidelines*, 2015, http://www.fao.org/nutrition/education/food-dietary-guidelines/home/en/. Accessed April 5, 2016.

Frey K, Ramsberger G: Comparison of outcomes before and after implementation of a water protocol for patients with cerebrovascular accident and dysphagia, *J Neurosci Nurs* 43(3):165, 2011.

Gaddey HL, Holder K: Unintentional weight loss in older adults, *Am Fam Physician* 89(9):718, 2014.

Garcia J, Chambers E: Managing dysphagia through diet modifications, *Am J Nurs* 110(11):26, 2010.

Garcia JM, et al: Quality of care issues for dysphagia: modification involving oral fluids, *J Clin Nurs* 19:1618, 2010.

Garon B, et al: Silent aspiration: results of 2,000 video fluoroscopic evaluations, *J Neurosci Nurs* 41(4):178, 2009.

Grodner M, et al: *Foundations and clinical applications of nutrition: a nursing approach*, ed 5, St Louis, 2012, Mosby.

Hammond K, Litchford M: Dietary and clinical assessment. In Mahan LK, Escott Stump S, et al, editors: *Krause's food nutrition and the nutrition care process*, ed 13, Philadelphia, 2012, Saunders.

Healthy People 2020: Healthy People.gov, *Nutrition and weight status*, 2014a, http://www.healthypeople.gov/2020/topics-objectives/topic/nutrition-and-weight-status. Accessed April 5, 2016.

Healthy People 2020: Food safety, 2014b, http://www.healthypeople.gov/2020/topics-objectives/topic/food-safety. Accessed April 5, 2016.

Hockenberry MJ, Wilson D: *Wong's nursing care of infants and children*, ed 10, St Louis, 2015, Mosby.

Kaspar K, Ekberg O: Identifying vulnerable patients: role of the EAT-10 and the multidisciplinary team for early intervention and comprehensive dysphagia care, *Nestle Nutr Inst Workshop Ser* 72:19, 2012.

Kyle G: Managing dysphagia in older people with dementia, *Br J Community Nurs* 16(1):6, 2011.

Lancaster J: Dysphagia: its nature, assessment and management, *Br J Community Nurs* S28–S32, 2015.

Litchford M: Clinical: biochemical assessment. In Mahan LK, Escott-Stump S, et al, editors: *Krause's food nutrition and the nutrition care process*, ed 13, Philadelphia, 2012, Saunders.

Mayo Clinic: *Diseases and conditions: dysphagia*, 2014, http://www.mayoclinic.org/diseases-conditions/dysphagia/basics/symptoms/con-20033444. Accessed April 5, 2016.

Meiner S: *Gerontologic nursing*, ed 5, St Louis, 2015, Mosby.

Metheny N: Preventing aspiration in older adults with dysphagia, *Try This: Best Practices in Nursing Care to Older Adults*, Issue No. 20, revised 2012. https://consultgeri.org/try-this/general-assessment/issue-20. Accessed April 5, 2016.

Metheny NA, Frantz RA: Head-of-bed elevation in critically ill patients: a review, *Crit Care Nurs* 33(3):53, 2013.

National Cancer Institute (NCI): *Oral complications of chemotherapy and head/neck radiation—for health professionals (PDQ®): oral mucositis*, 2014, http://www.cancer.gov/about-cancer/treatment/side-effects/mouth-throat/oral-complications-hp-pdq#section/_337. Accessed April 5, 2016.

National Dysphagia Diet Task Force (NDDTF): *National dysphagia diet: standardization for optimal care*, Chicago, 2002, American Dietetic Association.

National Heart, Lung, and Blood Institute (NHLBI): *Obesity education initiative*, 2012, http://www.nhlbi.nih.gov/health/health-topics/topics/obe/diagnosis. Accessed April 5, 2016.

National Heart, Lung, and Blood Institute (NHLBI): *What are the signs of iron-deficiency anemia?* 2014, http://www.nhlbi.nih.gov/health/health-topics/topics/ida/signs. Accessed April 5, 2016.

National Heart, Lung, and Blood Institute (NHLBI): *Calculate your body mass index*, n.d., http://www.nhlbi.nih.gov/health/educational/lose_wt/BMI/bmicalc.htm. Accessed April 5, 2016.

National Stroke Association: *Dysphagia*, nd, http://www.stroke.org/we-can-help/survivors/stroke-recovery/post-stroke-conditions/physical/dysphagia. Accessed August 3, 2016.

National Quality Forum (NQF): *National voluntary consensus standards for patient safety: a consensus report*, Washington, DC, 2010, NQF.

Nazarko L: Nutrition. Part 5: Dysphagia, *Br J Healthcare Assist* 3(5):228, 2009.

Ney D, et al: Senescent swallowing: impact, strategies, and interventions, *Nutr Clin Practice* 24:395, 2009.

Remig V, Weeden A: Medical nutrition therapy for neurologic disorders. In Mahan LK, Escott-Stump S, et al, editors: *Krause's food nutrition and the nutrition care process*, ed 13, Philadelphia, 2012, Saunders.

Steele CM, Cichero J: Physiological factors related to aspirational risk: systematic review, *Dysphagia* 29(3):295, 2014.

Sura L, et al: Dysphagia in the elderly: management and nutritional considerations, *Clin Interv Aging* 7:287, 2012.

Tanner D: Avoiding negative dysphagia outcomes, *Online J Issues Nurs* 19(2):6, 2014.

Terre R, Mearin F: Effectiveness of chin-down posture to prevent tracheal aspiration in dysphagia secondary to acquired brain injury: a videofluoroscopy study, *Neurogastroenterol Motil* 24(5):414, 2012.

The Joint Commission (TJC): *2015 Comprehensive accreditation manual for hospitals: the official handbook*, Oakbrook Terrace, IL, 2015, TJC.

The Joint Commission (TJC): *2016 National Patient Safety Goals (NPGs)*, 2016, TJC. http://www.jointcommission.org/standards_information/npsgs.aspx. Accessed April 5, 2016.

US Department of Agriculture (USDA): *ChooseMyPlate*, 2015, http://www.choosemyplate.gov/MyPlate. Accessed April 5, 2016.

US Department of Agriculture (USDA) and US Department of Health and Human Services (USDHHS): *Dietary guidelines for Americans*, 2015, http://health.gov/dietaryguidelines/2015-scientific-report/. Accessed April 5, 2016.

Walker K, et al: Swallowing problems (dysphagia) in multiple sclerosis: a provider's approach, *US Department of Veterans Affairs*, 2009, http://www.va.gov/MS/Veterans/symptom_management/Swallowing_Problems_Dysphagia_in_Multiple_Sclerosis_A_Provider_s_Approach.asp. Accessed April 5, 2016.

32 | Enteral Nutrition

OBJECTIVES

Mastery of content in this chapter will enable the nurse to:
- Assess patients who are to have enteral tubes inserted.
- Assess patients who are to receive enteral tube feedings.
- Demonstrate the ability to insert a small-bore feeding tube correctly.
- Discuss the rationale for methods to determine nasogastric or nasoenteric feeding tube placement.

- Discuss the reasons for risks of pulmonary complications during the insertion and maintenance of a feeding tube.
- Demonstrate the appropriate technique for irrigating a feeding tube.
- Demonstrate three appropriate techniques for administering enteral formulas.
- Evaluate a patient's tolerance of enteral feeding.

MEDIA RESOURCES

- evolve http://evolve.elsevier.com/Perry/skills
- Review Questions
- Audio Glossary

- **NSO** Nursing Skills Online
- Clinical Debrief and Review Questions Answers

PURPOSE

Enteral nutrition refers to the delivery of nutritional formulas through a tube that has been inserted into the gastrointestinal (GI) tract. Nasogastric (NG) feedings are delivered through a feeding tube introduced through the nose into the stomach. Nasointestinal (NI) feedings are delivered through a feeding tube introduced through the nose into the small intestine. Tubes are sometimes placed orally if a patient has trauma to the nose, cranial injury/surgery, or facial surgery. Candidates for tube feeding include patients who have adequate digestion and absorption but cannot ingest, chew, or swallow food safely or in adequate amounts.

STANDARDS OF CARE

- Bankhead R, et al., ASPEN, Enteral Nutrition Practice Recommendations, 2009—Enteral Tube Insertion and Maintenance, Enteral Feeding Guidelines
- Institute for Safe Medication Practices (ISMP), 2015—ENFit Enteral Devices
- The Joint Commission (TJC), 2016—Patient Identification

PRINCIPLES FOR PRACTICE

- The selection of an enteral feeding tube and placement method depends on the anticipated duration of feeding and other patient-related factors such as gastric emptying, GI anatomy, and risk for gastric reflux.

- Nasal tubes are associated with sinusitis, otitis, vocal cord paralysis, and pressure injuries to the nose and sinuses.
- The reflux of tube-feeding formula into the oropharynx can lead to aspiration into the lung.
- The Institute for Safe Medication Practices (ISMP) strongly recommends that liquid medication for patients with feeding tubes be prepared and dispensed in exact doses by pharmacy (ISMP, 2015).
- X-ray film verification is recommended to confirm correct placement of any blindly inserted enteral tube before its initial use for feedings or medication administration (Bourgault et al., 2015; Lemyze, 2010).
- Marking and documenting the exit site of an enteral tube at the time of radiographic confirmation of correct placement will be helpful in subsequent monitoring of the location of the tube during its use for feedings (McCarthy and Martindale, 2015).

PATIENT-CENTERED CARE

- The insertion and use of a feeding tube often raises emotional and psychological concerns. A patient and family caregiver need reassurance and encouragement throughout the insertion procedure and once the tube feeding is in progress.
- Nursing interventions such as oral hygiene and care of the nasal passage or tube insertion site promote patient comfort during tube feeding and can reduce complications.

- Although tube feedings offer life-sustaining treatment, artificial nutrition can never replace the social and symbolic benefits of sharing meals. Social, religious, and cultural events involve food; patients requiring long-term tube feeding may feel a sense of loss regarding their ability to participate in life activities.
- An interprofessional team approach can help patients and family caregivers use nutritional strategies to preserve or enhance quality of life. Involvement of a speech pathologist can evaluate the ability of a patient to swallow safely.
- Encourage patients who require long-term tube feedings to use resources available to them such as the Oley Foundation, which can provide them with education, outreach, and networking.
- Patients with living wills or other forms of advanced directives may refuse the use of artificial feeding via a feeding tube. An interprofessional approach that considers cultural, spiritual, and psychological dimensions of this issue should be considered based on the patient's treatment goals.

EVIDENCE-BASED PRACTICE

Evidence-based guidelines ensure correct technique for placing enteral feeding tubes, initiating and maintaining enteral nutrition, and reducing risks for feeding tube complications.

- Obtain radiographic confirmation of correct placement of any blindly inserted tube before its initial use for feeding or medication administration (Bankhead et al., 2009; Bourgault et al., 2015). The most common complication of blindly inserted feeding tubes is improper placement in the esophagus or pulmonary system (Bourgault et al., 2015).
- Feeding tubes are positioned into the small bowel to reduce the incidence of pulmonary aspiration of stomach contents. Research has not demonstrated this benefit consistently, but newer techniques for detecting aspiration provide some evidence that small-intestine feeding does reduce the incidence of pulmonary aspiration (Metheny et al., 2011).
- The testing of gastric pH is useful in distinguishing between gastric and small-bowel tube positons. This method is of minimal benefit during continuous feedings because enteral formula buffers the gastric pH (Gilbertson et al., 2011).
- Capnography and carbon dioxide (CO_2) detectors have been used to assess position of small-bore feeding tubes and can identify a tube placed in the airway by measuring CO_2 in expired air that directly reveals CO_2 being eliminated from the lungs. However, capnography does not verify proper position of the tube in the GI tract; therefore final tube placement should be

verified by an x-ray film (Krenitsky, 2011; Wallace and Gardner, 2015).
- Maintaining and monitoring tube location during enteral feeding and keeping the head-of-bed elevation at a minimum of 30 degrees (preferably 45 degrees) effectively reduces aspiration and subsequent pneumonia (Metheny and Frantz, 2013).
- Gastric residual volumes (GRVs) are measured routinely during tube feeding to identify risk for regurgitation and pulmonary aspiration of gastric contents. This technique involves withdrawing and measuring stomach contents at regular intervals during tube feeding. Feeding is stopped when GRVs exceed a specified level; however, studies have failed to demonstrate a consistent relationship between GRV and risk of pulmonary aspiration, regurgitation, or pneumonia (McCarthy and Martindale, 2015). Recommendations for stopping tube feeding for elevated GRVs range from 250 to 500 mL, but automatic cessation of feeding should not occur for GRV less than 500 mL in the absence of other signs of intolerance (Delegge, 2011; McCarthy and Martindale, 2015).

SAFETY GUIDELINES

- Be aware of factors that increase a patient's risk for complications related to feeding tube insertion: altered level of consciousness, abnormal clotting, or impaired gag or cough reflex.
- Know the purpose of the feeding and the intended location of the tip of the feeding tube.
- Take precautions to prevent microbial contamination of enteral formulas.
- Be aware of safety measures to prevent pulmonary aspiration of gastric contents and accidental tube displacement by patients.
- Consult with a pharmacist regarding a patient's medications and their route of delivery to determine if administration via feeding tube is appropriate.
- Use ENFit connector for all enteral nutrition sets, syringes, and feeding tubes to improve patient safety. The ENFit connector is not compatible with Luer-Lok connections or any other small-bore medical connectors and thus prevents misadministration of an enteral feeding or medication by the wrong route (ISMP, 2015; Kozeniecki and Fritzshall, 2015).
- A medical device–related pressure injury is a localized injury to the skin or underlying tissue that forms as a result of sustained pressure from a device. Choose the correct size of medical device(s) to fit the individual, cushion and protect the skin with dressings in high-risk areas (e.g., nasal bridge), and remove or move the device daily to assess skin (NPUAP, 2013).

◆ **SKILL 32.1**   **Inserting and Removing a Small-Bore Nasogastric or Nasoenteric Feeding Tube**

NSO *Nursing Skills Online Enteral Nutrition Module / Lessons 1 and 2*

Throughout this chapter nasally placed feeding tubes (8 to 12 French [Fr]) are referred to as *nasogastric (NG) tubes*; but some types of NG tubes, which are larger and more rigid, are used for gastric decompression instead of feeding (see Chapter 35). Small-bowel *nasointestinal (NI) tubes* such as nasojejunal (NJ) are also used for enteral tube feedings, and these are advanced into the jejunum of the small intestine by way of the nose. Feeding tubes are soft and flexible; many use a removable guidewire or stylet to provide stiffness during tube insertion. Although these wires

facilitate placement of a tube, they also add to the risk of pulmonary or esophageal injury during insertion. Nurses can also pass feeding tubes through the mouth (oral gastric tube), especially in critical care when the patient is also intubated or when contraindications to nasal placement such as a basilar skull fracture or facial trauma exist.

Placement of a feeding tube requires a health care provider's order. All candidates for NG or NI tube placement require an assessment of their coagulation status. Anticoagulation and bleeding disorders pose a risk for epistaxis during nasal tube placement; the health care provider may order platelet transfusion or other corrective measures before tube insertion.

Delegation and Collaboration

The skill of feeding tube insertion cannot be delegated to nursing assistive personnel (NAP). However, NAP may help with patient positioning and comfort measures during tube insertion.

Equipment

Insertion

- Small-bore NG or nasoenteric tube with or without stylet (select the smallest diameter possible to enhance patient comfort) (Fig. 32.1)
- 60-mL ENFit syringe
- Stethoscope, pulse oximeter, capnography (optional)
- Hypoallergenic tape, semipermeable (transparent) dressing, or tube fixation device
- Tincture of benzoin or other skin barrier protectant
- pH indicator strip (scale 1.0 to 11.0)
- Cup of water and straw or ice chips (for patients able to swallow)
- Water-soluble lubricant
- Emesis basin
- Towel or disposable pad
- Facial tissues
- Clean gloves
- Suction equipment in case of aspiration
- Penlight to check placement in nasopharynx

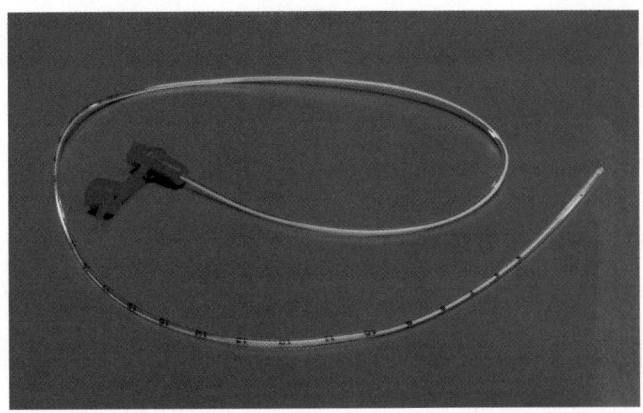

FIG 32.1 Small-bore feeding tube. (*Courtesy Kendall Brands, Mansfield, MA.*)

- Tongue blade
- Oral hygiene supplies

Removal
- Disposable pad
- Tissues
- Clean gloves
- Disposable plastic bag
- Towel

STEP	RATIONALE

ASSESSMENT

1. Verify health care provider's order for type of tube and enteric feeding schedule. Also check order to determine if health care provider wants prokinetic agent (e.g., metoclopramide) given before tube placement.	Health care provider's order is needed to insert feeding tube. Prokinetic agent given before tube placement may help advance tube into intestine.
2. Identify patient using at least two identifiers (e.g., name and birthday or name and medical record number), according to agency policy.	Ensures correct patient. Complies with The Joint Commission standards and improves patient safety (TJC, 2016).
3. Assess patient's knowledge of procedure.	Encourages cooperation, reduces anxiety, and minimizes risks. Identifies teaching needs.
4. Perform hand hygiene. Have patient close each nostril alternately and breathe. Examine each naris for patency and skin breakdown (apply clean gloves if drainage present).	Reduces transmission of microorganisms. Sometimes nares are obstructed or irritated, or septal defect or facial fractures are present. Place tube in most patent naris.
5. Review patient's medical history (e.g., for basilar skull fracture, nasal problems, nosebleeds, facial trauma, nasal-facial surgery, deviated septum, anticoagulant therapy, coagulopathy).	History of these problems may require you to consult with health care provider to change route of nutritional support. Passage of tube intracranially can cause neurological injury.

Clinical Decision Point *If a patient is at risk for intracranial passage of the tube, avoid the nasal route. Oral placement or placement under medical supervision using fluoroscopic direct visualization is preferable. Insertion of a gastrostomy or jejunostomy tube is another alternative.*

6. Assess patient's height, weight, hydration status, electrolyte balance, caloric needs and intake and output (I&O).	Provides baseline information to measure nutritional improvement after enteral feedings.
7. Assess patient's mental status (ability to cooperate with procedure, sedation), presence of cough and gag reflex, ability to swallow, critical illness, and presence of artificial airway.	These are risk factors for inadvertent tube placement into tracheobronchial tree (Krenitsky, 2011).

Clinical Decision Point *Recognize situations in which blind placement of a feeding tube poses an unacceptable risk for placement. Devices designed to detect pulmonary intubation such as CO_2 sensors or electromagnetic tracking devices enhance patient safety. Alternatively, to avoid insertion complications from blind placement in high-risk situations, clinicians trained in the use of visualization or imaging techniques should place tubes (AACN, 2010; Krenitsky, 2011).*

STEP	RATIONALE
8. Perform physical assessment of abdomen (see Chapter 6). Remove and dispose of gloves (if worn). Perform hand hygiene.	Absent bowel sounds, abdominal pain, tenderness, or distention may indicate medical problem contraindicating feedings.

NURSING DIAGNOSES

- Imbalanced nutrition: less than body requirements
- Impaired comfort
- Risk for aspiration

Related factors/Risk factors are individualized based on patient's condition or needs.

PLANNING

1. Expected outcomes following completion of procedure:	
• Tube is successfully placed in stomach or small intestine.	Proper position is essential before initiating feeding tube.
• Feeding tube remains patent.	Proper irrigation clears tube of formula residue (Bankhead et al., 2009).
• Patient has no respiratory distress (e.g., increased respiratory rate, coughing, poor color) or signs of discomfort or nasal trauma.	Correctly placed tube causes no interference with airway.
2. Explain procedure to patient, including sensations (e.g., burning in nasal passages) that will be felt during insertion.	Increases patient's cooperation with intubation procedure and helps lessen anxiety.
3. Explain to patient how to communicate during intubation by raising index finger to indicate gagging or discomfort.	Patient must have a way of communicating to alleviate stress and enhance cooperation.

IMPLEMENTATION

1. Perform hand hygiene. Prepare supplies at bedside.	Reduces transmission of microorganisms. Ensures organized procedure.
2. Stand on same side of bed as naris chosen for insertion and position patient upright in high-Fowler's position (unless contraindicated). If patient is comatose, raise head of bed as tolerated in semi-Fowler's position with head tipped forward, using a pillow chin to chest. If necessary have an NAP help with positioning of confused or comatose patients. If patient is forced to lie supine, place in reverse Trendelenburg's position.	Allows for easier manipulation of tube. Fowler's position reduces risk of aspiration and promotes effective swallowing. Forward head position helps with closure of airway and passage of tube into esophagus.
3. Apply pulse oximeter/capnograph and measure vital signs.	Provides baseline for objective assessment of respiratory status during tube insertion.
a. If patient has increase in end-tidal carbon dioxide or decrease in oxygen saturation, tube should not be inserted until you determine patient stability.	
4. Place bath towel over patient's chest. Keep facial tissues within reach.	Prevents soiling of gown. Insertion of tube frequently produces tearing.
5. Determine length of tube to be inserted and mark location with tape or indelible ink.	
a. Measure distance from tip of nose to earlobe to xyphoid process of sternum (see illustration). Mark this distance on tube with tape.	Length approximates distance from nose to stomach.
b. Measure distance from tip of nose to earlobe to mid-umbilicus for pediatric patient.	
c. Add 20 to 30 cm (8 to 12 inches) for NJ tubes.	Length approximates distance from nose to jejunum.

Clinical Decision Point *Tip of NG tube must reach stomach to avoid the risk for pulmonary aspiration, which occurs when tubes terminate in the esophagus.*

6. Prepare NG or NJ tube for intubation. NOTE: Do not ice tubes.	Iced tube becomes stiff and inflexible, causing trauma to nasal mucosa.
a. Obtain order for stylet tube and check agency policy for trained clinician to insert tube.	

STEP	RATIONALE
b. If tube has guidewire or stylet, inject 10 mL of water from ENFit syringe into tube	Aids in guidewire or stylet removal. Activates lubrication of tube for easier passage and ensures that tube is patent. ENFit devices will not be compatible with Luer connection or any other type of small-bore medical connector, thus preventing misadministration of an enteral feeding (ISMP, 2015).
c. If using stylet, make certain that it is positioned securely within tube. Inject 10 mL of water from ENFit syringe into tube.	Promotes smooth passage of tube into gastrointestinal (GI) tract. Improperly positioned stylet can cause tube to kink or injure patient. Ensures that tube is patent and aids in stylet removal. Once tube insertion is confirmed, have trained clinician remove stylet.
7. Prepare tube fixation materials. Cut hypoallergenic tape 10 cm (4 inches) long or prepare membrane dressing or other tube fixation device.	Used to secure tubing after insertion. Fixation devices allow tube to float free of nares, thus reducing pressure on nares, preventing device-related pressure injury (DRPI).
8. Apply clean gloves.	Reduces transmission of microorganisms.
9. *Option:* Dip tube with surface lubricant into glass of room-temperature water or apply water-soluble lubricant (see manufacturer directions).	Activates lubricant to facilitate passage of tube into naris and GI tract.
10. Hand alert patient a cup of water with straw (if able to swallow).	Patient is asked to swallow water to facilitate tube passage.
11. Explain next steps and gently insert tube through nostril to back of throat (posterior nasopharynx). This may cause patient to gag. Aim back and down toward ear (see illustration).	Natural contours facilitate passage of tube into GI tract.
12. Have patient take deep breath, relax, and flex head toward chest after tube has passed through nasopharynx.	Closes off glottis and reduces risk for tube entering trachea.
13. Encourage patient to swallow small sips of water. Advance tube as patient swallows. Rotate tube gently 180 degrees while inserting.	Swallowing facilitates passage of tube past oropharynx. Distinct tug may be felt as patient swallows, indicating that tube is following expected path.
14. Emphasize need to mouth breathe and swallow during insertion.	Helps facilitate passage of tube and alleviates patient's fears during procedure.
15. Do not advance tube during inspiration or coughing because it is more likely to enter respiratory tract. Monitor oximetry and capnography at this time.	Can cause tube to inadvertently enter patient's airway, which will be reflected in changes in oxygen saturation and/or capnography.
16. Advance tube each time patient swallows until desired length has been reached (see illustration).	Reduces discomfort and trauma to patient. Helps facilitate tube passage.

Clinical Decision Point *Do not force the tube or push against resistance. If patient starts to cough, experiences a drop in oxygen saturation, or shows other signs of respiratory distress, withdraw the tube into the posterior nasopharynx until normal breathing resumes.*

STEP	RATIONALE
17. Check for position of tube in back of throat using penlight and tongue blade.	Tube may be coiled, kinked, or entering trachea.
18. Temporarily anchor tube to nose with small piece of tape.	Movement of tube stimulates gagging. Assesses general position before anchoring tube more securely.

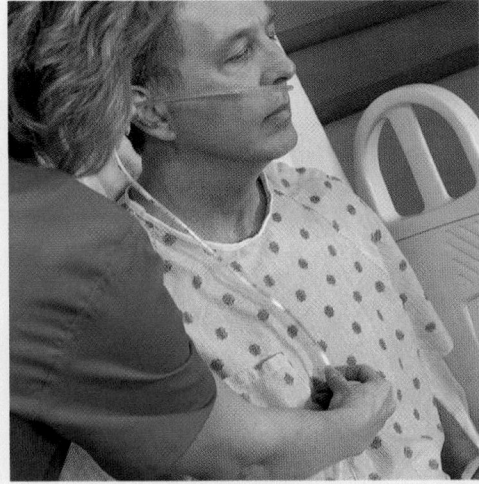

STEP 5a Measure to determine length of tube to insert.

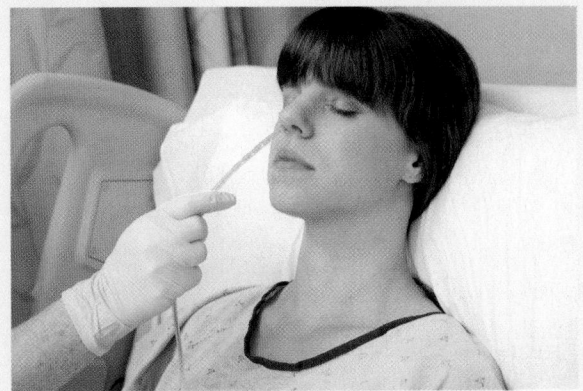

STEP 11 Insert tube through nostril to back of throat.

STEP	RATIONALE

19. Keep tube secure and check its placement by aspirating stomach contents to measure gastric pH (see Skill 32.2). Also measure amount, color, and quality of return.

Proper tube position is essential before initiating feeding.

Clinical Decision Point *Insufflation of air into tube while auscultating abdomen is not a reliable means to determine position of feeding tube tip (Bourgault et al., 2014; Simons and Abdallah, 2012).*

20. Anchor tube to patient's nose, avoiding pressure on nares. Mark exit site on tube with indelible ink. Select one of the following options for anchoring:
    a. Apply membrane dressing or tube fixation device:
      (1) Membrane dressing:
        (a) Apply tincture of benzoin or other skin protector to patient's cheek and area of tube to be secured.
        (b) Place tube against patient's cheek and secure tube with membrane dressing, out of patient's line of vision.
      (2) Tube fixation device:
        (a) Apply wide end of patch to bridge of nose (see illustration).
        (b) Slip connector around feeding tube as it exits nose (see illustration).

Marking tube can alert nurses to possible displacement of tube. Properly secured tube allows patient more mobility and prevents trauma to nasal mucosa.
Permits longer securement without need to change dressing. Allows membrane to adhere to skin.

Eliminates application of tape around naris. Decreases risk for patient's inadvertent extubation.

Secures tube and reduces friction on naris.

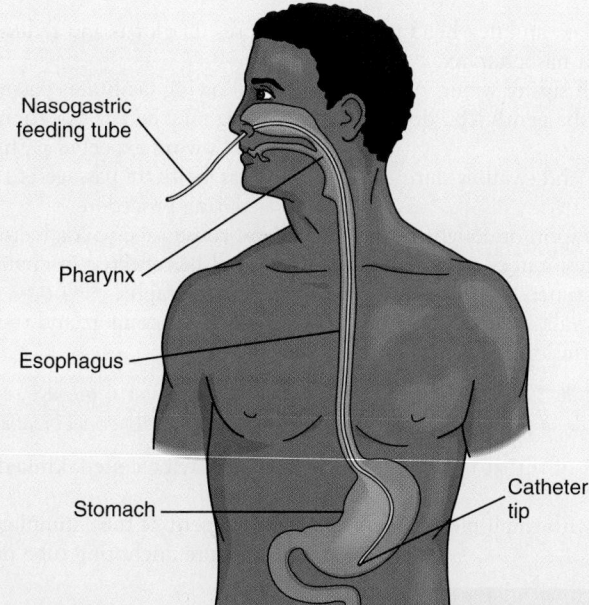

STEP 16 NG tube inserted through nasopharynx and esophagus into stomach.

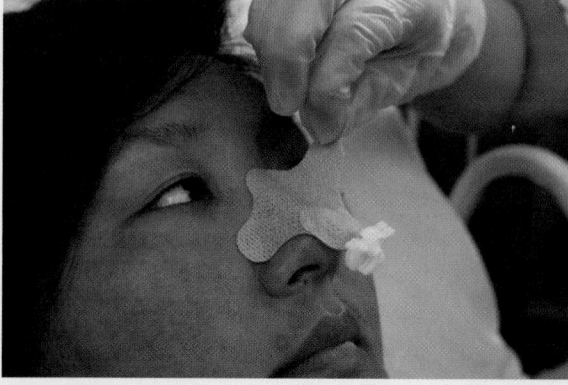

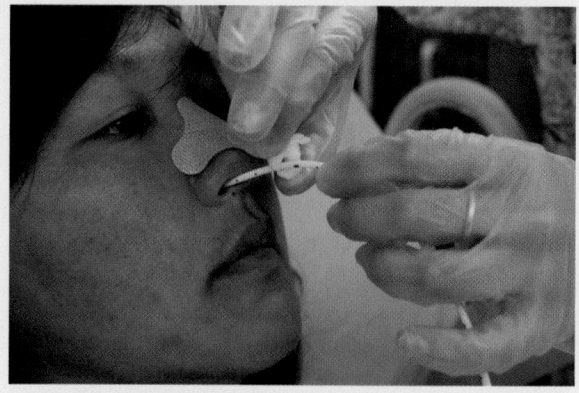

STEP 20a(2)(a) Apply tube fixation device to bridge of nose.

STEP 20a(2)(b) Slip connector around feeding tube.

STEP	RATIONALE

b. Apply tape:

Prevents pulling of tube. May require frequent change if tape becomes soiled.

(1) Apply tincture of benzoin or other skin adhesive on tip of patient's nose and allow it to become "tacky."

Helps tape adhere better. Protects skin.

(2) Remove gloves and tear two horizontal slits on each side of tape at ⅓ and ⅔ length. Do not split tape. Fold middle sections forward.

Creates a gap in tape that will allow tube to float and exert less pressure on naris.

(3) Tear vertical strip at bottom of tape. Print date and time on nasal part of tape.

Secures tube firmly.

(4) Place intact end of tape over bridge of patient's nose. Wrap each strip around tube as it exits (see illustration).

Tube is free floating in the naris with this taping method, resulting in movement of tube in pharynx. Securing tape to naris in this method reduces pressure on naris and risk for medical device–related pressure injury (Markowitz et al., 2013).

21. Fasten end of tube to patient's gown using clip (see illustration) or piece of tape. Do not use safety pins to secure tube to gown.

Reduces traction on naris if tube moves, which can cause medical device–related pressure injury. Safety pins become unfastened and cause injury to patients.

22. Help patient to comfortable position but keep head of the bed elevated at least 30 degrees (preferably 45 degrees) unless contraindicated (Metheny and Frantz, 2013). For intestinal tube placement, place patient on right side when possible until radiographic confirmation of correct placement is made.

Promotes patient comfort and lowers risk of aspiration should patient receive tube feeding. Placing patient on right side promotes passage of NI tube into small intestine.

23. Remove gloves and perform hand hygiene.

Reduces transmission of microorganisms.

Clinical Decision Point *Leave stylet in place until correct position is verified by x-ray film. Never try to reinsert a partially or fully removed stylet while feeding tube is in place. This can cause perforation of tube and injure patient.*

24. Contact radiology to obtain x-ray film of chest/abdomen.

X-ray film examination is most accurate method to determine feeding-tube placement (Bankhead et al., 2009; Bourgault et al., 2014).

25. Perform hand hygiene. Apply clean gloves and administer oral hygiene (see Chapter 18). Clean tubing at nostril with washcloth dampened in mild soap and water.

Promotes patient comfort and integrity of oral mucous membranes.

26. Remove gloves, dispose of equipment, and perform hand hygiene.

Reduces transmission of microorganisms.

27. Tube removal:

a. Verify health care provider's order for tube removal.

Health care provider's order is needed to remove feeding tube.

b. Gather equipment.

Ensures organized procedure.

c. Explain procedure to patient.

Encourages cooperation, reduces anxiety, and minimizes risks. Identifies teaching needs.

d. Perform hand hygiene. Apply clean gloves.

Reduces transmission of microorganisms.

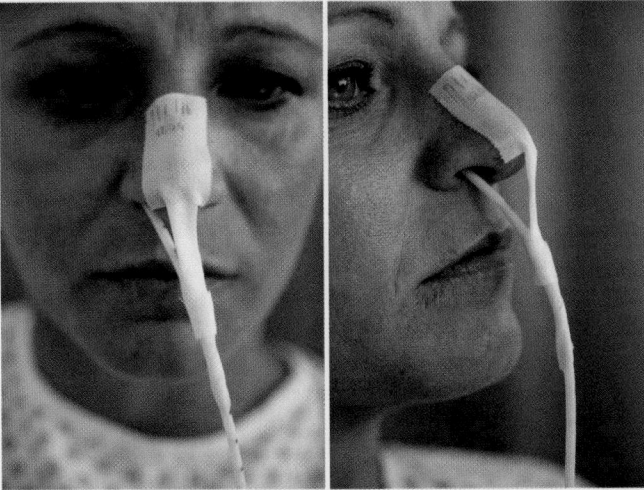

STEP 20b(4) A, Applying tape to anchor nasoenteral tube. **B,** Naris is free of pressure from tape and tube.

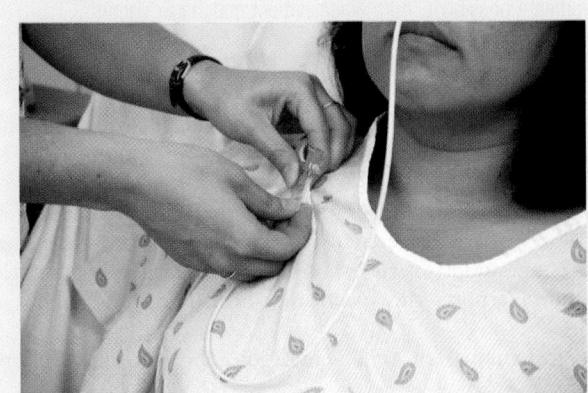

STEP 21 Fasten feeding tube to patient's gown.

STEP	RATIONALE
e. Position patient in high-Fowler's position unless contraindicated.	Reduces risk for pulmonary aspiration in event patient should vomit.
f. Place disposable pad or towel over patient's chest.	Prevents mucus and gastric secretions from soiling patient's clothing.
g. Disconnect tube from feeding administration set (if present) and clamp or cap end.	Prevents formula from spilling from tube as it is removed.
h. Remove tape or tube fixation device from patient's nose. Unclip tube from patient's gown.	Allows tube to be removed easily.
i. Instruct patient to take deep breath and hold it. Then as you kink end of tube securely (folding it over on itself), completely withdraw it by pulling it out steadily and smoothly onto towel or disposable bag. Dispose of it into appropriate receptacle.	Prevents inadvertent aspiration of gastric contents while tube is removed. Kinking prevents leakage of fluid from tube. Promotes patient comfort. Reduces transmission of microorganisms.
j. Offer tissues to patient to blow nose.	Clears nasal passages of remaining secretions.
k. Offer mouth care.	Promotes patient's comfort.
l. Remove and dispose of gloves; perform hand hygiene.	Reduces transmission of microorganisms.

EVALUATION

1. Observe patient's response to tube placement. Assess lung sounds; have patient speak; check vital signs; note any coughing, dyspnea, cyanosis, or decrease in oxygen saturation or capnography.

   Symptoms may indicate placement in respiratory tract. Auscultation of crackles, wheezes, dyspnea, or fever may be delayed response to aspiration. Capnography confirms tip not placed in trachea or lung.

2. Confirm x-ray film results with health care provider.

   Verifies position of tube before initiating enteral feeding.

3. Remove stylet after x-ray film verification of correct placement. Review agency policy regarding requirement of trained clinician for insertion.

   If placement needs adjustment, stylet is still in place.

4. Routinely check condition of nares, location of external exit site marking on tube, and color and pH of fluid aspirated from tube.

   Routine evaluation ensures no formation of medical device–related pressure injury and correct placement of tube.

5. After removal, assess patient's level of comfort.

   Provides for continued comfort of patient.

6. **Use Teach-Back:** "I want to be sure that I explained to you what you can do during insertion of the nasogastric tube so you can communicate with me. Tell me how you are going to do to communicate with me during tube insertion." Revise your instruction now or develop a plan for revised patient teaching if patient is not able to teach back correctly.

   Determines patient's level of understanding of instructional topic.

Unexpected Outcomes	Related Interventions
1. Aspiration of stomach contents into respiratory tract (delayed response or small-volume aspiration), evidenced by auscultation of crackles or wheezes, dyspnea, or fever.	• Report change in patient condition to health care provider; if there has not been a recent chest x-ray film, suggest ordering one. • Position patient on side to protect airway. • Suction nasotracheally and orotracheally. • Prepare for possible initiation of antibiotics.
2. Displacement of feeding tube to another site (e.g., from duodenum to stomach) possibly occurs when patient coughs or vomits.	• Aspirate GI contents and measure pH. • Remove displaced tube and insert and verify placement of new tube. • If there is question of aspiration, obtain chest x-ray film.

Recording and Reporting

• Record type and size of tube placed, location of distal tip of tube, patient's tolerance of procedure, condition of naris, and confirmation of tube position by x-ray film examination in nurses' notes in electronic health record (EHR) or chart.
• Record removal of tube, condition of naris, and patient's tolerance.
• Report any type of unexpected outcome and the interventions performed.
• Document your evaluation of patient learning.

Special Considerations
Teaching

• Instruct patient or family caregiver to offer oral hygiene frequently and keep patient's lips lubricated.
• Teach patient or family caregiver to report tension on feeding tube or displacement of tape or tube fixation device; instruct patient or caregiver to stabilize the tube and call for help.

Pediatric

• The distance from nose-to-ear-to–mid-umbilicus better predicts insertion length for gastric tube placement in neonates and children than traditional nose-to-ear-to-xyphoid measurements (Hockenberry and Wilson, 2015).

- X-ray film confirmation is the most accurate assessment of proper tube placement. Best bedside assessment of tube placement is to aspirate gastric contents for color and pH (Hockenberry and Wilson, 2015). When inserting a feeding tube in an infant, the heart rate and blood pressure may change in response to vagal stimulation.

Gerontological

- Ensure adequate lubrication of tube to decrease discomfort for the older adult because of the potential for decreased oral or nasopharyngeal secretions.

Home Care

- Assess patient's or family caregiver's ability to maintain a tube for a feeding program.
- Assess the environmental safety and sanitation of patient's home to determine potential for infection or injury.
- Teach patient or family caregiver how to assess tube placement (see Skill 32.2).
- Teach family caregiver correct method for securing a feeding tube and the routine care necessary to reduce pressure injuries.

◆ SKILL 32.2   Verifying Feeding Tube Placement

NSO *Nursing Skills Online Enteral Nutrition Module / Lesson 3*

Nurses insert small-bore feeding tubes nasally for intermittent or continuous feeding. It is possible for the tip of a feeding tube to move or migrate into a different location (e.g., from the stomach into the intestine or esophagus, from the intestine into the stomach). Although all tubes should be marked to document correct position, tube dislocation can sometimes occur without any external evidence that the tube has moved. The risk of aspiration of regurgitated gastric contents into the respiratory tract increases when the tip of the tube accidentally dislocates upward into the esophagus.

Following initial x-ray film verification of correct feeding tube position, you must monitor the tube to ensure that the tube tip remains in the intended site. Based on a patient's clinical condition and agency policies, you check feeding tube position at regular intervals (often every 4 to 6 hours) and before administering

formula or medications through the tube. Radiographic verification is impractical every 4 to 6 hours and costly, but the reports of routine chest and abdominal films should be monitored for reference to the feeding tube location. No single bedside method of monitoring tube position during feeding is completely reliable; there are a number of techniques to use in combination to detect feeding tube dislocation:

- Monitor the external length of the tube and observe the appearance, volume, and pH of fluid aspirated through it. The color of the fluid can help differentiate gastric from intestinal placement. Because most intestinal aspirates are stained by bile to a distinct yellow color and most gastric aspirates are not, the difference in color can often distinguish the sites (Fig. 32.2).

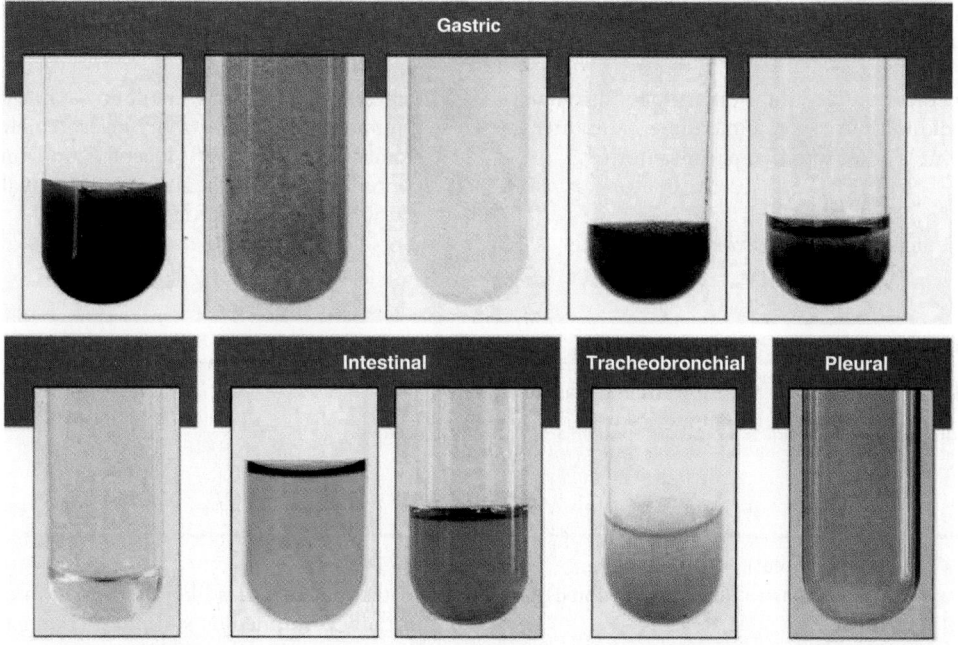

FIG 32.2 Typical color of aspirates from stomach, intestine, and airway. (*Used with permission from Metheny NA, et al: pH, color, and feeding tubes, RN 61:25, 1998.*)

- Testing the pH of an aspirate at the bedside using pH paper offers some information regarding the position of a feeding tube. However, the pH test has no value if a patient is receiving acid-suppression medication. Results are also less reliable during continuous feeding and should be used in combination with other indicators with careful assessment of a patient in the clinical setting (AACN, 2010; Lemyze, 2010; Simons and Abdullah, 2012).
- Obtain repeat x-ray film confirmation if bedside methods create any doubt regarding the location of a tube.

Delegation and Collaboration

The verification of tube placement is the responsibility of the nurse and cannot be delegated to nursing assistive personnel (NAP). The nurse directs the NAP to:
- Immediately inform the nurse if patient's respirations change or patient complains of shortness of breath, coughing, or choking.

- Immediately inform the nurse if the patient vomits or the NAP notices vomitus in patient's mouth during oral hygiene.
- Immediately inform the nurse if nasal skin irritation or excoriation is present.
- Immediately inform the nurse if a change in the external length of the tube occurs, which could indicate displacement of the tube.

Equipment
- 60-mL ENFit syringe
- Stethoscope
- Clean gloves
- pH indicator strip (scale of 1.0 to 11.0)
- Small medication cup

STEP	RATIONALE

ASSESSMENT

1. Review agency policy and procedures for frequency and method of checking tube placement. **Do not insufflate air into tube to check placement.**

2. Identify patient using at least two identifiers (e.g., name and birthday or name and medical record number) according to agency policy.

3. Observe for signs and symptoms of respiratory distress during feeding: coughing, choking, or reduced oxygen saturation.

4. Identify conditions that increase risk for spontaneous tube migration or dislocation: altered level of consciousness, agitation; retching, vomiting; nasotracheal suction.

5. Observe external part of tube for movement of ink or tape mark away from mouth or naris (see Skill 32.1).

6. Review patient's medication record for orders for continuous feeding, a gastric acid inhibitor (e.g., cimetidine, ranitidine, famotidine, nizatidine), or a proton pump inhibitor (e.g., omeprazole).

7. Review patient's medical record for history of prior tube displacement.

Maintains quality of patient care. Listening for air instilled through tube is unreliable (AACN, 2010; Bourgault et al., 2014).

Ensures correct patient. Complies with The Joint Commission standards and improves patient safety (TJC, 2016).

Once the tube has been correctly placed into gastrointestinal (GI) tract, movement into pulmonary system is unlikely. However, a tube that has been pulled back into esophagus can lead to regurgitation and aspiration of formula.

Feeding tubes may become dislocated by increases in intraabdominal pressure or coughing, but most frequently they are displaced when patient moves or during pulls on tube.

Increased external length of tube indicates that distal tip is no longer in correct position.

The presence of enteral formula in aspirated secretions diminishes usefulness of pH measurements by buffering pH of stomach. Similarly, H_2 receptor antagonists reduce acid content of secretions, also raising pH value (Bourgault et al., 2015, Simons and Abdallah, 2012).

Patients are at increased risk for repeated tube displacement.

NURSING DIAGNOSES

- Impaired gas exchange
- Risk for aspiration

Related factors/Risk factors are individualized based on patient's condition or needs.

PLANNING

1. Expected outcomes following completion of procedure:
   - Color, pH, and appearance of gastric aspirate are consistent with initial tube placement.

2. Explain procedure to patient.

Indicates that tube has likely remained in correct location, initially confirmed by x-ray film (Bourgault et al., 2015, Simons and Abdallah, 2012).

Patient has right to be informed regarding all procedures. Relieves anxiety.

STEP	RATIONALE

IMPLEMENTATION

1. Prepare equipment at patient's bedside, perform hand hygiene, and apply clean gloves.

2. Verify tube placement at following times:
   a. For intermittently tube-fed patients, test placement immediately before each feeding (usually a period of at least 4 hours will have elapsed since previous feeding) and before medications.

   b. Follow agency policy regarding when to test pH for patients receiving continuous tube feeding. AACN (2010) recommends that continuous feedings be stopped for several hours to obtain reliable pH readings; however, this is not appropriate for patient's therapeutic plan of care.

   c. Wait to verify placement at least 1 hour after medication administration by tube or mouth.

3. If tube feeding is infusing, turn off or place feeding on hold. Clamp or kink feeding tube and disconnect from feeding bag or for intermittent feedings remove plug at end of tube. Draw up 30 mL of air into a 60-mL ENFit syringe. Flush tube with 30 mL of air before attempting to aspirate fluid. Repositioning patient from side to side is helpful. In some cases more than one bolus of air is necessary.

4. Draw back on syringe slowly and obtain 5 to 10 mL of gastric aspirate (see illustration). Observe appearance of aspirate (see Fig. 32.2). Aspirates from nasogastric (NG) tubes of continuously tube-fed patients often look like curdled enteral formula. Gastric aspirates from intermittently tube-fed patients typically are not bile stained (unless intestinal fluid has refluxed into stomach) (AACN, 2010).

5. Gently mix aspirate in syringe. Expel few drops into clean medicine cup. Measure pH of aspirated GI contents by dipping pH strip into fluid or applying few drops of fluid to strip. Compare color of strip with color on chart (see illustration) provided by manufacturer.
   a. Gastric fluid from patient who has fasted for at least 4 hours usually has pH range of 5.0 or less.

   b. Fluid from tube in small intestine of fasting patient usually has pH greater than 6.0 (Bourgault et al., 2015).

RATIONALE

Reduces transmission of microorganisms. Organizes for procedure.

Each administration of feeding/medication can lead to pulmonary aspiration if tube is displaced. More frequent checking has been associated with increased clogging of small-bore tubes.

Feedings should not be stopped only for purpose of pH testing. pH testing may be helpful when feedings are interrupted for procedures or diagnostic studies (AACN, 2010; Bourgault et al., 2015).

Premature withdrawal of contents will remove unabsorbed medication, reducing dose delivered to patient.

Burst of air helps to aspirate fluid more easily. Smaller syringes generate unnecessarily high pressures inside tube.

It is often more difficult to aspirate fluid from small intestine than from stomach or smaller-size tube (AACN, 2010).

Drawing back quickly or using smaller syringe may cause tube to collapse.

Quantity is sufficient for pH testing.

Appearance of aspirate helps to assess position of tube.

Mixing ensures equal distribution of contents for testing. Most-accurate readings of gastric pH levels are provided by pH paper covering minimal range of from 1.0 to 11.0.

A pH value of pH 5.5 or below will exclude 100% of pulmonary placements and more than 93.9% of placements in small intestine (Metheny and Meert, 2004).

Intestinal contents are more basic than stomach contents. A pH greater than 6.0 indicates intestinal or pulmonary placement (Bourgault et al., 2015).

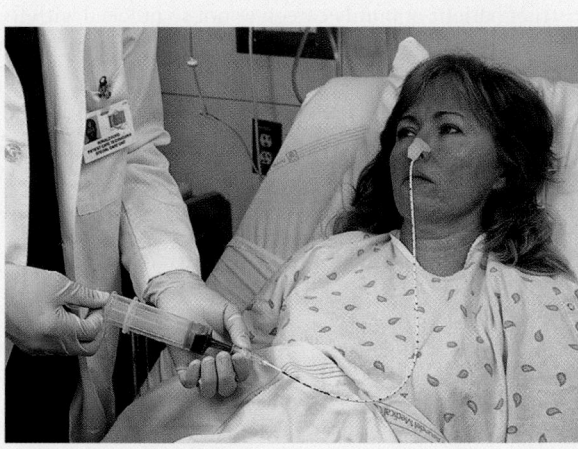

STEP 4 Obtain gastric aspirate.

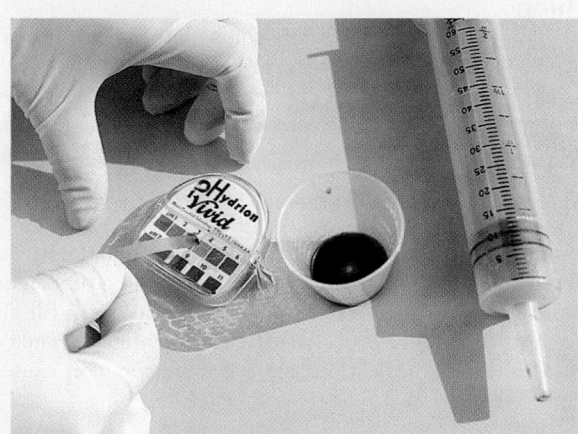

STEP 5 Compare color on test strip with color on pH chart.

STEP	RATIONALE
6. If after repeated attempts it is not possible to aspirate fluid from tube that was confirmed by x-ray film to be in desired position and if (1) there are no risk factors for tube dislocation, (2) tube has remained in original taped position, (3) patient is not in respiratory distress, assume that tube is correctly placed. Continue with irrigation, (AACN, 2010; Bourgault et al., 2015; Stepter, 2012).	Reports of routine chest or abdominal x-ray films can be used to monitor tube location. Repeat radiographic confirmation of tube position is indicated if external length of tube changes, tape holding tube comes loose, or patient coughs forcefully or vomits (AACN, 2010; Bankhead et al., 2009).
7. Irrigate tube (see Skill 32.3).	Keeps tube patent.
8. Remove and dispose of gloves and supplies in appropriate receptacle. Perform hand hygiene.	Reduces transmission of microorganisms.

EVALUATION

1. Observe patient for respiratory distress: persistent gagging, paroxysms of coughing, drop in oxygen (O_2) saturation, or respiratory patterns (e.g., rate and depth) that are inconsistent with baseline measures.	Indicates that tube may be displaced in respiratory tract.
2. Verify that external length of tube, pH, and appearance of aspirate are consistent with initial tube placement.	Indicates that tip of tube is likely to be positioned in same place as it was following x-ray film confirmation.
3. **Use Teach-Back:** "I want to go over what I explained earlier. Tell me why it is important for me to test gastric pH and the color of the gastric secretions before feedings." Revise your instruction now or develop a plan for revised patient or family caregiver teaching if patient or family caregiver is not able to teach back correctly.	Determines patient's and family caregiver's level of understanding of instructional topic.

Unexpected Outcomes

1. Red or brown coloring (coffee grounds appearance) of fluid aspirated from feeding tube indicates new or old blood, respectively, in GI tract.
2. Patient develops severe respiratory distress (e.g., dyspnea, decreased oxygen saturation, increased pulse rate) as a result of aspiration or tube displacement into lung.
3. Tube cannot be irrigated after testing.

Related Interventions

- If color is not related to medications recently administered, notify health care provider.
- Stop any enteral feedings.
- Notify health care provider.
- Obtain chest x-ray film as ordered.
- Reattempt to irrigate tube. Do not force fluid. If unsuccessful, notify health care provider.

Recording and Reporting

- Record and report pH and appearance of aspirate in nurses' notes in electronic health record (EHR) or chart.
- Document your evaluation of patient and family caregiver learning.

Special Considerations
Teaching

- Have family caregiver or patient demonstrate how to check tube placement while still in health care setting.
- Instruct patient to not pull or alter position of enteral tube.

Pediatric

- Decrease the amount of air insufflated according to patient's size (e.g., an infant may only need 1 mL of air, a small child 5 mL) before withdrawal of gastric secretions.

Home Care

- See Home Care, Skill 32.1.
- Instruct patient or family caregiver not to proceed with feedings or medication administration via the tube if there is any doubt as to its proper placement.

◆ SKILL 32.3   Irrigating a Feeding Tube

NSO *Nursing Skills Online Enteral Nutrition Module / Lesson 4*

Feeding tubes must remain patent to ensure that liquid nutritional formulas can pass through easily. All types of feeding tubes require routine irrigation to keep a tube patent. Inability to instill air or fluid suggests that a tube is occluded. Curdled enteral formula and improperly crushed medications are the most common causes of feeding tube occlusion.

Delegation and Collaboration

The skill of irrigating a feeding tube cannot be delegated to nursing assistive personnel (NAP). The nurse directs the NAP to:

- Report when a continuous tube feeding stops infusing.

Equipment

- 60-mL ENFit syringe
- Water (tap water or sterile [see agency policy], dated and initialed container at patient's bedside)
- Towel
- Clean gloves
- Stethoscope

STEP	RATIONALE

ASSESSMENT

1. Identify patient using at least two identifiers (e.g., name and birthday or name and medical record number), according to agency policy.

2. Perform hand hygiene and apply clean gloves. Inspect volume, color, and character of gastric aspirates (if obtainable) (see Skill 32.2). Remove and dispose of gloves and perform hand hygiene.

3. Assess bowel sounds.

4. Note ease with which tube feeding infuses through tubing.

5. Monitor volume of continuous enteral formula administered during shift and compare with ordered amount.

6. Refer to agency policies regarding routine irrigation or health care provider order.

Ensures correct patient. Complies with The Joint Commission standards and improves patient safety (TJC, 2016).

Excess volume of secretions (more than 250 mL) may indicate delayed gastric emptying.

Determines if peristalsis is present. Removal of tube will be delayed if peristalsis is not present. **NOTE:** Bowel sounds should be present if patient is receiving tube feedings.

Failure of formula to infuse as desired may indicate developing obstruction.

Indicates whether sufficient volume of feeding is infusing. Serves as baseline to determine tube patency.

Determines frequency of irrigations.

NURSING DIAGNOSES

- Deficient fluid volume
- Excess fluid volume
- Imbalanced nutrition: less than body requirements

Related factors are individualized based on patient's condition or needs.

PLANNING

1. Expected outcomes following completion of procedure:
   - Feeding tube remains patent.

   - Patient receives prescribed caloric intake.

2. Explain procedure to patient; stress that you are not removing tube.

3. Position patient in high-Fowler's (if tolerated) or semi-Fowler's position.

Irrigation fluid clears inner lumen of feeding tube of solids and secretions.

Feeding infuses without interruption.

Decreases patient anxiety.

Reduces reflux and risk for pulmonary aspiration during irrigation.

IMPLEMENTATION

1. Perform hand hygiene, prepare equipment at patient's bedside, and apply clean gloves.

2. Verify tube placement (see Skill 32.2) if fluid can be aspirated for pH testing.

3. Irrigate routinely before, between, and after final medication (before feedings are reinstituted); and before an intermittent feeding is administered.

4. Draw up 30 mL of water in ENFit syringe. Do not use irrigation fluids from bottles that are used on other patients. Patient should have individual bottle of solution.

Reduces transmission of microorganisms. Ensures organized approach to irrigation.

With tip of tube correctly placed in stomach or intestine, irrigation will not increase risk for pulmonary aspiration.

Certain formulas have properties that predispose to tube clogging. Irrigation prevents mixing of medications in tube, which may cause clogging.

This amount of solution will flush length of tube. Water is most effective agent for preventing tube clogging.

Clinical Decision Point *Do not use cola or fruit juices for flushing tubing.*

5. Change irrigation bottle every 24 hours. Irrigation trays, which hold both irrigation fluid and syringe, are considered open systems and may be more easily contaminated than sterile water bottles.
   NOTE: Be sure that syringe in tray has ENFit adaptor.

6. Kink feeding tube while disconnecting it from administration tubing or while removing plug at end of tube.

7. Insert tip of ENFit syringe into end of feeding tube. Release kink and slowly instill irrigation solution.

Ensures sterile solution. Sterile water is required for neonates and patients who are immune suppressed or critically ill (Bankhead et al., 2009; Hockenberry and Wilson, 2015).

Tap water may be appropriate in some clinical settings and in home care if municipal water supply is safe (Bankhead et al., 2009).

Prevents leakage of gastric secretions.

Infusion of fluid clears tubing.

STEP	RATIONALE
8. If unable to instill fluid, reposition patient on left side and try again.	Tip of tube may be against stomach wall. Changing patient's position may move tip away from stomach wall.
9. When water has been instilled, remove syringe. Reinstitute tube feeding or administer medication as ordered. Flush each medication completely through tube.	Tubing is clear and patent. Ensures that full dose reaches stomach and medications do not mix with formula.
10. Remove and discard gloves; dispose of supplies in appropriate receptacle. Perform hand hygiene.	Reduces transmission of microorganisms.

EVALUATION

1. Observe ease with which tube feeding instills through tubing.

2. Monitor patient's caloric intake.

3. **Use Teach-Back:** "I want to be sure that I explained to you and your wife why you need to flush your tube when you return home. Tell me why it is important to flush your tube." Revise your instruction now or develop a plan for revised patient or family caregiver teaching if patient or family caregiver is not able to teach back correctly.

Successfully irrigated tube is patent, allowing for free flow of solution.

Total enteral nutrition infuses without difficulty.

Determines patient's and family caregiver's level of understanding of instructional topic.

Unexpected Outcomes	Related Interventions
1. Tube cannot be irrigated and remains obstructed.	• Repeat irrigation; if unsuccessful, notify health care provider. • Tube may need to be removed, and a new tube placed.
2. Fluid and electrolyte imbalances occur. Insufficient irrigation can cause water deficiency; excessive irrigations can cause fluid volume excess.	• Notify health care provider of abnormal electrolyte levels or imbalanced intake and output.

Recording and Reporting

• Record time of irrigation, amount and type of fluid instilled in nurses' notes in electronic health record (EHR) or chart.
• Report if tubing has become clogged.
• Document your evaluation of patient and family caregiver learning.

Special Considerations
Pediatric

• Irrigation of a tube requires a smaller volume of solution in children: 1–2 mL for smaller tubes and 5–15 mL for larger tubes (Hockenberry and Wilson, 2015).

◆ **SKILL 32.4**   **Administering Enteral Nutrition: Nasoenteric, Gastrostomy, or Jejunostomy Tube**

NSO *Nursing Skills Online Enteral Nutrition Module / Lesson 5*

Enteral nutrition, or tube feeding, is a method for providing nutrients to patients who are not able to meet their nutritional requirements orally. As a rule candidates for enteral nutrition must have a sufficiently functional gastrointestinal (GI) tract to absorb nutrients. Examples of indications for enteral feeding include the following:

• Situations in which normal eating is unsafe because of high risk for aspiration: altered mental status, swallowing disorders, impaired gag reflex, dependence on mechanical ventilation, esophageal conditions (e.g., strictures or dysmotility), and delayed gastric emptying.
• Clinical conditions that interfere with normal ingestion or absorption of nutrients or create hypermetabolic states: surgical resection of oropharynx, proximal intestinal obstruction or fistula, pancreatitis, burns, and severe pressure injuries.
• Conditions in which disease- or treatment-related symptoms reduce oral intake: anorexia, nausea, pain, fatigue, shortness of breath, or depression.

Gastric feedings are the most common type of enteral nutrition, allowing tube-feeding formulas to enter the stomach and then pass gradually through the intestinal tract to ensure absorption. In contrast, small-bowel feeding occurs beyond the pyloric sphincter of the stomach, which theoretically reduces the risk for pulmonary aspiration, provided that feedings do not reflux back into the stomach (Metheny et al., 2011). To avoid bloating, cramping, and diarrhea, use of an enteral infusion pump controls the administration rate of small-bowel feedings and many continuous gastric feedings. Inadequate delivery of nutrients, potentially leading to caloric deficit or electrolyte disturbances, sometimes occurs because of frequent interruptions in feeding.

Aspiration is of concern for patients who receive enteral nutrition. Aspiration of enteral nutrition is a serious complication. Aspiration is the inhalation of oropharyngeal or gastric contents into the larynx and lower respiratory tract (Waybright et al., 2013). Efforts should be made to prevent or minimize aspiration. AACN (2012) recommends several expected practices to minimize the risk of aspiration in tube-fed patients:

• Maintain head-of-bed elevation at an angle of 30 to 45 degrees unless contraindicated.
• Use sedatives as sparingly as possible.
• For tube-fed patients, assess placement of the feeding tube at 4-hour intervals.

- For patients receiving gastric tube feedings, assess for GI intolerance to the feedings at 4-hour intervals.
- For tube-fed patients, avoid bolus feedings in those at high-risk for aspiration.

- Report any difficulty infusing the feeding or any discomfort voiced by patient.
- Report any gagging, paroxysms of coughing, or choking.
- Provide frequent oral hygiene.

Delegation and Collaboration

The skill of administration of nasoenteric tube feeding can be delegated to nursing assistive personnel (NAP) (refer to agency policy). A registered nurse (RN) or licensed practical nurse (LPN) must first verify tube placement and patency. The nurse directs the NAP to:
- Elevate head of bed to 30 to 45 degrees or sit patient up in bed or a chair unless contraindicated.
- Not adjust feeding rate; infuse the feeding as ordered.

Equipment

- Disposable feeding bag, tubing, or ready-to-hang system
- 60-mL or larger ENFit syringe
- Stethoscope
- Enteral infusion pump for continuous feedings
- pH indicator strip (scale 1.0 to 11.0)
- Prescribed enteral formula
- Clean gloves
- ENFit connector

STEP	RATIONALE

ASSESSMENT

1. Identify patient using at least two identifiers (e.g., name and birthday or name and medical record number), according to agency policy.	Ensures correct patient. Complies with The Joint Commission standards and improves patient safety (TJC, 2016).
2. Assess patient's clinical status to determine potential need for tube feedings: decreased level of consciousness, nutritional deficits, head or neck surgery, facial trauma, or impaired swallowing. Consult with nutrition support team and health care provider.	Identify candidates for enteral nutrition before they become nutritionally depleted. Health care provider order is necessary for feedings.
3. Assess patient for food allergies.	Prevents patient from developing localized or systemic allergic responses to feeding.
4. Perform physical assessment of abdomen, including auscultation for bowel sounds, before feeding (see Chapter 6).	Objective measures for assessing tolerance include changes in bowel sounds, expanding girth, tenderness and firmness on palpation, increasing nasogastric (NG) output, and vomiting (McCarthy and Martindale, 2015). Report findings to health care provider to determine if tube feeding can proceed safely (Bankhead et al., 2009).
5. Obtain baseline weight and review serum electrolytes and blood glucose measurement. Assess patient for fluid volume excess or deficit, electrolyte abnormalities, and metabolic abnormalities (e.g., hyperglycemia).	Enteral feedings should restore or maintain patient's nutritional status. Measures provide objective data and baseline to determine selection of formula and measure effectiveness of feedings.
6. Verify health care provider's order for type of formula, rate, route, and frequency.	Ensures that correct formula will be administered in appropriate volume. Enteral formulas are not interchangeable.

NURSING DIAGNOSES

- Imbalanced nutrition: less than body requirements
- Impaired swallowing
- Readiness for enhanced nutrition
- Risk for aspiration

Related factors/Risk factors are individualized based on patient's condition or needs.

PLANNING

1. Expected outcomes following completion of procedure:	
• Patient achieves established target for body weight over time.	Indicates that patient's nutritional status is maintained or improved.
• Patient has no sign of respiratory distress.	Feeding tube does not enter airway, and patient does not aspirate feeding.
• Patient remains or returns to fluid/electrolyte balance.	Scheduled feedings are administered as ordered.
• Patient is free of abdominal cramping.	Feeding administered without abdominal distention. Demonstrates tolerance of tube feeding.
2. Explain procedure to patient.	Decreases patient anxiety.

STEP	RATIONALE

IMPLEMENTATION

1. Perform hand hygiene. Apply clean gloves.

   Reduces transmission of microorganisms and potential contamination of enteral formula.

2. Verify correct formula and check expiration date; note integrity of container.

   Ensures that correct therapy is to be administered and checks integrity of formula.

3. Prepare formula for administration, following manufacturer guidelines.

   a. Have formula at room temperature.

   Cold formula causes gastric cramping and discomfort because liquid is not warmed by mouth and esophagus.

   b. Use aseptic technique to connect tubing to container as needed. Use proper ENFit connecter and avoid handling feeding system or touching can tops, container openings, spike, and spike port.

   Bag, connections, and tubing must be free of contamination to prevent bacterial growth (Bankhead et al., 2009).

   c. Shake formula container well. Clean top of canned formula with alcohol swab before opening it (Bankhead et al., 2009).

   Ensures integrity of formula; prevents transmission of microorganisms.

   d. For closed systems connect administration tubing to container. If using open system, pour formula from brick pack or can into administration bag (see illustration).

   Formulas are available in closed-system containers that contain a 24- to 48-hour supply of formula or in an open system, in which formula must be transferred from brick packs or cans to a bag before administration.

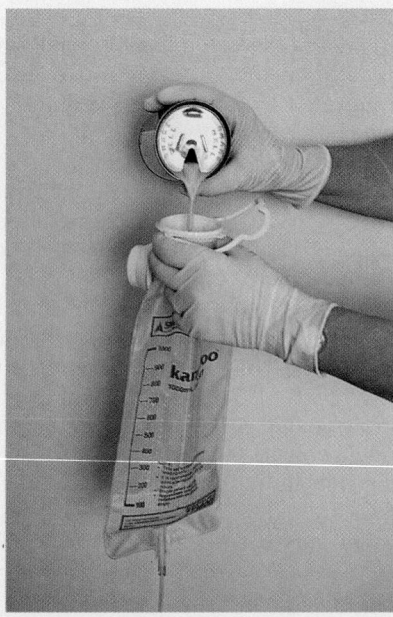

STEP 3d Pour formula into open feeding container.

4. Open roller clamp and allow administration tubing to fill. Clamp off tubing with roller clamp. Hang container on intravenous (IV) pole.

   Prevents introduction of air into stomach once feeding begins.

5. Place patient in high-Fowler's position or elevate head of bed at least 30 degrees (preferably 45 degrees). For patient forced to remain supine, place in reverse Trendelenburg's position, which raises head.

   Elevated head helps prevent pulmonary aspiration.

6. Verify tube placement (see Skill 32.2). Observe appearance of aspirate and note pH.

   Verifies if tip of tube is in stomach or intestine based on pH value.

   a. *Nasoenteric tube:* Attach ENFit syringe and aspirate gastric contents. Observe appearance of aspirate and note pH.

   Gastric fluid for patient who has fasted for at least 4 hours usually has pH of 1.0 to 4.0 (especially when patient is not receiving gastric acid inhibitor).

   b. *Gastrostomy tube:* Attach ENFit syringe and aspirate gastric contents. Observe appearance of aspirate and note pH.

   Continuous administration of tube feeding elevates pH (Simons and Abdullah, 2012).

STEP	RATIONALE
c. *Jejunostomy tube:* Attach syringe and aspirate intestinal secretions. Observe appearance; if significant amounts are returned or resemble gastric secretions, check pH.	Presence of intestinal fluid indicates that end of tube is in small intestine. If fluid tests acidic on pH test or looks like gastric fluid, tube may be displaced into stomach.
7. Check gastric residual volume (GRV) before each feeding (for bolus and intermittent feedings) and every 4 to 6 hours (for continuous feedings).	GRV determines if gastric emptying is delayed. Intestinal residual is usually very small. If residual volume is greater than 10 mL, displacement of tube into stomach may have occurred.
a. Draw up 10 to 30 mL air into ENFit syringe and connect to end of feeding tube. Inject air slowly into tube. Pull back slowly and aspirate total amount of gastric contents you can aspirate.	GRV may not be easy to obtain from small-bore feeding tube. 60-mL syringe prevents gastric tube collapse (Makic et al., 2011).
b. Return aspirated contents to stomach slowly unless volume exceeds 250 mL (see agency policy) (Metheny, 2010).	Prevents loss of nutrients and electrolytes in discarded fluid. Some questions exist regarding safety of returning high volumes of fluid into stomach (Metheny, 2010).
c. GRVs in range of 200 to 500 mL should raise concern and lead to implementation of measures to reduce risk of aspiration. Automatic cessation of feeding shouldn't occur for GRV less than 500 mL in absence of other signs of intolerance (McCarthy et al., 2015).	Raising cutoff value for GRV from lower number to higher number doesn't increase risk for regurgitation, aspiration, or pneumonia. Elevated GRV should raise concern and lead to measures to reduce risk of aspiration (McCarthy and Martindale, 2015).
d. Flush feeding tube with 30 mL water (see Skill 32.3).	Prevents clogging of tubing.
8. ENFit devices are to be used when administering enteral feedings.	These devices are not compatible with Luer-Lok connection. Use of ENFit prevents misadministration of enteral feeding or medication by wrong route such as IV tubing (ISMP, 2015).
9. Intermittent feeding (administered at certain times during the day):	
a. Pinch proximal end of feeding tube and remove cap. Connect distal end of administration set tubing to ENFit device on feeding tube and release tubing.	Prevents excessive air from entering patient's stomach and leakage of gastric contents. Ensures that feeding will be administered into correct tubing (ISMP, 2015).
b. Set rate by adjusting roller clamp on tubing (see illustration) or attach tubing to feeding pump. Allow bag to empty gradually over 30 to 45 minutes (length of time of a comfortable meal). Label bag with tube-feeding type, strength, and amount. Include date, time, and initials.	Gradual emptying of tube feeding reduces risk for abdominal discomfort, vomiting, or diarrhea induced by bolus or too-rapid infusion of tube feedings. Labeling provides means to determine when to change administration set and confirms that right patient is receiving feeding.

Clinical Decision Point *Use pumps designated for tube feeding, not IV fluids.*

STEP	RATIONALE
c. Immediately follow feeding with water (per health care provider's orders or agency policy). Cover end of feeding tube with cap when not in use. Keep bag as clean as possible. Change administration set every 24 hours.	Prevents tube from clogging. Prevents air from entering stomach between feedings and limits microbial contamination of system.
10. Continuous infusion method:	Method delivers prescribed hourly rate of feeding and reduces risk for abdominal discomfort.
a. Remove cap on tubing and connect distal end of administration set tubing to feeding tube using ENFit connector as in Step 9a.	Prevents excess air from entering patient's stomach and leakage of gastric contents.
b. Thread tubing through feeding pump; set rate on pump and turn on (see illustration).	Delivers continuous feeding at steady rate and pressure. Feeding pump alarms for increased resistance.
c. Advance rate of tube feeding (and concentration of feeding) gradually, as ordered.	Tube feeding can usually begin with full-strength formula. Conservative initiation and advancement of enteral nutrition depend on factors such as patient's age, medical condition, nutritional status, and expected patient tolerance (Kozeniecki et al., 2015).

Clinical Decision Point *Maximum hang time for formula is 12 hours in an open system; 24 to 48 hours in closed, ready-to-hang system (if it remains closed). Refer to manufacturer guidelines.*

STEP	RATIONALE

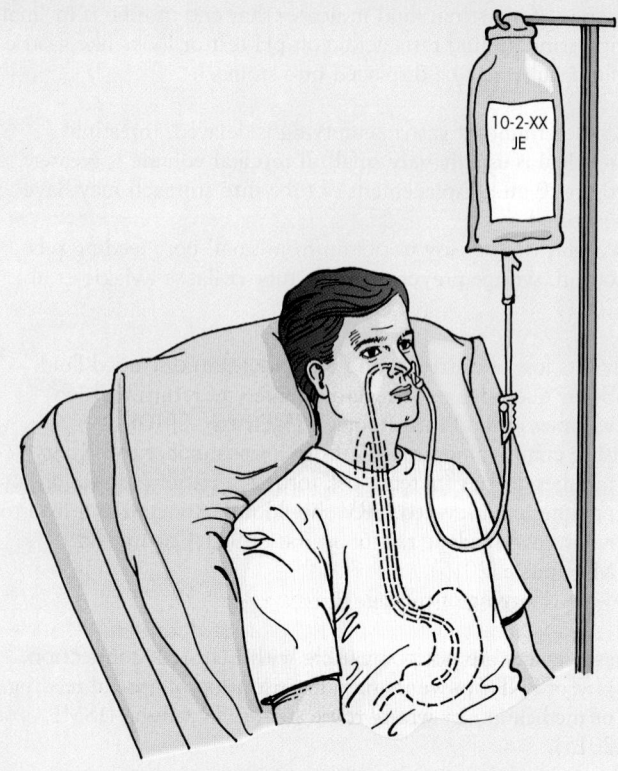

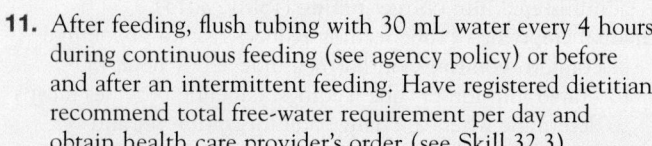

STEP 9b Administer intermittent feeding.

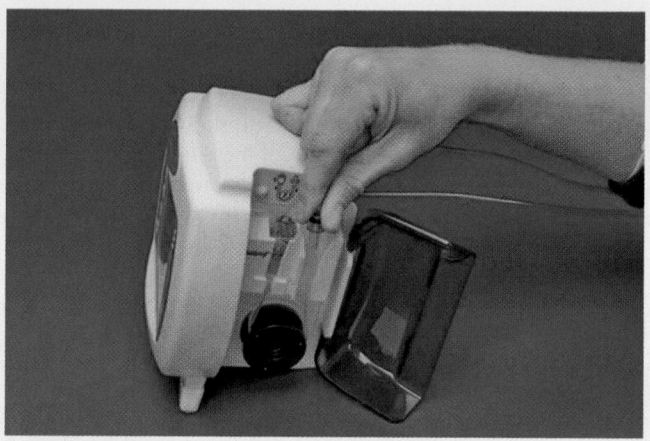

STEP 10b Connect tubing through infusion pump. (*Image used with permission Covidien. All rights reserved.*)

11. After feeding, flush tubing with 30 mL water every 4 hours during continuous feeding (see agency policy) or before and after an intermittent feeding. Have registered dietitian recommend total free-water requirement per day and obtain health care provider's order (see Skill 32.3).

Provides patient with source of water to help maintain fluid and electrolyte balance. Clears tubing of formula.

12. Rinse bag and tubing with warm water whenever feedings are interrupted. Use new administration set every 24 hours.

Rinsing bag and tubing with warm water clears old tube feedings and reduces bacterial growth.

13. Dispose of supplies and perform hand hygiene.

Reduces transmission of microorganisms.

EVALUATION

1. Measure GRV per policy, usually every 4 to 6 hours, and ask if nausea or abdominal cramping is present.

GI tolerance of tube feedings must be monitored closely to avoid complications.

2. Monitor intake and output at least every 8 hours and calculate daily totals every 24 hours.

Intake and output are indications of fluid balance, which can indicate fluid volume excess or deficit.

3. Weigh patient daily until maximum administration rate is reached and maintained for 24 hours; then weigh patient 3 times per week.

Slow weight gain is indicator of improved nutritional status; however, sudden gain of more than 2 lbs (0.9 kg) in 24 hours usually indicates fluid retention.

4. Monitor laboratory values as ordered by health care provider.

Determines correct administration of formula rate and strength.

5. Observe patient's respiratory status.

Change in respiratory status may indicate aspiration of tube feeding into respiratory tract. Symptoms may include coughing, dyspnea, tachypnea, change in oxygen saturation, crackles, and hoarseness.

6. Examine abdomen and auscultate bowel sounds.

Evaluates status of gastric emptying and peristalsis.

7. For gastrostomy tubes, inspect site for signs of impaired skin integrity and symptoms of infection, injury, or tightness of tube (see Procedural Guideline 32.1).

Enteral tubes often cause pressure and excoriation at insertion site.

8. Observe nasoenteral tube insertion site at least daily (see agency policy). Note skin integrity and look for edema under device, excoriation, or presence of injury.

Allows for early detection of excoriation than can progress to a medical device–related pressure injury.

STEP	RATIONALE
9. **Use Teach-Back:** "I want to be sure that I explained to you what you need to look for that may tell us you're not tolerating your tube feeding. Tell me two things that may tell us that you are not tolerating your tube feedings." Revise your instruction now or develop a plan for revised patient or family caregiver teaching if patient or family caregiver is not able to teach back correctly.	Determines patient's or family caregiver's level of understanding of instructional topic.

Unexpected Outcomes	Related Interventions
1. Feeding tube becomes clogged.	• Attempt to flush tube with water. • Special products are available for unclogging feeding tubes; do not use carbonated beverages and juices. • Hold feeding and notify health care provider. • Maintain patient in semi-Fowler's position. • Contact pharmacist to change medications to liquid form and flush before and after intermittent feedings and medications (Kozeniecki et al., 2015).
2. Patient develops large amount of diarrhea (more than three loose stools in 24 hours).	• Notify health care provider. • Consult dietitian about need to change formula to prevent malabsorption. • Identify and treat underlying medical/surgical issues and infections (Kozeniecki et al., 2015). • Provide perianal skin care after each stool. • Determine other causes of diarrhea (e.g., *Clostridium difficile* infection, contaminated tube feeding, medication containing sorbitol).
3. Patient develops nausea and vomiting.	• Administer antiemetic as ordered. • Use agents (ordered by health care provider) to increase gastric motility • Withhold tube feeding and notify health care provider. • Be sure that tube is patent; aspirate for residual.
4. Patient aspirates formula (auscultation of crackles or wheezes, dyspnea, or fever).	• Report change in condition to health care provider. • Position patient on side. • Suction nasotracheally or orotracheally.

Recording and Reporting

- Record amount and type of feeding, infusion rate, method of infusion, patient's response to tube feeding (e.g., GRV, cramping, bowel sounds, patency of tube, condition of skin at tube site) in nurses' notes in electronic health record (EHR) or chart.
- Record volume of formula and any additional water on intake and output form.
- Report type of feeding, status of feeding tube, patient's tolerance, and adverse outcomes.
- Document your evaluation of patient and family caregiver learning.

Special Considerations
Teaching

- Instruct patients and family caregivers not to reconnect lines that have separated but to seek clinical assistance.
- Teach patient and family caregiver that, if tolerated, patient should remain upright for 1 hour after feedings.
- Instruct patient or family caregiver that patient may express feelings of fullness, increased gas, belching, or diarrhea.
- Teach patient or family caregiver how to determine correct placement of feeding tube (see Skill 32.2).

Pediatric

- Preterm infants who are at risk for necrotizing enterocolitis frequently receive minimal enteral feeding (MEF) to limit stress on the GI tract. Breast milk is the preferred "formula" in this situation. MEF is usually administered slowly with a pump and supplemented with IV nutrition (Bankhead et al., 2009).

Gerontological

- Some older adults have decreased gastric emptying; therefore formula remains in the stomach longer than for younger patients. GRV checks are especially important in patients with impaired cognition to decrease the risk for pulmonary aspiration.

Home Care

- See Special Considerations, Skill 32.1.
- Instruct patient or family caregiver on technique for administering feedings in the home and proper storage and refrigeration of supplies.
- Instruct patient or family caregiver about any symptoms or discomfort that may occur during enteral feedings. Reinforce instruction to contact health care provider if symptoms of discomfort occur.
- Teach patient or family caregiver how to perform skin care around the gastrostomy or jejunostomy tube and signs and symptoms of infection at insertion site (see Procedural Guideline 32.1).

PROCEDURAL GUIDELINE 32.1 *Care of a Gastrostomy or Jejunostomy Tube*

Feeding tubes can be placed directly into the gastrointestinal (GI) tract through the abdominal wall in patients who cannot tolerate nasoenteric feeding tubes or require long-term enteral nutrition. The stomach (gastrostomy tube) and jejunum (jejunostomy tube) are the most common sites for long-term feeding tubes. Long-term tubes require endoscopic, radiological, or surgical placement. The insertion method used to place tubes may call for specific nursing interventions in the postinsertion period; but otherwise these tubes are used in a similar way to other feeding tubes. Feedings delivered via a gastrostomy tube are relatively safe to administer, provided the patient has normal gastric emptying. Gastrostomy tubes are often called G *tubes*; but they are also commonly referred to as percutaneous endoscopic gastrostomy (PEG) *tubes*, a term used to describe tubes placed endoscopically. Gastrostomy tubes range in size from 16 Fr to 28 Fr and exit through an incision in the upper left quadrant of the abdomen, where an internal bumper or balloon and an external bumper or disk hold the tube in place (Fig. 32.3).

Jejunostomy tubes are indicated when the risk of regurgitation and aspiration is especially high, as in cases of severely delayed gastric emptying or conditions such as pancreatitis that limit the use of the stomach for feeding. They can be placed directly into the small intestine in a surgical procedure or threaded through the stomach into the jejunum under fluoroscopy. Some jejunal tubes inserted through this transgastric approach are dual-channel devices that have openings in both the stomach and the small-intestine part of the tube. These *combination tubes,* as they are called, allow simultaneous gastric decompression and intestinal feeding for patients with impaired gastric emptying or upper-GI cancers. Each lumen of a combination tube is clearly labeled to distinguish between the gastric and the jejunal ports (Fig. 32.4).

Sometimes a jejunostomy tube is placed through an existing PEG tube. The percutaneous endoscopic jejunostomy (PEJ) tube is passed through the PEG tube and advanced into the jejunum (Fig. 32.5). The PEJ tube occupies the lumen of the PEG tube; this tube-through-a-tube design does not allow drainage of the stomach during small-intestine feeding. In the case of both combination tubes and PEJ tubes, you must know whether the

intended site for formula delivery is gastric or jejunal to ensure safe and effective nutritional care.

Delegation and Collaboration

Care of a PEG or PEJ tube cannot be delegated to nursing assistive personnel (NAP). However, there may be some exceptions (refer to nurse practice acts and agency policy). The nurse directs the NAP to:

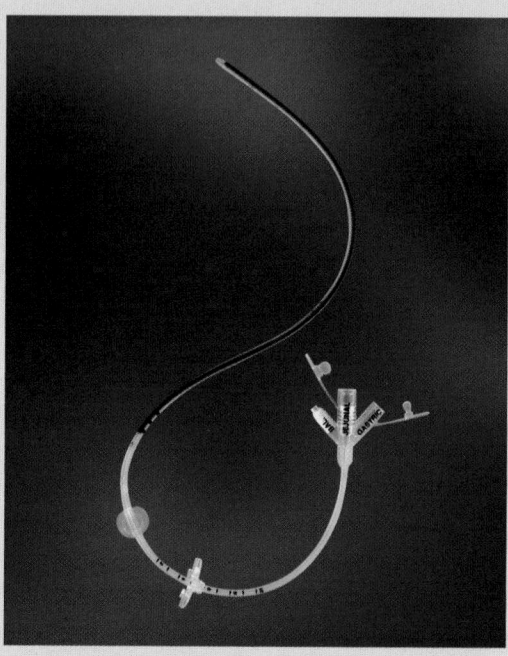

FIG 32.4 Dual lumen "combination tube" to allow jejunal feeding and gastric decompression. (*Image used with permission Kimberly-Clark Health Care. All rights reserved.*)

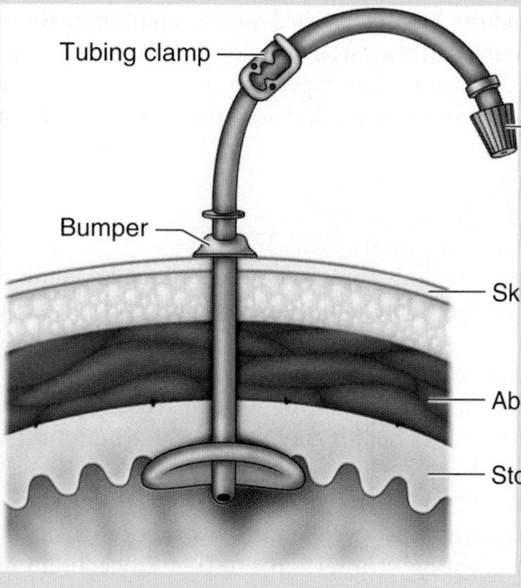

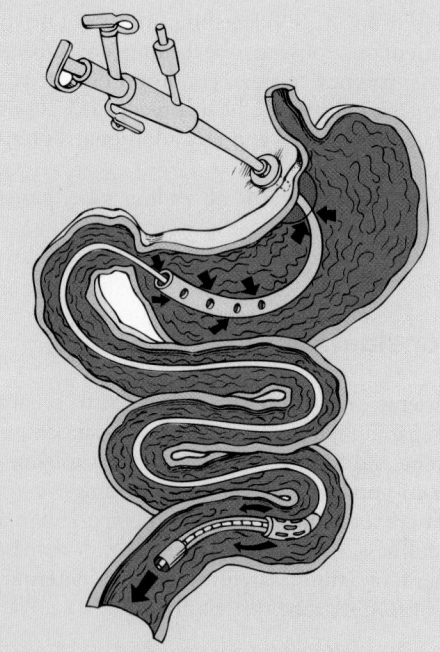

FIG 32.5 Endoscopic insertion of jejunostomy tube.

FIG 32.3 Placement of PEG tube into stomach.

PROCEDURAL GUIDELINE 32.1 *Care of a Gastrostomy or Jejunostomy Tube—cont'd*

- Inform the nurse of any patient complaints of discomfort at the insertion site.
- Inform the nurse of any drainage on the insertion site dressing.

Equipment
- Normal saline, dated and initialed container at patient's bedside
- 4 × 4–inch gauze
- Prepared drain-gauze dressing
- Tape
- Clean gloves

Procedural Steps
1. Determine whether exit site is left open to air or if a dressing is indicated. Check health care provider's order or verify agency policy.
2. Identify patient using at least two identifiers (e.g., name and birthday or name and medical record number), according to agency policy.
3. Perform hand hygiene and apply clean gloves.
4. Remove old dressing. Fold dressing with drainage contained inside; remove gloves inside out over dressing. Discard in appropriate container.
5. Assess exit site for evidence of tenderness, leakage, swelling, excoriation, infection, bleeding, or excessive movement (more than ¼ inch or 6 mm) of the tube in or out of the stomach.
6. Clean skin around stoma site with warm water and mild soap or saline (according to agency policy) with 4 × 4–inch gauze. (If drainage is present, apply clean gloves.) Clean starting next to the stoma site and work outwards using circular strokes.
7. Rinse and dry site completely.
8. Apply thin layer of protective skin barrier to exit site if indicated (e.g., site excoriated).
9. If dressing is ordered, place a drain-gauze dressing over external bar or disk. **NOTE:** Do not place dressing under external bar; this can cause gastric tissue erosion or internal abdominal wall pressure.
10. Secure dressing with tape.
11. Place date, time, and initials on new dressing.
12. Remove gloves and dispose of supplies in appropriate receptacle. Perform hand hygiene.
13. Evaluate condition of site routinely (see agency policy)
14. Document in nurse's notes in electronic health record (EHR) or chart appearance of exit site, drainage noted, and dressing application.
15. Report to health care provider any exit site complications.

◆ CLINICAL DEBRIEF

A 72-year-old male patient was admitted to the acute stroke unit following a cerebral hemorrhage. As a result of his stroke, he has left-sided paralysis and is sometimes not responsive to verbal commands. He recognizes his family and at times has spoken a few words. The patient has been made NPO. The nutrition support team has recommended that he have a small-bore nasogastric feeding tube inserted for nutritional support. A continuous tube feeding of Isosource HN has been ordered to run at 55 mL/h.

1. The patient is now ready for his nasogastric tube insertion. Place the following steps in correct order.
   1. Have patient swallow sips of water while advancing tube past nasopharynx.
   2. Perform hand hygiene.
   3. Tape or clip tube to gown to prevent pulling.
   4. Secure tube to nose.
   5. Measure to determine length of the tube to be inserted.
   6. Apply pulse oximeter and measure vital signs.
   7. Obtain x-ray film to determine proper tube placement.
2. Before the patient's first feeding, the nurse aspirates a gastric residual volume of 150 mL. What is the correct nursing action? (Select all that apply.)
   1. Consult the dietitian
   2. Stop the feeding immediately
   3. Continue tube feeding as ordered
   4. Discard the fluid withdrawn through the tube
   5. Continue to assess for feeding tolerance

3. The patient has received feedings for about 12 hours. Four hours ago the gastric residual volume (GRV) was 200 mL. The nurse is conducting rounds and finds the patient nauseated. Approximately 60 mL of vomitus is in the patient's emesis basin at the bedside. The nurse assesses the patient's abdomen to find it tender to touch and distended. Bowel sounds are decreased. The nurse aspirates 300 mL of gastric contents that has the appearance of formula. How does the nurse communicate this situation using SBAR?

◆ REVIEW QUESTIONS

1. Which of the following is the most reliable method of verifying the location of blindly inserted feeding tubes?
   1. pH testing of fluid withdrawn through the tube
   2. Auscultating over the epigastrium while instilling air through the tube
   3. Observing the color and appearance of fluid aspirated through the tube
   4. Obtaining x-ray confirmation of tube placement
2. A nurse is preparing to set up enteral nutrition on a patient. What does the nurse need to use for patient safety?
   1. A Luer-Lok syringe
   2. A regular catheter tip syringe
   3. An ENFit connector

3. Which responsibilities can a nurse delegate to NAP? (Select all that apply.)
1. Checking respirations or patient complaints of shortness of breath, coughing, or choking
2. Verifying tube placement
3. Performing oral hygiene
4. Inspecting skin around insertion site for irritation or excoriation

Ⓔ *Visit the Evolve site for a complete list of Clinical Debrief and Review Questions answers.*

REFERENCES

American Association of Critical Care Nurses (AACN): *Verification of feeding tube placement (blindly inserted)*, 2010, AACN, http://www.aacn.org/WD/Practice/Docs/PracticeAlerts/Verification_of_Feeding_Tube_Placement_05-2005.pdf. Accessed April 6, 2016.

American Association of Critical Care Nurses (AACN): Practice alerts 2012: prevention of aspiration, *Crit Care Nurse* 32(3):71, 2012.

Bankhead R, et al: Enteral nutrition practice recommendations, *JPEN J Parenter Enteral Nutr* 33(2):122, 2009.

Bourgault AM, et al: Factors influencing critical care nurses adoption of the AACN practice alert on verification of feeding tube placement, *Am J Crit Care* 23:2, 2014.

Bourgault AM, et al: Methods used by critical care nurses to verify feeding tube placement in clinical practice, *Crit Care Nurse* 35:1, 2015.

Delegge DH: Managing gastric residual volumes in the critically ill patient: an update, *Curr Opin Clin Nutr Metab Care* 14:193, 2011.

Gilbertson HR, et al: Determination of practical pH cutoff level for reliable confirmation of nasogastric tube placement, *JPEN J Parenter Enteral Nutr* 35(4):540, 2011.

Hockenberry MJ, Wilson D: *Wong's nursing care of infants and children*, ed 10, St Louis, 2015.

Institute for Safe Medication Practices (ISMP): *Safety Alert: ENFit enteral devices are on their way...Important safety considerations for hospitals*, 2015, https://www.ismp.org/newsletters/acutecare/showarticle.aspx?id=105. Accessed August 29, 2016.

Kozeniecki M, Fritzshall R: Enteral nutrition for adults in the hospital setting, *Nutr Clin Pract* 30(5):634, 2015.

Krenitsky J: Blind bedside placement of feeding tubes: treatment or threat? *Pract Gastroenterol* 93(3):32, 2011.

Lemyze M: The placement of nasogastric tubes, *CMAJ* 82(8):802, 2010.

Makic MB, et al: Evidenced-based practice habits: putting more sacred cows out to pasture, *Crit Care Nurse* 31(2):38, 2011.

Markowitz J, et al: *Device-related pressure ulcers, American Association of Critical Care Nurses (AACN) Clinical Scene Investigator Academy*, 2013, http://www.aacn.org/wd/csi/docs/FinalProjects/IU%20Methodist%20ACC%20-%20Power%20Point%20Presentation.pdf. Accessed August 29, 2016.

McCarthy MS, Martindale RG: What's on the menu? Delivering evidence-based nutritional therapy, *Nursing* 45(8):36, 2015.

Metheny NA: Inconclusive evidence regarding the volume of gastric aspirate that can be safely reintroduced following residual volume measurements, *Evid Based Nurs* 13(3):71, 2010.

Metheny NA, et al: Relationship between feeding tube site and respiratory outcomes, *JPEN J Parenter Enteral Nutr* 35:346, 2011.

Metheny NA, Frantz RA: Head of bed elevation in critically ill patients: a review, *Crit Care Nurse* 33(3):53, 2013.

Metheny N, Meert KL: Monitoring feeding tube placement, *Nutr Clin Pract* 19(5):487, 2004.

National Pressure Ulcer Advisory Panel (NPUAP): *Best practices for prevention of medical device–related pressure ulcers*, 2013, http://www.npuap.org/wp-content/uploads/2013/04/Medical-Device-Poster.pdf. Accessed August 29, 2016.

Simons SR, Abdallah LM: Bedside assessment of enteral tube placement: aligning practice with evidence, *Am J Nurs* 112(2):40, 2012.

Stepter CR: Maintaining placement of temporary enteral feeding tubes in adults: a critical appraisal of the evidence, *Medsurg Nurs* 21(2):61, 2012.

The Joint Commission (TJC): *2016 National Patient Safety Goals*, Oakbrook Terrace, IL, 2016, The Commission. http://www.jointcommission.org/standards_information/npsgs.aspx. Accessed August 29, 2016.

Wallace SC, Gardner LA: Misplacements of enteral feeding tubes increase after hospitals switch brands, *Am J Nurs* 115:8, 2015.

Waybright RA, et al: Treatment of clinical aspiration: a reappraisal, *Am J Health Syst Pharm* 70(15):1291, 2013.

33 | Parenteral Nutrition

OBJECTIVES

Mastery of content in this chapter will enable the nurse to:
- Describe the purpose and components of parenteral nutrition (PN).
- Identify patients who are candidates for PN.
- Discuss risks associated with PN.

- List the monitoring procedures used for patients receiving PN.
- Identify measures used to prevent complications of PN.
- Demonstrate appropriate nursing care and use of safe precautions when caring for a patient receiving PN.

MEDIA RESOURCES

- evolve http://evolve.elsevier.com/Perry/skills
- Review Questions

- ▶ Video Clips
- Audio Glossary
- Clinical Debrief and Review Questions Answers

PURPOSE

Parenteral nutrition (PN) is a specialized form of nutritional support that is given intravenously by an infusion pump to patients who have significant gastrointestinal (GI) dysfunction. In addition, PN meets long-term nutritional needs with infusions at home if GI dysfunction is expected to be long term (months to years) (Box 33.1).

STANDARDS OF CARE

- American Society for Parenteral and Enteral Nutrition (ASPEN), 2012—Parenteral Nutrition Core Curriculum
- Infusion Nurses Society (INS), 2016—Infusion Nursing

PRINCIPLES FOR PRACTICE

- Peripheral parenteral nutrition (PPN) can be used for patients who are experiencing mild or moderate malnutrition for up to weeks as long as the formula has a final dextrose concentration of 5% to 10% and amino acid content of 3% (Alexander et al., 2014; Phillips, 2014).
- For patients with short-term GI dysfunction, the goal is to provide nutritional requirements while minimizing PN-related complications until patients can resume full oral diets or meet their needs with enteral tube feedings (McClave, 2012; Worthington and Gilbert, 2012).
- The type of catheter to use for administration of PN depends on patient factors and the expected length of PN therapy. The location of the catheter is defined on the basis of where the distal tip of the catheter lies. Concentrated PN solutions are diluted quickly when infused into a large-diameter central vein (Fig. 33.1).
- Patients who self-administer their PN solutions at home will require a central catheter, which may be an implanted subcutaneous port, a peripherally inserted central catheter (PICC), or a tunneled central access device (Fig. 33.2; see Chapter 29).

- Patients who require PN infusions do so for medical or surgical conditions that are often associated with GI losses (e.g., obstruction, diarrhea, fistula) and organ dysfunction; therefore electrolyte monitoring is paramount. Thus a typical laboratory panel relative to PN infusions would include a baseline assessment of electrolytes, serum proteins, complete blood count, triglyceride level, and liver function tests (Box 33.2).
- The components of the PN solution are amino acids, glucose, and lipids as energy sources, with the addition of electrolytes, minerals, trace elements, vitamins, and water. The addition of lipid emulsion to the PN solution results in a preparation called a *3:1*, *3-in-1*, or *total nutrition admixture (TNA)*.
- Because hyperglycemia has been linked to increased infection rates, monitoring blood glucose levels during a PN infusion is an important procedure.
- When the goal is to prepare a patient for a cyclic home infusion of PN, it is very important to monitor glucose levels approximately 2 hours after an infusion begins (peak level) and 2 hours after it ends (trough level) to evaluate the need for adding regular human insulin to the infusion bag.
- Since a PN solution is typically provided in response to GI dysfunction and to support nutritional needs, it is important for you to monitor data that describe patient progress (see Box 33.2). Measurement of intake and output is very important to document when a patient's GI function is changing and to provide information regarding the adequacy of fluid intake from the PN solution.

PATIENT-CENTERED CARE

- Include patient and family caregiver in decisions to maintain patient control, activity level, personal decision making, and socialization with friends and family.
- Nurses collaborate with nutrition support teams and health care providers in administering PN and monitoring patients' response to PN therapy. Although practice patterns vary across agencies,

Indications for Parenteral Nutrition

Nonfunctional GI Tract
- Small bowel resection
- Small bowel surgery or GI bleed
- Paralytic ileus
- Intestinal obstruction
- Trauma to abdomen, head, or neck
- Severe malabsorption
- Intolerant of slow rates of enteral tube feeding
- Chemotherapy, radiation therapy, bone marrow transplantation
- Severely catabolic patients when GI tract is not functioning for more than 7 days

Nonfunctional GI Tract
- Enterocutaneous fistula
- Inflammatory bowel disease
- Severe diarrhea
- Moderate-to-severe pancreatitis

Preoperative Parenteral Nutrition
- Preoperative bowel rest
- Severe malnutrition before surgery

Typical Monitoring and Laboratory Orders for Patients With Parenteral Nutrition

Monitor
- Fluid intake, urine and gastrointestinal output every 8 hours
- Vital signs every 4 hours
- Body weight at least 3 times weekly

Initial and Repeated Weekly
- Complete metabolic panel with sodium (Na), potassium (K), chloride (Cl), carbon dioxide (CO_2), glucose, calcium (Ca), phosphate (PO_4), magnesium (Mg), triglycerides, transaminases, liver function
- Complete blood count (CBC) with hemoglobin, hematocrit, white blood count (WBC), red blood cells (RBCs), lymphocyte count
- Serum proteins, often including albumin, transferrin, C-reactive protein, and/or prealbumin

Daily Until Stable
- Electrolyte panel daily until stable; then weekly
- Glucose every 6 hours until within normal limits for 48 hours; then daily
- Glucose in preparation for cyclic home parenteral nutrition (PN); monitor 2 hours after PN begins and 2 hours after PN ends; adjust insulin per orders

Monthly or Biannually
- Trace elements such as zinc, copper, manganese, selenium (depending on underlying condition such as gastrointestinal/malabsorption) and in times of short supply or rationing of trace elements because of national shortages and for long-term home PN
- Selected vitamins for long-term home PN patients

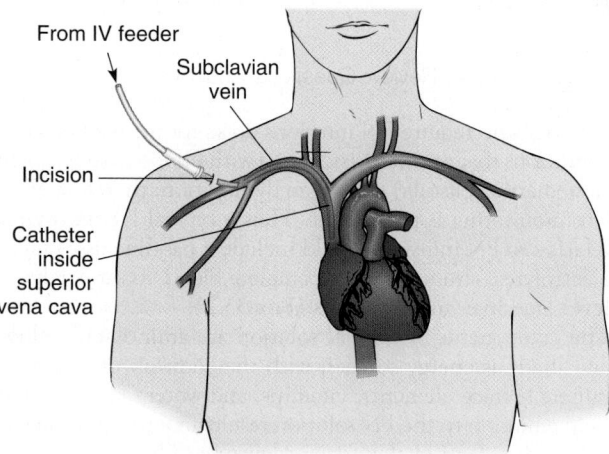

FIG 33.1 Placement of central venous catheter inserted into subclavian vein. *IV,* Intravenous. (*Courtesy Rolin Graphics.*)

typically dietitians or pharmacists provide advice on nutrition support goals and/or write PN orders in collaboration with health care provider.
- PN may pose concerns for members of ethnic groups or people with philosophical beliefs that include restriction of animal products. The components of PN are largely synthetic and do not contain pork. The lipid emulsion contains egg phospholipid, a product that may be objectionable to vegan patients.

EVIDENCE-BASED PRACTICE

When critically ill patients cannot tolerate enteral nutrition, PN provides an alternative route for nutritional delivery, including a decreased infection rate when it is initiated early versus later in their care (Malone, 2014). Key evidence-based practice guidelines for management of critically ill patients in intensive care units (ICU) include the following (Malone, 2014; Taylor et al., 2016):
- Enteral nutrition is preferred over PN for nutritional support (see Chapter 32).

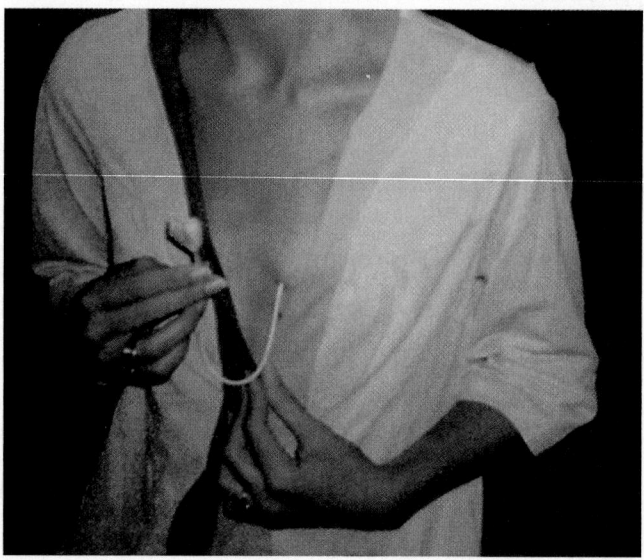

FIG 33.2 Tunneled catheter used for home central parenteral nutrition. (*From Morgan SL, Weinsier RL: Fundamentals of clinical nutrition, ed 2, St Louis, 1998, Mosby.*)

- If the patient was healthy before this critical illness, with no evidence of protein calorie malnutrition, use of PN should be reserved and initiated only after the first 7 days of hospitalization, when enteral nutrition is not available.
- PN should be initiated only if the duration is anticipated to be greater than or equal to 7 days.
- In patients stabilized on PN, efforts should be made to reintroduce oral or enteral nutrition.
- PN should not be terminated until greater than or equal to 60% of nutritional needs are being met by the oral or enteral route.

SAFETY GUIDELINES

- Although the use of PN has been an important technological advance that allowed improved care for patients with GI disorders, a number of complications have been associated with the therapy. The most frequent complication is catheter-related bloodstream infection (CRBSI), a risk that is found in both hospitalized patients and those with PN at home (Table 33.1). It is critically important that appropriate care of the vascular access device, dressing, and site are instituted to minimize CRBSI, including avoiding blood draws and interruption of the infusions (INS, 2016) (see Chapter 29).
- Central PN (CPN) using concentrated dextrose solutions should not be infused into a peripheral intravenous (IV) or midline catheter because of the increased risk for phlebitis. If only peripheral lines are available, the orders should clearly state that the administration route should be via a peripheral IV line so the compounding pharmacy will prepare PPN with a lower osmolarity (Table 33.2), which will require added fluid volume.
- PPN is used only for very short-term situations or when there is the need for very low caloric requirements because it is difficult to meet total nutrient requirements with PPN because of the limitation of dextrose concentration peripherally and the inability to meet caloric goals without large volumes.
- Many hospitals use PICCs, termed *PICC lines* (Fig. 33.3), which are placed by specially trained nurses or radiologists.
- Following central venous catheter insertion, do not initiate PN until placement of venous catheter tip is confirmed by a radiograph or through the use of electrocardiograph (ECG) tip verification technology (INS, 2016).
- Appropriate aseptic technique is needed when handling the central line, dressings, tubing, and the needleless end cap PN port (see Skill 29.6).

TABLE 33.1

Complications of Parenteral Nutrition

Problem	Cause	Symptoms	Immediate Action	Prevention
Pneumothorax	Tip of catheter enters pleural space during insertion, causing lung to collapse	Sudden chest pain, difficulty breathing, decreased breath sounds, cessation of normal chest movement on affected side, tachycardia	Per health care provider's order, the proper professional (CRNP, PA–C, or MD) may remove the central catheter. Administer oxygen via nasal cannula. Insert chest tube to remove air under water-seal drainage or dry one-way valve system.	Medical personnel should be properly trained to insert central catheters. Researchers suggest use of ultrasound when placing CVCs (Lamperti et al., 2012). Catheter should be secured properly to prevent migration, movement.
Air embolism	IV tubing disconnected; part of catheter system open or removed without being clamped	Sudden respiratory distress: decreased oxygen saturation levels, shortness of breath, coughing, chest pain, decreased blood pressure	Clamp catheter; position patient in left Trendelenburg's position; call health care provider; administer oxygen as needed (INS, 2016).	Make sure that all catheter connections are secure; clamp catheter when not in use. Never use a stopcock with a CVC. Unless contraindicated, instruct patient in Valsalva maneuver for tubing changes (INS, 2016).
Localized infection (exit site or tunnel)	Poor aseptic technique in removal of skin flora during site preparation and dressing care	*Exit site:* Erythema, tenderness, induration, or purulence within 2 cm (0.8 inches) of skin at exit site. *Tunnel:* Same as above but extends beyond 2 cm from exit site	Call health care provider. *Exit:* Apply warm compress, daily care of site, oral antibiotics. *Infection:* Collaborate with health care provider regarding removal of catheter (INS, 2016). *Tunnel:* Remove catheter.	Provide catheter site care using aseptic technique, visually inspect site (including cleaning site), applying new stabilization device, and applying sterile dressing (INS, 2016). Change transparent dressings at least every 5–7 days and gauze dressings every 48 hours (INS, 2016). Change dressing if damp, loosened, or soiled or when inspection of site is necessary (INS, 2016). Use chlorhexidine wipes to cleanse site. For adults, consider the use of chlorhexidine-impregnated dressings (INS, 2016).
Catheter-related sepsis or bacteremia	Catheter hub contamination; contamination of infusate; spread of bacteria through bloodstream from distant site	*Systemic:* Isolation of same microorganism from blood culture and catheter segment, with patient showing fever, chills, malaise, elevated white blood cell count	*Systemic:* Do not exceed hang time of 24 hours for PN that contains dextrose and amino acids either alone or with fat emulsion added as a 3-in-1 formulation (INS, 2016). Administer antibiotics intravenously; remove catheter by proper professional (CRNP, PA-C, or MD).	Use full sterile-barrier precautions during catheter insertion and dressing change. Consider the use of antibiotic-impregnated catheters (INS, 2016). Do not disconnect tubing unnecessarily. Replace IV tubing and filter every 24 hours. In some selected situations it is necessary to change administration sets with each new PN container (INS, 2016).

Continued

TABLE 33.1

Complications of Parenteral Nutrition—cont'd

Problem	Cause	Symptoms	Immediate Action	Prevention
Hyperglycemia	Possible blood-draw error, confirm with bedside glucose device; patient receiving too little insulin in PN solution; receiving steroids; new-onset infection	Excessive thirst, urination, blood glucose greater than 160 mg/ 100 dL, confusion	Call health care provider; may need to slow infusion rate (health care provider order).	Review medical history for blood drawn through central line with PN infusing (repeat peripheral blood draw or obtain fingerstick), glucose intolerance or diabetes, new infection, new medication such as steroids; keep rate as ordered; never increase PN to "catch up." Maintain blood glucose in range ordered by health care provider. Use aseptic technique and routine blood glucose monitoring.
Hypoglycemia	PN abruptly discontinued; too much insulin	Patient shaky, dizzy, nervous, anxious, hungry, blood glucose level <80 mg/100 dL	Call health care provider; if PN discontinued abruptly, may need to restart $D_{10}W$ at previous PN rate. If patient has oral intake, give ½ cup fruit juice. Perform blood glucose monitoring; retest in 15 to 30 min.	Decrease PN, "tapering" gradually until discontinued; blood glucose monitoring is used to ensure adequate insulin.

CRBSI, Catheter-related bloodstream infection; *CRNP*, certified registered nurse practitioner; *CVC*, central venous catheter; *ICU*, intensive care unit; *IV*, intravenous; *MD*, medical doctor; *PA-C*, physician's assistant–certified; *PN*, parenteral nutrition.

TABLE 33.2

Comparison of Central Versus Peripheral Parenteral Nutrition Orders

	Central Parenteral Nutrition	Peripheral Parenteral Nutrition
Osmolality	>600 mOsm	<600 mOsm
Route of administration	Central venous catheter	Small peripheral vein
Usual daily caloric intake	20–35 kcal/kg/day	5–10 kcal/kg/day
Usual daily volume (mL)	1000–2000	2000–3000
Fat emulsion	Minor caloric source	Major caloric source

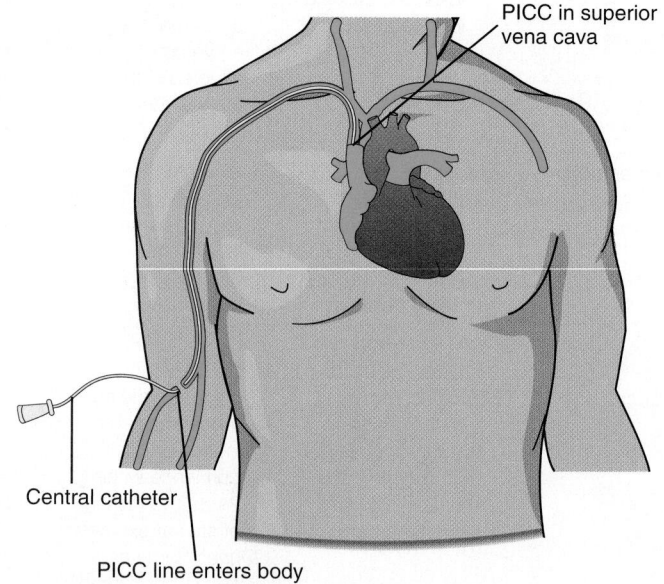

FIG 33.3 Peripherally inserted central catheter (PICC).

- PN without lipids can be infused using tubing with a 0.20-μm filter, and lipid-containing emulsions (3-in-1) can be infused using a larger 1.2-μm filter (INS, 2016). A filter is necessary because it prevents particulate matter or large droplets of lipid from reaching a patient, which could potentially result in a pulmonary embolism.
- In very malnourished patients, during a process termed *refeeding syndrome*, some electrolytes (e.g., potassium [K], magnesium [Mg] and phosphorus [P]) may shift intracellularly with glucose provided in the PN, potentially resulting in low serum levels with risk for arrhythmias and muscle weakness. Adequate electrolyte repletion should occur before the initiation of PN.

There is an increased risk of pulmonary edema and heart failure when initiating feeding in malnourished patients at greater risk of refeeding syndrome.

- Since there is a risk of bloodstream infection in patients with catheters, regular monitoring of temperature is important.

◆ SKILL 33.1   Administering Central Parenteral Nutrition

Administration of parenteral nutrition (PN) through a central line (CPN) requires the use of strict aseptic technique and application of critical thinking. Because of the composition of CPN fluids, patients can experience metabolic and fluid balance changes

quickly. In addition, the clinical condition of patients receiving CPN may be poor, especially when they have alterations in host defenses, severe underlying illnesses, and extremes of age. You will need to anticipate changes in a patient's condition that signal developing complications. Similarly, you need to use good judgment to maintain the intravenous (IV) system and ensure that it is functioning properly.

Delegation and Collaboration

The skill of administering CPN to a hospitalized patient cannot be delegated to nursing assistive personnel (NAP). The nurse directs the NAP to:

- Report when the pump alarms, shortness of breath, headaches, weakness, feeling shaky, or discomfort or bleeding at IV site.
- Perform fingerstick blood glucose monitoring as directed and report any abnormal results to the nurse.
- Report vital signs that are out of normal range to nurse.
- Measure urinary output and weigh patient per agency protocol.

Equipment

- PN solution (IV)
- Electronic infusion device (EID) with anti–free-flow control and alarms (INS, 2016)
- IV infusion tubing with Luer-Lok tip
- Appropriate IV filter (1.2-µm filter for three-in-one solutions or lipids containing a membrane that is particulate retentive and air eliminating; 0.20-µm filter for solutions that do not contain lipids) (INS, 2016)
- 5- to 10-mL syringe with sterile saline flush
- Bedside glucose monitoring kit
- Adhesive tape or tubing label
- Antimicrobial swab
- Clean gloves
- Stethoscope
- Medication administration record (MAR) or computer printout

STEP	RATIONALE

ASSESSMENT

STEP	RATIONALE
1. Assess indications of and risks for protein/calorie malnutrition: weight loss from baseline or ideal, muscle atrophy/weakness, edema, lethargy, failure to wean from ventilatory support, chronic illness, and nothing by mouth for more than 7 days. Confer with nutritional support team.	Clinical indications for PN. These baseline details provide a baseline from which change can be noted (Alexander et al., 2014).
2. Perform hand hygiene. Apply clean gloves as needed. Inspect condition of central vein access site for presence of inflammation, edema, and tenderness. Inspect tubing of access device for patency and kinking.	Reduces transmission of infection. Identifies early signs of infection, infiltration, or disruption in system integrity. Development of complication contraindicates infusion of fluids and indicates need to establish new IV site.
3. Assess vital signs, auscultate patient's lung sounds, inspect for edema of extremities, and measure weight.	Provides baseline for monitoring patient's response to fluid infusion and nutrients. Crackles in lungs are early indication of fluid volume excess.
4. Assess medical record for levels of serum albumin, total protein, transferrin, prealbumin, and triglycerides and check blood glucose level by fingerstick. Remove gloves and perform hand hygiene.	Provides baseline for measuring patient's nutritional status. In addition, nutritional baseline identifies patient's unique requirements, and PN admixture is tailored to patient's specific needs (Alexander et al., 2014). Reduces transmission of microorganisms. Serum glucose determines patient's baseline and tolerance to high levels of glucose in CPN solution.
5. Assess patient's medical history for factors influenced by CPN administration: electrolyte levels; renal, cardiac, and hepatic function. Assess for history of allergies.	Some patients require that CPN therapy be adapted by composition or volume (requires health care provider order) based on medical history. CPN includes constituents (e.g., medications) to which patient may be allergic.
6. Consult with health care provider and dietitian on calculation of calorie, protein, and fluid requirements for patient.	Provides multidisciplinary plan for patient's nutritional support.
7. Verify order for nutrients, minerals, vitamins, trace elements, electrolytes, added medications, and flow rate. Check for compatibility of added medications.	CPN is often ordered daily in hospital setting after review of laboratory values. In home setting orders may be obtained less frequently (e.g., weekly). Pharmacies that prepare parenteral solutions will check medication compatibility.
8. Assess patient's and family caregiver's knowledge of PN, including any previous experience with home management.	Determines level and extent of instruction required.

NURSING DIAGNOSES

- Deficient fluid volume
- Excess fluid volume
- Imbalanced nutrition: less than body requirements
- Knowledge deficit regarding PN purpose and home management
- Risk for infection
- Risk for unstable blood glucose level

Related factors/Risk factors are individualized based on patient's condition or needs.

STEP	RATIONALE

PLANNING

1. Expected outcomes following completion of procedure:
   - Patient's ideal weight gain is between 1 and 3 lbs (0.5 to 1.5 kg) per week.

   Weight is indicator of patient's nutritional status and determines fluid volume. Weight gain greater than 1 lb (0.5 kg)/day indicates fluid retention.

   - Blood glucose levels are maintained per health care provider's order for desired glucose range.

   Glucose levels needed for specific populations differ based on the degree of illness so a specific health care provider order is needed (McClave et al, 2016).

   - Central venous access device is patent; and site is free of pain, swelling, redness, or inflammation.

   Ensures that CPN is infusing into vein rather than into surrounding tissues and that there are no signs of an access device infection.

   - Patient is afebrile.

   Absence of systemic infection.

   - Patient and family caregiver are able to discuss purpose and steps for care of PN.

   Proper instruction informs patient and family caregiver and prepares for home care if needed.

2. Explain purpose of CPN to patient.

   Promotes understanding and reduces anxiety.

3. If CPN solution is refrigerated, remove from refrigeration 1 hour before infusion.

   Ensures solution will be administered at room temperature.

IMPLEMENTATION

1. Perform hand hygiene.

   Reduces transmission of microorganisms.

2. Check label on CPN bag with health care provider's order on MAR or computer printout and patient's name. Also check any additives and note solution expiration date.

   Prevents medication error. *This is the first check for accuracy.*

3. Inspect 2:1 CPN solution for particulate matter; inspect 3:1 CPN solution for separation of fat into layer.

   Presence of particulate matter or fat emulsion separation requires that solution be discarded.

4. Before leaving medication room, check IV solution second time using six rights of medication administration (see Chapter 20). Check label of CPN bag against MAR or computer printout.

   This is the second check for accuracy.

5. Identify patient using at least two identifiers (e.g., name and birthday or name and medical record number) according to agency policy. Compare identifiers with information on patient's MAR or medical record.

   Ensures correct patient. Complies with The Joint Commission standards and improves patient safety (TJC, 2016).

6. Take CPN solution to patient in advance of previous solution emptying. Compare names of solution and additives with MAR at bedside.

   This is the third check for accuracy.

7. Apply clean gloves. Prepare IV tubing for CPN solution:
   a. Attach appropriate filter to IV tubing.
   b. Prime tubing with CPN solution, making sure that no air bubbles remain, and turn off flow with roller clamp (see Chapter 29). Some infusion pumps and IV tubing require that priming be done on pump rather than by gravity.

   Maintains sterility of solution. Air introduced into central circulation could result in air embolus, a fatal IV complication.

8. Wipe end port of central vascular access device (CVAD) with alcohol swab, allow to dry, then attach syringe of 0.9% normal saline (NS) solution to needleless port, aspirate for blood return, and flush saline per agency policy.

   Scrubbing hub decreases microorganisms (INS, 2016; Alexander et al., 2014). Determines patency of IV device before infusing CPN.

9. Remove syringe. Connect Luer-Lok end of CPN IV tubing to end port of CVAD; for multilumen lines label tubing used for CPN.

   Ensures that tubing is securely connected to IV line. Dedicated line should be used for multilumen devices. Labeling of high-risk catheters prevents connection with inappropriate tube or catheter (TJC, 2016).

10. Place IV tubing in EID. Open roller clamp. Set and regulate flow rate as ordered (see illustration).

    CPN flow rates are ordered to meet patient's metabolic and electrolyte needs. Maintaining rates prevents electrolyte imbalances.

    a. *Continuous infusion (optional):* Flow rate is immediately set at ordered rate and given over 24-hour period.

    Ensures that blood glucose levels are maintained to prevent hypoglycemia or hyperglycemia (Alexander et al., 2014).

STEP	RATIONALE

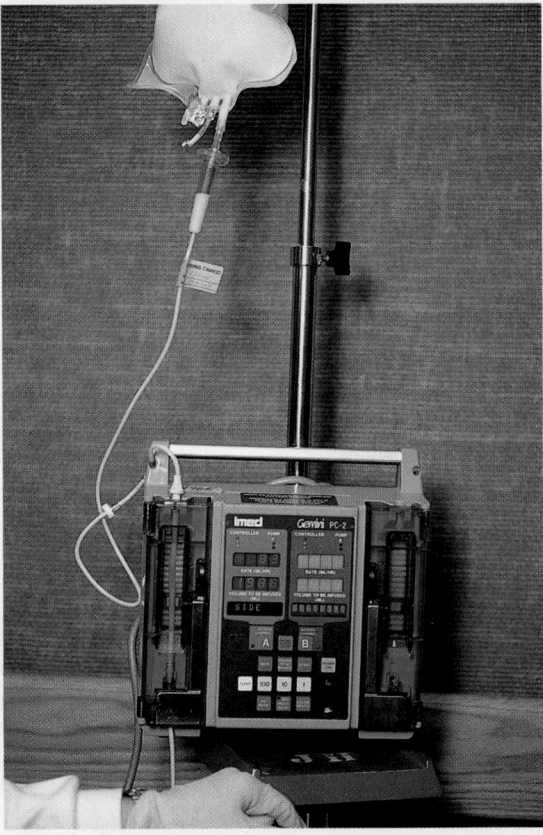

STEP 10 Parenteral nutrition solution infusing via infusion pump.

b. *Cycle infusion (optional):* Flow rate is initiated at about 40 to 60 mL/hr, and the rate is gradually increased until patient's nutritional needs are met. Before completion of infusion, rate is decreased at about the same milliliter per hour until the CPN is completed. The infusion is usually given over a shorter time frame (12 to 18 hours).

Infusion rates are usually increased and decreased to prevent hypoglycemia or hyperglycemia (Alexander et al., 2014).

11. Infuse all IV medications or blood through alternative IV site or multilumen device. Do not obtain blood samples or central venous pressure readings through same lumen used for CPN.

Prevents drug incompatibility and IV device occlusion (Alexander et al., 2014).

12. Do not interrupt CPN infusion (e.g., during showers, transport to procedure, blood transfusion) and be sure that rate does not exceed ordered rate.

Prevents development of catheter-related bacteremia (INS, 2016; Alexander et al., 2014).

13. CPN containing dextrose and amino acids alone or with fat emulsion added as a 3:1 formulation should have a hang time not to exceed 24 hours. Fat emulsions alone should have a hang time not to exceed 12 hours.

Prevents bacterial infection and deterioration of emulsion (INS, 2016; Alexander et al., 2014).

14. Change IV administration sets for CPN every 24 hours and immediately on suspected contamination. Discard used supplies and perform hand hygiene.

Reduces transmission of infection.

EVALUATION

1. Monitor and document flow rate according to agency policy and procedure. If infusion is not running on time, do not attempt to catch up.

Too-rapid or too-slow infusion could result in metabolic disturbances such as hyperglycemia and fluid overload.

2. Monitor fluid intake and urine and gastrointestinal (GI) fluid output every 8 hours.

Prevents fluid imbalance from too-slow or too-rapid infusion.

3. Measure vital signs every 4 hours.

Monitors for fluid overload response.

STEP	RATIONALE
4. Obtain initial weight and then weigh at least 3 times weekly.	Routine measurement of weights will reflect a gain/loss resulting either from caloric intake or fluid retention. Gradual weight gain, if weight gain is the goal, indicates adequate tolerance.
5. Evaluate for fluid retention; palpate skin of extremities; auscultate lung sounds.	Weight gain in excess of 1 lb (0.5 kg)/day, dependent edema, lung crackles, and intake greater than output per each 24-hour period indicate fluid retention.
6. Monitor patient's glucose levels every 6 hours or as ordered and other laboratory parameters daily or as ordered.	Maintenance of normal electrolyte levels, satisfactory fluid balance, acceptable serum glucose levels, and improvement in serum proteins indicate adequate tolerance to PN.
7. Inspect central venous access site for signs and symptom of swelling, inflammation, drainage, redness, warmth, tenderness or edema.	Determines IV patency and absence of infection, infiltration, or phlebitis.
8. Monitor for temperature, elevated white blood cell count, and malaise.	Signs of systemic infection.
9. **Use Teach-Back:** "I want to be sure I explained what can happen with your central parenteral nutrition. What signs and symptoms should you report to the nurse or doctor?" Revise your instruction now or develop a plan for revised patient or family caregiver teaching if patient or family caregiver is not able to teach back correctly.	Determines patient's or family caregiver's level of understanding of instructional topic.

Unexpected Outcomes

1. There is redness, swelling, and tenderness around central venous access site, indicating possible exit site infection.

2. Patient develops fever, malaise, and chills, indicating systemic infection.

3. Serum glucose level is greater than 150 mg/dL or target set by health care provider.

Related Interventions

- Notify health care provider.
- Apply warm compress and initiate daily site care as ordered.
- Systemic antibiotic therapy may begin.
- Check exit site for signs of infection.
- Notify health care provider and consult about need to obtain cultures of exit site or blood.
- Systemic antibiotic therapy may begin.
- Notify health care provider.
- Indicates intolerance to glucose load in CPN solution.
- May indicate new-onset infection.
- Verify that blood was not drawn with PN infusing or that proper procedures to interrupt PN and discard first blood draw was followed.
- Possible need for addition of insulin to CPN, modification of CPN solution, or sliding-scale insulin coverage.

Recording and Reporting

- Record condition of CVAD, rate and type of infusion, catheter lumen used for infusion, intake and output (I&O), blood glucose levels, vital signs, and weights in nurses' notes in electronic health record (EHR) or chart.
- If signs of infection, occlusion, fluid retention, or infiltration occur, notify the health care provider.
- Document your evaluation of patient and family caregiver learning.

Special Considerations
Teaching

- Instruct patient and family caregiver in the purpose and goals of CPN. Keep them informed about daily care of central line.
- Inform patient of signs of central line infection to report to the nurse.

Pediatric

- Consider children's developmental needs when they are on long-term CPN. Perform regular assessments of development to determine child's progress. Implement interventions to encourage expected milestones (Hockenberry and Wilson, 2015).

Gerontological

- Some older adults have impaired ability to tolerate higher fluid volumes because of cardiac or renal impairment.

Home Care

- Patients requiring long-term CPN benefit from a referral to a home nutrition therapy team.
- Patients should have a home safety and physical, nutritional, and psychological needs assessment (INS, 2016).
- Patients receiving home CPN may have a peripherally inserted central catheter (PICC) line or a tunneled or implanted catheter (see Fig. 33.2) to reduce the possibility of infection. Patients or family caregivers need to learn to perform catheter site care, dressing changes, techniques for connecting and disconnecting PN solutions, and infusion pump management.
- Some patients receive home CPN at night during sleep (cyclic CPN) to allow the freedom to leave home during the day. Some patients may also take an oral diet as tolerated, although their impaired GI function limits nutrient absorption. Encourage food/fluid intake for pleasure but monitor for diarrhea or increased output if eating to assess for dehydration.

- Teach patient and family caregiver to monitor patient's temperature, weight, I&O, and serum glucose level and recognize signs and symptoms of PN-related complications.
- Teach patient and family caregiver about actions to take in case of emergency or unexpected outcomes such as telephoning the health care provider or home infusion provider or going to the hospital, depending on the circumstances.

- If home CPN patients require insulin in their CPN, they will need a home glucose monitoring device and instruction in its use.
- Patient teaching for home CPN administration will be given by home infusion nurses after discharge or may be initiated in the hospital and continued at home.

◆ SKILL 33.2 **Administering Peripheral Parenteral Nutrition With Lipid (Fat) Emulsion**

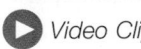 *Video Clip*

The administration of peripheral parenteral nutrition (PPN) requires a lower dextrose content and is more appropriate for short-term use until central access can be achieved or the patient can be fed orally or enterally. Patients with elevated nutritional requirements from hypermetabolic illnesses or conditions and patients with fluid restrictions are not suitable candidates (Worthington and Gilbert, 2012). This therapy is for short-term use, usually for 2 weeks or less. The PPN solution uses lower concentrations of dextrose and amino acids to reduce the osmolality (see Table 33.2) and decrease the risk for phlebitis. Adding lipid emulsion provides a source of calories with minimal impact on the osmolality. A lipid emulsion must be administered through vented intravenous (IV) tubing as a primary IV infusion or a piggyback.

This skill describes a piggyback administration of PPN. Administration sets (including piggybacks) used for fat emulsions are changed every 24 hours and immediately on suspected contamination (Alexander et al., 2014). The administration set must have a Luer-Lok design. Indications for PPN include the following:

- *Adequate peripheral access:* Despite its lower osmolality, PPN tends to cause phlebitis and often requires frequent changes in the access location. A midline catheter may be an alternative to the typical short-peripheral catheter.
- *Ability to tolerate larger volumes of fluid:* Because of the lower concentration of dextrose in PPN, a larger volume of fluid is required to attain adequate calories. Some patients with impaired renal or cardiac function do not tolerate PPN.
- *Ability to tolerate lipid emulsions:* Lipid is the most calorically dense nutrient. A 1-L amount of 10% dextrose without lipid

provides only 340 kcal. A 250-mL amount of 20% lipid solution provides 500 kcal.

Delegation and Collaboration

The skill of administering PPN for a hospitalized patient cannot be delegated to nursing assistive personnel (NAP). The nurse directs the NAP to:

- Report patient complaint of burning, pain, or redness at peripheral IV site.
- Report to nurse infusion pump alarms or moist IV site dressing.
- Report to nurse patient complaints of shortness of breath and change in vital signs.

Equipment

- PPN solution
- Lipid emulsion in glass container or in a separate chamber of the parenteral nutrition (PN) bag
- IV tubing for PPN with 0.20-µm filter for amino acid/dextrose solution
- IV tubing with a 1.2-µm filter for fat emulsion
- Bedside glucose monitoring kit
- Antimicrobial swab
- Electronic infusion pump with anti–free-flow control and alarms (INS, 2016)
- Clean gloves
- Medication administration record (MAR) or computer printout
- Stethoscope

STEP	RATIONALE

ASSESSMENT

1. Review medical record and assess patient for hypertriglyceridemia. Obtain orders for serum triglyceride level before initiation of PPN and weekly.

2. Perform hand hygiene, and apply clean gloves. Select or initiate appropriate functional IV site to administer PPN and lipid emulsion. Assess its patency and function (see Chapter 29).

3. Obtain blood glucose level by fingerstick.

4. Assess patient's fluid status by monitoring for edema in extremities, lung sounds, or fluid intake greater than fluid output.

5. Obtain patient's weight and vital signs. Remove gloves and perform hand hygiene.

Determines patient's ability to metabolize lipid.

PPN may cause phlebitis; therefore appropriate vein selection is important.

Provides baseline to determine tolerance to glucose infusion.

Fluid intake that is given with PPN may cause fluid overload in elderly patients or those who have impaired renal or cardiac function.

Provides baseline information to determine effectiveness and tolerance of PPN solution. Reduces transmission of microorganisms.

STEP	RATIONALE1
6. Check health care provider's order against MAR for volume of fat emulsion, PPN solution, and administration time for fat emulsion. Then check name of solution on label with MAR.	Health care provider must order fat emulsions and PPN. Fat emulsions may cause adverse symptoms if infused too rapidly as separate infusion. Infusion time is normally at least 8 hours. Fat emulsions should hang no longer than 12 hours as separate infusion from original container. *This is the first check for accuracy.*
7. Read label of fat emulsion solution.	Lipid emulsions are white and opaque; thus be sure to avoid confusing enteral tube–feeding formula with parenteral lipids.
8. Assess patient's and family caregiver's knowledge of PPN.	Determines level and extent of instruction required.

NURSING DIAGNOSES

- Excess fluid volume
- Imbalanced nutrition: less than body requirements
- Risk for infection
- Risk for unstable blood glucose level

Related factors/Risk factors are individualized based on patient's condition or needs.

PLANNING

1. Expected outcomes following completion of procedure:	
• Triglyceride level is <250 mg/dL in most patients.	Indicates adequate clearance of lipid.
• Blood glucose levels are maintained per health care provider's order for desired glucose range.	Glucose levels needed for specific populations differ based on the degree of illness, so a specific health care provider order is needed (McClave et al., 2016).
• Venipuncture site is free of phlebitis, pain, swelling, redness, and inflammation.	Ensures proper administration and monitoring of PPN with lipids.
• Patient does not show signs of systemic infection (e.g., elevated temperature).	Temperature is indication of possible systemic infection related to PN.
• Patient does not show signs of allergy to lipids.	Monitoring infusion requires observation for allergic response to infusion.
• Patient and family caregiver are able to explain purpose of PPN and complications to observe for.	Proper instruction informs patient and family caregiver.
2. Explain purposes of PPN and fat emulsion.	Promotes understanding and reduces anxiety.
3. Place patient in comfortable position for IV line insertion or initiation of infusion.	When patients are comfortable, they tolerate procedures more readily.
4. If PPN solution is refrigerated, remove from refrigeration 1 hour before infusion.	Solution should be removed from refrigeration before administration (Alexander et al., 2014).

IMPLEMENTATION

1. Perform hand hygiene.	Reduces transmission of microorganisms.
2. Compare label of PPN bag and lipid emulsion bottle with MAR or computer printout; check for correct additives and solution expiration date. Also check patient's name.	Prevents medication error. *This is the second check for accuracy.*
3. Examine lipid solution for separation of emulsion into layers or fat globules or presence of froth.	Do not administer if these elements appear.
4. Identify patient using at least two identifiers (e.g., name and birthday or name and medical record number) according to agency policy. Compare identifiers with information on patient's MAR or medical record.	Ensures correct patient. Complies with The Joint Commission standards and improves patient safety (TJC, 2016).
5. Compare identifiers with information on solution bag label and patient's MAR or medical record at the bedside.	Ensures patient receives correct infusion. *This is the third check for accuracy.*
6. Measure patient's vital signs.	Provides baseline assessment. Immediate allergic reaction can develop once infusion begins.
7. Apply clean gloves. Prepare IV tubing for PPN solution; run solution through tubing to remove excess air. Turn roller clamp to "off" position. Some infusion pumps and tubing require priming through infusion pump. Add sterile capped needle or place sterile cap on end of tubing. Follow same procedure with separate infusion set for lipid infusion.	To prevent air from entering vascular system, clear all tubing.

STEP	RATIONALE
8. Wipe end port of peripheral IV infusion tubing with antimicrobial swab and allow to dry. Connect needleless connector at end of PPN tubing to end port of patient's functional peripheral IV line. Gently disconnect old PPN tubing from IV site and insert adapter of new PPN infusion tubing. Open roller clamp on new tubing. Allow solution to run to ensure that tubing is patent; regulate IV drip rate using electronic infusion pump.	Prevents disruption of existing IV infusion and ensures patent infusion. Pump will deliver infusion at prescribed rate.
9. Clean needleless peripheral line tubing injection cap with antimicrobial swab.	Removes surface organisms at injection site and prevents organisms from entering blood system.
10. Attach fat emulsion infusion tubing to injection cap of IV line. Y-connector may be used if patient is receiving separate PPN and lipid infusions. Label tubing.	Fat emulsions cannot infuse through a 0.20-μm IV filter. Refer to agency policy; if larger 1.2-μm filter is used, lipids may be infused using a Y-connector (INS, 2016; Alexander et al., 2014). Labeling high-risk catheters prevents connection with an inappropriate tube or catheter (TJC, 2016).
11. Open roller clamp completely on fat emulsion infusion and check flow rate on infusion pump.	Initial slow infusion allows you to observe for allergic response.
12. Infuse lipids initially at 1 mL/min for adults and 0.1 mL/min for child for first 15 to 30 minutes; increase rate as ordered.	Up to 2.5 g fat/kg per day may be infused, but current practice is generally to give <1 g fat/kg body weight per day in adults.
13. Begin PPN at ordered rate. 20% fats are infused over at least 8 hours. All lipids can hang for 12 hours as a separate infusion.	Rate of PPN administration does not need to be increased gradually. Lower concentration of dextrose allows most patients to tolerate full administration rate without difficulty.
14. Remove and discard gloves and supplies and perform hand hygiene.	Reduces transmission of microorganisms.

EVALUATION

1. Monitor flow rate routinely hourly or more frequently if necessary.	Too-rapid or too-slow infusion could result in metabolic disturbances such as hyperglycemia.
2. Measure vital signs and patient's general comfort level every 10 minutes for first 30 minutes, then vital signs every 4 hours.	Monitors patient for lipid allergy.
3. Monitor patient's laboratory values (e.g., triglycerides, liver function tests) daily and perform blood glucose monitoring as ordered. Measure serum lipids 4 hours after discontinuing infusion.	Provides objective data to measure response to therapy (e.g., ability of liver to metabolize lipids). Measurement of lipids too soon after infusion will yield incorrect blood values.
4. Monitor temperature every 4 hours and regularly inspect venipuncture site for signs of phlebitis or infiltration.	Determines onset of fever, a complication of intolerance to fat emulsion or sepsis. Determines integrity of IV system.
5. Evaluate patient's weight, intake and output (I&O), condition of peripheral extremities (for edema), and breath sounds.	Weight gain, I&O imbalance, peripheral edema, and crackles in lungs indicate fluid retention.
6. **Use Teach-Back:** "I want to be sure I explained your peripheral parenteral nutrition. Why are you receiving this type of nutrition?" Revise your instruction now or develop a plan for revised patient or family caregiver teaching if patient or family caregiver is not able to teach back correctly.	Determines patient's or family caregiver's level of understanding of instructional topic.

Unexpected Outcomes

1. There is intolerance to fat emulsion, as evidenced by increased triglyceride levels, increased temperature (3° to 4° F), chills, flushing, headache, nausea and vomiting, diaphoresis, muscle ache, chest and back pain, dyspnea, pressure over eyes, vertigo.

2. See Unexpected Outcomes and Related Interventions for Skill 33.1.

Related Interventions

- Turn PPN infusion off.
- Inform health care provider.
- Prepare to treat anaphylactic reaction according to health care provider's orders.
- Record lipid allergy in patient's medical record.

Recording and Reporting

- Record condition of IV site, type of solutions, rate and status of infusion, catheter lumen used for infusion, I&O, blood glucose levels, vital signs, weights, and other assessment findings in nurses' notes in electronic health record (EHR) or chart on the appropriate flow sheets.
- Record any adverse reactions in nurses' notes in EHR or chart.
- If signs of fat intolerance, infection, occlusion, fluid retention, or infiltration occur, notify the health care provider.
- Document your evaluation of patient and family caregiver learning.

Special Considerations

Teaching
- PPN administration does not typically occur in the home unless patient is in need of long-term nutritional support.

Pediatric
- See Skill 33.1.

Gerontological
- Some older adults may have fragile peripheral veins or poor fluid tolerance because of cardiac or renal dysfunction, making PPN undesirable.

Home Care
- See Skill 33.1.

◆ CLINICAL DEBRIEF

A 43-year-old patient is admitted to the hospital with a severe exacerbation of Crohn's disease. He lost 10 lbs (4.5 kg) in the last 3 weeks and suffers recurrent abdominal pain, cramping, and loose stools. He is unable to tolerate food orally, becoming easily nauseated. He is to receive bowel rest and nutritional support with central parenteral nutrition (CPN). The health care provider inserted a central line for 3 : 1 parenteral nutrition (PN) therapy.

1. Identify four physical parameters that can change quickly and should be part of your baseline assessment before initiating CPN.
2. On the third day after central line insertion, the patient develops a fever and fatigue, preferring to stay in bed. What might the fever indicate, and what could be its source?
3. Two days after beginning CPN infusion, the patient experiences a 5-lb (2-kg) weight gain. He comments, "I'm gaining back some of the weight I lost." What would be your response? What would you include in a nursing assessment?
4. The nurse takes the patient's vital signs: HR 100, RR 20 with bilateral rales, BP 130/86. Patient denies SOB on exertion. Using SBAR, show how you would communicate with the health care team about this patient.

◆ REVIEW QUESTIONS

1. A patient is being switched from a standard intravenous (IV) solution to peripheral parenteral nutrition (PPN). Which reason(s) should the nurse give the patient about why a large-diameter vein needs to be used for the infusion? (Select all that apply.)
    1. The fluid is very hyperosmolar.
    2. The fluid cannot flow through smaller veins.
    3. Peripheral veins become very irritated because of the content of the fluid.
    4. The patient will have the infusion for an extended amount of time, which will allow for the use of both of his hands without an IV line in them.
    5. Large veins allow the solution to infuse at an increased rate needed for PPN.
2. A patient with which of the following is a good candidate for short-term PPN? (Select all that apply.)
    1. Anastomotic leak
    2. Intestinal obstruction
    3. Severe mucositis
    4. Severe malnutrition before surgery
    5. Pneumonia

3. Place the three checks for accuracy before administering central parenteral nutrition (CPN) in the correct order.
    1. Before leaving medication room, check intravenous (IV) solution a second time using the six rights of medication administration (see Chapter 20). Check label of CPN bag against medication administration record (MAR) or computer printout.
    2. Identify patient using at least two identifiers (e.g., name and birthday or name and medical record number), according to agency policy. Compare name of CPN solution and additives on label of bag with information on patient's MAR or medical record at bedside.
    3. When preparing CPN solution, check label on CPN bag with health care provider's order on MAR or computer printout and patient's name.

ⓔ *Visit the Evolve site for a complete list of Clinical Debrief and Review Questions answers.*

REFERENCES

Alexander M, et al: *Core curriculum for infusion nursing*, ed 4, Philadelphia, 2014, Lippincott, Williams & Wilkins.

Hockenberry MJ, Wilson D: *Wong's nursing care of infants and children*, ed 10, St Louis, 2015, Mosby.

Infusion Nurses Society (INS): Infusion therapy standards of practice, *J Intraven Nurs* 39(Suppl 1):S1, 2016.

Lamperti M, et al: International evidence-based recommendations on ultrasound-guided vascular access, *Intensive Care Med* 38(7):1105, 2012.

Malone A: Clinical guidelines from the American society for parenteral and enteral nutrition: best practice recommendations for patient care, *J Infus Nurs* 37(3):179, 2014.

McClave S: *American Society for Parenteral and Enteral Nutrition (ASPEN): Adult nutrition support core curriculum*, ed 2, 2012, ASPEN.

McClave S, et al: Guidelines for the provision and assessment of nutrition support therapy in the adult critically ill patient: Society of Critical Care Medicine (SCCM) and American Society for Parenteral and Enteral Nutrition (ASPEN), *JPEN J Parenter Enteral Nutr* 40(2):159, 2016.

Phillips L: *Manual of IV therapeutics: evidence-based practice for infusion therapy*, ed 6, Philadelphia, 2014, FA Davis.

Taylor B, et al: Guidelines for the provision and assessment of nutrition support therapy in the adult critically ill patient: Society of Critical Care Medicine (SCCM) and American Society for Parenteral and Enteral Nutrition (ASPEN), *Crit Care Med* 44(2):390, 2016.

The Joint Commission (TJC): *2016 National Patient Safety Goals*, Oakbrook Terrace, IL, 2016, The Commission. http://www.jointcommission.org/standards_information/npsgs.aspx. Accessed April 7, 2016.

Worthington PH, Gilbert KA: Parenteral nutrition: risks, complications, and management, *J Infus Nurs* 35(1):52, 2012.

34 | Urinary Elimination

OBJECTIVES

Mastery of content in this chapter will enable the nurse to:

- Discuss nursing interventions that promote normal micturition when toilet access is compromised or after a catheter is removed.
- Discuss the relationship between fluid balance and urinary elimination.
- Describe how to use patient-centered care principles when caring for patients with elimination alterations.
- Describe ways to provide for patient safety when managing elimination needs.

- Identify factors that increase risk for catheter-associated urinary tract infection (CAUTI).
- Perform the following skills: place and remove urinal, insert urinary catheter, care for an indwelling urinary catheter, measure postvoid residual (PVR) with catheterization and bladder scan, irrigate a catheter, remove an indwelling catheter, apply a condom catheter, and care for a suprapubic catheter.

MEDIA RESOURCES

- evolve http://evolve.elsevier.com/Perry/skills
- Review Questions
- ▶ Video Clips
- Case Studies

- Audio Glossary
- **NSO** Nursing Skills Online
- Clinical Debrief and Review Questions Answers

PURPOSE

A basic human function is urinary elimination, a function that can be compromised by a wide variety of illnesses and conditions. It is the role of a nurse to support bladder emptying as needed by helping the patient in toileting, which may include use of a commode, urinal, or bedpan. During acute illness a patient may require urinary catheterization for close monitoring of urine output or to facilitate bladder emptying when bladder function is compromised. Some patients require long-term indwelling catheters, urethral or suprapubic, when the bladder fails to empty effectively. The nurse also implements measures to minimize risk for infection when bladder function is impaired or urinary drainage tubes are required.

STANDARDS OF CARE

- Meddings J, Agency for Healthcare Research and Quality (AHRQ), 2013—Reducing Urinary Catheter Use

- The Joint Commission (TJC), 2016—Patient Safety Goals—Urinary Catheter Removal and Patient Identification

PRINCIPLES FOR PRACTICE

- Adequate oral intake is essential for bladder health, especially if a patient has an indwelling urinary catheter. Some patients with urinary problems limit fluid intake because of fear of incontinence and/or increased urinary frequency. Explain the importance of fluid intake in maintaining urinary health.
- Know the average output range for a patient. Adult urinary output averages 2200 to 2700 mL in 24 hours. An hourly output of less than 30 mL/hr for 2 hours identifies the need for further assessment.
- Know the signs of dehydration and fluid overload (Table 34.1). Start measurement of intake and output (I&O) when there is an actual or anticipated change in fluid balance.

TABLE 34.1

Signs of Fluid Volume Deficit and Fluid Volume Excess

Eyes	*FVD:* Sunken eyes, dry conjunctivae, decreased or absence of tearing *FVE:* Periorbital edema, blurred vision, papilledema
Mouth	*FVD:* Sticky, dry mucous membrane; dry, cracked lips; decreased saliva; increased viscosity of saliva; furrowed, shrunken tongue *FVE:* Excessive salivation
Skin	*FVD:* Increased skin temperature; dry, scaly skin; poor turgor *FVE:* Edema, anasarca
Cardiovascular	*FVD:* Increased pulse rate, weak pulse, hypotension, decreased pulse volume/pressure, decreased capillary filling, increased hematocrit, flat neck veins *FVE:* Bounding pulse rate, blood pressure normal with or without orthostatic changes, third heart sound (S_3), distended neck veins
Gastrointestinal	*FVD:* Sunken abdomen *FVD:* or *FVE:* Vomiting, diarrhea, abdominal cramps
Renal	*FVD:* Oliguria or anuria, increased urine specific gravity (normal, 1.010 to 1.030) *FVE:* Decreased urine specific gravity, diuresis (if kidneys are normal)

FVD, Fluid volume deficit; *FVE,* fluid volume excess.

- Assess a patient's most recent serum electrolyte measurements. Abnormal values reflect alterations in fluid balance that can lead to deterioration in patients' health.
- Weigh a patient to determine fluid status. Ask him or her to empty the bladder. Weigh with the same scale; at the same time of day; and with comparable articles of clothing, including bed linen if bed weights are necessary.

PATIENT-CENTERED CARE

- The personal level of touch required when you help patients with problems in urinary elimination requires you to understand their values and preferences.
- Determine how patients feel about having to undergo procedures such as catheterization. Try to adapt procedures to minimize the invasive nature of catheterization and maintain a patient's dignity and respect.
- When caring for patients from divergent cultures, it is important to incorporate into the plan of care sensitivity and awareness of factors that may impact how you deal with urinary elimination problems.
- Variations within a cultural group are common. Assess each patient and care for him or her as an individual. Many cultures have specific beliefs and practices related to elimination, privacy, and gender-specific care. For example:
  - Some cultures emphasize female modesty and prohibit nonrelated males and females from touching; provide for a same-gender caregiver.

- Some cultures emphasize interdependence over independence; thus family presence at the bedside for important decision making is common.
- Privacy is important in many cultures; thus careful attention to draping is important.

EVIDENCE-BASED PRACTICE

Major recommendations in evidence-based guidelines to reduce catheter-related problems and infection include reducing inappropriate catheter use and removing catheters as soon as possible (Fekete et al., 2015; Lo et al., 2014; Meddings et al., 2013; TJC, 2016). Evidence-based interventions for the prevention of CAUTI include the following:

- Use aseptic catheter insertion with sterile equipment (Fekete et al., 2015; TJC, 2016).
- Use only trained, dedicated personnel to insert urinary catheters (Lo et al., 2014).
- Use smallest catheter possible.
- Remove catheter as soon as possible (Meddings et al., 2013).
- Secure indwelling catheters to prevent movement and pulling on the catheter.
- Maintain a closed urinary drainage system.
- Maintain an unobstructed flow of urine through the catheter, drainage tubing, and drainage bag.
- Keep the urinary drainage bag below the level of the bladder at all times.
- When emptying the urinary drainage bag, use a separate measuring receptacle for each patient. Do not let the drainage spigot touch the receptacle.
- Perform routine perineal hygiene daily and after soiling.
- Quality improvement/surveillance programs should be in place that alert providers that a catheter is in place and include regular educational programming about catheter care.

SAFETY GUIDELINES

- Regularly assess and determine patients' functional status such as their ability to safely stand and/or transfer to a toilet or commode, their ability to follow and understand directions, and their motivation to help in self-care activities such as using a toilet, commode, or urinal.
- Evaluate a patient's normal pattern of micturition. Patients taking diuretic medications should have a toilet, commode, and/or urinal close to their bed or chair. Respond to any request for toileting assistance in a prompt manner to lessen the chance of patients falling as they try to reach a toilet.
- Consider a patient's age when assessing voiding habits. Toilet training and enuresis are concerns for toddlers and preschoolers. Frail older adults are at higher risk for incontinence because of multiple health care problems and associated physiological changes.
- Patients who need help with elimination should have a call bell within easy reach and the offer for help at regular intervals, especially in the morning after awakening, after meals, and before bedtime.
- Maintain aseptic technique when catheterizing a patient to prevent CAUTI (Fekete et al., 2015).

PROCEDURAL GUIDELINE 34.1 *Assisting With Use of a Urinal*

▶ *Video Clip*

A urinal is a container that collects and holds urine when access to a toilet is restricted. Patients who may need a urinal include those who have compromised mobility, severe dyspnea, or other illnesses that make walking to a bathroom impossible or excessively painful. In some instances a male patient may be able to stand at the bedside and use a urinal. Most urinals are used by men, but there are specially designed urinals for women (Fig. 34.1). The female urinal has a larger opening at the top with a defined rim, which helps position the urinal closely against the genitalia.

Delegation and Collaboration
The skill of assisting a patient with a urinal can be delegated to nursing assistive personnel (NAP). The nurse directs the NAP to:
- Help the patient with special needs or adaptations such as a need to hold a urinal for a patient.
- Provide personal hygiene as necessary after urination.
- Report immediately any changes in urine color, clarity, and odor; development of incontinence (involuntary loss of urine); patient reports of dysuria, which could indicate an infection; and any changes in the frequency and amount of urine.

Equipment
- Urinal
- Clean gloves
- Graduated cylinder (used for measuring volume if on intake and output (I&O)
- Supplies for diagnostic urine tests and specimen collection (see Chapter 7).
- Wash basin, washcloths, towels, and soap
- Toilet tissue

Procedural Steps
1. Assess patient's normal urinary elimination habits, including any episodes of incontinence.
2. Determine how much help is needed to place and remove the urinal. (Ask the patient or observe previous use.)
3. Review health care provider orders to determine if a urine specimen is to be collected.
4. Perform hand hygiene.

5. Explain procedure to patient.
6. Provide privacy by closing bedside curtain and room door.
7. Assess for a distended bladder by inspecting the lower one third of the abdomen or palpating gently above symphysis pubis.
8. Apply clean gloves.
9. Help patient into appropriate position: for a male patient on side, back, sitting with head of bed elevated, or in standing position; for a female patient lying supine. If needed, place an absorbent pad under patient's buttocks to protect bed linens from accidental spills.

Clinical Decision Point *Before having a patient stand to void, assess lower-extremity strength and mobility and assess blood pressure for orthostatic hypotension (Chapter 5), especially if there has been a period of prolonged bed rest.*

10. If possible, a male patient should hold urinal and position penis in urinal. If needed, help patient by positioning penis completely in urinal and holding urinal in place or by helping him hold urinal. Ensure that the urinal is placed dependent of the flow of urine.
11. Help a female patient by positioning the urinal against the genitalia and stabilizing it to keep it in position and dependent of urine flow.
12. Cover patient with bed linens and place the call bell within reach. If possible, give patient further privacy by leaving the bedside after ensuring that he or she is in a safe and comfortable position. Remove gloves and perform hand hygiene.
13. After patient has finished voiding, apply gloves and remove urinal and assess characteristics of the urine for color, clarity, odor, and amount. Help him or her wash and dry penis or genitalia.
14. Measure urine and record output on I&O record, if needed (see Chapter 6).
15. Empty and clean urinal. Return urinal to patient for future use.
16. Help patient perform hand hygiene as needed.
17. Remove and dispose of gloves; perform hand hygiene.

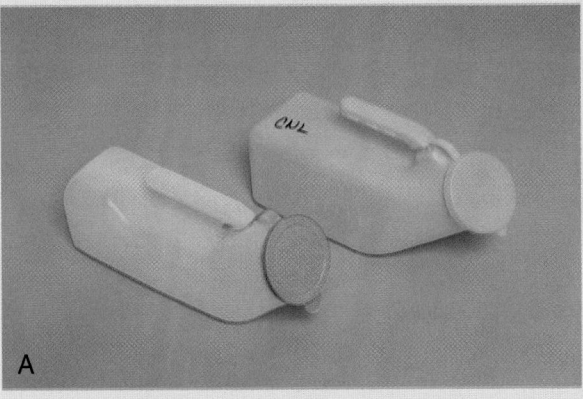
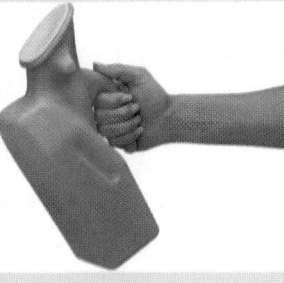

FIG 34.1 A, Male urinals. **B,** Female urinal. (**B** *Courtesy Briggs Medical Service Co.*)

✦ SKILL 34.1   Insertion of a Straight or an Indwelling Urinary Catheter

NSO *Nursing Skills Online Urinary Catheterization Module / Lessons 1 and 2*

Urinary catheterization is the placement of a tube through the urethra into the bladder to remove urine. This is an invasive procedure that requires a medical order and sterile technique (Lo et al., 2014). Urinary catheterization may be short term (2 weeks or less) or long term (more than 2 weeks) (Geng et al., 2012). Conditions that require use of urinary catheters include the need to monitor urine output, relief of urinary obstruction, postoperative care, or a bladder that empties inadequately as a result of a neurological condition. Excessive accumulation of urine in the bladder increases the risk for urinary tract infection (UTI) and can cause backward flow of urine up the ureters to the kidneys, causing kidney infection and/or damage. Urinary incontinence, an involuntary leakage of urine, may require indwelling catheterization if the leaking urine interferes with wound healing. Intermittent catheterization is used to measure postvoid residual (PVR) when a bladder scanner is not available or as a way to manage chronic urinary retention.

The steps for inserting an indwelling and a single-use straight catheter are the same. The difference lies in the inflation of a balloon to keep the indwelling catheter in place and the presence of a closed drainage system. Urinary catheters are made with one to three lumens (Fig. 34.2). Single-lumen catheters (see Fig. 34.2A) are used for intermittent catheterization (i.e., the insertion of a catheter for one-time bladder emptying). Double-lumen catheters, designed for indwelling catheters, provide one lumen for urinary drainage and a second lumen to inflate a balloon that keeps the catheter in place (see Fig. 34.2B). Triple-lumen catheters (see Fig. 34.2C) are used for continuous bladder irrigation or when it becomes necessary to instill medications into the bladder. One lumen drains the bladder, a second lumen is used to inflate the balloon, and a third lumen delivers irrigation fluid into the bladder.

A health care provider chooses a catheter on the basis of factors such as latex allergy, history of catheter encrustation, and susceptibility to infection. Indwelling catheters are made of latex or silicone. Some have special coatings that reduce urethral irritation and encrustation. Silver-coated catheters have been used as a measure to reduce infection; but efficacy data have been inconsistent, and the silver-coated catheter use is not common because of the increased cost of the catheters (Beattie and Taylor, 2010; Muzzi-Bjornson and Macera, 2011). Straight or intermittent catheters are made of rubber (softer and more flexible) or polyvinyl chloride. Patients who self-catheterize have a large selection of catheters: some with special coatings that do not require lubrication and others that are self-contained systems consisting of a lubricated catheter and packaged with a connected drainage bag.

The size of a urinary catheter is based on the French (Fr) scale, which reflects the internal diameter of the catheter. Most adults with an indwelling catheter should have a size 14 to 16 Fr to

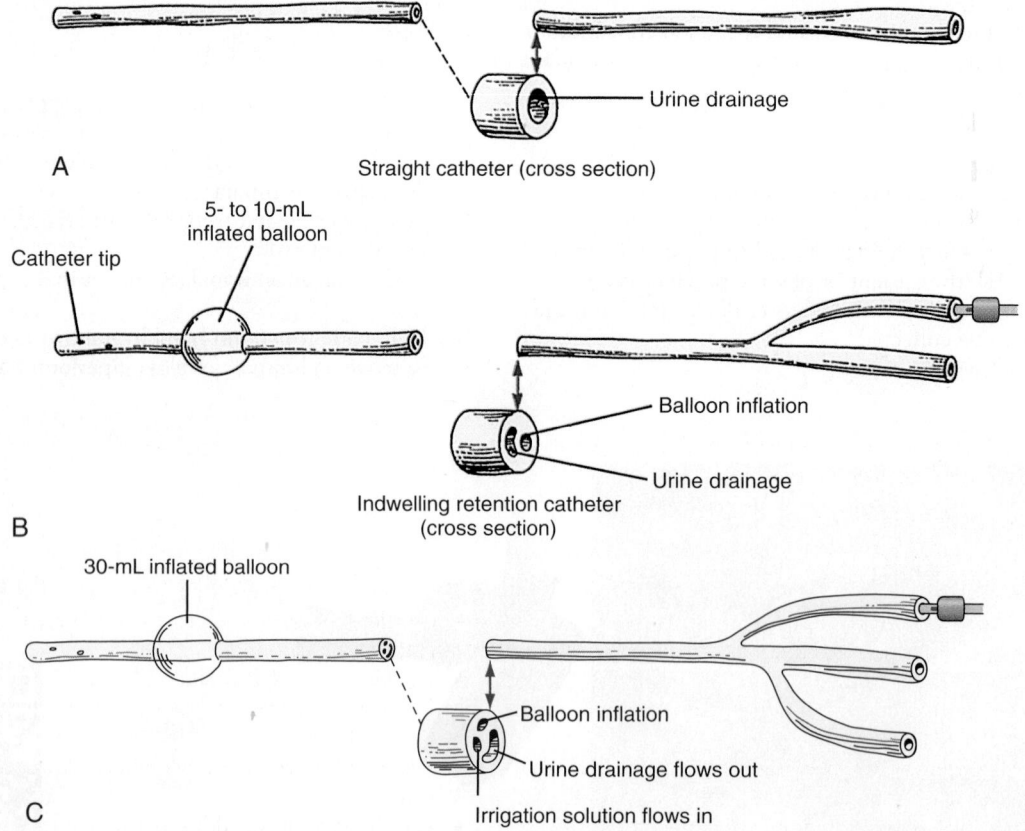

FIG 34.2 A, Single-lumen or straight catheter (cross section). **B,** Double-lumen or indwelling retention catheter (cross section). **C,** Triple-lumen catheter for continuous closed irrigation (cross section).

minimize trauma and risk for infection. Older women or older men with an enlarged prostate may need a smaller size (12 to 14 Fr). A coudé catheter is also available for men with an enlarged prostate with a urinary obstruction; it has a slightly bent tip designed to navigate past the obstruction. Larger-catheter diameters increase the risk for trauma to the bladder neck and urethra (Geng et al., 2012). However, larger sizes such as a 20 or 22 Fr are needed in special circumstances such as after urologic surgery or in the presence of gross hematuria. Smaller sizes are needed such as a 5 to 6 Fr for infants and an 8 to 10 Fr for children.

Indwelling catheters come in a variety of balloon sizes from 3 mL (for a child) to 30 mL for continuous bladder irrigation (CBI). The size of the balloon is usually printed on the catheter port (Fig. 34.3). The recommended balloon size for an adult is a 5-mL balloon (filled with 10 mL). Long-term use of larger balloons (30-mL) has been associated with increased patient discomfort, irritation, and trauma; increased risk of catheter expulsion; and incomplete emptying of the bladder because of urine that pools below the level of the catheter drainage lumen (Geng et al., 2012).

For patients requiring long-term catheterization (i.e., urinary retention or critical illness), catheter changes should be individualized, not routine (Geng et al., 2012). Catheters should be changed for leaking or blockage and before obtaining a sterile specimen for urine culture (Geng et al., 2012). Long-term catheterization should be avoided because of its association with urinary tract infections (UTIs). Every effort should be made to remove catheters as soon as the patient can void (Lo et al., 2014).

An indwelling catheter is attached to a urinary drainage bag to collect the continuous flow of urine. Always hang the bag below the level of the bladder on the bedframe or a chair so urine drains down, out of the bladder. The bag should never touch the floor. When a patient ambulates, carry the bag below the level of his or her bladder. The only exception to this rule is when a catheter is attached to a specially designed drainage bag (belly bag) that is worn across the abdomen. A one-way valve prevents the back flow of urine into the bladder.

Delegation and Collaboration

The skill of inserting a straight or indwelling urinary catheter cannot be delegated to nursing assistive personnel (NAP). The nurse directs the NAP to:

- Help the nurse with patient positioning, focus lighting for the procedure, maintain privacy, empty urine from collection bag, and help with perineal care.
- Report post-procedure patient discomfort or fever to the nurse.
- Report abnormal color, odor, amount of urine in drainage bag and if the catheter is leaking or causes pain.

Equipment

- Catheter kit (Fig. 34.4) containing sterile items: (**NOTE:** Catheter kits vary.)
  - Straight catheterization kit: single-lumen catheter, drapes (one fenestrated—has an opening in the center), sterile gloves, lubricant, cleaning solution incorporated in an applicator or to be added to cotton balls, and specimen container
  - Indwelling catheterization kit: drapes (one fenestrated—has an opening in the center), gloves, lubricant, antiseptic cleaning solution incorporated in an applicator or to be added to cotton balls, specimen container, and a prefilled syringe with sterile water (to inflate balloon). Some kits

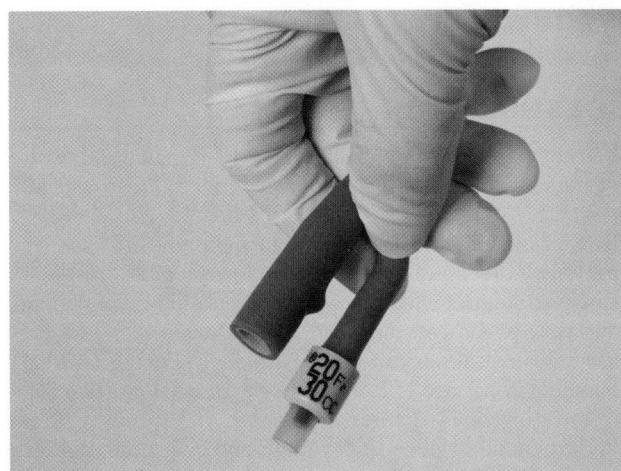

FIG 34.3 Size of catheter and balloon printed on catheter inflation valve.

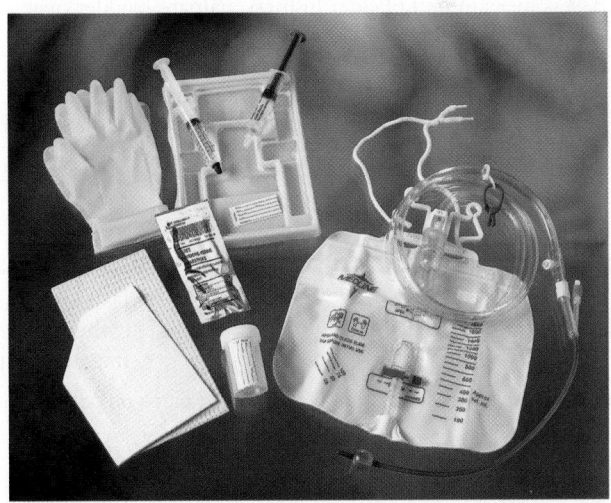

FIG 34.4 Indwelling catheterization kit includes drainage device, specimen cup, sterile drapes, sterile gloves, indwelling catheter, cleaning solution, sterile saline, sterile cotton balls, forceps, and lubricant. (*Image used with permission Medline Industries. All rights reserved.*)

contain a catheter with attached drainage bag; others contain only a catheter; others have no catheter.

- Sterile drainage tubing and bag (if not included in indwelling catheter insertion kit)
- Device to secure catheter (catheter strap or other device)
- Extra sterile gloves and catheter (*optional*)
- Clean gloves
- Basin with warm water, washcloth, towel, and soap for perineal care
- Flashlight or other additional light source
- Bath blanket, waterproof absorbent pad
- Measuring container for urine

STEP	RATIONALE

ASSESSMENT

1. Identify patient using two identifiers (e.g., name and birthday or name and medical record number), according to agency policy.	Ensures correct patient. Complies with The Joint Commission standards and improves patient safety (TJC, 2016).
2. Review patient's medical record, including health care provider's order and nurses' notes. Note previous catheterization, including catheter size, response of patient, and time of catheterization.	Identifies purpose of inserting catheter (such as for measurement of PVR, preparation for surgery, or specimen collection) and potential difficulty with catheter insertion.
3. Review medical record for any pathological condition that may impair passage of catheter (e.g., enlarged prostate gland in men, urethral strictures).	Obstruction of urethra may prevent passage of catheter into bladder.
4. Perform hand hygiene. Ask patient and check medical record for allergies.	Reduces transmission of microorganisms. Identifies allergy to antiseptic, tape, latex, and lubricant.
5. Assess patient's weight, level of consciousness, developmental level, ability to cooperate, and mobility.	Determines positioning for catheterization; indicates how much help is needed to properly position patient, ability of patient to cooperate during procedure, and level of explanation needed.
6. Assess patient's gender and age.	Determines catheter size.
7. Assess patient's knowledge, prior experience with catheterization, and feelings about procedure.	Reveals need for patient instruction and/or support.
8. Assess for pain and bladder fullness. Palpate bladder over symphysis pubis or use bladder scanner (if available) (see Procedural Guideline 34.2).	Palpation of full bladder causes pain and/or urge to void, indicating full or overfull bladder.
9. Perform hand hygiene and apply clean gloves. Inspect perineal region, observing for perineal anatomical landmarks, erythema, drainage or discharge, and odor. Remove gloves and perform hand hygiene.	Assessment of female perineal landmarks improves accuracy and speed of catheter insertion.

NURSING DIAGNOSES

- Acute pain
- Anxiety

- Deficient knowledge regarding catheterization procedure
- Impaired urinary elimination

- Risk for infection
- Urinary retention

Related factors/Risk factors are individualized based on patient's condition or needs.

PLANNING

1. Expected outcomes following completion of procedure:	
• Patient's bladder is not palpable.	Bladder successfully emptied.
• Patient verbalizes absence of abdominal discomfort or bladder pressure/fullness.	Catheterization and free flow of urine through catheter relieve bladder distention and discomfort.
• Patient has urine output of at least 30 mL/hr as measured in urinary drainage bag.	Verifies presence of catheter in bladder, catheter patency, and adequate kidney function.
• Patient verbalizes purpose and expectations about procedure.	Reflects patient understanding of procedure.
2. Explain procedure to patient.	Promotes cooperation.
3. Arrange for extra personnel to help as necessary. Organize supplies at bedside.	Some patients are unable to assume positioning independently for procedure. Ensures more efficient procedure.

IMPLEMENTATION

1. Check patient's plan of care for size and type of catheter (if this is a reinsertion). Use smallest-size catheter possible.	Ensures that patient receives correct size and type of catheter. Larger catheter diameters increase the risk for urethral trauma (Lo et al., 2014). Small catheter allows for adequate drainage of periurethral glands.
2. Perform hand hygiene.	Reduces transmission of microorganisms.
3. Provide privacy by closing room door and bedside curtain.	Promotes comfort and protects patient confidentiality.

STEP	RATIONALE
4. Raise bed to appropriate working height. If side rails in use, raise side rail on opposite side of bed and lower side rail on working side.	Promotes good body mechanics. Use of side rails in this manner promotes patient safety.
5. Place waterproof pad under patient.	Prevents soiling bed linen.
6. Apply clean gloves. Clean perineal area with soap and water, rinse, and dry (see Chapter 18). Use gloves to examine patient and identify urinary meatus. Remove and discard gloves. Perform hand hygiene.	Hygiene before initiating aseptic catheter insertion removes secretions, urine, and feces that could contaminate sterile field and increase risk for catheter-associated urinary tract infection (CAUTI).

Clinical Decision Point *Obtain help to position and support weak, frail, obese, or confused patients.*

STEP	RATIONALE
7. Position patient:	
a. Female patient:	
(1) Help to dorsal recumbent position (on back with knees flexed). Ask patient to relax thighs so you can rotate hips.	Exposes perineum and allows hip joints to be externally rotated.
(2) Alternate female position: Position side-lying (Sims') position with upper leg flexed at knee and hip. Support patient with pillows if necessary to maintain position.	Alternate position is more comfortable if patient cannot abduct leg at hip joint (e.g., patient has arthritic joints or contractures).
b. Male patient:	
(1) Position supine with legs extended and thighs slightly abducted.	Comfortable position for patient aids in visualization of penis.
8. Drape patient:	Protects patient dignity by avoiding unnecessary exposure of body parts.
a. Female patient:	
(1) Drape with bath blanket. Place blanket diamond fashion over patient, with one corner at patient's midsection, side corners over each thigh and abdomen, and last corner over perineum (see illustration).	
b. Male patient:	
(1) Drape patient by covering upper part of body with small sheet or towel; drape with separate sheet or bath blanket so only perineum is exposed (see illustration).	

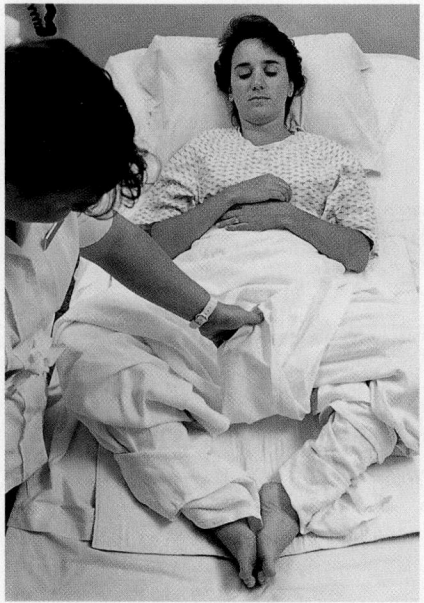

STEP 8a(1) Female patient draped and in dorsal recumbent position.

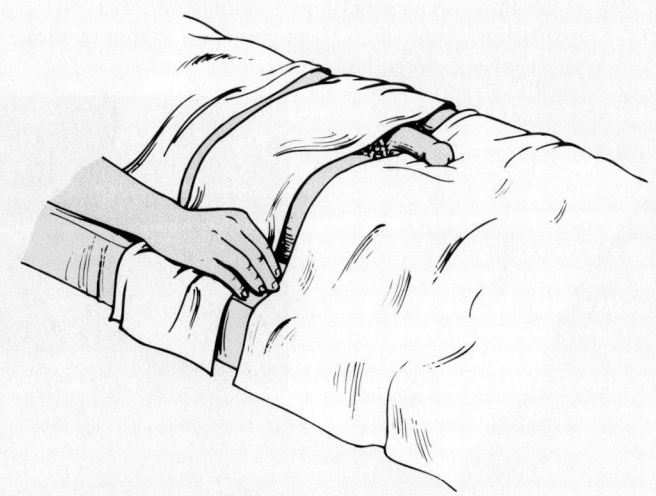

STEP 8b(1) Drape male patient with blankets.

STEP	RATIONALE
9. Position light to illuminate genitals or have assistant available to hold light source to visualize urinary meatus.	Adequate visualization of urinary meatus helps with speed and accuracy of catheter insertion.
10. Open outer wrapping of catheterization kit. Place inner wrapped catheter kit tray on clean, accessible surface such as bedside table or, if possible, between patient's open legs. Patient size and positioning dictate exact placement.	Provides easy access to supplies during catheter insertion.
11. Open inner sterile wrap covering tray containing catheterization supplies using sterile technique (see Chapter 10). Fold back each flap of sterile covering one at a time, with last flap opened toward patient.	Sterile wrap serves as sterile field.
a. Indwelling catheterization open system: Open separate package containing drainage bag, check to make sure that clamp on drainage port is closed, and place drainage bag and tubing in easily accessible location. Open outer package of sterile catheter, maintaining sterility of inner wrapper (see Chapter 10).	Open drainage bag systems have separate sterile packaging for sterile catheter, drainage bag and tubing, and insertion kit.
b. Indwelling catheterization closed system: All supplies are in sterile tray and arranged in sequence of use.	Closed drainage bag systems have catheter preattached to drainage tubing and bag.
c. Straight catheterization: All needed supplies are in sterile tray that contains supplies and can be used for urine collection.	
12. Apply sterile gloves.	Maintains surgical asepsis.
13. *Option:* Apply sterile drape with ungloved hands when drape is packed as first item. Touch only edges of drape. Then apply sterile gloves.	Maintains surgical asepsis.
14. Drape perineum, keeping gloves and working surface of drape sterile.	Sterile drapes provide sterile field over which you will work during catheterization.
a. Drape female:	
(1) Pick up square sterile drape touching only edges (2.5 cm [1 inch]).	
(2) Allow drape to unfold without touching unsterile surfaces. Allow top edge of drape (2.5 to 5 cm [1 to 2 inches]) to form cuff over both hands.	When creating cuff over sterile gloved hands, sterility of gloves and workspace is maintained.
(3) Place drape with shiny side down on bed between patient's thighs. Slip cuffed edge just under buttocks as you ask patient to lift hips. Take care not to touch contaminated surfaces with sterile gloves. If gloves are contaminated, remove and apply new pair.	
(4) Pick up fenestrated sterile drape out of tray. Allow drape to unfold without touching unsterile surfaces. Allow top edge of drape to form cuff over both hands. Apply drape over perineum so that opening is over exposed labia (see illustration).	Opening in drape creates sterile field around labia.

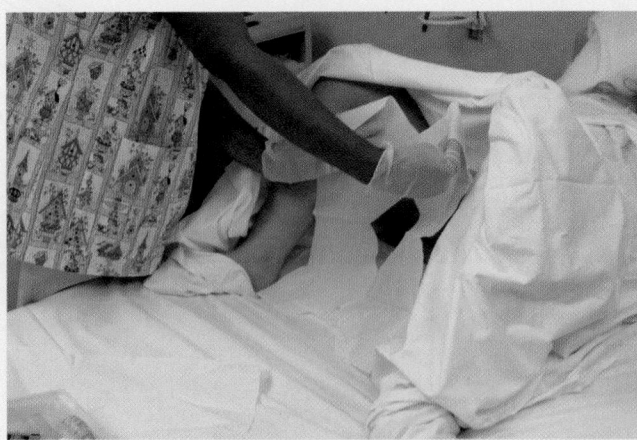

STEP 14a(4) Place sterile fenestrated drape (with opening in center) over female's perineum.

STEP	RATIONALE

b. Drape male:

(1) Use of square drape is optional; you may apply fenestrated drape instead.

(2) Pick up edges of square drape and allow to unfold without touching unsterile surfaces. Place over thighs, with shiny side down, just below penis. Take care not to touch contaminated surfaces with sterile gloves.

(3) Place fenestrated drape with opening centered over penis (see illustration).

15. Move tray closer to patient. Arrange remaining supplies on sterile field, maintaining sterility of gloves. Place sterile tray with cleaning solution (premoistened swab sticks or cotton balls, forceps, and solution), lubricant, catheter, and prefilled syringe for inflating balloon (indwelling catheterization only) on sterile drape.

Provides easy access to supplies during catheter insertion and helps to maintain aseptic technique. Appropriate placement is determined by size of patient and position during catheterization.

a. If kit contains sterile cotton balls, open package of sterile antiseptic solution and pour over cotton balls. Some kits contain package of premoistened swab sticks. Open end of package for easy access (see illustration and Fig. 34.4).

Use of sterile supplies and antiseptic solution reduces risk of CAUTI (Geng et al., 2012; Gould et al., 2010).

b. Open sterile specimen container if specimen is to be obtained (see Chapter 7).

Makes container accessible to receive urine from catheter if specimen is needed.

c. For indwelling catheterization, open sterile wrapper of catheter and leave catheter on sterile field. If part of closed system kit, remove tray with catheter and preattached drainage bag and place on sterile drape. Make sure that clamp on drainage port of bag is closed. If needed and if part of sterile tray, attach catheter to drainage tubing.

Indwelling catheterization trays vary. Some have preattached catheters; others need to be attached but are part of the sterile tray; others do not have catheter or drainage system as part of tray.

d. Open packet of lubricant and squeeze out on sterile field. Lubricate catheter tip by dipping it into water-soluble gel 2.5 to 5 cm (1 to 2 inches) for women and 12.5 to 17.5 cm (5 to 7 inches) for men (see illustration).

Lubrication minimizes trauma to urethra and discomfort during catheter insertion.
Male catheter needs enough lubricant to cover length of catheter inserted.

Clinical Decision Point *Pretesting a balloon on an indwelling catheter by injecting fluid from the prefilled sterile water syringe into the balloon port is no longer recommended. Testing the balloon may distort and stretch it and lead to damage, causing increased trauma on insertion.*

16. Clean urethral meatus:

a. Female patient:

(1) Separate labia with fingers of nondominant hand (now contaminated) to fully expose urethral meatus.

Optimal visualization of urethral meatus is possible.

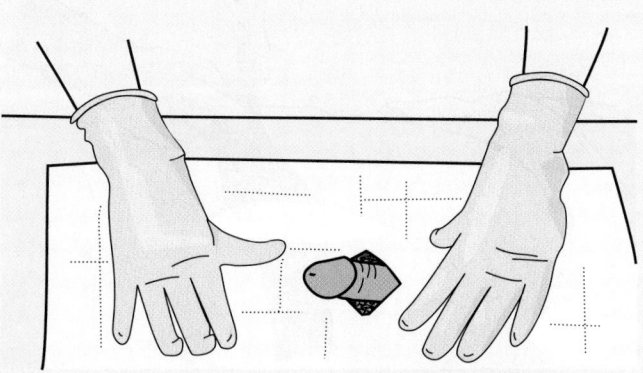

STEP 14b(3) Drape male with fenestrated drape.

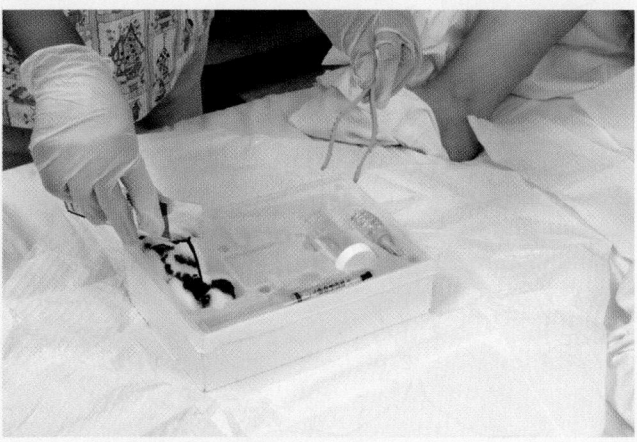

STEP 15a Sterile kit includes antiseptic swabs.

STEP	RATIONALE

(2) Maintain position of nondominant hand throughout procedure.

Closure of labia during cleaning means that area is contaminated and requires cleaning procedure to be repeated.

(3) Holding forceps in dominant hand, pick up one moistened cotton ball or pick up one swab stick at a time. Clean labia and urinary meatus from clitoris toward anus. Use new cotton ball or swab for each area that you clean. Clean by wiping far labial fold, near labial fold, and directly over center of urethral meatus (see illustration).

Front-to-back cleaning moves from area of least contamination toward highly contaminated area. Follows principles of medical asepsis (see Chapter 9). Dominant gloved hand remains sterile.

b. Male patient:

(1) With nondominant hand (now contaminated) retract foreskin (if uncircumcised) and gently grasp penis at shaft just below glans. Hold shaft of penis at right angle to body. This hand remains in this position for remainder of procedure.

When grasping shaft of penis, avoid pressure on dorsal surface to prevent compression of urethra.

Losing grasp during cleaning means that area is contaminated and requires cleaning procedure to be repeated.

(2) Using uncontaminated dominant hand, clean meatus with cotton balls/swab sticks, using circular strokes, beginning at meatus and working outward in spiral motion.

Circular cleaning pattern follows principles of medical asepsis (see Chapter 9).

(3) Repeat cleaning 3 times using clean cotton ball/swab stick each time (see illustration).

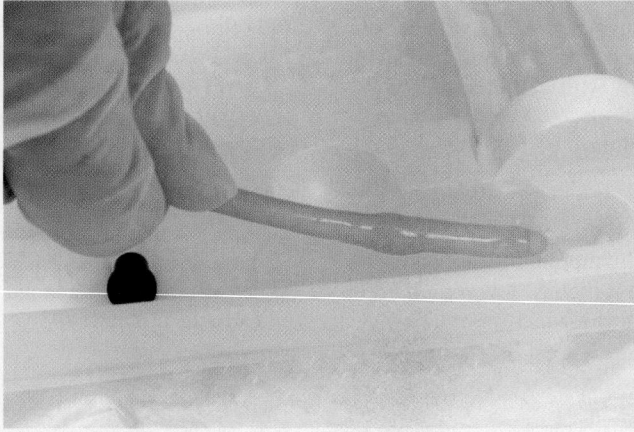

STEP 15d Lubricate catheter.

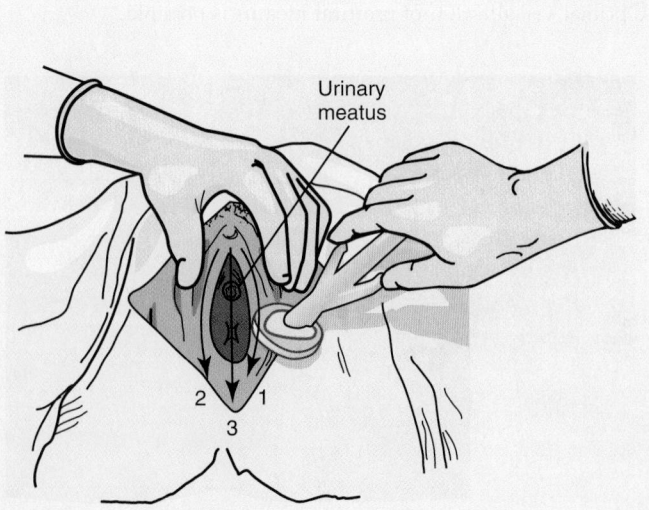

STEP 16a(3) Clean female perineum.

Urinary meatus

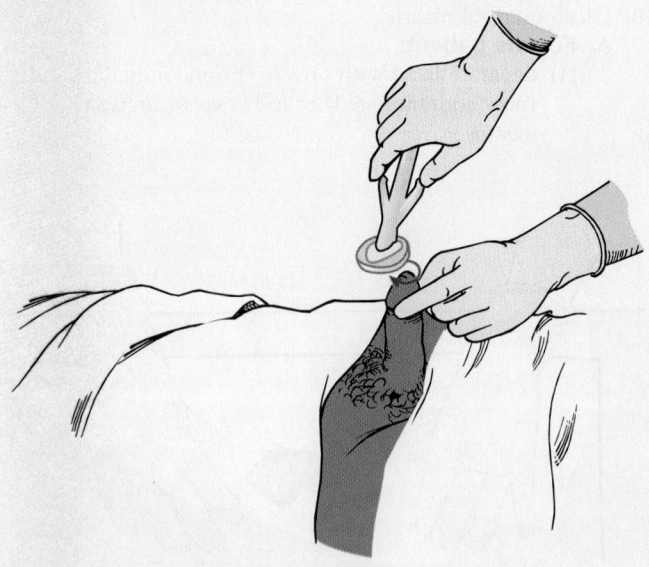

STEP 16b(3) Clean male urinary meatus.

STEP	RATIONALE

17. Pick up and hold catheter 7.5 to 10 cm (3 to 4 inches) from catheter tip with catheter loosely coiled in palm of hand. If catheter is not attached to drainage bag, make sure to position urine tray so end of catheter can be placed there once insertion begins.

Holding catheter near tip allows for its easier manipulation during insertion. Coiling catheter in palm prevents distal end from striking nonsterile surface.

18. Insert catheter. Explain to patient that feeling of burning, pinching, or pressure may be experienced as catheter is inserted into urethra. This sensation is normal and will go away quickly.

Helps to minimize patient anxiety.

   a. Female patient:

     (1) Ask patient to bear down gently and slowly insert catheter through urethral meatus (see illustration).

Bearing down may help visualize urinary meatus and promotes relaxation of external urinary sphincter, aiding in catheter insertion.

     (2) Advance catheter total of 5 to 7.5 cm (2 to 3 inches) or until urine flows out of catheter. When urine appears, advance catheter another 2.5 to 5 cm (1 to 2 inches). Do not use force to insert catheter.

Urine flow indicates that catheter tip is in bladder or lower urethra.

     (3) Release labia and hold catheter securely with nondominant hand.

Prevents accidental expulsion of catheter from the patient's bladder.

   b. Male patient:

     (1) Lift penis to position perpendicular (90 degrees) to patient's body and apply gentle upward traction (see illustration).

Straightens urethra to ease catheter insertion.

     (2) Ask patient to bear down as if to void and slowly insert catheter through urethral meatus.

Relaxation of external sphincter aids in insertion of catheter.

     (3) Advance catheter 17 to 22.5 cm (7 to 9 inches) or until urine flows out end of catheter.

Length of male urethra varies. Flow of urine indicates that tip of catheter is in bladder or urethra but not necessarily that balloon part of indwelling catheter is in bladder.

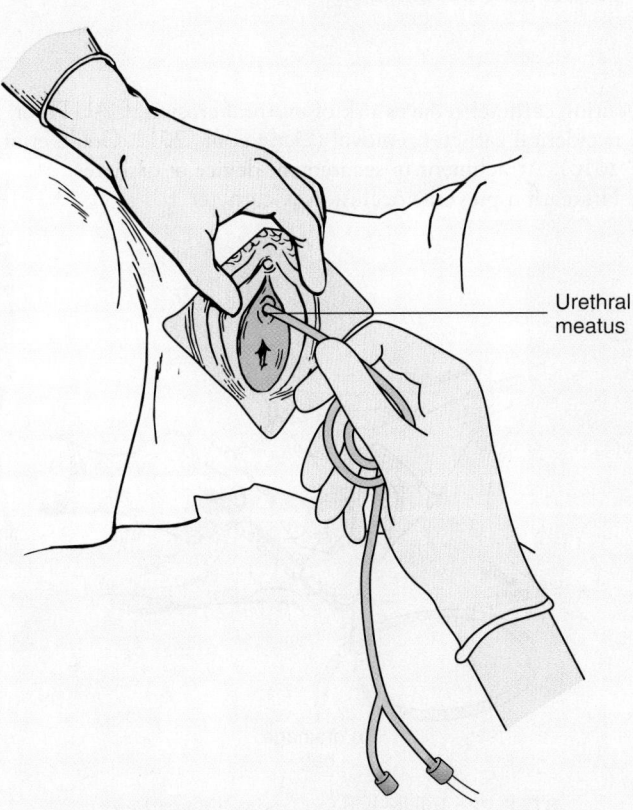

Urethral meatus

STEP 18a(1) Insert catheter into female urinary meatus.

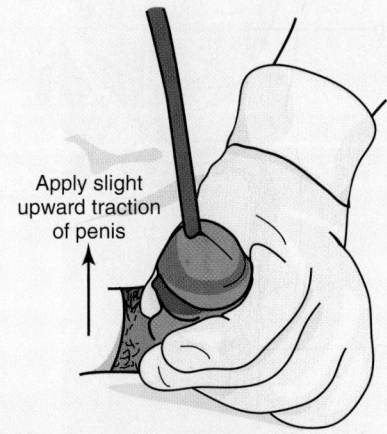

Apply slight upward traction of penis

STEP 18b(1) Insert catheter into male urinary meatus.

STEP	RATIONALE
(4) Stop advancing with straight catheter. When urine appears in indwelling catheter, advance it to bifurcation (inflation and deflation ports exposed) (see illustration).	Further advancement of catheter to bifurcation of drainage and balloon inflation port ensures that balloon part of catheter is not still in prostatic urethra (Méndez-Probst et al., 2012).
(5) Lower penis and hold catheter securely in nondominant hand.	Prevents accidental expulsion of catheter from the patient's bladder.
19. Allow bladder to empty fully unless agency policy restricts maximum volume of urine drained (see agency policy).	There is no definitive evidence regarding whether there is benefit in limiting maximal volume drained.
20. Collect urine specimen as needed (see Chapter 7). Fill specimen container to 20 to 30 mL by holding end of catheter over cup.	Sterile specimen for culture analysis can be obtained.
a. Label and bag specimen according to agency policy. Label specimen in front of patient. Send to laboratory as soon as possible.	Fresh urine specimen ensures more accurate findings. Labeling ensures that diagnostic results will be connected to correct patient.
21. Straight catheterization: When urine stops flowing, withdraw catheter slowly and smoothly until removed.	Minimizes trauma to urethra.
22. Inflate catheter balloon with amount of fluid designated by manufacturer.	Indwelling catheter balloon should not be underinflated. Underinflation causes balloon distortion and potential bladder damage (Geng et al., 2012).
a. Continue to hold catheter with nondominant hand.	Holding on to catheter before inflating balloon prevents expulsion of catheter from urethra.
b. With free dominant hand, connect prefilled syringe to injection port at end of catheter.	
c. Slowly inject total amount of solution (see illustration).	Full amount of solution needed to inflate balloon properly.

Clinical Decision Point *If patient complains of sudden pain during inflation of a catheter balloon or when resistance is felt when inflating the balloon, stop inflation, allow the fluid from the balloon to flow back into the syringe, advance catheter farther, and reinflate balloon. The balloon may have been inflating in the urethra. If pain continues, remove catheter and notify health care provider.*

STEP	RATIONALE
d. After inflating catheter balloon, release catheter from nondominant hand. *Gently* pull catheter until resistance is felt. Then advance catheter slightly.	By moving catheter slightly back into bladder, pressure on bladder neck is avoided.
e. Connect drainage tubing to catheter if it is not already pre-connected.	
23. Secure indwelling catheter with catheter strap or other securement device. Leave enough slack to allow leg movement. Attach securement device at tubing just above catheter bifurcation.	Securing catheter reduces risk of urethral erosion, CAUTI, or accidental catheter removal (Geng et al., 2012; Gould et al., 2010). Attachment of securement device at catheter bifurcation prevents occlusion of catheter.

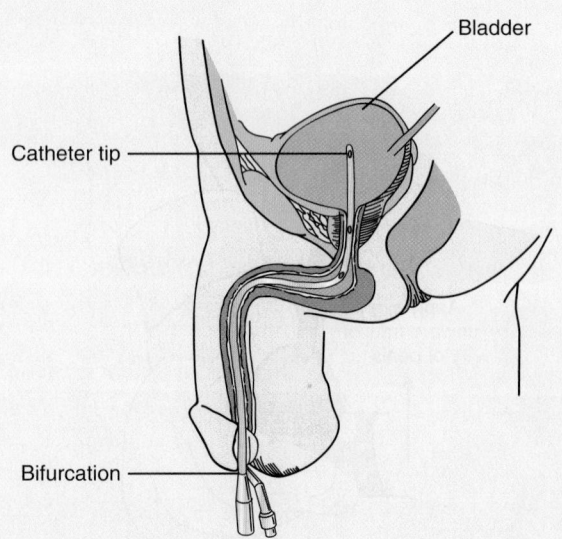

STEP 18b(4) Male anatomy with correct catheter insertion to bifurcation.

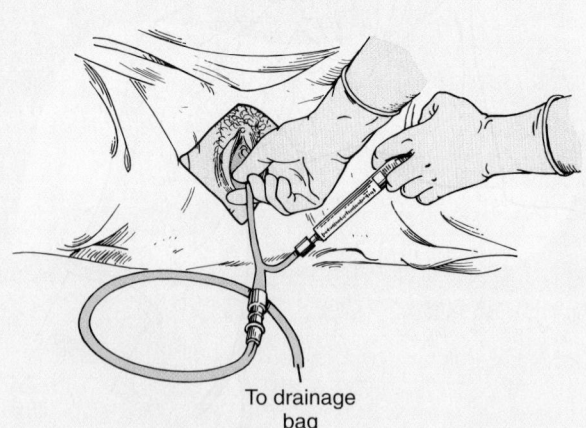

STEP 22c Inflate balloon (indwelling catheter).

STEP	RATIONALE

a. **Female patient:**

  (1) Secure catheter tubing to inner thigh, allowing enough slack to prevent tension (see illustration).

b. **Male patient:**

  (1) Secure catheter tubing to upper thigh (see illustration) or lower abdomen (with penis directed toward chest). Allow slack in catheter so movement does not create tension on catheter.

Anchoring catheter reduces traction on urethra and minimizes urethral injury (Geng et al., 2012).

  (2) If retracted, replace foreskin over glans penis.

Leaving foreskin retracted can cause discomfort and dangerous edema.

24. Clip drainage tubing to edge of mattress. Position drainage bag lower than bladder by attaching to bedframe. Do not attach to side rails of bed (see illustration).

Drainage bags that are below level of bladder ensure free flow of urine, thus decreasing risk for CAUTI (Geng et al., 2012; Gould et al., 2010). Bags attached to movable objects such as side rail increase risk for urethral trauma because of pulling or accidental dislodgement.

25. Check to ensure that there is no obstruction to urine flow. Coil excess tubing on bed and fasten to bottom sheet with clip or other securement device.

Obstruction to flow of urine increases risk for CAUTI (Geng et al., 2012; Gould et al., 2010).

26. Provide hygiene as needed. Help patient to comfortable position.

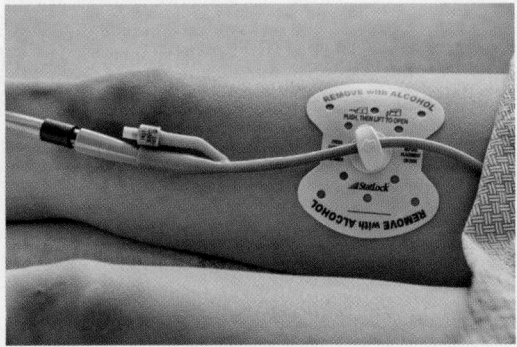

STEP 23a(1) Secure indwelling catheter on female with adhesive securement device.

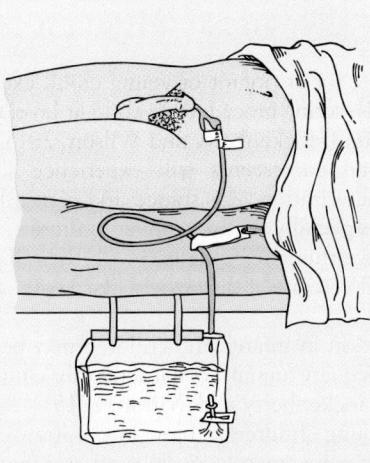

STEP 23b(1) Secure indwelling catheter on male with tape.

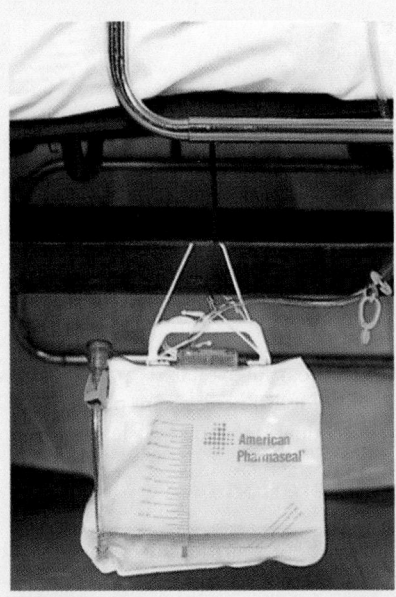

STEP 24 Drainage bag below level of bladder.

STEP	RATIONALE
27. Dispose of supplies in appropriate receptacles.	
28. Measure urine and record.	Provides baseline for urine output.
29. Remove gloves and perform hand hygiene.	Reduces transmission of infection.

EVALUATION

1. Palpate bladder for distention or use bladder scan (see Procedural Guideline 34.2) as per agency protocol.	Determines if distention is relieved.
2. Ask patient to describe level of comfort.	Determines if patient's sensation of discomfort or fullness has been relieved.
3. Indwelling catheter: Observe character and amount of urine in drainage system.	Determines if urine is flowing adequately.
4. Indwelling catheter: Determine that there is no urine leaking from catheter or tubing connections.	Prevents injury to patient's skin and ensures closed sterile system.
5. **Use Teach-Back:** "I want to be sure I explained clearly about your urinary catheter and some things you can do to ensure the urine flows out of the catheter. Tell me what you can do to keep the urine flowing." Revise your instruction now or develop plan for revised patient teaching if patient is not able to teach back correctly.	Determines patient's level of understanding of instructional topic.

Unexpected Outcomes	Related Interventions
1. Catheter goes into vagina.	• Leave catheter in vagina. • Clean urinary meatus again. Using another catheter kit, reinsert sterile catheter into meatus (check agency policy). **NOTE:** If gloves become contaminated, start procedure again. • Remove catheter in vagina after successful insertion of second catheter.
2. Sterility is broken during catheterization by nurse or patient.	• Replace gloves if contaminated and start over. • If patient touches sterile field but equipment and supplies remain sterile, avoid touching that part of sterile field. • If equipment and/or supplies become contaminated, replace with sterile items or start over with new sterile kit.
3. Patient complains of bladder discomfort, and catheter is patent as evidenced by adequate urine flow.	• Check catheter to ensure that there is no traction on it. • Notify health care provider. Patient may be experiencing bladder spasms or symptoms of UTI. • Monitor catheter output for color, clarity, odor, and amount.

Recording and Reporting

• Record and report the reason for catheterization, type and size of catheter inserted, amount of fluid used to inflate balloon, specimen collection (if applicable), characteristics and amount of urine, patient's response to procedure, and any education in nurses' notes in electronic health record (EHR) or chart.
• Record amount of urine on intake and output (I&O) flow sheet record in the EHR or chart.
• Report persistent catheter-related pain, inadequate urine output, and discomfort to health care provider.
• Document your evaluation of patient learning.

Special Considerations
Teaching

• Discuss with the patient routine care of the catheter and drainage system, which includes avoiding any kinking in the drainage tubing, keeping the drainage bag dependent, avoiding pulling on the catheter, and daily hygiene.

• Explain that adequate fluid intake helps prevent catheter blockage.

Pediatric

• When caring for an infant or young child, explain procedures to parents. Describe procedure to child at level the child is able to understand (Hockenberry and Wilson, 2015).
• Children and adolescents will experience some discomfort during catheterization. Assistance and gentle holding may be necessary, especially with younger children. Most children prefer to have the parents remain with them during the procedure. Ask adolescents if they would like a parent to remain with them.
• Catheterization in infants and children may be made easier by use of an adequate amount of catheter lubricant containing 2% lidocaine (Hockenberry and Wilson, 2015).
• Teaching young children to blow into a straw or pinwheel can help to relax pelvic muscles during catheter insertion (Hockenberry and Wilson, 2015).

Gerontological

- The urethral meatus of an older woman may be difficult to identify because of urogenital atrophy.
- Symptoms of a UTI in an older adult may be difficult to recognize and may only be indicated by a change in mental status or fever (Caterino et al., 2012).
- Older adults have an increased risk for UTI related to increased prevalence of chronic disease such as diabetes and prostatic hypertrophy and higher prevalence of incontinence.
- The presence of a urinary catheter and its drainage tubing and bag can interfere with the already compromised mobility of the older adult.

Home Care

- Patients who are at home may use a leg bag during the day and switch to a larger-volume bag at night. If a patient changes from a large-volume bag to a leg bag, instruct him or her in the importance of handwashing and cleaning the connection ports with alcohol before changing bags.
- Teach patients and/or caregivers how to properly position the drainage bag; empty the urinary drainage bag; and observe urine color, clarity, odor, and amount.
- Educate patients and/or family caregivers about the signs of UTI and troubleshooting techniques for a leaking catheter.
- Arrange for home delivery of catheter supplies, always ensuring that there is at least one extra catheter, insertion kit, and drainage bag in the home.

◆ SKILL 34.2   Care and Removal of an Indwelling Catheter

NSO *Nursing Skills Online Urinary Catheterization Module / Lesson 3*   *Video Clip*

Providing regular perineal hygiene, preventing catheter-related trauma, and removing indwelling catheters as soon as possible are important interventions to reduce risk of catheter-associated urinary tract infection (CAUTI) (Gould et al., 2010; Lo et al., 2014; Meddings et al., 2013). Prolonged indwelling catheterization is a major risk factor for CAUTI. When removing an indwelling catheter, it is important to ensure that the catheter balloon is fully deflated to minimize trauma to the urethra. Often clinicians clamp catheter tubing before removal in the belief that the practice allows the bladder to fill and obtain bladder tone. However, evidence is unclear that the practice of clamping a catheter before removal will improve bladder function after removal (Geng et al., 2012; Gould et al., 2010).

All patients should have their voiding monitored after catheter removal for at least 24 to 48 hours by using a voiding record or bladder diary. Record the time and amount of each voiding, including any incontinence, in the diary. Use a bladder scan (see Procedural Guideline 34.2) or ultrasound to monitor bladder functioning by measuring postvoid residual. Abdominal pain and distention, a sensation of incomplete emptying, incontinence, constant dribbling of urine, and voiding in very small amounts can indicate inadequate bladder emptying requiring intervention.

The risk of urinary tract infection (UTI) increases with the use of an indwelling catheter. Symptoms of infection can develop 2 or more days after catheter removal. Inform patients of the risk for infection, prevention measures (e.g., perineal hygiene), and signs and symptoms that need to be reported to the primary care provider.

Delegation and Collaboration

The skill of performing routine catheter care can be delegated to nursing assistive personnel (NAP). The skill of removing an indwelling catheter can be delegated to NAP (see agency policy);

however, the nurse must first assess a patient's status and verify the order. The nurse directs the NAP to:

- Report characteristics of the urine (color, clarity, odor, and amount) before and after removal.
- Report the condition of the patient's genital area (e.g., color, rashes, open areas, odor, soiling from fecal incontinence, trauma to tissues around urinary meatus).
- If allowed to remove catheter, check size of balloon and syringe needed to deflate balloon and report if balloon does not deflate and if there is bleeding after removal.
- Report time and amount of first voiding after catheter is removed.
- Report patient complaints of fever, chills, burning, flank pain, back pain, and blood in the urine.
- Report patient complaints of dysuria, hematuria, urgency, frequency, lower abdominal pain, change in mental status, and lethargy.

Equipment

Catheter Care
- Clean gloves
- Waterproof pad
- Bath blanket
- Soap, washcloth, towel, and basin filled with warm water. *Option:* Chlorhexidine 2% cloth

Removing a Catheter
- 10-mL or larger syringe without needle (Information on balloon size [mL] is printed directly on balloon inflation valve [see Fig. 34.3].)
- Graduated cylinder to measure urine
- Toilet, bedside commode, urine "hat," urinal, or bedpan
- Bladder scanner (if indicated)

STEP	RATIONALE

ASSESSMENT

STEP	RATIONALE
1. Identify patient using two identifiers (e.g., name and birthday or name and medical record number), according to agency policy.	Ensures correct patient. Complies with The Joint Commission standards and improves patient safety (2016).
2. Perform hand hygiene.	Reduces transmission of microorganisms.

STEP	RATIONALE
3. Assess need for catheter care:	
a. Observe urinary output and urine characteristics.	Reduces transmission of microorganisms. Sudden decrease in urine output may indicate occlusion of catheter. Cloudy, foul-smelling urine associated with other systemic symptoms may indicate CAUTI.
b. Assess for history or presence of bowel incontinence.	Most common bacteria to cause CAUTI are *Escherichia coli*, a major colonizer of the bowel; thus fecal incontinence increases risk for CAUTI (Gould et al., 2010; Lo et al., 2014).
c. Observe for any discharge, redness, bleeding, or presence of tissue trauma around urethral meatus (this may be deferred until catheter care).	Indicates inflammatory process, possible infection, or erosion of catheter through urethra.
d. Assess patient's knowledge of catheter care.	Determine need for patient education related to catheter care.
4. Assess need for catheter removal:	
a. Review patient's medical record, including health care provider's order and nurses' notes. Note length of time catheter was in place.	Catheters in place for more than a few days cause higher risk for catheter encrustation and UTI.
b. Assess patient's knowledge and prior experience with catheter removal.	Reveals need for patient instruction and/or support.
c. Assess urine color, clarity, odor, and amount. Note any urethral discharge, irritation of genital region, or trauma to urinary meatus (this may be deferred until just before removal).	May be indicator of inflammation or UTI and source of discomfort during catheter removal.
d. Determine size of catheter inflation balloon by looking at balloon inflation valve.	Determines size of syringe needed to deflate balloon and amount of fluid expected in syringe after deflation.

NURSING DIAGNOSES

- Deficient knowledge regarding catheter care
- Impaired urinary elimination
- Risk for infection

Related factors/Risk factors are individualized based on patient's condition or needs.

PLANNING

1. Expected outcomes following catheter care:	
• Genital area is free of secretions, fecal matter, and irritation.	Basic hygiene, especially after bowel movements, reduces risk for CAUTI (Gould et al., 2010; Lo et al., 2014).
• Patient verbalizes feeling of comfort.	Cleaning relieves local discomfort from irritation of catheter.
2. Expected outcomes after catheter removal:	
• Patient voids at least 150 mL with each voiding no more than 6 to 8 hours after removal.	Indicates return of voluntary bladder function without urinary retention.
• Patient verbalizes feeling of complete bladder emptying and absence of discomfort.	
• Patient identifies signs and symptoms of UTI.	Indicates patient learning.
3. Explain procedure to patient. Discuss signs and symptoms of UTI. If applicable, teach patient how to perform catheter hygiene.	Reduces anxiety and promotes cooperation. Self-care supports patient's sense of autonomy.

IMPLEMENTATION

1. Close room door and bedside curtain.	Provides patient privacy.
2. Perform hand hygiene.	Reduces transmission of microorganisms.
3. Raise bed to appropriate working height. If side rails are raised, lower side rail on working side.	Promotes use of proper body mechanics.
4. Organize equipment for perineal care and/or removal of catheter.	Increases efficiency of procedure.
5. Position patient with waterproof pad under buttocks and cover with bath blanket, exposing only genital area and catheter (see Skill 34.1).	Shows respect for patient dignity by only exposing genital area and catheter.

STEP	RATIONALE

a. Female in dorsal recumbent position.

b. Male in supine position.

6. Apply clean gloves.

Reduces transmission of infection.

7. Remove catheter securement device while maintaining connection with drainage tubing.

Provides ability to easily clean around catheter and to remove it.

8. **Catheter care:**

a. *Female:* Use nondominant hand to gently separate labia to fully expose urethral meatus and catheter. Maintain position of hand throughout procedure.

Provides full visualization of urethral meatus. Full separation of labia prevents contamination of meatus during cleaning.

b. *Male:* Use nondominant hand to retract foreskin if not circumcised and hold penis at shaft just below glans. Maintain hand position throughout procedure.

Retraction of foreskin provides full visualization of urethral meatus.

Clinical Decision Point *Accidentally closing labia or dropping penis during cleaning requires procedure to be repeated.*

c. Grasp catheter with two fingers to stabilize it.

Prevents unnecessary traction on catheter.
Pulling on catheter is cause of discomfort for patient and can damage urethra and bladder neck.

d. Assess urethral meatus and surrounding tissues for inflammation, swelling, discharge, or tissue trauma and ask patient if burning or discomfort is present.

Determines frequency and type of ongoing care required. Indicates possibility of CAUTI or catheter erosion through urethra.

e. Provide perineal hygiene using mild soap and warm water (see Chapter 18). *Option:* Use chlorhexidine 2% cloth.

Antiseptic cleaners have not been proven conclusively to decrease risk for CAUTI (Gould et al., 2010). Use of chlorhexidine poses minimal risk for perineal irritation.

f. Using clean washcloth, clean catheter.

(1) Starting close to urinary meatus, clean catheter in circular motion along its length for about 10 cm (4 inches), moving away from body (see illustration). Remove all traces of soap. *For male patients:* Reduce or reposition foreskin after care.

Reduces presence of secretions or drainage on outside catheter surface.

g. Reapply catheter securement device. Allow slack in catheter so movement does not create tension on it.

Securing indwelling catheter reduces risk of urethral trauma, urethral erosion, CAUTI, or accidental removal (Cipa-Tatum et al., 2011; Gould et al., 2010).

9. Routinely check drainage tubing and bag.

a. Catheter is secured to upper thigh (for women) or abdomen (for men).

Maintains unobstructed flow of urine out of bladder (Gould et al., 2010).

b. Tubing is coiled and secured onto bed linen.

c. Tubing is not looped or positioned above level of bladder.

d. Tubing is not kinked or clamped.

e. Drainage bag is positioned below level of bladder with urine flowing freely into bag.

f. Drainage bag is not overfull. Empty drainage bag when ½ full.

Overfull drainage bag creates tension and pulls on catheter, resulting in trauma to urethra and/or urinary meatus (Cipa-Tatum et al., 2011).

10. **Catheter removal:**

(Follow Step 8 before catheter removal.)

a. Move syringe plunger up and down to loosen and then pull it back to 0.5 mL. Insert hub of syringe into inflation valve (balloon port). Allow balloon fluid to drain into syringe by gravity. Syringe should fill. Make sure that entire amount of fluid is removed by comparing removed amount to volume needed for inflation.

Partially inflated balloon can traumatize urethral wall during removal. Passive drainage of catheter balloon prevents formation of ridges in balloon. These ridges can cause discomfort or trauma during removal.

b. Pull catheter out smoothly and slowly. Examine it to ensure that it is whole. Catheter should slide out easily. Do not use force. If you note any resistance, repeat Step 10a to remove remaining water.

Nonwhole catheter means that pieces of catheter may still be in bladder. Notify health care provider immediately.

c. Wrap contaminated catheter in waterproof pad. Unhook collection bag and drainage tubing from bed.

Promotes patient comfort and safety.

STEP	RATIONALE

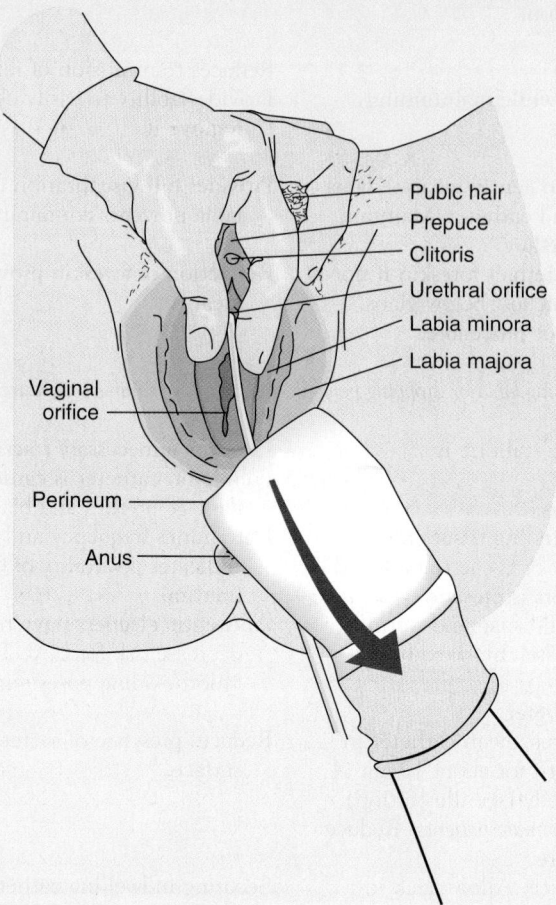

Labels on diagram:
- Pubic hair
- Prepuce
- Clitoris
- Urethral orifice
- Labia minora
- Labia majora
- Vaginal orifice
- Perineum
- Anus

STEP 8f(1) Clean catheter starting at meatus and moving downward while holding it securely.

d. Empty, measure, and record urine present in drainage bag (see Chapter 6).	Documents urinary output.
e. Encourage patient to maintain or increase fluid intake (unless contraindicated).	Maintains normal urine output.
f. Initiate voiding record or bladder diary. Instruct patient to tell you when need to empty bladder occurs and that all urine needs to be measured. Make sure that patient understands how to use collection container.	Evaluates bladder function.
g. Explain that many patients experience mild burning, discomfort, or small-volume voiding with first voiding, which soon subsides.	Burning results from urethral irritation.
h. Inform patient to report any signs of UTI.	
i. Ensure easy access to toilet, commode, bedpan, or urinal. Place urine "hat" on toilet seat if patient is using toilet. Place call bell within easy reach.	Reduces incidence of falls during toileting. Urine hat collects first voided urine.
11. Reposition patient as necessary. Provide hygiene as needed. Lower level of bed and position side rails accordingly.	Promotes patient comfort and safety.
12. Dispose of all contaminated supplies in appropriate receptacle, remove gloves, and perform hand hygiene.	Reduces transmission of microorganisms.

STEP	RATIONALE

EVALUATION

1. Inspect catheter and genital area for soiling, irritation, and skin breakdown. Ask patient about discomfort.

   Determines if area is cleaned properly and/or if patient has any irritation.

2. Observe time and measure amount of first voiding after catheter removal.

   Indicates return of bladder function after catheter removal.

3. Evaluate patient for signs and symptoms of UTI.

   Any patient who has a catheter or has had a catheter removed recently is at risk for UTI.

4. **Use Teach-Back:** "I want to be sure I explained clearly the signs of a urinary tract infection and some things you should do to prevent infection. In your own words, tell me ways you can prevent a urinary tract infection." Revise your instruction now or develop plan for revised patient teaching if patient is not able to teach back correctly.

   Determines patient's level of understanding of instructional topic.

Unexpected Outcomes

1. Water from inflation balloon does not return into syringe.

2. Patient has cloudy urine, foul urine odor, fever, chills, dysuria, flank pain, back pain, hematuria, urgency, frequency, lower abdominal pain, change in mental status, and lethargy (Medline Plus, 2016).

3. Patient is unable to void after catheter removal, has sensation of not emptying, strains to void, or experiences small voiding amounts with increasing frequency.

Related Interventions

- Reposition patient; ensure that catheter is not pinched or kinked.
- Remove syringe. Attach new syringe and allow enough time for passive emptying.
- Attempt to empty balloon by gently pulling back on syringe plunger.
- If catheter balloon does not deflate, *do not* cut balloon inflation valve to drain water. Notify health care provider.
- Assess for bladder distention and tenderness.
- Monitor vital signs and urine output.
- Report findings to health care provider; signs and symptoms may indicate UTI.
- Consult with health care provider for order to remove catheter.
- Assess for bladder distention.
- Help to normal position for voiding and provide privacy.
- Perform bladder ultrasound or scan (see Procedural Guideline 34.2) to assess for excessive urine volume in bladder.
- If patient is unable to void within 6 to 8 hours of catheter removal and/or experiences abdominal pain, notify health care provider.

Recording and Reporting

- Record time for catheter care and appearance of urine; describe condition of meatus and catheter in nurses' notes in electronic health record (EHR) or chart.
- Record and report time of catheter removal; amount of water removed from balloon; condition of urethral meatus and catheter; the time, amount, and characteristics of first voided urine in nurses' notes in EHR or chart.
- Record teaching related to catheter care, catheter removal, and fluid intake in nurses' notes in EHR or chart.
- Report hematuria, fever, dysuria, inability or difficulty voiding, and any new incontinence after a catheter is removed to health care provider.
- For patient continuing to have catheter in place, report signs of UTI to health care provider.

Special Considerations
Teaching

- Unless contraindicated, patients with a catheter should drink at least 2200 mL of fluid per day to promote continuous flushing of the bladder and prevent sediment from collecting in the catheter tubing.
- Instruct patient to hold collection bag below the level of the bladder when ambulating.
- Instruct patient not to disconnect the catheter from the collection tubing and bag.

Pediatric

- During catheter removal do not force catheter out of bladder if you meet resistance. When excessive tubing has been inserted in bladder, there have been occurrences of knotting of the tube (Hockenberry and Wilson, 2015).

Gerontological

- Older adults may exhibit atypical signs and symptoms of CAUTI such as a change in mental status attributed to delirium. A change in mental status may include confusion, agitation, and/or lethargy.
- In contrast to UTI, asymptomatic bacteriuria (ASB) is more common in older adults than in younger adults. Nursing home residents often suffer from significant cognitive deficits, impairing their ability to communicate, and from chronic genitourinary symptoms (e.g., incontinence, urgency, and frequency), which make the diagnosis of symptomatic UTI in this group particularly challenging. Furthermore, when infected, nursing home residents are more likely to present with nonspecific symptoms of UTI, such as anorexia, confusion, and a decline in functional status; fever may be absent or diminished (Rowe and Manisha, 2013).

Home Care

- Assess patient and family caregiver for ability and motivation to participate in routine catheter care.

PROCEDURAL GUIDELINE 34.2 *Bladder Scan and Catheterization to Determine Residual Urine*

A bladder scanner (Fig. 34.5) is a noninvasive device that creates an ultrasound image of the bladder for measuring the volume of urine in the bladder. The device makes calculations to report accurate urine volumes, especially lower volumes. Use a bladder scanner to assess bladder volume whenever inadequate bladder emptying is suspected such as after the removal of indwelling urinary catheters, in the evaluation of new-onset incontinence, and after urologic surgery. The most common use for the bladder scan is to measure postvoid residual (PVR) (i.e., the volume of urine in the bladder after a normal voiding). To obtain the most reliable reading, measure PVR within 5 to 15 minutes of voiding (Huether et al., 2017). A volume less than 50 mL is considered normal. Two or more PVR measurements greater than 100 mL require further investigation. If a bladder scanner is not available, obtain a PVR by measuring urine emptied from the bladder after a straight catheterization.

Delegation and Collaboration

The skill of measuring bladder volume by bladder scan can be delegated to nursing assistive personnel (NAP). The nurse must first determine the timing and frequency of the bladder scan measurement and interpret the measurements obtained. The nurse also assesses the patient's ability to toilet before measuring PVR and the abdomen for distention if urinary retention is suspected. The nurse directs the NAP to:

- Follow manufacturer recommendations for the use of the device.
- Measure PVR volumes within 5 to 15 minutes after helping the patient to void.
- Report and record bladder scan volumes.

Equipment
- Bladder scanner (follow manufacturer instructions for use)
- Ultrasound gel
- Cleaning agent for scanner head such as an alcohol pad
- Urethral catheterization tray with single-use catheter for straight/intermittent catheterization (see Skill 34.1).
- Paper towel or washcloth

Procedural Steps

1. Identify patient using at least two identifiers (e.g., name and birthday or name and medical record number), according to agency policy (TJC, 2016).
2. Assess intake and output (I&O) record to determine urine output trends and check the plan of care to verify correct timing of the bladder scan measurement.
3. Perform hand hygiene and apply clean gloves.
4. Provide privacy by closing room door and bedside curtain.
5. Discuss procedure with patient. If measurement is for PVR, ask patient to void and measure voided urine volume. Measurement should be within 5 to 15 minutes of voiding.
6. Measure PVR with the bladder scan.
   a. Help patient to supine position with head slightly elevated. Raise bed to appropriate working height. If side rails are raised, lower side rail on working side.
   b. Expose patient's lower abdomen.
   c. Turn on scanner per manufacturer guidelines.
   d. Set gender designation per manufacturer guidelines. Women who have had a hysterectomy should be designated as male.
   e. Wipe scanner head with alcohol pad or other cleaner and allow to air dry.
   f. Palpate patient's symphysis pubis (pubic bone). Apply generous amount of ultrasound gel (or if available a bladder scan gel pad) to midline abdomen 2.5 to 4 cm (1 to 1.5 inches) above symphysis pubis.
   g. Place scanner head on gel, ensuring that scanner head is oriented per manufacturer guidelines.
   h. Apply light pressure, keep scanner head steady, and point it slightly downward toward bladder. Press and release the scan button (see illustration).

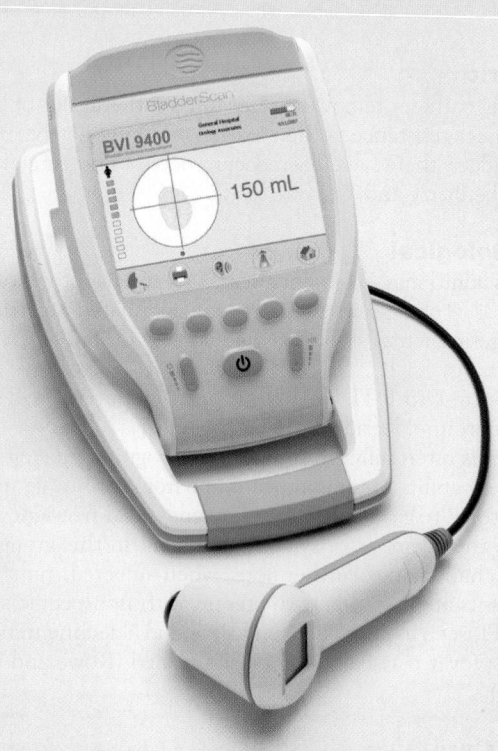

FIG 34.5 Bladder scanner with image.

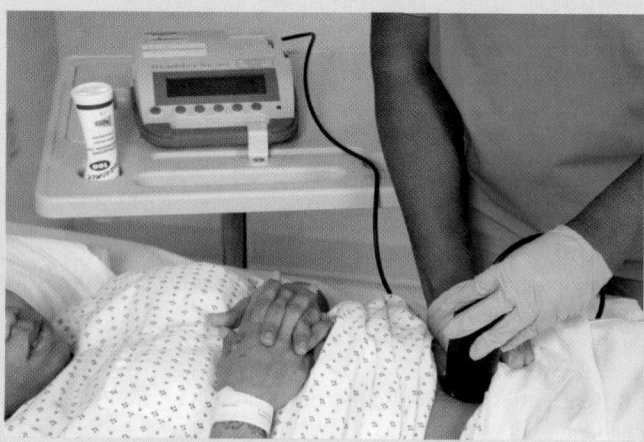

STEP 6h Placement of bladder scan head.

PROCEDURAL GUIDELINE 34.2 *Bladder Scan and Catheterization to Determine Residual Urine—cont'd*

   i. Verify accurate aim (refer to manufacturer guidelines). Complete scan and print image (if needed).

7. Remove ultrasound gel from patient's abdomen with paper towel or moist cloth.

8. Remove ultrasound gel from scanner head and wipe with alcohol pad or other cleaner; allow to air-dry.

9. Help patient to comfortable position. Lower bed and replace side rails accordingly.

10. Remove gloves and perform hand hygiene.

11. Measure PVR after using straight/intermittent catheterization (see Skill 34.1). Compare results with pre-voiding scan; urine volume should be less.

12. Review health care provider's order to determine how often to assess residual urine.

13. Review I&O record to determine urine output trends.

◆ SKILL 34.3   Performing Closed Urinary Catheter Irrigation

To maintain the patency of indwelling catheters, it is sometimes necessary to irrigate or flush a catheter with sterile solution. However, irrigation poses a risk for causing a urinary tract infection and thus must be done maintaining a closed urinary drainage system. In some instances the health care provider will determine that irrigations are needed to keep a catheter patent, such as after genitourinary surgery when there is a high risk for catheter occlusion from blood clots.

Closed catheter irrigation provides intermittent or continuous irrigation of a urinary catheter without disrupting the sterile connection between the catheter and the drainage system (Fig. 34.6). Continuous bladder irrigation (CBI) is an example of a continuous infusion of a sterile solution into the bladder, usually using a three-way irrigation closed system with a triple-lumen catheter. CBI is frequently used following genitourinary surgery to keep the bladder clear and free of blood clots or sediment.

Delegation and Collaboration

The skill of a closed catheter irrigation cannot be delegated to nursing assistive personnel (NAP). The nurse directs the NAP to:

- Report if the patient complains of pain, discomfort, or leakage of fluid around the catheter.
- Monitor and record intake and output (I&O); report immediately any decrease in urine output.
- Report any change in the color of the urine, especially the presence of blood clots.

Equipment

- Sterile irrigation solution at room temperature (as prescribed)
- Antiseptic swabs
- Clean gloves

Closed Intermittent Irrigation

- Antiseptic swabs
- Sterile irrigation solution at room temperature as prescribed
- Sterile container

- Syringe to access system: Luer-Lok syringe for needleless access port (per manufacturer instructions)
- Screw clamp or rubber band (used to temporarily occlude catheter as irrigant is instilled)

Closed Continuous Irrigation

- Antiseptic swabs
- Sterile irrigation solution at room temperature as prescribed
- Irrigation tubing with clamp to regulate irrigation flow rate
- Y connector (optional) to connect irrigation tubing to double-lumen catheter
- Intravenous (IV) pole (closed continuous or intermittent)

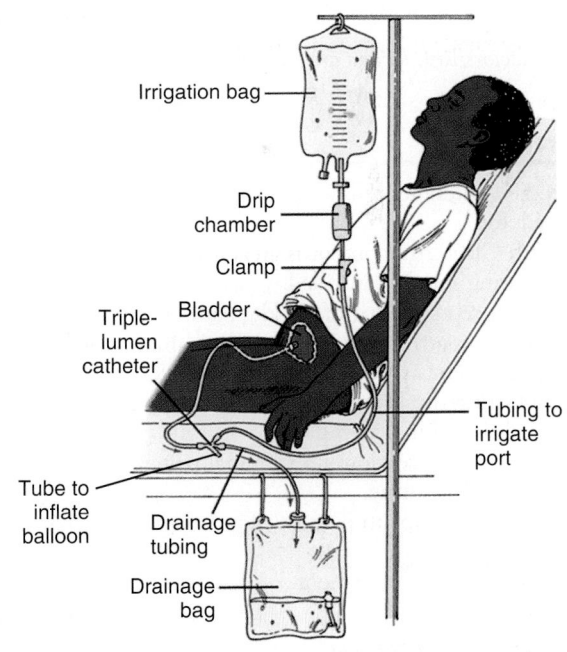

FIG 34.6 Closed continuous bladder irrigation.

STEP	RATIONALE

ASSESSMENT

1. Identify patient using two identifiers (e.g., name and birthday or name and medical record number), according to agency policy.

Ensures correct patient. Complies with The Joint Commission standards and improves patient safety (2016).

STEP	RATIONALE
2. Verify in medical record: **a.** Order for irrigation method (continuous or intermittent), type (sterile saline or medicated solution), and amount of irrigant.	Health care provider's order is required to initiate therapy. Frequency and volume of solution used for irrigation may be in the order or standardized as part of agency policy.
b. Type of catheter in place (see Fig. 34.2).	Single- and double-lumen catheters are used with open irrigation. Triple-lumen catheters are used for both intermittent and continuous closed irrigation.
3. Perform hand hygiene. Palpate bladder for distention and tenderness or use bladder scan (see Procedural Guidelines 34.2).	Reduces transmission of microorganisms. Bladder distention indicates that flow of urine may be blocked from draining.
4. Assess patient for abdominal pain or spasms, sensation of bladder fullness, or catheter bypassing (leaking).	May indicate overdistention of bladder caused by catheter blockage. Offers baseline to determine if therapy is successful.
5. Observe urine for color, amount, clarity, and presence of mucus; clots; or sediment.	Indicates if patient is bleeding or sloughing tissue, which would require increased irrigation rate or frequency of catheter irrigation.
6. Monitor I&O. If CBI is being used, amount of fluid draining from bladder should exceed amount of fluid infused into bladder.	If output does not exceed irrigant infused, catheter obstruction (i.e., blood clots, kinked tubing) should be suspected, irrigation stopped, and prescriber notified (Lewis et al., 2017).
7. Assess patient's knowledge regarding purpose of performing catheter irrigation.	Reveals need for patient instruction/support.

NURSING DIAGNOSES

- Acute pain
- Deficient knowledge regarding closed catheter irrigation
- Impaired urinary elimination
- Risk for infection

Related factors/Risk factors are individualized based on patient's condition or needs.

PLANNING

1. Expected outcomes following completion of this procedure:	
• With CBI: Urine output is greater than volume of irrigating solution instilled.	Indicates patency of drainage system, allowing for drainage of urine and irrigating solution.
• Patient reports relief of bladder pain or spasms.	Indicates bladder emptying.
• Urine output has decreased with an absence of blood clots and sediment. (**NOTE:** Urine will be bloody following bladder/urethral surgery, gradually becoming lighter and blood tinged in 2 to 3 days.)	Indicates that catheter is at decreased risk for occlusion with blood clots.
• Absence of fever, lower abdominal pain, cloudy and/or foul-smelling urine.	Signs of UTI are not present.
• Patient can explain purpose of procedure and what to expect.	Demonstrates learning.
2. Explain procedure to patient.	Reduces anxiety and promotes cooperation.

IMPLEMENTATION

1. Perform hand hygiene.	Reduces transmission of microorganisms.
2. Provide privacy by closing room door and bedside curtain.	Protects patient comfort and self-esteem.
3. Raise bed to appropriate working height. If side rails are raised, lower side rail on working side.	Promotes use of good body mechanics. Position provides access to catheter and promotes patient dignity as much as possible.
4. Position patient supine and expose catheter junctions (catheter and drainage tubing).	Position provides access to catheter and promotes patient dignity as much as possible.
5. Remove catheter securement device.	Eases access to catheter parts.
6. Organize supplies according to type of irrigation prescribed. Apply clean gloves.	Ensures an efficient procedure.

STEP	RATIONALE

7. Closed continuous irrigation:

a. Close clamp on new irrigation tubing and hang bag of irrigating solution on IV pole. Insert (spike) tip of sterile irrigation tubing into designated port of irrigation solution bag using aseptic technique (see illustration).

Prevents air from entering tubing. Air can cause bladder spasms. Technique prevents transmission of microorganisms.

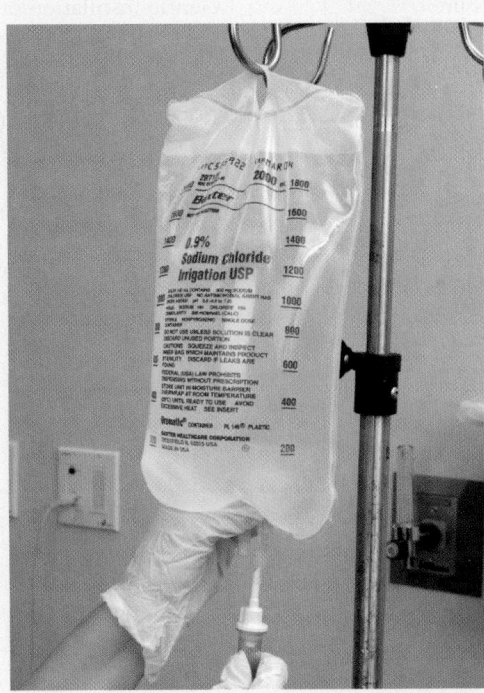

STEP 7a Spiking bag of sterile irrigation solution for continuous bladder irrigation.

b. Fill drip chamber half full by squeezing chamber. Remove cap at end of tubing, and then open clamp and allow solution to flow (prime) through tubing, keeping end of tubing sterile. Once fluid has completely filled tubing, close clamp and recap end of tubing.

Priming tubing with fluid prevents introduction of air into bladder.

c. Using aseptic technique, remove cap and connect end of tubing securely to port for infusing irrigation fluid into double/triple–lumen catheter.

Reduces transmission of microorganisms.

d. Adjust clamp on irrigation tubing to begin flow of solution into bladder. If set volume rate is ordered, calculate drip rate and adjust rate at roller clamp. If urine is bright red or has clots, increase irrigation rate until drainage appears pink (according to ordered rate or agency protocol).

Continuous drainage is expected. It helps to prevent clotting in presence of active bleeding in bladder and flushes clots out of bladder.

e. Observe for outflow of fluid into drainage bag. Empty catheter drainage bag as needed.

Discomfort, bladder distention, and possible injury can occur from overdistention of bladder when bladder irrigant cannot adequately flow from bladder. Bag will fill rapidly and may need to be emptied every 1 to 2 hours.

8. Closed intermittent irrigation:

Fluid is instilled through catheter in a bolus, flushing system. Fluid drains out after irrigation is complete.

a. Pour prescribed sterile irrigation solution into sterile container.

b. Draw prescribed volume of irrigant (usually 30 to 50 mL) into sterile syringe using aseptic technique. Place sterile cap on tip of needleless syringe.

Ensures sterility of irrigating fluid.

STEP	RATIONALE
c. Clamp catheter tubing below soft injection port with screw clamp (or fold catheter tubing onto itself and secure with rubber band).	Occluding catheter tubing below point of injection allows irrigating solution to enter catheter and flow into bladder.
d. Using circular motion, clean catheter port (specimen port) with antiseptic swab.	Reduces transmission of microorganisms.
e. Insert tip of needleless syringe using twisting motion into port.	Ensures that catheter tip enters lumen of catheter.
f. Inject solution using slow, even pressure.	Gentle instillation of solution minimizes trauma to bladder mucosa.
g. Remove syringe and clamp (or rubber band), allowing solution to drain into urinary drainage bag. (**NOTE:** Some medicated irrigants may need to dwell in bladder for prescribed period, requiring catheter to be clamped temporarily before being allowed to drain.)	Allows drainage to flow out by gravity. Medications must be instilled long enough to be absorbed by lining of bladder. Clamped drainage tubing and bag should not be left unattended.
9. Anchor catheter with catheter securement device (see Skill 34.1).	Prevents trauma to urethral tissue caused by pulling catheter.
10. Help patient to safe and comfortable position. Lower bed and place side rails accordingly.	Promotes patient comfort and safety.
11. Dispose of all contaminated supplies in appropriate receptacle, remove gloves, and perform hand hygiene.	Reduces transmission of microorganisms.

EVALUATION

1. Measure actual urine output by subtracting total amount of irrigation fluid infused from total volume drained into basin.	Determines accurate urinary output.
2. Review I&O flow sheet to verify that hourly output into drainage bag is in appropriate proportion to irrigating solution entering bladder. Expect more output than fluid instilled because of urine production.	Determines urinary output in relation to irrigation.
3. Inspect urine for blood clots and sediment and be sure that tubing is not kinked or occluded.	Decrease in blood clots means that therapy is successful in maintaining catheter patency. System is patent.
4. Evaluate patient's comfort level.	Indicates catheter patency by absence of symptoms of bladder distention.
5. Monitor for signs and symptoms of infection.	Patients with indwelling catheters remain at risk for infection.
6. **Use Teach-Back:** "I want to be sure I explained clearly about the irrigation of your catheter. Tell me in your own words the reason we are doing the irrigation." Revise your instruction now or develop plan for revised patient teaching if patient is not able to teach back correctly.	Determines patient's level of understanding of instructional topic.

Unexpected Outcomes	Related Interventions
1. Irrigating solution does not return (closed intermittent irrigation) or is not flowing at prescribed rate (CBI).	• Examine tubing for clots, sediment, and kinks. • Notify health care provider if irrigant does not flow freely from bladder, patient complains of pain, or bladder distention occurs.
2. Drainage output is less than amount of irrigation solution infused.	• Examine drainage tubing for clots, sediment, or kinks. • Inspect urine for presence of or increase in blood clots and sediment. • Evaluate patient for pain and distended bladder. • Notify health care provider.
3. Bright-red bleeding with the irrigation (CBI) infusion wide open.	• Assess for hypovolemic shock (vital signs, skin color and moisture, anxiety level). • Leave irrigation infusion wide open and notify health care provider. • Examine drainage tubing for clots, sediment, or kinks.
4. Patient experiences pain with irrigation.	• Evaluate urine for presence of or increase in blood clots and sediment. • Evaluate for distended bladder. • Notify health care provider.

Recording and Reporting

- Record irrigation method, amount and type of irrigation solution, amount returned as drainage, characteristics of output, urine output, and patient tolerance to procedure in nurses' notes in electronic health record (EHR) or chart.
- Report catheter occlusion, sudden bleeding, infection, or increased pain to health care provider.
- Record I&O on appropriate flow sheet.
- Document your evaluation of patient learning.

Special Considerations
Teaching

- Instruct patient and family caregiver to observe urine daily for changes in color, presence of mucus or blood, and odor.
- Inform patients that bleeding is common after many urologic procedures and to expect bright red–tinged urine during the first 48 hours after surgery, followed by a change in urine ranging from pink-tinged to clear.
- Instruct patient to maintain adequate oral intake of 2 L/day (unless contraindicated).

Home Care

- Patients and family caregivers can be taught to perform catheter irrigations with adequate support, demonstration/return demonstration, and written instructions.
- Teach patients and family caregivers to observe urine color, clarity, odor, and amount.
- Arrange for home delivery and storage of catheter/irrigation supplies.
- Teach patients and family caregivers signs of catheter obstruction or UTI.

◆ SKILL 34.4   Applying a Condom-Type External Catheter

NSO *Nursing Skills Online Urinary Catheterization Module / Lesson 6*

The external urinary catheter, also called a *condom catheter* or *penile sheath*, is a soft, pliable condom-like sheath that fits over the penis, providing a safe and noninvasive way to contain urine. Most external catheters are made of soft silicone that reduces friction. The silicone is clear, allowing for easy visualization of skin under the catheter. Latex catheters are still available and used by some patients. It is important to verify that a patient does not have a latex allergy before applying this type of catheter.

Condom-type external catheters are held in place by an adhesive coating of the internal lining of the sheath, a double-sided self-adhesive strip, brush-on adhesive applied to the penile shaft, or in rare cases an external strap. The catheter may be attached to a small-volume (leg) drainage bag or a large-volume (bedside) urinary drainage bag, both of which need to be kept lower than the level of the bladder. The condom-type external catheter is suitable for incontinent patients who have complete and spontaneous bladder emptying. The catheters come in a variety of styles and sizes. For the best fit and correct application it is important to refer to manufacturer guidelines. Condom-type external catheters are associated with less risk for urinary tract infection (UTI) than indwelling catheters; thus they are an excellent option for the male with urinary incontinence. Other externally applied catheters are available for men who cannot be fitted for a condom-type external catheter. One type attaches to the glans penis using hydrocolloid strips that stay in place for multiple days and allows straight catheterization. Another option available is a reusable condom-like device that is held in place by specially designed underwear.

Delegation and Collaboration

Assessment of the skin of a patient's penile shaft and determination of a latex allergy are done by a nurse before catheter application. The skill of applying a condom catheter can be delegated to nursing assistive personnel (NAP), depending on agency policy. The nurse directs the NAP to:

- Follow manufacturer directions for applying the condom catheter and securing device.
- Monitor urine intake and output (I&O) and record if applicable.
- Immediately report any redness, swelling, or skin irritation or breakdown of glans penis or penile shaft.

Equipment

- Condom catheter kit (condom sheath of appropriate size, securement device [internal adhesive or strap], skin preparation solution [per manufacturer directions])
- Urinary collection bag with drainage tubing or leg bag and straps
- Basin with warm water and soap
- Towels and washcloth(s)
- Bath blanket
- Clean gloves
- Scissors, hair guard, or paper towel

STEP	RATIONALE

ASSESSMENT

1. Identify patient using two identifiers (e.g., name and birthday or name and medical record number), according to agency policy.	Ensures correct patient. Complies with The Joint Commission standards and improves patient safety (TJC, 2016).
2. Review medical record and assess urinary pattern, ability to empty bladder effectively, and degree of urinary continence.	Incontinent patients are at risk for skin breakdown and thus candidates for condom catheter.
3. Review medical record for history of allergy to rubber or latex. Check patient's allergy wristband.	Condoms are made of latex and can cause serious skin reaction.

STEP	RATIONALE
4. Perform hand hygiene and apply clean gloves. Assess skin of penis for rashes, erythema, and/or open areas. (This may be deferred until just before catheter application.) Remove gloves and perform hand hygiene.	Reduces transmission of microorganisms. Provides baseline to compare changes in condition of skin after application of condom catheter.

Clinical Decision Point *Apply condom catheters only when the skin on the penile surface is intact.*

STEP	RATIONALE
5. Assess patient's mental status, knowledge of purpose of using condom-type catheter, and ability to apply device. It may be appropriate to include family caregiver in assessment.	Identifies patient learning needs and if self-application can be taught or if family member needs to be included in instruction.
6. Verify patient's size and type of condom catheter from plan of care or use manufacturer measuring guide to measure length and diameter of penis in flaccid state (apply gloves for measurement).	Identifies proper size of catheter needed. Penile shaft should be at least 2 cm (0.8 inch) in length to ensure successful application. If too small, condom catheter may fall off and compress urethra, stopping urine flow or causing local tissue trauma; if too big, catheter may leak or fall off (Kyle, 2011).

NURSING DIAGNOSES

- Deficient knowledge regarding catheter application and care
- Risk for impaired skin integrity
- Stress urinary incontinence (male)
- Total urinary incontinence

Related factors/Risk factors are individualized based on patient's condition or needs.

PLANNING

1. Expected outcomes following completion of procedure:	
• Patient's skin is free from urine wetness.	Catheter is applied correctly.
• Glans and penile shaft are free of skin irritation or breakdown.	Catheter is secure and not too tight.
• Patient explains purpose of procedure and what to expect.	Helps to minimize anxiety and promotes cooperation.
2. Explain procedure to patient.	Reduces anxiety and promotes cooperation.

IMPLEMENTATION

1. Identify patient using two identifiers (e.g., name and birthday or name and medical record number), according to agency policy.	Ensures correct patient. Complies with The Joint Commission standards and improves patient safety (TJC, 2016).
2. Perform hand hygiene.	Reduces transmission of microorganisms.
3. Provide privacy by closing room door and bedside curtain.	Promotes patient comfort and self-esteem.
4. Raise bed to appropriate working height. Lower side rail on working side.	Promotes use of good body mechanics.
5. Prepare urinary drainage collection bag and tubing (large-volume drainage bag or leg bag). Clamp off drainage bag port. Place nearby ready to attach to condom after applied.	Provides easy access to drainage equipment after applying condom catheter.
6. Help patient to supine or sitting position. Place bath blanket over upper torso. Fold sheets so only penis is exposed.	Respects patient dignity; draping prevents unnecessary exposure of body parts.
7. Apply clean gloves. Provide perineal care (see Chapter 18). Dry thoroughly before applying device. In uncircumcised male ensure that foreskin has been replaced to normal position before applying condom catheter. Do not apply barrier cream.	Prevents skin breakdown from exposure to secretions. Removes any residual adhesives. Perineal care minimizes skin irritation and promotes adhesion of new external catheter. Barrier creams prevent sheath from adhering to penile shaft.
8. Clip hair at base of penis as necessary before application of condom sheath. Some manufacturers provide hair guard that is placed over penis before applying device. Remove hair guard after applying catheter. An alternative to hair guard is to tear a hole in a paper towel, place it over penis, and remove after application of device.	Hair adheres to condom and is pulled during condom removal or may get caught in adhesive as external catheter is applied.

STEP	RATIONALE

Clinical Decision Point *The pubic area should not be shaved because it may increase risk for skin irritation.*

9. Apply condom catheter. With nondominant hand grasp penis along shaft. With dominant hand, hold rolled condom sheath at tip of penis with head of penis in cone. Smoothly roll sheath onto penis. Allow 2.5 to 5 cm (1 to 2 inches) of space between tip of glans penis and end of condom catheter (see illustration).

Excessive wrinkles or creases in external catheter sheath after application may mean that patient needs smaller size.

10. Apply appropriate securement device as indicated in manufacturer guidelines.

Condom must be secured firmly so it is snug and stays on but not tight enough to cause constriction of blood flow. Application of gentle pressure ensures adherence of adhesive with penile skin.

    a. Self-adhesive condom catheters: After application apply gentle pressure on penile shaft for 10 to 15 seconds to secure catheter.

    b. Outer securing strip-type condom catheters: Spiral wrap penile shaft with strip of supplied elastic adhesive. Strip should not overlap itself. Elastic strip should be snug, not tight (see illustration).

Using spiral wrap technique allows supplied elastic adhesive to expand so blood flow to penis is not compromised.

Clinical Decision Point *Never use regular adhesive tape to secure a condom catheter. Constriction from tape can reduce blood flow to tissues.*

11. Remove hair guard if used. Connect drainage tubing to end of condom catheter. Be sure that condom is not twisted. If using large drainage bag, place excess tubing on bed and secure to bottom sheet.

Allows urine to be collected and measured. Keeps patient dry. Twisted condom obstructs urine flow, causing urine pooling, skin irritation; and weakening and deterioration of adhesive, causing catheter to come off.

12. Help patient to safe, comfortable position. Lower bed and place side rails accordingly.

Promotes safety and comfort.

13. Dispose of contaminated supplies, remove gloves, and perform hand hygiene.

Reduces spread of microorganisms.

14. Remove and reapply daily following Steps 9 to 11 unless an extended-wear device is used. To remove condom, wash penis with warm, soapy water and gently roll sheath and adhesive off penile shaft.

Prevents trauma and irritation to penile sheath.

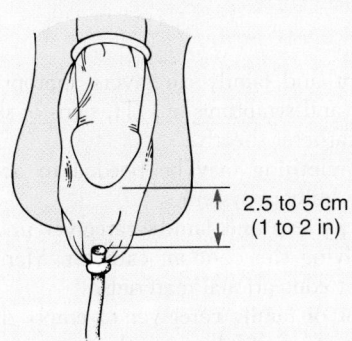

STEP 9 Condom catheter.

2.5 to 5 cm (1 to 2 in)

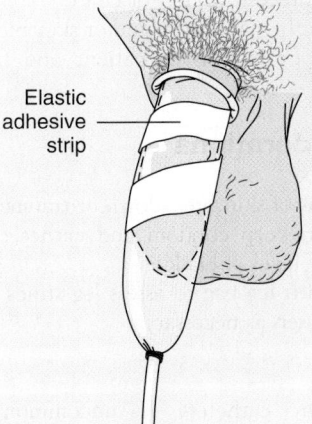

Elastic adhesive strip

STEP 10b Spiral application of adhesive strip.

EVALUATION

1. Observe urinary drainage.

Twisted condom prevents urine from draining into collection bag.

2. Inspect penis with condom catheter in place within 15 to 30 minutes after application. Assess for swelling and discoloration and ask patient if there is any discomfort.

Determines if condom is applied too tightly, impeding circulation to penis.

STEP	RATIONALE
3. Inspect skin on penile shaft for signs of breakdown or irritation at least daily, when performing hygiene, and before reapplying condom.	Changing external catheter decreases chance of infection.
4. **Use Teach-Back:** "I want to be sure I explained clearly about your external condom catheter and some things you can do to prevent it from falling off. Tell me how you can help keep the catheter on without it slipping off." Revise your instruction now or develop a plan for revised patient or family caregiver teaching if patient or family caregiver is not able to teach back correctly.	Determines patient's and family caregiver's level of understanding of instructional topic.

Unexpected Outcomes

1. Skin around penis is erythematous, ulcerated, or denuded.

2. Penile swelling or discoloration occurs.

3. Condom catheter does not stay on.

Related Interventions

- Check for latex allergy or allergy to skin preparation or adhesive device.
- Remove condom and notify health care provider.
- Do not reapply until penis and surrounding tissue are free from irritation.
- Ensure that condom is not twisted and urine flow is unobstructed after application.
- Remove external catheter.
- Notify health care provider.
- Reassess current condom size. See manufacturer size chart.
- Ensure that catheter tubing is anchored and that patient understands to not pull or tug on catheter.
- Reassess condom catheter size. Refer to manufacturer guidelines for sizing.
- Observe whether condom catheter outlet is kinked and urine is pooling at tip of condom, bathing penis in urine; reapply as necessary and avoid catheter obstruction.
- Assess need for another brand of external catheter (i.e., one that is self-adhesive).

Recording and Reporting

- Record condom application; condition of penis, skin, and scrotum; urinary output; and voiding pattern in nurses' notes in electronic health record (EHR) or chart.
- Report penile erythema, rashes, and/or skin breakdown.
- Document your evaluation of patient and family caregiver learning.

Special Considerations
Teaching

- Teach about signs of skin breakdown or trauma.
- Teach patient to keep condom and catheter kink free and positioned below level of bladder.
- Teach patient with leg bag to assess leg straps periodically for tightness and loosen as necessary.

Pediatric

- Use of condom catheters is uncommon in children. When used in adolescents, take precautions to minimize embarrassment.

Gerontological

- Evaluate patients with neuropathy carefully before applying a condom catheter. Patient may not feel sensation of pressure from condom device. Assess penile skin at more frequent intervals, at least twice daily.
- Condom catheters are not recommended in patients with prostatic obstruction.

Home Care

- Teach patient and family caregivers appropriate assessments such as signs and symptoms of UTI, signs of skin irritation, or poor-fitting catheter sheath.
- Loose-fitting clothing may be needed to accommodate the catheter and drainage system.
- Ensure that patient and family caregiver understand correct steps in applying the condom catheter. Manufacturers often supply patient educational materials.
- Teach patient or family caregiver to empty drainage bag frequently when one-half full to avoid unnecessary tension on the catheter that can lead to problems keeping the catheter intact.

◆ SKILL 34.5 Suprapubic Catheter Care

A suprapubic catheter is a urinary drainage tube inserted surgically into the bladder through the abdominal wall above the symphysis pubis (Fig. 34.7). The catheter may be sutured to the skin, secured with an adhesive material, or retained in the bladder with a fluid-filled balloon similar to an indwelling catheter.

Suprapubic catheters are placed when there is blockage of the urethra (e.g., enlarged prostate, urethral stricture, after urologic surgery) and when a long-term urethral catheter causes irritation or discomfort or interferes with sexual functioning.

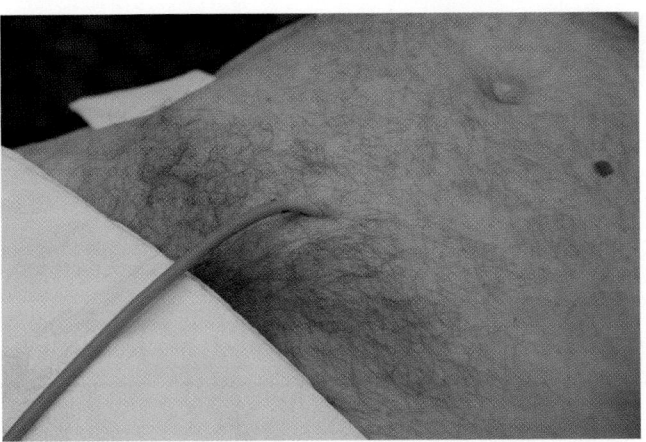

FIG 34.7 Suprapubic catheter without a dressing.

Delegation and Collaboration

The skill of caring for a newly established suprapubic catheter cannot be delegated to nursing assistive personnel (NAP); however,

care of an established suprapubic catheter may be delegated (refer to agency policy). The nurse directs the NAP to:

- Report patient's discomfort (bladder fullness, abdominal pain, skin irritation) related to the suprapubic catheter.
- Empty drainage bag and document urinary output on intake and output (I&O) record.
- Report any change in the amount and character of the urine.
- Report any signs of redness, foul odor, or drainage around catheter insertion site.

Equipment

- Clean gloves (sterile may be needed in some cases, see agency policy)
- Cleaning agent (sterile normal saline solution)
- Sterile cotton-tipped applicators
- Sterile surgical drainage gauze (split gauze)
- Sterile gauze dressing
- Washcloth, towel, soap, and water
- Tape
- Velcro tube holder or tube stabilizer (*optional*)

STEP	RATIONALE

ASSESSMENT

1. Identify patient using two identifiers (e.g., name and birthday or name and medical record number), according to agency policy.

Ensures correct patient. Complies with The Joint Commission standards and improves patient safety (2016).

2. Assess urine in drainage bag for amount, clarity, color, odor, and sediment.

Abnormal findings indicate potential complications such as urinary tract infection (UTI), decreased urinary output, and catheter occlusion.

3. Perform hand hygiene and apply clean gloves. Observe dressing for drainage and intactness.

Reduces transmission of infection. Drainage indicates potential complication such as infection. Dressing may become nonocclusive because of tape choice or drainage.

4. Assess catheter insertion site (may be deferred until you clean site) for signs of inflammation (i.e., pain, erythema, edema, and drainage) and for growth of overgranulation tissue. Ask patient if there is any pain at site; if so, have him or her rate on scale of 0 to 10. Remove gloves and perform hand hygiene.

If insertion is new, slight inflammation may be expected as part of normal wound healing but can also indicate infection. Overgranulation tissue can develop at insertion site as reaction to catheter. In some instances intervention may be needed (Geng et al., 2012). Reduces transmission of microorganisms.

5. Assess for elevated temperature and chills.

Increased temperature may indicate UTI or skin site infection.

6. Assess patient's knowledge of purpose of catheter and its care.

Determines level of instruction/support required.

7. Check for allergies.

Patient may be sensitive to tape, latex, or antiseptic solution.

NURSING DIAGNOSES

- Acute pain
- Deficient knowledge regarding catheter care
- Impaired skin integrity
- Impaired urinary elimination
- Risk for infection

Related factors/Risk factors are individualized based on patient's condition or needs.

PLANNING

1. Expected outcomes following completion of procedure:
   - Patient verbalizes no pain or discomfort at insertion site and over bladder.

   Patent catheter system keeps bladder empty and patient comfortable.

   - Urine output is 30 mL or greater per hour.

   Indicates that catheter is patent.

   - Urine remains clear without foul odor, and patient is afebrile.

   Indicates that patient is free of catheter-associated urinary tract infection (CAUTI).

STEP	RATIONALE

- Catheter exit site is free of infection (i.e., erythema, edema, drainage, tenderness). — Indicates absence of infection and irritation of skin.
- Patient and/or family caregiver can explain purpose of and methods for catheter care. — Evaluates learning.
2. Explain procedure to patient and/or family caregiver. — Reduces anxiety and promotes cooperation. Patients with suprapubic catheter frequently rely on family caregivers for support.

IMPLEMENTATION

1. Perform hand hygiene. — Reduces transmission of infection.
2. Provide privacy by closing room door and bedside curtain. — Promotes comfort and patient's self-esteem.
3. Raise bed to appropriate working height. If side rails are raised, lower side rail on working side. — Promotes use of good body mechanics.
4. Prepare supplies and open gauze packets in same manner as for applying dry dressing (see Chapter 41). — Keeps dressing sterile until application.
5. Apply clean gloves. Loosen tape and remove existing dressing. Note type and presence of drainage. Remove gloves and perform hand hygiene. — Provides baseline for condition of suprapubic wound. Reduces transmission of infection from dressing.
6. **Clean insertion site using sterile aseptic technique for newly established catheter:** Option is used less frequently; review agency policy or consider individual patient need. In some agencies, clean gloves are appropriate. — Catheter site is made surgically and therefore is treated similarly to other incisions as designated by agency policy. Confirm if using either medical aseptic or sterile technique is recommended.
   a. Apply sterile gloves.
   b. Without creating tension, hold catheter up with nondominant hand while cleaning. Use sterile gauze moistened in saline and clean skin around insertion site in circular motion, starting near insertion site and continuing in outward widening circles for approximately 5 cm (2 inches) (see illustration). — Moves from area of least contamination to area of most contamination. Tension on catheter may cause discomfort or damage to wall of bladder or catheter to slip out of place.
   c. With fresh, moistened gauze, gently clean base of catheter, moving up and away from site of insertion (proximal to distal). — Removes microorganisms that reside on any drainage that adheres to tubing.
   d. Once insertion site is dry, use sterile gloved hand to apply drain dressing (split gauze) around catheter (see illustration). Tape in place. — Collects drainage that develops around catheter insertion site.
7. **Clean long-term/established catheter:**
   a. Apply clean gloves.
   b. Without creating tension, hold catheter erect with nondominant hand while cleaning. Clean with soap and water in circular motion, starting near catheter insertion site and continuing in outward widening circles for approximately 5 cm (2 inches). — Cleaning and drying suprapubic insertion site requires general hygienic measures; dressing is option if drainage is not present.

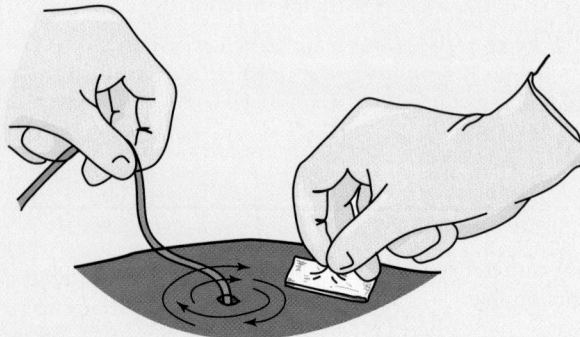

STEP 6b Clean around suprapubic catheter in circular pattern.

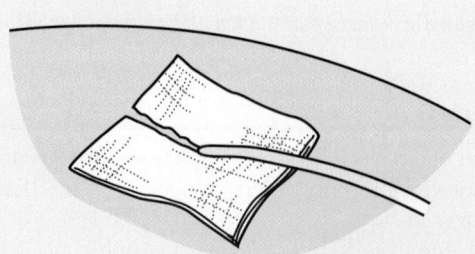

STEP 6d Split drain dressing for superpubic catheter.

STEP	RATIONALE
c. With a fresh washcloth or gauze, gently clean base of catheter, moving up and away from site of insertion (proximal to distal).	Removes microorganisms that reside in any drainage that adheres to tubing.
d. *Option:* Apply drain dressing (split gauze) around catheter and tape in place.	
8. Secure catheter to lateral abdomen with tape or Velcro multipurpose tube holder.	Secures catheter and reduces risk of excessive tension on suture and/or catheter.
9. Coil excess tubing on bed. Keep drainage bag below level of bladder at all times.	Maintains free flow of urine, thus decreasing risk for CAUTI (Gould et al., 2010).
10. Dispose of all contaminated supplies in appropriate receptacle, remove gloves, and perform hand hygiene.	Reduces transmission of microorganisms.

EVALUATION

1. Ask patient to rate pain or discomfort from suprapubic catheter on scale of 0 to 10.	Determines if bladder is draining and patient is free of infection.
2. Monitor for signs of infection (e.g., fever, elevated white blood count) and observe urine for clarity, sediment, unusual color, or odor.	Suprapubic catheters increase risk for UTI.
3. Observe catheter insertion site for erythema, edema, discharge, tenderness. Check dressing at minimum of every 8 hours.	Indicators of an insertion site infection.
4. Use Teach-Back: "I want to be sure I explained clearly about the care of your suprapubic catheter. Tell me about some of the things you need to do to care for it at home." Revise your instruction now or develop plan for revised patient or family caregiver teaching if patient or family caregiver is not able to teach back correctly.	Determines patient's and family caregiver's level of understanding of instructional topic.

Unexpected Outcomes	Related Interventions
1. Patient develops symptoms of UTI or catheter site infection.	• Increase fluid intake to at least 2200 mL in 24 hours (unless contraindicated).
	• Monitor vital signs, I&O; observe amount, color, consistency of urine; assess site.
	• Notify health care provider.
2. Suprapubic catheter becomes dislodged.	• Cover site with sterile dressing.
	• Notify health care provider. If newly established catheter, it will need to be reinserted immediately.
3. Skin surrounding catheter exit site becomes red or irritated and/or develops open areas.	• Notify health care provider.
	• Change dressing (if used) more frequently to keep site dry.
	• Consult with wound care nurse.

Recording and Reporting

- Record and report character of urine and type of dressing change, including assessments of insertion site and patient's comfort level with the catheter and dressing change in nurses' notes in electronic health record (EHR) or chart.
- Record urine output on I&O flow sheet. When there is both a suprapubic and urethral catheter, record outputs from each catheter separately.
- Document your evaluation of patient and family caregiver learning.
- Report any signs of UTI or insertion site infection to health care provider.

Special Considerations
Teaching

- If not contraindicated, encourage patients to consume a minimum of 2200 mL of fluids daily.

- Teach patient to keep the drainage bag lower than the bladder and to keep tubing free of kinks.

Home Care

- Teach patients and/or family caregivers how to clean and apply a dressing (if applicable) using clean technique.
- Caution patients and family caregivers about avoiding the use of powders or creams around the catheter unless specifically instructed to do so.
- Teach patients and family caregivers how to properly position the drainage bag; empty the urinary drainage bag; and observe urine color, clarity, odor, and amount.
- Arrange for home delivery of catheter supplies, always ensuring that there is at least one extra catheter and drainage bag in the home.
- Teach patient and family caregiver signs of catheter obstruction, UTI, and wound infection.

◆ CLINICAL DEBRIEF

You are caring for an 80-year-old woman of Middle Eastern heritage with a history of a stroke, type 2 diabetes mellitus, urinary retention, urinary incontinence, and recurrent urinary tract infections (UTIs). The health care provider has ordered measurement of postvoid residual (PVR) by either straight catheterization or bladder scan. There is also an order for an indwelling catheter if the PVR exceeds 400 mL. The patient's husband will not allow anyone to insert a catheter except her family.

1. Which assessments would be pertinent for this patient?
2. Explain why an assessment of PVR is important for this patient?
3. When measuring PVR, should the nurse use the bladder scanner, or should a straight catheterization be performed? Give the rationale for your answer.
4. Explain the teaching that would be appropriate when assessing PVR urine.
5. Using SBAR, show how you would communicate with the health care team about this patient.

◆ REVIEW QUESTIONS

1. Place the following steps for insertion of an indwelling catheter in a female patient in appropriate order.
   1. Insert and advance catheter.
   2. Lubricate catheter.
   3. Inflate catheter balloon.
   4. Clean urethral meatus with antiseptic.
   5. Drape patient with the sterile square and fenestrated drapes.
   6. When urine appears, advance another 2.5 to 5 cm (1 to 2 inches).
   7. Prepare sterile field and supplies.
   8. Gently pull catheter until resistance is felt.
   9. Attach drainage tubing.
2. The nurse is preparing to remove an indwelling urinary catheter. Which nursing interventions should the nurse implement? (Select all that apply.)
   1. Attaching a 3-mL syringe to the inflation port
   2. Allowing the balloon to drain into the syringe by gravity
   3. Initiating a voiding record/bladder diary
   4. Pulling catheter quickly
   5. Clamping the catheter before removal
3. Which nursing interventions are appropriate in the care of a patient with a newly inserted suprapubic catheter? (Select all that apply.)
   1. Using sterile technique, clean the skin close to the catheter with a circular motion.
   2. Wipe away any drainage on the catheter by wiping down the catheter toward the insertion site.
   3. Inspect the insertion site for erythema, edema, discharge, or tenderness.
   4. Secure the catheter to abdomen with tape or a tube-holder device.
   5. Apply upward tension to the catheter when cleaning the site and tubing.

ⓔ *Visit the Evolve site for a complete list of Clinical Debrief and Review Questions answers.*

REFERENCES

Beattie M, Taylor J: Silver alloy vs. uncoated urinary catheters: a systematic review of the literature, *J Clin Nurs* 20(15):2098, 2010.

Caterino JM, et al: Age, nursing home residence, and presentation of urinary tract infection in US emergency departments, 2001-2008, *Acad Emerg Med* 19(10):1173, 2012.

Cipa-Tatum J, et al: Urethral erosion: a case for prevention, *J Wound Ostomy Continence Nurs* 38(5):581, 2011.

Fekete T, et al: *Catheter-associated urinary tract infections in adults*, UpToDate, 2015. http://www.uptodate.com/contents/catheter-associated-urinary-tract-infection-in-adults. Accessed August 14, 2016.

Geng V, et al: *Catheterisation: indwelling catheters in adults: urethral and suprapubic*, European Association of Urology Nurses, 2012. https://www.guideline.gov/content.aspx?id=36631. Accessed August 14, 2016.

Gould CV, et al: Guideline for prevention of catheter-associated urinary tract infections 2009, *Infect Control Hosp Epidemiol* 31(4):319, 2010.

Hockenberry MJ, Wilson D: *Wong's nursing care of infants and children*, ed 11, St Louis, 2015, Mosby.

Huether SE, et al: *Understanding pathophysiology*, ed 6, St Louis, 2017, Elsevier.

Kyle G: The use of urinary sheaths in male incontinence, *Br J Nurs* 20(6):338, 2011.

Lewis SL, et al: *Medical-surgical nursing: assessment and management of clinical problems*, ed 10, St Louis, 2017, Elsevier.

Lo E, et al: Strategies to prevent catheter-associated urinary tract infections in acute care hospitals: 2014 update, *Infect Control Hosp Epidemiol* 35(5):464, 2014.

Meddings J, et al: Reducing unnecessary urinary catheter use and other strategies to prevent catheter-associated urinary tract infections: brief update review. In Agency for Healthcare Research and Quality (AHRQ), editor: *Making health care safer II: an updated critical analysis of the evidence for patient safety practices*, 2013. http://www.ahrq.gov/research/findings/evidence-based-reports/ptsafetyuptp.html. Accessed April 8, 2016.

Medline Plus: *Catheter related UTI, US National Library of Medicine*, 2016. https://medlineplus.gov/ency/article/000483.htm. Accessed August 15, 2016.

Méndez-Probst CE, et al: Fundamentals of instrumentation and urinary tract drainage. In Wein A, et al, editors: *Campbell-Walsh urology*, ed 10, Philadelphia, 2012, Saunders.

Muzzi-Bjornson L, Macera L: Preventing infection in elders with long-term indwelling urinary catheters, *J Am Acad Nurse Pract* 23:127, 2011.

Rowe TA, Manisha J: Urinary tract infection in older adults, *Aging Health* 9(5):10, 2013. http://www.ncbi.nlm.nih.gov/pmc/articles/PMC3878051/. Accessed August 14, 2016.

The Joint Commission (TJC): *2016 National Patient Safety Goals*, Oakbrook Terrace, IL, 2016, The Commission. http://www.jointcommission.org/standards_information/npsgs.aspx. Accessed April 8, 2016.

35 | Bowel Elimination and Gastric Intubation

OBJECTIVES

Mastery of content in this chapter will enable the nurse to:
- Describe factors that promote and impede normal bowel elimination.
- Discuss methods to relieve constipation or impaction.
- Describe precautions to follow when administering an enema.
- Describe approaches for managing a patient's comfort during nasogastric tube insertion.
- Perform the following skills: helping a patient use a bedpan, digitally removing stool, administering an enema, and inserting and removing a nasogastric tube.

MEDIA RESOURCES

- evolve http://evolve.elsevier.com/Perry/skills
- Review Questions
- ▶ Video Clips
- Case Studies
- Audio Glossary
- **NSO** Nursing Skills Online
- Clinical Debrief and Review Questions Answers

PURPOSE

Regular elimination of bowel waste products is essential for normal body functioning. Alterations of bowel elimination often indicate early signs, symptoms, or problems in the gastrointestinal (GI) system or other body systems (Costilla and Foxx-Orenstein, 2014). A patient's overall lifestyle patterns, food and fluid intake, medications, functional status, and chronic conditions influence bowel function. To manage a patient's bowel elimination problems you need to understand factors that promote, impede, or alter normal bowel elimination.

Patients may require your help to meet bowel elimination needs (e.g., using a bedpan). If a patient is constipated, you will likely administer enemas or digitally remove impacted stool. If severe diarrhea exists, a fecal management system (FMS) protects a patient's perianal skin and collects contaminated fecal waste (Sammon et al., 2015). When patients undergo abdominal surgery, or experience an alteration in GI peristalsis, a nasogastric (NG) tube is inserted for gastric decompression (Tho et al., 2011).

STANDARDS OF CARE

- Emergency Nurses Association, 2015—Clinical Practice Guideline, Gastric Tube Placement Verification
- The Joint Commission, 2016—Patient Identification
- Wound, Ostomy and Continence Nurses (WOCN) Society, 2016—Guideline for Prevention and Management of Pressure Ulcers (Injuries)
- National Pressure Ulcer Advisory Panel, 2016—Change in Terminology from Pressure Ulcer to Pressure Injury
- National Pressure Ulcer Advisory Panel, 2014—Prevention and Treatment of Pressure Ulcers: Clinical Practice Guidelines

PRINCIPLES OF PRACTICE

- Chronic constipation is a functional GI disorder and a condition frequently encountered in clinical practice (Box 35.1). Approximately 30% of people encounter constipation during their lifetime, with the older adult most affected (DeGiorgio et al., 2015).
- Opioid-induced constipation occurs frequently in the palliative care population. Opioids stimulate μ-opioid receptors, which induce analgesia. However, activation of these receptors reduces gastric emptying; increases pyloric, anal, and biliary sphincter tone; reduces biliary track secretions; and increases water absorption from the bowel. All of these factors reduce delayed intestinal transit time, and constipation occurs (Prichard and Bharucha, 2015).
- Constipation is also a complication of acute stroke; and, because of motor and/or sensory impairments, these patients need structured bowel-retraining programs to achieve bowel health (Lim and Childs, 2013).
- Patients with severe diarrhea may often require a Fecal Management System (FMS) to protect the perianal skin from

Common Causes of Constipation

- Irritable bowel syndrome: constipation predominant
- Chronic illnesses (e.g., Parkinson's disease, diabetes, connective tissue disorders, autoimmune disorders, hypothyroidism, pregnancy, depression, eating disorders (Costilla and Foxx-Orenstein, 2014)
- Low-fiber diet high in animal fats (e.g., meats, dairy products, eggs), refined sugars (rich desserts), and low fluid intake, which slow peristalsis (Ball et al., 2015; Touhy and Jett, 2014)
- Medications: Antihypertensives, anticonvulsants, antidepressants, antacids, iron supplements, opioid medications (Costilla and Foxx-Orenstein, 2014; Prichard and Bharucha, 2015)
- Laxative misuse (Burchum and Rosenthal, 2016)
- Older adults: Slowed peristalsis, loss of abdominal muscle elasticity, reduced intestinal mucus secretion, and often eating low-fiber foods (Ball et al., 2015; Touhy and Jett, 2014)
- Neurological conditions that block nerve impulses to the colon (e.g., spinal cord injury, tumor) (Lewis et al., 2017)
- Colonic action slowed by medications such as anticholinergics, antispasmodics, anticonvulsants, antidepressants, antihistamines, antihypertensives, antiparkinsonism drugs, bile acid sequestrants, diuretics, antacids, iron supplements, calcium supplements (Burchum and Rosenthal, 2016; Carrington et al., 2012)

breakdown, pressure injury formation, and fecal containment (Knowles et al., 2014; WOCN, 2016).

- Postoperative ileus and severe abdominal distention, with or without nausea and/or vomiting, is an indication of failure for the return of adequate bowel function. This causes patient discomfort, increases recovery time, and increases length of stay. When a postoperative ileus occurs, often an NG tube may need to be inserted (Sanfilippo and Spoletini, 2015).

PATIENT-CENTERED CARE

- Show respect for a patient's privacy, provide necessary comfort and hygiene measures, and attend to his or her emotional needs when performing required skills.
- When caring for patients with elimination issues from other cultural and ethnic groups, modify nursing interventions to meet their elimination needs. Provide for culturally sensitive hygiene needs. For example, hand hygiene can be practiced for hygienic reasons, ritual reasons during religious ceremonies, and symbolic reasons in specific everyday life situations (WHO, 2009).
- Determine patient's normal pattern of bowel elimination and accommodate that pattern while the patient is in a health care setting. Determine the time a patient normally has a bowel movement and the amount of help needed.
- Consider developmental changes that affect bowel functioning throughout the life span. For example, an older adult who becomes less active and has decreased muscle tone and changes in eating patterns is at higher risk for experiencing constipation (Huether and McCance, 2017).

EVIDENCE-BASED PRACTICE

- Research studies continue to investigate methods to correctly verify NG tube placement. This is crucial to avoid tube position complications. Radiographic verification of placement of tube immediately following insertion is the gold standard and provides a clear and measurable placement of the tube. Likewise, aspiration of gastric contents and pH measurement of pH ≤ 5

are used in subsequent verifications for tube placement (ENA, 2015; Tho et al., 2011).

- A study involving testing of a gastric pH electrode catheter (RightSpot) has shown it to be sensitive and specific for determination of intragastric pH (Lambert et al., 2013). The determination was found to be less than or greater than 4.5 as commonly used for nasogastric tubes. This catheter has the potential to provide health care providers with real-time assessment of pH to document NG tube placement and/or migration (Lambert et al., 2013).
- Pressure applied to the mucous membranes lining the GI tract can cause ischemia and medical device–related pressure injuries (MDRPIs) (NPUAP, 2012; Pittman et al., 2015). The resultant pressure injury generally conforms to the pattern or shape of the device (NPUAP, 2012).
  - NG and nasoenteral tubes can cause tissue necrosis, skin breakdown, and pressure on the intubated nares. NG tube fixation methods that remove pressure from the nares help to reduce the risk for MDRPI (NPUAP, 2012: Pittman et al., 2015; WOCN, 2016).
  - Indwelling FMSs are effective in protecting perianal skin from fecal enzyme irritation and subsequent breakdown. However, there is a risk for rectal mucosa necrosis and tearing secondary to the cuff, which is placed internally (Sammon et al., 2015; Whiteley and Sinclair, 2014).
- Methods to reduce MDRPI related to bowel elimination and gastric decompression include:
  - Conduct routine and ongoing assessment of nares and secondary pressure sites underlying medical devices and implement skin-care practices such a taping method to reduce risk for MDRPI (NPUAP, 2016b; Pittman et al., 2015; WOCN, 2016).
  - Frequently removing tape or fixation device to inspect underlying skin and provide skin care (Pittman et al., 2015).
  - Place thin foam or breathable dressings under medical devices (NPUAP, 2016b).
  - Positioning NG drainage tubing in such a manner as to not cause secondary pressure on the nares from the weight of the drainage tubing itself (NPUAP, 2012).
  - Verifying that immobile patient is not lying on drainage tubing.
  - For patients who have an FMS, routinely assessing anal and perianal areas for redness, blistering, edema, or breaks in skin integrity (Whiteley and Sinclair, 2014).

SAFETY GUIDELINES

- Promote comfort when a patient uses a bedpan. Encourage patient to use the bathroom when able.
- Answer the call light promptly to prevent a patient from attempting to get out of bed without help. This is a common factor related to patient falls.
- Patients with neurological sensory and/or motor deficits are prone to constipation. Place them on an individualized bowel training schedule and offer help with toileting at these intervals (Lim and Childs, 2013).
- Design and follow individualized bowel management protocols to reduce patient's risk for constipation and diarrhea secondary to the illness process, medications, and/or lack of activity (Knowles et al., 2014).
- When digital removal of impacted fecal material is ordered, obtain patient baseline vital signs and periodically monitor heart rate during the procedure. Digital removal of fecal impaction

stimulates the vagus nerve, which can cause a drop in heart rate (Ball et al., 2015; Solomons and Woodward, 2013).
- Follow agency policies to verify correct placement of NG tubes, which includes radiographic verification after insertion and subsequent pH verification, pH ≤5 (Tho et al., 2011).

- When a patient with an NG tube complains of nausea or vomits, assess both placement and patency of tube. Reposition and irrigate tube as needed (Tho et al., 2011).
- When handling fecal matter, always use standard precautions.

◆ SKILL 35.1 Providing a Bedpan

A patient restricted to bed must use a bedpan for bowel elimination. Two types of bedpans are available (Fig. 35.1). The regular and most commonly used bedpan has a curved, smooth upper end and a tapered lower end. The upper end (wide end) of the regular pan fits under a patient's buttocks toward the sacrum, with the lower end (tapered end) fitting just under the upper thighs toward the foot of the bed. A fracture pan, designed for patients with body or leg casts or those who are restricted from raising their hips (e.g., following total hip joint replacement), slips easily under a patient. The shallow upper end of the pan with a flat, wide rim fits under a patient's buttocks toward the sacrum, with the deep lower open end toward the foot of the bed.

Delegation and Collaboration

The skill of providing a bedpan can be delegated to nursing assistive personnel (NAP). The nurse instructs the NAP to:
- Correctly position patients with mobility restrictions or those who have therapeutic equipment such as wound drains, intravenous (IV) catheters, or traction.
- Provide perineal and hand hygiene for patient as necessary after using a bedpan.

Equipment

- Clean gloves
- Bedpan (regular or fracture) (see Fig. 35.1)
- Bedpan cover
- Toilet tissue
- Specimen container (if necessary); plastic bag clearly labeled with date, patient's name, and identification number
- Basin, washcloths, towels, and soap
- Waterproof, absorbent pads (if necessary)
- Clean drawsheet (if necessary)
- Stethoscope

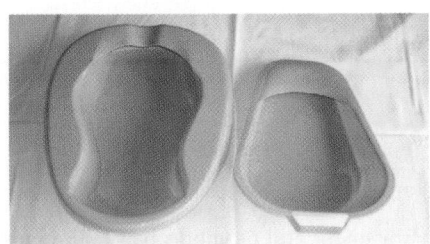

FIG 35.1 Types of bedpans. *Left*, Regular bedpan. *Right*, Fracture bedpan.

STEP	RATIONALE

ASSESSMENT

1. Assess patient's normal bowel elimination habits: routine pattern, character of stool, effect of certain foods/fluids and eating habits on bowel elimination, effect of stress and level of activity on normal bowel elimination patterns, current medications, and normal fluid intake.

Managing patient's elimination problems depends on thorough understanding of normal elimination and factors that create alterations. Peristalsis is strongest during the hour after first meal of the day. Anticipate when to offer bedpan.

2. Perform hand hygiene. Auscultate abdomen for bowel sounds and palpate lower abdomen for distention.

Normal bowel sounds occur irregularly at rate of 5 to 35 per minute. Presence of feces in colon, often mistaken for an abdominal mass, can be felt as a soft, rounded, boggy mass in the cecum and ascending, descending, or sigmoid colon (Ball et al., 2015).

3. Assess patient to determine level of mobility, including ability to sit upright and lift hips or turn.

Determines if patient can help in positioning on bedpan or if help is needed. Determines whether to use regular or fracture bedpan. Older adults, obese patients, patients who have had hip or knee surgery or spinal injury, and debilitated patients often require assistance of two or more nurses to help them onto or off bedpan.

4. Assess patient's level of comfort. Ask about presence of rectal or abdominal pain, presence of hemorrhoids, or irritation of skin surrounding anus.

Pain limits patient's ability to help with positioning. Rectal or abdominal pain reduces patient's ability to bear down during defecation.

5. Apply clean gloves. Inspect condition of perianal and perineal skin. Remove gloves and perform hand hygiene.

Repeated diarrhea can cause perineal and perianal skin irritation and skin breakdown (Sammon et al., 2015).

6. Determine need for stool specimen.

Provides opportunity to obtain specimen container before placing patient on bedpan.

STEP	RATIONALE

NURSING DIAGNOSES

- Acute pain
- Bowel incontinence
- Chronic pain
- Diarrhea

- Impaired physical mobility
- Perceived constipation
- Risk for constipation
- Chronic functional constipation

- Toileting self-care deficit
- Risk for frail elderly syndrome

Related factors/Risk factors are individualized based on patient's condition or needs.

PLANNING

STEP	RATIONALE
1. Expected outcomes following completion of procedure:	
• Perianal skin is clean and intact.	Hygiene technique after defecation keeps perianal skin clear of fecal secretions.
• Patient eliminates without pain or discomfort.	Patient is positioned comfortably on bedpan.
2. Explain procedure to patient, including self-help tips (e.g., how to use a trapeze, how to move hips).	Promotes independence, reduces anxiety, and helps patient to assist during procedure.
3. Obtain help from additional nursing personnel as warranted.	Adequate personnel resources minimize muscle strain for you and patient. Reduces patient's discomfort.

IMPLEMENTATION

STEP	RATIONALE
1. Perform hand hygiene.	Reduces transmission of microorganisms.

Clinical Decision Point *Use a fracture pan if the patient had a total hip replacement. An abduction pillow must be placed between the legs when turning to prevent dislocation of new joint.*

STEP	RATIONALE
2. Provide privacy by closing curtains around bed or door of room.	Reduces embarrassment and promotes bowel elimination.
3. Raise side rail on opposite side of bed.	Protects patient from falling out of bed. Patient can grasp side rail to move about in bed and onto bedpan.
4. Raise bed horizontally according to your height.	Promotes use of good body mechanics and minimizes muscle strain for you and patient.
5. Have patient assume supine position.	Position eases eventual pan placement.

Clinical Decision Point *Observe for the presence of drains, dressings, IV fluids, and traction. These devices make it difficult for a patient to help with positioning, and you will likely need more personnel to help place him or her on a bedpan.*

STEP	RATIONALE
6. Place patient who can help on bedpan.	
a. Apply clean gloves. Raise head of patient's bed 30 to 60 degrees.	Prevents hyperextension of back and provides support to upper torso when patient raises hips. Sitting position promotes defecation.
b. Remove upper bed linens so they are out of the way but do not expose patient.	Prevents embarrassment to patient; demonstrates respect for patient's sense of dignity (Touhy and Jett, 2014).
c. Have patient flex knees and lift hips upward.	If legs, upper torso, and arms are supporting body weight, little effort should be required of patient.
d. Place your hand that is closest to patient's head palm up under patient's sacrum to help lift. Ask patient to bend knees and raise hips. As patient raises hips, use other hand to slip bedpan under him or her (see illustrations). Be sure that open rim of bedpan is facing toward foot of bed. Do not force pan under patient's hips. (*Optional:* Have patient use overhead trapeze frame to raise hips.)	Positions bedpan high under buttocks so feces enters pan. Incorrect placement of bedpan causes discomfort for patient and spillage of contents. If legs, upper torso, and arms are supporting body weight, little effort should be required of patient. Forcing bedpan under patient increases risk for friction injury to underlying skin and tissues.
e. *Optional:* If using fracture pan, slip it under patient as hips are raised (see illustration). Be sure that deep, open, lower end of bedpan is facing toward foot of bed.	Patient requires less maneuvering and does not have to lift hips.

STEP	RATIONALE

7. Place patient who is immobile or has mobility restrictions on bedpan.

   a. Apply clean gloves. Lower head of bed flat or raise head slightly (if tolerated by medical condition).

Helps patient who cannot lift hips, who must remain flat, or who medically is not permitted to lift hips to roll onto bedpan.

   b. Remove top linens as necessary to turn patient while minimizing exposure.

Prevents embarrassment to patient; demonstrates respect for patient's sense of dignity.

   c. Help patient roll onto side with back toward you. Place bedpan firmly against patient's buttocks and down into mattress. Be sure that open rim of bedpan is facing toward foot of bed (see illustrations).

Incorrect placement causes discomfort to patient and spillage of contents.

Clinical Decision Point *If patient has had total hip replacement, use a fracture pan; make sure that abduction pillow remains between the patient's legs while he or she is transferring to and from and using the fracture pan.*

   d. Keep one hand against bedpan; place other around far hip of patient. Ask patient to roll back onto bedpan, flat in bed. Do not force pan under patient.

Using minimal exertion, this places patient squarely on pan. Avoid forcing bedpan under patient to decrease risk for friction injury to underlying skin and tissues.

   e. Raise patient's head 30 degrees or to a comfortable level (unless contraindicated).

Patient assumes sitting position unless condition necessitates maintaining flat position.

   f. Have patient bend knees (unless contraindicated).

Relieves stress on back.

8. Maintain patient's comfort, privacy, and safety. Cover patient for warmth. Place small pillow or rolled towel under lumbar curve of back. Leave room but stay close by.

Provides added comfort. Pain reduces or eliminates urge to defecate, which will result in bowel elimination problems.

9. Have call bell and toilet tissue within reach for patient.

Promotes safety by preventing patient from reaching over edge of bed for objects out of reach.

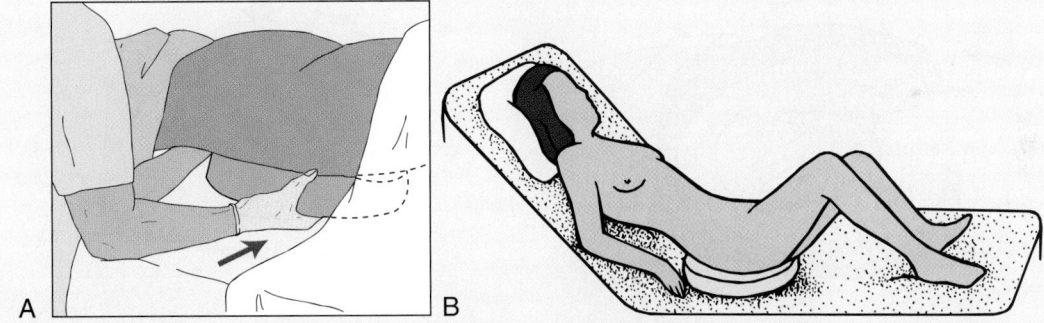

STEP 6d A, Placing bedpan under patient's hips. **B,** Correct positioning for placing mobile patient on bedpan.

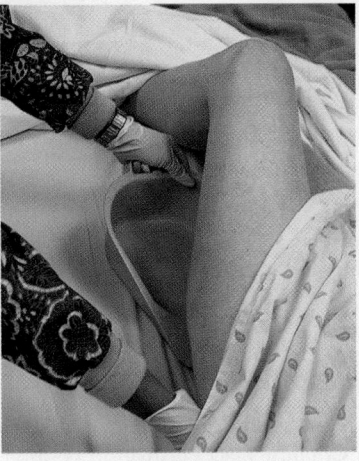

STEP 6e Patient lifts hips as fracture pan is positioned.

STEP	RATIONALE
10. Ensure that bed is in lowest position and raise upper side rails.	Promotes patient safety and enables patient to reposition pan as needed.
11. Remove and discard gloves and perform hand hygiene.	Reduces transmission of microorganisms.
12. Allow patient to be alone but monitor status and respond promptly.	Reassures patient. Removing bedpan in timely manner prevents pressure injuries.
13. Perform hand hygiene and apply clean gloves.	Reduces transmission of microorganisms.
14. **Remove bedpan:**	
a. Place patient's bedside chair close to working side of bed.	Provides area to place bedpan and contents on chair after removal from patient to prevent accidental spilling of full bedpan on bed surface.
b. Maintain privacy; determine if patient is able to wipe own perineal area. If you clean perineal area, apply clean gloves and use several layers of toilet tissue or disposable washcloths. For female patients clean from mons pubis toward rectal area.	Maintains respect for privacy. Cleans from clean to dirty area of perineum.
c. Deposit contaminated tissue in bedpan if no specimen or intake and output (I&O) is needed. Remove gloves and perform hand hygiene.	Toilet tissue contaminates specimen and affects accurate output measurement.
d. For mobile patient: Apply clean gloves. Ask patient to flex knees, placing body weight on lower legs, feet, and upper torso; lift buttocks up from bedpan. At same time place hand farthest from patient on side of bedpan to support it (prevent spillage) and place other hand (closest to patient) under sacrum to help lift. Have patient lift and remove bedpan. Place bedpan on draped bedside chair and cover.	Avoids pulling or forcing pan from under hips because this action pulls skin and causes tissue injury.

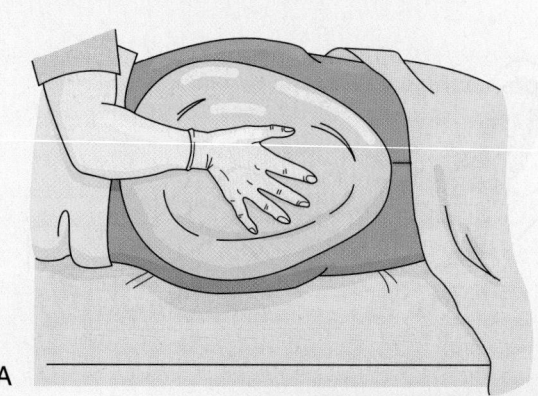
A

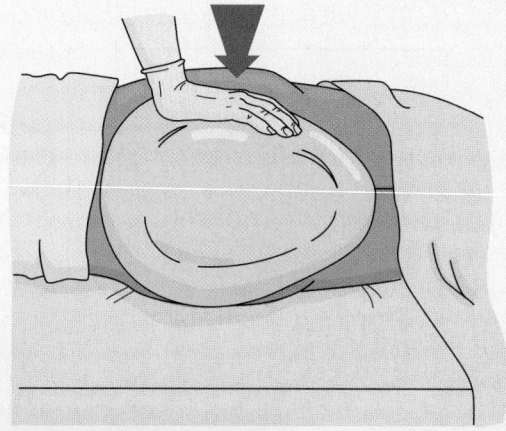
B

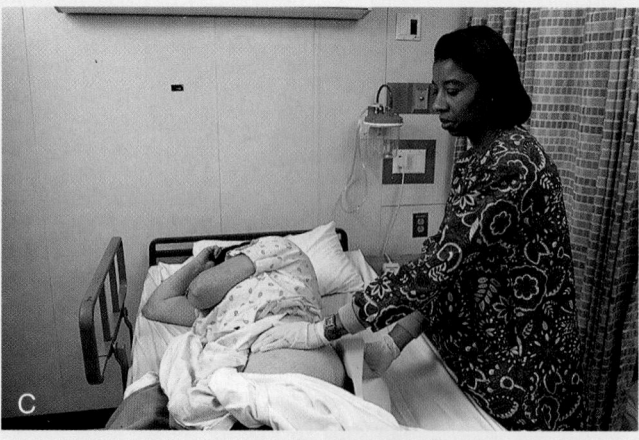
C

STEP 7c A, Position patient on one side and place bedpan firmly against buttocks. **B,** Push down on bedpan and toward patient. **C,** Nurse places bedpan in position. (*A and B from Sorrentino SA: Mosby's textbook for nursing assistants, ed 7, St Louis, 2009, Mosby.*)

STEP	RATIONALE
e. For immobile patient: Apply clean gloves. Lower head of bed. Help patient roll onto side away from you and off bedpan. Hold bedpan flat and steady while patient is rolling off; otherwise spillage will occur. Place bedpan on draped bedside chair and cover.	Reduces spread of microorganisms. Reduces spread of offensive odors.
15. Allow patient to perform hand hygiene. Change soiled linens, remove and dispose of gloves, and return patient to comfortable position.	Reduces chance of skin breakdown when bedridden patient lies on dry, wrinkle-free linens.
16. Place bed in its lowest position. Ensure that call bell, phone, drinking water, and desired personal items (e.g., books) are within easy access.	Promotes comfort and reduces risk for injury to patient. Patients often fall when reaching for items.
17. *Option:* Obtain stool specimen as ordered (see Skill 7.2). Wear clean gloves when emptying contents of bedpan into toilet or in special receptacle in utility room. Use spray faucet attached to most institution toilets to rinse bedpan thoroughly. Use disinfectant if required by agency; store pan. Remove gloves.	If bedpan becomes very soiled, replace with clean one.
18. Perform hand hygiene.	Reduces transmission of microorganisms.

EVALUATION

1. Assess characteristics of stool. Note color, odor, consistency, frequency, amount, shape (see Fig. 35.2), and constituents. Assess characteristics of urine if patient voided in bedpan.	Helps to identify significant changes or findings.
2. Evaluate patient's ability to use bedpan.	Provides continual assessment of patient's self-toileting ability.
3. Inspect patient's perianal area and surrounding skin while removing bedpan.	Liquid stool predisposes patient to skin breakdown (Sammon et al., 2015).
4. **Use Teach-Back:** "Since your leg is immobilized, I want to make sure you're comfortable getting off and on the bedpan by using the trapeze to pull your torso off the bed. Show me how you will position your arms on the trapeze." Revise your instruction now or develop a plan for revised patient or family caregiver teaching if patient or family caregiver is not able to teach back correctly.	Determines patient's and family caregiver's level of understanding of instructional topic.

Unexpected Outcomes	**Related Interventions**
1. Patient is unable to successfully use bedpan.	• If patient's mobility allows, obtain order for use of bedside commode.
2. Patient is incontinent of stool. Avoid use of adult briefs for bedridden patient.	• Establish regular schedule of offering bedpan. Adult briefs mask toileting needs and may potentiate skin breakdown called *incontinence-associated dermatitis (IAD)* (Sammon et al., 2015). • Discuss with staff need to answer patient's request for toileting help promptly and use toileting schedule. • Administer perianal skin care using moisture barrier.
3. Patient develops irritation and breakdown of skin around perianal area.	• Reassess perianal skin with each bowel movement and each position change.

Recording and Reporting

- Record the type of help needed and if patient tolerates getting on/off bedpan, character and amount of stool, and urine output if patient also voids on flow sheet or in nurses' notes in electronic health record (EHR) or chart.
- Document your evaluation of patient and family caregiver learning.
- Complete laboratory requisition if you collected stool or urine specimen and send to laboratory. Record the type of specimen sent.

Special Considerations
Pediatric

- Constipation in early childhood results from environmental changes such as being hospitalized and reluctance to use a bedpan. Toilet-trained children often regress during hospitalization (Hockenberry and Wilson, 2015).
- Repeated withholding of stool leads to stretching or dilating of the rectum and decreases the sensation or "urge" to defecate (Hockenberry and Wilson, 2015).

Gerontological

- Older adults have some loss of sphincter control and often require a quick response when requesting a bedpan (Ball et al., 2015).
- Incidence of constipation is greater because there is impaired rectal sensation to defecate. As a result, the older adult does not perceive the need to defecate.

- With increased age transit time through the bowel increases, causing a normal lengthening of the time between bowel movements (Ball et al., 2015).

◆ SKILL 35.2 **Removing Fecal Impaction Digitally**

Fecal impaction is the inability to pass a collection of hard stool. This condition occurs in all age-groups. Physically and mentally incapacitated individuals and institutionalized older adults are at greatest risk. Patients with acute stroke and spinal cord injuries are also at greater risk for fecal impaction (Lim and Childs, 2013; Solomons and Woodward, 2013).

Functional constipation is defined as including two or more of the following factors for at least 3 months: (1) straining with defecation at least one fourth of the time, (2) lumpy or hard stools (or both) one fourth of the time (Fig. 35.2), (3) sensation of anorectal blockage at least one fourth of the time, (4) loose stools rarely present without the use of laxatives, or (5) three or fewer bowel movements in a week (Costilla and Foxx-Orenstein, 2014; Wald, 2015).

Symptoms of fecal impaction include constipation, rectal discomfort, anorexia, nausea, vomiting, abdominal pain, abdominal bloating, diarrhea (leaking around the impacted stool), and urinary frequency (Ness, 2013). Prevention is the key to managing fecal impaction. With newer bowel management techniques such as transanal irrigation, digital removal of fecal material is not needed (Ness, 2013). However, once impaction occurs, digital removal of stool is the only alternative.

Delegation and Collaboration

The skill of removing a fecal impaction digitally cannot be delegated to nursing assistive personnel (NAP). The nurse instructs the NAP to:

- Help the nurse position a patient for the procedure. Monitor heart rate as nurse removes impaction.
- Observe the stool for color, consistency, rectal bleeding, or bloody mucus and report immediately to the nurse.
- Provide perineal care following each bowel movement.

Equipment

- Clean gloves
- Water-soluble local anesthetic lubricant (**NOTE:** Some agencies require use of water-soluble lubricant without anesthetic)

- Waterproof, absorbent pads
- Bedpan
- Bedpan cover (optional)
- Bath blanket
- Basin, washcloths, towels, and soap
- Vital sign equipment
- Stethoscope

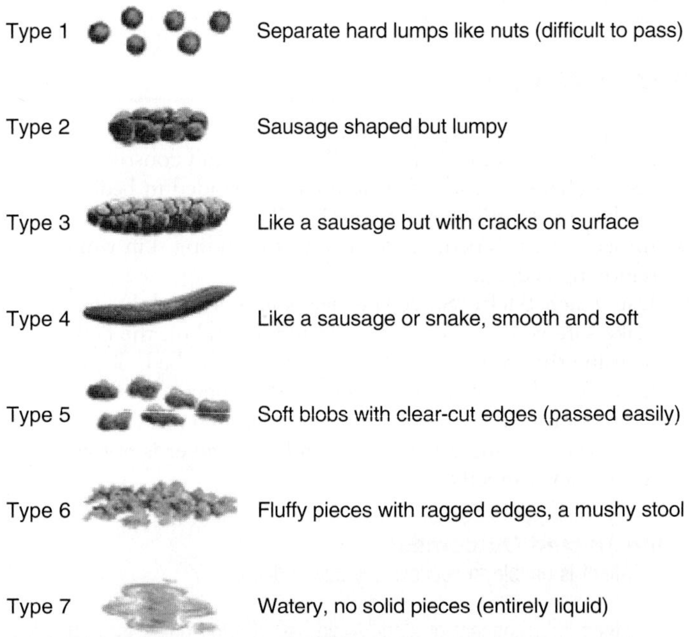

Type 1   Separate hard lumps like nuts (difficult to pass)

Type 2   Sausage shaped but lumpy

Type 3   Like a sausage but with cracks on surface

Type 4   Like a sausage or snake, smooth and soft

Type 5   Soft blobs with clear-cut edges (passed easily)

Type 6   Fluffy pieces with ragged edges, a mushy stool

Type 7   Watery, no solid pieces (entirely liquid)

FIG 35.2 Bristol stool form scale. (*From O'Donnell LJ, Virjee J, Heaton KW: Detection of pseudodiarrhoea by simple clinical assessment of intestinal transit rate, Br Med J 300:439, ©1990. Reprinted with permission of the BMJ Publishing Group.*)

STEP	RATIONALE

ASSESSMENT

1. Identify patient using at least two identifiers (e.g., name and birthday or name and medical record number) according to agency policy.

   Ensures correct patient. Complies with The Joint Commission standards and improves patient safety (TJC, 2016).

2. Ask patient about normal and current bowel elimination pattern, including frequency and characteristics of stool; use of laxatives, enemas, and other medications; level of exercise; urge to defecate but inability to do so; feelings of incomplete emptying; and sensations of bloating, cramping, and excessive gas.

   Information provides data in determining contributing factors and preventive measures. Large fecal mass causes rectal distention and increases perception of urge to evacuate rectum (DeGiorgio et al., 2015).

STEP	RATIONALE
3. Inspect patient's abdomen for distention.	Observation identifies distended or asymmetrical areas, which are then investigated on auscultation or palpation. Distention contributes to constipation.
4. Auscultate all four quadrants for presence of bowel sounds.	Hypoactive bowel sounds may result from partial obstruction of the gastrointestinal (GI) tract (Ball et al., 2015).
5. Palpate patient's abdomen for distention, discomfort, or masses.	Symptoms are related to accumulation of stool in intestinal tract. Palpable mass may be felt with severe constipation (Ball et al., 2015).
6. Measure patient's current vital signs and comfort level on a pain scale of 0 to 10.	Provides baseline measurement. Sacral branch of vagus nerve is stimulated during digital stimulation; this stimulation results in reflex slowing of heart rate (Ball et al., 2015).

> **Clinical Decision Point** *Because of the potential to stimulate the sacral branch of the vagus nerve, patients with a history of dysrhythmias or heart disease have a greater risk for changes in heart rhythm. Monitor patient's pulse before and during procedure. This procedure is often contraindicated in cardiac patients; if in doubt, verify with the health care provider.*

STEP	RATIONALE
7. If patient has a spinal cord injury (SCI), review his or her routine for digital removal of stool; and, if this is part of the patient's routine bowel care, it is essential not to interrupt the routine (Ness, 2013).	Level of SCI and severity of injury affect pattern of constipation. Injuries to cervicothoracic vertebrae increase frequency of constipation. In these patients, digital removal of stool is a routine intervention for bowel health and should not be interrupted (Solomons and Woodward, 2013).
8. Perform hand hygiene and apply clean gloves. Observe consistency of stool (see Fig. 35.2), seepage of liquid stool, or continued passage of small amounts of hard stool. Observe anal area for signs of irritation or hemorrhoids. Remove gloves and perform hand hygiene.	Seepage of stool is symptomatic of an impaction high in colon. Patient may be able to pass small pieces of hard stool or liquid fecal material around impacted mass (Wald, 2015). Leakage of fecal contents causes skin irritation and increases risk for pressure injury formation (Sammon et al., 2015).
9. Determine if patient is receiving anticoagulant therapy or has a past history of rectal surgery.	Procedure may be contraindicated. Manipulation of rectum can cause bleeding, which is prolonged with anticoagulants (Burchum and Rosenthal, 2016).
10. Check patient's record for health care provider's order for digital removal of impaction and use of anesthetic lubricant.	Obtain written order before performing procedure because this procedure involves excessive stimulation of vagus nerve.

NURSING DIAGNOSES

- Acute pain
- Chronic functional constipation
- Diarrhea

Related factors are individualized based on patient's condition or needs.

PLANNING

1. Expected outcomes following completion of procedure:	
• Impacted stool is removed successfully.	Indicates that rectum is clear of stool.
• Patient is free of abdominal or rectal discomfort.	Fecal impaction causes direct pain to rectum and indirect abdominal discomfort through abdominal distention (Ness, 2013).
• Vital signs remain within patient's baseline.	Indicates absence of vagal stimulation.
2. Explain procedure to patient.	Information reduces anxiety and encourages patient participation in therapeutic elimination protocol.
3. Perform hand hygiene. Arrange supplies at bedside.	Ensures access to supplies during procedure.

IMPLEMENTATION

1. Obtain help to change patient's position if necessary. Raise bed horizontally to comfortable working height.	Promotes patient safety and use of good body mechanics.
2. Pull curtains around bed or close door to room.	Maintains patient's sense of privacy and prevents unnecessary exposure of body parts.
3. Lower side rail on patient's right side. Keeping far side rail raised, help patient to left side-lying position with knees flexed and back.	Promotes patient safety. Provides access to rectum. Side-lying position promotes rectal sphincter relaxation.

STEP	RATIONALE
4. Drape patient's trunk and lower extremities with bath blanket and place waterproof pad under patient's buttocks.	Maintains patient's sense of privacy and prevents unnecessary exposure of body parts.
5. Perform hand hygiene, apply clean gloves, and place bedpan next to patient.	
6. Lubricate gloved index finger and middle finger of dominant hand with anesthetic lubricant.	Prevents transmission of microorganisms. Reduces discomfort and permits smooth insertion of finger into anus and rectum.
7. Instruct patient to take slow deep breaths during procedure. Gradually and gently insert gloved index finger and feel anus relax around finger. Insert middle finger.	Slow deep breaths help to relax patient. Gradual insertion of index finger helps to dilate anal sphincter.
8. Gradually advance fingers slowly along rectal wall toward umbilicus.	Guiding finger toward rectal wall follows natural direction of colon, allowing for access to impacted stool high in rectum (Ness, 2013).
9. Gently loosen fecal mass by moving fingers in scissors motion to fragment fecal mass. Work fingers into hardened mass.	Loosening and penetrating mass allows for removal of stool in small pieces, resulting in less discomfort to patient.
10. Work stool downward toward end of rectum. Remove small sections of feces and discard into bedpan.	Prevents need to force finger up into rectum and minimizes trauma to mucosa.
11. Observe patient's response and periodically assess heart rate and look for signs of fatigue.	Vagal stimulation slows heart rate and causes dysrhythmias. Procedure often exhausts patient.

Clinical Decision Point *Stop procedure if heart rate drops or rhythm changes from patient's baseline or if patient has dyspnea or complaints of palpitations.*

STEP	RATIONALE
12. Continue to clear rectum of feces and allow patient to rest at intervals.	Rest improves patient's tolerance of procedure, allowing heart rate to return to normal.
13. After removal of impaction, perform perineal hygiene (see Procedural Guideline 18.1).	Promotes patient's sense of comfort and cleanliness.
14. Remove bedpan and inspect feces for color and consistency. Dispose of feces in toilet.	Reduces transmission of microorganisms.
15. If needed, help patient to toilet or clean and store bedpan. (Procedure may be followed by enema or cathartic.)	Removal of impaction stimulates defecation reflex.
16. Remove gloves by turning them inside out and discarding in proper receptacle. Perform hand hygiene.	Reduces transmission of microorganisms.

EVALUATION

1. Apply clean gloves, perform rectal examination for stool, and observe anal and perianal area for irritation or skin breakdown. Remove and dispose of gloves; perform hand hygiene.	Determines if rectum is clear. Fecal material, especially diarrhea, causes irritation to perianal tissues (Sammon et al., 2015).
2. Reassess vital signs and compare to baseline value. Continue to monitor patient for 1 hour for bradycardia.	Determines extent of vagal stimulation.
3. Auscultate bowel sounds.	Determines presence of peristaltic activity.
4. Palpate abdomen to determine if it is soft and nontender.	Discomfort is relieved.
5. **Use Teach-Back:** "I want to make sure you include the high-fiber foods and fluids that we recommended for your diet to help increase the passage of stool. Tell me which foods you will add to your diet." Revise your instruction now or develop a plan for revised patient or family caregiver teaching if patient or family caregiver is not able to teach back correctly.	Determines patient's and family caregiver's level of understanding of instructional topic.

Unexpected Outcomes	Related Interventions
1. Patient experiences trauma to rectal mucosa as evidenced by rectal bleeding.	• Assess anal and perianal region for source of bleeding. • Stop procedure if bleeding is excessive and notify health care provider.
2. Patient experiences bradycardia (heart rate <60 per minute), decrease in blood pressure, and decrease in level of consciousness as result of vagus nerve stimulation.	• Stop procedure and measure vital signs. • Notify health care provider and remain with patient.
3. Patient has seepage of liquid stool after procedure complete.	• Assess patient for continuing impaction. • Notify health care provider for possible suppository or enema. • Increase patient's fluid intake and dietary fiber.

Recording and Reporting

- Record patient's tolerance to procedure, amount and consistency of stool removed, vital signs, and adverse effects on flow sheet or in nurses' notes in electronic health record (EHR) or chart.
- Record patient's and family caregiver's understanding through teach-back about the types of high-fiber foods to reduce the frequency of constipation.
- Report any changes in vital signs and adverse effects to health care provider.

Special Considerations

Pediatric

- Do not digitally remove stool in a pediatric patient because of the risk for anal fissures and pain that trigger stool withholding (Hockenberry and Wilson, 2015).

- Dietary changes with high fiber, increased fluid intake, and absorbable and nonabsorbable carbohydrates (e.g., sorbitol in prune, pear, and apple juices) can help alleviate constipation in children (Nurko and Zimmerman, 2014).

Gerontological

- Many older adults are especially prone to dysrhythmias and other problems related to vagal stimulation; monitor heart rate and rhythm closely (Ball et al., 2015).
- For older adults, instituting a diet adequate in dietary fiber (6 to 10 g per day) adds bulk, weight, and form to stool and improves defecation (DeGiorgio et al., 2015).
- Laxative use for chronic constipation in older adults must be individualized to patient's cardiac and renal co-morbidities, drug interactions, and side effects (DeGiorgio et al., 2015).

◆ SKILL 35.3   Administering an Enema

NSO *Nursing Skills Online Bowel Elimination/Ostomy Care Module / Lesson 2* 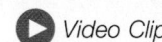 *Video Clip*

An enema is the instillation of a solution into the rectum and sigmoid colon to promote defecation by stimulating peristalsis. Typically enemas treat constipation or empty the bowel before diagnostic procedures or certain types of abdominal surgery. The volume or type of fluid that breaks up the fecal mass stretches the rectal wall and initiates the defecation reflex. Table 35.1 summarizes common types of enemas.

Cleansing enemas promote complete evacuation of feces from the colon. They act by stimulating peristalsis through infusion of large volumes of solution. Oil-retention enemas act by lubricating the rectum and colon, allowing feces to absorb oil and become softer and easier to pass.

Medicated enemas contain pharmacological therapeutic agents. Some are prescribed to reduce dangerously high serum potassium levels (e.g., sodium polystyrene sulfonate enema) or to reduce bacteria in the colon before bowel surgery (e.g., neomycin enema).

Delegation and Collaboration

The skill of administering an enema can be delegated to nursing assistive personnel (NAP). **NOTE:** If a medicated enema is ordered, then it must be administered by a nurse. The nurse instructs the NAP about:

- How to properly position patients who have mobility restrictions or therapeutic equipment such as drains, intravenous (IV) catheters, or traction.
- Informing the nurse immediately about patient's new abdominal pain (*exception:* a patient reports cramping) or rectal bleeding.
- Informing the nurse immediately about the presence of blood in the stool or around the rectal area or any change in vital signs.

Equipment

- Clean gloves
- Water-soluble lubricant

TABLE 35.1

Types of Enemas

Type of Enema	Description and Implications
Tap-water (hypotonic) enema	Do not repeat after first installation because water toxicity or circulatory overload can develop.
Physiological normal saline	Safest enema to administer. Infants and children can tolerate only this type because of their predisposition to fluid imbalance.
Hypertonic solution (e.g., commercially prepared Fleet enema)	Useful for patients who cannot tolerate large volumes of fluid.
Harris flush enema	A return-flow enema that helps to expel intestinal gas. Administer small amount (100–200 mL) of enema solution into patient's rectum and colon. Lower the enema container to allow the total volume of solution to flow back. The repeated back-and-forth administration and return of the fluid reduces flatus and promotes return of peristalsis.
Soapsuds enema (SSE)	Pure castile soap added to either tap water or normal saline. Use only pure castile soap. Recommended ratio of pure soap to solution is 5 mL (1 teaspoon) to 1000 mL (1 quart) warm water or saline. Add soap to enema bag after water is in place to reduce excessive suds.
Oil-retention enema	Oil-based solution. The colon absorbs a small volume, which softens stool for easier evacuation.
Carminative solution	Relieves gaseous distention. Example: MGW solution, which contains 30 mL of magnesium, 60 mL of glycerin, and 90 mL of water.

- Waterproof, absorbent pads
- Toilet tissue
- Bedpan, bedside commode, or access to toilet
- Bath blanket
- Basin, washcloths, towel, and soap
- Stethoscope

Enema Bag Administration
- Enema container with tubing and clamp (Fig. 35.3)
- IV pole

- Appropriate-size rectal tube (adult: 22 to 30 Fr; child: 12 to 18 Fr)
- Correct volume of warmed (tepid) solution (adult: 750–1000 mL; adolescent: 500–700 mL). For pediatric patients the weight of the child usually determines the volume for the enema, usually 5–10 mL/kg (Nurko and Zimmerman, 2014).

Prepackaged Enema
- Prepackaged enema container with lubricated rectal tip (Fig. 35.4)

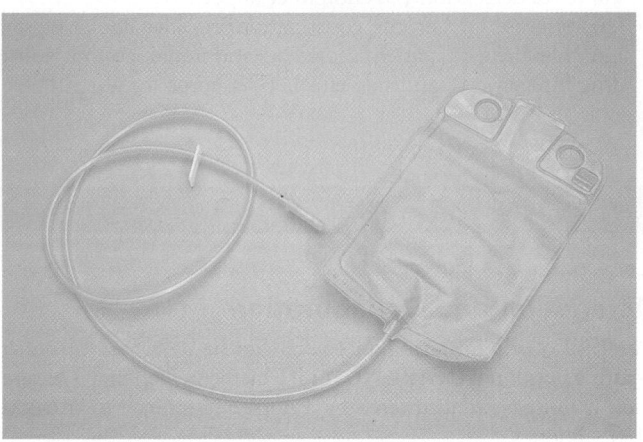

FIG 35.3 Enema bag with tubing.

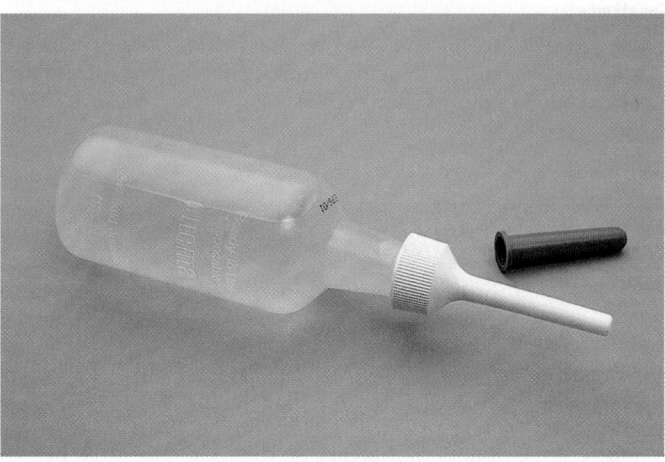

FIG 35.4 Prepackaged enema container with rectal tip and cap.

STEP	RATIONALE

ASSESSMENT

1. Identify patient using at least two identifiers (e.g., name and birthday or name and medical record number) according to agency policy).
   Ensures correct patient. Complies with The Joint Commission standards and improves patient safety (TJC, 2016).

2. Review health care provider's order for enema and clarify reason for administration.
   Order by health care provider is usually required for hospitalized patient. Order states which type of enema patient will receive.

3. Assess last bowel movement, normal versus most recent bowel pattern, presence of hemorrhoids, and presence of abdominal pain or cramping.
   Determines need for enema and type of enema used. Also establishes baseline for bowel function. Hemorrhoids may obscure rectal opening and cause discomfort or bleeding during evacuation.

4. Assess patient's mobility and ability to turn and position on side.
   Determines if assistance is needed for positioning patient.

5. Inspect abdomen for presence of distention and auscultate for bowel sounds.
   Establishes baseline for determining effectiveness of enema.

6. Assess patient for allergy to any active ingredients of Fleet enema.
   Reduces risk for allergic reaction.

7. Determine patient's level of understanding of purpose of enema.
   Allows for planning appropriate teaching measures.

Clinical Decision Point *"Enemas until clear" order means that you repeat enemas until patient passes fluid that is clear of fecal matter. The fluid the patient passes may also be tinted and have small flecks of fecal matter. Check agency policy, but usually patient should receive only three consecutive enemas to avoid disruption of fluid and electrolyte balance. It is essential to observe contents of solution passed.*

NURSING DIAGNOSES

- Acute pain
- Constipation
- Risk for constipation
- Chronic functional constipation

Related factors/Risk factors are individualized based on patient's condition or needs.

STEP	RATIONALE

PLANNING

1. Expected outcomes following completion of procedure:
   - Stool is evacuated.
   - Enema return is clear.
   - Abdomen is flat, nontender, with no distention.

2. Perform hand hygiene. Arrange supplies at bedside.

Solution clears rectum and lower colon of stool.
Indicates that all solid fecal material in colon has passed.
Gas and feces are expelled.
Ensures access to supplies during procedure.

IMPLEMENTATION

1. If enema is medicated, the skill may or may not be delegated to a NAP (see agency policy). Check accuracy and completeness of each medication administration record (MAR) with health care provider's written order. Check patient's name, type of enema, and time for administration. Compare MAR with label of enema solution.

The order is most reliable source and only legal record of drugs or procedure that patient is to receive. Ensures that patient receives correct enema.

2. Provide privacy by closing curtains around bed or closing door.

Reduces embarrassment for patient.

3. Place bedpan or bedside commode in easily accessible position. If patient will be expelling contents in toilet, ensure that toilet is available and place patient's nonskid slippers and bathrobe in easily accessible position.

Bedpan is used if patient is unable to get out of bed. Nonskid slippers help prevent patient who may be rushing to bathroom from falling. Extra gown provides modesty for patient.

4. Perform hand hygiene.

Reduces transmission of microorganisms.

5. With side rail raised on patient's right side and bed raised to appropriate working height, help patient turn onto left side-lying (Sims') position with right knee flexed. Encourage patient to remain in position until procedure is complete. Place a child in the dorsal recumbent position.

Allows enema solution to flow downward by gravity along natural curve of sigmoid colon and rectum, thus improving retention of solution.

Clinical Decision Point *Patients with poor sphincter control require placement of a bedpan under the buttocks. Administering enema with patient sitting on toilet is unsafe because curved rectal tubing can abrade rectal wall.*

6. Apply clean gloves and place waterproof pad, absorbent side up, under hips and buttocks. Cover patient with bath blanket, exposing only rectal area, clearly visualizing anus.

Pad prevents soiling of linen. Blanket provides warmth, reduces exposure of body parts, and allows patient to feel more relaxed and comfortable.

7. Separate buttocks and examine perianal region for abnormalities, including hemorrhoids, anal fissure, and rectal prolapse.

Findings influence approach for inserting enema tip. Prolapse contraindicates enema.

8. Administer enema.
   a. Administer prepackaged disposable enema:
   (1) Remove plastic cap from tip of container. Tip may already be lubricated. Apply more water-soluble lubricant as needed.

   Lubrication provides for smooth insertion of rectal tube without causing rectal irritation or trauma. With presence of hemorrhoids, extra lubricant provides added comfort.

   (2) Gently separate buttocks and locate anus. Instruct patient to relax by breathing out slowly through mouth.

   Breathing out promotes relaxation of external rectal sphincter.

   (3) Expel any air from enema container.

   Introducing air into colon causes further distention and discomfort.

   (4) Insert lubricated tip of container gently into anal canal toward umbilicus (see illustration).
   Adult: 7.5–10 cm (3–4 inches)
   Adolescent: 7.5 cm–10 cm (3–4 inches)
   Child: 5–7.5 cm (2–3 inches)
   Infant: 2.5–3.75 cm (1–1½ inches)

   Gentle insertion prevents trauma to rectal mucosa.

Clinical Decision Point *If pain occurs or you feel resistance at any time during procedure, stop and discuss with health care provider. Do not force insertion.*

STEP	RATIONALE

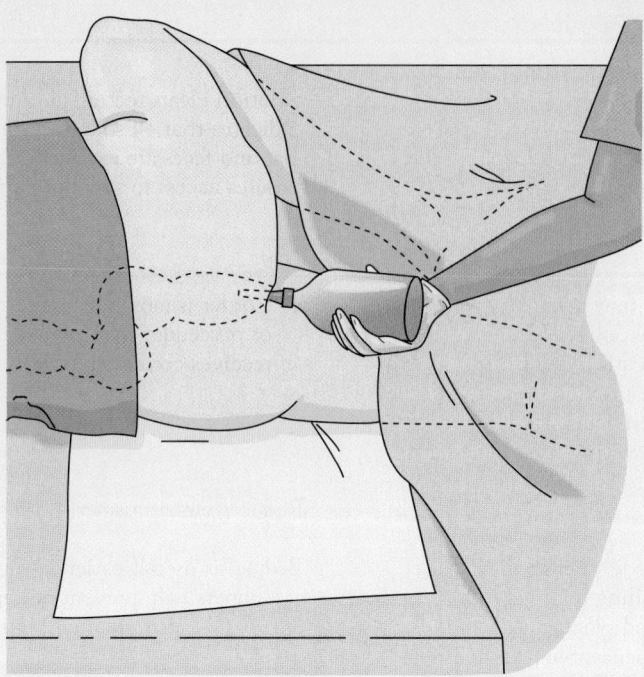

STEP 8a(4) With patient in left lateral Sims' position, insert tip of commercial enema into rectum. (*From Sorrentino SA: Mosby's textbook for nursing assistants, ed 7, St Louis, 2009, Mosby.*)

STEP	RATIONALE
(5) Roll plastic bottle from bottom to tip until all of solution has entered rectum and colon. Instruct patient to retain solution until urge to defecate occurs, usually 2 to 5 minutes.	Prevents instillation of air into colon and ensures that all content enters rectum. Hypertonic solutions require only small volumes to stimulate defecation.
b. Administer enema in standard enema bag:	
(1) Add warmed prescribed type of solution and amount to enema bag. Warm tap water as it flows from faucet. Place saline container in basin of warm water before adding saline to enema bag. Check temperature of solution by pouring small amount of solution over inner wrist.	Hot water burns intestinal mucosa. Cold water causes abdominal cramping and is difficult to retain.
(2) If soapsuds enema (SSE) is ordered, add castile soap after water.	Reduces suds in enema bag.
(3) Raise container, release clamp, and allow solution to flow long enough to fill tubing.	Removes air from tubing.
(4) Reclamp tubing.	Prevents further loss of solution.
(5) Lubricate 6–8 cm (2½–3 inches) of tip of rectal tube with lubricant.	Allows smooth insertion of rectal tube without risk for irritation or trauma to mucosa.
(6) Gently separate buttocks and locate anus. Instruct patient to relax by breathing out slowly through mouth. Touch patient's skin next to anus with tip of rectal tube.	Breathing out and touching skin with tube promotes relaxation of external anal sphincter.
(7) Insert tip of rectal tube slowly by pointing it in direction of patient's umbilicus. Length of insertion varies (see Step 8a[4]).	Careful insertion prevents trauma to rectal mucosa from accidental lodging of tube against rectal wall. Insertion beyond proper limit can cause bowel perforation.

Clinical Decision Point *If tube does not pass easily, do not force. Consider allowing a small amount of fluid to infuse and then try to reinsert the tube slowly. The instillation of fluid relaxes the sphincter and provides additional lubrication. If impaction is present, remove it (see Skill 35.2) before administering the enema.*

STEP	RATIONALE
(8) Hold tubing in rectum constantly until end of fluid instillation.	Prevents expulsion of rectal tube during bowel contractions.

STEP	RATIONALE
(9) Open regulating clamp and allow solution to enter slowly with container at patient's hip level.	Rapid infusion stimulates evacuation of tubing and can cause cramping.
(10) Raise height of enema container slowly to appropriate level above anus: 30–45 cm (12–18 inches) for high enema; 30 cm (12 inches) for regular enema (see illustration); 7.5 cm (3 inches) for low enema. Instillation time varies with volume of solution administered (e.g., 1 L may take 10 minutes). You may use an IV pole to hold an enema bag once you establish a slow flow of fluid.	Allows for continuous, slow instillation of solution. Raising container too high causes rapid instillation and possible painful distention of colon. High pressure causes rupture of bowel in infant.

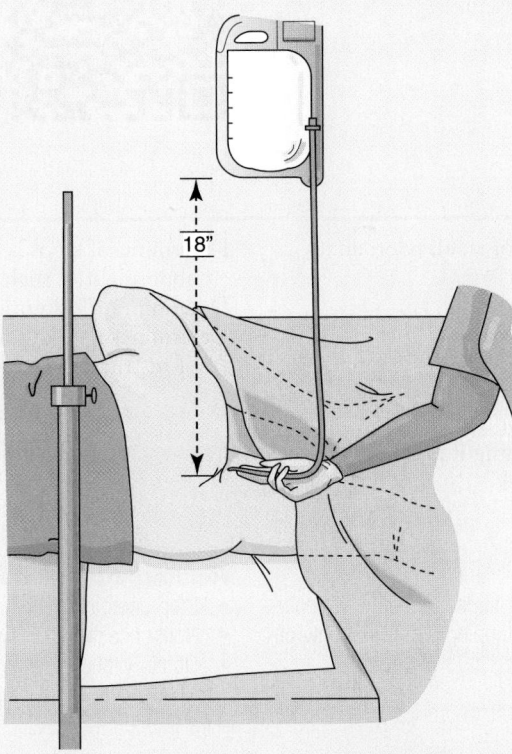

STEP 8b(10) IV pole is positioned so bottom of enema bag is 45 cm (18 inches) above anus. (*From Sorrentino SA: Mosby's textbook for nursing assistants, ed 7, St Louis, 2009, Mosby.*)

Clinical Decision Point *Temporary cessation of infusion minimizes cramping and promotes ability to retain solution. Lower container or clamp tubing if patient complains of cramping or if fluid escapes around rectal tube.*

(11) Instill all solution and clamp tubing. Tell patient that procedure is completed and that you will remove tubing.	Prevents entrance of air into rectum. Patients may misinterpret sensation of removing tube as loss of control.
9. Place layers of toilet tissue around tube at anus and gently withdraw rectal tube and tip.	Provides for patient's comfort and cleanliness.
10. Explain to patient that some distention and abdominal cramping are normal. Ask him or her to retain solution as long as possible until urge to defecate occurs. This usually takes a few minutes. Stay at bedside. Have patient lie quietly in bed if possible. (For infant or young child gently hold buttocks together for few minutes.)	Solution distends bowel. Length of retention varies with type of enema and patient's ability to contract rectal sphincter. Longer retention promotes stimulation of peristalsis and defecation.
11. Discard enema container or disposable bag and tubing in proper receptacle. Remove gloves and perform hand hygiene.	Reduces transmission and growth of microorganisms.

STEP	RATIONALE
12. Help patient to bathroom or commode if possible. If using bedpan, apply clean gloves and help patient to as near a normal position for evacuation as possible (see Skill 35.1).	Normal squatting position promotes defecation.
13. Observe character of stool and solution (caution patient against flushing toilet before inspection).	Determines if enema was effective.
14. Help patient as needed to wash anal area with warm soap and water (use gloves for perineal care).	Fecal contents irritate skin. Hygiene promotes patient's comfort.
15. Remove and discard gloves and perform hand hygiene.	Reduces transmission of microorganisms.

EVALUATION

1. Inspect color, consistency, and amount of stool; odor; and fluid passed.
2. Assess for abdominal distention.
3. **Use Teach-Back:** "I want to be sure I explained clearly how to position yourself in bed if you need to administer a Fleet enema to yourself. Explain to me how you would position yourself." Revise your instruction now or develop a plan for revised patient or family caregiver teaching if patient or family caregiver is not able to teach back correctly.

Determines if stool is evacuated or fluid is retained. Note abnormalities such as presence of blood or mucus.
Determines if distention is relieved.
Determines patient's and family caregiver's level of understanding of instructional topic.

Unexpected Outcomes	Related Interventions
1. Severe abdominal cramping, bleeding, or sudden abdominal pain develops and is unrelieved by temporarily stopping or slowing flow of solution.	• Stop enema. • Notify health care provider. • Obtain vital signs.
2. Patient is unable to hold enema solution.	• If this occurs during installation, slow rate of infusion.

Recording and Reporting

• Record the type and volume of enema given, time of administration, characteristics of results, and patient's tolerance of the procedure on flow sheet or in nurses' notes in electronic health record (EHR) or chart.
• Record patient's and family caregiver's understanding through teach-back for self-administration of a Fleet enema in nurses' notes in EHR or chart.
• Report the failure of patient to defecate and any adverse effects to health care provider.

Special Considerations
Pediatric

• The use of oral stool softeners is the initial recommended treatment of constipation in children (Nurko and Zimmerman, 2014).

• Children and infants usually do not receive prepackaged hypertonic enemas because hypertonic solutions cause rapid fluid shift (Hockenberry and Wilson, 2015).

Gerontological

• Caution is necessary when enemas are ordered "until clear" in older adults. Some older adults become tired, are at risk for fluid and electrolyte imbalances, and experience changes in vital signs (Touhy and Jett, 2014).
• Some older adults may have difficulty retaining fluid. The nurse may gently hold buttocks together to help with retention of fluid (DeGiorgio et al., 2015).

Home Care

• Assess patient's and family caregiver's ability and motivation to administer enema and provide instruction as needed.

PROCEDURAL GUIDELINE 35.1 *Applying a Fecal Management System*

A fecal management system (FMS) protects the perineum from fecal enzymes and prevents feces from spreading to wounds (Cooper, 2013; Whiteley and Sinclair, 2014). In addition, the FMS is useful for patients with severe fecal incontinence such as those with *Clostridium difficile*–associated diarrhea. FMS systems are latex-free, indwelling rectal catheters, with a low-pressure balloon to hold the catheter in place in the rectum and a soft, flexible drainage tubing attached to a containment device. These systems have an irrigation port to maintain patency of the catheter and promote fecal drainage. Risks associated with use of this indwelling device include rectal necrosis, loss of rectal tone, pressure injury, or fistula formation (Sammon et al., 2015; Whiteley and Sinclair, 2014). Consultation with a health care provider is recommended to discuss options for patients; certain situations contraindicate the use of a FMS (Box 35.2).

Delegation and Collaboration

The skill of applying a topical (external) fecal containment device cannot be delegated to nursing assistive personnel (NAP). The NAP can assist the nurse by helping to position a patient during device application. The nurse instructs the NAP to:
- Report to the nurse any instances of leakage or change in appearance of skin around device noted during routine care.
- Report to the nurse immediately any increase in patient's rectal pain or sensation of pressure or rectal bleeding.

Equipment

FMS, also called fecal containment device (FCD) kit (Fig. 35.5).
- Clean gloves
- Protective bed pad
- Bath basin

Procedural Steps

1. Identify patient using at least two identifiers (e.g., name and birthday or name and medical record number) according to agency policy (TJC, 2016).
2. Review medical record for contraindications for use of an FMS (see Box 35.2).
3. Assess for frequency and amount of diarrhea over the last 24–48 hours.
4. Assess patient for allergy to silicone. Note that these devices are latex free (Whiteley and Sinclair, 2014).

5. Perform hand hygiene and apply clean gloves. Perform perineal hygiene; and observe patient's anal region for swelling, hemorrhoids, redness, irritation, or drainage. Presence of these findings may contraindicate placement of the device or may indicate need for other interventions to the perianal skin.
6. Change gloves and perform digital rectal examination to ensure that there is no rectal impaction. Remove and discard gloves.
7. Perform hand hygiene and apply new clean gloves.
8. Apply the FMS.
   a. Prepare system by connecting collection bag to catheter tube assembly.
   b. Deflate cuff, usually done with 60-mL syringe supplied in the kit.
   c. Fill 60-mL syringe with 45 mL of tap water and attach syringe to inflation port. *DO NOT* inflate at this time. Inflation port is color coded.
   d. Position patient in left knee-chest position. This position helps to maximize sphincter relaxation.
   e. Place protective bedpad under patient's dependent hip.
   f. Fold cuff according to manufacturer directions and lubricate cuff. Note that folded cuff should be the size of your index finger.
   g. Generously lubricate anal sphincter.
   h. Gently separate patient's buttocks (NAP can assist), exposing perianal area for entire procedure. Make sure that perianal area is clean and dry. It may be necessary to perform perineal hygiene again.
   i. Insert cuff using index finger as a guide. Once the cuff is in the rectal vault, it will open to its original shape.
      (1) Inflate cuff with 45 mL water by slowly depressing syringe plunger; the cuff will inflate. *Use the pilot balloon as a guide: If the balloon indicates overinflation or underinflation, withdraw all fluid from the cuff, reposition it in the rectal vault, and reinflate.*
      (2) Remove syringe from injection port and gently pull on the catheter to ensure that cuff seats against rectal floor.

BOX 35.2

Contraindications for Use of Fecal Management Systems

- Suspected or confirmed anal pathology
- Pediatric population
- Existing poor anal sphincter
- Anorectal stricture or stenosis
- Anorectal surgery
- Colorectal surgery in the preceding 12 months
- Severe hemorrhoids
- Rectal tumor
- Fecal impaction
- Allergy or sensitivity to silicone
- Inflammatory processes of the rectum: Crohn's disease, radiation proctitis
- Anticoagulated patients

From Whiteley, I, Sinclair G: Faecal management systems for disabling incontinence or wounds: literature review, *Br J Nurs* 23(16):881, 2014.

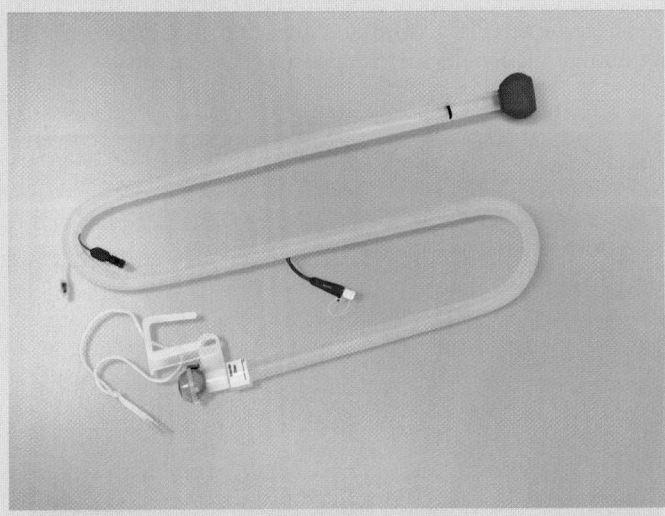

FIG 35.5 DIGNICARE® Stool Management System. (*Copyright © 2016 C.R. Bard, Inc. Used with permission.*)

Continued

PROCEDURAL GUIDELINE 35.1 *Applying a Fecal Management System*—cont'd

j. Note position of indicator line in relation to patient's anus. Changes in indicator line position may indicate need for cuff to be repositioned. Remove gloves and perform hand hygiene.

9. Irrigate cuff as needed: Fill syringe with 45 mL of tap water and attach to clear irrigation port. Observe flow; but, if leakage occurs, cuff may need repositioning (see manufacturer instructions).

Clinical Decision Point *If the catheter tubing is obstructed with fecal contents, irrigate the catheter. Attach a filled syringe to the FLUSH port and irrigate. Ensure that the flush port remains parallel to the catheter to prevent kinking.*

10. If stool sampling is needed, use sample port (see Fig. 35.5). Apply clean gloves, open sample port, and either tilt or milk catheter tubing to collect sample or insert a slip-tip catheter to withdraw fecal material. Close sample port when finished. Remove gloves and perform hand hygiene.

11. Replace collection bag as needed. Perform hand hygiene and apply clean gloves.
  a. Disconnect drainage tubing from collection bag.
  b. If necessary, attach bag plug into collection bag hub.
  c. Connect new bag to tubing.
  d. Dispose of fecal contents per agency policy. Remove gloves and perform hand hygiene.

12. Remove FMS. Perform hand hygiene and apply clean gloves.
  a. Attached depressed syringe 60 mL to cuff infusion port and slowly withdraw all water.
  b. Once cuff is deflated, grasp catheter as close to patient as possible and slowly slide out of anus.
  c. Dispose of FMS according to agency policy, remove gloves, and perform hand hygiene.

13. Position patient in comfortable position and perform any hygiene as needed.

14. Monitor patient for diarrhea and record amounts on intake and output (I&O) record every shift.

15. Record application of device and appearance of skin in nurses' notes in electronic health record (EHR) or chart.

◆ SKILL 35.4 **Insertion, Maintenance, and Removal of a Nasogastric Tube for Gastric Decompression**

There are times following major surgery or with conditions affecting the gastrointestinal (GI) tract when normal peristalsis is altered temporarily. Because peristalsis is slowed or absent, a patient cannot eat or drink fluids without causing abdominal distention. The temporary insertion of a nasogastric (NG) tube into the stomach serves to decompress the stomach, keeping it empty until normal peristalsis returns.

An NG tube is a hollow, pliable tube inserted through a patient's nasopharynx into the stomach. It allows for the removal of gastric secretions and the introduction of solutions into the stomach. Sometimes an NG tube is used for enteral feedings, but a softer small-bore feeding tube is preferred for feeding purposes (see Chapter 32). The Levin and Salem sump tubes are the most common for stomach decompression. The Levin tube is a single-lumen tube with holes near the tip (Fig. 35.6). You connect it to a drainage bag or an intermittent suction device to drain stomach secretions.

The Salem sump tube is preferable for stomach decompression. The tube has two lumens: one for removal of gastric *contents* and one to provide an air vent, which prevents suctioning of gastric mucosa into eyelets at the distal tip of a tube. A blue "pigtail" is the air vent that connects with the second lumen (Fig. 35.7). When the main lumen of the sump tube is connected to suction, the air vent permits free, continuous drainage of secretions. ***Never clamp off the air vent, connect to suction, or use for irrigation.***

Insertion of an NG tube is uncomfortable, with patients experiencing a burning sensation as the tube passes through the sensitive nasal mucosa. Following tube insertion, keep patient comfortable and observe skin around his or her nares because the tube is a constant irritation to mucosa and has the potential to cause a medical device–related pressure injury (MDRPI). Prevention of MDRPI is critical. You need to routinely assess the condition

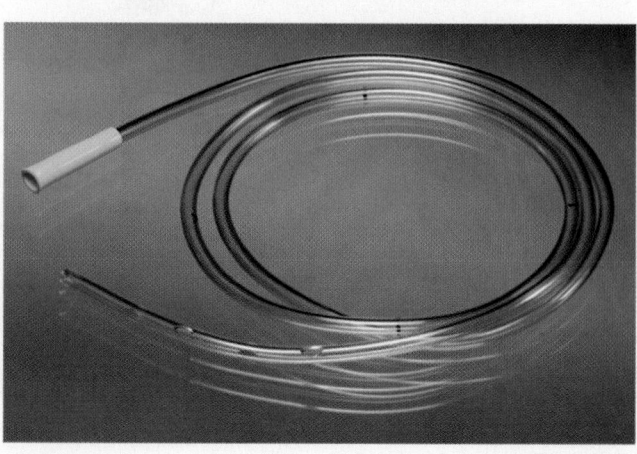

FIG 35.6 Levin tube. (*Courtesy Bard Medical, Covington, GA.*)

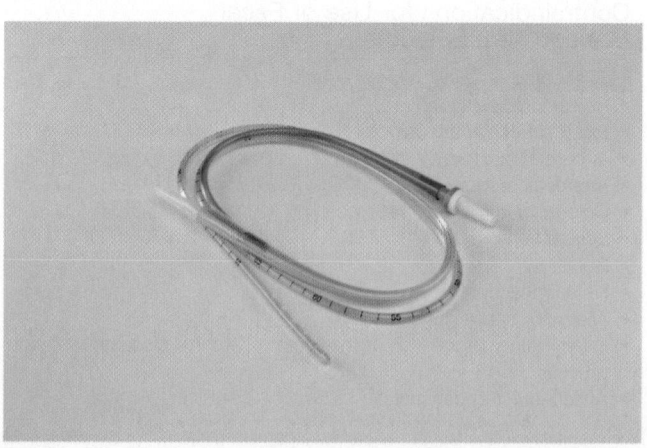

FIG 35.7 Salem sump tube. (*Courtesy Covidien, Mansfield, MA.*)

of the nares and mucosa for inflammation, blistering, and excoriation (Pittman et al., 2015).

Delegation and Collaboration

The skill of inserting and maintaining an NG tube cannot be delegated to nursing assistive personnel (NAP). The nurse instructs the NAP to:

- Measure and record the drainage from an NG tube.
- Provide oral and nasal hygiene measures.
- Perform selected comfort measures such as positioning or offering ice chips if allowed.
- Anchor the tube to patient's gown during routine care to prevent accidental displacement.
- Immediately report to the nurse any signs of redness or irritation to nares.

Equipment

- 14- or 16-Fr NG tube (Smaller-lumen catheters are not used for decompression in adults because they must be able to remove thick secretions.) (*Option:* A dual-purpose tube, one that is used for both gastric decompression and enteral feedings, may be ordered for selected patients.)

- Water-soluble lubricant
- pH test strips (measure gastric aspirate acidity); use paper with a range of at least 1.0–11.0 or higher
- Tongue blade
- Flashlight
- Emesis basin
- Asepto bulb or catheter-tipped syringe
- 2.5-cm (1-inch) wide hypoallergenic tape or commercial fixation device
- Safety pin and rubber band
- Clamp, drainage bag, or suction machine with pressure gauge if wall suction is to be used
- Towel
- Glass of water with straw
- Facial tissues
- Normal saline
- Tincture of benzoin (*optional*)
- Suction equipment
- Stethoscope
- Clean gloves

STEP	RATIONALE

ASSESSMENT

STEP	RATIONALE
1. Identify patient using at least two identifiers (e.g., name and birthday or name and medical record number) according to agency policy.	Ensures correct patient. Complies with The Joint Commission standards and improves patient safety (TJC, 2016).
2. Perform hand hygiene (apply clean gloves if risk of body fluid exposure). Inspect condition of patient's nares and nasal and oral cavity.	Documents if skin on nares is intact or irritated before NG tube insertion. Determines need for special nursing hygiene measures after tube placement.
3. Ask if patient has history of nasal surgery or congestion and allergies and note if deviated nasal septum is present.	Alerts nurse to potential obstruction. Insert tube into *uninvolved* nasal passage. Procedure may be contraindicated if surgery is recent.
4. Auscultate for bowel sounds. Palpate patient's abdomen for distention, pain, and rigidity. Remove and discard gloves if applied and perform hand hygiene.	In presence of diminished or absent bowel sounds, auscultate abdomen at least 1 minute in each quadrant (Ball et al., 2015). Documents baseline for any abdominal distention, gastrointestinal (GI) ileus, and general GI function, which later serves as comparison once tube is inserted.
5. Assess patient's level of consciousness and ability to follow instructions.	Determines patient's ability to help in procedure.

Clinical Decision Point *If patient is confused, disoriented, or unable to follow commands, get help from another staff member to insert the tube.*

STEP	RATIONALE
6. Determine if patient had previous NG tube and, if so, which naris was used.	Patient's previous experience complements any explanations and prepares patient for NG tube placement.
7. Verify health care provider order for type of NG tube to be placed and whether tube is to be attached to suction or drainage bag.	Requires order from health care provider. Adequate decompression depends on NG suction.

NURSING DIAGNOSES

- Acute pain
- Deficient knowledge regarding purpose of gastric decompression
- Dysfunctional gastrointestinal motility
- Impaired oral mucous membrane
- Risk for impaired skin integrity

Related factors/Risk factors are individualized based on patient's condition or needs.

STEP	RATIONALE

PLANNING

1. Expected outcomes following completion of procedure:
  - Abdomen is soft, nontender, and without distension.

  - Nares and nasal mucosa remain intact, clear, without abrasions or excoriation.
  - Patient's level of comfort improves or remains the same.

Correctly positioned NG tube remains patent, drains gastric secretions, and relieves gastric distention.
Ensures absence of irritation or pressure injury formation from NG tube.
Correctly inserted NG tube prevents abdominal discomfort from progressing.

2. Inform patient that procedure may make him or her gag and there will be a burning sensation in nasopharynx as tube is passed. Develop hand signal with patient.

Increases patient's cooperation and ability to anticipate nurse's action. If patient is unable to tolerate procedure, use of hand signal will alert nurse.

3. Perform hand hygiene and arrange supplies at bedside.

Ensures access to supplies during procedure.

IMPLEMENTATION

1. Position patient upright in high-Fowler's position unless contraindicated. If patient is comatose, raise head of bed as tolerated in semi-Fowler's position with head tipped forward, chin to chest.

Promotes patient's ability to swallow during procedure. Good body mechanics prevent injury to you or patient.

2. Place bath towel over patient's chest; give facial tissues to patient. Allow to blow nose if necessary. Place emesis basin within reach.

Prevents soiling of patient's gown. Tube insertion through nasal passages may cause tearing and coughing with increased salivation.

3. Pull curtain around bed or close room door.

Provides privacy.

4. Wash bridge of nose with soap and water or alcohol swab. Dry thoroughly.

Removes oils from nose to allow fixation devices to adhere completely.

5. Stand on patient's right side if right-handed, left side if left-handed. Lower side rail.

Allows easiest manipulation of tubing.

6. Instruct patient to relax and breathe normally while occluding one naris. Then repeat this action for other naris. Select nostril with greater airflow.

Tube passes more easily through naris that is more patent.

7. Measure distance from tip of patient's nose to earlobe to xiphoid process of sternum (see illustration).

Length approximates distance from nose to stomach. The NEX (nose-earlobe-xiphoid) method is commonly used in clinical settings.

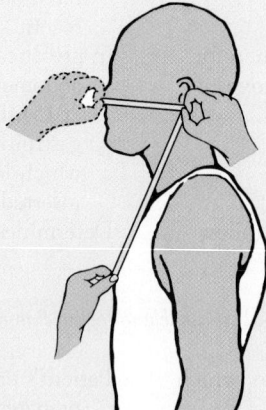

STEP 7 Determine length of tube to be inserted.

8. With small piece of tape placed around tube, mark length that will be inserted.

Indicates length of tube you will insert.

9. Prepare materials for tube fixation. Tear off a 7.5–10 cm (3–4 inch) length of hypoallergenic tape or open membrane dressing or other fixation device (see Step 24a[2]).

Fixation devices allow tube to float free of nares, thus reducing pressure on nares and preventing MDRPIs (Pittman et al., 2015).

10. Perform hand hygiene and apply clean gloves.

Reduces transmission of infection.

11. Apply pulse oximetry/capnography device and measure vital signs. Monitor oximetry/capnography during insertion.

Provides objective assessment of respiratory status before and during tube insertion.

STEP	RATIONALE
12. *Option:* Dip tube with surface lubricant into glass of room temperature water or lubricate 7.5–10 cm (3–4 inches) end of tube with water-soluble lubricant (see manufacturer directions).	Water activates lubricant, minimizes friction against nasal mucosa, and aids in insertion of tube. Water-soluble lubricant is less toxic than oil-base lubricant if aspirated.
13. Hand an alert patient a cup of water if able to hold cup and swallow. Explain that you are about to insert tube.	Swallowing water facilitates tube passage. Explanation decreases patient anxiety and increases patient cooperation.
14. Explain next steps. Insert tube gently and slowly through naris to back of throat (posterior nasopharynx). Aim back and down toward patient's ear.	Natural contour facilitates passage of tube into GI tract and reduces gagging.
15. Have patient relax and flex head toward chest after tube is passed through nasopharynx.	Closes off glottis and reduces risk of tube entering trachea.
16. Encourage patient to swallow by taking small sips of water when possible. Advance tube as patient swallows, Rotate tube gently 180 degrees while inserting.	Swallowing facilitates passage of tube past oropharynx. A tug may be felt as patient swallows, indicating that tube is following desired path.
17. Emphasize need to mouth breathe during procedure.	Helps facilitate passage of tube and alleviates patient's anxiety and fear during procedure.
18. Do not advance tube during inspiration of coughing because it will likely enter respiratory tract. Monitor oximetry/capnography.	When tube inadvertently enters airway, changes in oxygen saturation or end-tidal CO_2 (capnography) occur.
19. Advance tube each time patient swallows until you reach desired length.	Reduces discomfort and trauma to patient.

Clinical Decision Point Do not force NG tube. If patient starts to cough or has a drop in O_2 saturation or an increased CO_2, withdraw tube into the posterior nasopharynx until normal breathing resumes.

STEP	RATIONALE
20. Using penlight and tongue blade, check to be sure that tube is not positioned in back of throat.	Tube could become coiled, kinked, or enter trachea.
21. Temporarily anchor tube to nose with small piece of tape.	Securing tube prevents movement of tube and subsequent gagging. Allows for verification of tube placement.
22. Verify tube placement. Check agency policy for recommended methods of checking tube placement.	
a. Follow order for bedside x-ray film and notify radiology for examination of chest and abdomen.	Radiography is gold standard for verification of initial placement of tube (Tho et al., 2011). This must be done before any medication or liquid is administered (ENA, 2015).
b. While waiting for x-ray film to be performed, follow these procedures: Attach Asepto or catheter-tipped syringe to end of tube. Aspirate gently back on syringe to obtain gastric contents, observing amount, color, and quality of return (see illustration).	Observation of gastric contents is useful to determine initial tube placement. Gastric contents are usually green but are sometimes off-white, tan, bloody, or brown in color. Other common aspirate colors include yellow or bile stained (duodenal placement) or possibly saliva-appearing (esophagus) (Walthen and Peyton, 2014).
c. Use pH test paper to measure aspirate for pH with color-coded pH paper. Be sure that paper range of pH is at least from 1.0 to 11.0 (see illustration).	Evidence supports pH test to be used as indicator for placement (Walthen and Peyton, 2014; Tho et al., 2011). A pH 1.0 to 4.0 is a good indicator of gastric placement (Walthen and Peyton, 2014).
23. Anchor tube with a fixation device, avoiding pressure on the nares. Select one of the following fixation methods.	Proper anchoring and marking of tube helps prevent migration of tube and pressure injury formation.
a. Apply tape.	
(1) Apply tincture of benzoin or other skin adhesive on bridge of patient's nose and allow it to become "tacky."	Helps tape adhere better. Protects underlying skin.
(2) Tear small horizontal slits at ⅓ and ⅔ length of tape without splitting tape (see illustration). Fold middle sections toward one another to form a closed strip.	The strip holds tubing to lessen rubbing against soft palate and naris.
(3) Print date and time on tape and place top end of tape over bridge of patient's nose.	
(4) Wrap bottom end of tape around tube as it exits nose (see illustration).	

STEP	RATIONALE

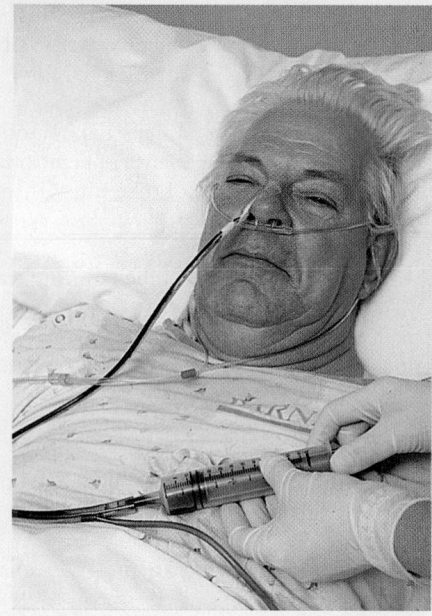

STEP 22b Aspiration of gastric contents.

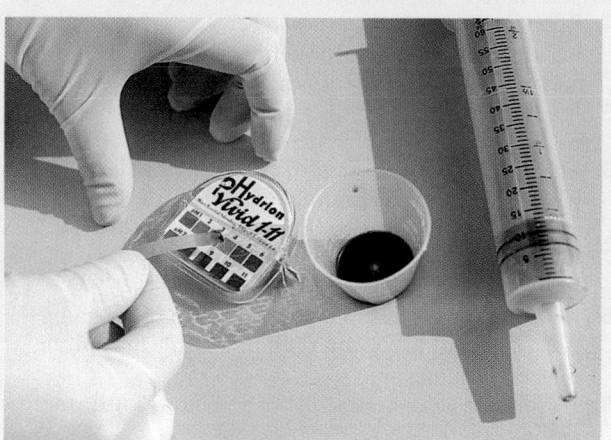

STEP 22c Checking pH of gastric aspirate.

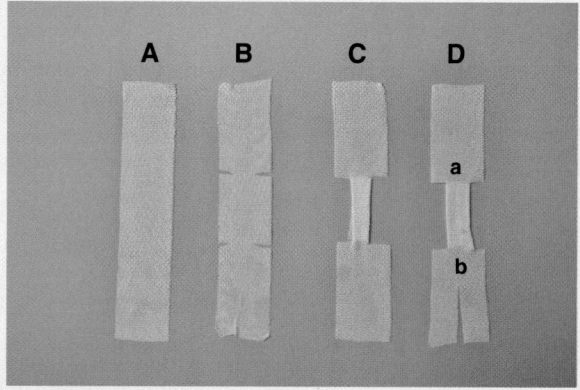

STEP 23a(2) Taping method. **A,** Start with piece of tape. **B,** Make two slits on both sides of tape. **C,** Fold middle section inward. **D,** Tear a new slit in bottom of tape. Top part (a) should attach to patient's nose; bottom part (b) should be wrapped around tube.

STEP	RATIONALE
b. Apply tube fixation device using shaped adhesive patch (see manufacturer directions).	Secures tube and reduces friction on nares.
(1) Apply wide end of patch to bridge of nose (see illustration).	
(2) Slip connector around tube as it exits nose (see illustration).	
24. Fasten end of nasogastric tube to patient's gown with piece of tape (see illustration). Do not use safety pins to fasten tube to gown.	Anchors tubing to prevent pulling on nose.
25. Keep head of bed elevated at least 30 degrees (preferably 45 degrees) unless contraindicated (Metheny and Franz, 2013).	Reduces risk for aspiration of stomach contents.

Clinical Decision Point *If inserting a Salem sump tube, keep the pigtail of the tube above level of the stomach. This prevents a siphoning action that clogs the tube.*

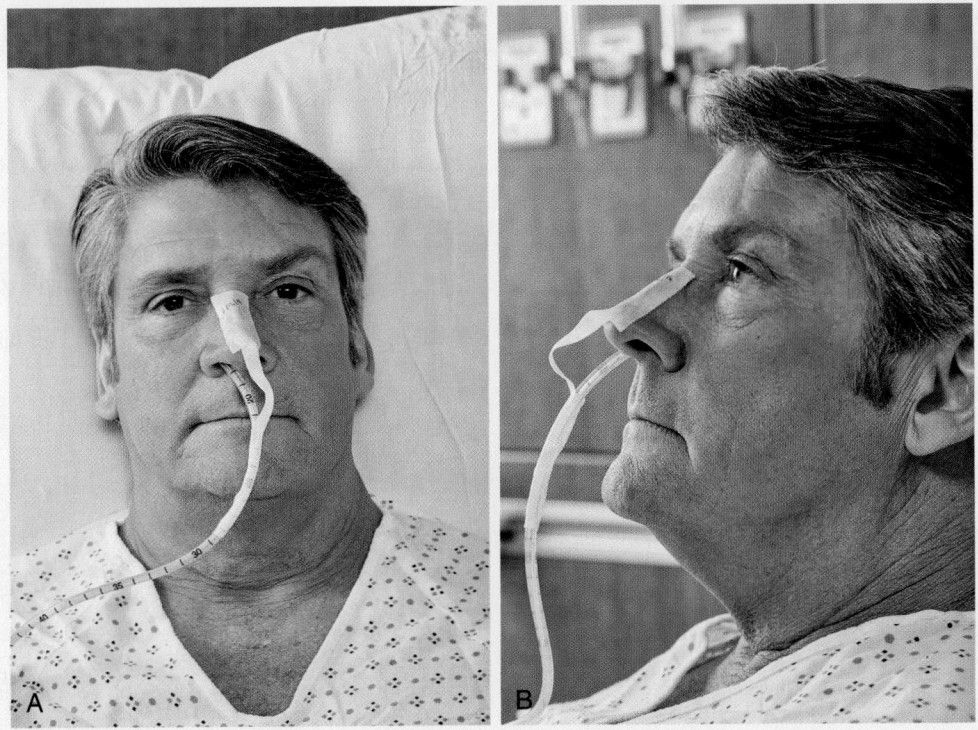

STEP 23a(4) A, Tape applied to anchor nasogastric tube. **B,** Nares are free of pressure from tape and tube.

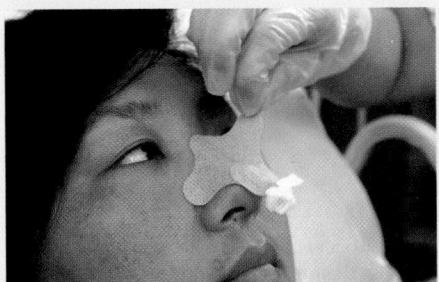

STEP 23b(1) Apply patch to bridge of nose.

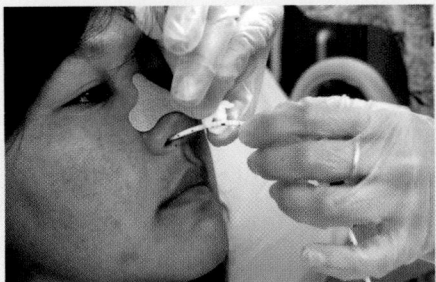

STEP 23b(2) Slip connector around NG tube.

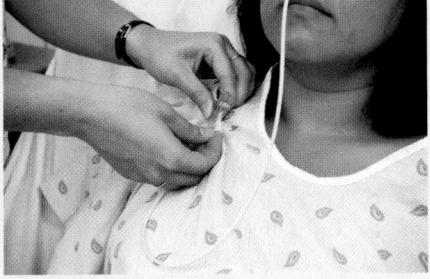

STEP 24 Fasten NG tube to patient gown.

STEP	RATIONALE
26. Assist radiology as needed in obtaining ordered x-ray film of chest and abdomen.	X-ray verification is the gold standard for NG tube verification (Stewart, 2014; Tho et al., 2011).
27. Remove gloves, perform hand hygiene, and help patient to comfortable position.	Reduces transmission of microorganisms.
28. Once placement is confirmed, measure amount of tube that is external and mark exit of tube at nares with indelible marker as guide for any tube displacement. Record this information in nurses' notes in electronic health record (EHR) or chart.	The mark alerts nurses and other health care providers to possible tube displacement, which will require confirmation of tube placement.

Clinical Decision Point *Never reposition an NG tube of a gastric surgical patient since positioning can rupture the suture line.*

STEP	RATIONALE
29. Attach NG tube to suction as ordered.	Suction setting is usually ordered low intermittent, which decreases gastric irritation from NG tube.

STEP	RATIONALE

Clinical Decision Point *If lumen of tube is narrow and secretions are thick, NG will not drain as desired. Irrigate tube (see Step 30). Consult with health care provider for higher suction setting if unable to irrigate tube because of thick secretions.*

30. NG tube irrigation:

a. Perform hand hygiene and apply clean gloves.	Reduces transmission of microorganisms.
b. Check for tube placement in stomach by disconnecting NG tube, connecting irrigating syringe, and aspirating contents (see Step 22b). Temporarily clamp NG tube or reconnect to connecting tube and remove syringe.	Prevents accidental entrance of irrigating solution into lungs.
c. Empty syringe of aspirate and use it to draw up 30 mL of normal saline.	Use of saline minimizes loss of electrolytes from stomach fluids.
d. Disconnect NG from connecting tubing and lay end of connection tubing on towel.	Reduces soiling of patient's gown and bed linen.
e. Insert tip of irrigating syringe into end of NG tube. Remove clamp. Hold syringe with tip pointed at floor and inject saline slowly and evenly. Do not force solution.	Position of syringe prevents introduction of air into vent tubing, which causes gastric distention. Solution introduced under pressure causes gastric trauma.

Clinical Decision Point *Do not introduce saline through blue "pigtail" air vent of Salem sump tube.*

f. If resistance occurs, check for kinks in tubing. Turn patient onto left side. Repeated resistance should be reported to health care provider.	Tip of tube may lie against stomach lining. Repositioning on left side may dislodge tube away from stomach lining. Buildup of secretions causes distention.
g. After instilling saline, immediately aspirate or pull back slowly on syringe to withdraw fluid. If amount aspirated is greater than amount instilled, record difference as output. If amount aspirated is less than amount instilled, record difference as intake.	Irrigation clears tubing so stomach should remain empty. Measure and document amount of irrigant fluid inserted in tube as intake.
h. Use an Asepto syringe to place 10 mL of air into blue pigtail.	Ensures patency of air vent.
i. Reconnect NG tube to drainage or suction. (Repeat irrigation if solution does not return.)	Reestablishes drainage collection; may repeat irrigation or repositioning of tube until NG tube drains properly.

31. Removal of NG tube:

a. Verify order to remove NG tube.	A health care provider order is required for procedure.
b. Auscultate abdomen for presence of bowel sounds.	Verifies return of peristalsis.
c. Explain procedure to patient and reassure that removal is less distressing than insertion.	Minimizes anxiety and increases cooperation. Tube passes out smoothly.
d. Perform hand hygiene and apply clean gloves.	Reduces transmission of microorganisms.
e. Turn off suction and disconnect NG tube from drainage bag or suction. With irrigating syringe, insert 20 mL of air into lumen of NG tube. Remove tape or fixation device from bridge of nose and patient's gown.	Have tube free of connections before removal. Clears gastric fluids from tube to prevent aspiration of contents or soiling of clothing and bedding.
f. Hand patient facial tissue; place clean towel across chest. Instruct patient to take and hold breath as tube is removed.	Some patients wish to blow nose after tube is removed. Towel keeps gown from soiling. Temporary airway obstruction occurs during tube removal.
g. Clamp or kink tubing securely and pull tube out steadily and smoothly into towel held in other hand while patient holds breath.	Clamping prevents tube contents from draining into oropharynx. Reduces trauma to mucosa and minimizes patient's discomfort. Towel covers tube, which is an unpleasant sight. Holding breath helps to prevent aspiration.
h. Inspect intactness of tube.	
i. Measure amount of drainage and note character of content. Dispose of tube and drainage equipment into proper container.	Provides accurate measure of fluid output. Reduces transfer of microorganisms.
j. Clean nares and provide mouth care.	Promotes comfort.
k. Position patient comfortably and explain procedure for drinking fluids if not contraindicated. Instruct patient to notify you if nausea occurs.	Sometimes patients are not allowed anything by mouth (NPO) for up to 24 hours. When fluids are allowed, orders usually begin with small amount of ice chips each hour and increase as patient is able to tolerate more.

STEP	RATIONALE
32. For all procedures, clean equipment and return to proper place. Place soiled linen in utility room or proper receptacle.	Proper disposal of equipment prevents spread of microorganisms and ensures proper exchange procedures.
33. Remove and discard gloves and perform hand hygiene.	Reduces transmission of microorganisms.

EVALUATION

1. Observe amount and character of contents draining from NG tube. Ask if patient feels nauseated.	Determines if tube is decompressing stomach of contents.
2. Auscultate for presence of bowel sounds. Turn off suction while auscultating.	Sound of suction apparatus is sometimes misinterpreted as bowel sounds.
3. Palpate patient's abdomen periodically. Note any distention, pain, and rigidity.	Determines success of abdominal decompression and return of peristalsis.
4. Inspect condition of nares and nose.	Evaluates onset of skin and tissue irritation.
5. Observe position of tubing.	Prevents tension applied to nasal structures.
6. Explain that it is normal if patient feels sore throat or irritation in pharynx.	Result of tube irritation.
7. Use Teach-Back: "I need to be sure I explained why you need the NG tube and the importance of letting me know if you are nauseated. Tell me why it is important for me to know if you feel nauseated?" Revise your instruction now or develop a plan for revised patient or family caregiver teaching if patient or family caregiver is not able to teach back correctly.	Determines patient's and family caregiver's level of understanding of instructional topic.

Unexpected Outcomes	Related Interventions
1. Patient complains of nausea, or patient's abdomen is distended and painful.	• Assess patency of tube. NG tube may be occluded or no longer in stomach. • Irrigate tube. • Verify that suction is on as ordered. • Notify health care provider if distention is unrelieved.
2. Patient develops irritation or erosion of skin around naris.	• Provide frequent skin care to area. • Use taping method designed to reduce MDRPI (see taping methods Step 23 a and b). • Consider switching tube to other naris.
3. Patient develops signs and symptoms of pulmonary aspiration: fever, shortness of breath, or pulmonary congestion.	• Perform complete respiratory assessment. • Notify health care provider. • Obtain chest x-ray film examination as ordered.

Recording and Reporting

- Record length, size, and type of gastric tube inserted and in which naris it was inserted. In addition, record patient's tolerance of procedure, confirmation of tube placement, location of distal tip of tube, character of gastric contents, pH value, results of radiography, whether the tube is clamped or connected to drainage bag or to suction, and amount of suction supplied on flow sheet or in nurses' notes in electronic health record (EHR) or chart.
- Record patient's and family caregiver's understanding through teach-back of what to report to nurse and purpose of NG tube in nurses' notes in EHR or chart.

- Record difference between amount of normal saline instilled and amount of gastric aspirate removed on intake and output (I&O) sheet. Record the amount and character of contents draining from NG tube, every shift.
- Record removal of tube "intact," patient's tolerance of procedure, and final amount and character of drainage.

Special Considerations
Gerontological

- Check for ill-fitting dentures and remove them for patient's safety and comfort during the insertion.
- Oral and nasal mucosal drying is sometimes present. Adequately lubricate the tube for insertion.

◆ CLINICAL DEBRIEF

A 66-year-old man with a history of severe osteoarthritis is hospitalized following a total right knee replacement performed 2 days ago. At present he is allowed touch-down weight bearing on his right leg. His last bowel movement was the day before surgery; thus he has gone 3 days without a bowel movement. Since surgery he received opioid pain medication through his intravenous (IV) line and began taking oral pain medication last night. His abdomen is nontender and slightly distended, with active bowel sounds in all four quadrants. He attempted a bowel movement with a great deal of straining and expelled small, hard, brown stool. You've talked to the health care provider and obtained orders for a Fleet enema.

1. You have explained the enema procedure to the patient and have prepared your supplies. You need to provide a bedpan or commode for him to expel the fecal material following the enema. Make your selection of the type of bedpan or use of commode and provide the rationale.

2. What is the expected outcome of the Fleet enema? Which, if any, instructions will you give to the nursing assistive personnel (NAP)?

3. Two days later the patient has the same symptoms as before receiving the enema. He has still not had a bowel movement. This time he has liquid stool seeping from the rectum. Using SBAR, show how you would communicate with the health care team about this patient?

◆ REVIEW QUESTIONS

1. The nurse is caring for a patient who needs to use a bedpan. Which of the following comfort measures should the nurse use for proper positioning and general comfort? (Select all that apply.)
   1. Keep the head of the bed flat.
   2. Place toilet tissue within reach.
   3. Stay with patient while he or she is using bedpan.
   4. Place a small pillow under lumbar curve in the back.
   5. Place the head of the bed at 45-degree angle.

2. The nurse has several activities to perform. Which can be delegated to the NAP? (Select all that apply.)
   1. Administering a tap-water enema
   2. Removing a fecal impaction
   3. Placing a patient on a bedpan
   4. Inserting a nasogastric (NG) tube
   5. Providing oral care for a patient with a NG tube

3. Your patient is to have a nasogastric (NG) tube inserted. Place the following steps in correct order.
   1. Measure distance to insert tube from tip of nose, to earlobe, and to xiphoid process.
   2. Verify order for the NG tube.
   3. Tape tube to nose.
   4. Perform hand hygiene and apply clean gloves.
   5. Identify patient using at least two identifiers.
   6. Pass the tube along the floor of nasal passage, then just past nasopharynx.
   7. Instruct patient to flex head forward and swallow while advancing the tube.

ⓔ *Visit the Evolve site for a complete list of Clinical Debrief and Review Questions answers.*

REFERENCES

Ball J, et al: *Seidel's guide to physical examination*, ed 8, St Louis, 2015, Mosby.

Burchum J, Rosenthal L: *Lehne's Pharmacology for nursing care*, ed 9, St Louis, 2016, Saunders.

Carrington R, et al: Pharmacologic management of osteoarthritis-related pain in older adults, *Am J Nurs* 112(3):S38, 2012.

Cooper KL: Evidence-based prevention of pressure ulcers in the intensive care units, *Crit Care Nurse* 33(6):57, 2013.

Costilla VC, Foxx-Orenstein AE: Constipation: understanding mechanisms and management, *Clin Geriatr Med* 30:107, 2014.

DeGiorgio R, et al: Chronic constipation in the elderly: a primer for the gastroenterologist, *BMC Gastroenterol* 5:130, 2015.

Emergency Nurses Association (ENA): *Clinical Practice Guideline: gastric tube placement verification*, 2015, https://www.ena.org/practice-research/research/CPG/Documents/GastricTubeCPG.pdf. Accessed February 13, 2016.

Hockenberry MJ, Wilson D: *Wong's nursing care of infants and children*, ed 10, St Louis, 2015, Mosby.

Huether S, McCance K: *Understanding pathophysiology*, ed 6, St Louis, 2017, Mosby.

Knowles S, et al: Evaluation of the implementation of a bowel management protocol in intensive care: effect on clinical practices and patient outcomes, *J Clin Nurs* 23:176, 2014.

Lambert CR, et al: Validation of the Right Spot Device™ for determination of gastric pH during nasogastric tube placement, *Int J Emerg Med* 6:28, 2013.

Lewis S, et al: *Medical-surgical nursing: assessment and management of clinical problems*, ed 10, St Louis, 2017, Elsevier.

Lim SF, Childs C: A systematic review of the effectiveness of bowel management strategies for constipation in adults with stroke, *Int J Nurs Stud* 50:1004, 2013.

Metheny NA, Franz RA: Head-of-bed elevation in critically ill patients: a review, *Crit Care Nurse* 33(3):53, 2013.

National Pressure Ulcer Advisory Panel (NPUAP): *Mucosal pressure ulcers: an NPUAP position statement*, 2012, http://www.npuap.org/wp-content/uploads/2012/03/Mucosal_Pressure_Ulcer_Position_Statement_final.pdf. Accessed February 13, 2016.

National Pressure Ulcer Advisory Panel (NPUAP): *National Pressure Ulcer Advisory Panel (NPUAP) announces a change in terminology from pressure ulcer to pressure injury and updates the stages of pressure injury*, 2016a, http://www.npuap.org/national-pressure-ulcer-advisory-panel-npuap-announces-a-change-in-terminology-from-pressure-ulcer-to-pressure-injury-and-updates-the-stages-of-pressure-injury/. Accessed June 7, 2016.

National Pressure Ulcer Advisory Panel (NPUAP): *Pressure injury prevention points*, 2016b, http://www.npuap.org/wp-content/uploads/2016/04/Pressure-Injury-Prevention-Points-2016.pdf. Accessed June 7, 2016.

Ness W: Digital removal of faeces, *Nurs Times* 109:17, 2013.

Nurko S, Zimmerman LA: Evaluation and treatment of constipation in children and adolescents, *Am Fam Physician* 90(2):82, 2014.

Pittman J, et al: Medical device–related hospital-acquired pressure ulcers, *J Wound Ostomy Continence Nurs* 42(2):151, 2015.

Prichard D, Bharucha A: Management of opioid-induced constipation for people in palliative care, *Int J Palliat Nurs* 21(6):272, 2015.

Sammon MA, et al: Randomized controlled study of the effects of 2 fecal management systems on incidence of anal erosion, *J Wound Ostomy Continence Nurs* 42(3):279, 2015.

Sanfilippo F, Spoletini G: Perspectives on the importance of postoperative ileus, *Curr Med Res Opin* 31:675, 2015.

Solomons J, Woodward S: Digital removal of faeces in the bowel management of patients with spinal cord injury: a review, *Br J Neurosci Nurs* 9(5):216, 2013.

Stewart ML: Interruptions in enteral nutrition delivery in the critically ill patients and recommendations for clinical practice, *Crit Care Nurse* 34:14, 2014.

The Joint Commission (TJC): *National Patient Safety Goals*, Oakbrook Terrace, IL, 2016, The Commission. http://www.jointcommission.org/standards_information/npsgs.aspx. Accessed February 13, 2016.

Tho PC, et al: Implementation of the evidence-review on best practice for confirming the correct placement of nasogastric tube in patients in an acute care hospital, *Int J Evid Based Healthc* 9(1):51, 2011.

Touhy T, Jett K: *Ebersole and Hess' gerontological nursing and healthy aging*, ed 4, St Louis, 2014, Mosby.

Wald A: Constipation: pathophysiology and management, *Curr Opin Gastroenterol* 31(1):45, 2015.

Walthen B, Peyton C: Pediatric nasogastric tube placement, *Nurs Crit Care* 9(3):14, 2014.

Whiteley I, Sinclair G: Faecal management systems for disabling incontinence or wounds: literature review, *Br J Nurs* 23(16):881, 2014.

World Health Organization (WHO): *WHO Guidelines on hand hygiene in health care: first global patient safety challenge: clean care is safer care*, Geneva Switzerland, 2009, World Health Organization Press.

Wound Ostomy and Continence Nurses (WOCN) Society: *Guideline for prevention and management of pressure ulcers (injuries)*, ed 2, Mount Laurel, NJ, 2016, WOCN Society.

OBJECTIVES

Mastery of content in this chapter will enable the nurse to:
- Identify the types of fecal and urinary diversions.
- Explain the differences in consistency of effluent based on the type of ostomy.

- Pouch a fecal or a urinary diversion.
- Describe methods used to maintain integrity of the peristomal skin.
- Catheterize a urinary diversion.

MEDIA RESOURCES

- evolve http://evolve.elsevier.com/Perry/skills
- Review Questions
- ▶ Video Clips

- Audio Glossary
- **NSO** Nursing Skills Online
- Clinical Debrief and Review Questions Answers

PURPOSE

With certain diseases or conditions a surgically created opening in the abdominal wall, called a *stoma*, is necessary to allow for the passage of urine or fecal matter. It is essential that a pouch be placed over a stoma correctly so the output from the stoma is contained, the skin around the stoma is protected, and a patient is free from odor or leakage.

STANDARDS OF CARE

- WCET International Ostomy Guideline, World Council of Enterostomal Therapists, 2014—Cultural Implications
- Ostomy Management: Core Curriculum, Wound Ostomy Continence Nurses Society, 2016—Principles of Ostomy Care and Management
- The Joint Commission, 2016—National Patient Safety Goals

PRINCIPLES FOR PRACTICE

- An ostomy, such as a colostomy or ileostomy, is an artificial opening in an organ of the body, created during an operation. For example, a stoma in the large intestine or colon is called a *colostomy* (Fig. 36.1), which is usually placed in the descending colon and results in a stool similar to that normally passed through the rectum.
- A stoma placed in the transverse or ascending colon is an ileostomy, which drains fecal effluent that is watery-to-thick and contains some digestive enzymes (Fig. 36.2).
- The character of the output of a bowel stoma (called *effluent*) is influenced by a patient's medications and hydration status and the foods eaten. Diet and fluid therapy are important therapies in managing ostomy effluent.

- If removal of the urinary bladder is necessary, a section of the ileum or small intestine is used to insert the ureters, creating an ileal conduit or a urostomy (Fig. 36.3) from which urine exits the body through the stoma.
- A patient with a colostomy, ileostomy, or ileal conduit has no sensation or control over the time or frequency of the output and must wear a pouch to collect effluent.
- There are surgical procedures that create continent internal fecal or urinary pouches, eliminating the need to wear an external pouch. An ileal pouch is an internal reservoir formed from a segment of the ileum that is then connected to the anal canal above the anal sphincter (Fig. 36.4A–B). A continent urinary reservoir (Fig. 36.5) is a reservoir created from the intestine. A small stoma on the abdominal wall allows access via a catheter inserted to empty urine from the pouch. These surgeries are less common than the urostomy.

PATIENT-CENTERED CARE

- A person with a newly created stoma for the elimination of urine or fecal matter from the body needs to be taught to care for his or her ostomy to regain autonomy in self-care for basic elimination. If a patient was not self-managing elimination before surgery, a family caregiver will need to be taught to provide this care.
- With any ostomy requiring a pouching system, a secure seal to prevent leakage of the effluent and protect the skin around the stoma (peristomal skin) is vital to helping patients resume normal activities and accept the changes in their bodies as a result of surgery (Salvadena, 2013).
- A reliable and effective pouching system is a very important factor in facilitating a patient's emotional adjustment to an ostomy (Carmel et al., 2016).

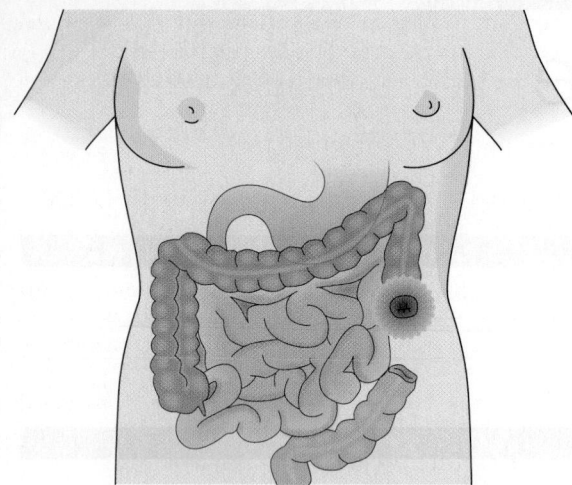

FIG 36.1 Sigmoid colostomy.

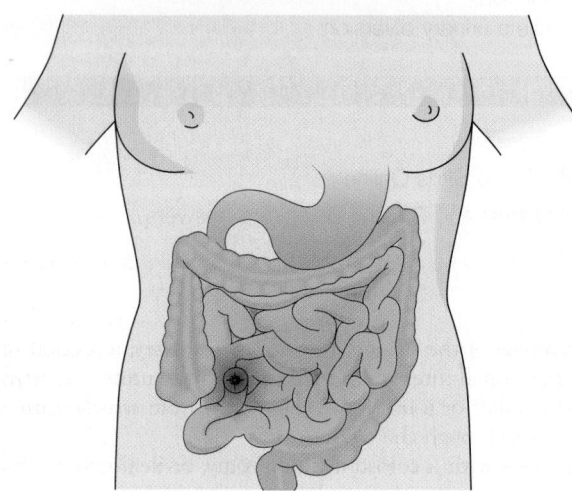

FIG 36.2 Ileostomy.

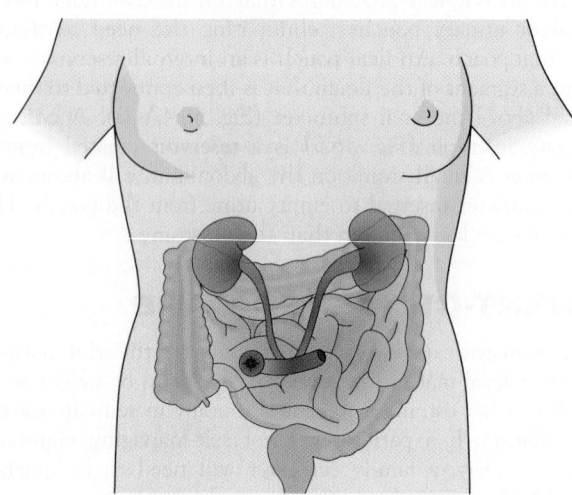

FIG 36.3 Urostomy (ileal conduit).

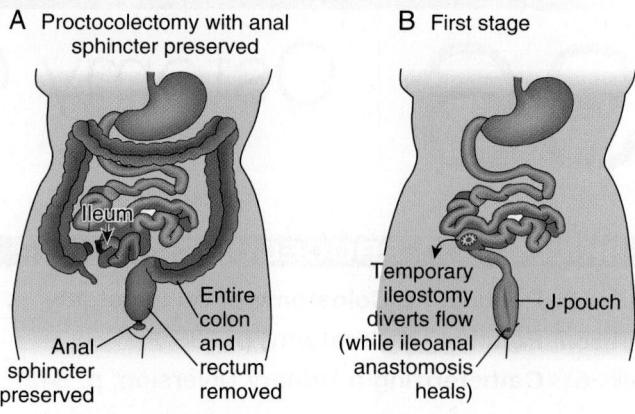

A Proctocolectomy with anal sphincter preserved

B First stage

FIG 36.4 Ileal pouch anal anastomosis.

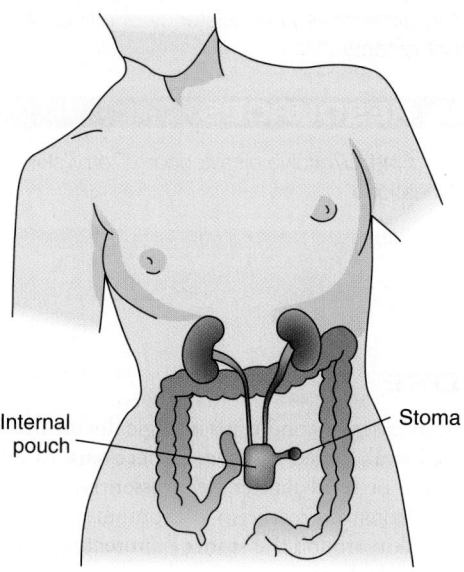

FIG 36.5 Continent urinary diversion.

- In addition to the stress of illness and surgical recovery, patients with ostomies face body image changes, fear of social rejection, concern about sexual function and intimacy, and the need for help with personal care (Carmel et al., 2016).
- Patients from some ethnic backgrounds and religious practices may find monitoring urinary or intestinal output from their stomas to be more invasive and embarrassing than patients from cultures that are more open about bodily functions (WCET, 2014). Discuss with patients their preferences.
- A nurse needs to consider the impact that caring for a person with an ostomy has on a family caregiver's quality of life (WCET, 2014).
- As you communicate with a patient during ostomy care, be sensitive and avoid communicating anything that the patient may interpret as disrespect or disgust. As always, prepare adequately for the procedure; seek necessary help; and maintain a calm, professional demeanor. Do not act offended by the odor or appearance of the effluent in the pouch or the appearance of the stoma. A negative reaction from caregivers only reinforces a patient's feelings that this alteration in bodily function makes him or her personally and socially unacceptable.
- When patients come to a hospital with an ostomy, encourage them to be able to resume self-care as soon as possible. Respect a patient's routine of care even if it differs from usual care in the agency. Offer educational materials to support the patient's adaptation to the new ostomy (ACS, 2016a; ACS, 2016b; ACS, 2016c).

EVIDENCE-BASED PRACTICE

There are evidence-based guidelines for proper stoma measurement and the role of an ostomy nurse in caring for patients.

- Before ostomy surgery a health care provider or ostomy care nurse should see a patient to mark a stoma site. Assessing a patient's abdomen while he or she is lying, sitting, and standing allows the nurse and the patient to find an optimal stoma location that will make it easy for the patient to see the stoma and apply a pouch with a reliable seal (Salvadena et al., 2015a, b).
- The WCET (2014) International Ostomy Guideline recommends that the site be marked on the abdomen away from abdominal scars, creases, skinfolds, or the belt line. Studies show that preoperative stoma site marking is crucial for improving patients' postoperative quality of life, promoting their independence, and reducing the rates of postoperative complications (Person et al., 2012).
- Having the support and care of a specialized ostomy nurse leads to better adjustment to an ostomy and improved health-related quality of life (Coca et al., 2015; Riemenschneider, 2015).

Whenever possible, refer a patient with a new ostomy to an ostomy nurse who has advanced, specialized training and may be certified as a Wound Ostomy Continence Nurse or CWOCN.

SAFETY GUIDELINES

- Change ostomy pouches when they are ⅓–½ full to avoid leakage, which can lead to chemical or enzymatic injury to the skin.
- Know the signs of a healthy stoma and surrounding skin:
  - *Color/moisture:* Stoma should be red or pink and moist. Report a gray, purple, black, or very dry stoma to the charge nurse or health care provider.
  - *Size:* In the 4 to 6 weeks after surgery, the stoma will likely decrease in size. Measure with each pouch change and adjust the size of the opening cut in the wafer.
  - *Peristomal skin:* It normally is intact with some reddening after the adhesive wafer is removed. Presence of blisters, a rash, or excoriated skin is abnormal.
- Wear gloves during pouch and stoma care to reduce exposure to and transmission of infectious microorganisms.

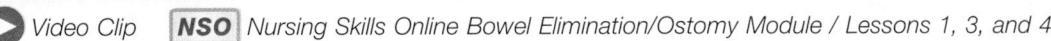

✦ SKILL 36.1   Pouching a Colostomy or an Ileostomy

▶ *Video Clip*   **NSO** *Nursing Skills Online Bowel Elimination/Ostomy Module / Lessons 1, 3, and 4*

Immediately after a fecal surgical diversion, it is necessary to place a pouch over a newly created stoma to contain effluent when the stoma begins to function. The pouch will keep a patient clean and dry, protect the skin from drainage, and provide a barrier against odor. A cut-to-fit, transparent pouching system is preferred because it will protect the peristomal skin, allow the stoma to be visualized, and accommodate changes in stoma size as swelling decreases after surgery.

Recognize the difference between a budded stoma (Fig. 36.6) and a flush or retracted stoma (Fig. 36.7). In the immediate postoperative period the stoma may be edematous, and the abdomen distended. These symptoms will resolve over a 4- to 6-week period after surgery, but during this time it will be necessary to revise the pouching system to meet the changing size of the stoma and the changes in body contours (Carmel et al., 2016).

There are many types of pouching systems. All have a protective layer that adheres to the skin, called a *skin barrier*, and a pouch. A one-piece pouching system (Fig. 36.8) has the two parts integrated together. A two-piece system (Fig. 36.9) has a separate skin barrier and pouch. The flush or retracted stoma may require a convex wafer (Fig. 36.10) for successful placement of a pouch. This type of skin barrier provides gentle pressure on the peristomal skin to push the stoma through the opening in the wafer. You apply the pouch to the skin barrier by attaching it to a flange (a plastic ring) on the barrier. You must use the skin barrier with a flange that fits the corresponding size pouch from the same manufacturer to avoid leakage between the skin barrier and the pouch. Some pouching systems have precut openings in the barrier for the stoma, whereas others need to be custom cut to size for a patient's stoma measurement. It is important to understand how to use each of these different pouching systems before applying them on patients (Carmel et al., 2016). The websites for the companies that make ostomy supplies have both patient and health care provider instructions that are helpful in understanding how to use the pouching systems (e.g., http://www.convatec.com; http://www.us.coloplast.com; and http://www.hollister.com).

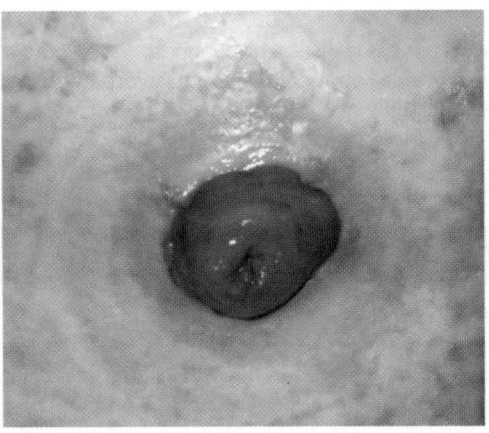

FIG 36.6 Budded stoma. (*Courtesy Jane Fellows.*)

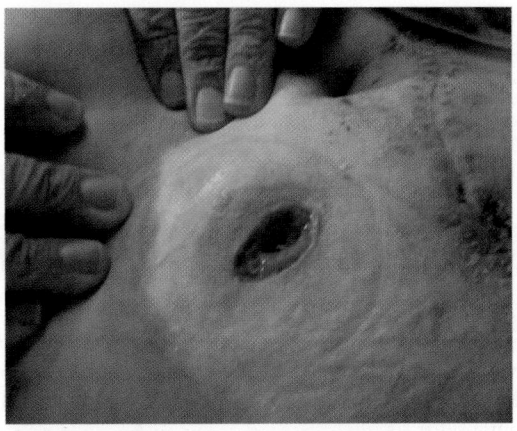

FIG 36.7 Retracted stoma. (*Courtesy Jane Fellows.*)

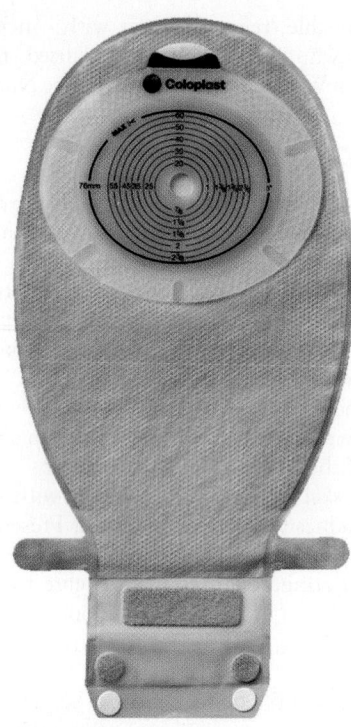

FIG 36.8 One-piece pouch with Velcro closure. (*Courtesy Coloplast, Minneapolis, MN.*)

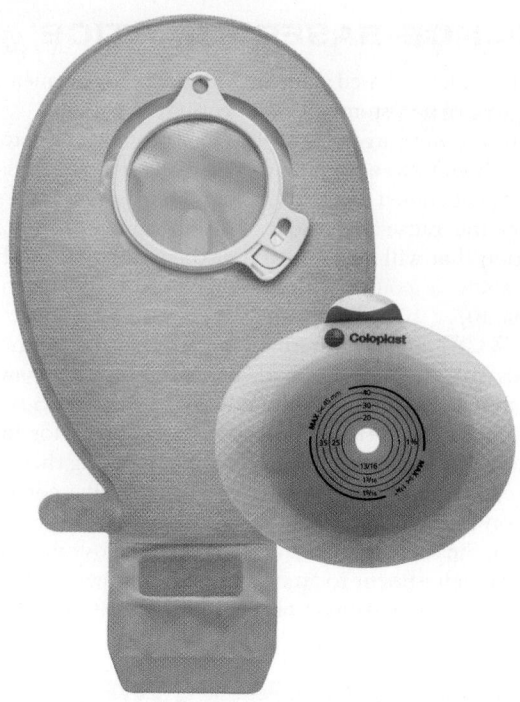

FIG 36.9 Two-piece pouching system with separate skin barrier and attachable pouch. (*Courtesy Coloplast, Minneapolis, MN.*)

Delegation and Collaboration

The skill of pouching a new ostomy should not be delegated to nursing assistive personnel (NAP). In some agencies care of an established ostomy (4 to 6 weeks or more after surgery) can be delegated to NAP. The nurse directs the NAP about:

- The expected amount, color, and consistency of drainage from an ostomy.
- The expected appearance of the stoma.
- Special equipment needed to complete a particular patient's pouching.
- The changes in a patient's stoma and surrounding skin integrity that should be reported.

Equipment

- Skin barrier/pouch—clear, drainable one-piece or two-piece, cut-to-fit or precut size
- Pouch closure device such as a clip if needed
- Ostomy measuring guide
- Adhesive remover (*optional*)
- Clean gloves
- Washcloth
- Towel or disposable waterproof barrier

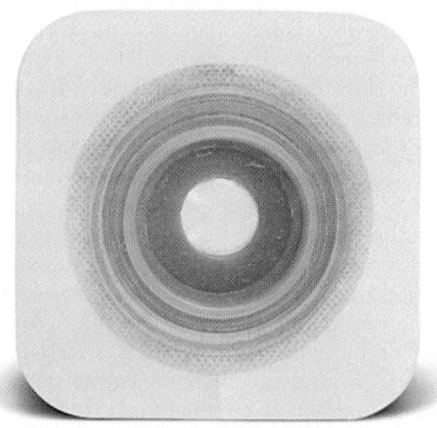

FIG 36.10 Convex skin barrier wafer. (*Used with permission Convatec, Inc. All rights reserved.*)

- Basin with warm tap water
- Scissors
- Waterproof bag for disposal of pouch
- Gown or goggles optional if there is any risk of splashing when emptying pouch

STEP	RATIONALE

ASSESSMENT

1. Identify patient using at least two identifiers (e.g., name and birthday or name and medical record number), according to agency policy.	Ensures correct patient. Complies with The Joint Commission standards and improves patient safety (TJC, 2016).
2. Perform hand hygiene and apply clean gloves.	Reduces transmission of microorganisms.

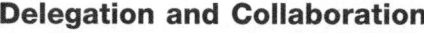

STEP	RATIONALE
3. Observe existing skin barrier and pouch for leakage and length of time in place. Pouch should be changed every 3 to 7 days, not daily (Carmel et al., 2016). If an opaque pouch is being used, remove it to fully observe stoma. Dispose of such a pouch in proper receptacle.	Assesses effectiveness of pouching system and detects potential for problems. To minimize skin irritation, avoid unnecessary changing of entire pouching system. When pouch leaks, skin damage from effluent causes more skin trauma than early removal of wafer.

Clinical Decision Point *Repeated leaking may indicate need for different type of pouch or addition of products such as stoma putty. If the pouch is leaking, change it. Taping or patching it to contain effluent leaves the skin exposed to chemical or enzymatic irritation.*

STEP	RATIONALE
4. Observe amount of effluent in pouch and empty it if it is more than $\frac{1}{3}-\frac{1}{2}$ full by opening the pouch and draining it into a container for measurement of output. Note consistency of effluent and record intake and output.	Weight of pouch may disrupt seal of adhesive on skin. Monitors fluid balance and bowel function after surgery. Normal colostomy effluent is soft or formed stool, whereas normal ileostomy effluent is liquid.
5. Observe stoma for type, location, color, swelling, presence of sutures, trauma, and healing or irritation of peristomal skin.	Stoma characteristics influence selection of an appropriate pouching system. Convexity in skin barrier is often necessary with a flush or retracted stoma.
6. Observe placement of stoma in relation to abdominal contours and presence of scars or incisions. Remove and dispose of gloves; perform hand hygiene.	Determines if current pouching system is effective or if new selection is needed. Abdominal contours, scars, or incisions affect type of system and adhesion to skin surface. Reduces transmission of microorganisms.
7. Explore patient's attitudes, perceptions, knowledge, and acceptance of stoma; discuss interest in learning self-care. Identify others who will be helping patient after leaving hospital.	Determines patient's willingness to learn. Facilitates teaching plan and timing of care to coincide with availability of family caregivers.

NURSING DIAGNOSES

- Alteration in body image
- Deficient knowledge regarding pouching of an ostomy
- Impaired skin integrity
- Readiness for enhanced knowledge
- Risk for impaired skin integrity

Related factors/Risk factors are individualized based on patient's condition or needs.

PLANNING

1. Expected outcomes following completion of procedure:	
• Stoma is red and moist; peristomal skin is intact and free of irritation; sutures are intact.	Normal findings in patient with postoperative ostomy that is healing.
• Stoma drains moderate amount of liquid or soft stool; and flatus is in pouch, which can be seen with bulging of pouch. (Flatus may not be observable if pouch has gas filter.)	Stoma is functioning normally. Snug seal around stoma has been attained. Flatus indicates return of peristalsis after surgery.
• Patient and/or family caregiver observe stoma and steps of procedure.	Reveals acceptance of alteration in body image and interest in self-care.
• Patient asks questions about procedure and attempts to help with pouch change.	Indicates readiness to learn and begin self-care.
2. Explain procedure to patient; encourage patient's interaction and questions.	Lessens patient's anxiety and promotes patient's participation.
3. Assemble equipment and close room curtains or door.	Optimizes use of time; provides privacy.

IMPLEMENTATION

1. Have patient assume semi-reclining or supine position (same position assumed during assessment and pouching). (NOTE: Some patients with established ostomies prefer to stand.) If possible, provide patient with mirror for observation.	When patient is semi-reclining, there are fewer skinfolds, which allows for ease of application of pouching system.
2. Perform hand hygiene and apply clean gloves.	Reduces transmission of microorganisms.
3. Place towel or disposable waterproof barrier under patient and across patient's lower abdomen.	Protects bed linen; maintains patient's dignity.

STEP	RATIONALE
4. If not done during assessment, remove used pouch and skin barrier gently by pushing skin away from barrier. Use adhesive remover to facilitate removal of skin barrier. Empty pouch and dispose of it in an appropriate receptacle. Measure output if needed. **NOTE:** There may be no output at time of first pouch change.	Reduces skin trauma. Improper removal of pouch and barrier can cause peristomal skin irritation or breakdown.
5. Clean peristomal skin gently with warm tap water using washcloth; do not scrub skin. If you touch stoma, minor bleeding is normal. Pat skin dry. Have washcloth handy for additional cleaning if there is output from the stoma while preparing pouch.	Soap leaves residue on skin, which may irritate skin. Pouch does not adhere to wet skin. Ileostomies have frequent output especially after eating.
6. Measure stoma (see illustration). Expect size of stoma to change for first 4 to 6 weeks after surgery.	Allows for proper fit of pouch that will protect peristomal skin.
7. Trace pattern of stoma measurement on pouch backing or skin barrier (see illustration).	Prepares for cutting opening in pouch.
8. Cut opening on backing or skin barrier wafer (see illustration). If using moldable or shape to fit barrier, use fingers to mold shape to fit stoma.	Customizes pouch to provide appropriate fit over stoma.
9. Remove protective backing from adhesive backing or wafer (see illustration).	Prepares skin barrier for placement.

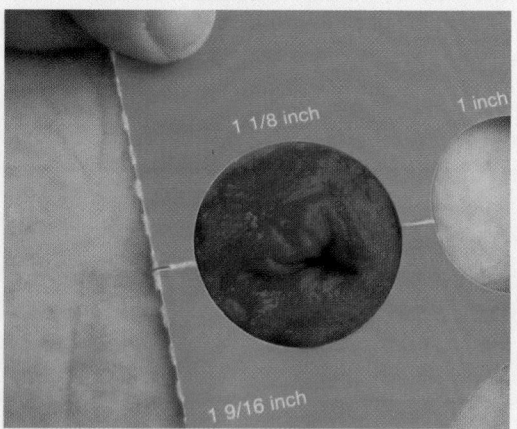

STEP 6 Measure stoma. (*Courtesy Coloplast, Minneapolis, MN.*)

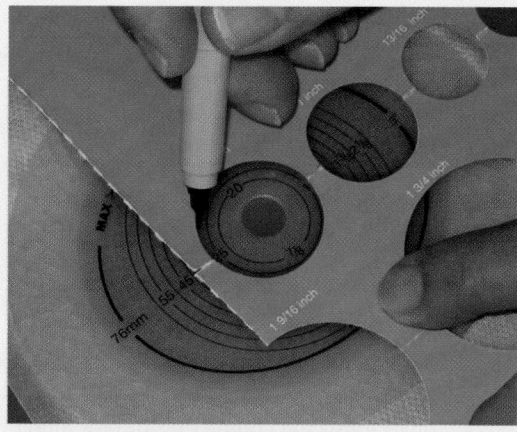

STEP 7 Trace measurement on skin barrier. (*Courtesy Coloplast, Minneapolis, MN.*)

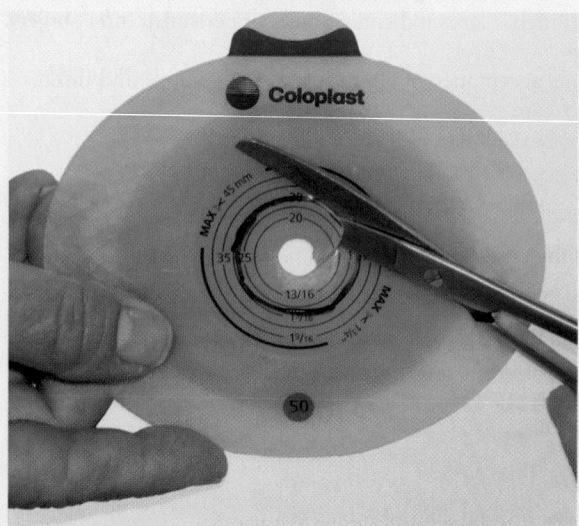

STEP 8 Cut opening in wafer. (*Courtesy Coloplast, Minneapolis, MN.*)

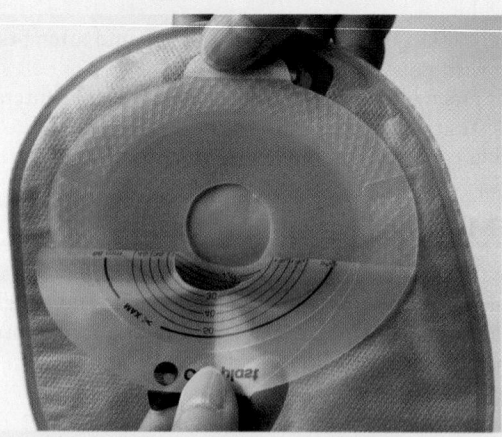

STEP 9 Remove protective backing. (*Courtesy Coloplast, Minneapolis, MN.*)

STEP	RATIONALE
10. Apply pouch over stoma (see illustration). Press firmly into place around stoma and outside edges. Have patient hold hand over pouch to apply heat to secure seal.	Pouch adhesives are heat and pressure sensitive and hold more securely at body temperature.

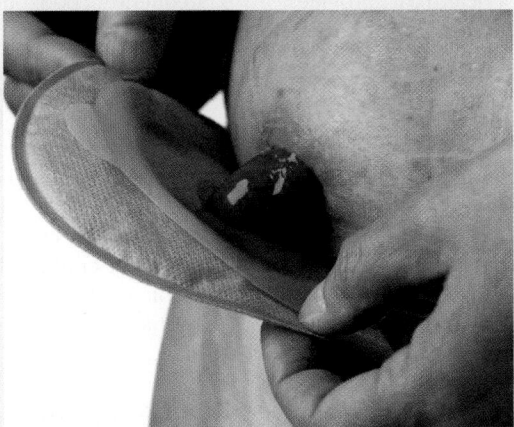

STEP 10 Apply pouch over stoma. (*Courtesy Coloplast, Minneapolis, MN.*)

STEP	RATIONALE
11. Close end of pouch with clip or integrated closure. Remove drape from patient. Help patient to assume comfortable position.	Ensures that pouch is secure. Contains effluent.
12. Remove and dispose of gloves and other disposables. Perform hand hygiene.	Reduces transmission of microorganisms.

EVALUATION

1. Observe condition of skin barrier and adherence of pouch to abdominal surface.

   Determines presence of leaks.

2. Observe appearance of stoma, peristomal skin, abdominal contours, suture line, and presence of any flatus during pouch change.

   Determines condition of stoma and peristomal skin and progress of wound healing.

3. Note if there is presence of any flatus during pouch change

   Determines if peristalsis is returning.

4. Observe patient's and family caregiver's willingness to view stoma and ask questions about procedure.

   Determines level of adjustment and understanding of stoma care and pouch application. Allows planning for future education needs and progress toward acceptance of altered body image.

5. **Use Teach-Back:** "I want to be sure you understand what is involved in changing your ostomy pouch. Tell me what you should do to prevent your skin from becoming irritated and the frequency with which you should empty your pouch." Revise your instruction now or develop a plan for revised patient or family caregiver teaching if patient or family caregiver is not able to teach back correctly.

   Determines patient's and family caregiver's level of understanding of instructional topic.

Unexpected Outcomes	Related Interventions
1. Skin around stoma is irritated, blistered, or bleeding or a rash is noted. May be caused by undermining of pouch seal by fecal contents, causing irritant dermatitis, or by adhesive removal causing skin stripping or fungal or other skin eruption.	• Remove pouch more carefully. • Change pouch more frequently or use different type of pouching system. • Consult ostomy care nurse. • Avoid use of acetone-based products.
2. Necrotic stoma is manifested by purple or black color, dry instead of moist texture, failure to bleed when washed gently, or tissue sloughing.	• Report to nurse in charge or health care provider. • Document appearance. • Obtain referral for ostomy care nurse.
3. Patient refuses to view stoma or participate in care.	• Allow patient to express feelings. • Encourage family support.

Recording and Reporting

- Record type of pouch and skin barrier applied, time of procedure, amount and appearance of effluent in pouch, location, size and appearance of stoma, and condition of peristomal skin in the electronic health record (EHR) or chart.
- Record patient and family caregiver's level of participation, teaching that was done, and response to teaching.
- Report any of the following to nurse and/or health care provider: abnormal appearance of stoma, suture line, peristomal skin, or character of output.

Special Considerations
Teaching

- Teach whenever doing a pouch change even if patient does not appear interested. Do not insist that patient look at stoma; allow time for adjustment.
- Include family caregiver in teaching to facilitate patient's readiness to learn.
- Some patients accept stoma with minimal emotional difficulty; some may never completely adjust to it. Individualize care according to patient's situation and circumstances (Riemenschneider, 2015).
- Give patient plain-language teaching materials that clearly state each step for a pouch change. Audiotaped or videotaped instructions are also available. Consider using materials that have illustrations for each step. For patients who do not speak English, provide a professional interpreter.
- Give patients a list of equipment and name, address, and phone number of a supplier.

Pediatric

- Select pediatric pouches designed especially for neonates, infants, and children. The pouches are smaller and have a more skin-sensitive adhesive on the barrier.
- Because most ostomy surgery done on neonates is for emergencies, often no time is available for preoperative selection of stoma site. The surgery is usually done because the neonate has necrotizing enterocolitis (NEC), Hirschsprung's disease, or congenital disorders (Bookout et al., 2011). The stomas frequently are temporary, with closure of the ostomy when the surgical repair has healed and the neonate is medically ready for surgery. Children and adolescents may have ostomy surgery for conditions such as cancer, inflammatory bowel disease, and trauma.

- Neonates may have multiple stomas on their tiny abdomens following corrective bowel surgeries. Select a cut-to-fit pouch that allows multiple stoma openings in skin barrier yet still fits on neonate's abdomen (Bookout et al., 2011).
- Because infants swallow air while sucking, it is normal to expect flatus. Make sure that pouch can accommodate increased amount of flatus after feeding or be prepared to release flatus frequently (Bookout et al., 2011).
- The skin of a preterm infant is not fully developed and is more absorbent than that of a full-term infant. Do not use skin sealants and adhesive removers unless they are approved for preterm-infant use (Bookout et al., 2011).
- As an infant grows in size, so does the stoma. Measure the stoma frequently and make appropriate adjustments in pouching and skin barrier size. Skin barriers for preterm infants must have flexibility to cover the infant's rounded abdominal contour (Bookout et al., 2011).
- Adolescents requiring an ostomy benefit from presurgical contact with other adolescents who have an ostomy (Bookout et al., 2011).

Gerontological

- Evaluate an older adult's cognitive status for understanding ostomy self-care instructions. Include a family caregiver in the care plan (if appropriate).
- Adapt care approaches for older patients who have impaired manual dexterity or limited vision. If a patient is unable to custom cut the size of the skin barrier, consider having barriers precut by an ostomy equipment supplier or using a precut pouching system.
- Costs of ostomy supplies and reimbursement are an issue for patients on fixed income if not covered by insurance.

Home Care

- Evaluate home toileting facilities and patients' ability to position to empty pouch directly into a toilet.
- A patient may shower without covering a pouch. A patient may take the pouch off in the shower to clean the peristomal skin if he or she wishes to do so and if cleared by health care provider.
- Patients should avoid storing pouches in extremely hot or cold locations. Temperature affects barrier and adhesive materials.

◆ SKILL 36.2   Pouching a Urostomy

Because urine flows continuously from an incontinent urinary diversion, placement of a pouch is more challenging than a fecal diversion. In the immediate postoperative period urinary stents extend out from a stoma (Fig. 36.11). A surgeon places the stents to prevent stenosis of the ureters at the site where the ureters are attached to the conduit. The stents will be removed during the hospital stay or at the first postoperative visit with the surgeon.

The stoma is normally red and moist. It is made from part of the intestinal tract, usually the ileum. A normal stoma protrudes above the skin. An ileal conduit is usually located in the right lower quadrant of a patient's abdomen. While the patient is in bed, the pouch may be connected to a bedside drainage bag to decrease the need for frequent emptying. When the patient goes home, a bedside drainage bag may be used at night to avoid having to get up to empty the pouch. Each type of urostomy pouch comes with

a connector for the bedside drainage bag (Fig. 36.12). Incorrect pouch placement, large volumes of urine in the pouch, or a urinary pouch without an antireflux valve promotes reflux of urine back into the urostomy and ureters, causing the risk of infection. You reduce the risk of reflux by attaching a urinary pouch to straight drainage when high urinary output is expected. A patient must understand the importance of draining the pouch frequently and using clean technique during stomal and skin care.

Delegation and Collaboration

The skill of pouching a new incontinent urinary diversion cannot be delegated to nursing assistive personnel (NAP). In some agencies care of an established urostomy (4 o 6 weeks or more after surgery) can be delegated to NAP. The nurse directs the NAP about:

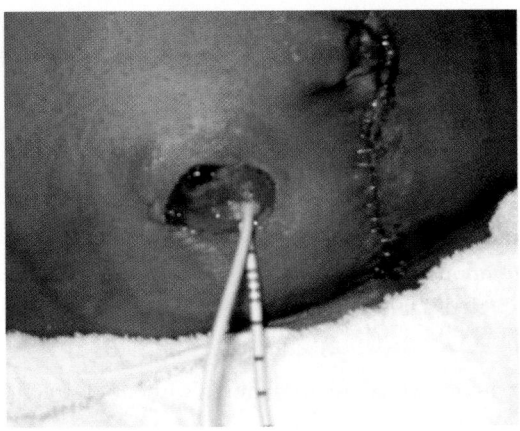

FIG 36.11 Urostomy stoma with stents in place. (*Courtesy Jane Fellows.*)

- Expected appearance of the stoma.
- Expected amount and character of the output and when to report changes.
- Change in patient's stoma and surrounding skin integrity that should be reported.
- Special equipment for a particular patient needed to complete procedure.

Equipment

- Urinary pouch (with antireflux flap and skin barrier; clear, drainable one- or two-piece, cut-to-fit or precut size
- Appropriate adapter for connection to bedside drainage bag
- Measuring guide

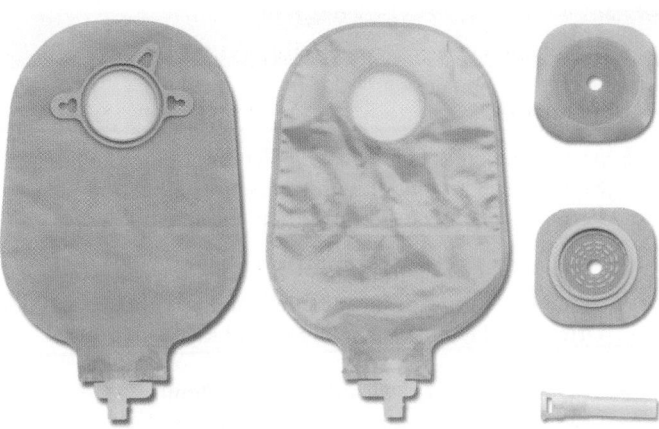

FIG 36.12 Urostomy pouching system with adapter to connect pouch to bedside drainage bag. (*Courtesy Hollister Inc, Libertyville, IL.*)

- Bedside urinary drainage bag
- Clean gloves
- Washcloth
- Towel or disposable waterproof barrier
- Basin with warm tap water
- Scissors
- Adhesive remover
- Absorbent wick made from gauze rolled tightly in the shape of a tampon
- Waterproof bag for disposal of pouch
- Mirror for patient to observe ostomy
- Gown and goggles optional if there is any risk of splashing when emptying pouch

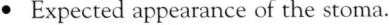

STEP	RATIONALE

ASSESSMENT

STEP	RATIONALE
1. Identify patient using at least two identifiers (e.g., name and birthday or name and medical record number), according to agency policy.	Ensures correct patient. Complies with The Joint Commission standards and improves patient safety (TJC, 2016).
2. Perform hand hygiene and apply clean gloves.	Reduces transmission of microorganisms.
3. Observe existing skin barrier and pouch for leakage and length of time in place. Pouch should be changed every 3 to 7 days, not daily (Carmel et al., 2016). If urine is leaking under wafer, change pouch.	Assesses effectiveness of pouching system and allows for early detection of potential problems. To minimize skin irritation, avoid changing entire pouching system unnecessarily. Repeated leakage may indicate need for different type of pouch to provide reliable seal.
4. Observe characteristics of urine in pouch or bedside drainage bag. Empty pouch if it is more than one-third to one-half full by opening valve and draining it into container for measurement.	There may be blood or large amounts of mucus in urine after surgery, but this should resolve in the first 1–2 weeks after surgery. Weight of pouch can disrupt seal. Urine from ileal conduit will contain mucus because of flow through intestinal segment.
5. Observe stoma for color, swelling, presence of sutures, trauma, and healing of peristomal skin. Assess type of stoma. Remove and dispose of gloves.	Consider stoma characteristics in selecting appropriate pouching system. Convexity in skin barrier is often necessary with flush or retracted stoma.
6. Explore patient's perceptions, acceptance and knowledge of stoma, and interest in learning self-care. Identify others who will be helping patient after leaving hospital.	Facilitates teaching plan and timing of care to coincide with availability of family caregivers.

NURSING DIAGNOSES

- Alteration in body image
- Deficient knowledge regarding care of a urostomy
- Impaired skin integrity
- Readiness for enhanced knowledge
- Risk for impaired skin integrity

Related factors/Risk factors are individualized based on patient's condition or needs.

STEP	RATIONALE

PLANNING

1. Expected outcomes following completion of procedure:
- Stoma is red and moist with stents protruding from it. Peristomal skin is free of irritation and intact. Sutures are intact.

  Normal findings for postoperative urinary diversion.

- Urine drains freely from stents or stoma.

  These are normal findings after surgery.

- Urine is yellow with mucus shreds and is without foul odor. Urine may be pink or contain small blood clots after surgery.

  Mucus shreds are normal when urine flows through intestinal segment.

- Volume of output is within acceptable limits (≥30 mL/h).

  Normal output reveals ureters draining without obstruction.

- Patient and family caregiver observe stoma and procedural steps.

  Shows adjustment to body image change and willingness to learn self-care.

- Patient asks questions about procedure and may help with pouch change.

  Indicates readiness to learn and begin self-care.

2. Explain procedure to patient; encourage his or her interaction and questions.

  Lessens patient's anxiety and promotes participation.

3. Assemble equipment and close room curtains or door.

  Optimizes use of time; provides privacy.

IMPLEMENTATION

1. Position patient in semi-reclining or supine position. If possible, provide patient with mirror for observation.

  When patient is semi-reclining, there are fewer skin wrinkles, which allows for ease of pouch application.

2. Perform hand hygiene and apply clean gloves.

  Reduces transmission of microorganisms.

3. Place towel or disposable waterproof barrier under patient and across patient's lower abdomen.

  Protects bed linen; maintains patient's dignity.

4. If not done during assessment, remove used pouch and skin barrier gently by pushing skin away from barrier. If stents are present, pull pouch gently around them and lay towel underneath. Empty pouch and measure output. Dispose of pouch in appropriate receptacle.

  Reduces risk for trauma to skin and for dislodging stents. Keeps urine from leaking onto skin. Urine output provides information about renal status and whether volume is within acceptable limits (≥30 mL/h).

5. Place rolled gauze at stoma opening. Maintain gauze at stoma opening continuously during pouch measurement and change.

  Using wick at stoma opening prevents peristomal skin from becoming wet with urine during pouch change.

6. While keeping rolled gauze in contact with stoma, clean peristomal skin gently with warm tap water and washcloth; do not scrub skin. If you touch stoma, minor bleeding is normal. Pat skin dry.

  Avoid soap. It leaves residue on skin, which can irritate it. Pouch does not adhere to wet skin.

7. Measure stoma (see illustration, Skill 36.1, Step 6). Expect size of stoma to change for first 4 to 6 weeks after surgery.

  Allows for proper fit of pouch that will protect peristomal skin.

8. Trace pattern on pouch backing or skin barrier (see illustration, Skill 36.1, Step 7).

  Prepares for cutting opening in pouch.

9. Cut opening in pouch (see illustration, Skill 36.1, Step 8). If using moldable or shape to fit barrier, use fingers to mold shape to fit stoma.

  Customizes pouch to provide appropriate fit over stoma.

10. Remove protective backing from adhesive backing or wafer surface. (see illustration, Skill 36.1, Step 9). Remove rolled gauze from stoma.

  Prepares pouch for application to skin.

11. Apply pouch (see illustration Skill 36.1, Step 10). Press adhesive barrier firmly into place around stoma and outside edges. Have patient hold hand over pouch 1 to 2 minutes to secure seal.

  Pouch adhesives are heat and pressure sensitive and will hold more securely at body temperature.

12. Use adapter provided with pouches to connect pouch to bedside urinary bag. Keep tubing below level of bag.

  Allows patient to rest without frequent emptying of pouch. Tubing position allows for collection and measurement of urine and prevents backflow of urine into stoma.

STEP	RATIONALE
13. Remove drape from patient. Help patient to assume comfortable position. Remove and dispose of gloves and other disposables; perform hand hygiene.	Reduces transmission of microorganisms. 

EVALUATION

1. Observe appearance of stoma, peristomal skin, and suture line during pouch change.	Determines condition of stoma and peristomal skin and progress of wound healing.
2. Evaluate character and volume of urinary drainage.	Determines if stoma and/or stents are patent. Character of urine reveals degree of concentration and whether there is possible urinary tract infection.
3. Observe patient's and family caregiver's willingness to view stoma and ask questions about procedure.	Determines level of adjustment and understanding of stoma care and pouch application.
4. Use Teach-Back: "I want to be sure you understand what is involved in changing your ostomy pouch. Let's review what we discussed. Tell me how often you should empty your pouch and how often you should change it." Revise your instruction now or develop a plan for revised patient or family caregiver teaching if patient or family caregiver is not able to teach back correctly.	Determines patient's and family caregiver's level of understanding of instructional topic.

Unexpected Outcomes	**Related Interventions**
1. Skin around stoma is irritated, blistered, or bleeding; or maceration is noted as result of chronic exposure to urine.	• Check stoma size and opening in skin barrier. • Resize skin barrier opening if necessary. • Remove pouch more carefully. • Consult ostomy care nurse.
2. No urine output for several hours, or output is less than 30 mL/h. Urine has foul odor.	• Increase fluid intake (if allowed). • Notify health care provider. • Obtain urine specimen for culture and sensitivity if ordered.
3. Patient and family caregiver are unable to observe stoma, ask questions, or participate in care.	• Consult ostomy care nurse. • Allow patient to express feelings. • Encourage family support.

Recording and Reporting

- Record type of pouch, time of change, condition and appearance of stoma/stents and peristomal skin, and character of urine in the electronic health record (EHR) or chart.
- Record urinary output on intake and output form.
- Record patient's and family caregiver's reaction to stoma and level of participation.
- Document your evaluation of patient and family caregiver learning.
- Report abnormalities in stoma or peristomal skin and absence of urinary output to nurse in charge or health care provider.

Special Considerations
Teaching

- Follow teaching considerations in Skill 36.1.
- Teach patients significance and importance of drinking 2 quarts of fluid daily to prevent urinary tract infections (UTIs) (Carmel et al., 2016). Explain that some mucus in urine is expected but patients should report any blood in their urine, excessively cloudy urine, chills, fever (38.3°C [101°F] or higher), and back (flank) pain to their health care provider.

Pediatric

- In neonates urinary diversions are less common than fecal ostomies.
- Select pediatric pouches designed especially for neonates, infants, and children; these pouches are smaller and have a more skin-sensitive adhesive on the barrier.

Gerontological

- Follow gerontological considerations in Skill 36.1.
- Older patients have decreased thirst and may not normally consume adequate fluids. Explain importance of fluid intake to promote healthy renal function and decrease risk for UTIs.

Home Care

- Follow home care considerations in Skill 36.1.
- Instruct patient that pouch can be connected to straight drainage at night. Make sure that patient understands that adapter will be needed to connect pouch to the bedside drainage bag (see Fig. 36.12).

◆ SKILL 36.3   Catheterizing a Urinary Diversion

Catheterization of a urinary diversion is the only method to obtain an accurate culture and sensitivity specimen to screen a patient for infection. When it is necessary to obtain a urine specimen from a urinary diversion, the best method is to insert a sterile catheter into the stoma. Obtaining a specimen of urine in a pouch does not provide an accurate finding because of the likely risk for contamination by microorganisms growing in the stagnant urine. With the use of strict aseptic technique, catheterization is relatively safe and easy. If a patient uses a two-piece system, remove the pouch from the skin barrier and replace it after catheterization without disturbing the skin barrier. If a patient uses a one-piece system, you have to remove the pouch to obtain the specimen and replace it with a new pouch after the procedure. To prevent trauma to the tissues, you need to understand how the stoma and implanted ureters are constructed for a patient (see Fig. 36.3).

Delegation and Collaboration

The skill of catheterizing a urinary diversion cannot be delegated to nursing assistive personnel (NAP). The nurse directs the NAP to:

- Inform nurse if patient complains of peristomal or flank pain (sign of kidney infection).
- Inform nurse if there is a change in color, odor, or amount of urine or if there is blood in the urine.

Equipment

- Urinary catheterization supplies (contained in prepackaged sterile catheter kit or may need to be gathered separately):
- 14- to 16-Fr sterile catheter
- Water-soluble lubricant
- Antiseptic swabs (e.g., povidone-iodine or chlorhexidine)
- Sterile gloves
- Sterile specimen container
- Absorbent gauze wick
- Bed protection barrier
- Towels
- Urinary pouch if needed
- Clean gloves

STEP	RATIONALE

ASSESSMENT

1. Identify patient using at least two identifiers (e.g., name and birthday or name and medical record number), according to agency policy.	Ensures patient safety. Complies with The Joint Commission standards and improves patient safety (TJC, 2016).
2. Observe for signs and symptoms of urinary tract infection (UTI): elevated temperature, chills, foul-smelling urine, and elevated white blood cell (WBC) count.	Determines need to perform catheterization to obtain sterile specimen from urinary diversion. Having urinary diversion poses risk for reflux of urine back to kidneys, resulting in infection.
3. Obtain health care provider's order for catheterization.	Invasive procedure requires health care provider's order.
4. Assess patient's understanding of need for procedure and how it is done.	Determines willingness to cooperate and reduces patient's anxiety.

NURSING DIAGNOSES

- Deficient knowledge regarding catheterization procedure
- Risk for infection
- Risk for injury: urinary tract

Related factors/Risk factors are individualized based on patient's condition or needs.

PLANNING

1. Expected outcomes following completion of procedure: • Urine specimen is not contaminated with bacteria during procedure.	Urine obtained correctly. Laboratory results are accurate.
• Patient describes risks for infection and techniques to prevent infection.	Demonstrates patient's learning.
2. Assemble equipment and close room curtain or door.	Optimizes use of time and provides privacy.
3. Explain procedure to patient, including sensations that will be felt. If possible, obtain specimen when patient is due to change pouch if using one-piece system.	Lessens anxiety and promotes patient's cooperation. Cleaning stoma and surrounding skin may cause cool sensation. Insertion of catheter may cause sensation of mild pressure, or it may not be felt at all. Changing pouch too frequently could result in skin trauma.

STEP	RATIONALE

IMPLEMENTATION

1. If possible, position patient sitting and drape towel across lower abdomen.

   Gravity facilitates flow of urine. Maintains patient's dignity. Towel absorbs urine.

2. Perform hand hygiene and apply clean gloves.

   Reduces transmission of microorganisms.

3. Remove pouch. If patient uses two-piece system, remove pouch but leave barrier attached to skin.

   Allows access to stoma.

4. Remove gloves and perform hand hygiene.

   Avoids contamination.

5. Open sterile catheterization set according to instructions or open needed equipment and place on sterile barrier using aseptic technique (see Chapter 9). If not using catheterization kit, place gauze pad on sterile field and squeeze small amount of lubricant onto gauze. Apply sterile gloves.

   Prepares sterile work field.

6. If needed, have patient hold absorbent gauze wick on stoma while you prepare catheterization supplies.

   Prevents leakage of urine on peristomal skin, linens, and clothing.

7. Clean surface of stoma with antiseptic swabs using circular motion from center outward. Use new swab each time; repeat twice. Allow chlorhexidine antiseptic to dry or wipe off excess antiseptic with dry sterile gauze or cotton ball.

   Removes surface bacteria. Chlorhexidene must dry to achieve antibacterial effect

Clinical Decision Point *If patient has stents in place, use antiseptic swab to clean the ends of the stents and place the stents in the sterile cup. Allow urine to drip into the cup until you obtain an adequate amount for a specimen. Then go directly to Step 13.*

8. Remove lid from sterile specimen container.

   Sterile container collects small volume of urine.

9. Lubricate tip of catheter with water-soluble lubricant, keeping catheter sterile.

   Facilitates passage of catheter through stoma.

10. With dominant hand gently insert catheter tip into stoma. Do not force catheter; redirect course as needed. Place distal end of catheter into specimen container. Have patient cough; massage abdomen near stoma or turn on his or her side.

    Use care to avoid trauma to conduit.
    Movement and coughing may facilitate flow of urine from conduit.

11. Hold container below level of stoma. If needed, wait several minutes to get adequate amount of urine.

    Culture and sensitivity studies only require 3 to 5 mL of urine (check agency policy).

12. Withdraw catheter slowly; place absorbent pad over stoma.

    Keeps skin dry.

13. Apply lid to specimen container.

    Prevents accidental spillage.

14. Reapply new pouch or reattach pouch if patient uses two-piece system (see Skill 36.2).

    Pouch is necessary to contain urine.

15. Dispose of used pouch and equipment properly.

    Avoids unpleasant odor in room.

16. Remove gloves; perform hand hygiene. Label specimen in presence of patient, place in biohazard bag, and send to laboratory at once.

    Ensures that laboratory results are assigned to correct patient. Labeling ensures acceptance and processing of specimen by laboratory. Urine that sits for long periods at room temperature will adversely affect laboratory results.

EVALUATION

1. Compare results of culture and sensitivity with expected findings. Mucus is normal finding if patient has ileal conduit.

   Determines presence of infection. If contamination appears likely, second specimen will be needed.

2. **Use Teach-Back:** "I want to be sure you understand the reason we needed to collect the urine. Tell me in your own words why we did this procedure to get urine from your stoma. What are the signs of a urinary tract infection when you have a urostomy?" Revise your instruction now or develop a plan for revised patient or family caregiver teaching if patient or family caregiver is not able to teach back correctly.

   Determines patient's and family caregiver's level of understanding of instructional topic.

Unexpected Outcomes

1. Unable to obtain urine specimen.

2. Skin or stoma reveals complications.

Related Interventions

- Reposition patient.
- If there is still no urine, push fluids and try again later.
- Inform health care provider if unable to obtain specimen on second attempt.
- Notify nurse and/or health care provider.
- Consult with ostomy care nurse about pouching system or skin barrier to use.

Recording and Reporting

- Record time specimen collected; patient's tolerance of procedure; and appearance of urine, skin, and stoma in the electronic record (EHR) or chart.
- Document your evaluation of patient and family caregiver learning.
- Report results of laboratory test to nurse in charge or health care provider.

Special Considerations
Teaching

- Explain common symptoms of UTI: flank pain, dark or bloody urine, foul-smelling urine, fever (38.3°C [101°F] or higher), confusion to patient and family caregiver.
- Encourage patient to notify health care provider if symptoms of infection develop.
- Reinforce importance of fluid intake (2 L/day).

♦ CLINICAL DEBRIEF

You are assigned to care for a 28-year-old fashion designer with a 10-year history of ulcerative colitis with an increase in bleeding, pain, and frequent episodes of diarrhea. Her health care provider has tried to control her symptoms with medications, but this has been unsuccessful in the last year. She has been admitted to the hospital for a colectomy with ileal pouch anal anastomosis and J-pouch construction (see Fig. 36.4). She will have a temporary ileostomy. An ostomy nurse has been consulted for stoma site marking and preoperative education.

1. Why is the consultation necessary?
2. When the patient returns from surgery, the nurse assesses her abdomen and finds that it is firm and distended, which would be expected after abdominal surgery. She has several sites on her abdomen where the laparoscopes were inserted; each has been closed with two staples, and no dressings are present on these sites. An ostomy pouch is placed on the right side of her abdomen. The stoma is visible through this pouch; it is red and round and protrudes above the abdomen. No output is present in the pouch. Using SBAR, show how the nurse communicates her assessment with the other health care providers.
3. On the first postoperative day Julie asks how often her pouch should be emptied and how frequently it will have to be changed. What should you tell her?

♦ REVIEW QUESTIONS

1. The nurse has inserted a catheter into a patient's urinary stoma, but only a few drops of urine have drained. Which actions should the nurse perform to try to obtain an adequate sample? (Select all that apply.)
   1. Remove the catheter and obtain urine from the pouch.
   2. Gently insert the catheter further into the stoma.
   3. Massage the patient's abdomen.
   4. Have the patient turn on his or her side.
   5. Attempt to intubate the stoma with a larger-size catheter.
2. A recent postoperative patient with an ileostomy notes a raw, weeping area of the skin around the stoma. Which actions are most appropriate in this situation? (Select all that apply.)
   1. Cleaning the area with alcohol to help dry the raw skin
   2. Consulting an ostomy care nurse
   3. Reviewing the pouch change procedure with the patient
   4. Having the patient continue his or her usual skin care regimen of cleaning gently with water and placing the pouch over the raw, moist skin
   5. Recommending that the patient measure the stoma again and cut a new pattern because the stoma may have changed size since surgery

3. Place the steps for an ostomy pouch change in the correct order.
   1. Close the end of the pouch.
   2. Measure the stoma.
   3. Cut the hole in the wafer.
   4. Press the pouch into place over the stoma.
   5. Remove the old pouch.
   6. Trace the correct measurement onto the back of the wafer.
   7. Observe the stoma and the skin around it.
   8. Clean and dry the peristomal skin.

ⓔ *Visit the Evolve site for a complete list of Clinical Debrief and Review Questions answers.*

REFERENCES

American Cancer Society (ACS): *Colostomy: a guide*, Atlanta, GA, 2016a, ACS. http://www.cancer.org/treatment/treatmentsandsideeffects/physicalsideeffects/ostomies/colostomyguide/index. Accessed March 6, 2016.

American Cancer Society (ACS): *Ileostomy*, Atlanta, GA, 2016b, ACS. http://www.cancer.org/treatment/treatmentsandsideeffects/physicalsideeffects/ostomies/ileostomyguide/index. Accessed March 6, 2016.

American Cancer Society (ACS): *Urostomy*, Atlanta, GA, 2016c, ACS. http://www.cancer.org/treatment/treatmentsandsideeffects/physicalsideeffects/ostomies/urostomyguide/index. Accessed March 6, 2016.

Bookout K, et al: *Pediatric ostomy care: best practice for clinicians*, Mt Laurel, NJ, 2011, WOCN.

Carmel JE, et al, editors: *Wound, Ostomy, Continence Nurses Society Core Curriculum: ostomy management*, Philadelphia, PA, 2016, Wolters Kluwer.

Coca C, et al: The impact of specialty nursing care on health-related quality of life in persons with ostomies, *J Wound Ostomy Continence Nurs* 42(3):257, 2015.

Person R, et al: The impact of preoperative stoma site marking on the incidence of complications, quality of life, and patient's independence, *Dis Colon Rectum* 55(7):783, 2012.

Riemenschneider K: Uncertainty and adaptation among adults living with incontinent ostomies, *J Wound Ostomy Continence Nurs* 42(4):361, 2015.

Salvadena G: The incidence of stoma and peristomal complications during the first 3 months after ostomy creation, *J Wound Ostomy Continence Nurs* 40(4):400, 2013.

Salvadena G, et al: WOCN Society and ASCRS position statement on preoperative stoma site marking for patients undergoing colostomy or ileostomy surgery, *J Wound Ostomy Continence Nurs* 42(3):249, 2015a.

Salvadena G, et al: WOCN Society and AUA position statement on preoperative stoma site marking for patients undergoing urostomy surgery, *J Wound Ostomy Continence Nurs* 42(3):253, 2015b.

The Joint Commission (TJC): *2016 Critical Access Hospital—National Patient Safety Goals*, http://www.jointcommission.org/standards_information/npsgs.aspx. Accessed December 27, 2015.

WCET International Ostomy Guideline, World Council of Enterostomal Therapists, June, 2014, http://www.wcetn.org/assets/Publications/wcet_april-june_2014f%20iog%20recommandations.pdf. Accessed February 8, 2016.

37 | Preoperative and Postoperative Care

SKILLS AND PROCEDURES

Skill 37.1 **Preoperative Assessment, p. 947**

Skill 37.2 **Preoperative Teaching, p. 951**

Skill 37.3 **Physical Preparation for Surgery, p. 960**

Skill 37.4 **Providing Immediate Anesthesia Recovery in the Postanesthesia Care Unit, p. 964**

Skill 37.5 **Providing Early Postoperative and Convalescent Phase Recovery, p. 972**

OBJECTIVES

Mastery of content in this chapter will enable the nurse to:

- Explain how to integrate patient-centered care into preoperative and postoperative care.
- Describe the physical preparations needed for a patient facing surgery.
- Identify risk factors that have a potential for affecting a patient's clinical outcomes postoperatively.
- Discuss cultural differences that might affect the implementation of preoperative and postoperative procedures.

- Describe the benefits of structured preoperative teaching.
- Explain the rationale for each of the postoperative exercises.
- Successfully teach a patient to perform postoperative exercises.
- Discuss the differences in nursing assessment during the immediate postoperative period and the convalescent phase of recovery.
- Conduct an assessment of a postoperative patient.

MEDIA RESOURCES

- evolve http://evolve.elsevier.com/Perry/nursinginterventions
- Audio Glossary
- Checklists
- Case Studies

- Review Questions
- ▶ Video Clips
- Clinical Debrief and Review Questions Answers

PURPOSE

Surgical care of patients is in a continuous state of technological advancement. As a result, patients have shortened lengths of stay because of less invasive surgery and less time spent in a hospital. During the preoperative phase the nursing role focuses on physical, psychological, sociocultural, and spiritual preparation while also validating existing information, reinforcing patient education, and providing nursing care to prepare the patient and significant other for the surgical experience (ASPAN, 2015). During the postoperative phase, when a patient returns from the operating room (OR), the nurse initially is responsible for completing a thorough assessment of the patient's physical and mental status while also providing continuous monitoring of his or her condition and ongoing education during the recovery process.

STANDARDS OF CARE

- Association of PeriOperative Nurses (AORN), 2012, 2015— Perioperative Nursing Practice Standards; Interprofessional Collaboration, Communication and Handoff Report; Patient Education

- American Society of PeriAnesthesia Nurses (ASPAN), 2015— Interprofessional Collaboration, Communication and Hand-Off Report
- The Joint Commission (TJC), 2016—Prevention Postoperative Infections; Safe Medication Administration in Perioperative Patients; Safe Patient Identification

PRINCIPLES FOR PRACTICE

- A variety of diagnostic tests are coordinated before surgery to ensure that the surgeon and anesthesia care providers have the information needed to determine a patient's risks during surgery and the postoperative period.
- The American Society of PeriAnesthesia Nurses (ASPAN, 2015; Schick and Windle, 2016) identifies levels of care provided to the surgical/procedural patient, including preprocedure, postanesthesia phase I, postanesthesia phase II, and extended care. Once a patient's condition stabilizes, the nurse focuses efforts on returning the patient to a functional level of wellness as soon as possible within the limitations created by surgery.
- The speed of a patient's recovery depends on how effectively the nurse anticipates potential complications, initiates necessary

supportive and preventive therapies, and actively involves the patient and family in the recovery process.

- Preoperative and postoperative patient education improves outcomes after surgery. The shift in how surgical services are now provided poses special challenges to meet patients' educational needs in a reduced time frame. Because a majority of patients undergo surgery in an ambulatory setting, it is essential that they receive adequate information to ensure that they or their family caregivers can manage postoperative care activities in the home setting.
- American Society of PeriAnesthesia Nurses (ASPAN, 2015) advocates for an ethical culture of accountability and safety with a systems analysis approach when exploring errors and unsafe practice. In addition, the society encourages reviewing errors/unsafe practices in a nonpunitive manner.

PATIENT-CENTERED CARE

- Engaging and involving patients and their significant others in their care results in safer and more patient-centered care (Spruce, 2015).
- To provide culturally competent care to a surgical patient, the nurse should begin by assessing the family to determine not only who should be involved but also who legally is responsible for making decisions and giving consent for surgery.
- To better understand the culture and needs of the patient, the nurse may be required to request very specific information from the patient, family, or religious leader.
- When providing preoperative teaching, include family caregivers. The use of professional interpreters for patients who do not speak English is beneficial and necessary in providing competent informed patient care.
- Before surgery it is important to accommodate a patient's religious and cultural needs and adapt the patient's care to encompass his or her practices and beliefs whenever possible. Identify cultural and religious beliefs and practices that may affect patients' and/or family caregivers' reactions to the surgical experience such as diet; pain; blood transfusions; and disposal of body parts, including hair.
- Both before and after surgery it will be helpful to assess patient preferences for pain medication. Many patients believe that pain medication leads to addiction and will attempt to endure the pain without medication. Cultures that value men being in control of their emotions may prevent members from verbalizing pain.
- Some religions and/or cultures may request to wear articles such as jewelry, medallions, or undergarments. To accommodate the needs and deliver patient-centered care, nurses may need to allow such articles (e.g., medals, underclothing) to be worn until just before surgery. If articles are removed, nurses must ensure that they are returned promptly after surgery.

EVIDENCE-BASED PRACTICE

Recent evidence-based research (Magill et al., 2014) estimates that 4% of all inpatients in acute care agencies in the United States develop hospital-associated infections. In this study of 183 hospitals, approximately 648,000 patients developed hospital-associated infections. The most prevalent infections noted were surgical site infections (SSIs) (21.8%), pneumonia (21.8%), gastrointestinal infections (17.1%), and device-related infections (25.6%).

Evidence-based guidelines have been identified to reduce SSIs (CDC, 2015; Diaz and Newman, 2015; Magill et al., 2014):

- Follow Centers for Disease Control and Prevention (CDC, 2015) guidelines for proper hand hygiene and cleaning and disinfection of equipment.
- Do not remove hair unless it will interfere with the operation and remove it using only electric clippers if possible.
- Give the correct antibiotic before surgery and at the appropriate time.
- Maintain blood glucose level after surgery, especially for patients undergoing cardiac surgery.
- Maintain normothermia (core temperature range of 36°C to 38°C [96.8°F to 100.4°F]).
- Patients receiving beta-blocker medication before surgery must maintain their regimen throughout the perioperative period.
- Follow proper insertion and maintenance practices for all devices inserted (e.g., foley catheters, intravenous lines).
- Insert urinary catheter devices only when necessary and leave them in only as long as is necessary.

There are also strict guidelines for use of antibiotics (Diaz and Newman, 2015). The goal of prophylactic antibiotic therapy is to select the most effective antibiotics for maximum coverage and administer them when they are most beneficial to protect patients from infection with as little risk as possible:

- Overall it is recommended that prophylactic antibiotics be given as close to the time of incision as possible (within 60 minutes) and not be given for longer than 24 hours after surgery.
- Vancomycin and fluoroquinolones (i.e., ciprofloxacin, levofloxacin) may be given up to 2 hours before incision because of their longer infusion times. Antibiotic use after incision closure does not reduce infection rates; and, when the antibiotics are continued, infections are more likely to be caused by a resistant organism (CDC, 2015).
- Prophylactic antibiotics should be discontinued within 24 hours after the end of surgery in most cases.

SAFETY GUIDELINES

- Know the type and nature of any previous surgery. Anatomical and physiological alterations affect a patient's risk for operative problems.
- Identify the factors and conditions that increase a patient's risks during surgery. Preoperative preparation and postoperative care depend on knowledge of these risk factors.
- Know the rationale for and extent of impending surgery. Each type of surgical procedure requires a different type of nursing care and allows you to anticipate potential complications correctly.
- Ensure that the patient has signed the informed consent. Although the nurse is witnessing a patient's signature only and not his or her knowledge, there is an obligation to advocate for the patient should the patient and/or family not be fully informed about the surgical procedure. Informed consent is required by law to help protect patient's rights, their autonomy, and their privacy. The surgeon should give the patient information about the extent and type of surgery; alternative therapies; and usual risks, benefits, and consequences of not having surgery. See agency policy regarding consent (Table 37.1).
- Complete the preoperative checklist. Include the global initiative of the World Health Organization (WHO) Surgical Safety Checklist (WHO, 2008).
- Administer pain-relief therapies according to a patient's perioperative needs. Pain can slow a surgical patient's recovery.
- Restrict patient activity after administration of preoperative and postoperative sedatives to minimize the risk for patient falls.

TABLE 37.1

Information Needed for Informed Consent

Parameters	Examples
Name of procedure/surgery	Abdominal hysterectomy under general anesthesia
Description of procedure/surgery	Removal of uterus only through an incision in the abdominal wall at the top of the pubic hairline; done while unconscious
Person performing procedure/surgery	Dr. Richard Jones assisted by Dr. William Smith
Benefits of procedure/surgery	To remove uterus with fibroids and stop excessive bleeding Abdominal route necessary because of anticipated adhesions from prior abdominal surgery
Potential risks and adverse effects of procedure/surgery	Risk of hemorrhage and infection from surgery; risk of excessive sedation and allergic reaction to drugs used with general anesthesia; accidental damage to bladder, intestines, and/or nerves controlling these organs
Approximate length of time for procedure/surgery	About 1 hour; 1 to 2 hours in postanesthesia care unit (PACU)
Approximate length of time needed for recovery	3 to 4 days on surgical unit; 4 to 6 weeks before resuming physically stressful work
Alternative treatments	Removal of uterus vaginally; radiation to shrink fibroids
Consequences of refusing treatment	Continuation of pain and vaginal bleeding, risk for developing anemia; after menopause fibroids should regress

◆ SKILL 37.1   Preoperative Assessment

A thorough preoperative nursing assessment of a patient's physiological and psychological condition allows a nurse to identify patient risks and plan for care during and after surgery. The assessment documents baseline data for future comparisons to determine the effect of instruction and whether complications develop during the perioperative period. Many health care agencies have a designated department devoted to completing thorough preoperative screening and testing. Laboratory tests, electrocardiograms (ECGs), chest x-ray films, and other tests are often obtained in these agencies 1 to 2 weeks in advance of the scheduled surgical procedure. Perioperative staff performs a thorough assessment and reviews the test results to identify any potential abnormalities that may need further evaluation and treatment before surgery.

The nurse assesses patients again 1 to 2 hours before the scheduled time of surgery to ensure that there are no changes to their medical condition. Advanced planning allows time for nurses to follow up on any unexpected outcomes. Before beginning this assessment, establish a trusting relationship with the patient. It is not unusual for the patient to remember and report at this time facts that were not previously told to the surgeon. Provide the patient privacy and a location free of interruption to encourage open communication. Initiate a preprocedure check list, beginning with the decision to perform a procedure, maintained with ongoing

data collection and assessment, and verified immediately before moving the patient to the procedure room (TJC, 2016). Typically the surgeon, anesthetist, or nurse completes an assessment and the patient signs a consent form. Current test results and notices of any special considerations during the procedure such as a need for blood products or special equipment should be available.

Delegation and Collaboration

The skill of preoperative assessment cannot be delegated to nursing assistive personnel (NAP). The nurse instructs the NAP to:
- Obtain vital signs and weight and height measurements.

Equipment
- Stethoscope
- Blood pressure monitoring equipment
- Pulse oximetry
- Thermometer
- Watch or clock with a second hand
- Method to measure height and weight
- Access to laboratory, ECG, x-ray films, and other diagnostic equipment as needed
- Preprocedure checklist
- Preoperative assessment form

STEP	RATIONALE

ASSESSMENT

1. Identify patient using at least two identifiers (e.g., name and birthday or name and medical record number), according to agency policy.

Ensures correct patient. Complies with The Joint Commission standards and improves patient safety (TJC, 2016).

2. Perform hand hygiene. Prepare equipment and room for assessment.

Reduces transmission of infection. Makes assessment more efficient.

3. Determine if patient has any communication impairment (e.g., blindness, hearing loss), is able to read and understand English, and is mentally competent. For example, give patient an informational brochure and have him or her explain part of the contents. Obtain a professional interpreter if needed.

Patient may not fully comprehend a diagnosis, understand proposed treatment, or effectively consider alternatives that are presented without effective communication. Relying on a family member as an interpreter cannot guarantee the accuracy of explanations.

STEP	RATIONALE
4. Assess patient's understanding of the intended surgery and anesthesia. Ask patient to offer a description rather than asking a simple yes or no question (e.g., "Tell me in your own words what your surgery will involve "). Ask about patient's and family caregiver's expectations of surgery and care. Include questions concerning fears, cultural practices, and religious beliefs if applicable.	Patients may have misconceptions and incomplete knowledge. Asking about fears, cultural practices, and religious beliefs allows you to anticipate priorities of patient and family caregiver and adapt your plan so you can give appropriate instruction and support.
5. Ask if patient has an advance directive (see Chapter 17).	Advance directives protect patient's rights by communicating patient's treatment preferences if he or she is unable to communicate.
6. Collect nursing history and identify surgical risk factors:	Allows for anticipation of possible complications and planning for interventions to reduce patient risks.

Clinical Decision Point *If patient is having emergency surgery, focus on assessment of primary body system affected.*

a. Condition requiring surgery.	Allows you to anticipate postoperative needs and possible complications.
b. Chronic illnesses and associated risks (e.g., hypertension—bleeding, and stroke; postoperative respiratory depression and arrest; asthma—impaired ventilation; hiatal hernia—aspiration; diabetes mellitus—poor wound healing; methicillin-resistant *Staphylococcus aureus*—impaired wound healing and sepsis).	Some chronic conditions increase risk of complications from surgery and anesthesia.
c. Determine if patient has obstructive sleep apnea (OSA). Many agencies use the STOP-Bang assessment tool: STOP • Do you SNORE loudly (louder than talking or loud enough to be heard through closed doors)? • Do you often feel TIRED, fatigued, or sleepy during the daytime? • Has anyone OBSERVED you stop breathing during your sleep? • Do you have or are you being treated for high blood PRESSURE? BANG • BMI more than 35 kg/m^2 • AGE over 50 years old • NECK circumference >16 inches (40 cm) • GENDER: Male *Any question answered *Yes* is a risk factor	In the surgical population, a STOP-Bang score of 5–8 identifies patients with high probability of moderate/severe obstructive sleep apnea (OSA). The STOP-Bang score helps the health care team to stratify patients for unrecognized OSA, practice perioperative precautions, or triage patients for diagnosis and treatment (Chung et al., 2016). Patients with OSA will require special anesthesia precautions. Patients with OSA are often sensitive to sedative medications, especially if the OSA is untreated. Even minimal sedation can cause airway obstruction and ventilatory arrest, thus requiring close monitoring postoperatively (Ogan and Plevak, n.d.)
d. Last menstrual period (for female patients in childbearing years).	Anesthetic agents and other medications could injure fetus.
e. Previous hospitalizations.	Determines if patient is familiar with hospital procedures.
f. Full medication history, including prescription, over-the-counter (OTC), and herbal remedies and date and time of last doses.	Patient may not report OTC medications and herbal remedies unless specifically asked. All may interact with anesthetic agents or other medications given during surgery. Patient may be instructed to take any routine blood pressure, cardiac, or seizure medications. Changes in dosages of oral diabetic agents or insulin may be ordered.
g. Previous experience with surgery and anesthesia; have patient clarify if any undesirable outcomes occurred.	Information helps to prevent recurrent problems with planned surgery.
h. Family history of complications from surgery or anesthesia.	Family history of reactions to anesthetic agents may indicate familial condition such as malignant hyperthermia, which is life threatening.
i. Allergies to medications, food, or tape, including specific questions about natural rubber latex. Ask patients if they have had any problem with medication or anything placed on their skin.	Allergies to medications or latex can be life threatening. Prevention of latex allergy in sensitized patients requires specific precautions. Often patients with latex allergies are scheduled as first case of the day. In addition, many patients do not understand that rubber and latex are the same. Using both words helps obtain accurate information.

STEP	RATIONALE
j. Physical impairment (e.g., paralysis, reduced range of motion of extremity).	Physical impairments may cause limited mobility and situations that could lead to problems with positioning and risk for pressure injury formation. Communicate this information to the operating room (OR) nurse because these patients may need special positioning or OR bed surfaces.
k. Prostheses and implants (e.g., implantable medication-delivery pump, dentures, hearing aid, pacemaker, internal defibrillator, hip prosthesis).	These devices could become damaged or malfunction from electrical equipment used during surgery. Report this information to the OR nurse.
l. Smoking, alcohol, and drug use.	Preoperative alcohol consumption is associated with an increased risk of general postoperative morbidity, general infections, wound complications, pulmonary complications, prolonged stay at the hospital, and admission to an intensive care unit (Eliasen et al, 2013). Preoperative use of illicit drugs can lead to pulmonary complications, poor pain control, and withdrawal symptoms. Smoking can lead to cardiopulmonary complications.
m. Occupation.	Anticipates how postoperative restrictions will affect patient's return to work.
7. Obtain patient's weight, height, and vital signs (see Chapters 5 and 6).	Height and weight are used to calculate drug dosages. Vital signs provide a baseline for postoperative comparison.

Clinical Decision Point *Many patients with OSA are morbidly obese, placing them at increased risk for aspiration of acidic gastric fluid at the time of induction of anesthesia. For this reason, many of these patients receive medications to suppress gastric acid production, neutralize the acid, or stimulate emptying of the stomach. Consult with physician regarding order for acid-suppressing medication*

8. Assess patient's respiratory status, including auscultation of lungs, adventitious sounds, character and rate of respirations, oxygen saturation, ability to breathe lying flat, use of oxygen or continuous positive airway pressure (CPAP) at home, and chest x-ray film report.	Poor respiratory condition can affect patient's response to general anesthesia. Use of CPAP may indicate that patient has OSA, a condition that poses risks after surgery.
9. Auscultate heart sounds and evaluate patient's circulatory status, including apical pulse, ECG report, and peripheral pulses (see Chapter 6).	Screens for possible cardiac problems that may contraindicate surgery. Circulation may be factor in positioning patient on OR table.
10. Assess for patient's risk for postoperative thrombus formation (e.g., older adults, immobilized patients, patients with personal or family history of blood clots, use of birth control pills, hormones). Ask patient about any leg pain. Observe calves for swelling, warmth, and redness; observe calves for symmetry; and palpate pedal pulses.	Circulation slows after general anesthesia, increasing tendency for blood clot formation. Immobilization during surgical procedure promotes venous stasis. Manipulation and positioning can cause accidental trauma to leg veins.

Clinical Decision Point *Homans' sign is not always present when a deep vein thrombosis (DVT) exists (Schick and Windle, 2016). If you suspect a thrombus, notify the surgeon and refrain from manipulating the extremity any further. Surgery will usually need to be postponed. Antiembolism stockings or venous flexus foot pump (Fig. 37.1) may be ordered for patients at risk for thrombus formation (see Chapter 12).*

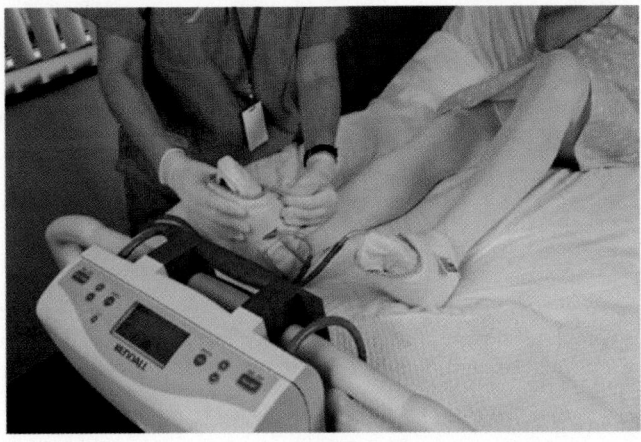

FIG 37.1 Venous plexus foot pump with bedside controls. (*Courtesy Tyco Healthcare Group LP.*)

STEP	RATIONALE
11. Complete a gastrointestinal assessment; identify time of patient's last intake of food or drink (see Chapter 6).	With patient under general anesthesia, the esophageal sphincter relaxes, and the stomach contents can be aspirated.
12. Complete neurological assessment; determine patient's neurological status, including level of consciousness (LOC), cognitive function, and sensation, and note neurological deficits (see Chapter 6).	Patient's neurological status affects attentiveness to instruction. Offers important baseline for postoperative evaluation.
13. Assess patient's musculoskeletal system, including range of motion (ROM) of joints (see Chapter 6).	If range of motion (ROM) is limited, extra care is needed to prevent injury related to positioning in surgery.
14. Examine patient's skin; identify any breaks in skin integrity and determine level of hydration (see Chapter 6). Pay particular attention to area of body on which patient will be positioned.	If skin is thin, broken, or bruised, extra padding is needed in surgery. Hydration may affect skin integrity.
15. Assess patient's emotional status, including level of anxiety, coping ability, and family caregiver support. Assess potential for abuse from a partner or family member.	If patient has high level of anxiety or fear, consultation with social worker, pastoral care, or advanced practice nurse might be useful.
16. Review results of laboratory tests, including complete blood count, electrolytes, urinalysis, and other diagnostic tests.	Laboratory work provides an assessment of major body systems.

NURSING DIAGNOSES

- Deficient knowledge regarding preoperative plan of care
- Risk for impaired skin integrity
- Risk for infection
- Risk for perioperative positioning Injury

Related factors/Risk factors are individualized based on patient's condition or needs.

PLANNING

1. Expected outcomes following completion of procedure:	
• Patient provides appropriate preoperative information required to establish plan of care.	Identifies patient's knowledge of preoperative plan of care.
• Patient remains alert and appropriately responsive to assessment questions.	Identifies patient readiness to learn.
• Patient does not incur any injury during preoperative preparation in OR.	Precautions taken as a result of assessment findings prevent positional and skin injury.

IMPLEMENTATION

1. Communicate to preoperative team risk factors that have the potential for making the patient vulnerable to complications intraoperatively.	Limitations in mobility and sensation should affect how patient is positioned for surgery. Presence of OSA and any cardiopulmonary abnormalities can influence anesthesia approach.

Clinical Decision Point *Even though the surgeon and anesthesia provider will conduct separate assessment, your findings may reveal surgical risk factors not identified previously.*

2. Based on the patient's cognitive status, experience, and nature of planned surgery, present preoperative instruction to patient and family caregiver (see Skill 37.2).	Assessment findings influence approach to instructions and topics to discuss.

EVALUATION

1. Determine if patient information is complete so plan of care can be established. Validate unclear information with family caregiver.	Provides preoperative baseline of assessment data.
2. Evaluate patient's ability to cooperate (e.g., makes eye contact, answers appropriately).	Establishes patient's ability to participate in assessment.

STEP	RATIONALE
3. **Use Teach-Back**: "I want to be sure I explained what you need to know about your intended surgery and anesthesia. Tell me when your surgery is scheduled and the reason you are having surgery." Revise your instruction now or develop a plan for revised patient or family caregiver teaching if patient or family caregiver is not able to teach back correctly.	Determines patient's and family caregiver's level of understanding of instructional topic.

Unexpected Outcomes	**Related Interventions**
1. Patient does not understand what surgery will be performed.	• Notify surgeon.
2. Patient reports allergy to latex.	• Remove all supplies containing latex from patient's room.
	• Post latex precautions sign one door or stretcher.
	• Notify surgeon, anesthesia provider, and OR nurse.

Recording and Reporting

- Document findings on the preoperative part of the nurses' detailed preoperative notes or other designated agency form in electronic health record (EHR) or chart.
- Report abnormal laboratory values or other concerns to the surgeon or anesthesiologist.
- Document your evaluation of patient and family caregiver learning.

Special Considerations
Pediatric

- Consider a child's developmental level when performing preoperative assessment and preoperative preparation (e.g., use stories, films, books, tours, toys, and games) (Hockenberry and Wilson, 2015).

Gerontological

- Age-related changes may result in diminished short-term memory. Additional assessment and teaching may be necessary.
- An older adult may have some limitation in ROM. If this limitation is significant, notify the OR nurse so surgical position can be modified.

 SKILL 37.2   Preoperative Teaching

▶ *Video Clip*

With shortened hospital lengths of stay and growth in ambulatory surgical procedures, there is a greater demand for patient preparation and support. Patient education must go beyond simply providing information because patients and families must be prepared to assume more preoperative and postoperative responsibilities. Preoperative patient teaching involves helping a patient understand and prepare mentally for the surgical experience. Effective education focuses on each patient's individual needs and leads to empowered patients who have sufficient knowledge that meets their needs, expectations, or preferences.

In the past patients received preoperative teaching the day or evening before surgery when patients were most anxious. Health care cost reduction practices now have most patients entering the hospital or ambulatory care center the morning of surgery. Preoperative teaching is not effective at this time because of patient anxiety and stress related to surgical preparation (Stannard and Krenzischek, 2012). Many health care agencies now provide outpatient education programs to prepare patients and their family caregivers for a specific surgery. For example, patients who require a total knee replacement go to preoperative preparation classes with other patients requiring the same surgery. Effective preoperative teaching increases patient satisfaction, promotes psychological well-being, and may decrease complications leading to an increased length of stay (Lewis et al., 2017). Plan your teaching based on the preoperative assessment. Make every attempt to ensure the patient's privacy. Select the best learning method for the patient. In many settings videotape and written materials are available to help you. Whenever possible, have the family caregivers responsible for the patient's care after surgery present. Later the family caregivers serve as coaches and help the patient perform exercises. Plan to have the patient demonstrate expected postoperative skills to allow for practice and facilitate understanding.

Patients and their families are often anxious about impending surgery, which hinders learning. Speak in a clear, slow voice to reduce the patient's anxiety and promote understanding. You may need extra time for teaching and reinforcement to ensure patient understanding. After surgery high anxiety can lead to negative psychological and physiological outcomes. Preoperative information about expected perioperative sensations decreases the distress associated with surgery. By teaching and setting expectations before surgery (pain level, average length of surgery), the patient and the nurse can make a significant contribution to success in the postoperative recovery phase.

Delegation and Collaboration

The skills of preoperative teaching cannot be delegated to nursing assistive personnel (NAP). NAP can reinforce and help patients perform postoperative exercises. The nurse instructs the NAP about:

- Any precautions or safety issues unique to the patient (e.g., fall precautions, mobility limitations, bleeding precautions, weight-bearing issues, dietary concerns).

- Informing the nurse of any identified concerns (e.g., patient is unable to perform the exercises correctly).

Equipment
- Stretcher or bed
- Pillow
- Incentive spirometer
- Preoperative education flow sheet
- Positive expiratory pressure (PEP) device
- Stethoscope

STEP	RATIONALE

ASSESSMENT

1. Identify patient using at least two identifiers (e.g., name and birthday or name and medical record number), according to agency policy.	Ensures correct patient. Complies with The Joint Commission standards and improves patient safety (TJC, 2016).
2. Ask about patient's previous experiences with surgery and anesthesia.	This allows you to individualize teaching and address specific patient concerns.
3. Determine if patient and family caregiver understand surgery.	This information determines if correction of misunderstanding is necessary.
4. Identify patient's cognitive level, language, and culture. If patient does not speak English, have a professional interpreter to assist you.	These factors may alter patient's ability to understand meaning of surgery and can affect postoperative healing course if there are mixed messages or misunderstanding.
5. Assess patient's risk for postoperative respiratory complications (see Skill 37-1). Check nursing history for patient's height and age.	General anesthesia predisposes patient to respiratory problems (see Chapters 23 and 25). Presence of underlying respiratory conditions or patient's inability to perform postoperative respiratory exercises increases patient's risk for pulmonary complications. Height and age are used to set incentive spirometer parameters.
6. Assess patient's anxiety related to surgery.	Directs you to provide additional emotional support and indicates patient's readiness to learn.
7. Assess family caregiver's willingness to learn and support patient following surgery.	Family caregiver's presence after surgery can be potential motivating factor for patient recovery. In addition, caregiver can coach patient through postoperative exercise and observe for any postoperative problems.
8. Assess patient's medical orders.	Preoperative and postoperative orders often require adaptations in way patient performs exercises.

NURSING DIAGNOSES

- Anxiety
- Deficient knowledge regarding postoperative exercises

Related factors are individualized based on patient's condition or needs.

PLANNING

1. Expected outcomes following completion of procedure:	
• Patient demonstrates eye contact and asks and answers questions appropriately.	Identifies patient's readiness to learn.
• Patient correctly performs splinting, turning and sitting, breathing exercises, and leg exercises.	Patient will be prepared to participate in postoperative exercises following surgery.
• Family identifies location of waiting room and time frame when they can expect status on their family member.	Family anxiety may be reduced with preoperative expectations clearly provided.
• Family caregivers verbalize ability to help prepare patient at home before surgery.	Family caregivers are able to assist patient with necessary preparations before surgery at home.
• Family caregivers provide emotional support for patient before surgery.	Both patient and family have support for surgery.

IMPLEMENTATION

1. Perform hand hygiene. Inform patient and family caregiver of date, time, and location of surgery; anticipated length of surgery; additional time in postanesthesia recovery area; and where to wait.	Reduces transmission of infection. Accurate information helps reduce stress associated with surgery.

STEP	RATIONALE
2. Answer questions patient and family caregiver ask.	Responding to patient and family caregiver questions helps to decrease anxiety and demonstrates your concern for them.
3. Instruct patient about preoperative bowel or skin preparations as needed. Check medical orders and agency policy regarding number of preoperative showers and agent to be used for each shower (2% chlorhexidine gluconate is used most often). Following each preoperative shower, instruct patient to rinse the skin thoroughly and dry with a fresh, clean, dry towel. Patient should don clean clothing.	Proper skin preparation is critical element in preventing surgical site infections (SSIs). Rinsing skin removes residual antiseptic preparation that may cause skin irritation. After use, towels contain microorganisms that can grow in presence of moisture. Using fresh towel after each shower and donning clean clothing minimizes risk of reintroducing microorganisms to clean skin (AORN, 2015; Graling and Vasaly, 2013).
4. Instruct patient about extent and purpose of food and fluid restrictions for period specified before surgery (e.g., no clear liquids at least 2 hours before surgery, no light meal [e.g., toast and a clear liquid] 6 hours or more before surgery, no meat or fried foods 8 hours before surgery, unless otherwise specified by surgeon or anesthesiologist) (ASA, 2011).	During general anesthesia muscles relax; and gastric contents can reflux into esophagus, leading to aspiration. Anesthetic eliminates patient's ability to gag.
5. Describe perioperative routines (e.g., time-out, site marking, intravenous [IV] therapy, urinary catheterization, enema, hair clipping or removal, laboratory tests, transport to operating room [OR]).	Allows patient to anticipate and recognize routine procedures, reducing anxiety.
6. Describe planned effect of preoperative medications.	Provides information about what to expect, decreasing anxiety.
7. Review which routine medications patient needs to discontinue before surgery.	Some medications are discontinued before surgery to minimize effects that can cause surgical risks. For example, anticoagulants may increase bleeding and are usually discontinued several days before surgery. Insulin dosages are usually adjusted because of reduced intake of food before surgery.
8. Describe perioperative sensations (e.g., blood pressure cuff tightening, electrocardiogram [ECG] leads, cool room, and beep of monitor).	Misconceptions and concerns about anesthesia have been ranked high among preoperative patients.
9. Describe pain-control methods to be used after surgery. Many patients have a patient-controlled analgesia (PCA) pump (see Chapter 16).	Patients are fearful of postoperative pain. Explaining pain-management techniques reduces this fear. Establishes what pain is acceptable, knowing that they will not be pain-free, but their pain will be managed.
10. Describe what patient will experience after surgery (e.g., where patient will be on awakening, frequent vital signs, catheters, drains, tubes, alternating pressure from sequential compression device, postoperative exercises).	Provides concrete description of what patient can expect after surgery so patient is prepared.
11. **Teach turning:**	
a. Instruct patient on turning and sitting up (especially suited for abdominal and thoracic surgery):	Promotes circulation and ventilation.
(1) Turn onto right side: Have patient assume supine position and move to side of bed (in this case left side) if permitted by surgery. Instruct patient to move by bending knees and pressing heels against mattress to raise and move buttocks (see illustration). Top side rails on both sides of bed should be in up position.	Positioning begins on side of bed so turning to other side does not cause patient to roll toward edge of bed. Buttocks lift prevents shearing force against sheets. If patient's bed has a turn-assist feature, use it to help position him or her.
(2) Have patient splint incision with right hand or with right hand with pillow over incisional area; keep right leg straight and flex left knee up (see illustration); grab right side rail with left hand, pull toward right, and roll onto right side. Reverse process to turn to left side.	Supports incision and decreases discomfort while turning.

STEP	RATIONALE
(3) Instruct patient to turn every 2 hours from side to side while awake. Often patient requires assistance with turning after surgery.	Reduces risk of vascular, pulmonary, and pressure injury complications.

Clinical Decision Point *Some patients, such as those who have had back surgery or vascular repair, are restricted from flexing their legs after surgery. Some patients are restricted from turning or may need help for positioning (see Chapter 11).*

(4) Sit up on right side of bed. Elevate head of bed and have patient turn onto right side. While lying on right side, patient pushes on mattress with left arm and swings feet over edge of bed with nurse's help. To sit up on left side of bed, reverse this process.	Sitting position lowers diaphragm to permit fuller lung expansion.

Clinical Decision Point *Caution patient to always ask for assistance, particularly first time sitting up on side of bed, to reduce risk of a fall.*

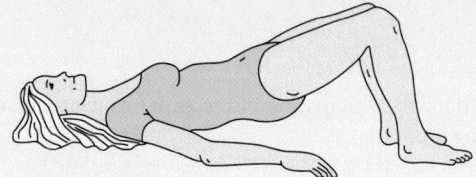

STEP 11a(1) Buttocks lift for moving to side of bed.

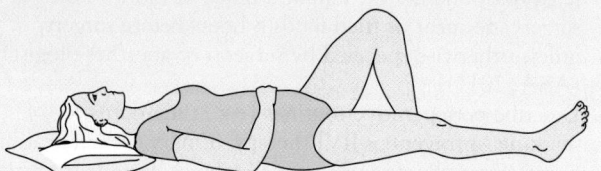

STEP 11a(2) Leg position when turning to right.

12. Teach coughing and deep breathing:	Patient may be unable or reluctant to deep breathe because of weakness or pain, resulting in secretions remaining in base of lungs. Collection of secretions increases risk of pulmonary atelectasis and pneumonia.
a. Help patient to high-Fowler's position in bed with knees flexed, or have patient sit on side of bed or chair in upright position.	Sitting position facilitates diaphragmatic expansion.
b. Instruct patient to place palms of hands across from one another lightly along lower border of rib cage or upper abdomen (see illustration).	This allows patient to feel rise and fall of abdomen during deep breathing.
c. Have patient take slow, deep breaths, inhaling through nose. Explain that patient will feel normal downward movement of diaphragm during inspiration. Demonstrate as needed.	Helps to prevent hyperventilation or panting. Slow deep breath allows for more complete lung expansion.

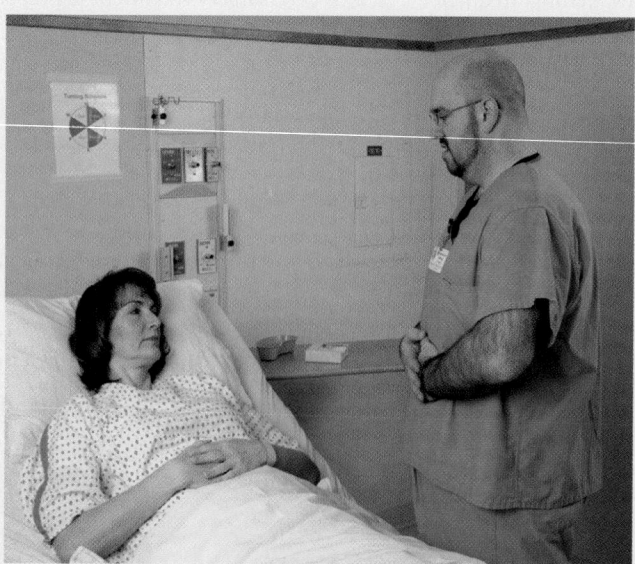

STEP 12b Deep-breathing exercise—placement of hands on upper abdomen during inhalation.

STEP	RATIONALE
d. Have patient avoid using chest and shoulder muscles while inhaling.	Increases unnecessary energy expenditure and does not promote full lung expansion.
e. Have patient take slow, deep breath; hold for count of 3 seconds; and slowly exhale through mouth as if blowing out candle (pursed lips).	Resistance during exhalation helps to prevent alveolar collapse.
f. Have patient repeat breathing exercise 3 to 5 times.	Repetition reinforces learning.
g. Have patient take two slow, deep breaths, inhaling through nose and exhaling through pursed lips.	Deep breaths expand lungs fully so air moves behind mucus to facilitate coughing.
h. Have patient inhale deeply a third time and hold breath to count of 3. Cough fully for two to three consecutive coughs without inhaling between coughs.	Deep breathing moves up secretions in respiratory tract to stimulate cough reflex without voluntary effort on part of patient (Lewis et al., 2017).
i. Caution patient against just clearing throat.	Clearing throat does not remove mucus from deeper airways.
j. Have patient practice several times. Instruct patient to perform turning, coughing, and deep breathing every 2 hours. Have family caregiver coach patient to exercise.	Ensures mastery of technique. Frequent pulmonary exercises and movement decrease risk of postoperative pneumonia (Lewis et al., 2017).
13. Teach use of an incentive spirometer (see also Skill 23.3):	Provides visual aid of respiratory effort. Encourages deep breathing to loosen secretions in lung bases.
a. Position patient in sitting position in chair or in reclining position with head of bed elevated at least 45 degrees in bed.	Facilitates diaphragm lowering and lung expansion.
b. Either set or indicate to patient on the incentive spirometer device scale the volume level to be reached with each breath (targeted tidal volume). Use manufacturer directions to set volume.	Establishes goal of volume level necessary for adequate lung expansion. Manufacturers determine target on basis of patient height and age.
c. Explain to patient how to place mouthpiece of incentive spirometer so lips completely cover mouthpiece (see illustration). Have patient demonstrate until position is correct.	Validates patient's understanding of instructions, evaluates psychomotor skills and lets patient ask questions.
d. Instruct patient to exhale completely, then position mouthpiece so lips completely cover it, and inhale slowly, maintaining constant flow through unit until reaching goal volume (see illustration).	Promotes complete inflation of lungs and minimizes atelectasis.
e. Once maximum inspiration is reached, have patient hold breath for 2 to 3 seconds and exhale slowly.	Promotes alveolar inflation.
f. Instruct patient to breathe normally for short period between each of the 10 breaths taken on incentive spirometer. Repeat every hour while awake.	Prevents hyperventilation and fatigue.
14. Teach PEP therapy and "huff" coughing:	
a. Set PEP device for setting ordered.	Higher settings require more effort.
b. Instruct patient to assume semi-Fowler's or high-Fowler's position in bed or to sit in a chair and place nose clip on patient's nose (see illustration).	Promotes optimum lung expansion and expectoration of mucus.

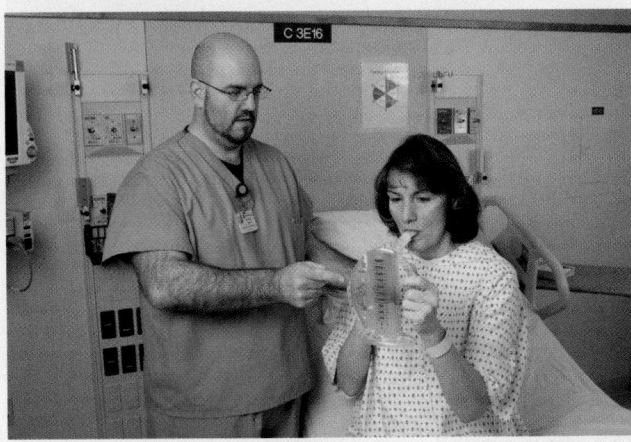

STEP 13c Patient demonstrates incentive spirometry.

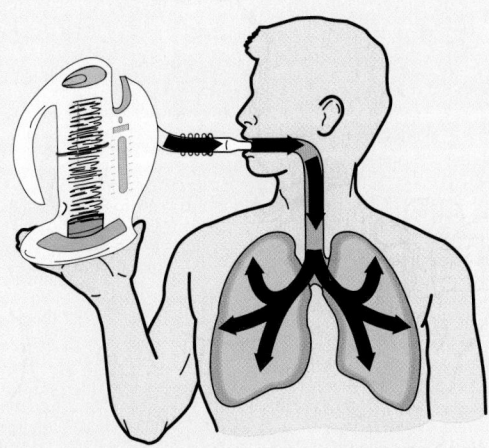

STEP 13d Diagram of use of incentive spirometer.

STEP	RATIONALE
c. Have patient place lips around mouthpiece. Instruct patient to take full breath and exhale 2 or 3 times longer than inhalation. Repeat pattern for 10 to 20 breaths.	Ensures that patient does all breathing through mouth. Ensures that patient uses device properly.
d. Remove device from mouth and have patient take slow, deep breath and hold for 3 seconds.	Promotes lung expansion before coughing.
e. Instruct patient to exhale in quick, short, forced "huffs." Repeat exercise every 2 hours while awake.	"Huff" coughing, or forced expiratory technique, promotes bronchial hygiene by increasing expectoration of secretions.
15. Teach controlled coughing:	Deep breaths expand lungs fully so air moves behind mucus and facilitates effective coughing.
a. Explain importance of maintaining upright position.	Position facilitates diaphragm excursion and enhances thorax and abdominal expansion.
b. Demonstrate coughing. Take two slow, deep breaths, inhaling through nose and exhaling through (pursed lips) mouth.	Consecutive coughs help remove mucus more effectively and completely than one forceful cough.
c. Inhale deeply a third time and hold breath to count of three. Cough fully for two to three consecutive coughs without inhaling between coughs (see illustration). (Tell patient to push all air out of lungs.)	Clearing throat does not remove mucus from deeper airways. Full, forceful cough is most effective in removing mucus.
d. Caution patient against just clearing throat instead of coughing deeply.	Clearing throat does not remove mucus from deeper airways.
e. If surgical incision is either thoracic or abdominal, teach patient to place either hands or pillow over incisional area and place hands over pillow to splint incision (see illustration). During breathing and coughing exercises, press gently against incisional area for splinting and support.	Surgical incision cuts through muscles, tissues, and nerve endings. Deep-breathing and coughing exercises place additional stress on suture line and cause discomfort. Splinting incision with hands or pillow provides firm support and reduces incisional pulling and pain.
f. Patient continues to practice coughing exercises, splinting imaginary incision (see illustration). Instruct patient to cough 2 to 3 times every 2 hours while awake.	Deep coughing with splinting effectively expectorates mucus with minimal discomfort.
g. Instruct patient to examine sputum for consistency, odor, amount, and color changes and notify a nurse if any changes are noted.	Sputum consistency, odor, amount, and color changes indicate presence of pulmonary complication such as pneumonia.

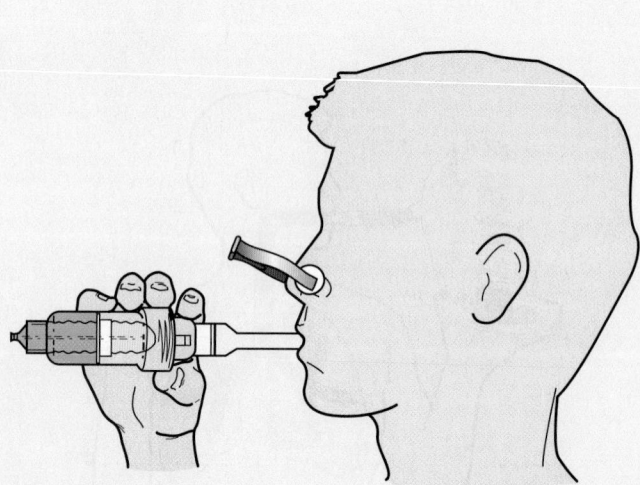

STEP 14b Diagram of use of positive expiratory pressure device.

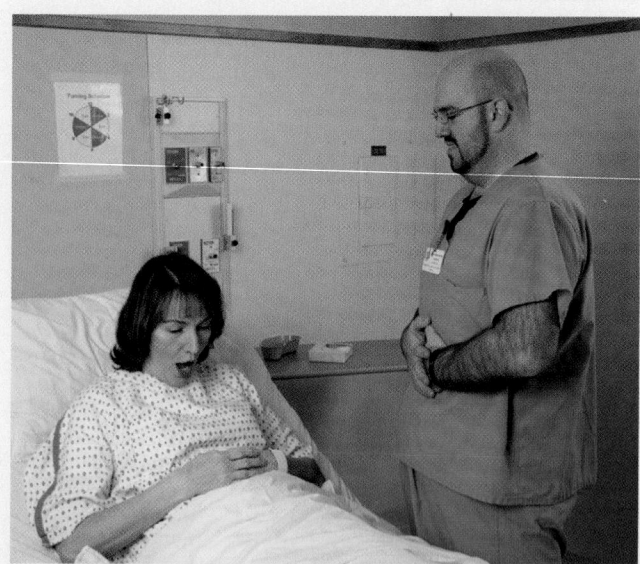

STEP 15c Controlled coughing with placement of hands on upper abdomen.

STEP	RATIONALE

16. Teach leg exercises:

a. Instruct and encourage patient in leg exercises to be performed every 1 to 2 hours while awake: ankle rotation, dorsiflexion and plantar flexion, leg extension and flexion, and straight leg raises.

Leg exercises facilitate venous return from lower extremities and reduce risk of circulatory complications such as venous thrombus.

b. Position patient supine.

c. Instruct patient to rotate each ankle in complete circle and draw imaginary circles with big toe 5 times (see illustration).

Promotes joint mobility.

d. Alternate dorsiflexion and plantar flexion while instructing patient to feel calf muscles tighten and relax. Repeat 5 times (see illustration).

Helps maintain joint mobility and promote venous return to prevent thrombus formation.

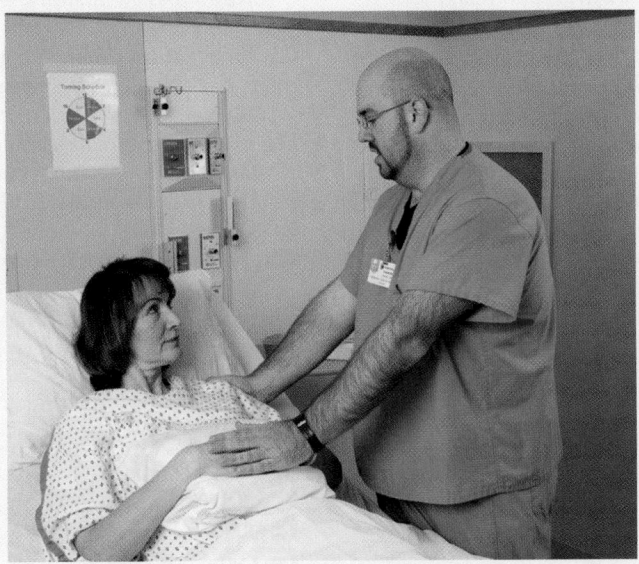

STEP 15e Patient splinting abdomen with pillow.

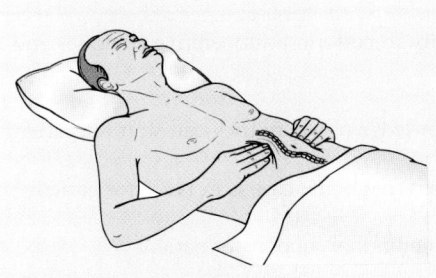
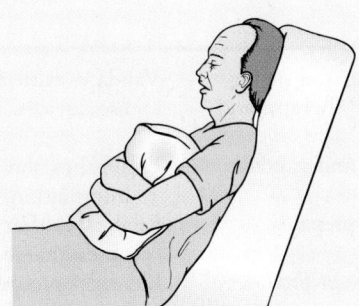
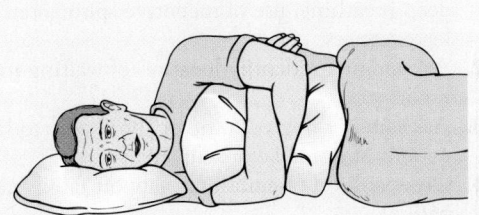

STEP 15f Techniques for splinting incisions.

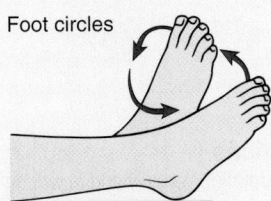

Foot circles

STEP 16c Foot circles. (*From Lewis S et al: Medical-surgical nursing: assessment and management of clinical problems, ed 9, St Louis, 2014, Mosby.*)

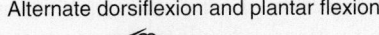
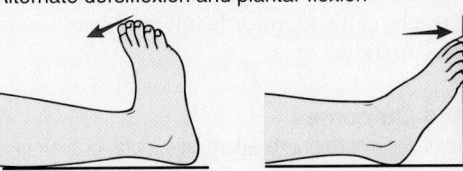

Alternate dorsiflexion and plantar flexion

STEP 16d Alternate dorsiflexion and plantar flexion. (*From Lewis S et al: Medical-surgical nursing: assessment and management of clinical problems, ed 9, St Louis, 2014, Mosby.*)

STEP	RATIONALE

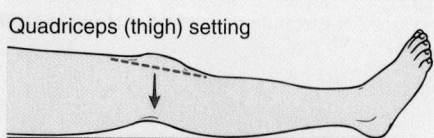

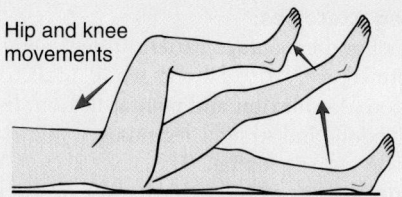

STEP 16e Quadriceps (thigh) setting. (*From Lewis S et al: Medical-surgical nursing: assessment and management of clinical problems, ed 9, St Louis, 2014, Mosby.*)

STEP 16f Hip and knee movements. (*From Lewis S et al: Medical-surgical nursing: assessment and management of clinical problems, ed 9, St Louis, 2014, Mosby.*)

    e. Perform quadriceps setting by tightening thigh and bringing knee down toward mattress and relaxing. Repeat 5 times (see illustration).

    f. Instruct patient to alternate raising legs straight up from bed surface. Leg should be kept straight. Repeat 5 times (see illustration).

17. Have patient continue to practice exercises before surgery at least every 2 hours while awake. Teach patient to coordinate turning and leg exercises with diaphragmatic breathing and use of incentive spirometer.

18. Verify that patient's expectations of surgery are realistic. Correct expectations as needed.

19. Reinforce therapeutic coping strategies. If ineffective, encourage alternatives.

Quadriceps-setting exercises contract muscles of upper legs, maintain knee mobility, and improve venous return to heart.

Causes quadriceps muscle contraction and relaxation, which help promote venous return (Lewis et al., 2017).

Leg exercises stimulate circulation, which prevents venous stasis to help prevent formation of deep vein thrombosis (DVT) (Lewis et al., 2017).

Can prevent postoperative anxiety or anger.

Therapeutic coping strategies promote postoperative compliance and recovery.

EVALUATION

1. Observe patient demonstrating splinting, turning and sitting, deep breathing, use of incentive spirometer, PEP therapy, and leg exercises.

2. Ask family to identify location of waiting room and validate if correct.

3. Ask family caregiver if he or she is able to help prepare patient at home before surgery.

4. Observe level of emotional support family caregiver provides patient.

5. **Use Teach-Back:** "I want to be sure I explained what you need to know about getting ready for surgery. Tell me which medications you should not take before surgery?" Revise your instruction now or develop a plan for revised patient or family caregiver teaching if patient or family caregiver is not able to teach back correctly.

Validates patient's ability to perform postoperative exercises and use devices.

Establishes family's knowledge of where they can wait for patient information.

Establishes that postoperative home care is in place for patient on discharge.

Identifies preoperative emotional support for patient.

Determines patient's and family caregiver's level of understanding of instructional topic.

Unexpected Outcomes
1. Patient identifies incorrect procedure, site, date, or time of surgery.

2. Patient incorrectly performs one of the postoperative exercises.

Related Interventions
- Provide correct information verbally and in writing for patient and family caregiver.
- Explain and demonstrate correct exercise technique.
- Explain importance of the postoperative exercise as it pertains to patient recovery.
- Instruct patient to repeat demonstration.

Recording and Reporting

- Document all preoperative patient and family caregiver teaching in the nurses' notes in electronic health record (EHR) or chart and their response to teaching.

Special Considerations
Teaching

- Nurses are responsible for ensuring that patient education material is clear, concise, in plain language, patient centered and based on the patients' needs and abilities. In addition, the nurse must evaluate the effectiveness of the teaching (Box 37.1) (Schick and Windle, 2016).

Pediatric

- Use an age-appropriate level of communication and provide simple explanations using familiar terms.
- The use of pictures, models, equipment, and play rather than verbal explanations increases learning in preschool and school-age children.

Gerontological

- Physiological changes that occur with aging may require admission to hospital before surgery for additional diagnostic tests and stabilization of condition (Table 37.2).
- Age-related changes in the central nervous system may diminish short-term memory. Additional time and reinforcement may be necessary for older adults to learn and comprehend information (Spry and Goodman, 2013). The greater the number of different exposures to new material, the higher the probability that the material will be learned.
- Reinforce teaching with verbal explanations, audiovisual resources, pamphlets, and demonstrations. Consider sight and hearing deficits when providing both written and verbal instructions (Spry and Goodman, 2013).

Home Care

- Review coughing, deep breathing, abdominal splinting, relaxation, leg exercises, and ambulation before admission to hospital or surgical clinic and after discharge.

BOX 37.1

The Joint Commission Patient and Family Education Standards

Education provided is appropriate to the patient's needs. The assessment of learning needs addresses cultural and religious beliefs, emotional barriers, desire to learn, physical or cognitive limitations, and barriers to communication as appropriate. When called for by the age of the patient and the length of stay, the hospital assesses and provides for patient's education needs. Patients are educated about:

- The plan for care, treatment, and services (i.e., postoperative monitoring).
- Basic health practices and safety (i.e., out of bed [OOB] only with help).
- The safe and effective use of medication (i.e., the patient is only one allowed to self-administer patient-controlled analgesia [PCA]).

- Nutrition interventions, modified diets, or oral health (i.e., progression of diet after surgery).
- Safe and effective use of medical equipment or supplies when provided by the hospital (i.e., incentive spirometer).
- Pain—Understanding pain, the risk for pain, the importance of effective pain management, the pain-assessment process, and methods for pain management (i.e., reporting pain, frequency of medications, nonpharmacological pain-relief techniques).
- Habilitation or rehabilitation techniques to help the patient reach the maximum independence possible (i.e., early ambulation).

Modified from The Joint Commission (TJC): *Accreditation manual for hospitals*, Chicago, 2011, The Commission; and Schick L, Windle P: *PeriAnesthesia nursing core curriculum: preprocedure, phase I and phase II PACU nursing*, ed 3, St Louis, 2016, Saunders.

TABLE 37.2

Physiological Factors That Place Older-Adult Patients at Risk for Surgery

Alterations	Surgery Risks	Nursing Implications
Cardiovascular		
Degenerative change in myocardium and valves	Reduced cardiac reserve	Assess baseline vital signs.
Rigidity of arterial walls and reduction in sympathetic and parasympathetic innervation to heart	Predisposes patient to postoperative hemorrhage and rise in systolic and diastolic blood pressure	Maintain adequate fluid balance to minimize stress to heart. Ensure that blood pressure is adequate to meet circulatory demands.
Increase in calcium and cholesterol deposits within small arteries; arterial walls thickened	Predisposes patient to clot formation in lower extremities	Teach patient techniques for performing leg exercises and proper turning. Apply bilateral antiembolism stockings, sequential compression devices (SCDs) (see Chapter 12).
Integumentary System		
Decreased subcutaneous tissue and increased fragility of skin	Prone to pressure injuries and skin tears	Assess skin every 4 hours; pad all bony prominences during surgery. Turn or reposition (see Chapter 39).

Continued

TABLE 37.2

Physiological Factors That Place Older-Adult Patients at Risk for Surgery—cont'd

Alterations	Surgery Risks	Nursing Implications
Pulmonary		
Rib cage stiffens and enlarges	Reduced vital capacity	Teach patient proper technique for coughing and deep-breathing exercises and use of incentive spirometer.
Reduced diaphragm excursion	Greater residual capacity or volume of air left in lung after normal breath increases, reducing amount of new air brought into lungs with each inspiration	Encourage deep breathing. Use incentive spirometer to enhance exhalation.
Lung tissue less distensible; alveoli enlarged	Reduced blood oxygenation	Assess oxygen saturation via oximetry (SpO_2).
Renal		
Reduced blood flow to kidneys	Blood loss that causes decrease in circulation to the kidney	Monitor urinary output and laboratory data (i.e., blood urea nitrogen [BUN], creatinine).
Reduced glomerular filtration rate and excretory times	Limits ability to remove drugs or toxic substances	Assess for adverse effects of medications.
Reduced bladder capacity	Increase in voiding frequency; larger amount of urine stays in the bladder after voiding. Sensation of need to void may not occur until bladder is filled	Instruct patient to notify nurse immediately when sensation of bladder fullness develops. Keep call light or bedpan within easy reach.
Neurological		
Sensory losses, including reduced tactile sense, increased pain tolerance	Patient less able to respond to early warning signs of surgical complications	Inspect bony prominences for signs of pressure.
Decreased reaction time	Patient becomes confused easily after anesthesia	Orient patient to surrounding environment. Observe for nonverbal signs of pain. Maintain safe environment. Institute fall precautions.
Metabolic		
Lower basal metabolic rate	Reduced total oxygen consumption and nutritional needs	Ensure adequate nutritional intake once diet is resumed.
Reduced number of red blood cells and hemoglobin levels	Reduces ability to carry adequate oxygen to tissues	Administer necessary blood products. Assess for adequacy of oxygenation, fatigue, and infection.
Change in total amounts of body potassium and water volume	Greater risk for fluid or electrolyte imbalance	Monitor electrolyte levels.

◆ **SKILL 37.3**   **Physical Preparation for Surgery**

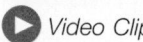 *Video Clip*

Preparing a patient for surgery involves activities and procedures that help to decrease anxiety, ensure patient safety, and decrease the risk for perioperative complications. The type of surgery determines the preparation required before surgery (e.g., low-residue and clear-liquid diets, enemas, cathartics, and oral antibiotics are for patients who undergo bowel surgery). Smoking cessation should be encouraged, and patients should be offered nicotine substitutes.. Nicotine delays wound healing, increases the risk of infection while also increasing the risk for venous thromboembolism (VTE) (Rothrock, 2015). Patients whose blood work indicates a low hemoglobin level and/or abnormal electrolyte levels or coagulopathies often require inpatient therapy before surgery.

Because many patients are admitted on the day of surgery, much of the preoperative preparation is often the responsibility of the patient or the primary caregiver. Therefore it is important that a preadmission nurse or nurse in the surgeon's practice provide adequate instructions. Patient teaching should include any food and fluid restrictions; which medications, if any, are permitted on the morning of surgery; and the need for surgical site preparation the evening before surgery (see Skill 37-2). It is also important to

include action that a patient will need to take if he or she omits any of these procedures by mistake. Written instructions are a useful adjunct to teaching because a patient and/or family caregiver can refer to them for any points that are unclear or forgotten. Videos and pamphlets are also useful adjuncts in preparing patients and their families.

The revised Joint Commission standards (2016) incorporated in the National Patient Safety Goals (NPSGs) implemented the Universal Protocol for Preventing Wrong Site, Wrong Procedure, Wrong Person surgery. This protocol was implemented as an added safety measure to ensure that the correct person, procedure, and surgical site are verified at the time of scheduling the procedure, on admission or entry into the agency, and each time the responsibility for care of the patient is transferred to another caregiver. A final verification check involving the entire surgical team occurs immediately before the start of the procedure. If the case involves laterality (right versus left), multiple structures (e.g., fingers, toes, lesions), or multiple levels (e.g., spine), the final verification should include a site marking by the person performing the procedure. The site markings need to be visible after the patient has been prepared and draped. Involve patients in this process when they are awake and aware. Immediately before starting the procedure a "time-out" is called. The entire operative team, using active communication, verifies correct patient identity, correct side and site, agreement on the procedure to be done, correct patient position, and availability of correct implants and any special equipment or special requirements. This final verification process should be documented.

Delegation and Collaboration

The skill of coordinating the patient's preparation for surgery cannot be delegated to nursing assistive personnel (NAP). However, the NAP may administer an enema or a douche; obtain vital signs in stable patients; apply antiembolism stockings; and help patients remove clothing, jewelry, and prostheses. The nurse instructs the NAP about:

- Using basic infection control practices and proper precautions when preparing a patient for surgery.
- Observing and using precautions if the patient has an intravenous (IV) catheter or other invasive devices in place.

Equipment

NOTE: Equipment varies by procedure ordered.
- Vital sign equipment: stethoscope, blood pressure (BP) cuff, thermometer, pulse oximeter
- Oxygen equipment
- Suction equipment as ordered
- Hospital gown
- IV solution and administration set (see Chapter 29)
- Skin-cleaning solution
- Compression (antiembolism) stockings (see Chapter 12)
- Intermittent compression devices (ICD)
- Venous foot pump
- Urinary catheterization kit (see Chapter 34)
- Preoperative checklist
- Medications (e.g., sedative)
- Clean gloves

STEP	RATIONALE

ASSESSMENT

1. Identify patient using at least two identifiers (e.g., name and birthday or name and medical record number), according to agency policy.

Ensures correct patient. Complies with The Joint Commission standards and improves patient safety (TJC, 2016).

2. Complete preoperative assessment (see Skill 37.1).
3. Assess and record patient's heart rate, blood pressure, respiratory rate, oxygen saturation, and temperature.

Provides all baseline assessment data for surgical team. Provides baseline for patient's preoperative status.

4. If patient is same-day admit or ambulatory patient, validate that admission preparations were completed as ordered. Specific preparations to review include NPO status, administration of medications, skin preparation, and bowel preparation if applicable.

Failure to complete preparation could lead to perioperative or postoperative complications and may necessitate postponement or cancellation of surgery.

5. Ask if patient has advance directive. If so, place it in his or her medical record.

Document conveys patient's wishes if life support measures are necessary.

NURSING DIAGNOSES

- Acute pain
- Anxiety
- Deficient knowledge regarding the surgical experience
- Fear
- Impaired oral mucous membrane

- Impaired physical mobility
- Ineffective airway clearance
- Ineffective breathing pattern
- Ineffective tissue perfusion
- Risk for aspiration
- Risk for delayed surgical recovery

- Risk for impaired skin integrity
- Risk for infection
- Risk for perioperative-positioning injury

Related factors/Risk factors are individualized based on patient's condition or needs.

PLANNING

1. Expected outcomes following completion of procedure:
   - Patient can state which surgical procedure is being performed and risks and benefits of surgery.

   Identifies readiness to sign informed consent.

   - Patient states that anxiety is decreased.

   Decreased anxiety increases participation.

IMPLEMENTATION

1. Perform hand hygiene. Help patient put on hospital gown and remove personal items. Patients are often anxious before surgery. Before any procedure, decrease anxiety by explaining how equipment or preparation will feel (e.g., cold, tight) before touching patient.

Reduces transmission of infection. Allows patient to orient to surroundings and understand presurgical procedures.

STEP	RATIONALE
2. Instruct patient to remove makeup, nail polish, hairpins, and jewelry.	Hair appliances and jewelry anywhere on body may become dislodged and cause injury during positioning and intubation. Rings decrease circulation in fingers. Makeup, nail polish, and false nails impede assessment of skin and oxygenation. In addition, acrylic nails harbor pathogenic organisms (Rothrock, 2015).
3. Ensure that money and valuables have been locked up or given to a family caregiver.	Patient may not return to same location after surgery. Prevents valuables from being misplaced or lost.
4. Ensure that patient has followed appropriate fluid and food restrictions per surgeon or anesthesiologist order (see Skill 37.2).	Extent and type of restriction vary by agency and health care provider. Under general anesthesia sphincters in the stomach relax, and contents can reflux into esophagus and trachea.
5. Verify presence of allergies and ensure that allergy/sensitivity band or other safety armbands are present.	Alerts surgeons and health care team to potential allergies, risk of falls.
6. Verify that patient has followed instructions about omission or ingestion of medications as instructed.	Missed or inaccurate dosage could precipitate complications.
7. Verify that bowel preparation (e.g., laxative, cathartic, enema) has been completed by patient or family caregiver at home if ordered.	Proper bowel evacuation needed for surgery to be performed.

Clinical Decision Point *In some situations additional enemas and/or cathartics are ordered. Emptying the bowel is necessary for bowel surgery and to decrease the risk of postoperative ileus. Enemas are used when surgery is near the lower intestine.*

STEP	RATIONALE
8. Ensure that medical history and physical examination results are in patient's record.	Ensures that pertinent laboratory and diagnostic test results are available and that all preoperative preparations are completed (Nagelhout and Plaus, 2014).
9. Verify that surgical consent, anesthesia consent, and consent for blood transfusion are complete. The name of procedure; name of surgeon; date; name of person authorized to obtain surgical consent; signature of surgeon (or authorized person) obtaining consent, anesthesia provider delivering anesthesia, and witness (often the nurse); and patient's signature all should be present.	Ensures patient's agreement to undergo intended procedure. In most settings surgeon obtains consent, and nurse verifies that it is complete and consistent with patient's understanding (refer to agency policy).
10. Ensure that necessary laboratory work, electrocardiogram (ECG), and chest x-ray film studies are completed and results are on chart.	Diagnostic test results may indicate medical problem and provide data for postoperative comparison.
11. Verify that blood type and cross-match are completed if ordered by surgeon and that blood transfusions are available as needed.	In many cases surgery cannot begin without availability of blood units.
12. Instruct patient to void.	Prevents risk of bladder distention or rupture during surgery.
13. Start IV line; refer to unit standards or surgeon's orders (see Chapter 29).	IV line provides access for fluids and medications to be administered when in operating room (OR).
14. Administer preoperative medications as ordered (e.g., preoperative antibiotics, prophylactic agents).	Preoperative medications are used for various reasons and should be administered as ordered for maximum effectiveness.
15. Apply compression stockings (see Chapter 12).	Compression stockings promote circulation during periods of immobilization, reducing risk of embolism.
16. Apply intermittent compression devices (ICDs) if ordered. **NOTE:** ICDs may or may not be used in combination with compression stockings. Verify order.	ICDs push blood from superficial veins into deep veins, decreasing venous stasis.

Clinical Decision Point *ICDs do not provide effective deep vein thrombosis (DVT) prophylaxis if the device is not applied correctly or if the patient does not wear the device continuously except during bathing, skin assessment, and ambulation. ICDs are not to be worn when a patient has an active DVT because of risk of pulmonary embolism.*

STEP	RATIONALE
17. Perform hand hygiene. Apply clean gloves. Clean and prepare surgical site if ordered.	Cleaning with antimicrobial soap decreases bacterial flora on skin.
18. Perform hand hygiene. Insert urinary catheter if ordered (see Chapter 34). **NOTE:** There are times when urinary catheter is placed in OR.	Maintains bladder decompression and provides for monitoring output during surgery.

STEP	RATIONALE
19. Allow patient to wear eyeglasses or hearing aid as long as possible before surgery so patient is able to sign consents and read materials. Remove contact lenses, eyeglasses, hairpieces, and dentures just before surgery (see checklist completed before surgery noting that all items are removed before proceeding to OR).	These aids facilitate patient cooperation by ensuring that patient has clear vision and maximal auditory perception throughout preoperative phase.
20. Place cap over patient's head and hair.	The cap contains hair and minimizes OR contamination during surgery. Plastic or reflective caps reduce heat loss during surgery.
21. Place patient on bed rest with call light within reach and inform him or her not to get out of bed without help. Allow family members to remain at bedside until patient is transferred to surgical area. Maintain quiet and relaxing environment.	There is increased chance of injury by trying to ambulate to void when patient is sedated and unattended.
22. Help patient onto stretcher for transport to OR.	Some ambulatory surgery patients walk to OR.

EVALUATION

1. Have patient describe surgical procedure and its benefits and risks.	Confirms level of knowledge needed to sign informed consent.
2. Have patient repeat preoperative instructions.	Provides evidence that patient understands instructions.
3. Monitor patient for signs and symptoms of anxiety and ask how patient and family are feeling.	Increased heart rate and blood pressure, dilated pupils, dry mouth, increased sweating, and muscle rigidity or shaking are responses to stress and anxiety. Asking patient about feelings gives permission to express concerns, which can be further explored.
4. **Use Teach-Back:** "I want to be sure you are ready for surgery. Tell me what you expect to happen once you get to the recovery room." Revise your instruction now or develop a plan for revised patient or family caregiver teaching if patient or family caregiver is not able to teach back correctly.	Determines patient's and family caregiver's level of understanding of instructional topic.

Unexpected Outcomes	Related Interventions
1. Patient is unable to give consent, and family member is unavailable.	• In emergency situations obtain telephone consent from next of kin. Two people must witness oral consent (according to agency policy).
	• Document explanation of situation and fact that oral consent was obtained and witnessed.
	• At earliest opportunity, person giving oral consent must sign written consent. Signed telegram or signed fax may also be considered oral consent. Follow agency policy.
2. Patient did not remain NPO, which may place him or her at risk for aspiration and may indicate that he or she did not understand instructions or forgot.	• Notify surgeon and anesthesiologist. Surgery may be postponed or cancelled.
3. Informed consent has not been signed and witnessed. Surgeon and anesthesiologist did not provide information and/or ensure that consent forms were signed.	• Patient is not ready for surgery. Patient must sign consent before administration of preoperative medications or any medication that alters central nervous system. Notify physician/surgeon/anesthesiologist.

Recording and Reporting

- Document preoperative physical preparation on preoperative checklist in the electronic health record (EHR) or chart.
- Record disposition of patient valuables/belongings (i.e., whether locked up according to agency policy or sent with family) in the EHR or chart.
- Report lack of signed and witnessed consent form or failure of patient to maintain NPO status and action taken.
- Document your evaluation of patient and family caregiver learning.

Special Considerations
Pediatric

- Give the child as many choices related to procedures as possible.
- Keep parent-child separation to the minimum time possible. When a parent cannot be present, it is important to leave a favorite possession with the child.

Gerontological

- Because of cognitive, sensory, or physical impairments, it may take an older patient increased time to dress for surgery and complete needed physical preparation.

◆ SKILL 37.4 **Providing Immediate Anesthesia Recovery in the Postanesthesia Care Unit**

The first phase of postoperative care takes place during the immediate recovery period. This phase extends from the time the patient leaves the operating room (OR) to the time he or she is stabilized in the postanesthesia care unit (PACU), meets discharge criteria, and is transferred to the nursing unit.

The first 1 to 2 hours are the most critical for assessing the aftereffects of anesthesia, including airway clearance, cardiovascular complications, temperature control, and neurological function (Table 37.3). A patient's condition can change rapidly; assessments must be timely, knowledgeable, and accurate. You need to be aware

---

TABLE 37.3

Postanesthesia Monitoring and Management of Complications

Condition	Interventions
Airway	
Mechanical obstruction: Decreased LOC and muscle relaxants, resulting in flaccid muscles and tongue blocking airway	Hyperextend neck; pull mandible forward; use nasal or oral airway; encourage deep breathing.
Retained thick secretions: Irritation from anesthesia; anticholinergic medications; history of smoking	Suction; encourage coughing.
Laryngospasm: Stridor from excessive secretions or airway irritation	Encourage to relax and breathe through the mouth. If extreme, it may require positive-pressure ventilation with oxygen, small dose of muscle relaxant (ordered by anesthesiologist), and intubation.
Laryngeal edema: Allergic reaction, irritation from ET tube, fluid overload	Administer humidified oxygen, antihistamines, steroids, sedatives; in some cases perform reintubation.
Bronchospasm: Preexisting asthma, anesthetic irritation (expiratory wheeze)	Administer bronchodilators as ordered.
Aspiration: Vomiting from hypotension, accumulated gastric secretions and delayed gastric emptying, pain, fear, position changes	Position on side; suction airway; administer antiemetic as ordered.
Breathing: Hypoventilation/Hypoxemia	
CNS depression: Anesthesia, analgesics, muscle relaxants (respiratory rate shallow)	Encourage to cough and deep breathe; use mechanical ventilator; administer narcotic antagonist and muscle-relaxant reversal agent.
Mechanical restriction: Obesity, pain, tight cast or dressings, abdominal distention	Reposition; give analgesic; loosen cast or dressings; implement measures to reduce gastric distention (e.g., NG intubation, NG suction).
Circulation	
Hypovolemia: Blood loss, dehydration	Administer IV fluids or blood replacement.
Hypotension: Anesthesia/drug effects, vasodilation (possibly from spinal anesthesia), narcotics	Elevate legs; give oxygen, IV fluids, or blood replacement; administer vasopressors; monitor I&O, stimulation, hemoglobin, and hematocrit.
Cardiac failure: Preexisting cardiac disease; circulatory overload; excessive/too-rapid fluid replacement	Provide digitalization and diuretics; monitor ECG.
Cardiac arrhythmias: Hypoxemia; MI; hypothermia; imbalance of potassium, calcium, magnesium	Provide IV fluid replacement; monitor ECG and urine output; identify and treat cause.
Hypertension: Pain, distended bladder, preexisting hypertension, vasopressor drugs	Compare with preoperative baseline; identify and determine cause.
Compartment syndrome: Pressure from edema causing enough compression to obstruct arterial and venous circulation resulting in ischemia, permanent numbness, loss of function; forearm and lower leg most common sites	Obtain compartment pressures to diagnose and elevate extremity no higher than heart level; remove or loosen bandage or cast to relieve compression; if left untreated, amputation may be required. Do not apply ice.

CNS, Central nervous system; *ECG,* electrocardiogram; *ET,* endotracheal; *I&O,* intake and output; *IV,* intravenous; *LOC,* level of consciousness; *MI,* myocardial infarction; *NG,* nasogastric.

TABLE 37.4

Focused Assessment of Patient Problems Related to Anesthesia Type

Anesthesia Type	Focused Assessment
General	Hypotension; changes in heart rate or rhythm; lowered body temperature; respiratory depression; emergence delirium in the form of shivering, trembling, confusion, or hallucinations
Spinal	Headache, hypotension, decreased cardiac output, cyanosis, difficulty breathing
Local	Skin rash; allergic reaction with edema of the face, lips, mouth, or throat; restlessness; bradycardia; hypotension; ischemic necrosis at injection site
Conscious sedation	Respiratory depression, bradycardia, hypotension, nausea and vomiting
Epidural	Cyanosis, breathing difficulties, decreased heart rate, irregular heart rate, pale skin color, nausea and vomiting

Data from Lilley LL, Collins SR, Snyder JS: *Pharmacology and the nursing process,* ed 7, St Louis, 2014, Mosby; and Rothrock JC: *Alexander's care of the patient in surgery,* ed 15, St Louis, 2015, Mosby.

TABLE 37.5

Aldrete Score for Postanesthesia Monitoring

		Score
Activity (moving voluntarily on command)	4 extremities	2
	2 extremities	1
	0 extremities	0
Respiration	Able to deep breathe and cough freely	2
	Dyspnea, shallow or limited breathing	1
	Apneic	0
Circulation	BP + 20 mm Hg of presedation level	2
	BP + 20–50 mm Hg of presedation level	1
	BP + 50 mm Hg of presedation level	0
Consciousness	Fully awake	2
	Arousable on having name called	1
	Not responding	0
Color	Normal	2
	Pale, dusky, blotchy, jaundiced, or other change	1
	Cyanotic	0

From American Society of PeriAnesthesia Nurses (ASPAN): *2015-2017 perianesthesia nursing standards, practice recommendations and interpretive statements,* Cherry Hill, NJ, 2015, ASPAN; Phillips NM, et al: Post-anaesthetic discharge scoring criteria: key findings from a systematic review, *Int Evid Based Healthc* 11(4):275, 2013.
BP, Blood pressure.

of the common complications and problems associated with the specific types of anesthesia (Table 37.4). Quick judgment regarding the most appropriate interventions is essential. A patient is usually ready for discharge to the general unit when specific standardized criteria are met. The Aldrete score is one of several scoring systems for assessment (Table 37.5). It uses parameters of activity, respiration, circulation, consciousness, and oxygen saturation. A score of 8 or less indicates that additional monitoring is required. A score of 10 indicates full recovery of the patient.

Recovery from ambulatory surgery requires the same assessments. However, the depth of general anesthesia may be less because the surgery is less involved and of shorter duration. Some patients have only intravenous (IV) conscious sedation, and intensive monitoring is required for a shorter time period. As soon as the patient is stable and alert, give instructions for home care to the patient and caregiver, including demonstrations and written instructions.

Delegation and Collaboration

The skill of initiating immediate anesthesia recovery of a patient cannot be delegated to nursing assistive personnel (NAP). The NAP may provide basic comfort and hygiene measures. The nurse instructs the NAP by:

- Explaining any restrictions for how to provide comfort measures (e.g., repositioning, turning, applying warming blanket).
- Offering instruction in providing needed supplies.
- NOTE: NAP may be allowed to do more in ambulatory surgery recovery such as provide initial PO liquids.

Equipment

- Equipment for physical assessment
- Various types and sizes of artificial airways
- Constant and intermittent suction
- Oxygen equipment such as mask, oxygen regulator and tubing, and positive-pressure delivery system
- Pulse oximeter
- End-tidal carbon dioxide (CO_2) monitor
- Blood pressure (BP) monitoring equipment
- Adjustable lighting
- Electrocardiogram (ECG) monitor
- Arterial blood gas supplies
- Bladder scanner
- Bedside portable ultrasound to assess pulses
- Thermoregulation equipment, including thermometers, blanket warmers, and cooling blankets
- IV supplies (if ordered) (see Chapter 29)
- Adult and pediatric emergency cart with defibrillator
- Stock supplies (e.g., facial tissues, dressings, bedpans, urinals, emesis basins)
- Personal protective equipment
- Latex-free supplies and equipment

STEP	RATIONALE

ASSESSMENT

1. Identify patient using at least two identifiers (e.g., name and birthday or name and medical record number), according to agency policy.

Ensures correct patient. Complies with The Joint Commission standards and improves patient safety (TJC, 2016).

STEP	RATIONALE
2. Receive hand-off report from circulating nurse and anesthesia provider, including procedure performed, range of vital signs, any complications, estimated blood loss (EBL), other fluid loss, fluid replacement during surgery, type of anesthesia, medications given, type of airway and size, extent of surgical wound, restrictions to movement of position during surgery, and any preoperative medical and/or nursing diagnoses.	Determines patient's general status and allows you to anticipate type of assessment needed, the need for special equipment, potential treatment measures, and nursing care interventions in PACU.
3. On patient's arrival in PACU, review surgeon's orders.	Allows you to focus on priority interventions; assists you in organizing your care.
4. Consider type of surgical procedure, restrictions to movement, and type of anesthesia used.	Influences type of assessments necessary, type of complications for which to observe, and specific nursing interventions needed.
5. Perform hand hygiene. Perform thorough patient assessment, including vital signs; pulse oximetry; pain and assessment of body systems to include respiratory, cardiac, neurological, gastrointestinal (GI), genitourinary (GU), metabolic, and fluid status. Assess patient's surgical site and drains, skin integrity, safety, and anxiety level.	Reduces transmission of infection. Provides baseline for ongoing postoperative evaluations. Identifies priority nursing interventions.
6. Take vital signs and monitor pulse oximetry during initial stabilization (ASPAN, 2015).	Monitors patient stability.
7. Discharge from phase I level of care is based on specific criteria, not a time limit. Criteria should address assessment of airway patency, oxygenation, hemodynamic stability, thermoregulation, neurological stability, intake and output, tube patency, dressings, pain and comfort management, and postanesthesia scoring system if used. Each agency defines frequency of assessment.	Discharge instructions are developed in consultation with anesthesia department.

Clinical Decision Point *Be sure to turn patient on side (when possible) to observe underlying skin and accumulation of blood or serous drainage not visible otherwise.*

NURSING DIAGNOSES

- Acute confusion
- Acute pain
- Deficient fluid volume
- Excess fluid volume
- Impaired gas exchange
- Impaired physical mobility
- Impaired skin integrity
- Impaired spontaneous ventilation
- Impaired swallowing
- Impaired verbal communication
- Ineffective airway clearance
- Ineffective breathing pattern
- Ineffective protection
- Ineffective thermoregulation
- Ineffective tissue perfusion
- Risk of aspiration
- Risk of urinary retention

Related factors/Risk factors are individualized based on patient's condition or needs.

PLANNING

1. Expected outcomes following completion of procedure:

• Patient's airway remains clear; respirations are deep, regular, and within normal limits by time of transfer. Oxygen saturation remains greater than 95%.	No occurrence of pulmonary changes except those expected from effects of anesthetic or analgesic.
• Patient's BP, pulse, and temperature remain within previous baseline or normal expected range by time of transfer.	No occurrence of cardiovascular, pulmonary, or thermoregulatory changes except those expected from effects of anesthetic or analgesic.
• Dressings are clean, dry, and intact by discharge from recovery.	Indicates wound stabilization without signs of bleeding or infection.
• Intake and output (I&O) is within expected parameters by discharge from recovery.	Adequate urinary elimination maintained. Fluid intake (IV and/or by mouth [PO]) adequately maintained.
• Patient reports relief of discomfort after analgesia or other pain-relief measures by time of transfer from immediate recovery area (usually 1 to 2 hours).	Pain-relief measures effectively alter patient's reception or perception of pain.
• Patient's postoperative assessments are within expected normal postoperative parameters.	Patient stable and may be prepared for next phase of postoperative recovery.

STEP	RATIONALE

2. Perform hand hygiene and prepare equipment for continued monitoring and care activities.

Reduces transmission of infection.

IMPLEMENTATION

1. While receiving hand-off report as patient enters PACU on stretcher/bed, immediately attach oxygen tubing to regulator, hang IV fluids, and check IV flow rates. Connect any drainage tubes to gravity drainage or continuous or intermittent suction as ordered. Attach cardiac monitor. Ensure that indwelling catheter and bag are in drainage position and patent.

Maintaining oxygenation and circulation are two priorities. Inhaled oxygen improves percentage of oxygen delivered to alveoli. IV fluids maintain circulatory volume and provide route for emergency drugs. Drainage tubes must remain patent and in proper position to allow fluid to drain.

2. Continue ongoing assessment of all vital signs every 5 to 15 minutes until patient stabilizes or more frequently if clinically indicated (ASPAN, 2015) (see agency protocol). Compare findings with patient's baseline. Provide warm blankets as needed for patient comfort.

Vital signs reveal onset of postoperative complications from surgery or anesthesia (e.g., respiratory depression, hypo-hyperthermia, pulse irregularity, or hypotension). Acute blood loss may lead to hypovolemic shock with signs of reduced BP, elevated heart and respiratory rates, pale skin, and restlessness. General anesthetic may affect temperature-regulating center, and lower metabolic rate causes hypothermia. Malignant hyperthermia is rare inherited condition that develops after receiving an anesthetic and is medical emergency (Rothrock 2015; Schick and Windle, 2016).

Clinical Decision Point *If patient underwent a short procedure under procedural sedation, check agency policy for sedation recovery guidelines. The perianesthesia registered nurse (RN) monitoring a patient who receives procedural sedation/analgesia should have no other responsibilities that compromise continuous patient monitoring (AORN, 2015; ASPAN, 2015). Monitor oxygenation until patients are no longer at risk for hypoxemia. Monitor ventilation and circulation at regular intervals until patients are suitable for discharge (ASPAN, 2015).*

3. Maintain patent airway after general anesthesia:
   a. Position patient on side with head facing down and neck slightly extended (see illustration). Never position patient with hands over chest (reduces chest expansion).

Ensures appropriate oxygenation.
Extension prevents occlusion of airway at pharynx. Downward position of head moves tongue forward; and mucus or vomitus can drain out of mouth, preventing aspiration.

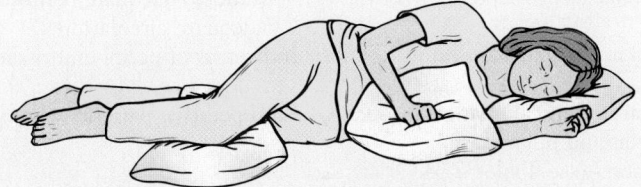

STEP 3a Position of patient during recovery from general anesthesia.

Clinical Decision Point *Always stay with a sedated patient until respirations are well established. Patients with an artificial airway may gag and vomit, become restless, or stop breathing. Closely monitor patients with a history of obstructive sleep apnea.*

   b. Place small folded towel or small pillow under patient's head. If patient is restricted to supine position, elevate head of bed approximately 10 to 15 degrees, extend neck, and turn head to side. Have emesis basin available if patient becomes nauseated.

Supports head in extended position. Prevents aspiration if patient should vomit.

Clinical Decision Point *If patient is not able to extend neck, turn head to side if possible; suction oropharynx (see Chapter 25) frequently.*

   c. Encourage patient to cough and deep breathe on awakening and every 15 minutes.

Promotes lung expansion and expectoration of mucus secretions.

   d. Suction artificial airway and oral cavity as secretions accumulate.

Clears airway of secretions.

STEP	RATIONALE

e. Once gag reflex returns, have patient spit out oral airway (see illustration). Do not tape oral airway.

Indicates that patient can clear airway independently. If airway is taped, patient will gag and may obstruct airway.

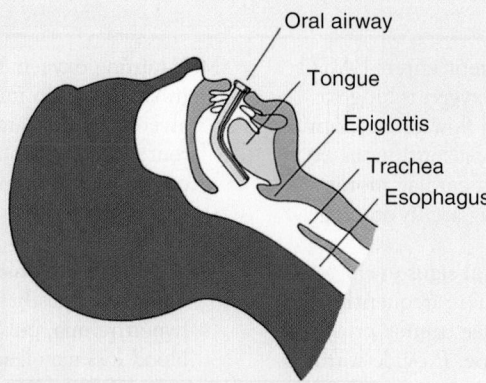

Oral airway
Tongue
Epiglottis
Trachea
Esophagus

STEP 3e Oral airway position before removal.

f. Avoid rapid position changes in patients who had spinal anesthesia, which can cause changes in patient's BP. Good body alignment is needed. Maintain IC infusion. Encourage fluid intake (only if patient is able to take fluids, such as with ambulatory surgery).

Rapid movements are avoided so as not to cause spinal headache from loss of cerebrospinal fluid. Increased IV or PO fluids help body replace cerebrospinal fluid.

Clinical Decision Point *Because of shorter half-life of drugs used today, many patients have oral airway removed before leaving the OR. PACU nurse must assess that respiratory effort is adequate; otherwise airway may need to be replaced, and patient may need a ventilator.*

4. Call patient by name in normal tone of voice. If there is no response, attempt to arouse patient by touching or gently moving a body part. Explain that surgery is over and patient is in recovery area.

Determines patient's level of consciousness and ability to follow commands.

5. Assess circulatory perfusion by inspecting color of nail beds, mucous membranes, and skin. Palpate for skin temperature. Test for capillary refill (see Chapter 6).

Pink or normal color of skin, nail beds, and mucous membranes and brisk (3 seconds or less) capillary refill indicate adequate perfusion. Warm extremities reveal adequate circulation.

6. Inspect color of nail beds and skin. Palpate for skin temperature.

Indicators of peripheral tissue perfusion.

7. Assess closely for any behavioral or clinical changes reflecting potential cardiovascular and pulmonary complications of general anesthesia (see Table 37.3) Monitor laboratory findings.

Postoperative patients who are sedated often become hypoxic.

8. If patient had general anesthesia: As patient arouses, introduce yourself and orient him or her to surroundings.

9. Monitor sensory, circulatory, pulmonary, and neurological responses after spinal or epidural anesthesia:

Reflects return of spinal function.

   a. Monitor for hypotension, bradycardia, and nausea and vomiting.

Blockage of sympathetic nervous system results in vasodilation of major vessels and systemic hypotension.

   b. Maintain adequate IV infusion.

Maintains BP by increasing fluid volume and fills temporarily expanded vascular space.

   c. Keep patient supine or with head slightly elevated and maintain position.

Minimizes risk of postspinal anesthesia headache from leakage of spinal fluid at injection site, with increased pressures caused by elevation of upper body. Headache is more common with spinal than epidural anesthesia (Lewis et al., 2017).

   d. Observe patients in PACU until they regain movement in extremities.

Patients fear permanent loss of function.

STEP	RATIONALE
e. Assess respiratory status, level of spinal sensation, and mobility in lower extremities. Drowsiness will be apparent after IV sedation. Level of anesthesia depends on location of sensation change. Have patient close eyes and use alcohol wipe to test sensation along sensory dermatomes. Have patient identify if warm or cold. *If patient had spinal anesthesia:* Remind him or her that loss of extremity sensation and movement is normal and will return in several hours.	Spinal block is set within 20 minutes of onset. However, if level of anesthesia moves above sixth thoracic vertebra (T6), respiratory muscles are affected. Patients often feel short of breath and may require mechanical ventilation if respiratory muscles are severely affected.
10. Monitor source of intake and output:	
a. Observe dressing and drains for any evidence of bright red blood. Inspect surgical incision for swelling or discoloration. Note condition of surgical dressing, including amount, color, odor, and consistency of drainage. Mark dressing with circle around drainage using black pen. Place time of marking and check area every 10 to 15 minutes, marking any changes and noting vital signs.	Determines extent of fluid loss and condition of underlying wound. Size, location, and depth of wound influence amount of drainage.
b. Reinforce pressure dressing or change simple dressing if ordered (see Chapter 41). Continue to monitor condition of incision, surrounding tissue, and amount and color of any drainage if incision is exposed or covered with transparent dressing.	Pressure dressing should not be removed because it helps to maintain hemostasis (termination of bleeding) and absorb drainage. Changing dressings immediately after surgery can disrupt wound edges and aggravate drainage. First dressing changes most often occur 24 hours after surgery and are usually done by surgeon. Minor surgical wounds may not have dressings but simply skin closure; or wounds may be covered with transparent dressing, which allows for observation of incision and surrounding tissue (Rothrock, 2015).
c. Inform surgeon of unexpected bloody drainage and reinforce dressing as indicated. Apply direct pressure. Also look underneath patient for any pooling of bloody drainage. Monitor for decreased BP and increased pulse.	Progressive increase or changes in characteristics of drainage warrant call to surgeon because they could indicate hemorrhage (Lewis et al., 2017; Schick and Windle, 2016). Hemorrhage from surgical wound is most likely within first few hours, indicating inadequate hemostasis during surgery. As dressing becomes saturated, blood often oozes down patient's side and collects underneath him or her.
d. Inspect condition and contents of any drainage tubes and collecting devices. Note character and volume of drainage.	Determines patency of drainage tube and extent of wound drainage.
e. Observe amount, color, and appearance of urine from indwelling Foley catheter (if present).	Urine output of less than 30 mL/h is sign of decreased renal perfusion or altered renal function.
f. If nasogastric (NG) tube is present, assess drainage. If not draining, check placement and irrigate if necessary with normal saline (see Chapter 35).	Maintains patency of tube to ensure gastric decompression. Expected drainage is dark or pale, yellow, or green and 100 to 200 mL/h. Bloody drainage occurs after some surgeries.
g. Monitor and maintain IV fluid rates. Observe IV site for signs of infiltration (see Chapter 29).	Provides adequate hydration and circulatory function.
11. Promote comfort:	
a. Provide mouth care by placing moistened washcloth to lips, swabbing oral mucosa with dampened swab or soft toothbrush, or applying petrolatum to lips.	Mouth is dry from NPO status and preoperative anticholinergics such as atropine.
b. Provide warm blanket or active rewarming therapy to promote warmth and minimize shivering.	General anesthesia impairs thermoregulation, OR environment is cold, and exposure of body cavity results in internal heat loss. Shivering increases oxygen consumption, predisposes patient to arrhythmias and hypertension, impairs platelet function, alters drug metabolism, impairs wound healing, and increases hospitalization costs because of cumulative adverse outcomes (ASPAN, 2015).
c. Help with position changes and provide supportive pillows.	Improves ventilation and circulation.

STEP	RATIONALE
12. Continue monitoring pain as patient awakens and until transfer to surgical unit or discharge, including quality, severity, and location (see Chapter 16). Do not assume that all postoperative pain is incisional pain.	Pain is often not directly related to surgical procedure (e.g., chest pain [myocardial infarction or pulmonary embolism] or muscle pain [trauma from positioning]). Referred pain (in shoulder) often occurs after laparoscopy. Systematic assessment of pain helps patients achieve functional status.
a. Provide pain medication as ordered and when vital signs have stabilized.	Promotes patient comfort.
13. Explain patient's condition to patient and inform of plans for transfer to nursing unit or discharge.	Decreases anxiety that can interfere with recovery process.
14. When patient's condition stabilizes, contact anesthesiologist to approve transfer to nursing unit or release to home.	Surgeon is responsible for authorizing transfer or discharge.
15. Before discharge to home from ambulatory surgery unit, provide verbal and written instructions (Box 37.2).	Patients and home care providers must be aware of potential complications and follow-up care.

Clinical Decision Point *If patient is to be discharged to home, ensure that patient has someone to drive him or her home and observe him or her for signs and symptoms of complications. Review with patient and driver reportable signs and symptoms and emergency care needed.*

EVALUATION

1. Compare all vital sign assessment measurements with patient's baseline and expected normal levels.

   Evaluates patient's respiratory, cardiovascular, and thermoregulatory status throughout recovery.

2. Inspect surgical wound and dressings for drainage. Be sure to assess for wound drainage under patient.

   Provides data to measure progress of wound healing.

3. Measure I&O. Urine output should be at least 30 to 50 mL/h.

   Indicates onset of fluid imbalances.

4. Auscultate bowel sounds and ask if patient has passed flatus.

   Allows you to evaluate return of peristalsis and diet tolerance.

5. Measure patient's perception of pain after implementing pain-relief measures such as positioning and use of analgesics.

   Determines level of comfort achieved and effectiveness of pain-relief measures.

6. Complete system-specific physical assessments as appropriate according to patient's unique type of surgery (e.g., craniotomy—neurological assessment; neck surgery—airway status; vascular surgery—circulation and bleeding; orthopedic surgery—neurovascular status and immobility or positioning).

   Allows you to monitor course of recovery.

7. **Use Teach-Back:** "I want to be sure you know what to expect when you go home. Tell me the signs and symptoms to expect if you were to get an infection?" Revise your instruction now or develop a plan for revised patient or family caregiver teaching if patient or family caregiver is not able to teach back correctly.

   Determines patient's and family caregiver's level of understanding of instructional topic.

Unexpected Outcomes

1. Patient exhibits respiratory depression (pulse oximetry <95%, respiratory rate <10 breaths/min or shallow).

Related Interventions

- Promptly report to surgeon.
- Administer oxygen as ordered by nasal cannula. Give patients with chronic obstructive pulmonary disease (COPD) 2 L/min or less of oxygen.
- Encourage deep breathing every 5 to 15 minutes.
- Position to promote chest expansion (on side or semi-Fowler's).
- Administer prescribed medications (e.g., epinephrine, muscle relaxant, narcotic reversal agent).

BOX 37.2

Postanesthesia and Ambulatory Surgery Discharge Criteria

Postanesthesia Discharge Criteria

- Patient awake (or returns to baseline)
- Vital signs stable
- No excess bleeding or drainage
- No respiratory depression
- SaO$_2$ greater than 90%
- Pain controlled
- Report given

Ambulatory Surgery Discharge Criteria

- All postanesthesia care unit (PACU) discharge criteria met
- No intravenous (IV) narcotics for last 30 minutes
- Minimal nausea and vomiting
- Pain controlled
- Voided (if appropriate to surgical procedure/orders)
- Able to ambulate if age appropriate and not contraindicated
- Responsible adult present to accompany patient
- Discharge instructions given and understood

STEP	RATIONALE
2. Patient exhibits signs of hypovolemia related to internal or incisional hemorrhage.	• Elevate patient's legs enough to maintain downward slope toward trunk of body. Do not lower head past flat position because this position increases respiratory effort and potentially decreases cerebral perfusion.
	• Promptly report patient's present status to surgeon.
	• Administer oxygen at 6 to 10 L/min by mask per order.
	• Increase rate of IV fluid or administer blood products as ordered.
	• Monitor BP and pulse every 5 to 15 minutes.
	• Apply pressure dressings as follows per order:
	• *Abdominal dressing:* Cover bleeding area with several thicknesses of gauze compresses and place tape 7 to 10 cm (3 to 4 inches) beyond width of dressing with firm, even pressure on both sides close to bleeding source. Maintain pressure as you tape entire dressing to maximize pressure at source of bleeding.
	• *Dressing on extremity:* Apply rolled gauze, pressing gauze compress over bleeding site. Do not continue tape around entire extremity.
	• *Dressing in neck region:* Cover with several thicknesses of gauze and place tape 7 to 10 cm (3 to 4 inches) beyond width of dressing. Apply with pressure, but do not occlude carotid artery or airway. Assess every 5 to 15 minutes for carotid pulse and evidence of airway obstruction.
	• Patient remains NPO because it is often necessary to return to surgery for control of bleeding.
3. Patient complains of severe incisional pain.	• Administer analgesics; reassess and provide analgesia before pain is severe.
	• Pain sometimes lowers BP; analgesia may restore vital signs to normal. Monitor vital signs carefully.
	• For patients with patient-controlled analgesia (PCA), be sure that patient is using device correctly. Warn family caregiver not to manipulate PCA.
	• *Orthopedic surgery:* Earliest symptom of compartment syndrome in extremity is pain unrelieved by analgesics. Other symptoms include numbness, tingling, pallor, coolness, and absent peripheral pulses. Surgeon *must* be notified. Do not elevate extremity above level of heart because this increases venous pressure. Application of ice is contraindicated because vasoconstriction will occur (Lewis et al., 2017).

Recording and Reporting

• Document in nurses' notes in electronic health record (EHR) or chart patient's arrival time at PACU; include vital signs and other physical parameters, level of consciousness (LOC), and pain severity. Also include condition of dressings and tubes, character of drainage, and all nursing measures initiated.

• Record vital signs and I&O on appropriate flow sheets.

• Report any abnormal assessment findings and signs of complications to surgeon.

• Document your evaluation of patient and family caregiver learning.

Special Considerations
Teaching

• If patient had spinal or epidural anesthetic, remind family or significant other that loss of extremity movement is normal for several hours.

• Reinforce preoperative teaching regarding coughing, deep breathing, leg exercises, and information concerning ambulation and pain control.

• Patient teaching for ambulatory surgical patients
  • Surgeon's office and surgery center telephone number (24-hour answer)
  • Follow-up appointment, date, time
  • Review of prescribed medications
  • Guidelines related to specific surgery
  • Dressing and wound care
  • Pain control
  • Activity restrictions
  • Guidelines related to possible effects of anesthesia
  • Dietary restrictions
  • Activity restrictions
  • Signs and symptoms of complications

Pediatric

• Maintenance of body temperature in infants and children after surgery is a priority because of their immature temperature-control mechanisms.

• Infants and children normally have higher metabolic rates and differences in physiological makeup than adults, resulting in greater oxygen, fluid, and calorie needs.

• Vomiting is a major concern in young children because of increased risk for fluid and electrolyte imbalances and risk for aspiration. Vomiting is also more likely because surgery in children is often necessitated by accidental injuries without benefit of NPO status.

Gerontological

- The ability of older adults to tolerate surgery depends on the extent of physiological changes that have occurred with aging, the presence of any chronic diseases, and the duration of the surgical procedure.
- When communicating with older adults, be aware of any auditory, visual, or cognitive impairment that may be present.

Home Care

- Teach ambulatory surgery patient and primary caregiver about any postoperative exercises, home modifications, or activity limitations.
- If patient is discharged with dressing changes, suggest that bedroom or bathroom is usually ideal for procedure.
- Assess need for a home health care referral.

◆ SKILL 37.5 **Providing Early Postoperative and Convalescent Phase Recovery**

The second phase of recovery is the postoperative convalescent period. ASPAN defines the phase II level of care as the period when the nursing roles focus on preparation for care in the home or an extended care environment. This period extends from the time a patient is discharged from the postanesthesia care unit (PACU) to the time he or she is discharged from the inpatient hospital. Outpatient surgical patients undergo convalescence at home. All patients who have undergone surgical procedures have similar postoperative needs. However, nursing care becomes very individualized and depends on the nature of a patient's surgery, preexisting medical conditions, the onset of complications, and the speed of recovery. Not all surgical patients recover at the same rate. During the convalescent period you begin preparation for discharge and actively include the patient, family, and significant others in the process. The nurse promotes the patient's independence, educates the patient and/or family caregiver about any limitations imposed by surgery, and provides resources needed for the patient to assume an improved state of wellness.

Delegation and Collaboration

The skill of providing early postoperative and convalescent phase recovery cannot be delegated to nursing assistive personnel (NAP). NAP may obtain vital signs (if patient is stable), apply nasal cannula or oxygen mask (but not adjust oxygen flow), and provide hygiene or repositioning for comfort. The nurse instructs the NAP by:
- Explaining how often to take vital signs.
- Reviewing specific safety concerns and what to observe and report back to the nurse.

- Explaining any precautions that affect how to provide basic hygiene and comfort measures.

Equipment

- Postoperative bed (recliner for day surgery recovery)
- Stethoscope, sphygmomanometer, thermometer
- Intravenous (IV) fluid poles and infusion pumps as needed
- Emesis basin
- Washcloth and towel
- Waterproof pads
- Equipment for oral hygiene
- Pillows
- Facial tissue
- Oxygen equipment and bag-valve-masks and emergency cart with defibrillator available for adult and children
- Suction equipment (to suction airway)
- Dressing supplies
- Intermittent suction (to connect to nasogastric [NG] or wound drainage tubes)
- Orthopedic appliances (if needed)
- Clean gloves
- Personal protective equipment as indicated
- Malignant hyperthermia cart (Rothrock, 2015; Schick and Windle, 2016)
- Latex-free supplies and equipment
- Transport equipment, including wheelchairs and carts

STEP	RATIONALE

ASSESSMENT

1. Obtain phone report from PACU nurse summarizing patient's current status.	Allows you to prepare hospital room with necessary supplies and equipment for patient's special needs.
2. Identify patient using at least two identifiers (e.g., name and birthday or name and medical record number), according to agency policy.	Ensures correct patient. Complies with The Joint Commission standards and improves patient safety (TJC, 2016).
3. On patient's arrival on nursing unit, collect more detailed hand-off report from nurse accompanying patient.	Detailed report helps nurse plan appropriate assessment and nursing care measures. Data provide baseline to detect any change in patient's condition.
4. Review patient's chart for information pertaining to type of surgery; complications; medications administered; preoperative medical risks; baseline vital signs, including PACU vitals; and patient's usual medications given/not given before surgery.	Nature of surgery, intraoperative complications, and presence of medical risks dictate complications for which to observe. Vital signs provide means to detect postoperative changes. List of patient's usual medications may necessitate call to surgeon for orders concerning timing and dose of drugs not given before surgery.
5. Review postoperative medical orders.	Offers additional guidelines for type of care to provide.
6. Assess patient's and family's knowledge and expectations of surgical recovery.	Patient will be better prepared to participate in care.

STEP	RATIONALE

NURSING DIAGNOSES

- Acute confusion
- Acute pain
- Deficient fluid volume
- Deficient knowledge regarding postoperative care
- Excess fluid volume

- Impaired gas exchange
- Impaired physical mobility
- Impaired skin integrity
- Impaired verbal communication
- Ineffective airway clearance
- Ineffective breathing pattern

- Ineffective protection
- Ineffective tissue perfusion
- Nutrition imbalance, less than body requirements
- Risk of aspiration
- Risk of urinary retention

Related factors/Risk factors are individualized based on patient's condition or needs.

PLANNING

1. Expected outcomes following completion of procedure:
- Patient's breath sounds remain clear bilaterally.

  No occurrence of pulmonary changes except those expected from effects of anesthetic or analgesic.

- Patient's vital signs remain within normal limits consistent with preoperative baseline.

  No occurrence of cardiovascular, pulmonary, or thermoregulatory changes except those expected from effects of anesthetic or analgesic.

- Incision wound edges are well approximated; no drainage is noted.

  Indicates wound healing without signs of bleeding or infection.

- Fluid balance is evident by I&O records.

  Adequate urinary elimination maintained. Fluid intake (IV and/or by mouth [PO]) adequately maintained.

- Patient describes pain as less than 4 on scale of 0 to 10 while engaged in moderate activity by discharge.

  Pain-relief measures effectively alter patient's reception or perception of pain.

- Normal bowel sounds are present after bowel surgery or general anesthesia within 48 to 72 hours after surgery.

  Indicates return of GI function.

- Patient or family caregiver describes signs that indicate complications that need to be reported, dietary modifications, and activity restrictions in the home. Identifies plans for follow-up visit and demonstrates incision care.

  Involves patient in plan of care and minimizes anxiety. As recovery progresses, patient is able to make more choices regarding how procedures should be performed. Family caregiver can serve as coach or provide direct assistance and help patient remember explanations given.

2. Perform hand hygiene and arrange equipment at bedside.

Reduces transmission of infection. Improves efficiency of care activity.

3. If patient is being transported by stretcher, prepare for transfer with bed in high position (level with stretcher), with sheet folded to side and room for stretcher to be placed beside bed easily (see Chapter 11).

Arrangement of equipment facilitates safety and smooth transfer process.

IMPLEMENTATION

1. Early Recovery Initial Postoperative Care

a. Help transport staff, using slide board, to move patient from stretcher to bed (see Chapter 11). Identify patient using at least two identifiers (e.g., name and birthday or name and medical record number), according to agency policy.

Ensures safe patient handling. Ensures correct patient. Complies with The Joint Commission standards and improves patient safety (TJC, 2016).

b. Attach any existing oxygen tubing, position IV fluids, verify IV flow-rate settings on infusion pump, and check drainage tubes (e.g., Foley catheter or wound drainage).

Maintains patency of IV and integrity of drainage tubing.

c. Maintain airway. If patient remains sleepy or lethargic, keep head extended and support in side-lying position (see Chapter 25).

Minimizes chances of aspiration and obstruction of airway with tongue.

d. Conduct initial assessment of level of consciousness (LOC) and vital signs and compare findings with vital signs in recovery area and patient's baseline values. Continue monitoring as ordered.

Patient's status may change during transfer. Movement of patient and pain level influence stability of vital signs. Change in vital signs may reveal onset of postoperative complications.

e. Encourage coughing, deep breathing, and use of incentive spirometry and PEP device (see Skill 37.2) to prevent atelectasis.

Anesthesia, medications, and intubation irritate airways, resulting in secretions and atelectasis. Coughing and use of devices expands chest, aerates lungs, and mobilizes secretions.

STEP	RATIONALE
f. Assess gastrointestinal system (GI) for return of bowel sounds.	Indicates return of GI function.
g. If NG tube is present, check placement and irrigate (see Chapter 35). Connect to proper drainage device. Connect all other drainage tubes to appropriate suction or collection device. Secure to prevent tension on tubing.	Transfer and movement may dislodge tubes, which would interfere with drainage.
h. Assess patient's surgical dressing for appearance, presence, and character of drainage. Unless contraindicated by surgeon, outline drainage along edges with pen and reassess in 1 hour for change. If no dressing is present, inspect condition of wound (see Chapter 40).	Wound can hemorrhage quickly during early postoperative period. Observations of wound and dressings provide data to measure progress of wound healing.

Clinical Decision Point *If unable to change dressing, mark area of drainage and label with time, date, and initials. Record frequency of reinforcement. Never use felt-tip marker to mark dressing because ink can bleed into gauze, contaminating incision site.*

STEP	RATIONALE
i. Palpate abdomen for bladder distention or use bladder ultrasound when available. If Foley catheter is present, check placement. Ensure that it is draining freely and properly secured. Patient may have continuous bladder irrigations or suprapubic catheter (see Chapter 34).	Anesthesia often contributes to urinary retention. Urinary stasis increases risk for urinary tract infection.
j. If no urinary drainage system is present, explain that voiding within 8 hours after surgery is expected. Male patients may void successfully if allowed to stand.	Anesthetics and analgesics depress sensation of bladder fullness. Patient may still have no sensations below level of spinal or epidural anesthetic.
k. Measure all sources of fluid intake and output (I&O) (including estimated blood loss during surgery).	Altered fluid and electrolyte balance is potential complication of major surgery.
l. Describe purpose of equipment and frequent observations to patient and significant others.	Unfamiliar sights (e.g., equipment, patient's appearance) often provoke anxiety.
m. Position patient for comfort, maintaining correct body alignment. Avoid tension on surgical wound site.	Reduces stress on suture line. Helps patient relax and promotes comfort.
n. Place call light within reach and raise side rails (one of two or three of four). Instruct patient to call for help to get out of bed.	Promotes patient's safety as effects of anesthesia continue to diminish. Raising all side rails may be considered physical restraint.
o. Assess patient's level of pain on age-appropriate pain scale. Assess last time analgesic was given. Patient-controlled analgesia (PCA) may be used for pain control (see Chapter 16). Medicate patient as ordered either around the clock or prn as ordered during first 24 to 48 hours. Explain to patient how you plan to control pain; review orders of what is prescribed and frequency.	Determines level of discomfort. Adequate pain control is needed to permit patient to participate with breathing exercises, coughing, and ambulation.
2. Continued Postoperative Care	
a. Assess vital signs at least every 4 hours or as ordered.	Temperature greater than 38°C (100.4°F) in first 48 hours may indicate atelectasis, the normal inflammatory response, or dehydration. Temperature greater than 37.8°C (100°F) on third day or after often indicates wound infection, pneumonia, or phlebitis (Lewis et al., 2017). Altered blood pressure or pulse is associated with cardiovascular complications (see Table 37.3).
b. Closely monitor progress of wound healing and change dressings as ordered.	Wound infection occurs most often within 3 to 6 days after surgery. Wound dehiscence occurs most often 3 to 11 days after surgery (see Chapter 40).
c. Monitor drainage (see illustration A) and maintain wound drainage devices such as Jackson-Pratt, Hemovac, or Penrose drains. Jackson-Pratt and Hemovac drainage systems must be emptied when they are half full of drainage or air and recharged (compressed to discharge air) (see illustration B).	Wound drainage devices promote healing from inside to outside and relieve pressure on suture line. Compressing flexible closed container and then plugging drainage hole creates negative suction pressure.

STEP	RATIONALE

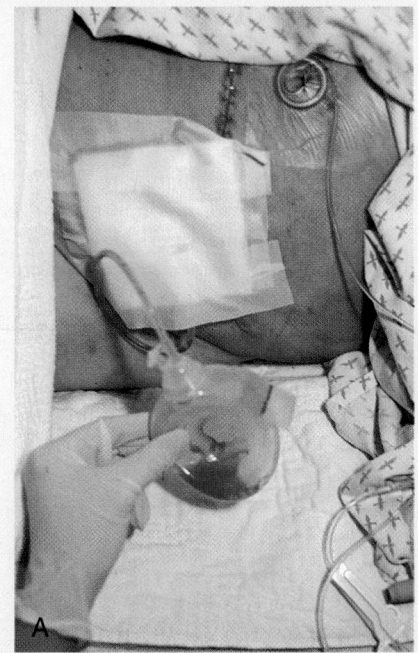 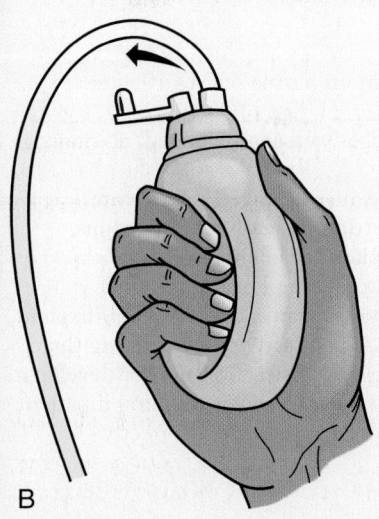

STEP 2c A, Note color of drainage from device. **B,** Charging Jackson-Pratt drainage system.

d. Provide oral care at least every 2 hours as needed. If permitted, offer ice chips.

Medication such as anticholinergic given before surgery makes mouth dry. Oral care and ice chips promote comfort.

e. Encourage patient to turn, cough, deep breathe, and use incentive spirometer and PEP device at least every 2 hours (see Skill 37.2).

Promotes adequate ventilation and minimizes hypoventilation and atelectasis. Especially necessary for patients with a history of smoking, pneumonia, or chronic obstructive pulmonary disease (COPD) or patients who are confined to bed rest.

f. Monitor function of sequential compression devices. If ordered, apply elastic stockings to lower extremities (see Chapter 12). Explain to patient that compression device will inflate and deflate intermittently.

Stockings increase venous return (Elisha et al., 2015). Explanation decreases anxiety and fosters cooperation.

g. Promote ambulation and activity as ordered (see Chapter 12). Assess vital signs before and after activity to assess tolerance. Patients often are encouraged to be up in chair the evening of surgery or next morning and progress to walking in room or hallway.

Ambulation is most significant nursing intervention to prevent postoperative complications. Mobility promotes circulation, lung expansion, and peristalsis. Postural hypotension is caused by sudden position changes.

h. Progress from clear liquids to regular diet as tolerated if nausea and vomiting do not occur.

Nausea and vomiting are associated with anesthesia and surgery. IV fluids are usually discontinued when oral intake is tolerated. Some patients must be NPO for several days until flatus returns or bowel sounds are heard.

i. Include patient and family caregiver in decision making; answer questions as they arise.

Promotes patient's sense of control and independence and improves self-esteem.

j. Provide opportunity for patients who must adjust to change in body appearance or function to verbalize feelings.

Radical surgery, amputation, or inoperable cancer often results in anxiety and depression. Grief response to loss of body organ is common and should be expected.

3. Convalescent Phase

a. Assess patient's home environment for safety, cleanliness, and availability of community resources and help for patient. (**NOTE:** In many settings this is done by a case manager and not a staff nurse. Use the information to revise any teaching you provide.)

Provides information about patient's need for home care. Verifies patient's and caregiver's level of knowledge and any additional teaching needs for discharge. Helps to promote uncomplicated discharge and patient's independence and participation in care.

b. Provide instruction on care activities that patient or family caregiver will perform at home (e.g., dressing change, medication administration, exercises, IV therapy).

Enables patient to achieve self-care at home.

c. Keep patient and family caregiver informed of progress made toward recovery. Explain time expected for discharge from hospital. Provide answers to individual patient questions or concerns.

Decreases anxiety and helps patient know what to anticipate to participate in discharge planning.

STEP	RATIONALE

EVALUATION

1. Auscultate breath sounds bilaterally.
2. Monitor trends in vital signs.
3. Evaluate I&O records. Assess time of patient's first postoperative urination.
4. Auscultate bowel sounds.
5. Ask patient to describe pain on a scale of 0 to 10 after moderate activity.
6. Inspect incision (wound edges well approximated, no drainage noted).
7. Have patient or family caregiver describe incision care, dietary modifications or restrictions, activity restrictions, medication schedule, and plans for follow-up visit.
8. **Use Teach-Back:** "I want to be sure I explained what you need to know about your postoperative activity level. Explain for me how you will increase your activity level during the first week at home." Revise your instruction now or develop a plan for revised patient or family caregiver teaching if patient or family caregiver is not able to teach back correctly.

Determines status of airways.
Provides data to measure progress of postoperative status.
Indicates onset of urination.

Allows you to evaluate return of peristalsis and diet tolerance.
Determines level of comfort achieved and effectiveness of pain-relief measures.
Provides data to measure progress of wound healing.

Identifies need for further teaching.

Determines patient's and family caregiver's level of understanding of instructional topic.

Unexpected Outcomes	Related Interventions
1. Vital signs are above or below patient's baseline or expected range. Initially this could be related to anesthesia effects, pain, hypovolemic shock, airway obstruction, fluid and electrolyte imbalance, or hypothermia.	• Identify contributing factors. • Notify surgeon.
2. Patient complains of severe incisional pain.	• Report to surgeon; discuss alternative analgesic option. • Try nonpharmacological pain control measures (see Chapter 16).

Recording and Reporting

- Document patient's arrival at nursing unit; describe vital signs, assessment findings, and all nursing measures initiated in nurses' notes in electronic health record (EHR) or chart.
- Continue to document these factors every 4 hours or more frequently as patient's condition warrants.
- Record vital signs and I&O on appropriate flow sheet.
- Report any abnormal assessment findings and signs of complications to surgeon.
- Document your evaluation of patient and family caregiver learning.

Special Considerations
Teaching

- Instruct patient and primary caregiver to identify signs and symptoms and appropriate actions to take for infection, respiratory, circulatory, or GI difficulties and wound disruptions.
- Provide important phone numbers to patient and primary caregiver for use in emergency and follow-up care on discharge.
- Teach patient about appropriate wound care, diet recommendations, and activity restrictions.

Pediatric

- Assessment of a child's perceptions of the surgical experience enforces positive experiences and clarifies misconceptions. Drawing and storytelling are effective methods that allow children to share their thoughts and feelings (Hockenberry and Wilson, 2015).

- Use appropriate pain assessment tools to determine child's pain level.

Gerontological

- Older adults often experience a longer and more difficult postoperative recovery. Assess carefully for the development of postoperative complications.
- Assess for postoperative delirium and changes in mental status along with potential causes.
- Older adults may not request pain medication because they believe it should be tolerated as an expected effect of surgery (Lewis et al., 2017).

Home Care

- Teach patient and family caregiver about postoperative exercises, home modifications, activity limitations, wound dressing care, medications, and nutritional needs.
- If patient is discharged with dressing changes, the bedroom or bathroom is usually ideal for the procedure. Have patient and family caregiver perform return demonstration of dressing change.
- Make referral to home health services if patient and family caregiver will have difficulty providing the expected level of care needed.
- Patients having surgery performed in ambulatory surgery centers must be accompanied by a family member or friend to allow for discharge after the procedure (see Box 37.2).

◆ CLINICAL DEBRIEF

You are assigned to care for a 52-year-old African-American female patient who is 5 feet tall and weighs 250 lbs (113.6 kg). She is married with three adult children and is employed as an attorney. You just received her from the postanesthesia care unit (PACU) following an abdominal hysterectomy for fibroid tumors and a bladder neck suspension. Her previous medical history includes 30-year, 2-pack-per-day cigarette smoking and type 2 diabetes; and she has been on birth control pills for 20 years. She has an abdominal dressing that has a small amount of shadowing on it, is on oxygen at 2 L via nasal cannula, and has both a Foley catheter and a suprapubic catheter draining pink-tinged urine. She has an intravenous (IV) infusion of $D_5 \frac{1}{2}$ normal saline (NS) infusing at 125 mL/h and a morphine patient-controlled analgesia (PCA) device. She received Ancef IV piggyback approximately 45 minutes before her incision was made and is to receive her second dose 8 hours later.

1. Which postoperative complications is this patient at risk for developing, and what are the nursing implications? Provide the rationale.
2. What postoperative teaching should be included, and who should be included in the teaching?
3. On postoperative day 2 the patient appears anxious and has a pulse oxygenation of 82%. On assessment her left lung sounds are diminished when compared to the right. She also complains that her left leg is painful and swollen. Using SBAR, show how you would communicate with the health care team about this patient.

◆ REVIEW QUESTIONS

1. Prevention of surgical site infections (SSIs) requires numerous actions by both the surgical team and the patient. Select the measures that are used to reduce SSIs. (Select all that apply.)
   1. Discharge patient from the hospital as soon as possible.
   2. Give prophylactic antibiotic therapy as close to the time of incision as possible.
   3. Shave excess hair with a razor just before the surgery begins.
   4. Control hyperglycemia in patients with and without diabetes.
   5. Give a shower or bath after the preoperative enema is evacuated.
2. There are numerous measures to prevent venous thromboembolism during the postoperative period. Which intervention would be most appropriate before the surgery begins? (Select all that apply.)
   1. Performing an assessment for Homans' sign
   2. Ensure bilateral lower-extremity sequential compression devices are on and functioning
   3. Teaching patient coughing and breathing techniques
   4. Instructing patient how to ambulate after surgery
   5. Teaching patient how to do leg exercises
3. Which assignment would the registered nurse (RN) delegate to the nursing assistive personnel (NAP)? (Select all that apply.)
   1. Managing the postoperative care of the patient
   2. Initial assessments on arrival to the PACU
   3. Emptying the Foley catheter
   4. Caring for the patient requiring monitoring and providing comfort measures
   5. Assessing the intravenous (IV) site.

ⓔ *Visit the Evolve site for a complete list of Clinical Debrief and Review Questions answers.*

REFERENCES

American Society of Anesthesiologists (ASA) Committee: Practice guidelines for preoperative fasting and the use of pharmacologic agents to reduce the risk of pulmonary aspiration: application to healthy patients undergoing elective procedures: an updated report by the American Society of Anesthesiologists Committee on Standards and Practice Parameters, *Anesthesiology* 114(3):495, 2011.

American Society of PeriAnesthesia Nurses (ASPAN): *2015-2017 perianesthesia nursing standards, practice recommendations and interpretive statements*, Cherry Hill, NJ, 2015, ASPAN.

Association of periOperative Registered Nurses (AORN): *Position statement: one perioperative registered nurse circulator dedicated to every patient undergoing a surgical or other invasive procedure*, 2012, The Association. http://www.aorn.org/aorn-org/guidelines/clinical-resources/position-statements. Accessed August 1, 2016.

Association of periOperative Registered Nurses (AORN): *Perioperative standards and recommended practices*, Denver, CO, 2015, AORN.

Centers for Disease Control and Prevention (CDC): *Infection control standards for The Joint Commission*, updated 2015. www.cdc.gov/ncidod/dhqp/hai.html. Accessed August 1, 2016.

Chung F, et al: STOP-Bang Questionnaire: a practical approach to screen for obstructive sleep apnea, *Chest* 149:631–638, 2016.

Diaz V, Newman J: Surgical site infection and prevention guidelines: a primer for certified registered nurse anesthetists, *AANA J* 83(1):2015.

Eliasen MI, et al: Preoperative alcohol consumption and postoperative complications: a systematic review and meta-analysis, *Ann Surg* 258(6):930–942, 2013.

Elisha S, et al: Venous thromboembolism: new concepts in perioperative management, *AANA J* 83(3):211, 2015.

Graling PR, Vasaly FW: Effectiveness of 2% CHG cloth bathing for reducing surgical site infections, *AORN J* 97(5):547, 2013.

Hockenberry MJ, Wilson D: *Wong's nursing care of infants and children*, ed 10, St Louis, 2015, Mosby.

Lewis S, et al: *Medical-surgical nursing: assessment and management of clinical problems*, ed 10, St Louis, 2017, Elsevier.

Magill S, et al: Multistate point-prevalence survey of health care-associated infections, *N Engl J Med* 370(13):1198, 2014.

Nagelhout JJ, Plaus KL: *Nurse anesthesia*, ed 5, St Louis, 2014, Saunders.

Ogan OU, Plevak DJ: *Anesthesia safety always an issue with obstructive sleep apnea*, The American Sleep Apnea Association, nd. http://www.apsf.org/newsletters/html/1997/summer/sleepapnea.html. Accessed August 6, 2016.

Rothrock J: *Alexander's care of the patient in surgery*, ed 15, St Louis, 2015, Mosby.

Schick L, Windle P: *PeriAnesthesia nursing core curriculum: preoperative, phase I and phase II PACU nursing*, ed 3, St Louis, 2016, Saunders.

Spruce L: Back to basics: patient and family engagement, *AORN J* 102(1):34, 2015.

Spry C, Goodman T: *Essentials of perioperative nursing*, ed 4, Gaithersburg, MD, 2013, Aspen.

Stannard D, Krenzischek D: *Perianesthesia nursing care: a bedside guide for safe recovery*, Sudbury, MA, 2012, Jones & Bartlett Learning.

The Joint Commission (TJC): *2016 National Patient Safety Goals*, Oakbrook Terrace, IL, 2016, The Commission. http://www.jointcommission.org/standards_information/npsgs.aspx. Accessed April 13, 2016.

World Health Organization (WHO): *Surgical safety checklist*, 2008. http://www.who.int/patientsafety/safesurgery/tools_resources/SSSL_Checklist_finalJun08.pdf?ua=1. Accessed April 13, 2016.

38 | Intraoperative Care

OBJECTIVES

Mastery of content in this chapter will enable the nurse to:
- Describe the meaning of a sterile conscience.
- Describe the roles of a registered nurse in the operating room.
- Identify guidelines for use of sterile technique in the operating room.

- Perform surgical hand antisepsis correctly.
- Describe how to correctly don a sterile surgical gown.
- Apply sterile gloves using the closed technique.

MEDIA RESOURCES

- evolve http://evolve.elsevier.com/Perry/skills
- Review Questions

- Audio Glossary
- Clinical Debrief and Review Questions Answers

PURPOSE

Nurses practicing in the operating room (OR) support patients' surgical experiences from the preoperative phase throughout the intraoperative period and into the various postoperative phases (see Chapter 37). Perioperative nurses exercise judgment, critical thinking, and interpersonal communication skills while also using the nursing process to ensure that patients receive appropriate nursing care throughout their surgical experience (AORN, 2015).

STANDARDS OF CARE

- Association of PeriOperative Nurses (AORN), 2015—Guidelines for Perioperative Practices: Registered Nurse Circulator Responsibilities
- The Joint Commission (TJC), 2016—2016 Patient Safety Goals; Prevent Mistakes in Surgery; Prevent Postoperative Infections
- World Health Organization (WHO), 2009; The Joint Commission (TJC), 2016—Surgical Checklist/Time-Out

PRINCIPLES FOR PRACTICE

- The interprofessional surgical team includes the surgeon (doctor of medicine [MD] or doctor of osteopathy [DO]), physician's assistant (PA), registered nurse first assistant (RNFA) (Box 38.1), certified registered nurse anesthetist (CRNA) and/or physician anesthesiologist (MD or DO), circulating nurse (RN), and scrub nurse/technician (RN, licensed practical nurse [LPN], (Box 38.2) or certified surgical technologist [CST]).

- The intraoperative phase begins when a patient enters the operating room (OR) suite and ends with admission to the postanesthesia care unit (PACU).
- A circulating nurse (Box 38.3) is an RN who both manages and collaborates closely with the interprofessional team while using the nursing process to guide the patient through the intraoperative phase (Rothrock, 2015). He or she is a "nonsterile" member of the surgical team who assumes responsibility and accountability for maintaining patient safety and continuity of quality care. This includes supervising the conduct of the scrub technician and delegating tasks to licensed and nursing assistive personnel (NAP) as appropriate. The circulating nurse also assists the first assistant, scrub nurse/technician, and surgeon.
- It is essential that perioperative nurses develop a sterile conscience, always knowing the location of a sterile field and what items are sterile versus nonsterile. A sterile conscience requires knowledge of the principles of aseptic technique; self-discipline; good communication skills to identify, address, and correct any breaks in sterile technique; and the maturity to overcome personal preferences.
- While a patient is in the OR and the OR team is gowned and gloved, it is recommended that a surgical safety checklist or the World Health Organization (WHO) checklist be completed (WHO, 2009) (Fig. 38.1). The WHO checklist identifies three phases of an operation, each corresponding to a specific period in the normal flow of work: before the induction of anesthesia ("sign in"), before the incision of the skin ("time-out"), and before the patient leaves the operating room ("sign out"). In each phase a checklist coordinator must confirm that the surgery

BOX 38.1

Role and Responsibilities of a Registered Nurse First Assistant

The registered nurse first assistant (RNFA) role is an expansion of the traditional perioperative nursing role, and areas of responsibility overlap. Responsibilities specific to the practice of first assisting include:

- Participating in "time-out" procedure with other surgical team members (safety measure taken to ensure correct patient, correct procedure, correct site and side, correct patient position, and correct implants/equipment present) (TJC, 2016).
- Providing surgical exposure (assisting in retracting tissues and suctioning surgical field).
- Providing hemostasis (control of bleeding).
- Handling and/or cutting tissue.
- Using surgical instruments/medical devices and suturing.
- Performing wound closure.
- Applying human anatomical and physiological considerations in practice; recognizing structure, function, and location of tissues and organs; manipulating tissues accordingly to avoid injury.
- Ensuring preoperative and postoperative patient management in collaboration with other health care providers.

From Association of periOperative Registered Nurses (AORN): *AORN standards and recommended practices for perioperative nursing—position statement: AORN official statement on RN first assistants,* Denver, 2015, The Association.

BOX 38.2

Role of the Scrub Nurse

- Helps circulating nurse prepare the OR and open supplies
- Performs surgical hand antisepsis and dons sterile gown and gloves
- Prepares sterile field with procedure-appropriate supplies and instruments, verifying that all are in working order
- Participates in "time-out" procedure with other surgical team members (safety measure taken to ensure correct patient, correct procedure, correct site and side, correct patient position, and correct implants/equipment present) (TJC, 2016)
- Performs sponge, sharps, and instrument counts with circulating nurse before incision is made, at the beginning of wound closure, and at the end of the surgical procedure
- Labels all liquids and/or medications on sterile field with sterile marking pen when liquid or medication is out of the original container or package
- Gowns and gloves surgeons and assistants as they enter the OR
- Assists surgeons with sterile draping of patient
- Keeps sterile field orderly and monitors progress of procedure and any breaks in aseptic technique
- Passes sterile instruments and supplies to surgeons and assistants
- Handles surgical specimens per agency policy
- Constantly monitors location of all sponges and sharps in the sterile field

OR, Operating room.

BOX 38.3

Role of the Circulating Nurse

- Incorporates nursing process in plan of care
- Organizes and prepares OR before start of surgical procedure; checks to see that equipment works properly
- Gathers supplies for surgical procedure and opens sterile supplies for scrub nurse/technician
- Counts sponges, sharps, and instruments with scrub nurse/technician before incision is made, at the beginning of wound closure, and at the end of the surgical procedure
- Ensures that all liquids and/or medications on the sterile field are labeled with sterile marking pen when liquid or medication is out of the original container or package
- Sends for patient at appropriate time
- Conducts preoperative patient assessment, including the following:
  - Explaining role and identifies patient
  - Reviewing medical record and verifies procedure and consents
  - Confirming dentures and prostheses removed
  - Confirming patient's allergies, nothing by mouth (NPO) status, laboratory values, ECG, x-ray film studies, skin condition, circulatory and pulmonary status
- Safely helps patient to operating table and positions patient according to surgeon preference and procedure type, using safety precautions (e.g., safety belt, securing arms, padding bony prominences)
- Participates in "time-out" procedure with other surgical team members (safety measure taken to ensure correct patient, correct procedure, correct site and side, correct patient position, and correct implants/equipment present) (TJC, 2016)
- Applies conductive pad to patient if electrocautery used; may prepare patient's skin; may apply ECG electrodes
- Applies antiembolism stockings and sequential compression device per physician order
- Explains briefly to patient what the circulating nurse and the scrub nurse/technician are doing
- Assists surgical team by tying gowns and arranging equipment
- Assists anesthesia personnel during induction and extubation
- Continuously monitors procedure for any breaks in aseptic technique and anticipates needs of the team; opens additional sterile supplies for scrub nurse/technician
- Handles surgical specimens per agency policy
- Documents on perioperative nurses' notes
- Communicates to family and PACU personnel during the surgical procedure

ECG, Electrocardiogram; *OR,* operating room; *PACU,* postanesthesia care unit.

procedure from start to finish. It is during the time-out that the team members agree at a minimum that the correct patient has been identified and the correct procedure is scheduled to be done. The time-out is documented before the procedure begins (TJC, 2016).

PATIENT-CENTERED CARE

- The patient may be unsure of what to expect and have concerns regarding pain, disfigurement, and length of recovery. It is a nurse's responsibility to provide this information and encourage questions.
- Care of the surgical patient requires specialized knowledge when the nurse is required to closely monitor a patient's intraoperative response to the experience.
- Patient needs vary based on preoperative health, type of surgical procedure, and cultural and religious beliefs. Nurses obtain information regarding culture and religious preferences that

team has completed the listed tasks before it proceeds with the operation.

- The surgical checklist verifies the patient's identity, ascertains if the patient has any allergies, checks if the surgical site is marked and verifies the site marking, and asks the patient if he or she has any questions (TJC, 2016; WHO, 2009).
- A time-out is conducted immediately before starting any invasive procedure or making an incision (TJC, 2016). Time-outs are standardized by each agency, initiated by a designated member of the team, and involve all the immediate members of the surgical/procedure team who will be participating in the

Surgical Safety Checklist

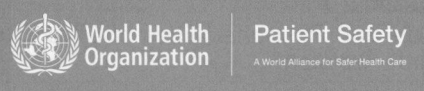

Before induction of anaesthesia

(with at least nurse and anaesthetist)

Has the patient confirmed his/her identity, site, procedure, and consent?
☐ Yes

Is the site marked?
☐ Yes
☐ Not applicable

Is the anaesthesia machine and medication check complete?
☐ Yes

Is the pulse oximeter on the patient and functioning?
☐ Yes

Does the patient have a:

Known allergy?
☐ No
☐ Yes

Difficult airway or aspiration risk?
☐ No
☐ Yes, and equipment/assistance available

Risk of >500ml blood loss (7ml/kg in children)?
☐ No
☐ Yes, and two IVs/central access and fluids planned

Before skin incision

(with nurse, anaesthetist and surgeon)

☐ **Confirm all team members have introduced themselves by name and role.**

☐ **Confirm the patient's name, procedure, and where the incision will be made.**

Has antibiotic prophylaxis been given within the last 60 minutes?
☐ Yes
☐ Not applicable

Anticipated Critical Events

To Surgeon:
☐ What are the critical or non-routine steps?
☐ How long will the case take?
☐ What is the anticipated blood loss?

To Anaesthetist:
☐ Are there any patient-specific concerns?

To Nursing Team:
☐ Has sterility (including indicator results) been confirmed?
☐ Are there equipment issues or any concerns?

Is essential imaging displayed?
☐ Yes
☐ Not applicable

Before patient leaves operating room

(with nurse, anaesthetist and surgeon)

Nurse Verbally Confirms:
☐ The name of the procedure
☐ Completion of instrument, sponge and needle counts
☐ Specimen labelling (read specimen labels aloud, including patient name)
☐ Whether there are any equipment problems to be addressed

To Surgeon, Anaesthetist and Nurse:
☐ What are the key concerns for recovery and management of this patient?

This checklist is not intended to be comprehensive. Additions and modifications to fit local practice are encouraged.   Revised 1 / 2009   © WHO, 2009

FIG 38.1 The WHO surgical safety checklist. (*Used with permission, World Health Organization.*)

may affect acceptance of education, blood administration, and surgical interventions.

- Information is communicated to the interprofessional team to ensure comprehensive intraoperative care.

EVIDENCE-BASED PRACTICE

Decreased glove perforation results in decreased surgical site infection and also protects the health care provider from exposure to bloodborne pathogens (AORN, 2015). Evidence-based research offers the following gloving guidelines:

- Double gloving is superior to single gloving.
- There is a significant reduction in the perforation of the innermost layers when double gloving is compared to single gloving (AORN, 2015; Childs, 2013; Korniewicz and El-Masri, 2012).
- In addition, double gloving and using the perforation indicator system (lighter pair of gloves worn over a darker pair) helps a health care provider better identify glove failure (Diaz, 2015).

Current evidence-based research links perioperative hypothermia with an increase in morbidity and mortality. Specifically, hypothermia can put the patient at an additional risk of surgical site infection, cardiac arrhythmias, changes in medication metabolism, and increased incidence of surgical bleeding. Patients at risk for hypothermia include the elderly, low body weight, metabolic disorders,

cold surgical environment and/or the use of cold infusions, and open-cavity surgical procedures (ASPAN, 2014; AORN, 2015; Schick and Windle, 2016).

- Interventions effective in preventing hypothermia include forced-air warming. Commencement of active warming preoperatively and monitoring it throughout the intraoperative period is effective. Combined strategies, including preoperative commencement of warming and the use of warmed fluids plus forced-air warming, are also effective (Moola and Lockwood, 2011).

OR personnel are responsible for adhering to specific infection control practices based on individualized agency guidelines. Basic evidence-based infection control practices include the following:

- Hand hygiene should be performed when OR staff arrive at the health care agency, before and after patient contact, before and after donning gloves and other personal protective equipment, before and after eating, before leaving the health care agency, and when visibly soiled (AORN, 2015).
- Hand scrub using alcohol-based hand-rub products should be approved by the infection control committee of the organization and should demonstrate a persistent and cumulative effect. The user must be made aware of and follow the manufacturer written instructions regarding storage, dispensing, technique, and amount of product required (AORN, 2015).

- Use approved brushless, alcohol-based surgical hand-rub products (with added emollients) that limit damage to the user's skin, improve adherence to hand antisepsis protocols, simplify application technique, and reduce material waste (i.e., water, brushes, and packaging) (Rothrock, 2015).
- Fingernails should be no longer than $\frac{1}{4}$ inch in length, and nail polish should not be chipped. Avoid use of any nail enhancements (artificial nails, acrylics, tips, and gels) (AORN, 2015).

SAFETY GUIDELINES

- Landers (2015) recommends an initiative to reduce intraoperative errors: using a time-out, decreasing distractions, non-punitive error reporting, and increasing staff ratios and education.
- All items used within a sterile field must be sterile.
- Gowns used by scrub people must be sterile before donning. Once in place, gowns are sterile from the front chest and shoulders to table level and on the sleeves to 5 cm (2 inches) above the elbow.
- Sterile people must keep their hands in view, above waist level and below neckline, to avoid contamination.
- When wearing a sterile gown, do not fold arms with hands tucked in the axillary region. This area is not considered sterile once you have donned the gown. Perspiration can lead to strike through, or contamination that occurs when moisture permeates a sterile barrier.
- Sterile-draped tables are sterile only at table level. Sides of the drape extending below table level are unsterile.
- All personnel moving around or within a sterile field must do so in a manner consistent with maintaining the sterility of that field. Scrubbed persons move from sterile areas to other sterile areas, contacting a sterile field only with sterile gowns and gloves. Unscrubbed people always stay at least 30 cm (12 inches) away from the sterile field while keeping it in constant view; they touch only unsterile areas.
- Group all sterile supplies and equipment around the sterile-draped patient.
- Unsterile people must avoid reaching over the sterile field.
- Scrubbed people remain close to the sterile field. When changing position, turn face to face or back to back.

◆ **SKILL 38.1** | **Surgical Hand Antisepsis**

In the operating room (OR) setting it is imperative that you achieve surgical hand antisepsis through effective surgical scrub or antiseptic hand rub (AORN, 2015). To reduce patient risk for acquiring postoperative infections, use of an antimicrobial preparation for hand antisepsis is an integral part of the presurgical scrubbing procedure for OR personnel. Although the skin cannot be sterilized, you can reduce the number of microorganisms greatly by chemical, physical, and mechanical means.

Through the use of an antimicrobial agent and sterile brushes or sponges, the surgical hand scrub removes debris and transient microorganisms from the nails, hands, and forearms; reduces the resident microbial count to a minimum; and inhibits rapid/rebound growth of microorganisms (AORN, 2015). Evidence suggests that completing a brushless hand-rub technique using approved hand-hygiene products, with or without water, is an alternative to the traditional hand scrub with a brush with the same microbial efficacy (AORN, 2015). Both hand-antiseptic methods are currently used in OR settings.

The AORN (2015) recommends a 3- to 5-minute hand and arm scrub with an approved antimicrobial agent for all surgical procedures. Surgical hand-scrub procedure for all staff using either the anatomical timed scrub or the counted-stroke method should be standardized (AORN, 2015) (see agency policy). Some procedures, described as clean procedures (e.g., laryngoscopy and proctoscopy), require performing hand hygiene but not necessarily surgical hand antisepsis.

Delegation and Collaboration

The skill of surgical hand antisepsis can be delegated to a surgical technologist or licensed practical nurse. The registered nurse routinely observes surgical hand antisepsis for staff compliance.

Equipment

- Deep sink with foot or knee controls for dispensing water and soap
- Antimicrobial agent approved by agency (dispenser with foot controls)
- Surgical scrub brush with plastic nail file
- Paper face mask, cap or hood, surgical shoe covers
- Protective eyewear/face shield
- Sterile towel
- Sterile pack containing sterile gown

STEP	RATIONALE

ASSESSMENT

1. Determine type and length of time for hand hygiene (see agency policy).

Guidelines vary regarding ideal time needed for surgical scrub.

2. Remove bracelets, rings, and watches.

Jewelry harbors and protects microorganisms from removal. Skin under rings has been shown to harbor more pathogens and should not be worn (AORN, 2015).

3. Inspect fingernails, which must be short ($\frac{1}{4}$ inch), clean, and healthy. Nail polish that is chipped should be removed before entering surgical area. Never wear artificial nails or extenders.

Long nails and chipped or old polish harbor greater numbers of bacteria (AORN, 2015). Long fingernails can puncture gloves, causing contamination. Artificial nails harbor gram-negative microorganisms and fungus (AORN, 2015).

STEP	RATIONALE

4. Inspect condition of cuticles, hands, and forearms for presence of abrasions, cuts, or open lesions.

Cuts, abrasions, exudative lesions, fresh tattoos, or hangnails tend to ooze serum, which may contain pathogens. Individuals with these conditions should not have patient contact until conditions heal (AORN, 2015).

NURSING DIAGNOSIS

- Risk for infection

Risk factors are individualized based on patient's condition or needs.

PLANNING

1. Expected outcomes following completion of procedure:
- Patient does not develop signs of surgical site infection.

Indicates that microorganisms are not transferred to patient and sterile field.

IMPLEMENTATION

1. Don surgical shoe covers, cap or hood, face mask, and protective eyewear.

Protective eyewear prevents exposure to blood or body fluids splashing from sterile field, which causes risk for infection (e.g., human immunodeficiency virus [HIV], hepatitis B virus [HBV]).

Clinical Decision Point *Laser surgery requires special protective eyewear to prevent eye damage from stray laser energy.*

2. Perform prescrub wash at beginning of work shift.
  a. Turn water on using foot or knee control and adjust to comfortable temperature.
  b. Wet hands thoroughly with water. Follow manufacturer directions for application of soap.
  c. Rub hands, covering all surfaces with lather, including backs of hands, fingertips, inner webs, and palms, washing for at least 15 seconds.
  d. Rinse hands well. Dry hands thoroughly with disposable towel and discard towel.
3. Surgical hand scrub (with sponge):
  a. Turn on water using foot or knee control. Clean under nails of both hands with disposable nail pick or cleaner (see illustration). Rinse hands and forearms under running water.

Prevents contamination of hands after scrub.

A short prescrub wash/rinse at least 15 seconds at beginning of work shift removes gross debris and superficial microorganisms (AORN, 2015).
Rinsing removes all soap and remaining debris.

Removes dirt and organic materials that harbor microorganisms.

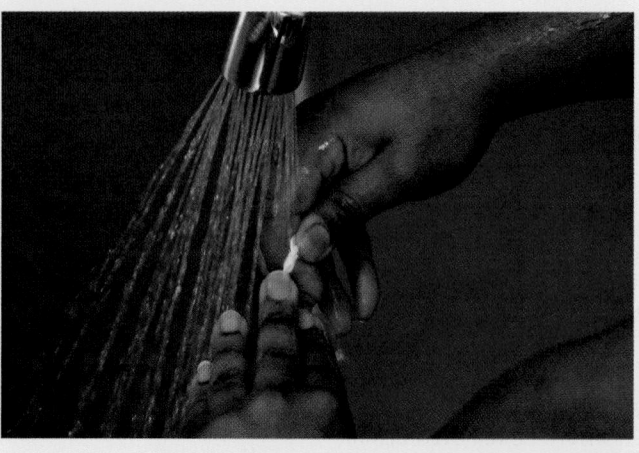

STEP 3a Clean under fingernails.

STEP	RATIONALE
b. Dispense antimicrobial scrub agent according to manufacturer instructions. Apply agent to wet hands and forearms with soft, nonabrasive sponge.	Ensures removal of resident microorganisms on all surfaces of hands and arms (AORN, 2015).
c. Time a 3- to 5-minute scrub (follow manufacturer instructions). Visualize each finger, hand, and arm as having four sides (see illustrations). Wash all four sides effectively, keeping hand elevated, elbow down. Repeat for other hand, fingers, and arm.	Times vary by product. Scrubbing all surfaces ensures removal of resident microorganisms on hands and arms (AORN, 2015). Keeping hands elevated and elbows down prevents microorganisms from flowing back onto hands.
d. Avoid splashing surgical attire. Discard sponges in appropriate container.	
e. Rinse hands and arms, running water from fingertips to elbows in one continuous motion, holding hands higher than elbows and away from surgical site (see illustration).	Hands remain cleanest part of upper extremities.
f. Turn off water using foot or knee controls and back into OR holding hands higher than elbows and away from surgical attire.	
g. Approach sterile setup and grasp sterile towel, taking care not to drip water on sterile field (see illustration).	Water contaminates field.
h. Keeping hands and arms above waist and outstretched, carefully grasp one end of sterile towel to dry one hand thoroughly, moving from fingers to elbow in rotating motion (see illustration).	Avoids sterile towel contacting unsterile scrub attire and transferring contamination to hands. Dries skin from cleanest (hands) to least clean (elbows).

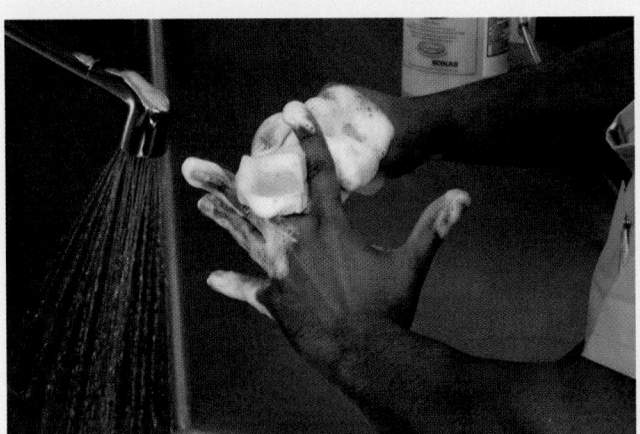 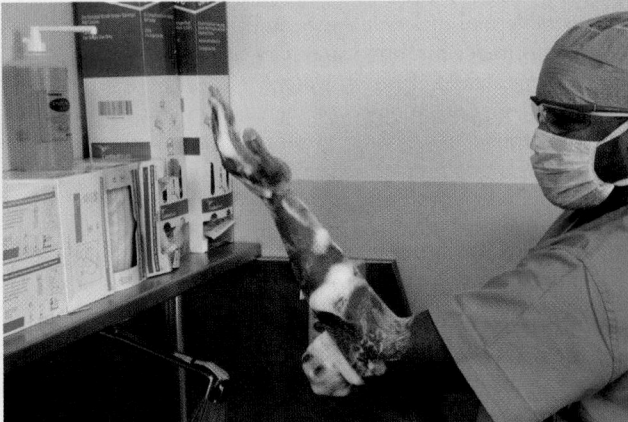

STEP 3c A, Scrub sides of fingers. **B,** Scrub forearms.

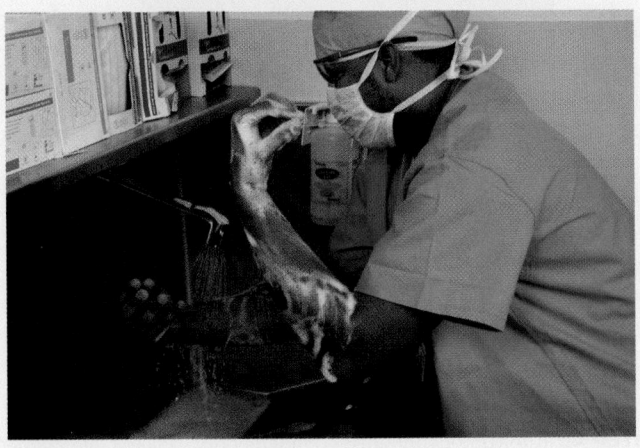 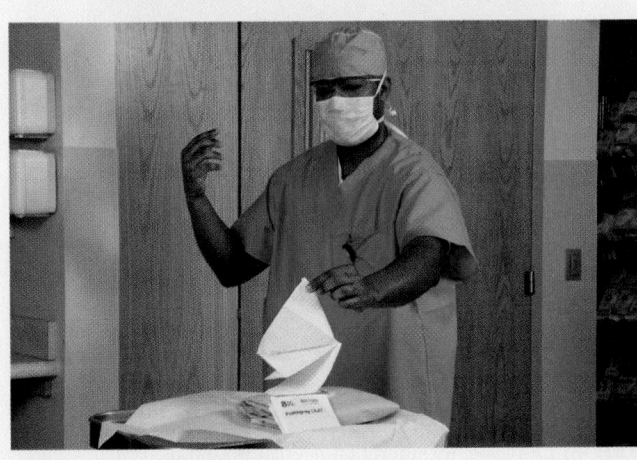

STEP 3e Rinse arms.   **STEP 3g** Grasp sterile towel.

STEP	RATIONALE

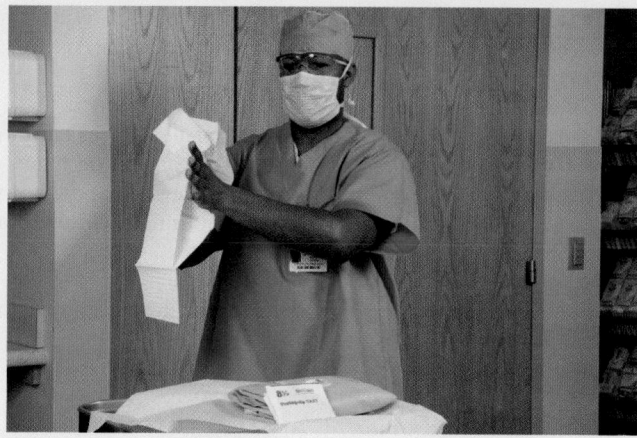

STEP 3h Dry hands thoroughly.

i. Use opposite end of towel to dry other hand.

Avoids transfer of microorganisms from elbow to opposite hand.

j. Drop towel into linen hamper or into circulating nurse's hand.

4. Perform spongeless surgical hand scrub with alcohol-based hand-rub product:

a. After prescrub wash (Step 2), turn on water using foot or knee control. Clean under nails of both hands with disposable nail pick or cleaner and rinse hands and forearms under running water. Dry hands thoroughly with paper towel. Turn off water.

b. Dispense manufacturer-recommended amount of antimicrobial agent hand preparation (see illustration). Apply agent to hands and forearms according to manufacturer instructions for application, recommended volume, and specified time.

Promotes reduction in microorganisms on all surfaces of hands and arms (AORN, 2015).

c. Repeat antimicrobial product application if indicated in manufacturer instructions.

d. Rub thoroughly until completely dry (see illustration). Proceed to OR to don gloves.

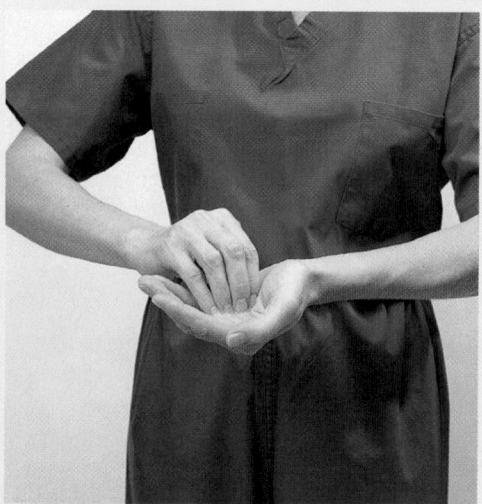

STEP 4b Dispense antimicrobial agent into hands. (*Photo Courtesy 3M Health Care.*)

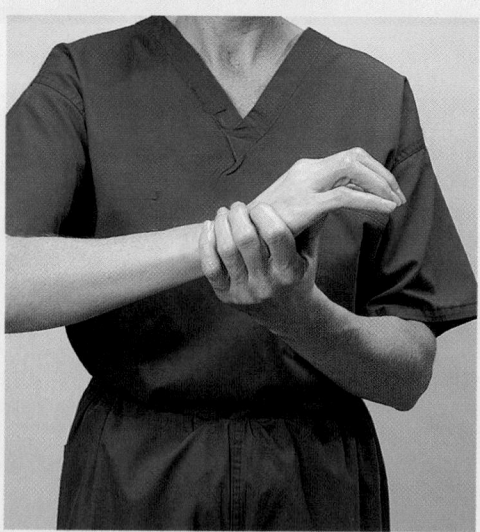

STEP 4d Rub thoroughly until completely dry. (*Photo Courtesy 3M Health Care.*)

STEP	RATIONALE

EVALUATION

1. Monitor patient after surgery for signs of surgical site infection (usually occurs 2 to 3 days after surgery).

Signs of infection include redness, heat, swelling, pain, and **purulent** drainage.

Unexpected Outcomes	**Related Interventions**
1. Redness, heat, swelling, pain, or purulent drainage may develop at surgical site, which often indicates wound infection.	• Individualize interventions based on patient's situation (e.g., wound care, antibiotic therapy).

Recording and Reporting

• No recording is required for surgical hand antisepsis. Record area and description of surgical site after surgery to provide baseline for monitoring wound.

♦ SKILL 38.2   Donning a Sterile Gown and Closed Gloving

Immediately following surgical hand antisepsis, apply a sterile gown and then apply sterile gloves. All members of the surgical team must prepare in this manner before entering the sterile field. Once applied, the surgical gown is considered sterile in the front from chest to waist or table level. The sleeves are considered sterile from 5 cm (2 inches) above the elbow to fingertips. The back of the gown is not considered sterile when worn. Surgical gowns should cover all garments worn underneath. All sterile gowns that are free of tears, punctures, strain, and abrasion provide an effective barrier against microorganisms, particulates, and fluids passing between unsterile and sterile areas (AORN, 2015).

Use the closed-glove method to apply gloves when you enter the sterile field. If a glove becomes contaminated during the surgery, the circulating nurse, wearing protective unsterile gloves, grasps the outside of the glove and pulls it off inside out, leaving the stockinette cuff of the gown in place. Another sterile team member assists in regloving. The open method can be used when only one glove has been contaminated. In some settings the scrub nurse will wear two pairs of sterile gloves. If both of the scrub nurse/

technician's gloves become contaminated, the gown is removed first, then the gloves are removed, and then the nurse regowns and regloves using the closed-glove method.

Delegation and Collaboration

The skills of donning a sterile gown and closed gloving can be delegated to a surgical technologist or licensed practical nurse. The registered nurse routinely observes sterile gown application and closed gloving for staff compliance.

Equipment

• **Package** of proper-size sterile gloves (latex-free if sensitivity or allergy present)
• **Sterile** pack containing sterile gown
• **Clean,** flat, dry surface (table or Mayo stand) on which to open gown and gloves
• **Paper** face masks, cap or hood, surgical shoe covers
• **Protective** eyewear/face shield

STEP	RATIONALE

ASSESSMENT

1. Select proper size and type of sterile gloves. Select latex-free gloves if you know that patient or any surgical personnel in room are latex sensitive.

Proper fit ensures ease of handling instruments and supplies. Prevents latex allergic response.

Clinical Decision Point *Know your agency policy because double gloving may be recommended to reduce the risk for glove perforation during a surgical procedure (AORN, 2015; Korniewicz and El-Masri, 2012).*

2. Select proper size and type of sterile surgical gown.

Ill-fitting gown impedes movement of extremities.

NURSING DIAGNOSIS

• Risk for infection

Risk factors are individualized based on patient's condition or needs.

STEP	RATIONALE

PLANNING

1. Expected outcomes following completion of procedure:
   • Patient does not develop signs of surgical site infection.

Nurse maintains aseptic technique and does not contaminate gown or gloves.

IMPLEMENTATION

1. **Donning sterile gown:**
   a. Open sterile gown and glove package on clean, dry, flat surface. Scrub nurse (before scrubbing hands) or circulating nurse can do this for you, preferably on small table separate from sterile field containing sterile instruments and supplies.

   Provides sterile area for gloving.

   b. Perform surgical hand antisepsis (see Skill 38.1). Dry hands thoroughly.

   c. Pick up gown (folded inside out) from sterile package, grasping inside surface at collar.

   Hands are not completely sterile. Inside surface of gown will contact surface of skin and thus is considered contaminated.

   d. Lift folded gown directly upward and step back, away from table.

   Prevents gown from touching unsterile object.

   e. Locate neckband; with both hands grasp inside front of gown just below neckband.

   Clean hands may touch inside of gown without contaminating outer surface.

   f. Keeping gown at arm's length away from body; allow it to unfold with inside of gown toward body. Do not touch outside of gown or allow it to touch floor.

   Outside of gown remains sterile.

   g. With hands at shoulder level, slip both arms into armholes simultaneously (see illustration). Do not allow hands to move through cuff opening. Have circulating nurse pull gown over shoulders by reaching inside arm seams. Pull gown on, leaving sleeves covering hands.

   Careful application prevents contamination. Gown covers hands to prepare for closed gloving.

   h. Have circulating nurse tie gown at neck and waist (see illustration). If gown is wraparound style, do not touch sterile front flap until scrub nurse/technician has gloved (see Step 3b).

   Secures gown without contaminating it.

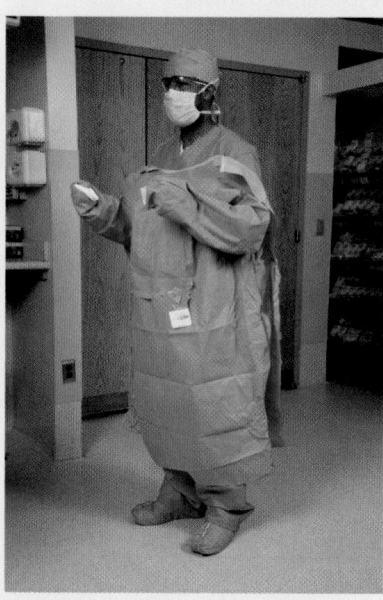

STEP 1g Place arms in sleeves.

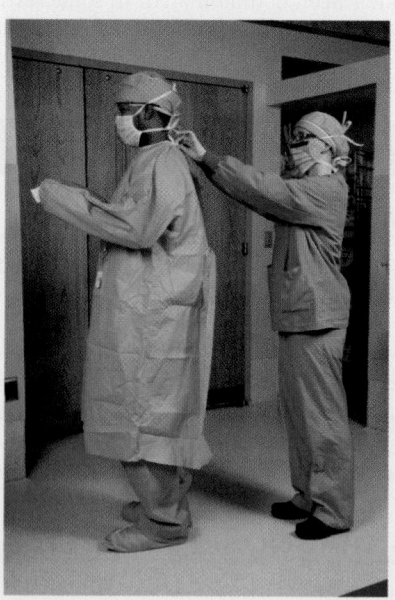

STEP 1h Circulating nurse ties scrub gown.

STEP	RATIONALE

2. Applying gloves using closed-glove method:

   a. With hands covered by gown cuffs and sleeves, open inner sterile glove package (see illustration).

                               Sterile gown cuff touches sterile glove surface.

   b. Grasp folded cuff of glove for dominant hand with nondominant hand.

                               Sterile gown touches sterile glove.

   c. Extend covered dominant hand and forearm forward with palm up and place palm of glove against palm of dominant hand. Glove fingers point toward elbow.

                               Positions glove for application over cuffed hand, keeping glove sterile.

   d. While holding glove cuff through gown with dominant hand on which it was placed, grasp back of glove cuff with nondominant hand and turn glove cuff over end of dominant hand and gown cuff (see illustration).

                               Positions glove over gown for hand insertion.

   e. Grasp top of glove and underlying gown sleeve with covered nondominant hand. Carefully extend fingers into glove, being sure that cuff of glove covers cuff of gown.

   f. Glove nondominant hand in same manner with gloved, dominant hand (see illustration A). Keep hand inside sleeve. Be sure that fingers are fully extended into both gloves (see illustration B).

                               Gloves remain sterile.

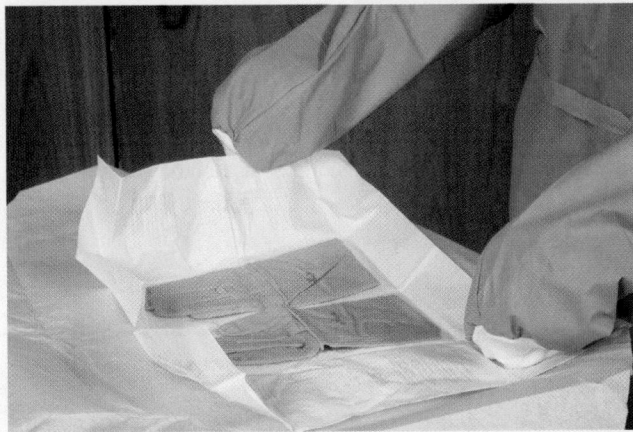

STEP 2a Scrub nurse opens glove package.

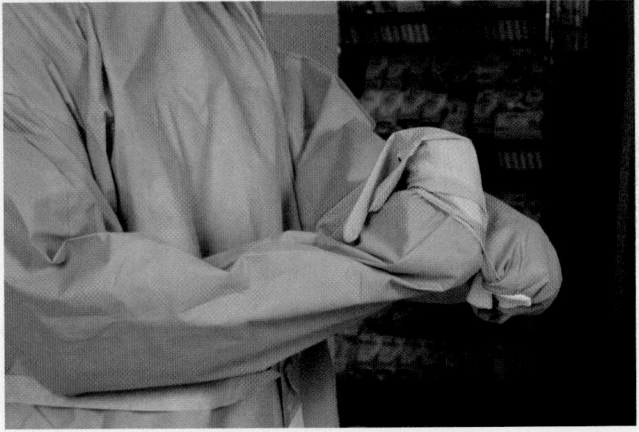

STEP 2d Glove applied as hands remain inside cuffs.

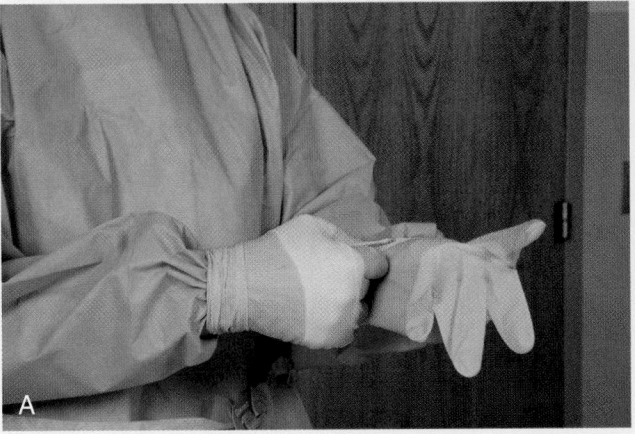

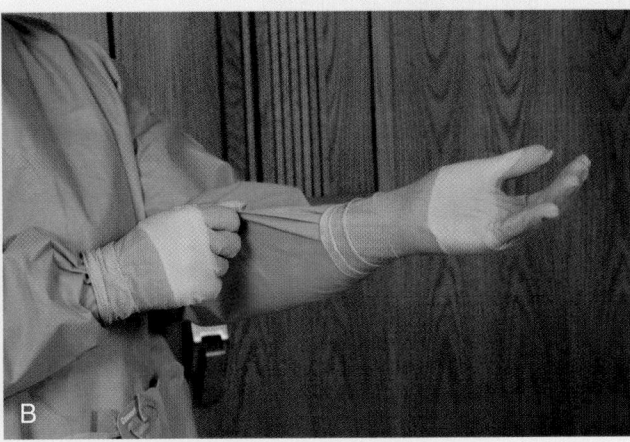

STEP 2f A, Second glove applied. **B,** Gloved fingers extended.

STEP	RATIONALE

3. **Donning wraparound gown:**

   a. Grasp sterile front flap/paper tab with gloved hands and untie.

Front of gown is sterile.

   b. Pass sterile paper tab to member of sterile surgical team or to nonsterile team member (e.g., circulating nurse) (see illustration). Keep gown tie in right hand. Circulating nurse stands still as scrub nurse/technician turns.

Nonsterile team member uses caution not to touch sterile tie when taking sterile paper tab while scrub nurse/technician turns.

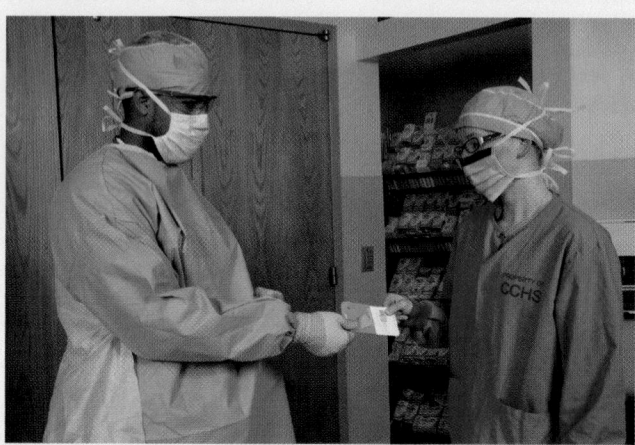

STEP 3b Paper tap on disposable gown is passed to circulating nurse.

   c. Allowing margin of safety, turn to left one-half turn, covering back with extended gown flap. Retrieve sterile tie only from team member and secure both ties in place.

Maneuver covers entire body with gown.
Nonsterile team member pulls off paper tab and discards.

EVALUATION

1. Monitor patient after surgery for signs of surgical site infection (usually occurs 2 to 3 days after surgery).

Signs of infection include redness, heat, swelling, pain, and purulent drainage.

Unexpected Outcomes	Related Interventions
1. Redness, heat, swelling, pain, or purulent drainage develops at surgical site, which often indicates wound infection.	• Individualize interventions based on patient's situation (e.g., wound care, antibiotic therapy).

Recording and Reporting

- No recording is required for sterile gowning and gloving. Record area and description of surgical site after surgery to provide baseline for monitoring wound.

◆ CLINICAL DEBRIEF

You are the circulating nurse in the general operating room, and your first case scheduled at 0730 is an 82-year-old female undergoing an exploratory laparotomy with lysis of adhesions. You're organized and have checked the supplies and equipment in the room. Anesthesia and the surgeon are ready and available in the room while the scrub nurse is performing a surgical hand scrub. When the patient arrives, you introduce yourself and review the chart. The patient's chart states that she is 5'1" and is 96.8 lbs (44 kg). When you interview her and review her past medical history, she verifies the information in her chart, stating that she has hypothyroidism.

1. In thinking about risk factors, what are your main concerns?
2. What are the complications associated with hypothermia?
3. What should the circulating nurse be anticipating regarding intraoperative irrigations and infusions?
4. When you look closer at the patient's chart you note, that the "on call to OR antibiotic," cefazolin 1 g IV, that has been ordered to infuse within 60 minutes of the time of the incision has not been administered and was never sent with the patient on transfer to the operating room. Using SBAR, note to whom you would address this issue and in addition, show how you would communicate with the interprofessional team regarding this patient situation.

◆ REVIEW QUESTIONS

1. You are performing a beginning of shift prescrub wash. Place the steps of the prescrub in the correct order.
   1. Wet hands and apply soap.
   2. Rinse well to remove all soap.
   3. Dry with disposable towel.
   4. Turn on water using foot or knee control.
   5. Rub hands covering all surfaces for at least 15 seconds.
2. Many individuals play a vital role as part of the surgical team. What is included in the responsibilities of the circulating nurse? (Select all that apply.)
   1. Conducting perioperative assessments
   2. Reviews medical records for accuracy and completeness
   3. Performing the surgical hand scrub and donning a sterile gown and gloves

   4. Participates in "time out"
   5. Maintain patient safety and continuity of care throughout the perioperative period
3. AORN (2015) suggests guidelines to reduce the incidence of contamination between surgical personnel and patients. Which specific guidelines are included? (Select all that apply.)
   1. Fingernails should be no longer than ¼ inch.
   2. No acrylic tips or gels should be worn.
   3. No rings or bracelets should be worn.
   4. If watch is worn, it should be removed before surgical scrub.
   5. Hand hygiene should be completed as needed.

e *Visit the Evolve site for a complete list of Clinical Debrief and Review Questions answers.*

REFERENCES

American Society of PeriAnesthesia Nurses (ASPAN): *2015-2017 PeriAnesthesia nursing standards, practice recommendations and interpretive statements,* Cherry Hill, NJ, 2014, ASPAN.

Association of periOperative Registered Nurses (AORN): *Guidelines for perioperative practices,* Denver, 2015, The Association.

Childs T: Risk of exposure to bloodborne pathogens: an integrative approach, *AORN J* 98(6):586, 2013.

Diaz V: Surgical site infections and preventions guidelines: a primer for certified registered nurse anesthetists, *AANA J* 83(1):63, 2015.

Korniewicz D, El-Masri M: Exploring the benefits of double gloving during surgery, *AORN J* 95(3):328, 2012.

Landers R: Reducing surgical errors: implementing a three-hinge approach to success, *AORN J* 101(6):657, 2015.

Moola S, Lockwood C: Effectiveness of strategies for the management and/or prevention of hypothermia within the adult perioperative environment, *Int J Evid Based Healthc* 9(4):337, 2011.

Rothrock J: *Alexander's care of the patient in surgery,* ed 15, St Louis, 2015, Mosby.

Schick L, Windle P, editors: *Perianesthesia nursing core curriculum,* St Louis, 2016, Saunders.

The Joint Commission (TJC): *2016 National Patient Safety Goals,* 2016, Oakbrook Terrace, IL, http://www.jointcommission.org/standards_information/npsgs.aspx. Accessed April 9, 2016.

World Health Organization (WHO): *Surgical safety checklist,* 2009, http://www.who.int/patientsafety/safesurgery/checklist/en/. Accessed April 9, 2016.

SKILLS AND PROCEDURES

Skill 39.1 **Risk Assessment, Skin Assessment, and Prevention Strategies, p. 995**

Skill 39.2 **Treatment of Pressure Injuries, p. 1003**

OBJECTIVES

Mastery of content in this chapter will enable the nurse to:
- Describe patient and pressure injury characteristics to include in an assessment.
- Describe guidelines for prevention of pressure injuries.
- Discuss the use of risk assessment tools in the assessment of pressure injuries.
- Identify risk factors for development of pressure injuries.
- Identify outcome criteria for patients at risk for pressure injuries or impaired skin integrity.

- Discuss indications for the use of topical agents in the treatment of pressure injuries.
- Use correct topical agents in the management of a pressure injury.
- Discuss teaching needs of patient and family caregiver regarding pressure injury prevention and treatment.

MEDIA RESOURCES

- evolve http://evolve.elsevier.com/Perry/skills
- Review Questions
- ▶ Video Clips
- Case Studies

- Audio Glossary
- NSO Nursing Skills Online
- Clinical Debrief and Review Questions Answers

PURPOSE

Prevention of pressure injuries is essential to safe patient care. Comprehensive skin assessment identifies factors increasing patient's risk for a pressure injury. Once a pressure injury occurs, there are specific treatments to promote healing. A pressure injury is localized damage to the skin and/or underlying soft tissue, usually over a bony prominence or related to placement of a medical device. The injury can present as intact skin or an open injury and may be painful. The injury occurs as a result of intense and/or prolonged pressure or pressure in combination with shear. The tolerance of soft tissue for pressure and shear may also be affected by microclimate, nutrition, perfusion, co-morbidities, and condition of the soft tissue. The term *pressure injury* replaces *pressure ulcer* in the National Pressure Ulcer Advisory Panel Pressure Injury Staging System as of April 2016. The updated staging definitions and the use of the term *pressure injury* were presented at a consensus meeting where over 400 professionals were guided to consensus on the updated definitions through an interactive discussion and voting process. The change in terminology more accurately describes pressure injuries to both intact and ulcerated skin. In the previous staging system, stage 1 and deep tissue injury described injured intact skin, whereas the other stages described open injuries. This led to confusion because the definitions for each of the stages referred to the injuries as pressure ulcers (http://www.npuap.org/national-pressure-ulcer-advisory-panel-npuap-announces-a-change-in-terminology-from-pressure-ulcer-to-pressure-injury-and-updates-the-stages-of-pressure-injury). This chapter will have some references to pressure ulcers because this was the terminology when the cited literature was published; however, the majority of this text will use the updated term pressure injury.

STANDARDS OF CARE

- National Pressure Ulcer Advisory Panel (NPUAP), European Pressure Ulcer Advisory Panel (EPUAP) and Pan Pacific Pressure Injury Alliance (PPPIA), 2014—Prevention and Treatment of Pressure Ulcers
- The Joint Commission, 2016—National Patient Safety Goals
- Wound Ostomy and Continence Nurses (WOCN) Society, 2016—Guideline for Prevention and Management of Pressure Ulcers (Injuries)
- National Pressure Ulcer Advisory Panel (NPUAP), 2016—National Pressure Ulcer Advisory Panel Announces a Change in Terminology from Pressure Ulcer to Pressure Injury and Updates the Stages of Pressure Injury

PRINCIPLES FOR PRACTICE

- Pressure injuries occur from unrelieved prolonged soft tissue compression, which interferes with the blood flow to the tissue; if this compression continues for a prolonged period of time, the tissue dies from lack of blood flow, or tissue ischemia. Ischemia develops when pressure on the skin is greater than vascular pressure inside the vessels, causing the vessels to collapse and decreasing tissue perfusion.
- The most common sites for the development of pressure injuries are over bony prominences and can include the sacrum, coccyx,

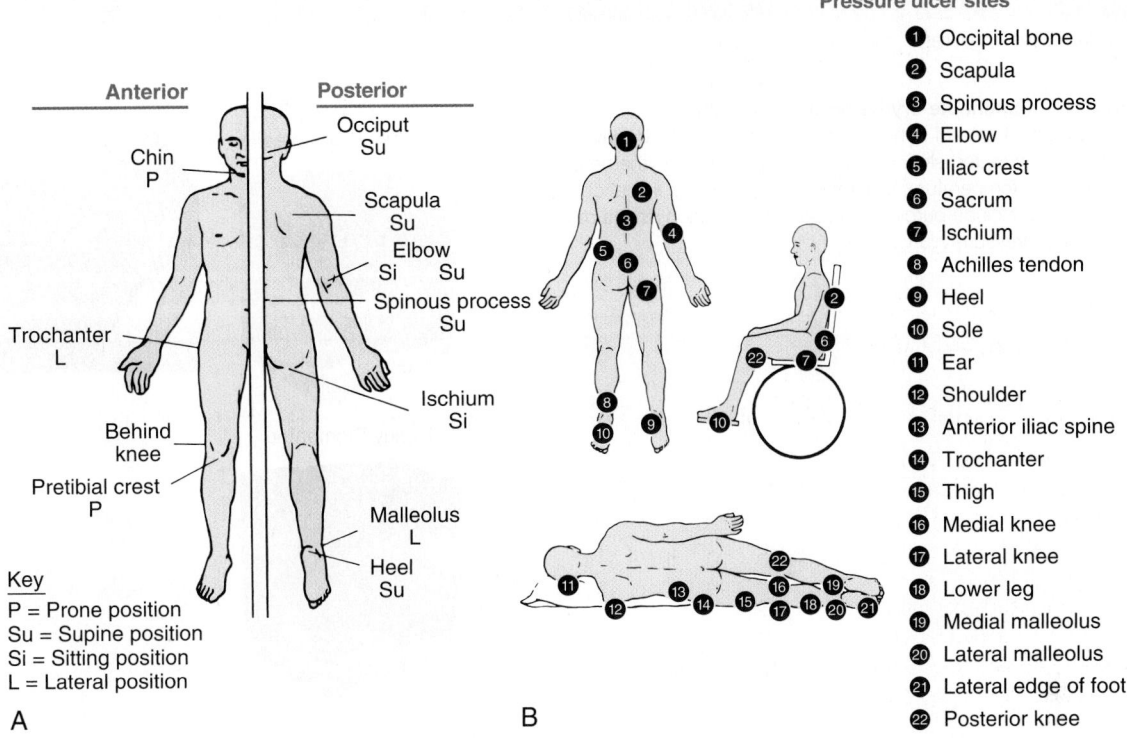

FIG 39.1 A, Bony prominences most frequently underlying pressure injuries. **B,** Pressure injury sites. *(From Trelease CC: Developing standards for wound care, Ostomy Wound Manage 26:50, 1988.)*

ischial tuberosities, greater trochanters, heels, scapulas, iliac crests, and lateral and medial malleoli (Pieper, 2016). Fig. 39.1 shows pressure points over bony prominences where pressure injuries can develop in sitting or lying positions.

- Pressure injury can occur on any area of skin subjected to pressure over nonbony locations from a poorly positioned or ill-fitting device or incorrect device use. These types of skin injuries are called *medical device–related pressure injuries (MDRPIs)*. They have been defined as those that result from devices designed and applied for diagnostic or treatment purposes and generally conform to the shape of the device (WOCN, 2016).
- MDRPIs are pressure injuries that cause pain, loss of function, increased length of stay, and increased health care costs. Timely assessment of risk for or actual MDPRI provides for prompt prevention or treatment (Pittman et al., 2015; Schallom et al., 2015).
- Factors such as incontinence and shear contribute to pressure injury formation. Chronic moisture from fecal and urinary incontinence compromises the protective barrier of the skin and may overhydrate it, making skin more susceptible to breakdown. Shear can damage the skin in one of two ways: sheer stress defined as the force per unit area exerted parallel to the plane of interest and shear strain defined as the distortion or deformation of tissue as a result of shear stress (NPUAP, EPUAP, PPPIA, 2014).
- Shear stress can result in skin tears (shearing of the epidermal layer from the dermal layer such as inappropriate tape removal) or in deep damage such as pressure injuries. Shear strain occurs when the subcutaneous tissue shears against the dermal layer, distorting the blood vessels (e.g., when the patient slides down in bed; deep tissue injury can occur in these instances) (Doughty and Sparks-Defriese, 2016).

- Other risk factors that can contribute to the development of pressure injuries include immobility, loss of sensory perception, decrease in activity, and malnutrition.
  - Immobility often restricts a patient's ability to change and control body position, thus increasing the pressure over bony prominences.
  - Loss of sensory perception decreases the individual's ability to respond to increased, prolonged pressure in an area of the body and change positions accordingly.
  - Level of activity refers to the person's normal physical movement. A person who is bed bound is at greater risk for skin breakdown than a person who is fully or partially mobile.
  - Research indicates that malnutrition contributes to the development of pressure injuries (WOCN, 2016).
- Pressure injuries pose serious risks to a patient's health. A break in the skin, seen in categories/stages 2 to 4 pressure injuries (Box 39.1), eliminates the first line of defense of the body against infection.
- Reports vary as to the number of patients who are at risk for and develop pressure injuries, but the number of patients who develop them is significant. Patients are now older and sicker, are hospitalized for shorter periods of time, and are discharged to home or intermediate or long-term care facilities at a more acute stage of illness (Pieper, 2016). These changes contribute to an increased number of patients at risk for developing pressure injuries. Thus it is critical to respond with an aggressive preventive approach. As a nurse you must identify the factors that place your patients at risk for the development of pressure injuries. Once you identify these factors, begin interventions to reduce or relieve the negative effects of each factor.
- When a pressure injury develops, explore the factors that contributed to skin breakdown, vigorously attempt to minimize the effects of these variables, and use current wound-healing

BOX 39.1

Staging of Pressure Injuries

Stage 1

Pressure Injury: Nonblanchable erythema of intact skin

Intact skin with a localized area of nonblanchable erythema, which may appear differently in darkly pigmented skin. Presence of blanchable erythema or changes in sensation, temperature, or firmness may precede visual changes. Color changes do not include purple or maroon discoloration; these may indicate deep tissue pressure injury.

Lightly Pigmented

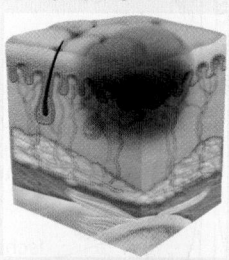 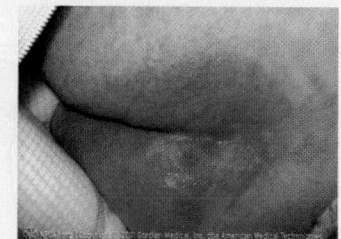

Darkly Pigmented

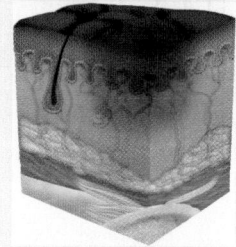

Stage 2

Pressure Injury: Partial-thickness skin loss with exposed dermis

Partial-thickness loss of skin with exposed dermis. The wound bed is viable, pink or red, and moist and may also present as an intact or ruptured serum-filled blister. Adipose (fat) and deeper tissues are not visible. Granulation tissue, slough, and eschar are not present. These injuries commonly result from adverse microclimate and shear in the skin over the pelvis and shear in the heel. This stage should not be used to describe moisture-associated skin damage (MASD), including incontinence-associated dermatitis (IAD), intertriginous dermatitis (ITD), medical adhesive–related skin injury (MARSI), or traumatic wounds (skin tears, burns, abrasions).

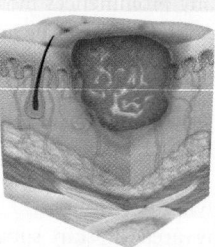 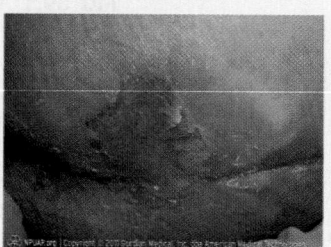

Stage 3

Pressure Injury: Full-thickness skin loss

Full-thickness loss of skin, in which adipose (fat) is visible in the injury and granulation tissue and epibole (rolled wound edges) are often present. Slough and/or eschar may be visible. The depth of tissue damage varies by anatomical location; areas of significant adiposity can develop deep wounds. Undermining and tunneling may occur. Fascia, muscle, tendon, ligament, cartilage, and/or bone are not exposed. If slough or eschar obscures the extent of tissue loss, this is an Unstageable Pressure Injury.

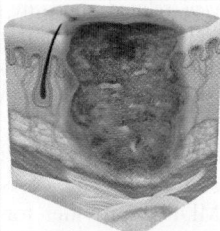 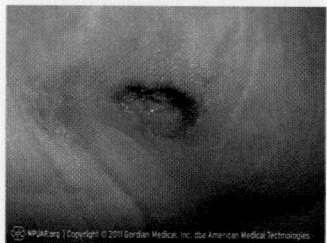

Stage 4

Pressure Injury: Full-thickness skin and tissue loss

Full-thickness skin and tissue loss with exposed or directly palpable fascia, muscle, tendon, ligament, cartilage, or bone in the injury. Slough and/or eschar may be visible. Epibole (rolled edges), undermining, and/or tunneling often occur. Depth varies by anatomical location. If slough or eschar obscures the extent of tissue loss, this is an unstageable pressure injury.

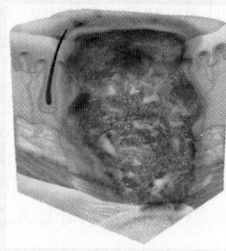 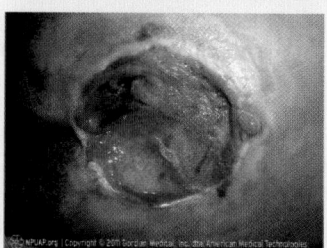

BOX 39.1

Staging of Pressure Injuries—cont'd

Deep Tissue Pressure Injury

Persistent nonblanchable deep red, maroon, or purple discoloration

Intact or nonintact skin with localized area of persistent nonblanchable deep red, maroon, or purple discoloration or epidermal separation revealing a dark wound bed or blood-filled blister. Pain and temperature change often precede skin color changes. Discoloration may appear differently in darkly pigmented skin. This injury results from intense and/or prolonged pressure and shear forces at the bone-muscle interface. The wound may evolve rapidly to reveal the actual extent of tissue injury or may resolve without tissue loss. If necrotic tissue, subcutaneous tissue, granulation tissue, fascia, muscle, or other underlying structures are visible, this indicates a full-thickness pressure injury (unstageable, stage 3 or 4). Do not use *deep tissue pressure injury (DTPI)* to describe vascular, traumatic, neuropathic, or dermatological conditions.

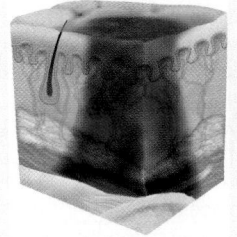
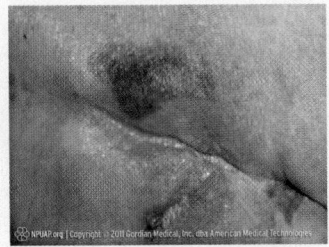

Unstageable Pressure Injury

Obscured Full-Thickness Skin and Tissue Loss: full-thickness skin and tissue loss in which the extent of tissue damage within the injury cannot be confirmed because it is obscured by slough or eschar. If slough or eschar is removed, a stage 3 or 4 pressure injury will be revealed. Stable eschar (i.e., dry, adherent, intact without erythema or fluctuance) on the heel or ischemic limb should not be softened or removed.

Dark Eschar

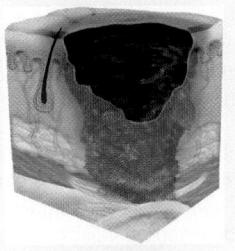
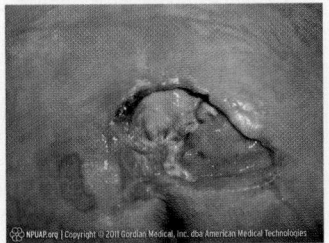

Slough Eschar

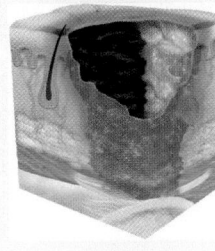

Used with permission of the National Pressure Ulcer Advisory Panel, (NPUAP), European Pressure Ulcer Advisory Panel (EPUAP) and Pan Pacific Pressure Injury Alliance (PPPIA): *Prevention and treatment of pressure ulcers: quick reference guide,* July 22, 2016.

principles in the management of injuries (see Chapters 40 and 41).

PATIENT-CENTERED CARE

- Pressure injuries and the associated treatments affect patients' lives emotionally, mentally, physically, and socially. Patients are aware of the amount and quality of care they receive, including levels of comfort during dressing changes and the timing of interventions. The presence of a pressure injury increases hospital stays, rates of readmissions, and health care costs (WOCN, 2016). Given that it affects a patient's quality of life, providing culturally appropriate information about treatment and wound-healing expectations is an important aspect of care.

- When planning care for a patient, consider issues such as skin tones, patient and family caregiver education, and the social effects of a pressure injury. Skin assessment depends on skin color, and detection becomes a challenge in dark-skinned patients (Nix, 2016). For example, redness in a dark-skinned patient is difficult to determine without the use of palpation and a comparison to other, nonaffected body parts (Box 39.2).

- When providing pressure injury care, remember that in some cultures hair has significance and should not be shaved. When shaving is absolutely necessary to prevent pain or trauma from taping hair around an injury, you may need the help of a patient's family or cultural elder.

- When you educate patients and family caregivers, consider their primary language and reading ability when using printed materials. Use pictures to determine if reading skills are adequate for printed educational materials.

- Consider how the presence of a pressure injury will affect the patient's social situation (e.g., if a wound would prevent a patient from socializing in the community). The presence of a pressure injury can also cause pain and resultant disability, which affect family dynamics.

EVIDENCE-BASED PRACTICE

- Risk assessment is a central component of clinical practice aimed at identifying individuals susceptible to pressure injuries to target appropriate interventions and prevent pressure injury development (NPUAP, EPUAP, PPPIA, 2014; WOCN, 2016):

BOX 39.2

Patient-Centered Care for Skin Assessment of Pressure Injuries: Patients With Darkly Pigmented Skin

Patients with darkly pigmented skin cannot be assessed for pressure injury risk by examining only skin color. Changes in sensation, temperature, or tissue consistency may precede visual skin changes (WOCN, 2016).

1. Use natural lighting, but note that visual inspection techniques to identify pressure injuries are ineffective in darkly pigmented skin. Skin inspection techniques for individuals with darkly pigmented skin must include assessment of temperature, edema, and changes in tissue consistency as compared with the surrounding skin (WOCN, 2016).
2. Assess localized skin color changes. Any of the following may appear:
   - Color remains unchanged when pressure is applied.
   - Color changes occur at site of pressure, which differ from patient's usual skin color.
   - If patient previously had a pressure injury, that area of skin may be lighter than original color.
   - Localized area of skin may be purple/blue or violet instead of red. Purple or maroon discoloration may indicate deep tissue injury (WOCN, 2016).
3. Circumscribed area of intact skin may be warm to touch. As tissue changes color, intact skin will feel cool to touch. **NOTE:** Gloves may decrease sensitivity to changes in skin temperature.
   - Localized heat (inflammation) is detected by making comparisons to surrounding skin. Localized area of warmth eventually will be replaced by area of coolness, which is a sign of tissue devitalization.
4. Edema may occur with induration of more than 15 mm in diameter and may appear taut and shiny.
5. Palpate tissue consistency in surrounding tissues to identify any changes in tissue consistency between area of injury and normal tissue.
6. Patient complains of discomfort at a site that is predisposed to pressure injury development (e.g., bony prominence, under medical devices).

Adapted from Nix DP: Skin and wound inspection and assessment. In Bryant RA, Nix DP, editors: *Acute and chronic wounds: current management concepts*, ed 5, St Louis, 2016, Mosby; Wound Ostomy and Continence Nurses Society (WOCN): *Guideline for prevention and management of pressure ulcers, WOCN clinical practice guideline series*, Mt. Laurel, NJ, 2016, WOCN Society.

- Ensure that a complete skin assessment is part of the risk assessment screening policy in place in all health care settings (NPUAP, EPUAP, PPPIA, 2014; WOCN, 2016). Ongoing skin assessment is necessary to detect early signs of pressure damage.
- Skin integrity bundles that identify key areas of assessment, skin-care measures, repositioning, and pressure-reducing strategies are effective in reducing frequency and severity of pressure injuries in critically ill patients. These bundles provide health care providers with specific preventive and treatment measures for a select group of high-risk patients (Coyer et al., 2015)
- Use risk assessment scores to further improve identification of at-risk patients such as patients with nonblanchable erythema, urogenital disorders, and higher body temperatures (Demarre et al., 2015).
- In individuals at risk of pressure injuries, conduct a comprehensive skin assessment as soon as possible, but within 8 hours of admission (or first visit in community settings), as part of every risk assessment, ongoing based on the clinical setting and the individual's degree of risk, and before the individual's discharge (NPUAP, EPUAP, PPPIA, 2014; WOCN, 2016).

- The use of dressings such as hydrocolloid as part of pressure injury prevention help reduce the incidence of MDRPI in at-risk patients (Clark et al., 2014).
- Medical devices are commonly used in hospital settings and can create pressure. Humidity and heat develop between the device and the skin, changing the microclimate of the skin. Prompt and routine assessment of skin under the device helps to reduce the risk for pressure injury, identifies early stages of skin breakdown, and prompts interventions (Black et al., 2010; Pittman et al., 2015).

SAFETY GUIDELINES

- Routinely assess patients for individual risks for development of pressure injuries. Select and use a risk assessment tool. The Braden Scale and the Norton Scale are the most extensively studied in the adult population and have been found valid (WOCN, 2016). **Note:** Evidence is lacking to conclude that the use of risk assessment scales reduces the incidence of pressure injuries (WOCN, 2016).
- Perform pressure injury risk assessment on all patients who have one or more risk factors when admitted to an acute care facility, home care, hospice, or extended care facility (NPUAP, EPUAP, PPPIA, 2014; WOCN, 2016). The use of scales has been found to be a better risk predictor than nurses' clinical judgment alone (Pancorbo-Hidalgo et al., 2006).
- Assess and inspect skin on a schedule based on the acuity of the patient and on an awareness of when pressure ulcers occur in a particular clinical setting (Stechmiller et al., 2008; WOCN, 2016). Note all pressure points; document results.
- Position patients to redistribute the amount and duration of pressure to prevent ischemic tissue injury. The development of pressure injuries—especially stages 3 and 4 and any unstageable ulcers—in a care setting is a serious reportable event. These events are called "never" events; and the Department of Health and Human Services (DHHS), Centers for Medicare and Medicaid Services (CMS) will not financially reimburse acute care hospitals if a patient acquires one of these injuries during hospitalization (DHHS, 2009).
  - Turn and reposition a patient often to redistribute pressure from the superficial capillaries and allow tissues to compensate for temporary ischemia. Use safe patient-handling measures to turn and reposition patients every 1 to 2 hours as their condition allows. Proper positioning helps minimize formation of pressure injuries (see Chapter 11).
  - Specialized beds, overlays, and mattresses (see Chapter 13) redistribute pressure over the entire body surface to prevent excess pressure over bony prominences. By distributing pressure evenly over a patient's body surface, less pressure is applied at the skin level. Place patients at high risk for pressure injury formation on these devices as soon as possible. Consider the use of a chair cushion to redistribute pressure when a patient is seated.
- Clean patients who are incontinent of stool or urine as soon as possible. Prolonged skin moisture and wetness from urinary and fecal incontinence is a risk factor for skin breakdown (Thayer et al., 2016). Protect areas subjected to repeated episodes of incontinence with a barrier ointment or barrier paste. Fecal containment devices are available (see Chapter 35).
- Use approaches to minimize friction and shear. Use lift sheets when repositioning patients to reduce rubbing skin against sheets. Raise the head of the bed no more than 30 degrees

(unless medically contraindicated) to prevent sliding and shear injury (WOCN, 2016).

- Adequate nutrition helps to prevent and treat pressure injuries (WOCN, 2016). A diet high in protein with enough calories, vitamins, and minerals helps maintain normal tissue status and promotes healing. With tissue injury the body needs more calories for healing; nutrient deficiencies may result in impaired or delayed healing. Make sure that monitoring the nutritional status is part of your total assessment (WOCN, 2016).

✦ SKILL 39.1 **Risk Assessment, Skin Assessment, and Prevention Strategies**

NSO *Nursing Skills Online Wound Care Module / Lessons 1 and 2*

The goal in preventing the development of pressure injuries is early identification of an at-risk patient and the implementation of prevention strategies. The *Guideline for Prevention and Management of Pressure Injuries* represents findings from an extensive literature review on the prevention and management of pressure injuries (WOCN, 2016). The panel then identifies the best available evidence in their prevention and management. The overall management goals suggested by WOCN (2016) include the following:

- Identify individuals at risk for developing pressure injuries and initiate an early prevention program.
- Implement appropriate strategies/plans to:
  - Attain/maintain intact skin.
  - Prevent complications.
  - Promptly identify or manage complications.
  - Involve patient and family caregiver in self-management.
- Implement cost-effective strategies/plans that prevent and treat pressure injuries.

The current recommendation is to perform a pressure injury risk assessment on entry to a health care setting and to repeat this on a regularly scheduled basis or when there is a significant change in an individual's condition (WOCN, 2016). For example, if a patient who was ambulatory becomes bed bound because of a surgical procedure, this person is potentially at higher risk for skin breakdown than when first admitted when ambulatory. Use risk assessment tools such as the Braden Scale or the Norton Scale (WOCN, 2016).

The Braden Scale (Table 39.1) is a reliable clinical assessment tool for prediction of pressure injuries. It has six parameters: sensory perception (ability to respond meaningfully to pressure-related discomfort), moisture (degree to which skin is exposed to moisture), activity (degree of physical activity), mobility (ability to change and control body position), nutrition (usual food intake pattern), and friction and shear (Ayello and Braden, 2002; Braden and Bergstrom, 1989, 1994). Risk cutoff scores vary for specific patient populations (Table 39.2). The Norton Scale, developed in 1962, includes five risk factors: physical condition, mental state, activity, mobility, and incontinence (Norton et al., 1975). It is important to understand how to interpret the meaning of a patient's total score on whichever scale you use.

TABLE 39.1

Braden Scale for Predicting Pressure Ulcer Risk*

Sensory Perception

Ability to respond meaningfully to pressure-related discomfort	1. *Completely limited:* Unresponsive (does not moan, flinch, or grasp) to painful stimuli because of diminished level of consciousness or sedation *or* Limited ability to feel pain over most of body	2. *Very limited:* Responds only to painful stimuli Cannot communicate discomfort except by moaning or restlessness *or* Has a sensory impairment that limits the ability to feel pain or discomfort over half of body	3. *Slightly limited:* Responds to verbal commands but cannot always communicate discomfort or need to be turned *or* Has some sensory impairment, which limits ability to feel pain or discomfort in one or two extremities	4. *No impairment:* Responds to verbal commands Has no sensory deficit that would limit ability to feel or voice pain or discomfort

Moisture

Degree to which skin is exposed to moisture	1. *Constantly moist:* Skin kept moist almost constantly by factors such as perspiration and urine Dampness detected every time patient is moved or turned	2. *Very moist:* Skin often but not always moist Linen must be changed at least once a shift	3. *Occasionally moist:* Skin occasionally moist, requiring extra linen change approximately once a day	4. *Rarely moist:* Skin usually dry; linen requires changing only at routine intervals

Activity

Degree of physical activity	1. *Bedfast:* Confined to bed	2. *Chairfast:* Ability to walk severely limited or nonexistent Cannot bear own weight and/or must be helped into chair or wheelchair	3. *Walks occasionally:* Walks occasionally during day but for very short distances with or without help Spends most of each shift in bed or chair	4. *Walks frequently:* Walks outside room at least twice a day and inside room at least once every 2 hours during waking hours

Continued

TABLE 39.1

Braden Scale for Predicting Pressure Ulcer Risk*—cont'd

Mobility

Ability to change and control body position	1. *Completely immobile:* Does not make even slight changes in body or extremity position without help	2. *Very limited:* Makes occasional slight changes in body or extremity position but unable to make frequent or significant changes independently	3. *Slightly limited:* Makes frequent, although slight, changes in body or extremity position independently	4. *No limitations:* Makes major and frequent changes in position without help

Nutrition

Usual food intake pattern	1. *Very poor:* Never eats a complete meal Rarely eats more than one third of any food offered Eats two servings or less of protein (meat or dairy products) per day Takes fluids poorly; does not take a liquid dietary supplement *or* Is NPO and/or maintained on clear liquids or IV infusions for more than 5 days	2. *Probably inadequate:* Rarely eats a complete meal and generally eats only about half of any food offered Protein intake includes only three servings of meat or dairy products per day Occasionally takes a dietary supplement *or* Receives less than optimal amount of liquid diet or tube feeding	3. *Adequate:* Eats over half of most meals Eats a total of four servings of protein (meat, dairy products) each day Occasionally refuses a meal but usually takes a supplement when offered *or* Is on a tube-feeding or TPN regimen that probably meets most of nutritional needs	4. *Excellent:* Eats most of every meal Never refuses a meal Usually eats a total of four or more servings of meat and dairy products Occasionally eats between meals Does not require supplementation

Friction and Shear

	1. *Problem:* Requires moderate-to-maximum help to move Complete lifting without sliding against sheets impossible Frequently slides down in bed or chair; repositioning with maximal help Spasticity, contractions, or agitation leads to almost constant friction	2. *Potential problem:* Moves feebly or requires minimal help During a move skin probably slides to some extent against sheets, chair, restraints, or other devices Maintains relatively good position in chair or bed most of the time but occasionally slides down	3. *No apparent problem:* Moves in bed and chair independently and has sufficient muscle strength to sit up completely during move Maintains good position in bed or chair	

Adapted from Barbara Braden, PhD, RN, Creighton University School of Nursing, Omaha, NE.
IV, Intravenous; *NPO,* nothing by mouth; *TPN,* total parenteral nutrition.
*Score patient in each of the six subscales. Maximum score is 23, indicating little or no risk. A score of ≤16 indicates "at risk"; ≤9 indicates very high risk.

Inspect patient's skin and bony prominences at least daily. Remove medical devices or tape securing these devices, shoes, socks, antiembolic stockings, and heel and elbow protectors for the skin inspection (Black et al., 2010). Inspect all bony prominences, including back of head, shoulders, rib cage, elbows, hips, ischium, sacrum, coccyx, knees, ankles, and heels (see Fig. 39.1). Palpate any reddened or discolored areas with a gloved finger to determine if the erythema (redness of the skin caused by dilation and congestion of the capillaries) blanches (lightens in color). Blanching is normal. If you palpate an area that does not blanch (abnormal reactive hyperemia), this area is a site for potential skin breakdown.

Delegation and Collaboration

The skill of pressure injury risk assessment cannot be delegated to nursing assistive personnel (NAP). The nurse instructs the NAP to:

TABLE 39.2

Pressure Ulcer Braden Risk Scores by Patient Population

Patient Population	High Level of Risk for Pressure Injury Development if Below These Scores
General population	≤16
Intensive care unit patients	≤15
Older adults	≤18
Black and Latino patients	≤18

Data from Ayello E: Predicting pressure ulcer risk, *Best Pract Nurs Care Older Adult* 5:1, 2012; Bergstrom N, Braden BJ: Predictive validity of the Braden Scale among black and white subjects, *Nurs Res* 51(6):398, 2002; Braden BJ, Bergstrom N: Clinical utility of the Braden Scale for predicting pressure sore risk, *Decubitus* 2(3):44, 1989.

- Frequently change patient's position and specific positions individualized for the patient.
- Report any redness or break in the patient's skin.
- Report any abrasion from medical devices.

Equipment

- Risk assessment tool (Use agency-approved tool, see agency policy.)
- Documentation record
- Pressure-redistribution mattress, bed, and/or chair cushion
- Positioning aids
- Clean gloves

STEP	RATIONALE

ASSESSMENT

1. Identify patient using at least two identifiers (e.g., name and birthday or name and medical record number), according to agency policy.

   Ensures correct patient. Complies with The Joint Commission standards and improves patient safety (TJC, 2016).

2. Review medical record to assess patient's risk for pressure injury formation:

   Determines need to administer preventive care and identifies specific factors that place patient at risk (NPUAP, EPUAP, PPPIA, 2014).

   a. Paralysis or immobilization caused by restrictive devices

   Patient is unable to turn or reposition independently to relieve pressure.

   b. Presence of medical device such as nasogastric (NG) tube, oxygen equipment, artificial airways, drainage tubing, or mechanical devices (Doughty and McNichols, 2016).

   Medical devices have potential to exert pressure on patient's nares or ears or on tissue adjacent to devices such as artificial airways and drainage tubes (Pittman et al., 2015).

   (1) If not medically contraindicated, remove medical device to observe and palpate skin and tissues under and around each medical device

   Pressure area assumes same configuration as medical device (WOCN, 2016; Schallom et al., 2015).

   c. Sensory loss (e.g., hemiplegia, spinal cord injury)

   Patient is unable to feel discomfort from pressure and does not independently change position.

   d. Circulatory disorders (e.g., peripheral vascular diseases, vascular changes from diabetes mellitus, neuropathy)

   Reduce perfusion of tissue layers of skin.

   e. Fever

   Increases metabolic demands of tissues.
   Accompanying diaphoresis leaves skin moist.

   f. Anemia

   Decreased hemoglobin level reduces oxygen-carrying capacity of blood and amount of oxygen available to tissues.

   g. Malnutrition

   Inadequate nutrition leads to weight loss, muscle atrophy, and reduced tissue mass.
   Nutrient deficiencies result in impaired or delayed healing (Stotts, 2016).

   h. Fecal or urinary incontinence

   Skin becomes exposed to moist environment that contains bacteria. Excessive moisture macerates skin (Gray et al., 2011).

   i. Heavy sedation and anesthesia

   Patient is not mentally alert and does not turn or change position independently. Sedation alters sensory perception.

   j. Age

   Neonates and very young children are at high risk, with the head being most common site of pressure injury occurrence (WOCN, 2016).
   There is loss of dermal thickness in older adults, impairing ability to distribute pressure (Pieper, 2016).

   k. Dehydration

   Results in decreased skin elasticity and turgor.

   l. Edema

   Edematous tissues are less tolerant of pressure, friction, and shear.

   m. Existing pressure injuries

   Limit surfaces available for position changes, placing available tissues at increased risk.

   n. History of pressure injury

   Tensile strength of skin from previously healed pressure injury is 80% or less; therefore this area cannot tolerate pressure as much as undamaged skin (Doughty and Sparks-Defriese, 2016).

3. Select agency-approved risk assessment tool such as the Braden Scale or Norton Scale. Perform risk assessment when patient enters health care setting and repeat on regularly scheduled basis or when there is significant change in patient's condition (WOCN, 2016).

   Valid and reliable risk assessment tools evaluate patient's risk for developing a pressure injury. Identifying risk factors that contribute to the potential for skin breakdown allows you to target specific interventions for decreasing risk for skin breakdown.

STEP	RATIONALE
4. Obtain risk score (see Tables 39.1, 39.2, and 39.3) and evaluate its meaning based on patient's unique characteristics.	Risk cutoff score depends on instrument used. Score involves identifying risk factors that contributed to it and minimizing these specific deficits (Ayello, 2012).
5. Perform hand hygiene. Assess condition of patient's skin over regions of pressure (see Fig. 39.1). Apply gloves as needed with open and/or draining wounds.	Body weight against bony prominences places underlying skin at risk for breakdown.
a. Inspect for skin discoloration (see Box 39.2 for patients with darkly pigmented skin) and tissue consistency (firm or boggy feel) and/or palpate for abnormal sensations (Nix, 2016).	Indicates that tissue was under pressure; hyperemia is a normal physiological response to hypoxemia in tissues.
b. Palpate discolored area on skin and under and around medical devices, release your fingertip, and look for blanching.	If on palpation an area of redness blanches (lightens in color), this indicates normal reactive hyperemia; tissue is not at risk for skin breakdown. Tissue that does not blanch when palpated indicates abnormal reactive hyperemia; indication of possible ischemic injury.
c. Inspect for pallor and mottling.	Persistent hypoxia in tissues that were under pressure; an abnormal physiological response.
d. Inspect for absence of superficial skin layers.	Represents early pressure injury formation; usually a partial-thickness wound that may have resulted from friction and/or shear.
e. Inspect for changes in skin temperature, edema, and tissue consistency, especially in individuals with darkly pigmented skin.	Localized heat, edema, and induration have been identified as warning signs for pressure injury development. Because it is not always possible to observe changes in skin color on darkly pigmented skin, these additional signs should be considered in assessment (NPUAP, EPUAP, PPPIA, 2014).
f. Inspect for wound drainage	Wound drainage increases risk for skin breakdown because it is caustic to skin and underlying tissues.
	Tubing from drainage devices (e.g., Jackson-Pratt, Hemovac) causes pressure under device and on adjacent skin (Black et al., 2015).
6. Assess skin and tissue around and beneath medical devices every nursing shift for additional areas of potential pressure injury resulting from medical devices (Black et al., 2015) (Table 39.4).	Patients at high risk have multiple sites for pressure necrosis from medical devices in areas other than bony prominences (Coyer et al., 2014; Makic, 2015).
	Pressure points around medical devices (e.g., oxygen cannula and masks, drainage tubing) can cause pressure injury to underlying tissue and become full-thickness pressure injuries (Black et al., 2015; Pittman et al., 2015; Schallom et al., 2015).
a. Nares: NG tube, oxygen cannula	Pressure to nares occurs from tape and other materials used to secure NG tube.
b. Ears: oxygen cannula, pillow	Patients' ears and tips of nares are at risk for pressure from nasal cannula (Black et al., 2015; Schallom et al 2015).
c. Tongue and lips: oral airway, endotracheal (ET) tube	Pressure results from artificial airway and materials used to secure airway (Black et al., 2015).
d. Forehead: pulse oximetry device	

TABLE 39.3

Guidelines for Pressure Injury Risk Assessment

Level of Care	Initial	Reassessment
Acute care	Within 8 hours of admission (NPUAP, EPUAP, PPPIA, 2014)	• On a defined schedule (e.g., every 24 to 48 hours) • Whenever major change in patient's condition occurs
Critical care	On admission	• Every 24 hours (Ayello, 2012)
Long-term care	On admission	• Weekly for first 4 weeks after admission • Routinely on quarterly basis • Whenever patient's condition changes or deteriorates
Home care	On admission	• Every registered nurse visit

STEP	RATIONALE
e. Drainage or other tubing	Stress and pressure against tissue at exit site or from tubing lying under any part of patient's body (Black et al., 2015).
f. Indwelling urethral (Foley) catheter	For female patients catheter can put pressure on labia, especially when edematous. For male patients pressure from catheter not properly anchored can put pressure on tip of penis and urethra (Black et al., 2015).
g. Orthopedic and positioning devices such as casts, neck collars, splints	Applied devices have potential to cause pressure to underlying and adjacent skin and tissue (Black et al., 2015).
h. Compression stockings	Compression stockings have potential to cause pressure, especially if they fit poorly or are rolled down (Black et al., 2015).
i. Immobilization device and restraints	If device is too tight or poorly placed or if patient strains, pressure points occur under it.

TABLE 39.4

Strategies to Prevent Medical and Immobilization Device–Related Pressure Injuries

Device	Pressure Areas	Prevention Strategies*
Nasogastric tubes	Nares Skin on nasal bridge	Secure tube using pressure-relieving techniques, which direct the pressure from the tube away from the nares (see Chapters 32 and 35). Reposition tube.
Endotracheal tubes	Lips Tongue	Remove securing device daily and inspect for pressure injury (Branson et al., 2014). Rotate tube every shift or more often.
Nasotracheal tube	Nose/nasal bridge Nares	Remove securing device daily and inspect for pressure injury (Branson et al., 2014). Reposition.
Tracheostomy tubes	Front of neck and stoma site Back of beck	Remove securing device daily. Increase stoma care. Apply dressing to back of neck.
Oxygen cannula and tubing	Ears Nose	Apply dressing to external ear. Periodically remove cannula to relieve pressure and inspect for pressure injury (Schallom et al,, 2015).
Noninvasive positive-pressure ventilation (NIPPV)/bi-level positive airway pressure (BiPAP)	Forehead Nose/nasal bridge	Pretreat bridge of nose with dressing before application of mask. If possible, remove mask for a few minutes.
Drainage tubing	Area immediately next to drainage tube Adjacent area during patient position changes	Apply appropriate dressing around drainage tube. Check tubing placement with each position change. Instruct patient not to lie on the tubing (Pittman et al., 2015).
Indwelling catheter	Thighs Female: urethra, labia Male: tip of penis	Provide meticulous perineal care. Anchor and secure catheter to reduce pressure.
Orthopedic devices	All areas where device comes in contact with patient's skin and tissues	When possible and not contraindicated, inspect under the device.
Neck collar	Neck and occipital region Scalp	Remove hard collars as soon as possible and replace with softer collar (Black et al., 2015). Inspect scalp daily.
Compression stockings	Calf Behind knee Heel Toes	Verify proper fit. To reduce pressure and risk of injury to skin and underlying tissue, remove stockings twice daily for at least 1 hour (Black et al., 2015).
Immobilization devices	Wrists Ankles	Apply dressing between patient's skin and immobilizer (Black et al., 2015). Verify space beetween immobilizer and patient's skin. With assistive personnel present, remove restraints one at a time to inspect skin.

*In addition to routine inspection and cleaning of skin under and around medical device.

STEP	RATIONALE
7. Observe patient for preferred positions when in bed or chair.	Preferred positions result in weight of body being placed on certain bony prominences.
	Presence of contractures may result in pressure exerted in unexpected places.
8. Observe ability of patient to initiate and help with position changes.	Potential for friction and shear increases when patient is completely dependent on others for position changes.
9. Assess patient's and family caregiver's understanding of what a pressure injury is and the individual risks for patient to develop pressure injuries.	Determines baseline knowledge for pressure injury risk and identifies areas for patient teaching.

NURSING DIAGNOSES

- Deficient knowledge regarding pressure injury prevention
- Imbalanced nutrition: less than body requirements

- Impaired physical mobility
- Impaired skin integrity

- Ineffective peripheral tissue perfusion
- Risk for impaired skin integrity

Related factors/Risk factors are individualized based on patient's condition or needs.

PLANNING

1. Expected outcomes following completion of procedure:	
• Risk factors are identified.	Establishes baseline for future assessment.
• Patient experiences no change from baseline skin assessment.	Prevention guidelines prevent occurrence or worsening of pressure injury.
• Skin is intact with no evidence of erythema or no signs of breakdown.	Prevention strategies reduce risk factors.
• Patient and family caregiver learn patient's personal risk factors for pressure injury.	Demonstrates learning.
2. Explain procedure(s) and purpose to patient and family caregiver.	Relieves anxiety and provides opportunity for education.

IMPLEMENTATION

STEP	RATIONALE
1. Implement prevention guidelines adapted from WOCN Society *Guideline for Prevention and Management of Pressure Ulcers* (2016).	Reduces patient's risk for developing pressure injury.
2. Close room door or bedside curtain and perform hand hygiene.	Maintains patient privacy.
3. If patient has open, draining wounds, apply clean gloves.	Use of standard precautions prevents accidental exposure to body fluids.
4. Following initial assessment, continue to inspect skin at least once a day.	
a. Observe patient's skin; pay particular attention to bony prominences and areas around and under medical devices and tubes. If you find reddened area, gently press area with gloved finger to check for blanching. If area does not blanch, suspect tissue injury and recheck in 1 hour. Any discoloration may vary from pink to a deep red.	Routine skin inspection is fundamental to risk assessment and in selecting interventions to reduce risk (WOCN, 2016). Persistent redness when lightly pigmented skin is pressed can indicate tissue injury. If area of redness blanches (lightens in color), it indicates that skin is not at risk for breakdown.

Clinical Decision Point *Do not massage reddened areas because doing so may cause additional tissue trauma. Reddened areas indicate blood vessel damage, and massaging can further damage the vessel (Bryant and Nix, 2016).*

b. If patient has darkly pigmented skin, look for color changes that differ from his or her normal skin color.	Darkly pigmented skin may not blanch. A change in color may occur at the site of pressure; this change in color differs from patient's usual skin color (NPUAP, EPUAP, PPPIA, 2014) (see Box 39.2).
5. Each shift, check all treatment and assistive devices (catheters, feeding tubes, casts, braces) for potential pressure points (see Table 39.4).	Pressure from these devices increases risk on bony prominences and other areas.

STEP	RATIONALE
a. Verify that device is correctly sized, positioned, and secured.	Incorrect size, placement, and securing of medical device can cause excessive pressure and rubbing by device on underlying skin (Makic, 2015).
b. Consider shielding underlying at-risk skin with protective dressing (silicone, hydrocolloid).	These dressings absorb moisture from body and reduce pressure to underlying skin (Black et al., 2015; Makic, 2015).

Clinical Decision Point *Inspect skin around and beneath orthopedic devices (e.g., cervical collar, braces, or cast). Note any abrasions or warmth in areas where devices can rub against the skin (Pittman et al., 2015; Schallom et al., 2015).*

6. Remove and dispose of gloves; perform hand hygiene.	Reduces transmission of microorganisms.
7. Review patient's pressure injury risk assessment score.	Risk scores aid in identifying interventions to lessen or eliminate present risk factors.
8. If immobility, inactivity, or poor sensory perception is a risk factor(s) for patient, consider one of the following interventions:	Immobility and inactivity reduce patient's ability or desire to independently change position. Poor sensory perception decreases patient's ability to feel sensation of pressure or discomfort.
a. Reposition patient on schedule basis and frequently assess individual's skin condition to help identify early signs of pressure damage. If skin changes occur, reevaluate the plan.	Reduces duration and intensity of pressure. Some patients may require more frequent repositioning (NPUAP, EPUAP, PPPIA, 2014; WOCN, 2016).
b. When patient is in side-lying position in bed, use 30-degree lateral position (see illustration). Avoid 90-degree lateral position.	Reduces direct contact of trochanter with support surface.
c. When needed, use pillow bridging (see illustration).	Use of pillows prevents direct contact between bony prominences.

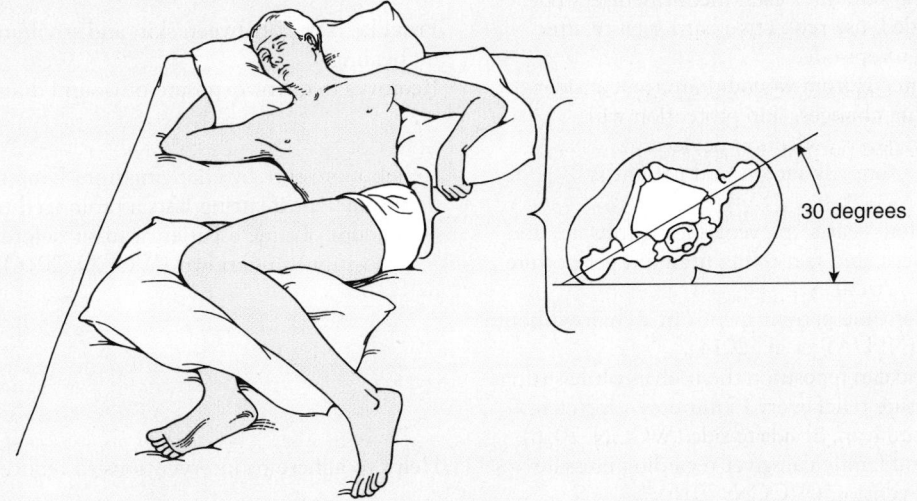

30 degrees

STEP 8b Thirty-degree lateral position with pillow placement.

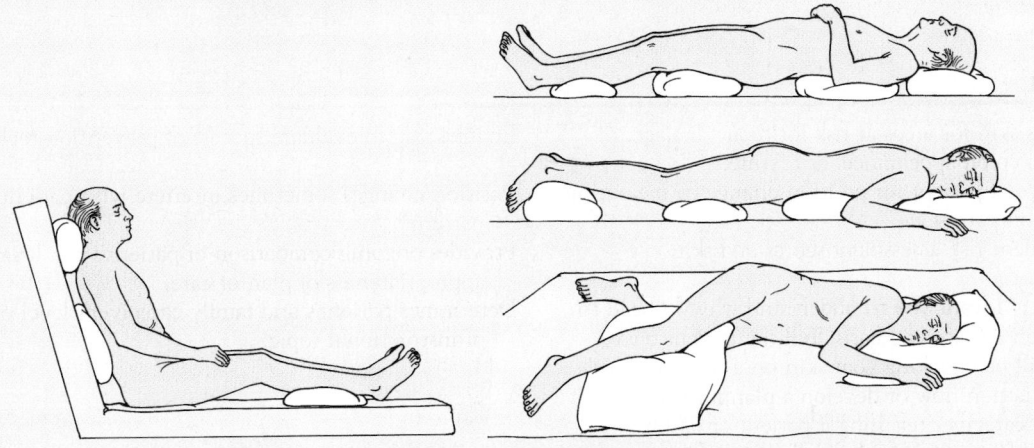

STEP 8c Pillow bridging.

STEP	RATIONALE
d. Place patient (when lying in bed) on pressure-redistribution surface.	Reduces amount of pressure exerted on tissues.
e. Place patient (when in chair) on pressure-redistribution device and shift points under pressure at least every hour (WOCN, 2016).	Reduces amount of pressure on sacral and ischial areas.
9. If friction and shear are identified as risk factors, consider the following interventions:	Friction and shear damage underlying skin.
a. Use safe patient handling guidelines to reposition patient (see Chapter 11). For example, use slide board to transfer patient from bed to stretcher.	Proper repositioning of patient prevents creating shear from dragging patient along sheets. Slide board provides slippery surface to reduce friction. Use of lift team when appropriate raises patient's skin off sheets.
b. Ensure that heels are free from surface of bed by using a pillow under calves to elevate heels or use a heel-suspension device; knees should be in 5- to 10-degree flexion (WCON, 2016; Baath et al., 2016).	"Floating" heels from bed surface offload the heel completely and redistribute the weight of the leg along the calf without applying pressure on the Achilles tendon (Baath et al., 2016).
c. Maintain head of the bed at 30 degrees or lower or at the lowest degree of elevation consistent with patient's condition (do not lower HOB if patient is at risk for aspiration) (WOCN, 2016).	Decreases potential for patient to slide toward foot of bed and incur shear injury.
10. If patient receives low score on moisture subscale, consider one of the following interventions:	Continual exposure of body fluids on patient's skin increases risk for skin breakdown and pressure injury development.
a. Apply clean gloves. Clean and dry the skin as soon as possible after each incontinent episode (WOCN, 2016). Apply moisture barrier ointment to perineum and surrounding skin after each incontinent episode.	Friction and shear are enhanced in the presence of moisture. Protects skin from fecal or urinary incontinence.
b. If skin is denuded, use protective barrier paste after each incontinent episode.	Provides barrier between skin and stool/urine, allowing for healing.
c. If moisture source is from wound drainage, consider frequent dressing changes, skin protection with protective barriers, or collection devices.	Removes frequent exposure of wound drainage from skin.
11. If friction and shear are risk factors and patient is chairbound:	Relief of pressure by changing from lying to sitting position is insufficient if sitting lasts a prolonged time. The maximum amount of time a patient can sit before there is a need to reposition is unknown (WOCN, 2016).
a. Tilt patient's chair seat to prevent sliding forward, and support arms, legs, and feet to maintain proper posture (NPUAP et al., 2014).	
b. Limit amount of time patient spends in a chair without pressure relief (NPUAP et al., 2014).	
c. For patients who can reposition themselves while sitting, encourage pressure relief every 15 minutes using chair push-ups, forward lean, or side to side (WOCN, 2016).	
12. Educate patient and family caregiver regarding pressure injury risk and prevention (WOCN, 2016).	Helps to adhere to interventions to reduce pressure injury risk.
13. Remove gloves and discard in appropriate receptacle. Perform hand hygiene.	Reduces transmission of microorganisms.

EVALUATION

1. Observe patient's skin for areas at risk for tissue damage, noting change in color, appearance, or texture.	Enables you to evaluate success of prevention techniques.
2. Observe tolerance of patient for position change by measuring level of comfort on pain scale.	Position changes sometimes interfere with patient's sleep and rest pattern.
3. Compare subsequent risk assessment scores and skin assessments.	Provides ongoing comparison of patient's risk level to facilitate appropriateness of plan of care.
4. **Use Teach-Back:** "I want you to understand why we need to assess your skin on an ongoing basis. Tell me in your own words why we will be checking your skin on a regular basis?" Revise your instruction now or develop a plan for revised patient or family caregiver teaching if patient or family caregiver is not able to teach back correctly.	Determines patient's and family caregiver's level of understanding of instructional topic.

STEP	RATIONALE

Unexpected Outcomes

1. Skin becomes mottled, reddened, purplish, or bluish.

2. Areas under pressure develop persistent discoloration, induration, or temperature changes.

Related Interventions

- Refer patient to wound, ostomy, and continence nurse (WOCN); dietitian; clinical nurse specialist (CNS); nurse practitioner (NP) and/or physical therapist as necessary. Reevaluate position changes and bed surface.
- Refer patient to WOCN; dietitian; CNS; NP; and/or physical therapist as necessary.
- Modify patient's positioning and turning schedule.

Recording and Reporting

- Record on flow sheet in nurses' notes in electronic health record (EHR) or chart any skin changes, patient's risk score, and skin assessment. Describe positions, turning intervals, pressure-redistribution devices, and other prevention measures. Note patient's response to the interventions.
- Record your evaluation of patient's and family caregiver's understanding of the need for frequent skin and pressure injury assessment education.
- Report need for additional consultations for the high-risk patient to health care provider.

Special Considerations
Teaching

- Help patient and family caregiver understand multiple factors involved in preventing and treating pressure injuries.
- Explain and demonstrate positioning options to achieve pressure redistribution.
- Explain the purpose and maintenance of pressure-redistribution devices (see Chapter 13).
- When teaching patients to change position for pressure redistribution, suggest using television programming and commercial intervals or a watch with an alarm as reminders.

Pediatric

- Infants and young children in diapers are at risk for skin breakdown.

Gerontological

- Reevaluate sitting posture and position because body weight and muscle tone change with age.
- In older adults the dermis is not as thick. Skin over the legs and forearms is especially thin. There is less subcutaneous tissue, leading to less padding protection over bony prominences; and the time for epidermal regeneration is diminished, leading to slower healing (Wysocki, 2016).

Home Care

- Identify community resources such as neighbors and relatives to provide help if patient needs help with position changes.
- Closely monitor home care patients for pressure injury development if they have any of the following risk factors: wheelchair or bed dependence, incontinence, anemia, fracture, and/or skin drainage.
- Remind patient and family caregiver that position changes need to occur while a patient is sitting in a chair. Consider shifts in position every 15 minutes. Small shifts such as moving or repositioning the legs redistributes pressure over bony prominences (WOCN, 2016).

◆ **SKILL 39.2**   **Treatment of Pressure Injuries**

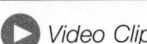 *Video Clip*

The principles of managing patients with pressure injuries include systematic support of patients, reduction or elimination of the cause of skin breakdown, and management that provides an environment conducive to healing. Once you find the cause of the pressure injury, take steps to control or eliminate it. For example, if the injury is related to unrelieved pressure, choose the appropriate pressure-redistribution surface, develop a turning schedule, reposition tubing from medical equipment, or choose the appropriate chair pad. Next assess the patient's wound-healing abilities: cardiovascular and pulmonary function, nutritional status, and conditions that interfere with wound healing such as diabetes, steroid administration, and immunosuppression (Doughty and Sparks-Defriese, 2016). Wound assessment tools such as the Bates-Jensen Wound Assessment Tool (BWAT) (Nix, 2016) and the Pressure Ulcer Scale for Healing (PUSH) tool can help to determine the individual treatment goals for different pressure injuries.

The best environment for wound healing is moist and free of necrotic tissue and infection. Perform a thorough assessment of the wound and the periwound skin before initiating wound therapy. No specific studies demonstrate the benefit of using one cleaner over another for pressure injuries. In most cases water or saline is sufficient for cleansing a clean wound (WOCN, 2016). Hydrogen peroxide was once widely used but is now known to cause tissue damage. When a wound is contaminated with debris, necrotic tissue, or heavy drainage, use a cleaner that is noncytotoxic to healthy tissue. If the tissue in the wound is devitalized, consult with a patient's health care provider to consider debridement, which is the removal of devitalized tissue. Debridement is accomplished by the choice of dressing and the use of enzyme preparations or surgical or laser techniques. The choice of the type of debridement depends on a patient's overall condition, the condition of the wound, and the type of devitalized tissue (WOCN, 2016).

Choose wound dressings to meet the characteristics of the wound bed (Rolstad et al., 2016). The type of dressings to use will change as the pressure injury characteristics change; frequent wound assessment is key. The choice of a wound dressing depends on the type of wound tissue in the base of the wound, the amount of wound drainage, the presence or absence of infection, the location of the wound, the size of the wound, the ease of use, cost-effectiveness, and patient comfort. Categories of wound dressings include transparent films, hydrocolloids, hydrogels, foams, calcium alginates, gauze, and antimicrobial dressings (see Chapter 41).

Advanced wound-care therapies used in select cases include growth factors, electrical stimulation, and negative-pressure wound therapy. Growth factors occur naturally in wound fluid; they regulate cell proliferation and differentiation and are considered in the treatment of category/stage 3 and 4 pressure injuries that have delayed healing (NPUAP, EPUAP, PPIAA, 2014). Electrical stimulation induces intermittent muscle contractions and reduces the risk of pressure injury development in individuals with spinal cord injury by increasing muscle mass, improving blood flow and oxygenation (NPUAP, EPUAP, PPIAA, 2014). Negative-pressure wound therapy (NPWT) applies subatmospheric (negative) pressure to the wound bed through suction to facilitate healing and collect wound fluid (Netsch, 2016) (see Chapter 40).

Delegation and Collaboration

The skill of treating pressure injuries and dressing changes cannot be delegated to nursing assistive personnel (NAP). The nurse instructs the NAP to:

* Report immediately to the nurse pain, fever, or any wound drainage to the nurse.
* Report immediately to the nurse any change in skin integrity.
* Report any potential contamination to existing dressing such as patient incontinence or dislodgement of the dressing.

Equipment

* Protective equipment: clean gloves, goggles, cover gown (if splash is a risk)
* Sterile gloves (optional)
* Plastic bag for dressing disposal
* Measuring device
* Sterile cotton-tipped applicators (check agency policy for use of sterile applicators)
* Topical agent (as ordered)
* Cleaning agent (as ordered)
* Sterile solution container
* Dressing of choice based on patient wound characteristics (Table 39.5)
* Hypoallergenic tape (if needed)
* Documentation records
* Scale for assessing wound healing
* Wash basin

TABLE 39.5

Dressings by Pressure Injury Stage

Pressure Injury Stage	Pressure Injury Status	Dressing	Comments*	Expected Change	Adjuvants
1	Intact	None Transparent dressing Hydrocolloid	Allows visual assessment. Protects from shear. Do not use in presence of excessive moisture. Does not allow visual assessment.	Resolves slowly without epidermal loss over 7 to 14 days	Turning schedule. Support hydration. Nutritional support. Use pressure-redistribution bed or chair cushion.
2	Clean	Composite film Hydrocolloid Hydrogel	Limits shear. Change when seal of dressing breaks; maximal wear time 7 days. Provides moist environment.	Heals through reepithelialization	See previous stage. Manage incontinence.
3	Clean	Hydrocolloid Hydrogel covered with foam dressing Calcium alginate Gauze Growth factors	Change when seal of dressing breaks; maximum wear time 7 days. Apply over wound to protect and absorb moisture. Use when there is significant exudate. Cover with secondary dressing. Use with normal saline or other prescribed solution. Wring out excess solution; unfold to make contact with wound. Use with gauze per manufacturer instructions.	Heals through granulation and reepithelialization	See previous stages. Evaluate pressure-redistribution needs.
4	Clean	Hydrogel covered with foam dressing Calcium alginate Gauze	See stage 3: clean. Used with significant exudate; must cover with secondary dressing See stage 3: clean.	Heals through granulation, scar tissue development, and reepithelialization	Surgical consultation may be necessary for closure. See stages 1, 2, and 3.
Unstageable	Wound covered with eschar	Adherent film Gauze plus ordered solution Enzymes None	Facilitates softening of eschar. Delivers solution and wicks wound drainage. Breaks down eschar, providing debridement. Rarely, if eschar is dry and intact, no dressing is used, allowing eschar to act as physiological cover.	Eschar lifts at edges as healing progresses Eschar loosens over time.	See previous stages. Surgical consultation may be considered for debridement. May be considered for slow debridement.

*As with *all* occlusive dressings, wounds should not be clinically infected.

STEP	RATIONALE

ASSESSMENT

1. Identify patient using at least two identifiers (e.g., name and birthday or name and medical record number), according to agency policy.

   Ensures correct patient. Complies with The Joint Commission standards and improves patient safety (TJC, 2016).

2. Assess patient's level of comfort on pain scale of 0 to 10. If patient is in pain, determine if prn pain medication has been ordered and administer.

   Dressing change should not be traumatic for patient; evaluate wound pain before, during, and after wound-care management (Hopf et al., 2016).

3. Determine if patient has allergies to topical agents.

   Topical agents could contain elements that cause localized skin reactions.

4. Review order for topical agent(s) and/or dressings.

   Ensures administration of proper medication and treatment.

Clinical Decision Point *Determine if the order is consistent with established wound care guidelines and outcomes for a patient. If the order is not consistent with guidelines or varies from the identified outcome for a patient, review with the health care team.*

5. Close room door or bedside curtains.

   Provides privacy.

6. Position patient to allow dressing removal and position plastic bag for dressing disposal.

   Provides an accessible area for dressing change. Proper disposal of old dressing promotes proper handling of contaminated waste.

7. Perform hand hygiene and apply clean gloves. Remove and discard old dressing.

   Reduces transmission of microorganisms and prevents accidental exposure to body fluids.

8. Assess patient's wounds using wound parameters and continue ongoing wound assessment per agency policy. **NOTE:** This may be done during wound care procedure.

   Determines effectiveness of wound care and guides treatment plan of care (WOCN, 2016).

   a. *Wound location:* Describe body site where wound is located.

   b. *Stage of wound:* Describe extent of tissue destruction (see Box 39.1).

   Staging is way of assessing a pressure injury based on depth of tissue destruction. Wounds are documented as unstageable if wound base is not visible (NPUAP, EPUAP, PPPIA, 2014).

   c. *Wound size:* Length, width, and depth of wound are measured per agency protocol. Use disposable measuring guide for length and width. Use cotton-tipped applicator to assess depth (see illustration).

   Injury size changes as healing progresses; therefore longest and widest areas of wound change over time. Measuring width and length by measuring consistent areas provides consistent measurement (Nix, 2016).

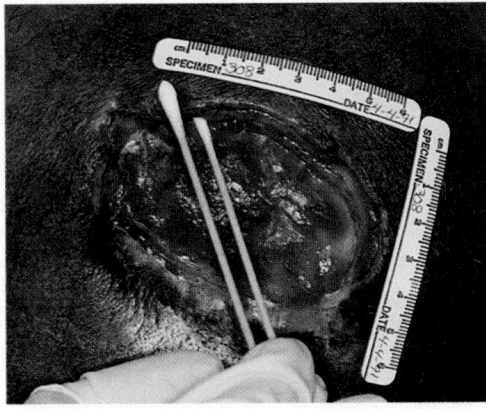

STEP 8c Measuring wound width, length, and undermining of skin.

   d. *Presence of undermining, sinus tracts, or tunnels:* Use sterile cotton-tipped applicator to measure depth and, if needed, a gloved finger to examine wound edges.

   Wound depth determines amount of tissue loss.

   e. *Condition of wound bed:* Describe type and percentage of tissue in wound bed.

   Approximate percentage of each type of tissue in wound provides critical information on progress of wound healing and choice of dressing. Wound with high percentage of black tissue requires debridement; yellow tissue or slough tissue may indicate presence of infection or colonization; and granulation tissue indicates that wound is moving toward healing.

   f. *Volume of exudate:* Describe amount, characteristics, odor, and color.

   Amount and type of exudate may indicate type and frequency of dressing changes (Bates-Jensen, 2016).

STEP	RATIONALE
g. *Condition of periwound skin:* Examine skin for breaks, dryness, and presence of rash, swelling, redness, or warmth. Modify assessment based on patient's skin color (see Box 39.2).	Impaired skin condition at edge of injury indicates progressive tissue damage. Maceration on periwound skin shows need to alter choice of wound dressing.
h. *Wound edges:* Examine edges for condition of tissue.	Gives information regarding epithelialization, chronicity, and etiology.
9. Assess periwound skin; check for maceration, redness, denuded tissue.	Skin condition determines if skin barrier needed.
10. Remove gloves and discard in appropriate receptacle. Perform hand hygiene.	Reduces transmission of microorganisms. Repeated hand hygiene is needed as you assess other pressure areas. Different organisms contaminate different wounds.
11. Assess for factors affecting wound healing: poor perfusion, immunosuppression, or preexisting infection.	Factors affect treatment and wound healing.
12. Assess patient's nutritional status (see Chapter 31). Clinically significant malnutrition is present if (1) serum albumin level is less than 3.5 g/dL, (2) lymphocyte count is less than 1800/mm^3, or (3) body weight decreases more than 15% (see illustration) (WOCN, 2016).	Delayed wound healing occurs in poorly nourished patients.

Clinical Decision Point *When you suspect malnutrition, consider a nutritional consultation to modify patient's diet to promote wound healing.*

13. Assess patient's and family caregiver's understanding of prevention, treatment, and factors contributing to recurrence of pressure injuries (WOCN, 2016).	Patient and family caregiver need to partner with health care providers to prevent further skin breakdown.

NURSING DIAGNOSES

- Deficient knowledge regarding pressure injury treatment plan
- Imbalanced nutrition: less than body requirements

- Impaired physical mobility
- Impaired skin integrity

- Ineffective tissue perfusion
- Pain (acute, chronic)

Related factors are individualized based on patient's condition or needs.

PLANNING

1. Expected outcomes following completion of procedure:	
• Injury drainage decreases.	Reflects decrease in inflammatory process and progress toward healing.
• Granulation tissue is present in wound base.	Evidence that wound is moving toward healing.
• Skin surrounding injury remains healthy and intact.	No additional damage is evident; dressing is appropriate to contain wound drainage.
• Nutritional intake meets caloric and nutrient targets.	Nutritional therapy provides adequate protein to support wound healing.
• Patient's overall skin remains intact and without further breakdown.	Patient remains at risk for further breakdown while existing injury heals.
• Patient or family caregiver able to describe signs of wound healing and wound deterioration.	Demonstrates learning.
2. Explain procedure to patient and family caregiver.	Preparatory explanations relieve anxiety, correct any misconceptions about injury and its treatment, and offer an opportunity for patient and family caregiver education.
3. Prepare the following equipment and supplies:	
a. Wash basin, warm water, equipment, and supplies	
b. Normal saline or other wound-cleaning agent in sterile solution container	Clean injury surface before applying topical agents and new dressing.

Clinical Decision Point *Use only noncytotoxic agents to clean pressure injuries.*

c. Prescribed topical agent:	
(1) Enzyme debriding agents. (Follow specific manufacturer directions for frequency of application.) *Or*	Enzymes debride dead tissue to clean injury surface. Enzymes are not applied to healthy tissue.

STEP	RATIONALE

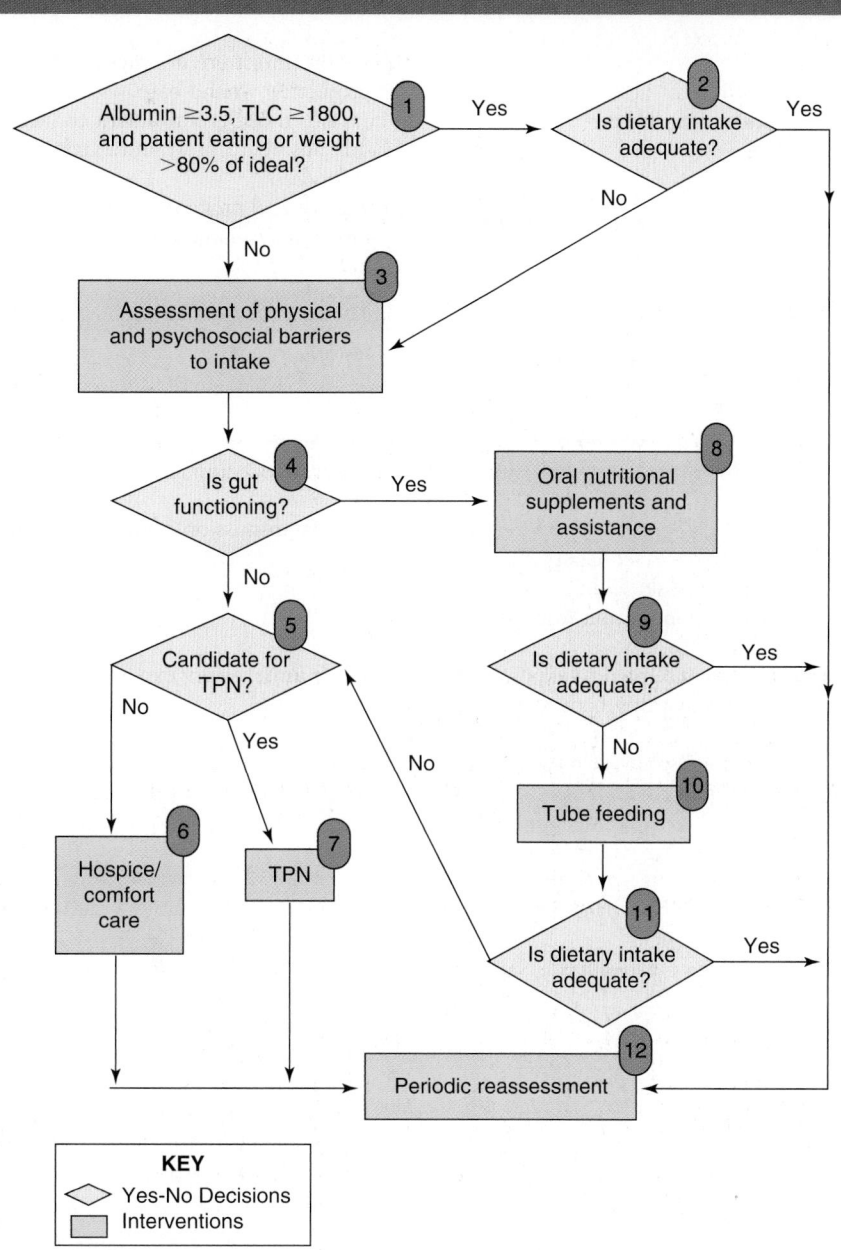

STEP 12 Nutritional assessment and support. *TLC,* Total lymphocyte count; *TPN,* total parenteral nutrition. (*From Bergstrom N et al: Treatment of pressure injuries, AHCPR Pub No. 95-0652, Rockville, MD, 1994, Agency for Health Care Policy and Research, Public Health Service, US Department of Health and Human Services.*)

(2) Topical antibiotics	Topical antibiotics decrease bioburden of wound and should be considered for use if no healing is noted after 2 to 4 weeks of optimal care (WOCN, 2016).
d. Select appropriate dressing based on pressure injury characteristics, principles of wound management, and patient care setting. Dressing options include (see Table 39.5) (see Chapter 41):	Dressing should maintain moist environment for wound while keeping surrounding skin dry (Rolstad et al., 2016).
(1) Gauze—Apply as moist dressing, a dry cover dressing when using enzymes or topical antibiotics, or a means to deliver solution to wound (see Chapter 41)	Gauze delivers moisture to wound and is absorptive.
(2) Transparent film dressing—Apply over superficial injuries with minimal or no exudate and skin subjected to friction	Maintains moist environment and offers intact skin protection.

STEP	RATIONALE
(3) Hydrocolloid dressing	Maintains moist environment to facilitate wound healing while protecting wound base.
(4) Hydrogel—available in sheet or in tube	Maintains moist environment to facilitate wound healing.
(5) Calcium alginate	Highly absorbent of wound exudate in heavily draining wounds.
(6) Foam dressings	Protective and prevents wound dehydration; also absorbs moderate-to-large amounts of drainage.
(7) Silver impregnated dressings/gels	Controls bacterial burden in wound.
(8) Wound fillers	Fills shallow wounds, hydrates, and absorbs.
e. Obtain hypoallergenic tape or adhesive dressing sheet	Used to secure nonadherent dressing. Prevents skin irritation and tearing.

IMPLEMENTATION

1. Assemble supplies at bedside. Close room door or bedside curtains.	Organizes procedure and maintains patient privacy.
2. Perform hand hygiene and apply clean gloves. Open sterile packages and topical solution containers (see Chapter 10). Keep dressings sterile. Wear goggles, mask, and moisture-proof cover gown if potential for contamination from spray exists when cleaning wound.	Reduces transmission of microorganisms.
3. Remove bed linen and arrange patient's gown to expose injury and surrounding skin. Keep remaining body parts draped.	Prevents unnecessary exposure of body parts.
4. Clean wound thoroughly with normal saline or prescribed wound-cleaning agent (see Chapter 40) from least contaminated to most contaminated area. For deep injuries, clean with saline delivered with irrigating syringe as ordered. Remove gloves and discard.	Cleaning wound removes wound exudate and/or dressing residue and reduces surface bacteria.
5. Perform hand hygiene and apply clean or sterile gloves. (Refer to agency policy).	Maintains aseptic technique during cleaning, measuring, and applying dressings.
6. Apply topical agents to wound using cotton-tipped applicators or gauze as ordered:	
a. Enzymes	Follow manufacturer directions for method and frequency of application. Be aware of which solutions inactivate enzymes and avoid their use in wound cleaning.
(1) Apply small amount of enzyme debridement ointment directly to necrotic areas in pressure injury. *Do not apply enzyme to surrounding skin.*	Thin layer absorbs and acts more effectively than thick layer. Excess medication irritates surrounding skin (Rolstad et al., 2016). Proper distribution of ointment ensures effective action.

Clinical Decision Point *If using an enzymatic debriding agent, do not use wound-cleaning agents with metals.*

(2) Place moist gauze dressing directly over injury and tape in place. Follow specific manufacturer recommendation for type of dressing material to use to cover a pressure injury when using enzymes. Tape dressing in place.	Protects wound and prevents removal of ointment during turning or repositioning.
b. Antibacterials (e.g., bacitracin, metronidazole, and silver sulfadiazine).	Reduces bacterial growth.
7. Apply prescribed wound dressing:	
a. Hydrogel:	Hydrogel dressings are designed to hydrate and donate moisture to wound (Rolstad et al., 2016).
(1) Cover surface of injury with thick layer of amorphous hydrogel or cut sheet to fit wound base.	Provides moist environment to facilitate wound healing.
(2) Apply secondary dressing such as dry gauze; tape in place.	Holds hydrogel against wound surface because amorphous hydrogel (in tube) or sheet form does not adhere to wound and requires secondary dressing to hold it in place.
(3) If using impregnated gauze, pack loosely into wound; cover with secondary gauze dressing and tape.	A loosely packed dressing delivers gel to wound base and allows any wound debris to be trapped in gauze.

STEP	RATIONALE
b. Calcium alginate:	Alginate dressings absorb serous fluid or exudate, forming a nonadhesive hydrophilic gel, which conforms to shape of wound (Rolstad et al., 2016). Use in heavily draining wounds.
(1) Lightly pack wound with alginate using sterile cotton-tipped applicator or gloved finger.	The dressing swells and increases in size; tight packing can compromise blood flow to the tissues.
(2) Apply secondary dressing and tape in place.	
c. Transparent film dressing; hydrocolloid; and foam dressings (see Chapter 41)	

Clinical Decision Point *Use transparent dressings for autolytic debridement of noninfected superficial pressure injuries.*
Use a hydrocolloid to protect skin from friction. Some brands have custom shapes available for specific anatomical parts such as heel, elbows, and sacrum.

STEP	RATIONALE
8. Reposition patient comfortably off pressure injury.	Prevents pressure to injury.
9. Remove and dispose of gloves. Dispose of soiled supplies in appropriate receptacle. Perform hand hygiene.	Reduces transmission of microorganisms.

EVALUATION

1. Observe skin surrounding injury for inflammation, edema, and tenderness.	Determines progress of wound healing.
2. Inspect dressings and exposed injuries, observing for drainage, foul odor, and tissue necrosis. Monitor patient for signs and symptoms of infection: fever and elevated white blood cell (WBC) count.	Injuries can become infected.
3. Compare subsequent injury measurements, using one of the scales designed to measure wound healing such as PUSH Tool or BWAT Assessment.	Allows comparison of serial measurements to evaluate wound healing. Provides standard method of data collection that demonstrates wound progress or lack thereof.
4. Use Teach-Back: "I want to be sure that you understand why we will examine your pressure injury on an ongoing basis. Why we will measure your wound and look at the tissue type and surrounding skin each time we change your dressing?" Revise your instruction now or develop a plan for revised patient or family caregiver teaching if patient or family caregiver is not able to teach back correctly.	Determines patient's and family caregiver's level of understanding of instructional topic.

Unexpected Outcomes	Related Interventions
1. Skin surrounding injury becomes macerated.	• Reduce exposure of surrounding skin to topical agents and moisture. • Select dressing that has increased moisture-absorbing capacity.
2. Injury becomes deeper with increased drainage and/or development of necrotic tissue.	• Review current wound-care management. • Consult with multidisciplinary team regarding changes in wound-care regimen. • Obtain wound cultures (see Chapter 7). • Monitor for systemic signs and symptoms of poor wound healing such as abnormal laboratory results (WBC count, levels of hemoglobin/hematocrit, serum albumin, serum prealbumin, total proteins), weight loss, and fluid imbalances.
3. Pressure injury extends beyond original margins.	• Assess and revise current turning schedule. • Consider further pressure-redistribution devices.

Recording and Reporting

- Record type of wound tissue present in injury, injury measurements, periwound skin condition, character of drainage or exudate, type of topical agent used, dressing applied, and patient's response on flow sheet in nurses' notes in electronic health record (EHR) or chart.
- Document your evaluation of patient's and family caregiver's understanding of frequent observation and measuring of wound.
- Report any deterioration in injury appearance to nurse in charge or health care provider.

Special Considerations
Teaching

- Discuss treatment and identify individual(s) who will help with care at home.
- Discuss process of wound healing and expected wound appearance. For example, discuss patient's perception about appearance of the pressure injury. Sometimes eschar looks like a scab to a patient, and he or she needs to understand the difference. A scab is caused by exudate, and an eschar is dead tissue that the patient should not remove.
- Discuss with patient and family caregivers perceptions about size of pressure injury. Some wounds, especially after debridement, may appear larger and are very troublesome to patients and support people.
- Discuss with patient and family caregivers perceptions about treatment. Some patients and family caregivers believe that it is cruel for staff to keep turning and positioning a patient on a frequent basis.
- Review prevention guidelines to prevent further breakdown.
- Discuss options for maintaining good nutrition.

Gerontological

- Wound healing is often slower in older adults (Doughty and Sparks-Defriese, 2016).
- The normal reduction in the Langerhans cells in the older adult's epidermis causes a decrease in T-cell function and immunity.
- Because older skin has a slower and less intense inflammatory reaction, monitor older patients more closely for altered responses to skin irritants.

Home Care

- Consider family caregiver time when selecting a dressing. In the home care setting caregivers may sometimes choose more expensive dressing materials to reduce the frequency of dressing changes.
- Some patients have more time than financial resources. They may choose a less expensive treatment option (e.g., dressing material), especially if there is no third-party reimbursement. Another example is to teach the family caregiver to make a normal saline solution rather than buying it ready-made.
- Identify clean storage area for dressing supplies. Determine availability of required supplies. Discuss need for home care nurse.
- Discuss need for home pressure-redistribution surface or bed. Identify adaptive equipment needed to care for patient at home.
- Medicare regulations limit reimbursement of some types of support surfaces in the treatment of pressure injuries.

Long-Term Care

- Rehabilitation units often use a variety of support surfaces and beds.
- Some patients may be discharged to long-term care facilities that specialize in pressure injury and wound care.

◆ CLINICAL DEBRIEF

A 72-year-old African-American woman underwent a total left hip replacement. Her significant medical history includes rheumatoid arthritis and coronary artery disease. This is her first postoperative day, and she is resting in bed with an immobilizer (a foam wedge that is placed between her thighs to keep her hip in position) in place. Her skin is very moist, and she required a bath and change of linen during the night. She weighs 90.9 kg (200 lbs) and is approximately 5 feet 6 inches tall. Her pain assessment done while bed bound is a 5 on a scale of 1 to 10. A physical therapist is scheduled to see her today to help her get out of bed for the first time since surgery. When the physical therapist is not available, the patient is on bed rest. A daily skin risk assessment using the Braden Scale was completed. The scores were as follows: Sensory Perception (4); Moisture (2); Activity (2); Mobility (2); Nutrition (3); Friction and Shear (1). The daily skin assessment reveals a 2.5-cm (1-inch) round, right-heel injury; wound base red, partial-thickness depth; and a 2-cm (1-inch) red warm spot that does not blanch. There is no break in the skin located over the sacrum.

1. The Braden Scale risk assessment tool was used to determine the risk factors that place the patient at risk for skin breakdown; the subscales for which she was noted to be at risk include activity, mobility, and friction/shear. Which interventions would you put in place to reduce these risk factors?
2. At a skin inspection, the patient was found to have a partial-thickness injury tissue on her right heel and red, warm, nonblanchable spot over the sacral area. How would you chart the staging of these areas of

impaired skin integrity, and what would the appropriate topical treatment be?
3. At the next skin assessment in 24 hours, the sacral area has opened and has a red, moist, painful base. Using SBAR, show how you would communicate with the health care team about this patient.

◆ REVIEW QUESTIONS

1. A patient who is completely immobile scores low on the activity, mobility, and friction/shear Braden subscales. A red, intact, warm area is noted over the sacrum. Which interventions would be appropriate for the care of this patient? (Select all that apply.)
   1. Use a moisture-barrier ointment at least 3 times per day.
   2. Consult with the wound clinical nurse specialist about the most appropriate bed surface to redistribute pressure.
   3. Develop and implement a turning schedule commiserate with the patient's condition.
   4. Use a dressing to protect the sacrum and promote healing.
   5. Use safe patient handling to help reposition frequently.
   6. Massage the red area at each position change.
2. A patient in intensive care has an endotracheal tube (ET) inserted through the mouth for ventilation, an intravenous (IV) line in place, an abdominal incision that is dry and intact, and pillows under both calves. The patient weighs 145.45 kg (320 lbs) and is difficult to turn.

Which locations are at high risk for developing a pressure injury? (Select all that apply.)

1. Heels
2. Posterior bony prominences
3. Nose
4. Mouth
5. IV site

3. What are the correct steps in assessing a pressure injury and changing the pressure injury dressing?

1. Remove the old dressing; assess the amount, color, and character of the drainage if present.
2. Measure the wound diameter (length, width, and depth).
3. Assess the periwound skin.
4. Ask the patient about his or her pain level at previous dressing changes and medicate as indicated.
5. Clean the wound base and the surrounding skin with prescribed solution.
6. Bring wound dressings to bedside.
7. Describe the wound base and stage.
8. Replace the dressing.

ⓔ *Visit the Evolve site for a complete list of Clinical Debrief and Review Questions answers.*

REFERENCES

Ayello E: Predicting pressure ulcer risk, *Best Pract Nurs Care Older Adult* 5:1, 2012.

Ayello EA, Braden B: How and why do pressure ulcer risk assessment, *Adv Wound Care (New Rochelle)* 15(3):125, 2002.

Baath C, et al: Prevention of heel pressure ulcers among older patients from ambulance care to hospital discharge: A multi centre randomized controlled trial, *Appl Nurs Res* 30:170, 2015.

Bates-Jensen BM: Assessment of the patient with a wound. In *Core curriculum: wound management*, Philadelphia, PA, 2016, Wolters Kluwer.

Black J, et al: Medical device–related pressure ulcers in hospitalized patients, *Int Wound J* 7:358, 2010.

Black J, et al: Use of wound dressings to enhance prevention of pressure ulcers caused by medical devices, *Int Wound J* 12:322, 2015.

Braden BJ, Bergstrom N: Clinical utility of the Braden scale for predicting pressure sore risk, *Decubitus* 2(3):44, 1989.

Braden BJ, Bergstrom N: Predictive utility of the Braden scale for predicting pressure sore risk, *Res Nurs Health* 17:459, 1994.

Branson RD, et al: Management of the artificial airway, *Respir Care* 59(6):974–990, 2014.

Bryant RA, Nix DP: Developing and maintaining a pressure ulcer prevention program. In Bryant RA, Nix DP, editors: *Acute and chronic wounds: current management concepts*, ed 5, St Louis, 2016, Mosby.

Clark M, et al: Systematic review of the use of prophylactic dressings in the prevention of pressure ulcers, *Int Wound J* 11:460, 2014.

Coyer FM, et al: A prospective window into medical device–related pressure ulcers in intensive care, *Int Wound J* 11(6):656, 2014.

Coyer FM, et al: Reducing pressure injuries in critically ill patients by using a patient skin integrity care bundle (InSpire), *Am J Crit Care* 24:199, 2015.

Demarre L, et al: Factors predicting the development of pressure ulcers in an at-risk population who receive standardized preventive care: secondary analysis of a multicenter randomized controlled trial, *J Adv Nurs* 71(2):391, 2015.

Department of Health and Human Services (DHHS), Centers for Medicare & Medicaid Services: *State Medicaid director letter*, 2009, https://downloads.cms.gov/cmsgov/archived-downloads/SMDL/downloads/smd073108.pdf. Accessed April 10, 2016.

Doughty DB, Sparks-Defriese B: Wound-healing physiology. In Bryant RA, Nix DP, editors: *Acute and chronic wounds: current management concepts*, ed 5, St Louis, 2016, Mosby.

Doughty DB, McNichols LL: General concepts related to skin and soft tissue injury caused by mechanical factors. In *Core curriculum: wound management*, Philadelphia, PA, 2016, Wolters Kluwer.

Gray M, et al: Moisture-associated skin damage: overview and pathophysiology, *J Wound Ostomy Continence Nurs* 38(3):233, 2011.

Hopf H, et al: Managing wound pain. In Bryant RA, Nix DP, editors: *Acute and chronic wounds: current management concepts*, ed 5, St Louis, 2016, Mosby.

Makic MB: Medical device–related pressure ulcers and intensive care, *J Perianesth Nurs* 30(4):336, 2015.

National Pressure Ulcer Advisory Panel (NPUAP): *National Pressure Ulcer Advisory Panel announces a change in terminology from pressure ulcer to pressure injury and updates the stages of pressure injury*, April 2016. https://www.npuap.org/national-pressure-ulcer-advisory-panel-npuap-announces-a-change-in-terminology-from-pressure-ulcer-to-pressure-injury-and-updates-the-stages-of-pressure-injury/. Accessed October 29, 2016.

National Pressure Ulcer Advisory Panel (NPUAP), European Pressure Ulcer Advisory Panel (EPUAP) and Pan Pacific Pressure Injury Alliance (PPPIA): Haesler Emily, editor: *Prevention and treatment of pressure ulcers: quick reference guide*, Perth, Australia, 2014, Cambridge Media.

Netsch D: Refractory wounds. In *Core curriculum: wound management*, Philadelphia, PA, 2016, Wolters Kluwer.

Nix DP: Skin and wound inspection and assessment. In Bryant RA, Nix DP, editors: *Acute and chronic wounds: current management concepts*, ed 5, St Louis, 2016, Mosby.

Norton D, et al: *An investigation of geriatric nursing problems in hospital*, Edinburgh, 1962, reissue 1975, Churchill Livingstone.

Pancorbo-Hidalgo PL, et al: Risk assessment scales for pressure ulcer prevention: a systematic review, *J Adv Nurs* 54(1):94, 2006.

Pieper B: Pressure ulcers: impact, etiology, and classification. In Bryant RA, Nix DP, editors: *Acute and chronic wounds: current management concepts*, ed 5, St Louis, 2016, Mosby.

Pittman J, et al: Medical device–related hospital-acquired pressure ulcers, *J Wound Ostomy Continence Nurs* 42(2):151, 2015.

Rolstad BS, Bryant RA, et al: Topical management. In Bryant RA, Nix DP, editors: *Acute and chronic wounds: current management concepts*, ed 5, St Louis, 2016, Mosby.

Schallom M, et al: Pressure ulcer incidence in patients wearing nasal-oral versus full-face noninvasive ventilation masks, *Am J Crit Care* 24(4):349, 2015.

Stechmiller JK, et al: Guidelines for prevention of pressure ulcers, *Wound Repair Regen* 16:151, 2008.

Stotts N: Nutritional assessment and support. In Bryant RA, Nix DP, editors: *Acute and chronic wounds: current management concepts*, ed 5, St Louis, 2016, Mosby.

Thayer DM, et al: Top down injuries: prevention and management of moisture-associated skin damage, medical adhesive–related skin injury and skin tears. In *Core curriculum: wound management*, Philadelphia, PA, 2016, Wolters Kluwer.

Theisen S, Drabik A, et al: Pressure ulcers in older hospitalised patients and its impact on length of stay: a retrospective observational study, *J Clin Nurs* 21(3):380, 2012.

The Joint Commission (TJC): *2016 National Patient Safety Goals*, 2016, The Commission, http://www.jointcommission.org/standards_information/npsgs.aspx. Accessed April 10, 2016.

Wound Ostomy and Continence Nurses (WOCN) Society: *Guideline for prevention and management of pressure ulcers*, WOCN clinical practice guidelines series, Mount Laurel, NJ, 2016, The Society.

Wysocki A: Anatomy and physiology of skin and soft tissue. In Bryant R, Nix D, editors: *Acute and chronic wounds: current management concepts*, ed 5, St Louis, 2016, Mosby.

40 | Wound Care and Irrigation

OBJECTIVES

Mastery of content in this chapter will enable the nurse to:
- Discuss the response of the body during each stage of the wound-healing process.
- Differentiate between primary- and secondary-intention wound healing.
- Explain factors that promote or impair normal wound healing.

- Perform a wound assessment.
- Perform a wound irrigation.
- Remove sutures or staples.
- Demonstrate care of a wound-drainage system.
- Demonstrate care related to negative-pressure wound therapy.

MEDIA RESOURCES

- evolve http://evolve.elsevier.com/Perry/skills
- Review Questions
- ▶ Video Clips

- **NSO** Nursing Skills Online
- Clinical Debrief and Review Questions Answers

PURPOSE

Proper wound care is necessary to promote healing that results in an intact skin layer. Intact skin is the first line of defense of the body against invasion by infectious microorganisms. The skin defends the body in other ways by serving as a sensory organ for pain, touch, and temperature; and it has an acid pH, which is often called the *acid mantle*. It also plays a major role in thermoregulation, metabolism, immunity, and fluid balance regulation (Bryant and Nix, 2016a).

STANDARDS OF CARE

- National Pressure Ulcer Advisory Panel (NPUAP), European Pressure Ulcer Advisory Panel (EPUAP) and Pan Pacific Pressure Injury Alliance (PPPIA), 2014—Prevention and Treatment of Pressure Ulcers
- National Pressure Ulcer Advisory Panel (NPUAP), 2016—National Pressure Ulcer Advisory Panel Announces a Change in Terminology from Pressure Ulcer to Pressure Injury and Updates the Stages of Pressure Injury
- The Joint Commission (TJC), 2016—National Patient Safety Goals

- Wound Ostomy and Continence Nurses (WOCN) Society, 2016—Guideline for Prevention and Management of Pressure Ulcers (Injuries)

PRINCIPLES FOR PRACTICE

- The skin is the largest external organ. It has two layers: the epidermis and the dermis (Fig. 40.1). The epidermis has five layers.
  - Stratum corneum, the outermost layer, consists of flattened dead keratinized cells. Stratum corneum prevents dehydration of underlying cells and is a physical barrier to the entry of certain chemicals.
  - The next layers of the epidermis are the stratum lucidum, stratum granulosum, and stratum spinosum.
  - Stratum germinativum, the innermost layer, is sometimes called the *basal layer*. Important features of the stratum germinativum are the epidermal protrusions, or "peaks and valleys" that point downward into the dermis. These provide resiliency and integrity to the skin structure. Melanocytes, the cells that give the skin its color, are also in this layer.
- The area that separates the epidermis from the dermis is called the *dermoepidermal junction* or the *basement membrane zone.*

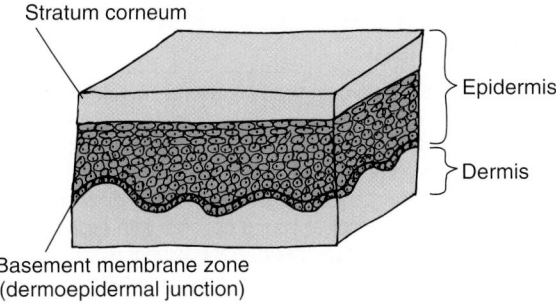

FIG 40.1 Diagram of layers of skin and subcutaneous tissue.

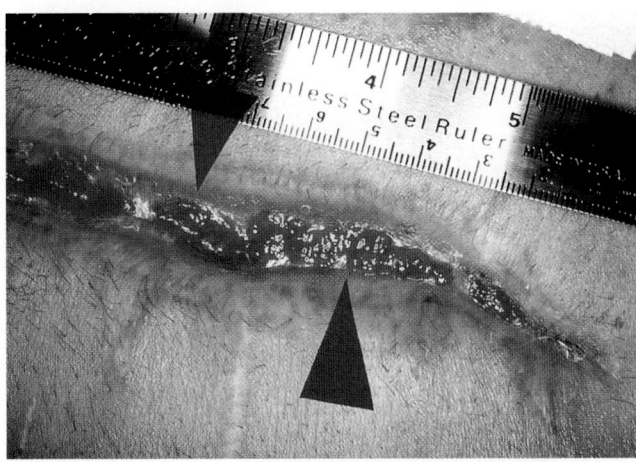

FIG 40.2 Surgical wound with epithelialization occurring: epithelial healing ridge apparent. (*From Bryant RA, Nix DP, editors:* Acute and chronic wounds: current management concepts, *ed 3, St Louis, 2007, Mosby.*)

- Beneath the epidermis is the dermis. Collagen (a tough fibrous protein layer), blood vessels, and nerves compose the dermal layer. Collagen composes about 70% of the dermis and is extremely important in wound healing. The dermis restores the physical properties of the skin and its structural integrity. Restoration of both the epidermal and dermal layers is necessary to promote healing. Risk for local or systemic infection, impaired circulation, and breakdown of tissue directly impairs the wound-healing ability of the skin layers (Doughty and Sparks-Defriese, 2016).
- Wounds should be assessed on a scheduled basis to determine if the wound is moving toward healing. If the assessment finds that the wound is not progressing as expected, the plan of care can be changed to facilitate wound healing (Procedural Guideline 40.1).
- A thorough wound assessment includes the identification of the type of wound healing (e.g., primary, secondary, or tertiary intention) and the type of tissue in the wound base; these parameters will be used to base the proper wound intervention.
- The healing process proceeds in a series of events, generally described as *phases*. In a full-thickness wound the phases are hemostasis, inflammation, proliferation, and remodeling (Box 40.1).
- During the proliferative stage fibroblasts are at the site of injury. These fibroblasts increase synthesis of collagen, which forms the healing ridge that can be palpated under an intact healing incision by days 5 to 9 (Fig. 40.2) (Doughty and Sparks-Defriese, 2016).
- Wound healing occurs by primary, secondary, and tertiary intention (Fig. 40.3).
  - Healing by primary intention occurs when the edges of a clean surgical incision remain close together. The wound heals quickly, and tissue loss is minimal or absent (Doughty and Sparks-Defriese, 2016). The skin cells regenerate quickly, and capillary walls stretch across under the suture line to form a smooth surface as they join.
  - Wounds that are left open and allowed to heal by scar formation are classified as healing by secondary intention (Beitz, 2016). There is tissue loss and open wound edges. Granulation tissue gradually fills in the area of the defect (Fig. 40.4). This process is typical of severe laceration or massive surgical intervention with skin loss.
  - In secondary intention there is a gap between the edges. Connective tissue develops, which supports new capillaries. This form of healing results in the formation of scar tissue to close the wound. The slowness of this process places a patient at greater risk for infection because there is no epidermal barrier until later in the healing process.

Phases of Wound Healing (Full-Thickness Wounds)

Hemostasis Phase

Blood vessels constrict; clotting factors activate coagulation pathways to stop bleeding. Clot formation seals the disrupted vessels so blood loss is controlled and acts as a temporary bacterial barrier. Platelets release growth factors, which attract cells needed to begin the repair process.

Inflammatory Phase

Vasodilation occurs, allowing plasma and blood cells to leak into the wound, noted as edema, erythema, and exudate. Leukocytes (white blood cells) arrive in the wound to begin wound cleanup. Macrophages, a type of white blood cell, appear and begin to regulate the wound repair. The result of the inflammatory phase is a clean wound bed in a patient with a noncomplicated wound.

Proliferative Phase

Epithelialization (the construction of new epidermis) begins. At the same time new granulation tissue is formed. New capillaries (angiogenesis) are created, restoring the delivery of oxygen and nutrients to the wound bed. Collagen is synthesized and begins to provide strength and structural integrity to the wound. Contraction, which occurs in open wounds, reduces the size of the wound.

Maturation (Remodeling) Phase

Collagen is remodeled to become stronger and provide tensile strength to the wound. Outer appearance in an uncomplicated wound will be that of a well-healed scar.

Data from Doughty DB, Sparks-Defriese B: Wound healing physiology. In Bryant RA, Nix DP, editors: *Acute and chronic wounds: current management concepts*, ed 5, St Louis, 2016, Mosby.

- Healing by tertiary intention is sometimes called *delayed primary intention* or *closure*. It occurs when surgical wounds are not closed immediately but left open for 3 to 5 days to allow edema or infection to diminish. Then the wound edges are sutured or stapled closed (Doughty and Sparks-Defriese, 2016).
- The percentage and type of tissue in the wound bed healing by secondary intention provide insight into the severity and duration of the wound, the extent to which it is progressing toward healing, and the effectiveness of current interventions (Nix,

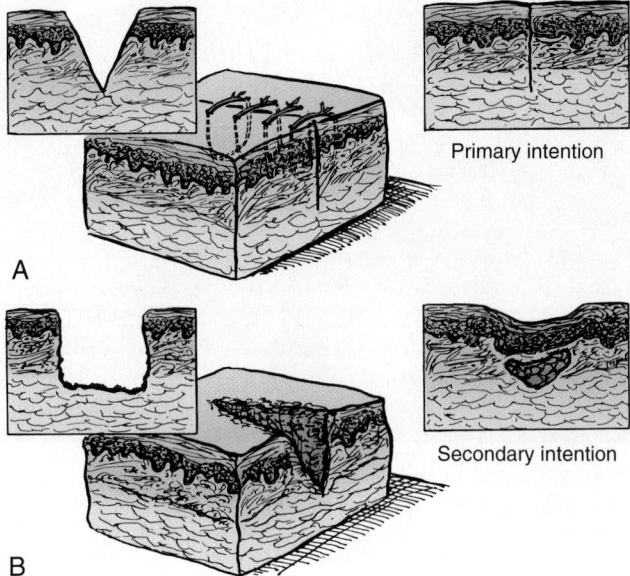

FIG 40.3 Wound healing by primary intention such as with a surgical incision. **A,** Wound healing edges are pulled together and approximated with sutures, staples, or adhesive tapes; and healing occurs by connective tissue deposition. **B,** Wound healing by secondary intention. Wound edges are not approximated, and healing occurs by granulation tissue formation and contraction of the wound edges. (*From Bryant RA, Nix DP, editors: Acute and chronic wounds: current management concepts, ed 5, St Louis, 2016, Mosby.*)

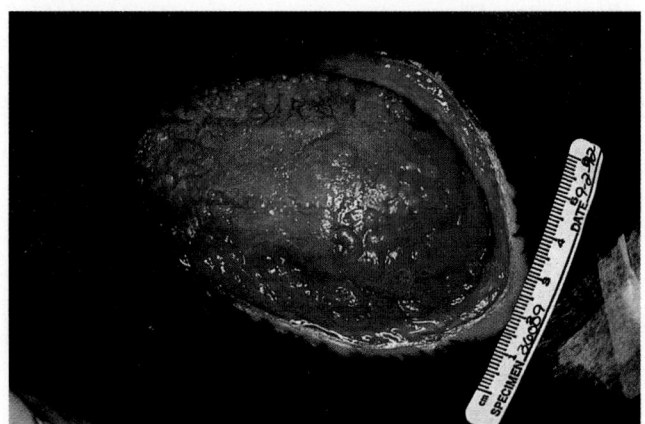

FIG 40.4 Open wound with granulation tissue.

2016). Viable tissue is normally red to pink in color and moist in appearance (Table 40.1). This type of tissue is called *granulation tissue* and indicates a wound moving toward healing. Black, brown, or tan tissue in the wound is slough or eschar and should be removed, or wound healing will be delayed.

- The location, severity, and extent of the injury and the tissue layer or layers involved all affect the wound-healing process (Doughty and Sparks-Defriese, 2016). In addition, there are underlying factors that prevent the ability of cells and tissues to regenerate, return to normal structure, or resume normal functioning (Box 40.2).
  - Partial-thickness wounds (loss of tissue limited to epidermis and possible partial loss of the dermis) heal by the process of regeneration.

TABLE 40.1	
Wound Color/Tissue	
Black/brown wounds/ eschar	Black or brown tissue is eschar, which represents full-thickness tissue destruction. Black is used to describe necrotic tissue or desiccated tissue such as tendon. It is also related to gangrenous lesions secondary to peripheral vascular disease.
	If the goal for a wound covered with eschar is debridement, sharp debridement is used to quickly remove the tissue, chemical debridement is used to soften the tissue for removal, or a moist dressing is also considered to loosen the tissue. The method of debridement depends on the overall goal for the patient.
Yellow wounds/ slough	Yellow tissue represents nonviable tissue and in some cases the presence of an infection. Slough tissue can be yellow; cream colored; or gray slough, which is usually accompanied by purulent drainage.
	For patients with a low infection risk, the use of moisture-retentive dressings enhances debridement of the yellow/slough tissue. Moisture-retentive dressings may include moist dressings, hydrocolloids, hydrogels, or alginates. If the wound is infected, topical antimicrobials are used.
Red wounds/ granulation	Red tissue represents the presence of granulation tissue. The red color is the result of an increasing amount of new blood vessels in the wound and is considered healthy.
	The goal in management of a red granulated wound is to select a dressing that maintains a clean and moist wound environment and minimizes damage to healing tissue.

BOX 40.2
Factors That Influence Wound Healing

- Hypovolemia, hypotension, vasoconstriction, edema, and hypoxia negatively affect wound healing because adequate perfusion and oxygenation are necessary for new vessel development, collagen synthesis, and development of tensile strength.
- An adequate nutritional status is critical for collagen synthesis, tensile strength, and immune function.
- Wound infection prolongs the inflammatory response, and the microorganisms use nutrients and oxygen needed for wound repair.
- A patient with diabetes mellitus may have impaired wound healing because of abnormal and prolonged inflammation, reduced collagen synthesis, and impaired epithelial migration. Hyperglycemia is associated with compromised neutrophil function and impaired migration.
- Corticosteroid therapy or the use of other immunosuppressive agents such as chemotherapy increases the patient's susceptibility to infection.
- Advanced age can contribute to a diminished proliferation of cells critical to repair.

From Doughty DB, Sparks-Defriese B: Wound healing physiology. In Bryant RA, Nix DP, editors: *Acute and chronic wounds: current management concepts*, ed 5, St Louis, 2016, Mosby.

- Full-thickness wounds (total loss of skin layers and some deeper tissues) heal by scar formation.
- Negative-pressure wound therapy (NPWT) is a wound-care treatment that uses subatmospheric (negative) pressure to a wound through suction to facilitate healing and collect wound

fluid (Netsch, 2016). NPWT enhances wound healing by the following: elimination of chronic wound exudate; maintenance of a moist wound surface; reduction in edema with resultant improvement in perfusion; macrodeformation (traction on the side of the wound), which promotes wound contraction; micordeformation; and mechanical stretch on the cells in the wound bed, which changes cell shape and the activated intracellular process that promote healing (Netsch et al., 2016).

PATIENT-CENTERED CARE

- When caring for patients from other cultures who have acute or chronic wounds, it is important to understand their cultural beliefs and practices and how these might impact wound care. For example, dressing materials containing animal-derived products such as collagen and honey may be in conflict with a patient's religious ideology (Boyer, 2013).
- In general, using gender-congruent caregivers and having the family caregiver and a professional translator help with translation and care issues relieves some of the patient's anxiety.
- In some cultures the meaning of blood and secretions is perceived as dirty; thus it would be advisable to promptly change stained bed linens and gowns. Since some cultures believe that blood is the life force, you should explain the presence of blood-stained secretions and drainage thoroughly.
- In some cultures, their doctrine prohibits the consumption of porcine products, and these types of products may be unacceptable for wound care (Boyer, 2013).
- Be sure to recognize family caregivers when giving explanations about the nursing care regimen. In collectivist cultures presence of family members at the bedside is customary. Among some cultures it is important to recognize that they may not be comfortable exposing body parts to a member of the opposite sex (Padela and del Pozo, 2011).
- Remind patients that traditional home remedies and practices need to be avoided because they may increase the risk for infection in open wounds.

EVIDENCE-BASED PRACTICE

- Nonviable tissue in a wound can delay wound healing and contribute to wound infection. Debridement, the removal of nonviable tissue from the wound, is an essential objective of topical therapy and a critical component of optimal wound management (Ramundo, 2016).
- Methods of debridement include enzymatic, mechanical, autolytic, or sharp. The type of debridement chosen depends on the condition of the wound, goal of wound treatment, and the patient's overall condition (NPUAP, EPUAP, PPPIA, 2014; WOCN, 2016).
- Enzymatic debridement is the topical application of enzymes such as collagenase over the necrotic tissue. Collagenase digests the necrotic tissue by dissolving the collagen in the dead tissue (NPUAP, EPUAP, PPPIA, 2014). When collagenase is used on a wound, the necrotic tissue is covered with the collagenase, and a moisture-retentive dressing can be used to soften the tissue (Ramundo, 2016).
- The type of suture material does not increase the risk for surgical site infection (SSI) or postoperative wound complications, as long as the primary repair approximates the wound edges and the incision is adequately perfused (Hemming et al., 2013).

SAFETY GUIDELINES

- Do not remove an initial surgical dressing for direct wound inspection until the health care provider writes an order for removal.
- Provide analgesia 30 minutes before a dressing change when possible.
- Healed skin from a prior injury or ulceration is weaker than skin that has never had an injury.
- Know a patient's age. With aging vascular changes occur, collagen tissue is less pliable, and scar tissue is tighter. Because the dermoepidermal junction becomes flatter in older adults, their skin tears more easily from mechanical trauma of tape removal.
- Know a patient's nutritional status. Tissue repair and infection resistance are directly related to adequate nutrition, including proteins, carbohydrates, lipids, vitamins, and minerals. Patients who are malnourished are at increased risk for wound infections and wound infection–related sepsis (Stotts, 2016a).
- Understand the risks of obesity. Inadequate vascularization decreases delivery of nutrients and cellular elements required for healing. The patient is at greater risk for wound infection and dehiscence or evisceration (Beitz, 2014).
- When a drain is present, clean the drain site using a circular stroke, starting with the area immediately next to the drain (Fig. 40.5). Using a new swab, clean immediately next to the drain and attempt to clean a little farther out from the drain.
- Identify factors that decrease oxygenation such as decreased hemoglobin level, smoking, and underlying cardiopulmonary conditions. Adequate oxygenation at the tissue level is essential for white blood cell activity and phagocytosis, fibroblast proliferation and collagen synthesis, and re-epithelialization (Doughty and Sparks-Defriese, 2016). Tissue repair is negatively influenced by a hematocrit value below 33% and a hemoglobin value below 10 g/100 mL. Hemoglobin level and oxygen release to tissues are reduced in smokers.
- Know the types of medications prescribed. Steroids reduce the inflammatory response and slow collagen synthesis. Cortisone depresses fibroblast activity and capillary growth. Chemotherapy depresses bone marrow production of white blood cells and impairs immune function.
- Identify the presence of chronic diseases or chronic trauma such as diabetes mellitus or radiation. Decreased tissue perfusion and failure to release oxygen to tissues result from diabetes mellitus.

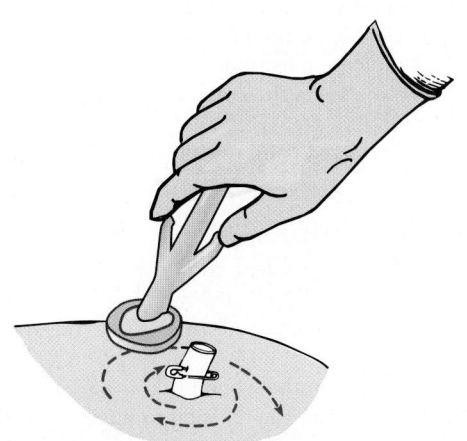

FIG 40.5 Cleaning drain site.

PROCEDURAL GUIDELINE 40.1 *Performing a Wound Assessment*

NSO *Nursing Skills Online Wound Care Module / Lesson 1*   ▶ *Video Clip*

Wound assessment provides the baseline for planning and evaluating the wound-care plan. Normal wound healing occurs in an organized fashion, and evaluating the wound status provides an ongoing assessment of wound healing and helps to determine wound treatments. The frequency of wound assessment depends on the patient's overall condition, policy of the health care setting, type of dressings used, and overall patient goals (Nix, 2016). Acute care settings generally require wound assessment daily or with each dressing change. Long-term care facilities may require an initial admission wound assessment and weekly assessment for chronic wounds. Check agency policy for frequency of wound assessment and specific wound assessment tool.

Routine wound assessments provide valuable information regarding the status of the wound. For example, is wound healing progressing as expected, or is it delayed? Is there new drainage? Wound size may increase in a wound with necrotic tissue. Removal of the necrotic tissue may result in a larger wound and is an expected finding. An increase in the amount and consistency of the drainage and new presence of odor may indicate a wound infection; and a wound culture is often necessary to support appropriate antibiotics.

The following parameters are included in a wound assessment:

- *Location:* Note the anatomical position of the wound.
- *Type of wound:* If possible, note the etiology of the wound (i.e., surgical, pressure, trauma).
- *Extent of tissue involvement:* Full-thickness wound involves both the dermis and epidermis. Partial-thickness wound involves only the epidermal layer. If it is a pressure injury, use the staging system of the National Pressure Ulcer Advisory Panel (NPUAP, 2016; see Chapter 39).
- *Type and percentage of tissue in wound base:* Describe the type of tissue (i.e., granulation, slough, eschar) and the approximate amount.
- *Wound size:* Follow agency policy to measure wound dimensions, which includes width, length, and depth.
- *Wound exudate:* Describe the amount, color, and consistency. Serous drainage is clear like plasma; sanguineous or bright red drainage indicates fresh bleeding; serosanguineous drainage is pink; and purulent drainage is thick and yellow, pale green, or white.
- *Presence of odor:* Note the presence or absence of odor, which may indicate infection.
- *Periwound area:* Assess the color, temperature, and integrity of the skin.
- *Pain:* Use a validated pain assessment scale to evaluate pain.

Delegation and Collaboration

The skill of wound assessment cannot be delegated to nursing assistive personnel (NAP). It is the nurse's responsibility to assess and document wound characteristics. The nurse directs the NAP to:

- Report drainage from the wound that is present on sheets or as strike-through from the dressing to nurse for further assessment.
- Report the presence of odor in the area of the wound.
- Report any dressing that is no longer adherent

Equipment

- Protective equipment: clean gloves, gown, and goggles if splash/spray risk exists
- Agency tool to document assessment: measuring guide
- Cotton-tipped applicator
- Dressing supplies as ordered
- Disposable waterproof biohazard bag

Procedural Steps

1. Identify patient using at least two identifiers (e.g., name and birthday or name and medical record number) according to agency policy.
2. Examine the medical record for the last wound assessment to use as a comparison for this wound assessment. Review the record to determine the etiology of the wound.
3. Determine agency-approved wound assessment tool and review the frequency of assessment. Examine the last wound assessment to use as comparison for this assessment.
4. Assess comfort level or pain on a scale of 0 to 10 and identify symptoms of anxiety. Offer pain medication if indicated.
5. Perform hand hygiene. Close room door or bed curtains and position patient.
   a. Position comfortably to permit observation of wound in well-lighted room.
   b. Expose only the area of the wound.
6. Explain procedure of wound assessment to patient.
7. Form a cuff on waterproof biohazard bag and place near bed.
8. Apply clean gloves and remove soiled dressings.
9. Examine dressings for quality of drainage (color, consistency), presence or absence of odor, and quantity of drainage (note if dressings were saturated, slightly moist, or had no drainage). Discard dressings in waterproof biohazard bag. Discard gloves.
10. Perform hand hygiene and apply clean gloves.
11. Inspect wound and determine type of wound healing (e.g., primary or secondary intention).
12. Use agency-approved assessment tool and assess the following:
    a. Wound healing by primary intention (surgical wound):
       (1) Assess anatomical location of wound on body.
       (2) Note if incisional wound margins are approximated or closed together. The wound edges should be together with no gaps.
       (3) Observe for presence of drainage. A closed incision should not have any drainage.
       (4) Look for evidence of infection (presence of erythema, odor, or wound drainage).
       (5) Lightly palpate along incision to feel a healing ridge (see Fig. 40.2). The ridge will appear as an accumulation of new tissue presenting as firmness beneath the skin, extending to about 1 cm ($\frac{1}{2}$ inch) on each side of the wound between 5 and 9 days after the incision had been created. This is an expected positive sign (Doughty and Sparks-Defriese, 2016).

PROCEDURAL GUIDELINE 40.1 *Performing a Wound Assessment—cont'd*

b. Wound healing by secondary intention (e.g., pressure injury or contaminated surgical or traumatic wound:

(1) Assess anatomical location of wound.

(2) Assess wound dimensions: Measure size of wound (including length, width, and depth) using a centimeter measuring guide. Measure length by placing a ruler over wound at the point of greatest length (or head to foot). Measure width from side to side (Nix, 2016) (see illustration). Measure depth by inserting cotton-tipped applicator in area of greatest depth and placing a mark on applicator at skin level. Discard measuring guide and cotton-tipped applicator in a biohazard bag.

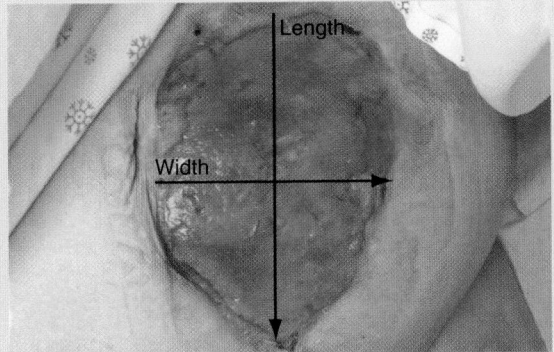

STEP 12b(2) Measuring wound length and width.

(3) Assess for undermining: Use cotton-tipped applicator to gently probe wound edges. Measure depth and note location using the face of a clock as a guide. The 12 o'clock position (top of wound) would be the head of patient, and the 6 o'clock position would be the bottom of the wound toward patient's feet. Document the number of centimeters that area extends from wound edge (e.g., underneath intact skin).

(4) Assess extent of tissue loss: If wound is a pressure injury, determine the deepest viable tissue layer in wound bed and determine stage. If necrotic tissue does not allow visualization of base of wound, the stage cannot be determined. If the wound is not a pressure injury, determine if there is partial-thickness loss (epidermis and part of the dermis) or full-thickness loss (loss of both the epidermis and the dermis). If it is a pressure injury, use the staging system of the National Pressure Ulcer Advisory Panel (NPUAP, 2016).

(5) Observe tissue type, including percentage of granulation, slough, and necrotic tissue.

(6) Note presence of exudate: amount, color, consistency and odor. Indicate amount of exudate by using part of dressing saturated (completely or partially saturated or in terms of quantity (e.g., scant, moderate, or copious).

(7) Note if wound edges are rounded toward wound bed; this may be an indication of delayed wound healing. Describe presence of epithelialization at wound edges (if present) because this indicates movement toward healing.

Clinical Decision Point *Compare the wound assessment to previous assessment and determine progress toward healing. If there is no movement toward healing or if you notice deterioration, consider a wound-care consultation. Lack of wound healing is often related to infection. Notify health care provider and wound, ostomy, continence nurse (WOCN) or wound-care team.*

13. Inspect the periwound skin, including color, texture, and temperature; and describe skin integrity (e.g., open macerated areas, blistering). Periwound assessment provides clues about the effectiveness of wound treatment and possible wound extension (Nix, 2016).

14. Apply dressings per order. Place time, date, and initials on new dressing.

15. Reassess patient's pain and level of comfort, including pain at wound site, using a scale of 0 to 10, after dressing is applied.

16. Discard biohazard bag, soiled supplies, and gloves per agency policy. Perform hand hygiene.

17. Record wound assessment findings and compare assessment with previous wound assessments to monitor wound healing.

◆ SKILL 40.1 Performing a Wound Irrigation

 Video Clip

Wound irrigation cleans open surgical or chronic wounds such as pressure injuries. Typically the irrigation of an open wound involves the use of clean gloves. Review the health care provider's order to determine if a sterile solution is required. Sterile solutions may be necessary with new traumatic wounds (Graybill et al., 2016). Irrigation involves introducing the cleaning solution directly into the wound with a syringe, syringe and catheter, pulsed lavage device, or a handheld shower. A proper wound cleaning solution is one that does not harm the tissue and uses an adequate force to agitate and wash away surface debris and devitalized tissue that contain bacteria (Table 40.2) (Jaszarowski and Murphree, 2016).

When using a syringe, the tip remains 2.5 cm (1 inch) above the wound. If a patient has a deep wound with a narrow opening, attach a soft catheter to the syringe to permit the fluid to enter the wound. Pulsed lavage delivers kinetic and mechanical energy and suction (a form of subatmospheric pressure). When pulsed lavage

TABLE 40.2

Wound Cleaning Considerations

	Mechanical Force	
	High-Pressure	**Low-Pressure**
Wound base characteristics	Presence of necrotic tissue (eschar, fibrin slough), debris, or other particulate matter Significant bacterial burden Moderate/large amount of exudate	Presence of granulation tissue or new epithelial cells Non/minimum serous or serosanguinous exudate
Clinical outcome(s)	Loosen, soften, and remove devitalized tissue from wound Separate eschar from fibrotic tissue/fibrotic tissue from granulating base	Prevent trauma to viable wound tissue Remove wound-care product residue
Solution	Normal saline Volume of solution depends on size of wound	Normal saline Volume of solution depends on size of wound
Delivery systems	35-mL syringe/19-gauge angiocatheter	Pouring saline directly from bottle Bulb syringe Piston syringe

Adapted from Spear M: Wound cleansing: solutions and techniques, *Plast Surg Nurs* 31(1):29, 2011.

TABLE 40.3

Common Wound Dressing Categories

Category	Description/Function	Indications	Side Effects	Examples
Hydrogel	Composed of water or glycerin-based polymers Provides moisture to wound bed Autolytic debridement	Partial- and full-thickness wounds Dry-to-lightly exudate Necrotic wounds	Not indicated : Third-degree burns Heavily exudating wounds	Skintegrity Elasto-Gel Vigilon
Alginate	Highly absorptive products that are retentive gel or fiber-gelling dressings	Moderate-to-heavy wound exudate Full-thickness wounds	May contribute to wound desiccation if wound exudate is minimal and gel dries	Restore Calcicare SeaSorb Algisite M
Foams	Absorption Available in adhesive and nonadhesive forms	Absorption of moderate-to-heavy exudate	May promote wound dehydration	Biatain Hydrocell PolyMem
Gauze	Available in woven or nonwoven, cotton or synthetic, sterile and nonsterile	Protection of surgical wounds Moist-to-dry dressings Wound-packing material	May adhere to healthy tissue and cause injury on removal	Curity Gauze Sponges KERLIX Super Sponge KLING gauze rolls NU GAUZE packing strips
Hydrocolloids	Adhesive dressings that contain a gel-forming agent, mold to body contours Maintain moist environment by forming a gelatinous mass	Autolytic debridement Absorption of minimal-to-moderate exudate	Some products leave residue in wound on removal Potential for periwound maceration	DuoDERM Exuderm Replicare

Data from Bryant RA, Nix DP: Principles of wound healing and topical management. In Bryant RA, Nix D P, editors: *Acute and chronic wounds: current management concepts*, ed 5, St Louis, 2016b, Mosby.

is used, normal saline may be delivered between 4 and 15 psi (pressurized irrigation) through a mechanical apparatus. Suction (subatmospheric pressure) may be used to aspirate wound debris and remove microorganisms. The use of mechanical energy through a pressurized spray also helps with the removal of wound debris. Ambulatory patients often benefit from the use of a handheld shower for wound cleaning, holding the shower spray approximately 30 cm (12 inches) from the wound.

Delegation and Collaboration

The skill of wound irrigation cannot be delegated to nursing assistive personnel (NAP) unless it is an established chronic wound. It is the nurse's responsibility to assess and document wound characteristics. The nurse directs the NAP to:
- Notify the nurse when the wound is exposed so an assessment can be completed.
- Report to the nurse patient's pain, presence of blood, drainage.

Equipment

- Irrigant/cleaning solution (volume 1.5 to 2 times the estimated wound volume)
- Irrigation delivery system (per order), depending on amount of pressure desired:
- 35-mL syringe with a 19-gauge angiocatheter to facilitate optimum pressure for cleaning with minimal risk for tissue injury (Bryant and Nix, 2016b)
- Protective equipment: clean gloves, gown, and goggles if splash/spray risk exists
- Waterproof underpad if needed
- Dressing supplies (Table 40.3; and Table 41.1)
- Disposable waterproof biohazard bag
- Extra towels and padding (to use to protect bed)
- Wound assessment supplies (see Procedural Guideline 40.1)

STEP	RATIONALE

ASSESSMENT

1. Identify patient using at least two identifiers (e.g., name and birthday or name and medical record number) according to agency policy.

   Ensures correct patient. Complies with The Joint Commission standards and improves patient safety (TJC, 2016).

2. Review health care provider's order for irrigation of open wound and type of solution to be used.

   Open-wound irrigation requires medical order, including type of solution(s) to use.

3. Assess patient's level of comfort using pain scale of 0 to 10.

   Provides baseline to determine tolerance to procedure.

4. Review medical record for sign and symptoms related to patient's open wound.

   Provides ongoing data to indicate change in wound status (Nix, 2016).

   a. Extent of impairment of skin integrity, including size of wound

   b. Verify number of drains present

   Awareness of drain position facilitates safe dressing removal and determines need for special dressings.

   c. Drainage, including amount, color, consistency, and any odor noted

   Ongoing data; drainage should decrease in healing wound. When drainage increases, it is often related to infection (Doughty and Sparks-Defriese, 2016).

   d. Wound tissue color

   Color represents balance between necrotic and new scar tissue. Proper selection of wound-care products on basis of wound color facilitates removal of necrotic tissue and promotes new tissue growth (Nix, 2016).

   e. Culture reports

   Infected wound is colonized with bacteria. Culture reports identify type of bacteria and proper treatment. Ongoing wound cultures document resolution of infectious process (Stotts, 2016b).

5. Assess patient for history of allergies to antiseptics, solutions, medications, tapes, or dressing material.

   Known allergies suggest applying sample of prescribed wound treatment as skin test before flushing wound with large volume of solution or selecting different tape or dressing material.

6. Assess patient's and family caregiver's understanding of need for irrigation and signs of wound infection.

   Determines extent of instruction required.

NURSING DIAGNOSES

- Acute pain
- Deficient knowledge related to purpose of irrigation
- Impaired skin integrity
- Impaired tissue integrity
- Risk for infection
- Risk for injury

Related factors/Risk factors are individualized based on patient's condition or needs.

PLANNING

1. Expected outcomes following completion of procedure:
   - Patient states acceptable level of comfort on pain scale of 0 to 10 after wound irrigation.

     Premedication, gently administered irrigation, application of clean dressing, and repositioning patient ensure comfort.

   - Wound begins to demonstrate signs of healing; wound is free of excessive drainage, exudate, and inflammation.

     Healing progresses in absence of debris and presence of protective coating.

   - Skin integrity is maintained; no redness, edema, or inflammation noted in surrounding tissue.

     No further skin and tissue damage has resulted from wound irrigation.

   - Patient is able to describe signs of wound healing and infection.

     Demonstrates learning.

2. Perform hand hygiene. Administer analgesic at least 30 minutes before starting wound irrigation procedure.

   Promotes pain control and permits patient to move more easily and be positioned to facilitate wound irrigation (Krasner, 2016).

3. Explain procedure to patient and family caregiver about procedure. Describe signs of healing and infection during irrigation.

   Promotes cooperation and reduces anxiety.

4. Gather appropriate supplies for wound irrigation and dressing.

   Ensures an organized procedure.

5. Close room door or bed curtains, perform hand hygiene, and position patient.

   Maintains privacy; frequent hand hygiene reduces microorganisms.

STEP	RATIONALE

a. Position comfortably to permit gravitational flow of irrigating solution over wound and into collection receptacle (see illustration). | Directing solution from top to bottom of wound and from clean to contaminated area prevents further infection. Position patient during planning stage, keeping in mind bed surfaces needed for later preparation of equipment.

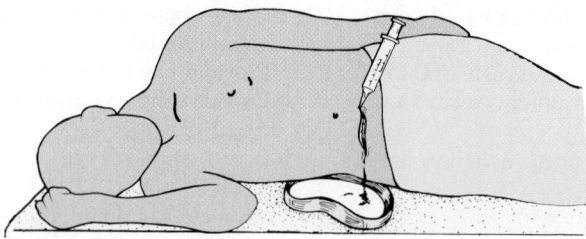

STEP 5a Patient position for wound irrigation.

b. Position patient so wound is vertical to collection basin. Irrigant should be room temperature. | Room-temperature solution increases comfort and reduces vascular constriction response in tissues.

c. Place padding or extra towel on bed under area where irrigation will take place. | Protects bedding from becoming wet.

IMPLEMENTATION

1. Perform hand hygiene. | While cleaning wound, use meticulous hand hygiene and proper infection control procedures before and after removing soiled dressings to limit risk for health care–acquired infection (Jaszarowski and Murphree, 2016).

2. Form cuff on waterproof biohazard bag and place near bed. | Cuffing helps to maintain large opening, thereby permitting placement of contaminated dressings without touching bag itself.

3. Apply gown, mask, goggles as indicated; apply clean gloves and remove old dressing. | Reduces transmission of microorganisms. Protects nurse from splashes or sprays of blood and body fluids.

4. Discard old dressing and gloves in biohazard bag. Perform hand hygiene. | Reduces transmission of microorganisms.

5. Apply clean or sterile gloves (check agency policy). Perform wound assessment and examine recent charted assessment of patient's open wound (see Procedural Guideline 40.1). | Provides ongoing wound-healing data. Use sterile precautions when sterile gloves are needed.

6. Expose area near wound only. | Provides privacy and prevents chilling of patient.

7. Irrigate wound with wide opening:

a. Fill 35-mL syringe with irrigation solution. | Irrigating wound uses mechanical force, which helps with separation and removal of necrotic debris and surface bacteria (Jaszarowski and Murphree, 2016). Flushing wound helps remove debris and facilitates healing by secondary intention.

b. Attach 19-gauge angiocatheter. | Catheter lumen delivers ideal pressure for cleaning and removing debris (Ramundo, 2016). Mechanical debridement may include irrigation, which can be done through use of 35-mL syringe with 19-gauge angiocatheter with irrigation pressures delivered between 4 and 15 psi (WOCN, 2016).

c. Hold syringe tip 2.5 cm (1 inch) above upper end of wound and over area being cleaned. | Prevents syringe contamination. Careful placement of syringe prevents unsafe pressure of flowing solution.

d. Using continuous pressure, flush wound; repeat Steps 7a to 7c until solution draining into basin is clear. | Flushing wound helps to remove debris; clear solution indicates removal of all debris.

8. Irrigate deep wound with very small opening:

a. Attach soft catheter to filled irrigation syringe. | Catheter permits direct flow of irrigant into wound. Expect wound to take longer to empty when opening is small.

b. Gently insert tip of catheter into opening about 1.3 cm (0.5 inch). | Prevents tip from touching fragile inner wall of wound.

Clinical Decision Point *Do not force catheter into the wound because this will cause tissue damage.*

STEP	RATIONALE
c. Using slow, continuous pressure, flush wound.	Use of slow mechanical force of stream of solution loosens particulate matter on wound surface and promotes healing (Ramundo, 2016).

Clinical Decision Point *Pulsatile high-pressure lavage is often the irrigation of choice for necrotic wounds. Pressure settings should be set per provider order, usually between 4 and 15 psi, and should not be used on skin grafts, exposed blood vessels, muscle, tendon, or bone. Use with caution if patient has coagulation disorder or is taking anticoagulants (Ramundo, 2016).*

STEP	RATIONALE
d. While keeping catheter in place, pinch it off just below syringe.	Avoids contamination of sterile solution
e. Remove and refill syringe. Reconnect to catheter and repeat until solution draining into basin is clear.	
9. Clean wound with handheld shower:	
a. With patient seated comfortably in shower chair or standing if condition allows, adjust spray to gentle flow; make sure that water is warm.	Useful for patients able to shower with help or independently. May be accomplished at home.
b. Shower for 5 to 10 minutes with shower head 30 cm (12 inches) from wound.	Ensures that wound is cleaned thoroughly.
10. When indicated, obtain cultures (see Chapter 7) after cleaning with nonbacteriostatic saline.	WOCN (2016) recommends using quantitative bacterial cultures (tissue biopsy or swab cultures). Most common type of wound cultures are swab technique, aspirated wound fluid, or tissue biopsy (Stotts, 2016b).

Clinical Decision Point *Obtain a wound culture if indicated by the presence of inflammation around the wound, purulent odor or drainage, new drainage, or a febrile patient.*

STEP	RATIONALE
11. Dry wound edges with gauze; dry patient after shower.	Prevents maceration of surrounding tissue from excess moisture.
12. Remove and dispose of gloves. Perform hand hygiene. Apply clean or sterile gloves (see agency policy). Apply appropriate dressing and label with time, date, and nurse's initials.	Reduces transmission of microorganisms. Maintains protective barrier and healing environment for wound.
13. Remove mask, goggles, and gown.	Prevents transfer of microorganisms.
14. Dispose of equipment and soiled supplies; remove and dispose of gloves. Perform hand hygiene.	Reduces transmission of microorganisms.
15. Help patient to comfortable position.	

EVALUATION

1. Have patient rate level of comfort on scale of 0 to 10.	Patient's pain should not increase as result of wound irrigation.
2. Monitor type of tissue in wound bed.	Identifies wound healing progress and determines type of wound cleaning and dressing needed.
3. Inspect dressing periodically (see agency policy).	Determines patient's response to wound irrigation and need to modify plan of care.
4. Evaluate periwound skin integrity.	Determines if extension of wound has occurred or signs of infection are present (warm red periwound skin).
5. Observe for presence of retained irrigant.	Retained irrigant is medium for bacterial growth and subsequent infection.
6. **Use Teach-Back:** "I want to be sure that I explained why the wound was irrigated today. Tell me why it is important to irrigate your wound." Revise your instruction now or develop plan for revised patient or family caregiver teaching if patient or family caregiver is not able to teach back correctly.	Determines patient's and family caregiver's level of understanding of instructional topic.

STEP	RATIONALE
Unexpected Outcomes	**Related Interventions**
1. Bleeding or serosanguinous drainage appears.	• Flush wound during next irrigation using less pressure.
	• Notify health care provider of bleeding.
2. Increased pain or discomfort occurs.	• Decrease force of pressure during wound irrigation.
	• Assess patient for need for additional analgesia before wound care.
3. Suture line opening extends.	• Notify health care provider.
	• Reevaluate amount of pressure to use for next wound irrigation.

Recording and Reporting

• Record wound assessment before and after irrigation; amount, color, and odor of drainage on dressing removed; amount and type of solution used; irrigation device used; patient's tolerance of the procedure; and type of dressing applied after irrigation on flow sheet in nurses' notes in electronic health record (EHR) or chart.

• Record patient's and family caregiver's understanding through teach-back for reasons for wound irrigations.

• Immediately report to the health care provider any evidence of fresh bleeding, sharp increase in pain, retention of irrigant, or signs of shock.

Special Considerations
Teaching

• Instruct patient and family caregiver regarding wound-care technique, observe them doing a return demonstration, and provide written instructions.

• Explain the need for specialized supplies such as irrigating solutions and dressings and the need to maintain asepsis when performing care.

• Teach patient and family caregiver signs of healing wound, improper wound healing, and wound infection.

Pediatric

• Some pediatric patients are very frightened. They might verbally and physically try to prevent the nurse from cleaning the wound. Having the child take active part in the procedure or working out his or her feelings about wound irrigation with play therapy on a doll with a wound helps the child to be more cooperative.

• Neonatal skin is immature and easily damaged from pressure and wound-care products. Check that products are approved for use with this population. Remember that in neonates the skin readily absorbs products.

Gerontological

• Wound irrigations are traumatic, frightening, and painful to some older patients. Assess patient's cooperation before irrigating wound. Be aware of patient's cognitive level of understanding when performing wound irrigation.

Home Care

• Assess patient's home environment to determine adequacy of resources for performing wound care; check especially for adequate lighting, running water, and storage of supplies.

• Plan wound care in conjunction with patient's total rehabilitation goals. The objective of wound-care management in a subacute care setting is to return the patient to his or her home environment.

• Provide support for patient and caregiver during the wound-healing process. Chronic wounds do not heal properly and do not close in a timely manner (Doughty and Sparks-Defriese, 2016).

• Some patients need to receive wound-care management in an outpatient wound-care clinic. Be sure that patient has directions to clinic and knows where to park and where to obtain dressing supplies.

• Solutions to use for irrigation in the home include potable tap water, distilled water, cooled boiled water, and normal saline (WOC, 2016). Teach patient and family caregiver how to make normal saline, especially if cost is an issue. You make normal saline by using 8 teaspoons of salt in 1 gallon of distilled water; keep it refrigerated for 1 month. The saline solution should be allowed to reach room temperature before use.

◆ SKILL 40.2   Removing Sutures and Staples

Agency policy determines whether *only* a health care provider *and* nurse may remove sutures and staples. The health care provider must determine and order removal of all sutures or staples at one time or removal of every other suture or staple as the first phase, with the remainder removed in the second phase.

Sutures and staples generally are removed within 7 to 14 days after surgery if healing is adequate (Whitney, 2016). Retention sutures usually remain in place 14 to 21 days. Timing the removal of sutures and staples is important. They must remain in place long enough to ensure initial wound closure with enough strength to support internal tissues and organs. Sutures left in longer than 14 days generally leave suture marks (Whitney, 2016).

Sutures are threads of wire or other materials used to sew body tissues together. They come in different sizes and are absorbent or nonabsorbent. They are placed within tissue layers in deep wounds and superficially as the final means for wound closure. The choice of suture technique depends on the type and anatomical location of the wound, thickness of the skin, degree of tension, and desired cosmetic effect (Fig. 40.6) (Whitney, 2016). A patient's history of wound healing, site of wound, tissues involved, and the purpose of the sutures determine the suture material selected. For example, a patient with repeated abdominal surgeries might require wire sutures for greater strength to promote wound closure.

Staples are stainless-steel wires, are quick to use, and provide strength. The location of the incision sometimes restricts their use because there must be adequate distance between the skin and structures that lie below the skin, including bone and vascular structures. They are used for skin closure of abdominal incisions

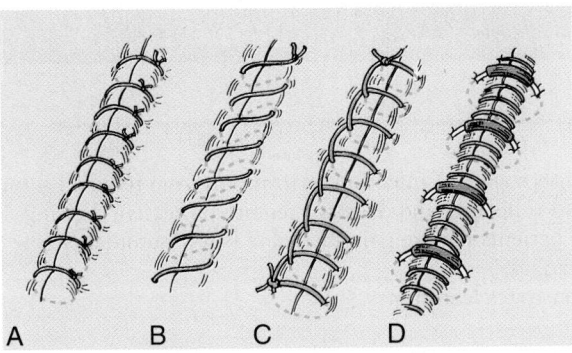

FIG 40.6 Types of sutures. **A,** Intermittent. **B** and **C,** Continuous. **D,** Blanket.

and orthopedic surgery when appearance of the incision is not critical. Removal requires a sterile staple extractor and aseptic technique.

If there is any sign of suture line separation during the removal process, the remaining sutures/staples are left in place, and a description is documented and reported to the health care provider.

In some cases these are removed several days to 1 week later. After sutures/staples are removed, the nurse applies Steri-Strips over the incision to provide support. The strips loosen over time (5 to 7 days) and can be removed when half of the strip is no longer attached to the skin.

Delegation and Collaboration

The skill of staple and/or suture removal cannot be delegated to nursing assistive personnel (NAP). The nurse directs the NAP to:

- Report to the nurse drainage, bleeding, swelling at the incision site or an elevation in patient's temperature.
- Report to the nurse patient's complaints of pain.
- Provide special hygiene practices following suture removal.

Equipment

- Disposable waterproof biohazard bag
- Sterile suture removal set (forceps and scissors) or sterile staple extractor
- Sterile antiseptic swabs
- Gauze pads
- Steri-Strips or butterfly adhesive strips
- Clean gloves (sterile gloves optional)

STEP	RATIONALE

ASSESSMENT

1. Identify patient using at least two identifiers (e.g., name and birthday or name and medical record number) according to agency policy.

Ensures correct patient. Complies with The Joint Commission standards and improves patient safety (TJC, 2016).

2. Review patient's medical record for the following information:
   a. Check health care provider's order.
   b. Review specific directions related to suture or staple removal.
   c. Determine history of conditions that may pose risk for impaired wound healing: advanced age, cardiovascular disease, diabetes, immunosuppression, radiation, obesity, smoking, poor nutrition, and infection.

Health care provider's order is required for removal of sutures.
Indicates specifically which sutures are to be removed (e.g., every other suture).
Preexisting health disorders affect speed of healing and sometimes result in dehiscence.

3. Assess patient for history of allergies.
4. Assess patient's comfort level on pain scale of 0 to 10.

Determines if patient is sensitive to antiseptic or latex.
Provides baseline of patient's comfort level to determine response to therapy.

5. Perform hand hygiene. Inspect incision for healing ridge and skin integrity of suture line for uniform closure of wound edges, normal color, and absence of drainage and inflammation. Apply clean gloves if necessary to palpate wound. Remove and dispose following assessment.

Indicates adequate wound healing for support of internal structures without continued need for sutures or staples (Whitney, 2016).

6. Assess patient's or family caregiver's knowledge of wound care and observations to make.

Determines extent of instruction required.

Clinical Decision Point *If wound edges are separated or signs of infection are present, the wound has not healed properly. Notify the health care provider because sutures or staples may need to remain in place and/or other wound care initiated.*

NURSING DIAGNOSES

- Acute pain
- Knowledge deficit regarding incision care
- Impaired skin integrity
- Risk for impaired skin integrity
- Risk for infection

Related factors/Risk factors are individualized based on patient's condition or needs.

STEP	RATIONALE

PLANNING

1. Expected outcomes following completion of procedure:
- All suture material or staples are removed.
- Suture line is intact.
- Patient states acceptable level of comfort on scale of 0 to 10 following removal of sutures or staples.
- Patient or family caregiver is able to describe wound care following suture removal.

2. Explain to patient how you will remove staples and that suture removal is usually not a painful procedure but patient may feel pulling or tugging of skin.

3. Administer prescribed analgesic if needed at least 30 minutes before procedure.

Removes source of infection or irritation from retained sutures.
Wound is healing and does not require protective dressings.
Some patients require pain medicine before suture or staple removal.
Demonstrates learning.

Gains patient cooperation and reduces anxiety.

Promotes patient comfort to help minimize movement during suture removal.

IMPLEMENTATION

1. Close curtains or room door.

Provides privacy.

Clinical Decision Point *For patient who is highly anxious or who has an extensive wound, consider need to administer analgesic 30 minutes before suture removal.*

2. Position patient comfortably while exposing suture line. Ensure that direct lighting is on suture line.

Aids visibility and correct placement of forceps or extractor during removal process, ultimately reducing soft tissue injury.

3. Perform hand hygiene.

Reduces transmission of microorganisms.

4. Place cuffed waterproof disposal bag within easy reach.

Provides for easy disposal of contaminated dressings and prevents passing items over sterile work area.

5. Prepare materials needed for suture/staple removal:
  a. Open sterile suture removal kit or staple extractor kit.
  b. Open sterile antiseptic swabs and place on inside surface of kit.
  c. Obtain gloves (sterile gloves if policy indicates).

Ensures an organized procedure.

6. Apply clean gloves. Carefully remove dressing; discard dressing and gloves in prepared refuse disposal bag.

Reduces transmission of infection.

7. Inspect incision and suture line (see illustration).

Determines adequacy of wound healing.

8. Perform hand hygiene. Apply clean or sterile gloves as required by agency policy.

Reduces transmission of infection.

9. Clean sutures or staples and healed incision with antiseptic swabs. Start at sides next to incision and then wipe across suture line using new antiseptic swab for each swipe.

Removes surface bacteria from incision and sutures or staples.

10. Remove staples:
  a. Place lower tips of staple extractor under first staple. As you close handles, upper tip of extractor depresses center of staple, causing both ends of staple to be bent upward and simultaneously exit their insertion sites in dermal layer (see illustration).

Avoids excess pressure to suture line and secures smooth removal of each staple.

  b. Carefully control staple extractor.
  c. As soon as both ends of staple are visible, move it away from skin surface (see illustration) and continue until staple is over refuse bag.

Avoids pressure on suture line and patient discomfort.
Prevents scratching tender skin surface with sharp pointed ends of staple for comfort and infection control.

  d. Release handles of staple extractor, allowing staple to drop into refuse bag.

Avoids contaminating sterile field with used staples.

  e. Repeat Steps a through d until all staples are removed.

11. Remove interrupted sutures:
  a. Place gauze few inches from suture line. Hold scissors in dominant hand and forceps (clamp) in nondominant hand.

Gauze serves as receptacle for removed sutures. Placement of scissors and forceps allows for efficient suture removal.

STEP	**RATIONALE**

Clinical Decision Point *Placement of scissors and forceps is very important. Avoid pinching the skin around the wound when lifting up the suture. Likewise avoid cutting the skin around the wound by accident when snipping the suture.*

b. Grasp knot of suture with forceps and gently pull up knot while slipping tip of scissors under suture near skin (see illustration).

Releases suture.

c. Snip suture as close to skin as possible at end distal to knot.

Clinical Decision Point *Never snip both ends of suture; there will be no way to remove the part of the suture situated below the surface.*

d. Grasp knotted end with forceps and in one continuous smooth action pull suture through from the other side (see illustration). Place removed suture on gauze.

Smoothly removes suture without additional tension to suture line.

Clinical Decision Point *Never pull exposed surface of any suture into tissue below epidermis. The exposed surface of any suture is considered contaminated.*

e. Repeat Steps a through d until you have removed every other suture.

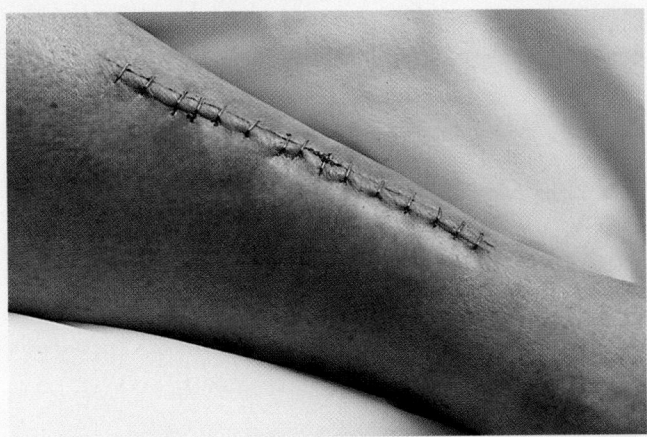

STEP 7 Suture line secured with staples.

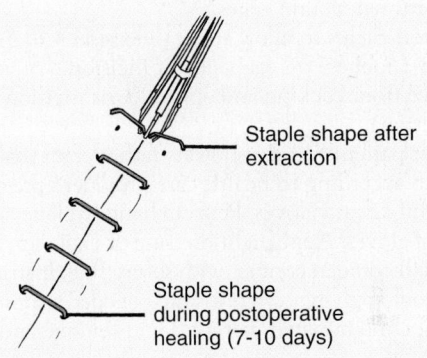

Staple shape after extraction

Staple shape during postoperative healing (7-10 days)

STEP 10a Staple extractor placed under staple.

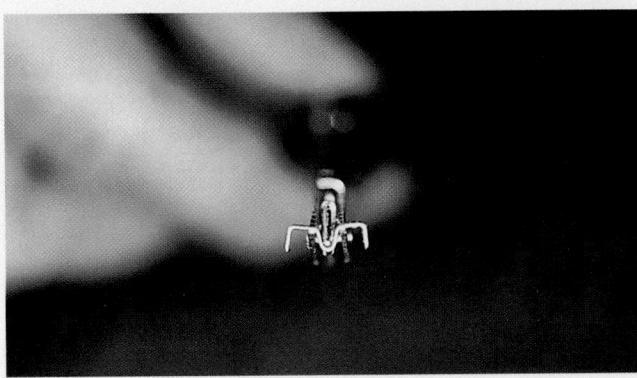

STEP 10c Metal staple removed by extractor.

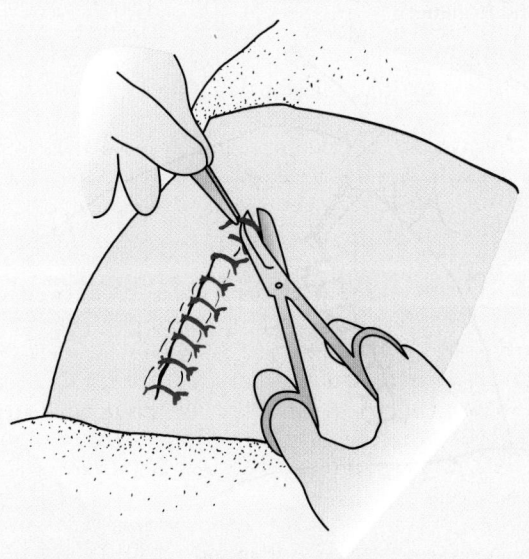

STEP 11b Removal of intermittent suture. Nurse cuts suture as close to skin as possible, away from knot.

STEP	RATIONALE
f. Observe healing level. Based on observations of wound response to suture removal and health care provider's original order, determine whether remaining sutures will be removed at this time. If so, repeat Steps a to d until you have removed all sutures.	Determines status of wound healing and if suture line will remain closed after all sutures are removed.
g. If any doubt, stop and notify health care provider.	
12. Remove continuous and blanket stitch sutures:	
a. Place sterile gauze a few inches from suture line. Grasp scissors in dominant hand and forceps in nondominant hand.	Gauze serves as receptacle for removed sutures. Placement of scissors and forceps allows for efficient suture removal.
b. Snip first suture close to skin surface at end distal to knot.	Releases suture.
c. Snip second suture on same side.	Releases interrupted sutures from knot.
d. Grasp knotted end and gently pull with continuous smooth action, removing suture from beneath skin. Place suture on gauze compress.	Smoothly removes sutures without additional tension to suture line. Prevents pulling of contaminated part of suture through skin.
e. Repeat Steps a to d in consecutive order until entire line is removed.	
13. Inspect incision to make sure that all sutures are removed and identify any trouble areas. Gently wipe suture line with antiseptic swab to remove debris and clean incision.	Reduces risk for further incision line separation.
14. Apply Steri-Strips if *any* separation greater than two stitches or two staples in width is apparent to maintain contact between wound edges.	Supports wound by distributing tension across wound and eliminates closure technique scarring.
a. Cut Steri-Strips to allow strips to extend 4 to 5 cm (1½ to 2 inches) on each side of incision.	
b. Remove from backing and apply across incision (see illustration).	
c. Instruct patient to take showers rather than soak in bathtub according to health care provider's preference.	Steri-Strips are not removed and are allowed to fall off gradually.
15. Remove and discard gloves. Perform hand hygiene and apply new pair of gloves. Apply light dressing or expose to air if no clothing will come in contact with suture line. Instruct patient about applying own dressing if needed at home.	Healing by primary intention eliminates need for dressing.
16. Discard all contaminated materials and remove and dispose of gloves.	Reduces transmission of infection.
17. Dispose of sharps (disposable staple extractor and/or scissors) in designated sharps disposal bin and perform hand hygiene.	Reduces transmission of infection. Provides a safe environment because instruments are sharp and contaminated.

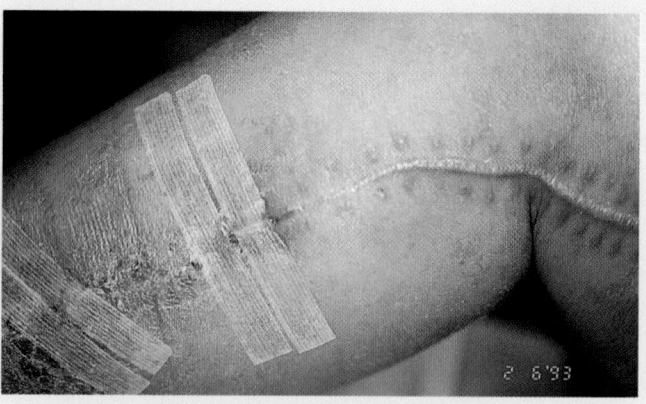

STEP 11d Nurse removes suture and never pulls contaminated stitch through tissues.

STEP 14b Steri-Strips over incision.

STEP	**RATIONALE**

EVALUATION

1. Assess site where sutures or staples were removed; inspect condition of soft tissues, including skin. Look for any pieces of removed suture left behind.

Ensures that sources of infection have been removed.

2. Determine if patient has pain along incision.

Determines comfort level and can indicate if suture material remains in skin.

3. **Use Teach-Back:** "I want to be sure that I have adequately explained the signs of a wound or incision infection before you are discharged. Tell me the signs of infection and what you need to tell your health care provider if this happens?" Revise your instruction now or develop plan for revised patient or family caregiver teaching if patient or family caregiver is not able to teach back correctly.

Determines patient's and family caregiver's level of understanding of instructional topic.

Unexpected Outcomes	**Related Interventions**
1. Retained suture is present.	• Notify health care provider.
	• Instruct patient to notify health care provider if signs of suture line infection develop following discharge from agency.
2. Patient experiences wound separation or drainage secondary to healing problems.	• Leave remaining sutures or staples in place.
	• Place Steri-Strip closures across suture line.
	• Notify health care provider.

Recording and Reporting

- Record the time the sutures or staples were removed and the number of sutures or staples removed; document the cleaning of the suture line, appearance of the wound, level of healing of the wound, and type of dressing applied; document patient's response to suture or staple removal on flow sheet in nurses' notes in electronic health record (EHR) or chart.
- Record patient's and family caregiver's understanding through teach-back about why the sutures were removed today.
- Immediately report to the health care provider if suture line separation, dehiscence, evisceration, bleeding, or purulent drainage occurs.

Special Considerations
Teaching

- Teach patient to observe for any sign of separation of wound edges before removing remaining sutures/staples and inspect incision for continued healing.
- Reinforce instruction about resuming bathing and showering activities, preventing abdominal strain during defecation, and providing adequate nutrition and ambulation.

- Teach patient not to put additional stress on suture line from such activities as lifting or bending. Patients with abdominal surgery or injury need to avoid lifting heavy packages or equipment for several weeks.
- Instruct patient that sometimes there is a small amount of drainage from wound immediately after suture removal.

Pediatric

- Help is sometimes necessary to keep infants from moving during the suture removal procedure.
- Topical anesthetic solutions (e.g., lidocaine, EMLA) applied to intact skin may provide short-term (20 minutes) anesthesia (Krasner, 2016).

Gerontological

- Some older adults need reassurance about suture/staple removal procedure. Depending on their mental status, they may not understand the procedure.
- Older skin is often at higher risk for dehiscence after sutures/staples are removed.

♦ **SKILL 40.3** **Managing Wound Drainage Evacuation**

NSO *Nursing Skills Online Wound Care Module / Lesson 3*

If drainage accumulates in a wound bed, wound healing is delayed. Drainage is facilitated when the surgeon inserts either a closed- or an open-drain system, even if the amount of drainage is small. The drain is inserted directly through a small stab wound near the suture line into the area of the wound.

An open-drain system (e.g., a Penrose drain [Fig. 40.7]) removes drainage from the wound and deposits it onto the skin surface. A sterile safety pin is inserted through this drain, outside the skin, to prevent the tubing from moving into the wound.

A closed-drain system such as the Jackson-Pratt (JP) drain (Fig. 40.8) or Hemovac drain relies on the presence of a vacuum to withdraw accumulated drainage from around the wound bed into the collection device. A JP drain collects fluid that is in the range of 100 to 200 mL/24 h. A Hemovac or ConstaVac drainage system is used for larger amounts of drainage (500 mL/24 h). The collection device is connected to a clear plastic drain with multiple perforations. Drainage collects in a closed reservoir or a suction bladder. The closed system collects fluid but operates only if the

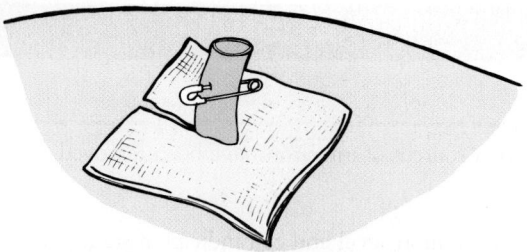

FIG 40.7 Penrose drain with drain-split gauze.

tubing is patent and a vacuum exists. If drainage device is half full, empty the chamber and measure the drainage. After measurement reestablish the vacuum and ensure that all drainage tubes are patent.

Delegation and Collaboration

The assessment of wound drainage and maintenance of drains and the drainage system cannot be delegated to NAP. However, you may delegate emptying a closed drainage container or pouch, measuring the amount of drainage, and reporting the amount on the patient's intake and output (I&O) record to NAP. The nurse directs the NAP by:

- Discussing any increase in frequency of emptying the drain other than once a shift.
- Instructing to report to the nurse any change in amount, color, or odor of drainage.
- Reviewing the intake and output (I&O) procedure.

Equipment

- Graduated measuring cylinder or specimen container
- Antiseptic wipes
- Gauze sponges, including split gauze sponges for drain site

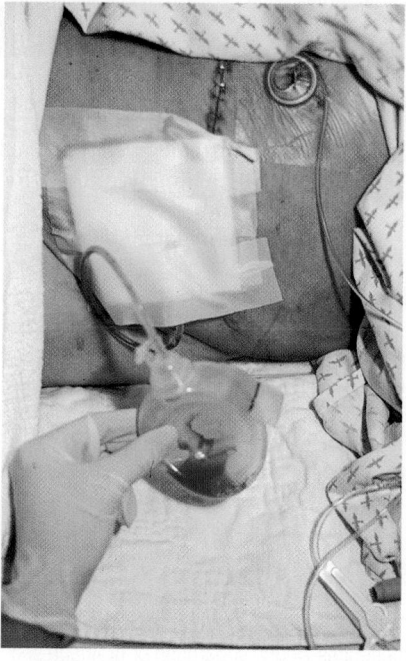

FIG 40.8 Jackson-Pratt wound drainage system.

- Sterile gauze dressings as needed
- Clean gloves
- Safety pin(s)
- Protective equipment: goggles, mask, and gown if risk of spray from drain is present
- Disposable drape or barrier
- *Optional:* Normal saline for cleaning insertion site

STEP	RATIONALE

ASSESSMENT

1. Identify patient using at least two identifiers (e.g., name and birthday or name and medical record number) according to agency policy.

   Ensures correct patient. Complies with The Joint Commission standards and improves patient safety (TJC, 2016).

2. Review medical record to identify presence, location, and purpose of closed wound drain and drainage system as patient returns from surgery.

   Drainage tubing is usually placed near wound through small surgical incision.

3. Perform hand hygiene. Apply clean gloves if there is a risk of contacting drainage. Assess drainage present on patient's dressing. Identify number of wound drain tubes and what each one will be draining. Label each drain tube with a number or label.

   Assigning labeling system to each drain helps with consistent documentation when patient has multiple drainage tubes.

4. Inspect system to determine presence of one straight tube or Y-tube arrangement with two tube insertion sites.

   Allows nurse to plan skin care and identifies quantity of sterile dressing supplies needed.

5. Inspect system to ensure proper functioning. Complete systematic inspection includes insertion site, drainage moving through tubing in direction of reservoir, patency of drainage tubing, airtight connection sites, and presence of any leaks or kinks in system. Remove and dispose of gloves. Perform hand hygiene.

   Properly functioning system maintains suction until reservoir is filled or drainage is no longer being produced or accumulated. Tension on drainage tubing increases injury to skin and underlying muscle.

6. Determine if drain tube needs self-suction, wall suction, or no suction by checking health care provider's orders.

   Some drain tubes such as Hemovac can be used with self-suction or wall suction.

Clinical Decision Point *Attach tape and a safety pin to drainage tubing with tape and pin to patient's gown so the suction device is below the level of the wound and does not pull on the insertion site.*

STEP	RATIONALE

7. Identify type of drainage containers that patient has.

Determines frequency for emptying drainage.

8. Assess patient's level of understanding of purpose of drainage system and precautions to take to avoid accidental removal.

Determines extent of instruction required.

NURSING DIAGNOSES

- Deficient knowledge regarding wound drain function.
- Impaired skin integrity
- Risk for infection
- Risk for injury

Related factors/Risk factors are individualized based on patient's condition or needs.

PLANNING

1. Expected outcomes following completion of procedure:
   - Wound healing continues.
   - Vacuum is reestablished.
   - Tubing is patent.
   - Patient describes precautions to avoid drain removal.
2. Explain procedure to patient.

Patient is comfortable, and wound drainage is collected.
Suction system is intact.
Fluid is draining away from wound area.
Demonstrates learning.
Promotes patient's cooperation and reduces anxiety.

IMPLEMENTATION

1. Close room door or bedside curtains.
2. Perform hand hygiene and apply clean gloves.
3. Place open specimen container or measuring graduate on bed between you and patient.
4. **Empty Hemovac or ConstaVac:**
   a. Maintain asepsis while opening plug on port indicated for emptying drainage reservoir.
      (1) Tilt suction container in direction of plug.
      (2) Slowly squeeze two flat surfaces together, tilting toward measuring container.
   b. Drain contents into measuring container (see illustration).
   c. Hold uncovered antiseptic swab in dominant hand. Place suction device on flat surface with open outlet facing upward; continue pressing downward until bottom and top are in contact (see illustration).

Provides privacy.
Reduces transmission of microorganisms.
Permits measuring and discarding of wound drainage.

Avoids entry of pathogens.
Vacuum will be broken, and reservoir will pull air in until chamber is fully expanded.
Drains fluid toward plug.
Prevents splashing of contaminated drainage. Squeezing empties reservoir of drainage.
Contents counted as fluid output (see Chapter 6).
Cleaning plug reduces transmission of microorganisms into drainage evacuation.

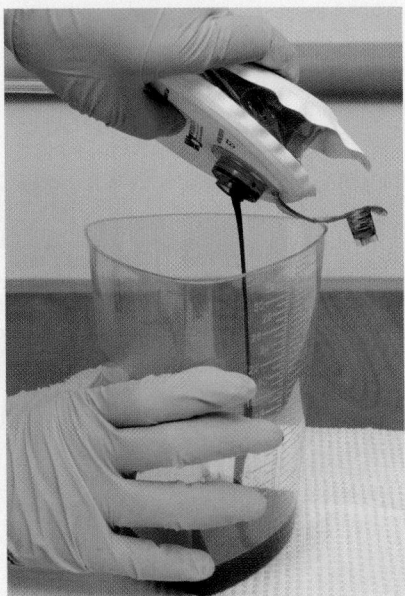

STEP 4b Hemovac contents drained into measuring container.

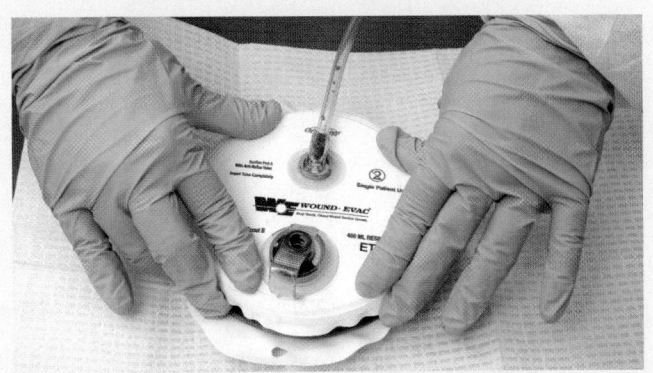

STEP 4c Hemovac compressed to create suction.

STEP	RATIONALE
d. Holding surfaces together with one hand and using antiseptic swab, quickly clean opening, plug with other hand, and immediately replace plug; secure suction device on patient's bed.	Compression of surface of Hemovac creates vacuum.
e. Check device for reestablishment of vacuum, patency of drainage tubing, and absence of stress on tubing.	Facilitates wound drainage and prevents tension on drainage tubing.
5. Empty Hemovac with wall suction:	Empties drainage and reestablishes suction to wound bed.
a. Turn off suction.	
b. Disconnect suction tubing from Hemovac port.	
c. Empty Hemovac as described in Step 4.	
d. Use an antiseptic swab to clean port opening and the end of suction tubing. Reconnect tubing to port.	Cleaning plug reduces transmission of microorganisms.
e. Set suction level as prescribed or on low if health care provider does not specify suction level.	Reestablishes wound suction.
6. Empty JP suction drain:	
a. Open port on top of bulb-shaped reservoir (see illustration).	Breaks vacuum for drain.
b. Tilt bulb in direction of port and drain toward opening. Empty drainage from device into measuring container (see illustration). Clean end of emptying port and plug with antiseptic wipe.	Reduces transmission of microorganisms.
c. Compress bulb over drainage container. While compressing bulb, replace plug immediately.	Reestablishes vacuum.
7. Place and secure drainage system below site with safety pin on patient's gown. Be sure that there is slack in tubing from reservoir to wound.	Pinning drainage tubing to patient's gown prevents tension or pulling on tubing and insertion site.
8. Note characteristics of drainage in measuring container: measure volume and discard by flushing in commode.	Contents count as fluid output.
9. Discard soiled supplies and remove and dispose of gloves. Perform hand hygiene.	Reduces transmission of microorganisms.
10. Apply clean gloves. Proceed with dressing change (see Chapter 41) around drain site and inspection of skin if indicated or ordered. Split-drain sponge dressings are often used around drain tubes (see illustration) and taped in place.	Prevents entrance of bacteria into surgical wound.
11. Discard contaminated materials and remove gloves. Perform hand hygiene.	Reduces transmission of microorganisms.

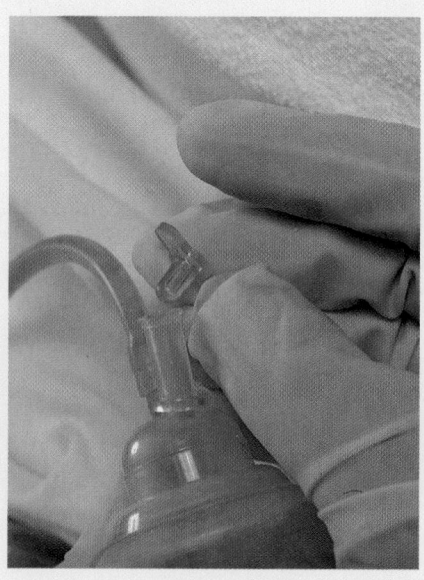

STEP 6a Opening port of Jackson-Pratt device.

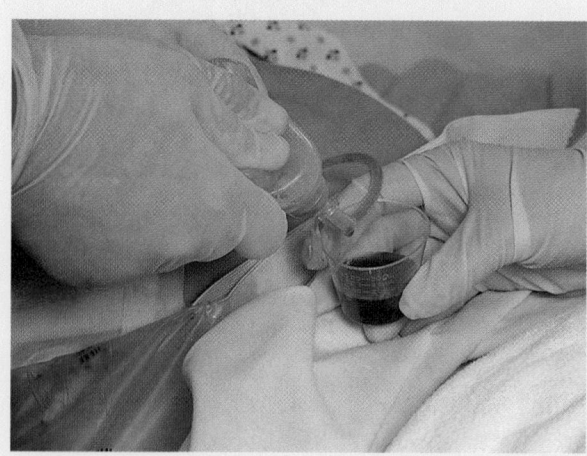

STEP 6b Emptying contents from Jackson-Pratt drainage device.

STEP	RATIONALE

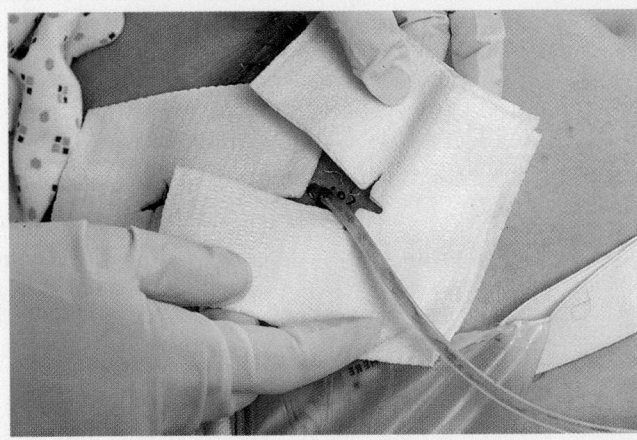

STEP 10 Applying split gauze dressing around Jackson-Pratt drain tube.

EVALUATION

1. Observe for drainage in suction device.	Indicates presence of vacuum, patency of tubing, and functioning of drainage suction device.

Clinical Decision Point *Inspect for clots or cellular debris. Clots or large collections of debris may block drainage flow. The Y-site in the drainage tubing is especially prone to clogging.*

2. Inspect wound for drainage or collection of drainage fluid under skin, causing seroma.	Drainage should not be significant under suture line. May indicate inadequate functioning of drainage suction device.
3. Measure drainage from drainage system, and record on I&O form every 8 to 12 hours and as needed for large drainage volume.	Determines status of wound healing. Collect diagnostic specimen in presence of unexpected purulence or pungent odor, report findings to health care provider, and record in progress note.
4. Use **Teach-Back:** "I want to be sure I explained clearly why it is important not to pull on your drain. Tell me what can happen if you pull the drain out accidentally." Revise your instruction now or develop a plan for revised patient or family caregiver teaching if patient or family caregiver is not able to teach back correctly.	Determines patient's and family caregiver's level of understanding of instructional topic.

Unexpected Outcomes	**Related Interventions**
1. Site where tube exits becomes infected.	• Notify health care provider about presence of signs of infection: purulent drainage, odor, reddened site, increased white blood cell count, and temperature elevation. • Use aseptic technique when changing dressings.
2. Bleeding appears in/or around drainage collector.	• Determine amount of bleeding and notify health care provider if excessive. • Assess for tension on patient's drainage tubing. • Secure tubing to prevent pulling and pain.
3. Patient experiences pain.	• Assess patient's level of pain. • Medicate patient. • Stabilize drainage tubing to reduce tension and pulling against incision. • Notify health care provider if signs of wound infection are present.
4. Drainage suction device is not accumulating drainage.	• Assess drainage tubing for clots. • Assess drainage system for air leaks or kinks. • Notify health care provider.

Recording and Reporting

- Record emptying the drainage suction device; reestablishing vacuum in suction device; amount, color, odor of drainage; dressing change to drain site; and appearance of drain insertion site on flow sheet in nurses' notes in electronic health record (EHR) or chart.
- Record amount of drainage on I&O record.
- Document your evaluation of patient and family caregiver learning.
- Immediately report a sudden change in amount of drainage, either output or absence of drainage flow, to the health care provider. Also report pungent odor of drainage or new evidence of purulence, severe pain, or dislodgement of the drainage tube to the health care provider.

Special Considerations
Teaching

- Instruct patient about anticipated postoperative drainage, expected progress of wound healing and drainage volume, and estimated date of removal of drain as volume diminishes.

- Teach patient or family caregiver how to empty and record amount of drainage. If patient is going home with drainage device, ask patient or family caregiver to record amount emptied and bring the recording to the next outpatient visit.

Pediatric

- Have parents help to prevent pediatric patients from dislodging drainage tubes.

Gerontological

- Be aware that older adults with large amounts of drainage will need additional fluid intake because they are more likely to become dehydrated.
- Take measures to prevent a confused patient from pulling out drain collector.

Home Care

- Provide written instructions in drain care. Include importance of measuring and documenting the amount of drainage. Patient should share the volume of drainage on a daily basis with the health care provider.

◆ SKILL 40.4 Negative-Pressure Wound Therapy

NSO *Nursing Skills Online Wound Care Module / Lesson 2*

Negative-pressure wound therapy (NPWT) is the application of a subatmospheric (negative) pressure to a wound through suction to facilitate healing and collect wound fluid (Netsch et al., 2016). The primary effects of negative pressure at the wound surface (Figures 40.9 and 40.10) Netsch, 2016) are as follows:

- Removing wound exudates
- Maintaining a moist wound surface
- Reducing edema with improved perfusion
- Macrodeformation (traction on the sides of the wound), which promotes wound contraction
- Microdeformation and mechanical stretch on the cells in the wound bed, which changes cell shape and activates intracellular processes to promote healing

Indications for NPWT include chronic, acute, traumatic, subacute, and dehisced wounds; partial-thickness burns; injuries (e.g. diabetic

and pressure); flaps and grafts once nonviable tissue is removed; and select high-risk postoperative surgical incisions (e.g., orthopedic, sternal). NPWT is also used in wounds with tunnels, undermining, or sinus tracts as long as the wound filler can fill the dead space and is easily retrieved (Netsch et al., 2016). Research also supports the use of an installation of wound- rinsing agents to facilitate healing in some chronic wounds (Matiasek et al., 2014).

Contraindications to NPWT include necrotic tissue with eschar present; untreated osteomyelitis; nonenteric and unexplored fistulas; malignancy in the wound; exposed vasculature; and exposed nerves, anastomotic site, or organs. Other safety precautions to consider are patients at high risk for bleeding or hemorrhage; patients taking anticoagulants; and patients requiring magnetic resonance imaging (MRI), hyperbaric chamber, or defibrillation (Netsch et al., 2016).

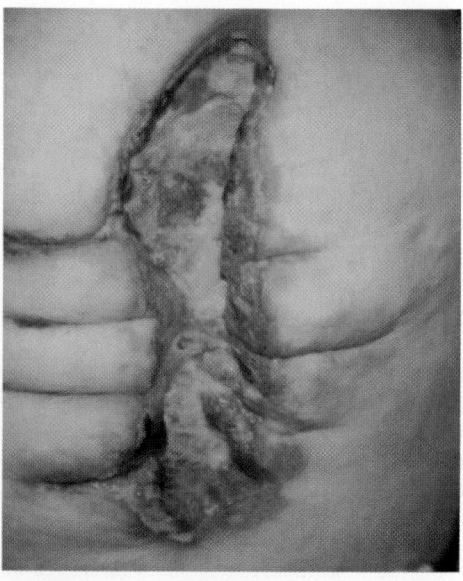

FIG 40.9 Dehisced wound before negative-pressure wound therapy. *(Courtesy KCI Licensing, San Antonio, TX)*.

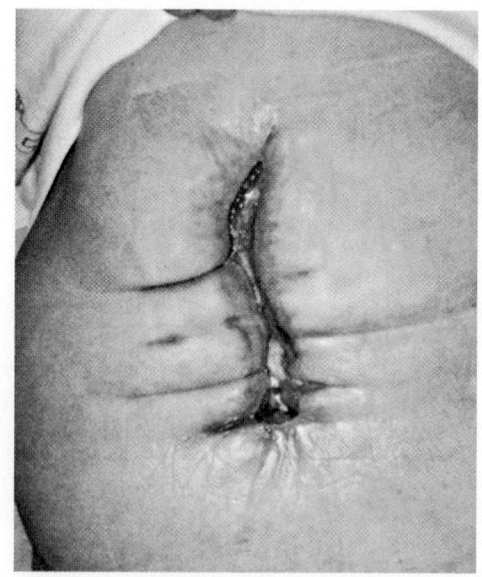

FIG 40.10 Dehisced wound after negative-pressure wound therapy. *(Courtesy KCI Licensing, San Antonio, TX)*.

There are a number of different NPWT systems, some of which are gauze or foam based; some are designed for acute care settings or for outpatient care (Netsch, 2016).

NPWT can be delivered intermittently or continuously. Research and review of evidence show improved microvascular blood flow and granulation tissue formation with intermittent versus continuous therapy delivered at 125 mm Hg (WOCN, 2016). However, for patients with severe pain, lower levels of pressure (75–80 mm Hg) can be used to reduce pain and discomfort without compromising effectiveness (NAPUAP-EPUAP, 2009; Netsch et al., 2016).

Delegation and Collaboration

The skill of NPWT cannot be delegated to nursing assistive personnel (NAP). The nurse directs the NAP to:
- Use caution in positioning or turning patient to avoid tubing displacement.
- Report any change in dressing shape or integrity to the nurse.
- Report any change in patient's temperature or comfort level to the nurse.
- Report any wound fluid leakage around the edges of the adhesive drape.

Equipment

- NPWT unit (requires health care provider's order) (For this skill the vacuum-assisted closure [V.A.C.] unit is used for illustration; several other systems are available, and their applications may differ. See manufacturer instructions.)
- NPWT dressing (gauze or foam, see manufacturer recommendations; transparent dressing, adhesive drape)
- NPWT suction device
- Tubing for connection between NPWT unit and NPWT dressing
- Three pairs of gloves, clean and sterile
- Scissors, sterile
- Waterproof biohazard bag for disposal
- Skin preparation/skin barrier protectant/hydrocolloid dressing/skin barrier
- Moist washcloths
- Linen bag
- Protective equipment: gown, mask, goggles (used when splashing from wound is a risk)

STEP	RATIONALE

ASSESSMENT

1. Identify patient using at least two identifiers (e.g., name and birthday or name and medical record number) according to agency policy.

Ensures correct patient. Complies with The Joint Commission standards and improves patient safety (TJC, 2016).

2. Review health care provider's orders for frequency of dressing change, amount of negative pressure, type of foam or gauze to use, and pressure cycle (intermittent or continuous).

Determines frequency of dressing change, negative-pressure setting, and special instructions. Health care provider's order is also necessary for reimbursement.

3. Review medical record for signs and symptoms related to condition of patient's wound.

Provides baseline to compare your findings with previous dressing change assessments and reflects wound-healing progress.

4. Assess patient's level of comfort on pain scale of 0 to 10.

Serves as baseline to measure response to dressing therapy.

5. Perform hand hygiene. Apply clean gloves. Assess location, appearance, and size of wound (see Procedural Guideline 40.1). Remove and dispose of gloves. Perform hand hygiene.

Provides information regarding status of wound healing, presence of complications, and proper type of supplies and help needed.

6. Assess patient's and family caregiver's knowledge of purpose of dressing and whether they will participate in dressing wound.

Identifies patient's learning needs. Prepares patient and family caregivers if dressing will need to be changed at home.

NURSING DIAGNOSES

- Acute pain
- Chronic pain
- Deficient knowledge regarding purpose of dressing
- Impaired skin integrity
- Risk for infection

Related factors/Risk factors are individualized based on patient's condition or needs.

PLANNING

1. Expected outcomes following completion of procedure:
   - Patient's wound shows evidence of healing as wound decreases in size with less drainage, redness, or swelling.

Dressing is effective in promoting healing and preventing infection.

   - Patient reports acceptable level of comfort on scale of 0 to 10 during and after dressing changes.

Analgesic and comfort measures effective in controlling pain.

   - Dressing remains intact with airtight seal and prescribed negative pressure.

Dressing is applied correctly and maintains negative pressure.

   - Patient or family caregiver demonstrates correct method of dressing changes.

Indicates that patient and family caregiver learning has occurred.

2. Explain procedure to patient and family caregiver.

Relieves anxiety and promotes understanding of healing process.

3. Administer prescribed analgesic as needed 30 minutes before dressing change.

Comfortable patient will be less likely to move suddenly, causing wound or supply contamination.

STEP	RATIONALE

IMPLEMENTATION

1. Close room door or cubicle curtains.	Provides for patient privacy and reduces transmission of organisms.
2. Position patient comfortably and drape to expose only wound site. Instruct patient not to touch wound or sterile supplies.	Promotes patient's cooperation and completion of procedure smoothly. Prevents contamination of sterile supplies.
3. Cuff top of disposable waterproof biohazard bag and place within reach of work area.	Cuff prevents accidental contamination of top of outer bag.
4. Perform hand hygiene and apply clean gloves. If risk for spray exists, apply protective gown, goggles, and mask.	Reduces transmission of infectious organisms from soiled dressings to nurse's hands.
5. Follow manufacturer directions for removal and replacement because each NPWT unit varies slightly with approach. Turn off NPWT unit by pushing therapy on/off button.	Deactivates therapy and allows for proper drainage of fluid in drainage tubing.
a. Keeping tube connectors attached to NPWT unit, raise tubing connectors; disconnect tubes from one another and drain fluids into drainage collector.	Prevents backflow of any drainage in tubing back into wound.
b. Before lowering, tighten clamp on canister tube and disconnect canister and dressing tubing at connection points.	Prevents drainage from exiting tubing when removed.
6. Remove transparent film by gently stretching it and slowly pull away from skin.	Prevents injury to wound tissue. Protects periwound skin breakdown from transparent adhesive.
7. Remove old dressing one layer at a time and discard in bag. Observe drainage on dressing. Use caution to avoid tension on any drains that are present.	Determines type and amount of dressings needed for replacement. Prevents accidental removal of drains.
8. Perform wound assessment. Observe surface area and tissue type, color, odor, and drainage within wound. Measure length, width, and depth of wound as ordered.	Measurement of wound is necessary to assess wound healing progression and justify continuation of NPWT for third-party payers (Netsch et al., 2016). Determines condition of wound and need for replacement of dressing.

Clinical Decision Point *This is a time when a wound-care nurse or physician might debride the wound. Debridement of eschar or slough, if present, should be performed for removal of devitalized tissue to prepare the wound bed (Netsch et al., 2016).*

9. Remove and discard gloves in waterproof bag. Avoid having patient see old dressing because sight of wound drainage may be upsetting. Perform hand hygiene.	Reduces transmission of microorganisms. Lessens patient anxiety during procedure.
10. Clean wound.	Irrigation removes wound debris and cleans wound bed. Cleaning periwound is essential for airtight seal.
a. Apply sterile or clean gloves, depending on agency policy and wound status.	
b. If ordered, irrigate wound with normal saline or other solution ordered by health care provider (see Skill 40.1). Gently blot periwound with gauze to dry thoroughly.	

Clinical Decision Point *Health care providers may order wound cultures routinely. However, when drainage looks purulent or has a foul odor or if there is a change in amount or color, obtain wound culture. This may be an indication that NPWT may need to be discontinued (Martindell, 2012).*

11. Apply skin protectant, barrier film, solid skin barrier sheet, or hydrocolloid dressing to periwound skin.	Maintains airtight seal needed for NPWT wound therapy (Netsch et al., 2016). Protects periwound skin from moisture-associated skin damage (Martindell, 2012).
12. Fill any uneven skin surfaces (e.g., creases, scars, and skinfolds) with skin-barrier product (e.g., paste, strip).	Further helps to maintain airtight seal (Netsch et al., 2016).
13. Remove and discard gloves. Perform hand hygiene.	Prevents transmission of microorganisms.
14. Depending on type of wound, apply sterile or new clean gloves (see agency policy).	Fresh sterile wounds require sterile gloves. Chronic wounds require clean technique (WOCN, 2016).

STEP	RATIONALE

15. Apply NPWT.

a. Prepare NPWT filler dressing. Consult with wound-care expert for appropriate type.

Filler dressing depends on NPWT used and can include foam or gauze dressings with or without antimicrobials such as silver. Type of dressing may be adjusted based on undermining, tunneling, or sinus tracts present (Netsch et al., 2016).

(1) Measure wound and select appropriate-size dressing.

Establishes baseline for wound size.
Black polyurethane (PU) foam has larger pores and is most effective in stimulating granulation tissue and wound contraction. White soft foam is denser with smaller pores and used when growth of granulation tissue needs to be restricted (Netsch et al., 2016; Martindell, 2012).

(2) Using sterile scissors, cut filler dressing foam to wound size, making sure to fit exact size and shape of wound, including tunnels and undermined areas.

Proper size of foam dressing maintains negative pressure to entire wound (Netsch et al., 2016).

Clinical Decision Point *In some instances an antimicrobial product such as sliver impregnated gauze or topical antibiotic is in order. These products help reduce the bioburden of the wound.*

b. Place filler dressing in wound following manufacturer instructions. Be sure that filler dressing is in contact with entire wound base, margins, and tunneled and undermined areas. Count number of filler dressings and document in patient's chart.

Maintains negative pressure to entire wound. Edges of foam dressing must be in direct contact with patient's skin.
Dressing count provides nurse who removes dressing with number of filler dressings that should be removed.

c. Place suction device per manufacturer instructions.

d. Apply NPWT transparent dressing over foam wound dressing.

(1) Trim dressing to cover wound and dressing so it will extend onto periwound skin approximately 2.5 to 5 cm (1 to 2 inches).

Prepares dressing of appropriate size for wound.

(2) Apply transparent dressing, keeping it wrinkle-free (see illustration).

Ensures that wound is properly covered and negative-pressure seal can be achieved (Box 40.3). Dressing should be airtight with no tunnels or gaps to ensure a good seal when suction is activated.

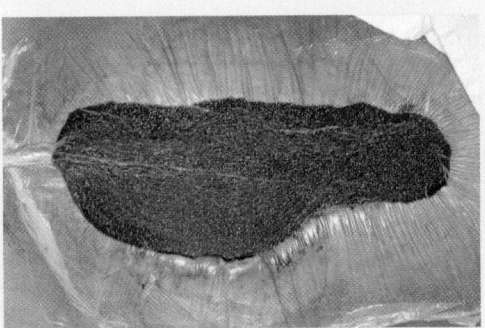

STEP 15d(2) Foam wound filler; transparent dressing over existing wound.

(3) Secure tubing to transparent film, aligning drainage holes to ensure occlusive seal. Do not apply tension.

Excessive tension may compress foam dressing and impede wound healing. It also produces shear force on periwound area (Kinetic Concepts International, 2013).

(4) Secure tubing several centimeters away from dressing, avoiding pressure points.

Drainage tubes over bony pressure prominences can cause medical device–related pressure injuries (Netsch et al., 2016; Pittman et al., 2015).

16. After wound is completely covered, connect tubing from dressing to tubing from canister and NPWT unit and set at ordered suction level.

Intermittent or continuous negative pressure can be administered at 80 to 125 mm Hg (Netsch et al., 2016; WOCN, 2016).

a. Remove canister from sterile packing and push unit until you hear click. **NOTE:** An alarm sounds if canister is not properly engaged.

STEP	RATIONALE
b. Connect dressing tubing to canister tubing. Make sure that both clamps are open.	
c. Place on level surface or hang from foot of bed. **NOTE:** Unit alarms and deactivates therapy if it is tilted beyond 45 degrees.	
d. Press power button (commonly this is a green-lit button) and set pressure as ordered.	
17. Inspect NPWT system.	
a. Verify that the system is on. This is different for each type of NPWT unit. For example, on some units the display screen shows "Therapy On." Check agency policy and procedure for specific information.	
b. Verify that all clamps are open and all tubing is patent.	
c. Examine system to be sure that seal is intact and therapy is working.	Negative pressure is achieved when a tight seal is present (Netsch, 2016).
d. If a leak is present, use strips of transparent film to patch areas around edges of wound.	
18. Record initials, date, and time on new dressing.	Provides reference for next dressing change.
19. Help patient to comfortable position. Patients may ambulate with NPWT.	Enhances patient comfort and relaxation.
20. Discard gloves and dispose of any dressing material. Perform hand hygiene.	Prevents transmission of microorganisms.

EVALUATION

1. Inspect condition of wound on ongoing basis; note drainage and odor.	Determines status of wound healing.
2. Ask patient to rate pain using scale of 0 to 10.	Determines patient's level of comfort following procedure.
3. Verify airtight dressing seal and correct negative-pressure setting.	Determines effective negative pressure being applied.
4. Measure wound drainage output in canister on regular basis.	Monitors fluid balance and wound drainage.
5. **Use Teach-Back:** "I want to be sure I explained clearly what your wound should look like as it is healing and the signs of infection before you are discharged. Explain to me what your wound will look like as it begins to heal." Revise your instruction now or develop plan for revised patient or family caregiver teaching if patient or family caregiver is not able to teach back correctly.	Determines patient's and family caregiver's level of understanding of instructional topic.

Unexpected Outcomes	Related Interventions
1. Wound appears inflamed and tender, drainage has increased, and odor is present.	• Notify health care provider. • Obtain wound culture. • Increase frequency of dressing changes.
2. Patient reports increase in pain.	• Patient may need more analgesia. • Instill normal saline to moisten foam and other filler dressings to allow them to loosen from granulation tissue. • If using black foam, switch to polyvinyl alcohol (PVA) white soft foam. • Decrease pressure setting. • Change from intermittent to continuous cycling. • Change type of NPWT system.
3. Negative-pressure seal has broken.	• Take preventive measures (see Box 40.3).
4. Wound hemorrhages.	• Stop NPWT immediately and notify health care provider.
5. Patient or family caregiver is unable to perform dressing change.	• Provide additional teaching and support. • Obtain services of home care agency.

BOX 40.3

Maintaining an Airtight Seal With Negative-Pressure Wound Therapy

To avoid loss of suction (negative pressure), the wound and dressing must stay sealed after therapy is initiated. Problem seal areas include wounds around joints; near skin creases and folds; and near moisture such as diaphoresis, wound drainage, and urine or stool. The following points may help to maintain an airtight seal:

- Clip hair on skin around wound (check agency policy).
- Fill uneven skin surfaces with a skin-barrier product such as paste or strips.
- Make sure that periwound skin surface is dry.
- Cut transparent film to extend 2.5 to 5 cm (1 to 2 inches) beyond wound perimeter.
- Frame periwound area with skin sealant, solid skin barrier, hydrocolloid, or transparent film dressing.
- Cut or mold transparent dressing to fit wound.
- Avoid wrinkles when applying transparent film.
- Identify any air leaks with a stethoscope and repair them with a sealant dressing (e.g., transparent dressing). Use only one or two additional layers for large leaks. Multiple layers reduce moisture vapor transmission and cause maceration of wound.
- Avoid adhesive remover because it leaves a residue that hinders film adherence.

Data from Netsch DS: Refractory wounds. In Wound Ostomy and Continence Nurses Society: *Core curriculum: wound management,* Philadelphia, 2016, Wolters Kluwer; Netsch DS et al: Negative-pressure wound therapy. In Bryant RA, Nix DP, editors: *Acute and chronic wounds: current management concepts,* ed 5, St Louis, 2016, Mosby.

Recording and Reporting

- Record appearance of wound, characteristics of drainage, placement of NPWT (type of dressing, pressure mode and setting), and patient response to dressing change on flow sheet in nurses' notes in electronic health record (EHR) or chart.
- Document your evaluation of patient and family caregiver learning.
- Report brisk, bright-red bleeding, evidence of poor wound healing, evisceration or dehiscence, and possible wound infection to health care provider immediately.

Special Considerations
Teaching

- Successful NPWT relies on patient's and family caregiver's cooperation with treatment. NPWT can be difficult to use when patient is unable to consciously cooperate (e.g., dementia) (Netsch et al., 2016).
- Patients and family caregivers need to learn how to administer analgesics appropriately. Patient tolerance of and adherence to NPWT are difficult if dressing changes are painful (Netsch et al., 2016).
- Educate patients and family caregivers about the signs and symptoms that indicate development of an infection and to report to health care provider immediately.
- Explain expected wound appearance with use of dressing. Instruct patient and caregiver in appearance of foam dressings.
- Teach patient and family caregiver points to follow to maintain negative-pressure seal.
- Explain frequency of dressing changes required. Often the dressing is not changed daily.

Pediatric

- NPWT therapy is not appropriate for fragile neonatal skin.
- Parents need to actively participate in NPWT treatment.

Gerontological

- Use skin-care practices to protect periwound tissue. Transparent film may be irritating to fragile skin. A skin protectant is one method to reduce the risk for tissue injury.
- Therapy may need to start with lower negative pressures such as −75 mm Hg and slowly titrate to more negative pressure.

Home Care

- Patient and family caregiver may benefit from visits from a home care agency to monitor initial treatments.
- Provide information to family caregiver regarding proper disposal of contaminated products.

◆ CLINICAL DEBRIEF

A patient is 6 days postoperative from a colon resection for a perforated diverticulum. She has been readmitted because of excessive drainage from her midline abdominal incision; on admission one half of the staples in her incision were removed by the admitting resident. The wound has been left to heal by secondary intention; moist saline gauze dressings will be applied every 12 hours. At admission she had a computed tomography (CT) scan that found a fluid accumulation that was drained in interventional radiology, and the drain was left and attached to a bulb syringe.

1. The abdominal wound will be healing by which type of wound healing, and what principle will guide the wound toward healing?
2. Name two types of wound irrigation that may be appropriate for the twice-daily irrigation order per the health care provider?
3. The patient was discharged with open wound and instructed to use twice-daily irrigation and to apply moist-to-dry wound dressing. Now the patient returns to the wound clinic 1 week after discharge. Patient complains of increased tenderness around the wound and some light yellow drainage. The nurse takes the patient's vital signs and notes a temperature of 38.7°C (101.6°F). Wound assessment reveals yellow, foul-smelling purulent drainage and red wound edges. Use SBAR documentation to communicate these findings to the health care team.

◆ REVIEW QUESTIONS

1. A patient has recently undergone a colon resection and has an abdominal wound healing by secondary intention. She is 4 days out from the surgical procedure and has had a moist saline gauze dressing changed twice a day. The NAP calls you to the room because of excessive drainage from under the abdominal wound dressing. Which of the following assessments will you plan to do on the basis of this finding? (Select all that apply.)
   1. Ask the NAP to obtain vital signs and note the temperature.
   2. Reinforce the dressing and call the surgical team.
   3. Remove dressings and assess how many of the dressings are soaked with drainage; note the drainage color consistency and any presence of odor.
   4. Suggest ambulation to help the wound drain additional fluid.
   5. Instruct the NAP to change the dressing as needed.
   6. Observe the wound tissue for color and presence of abnormal drainage and the periwound area for redness or warmth.

2. A patient has an extensive abdominal wound and is to have half of the staples removed and the incision cleaned. Place the steps in correct order for preparation and actual interaction with the patient.
1. Assess healing ridge and skin integrity of suture line.
2. Describe to patient how you will be removing staples.
3. Place upper tip of staple remover under staple to ease removal.
4. Assess patient for pain.
5. Lift up on staple when depressing the extractor handles.
6. Clean incision before removing staples, starting at sides next to incision.

3. The nurse notes approximately 60 mL of bright red drainage in the Jackson-Pratt drain 6 hours after surgery. Which two nursing interventions should be included in the care for this patient?
1. Emptying the drain in 24 hours
2. Shaking the bulb to thin the drainage
3. Calling the surgical service to report finding
4. Securing the drain above the level of the wound
5. Emptying the drain immediately and checking the volume again in 2 hours

ⓔ *Visit the Evolve site for a complete list of Clinical Debrief and Review Questions answers.*

REFERENCES

Beitz JM: Providing quality skin and wound care for the bariatric patient: an overview of clinical challenges, *Ostomy Wound Manage* 60(1):12, 2014.

Beitz JM: Wound healing. In Wound Ostomy and Continence Nurses Society, editor: *Core curriculum: wound management*, Philadelphia, 2016, Wolters Kluwer.

Boyer D: Cultural considerations for advanced wound care, *Adv Skin Wound Care* 26(3):110, 2013.

Bryant RA, Nix DP: Principles for practice development. In Bryant RA, Nix DP, editors: *Acute and chronic wounds: current management concepts*, ed 5, St Louis, 2016a, Mosby.

Bryant RA, Nix DP: Principles of wound healing and topical management. In Bryant RA, Nix DP, editors: *Acute and chronic wounds: current management concepts*, ed 5, St Louis, 2016b, Mosby.

Doughty DB, Sparks-Defriese B: Wound-healing physiology. In Bryant RA, Nix DP, editors: *Acute and chronic wounds: current management concepts*, ed 5, St Louis, 2016, Mosby.

European Pressure Ulcer Advisory Panel (EPUAP) and National Pressure Ulcer Advisory Panel (NPUAP): *Treatment of pressure ulcers: quick reference guide*, Washington, DC, 2009, NPUAP.

Graybill JC, et al: Traumatic wounds: bullets, blasts, and vehicle crashes. In Bryant RS, Nix DP, editors: *Acute and chronic wounds: current management concepts*, ed 5, St. Louis, 2016, Elsevier.

Hemming K, et al: A systematic review of systematic reviews and meta-analysis: staples versus sutures for surgical procedures, *PLoS ONE* 8(10):e75132, 2013.

Jaszarowski KA, Murphree RW: Wound cleansing and dressing selection. In Wound Ostomy and Continence Nurses Society, editor: *Core curriculum: wound management*, Philadelphia, 2016, Wolters Kluwer.

Kinetic Concepts International (KCI): *VAC therapy for wounds, product information*, San Antonio, TX, 2013, Kinetic Concepts International (KCI).

Krasner DL: Wound pain: impact and assessment. In Bryant RA, Nix DP, editors: *Acute and chronic wounds: current management concepts*, ed 5, St Louis, 2016, Mosby.

Martindell D: The safe use of negative-pressure wound therapy, *Am J Nurs* 112(6):61, 2012.

Matiasek J, et al: The combined use of NPWT and instillation using an octenidine-based wound rinsing solution: a case study, *J Wound Care* 23(11):590, 2014.

National Pressure Ulcer Advisory Panel (NPUAP), European Pressure Ulcer Advisory Panel (EPUAP) and Pan Pacific Pressure Injury Alliance (PPPIA), Haesler Emily, editors: *Prevention and treatment of pressure ulcers: quick reference guide*, Osborne Park, Western Australia, 2014, Cambridge Media.

National Pressure Ulcer Advisory Panel (NPUAP): *National Pressure Ulcer Advisory Panel announces a change in terminology from pressure ulcer to pressure injury and updates the stages of pressure injury*, April 2016, https://www.npuap.org/national-pressure-ulcer-advisory-panel-npuap-announces-a-change-in-terminology-from-pressure-ulcer-to-pressure-injury-and-updates-the-stages-of-pressure-injury/. Accessed October 29, 2016.

Netsch DS: Refractory wounds. In Wound Ostomy and Continence Nurses Society, editor: *Core curriculum: wound management*, Philadelphia, 2016, Wolters Kluwer.

Netsch DS, et al: Negative pressure wound therapy. In Bryant RA, Nix DP, editors: *Acute and chronic wounds: current management concepts*, ed 5, St Louis, 2016, Mosby.

Nix DP: Skin and wound assessment. In Bryant RA, Nix DP, editors: *Acute and chronic wounds: current management concepts*, ed 5, St Louis, 2016, Mosby.

Padela AL, del Pozo PR: Muslim patients and cross-gender interactions in medicine: an Islamic bioethical perspective, *J Medical Ethics* 37(1):40, 2011.

Pittman J, et al: Medical device–related hospital-acquired pressure ulcers, *JWOCN* 42(2):151, 2015.

Ramundo J: Wound debridement. In Bryant RA, Nix DP, editors: *Acute and chronic wounds: current management concepts*, ed 5, St Louis, 2016, Mosby.

Stotts NA: Nutritional assessment and support. In Bryant RA, Nix DP, editors: *Acute and chronic wounds: current management concepts*, ed 5, St Louis, 2016a, Mosby.

Stotts NA: Wound infection: diagnosis and management. In Bryant RA, Nix DP, editors: *Acute and chronic wounds: current management concepts*, ed 5, St Louis, 2016b, Mosby.

The Joint Commission (TJC): *2016 National Patient Safety Goals*, 2016, The Commission. http://www.jointcommission.org/standards_information/npsgs.aspx. Accessed April 10, 2016.

Whitney JD: Surgical wounds and incisional care. In Bryant RA, Nix DP, editors: *Acute and chronic wounds: current management concepts*, ed 5, St Louis, 2016, Mosby.

Wound Ostomy and Continence Nurses Society (WOCN): *Guideline for prevention and management of pressure ulcers (injuries)*, Mount Laurel, NJ, 2016, WOCN.

41 | Dressings, Bandages, and Binders

OBJECTIVES

Mastery of content in this chapter will enable the nurse to:
- Assess a wound correctly.
- Understand the purposes and techniques of dressings, bandages, and abdominal binders.
- Understand how to choose the correct dressing for a wound based on its characteristics.
- Apply dry, damp-to-dry, pressure, transparent, and synthetic dressings correctly.
- Apply an abdominal binder correctly.

MEDIA RESOURCES

- evolve http://evolve.elsevier.com/Perry/skills
- Review Questions
- ▶ Video Clips
- **NSO** Nursing Skills Online
- Clinical Debrief and Review Questions Answers

PURPOSE

Correct use of dressings, bandages, and binders support underlying tissues and promote wound healing. Knowledge and use of proper wound dressing techniques are essential nursing practices. Selection of the type of dressing is based on specific characteristics of the wound; the expected outcomes desired; and, for chronic wounds, the practicality and feasibility of performing the dressing changes by family caregivers in the home setting.

STANDARDS OF CARE

- CDC, 1999—Guideline for Prevention of Surgical Site Infection,
- National Pressure Ulcer Advisory Panel (NPUAP) and European Pressure Ulcer Advisory Panel (EPUAP), 2014—New 2014 Prevention and Treatment of Pressure Ulcers: Clinical Practice Guidelines
- The Joint Commission (TJC), 2016—National Patient Safety Goals

PRINCIPLES FOR PRACTICE

- Acute wounds go through a predictive process as they heal from the injury moving through the following: hemostasis, inflammation, proliferation (repair), and the maturation (remodeling) phase. Chronic wounds fail in this process, often remaining in the repair process (Ermer-Seltun and Rolstad, 2016).
- The TIME framework addresses barriers to wound healing and identifies key clinical assessments and treatment options (Chamanga et al., 2015; Ermer-Seltun and Rolstad, 2016; Mudge, 2015):
  - **Tissue management:** Removes nonviable, nonhealthy tissue from the wound bed. In addition, tissue management also reduces bioburden of the wound, which impedes wound healing. Wound debridement reduces bioburden and in turn reduces risk for wound infection. Tissue management also controls for hypergranulation and hypertrophic scar formation, both of which affect wound healing.
  - **Inflammation/infection:** Influenced by the presence of nonviable tissue, high bacterial loads, and impaired leukocytes. The goal is to identify and treat wound infection and inflammation promptly.
  - **Moisture:** When a wound surface is too wet or too dry, the repair process is delayed. The goal is to keep a wound surface moist, not wet.
  - **Edge:** Affects the integrity of the perimeter of the wound. A closed or compromised wound edge prevents resurfacing and wound repair. The goal is to have a proliferative wound edge.
- The key principles of a physiological wound environment are adequate moisture, temperature control, pH, and control of bacterial burden.

Dressing Characteristics and Outcomes

Characteristics

- Nontraumatic and able to absorb exudate; keeps wound bed moist and surrounding periwound tissues dry and intact
- Appropriate for infected wounds
- Can be removed without trauma, pain, or leaving dressing fragments in the wound
- Conforms to the body part for ease of movement
- Maintains stable physiological wound environment
- Easy to apply and remove with easy-to-follow patient/family caregiver instructions
- Cost-effective

Outcomes

- Reduces volume of exudate and amount of necrotic tissue
- Resolves or prevents periwound erythema
- Reduces wound dimensions or depth of sinus tract
- Reduces pain intensity during dressing changes

Data from Bryant RA, Nix DP: Principles of wound healing and topical management. In Bryant RA, Nix DP: *Acute and chronic wounds: current management concepts*, ed 5, St Louis, 2016, Mosby; Doughty DB, McNichol LL, editors: *Wound Ostomy and Continence Nurses Society Core Curriculum: wound management*, Philadelphia, 2016, Wolters Kluwer.

- Effective dressings control wound moisture and drainage, debride dead tissue, protect a wound, and reduce the spread of infection.
- Primary wound healing occurs when tissue is cut cleanly and margins are reapproximated (i.e., surgical incisions).
- Secondary wound healing occurs when skin is left open, healing from granulation tissue at the base of the wound combined with epithelialization from the sides.
- Select dressing material that has characteristics to promote wound healing (Box 41.1).

PATIENT-CENTERED CARE

- Numerous dressings and products are available for the management of acute and chronic wounds; select dressings to achieve individual patient care outcomes (Table 41.1).
- A priority in wound care management is patient comfort:
  - Select dressings that help to reduce pain. For example, moisture-retentive dressings have some ability to reduce wound-related pain (Hopf et al., 2016; Krasner, 2016).
  - Provide patients appropriate analgesic doses 30 minutes before a dressing change to maximize comfort when the dressing and tissues will be manipulated.
- Recommend pharmacological and nonpharmacological pain-relief measure before dressing changes, even when patients do not request them. These measures include but are not limited to reducing sensory stimulus during dressing change, allowing the patient to perform dressing change, and allowing for "time-outs" during painful dressing changes (Hopf et al., 2016).
- Provide an opportunity for family caregivers to be present during dressing changes. This allows them to see the actual dressing change, and it provides the patient comfort and emotional support (Bishop et al., 2013).
- Consider a patient's culture as an important variable to assess related to pain.

- If a patient's pain is from eroded or denuded skin around the margin of a wound, use skin sealants or barriers. Dressings alone do not offer skin protection (Bryant and Best, 2016).
- If a patient has a chronic wound, assess the patient's or family caregiver's knowledge about proper wound care. Patients might have preferences regarding the time of day to change a dressing or before or after a certain activity.
- If it is likely that the patient will continue to have the same type of dressing while at home, be sure to educate him or her and family caregiver on the proper techniques for changing it and disposing of medical waste.
- Patients may attribute different meanings to wounds and trauma, blood loss, and disposal of soiled dressings and linens. To provide patient-centered care, it is important to assess and try to understand the different meanings of blood and wounds and how they affect patients and their families.
- Dressing changes require respect for a patient's privacy. However, sometimes patients may have culturally specific needs such as the need for gender-congruent caregivers.

EVIDENCE-BASED PRACTICE

- Management of chronic wounds is a challenge. These wounds often have bacterial bioburden and slough. The *tissue, inflammation/infection, moisture,* and *edge* of wound (TIME) framework provides an organized approach to wound healing (Chamanga et al., 2015; Mudge, 2015).
- Wound cleaning with topical antimicrobial agents reduces the bioburden in chronic wounds and improves wound healing (Chamanga et al., 2015).
- Comprehensive wound assessment not only helps to predict pressure injury risk, but also identifies hard-to-heal wounds in a timely manner (Mudge, 2015).
- Polyurethane film dressings are effective in reducing surgical site infection in postoperative wounds and in turn reduce postoperative complications (Arroyo et al., 2015).
- Border silicone sacral dressing provides absorption and reduces friction, shear, and moisture by providing a barrier between the patient and the bed (Brindle and Wegelin, 2012).
- Multilayered soft, silicone foam dressings are effective in preventing pressure injuries (Santamaria el al., 2015).
- Application of silicone foam dressing to the sacrum every 3 days to reduce shearing forces, friction, and moisture in the sacral area of intensive care unit (ICU) patients diminished the incidence of pressure injuries (Walsh el al., 2012).

SAFETY GUIDELINES

- Know the type of wound to be dressed. Wounds related to vascular insufficiency, diabetes mellitus, pressure, trauma, and surgery are all very different and must have an individualized treatment plan. Not knowing the cause of a wound can have serious negative effects if you use treatments that are contraindicated for certain types of wounds (Bryant and Nix, 2016).
- Identify appropriate wound-cleaning agents. No agent is ideal for every situation; therefore verify the type and frequency of wound-cleaning agents (CDC, 1999).
- Know the expected amount and type of wound exudate or drainage (Box 41.2). Wounds with a large amount of drainage usually require more frequent dressing changes or need an absorptive dressing.

TABLE 41.1

Comparison of Wound Care Products

Product Category	Indications for Use	Contraindications	Advantages	Disadvantages	Frequency of Change (per Manufacturer Recommendations)
Gauze Dressings					
Cotton or synthetic material; woven or nonwoven construction	Protection of surgical incision Mechanical debridement (moist-to-dry) Secondary dressing for other wound products Packing wounds	Granulating wounds as primary treatment	Available in many sizes and forms Sterile and nonsterile	Moisture evaporates quickly, and dressing dries out Lint fibers may be left in wound and increase risk of infection Requires frequent dressing changes	Usually change 2 or 3 times per day as needed.
Transparent Films					
Adhesive membrane dressings; waterproof, impermeable to fluids and bacteria; allow oxygen and moisture vapor exchange	Shallow wounds Dry to minimally exudative wound Promote autolytic debridement Stage 1 or 2 pressure injuries As a secondary dressing to other products such as alginates and foam Selected to allow a 2.5 cm (1 inch) perimeter of intact surrounding skin	Not recommended for acutely infected wounds Third-degree burns	Easy to apply and remove without damage to underlying tissue Permit viewing of wound Create second skin; protect from friction Waterproof Create moist wound that softens thin slough and eschar Protective shield to external fluids and bacteria	May cause skin maceration May not adhere to moist areas May cause skin stripping if improperly removed	Change every 3 or 4 days or as needed. If using to facilitate autolytic debridement, change every 24 hours. Change when exudate extends beyond the edges of the wound on to periwound skin.
Hydrocolloids					
Adhesive dressings that contain gel-forming agents; mold to body contours; considered semiocclusive dressings	Partial- or full-thickness wound; shallow Minimal-to-moderate exudating wounds Clean stage 2 and noninfected shallow stage 2–4 pressure injuries Can be used in combination with absorbent powder or alginate	Third-degree burns, acutely infected wounds; arterial or diabetic ulcers (use with caution) Wounds with dry eschar Use with caution in people with diabetes mellitus or arterial disease	Available in many sizes Promote autolytic debridement of necrotic tissue Reduce pain Impermeable to fluids/bacteria Thermal insulator Easy to apply and remove	Potential for periwound maceration if dressing left in place too long Drainage (gelatinous mass) under dressing often mistaken for pus/infection Adhesive possibly too aggressive for fragile skin	Change every 2 to 5 days (Cowan, 2016).
Hydrogel					
Glycerin- or water-based dressings designed to maintain clean, moist wound; may also absorb small amount of exudate	Partial- or full-thickness wounds; shallow or deep Dry to lightly exudative wounds with or without clean granular wound base Shallow or deep wounds Wounds with undermining Necrotic wounds	Third-degree burns Wounds with heavy exudate	Nonadherent Cool and soothing Decrease pain Facilitates autolysis Conform to wound	Potential for maceration or candidiasis of periwound area	Change daily if adhesive sheets or wound fillers are not used. Change adhesive covers up to 3 times per week.

Continued

TABLE 41.1

Comparison of Wound Care Products—cont'd

Product Category	Indications for Use	Contraindications	Advantages	Disadvantages	Frequency of Change (per Manufacturer Recommendations)
Alginates					
Highly absorbent, nonwoven material that forms gel when exposed to wound drainage; fibrous product derived from brown seaweed	Moderate-to–heavily exudating wounds; shallow or deep Full-thickness wounds without depth Leg ulcers, donor sites, traumatic wounds	Third-degree burns Dry necrotic wounds Wounds covered with eschar In combination with hydrogels	Nonadhering, nonocclusive Hemostatic properties May be packed into tunneled areas Promote autolytic debridement in exudating wounds Highly absorbent	More expensive than gauze or gauze packing strips Not practical for large wounds Gelled material may be mistaken for purulence	Change daily or as often as needed, usually every 24 to 48 hours.
Foam Dressings					
Absorbent, nonadherent polyurethane or film-coated layer used to protect wounds and maintain moist healing environment	Moderate-to-heavily exudating wounds Partial- and full-thickness wounds; shallow and deep Stage 3–4 pressure injuries	Ischemic wound with dry eschar Third-degree burns Ischemic wounds with dry eschar	Highly absorbent while maintaining moist wound environment Often used as secondary dressing along with films and absorbers Many nonadherent to wound bed	Nonadhesive foams require secondary dressing Maceration of periwound may occur if dressing left on too long	Change every 24 hours or as needed.

Modified from Bryant RA, Nix DP: Principles of wound healing and topical management. In Bryant RA, Nix DP: *Acute and chronic wounds: current management concepts,* ed 5, St Louis, 2016, Mosby.

BOX 41.2

Types of Wound Drainage

Serous, which is a clear, watery plasma

Serosanguineous, which is a pale, red, more watery drainage than sanguineous drainage

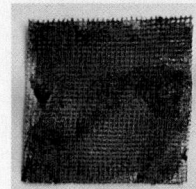

Sanguineous, which indicates fresh bleeding, bright red

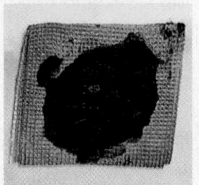

Purulent, which is a thick, yellow, green, tan, or brown drainage

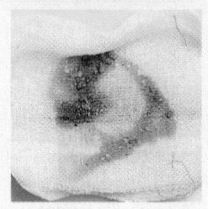

- Determine if wound-drainage devices are present in the wound to prevent their accidental dislocation when you remove the old dressing (see Skill 40.3).
  - Verify that any wound-drainage devices do not cause pressure on adjacent skin, which can result in medical-device pressure injury (MDPI) (Pittman et al., 2015).
- A wound is a break in skin integrity that increases a patient's risk for infection. Perform hand hygiene before and after a dressing change. This is beneficial in reducing the risk for surgical site infections in the postoperative phase (CDC, 1999).
- Use the appropriate type of gloves when changing a dressing.
- In the home setting, assess the patient's and family caregiver's knowledge of infection control practices and provide patient education as needed.

◆ SKILL 41.1   Applying a Dressing (Dry and Damp-to-Dry)

NSO   *Nursing Skills Online Wound Care Module / Lesson 4*

Dry gauze dressings are used for wound healing by primary intention with little drainage (Fig. 41.1). Dry dressings protect the wound from injury, reduce discomfort, and speed healing. Dry gauze dressings do not interact with wound tissues and cause little wound irritation (Bryant and Nix, 2016). These dressings are commonly used for abrasions and nondraining postoperative incisions (see Table 41.1). Telfa gauze dressings contain a shiny, nonadherent surface on one side that does not stick to a wound.

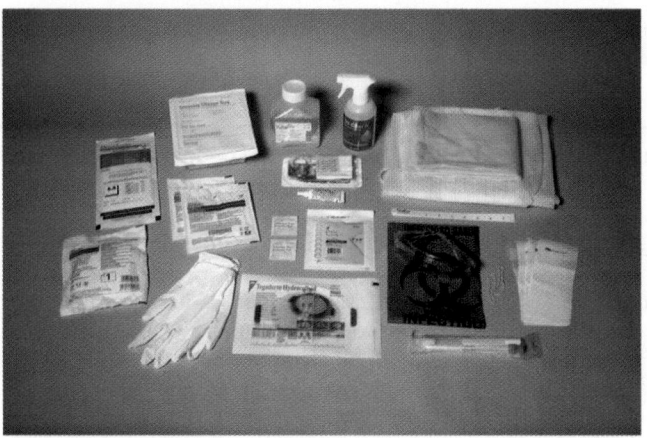

FIG 41.1 Dressing set with PPE and wound cleaners.

Principles for Packing a Wound

- Use the wound characteristics to decide which type of packing is appropriate.
- Make sure that the packing material can be safely used to pack a wound.
- Moisten the packing material with a noncytotoxic solution such as normal saline. Never use cytotoxic solutions (e.g., povidone-iodine) to pack a wound.
- If using woven gauze, fluff it before packing it into the wound.
- Loosely pack the wound.
- Do not let the packing material drag or touch the surrounding wound tissue before you put it into the wound.
- Fill all the wound dead space with the packing material.
- Pack the wound until you reach the wound surface; never pack the wound higher than the wound surface.

Drainage passes through the nonadherent surface to the outer gauze dressing.

Dry dressings have the disadvantage of moisture evaporating quickly, which can cause a dressing to dry out. As a result, frequent dressing changes are usually needed, and there are increased infection rates when compared with semiocclusive dressings (Bryant and Nix, 2016). Dry gauze may come impregnated with a variety of substances such as zinc oxide paste, iodinated agents, petrolatum, and crystalline sodium chloride. Impregnated gauze can hydrate a wound and absorb exudate or deliver antimicrobial agents.

Dry dressings are not appropriate for debriding wounds. When gauze adheres to drainage on a wound surface, the seal can pull off healthy tissue when the gauze is removed. If the old gauze dressing does adhere to a wound, moisten the dressing with sterile normal saline or sterile water before removing it to minimize wound trauma and pain.

Damp-to-dry dressings (also called *wet-to-dry* or *moist-to-dry*) are gauze moistened with an appropriate solution. A moist-to-dry dressing has a moist contact dressing layer that touches the wound surface. The moistened gauze increases the absorptive ability of the dressing to collect exudate and wound debris. When other forms of moisture-retentive dressings are not available, moist gauze is effective to mechanically debride the wound and promote wound healing (Bryant and Nix, 2016).

Recent advances in wound care have created a number of new debriding products used for debriding necrotic wounds. Autolytic debriding products are applied to wounds to allow enzymes to self-digest dead tissue. Enzymatic debriding agents applied directly to a wound bed act by digesting collagen in necrotic tissue (NPUAP-EPUAP, 2014; Ramundo, 2016). Both autolytic and enzymatic products are often used in combination with moist gauze but may also come as prepackaged dressings that do not require any additional gauze.

Some wounds require packing to promote healing. The purpose of packing a wound is to fill dead space and avoid the potential of abscess formation by a wound closing too soon (Bryant and Nix, 2016). Impregnated gauze is used when there is undermining (i.e., the destruction of tissue under intact skin around the wound perimeter) or wound tunneling (i.e., a channel has formed that extends from any part of the wound through subcutaneous tissue or muscle). Strip gauze is use to fill the narrow areas in the channel so the complete dressing can be removed easily during a dressing change. Damp gauze is used to pack exudative wounds. Box 41.3 summarizes principles for correctly packing a wound.

Open wounds require cleaning with each dressing change to remove surface bacteria and debris (Ramundo, 2016). Usually normal saline is the solution of choice, but commercially prepared wound cleaners are also appropriate. Use an irrigating catheter and/or syringe for cleaning if a wound is deep (see Chapter 40).

Delegation and Collaboration

The skill of applying dry and damp-to-dry dressings can be delegated to nursing assistive personnel (NAP) if the wound is chronic (see agency policy and Nurse Practice Act). The nurse is responsible for wound assessments, care of acute new wounds, wound care requiring sterile technique, and evaluation of wound healing. The nurse directs the NAP about:

- Any unique modifications of the dressing change such as the need for use of special tape or taping techniques to secure the dressing.
- Reporting pain, fever, bleeding, or wound drainage to the nurse immediately.

Equipment

- Clean gloves
- Sterile gloves (*optional*)
- Sterile dressing set (scissors, forceps) (*optional*, check agency policy)
- Sterile drape (*optional*)
- Sterile dressings: fine mesh gauze, 4 × 4–inch gauze, abdominal (ABD) pads
- Sterile basin (*optional*)
- Antiseptic ointment (as prescribed)
- Wound cleaner (as prescribed)
- Sterile normal saline or prescribed solution
  - Debriding gel as ordered
- Tape, Montgomery ties, or DuoDERM as needed (include nonallergenic tape if necessary)
  - Skin barrier (optional if using Montgomery ties)
- Protective waterproof underpad
- Biohazard bag
- Adhesive remover (*optional*)
- Measurement devices (*optional*): Cotton-tipped applicator, measuring guide, camera
- Personal protective equipment (PPE): gown, goggles, mask as needed
- Additional lighting if needed (e.g., flashlight, treatment light)

STEP	RATIONALE

ASSESSMENT

1. Identify patient using at least two identifiers (e.g., name and birthday or name and medical record number) according to agency policy.

2. Assess patient for allergies, especially antiseptics, tape, or latex; and acquire specific orders for dressing change.

3. Ask patient to rate level of pain using a pain scale of 0 to 10 and assess character of pain. Administer prescribed analgesic as needed 30 minutes before dressing change.

4. Assess size, location, and condition of wound. Review previous nurses' notes in electronic health record (EHR) or chart.

5. Assess patient's and family caregiver's knowledge of purpose of dressing change.

6. Assess need, readiness, and willingness for patient or family caregiver to participate in dressing wound.

7. Review medical orders for type of dressing.

8. Identify patients at risk for wound-healing problems, including aging, premature infant, obesity, diabetes mellitus, circulation disorders, nutritional deficit, immunosuppression, radiation therapy, high levels of stress, and use of steroids.

Ensures correct patient. Complies with The Joint Commission standards and improves patient safety (TJC, 2016).

Reduces risk for localized or systemic allergic reactions to these supplies.

Superficial wounds with multiple exposed nerves may be intensely painful, whereas deeper wounds with destruction of dermis should be less painful (Krasner, 2016). A comfortable patient is less likely to move suddenly, causing wound or supply contamination.

Serves as baseline to measure response to dressing therapy.

Helps to plan for proper dressing type and securement of supplies needed and if help is needed during dressing procedure.

Determines level of support and explanation required.

Identifies areas for patient education to prepare patient or family caregiver if dressing must be changed at home.

Indicates types of dressing supplies needed.

Physiological changes resulting from aging, chronic illness, poor nutrition, medications that affect wound healing, and cancer treatments have potential to affect wound healing (Doughty and Sparks-DeFriese, 2016).

NURSING DIAGNOSES

- Acute pain
- Chronic pain

- Deficient knowledge regarding need for dry or damp-to-dry dressing
- Impaired skin integrity

- Risk for infection
- Risk for caregiver role strain

Related factors/Risk factors are individualized based on patient's condition or needs.

PLANNING

1. Expected outcomes following completion of procedure:
   - Patient's wound shows evidence of healing by decrease in size and reduced drainage, redness, or swelling.
   - Patient reports pain less than previous assessment after dressing change.
   - Dressing remains clean, dry, and intact.

   - Patient or family caregiver explains purpose of dressing and method of dressing application.

2. Explain procedure to patient.

Indicates that wound is healing appropriately.

Indicates that patient has appropriate analgesia.

Indicates that proper application and securement are used for dressing.

Indicates understanding and that learning has occurred.

Decreases patient's anxiety.

IMPLEMENTATION

1. Close room or cubicle curtains. Perform hand hygiene.

2. Position patient comfortably and drape to expose only wound site. Instruct patient not to touch wound or sterile supplies.

3. Place disposable biohazard bag within reach of work area. Perform hand hygiene and apply clean gloves. Apply gown, goggles, and mask if risk for splashing exists.

4. Gently remove tape, bandages, or ties: use nondominant hand to support dressing and, with your dominant hand, pull tape parallel to skin and toward dressing. If dressing is over hairy area, remove in direction of hair growth. Get patient permission to clip or shave area (check agency policy). Remove any adhesive from skin.

Provides for privacy.

Draping provides access to wound while minimizing exposure. Dressing supplies become contaminated when touched by patient's hand.

Ensures easy disposal of soiled dressings.

Use of PPE reduces transmission of microorganisms.

Pulling tape toward dressing reduces stress on suture line or wound edges, irritation, and discomfort.

STEP	RATIONALE

5. With gloved hand or forceps remove dressing one layer at a time, observing appearance and drainage of dressing. Carefully remove outer secondary dressing first; then remove inner primary dressing that is in contact with wound bed. If drains are present, slowly and carefully remove dressings (see illustration) and avoid tension on any drainage devices. Keep soiled undersurface from patient's sight.

Purpose of primary dressing is to remove necrotic tissue and exudate. Appearance of drainage may be upsetting to patient. Avoids accidental removal of drain.

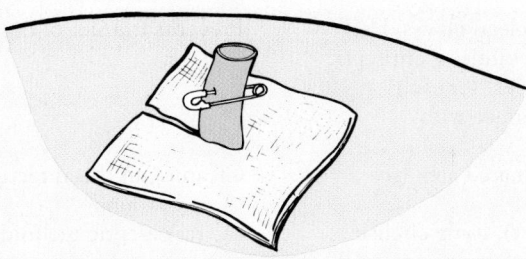

STEP 5 Penrose drain with split gauze.

   a. If bottom layer of damp-to-dry dressing adheres to wound, gently free dressing and alert patient of discomfort.

Damp-to-dry dressing should debride wound (The Wound Healing and Management Node Group, 2011).

   b. If dry dressing adheres to wound that is not to be debrided, moisten with normal saline and remove.

Prevents injury to wound surface and periwound during dressing removal.

6. Inspect wound and periwound for appearance, color, size (length, width, and depth), drainage, edema, presence and condition of drains, approximation (wound edges are together), granulation tissue, or odor (see Chapter 40). Use measuring guide or ruler to measure size of wound (see Chapter 40). Gently palpate wound edges for bogginess or patient report of increased pain.

Assesses condition of wound and periwound condition. Indicates status of healing.

7. Fold dressings with drainage contained inside and remove gloves inside out. With small dressings remove gloves inside out over dressing (see illustrations). Dispose of gloves and soiled dressing according to agency policy. Cover wound lightly with sterile gauze pad and perform hand hygiene.

Contains soiled dressings, prevents contact of nurse's hands with drainage, and reduces cross-contamination.

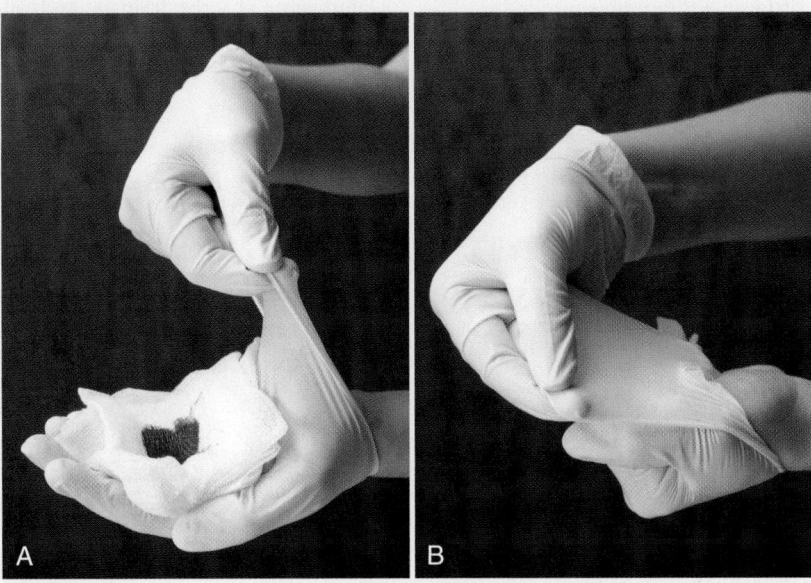

STEP 7 **A** and **B,** Dispose of soiled dressings by placing in gloved hand and pulling glove off over dressing and then off hand.

STEP	RATIONALE

8. Describe appearance of wound and any indicators of wound healing to patient.

> Wounds may be unsettling and frightening to patients. It helps patient to know that wound appearance is as expected and whether healing is taking place.

9. Create sterile field with sterile dressing tray or individually wrapped sterile supplies on over-bed table (see Chapter 10). Pour any prescribed solution into sterile basin.

> Sterile dressings remain sterile while on or within sterile surface. Preparation of all supplies before dressing change prevents break in technique during dressing change.

10. Clean wound (see Chapter 40):
   a. Perform hand hygiene and apply clean gloves. Use gauze or cotton ball moistened in saline or antiseptic swab (per health care provider order) for each cleaning stroke or spray wound surface with wound cleaner.

> Prevents transfer of organisms from previously cleaned area.

   b. Clean from least to most contaminated area (see Chapter 40) (see illustration).

> Cleaning in this direction prevents introduction of organisms into wound.

   c. Clean around any drain (if present), using circular strokes starting near drain and moving outward and away from insertion site (see illustration) (see Chapter 40).

> Correct aseptic technique in cleaning prevents contamination.

11. Use sterile dry gauze to blot wound bed in same manner as in Step 10.

> Drying reduces excess moisture, which could eventually harbor microorganisms.

12. Apply antiseptic ointment (if ordered) with sterile Q-tip or gauze, using same technique to apply as for cleaning. Dispose of gloves. Perform hand hygiene.

> Helps reduce growth of microorganisms.

13. Apply dressing (see agency policy):
   a. Dry sterile dressing:
      (1) Apply clean gloves (see agency policy).

> Some agencies or condition of wounds may require sterile gloves.

      (2) Apply loose woven gauze as contact layer (see illustration).

> Promotes proper absorption of drainage.

      (3) If drain is present, apply precut, split 4 × 4–inch gauze around drain.

> Secures drain and promotes drainage absorption at site.

      (4) Apply additional layers of gauze as needed.

> Ensures proper coverage and optimal absorption.

      (5) Apply thicker woven pad (e.g., Surgipad, abdominal [ABD] pad) (see illustration).

> This dressing is used on postoperative wounds when there is excessive drainage.

   b. Damp-to-dry dressing:
      (1) Apply sterile gloves (see agency policy).

> Reduces transmission of infection.

      (2) Place fine-mesh or loose 4 × 4–inch gauze in container of prescribed sterile solution. Wring out excess solution.

> Damp gauze absorbs drainage and, when allowed to dry, traps debris.

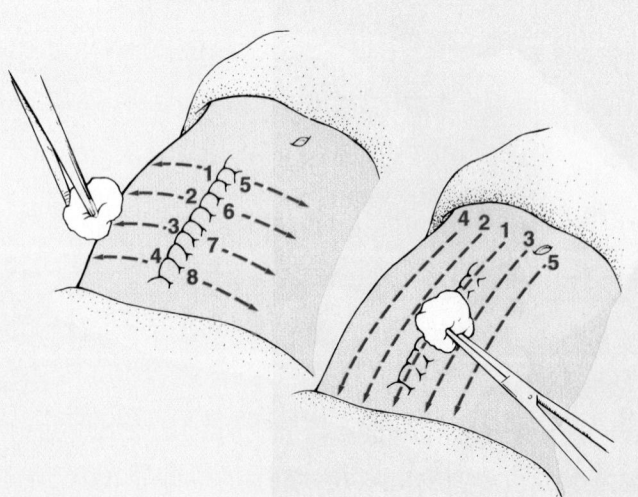

STEP 10b Methods for cleaning a wound; cleaning from least to most contaminated.

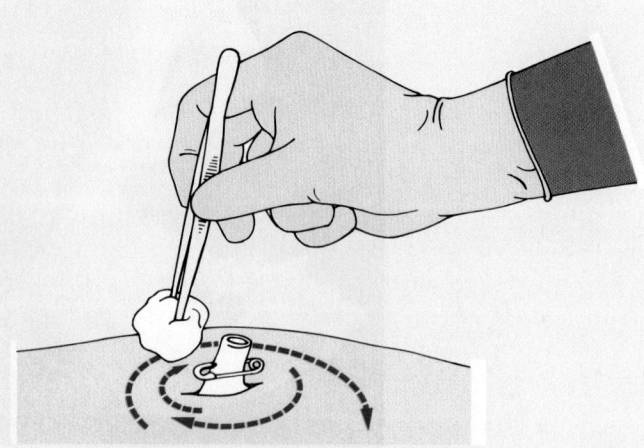

STEP 10c Cleaning around a drain site.

STEP	RATIONALE

> **Clinical Decision Point** *If using "packing strips," use sterile scissors to cut the amount of dressing that you will use to pack the wound. Do not let the packing strip touch the side of the bottle. Place packing strip in container of prescribed sterile solution. Wring out excess solution.*

(3) Apply damp fine-mesh or open-weave gauze as single layer directly onto wound surface. If wound is deep, gently pack gauze into wound with sterile gloved hand or forceps until all wound surfaces are in contact with moist gauze, including dead spaces from sinus tracts, tunnels, and undermining (see illustration A). Be sure that gauze does not touch periwound skin (see illustration B).

Inner gauze should be moist, not dripping wet, to absorb drainage and adhere to debris. When packing a wound, gauze should conform to base and side of wound (Rolstad et al., 2011). Wound is loosely packed to facilitate wicking of drainage into absorbent outer layer of dressing. Moisture that escapes dressing often macerates the periwound area.

> **Clinical Decision Point** *Be sure to count how many pieces of gauze are packed in the wound, especially deep wounds. This ensures that all gauze from previous dressing change are removed from the wound.*

> **Clinical Decision Point** *When packing the wound, do not overpack or underpack it (Bryant and Nix, 2016). Packing should fill the wound but should not be above the level of the skin.*

(4) Apply dry sterile 4 × 4–inch gauze over moist gauze.
(5) Cover with ABD pad, Surgipad, or gauze.

Dry layer pulls moisture from wound.
Protects wound from entrance of microorganisms.

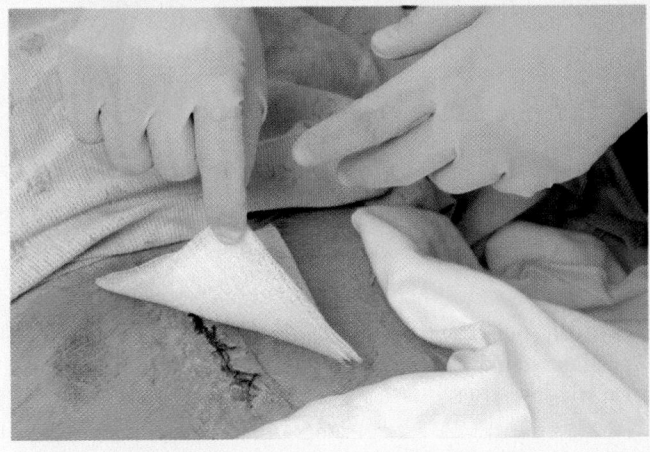

STEP 13a(2) Placing dry gauze dressing over simple wound.

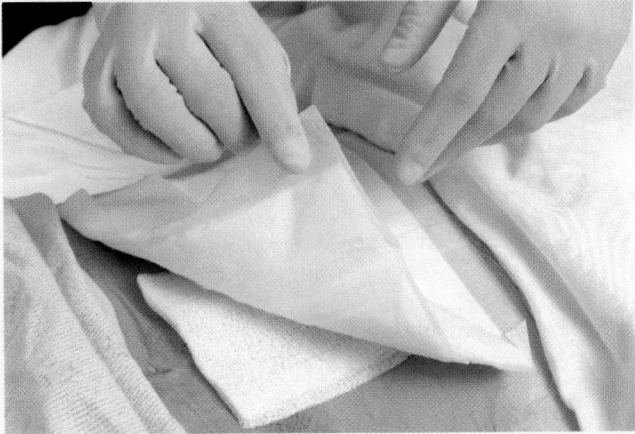

STEP 13a(5) Placing ABD pad over gauze dressing.

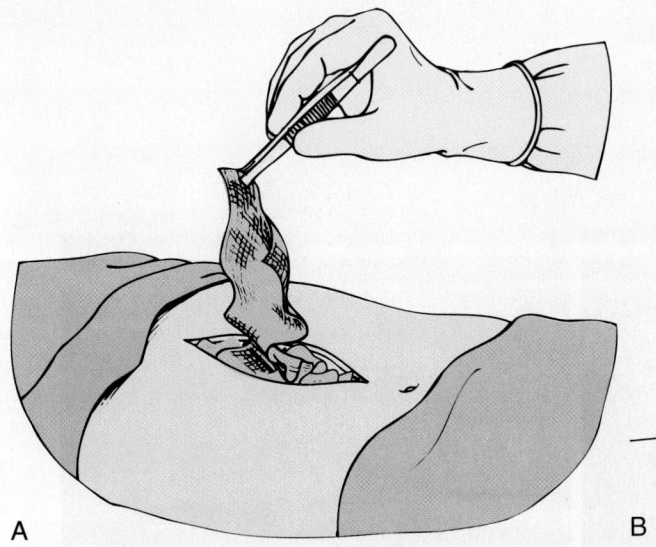
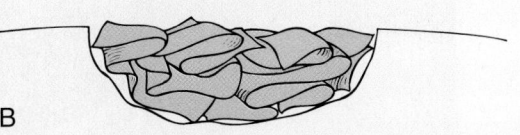

STEP 13b(3) A, Packing wound with fine-mesh gauze. **B,** Cross-section of deep wound packed loosely with gauze roll.

STEP	RATIONALE

14. Secure dressing.

    a. *Tape:* Apply tape 2.5 to 5 cm (1 to 2 inches) beyond dressing. Use nonallergenic tape when necessary.

    b. Montgomery ties (see illustrations).

        (1) Be sure that skin is clean. Application of skin barrier is recommended (see Chapter 39).

        (2) Expose adhesive surface of tape ends.

        (3) Place ties on opposite sides of dressing over skin or skin barrier.

        (4) Secure dressing by lacing ties across dressing snugly enough to hold it secure but without placing pressure on skin.

Supports wound and ensures placement and stability of dressing.

Prevents skin irritation. Ties allow for repeated dressing changes without removal of tape.

Skin barrier (stomahesive) protects intact skin from stretch and tension of adhesive tape.

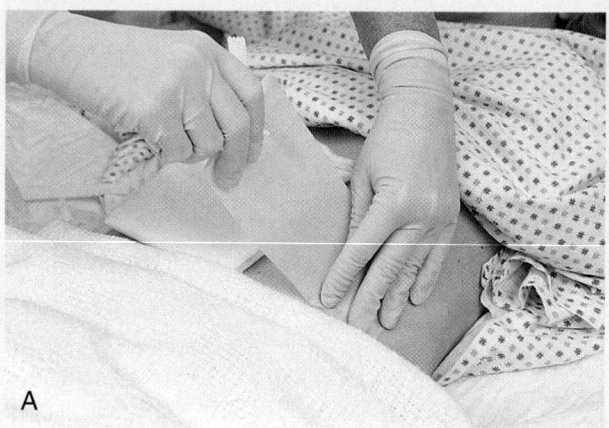
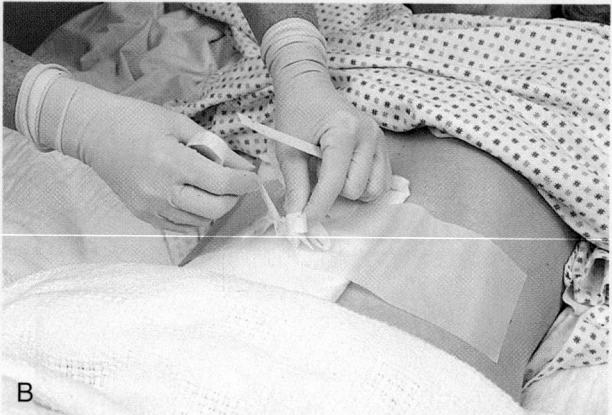

A   B

STEP 14b Montgomery ties. **A,** Each tie is placed at side of gauze dressing. **B,** Securing ties encloses dressing.

    c. For protective window:

        (1) Cut strip of stomahesive or hydrocolloid pad into 1-cm (½-inch) strips.

        (2) Use skin barrier to wipe areas of skin where strips will be applied.

        (3) Apply adhesive strips dressing to frame a "window" around the wound using four strips, one on each side, one on the top, and one on the bottom of the dressing material (see illustrations).

        (4) Apply dressing; secure tape ends to adhesive strips (see illustration).

A protective window is an alternative to Montgomery ties for smaller wounds. There is less skin irritation by placing tape on window strips.

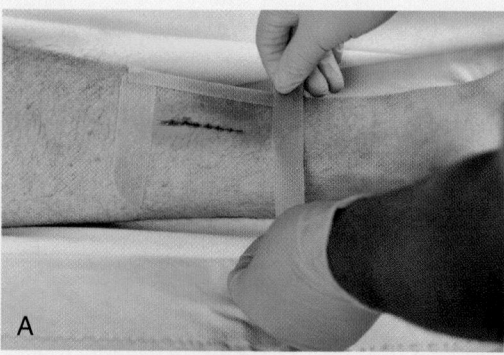
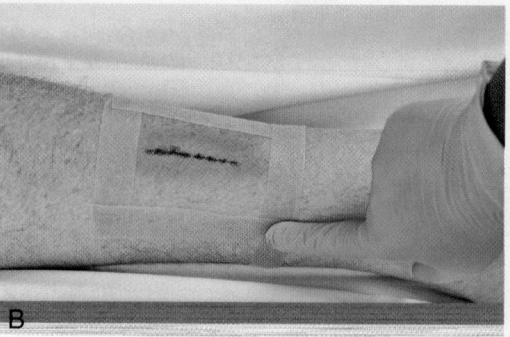

A   B

STEP 14c(3) Apply adhesive strips to frame a "window" around wound using four strips.

STEP	RATIONALE

   d. For dressing extremity, secure with roller gauze (see illustration) or elastic net.

Roller gauze conforms to contour of foot or hand.

15. Dispose of all dressing supplies. Remove cover gown and goggles; remove gloves inside out; dispose of them according to agency policy.

Reduces transmission of microorganisms. Clean environment enhances patient comfort.

16. Label tape over dressing with your initials and date dressing is changed.

Provides timeline for when next dressing change is to be scheduled.

17. Help patient to comfortable position.

Promotes patient's sense of well-being.

18. Perform hand hygiene.

Reduces transmission of microorganisms.

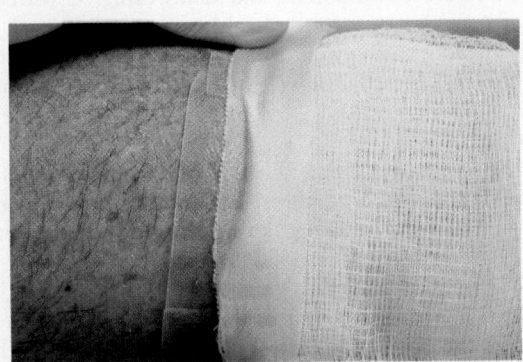

STEP 14c(4) Apply dressing; secure tape ends to adhesive strips.

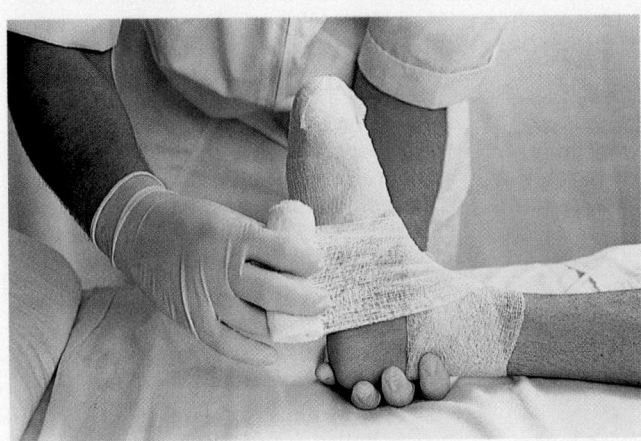

STEP 14d Wrap roller gauze around extremity to secure dressing.

EVALUATION

1. Observe appearance of wound for healing: measure size of wound; observe amount, color, and type of drainage and periwound erythema or swelling.

Determines rate of healing.

2. Ask patient to rate pain using a scale of 0 to 10.

Increased pain is often indication of wound complications such as infection or result of dressing pulling tissue.

3. Inspect condition of dressing at least every shift.

Determines status of wound drainage.

4. Use Teach-Back: "I want to be sure I explained why and how often you need to continue these dressing changes in the hospital and at home. Tell me why it is important to change your dressing and how often you will do this." Revise your instruction now or develop a plan for revised patient or family caregiver teaching if patient or family caregiver is not able to teach back correctly.

Determines patient's and family caregiver's level of understanding of instructional topic.

Unexpected Outcomes	Related Interventions
1. Wound appears inflamed and tender, drainage is evident, and/or odor is present.	• Monitor patient for signs of infection (e.g., fever, increased white blood cell count). • Notify health care provider. • Obtain wound cultures as ordered. • If there is yellow, tan, or brown necrotic tissue, notify health care provider to determine need for debridement (Table 41.2).
2. Wound bleeds during dressing change.	• Observe color and amount of bloody drainage. If excessive, may need to apply direct dressing. • Inspect area along dressing and directly underneath patient to determine amount of bleeding. • Obtain vital signs as needed. • Notify health care provider.

STEP	RATIONALE
3. Patient reports sensation that "something has given way under the dressing."	• Observe wound for increased drainage or dehiscence (partial or total separation of wound layers) or evisceration (total separation of wound layers and protrusion of viscera through wound opening). • If dehiscence or evisceration occurs, protect wound. Cover with sterile moist dressing. • Instruct patient to lie still. • Stay with patient to monitor vital signs. • Notify health care provider.

TABLE 41.2

Problems Associated With Wounds Requiring Debridement

Problem	Nursing Activities
Solutions used may be irritating to healthy skin around wound.	Protect healthy skin with protective barrier such as stomahesive or apply topical ointments such as zinc oxide. If zinc oxide is used, it should be removed with mineral oil. Avoid scrubbing the skin because scrubbing can cause harm to the epithelial layer.
Wound becomes excessively dry.	A continually moist dressing (with a health care provider's order) might be tried. Eliminate fine-mesh gauze and lightly pack wound with fluffy gauze dampened with prescribed solution.
Wound is deep, and retention of dressing in cavity is suspected.	Irrigate wound copiously with prescribed solution to loosen dressing for removal. Use continuous "ribbon" or strip of gauze to dress deep wounds.
Wound drainage is damaging healthy tissue.	Protect healthy tissue with skin barrier such as a hydrocolloid. Wounds with large amounts of drainage may benefit from occlusive drainage collection device.
Patient's skin is irritated by tape.	Use hydrocolloid under tape, Montgomery ties as needed, fabric tape that has multidirectional stretch; secure dressing with binder or wrap with roll gauze if on extremity.

Recording and Reporting

• Record appearance and size of wound, characteristics of drainage, presence of necrotic tissue, type of dressing applied, patient's response to dressing change, and level of comfort on flow sheet in nurses' notes in electronic health record (EHR) or chart.
• Record patient's and family caregiver's understanding through teach-back for effective dressing change.
• Report any unexpected appearance of wound drainage, accidental removal of drain, bright red bleeding, or evidence of wound dehiscence or evisceration.

Special Considerations
Teaching

• Explain expected wound appearance and risks of improper wound care. Provide patient and family caregiver with a written list of signs to report to the health care provider.
• After demonstrating wound care, allow patient or caregiver to perform dressing change with and without supervision.

Pediatric

• Some pediatric patients are fearful of dressing changes. Obtain patient's cooperation and/or have another person available to keep child from moving during dressing change procedure (Hockenberry and Wilson, 2015).
• Older children may need something to do during dressing changes. Listening to music or watching a video helps to relieve some of the boredom or stress during the procedure (Hockenberry and Wilson, 2015).

Gerontological

• Adhesive tape often irritates older adults' skin and causes skin tears. Use paper tape, nonallergenic tape, or wraps or mesh to prevent tape from contacting patient's skin.
• Another option is to create a stomahesive window. Cut strips of stomahesive into 1-cm (½-inch) strips. Use a skin barrier to wipe areas of intact skin where you will place strips. Apply the adhesive strips to two or four sides of the wound, framing it. Apply dressing. Apply tape to the stomahesive strips.
• Normal aging changes of skin and tissue and the inflammatory response may delay wound healing (Wysocki, 2016).

Home Care

• When the patient needs the same type of dressing while at home, be sure to educate him or her and family caregiver on the proper techniques for disposing of medical waste.
• Consider resources within the home, ability of a family caregiver, and the amount of time needed to change a particular dressing when selecting a dressing procedure in the home setting. More expensive dressings may be used to decrease frequency of dressing changes.
• Reimbursement for wound care requires a signed health care provider's order, treatment plan, and documentation of the actual care provided.

◆ SKILL 41.2 **Applying a Pressure Bandage**

A pressure bandage is a temporary treatment to control excessive, sudden, unanticipated bleeding. Hemorrhage may occur during surgical intervention (e.g., cardiac catheterization, arterial puncture, organ biopsy) or after surgery or be a life-threatening occurrence related to accidental trauma (e.g., stabbing, suicide attempt). Pressure dressings are essential to stopping the flow of blood and promoting clotting at the site until definitive action can be taken to stop the source.

Given the emergent nature of an acute bleeding episode, the aseptic techniques considered essential in most dressing applications are secondary to halting the bleeding. A pressure dressing applied in an emergency is usually temporary; the wound can be cleaned, and the dressing changed once the bleeding has been controlled.

Delegation and Collaboration

The skill of applying a pressure dressing in an emergency situation cannot be delegated to nursing assistive personnel (NAP). If application requires more than one person, the NAP can help. The nurse directs the NAP to:

- Assist the nurse as directed.

- Observe the pressure dressing during care activities to make sure that it remains in place and that there is no visible bleeding from the site.
- Observe underneath patient for bleeding after dressing has been applied.

Equipment

- Necessary dressings: Fine-mesh gauze, abdominal (ABD) pads, hemostatic dressings, roller gauze
- Adhesive tape; hypoallergenic if necessary
- Adhesive remover (optional)
- Clean gloves
- Personal protective equipment (PPE) (e.g., gown, goggles, mask) as needed
- Equipment for vital signs

STEP	RATIONALE

ASSESSMENT

1. If situation permits, identify patient using two identifiers (e.g., name and birthday or name and medical record number) according to agency policy.

Ensures correct patient. Complies with The Joint Commission standards and improves patient safety (TJC, 2016).

2. Anticipate patients at risk for unexpected bleeding, including traumatic injury, arterial puncture, donor graft site, postoperative incision, wounds after surgical debridement, and surgical patient with history of bleeding disorder.

Familiarity with conditions associated with unexpected bleeding allows you to rapidly respond to bleeding.

3. Assess location where hemorrhage occurred.

4. Assess patient for allergies to antiseptics, tape, or latex. If patient is nonresponsive and no history is available, use nonlatex or nonallergenic supplies.

Helps identify proper type and amount of supplies needed.
Prevents localized or systemic allergic reaction.

5. Quickly assess patient's anxiety level.

Determines need for education and positive reinforcement during procedure.

6. Assess patient's baseline vital signs before onset of hemorrhage.

If data are available, baseline vital signs indicate status of circulatory function.

NURSING DIAGNOSES

- Impaired skin integrity
- Risk for imbalanced fluid volume

Related factors/Risk factors are individualized based on patient's condition or needs.

PLANNING

1. Expected outcomes following completion of procedure:
   - Patient shows cessation of bleeding and no evidence of hematoma formation.
   - Patient maintains stable blood pressure and heart rate.
   - Distal circulation is maintained with intact pulses (distal to site of injury).

Hemostasis is achieved.
Hemodynamic stability is achieved with minimal blood loss.

IMPLEMENTATION

Phase I: Immediate Action—First Nurse

1. Identify external bleeding site. You will need to turn patient to observe underneath patients with large ABDs. **NOTE:** Wounds to groin area also can result in large amounts of blood loss, which is not always visible.

Quick identification increases response time to stop bleeding. Maintaining asepsis and privacy are considered only if time and severity of blood loss permit.

2. Apply immediate manual pressure to bleeding site.
3. Seek help.

Hemostasis maintained as supplies are prepared.
Bandage must be secured quickly. Situation could be life threatening.

STEP	RATIONALE

Phase II: Applying Pressure Bandage—Second Nurse

4. Quickly identify source of bleeding.
   - *Arterial bleeding* is bright red and gushes forth in waves, related to patient's heart rate; if vessel is very deep, flow is steady.
   - *Venous bleeding* is dark red and flows smoothly.
   - *Capillary bleeding* is oozing of dark red blood; self-sealing controls this bleeding.
5. Elevate affected body part (e.g., extremity) if possible.
6. First nurse continues to apply direct pressure as second nurse unwraps roller bandage and places within easy reach. Second nurse quickly cuts three to five lengths of adhesive tape and places them within reach; *do not clean wound.*
7. In simultaneous coordinated actions:
   a. Rapidly cover bleeding area with multiple thicknesses of gauze compresses. First nurse slips fingers out as other nurse exerts adequate pressure to continue controlling bleeding (see illustrations).

Determines method of application and supplies to use.

Helps slow rate of bleeding.

Pressure dressing controls bleeding temporarily. Preparation allows for securing pressure bandage quickly.

Gauze is absorbent. Layers provide bulk against which local pressure can be applied to bleeding site.

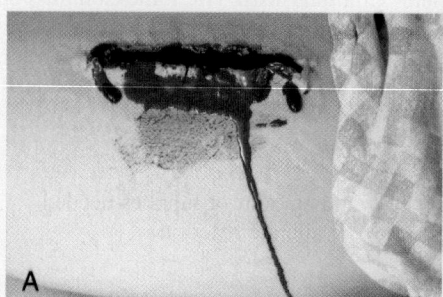 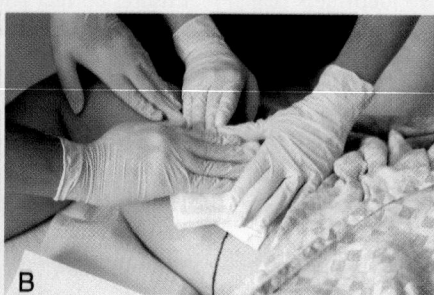 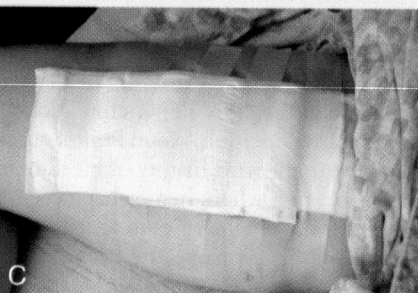

STEP 7a A, Bleeding wound. **B,** Nurses apply pressure dressing. **C,** Dressing applied.

b. Place adhesive strips 7 to 10 cm (3 to 4 inches) beyond width of dressing with even pressure on both sides of fingers as close as possible to central bleeding source. Secure tape on distal end, pull tape across dressing, and keep firm pressure as proximate end of tape is secured.

c. Remove fingers temporarily and quickly cover center of area with third strip of tape.

d. Continue reinforcing area with tape as each successive strip is overlapped on alternating sides of center strip. Keep applying pressure.

e. When pressure bandage is on extremity, apply roller gauze: apply two circular turns tautly on both sides of fingers that are pressing gauze. Compress over bleeding site. Simultaneously remove finger pressure and apply roller gauze over center. Continue with figure-eight turns. Secure end with two circular turns and strip of adhesive (see Procedural Guideline 41.1).

Tape exerts downward pressure, promoting hemostasis. To ensure blood flow to distal tissues and prevent tourniquet effect, adhesive tape must not be continued around entire extremity.

Provides pressure to source of bleeding.

Prevents tape from loosening.

Roller gauze acts as pressure bandage, exerting more even pressure over extremity.

Clinical Decision Point *Start pressure bandage from distal to proximal, working toward the heart. If bleeding continues, contact health care provider.*

EVALUATION

1. Observe dressing for control of bleeding.

2. Evaluate adequacy of circulation (distal pulse, skin characteristics).

Effective pressure bandage controls bleeding without blocking distal circulation.

Determines level of perfusion to distal body parts.

STEP	RATIONALE
3. Estimate volume of blood loss (e.g., count number of dressings used, weigh saturated dressing).	Helps to determine blood and fluid replacement needs.
4. Monitor vital signs.	Identifies patient's response to blood loss and early stages of hypovolemic shock.

Unexpected Outcomes

1. There is continued bleeding. Fluid and electrolyte imbalance, tissue hypoxia, confusion, hypovolemic shock, and cardiac arrest develop.

2. Pressure dressing is too tight and occludes circulation.

Related Interventions

- Notify health care provider.
- Reinforce or adjust pressure dressing.
- Initiate intravenous (IV) therapy per order.
- Place patient in Trendelenburg's position; provide covers for warmth.
- Monitor vital signs every 5 to 15 minutes (apical pulse, distal pulses, and blood pressure).
- Inspect areas distal to pressure dressing to ensure that circulation has not been occluded.
- Adjust dressing as needed.

Recording and Reporting

- Report immediately to health care provider present status of patient's bleeding control, time bleeding was discovered, estimated blood loss, nursing interventions (including effectiveness of applied pressure bandage), apical and distal pulses, blood pressure, mental status, signs of restlessness, and need for health care provider to administer to patient without delay.
- Record assessment, application of pressure dressing, and patient response on flow sheet in nurses' notes in electronic health record (EHR) or chart.

Special Considerations
Teaching

- Explain to patient and family caregiver (if present) need to monitor vital signs.
- Explain need for patient to remain quiet and stay in position to reduce bleeding.

Pediatric

- If family and health care providers can remain calm, a child may calm down and be more cooperative.

Gerontological

- Because of the normal changes of aging, the older adult has an increased risk for vascular and tissue changes distal to the pressure dressing. Evaluate skin and pulse distal to the pressure bandage frequently.

Home Care

- If patient is at risk for hemorrhage, instruct on the following:
  - How family caregiver or patient should apply pressure with clean towels or linen
  - Immediate activation of emergency system (9-1-1)
  - How to position patient by elevating affected body part (if extremity)
  - CAUTION: If a puncture wound occurs from a penetrating object (e.g., knife, toy, building materials), instruct family caregivers not to remove the object. Removal will cause more rapid blood loss and may damage underlying structures.
  - How to position patient to promote elevation of affected body part (if extremity) and relaxation

---

◆ SKILL 41.3 Applying a Transparent Dressing

NSO *Nursing Skills Online Wound Care Module / Lesson 4*

A transparent film dressing is a clear, adherent, nonabsorptive, polyurethane sheet, which is impermeable to fluids and bacteria (Bryant and Nix, 2016). Once it is applied, a moist exudate forms over the wound surface, which prevents tissue dehydration and allows for rapid, effective healing by speeding epithelial cell growth.

The dressings are appropriate for prophylaxis on high-risk intact skin (e.g., high friction areas), superficial wounds with minimal or no exudate, and eschar-covered wounds when autolysis is indicated and safe (NPUAP-EPUAP, 2014). Clinicians commonly use transparent dressings as the dressing of choice over an intravenous (IV) catheter insertion site. The synthetic permeable membrane acts as a temporary second skin, adheres to undamaged skin to contain exudate, minimizes wound contamination, and allows a wound to "breathe."

Delegation and Collaboration

The skill of applying a transparent dressing for select wounds can be delegated to nursing assistive personnel (NAP) (refer to agency policy). The assessment of the wound and care of sterile or new acute wounds cannot be delegated to NAP. The nurse directs the NAP about:

- Explaining how to adapt the skill for a specific patient.
- Reporting any signs of bleeding, drainage, infection, or poor wound healing immediately to the nurse.

Equipment

- Sterile gloves (*optional*)
- Dressing set (*optional*)
- Sterile saline or other cleansing agent (as ordered)

- Clean gloves
- Cotton swabs
- Biohazard bag for disposal
- Transparent dressing (size as needed)

- Sterile 4 × 4–inch gauze pads
- Skin-preparation materials (*optional*)
- Personal protective equipment (PPE) as needed

STEP	RATIONALE

ASSESSMENT

1. Identify patient using at least two identifiers (e.g., name and birthday or name and medical record number) according to agency policy.	Ensures correct patient. Complies with The Joint Commission standards and improves patient safety (TJC, 2016).
2. Assess location, appearance, and size of wound (see Chapter 40). Determine size of transparent dressing needed. Review previous nurses' notes in electronic health record (EHR) or chart.	Determines type of materials needed for dressing change. These dressings are applied over clean, debrided wounds that are not actively bleeding.
3. Review health care provider's orders for frequency and type of dressing change.	Health care provider orders frequency of dressing changes and special instructions.
4. Assess patient for allergies, especially antiseptics, tape, or latex.	Prevents local or systemic allergic reaction.
5. Ask patient to rate level of pain using pain scale of 0 to 10 and assess characteristics of pain. Administer prescribed analgesic as needed 30 minutes before dressing change.	Comfortable patient will be less likely to move suddenly, causing wound or supply contamination. Serves as baseline to measure response to dressing therapy.
6. Assess patient's knowledge of purpose of dressing.	Identifies patient's learning needs.
7. Assess patient's risks for impaired wound healing (e.g., aging, poor nutrition).	Physiological changes caused by aging, chronic illness, poor nutrition, medications, and cancer treatments have potential to affect wound healing (Doughty and Sparks-DeFriese, 2016).

NURSING DIAGNOSES

- Acute pain
- Impaired skin integrity
- Risk for infection

Related factors/Risk factors are individualized based on patient's condition or needs.

PLANNING

1. Expected outcomes following completion of procedure:	
• Wound heals *appropriately.*	Dressing effective in preventing infection and promoting healing.
• Patient experiences minimal discomfort during dressing change.	Adequate pain control achieved.
2. Explain procedure to patient.	Relieves anxiety and promotes understanding of healing process.
3. Position patient comfortably and to allow for access to dressing site.	Facilitates application of dressing.

IMPLEMENTATION

1. Close door or cubicle curtains; keep sheet or gown draped over body parts not requiring exposure.	Provides privacy and decreases transfer of microorganisms.
2. Expose wound site, minimizing exposure. Instruct patient not to touch wound or sterile supplies.	Dressing supplies become contaminated when touched by patient's hand.
3. Place biohazard bag within reach of work area.	Ensures easy disposal of soiled dressing.
4. Perform hand hygiene and apply clean gloves. Apply PPE (e.g., gown, mask, goggles as needed).	Reduces transmission of infectious organisms from soiled dressings to nurse's hands.
5. Remove old dressing by stretching film in direction parallel to wound rather than pulling.	Stretching action gently breaks dressing seal (Bryant and Nix, 2016). Reduces excoriation, tearing, or irritation of skin after dressing removal.
6. Dispose of soiled dressing in waterproof bag, remove gloves by pulling them inside out, dispose of them in waterproof bag, and perform hand hygiene.	Reduces transmission of microorganisms.
7. Prepare dressing supplies. **Use sterile supplies for new wounds (check agency policy).**	Reduces risk for break in sterile technique.
8. Pour saline or prescribed solution over 4 × 4–inch sterile gauze pads.	Maintains sterility of dressing.
9. Apply clean or sterile gloves (check agency policy).	Allows you to handle dressings.

STEP	RATIONALE
10. Clean wound and periwound area gently with 4 × 4–inch sterile gauze pads moistened in sterile saline or spray with wound cleaner. Clean from least to most contaminated area (see Skill 41.1).	Reduces introduction of organisms into wound.
11. Pat skin around wound; dry thoroughly with dry 4 × 4–inch sterile gauze pads.	Transparent dressing with adhesive backing does not adhere to damp surface (Bryant and Nix, 2016).
12. Inspect wound for tissue type, color, odor, and drainage; measure if indicated (see Chapter 40).	Provides baseline for monitoring wound healing.

Clinical Decision Point *If patient has thin or fragile skin, use a skin barrier on the skin around a wound before dressing application to protect patient's skin from further injury (Bryant and Best, 2016).*

STEP	RATIONALE
13. Remove gloves and perform hand hygiene.	Reduces transmission of microorganisms.

Clinical Decision Point *If wound has a large amount of drainage, choose another dressing that can absorb drainage.*

STEP	RATIONALE
14. Apply clean gloves, and apply transparent dressing according to manufacturer directions. *Do not stretch film during application and avoid wrinkles.*	Wrinkles provide tunnel for exudate drainage.
a. Remove paper backing, taking care not to allow adhesive areas to touch one another.	
b. Place film smoothly over wound without stretching (see illustrations).	Ensures coverage of wound. Prevents shearing of skin from dressing that is too tight. Stretching can also break wound seal.
c. Use your fingers to smooth and adhere dressing.	
d. Label dressing with date, your initials, and time of dressing change on outer label of dressing (see illustration).	Provides record for determining when to next change dressing.

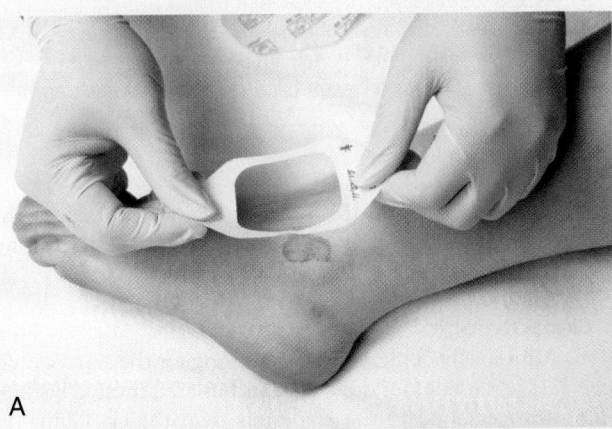 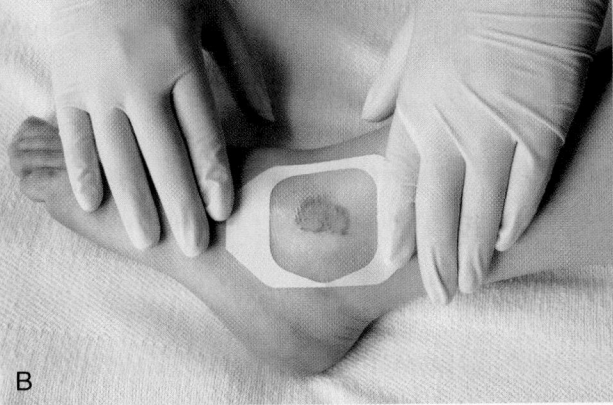

STEP 14b A, Transparent dressing placed over small wound on ankle. **B,** Place film smoothly without stretching.

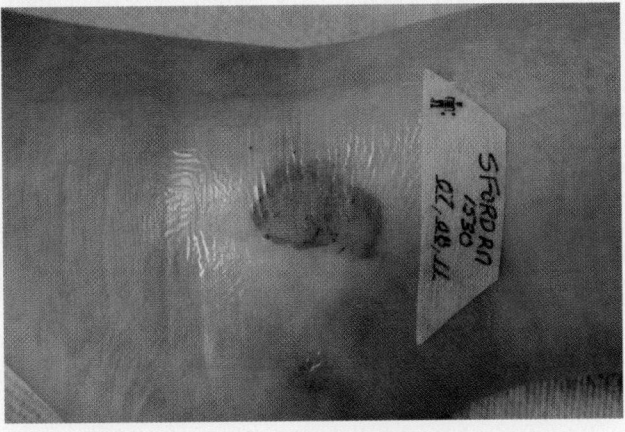

STEP 14d Transparent dressing correctly labeled.

STEP	RATIONALE
15. Discard soiled dressing materials properly. Remove gloves by pulling them inside out and discard in prepared bag. Perform hand hygiene.	Reduces transfer of microorganisms.
16. Help patient to comfortable position.	Enhances patient comfort and relaxation.

EVALUATION

1. Inspect appearance of wound and amount of drainage and measure size.
2. Inspect periwound areas.
3. Ask patient to rate pain using scale of 0 to 10.
4. **Use Teach-Back:** "I want to be sure you understand how to apply this transparent dressing since you will be using it at home. Show me how you will apply this dressing." Revise your instruction now or develop a plan for revised patient or family caregiver teaching if patient or family caregiver is not able to teach back correctly.

Clear dressing allows you to observe wound and status of wound healing.
Identifies any injury to surrounding skin.
Determines any change in pain during procedure.
Determines patient's and family caregiver's level of understanding of instructional topic.

Unexpected Outcomes
1. Wound is inflamed, tender; accumulation of fluid with white, opaque appearance and erythema of surrounding tissue; increased drainage or change in the color of drainage; necrosis; and/or odor is present.
2. Dressing does not stay in place.

3. Outer layer of patient's skin tears on removal of dressing.

Related Interventions
- Remove dressing and obtain wound culture according to agency policy.
- Different type of dressing may be required.
- Notify health care provider.
- Evaluate size of dressing used for adequate wound margin (2.5 to 3.75 cm [1 to 1½ inches]).
- Assess for increased drainage from wound.
- Dry patient's skin thoroughly before reapplication.
- Adhesive backing may be too strong for patient's skin.
- Consider other nonadhesive-backed transparent dressing.

Recording and Reporting
- Record appearance of wound, presence and characteristics of drainage, and presence of odor on flow sheet in nurses' notes in electronic health record (EHR) or chart.
- Record patient's and family caregiver's understanding through teach-back for effective application of dressing.
- Report any signs of infection to the health care provider.

Special Considerations
Teaching
- Explain need to change dressing should edges loosen.
- Explain to patient and family caregiver that collection of wound fluid under dressing is not "pus" but normal interaction of body fluids with dressing.

Pediatric
- Adhesive backing may cause skin tears on premature infants' immature skin (Hockenberry and Wilson, 2015).

- Children may find this procedure more tolerable if they know that the longer the dressing is left on, the easier it is to remove (Hockenberry and Wilson, 2015).

Gerontologic
- Adhesive backing may be too strong for the skin of older adults. Do not use a film dressing that has an adhesive backing with a stronger bond to the epidermis than the epidermis has to the dermis.

Home Care
- Wound may be cleaned in shower if approved by health care provider.
- Many types of transparent dressings exist. Explore types with patient and recommend type to which patient has easy access and finds easy to apply.

◆ SKILL 41.4 **Applying a Hydrocolloid, Hydrogel, Foam, or Alginate Dressing**

NSO *Nursing Skills Online Wound Care Module / Lesson 3*

Hydrocolloid dressings are a formulation of elastomeric, adhesive, and gelling agents. These dressings absorb drainage and hydrate and debride wounds. When in contact with wound drainage, the hydrocolloid forms a gel that promotes a moist environment and facilitates autolytic and enzymatic debridement. They promote statistically significant better wound healing outcomes compared with conventional gauze (Baranoski and Ayello, 2012; Bryant and Nix, 2016). The cushioning effect of a hydrocolloid adhesive dressing diminishes pain and protects the wound and periwound skin. This type of dressing conforms well to different body contours and protects the periwound from blister formation when a dressing over a joint (e.g., knee or hip) is flexed with movement (Siddique et al., 2011). Hydrocolloid dressings come in the form of granules, paste, or wafers.

Hydrogel dressings are glycerin- or water-based dressings designed to hydrate a wound, thus promoting moist wound healing and autolysis (Bryant and Nix, 2016). They have some absorptive properties. These dressings are similar to hydrocolloids and come in the form of sheets, amorphous gels, and impregnated gauze. The gel dressings are nonadherent and less painful to remove.

Polyurethane foam dressings are sheets of foamed polymers that contain small open cells capable of holding wound exudate away from a wound bed (Bryant and Nix, 2016). Foam dressings are not appropriate when there is wound tunneling because the dressing expands, which can enlarge the tunnel. The foam dressings protect the wound surface while maintaining a moist, insulated environment. Application directions for the different brands of foam dressings vary.

Alginate dressings create a moist environment and promote autolysis, granulation, and epithelization (Bryant and Nix, 2016). These dressings include calcium alginate materials, which are manufactured from natural material (seaweed) and known for their absorptive properties, forming a gel over the wound surface to contain exudate. The dressing may come as a sheet or rope that can be packed into a wound. You can safely pack deep tracking wounds with calcium-sodium alginate preparation, which allows easy removal with little risk for retained dressing deep in the wound cavity (Bryant and Nix, 2016).

Delegation and Collaboration

The skill of applying a hydrocolloid, hydrogel, foam, or alginate dressing cannot be delegated to nursing assistive personnel (NAP). The nurse directs the NAP to:
- Help position patient during dressing application.
- Immediately report to the nurse any pain, fever, bleeding, wound drainage, or slippage of dressing.

Equipment
- Sterile gloves (*optional*)
- Clean gloves

Dressing Set (*optional*)
- Sterile scissors (*optional*)
- Sterile drape (*optional*)
- Necessary primary dressings: gauze, hydrocolloid, hydrogel, foam, or alginate
- Secondary dressing of choice
- Sterile 4 × 4–inch gauze pads
- Sterile saline or other cleaning solution (as ordered)
- Skin barrier wipe
- Tape (nonallergenic paper or adhesive), ties as needed
- Measuring guide (tape measure, tracing paper, camera as needed)
- Adhesive remover
- Biohazard bag
- Debriding gel (as ordered)
- Sterile 4 × 4–inch gauze pads
- Irrigating solution as supplies if indicated (see Skill 41.1)
- Personal protective equipment (PPE) (e.g., gown, goggles, and mask as needed

STEP	RATIONALE

ASSESSMENT

1. Identify patient using at least two identifiers (e.g., name and birthday or name and medical record number) according to agency policy.
2. Assess for presence of allergies, especially antiseptics, tape, or latex.
3. Inspect location, size, and condition of wound.
4. Ask patient to rate pain using pain scale of 0 to 10 and assess character of pain. Administer prescribed analgesic as needed 30 minutes before dressing change.
5. Review health care provider's orders for frequency and type of dressing change. *Do not use alginate or absorptive dressings on nonexudative wounds.*
6. Review previous nurses' notes in electronic health record (EHR) or chart. Note possible need to use customized shape or size of dressing to fit difficult body parts (e.g., sacrum, heels, or elbows).
7. Assess patient's knowledge of purpose of dressing and determine need to include family caregiver in dressing wound.

Ensures correct patient. Complies with The Joint Commission standards and improves patient safety (TJC, 2016).

Prevents localized or systemic reaction to supplies.

Determines supplies and help needed.
Patient may require pain medication before dressing change. Allows for peak effect of drug during procedure.

Indicates type of dressing or application to use.

Customized shapes aid in patient-centered dressing selection and better dressing adherence.

Identifies patient's and family caregiver's learning needs.

NURSING DIAGNOSES

- Acute pain
- Chronic pain
- Deficient knowledge regarding application of hydrocolloid, hydrogel, foam, or alginate dressing.
- Impaired skin integrity
- Risk for infection

Related factors/Risk factors are individualized based on patient's condition or needs.

STEP	RATIONALE

PLANNING

1. Expected outcomes following completion of procedure:
   - Patient's wound shows evidence of healing as it becomes smaller in size/depth with less drainage, redness, or swelling.
   - Patient reports pain less than previously assessed level (scale of 0 to 10) during and after dressing change.
   - Dressing remains clean, dry, and intact.
   - Patient or family caregiver explains procedure correctly.
2. Explain procedure to patient or family caregiver.
3. Position patient comfortably to allow access to dressing site.

Rationale column:

Dressing effective in promoting healing.

Pain control achieved during dressing removal and reapplication.

Dressing applied correctly.
Indicates that learning has occurred.
Relieves anxiety and promotes understanding of healing process.
Facilitates application of dressing.

IMPLEMENTATION

1. Close room door or cubicle curtains.
2. Expose wound site and drape patient. Instruct patient not to touch wound or sterile supplies.

3. Place biohazard bag within reach of work area. Fold top of bag to make a cuff.
4. Perform hand hygiene and apply clean gloves. Apply appropriate PPE as needed if there is risk for splashing.
5. Using nondominant hand, gently remove tape, bandages, or ties of existing dressing. Pull tape parallel to skin and toward dressing. If dressing is over hairy areas, remove tape in direction of hair growth and get patient's permission to clip or shave area before applying new dressing (check agency policy). Remove any adhesive from skin.
6. With gloved hand or forceps, remove old dressing one layer at a time. Note amount and character of drainage (see illustration). Use caution to avoid tension on any drains.

Rationale column:

Provides for patient privacy.
Draping provides access to wound while minimizing exposure. Dressing supplies become contaminated when touched by patient's hand.
Ensures easy disposal of soiled dressings. Nurse should not reach across sterile field.
Reduces transmission of infectious organisms.

Pulling tape toward dressing reduces stress on wound edges, irritation, and discomfort.

Reduces irritation and possible injury to skin. Prevents accidental removal of drain.

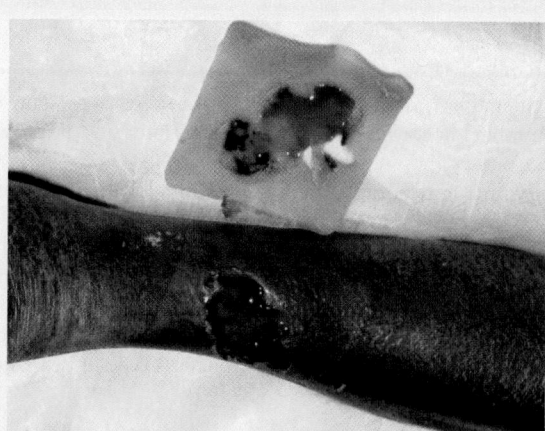

STEP 6 Hydrocolloid dressing after removal from venous injury. Purulent-appearing exudate is present on dressing and wound. This is expected with autolysis under the dressing and is not evidence of infection. (*From Bryant R, Nix D: Acute and chronic wounds: current management concepts, ed 5, St Louis, 2016, Mosby.*)

Clinical Decision Point *Check removal directions for specific brand of dressing used. Some brands need to have old dressing soaked, irrigated, or moistened for removal. If necessary, use adhesive remover to ease off dressing but avoid contact of adhesive remover with the wound.*

7. Fold dressings with drainage contained inside and remove gloves inside out. With small dressings, remove gloves inside out to enclose dressing (see Skill 41.1). Dispose of gloves and soiled dressing according to agency policy. Cover wound lightly with a sterile 4 × 4–inch gauze pad. Perform hand hygiene.

Rationale column:

Contains soiled dressings; prevents contact of nurse's hands with drainage; reduces cross-contamination.

STEP	RATIONALE

Clinical Decision Point *Hydrocolloid dressings interact with wound fluids and form a soft whitish-yellowish gel, which is sometimes hard to remove and may have a faint odor. A residual gel substance occurs in wound beds with some absorption dressings. This is a normal occurrence; do not confuse these findings with pus or purulent exudate, wound infection, or wound deterioration (Bryant and Nix, 2016).*

8. Prepare sterile field with sterile dressing kit or individually wrapped sterile supplies on over-bed table (see Chapter 10). Pour prescribed solution into sterile bowl.

   Creates sterile work area.

9. Remove gauze cover over wound.

10. Clean wound:

    a. Perform hand hygiene. Apply clean gloves. Sterile gloves are optional (see agency policy). Use 4 × 4–inch gauze cotton ball moistened in saline or an antiseptic swab (per health care provider order) for each cleaning stroke. *Option:* Spray wound surface with wound cleaner (see Chapter 40).

    Reduces introduction of organisms into wound. Cleaning and irrigating effectively remove residual dressing gel without injuring newly formed delicate granulation tissue in healing wound bed.

    b. Clean from least contaminated to most contaminated

    Cleaning in this direction prevents introduction of organisms into noncontaminated areas.

    c. Clean around any drain, using circular stroke starting near drain and moving outward away from insertion site (see Skill 41.1).

11. Use sterile dry gauze to blot dry wound bed and on skin around wound.

    Dressing will not adhere to damp surface. Periwound maceration can enlarge wound and impede healing.

12. Inspect appearance and condition of wound (see Chapter 40). Measure wound size and depth.

    Appearance and measurement indicate state of wound healing.

13. Remove gloves and perform hand hygiene,

    Reduces transmission of microorganisms.

14. Apply dressing (see manufacturer directions).

    Ensures proper application of dressing.
    Different brands of dressings require different application techniques.

    a. **Hydrocolloid dressings:**

    (1) Select proper size wafer, allowing dressing to extend onto intact periwound skin at least 2.5 cm (1 inch) (Bryant and Nix, 2016) (see illustration). Do not stretch dressing; avoid wrinkles and tenting.

    Hydrocolloid design prevents shear and friction from loosening edges and circumvents need for tape along dressing borders (Bryant and Nix, 2016).

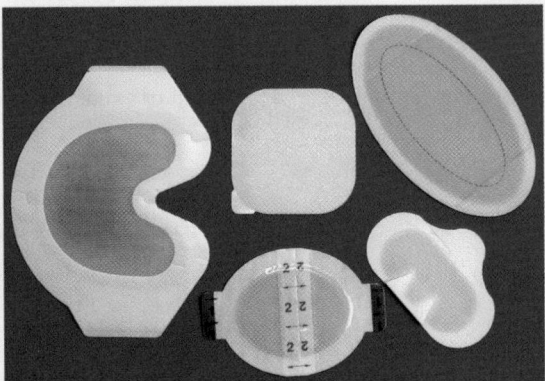

STEP 14a(1) Variety of sizes and shapes of hydrocolloid dressings. *(Courtesy Bonnie Sue Rolstad.)*

(2) For deep wound, apply hydrocolloid granules, impregnated gauze, or paste before the wafer.

Functions as filler material to ensure contact with all wound surfaces.

(3) Remove paper backing from adhesive side and place over wound. Do not stretch and avoid wrinkles or tenting. Hold dressing in place for 30 to 60 seconds after application.

Molds dressing at body temperature (Bryant and Nix, 2016).

(4) If cut from larger piece, tape edges with nonallergenic tape to avoid rolling or adherence to clothing.

STEP	RATIONALE

b. Hydrogel dressings:

(1) Apply skin barrier wipe to surrounding skin that will come in contact with any adhesive or gel.

Protects periwound skin. Because of high water content of gels, care must be taken to protect periwound skin through use of skin barrier (Bryant and Nix, 2016).

(2) Apply gel or gel-impregnated gauze directly into wound, spreading evenly over wound bed (see illustration). Fill wound cavity with gel about ⅓- to ½-full or pack gauze loosely, including any undermined or tunneled areas. Cover with moisture-retentive dressing or hydrocolloid wafer. *Option:* Hydrogel sheets composed of water should be cut to size of wound *only*.

Hydrogels hydrate and facilitate autolytic debridement of wounds. Filling wound cavity partially full allows for expansion with absorption of exudate (Bryant and Nix, 2016).

(3) Cut hydrogel sheet containing glycerin so it extends 2.5 cm (1 inch) out on to intact periwound skin. Cover with secondary moisture-retentive dressing if needed.

Protects skin around wound from maceration.

(4) Secure dressing with nonallergenic tape if secondary dressing is not self-adhering.

c. Foam dressings:

(1) Know removal and application characteristics of specific brand of foam dressing.

(2) Apply skin barrier wipe to surrounding skin that will come in contact with thin foam dressing adhesive.

Protects periwound skin from maceration or irritation from adhesive.

(3) Cut foam sheet to extend 2.5 cm (1 inch) out onto intact periwound skin. (Verify which side of foam dressing should be placed toward wound bed and which side should be facing away from it; check product instructions.)

Ensures proper absorption and keeps wound exudate away from wound bed (Bryant and Nix, 2016).

(4) Cut foam to fit around drain or tube.

(5) Cover with secondary dressing as necessary.

Some foam must be covered with secondary dressing (Bryant and Nix, 2016).

d. Alginate dressings:

(1) Cut sheet or rope to fit size of wound or loosely pack into wound space (see illustration), filling ½ to ⅔ full.

Highly absorptive product expands with absorption of serous fluid or exudate (Bryant and Nix, 2016).

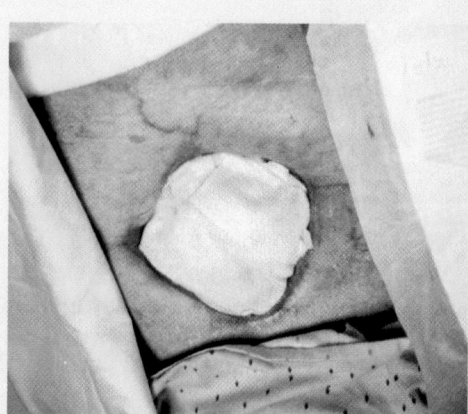

STEP 14b(2) Hydrogel-impregnated gauze used to maintain moist wound bed and fill dead space in this deep abdominal wound with undermining. *(From Bryant R, Nix D: Acute and chronic wounds: current management concepts, ed 5, St Louis, 2016, Mosby.)*

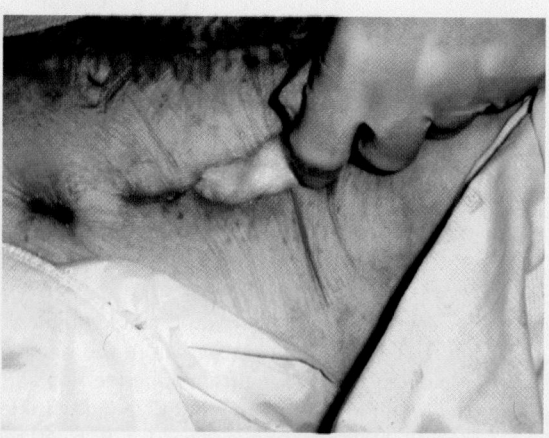

STEP 14d(1) Alginate dressing applied to fill dead space and absorb exudate in full-thickness abdominal wound. *(From Bryant R, Nix D: Acute and chronic wounds: current management concepts, ed 5, St Louis, 2016, Mosby.)*

STEP	RATIONALE

(2) Apply secondary dressing such as transparent film (see illustration) (see Skill 41.3), foam, or hydrocolloid.

Secondary dressing prohibits drainage on bed linens and clothing.

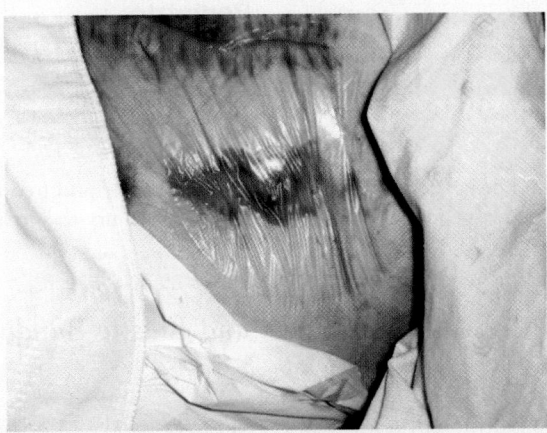

STEP 14d(2) Alginate dressing secured with secondary transparent dressing. *(From Bryant R, Nix D: Acute and chronic wounds: current management concepts, ed 5, St Louis, 2016, Mosby.)*

15. Label dressing with your initials and date dressing changed.

Provides timeline for next dressing change.

16. Discard soiled dressing materials properly. Remove gloves by pulling them inside out and discard in prepared bag. Perform hand hygiene.

Reduces transfer of microorganisms.

17. Help patient return to a comfortable position.

Enhances patient comfort and relaxation.

EVALUATION

1. Inspect appearance of wound: measure size of wound, observe amount and color of drainage; observe presence of periwound edema or erythema. Palpate around wound for tenderness.

Determines status of wound healing.

2. Evaluate patient's level of comfort.

Documents patient's level of comfort after procedure.

3. Inspect condition of dressing at least every shift or as ordered.

Determines integrity of wound dressing.

4. Use Teach-Back: "I want to be sure I explained why I need to use a foam dressing for your wound. Tell me why this foam dressing material is the best option for your wound." Revise your instruction now or develop a plan for revised patient or family caregiver teaching if patient or family caregiver is not able to teach back correctly.

Determines patient's and family caregiver's level of understanding of instructional topic.

Unexpected Outcomes	**Related Interventions**
1. Wound develops more necrotic tissue and increases in size.	• In rare instances some wounds do not tolerate hypoxia induced by hydrocolloid dressings. In these patients discontinue use. Notify health care provider. • Evaluate appropriateness of wound care protocol. • Evaluate for other factors impairing wound healing.
2. Dressing does not stay in place.	• Evaluate size of dressing used for adequate margin (2.5 to 3.75 cm [1 to 1½ inches]) or dry skin more thoroughly before reapplication. • Consider custom shapes for difficult body parts. "Picture frame" edges of hydrocolloid dressing using tape. • Dressing may be secured with roll gauze, tape, transparent dressing, or dressing sheet.
3. Periwound skin is macerated.	• Assess moisture control property of dressing or application technique. May need new type of dressing.

Recording and Reporting

- Record appearance of wound, color, size, characteristics of drainage, response to dressing change, condition of periwound skin, and patient's level of comfort on flow sheet in nurses' notes in electronic health record (EHR) or chart.
- Graph wound surface area or volume if wound is chronic.
- Record patient's and family caregiver's understanding through teach-back for proper wound dressing.
- Report signs of infection, necrosis, or deteriorating wound status to health care provider immediately.

Special Considerations
Teaching

- Explain expected wound appearance, fluid or gel accumulation in wound bed, and possible odor with use of specific dressing.

- Because application techniques can vary with different brands, tell patient and family caregiver not to purchase a brand different from the one for which the nurse gave instructions. If a different brand must be used, patient and caregiver should check with nurse for any additional instructions or modifications in application and removal techniques.

Pediatric

- See Pediatric Considerations for Skills 41.1, 41.2, and 41.3.

Gerontological

- See Gerontological Considerations for Skills 41.1, 41.2, and 41.3.
- Avoid early and frequent removal of a hydrocolloid dressing to reduce injury to surrounding intact skin.

PROCEDURAL GUIDELINE 41.1 *Applying Gauze and Elastic Bandages*

NSO *Nursing Skills Online Wound Care Module / Lesson 3* ▶ *Video Clip*

Gauze and elastic bandages secure or wrap hard-to-cover areas of the body such as dressings on extremities and amputation stumps. Bandages are a secondary dressing, providing protection, pressure, immobilization, and anchoring of underlying dressings or splints. There are numerous types of and applications for bandages. They are available in rolls of various widths and materials, including gauze, elastic, webbing, elasticized knit, and muslin. Gauze bandages are lightweight and inexpensive, mold easily around body contours, and permit air circulation to prevent skin maceration. Elastic bandages apply compression to a body part. Elastic compression to a lower extremity prevents edema by promoting the return of blood from the peripheral to the central circulation.

When applying a bandage, select a type of bandage turn (Table 41.3) and width, depending on the size and shape of the body

part to be bandaged. For example, 7.5-cm (3-inch)–wide bandages are commonly used for the adult leg.

Delegation and Collaboration

The skill of applying an elastic bandage for compression cannot be delegated to nursing assistive personnel (NAP). A nurse assesses the condition of any wound or dressing before applying a bandage. The skill of applying bandages to secure nonsterile dressings can be delegated to NAP (refer to agency policy). The nurse directs the NAP about:

- Modifying the bandage application such as with special taping.
- Reviewing what to observe and report back to the nurse (e.g., patient's complaint of pain, numbness, or tingling after application or changes in patient's skin color or temperature).

TABLE 41.3

Types of Bandage Turns

Type	Description	Purpose or Use
Circular turn	Bandage turn overlapping previous turn completely	Anchors bandage at first and final turn; covers small part (finger, toe)
Spiral turn	Bandage ascending body part with each turn overlapping previous one by one-half or two-thirds width of bandage	Covers cylindrical body parts such as wrist or upper arm
Spiral-reverse turn	Turn requiring twist (reversal) of bandage halfway through each turn	Covers cone-shaped body parts such as forearm, thigh, or calf; useful with nonstretching bandages such as gauze or flannel
Recurrent turn	Bandage first secured with two circular turns around proximal end of body part; half turn made perpendicular up from bandage edge; body of bandage brought over distal end of body part to be covered, with each turn folded back on itself	Covers uneven body parts such as head or stump

PROCEDURAL GUIDELINE 41.1 *Applying Gauze and Elastic Bandages*—cont'd

Equipment
- Correct width and number of gauze or elastic bandages
- Clips or adhesive tape
- Clean gloves if wound drainage is present
- *Option:* Pillow

Procedural Steps
1. Identify patient using at least two identifiers (e.g., name and birthday or name and medical record number) according to agency policy.
2. Review patient's medical record for specific orders related to application of gauze or elastic bandage. Note area to be covered, type of bandage required, frequency of change, and previous response to treatment.
3. Assess patient's level of comfort (pain scale of 0 to 10). Administer prescribed analgesic as needed before dressing change.
4. Observe adequacy of circulation by palpating temperature of skin and pulses, presence of edema, and sensation (distal to area to be bandaged). Observe skin color and movement of body part to be wrapped. **NOTE:** Impaired circulation may result in pain, coolness to touch when compared with the opposite side of the body, cyanosis or pallor of skin, diminished or absent pulses, edema or localized pooling, and numbness and/or tingling of body part.
5. Perform hand hygiene and apply clean gloves (if drainage or break in skin is present). Inspect skin of area to be bandaged for alterations in integrity as indicated by presence of abrasion, discoloration, or chafing. Pay close attention to areas over bony prominences.
6. Inspect the condition of any wound for appearance, size, and presence and character of drainage and be sure that it is covered with a proper dressing. If not, reapply dressing (check agency policy for type of gloves to use). Remove clean gloves and perform hand hygiene.
7. Assess for size of bandage:
   a. *Gauze or basic elastic bandage to secure a dressing:* Assess size of area to be covered. Each successive roll of gauze/elastic should overlap previous layer. Use smaller widths for upper extremities, larger widths for lower extremities.
   b. *Elastic bandage to provide simple compression:* Assess circumference of lower extremity before or shortly after patient gets out of bed in the morning or after patient has been in bed for at least 15 minutes. Select width that will cover and overlap without bulkiness.
8. Identify patient's and family caregiver's present knowledge level and ability to manipulate bandage if bandaging will be continued at home.
9. Close room door or curtains. Position patient comfortably in an anatomically correct supine position in bed.
10. Perform hand hygiene and apply clean gloves if drainage is present.
11. Apply gauze or elastic bandage to secure dressings:
    a. Elevate dependent extremity for 15 minutes before applying elastic bandage to promote venous return.
    b. Make sure that primary dressing over wound is securely in place.
    c. Begin elastic bandage application at the distal body part. Hold roll of bandage in your dominant hand and use other hand to lightly hold beginning layer.

d. Apply even tension during application and begin with two circular turns to anchor bandage. Continue to maintain even tension and transfer roll to dominant hand as you wrap bandage (see illustration).

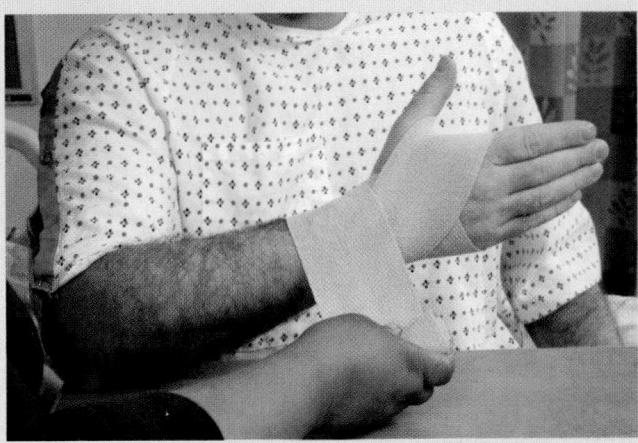

STEP 11d Hold elastic bandage in dominant hand and apply with circular turns.

e. Apply bandage from distal point toward proximal boundary (see illustration), using appropriate turns to cover various shapes of body parts (see Table 41.3). Roll gauze, overlapping each layer by one half to two thirds the width of the bandage.

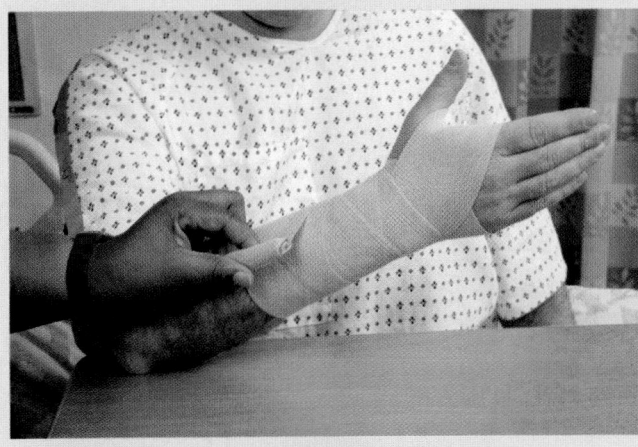

STEP 11e Apply bandage from distal to proximal.

f. Double check your tension and ensure that bandage is snug but not tight and that primary dressing or splint is positioned correctly. A tight bandage may cause numbness and tingling from impaired circulation and/or pressure on peripheral nerves.

g. While unrolling an elastic bandage, stretch bandage slightly. Explain to patient that smooth, even pressure will be applied to improve circulation, reduce swelling, immobilize body part, and provide pressure.

h. End bandage with two circular turns; secure end of gauze or elastic bandage to outside layer of bandage, not skin, with tape or clips (see illustration).

Continued

PROCEDURAL GUIDELINE 41.1 *Applying Gauze and Elastic Bandages—cont'd*

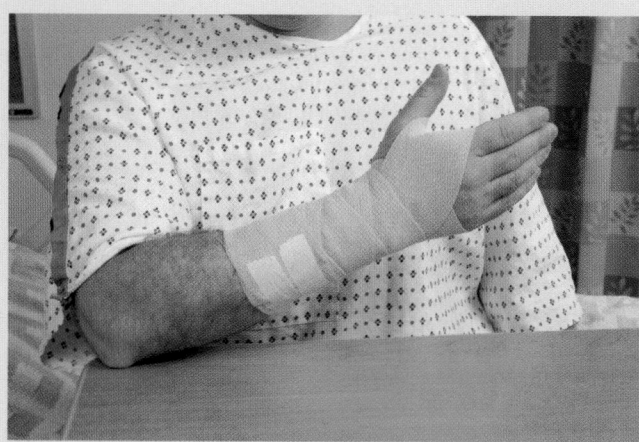

STEP 11h Secure with tape or closure device.

Clinical Decision Point *Keep toes or fingertips uncovered and visible for follow-up circulatory assessment, except in cases in which toes or fingers are treated because of wounds.*

12. Apply elastic bandage over stump (see illustrations):
    a. Elevate stump with pillow or support it with the help of another person.
    b. Secure bandage by wrapping it twice around proximal end of stump or person's waist (depending on size of stump)
    c. Make half turn with bandage perpendicular to its edge.
    d. Bring body of bandage over distal end of stump.

    e. Continue to fold bandage over stump, wrapping from distal to proximal points.
    f. Secure with metal clips, Velcro if provided, or tape.
13. Remove gloves if worn and perform hand hygiene.
14. Assess degree of tightness of bandage, wrinkles, looseness, and presence of drainage.
15. Evaluate distal circulation when bandage application is complete, at least twice during next 8 hours, and then at least every shift.
    a. Observe skin color for pallor or cyanosis.
    b. Palpate skin for warmth.
    c. Palpate distal pulses and compare bilaterally.
    d. Ask patient to rate any pain on scale of 0 to 10 and to describe any numbness, tingling, or other discomfort to evaluate for neurological and vascular changes.
16. Observe mobility of extremity.
17. **Use Teach-Back:** "I want to be sure I explained how to apply the elastic roll to your sprained ankle. Show me how you would apply this elastic roll to your ankle." Revise your instruction now or develop a plan for revised patient or family caregiver teaching if patient or family caregiver is not able to teach back correctly.
18. Record patient's level of comfort, circulation status, type of bandage applied, presence of swelling, and range of motion at baseline and after bandage application on flow sheet in nurses' notes in electronic health record (EHR) or chart.
19. Report any changes in neurological or circulatory status to health care provider.

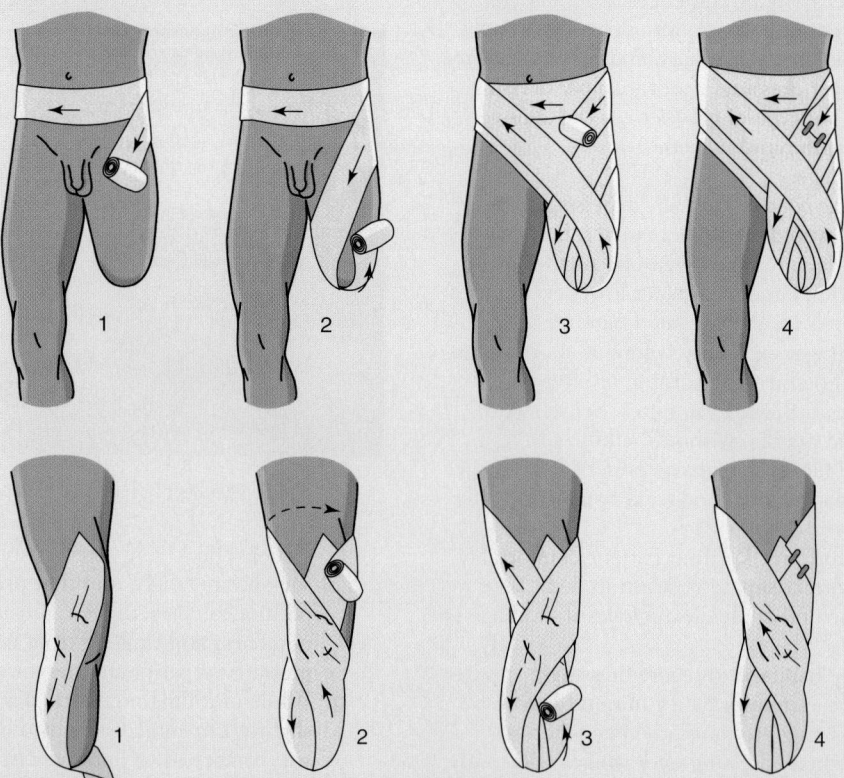

STEP 12 *Top,* Correct method for bandaging midthigh amputation stump. Note that bandage must be anchored around patient's waist. *Bottom,* Correct method for bandaging midcalf amputation stump. Note that bandage need not be anchored around waist. *(From Monahan F et al: Phipps' medical-surgical nursing: health and illness perspectives, ed 8, St Louis, 2006, Mosby.)*

PROCEDURAL GUIDELINE 41.2 *Applying an Abdominal Binder*

Binders are bandages made of large pieces of material specially designed to fit a specific body part. Most binders are made of elastic or cotton. The most common type is the abdominal binder. Breast binders are not used as often in current practice because sports bras are preferred for breast support following certain surgeries.

An abdominal binder supports large abdominal incisions that are vulnerable to tension or stress as a patient moves or coughs (Fig. 41.2). The binder also lessens pain in postoperative patients. In addition, abdominal binders provide a noninvasive intervention for enhancing recovery of walk performance, controlling pain, and improving patient's experience following major abdominal surgery (Gallagher, 2016). Binders support underlying muscles and large incisions, lessening muscle stress, which helps a patient move more freely without additional discomfort.

Delegation and Collaboration
The skill of applying a binder can be delegated to nursing assistive personnel (NAP). A nurse assesses the condition of any incision, the skin, and patient's ability to breathe before binder application. The nurse directs the NAP about:
- How to modify the skill such as special wrapping or manner of securing the binder.
- Reporting patient's complaint of pain, numbness, tingling, or difficulty breathing after applying abdominal binder or any changes in patient's skin color or temperature.

Equipment
- Clean gloves if wound drainage present
- Gauze bandage as needed
- Correct type and size of binder
- Closures for cloth binder

Procedural Steps
1. Identify patient using at least two identifiers (e.g., name and birthday or name and medical record number) according to agency policy.
2. Review medical record for order for binder (check agency policy).
3. Observe patient who needs support of thorax or abdomen; observe ability to breathe deeply, cough effectively, and turn or move independently.
4. Inspect skin for actual or potential alterations in integrity. Observe for irritation, abrasion, and skin surfaces that rub against one another.

5. Inspect any surgical dressing for intactness, presence of drainage, and coverage of incision. Change any soiled dressing before applying binder (using clean gloves).
6. Determine patient's level of comfort using scale of 0 to 10. Administer prescribed analgesic 30 minutes before dressing change.
7. Gather necessary data regarding size of patient and appropriate binder to use (see manufacturer guidelines) to ensure proper fit.
8. Determine patient's knowledge of purpose of binder.
9. Close curtains or room door.
10. Perform hand hygiene and apply clean gloves (if likely to contact wound drainage).
11. Apply abdominal binder:
    a. Position patient in supine position with head slightly elevated and knees slightly flexed.
    b. Help patient roll on side away from you toward raised side rail while firmly supporting abdominal incision and dressing with hands. Fanfold far side of binder toward midline of binder.
    c. Place binder flat on bed, right side up. Fanfold far side of binder toward midline of binder so patient can roll over with minimal effort.
    d. Place fanfolded ends of binder under patient.
    e. Instruct patient or help him or her roll over folded binder. For overweight patients consider asking nurse colleague to help.
    f. Unfold and stretch ends out smoothly on far side of bed. Then stretch out ends on near side of bed.
    g. Instruct patient to roll back into supine position.
    h. Adjust binder so supine patient is centered over binder, using symphysis pubis and costal margins as lower and upper landmarks.
    i. If patient is very thin, pad iliac prominences with gauze bandage.
    j. Close binder. Pull one end of binder over center of patient's abdomen. While maintaining tension on that end of binder, pull opposite end of binder over center and secure with Velcro closure tabs or metal fasteners. Provides continuous wound support and comfort.

Clinical Decision Point *After binder is in place, assess patient's ability to breathe deeply and cough effectively. When applied correctly, an abdominal binder over midline abdominal incisions should not have any effect on the patient's pulmonary function.*

12. Assess patient's comfort level and adjust binder as necessary.
13. Remove gloves and perform hand hygiene.
14. Ask patient to rate pain on scale of 0 to 10.
15. Remove binder and surgical dressing to assess skin and wound characteristics at least every 8 hours.
16. Evaluate patient's ability to ventilate properly, including deep breathing and coughing, every 4 hours to determine presence of impaired ventilation and potential pulmonary complications.
17. Record baseline and post binder condition of skin, circulation, integrity of underlying dressing, and patient's comfort level in nurses' notes in the electronic health record (EHR) or chart. Also record type of bandage applied.
18. Report any complications (e.g., pain, skin irritation, impaired ventilation) to nurse in charge.
19. Report reduced ventilation (e.g., pulse oximetry, pulmonary function tests) to health care provider immediately.

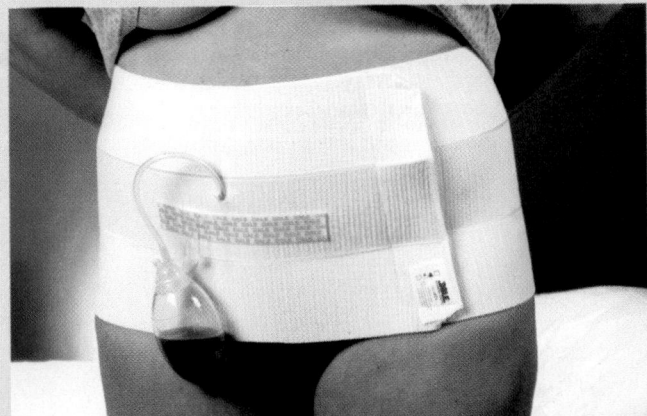

FIG 41.2 Abdominal binder with Velcro closures. (*Courtesy Dale Medical Products, Plainsville, MA.*)

◆ CLINICAL DEBRIEF

A 75-year-old male is postexploratory laparotomy with a total gastrectomy for gastric cancer. He is postoperative day 2 and has developed a fever of 38.5°C (101.3°F). There was purulent drainage coming from his midline incision and surrounding erythema. Approximately 5 cm (2 inches) of the incision was opened at bedside by removal of 10 staples.

1. Based on the type of wound and amount of wound drainage, which type of dressing would be appropriate?

2. On assessing the patient on postoperative day 3, you notice a large amount of bright red blood coming from the base of the open wound. How would you proceed, and which type of dressing would you choose?

3. Using SBAR, show how you communicate with the health care team about this patient.

◆ REVIEW QUESTIONS

1. Of the following dressings, which would be most appropriate for a shallow wound with minimal exudate? (Select all that apply.)
   a. Damp-to-dry gauze dressing
   b. Calcium alginate dressing
   c. Hydrogel dressing
   d. Transparent film dressing
   e. Hydrocolloid dressing

2. Match the following wound drainage with the appropriate definition:

Serous	a. Yellow, green, or brown drainage
Serosanguineous	b. Indicates fresh bleeding, bright red
Sanguineous	c. Pale, red, more watery drainage
Purulent	d. Clear, watery plasma

3. Which of the following are necessary to prepare the patient for changing the dressing on an open abdominal wound? (Select all that apply.)
   (a) Assessing size, location, and condition of wound
   (b) Explaining procedure to the patient
   (c) Reviewing all blood results
   (d) Asking patient to rate his or her pain level
   (e) Assessing patient for allergies

ⓔ *Visit the Evolve site for a complete list of Clinical Debrief and Review Questions answers.*

REFERENCES

Arroyo AA, et al: Open-label clinical trial comparing the clinical and economic effectiveness of using a polyurethane film surgical dressing with gauze surgical dressings in the care of postoperative surgical wounds, *Int Wound J* 12:285, 2015.

Baranoski S, Ayello E: Wound dressings: an evolving art and science, *Adv Skin Wound Care* 25(2):88, 2012.

Bishop S, et al: Family presence in the adult burn intensive care unit during dressing changes, *Crit Care Nurse* 33(1):14, 2013.

Brindle CT, Wegelin JA: Prophylactic dressing application to reduce pressure ulcer formation in cardiac surgery patients, *J Wound Ostomy Continence Nurs* 39(2):133, 2012.

Bryant RA, Best M: Management of draining wounds and fistulas. In Bryant RA, Nix DP, editors: *Acute and chronic wounds: current management concepts*, ed 5, St Louis, 2016, Mosby.

Bryant RA, Nix DP: Principles of wound healing and topical management. In Bryant RA, Nix DP, editors: *Acute and chronic wounds: current management concepts*, ed 5, St Louis, 2016, Mosby.

Centers for Disease Control and Prevention (CDC): *Guideline for prevention of surgical site infection*, 1999, http://www.cdc.gov/hicpac/pdf/guidelines/SSI_1999.pdf. Accessed March 2016.

Chamanga ET, et al: Chronic wound bed preparation using a cleansing solution, *Br J Nurs* 24(12):S30, 2015.

Cowan LJ: *Wound series part 2: approaches to treating common wounds*, 2016, https://ceufast.com/course/wound-series-part-2-approaches-to-treating-chronic-wounds. Accessed August 29, 2016.

Doughty D, Sparks-DeFriese B: Wound-healing physiology. In Bryant RA, Nix DP, editors: *Acute and chronic wounds: current management concepts*, ed 5, St Louis, 2016, Mosby.

Ermer-Seltun J, Rolstad BS: General principles of topical therapy. In Doughty DB, McNichol LL, editors: *Wound Ostomy and Continence Nurses Society Core Curriculum: wound management*, Philadelphia, 2016, Wolters Kluwer.

Gallagher S: Skin care needs of obese patient. In Bryant RA, Nix DP, editors: *Acute and chronic wounds: current management concepts*, ed 5, St Louis, 2016, Mosby.

Hockenberry MJ, Wilson D: *Wong's nursing care of infants and children*, ed 10, St Louis, 2015, Mosby.

Hopf HW, et al: Managing wound pain. In Bryant RA, Nix DP, editors: *Acute and chronic wounds: current management concepts*, ed 5, St Louis, 2016, Mosby.

Krasner DL: Wound pain: impact and assessment. In Bryant RA, Nix DP, editors: *Acute and chronic wounds: current management concepts*, ed 5, St Louis, 2016, Mosby.

Mudge EJ: Recent accomplishments in wound healing, *Int Wound J* 12:4, 2015.

National Pressure Ulcer Advisory Panel (NPUAP) and European Pressure Ulcer Advisory Panel (EPUAP): *New 2014 prevention and treatment of pressure ulcers: clinical practice guidelines*, 2014, http://www.npuap.org/resources/educational-and-clinical-resources/prevention-and-treatment-of-pressure-ulcers-clinical-practice-guideline/. Accessed March 2016.

Pittman J, et al: Medical device–related hospital-acquired pressure ulcers, *J Wound Ostomy Continence Nurs* 42(2):151, 2015.

Ramundo JM: Wound debridement. In Bryant RA, Nix DP, editors: *Acute and chronic wounds: current management concepts*, ed 5, St Louis, 2016, Mosby.

Rolstad BS, Bryant RA, et al: Topical management. In Bryant RA, Nix DP, editors: *Acute and chronic wounds: nursing management*, ed 4, St Louis, 2011, Mosby.

Santamaria N, et al: A randomized controlled trial of the effectiveness of soft silicone multi-layered foam dressings in the prevention of sacral and heel pressure ulcers in trauma and critically ill patients: the border trial, *Int Wound J* 12(3):302, 2015.

Siddique K, et al: Effectiveness of hydrocolloid dressing in postoperative hip and knee surgery: literature review and our experience, *J Perioper Pract* 21(8):275, 2011.

The Joint Commission (TJC): *2016 National Patient Safety Goals*, Oakbrook Terrace, IL, 2016, http://www.jointcommission.org/standards_information/npsgs.aspx. Accessed March 2016.

The Wound Healing and Management Node Group: Joanna Briggs Institute: Wet-to-dry saline moistened gauze for wound dressing, *Wound Pract Res* 19(1):48, 2011.

Walsh NS, et al: Use of sacral silicone border foam dressing as one component of a pressure ulcer prevention program in an intensive care unit setting, *J Wound Ostomy Continence Nurs* 39(2):146, 2012.

Wysocki AB: Anatomy and physiology of skin and soft tissue. In Bryant RA, Nix DP, editors: *Acute and chronic wounds: current management concepts*, ed 5, St Louis, 2016, Mosby.

42 | Therapeutic Use of Heat and Cold

OBJECTIVES

Mastery of content in this chapter will enable the nurse to:
- Identify the effects of heat and cold on a patient.
- Differentiate the types of injuries or conditions that benefit from heat and cold applications.
- Identify the risks to patients related to heat and cold applications.
- Explain common guidelines used to protect patients who receive heat and cold applications.
- Correctly apply heat and cold applications.

MEDIA RESOURCES

- evolve http://evolve.elsevier.com/Perry/skills
- Review Questions
- Audio Glossary
- Clinical Debrief and Review Questions Answers

PURPOSE

Local application of moderate heat and cold to body parts provides comfort and pain relief, reduces muscle spasm, improves mobility, and promotes healing. To use heat and cold therapies safely, you need to understand the physiological response and potential risk associated with heat or cold therapy. The choice of heat or cold therapy depends on the local responses desired, such as reducing local inflammation, wound healing, or control of body temperature.

STANDARDS OF CARE

American Physical Therapy Association (APTA), 2016—Scope of Practice

National Quality Forum (NQF), 2016—Patient Safety

The Joint Commission (TJC), 2016—National Patient Safety Goals

PRINCIPLES FOR PRACTICE

- Exposure to heat or cold causes both systemic and local responses (Table 42.1). Body temperature is affected by environmental and internal factors. When the skin is exposed to warm or hot temperatures, vasodilation and perspiration occur to promote heat loss. As perspiration evaporates from the skin, cooling occurs. When the skin is exposed to cool or cold temperatures, the systemic response includes vasoconstriction and piloerection to conserve heat. Shivering occurs in response to cooler temperatures, producing heat through skeletal muscle contraction.
- Sensory adaptation to local temperature extremes can occur quickly within the body. Eventually excessive heat causes a burning sensation, and excessive cold causes a numbing sensation before pain is sensed.
- An order for a heat or cold application is always necessary, and it should include the duration of the treatment and the desired temperature to be used when settings can be controlled.
- Cold vasoconstricts the vasculature in adjacent tissues and slows bleeding into damaged tissues. Application of cold therapy decreases the release of inflammatory mediators from the damaged tissues, which hinders protein release from the vasculature and decreases edema (da Costa Santos et al., 2015).
- Hypothermia and hyperthermia devices are used selectively for specific clinical conditions. They are designed to raise, lower, or maintain body temperature through heat or cold transfer between the device and the patient.

PATIENT-CENTERED CARE

- When explaining the use of warm and cold therapy to patients, the meaning and significance of the therapy can take on very different interpretations based on a patient's culture (Giger, 2017). Therefore it is important to assess the culture-specific applications of warm and cold principles for each patient and family caregiver:

- Assess how heat and cold are used normally in the care of the patient in the home.
- Reinforce the purpose of the therapy and identify patient concerns or questions.
- During the application of heat or cold therapy, the patient or his or her extremities may be exposed; maintain comfort and privacy by additional blankets, privacy curtains, and room doors. Some patients refuse exposure to reduce body temperature.
- Use cultural brokers such as family members and religious leaders to increase acceptance of critical therapies such as hypothermia or ice packs that contradict a patient's or family's beliefs and practices. Use a professional interpreter if patient speaks a second language.

EVIDENCE-BASED PRACTICE

- The application of ice or cryotherapy is one of the most widely used therapeutic modalities in the management of acute musculoskeletal injuries. Patients who used a numerical rating score for pain reported decrease in pain following application of ice on their neck. The use of cold therapy reduces the conduction of pain impulses, which occurs when the skin temperature is lowered (da Costa Santos et al., 2015; Maxwell and Sterling, 2013).

- Ice applied to soft tissue injuries is effective in initial pain control. Optimal ice-pack therapy is 10 minutes but may be adjusted according to individual needs and situation (Chu et al., 2013).
- Regional hypothermia along with adequate oral hygiene decreases the duration of chemotherapy-induced oral mucositis (Kadakia et al., 2014).
- Cold therapy decreases nerve conduction velocity, formation and accumulation of edema, and blood flow to injured tissues. As a result, these physiological effects are effective in reducing inflammation, pain, and acute swelling and can control hemorrhage and edema in soft tissue injuries (Ewell et al., 2014).
- Application of heat is useful in maintaining or improving range of joint motion following the acute phase of soft tissue injuries (Nakano et al., 2012).
- A combination of cold and heat therapy is effective in adults and children with musculoskeletal injuries to reduce inflammation and edema and improve joint function (Brooks et al., 2015).

SAFETY GUIDELINES

- Know your patient's risk for injury from heat or cold. Certain patients are more predisposed to injury than others (see Table 42.2).
- Exposed layers of skin are more sensitive to temperature variations than intact skin. Therefore protect damaged skin when applying hot or cold therapy.
- Do not microwave towels or medical products used for heat application.
- Know the temperature of the application being used. Many devices such as heating pads or water-flow pads (e.g., Aqua-K pads) have thermostats to regulate temperature. Always check the temperature of a device and of a moist compress applied directly to the skin.
- Burns and skin injuries sustained from hot or cold therapies are serious reportable events and are preventable (NQF, 2016). If they occur, they have functional implications for patients. In addition, because these are preventable events, there is a potential that the health care costs for these injuries will not be reimbursed to the health care agency.
- It is important to individualize care to meet a patient's needs and preferences. Remember that patient safety, comfort, and privacy are important when using warm or cold therapies.
- Consider patient age, skin and circulation, vital signs, ability to sense temperature, and ability to communicate before applying

TABLE 42.1

Pathophysiological Effects of Hot and Cold Applications

	Cold	Hot
Pain	↓	↓
Spasm	↓	↓
Metabolism	↓	↑
Blood flow	↓	↑
Inflammation	↓	↑
Edema	↓	↑
Extensibility	↓	↑

Data from da Costa Santos VN et al: Effect of cryotherapy on the ankle temperature in athletes: ice pack and cold water immersion, *Fisioter Mov* 28:1, 2015; Garner A, Fendius A: Temperature physiology, assessment and control, *Br J Neurosci Nurs* 6(8):397, 2011.

TABLE 42.2

Characteristics of Hot and Cold Application

	Examples of Conditions	Precautions	Adverse Outcomes
Cold application	Immediately after direct trauma such as sprain, strains, fractures, muscle spasms; after superficial lacerations or puncture wounds; after minor burns; chronic pain from arthritis, joint trauma; delayed-onset muscle soreness; inflammation	Circulatory insufficiency Cold allergy Diabetes mellitus	Cardiovascular effects (bradycardia) Raynaud's phenomenon Cold urticaria Nerve and tissue damage Slow wound healing Frostbite
Heat application	Inflamed or edematous body part; new surgical wound; infected wound; arthritis; degenerative joint disease; localized joint pain, muscle strains; low back pain; menstrual cramping; hemorrhoid, perianal, and vaginal inflammation; local abscess	Pregnancy Laminectomy sites Spinal cord Malignancy Vascular insufficiency Eyes, testes, heart	Burns Infections Increased pain Increased inflammation

TABLE 42.3

Warm Application: Moist versus Dry

Type	Advantages	Disadvantages
Moist application	Reduces drying of skin and softens wound exudate Conforms well to body area being treated Penetrates deeply into tissue layers Lessens sweating and insensible fluid loss	Can cause maceration of skin with prolonged exposure Cools rapidly because of moisture evaporation Creates greater risk for burns to skin because moisture conducts heat
Dry application	Less likely to burn skin Does not cause skin maceration Retains temperature longer because it is not influenced by evaporation	Increases insensible fluid loss through sweating Does not penetrate deep into tissue Causes increased drying of skin

heat or cold therapies. Certain patients such as the very young or very old or patients with paralysis, sensory impairment, or peripheral vascular diseases have a greater risk for injury from warm and cold applications (Table 42.2).

- When using heat or cold therapies, you can use either dry or moist applications. The selection depends on the expected outcome for the patient. Temperature travels from an external source such as a compress or heating pad to the surface of the skin. A substance that conducts temperatures poorly is a good insulator and thus a protector for skin and tissues. However, there are distinct advantages to using both dry and moist applications (Table 42.3).
- Extremities or perineal areas have decreased fat and underlying tissue and are more sensitive than others to temperature extremes. Modify the intensity of heat and cold when treating sensitive skin areas.
- Check the patient frequently during a heat or cold application. The condition of the skin indicates whether tissue injury is

occurring. Observe for signs of excessive redness, maceration, or blistering.

- Do not allow patients to adjust temperature settings.
- Position patients so they can move away from the temperature source. This decreases the risk for injuries from temperature exposure. The hospitalized patient should always have a call light within reach.
- Do not leave a patient unattended if he or she is unable to sense temperature changes or move away from the temperature source.
- If patients have diabetes mellitus or peripheral vascular diseases, it is important to use caution when applying hot or cold therapies. In addition, these patients require more frequent skin assessment during the treatment.
- Be aware of the impact that heat application has on a patient's vital signs. In particular, a Sitz bath causes localized vasodilation. If this vasodilation is significant, the patient's blood pressure may decrease, causing dizziness and increasing a patient's risk for falls.

◆ **SKILL 42.1**   **Application of Moist Heat (Compress and Sitz Bath)**

Moist heat is beneficial in increasing muscle and ligament flexibility, promoting relaxation and healing, and relieving muscle spasm and joint stiffness following the acute phase of a musculoskeletal injury (Nakano et al., 2012; Petrofsky et al., 2013). Factors to consider before application include level of temperature and duration of the heat therapy and the nature of the tissues being treated.

Warm compresses and commercial heat packs (Fig. 42.1) are examples of moist heat applications used for a variety of conditions. A warm compress is a section of sterile or clean gauze moistened with a prescribed heated solution (i.e., normal saline or sterile water) and applied directly to an affected area. Commercially packaged sterile, premoistened compresses are available in some agencies. They require the use of a special infrared lamp to heat. Plain sterile or clean gauze is heated by adding the gauze to a container of warmed solution. A commercial heat pack produces its own moisture by drawing moisture from humidity in the air and retaining it in the outer flannel cover of the hot pack.

Moist heat application also includes the use of warm baths, soaks, and Sitz baths. A warm bath or soak involves immersion of a body part into a warmed solution. Warm soaks and Sitz baths promote circulation, reduce edema and inflammation, promote muscle relaxation, debride wounds, and apply medicated solutions. If a body part is too large to immerse, you can soak it by wrapping it in a dressing saturated with the prepared, warmed solution.

Sitz baths use a special tub or chair basin that allows a patient to sit in water without immersing the legs, feet, and upper trunk (Fig. 42.2). Sitz basins are disposable and especially easy to use in

the home. Portable baths fit easily on top of toilets. Patients who have undergone perineal or rectal surgery, who have had an episiotomy during childbirth, or who have painful hemorrhoids or perineal inflammation benefit from a Sitz bath.

When preparing a soak or bath, remember that the heated solution is in direct contact with the patient's skin. Be sure to assess

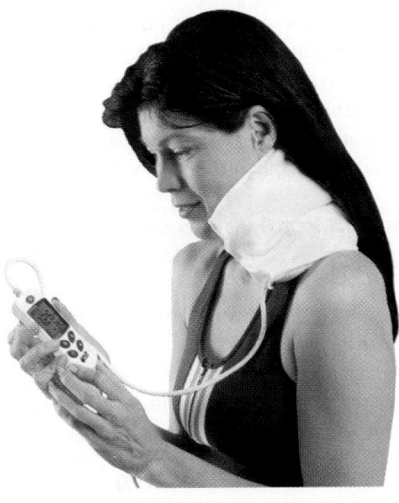

FIG 42.1 Digital moist-heat pack. (*Image used with permission from Theratherm, Chattanooga, a DJO Company. All rights reserved.*)

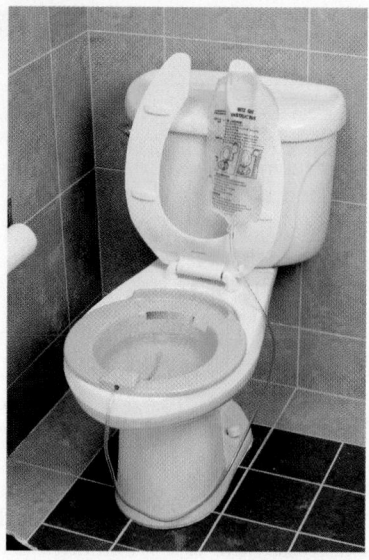

FIG 42.2 Disposable sitz bath. (*Used with permission, Briggs Corporation.*)

the patient's skin for any excessive redness or blistering after 10 to 15 minutes and check water temperature frequently to prevent burns. It is desirable to keep the solution temperature constant to enhance the therapeutic effects of the moist heat. Whenever you add heated solution to a soak basin or bath, remove the patient's body part and reimmerse once the solution has mixed and the temperature has been checked.

Delegation and Collaboration

The skill of applying moist heat can be delegated to nursing assistive personnel (NAP). However, in most settings the nurse applies any sterile applications. The assessment of the patient's condition and the skin and tissues in the area that is treated, evaluation of the patient's response, and explanation of the purpose of the treatment cannot be delegated. If there are risks or expected complications, this skill cannot be delegated. The nurse instructs the NAP about:

- Proper temperature of the application.
- Skin changes to immediately report to the nurse (e.g., burning, blistering, or excessive redness).
- Specific patient complaints and changes in vital signs to immediately report to the nurse (e.g., pain, dizziness or light-headedness, increased or decreased pulse, decreased blood pressure).
- Specific positioning and application time requirements based on agency policy and manufacturer instructions.
- Reporting when treatment is complete so an evaluation of the patient's response can be made.

Equipment

All Moist Heat Applications
- Prescribed analgesia (if ordered)
- Dry bath towel, bath blanket
- Warmed prescribed solution (i.e., normal saline) or commercially prepared compresses or commercial heat pack
- Biohazard waste bag
- Clean gloves
- Compress
- Clean basin
- Waterproof pad
- Ties or cloth tape
- Clean gauze or towel
- Options for moist heat application, depending on health care provider's order:
  - Sterile compress: sterile basin, sterile gauze, and sterile gloves
  - Aquathermia pad
  - Disposable sitz bath: prescribed solution and any topical medication after the soak

STEP	RATIONALE

ASSESSMENT

1. Identify patient using at least two identifiers (e.g., name and birthday or name and medical record number) according to agency policy.

   Ensures correct patient. Complies with The Joint Commission standards and improves patient safety (TJC, 2016).

2. Refer to health care provider's order for type of moist heat application, location and duration of application, desired temperature, and agency policies regarding temperature.

   Ensures safe practice by verifying specific location for therapy and type and duration of heat application.

3. Perform hand hygiene and assess skin around area to be treated. Perform neurovascular assessments for sensitivity to temperature and pain by measuring light touch, pinprick, and temperature sensation (see Chapter 6).

   Certain conditions alter conduction of sensory impulses that transmit temperature and pain, predisposing patients to injury from heat applications. Patients with diminished sensation to heat or cold must be monitored closely during treatment.

Clinical Decision Point *Patients with diabetes mellitus, vascular diseases, paralysis, peripheral neuropathy, certain cardiovascular medications, and rheumatoid arthritis are at greater risk for thermal injury (Kaplow, 2013).*

4. Refer to patient's medical record to identify any contraindications to moist heat application: unstable cardiac conditions, active bleeding, nitroglycerin or other therapeutic medicinal patch, acute inflammatory reactions, recent (<72 hours) musculoskeletal injury, and skin conditions such as eczema.

   Patients with certain cardiovascular conditions and who exhibit side effects of certain medications such as cardiac, hypertensive, and vasoactive medications may be at risk for sudden changes in blood pressure and blood flow caused by vasodilation. Heat causes vasodilation, which aggravates active bleeding, which can increase hemorrhage or bleeding into soft tissues adjacent to musculoskeletal injury (Kaplow, 2013). Vasodilation increases rate of medication absorption when direct heat is applied over medication patch.

STEP	RATIONALE
5. When treating a wound, apply clean gloves and assess it for size, color, drainage volume, pain (using pain scale, see Chapter 16), and odor (this may be deferred until dressing is removed [see Step 5c in Implementation] and heat is applied). Remove and discard gloves (if used).	Provides baseline to determine change in wound following heat application. Provides baseline for patient's comfort level.
6. Assess patient's blood pressure and pulse.	Establishes baseline to determine response to therapy.
7. Assess patient's ROM of affected part if being treated for muscle sprain.	Provides baseline to determine if ROM improves following therapy.
8. Assess patient's mobility: ability to position self for soak application, position self in bath, and sit up from bath.	Determines level of help needed to position patient for treatment.
9. Assess patient's level of consciousness and responsiveness (e.g., confusion, disorientation, dementia).	Patients with altered level of consciousness are unable to sense or report reduced sensation of discomfort.
10. Assess patient's and family caregiver's understanding of application and related safety factors.	Determines need for health teaching.

NURSING DIAGNOSES

- Acute pain
- Chronic pain
- Deficient knowledge regarding heat therapy
- Impaired physical mobility
- Impaired skin integrity
- Ineffective peripheral tissue perfusion
- Risk for injury

Related factors/Risk factors are individualized based on patient's condition or needs.

PLANNING

1. Expected outcomes following completion of procedure:	
• Affected area is pink and warm to touch immediately after heat application.	Vasodilation increases blood flow to site.
• After multiple applications, wound shows signs of healing (e.g., tissue granulation; reduced edema, inflammation, drainage).	Moist heat increases blood flow, enhances white blood cell infiltration, and removes waste products from cells (da costa Santos et al., 2015).
• Patient denies burning sensation.	Indicates temperature applied appropriately.

Clinical Decision Point *Note that in some situations heat applications cause pain signals to be overridden and decrease pain perception in cerebral cortex (Garner and Fendius, 2011).*

• Patient reports measurable increased mobility and decrease in pain in affected region.	Heat reduces edema/inflammation and relaxes stiff and strained muscles. Heat used in conjunction with physical therapy and/or exercise improved function and mobility (Bleakley and Costello, 2013).
• Blood pressure and pulse are within patient's normal range.	No systemic vascular changes occur. Goal of therapy is to achieve localized vascular response.
• Patient is able to self-apply therapy safely.	Measures level of learning; necessary for home care.
2. Assemble and prepare equipment and supplies.	Organization of supplies prevents unnecessary delays in procedure.
3. Explain steps of procedure and purpose to patient. Describe sensation that patient will feel such as warmth and wetness. Explain precautions to prevent burning.	Minimizes patient's anxiety and promotes cooperation during procedure.

IMPLEMENTATION

1. Close door if in private room and/or close bedside curtains.	Decreases drafts, thus decreasing transmission of microorganisms. Provides for privacy.
2. Perform hand hygiene and apply clean gloves.	Reduces transmission of microorganisms.
3. Position patient in bed, keeping affected body part in proper alignment. Expose body part to be covered with heat application and drape patient with bath blanket or towel as need.	Limited mobility in uncomfortable position causes muscular stress. Draping prevents cooling.
4. Place waterproof pad under patient (exception: do not do this with sitz bath or commercial heat pad).	Protects bed linen from moisture and soiling.

STEP	RATIONALE
5. Apply moist sterile compress:	
a. Heat prescribed solution to desired temperature by immersing closed bottle of solution in basin of very warm water.	Prevents burns by ensuring proper temperature of solution.
b. Prepare aquathermia pad if needed. Temperature is usually preset by manufacturer or bioengineering.	Prevents burning by using proper temperature.
c. Remove any present existing dressing covering wound. Inspect condition of wound and surrounding skin. Inflamed wound appears reddened, but surrounding skin is less red in color. Dispose of gloves and old dressings in biohazard bag.	Reduces transmission of microorganisms. Provides baseline to measure wound healing.

Clinical Decision Point *If skin surrounding wound is inflamed or reddened or has active bleeding or drainage, moist heat application may be contraindicated. Verify with health care provider.*

STEP	RATIONALE
d. Perform hand hygiene.	Reduces transmission of microorganisms.
e. Prepare compress.	Use of appropriate aseptic technique keeps gauze compress clean or sterile. Sterile compress is needed when applied to open wound.
(1) Pour warmed solution into container (if sterile asepsis is required, use sterile technique to add sterile gauze into warmed sterile solution to immerse gauze).	
(2) Open gauze. If applying sterile compress, open sterile supplies using sterile technique (see Chapter 10).	Sterile compress is needed when applied to open wound.
(3) Add gauze to container of solution to immerse gauze: use proper aseptic technique.	
(4) If using commercially prepared compress, follow manufacturer instructions for warming.	

Clinical Decision Point *To avoid injury to a patient, test temperature of sterile solution by applying a drop to your forearm (without contaminating solution). It should feel warm to the skin without burning.*

STEP	RATIONALE
f. Apply sterile gloves if dressing change is sterile; otherwise apply clean gloves.	Allows you to manipulate sterile dressing and touch open wound.
g. Pick up one layer of immersed gauze, wring out any excess solution, and apply it lightly to wound; avoid surrounding unaffected skin. *Option:* Apply commercial compress or heat pack over wound only; only use with clean wounds.	Excess moisture macerates skin and increases risk for burns and infection. Skin is sensitive to sudden change in temperature.
h. After a few seconds, lift edge of gauze to assess for redness.	Increased redness indicates burn. Burns and injuries from hot therapies are preventable events (NQF, 2016).
i. If patient tolerates compress, pack gauze snugly against wound. Be sure to cover all wound surfaces with warm compress.	Packing compress prevents rapid cooling from ambient air currents.
j. Cover moist compress with dry sterile dressing and bath towel. If necessary, pin or tie in place. Remove and dispose of gloves and perform hand hygiene.	Dry sterile dressing prevents transfer of microorganisms to wound via capillary action caused by moist compress. Towel insulates compress to prevent heat loss.
k. *Option:* When using gauze compress, apply aquathermia, commercial heat pack, or waterproof heating pad (see Skill 42.2) over towel. Keep it in place for desired duration of application.	Provides constant temperature to compress.
l. Leave compress in place for 20 minutes or less (per order or agency policy). If aquathermia pad or commercial heat pack is *not* used, change warm compress using sterile technique every 5 to 10 minutes or as ordered during duration of therapy.	Maintains constant temperature for best therapeutic benefit. Moist heat promotes transfer of heat to underlying subcutaneous tissues, which helps to reduce thermal injury to skin (Igaki et al., 2014). Time limit prevents risk of overexposure and injury to underlying skin.
m. After prescribed time, perform hand hygiene and apply clean gloves. Remove pad, towel, and compress. Evaluate wound and condition of skin and replace dry sterile dressing (using sterile gloves) as ordered.	Continued exposure to moisture macerates skin. Prevents entrance of microorganisms into wound site.

STEP	RATIONALE
n. Help patient to preferred comfortable position.	Maintains patient's comfort.
o. Dispose of equipment and soiled compress. Perform hand hygiene.	Reduces transmission of microorganisms.
6. Sitz bath or warm soak to intact skin or wound:	
a. Remove any existing dressing covering wound. Dispose of gloves and dressings in proper receptacle and perform hand hygiene.	Reduces transmission of microorganisms.
b. Inspect condition of wound and surrounding skin. Pay particular attention to suture line.	Provides baseline to determine response to warm soak.
c. When exudate or drainage is present, apply a new pair of clean gloves and clean intact skin around open area with clean cloth and soap and water. Sterile gloves and gauze may be needed to clean open wound (check agency policy). Dispose of gloves and perform hand hygiene.	Cleaning removes organisms so bath solution does not spread infection.
d. Fill sitz bath or bathtub in bathroom with warmed solution. Check temperature (check agency policy). *Option:* If using bag of normal saline, warm per agency policy.	Ensures proper temperature and reduces risk for burns.
e. Assist patient to bathroom to immerse body part in sitz bath, bathtub, or basin. Cover patient with bath blanket or towel as needed.	Prevents falls. Covering patient prevents heat loss through evaporation and maintains constant temperature.
f. Assess heart rate. Make sure that patient does not feel light-headed or dizzy and that call light is within reach.	Provides baseline to determine if vascular response to vasodilation occurs during treatment.
g. After 15 to 20 minutes remove patient from soak or bath; dry body parts thoroughly. (Wear clean gloves.)	Avoids chilling. Enhances patient's comfort.
h. Drain solution from basin or tub. Clean and place in proper storage area according to agency policy. Dispose of soiled linen and gloves; perform hand hygiene.	Reduces transmission of microorganisms.

EVALUATION

1. Inspect condition of body part or wound treated for evidence of healing. Observe skin color, temperature, edema, and sensitivity to touch.	Evaluates effectiveness of treatment and risk for potential injury.
2. Ask patient to describe level of comfort on pain scale of 0 to 10. Ask about any sensation of burning following treatment.	Determines if patient was exposed to temperature extreme, resulting in burn. Evaluates patient's subjective response to therapy.
3. Obtain blood pressure and pulse and compare with baseline.	Determines if systemic vascular response to vasodilation has occurred.
4. Evaluate ROM of affected body part.	Determines if edema or muscle spasm is relieved.
5. **Use Teach-Back:** "I want to be sure I demonstrated how to apply a warm moist compress so you can do this at home. Show me how you would apply this compress at home." Revise your instruction now or develop a plan for revised patient or family caregiver teaching if patient or family caregiver is not able to teach back correctly.	Determines patient's and family caregiver's level of understanding of instructional topic.

Unexpected Outcomes	Related Interventions
1. Patient's skin is reddened and sensitive to touch, either during treatment or 30 minutes after, or patient complains of burning.	• Discontinue moist application immediately. • Verify proper temperature or check device for proper functioning. • Notify health care provider and, if there is a burn, complete an incident or adverse event report (see agency policy).
2. Patient complains of burning and increased discomfort.	• Reduce temperature of compress. • Assess for skin breakdown. • Notify health care provider.

Recording and Reporting

- Record procedure, noting type, location, and duration of application; solution and temperature; condition of body part, wound, and skin before and after treatment; and patient's response to therapy on flow sheet in nurses' notes in electronic health record (EHR) or chart.
- Record preprocedure and postprocedure vital signs (as indicated).
- Document your evaluation of patient and family caregiver learning.
- Report any unexpected changes in condition of skin or wound to health care provider.

Special Considerations
Teaching

- If a patient needs to continue heat applications after discharge, have patient or family caregiver give a return demonstration before discharge.
- Teach patient how to gently pack wound to avoid discomfort.
- Family caregivers and patients need to learn and demonstrate the careful assessment that is needed for patients with reduced sensation to determine if temperature of compress is too hot.

Pediatric

- The skin of infants and children is thin and fragile and therefore easily damaged. Use special caution with application of heat in this population (Hockenberry and Wilson, 2015). Remain with children during procedure for safety.

- It is often helpful to incorporate play into the time a child is required to soak. Placing items with which the child can interact in the basin is helpful. Place clean boats or other similar clean water toys in the bath with a child who requires a bath soak. Adult supervision is necessary.

Gerontological

- Normal aging results in thinning and increased fragility of a patient's skin. If an older adult is receiving long-term steroid therapy or is malnourished, the skin becomes even more fragile. The thinning and increased fragility of an older adult's skin increases the risk for damaged skin. Skin also becomes less elastic and more prone to tears. As a result of chronic diseases, an older adult may have impaired circulation to a skin area or impaired sensation for pain or temperature (Touhy and Jett, 2014).
- Older adults who have lost subcutaneous tissue and fat have lost the insulating effect of these tissues and may experience alterations in thermoregulation and have an increased risk of injury from heat applications (Touhy and Jett, 2014).

Home Care

- When necessary, assess availability of family caregiver to help patient apply moist heat, family caregiver's understanding of purpose of procedure, and willingness of caregiver to comply with procedure and not leave patient unattended during therapy.
- Assess physical environment to determine adequacy of facilities for use by patient. Patient may need assistive devices to get in or out of a tub or a commode chair to set up a sitz bath.

◆ SKILL 42.2   Applying Aquathermia and Dry Heat

A water-flow pad such as an aquathermia pad, electric heating pads, and commercial heat packs (Fig. 42.3) are common forms of dry heat therapy. A new product, an air-activated wearable heat wrap, maintains a temperature of 40°C (104°F) and can be worn from 8 to 10 hours. The aquathermia pad (water-flow pad) used in health care settings consists of a waterproof rubber or plastic pad connected by two hoses to an electrical control unit that has a heating element and motor. Distilled water circulates through hollowed channels in the pad to the control unit where water is heated (or cooled).

Dry heat devices are applied directly to the surface of the skin. For this reason extra precautions need to be taken to prevent burns and skin and tissue injury (Igaki et al., 2014). A conventional heating pad uses dry heat and is often used in the home care setting. These devices are not used in health care settings. A cotton or flannel cloth must cover the heating pad. The pad has a temperature-regulating unit for high, medium, or low settings. Because it is so easy to readjust temperature settings on heating pads, instruct patients not to turn the setting higher once they have adapted to the temperature.

Delegation and Collaboration

The skill of applying aquathermia and dry heat can be delegated to nursing assistive personnel (NAP) (see agency policy). The nurse must assess and evaluate the condition of the skin and tissues in the area that is treated and explain the purpose of the treatment. If there are risks or expected complications, this skill cannot be delegated. The nurse instructs the NAP about:

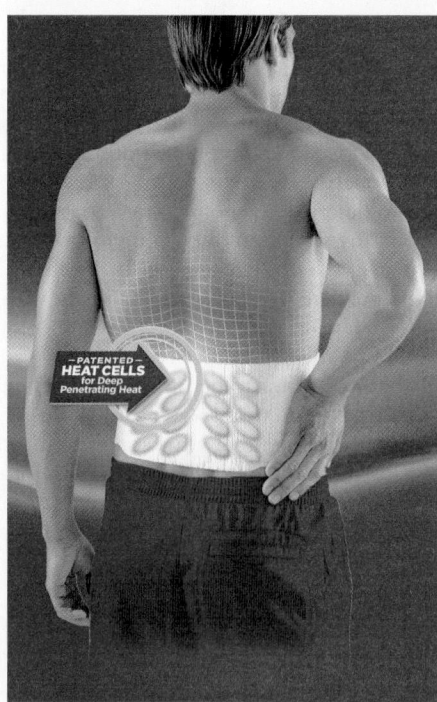

FIG 42.3 Dry heat wrap. (*Image used with permission, ThermaWrap, Pfizer Consumer Healthcare. All rights reserved.*)

- Specific positioning and time requirements to keep the application in place based on health care provider order or agency policy.
- What to observe and report immediately such as excessive redness and pain during application.
- Reporting to the nurse when treatment is complete so the patient's response can be evaluated.

Equipment

- Aquathermia or commercial heat pack
- Distilled water (for aquathermia pad)
- Bath towel or pillowcase
- Tape, ties, or gauze roll

STEP	RATIONALE

ASSESSMENT

1. Identify patient using at least two identifiers (e.g., name and birthday or name and medical record number) according to agency policy.

   Ensures correct patient. Complies with The Joint Commission standards and improves patient safety (TJC, 2016).

2. Refer to health care provider's order for location of application and duration of therapy. Agency policy usually sets recommended temperature for aquathermia pad.

   Order required to help ensure patient's safety. Preset temperature on device reduces risk of skin and tissue injury.

3. Perform hand hygiene and assess condition of skin and underlying tissue in area where you will apply pad for skin integrity. Assess for skin color, temperature, sensitivity to touch, blistering, and excessive dryness (see Chapter 6).

   Provides baseline to determine change in skin condition after heat application.

4. Ask patient to describe level of comfort on pain scale of 0 to 10. Assess range of motion (ROM) if patient is being treated for muscle sprain.

   Provides baseline to determine if pain relief or improved ROM is achieved.

5. Assess patient's level of consciousness and responsiveness.

   Patients with reduced level of consciousness are unable to sense or report reduced sensation or discomfort.

6. Check electrical plugs and cords for obvious fraying or cracking.

   Prevents injury from accidental electrical shock.

7. Determine patient's or family caregiver's knowledge of procedure, including steps for application and safety precautions.

   Heating pads frequently are used in home. Assessment determines extent of health teaching required.

NURSING DIAGNOSES

- Acute pain
- Chronic pain
- Deficient knowledge regarding heat application
- Impaired physical mobility
- Impaired skin integrity
- Ineffective peripheral tissue perfusion
- Risk for injury

Related factors/Risk factors are individualized based on patient's condition or needs.

PLANNING

1. Expected outcomes following completion of procedure:
   - Skin is pink and warm to touch after application.

     Vasodilation from heat exposure increases blood flow to affected part.

   - Patient reports less pain of inflamed tissues or strained muscles.

     Thermoreceptors, special temperature-sensitive nerve endings, are activated by changes in skin temperature.

   - Patient's ROM increases.

     Superficial heat increases joint mobility by increasing connective tissue extensibility, reducing pain, and tissue viscosity (Bleakley and Costello, 2013).

   - Patient correctly applies pad.

     Documents learning.

2. Prepare equipment and supplies.

   Organization of supplies prevents unnecessary delays in procedure.

3. Explain procedure and precautions.

   Improves likelihood of patient's adherence to therapy.

IMPLEMENTATION

1. Close door if in private room and/or close bedside curtains.

   Provides for patient's privacy.

2. Perform hand hygiene, apply clean gloves, and position patient to expose area being treated.

   Reduces transfer of microorganisms. Patient must be able to assume position for several minutes during application.

STEP	RATIONALE

3. Apply heat therapy.
   a. Aquathermia heating pad:
   (1) Cover or wrap area to be treated with single layer of bath towel or enclose pad with pillowcase.

Prevents heated surface from touching patient's skin directly and increasing risk for injury to patient's skin.

Clinical Decision Point *Do not pin wrap to pad because this may cause a leak in device.*

   (2) Place pad over affected area and secure with tape, tie, or gauze as needed (see illustration).

Pad delivers dry, warm heat to injured tissues. Pad should not slip onto different body part.

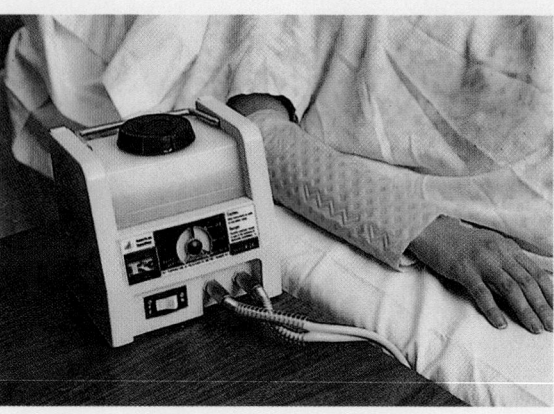

STEP 3a(2) Aquathermia pad.

   (3) Turn on aquathermia unit and check temperature setting. **NOTE:** Temperature of unit is usually set by agency's bioengineering department.

Prevents exposure of patient to temperature extremes.

   b. Apply commercially prepared heat pack: break pouch inside larger pack (follow manufacturer guidelines).

Activates chemicals within pack to warm outer surface.

Clinical Decision Point *Never position patient so he or she is lying directly on heating device. This position prevents dissipation of heat and increases risk for burns.*

4. Remove and dispose of gloves; perform hand hygiene.

Reduces transmission of microorganisms.

5. Monitor condition of skin over site every 5 minutes and ask patient about sensation of burning.

Determines if heat exposure is causing any burn, blistering, or injury to underlying skin.

6. After no more than 20 minutes (or time ordered by health care provider), perform hand hygiene, apply clean gloves, and remove pad and store.

Heat therapy may reduce pain and spasm and increase blood flow and compliance of soft tissue structures (Brooks et al., 2015).

7. Help patient return to preferred comfortable position, dispose of soiled linen and gloves, and perform hand hygiene.

Promotes relaxing environment. Reduces transmission of microorganisms.

EVALUATION

1. Inspect condition of skin for integrity, color, temperature, dryness, and blistering. Evaluate again 30 minutes following treatment.

Evaluates response of skin to heat exposure.

2. Evaluate ROM. Ask patient to rate pain on scale of 0 to 10.

Heat reduces edema and relieves pain from muscle stiffness and spasm (Bleakley and Costello, 2013; Nakano et al., 2012).

Clinical Decision Point *Do not have patient actively exercise muscle to evaluate results of therapy. Active exercise can aggravate muscle strain.*

3. Use Teach-Back: "I want to be sure I explained how to safely use a heating pad at home. Explain to me why a layer of cloth between the heating pad and your skin is important." Revise your instruction now or develop a plan for revised patient or family caregiver teaching if patient or family caregiver is not able to teach back correctly.

Determines patient's and family caregiver's level of understanding of instructional topic

STEP	RATIONALE

Unexpected Outcomes
1. See Skill 42.1, Unexpected Outcomes.
2. Body part remains painful to move.

3. Patient or family caregiver applies heat incorrectly or is unable to explain precautions.

Related Interventions

- Discontinue aquathermia pad or heat pack use.
- Observe for localized swelling.
- Notify health care provider.
- Reinstruct patient or family caregiver as necessary. Consider possible home health referral (if patient is eligible).

Recording and Reporting

- Record appearance and condition of skin, degree of ROM of affected part, type of application, temperature and duration of therapy, and patient's response on flow sheet in nurses' notes in electronic health record (EHR) or chart.
- Document your evaluation of patient and family caregiver learning.
- Report occurrence of increased pain, reduced ROM, burn, blistering, or other injury to the skin to health care provider.

Special Considerations
Teaching

- Highlight safety precautions during procedure so they are followed during application.
- Instruct patient and family caregiver not to use the highest setting and check frequently for redness or blistering on the skin exposed to the heating device.

Pediatric

- The skin of infants and children is thin and fragile and therefore easily damaged. Use special caution in this population (Hock-

enberry and Wilson, 2015). Remain with children during procedure for safety and effectiveness.

Gerontological

- Older adults are more at risk for burns because of loss of heat sensation. Check site frequently during all treatments.
- Older patients have thin, more fragile skin that is susceptible to burns.

Home Care

- Assess patient and primary caregiver as to their understanding, ability, and motivation to comply with procedure.
- Assess home environment for facilities (e.g., condition of electrical outlets and equipment) to comply with implementation of procedure.
- Discourage use of heating pad. However, if patient has limited resources and chooses to use pad at home, instruct on all safety precautions.

◆ SKILL 42.3 Application of Cold

A variety of cold (cryotherapy) modalities such as ice packs, moist cold compresses, chemical cold packs, electromechanical or compression devices, or cold-soak immersion of a body part are available. Cold therapy treats localized inflammatory responses that lead to edema, hemorrhage, muscle spasm, or pain (see Table 42.1). Improvement to joint mobility following cold therapy is related to facilitating, relieving pain, inhibiting muscle spasm, and reducing muscle tension (Petrofsky et al., 2013).

Cold exerts a profound physiological effect on the body, reducing inflammation caused by injuries to soft tissue and the musculoskeletal system (APTA, 2016). Cold is one step in the PRICE principle (i.e., the acronym used in treating sprains and strains [(ACSM, 2011; Maughan, 2016]). The overall goal of the PRICE principle is to limit the amount of swelling at the injury site and promote healing:

- P—Protect from further injury
- R—Restrict/Rest activity
- I—Apply Ice
- C—Apply Compression
- E—Elevate injured area

Vasoconstriction resulting from cold application reduces blood flow to the injured part and thus reduces fluid accumulation and slows bleeding and hematoma formation associated with trauma. The lower temperature also suppresses muscle spasm and produces a local anesthetic response (Petrofsky et al., 2013).

When used appropriately, cold applications significantly lessen pain; thus mobility is improved. Cold applications produce maximal

analgesia, control the inflammatory response, and decrease nerve conduction (da Costa Santos et al., 2015).

A cold compress usually consists of a commercial cold pack or a gauze dressing or washcloth that has been immersed in iced or chilled solution to achieve the desired temperature. The compress may be sterile or clean; however, a clean compress is most common. Any open wounds require sterile applications. There are many sizes or thicknesses of gauze, depending on the site of injury. For example, a cold compress to the eye requires thicker gauze that fits a small area to maintain a cold temperature. Thin gauze works more effectively for larger areas such as the face.

Ice bags and cold packs come in a variety of sizes to fit different body parts (Fig. 42.4). When a commercial ice bag or cold pack is unavailable, use a plastic bag or glove filled halfway with crushed ice. Squeeze the bag or glove to expel air, which hampers cold conduction. Wrap all of these items in a towel or cloth before application.

Electrically controlled continuous cold-flow therapy devices simultaneously provide cold and compression (e.g., Cryo/Cuff [Fig. 42.5]). Compression acts with cold to reduce the blood flow and edema formation while providing support to the soft tissues. The cooling pad has the advantage of delivering a constant cool temperature. Elevating the extremity during treatment further augments venous return. A person who undergoes treatment with one of these devices is simultaneously receiving all five components of the *p*rotection, *r*est, *i*ce, *c*ompression, and *e*levation (PRICE) method for managing this type of injury (APTA, 2016).

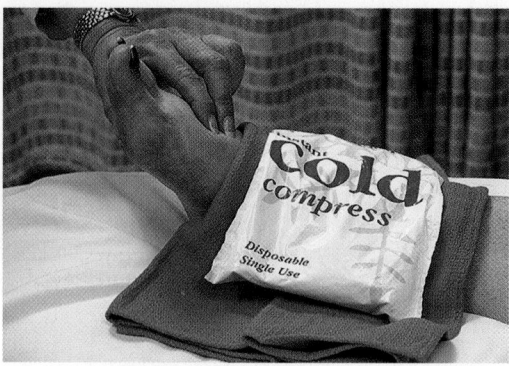

FIG 42.4 Commercial ice pack.

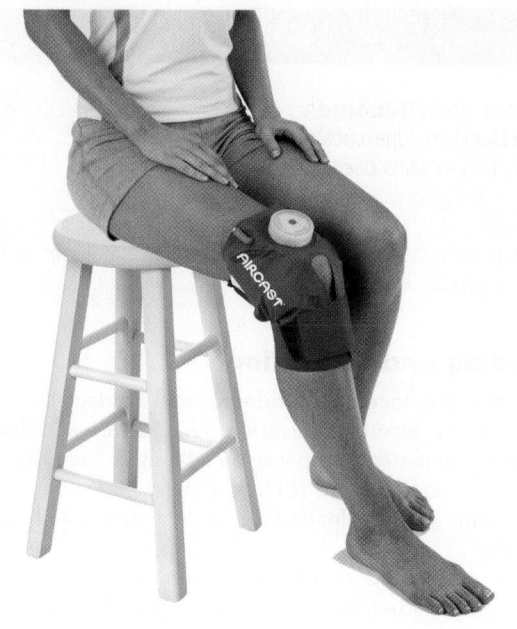

FIG 42.5 Cryo/Cuff includes integrated cooler. (*Image of AirCast Cryo/Cuff used with permission of DJO Global.*)

Delegation and Collaboration

The skill of applying cold applications can be delegated to nursing assistive personnel (NAP) in special situations (see agency policy). The nurse must assess and evaluate the patient and explain the purpose of the treatment. If there are risks or possible complications, this skill is not delegated. The nurse instructs the NAP to:

- Keep the application in place for only the length of time specified in the health care provider's order.
- Immediately report to the nurse any excessive redness on the skin, increase in pain, or decrease in sensation.
- Report when treatment is complete so a nurse can evaluate the patient's response.

Equipment

All Compresses, Bags, and Packs
- Clean gloves (if blood or body fluids are present)
- Cloth tape or ties or elastic wrap bandage
- Soft cloth cover: towel, pillowcase, or stockinette
- Bath towel or blanket and waterproof pad

Cold Compress
- Absorbent gauze (clean or sterile) folded to desired size
- Basin
- Prescribed solution at desired temperature

Ice Bag or Gel Pack
- Ice bag
- Ice chips and water or
- Reusable commercial gel pack (cold pack)
- Disposable commercial chemical cold pack

Electrically Controlled Cooling Device
- Cool water-flow pad or cooling pad and electrical pump
- Gauze roll or elastic wrap

STEP	RATIONALE

ASSESSMENT

STEP	RATIONALE
1. Identify patient using at least two identifiers (e.g., name and birthday or name and medical record number), according to agency policy.	Ensures correct patient. Complies with The Joint Commission standards and improves patient safety (TJC, 2016).
2. Refer to health care provider's order for type, location, and duration of application. Temperature of cooling pad will be ordered or preset.	Health care provider's order is required for all cold applications.
3. Perform hand hygiene and inspect condition of injured or affected part. Gently palpate area for edema (apply clean gloves if there is risk of exposure to body fluids).	Provides baseline for determining change in condition of injured tissues. Reduces transmission of microorganisms.

Clinical Decision Point *Keep injured part in alignment and immobilized. Movement can cause further injury to strains, sprains, or fractures.*

STEP	RATIONALE
4. Perform neurovascular check and inspect surrounding skin for integrity, circulation (presence of pulses), color, temperature, and sensitivity to touch (see Chapter 6).	Determines if patient is insensitive to cold extremes, which increases risk for injury.
5. Consider time elapsed since injury occurred.	Apply cold therapy as soon as possible after injury to reduce swelling, inflammation, tissue bleeding and pain (Brooks et al., 2015; Maughan, 2016; Maxwell and Sterling, 2013).
6. Ask patient to describe character of pain and rate severity on scale of 0 to 10 (or other pain scale when applicable) if able. Assess ROM of affected part if muscle sprain is involved.	Provides baseline for determining pain relief and ROM with therapy.

STEP	RATIONALE
7. Review medical history for conditions that contraindicate use of cold therapy: peripheral vascular diseases (e.g., Raynaud's disease, Buerger's disease), diabetic neuropathy, rheumatoid arthritis, frostbite.	These conditions increase risk for skin and tissue injury when exposed to cold.
8. Assess patient's level of consciousness and responsiveness.	Patients with reduced level of consciousness are unable to sense or report reduced sensation or discomfort.
9. Assess patient's or family caregiver's understanding and/or knowledge of procedure.	Cold applications are frequently used in the home. Determines extent of instruction required.

NURSING DIAGNOSES

- Acute pain
- Chronic pain

- Deficient knowledge regarding cold application
- Impaired physical mobility

- Ineffective peripheral tissue perfusion
- Risk for injury

Related factors/Risk factors are individualized based on patient's condition or needs.

PLANNING

1. Expected outcomes following completion of procedure:	
• Affected area is slightly pale and cool to touch.	Result of vasoconstriction.
• There is decreased edema and/or bleeding in tissues at site of injury.	Cold reduces blood flow to affected part by reducing protein extravasation from vasculature and subsequent edema formation (Brooks et al., 2015).
• Patient reports decreased pain as measured on scale of 0 to 10.	Cold decreases local swelling, reduces inflammatory response, and decreases nerve conduction and subsequent pain, creating localized analgesic effect (Brooks et al., 2015).
• Patient's ROM increases.	Cold reduces swelling.
• Patient or family caregiver correctly states how to apply cold and provides demonstration.	Documents learning.
2. Prepare equipment and supplies.	Organization prevents unnecessary delays.
3. Explain procedure and precautions.	Improves likelihood of patient's adherence to therapy.

IMPLEMENTATION

1. Close room door and bedside curtain. Perform hand hygiene and apply clean gloves.	Provides privacy for patient. Reduces spread of microorganisms.
2. Position patient carefully, keeping body part in proper alignment and only exposing area to be treated; drape patient with bath blankets.	Prevents further injury to body part. Avoids unnecessary exposure of body parts, maintaining patient's comfort and privacy.
3. Place towel or absorbent pad under area that you will treat.	Prevents soiling of bed linen.
4. Apply cold compress:	
a. Place ice and water in basin and test temperature on inner aspect of arm.	Extreme temperature can cause tissue damage.
b. Submerge gauze into basin filled with cold solution; wring out excess moisture.	Dripping gauze is uncomfortable to patient.
c. Apply compress to affected area, molding it gently over site.	Ensures that cold is directed over site of injury.
d. Remove, remoisten, and reapply to maintain temperature as needed.	
5. Apply ice pack or bag:	
a. Fill bag with water, secure cap, and invert.	Ensures that there are no leaks.
b. Empty water and fill bag two-thirds full with small ice chips and water.	Bag is easier to mold over body part when it is not full.
c. Express excess air from bag, secure bag closure, and wipe bag dry.	Excess air interferes with cold conduction. Allows bag to conform to area and promotes maximum contact.
d. Squeeze or knead commercial ice pack according to manufacturer's directions.	Releases alcohol-based solution to create cold temperature.
e. Wrap pack or bag with single layer of towel, pillowcase, or stockinette. Apply over injury. Secure with tape as needed.	Protects patient's tissue and absorbs condensation. Prevents direct exposure of cold against patient's skin.

STEP	RATIONALE

6. Apply commercial gel pack:
   a. Remove from freezer.
   b. Wrap pack with towel, pillowcase, or stockinette. Apply pack directly over injury.
   c. Secure with gauze, cloth tape, or ties as needed.

Protects patient's tissue and absorbs condensation. Prevents direct exposure of cold against patient's skin.

Clinical Decision Point *Do not reapply ice pack to red or bluish areas; continual use of ice pack makes ischemia worse.*

7. Apply electrically controlled cooling device:
   a. Prepare device following manufacturer's directions. Some devices are gravity-fed and require you to manually fill with iced water. Motorized units circulate chilled water.
   b. Make sure that all connections are intact and temperature, if adjustable, is set (see agency policy).
   c. Wrap cool-water flow pad in single layer of towel or pillowcase.
   d. Wrap cool pad around body part.
   e. Turn device on and check correct temperature. (NOTE: Temperature is usually preset in health care settings [check agency policy]).
   f. Secure with elastic wrap bandage, gauze roll, or ties.
8. Remove and dispose of gloves in proper container. Perform hand hygiene.
9. Check condition of skin every 5 minutes for duration of application.
   a. If area is edematous, sensation may be reduced; use extra caution during cold therapy and assess site more often.
   b. Numbness and tingling are common sensations with cold applications and indicate adverse reactions only when severe and coupled with other symptoms. Stop treatment when patient complains of burning sensation or skin begins to feel numb.
10. After 20 minutes (or as ordered by health care provider), perform hand hygiene, apply clean gloves, remove compress or pad, and gently dry off any moisture.

Ensures safe temperature application.

Prevents adverse reactions from cold such as burn or frostbite.

Ensures even application of cold temperature.
Ensures effective therapy. Preset temperature reduces risk of skin and tissue injury.

Ensures cold is distributed to correct body part.
Reduces transmission of microorganisms.

Determines if there are adverse reactions to cold (e.g., mottling, redness, burning, blistering, numbness).

When applying cold, skin will initially feel cold, followed by relief of pain. As cryotherapy continues, patient will feel burning sensation, then pain in skin, and finally numbness.

Drying prevents maceration of skin.

Clinical Decision Point *Areas with little body fat (e.g., knee, ankle, and elbow) do not tolerate cold as well as fatty areas (e.g., thigh and buttocks) do. For bony areas decrease time of cold application to lower range.*

11. Help patient to comfortable position.
12. Remove and dispose of supplies. Empty basin, if used, and dry. Dispose of soiled linen and gloves. Perform hand hygiene.

Maintains relaxing environment.
Reduces transmission of microorganisms.

EVALUATION

1. Inspect affected area for integrity, color, temperature, and sensitivity to touch. Reevaluate 30 minutes after procedure.
2. Palpate affected area gently of edema, bruising, and bleeding (apply gloves if there is risk of exposure to body fluids).
3. Ask patient to report pain level on scale of 0 to 10.
4. Measure ROM of affected body part.
5. **Use Teach-Back:** "I want to be sure I showed you how to apply an ice pack to your ankle. Show me how to apply an ice pack." Revise your instruction now or develop a plan for revised patient or family caregiver teaching if patient or family caregiver is not able to teach back correctly.

Determines reaction to cold application.

Determines level of edema.

Determines if pain has been relieved.
Determines if edema or muscle spasm is relieved.
Determines patient's and family caregiver's level of understanding of instructional topic.

STEP	RATIONALE
Unexpected Outcomes 1. Skin appears mottled, reddened, or bluish as a result of exposure to cold. 2. Patient complains of burning pain and numbness. 3. Patient or family caregiver is unable to describe or demonstrate therapy.	**Related Interventions** Stop treatment. Notify health care provider. Stop therapy. Notify health care provider. Provide further instruction and/or demonstration.

Recording and Reporting

- Record appearance and condition of skin and affected body part; procedure, including type, location, and duration of application; and patient's response on flow sheet in nurses' notes in electronic health record (EHR) or chart.
- Document your evaluation of patient and family caregiver learning.
- Report any sensations of burning, numbness, or unrelieved skin color changes to health care provider.

Special Considerations
Teaching

- Injuries requiring this type of therapy usually occur outside of acute care settings. Patients active in sports should know steps to take to minimize extent of injury.

Pediatric

- A greater metabolic rate and larger trunk in relation to the rest of the body make children more prone to hypothermia (Hockenberry and Wilson, 2015).
- Infants have an unstable temperature control mechanism; thus mottling of extremities is common and does not always indicate an adverse reaction (Hockenberry and Wilson, 2015).
- Cool soaks also decrease itching with some skin lesions. Use the same precautions and play techniques as with warm soaks.

Gerontological

- Older adults are more at risk for tissue damage because of altered responses to change in body temperature; therefore they need frequent skin assessment during treatment (Touhy and Jett, 2014).

◆ SKILL 42.4 Caring for Patients Requiring Hypothermia or Hyperthermia Blankets

A hypothermia or hyperthermia blanket raises, lowers, or maintains body temperature through conductive heat or cold transfer between the blanket and the patient (Fig. 42.6). When operated manually, the unit maintains a set temperature, regardless of the patient's temperature. Because you assess a patient's temperature using conventional thermometers, the temperature of the unit is adjusted manually to reach a different temperature setting. When operating in the automatic setting, the unit continually monitors a patient's temperature with a thermistor probe (rectal, skin, or esophageal).

Patients can have high, prolonged fevers from infectious neurological diseases, from side effects of anesthesia, and following severe brain injury (Bohman and Levine, 2014). Recent research

shows that induced hypothermia prevents or moderates neurological outcomes following neurosurgery, traumatic brain injury, and acute stroke (Bohman and Levine, 2014; Rittenberger and Callaway, 2016). Mild hypothermia (32°C to 34°C [89.6°F to 93.2°F]) in the first hours after an ischemic event and for 72 hours or until stabilization occurs helps prevent permanent damage.

Following severe trauma or major surgery such as cardiac surgery, thermoregulation is essential. Hypothermia causes vasoconstriction, shivering, increased oxygen demand, altered coronary blood flow, cardiac dysrhythmias, acid base imbalances, and impaired coagulation (Block et al., 2012; Kaplow, 2013). Therapeutic interventions designed to correct hypothermia and progressively raise body temperature are essential to improve patient outcomes by correcting three components: acid-base imbalances, body temperature, and coagulopathies. Each of these three components feed into one another and, if left uncorrected, result in death (Block et al., 2012).

Delegation and Collaboration

The skill of applying a hypothermia or hyperthermia blanket can be delegated to nursing assistive personnel (NAP) (see agency policy). The nurse is responsible for assessing and evaluating treatment and related patient education. If the patient is unstable and at risk for complications, this skill is not delegated. The nurse instructs the NAP to:

- Maintain proper temperature of the application throughout the treatment and discontinue the application as specified in the health care provider's order.
- Inform the nurse of any unexpected patient outcomes (e.g., shivering or redness to the skin).
- Report when treatment is complete so an evaluation of patient's response can be made.

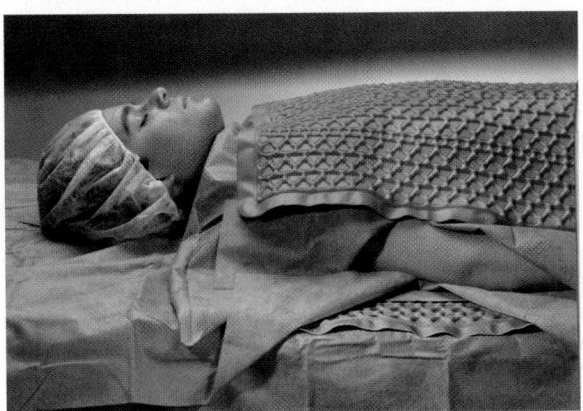

FIG 42.6 Hypothermia cooling blanket is applied over paper sheet before additional top sheet is applied to bed. *(Courtesy Cincinnati SubZero Maxi-Therm Hyper-Hypothermia Blanket.)*

Equipment

- Hypothermia or hyperthermia blanket with control panel and rectal probe
- Sheet or thin bath blanket
- Distilled water to fill the units if necessary
- Clean gloves
- Rectal thermometer

STEP	RATIONALE

ASSESSMENT

1. Identify patient using at least two identifiers (e.g., name and birthday or name and medical record number), according to agency policy.	Ensures correct patient. Complies with The Joint Commission standards and improves patient safety (TJC, 2016).
2. Refer to health care provider's order and check that patient's current body temperature indicates use of hypothermia or hyperthermia blanket.	Instituting therapy requires health care provider's order.
3. Perform hand hygiene. Obtain vital signs and assess neurological status, mental status, and peripheral circulation.	Establishes baseline data to use for comparison during therapy.
4. Verify that other less intensive measures cannot return patient's body temperature to normal.	Use of hypothermia or hyperthermia blanket is not without risk and should be instituted only when other measures are not effective.

Clinical Decision Point *Antipyretic therapy may be used in combination with a cooling blanket. Temperatures greater than 41°C (105.8°F) have detrimental effects in the neurological patient, children, and older adults (Cannon, 2013).*

5. Assess patient's skin on chest and extremities, paying close attention to bony prominences such as hands and feet.	These areas are more exposed to blanket and consequently are at greater risk for skin and tissue injury. Baseline data enable you to quickly determine if injury to skin or development of pressure injury is result of therapy.

NURSING DIAGNOSES

- Hyperthermia
- Hypothermia
- Impaired skin integrity
- Ineffective peripheral tissue perfusion
- Risk for injury

Related factors/Risk factors are individualized based on patient's condition or needs.

PLANNING

1. Expected outcomes following completion of procedure:	
• Temperature is within normal range.	Indicates that therapy is effective.
• Absence of shivering with hypothermia blanket.	Shivering increases metabolic rate and heat production but also increases oxygen consumption. In addition, shivering causes vasoconstriction, which can injure skin of distal body regions (Garner and Fendius, 2011; Rittenberger and Callaway, 2016).
• Skin is clear without signs of injury or burns.	Distal regions of patient's skin are at greatest risk for injury from blanket. Indicates that treatment is causing no adverse effects.
2. Explain procedure and precautions to patient or family caregiver.	Increases cooperation and reduces anxiety.
3. Prepare blanket according to agency policy and manufacturer instructions. Manufacturer instructions are usually located on machine.	Agencies have specific policies on maintaining equipment in functional order. Each type of blanket varies from one manufacturer to another.

IMPLEMENTATION

1. Perform hand hygiene and apply clean gloves. Position patient comfortably.	Reduces transmission of microorganisms.
2. Turn on blanket and observe that cool or warm light is on. Precool or prewarm blanket, setting pad temperature to desired level.	Verifies that blanket is set correctly to help reduce (cool) or increase (warm) patient's body temperature. Prepares blanket for prescribed therapy.
3. Verify that pad temperature limits are set at desired safety ranges.	Safety ranges prevent excessive cooling or warming. Blanket automatically shuts off when preset body temperature is achieved.

STEP	RATIONALE
4. Cover hypothermia or hyperthermia blanket with thin paper or cloth sheet or bath blanket.	Injuries from hot or cold therapies are preventable events (NQF, 2016). Thin sheet protects patient's skin from direct contact with blanket, thus reducing risk for injury to skin. Sheet or blanket covers plastic and provides insulation between patient and appliance.
5. Position hypothermia or hyperthermia blanket following manufacturer directions.	Provides distribution of blanket against patient's skin.
a. Wrap patient's hands and feet in gauze.	Reduces risk for thermal injury to distal areas of body.
b. Wrap scrotum with towels.	Protects sensitive tissue from direct contact with cold.
6. Lubricate rectal probe and insert into patient's rectum.	When using hypothermia or hyperthermia blanket, it is imperative that you monitor patient's core interior (rectal) temperature continuously.
7. Turn and position patient regularly to protect from pressure injury development and impaired body alignment (see Chapter 11). Keep linens free of perspiration and condensation.	Patient has increased risk for pressure injury development because of skin moisture created by blanket and patient's body temperature.
8. Double-check fluid thermometer on control panel of blanket before leaving room.	Verifies that pad temperature is maintained at desired level.
9. Remove gloves and perform hand hygiene.	Reduces transmission of microorganisms.

EVALUATION

1. Monitor patient's temperature and vital signs every 15 minutes during first hour and every 30 minutes of therapy thereafter.	Provides continuous evaluation of patient's response to therapy during initial and continual therapy.
2. Following initial evaluation of patient response to thermal regulation in Step 1, evaluate automatic temperature control every 30 minutes visually and every 4 hours by taking patient's rectal temperature.	Ensures removal of hypothermia or hyperthermia blanket when patient's temperature returns to desired level. Decreases risk for subnormal body temperature. Verifies accuracy of rectal probe and automatic temperature control device.
3. Observe skin for indications of burns, change in color, and other signs of injury.	Hypothermia and hyperthermia blankets have potential to cause skin injuries.
4. Observe patient for signs of shivering.	Early signs of shivering, which may harm patient, include electrocardiographic changes, facial muscle twitching, or hyperventilation.
5. Determine patient's level of comfort.	Therapy has potential to cause discomfort. Prompt assessment reduces risk for severe injuries.
6. **Use Teach-Back:** "I want to be sure I explained why this blanket is important for your loved one's care. Tell me why we are using the blanket?" Revise your instruction now or develop a plan for revised family caregiver teaching if family caregiver is not able to teach back correctly.	Determines family caregiver's level of understanding of instructional topic

Unexpected Outcomes	Related Interventions
1. Patient's core body temperature decreases or rises rapidly. This indicates that temperature is too extreme and might produce injury to patient.	• Adjust blanket temperature no more than 0.6°C (1°F) every 15 minutes to avoid complications.
2. Patient's core temperature remains unchanged.	• Patient may need hypothermic or hyperthermic treatment of sites such as axilla, groin, and neck in addition to those covered by blanket. • Discuss use of antipyretic with health care provider.
3. Patient begins to shiver. Shivering increases metabolic rate and heat production, causing patient's core body temperature to rise, and increases oxygen consumption.	• Adjust temperature to more comfortable range and assess if shivering decreases. • If shivering continues, stop treatment and notify health care provider.

Recording and Reporting

• Record baseline data: vital signs, neurological and mental status, status of peripheral circulation, and skin integrity when therapy was initiated. Include type of hyperthermia-hypothermia unit used; control settings (manual or automatic and temperature settings); date, time, duration; and patient's tolerance of treatment in nurses' notes in electronic health record (EHR) or chart.

• Chart on temperature graphic repeated measurements of vital signs to document response to therapy.

- Document your evaluation of family caregiver learning.
- Report any unexpected outcome to health care provider. Further treatment may be needed.

Special Considerations
Teaching
- Instruct patients and their families not to move patient off blanket.

Pediatric
- Infants have an unstable temperature-control mechanism; thus mottling of extremities is common and does not always indicate an adverse reaction (Hockenberry and Wilson, 2015).

Gerontological
- Some older adults are more at risk for tissue damage because of loss of cold sensation. Check patient frequently during all treatments (Touhy and Jett, 2014).

◆ CLINICAL DEBRIEF

You are assigned to care for a 58-year-old male patient with diabetes mellitus who is postoperative day 1 for total left knee arthroplasty. He has had diabetes mellitus type 1 since childhood and is regulated with insulin.

The surgeon has ordered an electronically controlled cold compression cuff to be applied to the left knee for 2 to 3 hours, followed by a 1- to 2-hour break with compression loosened. The patient is receiving pain medication by mouth every 4 hours for pain.

1. Place in correct order what you need to do to begin his cold application. Explain your choice(s).
   1. Refer to health care provider's order for location and duration of the application
   2. Explain the procedure and precautions to avoid injury to the skin
   3. Assess condition of injured or affected body part
   4. Assess current pain level
2. Because the patient has diabetes mellitus and some peripheral circulatory impairment, what is the major risk associated with cold application, and how would you assess for this risk?
3. After 24 hours of intermittent cold therapy using a compression cuff, the patient complains of a burning sensation and you observe a reddened 2-cm area and a blister on his skin under the compression cuff. Left leg is warm, normal color, with pulses present distal to compression cuff. Patient denies incisional pain. Incision is clean and intact. Using SBAR, show how you would communicate with the health care team about this patient.

◆ REVIEW QUESTIONS

1. Which of the following patients would be at risk for injury from heat application? (Select all that apply.)
   1. A patient with an acute ankle sprain
   2. A patient with a lot of body fat
   3. A patient being treated for anxiety
   4. A patient with peripheral vascular disease
   5. A patient with skin lesions
   6. A patient with altered sensation
2. The nurse is preparing to apply an electronically cooled device application to a patient's shoulder. Place the following steps in the correct sequence.
   1. Place cooling pad in a pillowcase or wrap in a towel.
   2. Assess patient's level of pain.
   3. Secure device with elastic bandage or roll.
   4. Turn device on and check correct temperature.
   5. Apply device to patient's shoulder.
3. A patient placed on a hypothermia blanket begins to shiver and also has an increased temperature. Both of these are a concern for this patient. Indicate which of the following body responses are associated with *Increased Temperature*.
   1. Increases patient's oxygen consumption
   2. Causes vasoconstriction
   3. Increases metabolic demand
   4. Increases amount of heat lost
   5. Increases body temperature

Ⓔ *Visit the Evolve site for a complete list of Clinical Debrief and Review Questions answers.*

REFERENCES

American College of Sports Medicine (ACSM): *Sprains, strains, and tears*, 2011, http://acsm.org/docs/brochures/sprains-strains-and-tears.pdf. Accessed February 8, 2016.

American Physical Therapy Association (APTA): *The physical therapist scope of practice*, 2016, http://www.apta.org/ScopeOfPractice/. Accessed August 20, 2016.

Bleakley CM, Costello JT: Do thermal agents affect range of movement and mechanical properties in soft tissues? A systematic review, *Arch Phys Med Rehabil* 94:140, 2013.

Block J, et al: Evidence-based thermoregulation for adult trauma patients, *Crit Care Nurs Q* 35:50, 2012.

Bohman L, Levine J: Fever and therapeutic normothermia in severe brain injury: an update, *Curr Opin Crit Care* 20:182, 2014.

Brooks G, et al: Musculoskeletal injury in children and skeletally immature adolescents: overview of treatment principles for nonoperative injuries, *UpToDate* 2015.

Cannon J: Perspective on fever: the basic science and conventional medicine, *Complement Ther Med* 21(Suppl 1):S54, 2013.

Chu CC, et al: Comparing the antiswelling and analgesic effects of three different ice pack therapy durations: a randomized controlled trial on cases with soft tissue injuries, *J Nurs Res* 21:186, 2013.

da Costa Santos V, et al: Effect of cryotherapy on the ankle temperature in athletes: ice pack and cold water immersion, *Fisioter Mov* 28:1, 2015.

Ewell M, et al: The use of focal knee joint cryotherapy to improve functional outcomes after total knee arthroplasty: review article, *PM R* 6:729, 2014.

Garner A, Fendius A: Temperature physiology, assessment and control, *Br J Neurosci Nurs* 6(8):397, 2011.

Giger J: *Transcultural nursing: assessment and interventions*, ed 7, St Louis, 2017, Mosby.

Hockenberry MJ, Wilson D: *Wong's nursing care of infants and children*, ed 10, St Louis, 2015, Elsevier.

Igaki M, et al: A study of the behavior and mechanism of thermal conduction in the skin under moist and dry heat conditions, *Skin Res Technol* 20:43, 2014.

Kadakia KC, et al: Supportive cryotherapy: a review from head to toe, *J Pain Symptom Manage* 47:1100, 2014.

Kaplow R: Safety of patients transferred from the operating room to the intensive care unit, *Crit Care Nurse* 33:86, 2013.

Maughan K: Ankle injury, *UpToDate* 2016. http://www.uptodate.com/contents/ankle-sprain. Accessed August 20, 2016.

Maxwell S, Sterling M: An investigation of the use of a numeric pain-rating scale with ice application to the neck to determine cold hyperalgesia, *Man Ther* 18:172, 2013.

Nakano J, et al: The effect of heat applied with stretch to increase range of motion: a systematic review, *Phys Ther Sport* 13:180, 2012.

National Quality Forum (NQF): *Patient safety 2015: final technical report*, Washington, DC, 2016, Author.

Petrofsky JS, et al: Effect of heat and cold on tendon flexibility and force to flex the human knee, *Med Sci Monit* 19:661, 2013.

Rittenberger J, Callaway C: Post-cardiac arrest management in adults, *UpToDate* 2016. http://www.uptodate.com/contents/post-cardiac-arrest-management-in-adults. Accessed August 20, 2016.

The Joint Commission: *2016 National Patient Safety Goals (NPGs)*, 2016, TJC. https://www.jointcommission.org/assets/1/6/2016_NPSG_HAP_ER.pdf. Accessed August 18, 2016.

Touhy TA, Jett KF: *Ebersole and Hess' Gerontological nursing & healthy aging*, ed 4, 2014, Elsevier.

Home Care Safety

OBJECTIVES

Mastery of content in this chapter will enable the nurse to:
- Identify clients at risk for safety problems and possible accidents in the home.
- Promote self-care of clients in the home.
- Describe the factors within a home environment that create risks for client injury.
- Perform a home safety risk assessment.

- Identify interventions that modify the home environment for physical safety.
- Identify interventions to reduce safety risks for clients with sensory, cognitive, and mental status alterations.
- Recommend strategies to ensure safe drug administration within the home.
- Perform a geriatric fall risk assessment.

MEDIA RESOURCES

- eVOlVe http://evolve.elsevier.com/Perry/skills
- Review Questions

- Clinical Debrief and Review Questions Answers

PURPOSE

Safety for clients in the home setting includes anticipating and preventing injuries (Berland et al., 2012). The CDC (2014a) describes a healthy home as one that is sited, designed, built, renovated, and maintained to support health. Injuries and violence impact one's sense of security and can affect an individual, the family, and the community. *Healthy People 2020* identifies injury and violence prevention as a topic area, with objectives geared toward preventing unintentional injuries (USDHHS, 2014). Home care safety begins before a client is discharged from a health care agency. A home care nurse and interprofessional team collaborate with the client to assess the home environment for risks, with a goal to select appropriate interventions for preventing unintentional injuries.

STANDARDS OF CARE

- Centers for Disease Control and Prevention (CDC), 2014—Medication Safety Program
- National Fire Protection Association (NFPA), 2013—Home Safety
- Quality and Safety Education for Nurses (QSEN), 2014—Pre-licensure KSAS
- US Department of Health and Human Services (USDHHS): *Healthy People 2020*, 2014—Injury and Violence Prevention

PRINCIPLES FOR PRACTICE

- The term "client" is used in home care settings due to the collaborative relationship with the interprofessional team.

- Home care safety involves communication among a client, family caregivers, and interprofessional home care providers.
- The ultimate goal is to create an environment in which a client and family caregiver can provide self-care safely and effectively.
- Insurance coverage, including Medicare, can be very limited for home care. Therefore the time spent in the home with the client must be well planned and used to the fullest.
- Clients living in socioeconomically disadvantaged areas may be at increased risk for injury as a result of violence or poor living conditions.
- Fall prevention is a critical aspect of care for older adults, especially in the community. Conduct a client history to assess for risk factors in the home and surrounding community and reasons for recent falls to plan appropriate interventions.

CLIENT-CENTERED CARE

- Respect a client's home. In home care nursing you are a guest. Take time to listen to a client's health concerns and apply the knowledge you have about the client to understand which interventions within the home are likely to be accepted by a client and the family caregiver.
- Communication is essential in home care and is a continuous process between you and a client. At the first meeting introduce yourself, explaining how you would like the client to address you, and ask the client how you should refer to him or her. If a language barrier exists, have a professional interpreter assist you.
- Collaborate with clients in assessing their home environments. Ask them if they are willing to give you a tour of their home

and explain the purpose. Do not focus on what is wrong (e.g., barriers or features in disrepair), point out why safety is an issue for the client (based on health condition), and explain why a change in a feature of the home will make him or her safer.

- Assess for culture-specific health-related beliefs that may impact a client's willingness to use home care services. For example, some clients may prefer to care for their older-adult family members in the home without outside help (Crist and Speaks, 2011).
- When assessing the availability of family caregivers in the home, recognize that families can value the role of caregivers in different ways. With the client's permission, include these family caregivers when performing the home safety assessment.
- Assess and provide support for informal and family caregivers; the presence or absence of these could be the difference between a client remaining in the home or being readmitted to an acute care facility (Buch and Nies, 2014).

- Barriers to safe care, including physical structure, access, and lack of qualified home care providers

With the increasing number of older adults living with dementia, Bekhet (2013) examined positive cognition and resourcefulness among family caregivers. Positive cognition is the ability to think in a positive way when faced with a challenging situation (e.g., caring for a client with dementia). An individual's resourcefulness has been tied to resilience. This study involved surveys of 80 family caregivers. The findings were encouraging in identifying strategies to help nurses and family caregivers deal with burden and develop healthy coping strategies:

- Family caregivers of people with dementia may benefit from positive cognition interventions such as programs to help family caregivers use positive self-talk, reframe situations positively, break a problem down to make it seem more manageable, and use relaxation techniques (Bekhet, 2013).
- Support family caregivers to practice these techniques so they can integrate them into their lives.

EVIDENCE-BASED PRACTICE

Home care safety addresses the physical environment and the clients and family caregivers who are the focus of care. Lang et al. (2014) conducted a qualitative study to examine the perceptions of safety in home care from the perspectives of the home care clients, family caregivers, and providers. Semi-structured interviews and two focus groups allowed for collection of data at multiple sites. Safety was explored in different ways, including functional, emotional, physical, and social safety, allowing for a multidimensional approach to care. Key findings highlighted six patterns related to safety concerns of all participants:

- The desire to remain at home and maintain some degree of independence, control, and normalcy
- Concerns for the ability to pay for portable oxygen supplies
- Growing burden and responsibility facing family caregivers as clients' conditions deteriorated
- Cleanliness of the home and ability to maintain the surroundings
- Deteriorating health of the family caregivers and impact of this on the client

SAFETY GUIDELINES

- Accident prevention begins with making timely and adequate home repairs (e.g., replacing loose floor tile, securing railings on stairwells). When clients do not have the resources for maintaining a safe home environment, a nurse's role is to help identify appropriate resources or services in the community.
- The nurse plays an important role in improving and maintaining a client's safety by collaborating with clients, family caregivers, and health care providers in the community in finding the best approaches for meeting a client's safety needs.
- The ultimate goal is to create an environment in which client and family can provide self-care safely and effectively.
- When helping a client change the home environment, retain as much of his or her independence and ability to provide self-care as possible.
- Ask if client and/or family caregiver has concerns or questions about safety and if he or she has any suggestions to improve safety (Mullin, 2010).
- Make modifications to the home environment only after considering client's physical strengths, remaining functional abilities, and resources for making change.

◆ **SKILL 43.1** **Home Environment Assessment and Safety**

The home environment should be a place where individuals feel healthy, comfortable, and safe. People want to be able to move about freely within their homes, regardless of the size of the home, and to have a sense of control over daily living routines. This requires maintaining personal space and a sense of privacy. As the home care nurse you can help a client maintain independence and reduce risk in the home environment by conducting a safety assessment.

Clients requiring home care often experience physical alterations (e.g., progressive physical changes of aging) that require changes in their home environment. For example, if a client has poor balance but good upper-arm strength, you may need to make modifications (e.g., install handrails on both sides of a staircase and in bathroom areas) so he or she can safely walk or move throughout the house, ascend and descend stairs, and enter and exit a bathtub or shower. Teaching a client to safely use assistive devices (e.g., walker or cane) helps him or her increase mobility and maintain independence (Fig. 43.1).

Respect the concept of personal space. Making changes too rapidly without a client's consent causes more problems than benefits. Appreciate the arrangement of a client's space within the home and do not move things or suggest modifications without permission. Provide a rationale to the client as to why the changes are beneficial and/or needed. Knowing the rooms that a client uses most frequently helps make the adjustments to create a safe environment.

Delegation and Collaboration

The skill of conducting an initial home safety assessment cannot be delegated to nursing assistive personnel (NAP). The nurse instructs the NAP to:

- Inform the nurse of suggestions for ways to make the home safer.

Equipment

- Home safety checklist

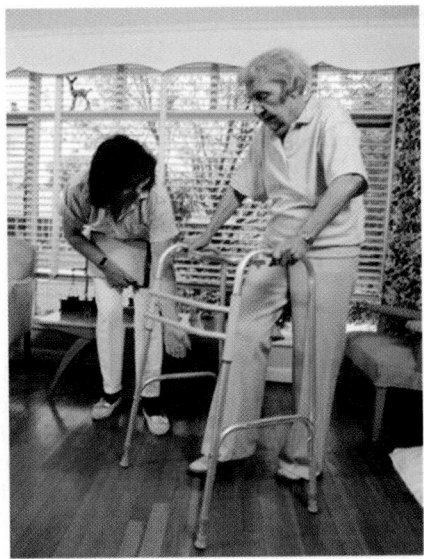

FIG 43.1 Use of walker may help client remain mobile.

STEP	RATIONALE

ASSESSMENT

1. Review risk factors that predispose clients to accidents within the home:

a. Known visual impairment

Reduced visual function alters client's balance, depth perception, or adaptation to dark or glaring light (Touhy and Jett, 2014).

b. Hearing impairment

Prevents client from hearing normal environmental sounds (e.g., call out by family member) clearly as source of orientation. Prevents clear perception of home-installed alarms (e.g., smoke alarm).

Interferes with communication for clients to hear and interpret what you are saying (Touhy and Jett, 2014).

c. Neuromuscular alterations (e.g., lower-extremity weakness, unsteady gait, impaired balance, poor ankle dorsiflexion)

Factors predispose clients to falls. Recurrent falls are associated with difficulty standing up from chair (Touhy and Jett, 2014).

d. Reduced energy or fatigue

Predisposes clients to falls.

e. Incontinence or nocturia

Frequent trips to bathroom often cause client with other deficits to accidentally trip or fall over barriers. Dementia does not cause incontinence, but it affects client's ability to find bathroom and recognize need to void (Touhy and Jett, 2014).

f. History of stroke, parkinsonism, delirium, seizures, dementia, syncope

These conditions present multiple reasons for falls, including impaired gait and coordination, visual changes, diminished cognition, pain, muscle weakness, and polypharmacy (Hill and Fauerbach, 2014).

Gait disorders make clients vulnerable to tripping and falling (Hill and Fauerbach, 2014). Age-related changes of neurological system include slowing of reaction time (Meiner, 2015).

g. Cardiopulmonary conditions: postural hypotension, arrhythmias, palpitations, difficulty breathing, or shortness of breath

Dizziness, fatigue and light-headedness predispose to falls (Touhy and Jett, 2014) and cause client to be unsteady and compensate for difficulties.

h. Medication usage and history, including polypharmacy and use of sedatives, antihypertensives, antidepressants, and diuretics

Use of multiple medications has been associated with falls. Medications that alter sensorium affect balance and judgment (Muir et al., 2010).

i. History of previous fall— obtain detailed description of previous fall

Increases risk for future fall. Helps identify circumstances that may lead to fall (Hill and Fauerbach, 2014).

STEP	RATIONALE

2. Determine if client has fallen in home or had other injuries within home. Be specific in your assessment. Use mnemonic SPLATT (Meiner, 2015):

- *Symptoms at time of fall*
- *Previous fall*
- *Location of fall*
- *Activity at time of fall*
- *Time of fall*
- *Trauma after fall*

Key symptoms are helpful in identifying cause of fall. Onset, location, and activity associated with fall provide further details on causative factors and how to prevent future falls.

SPLATT test allows client to explain symptoms in own words; it is important to understand circumstances around fall (Meiner, 2015).

3. Have client who has had a near fall or actual fall maintain a fall diary (Box 43.1).

Information in fall diary is very helpful in determining antecedents and consequences of falling (Meiner, 2015).

4. Conduct timed get-up-and-go (TGUG) test for basic mobility (see Skill 14.1).

Simple screening examination is very useful in detecting difficulties with balance or gait. Helps in diagnosis and treatment of underlying causes; refer to physical therapist for gait and progressive balance training (Touhy and Jett, 2014). TGUG time performance is associated with past history of falls, but its predictive ability for future falls remains limited (Beauchet et al., 2011).

5. Determine if client has fear of falling. Possible indicators include apprehension during ambulation (observed in facial expressions); sweating or trembling while ambulating; clutching people or objects while ambulating; reluctance to change position or ambulate; and new onset of wobbly, reduced mobility after fall.

Fear of falling occurs variably in older adults. Some clients may restrict mobility and participation in activities of daily living (ADLs) or instrumental activities of daily living (IADLs) because of fear of falling (Hill and Fauerbach, 2014).

Clinical Decision Point *In addition to client, include family caregivers as a resource in assessments because they may witness accident trends or patterns.*

6. Partner with client and family caregivers to conduct home safety assessment:

Provides comprehensive review of all areas within home that pose hazardous situations.

  a. Front and back entrances:

    (1) Are walkways to front/back door even and free from holes or cracks?

Entrances pose barriers in surfaces over which client must walk. Uneven pavement and holes may not be seen by client, causing tripping and falls.

    (2) Are home entrances, including walkways, well lit?

Poorly lit areas prevent individuals from seeing variations in walking surface.

    (3) Does client have nonskid strips/safety treads or bright-colored paint on outdoor steps? Which colors are most easily seen by client? Are these colors used?

Nonskid surfaces cause fewer slips on stairs. Color on steps permits individual to see edges, accommodating for any reduced depth perception.

    (4) Are doormats in good repair with nonskid backing and tapered edge?

Raised edges pose risk for tripping. Doormats without nonskid backing slide when stepped on, causing client to lose balance.

    (5) Are doors in good repair, and do they open and close easily? Can client open and close all doors easily?

Act of opening and closing door is difficult if grasp is weak. Tripping may occur during opening and cause fall.

    (6) Is there sturdy handrail on both sides of stairs leading to entrance?

Handrails provide greater support while ascending and descending stairs.

BOX 43.1

Fall/Near-Fall Diary

- Keep a notebook and create across the longest edge of the paper these headings: "Date," "Time of Fall," "Activity at Time of Fall," "Symptoms," and "Injury."
- As soon as possible after a fall, have client or family caregiver complete information under each heading.

- List emergency contact numbers at the bottom of the fall diary for client to call in case a fall results in serious injury.
- Instruct client to bring the diary to the health care provider's office at the next scheduled visit or share information with home care nurse on next home visit.

Modified from Meiner SE: *Gerontologic nursing*, ed 5, St Louis, 2015, Mosby.

STEP	RATIONALE
(7) Are steps in good condition with even, flat surfaces?	Uneven surfaces predispose to tripping.
(8) Are doorways and stairs free of clutter?	Reduces risk for tripping and/or falling.
b. Kitchen:	Kitchen is one of most hazard-oriented rooms in home. Poses serious hazards for fire.
(1) Does client wear clothing with short or close-fitting sleeves when cooking?	Short or close-fitting sleeves are less likely to accidentally catch on fire when person works at stove.
(2) Does client always stay in kitchen when cooking?	Lack of attention when using fire is risk.
(3) Does client have loud timer to signal when food is cooked?	Prevents burning food and risk for fire.
(4) Does client keep stove top and oven clean and grease free?	Grease is highly flammable.
(5) Are stove control dials easy to see and use?	Client may accidentally use higher flame than is necessary for cooking safely.
(6) Is charged, easy-to-use fire extinguisher close at hand?	Extinguisher should be ready for use at all times.

Clinical Decision Point *Have client demonstrate steps of how to use fire extinguisher.*

STEP	RATIONALE
(7) Are emergency numbers for police, fire, and poison control posted on or near telephone?	Emergency phone numbers and extinguisher ensure quick response if fire occurs.
(8) Can items in kitchen cabinets and shelves be reached without climbing on stool or chair?	Climbing on step stools or chairs creates risks for falls.
(9) Is there adequate lighting over sink, stove, and work areas?	Poor lighting makes it difficult to see control knobs or dials and provides inadequate illumination when using sharp knives or utensils (Touhy and Jett, 2014).
(10) Are kitchen throw rugs and mats slip resistant?	Rugs or mats that are not slip resistant can easily slide on tile or wood floors.
(11) Assess food safety: Are perishable foods in refrigerator and nonperishable foods safe to eat? Is food stored appropriately? Are expiration dates past? Is there evidence that food has spoiled? Does client know how to prepare and store food safely?	Proper food storage and preparation can prevent foodborne illnesses. One basic of food safety is cooking food to its proper temperature. Foods are properly cooked when they are heated for long enough time and at high enough temperature to kill harmful bacteria that cause foodborne illness (Foodsafety.gov, 2015). Eating foods that have spoiled or with expiration dates that have passed puts client at risk for foodborne illness (e.g., food poisoning).
c. Bathroom:	
(1) Can client unlock bathroom door from both sides of door?	Functional locks prevent person from being trapped in bathroom.
(2) Is tub or shower equipped with nonskid mats, abrasive strips, or surfaces that are not slippery?	Bathrooms are hazardous. Wet floors and tub or shower bottoms can be very slippery, creating risk for falls.
(3) Does bathroom floor have nonslip surface or rug with nonskid backing?	Slippery tile predisposes to falls (Touhy and Jett, 2014).
(4) Does client avoid using slippery bath oils when bathing?	Use of bath oils makes tub surface slippery and increases risk for falls.
(5) Do bathtub and shower have at least one grab bar or handrail placed where client can reach it?	Grab bars provide extra support while maneuvering into and out of tubs or showers. Grab bars placed correctly where client can safely reach them help to steady gait and lessen chance of falls (Meiner, 2015).
(6) Is client careful not to place towels on grab bars?	Some clients accidentally grab towel instead of bar when needing support. Towel can slip off bar.
(7) Does shower have stable stool or chair and handheld sprayer? Is shower easy to access (walk-in versus step-in to tub area)?	Shower stool allows client to sit while showering.
(8) Are cold and hot water faucets clearly marked, and is temperature on water heater 48.8° C (120° F) or lower?	Accidental burns can occur from exposure to hot water.
d. Bedroom:	
(1) Is night-light placed in bedroom and/or bath?	Older adults have altered night vision.
(2) Is working smoke detector just outside bedroom door?	Alarm situated just outside bedroom can awaken person early enough to escape fire.

STEP	RATIONALE
(3) Can client turn on light without having to get out of bed in dark? Is flashlight available at bedside? Flashlight can be attached to walker or cane (Touhy and Jett, 2014).	Getting out of bed without proper lighting or ability to adjust to light changes and reaching for necessary objects puts client at risk for falls.
(4) Is furniture arranged to provide clear path from bed to bathroom?	Obstructed path creates barrier that causes tripping and falls.
(5) Is phone with emergency numbers within easy reach of bed?	If clients develop physical symptoms while in bed, they need to be able to reach phone without having to get out of bed.
(6) Are other alarm systems available? Push buttons that call for help? Nursery listening devices for cognitively impaired or nonambulatory clients?	Alarm systems placed in readily accessible location can alert family caregivers when person requires immediate help. Bedside phone, cordless phone, intercom buzzer, or lifeline can be placed in readily accessible location (Touhy and Jett, 2014).
e. Living room/family room:	
(1) Are electrical or extension cords removed from under furniture and carpeting? Kept out of way of traffic?	Clients can easily trip or fall over electrical cords. Hidden cords are trip and fire hazards.
(2) Can client turn on light without having to walk into dark room?	Darkened room can disorient and prevent client from seeing uneven surfaces.
(3) Are hallways and walkways free from objects and clutter?	Objects and clutter in common walkway can cause client to trip, resulting in falls.
(4) Are loose area rugs securely attached to floor and not placed over carpeting? (For best safety, consider removing throw rugs.)	Loose edges of rugs are easy for persons to trip over (Touhy and Jett, 2014).
(5) Is furniture arranged in each room so client can walk around easily?	Furniture creates obstacles to walking in room.
(6) Is all furniture steady and without sharp edges?	Clients often use edge of furniture for support when standing.
f. Around the house:	
(1) Are all living areas and stairways well lit?	Adequate lighting helps people see any barriers or uneven walking surfaces.
(2) Is flooring or carpeting throughout house in good repair?	Frayed carpet or irregular surfaces can cause tripping and result in fall.
(3) Are all thresholds level with floor or no more than 1.27 cm (½ inch) in height?	Uneven thresholds can cause tripping.
(4) Is light switch at both top and bottom of stairs?	Prevents individual from having to walk part of stairs in dark.
(5) Does lighting produce glare or shadows on stairs or floor surfaces?	Older adults are sensitive to glare because their visual pathway becomes distorted.
(6) Do handrails run continuously from top to bottom of flights of stairs?	Handrails provide source of physical support when ascending and descending stairs.
(7) Are handrails securely attached to wall?	Handrails should be installed at least on one side of hallway or stairwell (Touhy and Jett, 2014).
(8) Are step coverings in good condition?	Loosened covering can cause tripping.
(9) Are guns kept in house? Are trigger locks installed on all guns? Are guns stored unloaded? Is ammunition in secure location?	Following gun safety standards decreases risk for injury and death related to gun use (NRA, 2015).
g. General fire safety:	
(1) Does client have properly working smoke detectors with fresh batteries?	Smoke alarms properly located, functioning well, and with batteries replaced twice a year can provide timely alert for fire.

Clinical Decision Point *Check to see when smoke-alarm battery was last changed; battery should be changed every 6 months. Instruct clients to change battery each time they change their house clocks for daylight savings.*

STEP	RATIONALE
(2) Does client have several emergency exit plans in case of fire?	Exit plan helps people anticipate route of escape when fire does occur. Exit should not have locks that are difficult to open or any physical barriers.
(3) Has family determined meeting place in event of emergency such as at mailbox in front of home?	Use of common emergency meeting location is efficient method for determining that all family members are safely out of house.
(4) Does client use portable space heaters? Are they kept at least 1 meter (3 feet) away from flammable items?	Heaters, furnaces, and chimneys pose risks for fire.
(5) Is furnace area free of things that can catch on fire?	Heating equipment was second-most common cause of home fire fatalities from 2007 through 2011 (NFPA, 2013).

STEP	RATIONALE
(6) Does qualified professional check furnace and chimney annually?	Buildup of creosote within chimney can catch on fire. Overheated motor in furnace can burn out and possibly cause fire.
(7) Does client who smokes report smoking in bed?	Smoking materials were fifth leading cause of home fire deaths in 2007 through 2011 (NFPA, 2013). Smoking in bed has added risk of client falling asleep while cigarette is lit.
h. General electrical safety:	
(1) Are electrical cords in good condition (i.e., not frayed, spliced, or cracked)?	Damaged cords can short circuit and lead to fire.
(2) Are electrical cords kept away from water?	Use of any appliance or device that is exposed to water creates risk for electrical shock.
(3) Does client use extension cord/outlet extenders with built-in circuit breaker or fuse?	Prevents overloading of circuit that can lead to fire.
(4) Do all wall outlets and switches have cover plates?	Prevents physical contact with wiring.
(5) Does client use light bulbs of correct wattage for each fixture?	Use of excessive wattage can lead to fire.
(6) Is main electrical fuse box for home easily accessible and clearly labeled?	In event of emergency, fuse box should be easy to access so proper circuit can be cut off.
i. Carbon monoxide prevention:	
(1) Are furnace flues checked regularly for patency?	Obstructed flues are common cause of carbon monoxide toxicity.
(2) Is there working carbon monoxide detector in home?	
7. Assess client's financial resources; determine monthly income used for ongoing expenses.	Determines potential for making repairs to home. Reveals need for low-cost community service support.
8. Assess client's and family caregiver's willingness to make changes. Has client accepted limitations that pose risk for injury? Determine how important functional independence is for client.	Some clients perceive attempts to improve safety within home as intrusive. If you show that necessary revisions to home environment will preserve independence, client will participate more willingly.

NURSING DIAGNOSES

- Anxiety
- Deficient knowledge regarding safety risks
- Impaired home maintenance
- Impaired memory
- Impaired physical mobility
- Ineffective health maintenance
- Risk for falls
- Risk for foodborne illness
- Risk for injury

Related factors/Risk factors are individualized based on client's condition or needs.

PLANNING

1. Expected outcomes following completion of procedure:	
• Client and/or family caregiver describes potential environmental risks within home that predispose to accidents.	Demonstrates client's and family caregiver's recognition of safety risks that are of greatest concern.
• Client and/or family caregiver initiate actions to correct environmental risks, making home safer.	Client sees value in altering living environment.
• Client remains free of injury.	Environmental barriers are reduced or removed to minimize injuries.
2. Prioritize with client and family caregiver environmental barriers that pose greatest risk.	Client's own physical and/or cognitive deficits make certain environmental risks more hazardous. Prioritization helps client make best choices.
3. Recommend calling in reliable contractor if major home repairs are necessary and acceptable to client and family.	Ensures that repairs are made safely and correctly.

IMPLEMENTATION

1. General home safety:	
a. Provide direct light source in areas where client reads, cooks, uses tools, or conducts hobby work. High-intensity light on object or surface that is involved works best.	Visual impairment in older adults usually is result of cataracts, macular degeneration, glaucoma, or diabetic retinopathy (Touhy and Jett, 2014).

Clinical Decision Point *Avoid fluorescent lighting because it creates excessive glare.*

STEP	RATIONALE
b. Consider satin and nonglossy finishes for walls, cabinets, and countertops in kitchen. Have sheer curtains or adjustable shades in other living areas.	Reduces glare for older adults.
c. Apply colored tape or paint to color code controls of stove, oven, dryer, toaster, and other appliances.	Clients with reduced visual acuity may adjust appliance to wrong setting, creating potential risk for fire or burning.
d. Consider installing lazy Susan or pull-out drawers with glide mechanisms in kitchen cabinets. Install C-ring handles in lower cabinets.	Makes access to food and kitchen supplies easier.
e. Install automatic door openers, level doorknob handles, and hook-and-chain locks.	Devices may be easier to grasp and use. Remote-controlled door locks can also provide additional security (Touhy and Jett, 2014).
2. Fall prevention steps:	
a. Paint edges of concrete stairs bright yellow, orange, or white.	Client can see edge of stairs more clearly.
b. Install treads with uniform depth of 22.5 cm (9 inches) and 22.5-cm (9-inch) risers (vertical face of steps).	If stairs are of uniform size, client does not have to continually adjust vision or stride.
c. Rearrange furniture to open up space through hallways and major rooms.	Creates unobstructed pathway for ambulation.
d. Reduce clutter within living areas (e.g., footstools, flower pots, extension cords, children's toys, stacked newspapers or magazines).	Mobility hazards resulting from clutter are especially risky at night.
e. Secure all carpeting, mats, and tile; place nonskid backing under small rugs and doormats. Remove throw rugs/mats in nonessential (dry) areas.	Reduces chance of client slipping when stepping on rug surface (Touhy and Jett, 2014).
f. Pad floor and use specialized tile that absorbs impact of falls.	Cushions person's fall.
g. Use low-rise beds, futon beds, or mattress on floor if not contraindicated.	Lowers distance to floor surface.
h. Have enough electrical outlets installed to be able to plug light or electronic device (e.g., television, video) into nearby outlet. Secure electrical cords against baseboards.	Prevents need to run extension cords across walkways.
i. Install nonskid strips on surface of bathtub and/or shower stall. Be sure that floor is clean and dry.	Reduces chances of slipping on tub/shower stall surface.
j. Have grab bar installed in studs at tub, toilet, and/or shower (see illustration). Have client select vertical or horizontal placement if choice available. Be sure that bar is different color than wall and easy to see.	Bar provides stability for maneuvering in bathroom (Touhy and Jett, 2014). Grab bars placed in correct place where client can safely reach them help to steady stance and gait and lessen chance of falls (Meiner, 2015).
k. Have handrails installed along side of any stairway (see illustration). Be sure that stairways are well lit, with switches at top and bottom of steps.	Ideally handrails on both sides of stairwell provide greatest stability for client. If entrance space does not allow this, install at least on one side to prevent fall from imbalance (Touhy and Jett, 2014). Older adults have difficulty seeing edges of stairs.
l. Install appropriate broad-beam lighting for outside walkways.	Provides full illumination.
m. Keep lighted phone easily accessible, next to client's bed.	Prevents client from having to get up out of bed, often in dark.
n. Install motion-sensor exterior lighting for walkways/driveway.	Reduces risk for client falls caused by dark surroundings.
o. Have client use padding or types of clothing that will cushion bony prominences, especially high-risk bony prominences (e.g., hips). Specially designed hip protectors are available.	Helps to absorb impact of falling body.
3. Prevent spread of infection	
a. Teach client and family caregiver cleaning practices to prevent spread of infection.	Ensures more consistent infection control practices in the home.
b. Instruct client not to share eating and drinking utensils.	Some infections are spread by saliva.
c. Instruct client to clean appliances and surfaces daily.	Regular cleaning prevents risk for contamination and spread of infection.

STEP	RATIONALE

d. Instruct client in safe food preparation and storage. Refer to guidelines in Foodsafety.gov. For example:

- 4–12 lb turkey can safely be thawed in refrigerator for 1–3 days or in cold water for 6–12 hours; cook poultry to 165°F.

Ensures safe thawing and cooking of foods (Foodsafety.gov, 2015).

- Bacon can be stored in refrigerator for 7 days and freezer for 1 month; hamburger and other ground meats can be stored in refrigerator for 1–2 days and in freezer for 3–4 months.

Safe storage times for food in refrigerator and freezer helps prevent foodborne illnesses (Foodsafety.gov, 2015).

4. Fire safety

a. Have smoke detectors installed near each bedroom, in kitchen, and in home basement. Be sure that detector is on each floor of home. Alarm should be close to alert client and family when sleeping.

Fires most frequently start in basement near furnace, dryer, or electrical wiring; kitchen; or living areas where there is extensive wiring.

b. Have client select fire extinguisher that is easy to handle and manipulate (see illustration). Ask him or her to read instructions and demonstrate its proper use.

Some older adults or clients with disabilities have difficulty gripping mechanisms on certain extinguishers.

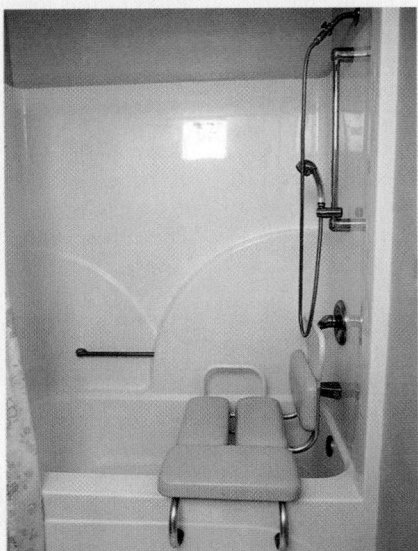

STEP 2j Grab bars and safety seat installed in shower.

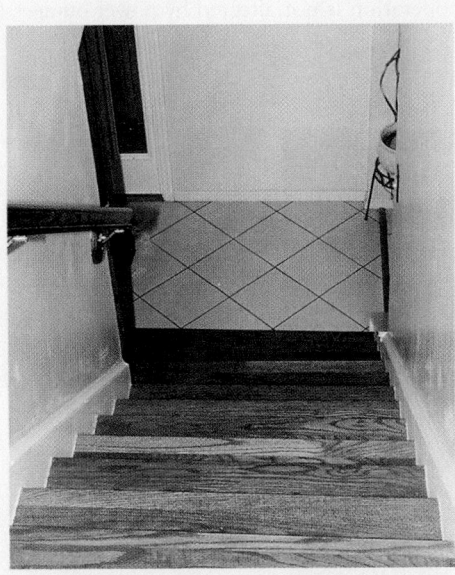

STEP 2k Handrails installed along stairways provide security for clients with visual, balance, and coordination problems.

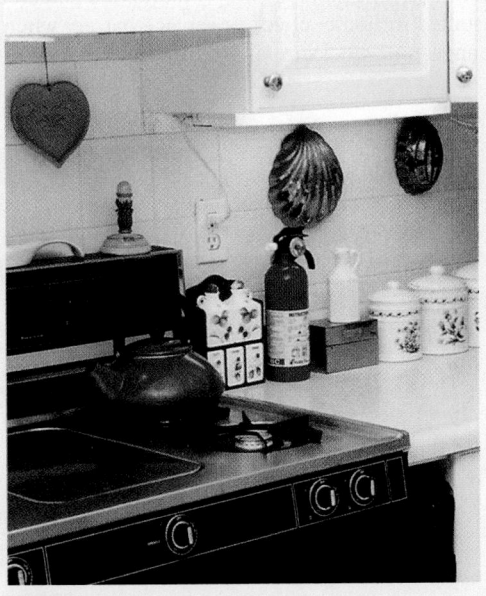

STEP 4b Fire extinguisher accessible in kitchen.

STEP	RATIONALE

c. Have area around furnace cleared of any flammable items.

Reduces risk for fire.

d. Instruct client to be sure that portable space heater has emergency shut off and that equipment housing and electrical cords are intact (Meiner, 2015).

Space heaters can be overturned by accident, which can cause fire; safety mechanism on newer models will turn unit off immediately (Meiner, 2015).

e. Have client make appointments for maintenance of furnace and chimney cleaning in appropriate season.

Furnace maintenance prevents short circuits and fires. Accumulation of creosote on chimney walls can lead to fire.

f. Have client check light-bulb wattage in all fixtures.

Ensures proper wattage being used; wattage that exceeds recommendation can cause fire.

g. Have client establish routine during cooking that keeps him or her in kitchen. Be sure that cooking range is clean and items such as potholders and towels are away from burners.

Food cooking on stove can easily boil over or begin to burn when unattended.

h. If client is a smoker, review need to keep ashtrays clean and emptied. Placing small amount of water or sand in bottom of ashtray is useful if client is visually impaired.

Clients with reduced vision may be unable to tell if cigarette, cigar, or match has extinguished.

i. Strongly discourage smoking in bed, smoking in chair when there is possibility of falling asleep, and smoking after taking medication that diminishes alertness. Instruct client/family caregiver to put cigarette or cigar out at first sign of feeling drowsy (Meiner, 2015).

Risks factors for burns and fire. Client's reaction time may be slower when tired.

j. Recommend that client install power strips or surge protectors for plugging in multiple appliances/devices.

Prevents risk for electrical short, which can cause fire.

5. Burn safety:

a. Have setting on hot water heater adjusted to 49°C (120°F) or lower.

Prevents scalding burns (Meiner, 2015).

b. Instruct client to always turn cold water on first.

Prevents direct exposure to hot water.

c. Install touch pads on lamps.

Light is easy to turn on without risk of touching hot light bulb.

d. Use color codes of red for hot and blue for cold on water faucets. (If client has difficulty distinguishing these colors, choose two that are easily distinguished.)

Prevents accidental burning from turning on wrong faucet.

6. Carbon monoxide safety:

a. Have condition of furnace venting checked annually just before turning on furnace.

Improper venting prevents escape of carbon monoxide, a poisonous gas that alters hemoglobin to prevent formation of oxyhemoglobin and reduces oxygen supply to tissues.

b. Caution clients against using gas stove or barbecue grill for heating inside home.

Both are sources of carbon monoxide (Meiner, 2015).

c. Have battery-operated carbon monoxide detector installed in home; check or replace battery when you change your clocks in fall and spring (see illustration).

Detector alarms when carbon monoxide reaches unsafe levels. Battery operation is not affected by power outages (Meiner, 2015).

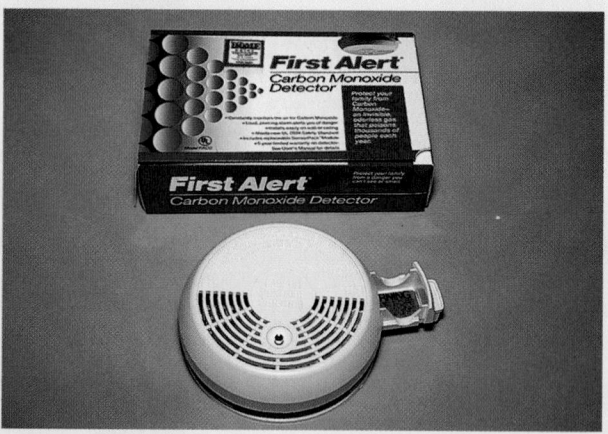

STEP 6c Carbon monoxide detector.

STEP	RATIONALE

7. Firearm safety:
  a. Teach client about dangers associated with keeping guns in home.
  b. If guns are in home, teach client to install trigger locks and store them unloaded in locked cabinet. Teach client to store ammunition in secured area separate from guns. Store keys in place inaccessible to children.
	Risk of suicide increases in homes with firearms (Edelman et al., 2014).
	Following gun safety standards decreases risk of injury and death related to gun use (Hockenberry and Wilson, 2015).

EVALUATION

1. Have client and family caregiver(s) identify safety risks revealed in home safety assessment.	Demonstrates what client recognizes as risk and its relative importance for changing.
2. During follow-up visit or call to home ask client to discuss plans for making any modifications and observe changes client has implemented.	Evaluates extent to which client sees risks as potentially harmful and complies with suggested changes.
3. During follow-up visits or calls ask if client has experienced any falls or other injuries within home.	Reveals if risks have been eliminated, depending on client's previous history of injury.
4. During subsequent home visits, reassess for progression of dementia.	Evaluates for potential new risks to client and caregiver.
5. Use Teach-Back: "I want to be sure I explained why you need to make modifications in your home. Tell me why this important." Revise your instruction now or develop a plan for revised client or family caregiver teaching if client or family caregiver is not able to teach back correctly.	Determines client's and family caregiver's level of understanding of instructional topic.

Unexpected Outcomes	Related Interventions
1. Client and family caregiver do not acknowledge risks identified from home safety assessment.	• Determine reason client is reluctant to make changes. Consider limited resources, disbelief concerning need to make changes, fear of loss of autonomy, or other reasons. • Review implications of risks to client's safety and welfare.
2. Client fails to make changes agreed on in previous plan.	• Determine reason for failure to make changes. • Help prioritize greatest risks. • Suggest making a single change and gauge client's response.
3. Client suffers fall or burn within home.	• Conduct assessment of contributing factors and conditions in environment at time of injury. • Make revisions based on assessment findings.

Recording and Reporting

- Retain copy of home safety assessment in client's home care record.
- Record any instruction provided, client's and family caregiver's response, and changes made within environment in nurses notes' electronic health record (EHR) or chart.

Special Considerations
Teaching

- Family caregivers will benefit from learning how to safely help client ambulate or transfer from bed to chair or wheelchair to chair, depending on client's mobility limitations (see Chapter 11).
- Instruct client and family caregiver about what to do in case client falls, including access to emergency help and how to prevent further injury.
- When appropriate, teach family caregiver and client how to use any emergency assistive devices (e.g., devices that are worn around client's neck and a special monitor connected to client's telephone). Clients summon help by pressing button on device if phone is inaccessible. Refer the family caregiver to local health care agencies and department of aging for options.
- Reinforce the importance of preserving client autonomy as much as possible with family caregivers.

Pediatric

- Caution parents when working in the kitchen to never pour hot liquids when an infant or young child is near.
- Remove all crib toys that are strung across crib or playpen when child begins to push up on hands or knees (4 to 7 months) (Hockenberry and Wilson, 2015).
- Install safety measures appropriate to developmental level (e.g., cabinet locks and gates).
- Do not let young children use the sink or tub without adult help; when child is in tub, stay with him or her.

Gerontological

- Use "aging in place" resources and designs to accommodate the needs of seniors or disabled individuals without having to completely redesign the home. Resources include community and government agencies and initiatives such as local councils on aging and the American Association of Retired Persons (AARP). Resources also focus on helping older adults to continue to live in the home of their choice, with a focus on quality of life. For example, install grab bars in bathrooms, movable cabinets under the sink so someone in a wheelchair can use the space, and light switches and electrical outlets at heights that can be reached easily.

- Place a bedside commode (with bedpan removed) over a conventional toilet seat. Commode level is usually higher than toilet and can also be moved near the bed for nighttime use.

◆ SKILL 43.2   Adapting the Home Setting for Clients With Cognitive Deficits

Clients with cognitive impairments and their family caregivers need help to make adaptations to preserve the client's abilities to function safely within their homes. An important aspect of safety is a person's ability to perform routine activities of daily living (ADLs) and instrumental activities of daily living (IADLs). This requires a client to make correct decisions about home-management activities. ADLs include a client's ability to bathe, dress, go to the toilet, transfer, and feed oneself. IADLs include the ability to use a telephone, prepare meals, travel, do housework, take medication, and shop. When there are cognitive limitations, a person's independence is threatened. Family caregivers often do not understand changes in a client's cognition and thus require help to determine whether a client is competent to stay at home safely.

Two common cognitive conditions affecting clients in the home are dementia and depression. Depression often results from social isolation (e.g., an older adult becomes homebound and has few visitors). Major depression is very common among elderly adults receiving home health care and is characterized by greater medical illness, functional impairment, and pain (Pickett et al., 2012). Clients with depression are less likely to adhere to medical regimens and do not care for themselves (e.g., poor diet, limited activity or exercise). Compared to other home health care clients, depressed clients have been shown to have higher risk of hospitalization, injury-producing falls, and higher health care costs (Pickett et al., 2012).

Dementia is a chronic generalized impairment of intellectual functioning that leads to a decline in the ability to perform basic ADLs and IADLs. It is characterized by a gradual, progressive, irreversible cerebral dysfunction. Alzheimer's disease is the most common form of dementia; as of 2015 there were 5.3 million Americans of all ages with Alzheimer's disease (Alzheimer's Association, 2015a). As it progresses, older adults become more dependent on family caregivers for help.

Alzheimer's disease causes problems with memory, thinking, or behavior; for some individuals with Alzheimer's disease there is a risk for wandering (Alzheimer's Association, 2015a). Wandering refers to moving about without having a definite place to go or a purpose. A wandering client may walk around the house trying repeatedly to carry out a task independently or try to leave his or her place of residence, necessitating family caregiver intervention to stop him or her. Family caregivers need to learn how to make the home safe to discourage wandering and prevent clients from leaving their homes unattended.

Delegation and Collaboration

The skill of adapting the home environment for clients with cognitive deficits cannot be delegated to nursing assistive personnel (NAP). The nurse is responsible for the assessment of cognitive function. The nurse directs the NAP to:

- Inform the nurse when there is a change in client's mood, memory, and ability to maintain the home or perform self-care.

Equipment

- Mini-Mental State Examination (MMSE)
- Short Geriatric Depression Scale (SGDS)
- Beck Depression Inventory (BDI)
- Calendar
- Paper for making lists
- Medication organizer (*optional*)
- Bulletin board or poster board (*optional*)
- Motion detector (*optional*)

STEP	RATIONALE

ASSESSMENT

1. Assess client over several short periods of time and be ready to adapt assessment if client has sensory disabilities.	Respects human dignity of client. Improves likelihood of gathering relevant data.
2. Be sure that room in which you meet with client and family is well lit with minimal outside noises or interruptions. Listen carefully and speak clearly and in normal tone of voice.	Optimal environment for assessment of client's cognitive and mental status provides more valid assessment.
3. Ask client to describe own level of health and have him or her describe how it affects ability to perform ADLs and IADLs. Ask family caregiver (if available) to confirm description. Screen for risky behaviors (e.g., medication nonadherence, unsupervised use of stove)	Question requires client to focus on one topic. Allows you to assess attention and concentration. Also determines if client is fully perceptive of physical and cognitive capabilities.

Clinical Decision Point *Be aware of your communication with the client and family caregivers. Do not make the client think that you are not listening to his or her views. The additional person supplements answers with client's consent, but the client remains the focus of the interview.*

STEP	RATIONALE
4. Ask how client is handling home-management responsibilities: "Tell me which bills you pay each month. Can you tell me what each one is for?" *Ability to perform ADLs:* "Can you tell me about your normal day? When do you get up, eat meals, dress? Tell me what you do to dress or bathe each morning."	Provides good comparison of client and family perceptions. Interaction helps to measure short-term memory, judgment, and problem solving.
5. Assess client's adherence to taking medications. Review number and type of medications being taken, client's understanding of purpose as prescribed (or as chosen for over-the-counter [OTC] medications), time of day taken, and dosages. Conduct pill count over course of a week (family caregiver may need to help). Also assess where client stores medications. Give special attention to pain medications, anticonvulsants, antihypertensives (especially beta-adrenergic blockers), diuretics, digoxin, aspirin, and anticoagulants. Have client or caregiver keep updated list of medications that can be brought to emergency department if needed. Ask to see medications and/or list used.	Depression and dementia can lead to poor medication adherence. Older adults frequently suffer drug interactions from polypharmacy (i.e., concurrent prescriptions for multiple medications). Some drugs and/or combinations of drugs place client at risk for side effects that increase chances of injury as result of physical or cognitive changes. Client-related factors such as disease-related knowledge, health literacy, and cognitive function; drug-related factors such as adverse effects and polypharmacy; and other factors, including client-provider relationship, are barriers to medication adherence (Walid et al., 2011). Keeping list of medications allows health care provider easy access to medication history.
6. Determine if client has family caregiver who helps with self-care or home-management responsibilities. What level of support does caregiver provide? How frequently is caregiver available? Does client perceive satisfaction in caregiver's support? What level of satisfaction does caregiver perceive? Does caregiver have access to and/or take advantage of respite care?	Relationship between family caregiver and client helps define how difficult it is to provide caregiving support. Role of family caregiver is often stressful, particularly if individual has other responsibilities such as parenting, work, or school. Determines availability of resource to client and quality of that support.
7. During discussion observe client's dress, nonverbal expressions, appearance, and cleanliness.	Conditions such as depression and dementia can result in client's inability to attend to personal appearance.

Clinical Decision Point *Do not confuse behavioral changes with lack of available resources to maintain hygiene. Also be aware of signs and symptoms of abuse or neglect (see Chapter 6). Report suspected abuse to appropriate social service agency.*

STEP	RATIONALE
8. Observe immediate home environment.	Behavioral changes associated with cognitive dysfunction are evident in disorderly home and inappropriate placement of objects (e.g., carton of orange juice placed inside kitchen cabinet instead of in refrigerator).
9. If you suspect cognitive or mental status change: a. Complete MMSE (e.g., Folstein's examination) for dementia.	Test screens orientation, attention and calculation, recall, language, and intelligence. The highest possible score is 30. If client scores 21 or less, it generally indicates that there is cognitive impairment that requires further evaluation (Meiner, 2015).
b. Complete SGDS for depression. (**NOTE:** Other depression scales such as the BDI are available.)	SGDS is recommended because it takes 5 minutes to administer and has been tested, validated, and used extensively for depression in older adults (Harvath and McKenzie, 2012).
10. If you suspect that client is at risk for wandering or is wandering, observe for following behaviors (family caregivers might provide information as well): • Repeated shadowing or seeking whereabouts of caregiver • Revisiting one destination many times • Inability to locate landmarks or getting lost in familiar setting • Going into unauthorized or private places • Searching for "missing" people or places • Walking with no apparent destination or purpose • Haphazard or continuous moving, walking, or pacing • Walking that cannot easily be redirected	Alerts family and caregivers to potential safety risks. When wandering extends outside safe environment, client is at increased risk for injury or death.
11. Assess which current environmental strategies family caregivers are using to deal with wandering (e.g., latches and alarms on doors, visual cues such as STOP signs, constant supervision, and wearing identification band).	Helps to determine level of intervention necessary. Allows for assessment of how family is dealing with issues of wandering and need for additional outside support.

STEP	RATIONALE
12. Assess family caregiver for signs and symptoms of stress.	Helps to determine if family caregiver is feeling burdened or overwhelmed and is in need of help.

NURSING DIAGNOSES

- Acute confusion
- Caregiver role strain
- Impaired home maintenance
- Impaired memory

- Ineffective health maintenance
- Ineffective role performance
- Risk for injury

- Self-care deficit (feeding, toileting, bathing/hygiene, dressing/grooming)
- Wandering

Related factors/Risk factors are individualized based on client's condition or needs.

PLANNING

1. Expected outcomes following completion of procedure:	
• Client is able to complete home management responsibilities within existing limitations.	Modifications are made that help client apply remaining cognitive functions.
• Client receives appropriate combination of medications for diagnosed conditions.	Assistive devices enable client to adhere to prescribed medication regimen.
• Client is able to perform self-care activities or receives appropriate help.	Interventions preserve client's autonomy and maximize his or her functionality.
• Family caregivers describe steps to take to minimize wandering.	Instruction prepares family caregivers with wandering-management strategies.
• Client experiences fewer episodes of wandering.	Wandering-management strategies are effective.
• Family caregiver identifies community resources for support.	Services available can include respite care, adult day care programs, and support groups.
2. If client has difficulty with self-care or fine-motor skills, refer family to occupational therapy, homemaker services, or respite care as appropriate.	Occupational therapists provide assistive devices and recommend self-care adaptations. Homemaker services provide added resource for meal preparation and home cleaning. Respite care provides family caregiver temporary rest away from continuous responsibilities.
3. Consider client's level of cognitive impairment when making changes in his or her living environment. Some clients may require only minor adaptations, and others will depend more on help of family caregivers.	Retention of client's independence and autonomy is ultimate goal.
4. Determine best time of day for approaches that result in desired response.	Some clients are more alert and responsive in morning versus afternoon or vice versa.

IMPLEMENTATION

1. If client has difficulty remembering when to perform tasks (e.g., paying bills, making appointments), help to create list or post reminder notes in conspicuous location (e.g., bulletin board, front of refrigerator).	Lists and organizers help client cope with memory loss and still safely perform activities.
2. If client has difficulty remembering when to take medicines, help to create list or reminder note, provide medication container organized by days of week, or recommend wristwatch with alarm or schedule of text messages to signal medication administration times.	There is no gold standard for improving medication adherence. Reminder systems have benefit if client or family caregiver is motivated and/or desire to adhere to them. Level of evidence for efficacy of reminders is low (AHRQ, 2012).
3. When client has difficulty completing tasks such as writing checks for bills or bringing groceries into home from store, reduce steps it takes to complete task. Consolidate steps or simplify task.	Prevents frustration in completing task and/or forgetting step that leads to task being unfinished.
4. If client has difficulty bathing, dressing, writing, and feeding, offer assistive devices (see illustrations).	Assistive eating devices have larger handles, cup handles, or plate edges to help with meals. Assistive dressing devices use Velcro, large zippers, and elastic to facilitate independence when dressing.

STEP	RATIONALE

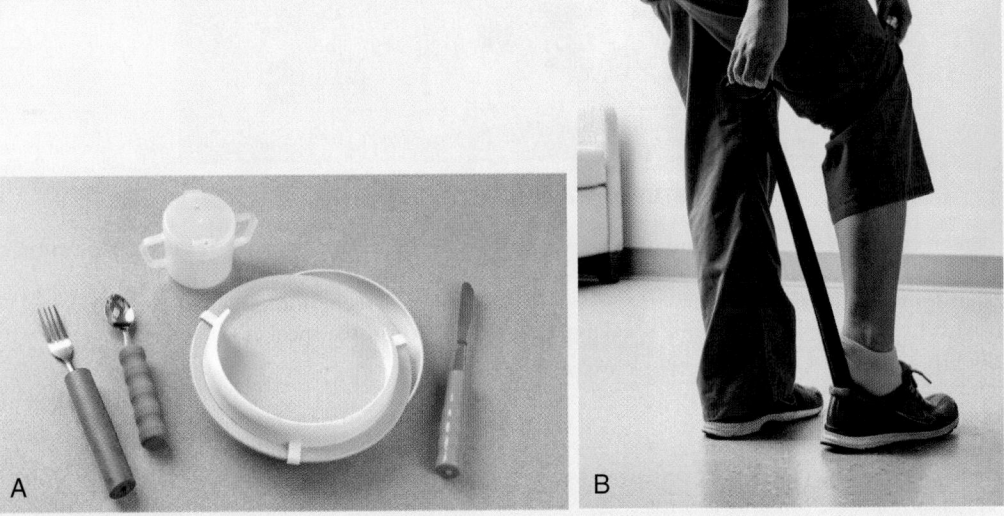

STEP 4 A, Assistive feeding devices. **B,** Assistive device to help put on shoes. (*Image used with permission ArcMate Manufacturing Corporation. All rights reserved.*)

5. Help client and family caregiver determine routine schedule for ADLs such as eating, bathing, daily exercise, home cleaning, and napping. Have large calendar posted in conspicuous area to write in appointments or special planned events.	Consistency creates sense of security and keeps client oriented to daily activities. Routines are important in providing security, but client also needs to have option of making changes as necessary (Touhy and Jett, 2014).
6. Instruct family caregiver to focus on client's abilities rather than disabilities. Use abilities in modifying approaches to perform daily activities (e.g., if client has limited use of right hand, try approaches that maximize use of left hand).	Retains client's autonomy and sense of self-worth.
7. Have family caregiver help set up activities so client can complete tasks (e.g., chopping vegetables before cooking, placing wash basin on table in bedroom for sponge bath, placing clothes to wear for day on bed, unpacking groceries on countertop for eventual storage, arranging food on plate with items in clockwise orientation [e.g., vegetables at 9, salad at 3, meat at 6]).	Helps client master task even though unable either physically or cognitively to perform all steps.
8. Discuss with client, family caregiver, pharmacist, and health care provider options for scheduling multiple medications:	Drugs sometimes cause physiological changes that create risk for injury.
a. Have medications that are likely to cause confusion prescribed to be given at bedtime.	Reduces risk for confusion during waking hours that contribute to disorientation and risk for falling.

Clinical Decision Point *Do not recommend this if client has nocturia because client will be at greater risk for falling.*

b. Space antihypertensives and antiarrhythmics at different times to minimize side effects.	These drugs cause blood pressure changes and dizziness, thus increasing risk for falls.
c. When possible reduce number of pain medications used.	Drugs create sedative effects, increasing risk for falls.
d. Have diuretics taken early in day and not at night.	Diuretic effect occurs during day while client is awake.
e. Discuss with health care provider possibility of taking medications at same time.	If safe and appropriate, taking medications at same time will alleviate problem of client remembering multiple administration times.
f. Discuss use of medication organizer and dispenser (see illustration).	Organizing medication in daily dispenser helps client and caregiver avoid medication errors of duplicating or missing medications.

STEP	RATIONALE

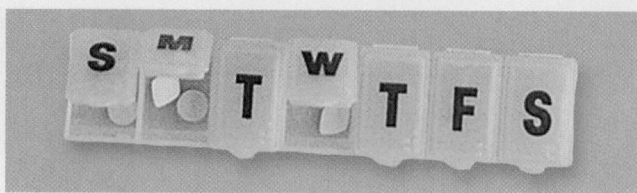

STEP 8f Weekly medication organizer.

9. Teach family caregiver how to use simple and direct communication:
   a. Sit or stand in front of client in full view.
   b. Face client with hearing impairment while speaking; do not cover mouth and do not speak in a loud tone.
   c. Use calm and relaxed approach.
   d. Use eye contact and touch.
   e. Speak slowly, in simple words and short sentences.
   f. Use nonverbal gestures that complement verbal messages.

Relays care and support through therapeutic communication techniques.
Promotes reception of verbal and nonverbal messages.
Client can see speaker's lips. Prevents voice distortion.

Helps to reinforce messages.
Enhances understanding of messages.
Provides clear messages.

10. Place clocks, calendars, and personal mementos (e.g., pictures, scrapbooks) throughout rooms within home. Enhance environment with addition of tactile boards or three-dimensional art.

Maintaining familiar surroundings maximizes cognitive function.

11. Have family caregiver routinely orient client to who family caregiver is and which activities he or she is going to complete.

This strategy is useful in clients with progressive dementia. Behavioral symptoms in later stages include delusions, agitation, and hallucinations (Alzheimer's Association, 2015a).

12. Be sure that client has regular naps or rest periods during day.

Fatigue adds to any mental status changes. Provides client energy to perform planned activities.

13. Have family caregiver encourage and support frequent visits by family and friends. Teach family caregiver how to use humor and reminiscing about favorite stories to promote social interaction.

Participation in social activities prevents boredom and restlessness.

14. Provide safe place for person to wander (e.g., large family room or fenced yard).

Reduces risk for injury and leaving residence (Touhy and Jett, 2014).

15. Recommend that family of wandering client install door locks or electronic guards.

Reduces chance of client exiting home unsupervised.

16. Create calm, safe setting that is appropriate for client's abilities (Alzheimer's Association, 2015a).

Prevents falls and minimizes behavioral symptoms.

17. Monitor client for personal comfort (e.g., hunger, thirst, constipation, full bladder, and comfortable temperature) (Alzheimer's Association, 2015a).

Reduces stimuli that prompt wandering.

18. Keep list of places to which client may wander (e.g., former homes or workplaces).

Client may seek a familiar place.

19. Consider having client wear GPS device to help manage location. Install motion detector near exit site, with portable alarm that can accompany family caregiver.

Alerts family caregiver to client's attempt to exit residence (Alzheimer's Association, 2015a).

20. Consider need for full-time care.

EVALUATION

1. During follow-up visits ask client to review home-management activities completed the morning of that day and previous day.

Determines client's ability to recall events and evaluates if client completed planned activities.

2. Review with client and family caregiver revised schedule for medication administration.

Evaluates understanding of regimen.

3. Check pill count you asked client/family caregiver to maintain for a week.

Tracking doses confirms if client is adherent to regimen.

4. Ask family caregiver to describe ways that will increase client's success in completing home-management and self-care activities.

Measures learning.

STEP	RATIONALE
5. Have family caregiver show schedules of daily routines and review specific approaches used. Observe environment for presence of reality orientation cues.	Determines family caregiver's success in applying information and making environmental changes.
6. Have family caregivers describe options for minimizing wandering.	Measures learning.
7. Have family caregivers report number of occurrences of wandering.	Determines if reduction in wandering has occurred.
8. **Use Teach-Back:** "I want to be sure I explained how you can help minimize your husband's wandering. Tell me some ways you can do this." Revise your instruction now or develop a plan for revised family caregiver teaching if family caregiver is not able to teach back correctly.	Determines family caregiver's level of understanding of instructional topic.

Unexpected Outcomes

1. Client is unable to complete ADLs/IADLs as planned.

2. Client experiences drug interaction from multiple medications.

3. Family caregiver is unable to describe/implement techniques that will improve client's orientation and ability to complete activities.

4. Family caregiver is unable to describe/implement strategies to decrease wandering.

5. Client's wandering increases.

6. Client misses medication doses or takes wrong dosage.

Related Interventions

- Further modifications are sometimes necessary.
- Reassess what occurred when task was not completed.
- Have family caregiver offer suggestions.
- Have health care provider evaluate client's medication regimen.
- Recommend feasibility of pharmacy consultation.
- Reinstruction and discussion are necessary.
- Support for family caregiver is sometimes necessary before caregiver can learn how to support someone else.
- Consider that family caregiver is not able to provide necessary support; need to analyze other options.
- Reinstruction and discussion are necessary.
- Family caregiver may not have resources available to adapt environment.
- Reconsider strategies used.
- Reassess factors prompting wandering.
- Review list of medications and method for administering (e.g., medication dispenser).
- Reconsider strategies to organize and schedule medications.
- Assess client for adverse effects (Meiner, 2015).

Recording and Reporting

- Record assessment of client's cognitive and mental status, recommended interventions, and client's and family caregiver's response in nurses' notes in electronic health record (EHR) or chart.
- Report to health care provider any change in client's behavior that reflects a decline in cognitive or mental status.

Special Considerations
Teaching

- Instruct family caregiver in signs and symptoms of dementia and depression. If client's functionality continues to decline, caregiver may choose to learn more ADL support skills (e.g., how to help with hygiene, dressing, transfer and turning, toileting).

Pediatric

- Children with cognitive impairment often are not aware of inherent dangers during play and other activities. Parental supervision is critical.

Gerontological

- Early diagnosis of the cause of dementia is best for the client and caregiver so prompt treatment can begin, the client can be included in treatment decisions as much as possible, and the caregiver has an understanding of the behavior (Alzheimer's Association, 2015a).
- Family caregivers will need access to respite programs, which will allow them planned time away from their caregiving role (Mueth, 2015).
- Consider that clients may not have family caregivers who are able or willing to care for them. Additional help of a contracted caregiver may be required if available; this may also affect client's ability to stay in his or her home and not be placed in assisted or skilled care.
- If wandering is an ongoing problem, have family caregiver provide current photographs of the client to local police. Recommend enrolling client in the national MedicAlert + Alzheimer's Association Safe Return program, which provides 24-hour emergency and wandering response services and support services for family and caregivers (Alzheimer's Association, 2015b). Local resources of informal caregivers (e.g., neighbors and members of the spiritual community) can also be explored to ensure safety for the client inside and outside of the home.

◆ SKILL 43.3   Medication and Medical Device Safety

The first time you visit a client's home you will review and list all of a client's medications and medication bottles. It is important to note drug name, dosage, frequency, and route and compare your list with any previous lists (e.g., known medications ordered by primary health care provider or other physicians and hospital discharge instructions). This process is known as medication reconciliation; the goal is to ensure that there are no errors or omissions in a client's medication regimen, while also assessing if there is any need for change in medications (IHI, 2015).

Clients in the home frequently manage the administration of medications and the use of medical devices such as syringes, blood glucose monitoring equipment, dressing supplies, and even intravenous (IV) devices. This includes administration, storage, and disposal of medications and medical devices. It is critical that a client administers medications correctly, uses devices properly, cleans equipment, and removes waste properly. Infection control is just one safety principle that a client and/or family caregiver must learn for the home setting. Make sure that clients know regulations regarding waste disposal and follow the procedures consistent with local and federal laws (e.g., place soiled dressings in securely fastened plastic bags before adding to regular trash and use trash containers with tight lids to avoid attracting animals).

One of a nurse's responsibilities within the home environment is to help a client with sensory, mobility, or cognitive deficits. Clients who require special consideration include those with acute sensory or neurological impairment; those with chronic illness such as diabetes or arthritis; and older adults, who frequently have physical limitations that make manipulating medical devices and dispensing medications difficult. For example, clients with arthritic hands are often unable to open medication containers because of weakness in the hands and the pain created by pressure on the joints.

Delegation and Collaboration

The skill of assessing for and monitoring medication and medical device safety cannot be delegated to nursing assistive personnel (NAP). The nurse directs the NAP to:
- Make suggestions that further ensure client safety regarding the use of basic infection control practices.
- Make suggestions as to how to properly dispose of sharps, needles, and contaminated supplies in the home.

Equipment

- Colored marking pens
- Labels
- Puncture-resistant sharps container or 2-L hard plastic bottle with cap
- Duct, masking, or adhesive tape
- Assistive devices (e.g., syringe magnifier)
- Medication organizers

STEP	RATIONALE

ASSESSMENT

1. Assess client's sensory, musculoskeletal, and neurological function (see Chapter 6), specifically hand strength, ability to read labels on containers, ability to read doses on syringe, ability to prepare medicine in a syringe.	Reveals any deficits that will affect preparation and use of medications or medical devices.
2. If family caregiver provides routine help, ask caregiver if there are any concerns about being able to care for client.	Assesses family caregivers' health. Can help educate family caregivers as to need for help and provide information to avoid injury (Clark, 2015).
3. Assess client's medication regimen and length of time that client has been receiving each drug. Ask client to describe doses taken daily for each medication. Query family caregiver if necessary.	Determines complexity of medication regimen and how familiar client or family caregiver is with regimen.
4. Assess client's and family caregiver's health literacy level (e.g., ask them to read a medication label out loud to you).	Helps to ensure that client and family caregiver can read and understand medication that client is taking. Helps prevent medication errors.

Clinical Decision Point *Be sure that medication labels are not confusing for a client. For example, the Spanish word for "eleven" is written as "once." A Spanish-speaking client could confuse a medication direction that requires them to take a medication 1 time a day as 11 times a day.*

5. Ask client to show you where medications are stored in home. Look at each container.	Determines condition and labeling of containers.
6. Assess temperature of storage area.	Medication should not be stored in extreme heat. Insulin should not be stored near extreme heat or cold (ADA, 2014).
7. Assess client's daily schedule for drug administration. Ask client to describe schedule and whether there are any problems in following that schedule.	Helps to reveal client's adherence to or misunderstanding of instructions.
8. If client self-administers injections, ask to see where he or she stores supplies and what he or she uses to dispose of used syringes and needles.	Determines sterility of equipment and whether method of disposal creates risk to client or family for needlestick injuries.

STEP	RATIONALE
9. If client uses glucose-monitoring device, ask to see where monitor, lancets, and glucose strips are stored. Also ask about how client disposes of lancets.	Allows you to examine cleanliness of equipment, sterility of lancets, and condition of glucose strips. Sharps should be disposed of in puncture-proof container.

NURSING DIAGNOSES

- Caregiver role strain
- Deficient knowledge regarding medication safety
- Ineffective health maintenance
- Noncompliance
- Risk for infection
- Risk for injury

Related factors/Risk factors are individualized based on client's condition or needs.

PLANNING

1. Expected outcomes following completion of procedure:	
• Client and family caregiver discuss principles of medication safety.	Client education includes information and techniques for safe medication administration.
• Client and family caregiver prepare medications independently.	Adaptations successfully accommodate client's and/or family caregiver's deficits in handling and manipulating equipment.
• Client and family caregiver identify correct conditions for storing medications, medical devices, and supplies.	Instruction focuses on ensuring infection control measures.
• Client and family caregiver dispose of used medical equipment and supplies correctly.	Appropriate receptacles and methods for disposal are made available and used.

IMPLEMENTATION

1. Teach client and family caregiver following principles to ensure that medications are safe to use:	
a. Never take medicine prescribed for another member of household (CDC, 2014b).	Medications must be of full strength and used for appropriate pharmacological reason to have therapeutic benefit.
b. Do not take any medicine more than 1 year old or past expiration date on container.	Expired medication is sometimes toxic or no longer effective.
c. Do not place different medicines in same container.	Prevents accidental "mix-up" of medications and medication error.
d. Do not place medications in pill containers different from their original ones.	Prevents accidental "mix-up" of medications and confusion as to expiration dates.
e. Always finish prescribed medication; do not save for future illness.	Prevents underdosing or inappropriate dosing.
f. Wash hands before and after administering/taking medication.	Contaminated hands are source of infection transmission.
2. Recommend approaches for preparation of medications:	
a. For clients with weakened grasp or pain of hands and fingers, have local pharmacist place medications in screw-top container.	Tops of childproof containers are difficult to remove, especially if hand and finger grasp is weakened.

Clinical Decision Point *If client has children or grandchildren who have easy access to medication storage area or client's purse, be sure that medications are stored in secure place.*

b. For clients with visual alterations, have pharmacy type larger labels on all medication containers.	Ensures that client is able to read drug name and dosage schedule clearly.
c. For clients who are legally blind, have Braille labels placed on medication containers.	Labels embossed with drug name, strength, and prescription numbers are easy to read for client trained in use of Braille.
d. For clients taking multiple medications, ask if they wish to try to introduce color-coding system. Use same color for drugs that client needs to take at same time. Mark tops of bottle caps with colored marking pen.	Technique helps client take correct drugs and doses at correct times of day. Best used when client is reliable in self-administration.
e. Provide specially designed syringes with large numerals or syringe magnifier for clients with visual alterations (see illustration).	Ensures that accurate dose of drug is prepared in syringe.

STEP	RATIONALE

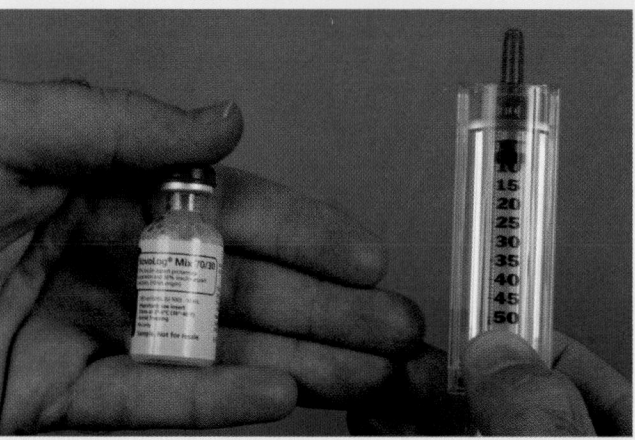

STEP 2e Syringe with magnifier.

STEP	RATIONALE
f. For clients who have difficulty manipulating syringes, offer spring-loaded needle insertion aid.	Delivers injection safely without manipulation of plunger.

Clinical Decision Point *Teach family caregivers what to do following a needlestick injury. Wash the affected area thoroughly with soap and water and dry. If client has acquired immunodeficiency syndrome (AIDS), hepatitis, or other communicable disease, caregivers should pursue appropriate laboratory testing.*

STEP	RATIONALE
g. Teach family caregivers how to properly draw up prescribed volume of medication into syringe. When necessary, have family caregiver prepare extra prefilled syringes for client's use when caregiver is absent.	Ensures that family caregiver knows proper preparation techniques and that client has access to injections. Watch client and/or family caregiver draw up and dispense medications to determine if more teaching is needed.
3. Recommend approaches for medication and supply storage:	
a. Store medications in safe, dry place, preferably in kitchen.	Moisture in bathroom may cause medications to decompose.
b. Keep liquid medications and parenteral drugs, especially insulin, in cool place.	Prevents decomposition of drug.

Clinical Decision Point *Although manufacturers recommend storing insulin in the refrigerator, injecting cold insulin can sometimes make the injection more painful. To avoid this, store the bottle of insulin being used at room temperature. Insulin kept at room temperature will last approximately 1 month. However, remember to store extra bottles in the refrigerator if a client buys more than one bottle at a time to save money (American Diabetes Association, 2014). If insulin is stored in refrigerator, be sure that drug is in a bin or container, away from food.*

STEP	RATIONALE
c. Keep medical supplies such as syringes, dressing supplies, and glucose meter in airtight container (e.g., plastic storage bin) and store in cool place such as bedroom closet.	Ensures that supplies are not exposed to moisture or other contaminants.
d. Instruct client and family caregiver to use new needle with each medication administration.	Multiple use of same needle puts client at risk for infection.
4. Review for client and family caregiver proper techniques for disposal of medications, "sharps," and disposable medical supplies:	Proper practices necessary to prevent client injury.
a. Discard unused parts of drugs or outdated drugs properly, using these guidelines from ISMP (2014):	
(1) DO NOT FLUSH unused medications. However, although rule of thumb is not to flush, the Food and Drug Administration (FDA) has determined that certain medications should be flushed because of their abuse potential. Read the instructions on your medication and talk to your pharmacist.	Recent environmental impact studies report that flushing medications down toilet could be having an adverse impact on environment (ISMP, 2014).

STEP	RATIONALE
(2) When tossing unused medications, protect children and pets by crushing solid medications or dissolve them in water (this applies for liquid medications as well) and mix with kitty litter, coffee grounds, or sawdust (e.g., any material that absorbs dissolved medication and makes it less appealing for pets or children to eat); place in sealed plastic bag BEFORE tossing in trash.	Ensures that no one in household uses drug not prescribed for their use or drugs that will be ineffective pharmacologically.
(3) Remove and destroy ALL identifying personal information (prescription label) from medication container.	Ensures safe disposal to prevent outsider from acquiring medications.
(4) Check for approved state and local collection programs or with area hazardous waste facilities.	In certain states you may be able to take your unused medications to your community pharmacy (ISMP, 2014).
b. Obtain sharps container from medical supply store or IV equipment supplier. (If finances are limited, have client use small-neck plastic bottle such as soda bottle.) Dispose of all needles and lancets in container.	Puncture-proof container prevents exposure to contaminated needlestick. Small-neck container makes it difficult for anyone to easily retrieve used needle or sharp.
c. Caution against filling sharps container to point where needles protrude out opening. Discard when three-fourths full, securing top with duct tape or adhesive tape.	Prevents needlesticks.
d. Store sharps container in area inaccessible to children.	Prevents injury to child.
e. Dispose of soiled dressings, used glucose testing reagent strips, and IV tubing in separate, sealed, plastic garbage bag. Place in second plastic bag (double bagged) and discard appropriately as trash.	Prevents contamination with other items in home. Minimizes chances of caregiver being exposed to infectious waste.
f. Consult local public health department or community authorities regarding proper way to dispose of waste, including some medications.	Most communities have strict guidelines for waste and medication disposal.

EVALUATION

1. Have client and/or family caregiver describe steps to take to ensure that medications are safe to use.	Demonstrates learning.
2. Observe client and/or caregiver prepare and administer medication dose.	Evaluates ability to physically manipulate medications and necessary equipment.
3. Observe home setting for location of medications and supplies.	Evaluates client's and/or family caregiver's adherence to recommendations.
4. Have client describe how sharps or medical equipment is discarded.	Demonstrates learning.
5. Do pill counts (pills remaining in containers) at successive intervals such as twice a week for 2 weeks.	Helps to verify that client takes correct number of medications over period of time.
6. Use Teach-Back: "I want to be sure I explained the importance of disposing of sharps appropriately. Tell me how to dispose of your lancets correctly and why this is important." Revise your instruction now or develop a plan or revised client or family caregiver teaching if client or family caregiver is not able to teach back correctly.	Determines client's and family caregiver's level of understanding of instructional topic.

Unexpected Outcomes	Related Interventions
1. Client and/or family caregiver is unable to recall principles for safe use of drugs.	• Reinstruction necessary, or client and caregiver need chance to ask more questions regarding benefit of precautions.
	• Offer simple, plain language and/or written instructions.
2. Client and/or family caregiver has difficulty or is unable to prepare and self-administer medication.	• Offer further help to set up equipment.
	• Offer assistive aids.
	• Reinstruct in steps used to prepare medication.

STEP	RATIONALE
3. Medications and medical devices are not stored in secure or appropriate location.	• Assess whether client chooses to store items conveniently rather than safely or has limited resources. • Reinstruction and discussion are necessary.
4. Sharps and disposable medical equipment are not disposed of properly.	• Provide reinstruction. • Arrange to provide appropriate containers.
5. Excess or insufficient number of pills found during pill count.	• Review with client and family caregiver daily drug prescribed. • Reevaluate use of dosage reminders. • Notify health care provider.

Recording and Reporting

• Record instructions and recommendations to client and family caregiver and results of return demonstrations in nurses' notes in electronic health record (EHR) or chart.
• Report to health care provider any unsafe situation.

Special Considerations
Teaching

• Instruct clients in care of linens. Instruct the client or family caregiver to avoid agitating the soiled linens and to handle them as little as possible (CDC, 2011).
• If linens are contaminated with microorganisms, they should be decontaminated by washing with soap/detergent and hot water.

Commercial washers may reach a temperature of 160°F; normal washing cycles using laundry chemicals suitable for lower temperatures in the home are usually adequate to clean linens (CDC, 2011).

Pediatric

• It is vital to keep medications and other equipment such as cleaning products out of the reach of children (Hockenberry and Wilson, 2015).
• All medicines and cleaning products should have child safety caps (Hockenberry and Wilson, 2015).
• If teaching self-management skills, include adult supervision and input. Never refer to medications as candy.

◆ CLINICAL DEBRIEF

A 79-year-old woman lives with her 84-year-old sister in a split-level four-bedroom home that she has owned for over 50 years. She has a history of metastatic bone cancer and was recently diagnosed with heart failure. In addition to taking multiple oral medications, she undergoes weekly intravenous chemotherapy for progression of her cancer. She has no other family closer than a 2-hour drive, and her older sister has advanced glaucoma and diminished hearing.

Both women refuse to move from their home, even at the urging of her three children to move closer to one of them. The client no longer drives, nor does her sister; and she is unable to climb the few steps needed to move beyond the lower living level of the home. She has begun to show signs of depression; and, when the nurse talks to her sister, the nurse recognizes that the sister is overwhelmed by the amount of care she needs to provide. Because of the client's immobility, she cannot reach the upstairs bathrooms, which contain showers, and she relies on her older sister to help care for her and maintain the house on a daily basis.

1. Give three examples for how the nurse might adapt the home setting to make it safer for the client and her sister.
2. Which equipment might the nurse bring to the home to perform the initial home assessment?
3. The client now lives in an assisted-living facility in a private room; you visit her at the facility and plan to meet with the health care team on site to give report. Her sister passed away the month before, and her children convinced her to move to the facility, believing she will be safer in this environment. Her apartment is on the second floor of the facility, and the dining/socialization areas are on the first floor. When you visit her, she appears to be confused as to why she is in the assisted-living facility and asks you when she can return "home." Using SBAR, show how you would communicate with the health care team at the assisted-living facility about this client.

◆ REVIEW QUESTIONS

1. A woman found wandering in her nightclothes is also dirty but does not appear to have any injuries. Which assessment topics would a home care nurse include to determine the client's physical and mental status? (Select all that apply.)
   1. The medications she is taking and who supervises her
   2. Any decrease in cognitive function seen within the past few months
   3. Whether she or someone else pays her bills
   4. Any history of wandering
   5. Whether the family has a current photograph available
   6. When she was last seen by her health care provider
2. An older adult with diabetes mellitus asks the home health nurse how to maintain her diabetic supplies. The nurse knows that teaching was successful when the client states the following: (Select all that apply.)
   1. "Insulin cannot harm my grandchildren; so I don't need to keep it locked up when they visit."
   2. "I keep the insulin vials in the kitchen freezer until about 2 hours before I need to use them."
   3. "I store extra bottles of insulin that I am not using in my refrigerator in the bin with the eggs so they will not break."
   4. "I can store my glucose meter and insulin syringes in an airtight bag when I'm not using them."
   5. "When my daughter comes to visit, I'll ask her to prepare extra prefilled syringes for me."
3. The nurse is visiting an elderly client who is recovering from hip replacement surgery at her home. Which of the following discoveries makes the nurse concerned that the client is at risk for falls? (Select all that apply.)

1. Handrails are present on one side of the staircase leading to the upstairs.
2. The outdoor steps are all one color, blending in with the sidewalk.
3. There are slip-resistant mats in the kitchen and bathroom.
4. The client is taking morphine tablets for pain every 8 hours.
5. The client has a history of previous falls in the past 6 months.

ⓔ *Visit the Evolve site for a complete list of Clinical Debrief and Review Questions answers.*

REFERENCES

Agency for Healthcare Research and Quality (AHRQ): *Closing the quality gap series: medication adherence interventions: comparative effectiveness*, 2012, http://effectivehealthcare.ahrq.gov/index.cfm/search-for-guides-reviews-and-reports/?productid=1249&pageaction=displayproduct. Accessed March 29, 2016.

Alzheimer's Association: *Alzheimer's and dementia basics*, 2015a, http://www.alz.org/alzheimers_disease_what_is_alzheimers.asp. Accessed March 29, 2016.

Alzheimer's Association: *MedicAlert + Alzheimer's Association safe return*, 2015b, http://www.alz.org/care/dementia-medic-alert-safe-return.asp. Accessed March 29, 2016.

American Diabetes Association (ADA): *Living with diabetes: insulin storage and syringe safety*, 2014, http://www.diabetes.org/living-with-diabetes/treatment-and-care/medication/insulin/insulin-storage-and-syringe-safety.html. Accessed March 29, 2016.

Beauchet O, et al: Timed get-up-and-go test and risk of falls in older adults: a systematic review, *J Nutr Health Aging* 15(10):933, 2011.

Bekhet AK: Effects of positive cognitions and resourcefulness on caregiver burden among caregivers of persons with dementia, *Int J Ment Health Nurs* 22(4):340, 2013.

Berland A, et al: Patient safety culture in home care: experiences of home-care nurses, *J Nurs Manag* 20(6):794, 2012.

Buch CL, Nies MA: Home health and hospice. In Nies MA, McEwen M, editors: *Community/public health nursing: promoting the health of populations*, ed 6, St Louis, 2014, Mosby.

Centers for Disease Control and Prevention (CDC): *Laundry: washing infected material*, 2011, http://www.cdc.gov/HAI/prevent/laundry.html. Accessed March 29, 2016.

Centers for Disease Control and Prevention (CDC): *Healthy homes*, 2014a, http://www.cdc.gov/healthyhomes/. Accessed March 29, 2016.

Centers for Disease Control and Prevention (CDC): *Medication safety program*, 2014b, http://www.cdc.gov/medicationsafety/. Accessed March 29, 2016.

Clark MJ: *Population and community health nursing*, ed 6, Hoboken, NJ, 2015, Pearson.

Crist JD, Speaks P: Keeping it in the family: when Mexican-American older adults choose not to use home healthcare services, *Home Healthc Nurse* 29(5):282, 2011.

Edelman CL, et al: *Health promotion throughout the lifespan*, ed 8, St Louis, 2014, Mosby.

Foodsafety.gov: *Keep food safe*, 2015, http://www.foodsafety.gov/keep/index.html. Accessed March 29, 2016.

Harvath T, McKenzie G: *Nursing standard of practice protocol: depression in older adults*, 2012, http://consultgerirn.org/topics/depression/want_to_know_more#ref16. Accessed August 17, 2016.

Hill E, Fauerbach LA: Falls and fall prevention in older adults, *J Legal Nurs Consult* 25(2):24, 2014.

Hockenberry MJ, Wilson DW: *Wong's nursing care of infants and children*, ed 10, St Louis, 2015, Mosby.

Institute for Healthcare Improvement (IHI): *Reconcile medications at all transition points*, 2015, http://www.ihi.org/resources/Pages/Changes/ReconcileMedicationsatAllTransitionPoints.aspx. Accessed May 29, 2016.

Institute for Safe Medication Practices (ISMP): *ConsumerMedSafety.org, Throw away your old medicines safely*, 2014, http://www.consumermedsafety.org/medication-safety-articles/item/580-throw-away-your-old-medicines-safely. Accessed March 29, 2016.

Lang A, et al: Researching triads in home care: perceptions of safety from home care patients, their caregivers, and providers, *HHC Management Practice* 26(2):59, 2014.

Meiner SE: Safety. In Meiner SE, editor: *Gerontologic nursing*, ed 5, St Louis, 2015, Mosby.

Mueth EC: Family influences. In Meiner SE, editor: *Gerontologic nursing*, ed 5, St Louis, 2015, Mosby.

Muir SW, et al: Modifiable risk factors identify people who transition from non-fallers to fallers in community-dwelling older adults: a prospective study, *Physiother Can* 62(4):358, 2010.

Mullin L: Keeping safety a priority in home care and hospice: one agency's journey, *Home Healthc Nurse* 28(2):63, 2010.

National Fire Protection Association (NFPA): *Home safety*, 2013, http://www.nfpa.org/standard_items/search_results?searchStr=home%20safety. Accessed March 29, 2016.

National Rifle Association (NRA): *NRA gun safety rules*, 2015, http://training.nra.org/nra-gun-safety-rules.aspx. http://www.nrahq.org/education/guide.asp. Accessed March 29, 2016.

Pickett Y, et al: Late-life depression in home healthcare, *Aging Health* 8(3):273, 2012.

Quality and Safety Education for Nurses (QSEN): *Pre-licensure KSAS*, 2014, http://qsen.org/competencies/pre-licensure-ksas/. Accessed March 29, 2016.

Touhy TA, Jett KF: *Ebersole and Hess' gerontological nursing & health aging*, ed 4, St Louis, 2014, Mosby.

US Department of Health and Human Services (USDHHS): *Healthy People 2020, injury and violence prevention*, 2014, http://www.healthypeople.gov/2020/topics-objectives/topic/injury-and-violence-prevention. Accessed March 29, 2016.

Walid FG, et al: A systematic review of barriers to medication adherence in the elderly: looking beyond cost and regimen complexity, *Am J Geriatr Pharmacother* 9(1):11, 2011.

44 | Home Care Teaching

OBJECTIVES

Mastery of content in this chapter will enable the nurse to:

- Identify factors that influence clients' abilities to learn and care for themselves at home.
- Discuss the collaborative nature of home care teaching with the client and/or family caregiver.
- Assess safety factors that may impair or prohibit a client's ability to perform skills in the home setting.
- Discuss situations and conditions that require a client and/or family caregiver to learn skills that support and achieve health maintenance.
- Choose evidence-based teaching strategies to use in the home setting.
- Implement and evaluate evidence-based learning strategies that support clients' ability to care for themselves in the home.

MEDIA RESOURCES

- evolve http://evolve.elsevier.com/Perry/skills
- Review Questions
- Audio Glossary
- Clinical Debrief and Review Questions Answers

PURPOSE

Many clients recover from or are treated for illnesses in their homes. In these situations clients assume greater responsibility for managing their own care and are supported by home care nurses. Home care nurses provide health education and resources by collaborating with a client or family caregiver to address the client's health needs, preferences, and values and incorporating their strengths, skills, and capacity (Nies and McEwen, 2015).

STANDARDS OF CARE

- American Nurses Association (ANA), 2014—Scope and Standards of Practice for Home Health Nursing
- The Joint Commission (TJC), 2016—National Patient Safety Goals: Home Accreditation Program

PRINCIPLES FOR PRACTICE

- Home care nurses thoroughly assess factors that affect a client's abilities and willingness to manage self-care. Determine what the clients want to know, how they learn, and what motivates them to learn new information (ANA, 2014).

- Client teaching is an essential part of nursing practice. Information needs to be relevant, current, and clearly presented (Jett, 2014).
- Home care nurses creatively adapt teaching strategies to meet each client's unique physical, psychosocial, and cultural needs (Marrelli, 2014).
- For collaboration to be successful, home care nurses identify who is involved in the client's care and establish mutual trust and respect through open and honest communication (Nies and McEwen, 2015).
- Consider principles of diversity when caring for clients in their homes. Respect each individual's cultural background and beliefs.
- Health education resources for clients and health care providers are available as part of the Home Health Quality Improvement campaign. Best-practice intervention packages use a variety of media sources such as YouTube, podcasts, and toolkits to improve care delivery and outcomes (HHQI, 2015).

CLIENT-CENTERED CARE

- Engage the client and /or family caregiver(s) as participants in care (Rosa et al., 2014).

- Clients must understand how to manage their health and illnesses, take discharge medications correctly and safely, and perform related care at home. In home care nurses help clients and family caregivers make well-informed decisions about their health practices (Parker et al., 2014).
- Teach-back is a way to confirm that client teaching is understood. Client understanding is confirmed when a client explains or demonstrates a topic back to the nurse (Tamura-Lis, 2013).
- Respectful communication includes addressing a client in an appropriate manner and using acceptable body language. For example, direct eye contact during an interview may be considered rude in some cultures (Jett, 2014).
- Reinforce verbal instructions with printed, client education information in preferred reading level language and use other audiovisual materials when possible (Eadie, 2014).

EVIDENCE-BASED PRACTICE

Clients are discharged sooner from hospitals and present with more complex health care needs. Thus the home care nurse is challenged to teach them and help them feel secure along with coordinating their care among the health care providers.

- A review of outcomes in home health care identified the importance of care coordination among providers when clients transition from acute care to home care. Client's health can be improved with quality and efficient coordination among these levels of care (Parker et al., 2014). Nurses possess the knowledge and skills to strengthen care coordination and improve client outcomes in home care and other nonacute settings (Camicia et al., 2014).
- One quality improvement project examined postacute clients' perception of discharge teaching and readiness for discharge. The findings suggest that interprofessional teaching and client engagement improve client satisfaction scores, clients' readiness for discharge, and perceptions of the usefulness of discharge instructions (Knier et al., 2015).
- Recent studies compared different teaching modalities to improve health outcomes with chronic diseases. It was determined that Internet education programs may improve client engagement and management of chronic diseases such as diabetes (Pereira et al., 2015).
- One study examined the incidence of adverse events and unplanned hospitalizations of clients who were receiving

home care. Clients who are prescribed multiple medications (polypharmacy) are at increased risk of adverse events; therefore a review of the client's medication list is recommended at every visit, along with education about potential medication side effects (Mager, 2014).

The National Institute of Health (2015) provides best-practice strategies from its health literacy research. Following is a list of pertinent findings about literacy and providers' communication.

- Clients who are struggling to understand health information may feel judged for not understanding.
- Regardless of education level, everyone is at risk for misunderstanding health education and client teaching material.
- Embarrassment may prevent clients from asking questions or seeking clarification from the health care provider.

SAFETY GUIDELINES

- Assess if a client in the home setting is able to safely perform a skill. If he or she is unable to execute a skill independently, identify a family caregiver who will provide it safely in the home setting.
- Assess and determine if the client has home medical equipment and knows how to use it properly for safe and successful self-care management.
- Include teaching interventions for other people in the household who positively or negatively influence the client's self-care management.
- Provide an opportunity for client and/or family caregivers to demonstrate skill.
- Assess environment and teach appropriate disposal of client care medical products. For example, after clients use needles and other sharps, place the items in sharps disposal containers. Containers are to be placed at a height that is not accessible to children and pets.
- An additional challenge facing home care nurses today is health literacy. Health literacy is the ability to get the health information you need and understand it (Eadie, 2014).
- It is estimated that over 35% of American adults have low health literacy (CHCS, 2015). Individuals with low health literacy are generally less likely to self-manage chronic conditions and use more resources.
- To improve health literacy, use simple and plain words when speaking to clients and providing written instructions (USDHHS, 2015).

◆ SKILL 44.1 Teaching Clients to Measure Body Temperature

An elevation in body temperature may be an early warning sign of serious health problems. Clients susceptible to temperature alterations (e.g., immunosuppressed clients) or their family caregivers need to know how to measure temperature correctly so clients can seek medical attention earlier. Parents need to know how to measure their children's temperature because children can develop high fevers very quickly; older adults or their family caregivers need to know the techniques for temperature measurement because older adults have impaired temperature-control mechanisms. Teach clients and family caregivers the skills of measuring body temperature and techniques to lower temperature when a fever occurs at home.

A variety of body temperature thermometers are currently available, including disposable single-use, electronic digital, noncontact,

temporal, and tympanic thermometers. The Environmental Protection Agency (EPA, 2014) recommends the use of non-mercury thermometers; and most states have banned the sale of mercury fever thermometers. If a mercury thermometer breaks or is not disposed of properly, the mercury vapor gets into the air, posing a major health risk in the home and community (EPA, 2014). Educate clients about the environmental hazards associated with mercury in the home and encourage them to purchase mercury-free thermometers.

Help a client choose the most appropriate thermometer to use in the home on the basis of his or her normal dexterity, vision, and financial resources. For example, a client with visual impairment from glaucoma or retinopathy is able to read a thermometer with a large digital display more easily. The need for an oral, rectal, or axillary temperature depends on the client's age and health status (see Chapter 5).

Delegation and Collaboration

The skill of teaching clients to measure body temperature cannot be delegated to nursing assistive personnel (NAP). The nurse instructs the NAP to:

* Inform the nurse of client or family caregiver concerns about measuring body temperature.

Equipment

* Thermometer
* Disposable probe cover (if needed)
* Water-soluble lubricant (for rectal measurements)
* Paper and pencil or pen or computer if frequent measurements are to be taken
* Disposable clean gloves (for rectal temperature taken by a family caregiver)

STEP	RATIONALE

ASSESSMENT

1. Identify client using at least two identifiers during first visit. Facial recognition can be used as one of two identifiers for ongoing visits.

2. Assess client's or family caregiver's ability to manipulate and read thermometer. Have client put on eyeglasses if necessary.

3. Assess client's knowledge of normal temperature range, symptoms of fever and hypothermia, and client's risk for body temperature alterations.

4. Assess client's ability to determine appropriate type of thermometer to be used in varying situations (see Chapter 5).

5. Assess client's learning readiness and ability to concentrate; consider presence of pain, nausea, or fatigue and client interest in instruction.

6. Assess client's or family caregiver's previous knowledge and experience in measuring temperature and maintaining thermometer. Have client or caregiver perform return demonstration if he or she indicates ability to measure temperature.

Ensures client safety (TJC, 2016).

Physical restrictions in handling or reading thermometer prevent client from being able to read thermometer and often require teaching caregiver instead of client.

Identifies client's ability to recognize alterations in body temperature and to initiate preventive health measures.

Determines knowledge of age-related or medical conditions that determine selection of temperature.

Presence of significant illness, frailty, or confusion affects client's ability to attend to teaching plan. Indicates need to rely on family caregiver for learning and implementation (if available) on short- or long-term basis.

Allows assessment of client's or caregiver's knowledge and use of safety precautions, aseptic technique, and time period for insertion.

NURSING DIAGNOSES

* Deficient knowledge regarding temperature measurement skill
* Ineffective thermoregulation
* Risk for imbalanced body temperature
* Risk for infection

Related factors/Risk factors are individualized based on client's condition or needs.

PLANNING

1. Expected outcomes following completion of procedure:
   * Client or family caregiver is able to correctly measure body temperature.
   * Client or family caregiver demonstrates proper cleaning and storage of equipment.
   * Client or family caregiver states normal temperature range and factors that affect temperature, signs and symptoms of fever and hypothermia, and measures to take with abnormal temperatures.
2. Select setting in home where client or family caregiver is most likely to measure temperature.
3. Select setting in home where client is most likely to measure temperature and is a good location for teaching session:
   a. Select room that is well lit with comfortable seating.
   b. Be sure that client is close and can see nurse clearly.
   c. Control sources of noise and distractions.

Indicates that skills are learned.

Prevents transfer of microorganisms and maintains integrity of thermometer.

Cognitive learning is achieved.

Considers client's preferences; is responsive to client's needs (Ashton and Oermann, 2014).

Improves likelihood of client and family caregiver being attentive to instruction.

Room environment needs to minimize existing sensory alterations. Comfortable environment free of distractions promotes client's attention.

STEP	RATIONALE
4. Discuss and demonstrate with client or family caregiver normal temperature ranges; instruct caregiver to remain with client during measurement if age or physical status requires.	Learning by doing; active engagement is more effective than passive models (Peter et al., 2015).

IMPLEMENTATION

STEP	RATIONALE
1. Demonstrate steps of thermometer preparation, insertion, and reading. Provide rationale for steps to client or family caregiver.	Observing and evaluation of demonstration is cornerstone of client-centered care (McBride and Andrews, 2013). It is measured through client's performance and ability to follow directions/instruction.
a. Instruct client to take oral temperature 20 to 30 minutes after smoking or ingesting hot or cold liquids or foods and to wait at least an hour after hot bath or vigorous exercise. Explain indications for selecting temperature site other than oral.	Waiting at least 15 minutes after drinking hot or cold liquids or foods improves accuracy of temperature reading (AAP, 2015).
b. Perform hand hygiene. Instruct family caregiver to wear clean, disposable gloves.	Client and family caregiver must be knowledgeable about infection prevention techniques.
c. Teach client or family caregiver proper way to position client for temperature measurement (see Chapter 5).	Improves accuracy of readings.
d. Demonstrate temperature measurement technique and have client or caregiver perform each step with guidance. Do not rush him or her.	Allows for correction of errors in technique as they occur and for discussion of potential consequences of errors.
e. Explain any special precautions in using thermometers: oral thermometer must be placed in sublingual pocket; rectal thermometers must be lubricated with water-soluble lubricant; use rectal thermometer only for measuring rectal temperatures; never force rectal thermometer into rectum.	Ensures accurate reading and avoidance of injury to client.
f. Discuss typical time frame needed for each type of temperature to register (based on thermometer type) and how to take reading.	Ensures accurate reading.
g. Teach proper method for removing, cleaning, and storing thermometer (when applicable) and select suitable storage location.	Prevents transmission of infection. Thermometer is stored properly so it does not break or become inaccurate when not in use.
2. Discuss common symptoms of fever: warm, dry, flushed skin; feeling warm; chills; piloerection; malaise; and restlessness.	Client or family caregiver needs to recognize onset of fever in self or family member for early detection and intervention.
3. Discuss common signs and symptoms of hypothermia: cool skin, uncontrolled shivering, loss of memory, and signs of poor judgment. Explain that people with inadequate home heating, older adults, or those unaware of potential dangers of cold conditions are at risk.	Client or family caregiver needs to recognize onset of hypothermia in self or family member for early detection and intervention (Sund-Levander and Grodzinsky, 2013).

Clinical Decision Point *Teach client to take temperature after chills/shivering subsides to obtain an accurate temperature.*

STEP	RATIONALE
4. Discuss importance of notifying health care provider when temperature elevations occur. Review common therapies for temperature reduction that are safe to perform at home, including when to use antipyretics; exposing skin to air; reducing room temperature; increasing air circulation; applying cool, moist compresses to skin (e.g., forehead); and drinking fluids (Hockenberry and Wilson, 2015).	Treating fever enhances client comfort. Lowering temperature can reduce risk of febrile seizures in children (Hockenberry and Wilson, 2015).
5. Provide set of written guidelines for client's reference at appropriate level of health literacy.	Clients prefer written materials that are clear and concise; bulleted lists are preferred to text blocks (NIH, 2015).
6. Give client or caregiver paper or digital logbook to time and record temperature if frequent monitoring is required. Instruct client to use written record to report temperatures to health care provider.	Keeping organized record of temperatures helps client validate and report temperature fluctuations to health care provider.

STEP	RATIONALE

EVALUATION

1. Have client or family caregiver independently demonstrate technique for temperature measurement, including body placement and ability to read thermometer three separate times.

   When psychomotor skill is performed with confidence and correctly, it demonstrates mastery of skill (Buscombe, 2013).

2. Ask client or caregiver to identify normal temperature range and influence of smoking and hot and cold liquids or foods on oral readings; discuss safety implications for temperature measurement.

   Measures cognitive learning and confirms understanding of information.

3. Have client or caregiver describe common signs and symptoms of fever and hypothermia and methods for control.

   Measures cognitive learning.

4. Watch client or caregiver clean and store equipment.

   Proper cleaning prevents bacterial growth, and proper storage preserves accuracy of thermometer.

5. Watch client record temperature values and times in log. Review client's log periodically to ensure that temperatures are being recorded correctly.

   Health care providers make changes in client care based on information provided by client. To ensure that changes are made appropriately, client needs to record accurate information.

6. **Use Teach-Back:** "I want to be sure I explained the importance of monitoring your temperature. Explain in your own words why it is important to know how to take your own temperature." Revise your instruction now or develop a plan for revised client or family caregiver teaching if client or family caregiver is not able to teach back correctly.

   Determines client's and family caregiver's level of understanding of instructional topic.

Unexpected Outcomes

1. Client or family caregiver is unable to measure temperature, clean and store thermometer correctly, or verbalize knowledge about fever and temperature measurement.

2. Client reports breaking mercury glass thermometer.

Related Interventions

- Ask client or caregiver to describe difficulties experienced while performing temperature measurement.
- Use a different teaching strategy.
- Plan for client to perform another return demonstration during next scheduled home care visit or plan to teach family caregiver.
- Teach client steps to dispose of thermometer safely (Box 44.1).

BOX 44.1

Steps to Take in the Event of a Mercury Spill

- If possible, close the room off from the rest of the house and increase ventilation in the affected room by opening windows or turning on a fan.
- Put on rubber, nitrile, or latex gloves. Do not touch mercury. Do not allow children to help clean up the spill. Remove all pets from the area.
- Pick up glass pieces, place them in a folded paper towel, and place glass and towel into plastic zip lock bag.
- Use a squeegee or cardboard to gather mercury beads. Use an eyedropper to collect or draw up visible mercury beads. Slowly and carefully squeeze mercury onto a damp paper towel. Place the paper towel in a zip lock bag and secure. Then put shaving cream on a small brush and "dot" the area or press duct tape in area to pick up smaller beads.

- Place mercury, material used to pick up mercury, and broken glass in a plastic zip lock bag. Triple bag the contaminated objects (place in a total of three sealed bags).
- Place gloves, mercury, and all other wastes into a trash bag. Secure and label the bag.
- Call local health department to determine where to dispose of mercury safely.
- If possible, keep windows open and room well ventilated for at least 24 hours after clean up.
- Instruct client not to use a vacuum cleaner, a broom, or household cleaners when cleaning up mercury spill. Also instruct client not to put mercury down the drain or place contaminated clothing into the washing machine.

Data from EPA: *Mercury releases and spills*, 2014, http://www.epa.gov/mercury/spills/index.htm#thermometer. Accessed April 13, 2016.

Recording and Reporting

- Record information taught and client's and family caregiver's return demonstration in home care record.
- Record temperature in home care record and home documentation system (e.g., log).
- Report high and low temperatures to health care provider.

Special Considerations
Teaching

- Instruct client or family caregiver to never force thermometer into rectum or use rectal thermometer after rectal surgery, when the client has a rectal disorder such as tumor or severe hemorrhoids, when the client has a low platelet count, or when it is difficult to position client for proper thermometer placement.

- Use caution in recommending aspirin or any other over-the-counter (OTC) drug or antipyretic medicine in clients whose conditions contraindicate their use (e.g., gastric ulcer, bleeding tendencies, allergic reactions, drug interactions, liver or kidney dysfunction). Encourage client to contact health care provider before using OTC antipyretics.
- Instruct client to never use sponging with isopropyl alcohol to lower fever because of neurotoxic effects (Hockenberry and Wilson, 2015).
- Always leave a phone number and instructions about how to reach home care nurse if needed.

Pediatric
- Stage of growth and development of child will determine site of measurement and type of equipment used (see Chapter 5).
- Different types of thermometers are available for use with children (e.g., temporal artery, tympanic). Reliability of these different thermometers varies; ensure that parents know how to use the equipment correctly and detect the signs and symptoms of a fever (Hockenberry and Wilson, 2015).

- Teach parents to take a child's temperature whenever he or she feels warm to the touch, even if the temperature was recently normal (Hockenberry and Wilson, 2015).
- Avoid aspirin in children under the age of 19 to prevent Reye's syndrome.

Gerontological
- Older adults' normal temperatures often range below 36.1°C (97°F); therefore a normal temperature range for adults sometimes reflects a fever in the older adult (Sund-Levander and Grodzinsky, 2013).
- Older adults are more sensitive to temperature changes and tend to demonstrate symptoms of delirium or dementia with variations of body temperature.
- Altered internal temperature regulation or dehydration occurs frequently in frail, debilitated clients. Temperature measurement becomes very important to prevent severe states of hypothermia or hyperthermia.
- Consider common age-related sensory changes in the older adult and direct teaching strategies to compensate for any alterations (e.g., a magnifying glass to read thermometer).

◆ SKILL 44.2   Teaching Blood Pressure and Pulse Measurement

Clients with a variety of illnesses such as cardiac, kidney, or vascular diseases are susceptible to wide variations in their blood pressure (BP) and pulse. They benefit from knowing how to assess their own BP and pulse because they are able to seek medical attention early when readings vary from their acceptable ranges. In addition, healthy people who exercise learn how their body responds to exercise and are able to determine appropriate exercise plans based on knowing what their pulse and BP are before, during, and after exercise.

Research related to home monitoring of BP has illustrated the importance of regular monitoring outside of acute care settings and medical offices so the health care provider can treat clients with hypertension appropriately (Crabtree and Stuart-Shor, 2014). If treatment is based on single readings during an office visit, health care providers do not see an accurate picture of a client's health. To gather this essential information about clients living at home, you will teach them to measure their BP and pulse regularly and interpret readings that are outside of their individualized normal values. For example, teach clients about factors that affect the accuracy of BP readings such as cuff placement, movement of the tubing, speaking during measurement, and position and movement of the extremity or body.

Aneroid sphygmomanometers are available to measure BP in the home (see Chapter 5). Aneroid manometers are safe, lightweight, compact, and portable. In the home many clients choose to use commercial automatic electronic BP devices. These devices may measure pulse rate and produce a BP measurement without needing to use a stethoscope. The devices involve placing a cuff around the arm, the wrist, or a fingertip. A reading is displayed electronically for the client. Electronic BP monitors are often easier to use, but their accuracy compared to manual BP monitoring is still a focus of debate. However, home monitoring of BP is still recommended because of the increased number of BP readings that can be obtained (Kantarci, 2013). It is essential for clients to

keep a record of all of their BP readings and compare those obtained by a health care provider with their electronic monitor to assess the accuracy of readings.

Additional factors that affect the accuracy of BP monitoring are cuff size and placement (Fallon, 2015). Have clients learn to place a cuff directly on their skin. BP cuffs that are too small tend to overestimate BP, whereas cuffs that are too large tend to underestimate it (Fallon, 2015). Not all electronic home BP monitors come with interchangeable cuff sizes, which can complicate BP monitoring at home. Help clients and family caregivers determine cuff size, calibration, and accuracy of electronic equipment before they determine which type of BP monitor to purchase.

Delegation and Collaboration
The skill of teaching clients to measure BP and pulse cannot be delegated to nursing assistive personnel (NAP). The nurse instructs the NAP to:
- Report concerns related to BP (e.g., episodes of suspected orthostatic hypotension) and measurements to the nurse.

Equipment
For Blood Pressure
- Sphygmomanometer or electronic BP reading device (Fig. 44.1) with bladder and cuff: Bladder should completely encircle arm without overlapping; cuff should be secure and fit snugly (Box 44.2).
- Stethoscope (two-headed teaching stethoscope is ideal) if using sphygmomanometer

For Pulse
- Wristwatch or clock with a second hand

For Both
- Log

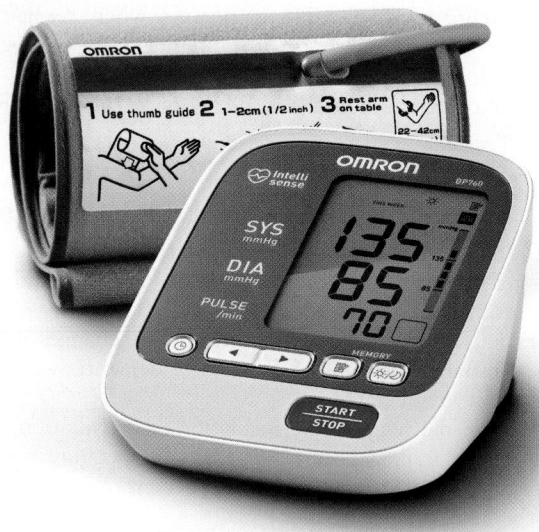

FIG 44.1 Home blood pressure monitoring device. (*Courtesy Omron Healthcare, Bannockburn, IL.*)

STEP	RATIONALE

ASSESSMENT

1. Identify client using at least two identifiers during first visit. Facial recognition can be used as one of two identifiers for ongoing subsequent visits.	Ensures client safety (TJC, 2016).
2. Assess client's or caregiver's psychomotor function: visual (see dial and clock) and auditory (hear Korotkoff sounds) acuity, ability to manipulate BP monitoring equipment, and ability to feel pulse.	Vision or hearing problems require use of equipment that has been adapted for these conditions (e.g., larger print) (Heiss, 2013). Other deficits may require caregiver to perform skills.
3. Assess client's or family caregiver's knowledge of normal BP and pulse range for client and the symptoms of high or low readings. (Consult with health care provider regarding normal range desired.)	Identifies client's or family caregiver's ability to know when to initiate preventive health measures and recognize alterations in BP and pulse.
4. Assess client's or family caregiver's knowledge of what BP and pulse measure, specific medical issues that affect them, and why awareness of variations is important to client's health.	Identifies client's or family caregiver's understanding of potential cause-and-effect relationships between variations in BP and pulse and health status.
5. Assess client's or family caregiver's previous knowledge and experience in measuring BP and pulse. Have client or caregiver perform return demonstration if he or she indicates ability to measure BP or pulse.	Allows nurse to assess client's or family caregiver's knowledge and skill performance.
6. Assess client's learning readiness and ability to concentrate; consider presence of pain, nausea, or fatigue and client interest in instruction.	Presence of significant illness, frailty, or confusion affects client's ability to attend to teaching plan. Indicates need to rely on family caregiver for learning and implementation (if available) on short- or long-term basis.
7. Assess home environment for favorable place to measure BP and pulse (e.g., quiet room with comfortable place to sit) along with quality of home BP equipment.	Ensures more accurate measurement (Jung et al., 2015).

NURSING DIAGNOSES

- Deficient knowledge regarding pulse/ BP measurement
- Ineffective health maintenance

Related factors are individualized based on client's condition or needs.

STEP	RATIONALE

PLANNING

1. Expected outcomes following completion of procedure:
- Client or family caregiver accurately measures BP and pulse.
- BP and pulse are within range expected for client's age and condition (see Chapter 5).
- Client or caregiver explains importance of measuring BP and pulse, common causes for changes, best time for measurement, and when to communicate with health care provider to evaluate changes in treatment regimen.

Learning has occurred.
Cardiovascular status is stable at level that is determined for client by his or her health care provider.
Measures cognitive learning.

2. Encourage client or family caregiver to perform measurements on routine schedule for long-term monitoring plan.

Daily activities and many extrinsic and intrinsic factors affect measurement fluctuations. Routine schedule allows for daily comparisons.

3. Encourage client to avoid exercise, caffeine, and smoking for 30 minutes before assessment to avoid inaccuracy.

These factors cause elevations in BP and pulse (AHA, 2015).

4. Have client or family caregiver perform measurement in comfortable position, with arm supported and feet flat on floor and in warm and quiet environment.

Maintains client's comfort during measurement. Systolic and diastolic BP increases with crossed-leg position (Frese et al., 2011).

IMPLEMENTATION

1. BP measurement:

a. Explain importance of having client sit quietly for 5 minutes with back supported and feet on floor before measurement. If client cannot sit in this position, select position that client can maintain.

Reduces anxiety that can falsely elevate BP readings (Fallon, 2015).
It is important for client to maintain same position for each reading.

b. Discuss with client or family caregiver best sites for assessing BP. For self-measurement brachial artery is almost always used. If client cannot sit in this position, select position that client can maintain. Explain to avoid applying cuff to arm with:
- Intravenous (IV) catheter with or without fluids infusing
- Arteriovenous shunt
- Breast or axillary surgery
- Trauma, inflammation, or disease

Most accessible sites are easiest to measure for accuracy of assessment. Appropriate site selection promotes accuracy in reading and minimizes potential for trauma. It is important for client to maintain same position for each reading. Application of pressure from inflated bladder temporarily impairs blood flow and compromises circulation in extremity that already has impaired circulation.

c. Demonstrate steps for measuring BP (see Chapter 5):

Eventual evaluation of psychomotor skill is measured through client's performance and ability to follow directions/instructions (Heiss, 2013).

(1) Use of sphygmomanometer and stethoscope:

(a) Teach palpating artery, positioning cuff, wrapping cuff, placing stethoscope, inflating and releasing cuff, listening for Korotkoff sounds.

Prepares client or family caregiver for measuring BP.

(b) Describe sounds of measurement and relationship to observation of gauge during BP reading. Caution client or family caregiver about level and length of time appropriate for cuff inflation.

Ensures accurate reading. Prolonged inflation of cuff impairs circulation to extremity.

(c) Teach client or family caregiver to routinely clean diaphragm and earpieces of stethoscope with rubbing alcohol or damp cloth.

Stethoscopes are frequently contaminated with microorganisms. Cleaning stethoscope routinely prevents transmission of microorganisms.

Clinical Decision Point *If client or family caregiver needs to use stethoscope to take BP, use double-headed teaching stethoscope to verify accuracy of reading or read BP 1 to 2 minutes after client's attempt to verify accuracy. If client is having difficulty hearing Korotkoff sounds, ensure that he or she is applying cuff appropriately and using the correct size cuff. Also determine correct use of equipment (e.g., cuff may have been deflated too quickly or too slowly; cuff may not have been pumped high enough for systolic readings).*

(2) Use of electronic BP monitor:

(a) Teach correct placement of cuff and use of electronic equipment for proper cuff inflation.

Using electronic equipment correctly helps ensure accurate BP readings.

STEP	RATIONALE

2. Pulse measurement:

    a. Discuss with client or family caregiver best sites for assessing pulse: radial and carotid.

Radial and carotid sites are accessible and usually easiest to palpate.

Clinical Decision Point *If carotid site is chosen, caution client against vigorously massaging neck while attempting to locate pulse or attempting to locate both arteries at the same time. Stimulation of carotid sinus leads to reflex slowing of heart rate from vagal stimulation. In addition, simultaneous occlusion of both carotid arteries decreases blood to brain, resulting in fainting.*

    b. Demonstrate steps for palpating pulse (see Chapter 5): position of artery on wrist or neck, how to locate artery, using fingertips for palpation, compressing artery, palpating pulse before counting, counting pulse, and calculating pulse rate (see illustration).

Eventual evaluation of psychomotor skill is measured through client's performance and ability to follow directions/instructions (Heiss, 2013).

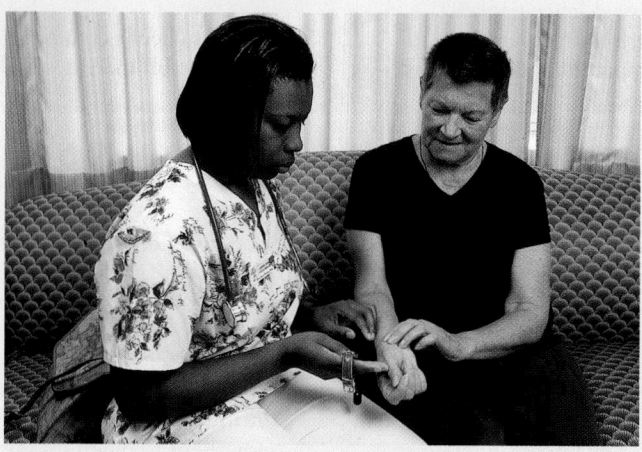

STEP 2b Nurse observing client checking radial pulse.

    (1) Instruct in use of gentle pressure; reinforce not to press hard over pulse site.

Pressing too hard may occlude artery.

    (2) Instruct in use of watch or clock with second hand to count pulse.

Ensures correct timing of pulse.

    (3) Instruct to count for full 60 seconds, starting with second hand at 12:00 position.

Consistent timing of procedure reduces confusion or forgetfulness about time period or starting point used for pulse measurement. Full 60-second count increases accuracy of measure.

3. Educate client or caregiver about normal desired BP and pulse ranges, purposes for monitoring, and when to take measurements (e.g., before and after taking cardiac or antihypertensive medications; before, during, and after exercise).

Client needs to be able to determine when values are not in desired ranges and when measurements need to be taken.

4. Describe symptoms that indicate need to perform BP and/or pulse measurement.

Promotes understanding of health status alterations that need medical intervention.

Clinical Decision Point *Discuss importance of notifying health care provider and withholding medications when abnormal values in BP or pulse occur (e.g., hypotension or bradycardia). Client needs to understand preventive measures to take and to follow health care provider's directions if alterations develop.*

5. Have client or caregiver attempt each step of skill on you or family member.

You can correct any errors in technique as they occur.

6. Observe client demonstrate techniques to measure pulse and BP on self. When measuring BP, do not allow multiple repetitive BP attempts on any one limb.

After developing confidence in measuring values in others, client is ready to measure own values. Making multiple repetitive BP attempts restricts circulation and alters measurement.

7. Teach client or family caregiver to monitor BP and pulse even if they remain in normal range.

Continuous monitoring provides important information that evaluates effectiveness of medications or other treatments.

STEP	RATIONALE
8. Provide client or family caregiver with printed instructions with written or pictorial guide or with videotape/DVD demonstration of procedure if possible.	Printed and audiovisual teaching materials help stimulate client's visual and auditory senses, which enhances learning (Heiss, 2013).
9. Give client or family caregiver log to record BP and pulse and time they were taken. In addition, client records whether or not medications that affect BP or pulse were taken. Instruct client to use written record to report readings to health care provider.	Keeping organized record of BP and pulse readings and medications empowers client and provides accurate information to health care providers.
10. Instruct client or family caregiver in proper care of equipment (e.g., storage, cleaning, and battery care).	Improper care and storage of equipment affects accuracy of measurement.

EVALUATION

1. Observe client or family caregiver demonstrate technique for BP and/or pulse measurement on at least three different occasions and verify that client adds information to logbook correctly.	Feedback through return demonstration of psychomotor learning is best means to evaluate learning.
2. Ask client or family caregiver if readings are within desired range and when to report abnormal readings to health care provider.	Determines client's ability to know when readings are within proper range and what to do when abnormal readings are obtained.
3. Ask client or family caregiver to describe reason for BP and pulse monitoring and any related medications (e.g., antihypertensives, antidysrhythmics) or treatment (e.g., diet and exercise).	Determines if client understands monitoring and related therapies.
4. Have client or family caregiver demonstrate proper care of equipment.	Demonstrates learning.
5. **Use Teach-Back:** "I want to be sure I explained the importance of monitoring your BP. Explain to me how your medications can affect your BP readings." Revise your instruction now or develop a plan for revised client or family caregiver teaching if client or family caregiver is not able to teach back correctly.	Determines client's and family caregiver's level of understanding of instructional topic.

Unexpected Outcomes	**Related Interventions**
1. Client or family caregiver is unable to measure BP or pulse (e.g., inability to manipulate equipment, visualize numbers on equipment or clock, hear BP sounds).	• Alter teaching plan to accommodate client's problems (e.g., use other types of equipment that are easier to manipulate, see, or hear). • Reinforce information taught and continue return demonstrations until client is able to perform skill. • Teach skill to different family caregiver.
2. Client or family caregiver has difficulty explaining purposes of measurement or implications of therapy.	• Review and reinforce information that client or caregiver does not understand.

Recording and Reporting

• Record teaching, client and family caregiver responses, and demonstration in home care record.
• Record BP and pulse in home care record and home documentation system (e.g., logbook).
• Report changes in readings of BP and/or pulse.

Special Considerations
Teaching

• Educate client about risks for hypertension, hypotension, or change in pulse rate (see Chapter 5).
• Ensure that client understands health care provider's recommendations for treatment regimen, including potential side effects and interactions of any medication therapies (e.g., clients taking thyroid medications might need to withhold them when BP is above normal range or pulse is above 100 beats/min). Confirm specific guidelines for BP and pulse with health care provider; document information in home care record; and provide clear, written instructions for the client.
• Always leave a phone number and instructions about how to reach home care nurse if needed.

Pediatric

• Readings (BP or pulse) are often inaccurate if an infant or child is anxious and uncooperative. BP is also inaccurate when the cuff size is inappropriate. Having others divert the child's attention or taking his or her BP or pulse while he or she is seated on the parent's lap usually helps calm the child (Hockenberry and Wilson, 2015).

- Young children will be more likely to cooperate if allowed to touch and/or play with equipment before procedure. Consider performing the procedure first on the parent or another person significant to child. This allows the child to observe that the procedure is safe.
- Use the radial pulse in children over 2 years of age. Femoral or brachial pulse is the best site for palpation of pulse for children under 2 years of age (Hockenberry and Wilson, 2015). When under the age of 1 year, use a stethoscope to obtain the apical heart.

Gerontological

- Musculoskeletal changes such as arthritis or other joint conditions may impair a client's ability to position limb comfortably and/or perform fine-motor skills required to measure BP and pulse (Jett, 2014).
- Older adults, especially those who are frail or who have lost upper-arm mass, require a smaller BP cuff.
- Home BP monitoring is not a replacement for BP monitoring by health care providers in older adults, but it can serve to provide more information to ensure the best treatment.

◆ SKILL 44.3 Teaching Intermittent Self-Catheterization

Most people urinate and empty their bladder 4 or 5 times a day (SUNA, 2010). However, some clients are not able to empty their bladder. Infections in the bladder or kidneys and damage to the kidneys sometimes result from incomplete emptying of the bladder. Clean intermittent self-catheterization (CISC) is a safe and effective way to empty the bladder. The client performs self-catheterization with clean technique, eliminating the need to wear gloves. Clients who use CISC have a variety of health problems that affect the neuromuscular control of the bladder (Wyndaele, 2014). Current practice supports CISC for use in the home to provide a means to completely empty the bladder, prevent urinary tract infections (UTIs), and prevent further bladder and kidney damage (Sheldon, 2013). Inadequate or excessive fluid intake, poor catheterization technique and catheter care, and traumatic catheterization can cause UTIs. Teaching proper self-catheterization technique is crucial in preventing infections (Sheldon, 2013).

Using CISC helps clients believe that they are more in control of their daily needs, which enhances their quality of life. It helps some clients become continent, maintain a positive body image, and experience less anxiety and embarrassment. In addition, CISC allows clients to express their sexuality and sustain satisfying relationships with significant others. However, the skill requires physical and manual dexterity, and clients must adhere to a regular schedule for it to be successful (Seth et al., 2014). When the client is unable to perform CISC independently, teach his or her family caregiver how to perform the skill. For clients with certain medical conditions (e.g., immunosuppressed clients), sterile or aseptic technique is the recommended method of self-catheterization rather than CISC (Newman and Willson, 2011).

Delegation and Collaboration

The skill of teaching intermittent self-catheterization cannot be delegated to nursing assistive personnel (NAP). The nurse instructs the NAP to:
- Record the amount of urine on the paper or digital logbook if the client is unable.
- Report to the nurse changes to the color, odor, and/or amount of urine.

Equipment

- Soap, water, and clean washcloth
- Mirror (optional)
- Urethral catheter (smallest size that is able to pass easily into the bladder and completely drain client's urine)
- Lubricant (e.g., water-soluble jelly) if catheter is uncoated
- Container for collection of urine (e.g., urinal)—not needed for clients emptying urine directly into toilet
- Mild soap (e.g., Ivory)
- Catheter storage item or container (e.g., brown paper bag, clean towel)
- Disposable clean gloves (for family caregiver)
- Log book (optional)

STEP	RATIONALE

ASSESSMENT

1. Identify client using at least two identifiers during first visit. Facial recognition can be used as one of two identifiers for ongoing subsequent visits.	Ensures client safety (TJC, 2016).
2. Review client's medical record, including order for CISC and nurses' notes. Gather information about voiding history, existing medical and surgical history, client's usual daily fluid intake, postvoid residual amounts, and daily voiding routine.	Determines reason for CISC, frequency of catheterization, and previous responses to client education.
3. Assess client's ability to perform CISC, including developmental level, level of consciousness, motor function, and psychosocial status.	Client must be physically able to reach urethra and move equipment as needed. Client who cannot see urethra can be taught to feel for proper location of urethral opening (Sheldon, 2013).
4. Assess client's or family caregiver's knowledge about CISC and observe performance of CISC if client has performed previously.	Effective client or caregiver education builds on previous knowledge; observation is effective way to assess performance of psychomotor skills (Heiss, 2013).

STEP	RATIONALE

NURSING DIAGNOSES

- Deficient knowledge regarding self-catheterization
- Impaired urinary elimination
- Readiness for enhanced urinary elimination
- Reflex urinary incontinence
- Urinary retention

Related factors are individualized based on client's condition or needs.

PLANNING

1. Expected outcomes following completion of procedure:
   - Client or family caregiver states signs and symptoms that indicate need for CISC.
   - Client or family caregiver correctly demonstrates how to perform CISC and clean and store equipment.
   - Client or family caregiver verbalizes signs and symptoms of complications of CISC (e.g., UTI, urethral bleeding, urethritis, stricture, creation of false passage) and when to contact health care provider (Newman and Willson, 2011).
2. Select setting in home that client or family caregiver will most likely use when performing CISC.
3. Help client or family caregiver select catheter that is easiest to use, causes least amount of trauma, and is most comfortable.

Indicates ability to identify appropriate times to use CISC.

Return demonstration of skill indicates learning (Heiss, 2013).

Urinary complications such as UTI can result in clients who use CISC (Bolinger and Engberg, 2013). Verbalization of signs and symptoms of complications helps clients or caregivers identify potential problems early and seek appropriate care.
Respecting client's needs, values, and choices is key in client-centered care (Heiss, 2013).
Variety of single-use and reusable catheters is currently available.

IMPLEMENTATION

1. Teach client or family caregiver how to perform appropriate hand hygiene using soap and water. If family caregiver is performing skill, have him or her apply pair of disposable clean gloves.
2. Perform hand hygiene. Help client get into comfortable position. Some men prefer to stand, whereas others prefer to sit. Female clients often need to try different positions to decide which position is most comfortable (SUNA, 2010). Position client in place that has adequate lighting.
3. Teach client or family caregiver how to clean urethral meatus:
   a. *For women:* Have client spread labia with one hand. Use other hand to clean urethral opening with a washcloth containing warm soapy water, and then use a clean moist washcloth to rinse. Have female clean in direction from urethral meatus toward rectum.
   b. *For men:* If client has not been circumcised, teach him to retract foreskin to expose urethral meatus. Teach client to hold penis perpendicular to body with one hand, use other hand to clean urethral opening with a washcloth containing warm soapy water, and then use a clean moist washcloth to rinse. Have male clean in circular motion from meatus outward.
4. Teach female client or family caregiver how to insert catheter:
   a. Catheter selection depends on client preference and includes single-use or reusable catheter.
   b. Using mirror, help client locate meatus. Explain that it is just below clitoris and just above vaginal opening.

Prevents risk for UTI and trauma, which can lead to urethral strictures (Sheldon, 2013). Prevents transmission of infection.

Reduces transmission of infection. Client needs adequate lighting to see meatus and equipment.

Retraction of labia allows for female urethral meatus to be cleaned, reducing risk for infection (Wilson, 2015). Reduces transmission of infection from rectal area to meatus.

Ensures cleaning of meatus and reduces risk for infection (SUNA 2010; Wilson, 2015).

Single-use catheter is disposed of after one use. Reusable catheter is cleaned and stored between uses (Newman and Willson, 2011).
Mirror helps female client visualize anatomy (Wilson, 2015).

Clinical Decision Point *If female client wants to learn how to find meatus while in a sitting position, teach touch technique by helping her use fingers to find her urethral opening (Wilson, 2015). Teach her to put one finger over the clitoris and another finger over the vaginal opening. Then help her use these two fingers to find the urethral opening. Another method is the tunnel technique. When women sit with their hips flexed forward, the labia create a "tunnel" that leads to the urethral opening. Teach the woman to slightly separate labia near the clitoris and angle the catheter backward into the urethral opening while placing a finger over the vaginal opening.*

STEP	RATIONALE
c. If an uncoated catheter is selected, have client lubricate tip of catheter with water-soluble jelly by rotating tip to spread lubricant around bottom 2.5 to 5 cm (1 to 2 inches) of catheter. Coated catheters do not require use of separate lubrication.	Lubrication reduces urethral trauma (SUNA, 2010). Coated catheter uses hydrophilic or other coatings that do not require use of separate lubricant (Sheldon, 2013).
d. Place outflow end of catheter into urine collection container or let hang over toilet bowl. Slowly and gently insert tip of catheter 5 to 10 cm (2 to 4 inches) into meatus until urine begins to flow.	Appearance of urine indicates that catheter tip is in bladder.

Clinical Decision Point *If client feels resistance at the internal sphincter, teach her to apply firm, gentle, steady pressure until muscles relax and allow catheter to pass (SUNA, 2010).*

STEP	RATIONALE
5. Teach male client or family caregiver how to insert catheter:	
a. Catheter selection depends on client preference and includes single-use or reusable catheter.	Client preference is important for adherence to CISC (Dean, 2015). Single-use catheter is disposed of after one use. Reusable catheter is cleaned and stored between use (Newman and Willson, 2011).
b. Lubricate tip of uncoated catheter with water-soluble jelly by rotating tip to spread lubricant around bottom 13 to 18 cm (5 to 7 inches) of catheter. Coated catheters do not require separate lubricant (Sheldon, 2013).	Lubrication reduces urethral trauma in uncoated catheters. Dry catheters may cause excoriations in urethra, which can lead to entry point for bacterial contamination (Newman and Willson, 2011).
c. Place outflow end of catheter into urine collection container or let hang over toilet bowl. Slowly and gently insert tip of catheter 15 to 20 cm (6 to 8 inches) into meatus until urine begins to flow. For uncircumcised male, retract foreskin before inserting catheter. Tell client that catheter often needs to be inserted all the way for urine to begin to flow.	Male urethra is longer than female urethra. Flow of urine indicates that catheter tip is in bladder.

Clinical Decision Point *Men may experience some resistance when the catheter reaches the prostatic urethra or the neck of the bladder. If client feels resistance, do not pull the catheter in and out. Teach him to apply firm, gentle, steady pressure to fatigue the external sphincter and cause muscle relaxation (SUNA, 2010).*

STEP	RATIONALE
6. Instruct client or family caregiver to hold catheter in place while urine flows into container or toilet.	Release of catheter during procedure often causes catheter to accidentally come out before bladder is completely emptied.
7. When urine flow stops, teach client to slowly and gently remove catheter. For uncircumcised male, bring foreskin back over glans penis. Then perform hand hygiene.	Removing catheter slowly allows pockets of urine that can accumulate at base of bladder to drain (SUNA, 2010).
8. Give client log to record amount of urine if needed.	Some clients need to keep track of their urinary output.
9. Single-use catheters are discarded after self-catheterization is complete (Sheldon, 2013). Instruct client to clean reusable catheter with mild soap (e.g., Ivory) and water immediately after use. Rinse catheter completely, allow to air dry, and store in clean, dry towel or brown paper bag.	Minimizes risk of UTIs.
10. Teach client or family caregiver to replace reusable catheters as directed by health care provider.	Appropriate disposal and replacement of equipment prevents complications of CISC.

EVALUATION

1. Observe client or family caregiver independently demonstrate technique for CISC.	Feedback through return demonstration of psychomotor skill is best means of evaluating learning of skill.
2. Ask client to identify plan for timing of CISC and steps to take when problems arise.	Measures client's cognitive learning and ability to problem solve.
3. Review client's log book and observe client enter information about urine output if indicated.	Confirms that client understands record keeping and importance of tracking urine output.
4. **Use Teach-Back:** "I want to be sure I explained the steps clearly for how to clean and store your catheter. Explain to me how to clean and store your reusable catheter." Revise your instruction now or develop a plan for revised client or family caregiver teaching if client or family caregiver is not able to teach back correctly.	Determines client's and family caregiver's level of understanding of instructional topic.

STEP	RATIONALE

Unexpected Outcomes

1. Client is unable to easily pass catheter into bladder.

2. Client states that he or she is having symptoms of UTI (e.g., intense urge to urinate; flank or abdominal pain, malaise, fever, chills).

Related Interventions

- Teach client not to force catheter into bladder.
- Tell client to go to nearest urgent care center or emergency department if bladder is full and client is unable to insert catheter.
- Consider initiating consultation with urologist.
- Inform client's health care provider of symptoms and anticipate treatment with antibiotic.

Recording and Reporting

- Record teaching, client and family caregiver responses, and demonstration in home care record.
- Record urine output in home care record and home documentation system (e.g., log book).
- Report signs and symptoms of UTIs and difficulty performing CISC to health care provider.

Special Considerations
Teaching

- It is common for clients who perform CISC routinely to have an abnormal urinalysis. Clients should only be treated for UTIs if they have symptoms of an infection (e.g., back pain, pelvic tenderness, malaise, confusion, foul-smelling urine, urgency) (Bolinger and Engberg, 2013).
- Always leave a phone number and instructions about how to reach home care nurse if needed.

Pediatric

- Children who are motivated and physiologically and developmentally ready are encouraged to learn how to catheterize themselves. Consult a pediatric urologist; children need special assessment (Dean, 2015).
- When teaching children to perform CISC, use developmentally appropriate teaching strategies. Urinary diversion requires special care (see Chapter 34).
- Concerns of children and adolescents who use CISC include leakage and being wet. They also are often concerned about what their peers know. Allow children to voice their concerns and help them problem solve what they will do in a variety of situations.

Gerontological

- CISC is very effective in older adults because it helps restore continence, decreases urinary urge and nocturia, and improves quality of life.
- Older adults may have difficulty performing CISC because of limited manual dexterity. Individualize care for a client's needs and functional abilities. Educate the client or family caregivers (Ebersole et al., 2015).

◆ SKILL 44.4 Using Home Oxygen Equipment

Medical oxygen is classified by the Food and Drug Administration (FDA) as a drug; therefore a prescription from a health care provider is required for home use (DHSS, 2015). The prescription includes the following components: drug/apparatus, dose, route of administration, and duration. The route of administration of oxygen in the home may include nasal cannula, face mask, tracheal mask, or tracheal catheter. Equipment selection needs to support as much client independence as feasible (Tiep et al., 2015)

Oxygen-conserving devices (OCDs) were introduced to reduce the weight of portable oxygen systems and extend operating time by not wasting oxygen through continuous flow. There are three types of OCDs:

- *Reservoir nasal cannula:* Stores oxygen in a small chamber during exhalation for subsequent delivery during early-phase inhalation.

- *Demand pulsing oxygen-delivery systems:* Deliver a burst of oxygen at the onset of inspiration; small oxygen pulses are very effective in oxygenating a client.
- *Transtracheal oxygen catheter:* Delivers oxygen directly through a catheter placed between the second and third tracheal rings (American Thoracic Society, 2015) (Table 44.1).

Oxygen sources in the home include liquid oxygen systems, compressed oxygen in tanks, or oxygen concentrators (Fig. 44.2A) (Lewis et al., 2017). Some oxygen tanks (e.g., compressed) are large and stationary. Portable tanks weighing more than 10 lbs are not designed to be carried and deliver oxygen for about 5 hours at 2 L/min. Ambulatory tanks weigh less than 10 lbs, are designed to be carried (Fig. 44.2B), and deliver oxygen for at least 4 hours at 2 L/min. Table 44.2 compares the different types of home oxygen-delivery systems.

TABLE 44.1

Oxygen Flow and Appropriate Uses for Oxygen-Delivery Devices

Device	Flow (L/min)	FiO2 Range (%)	Uses
Nasal cannula	1–6	24–44	Clients who require low concentrations of oxygen therapy
Simple face mask	6–12	35–50	Clients who require short-term oxygen therapy with moderate FiO2 needs
Oxygen-conserving cannula	8	Up to 30–50	Clients in need of long-term home therapy
Partial and nonrebreather mask	10-15	60–90	Clients in acute respiratory failure or in emergency situations

Data from Lewis S, et al: *Medical-surgical nursing: assessment and management of clinical problems*, ed 10, St Louis, 2017, Elsevier.

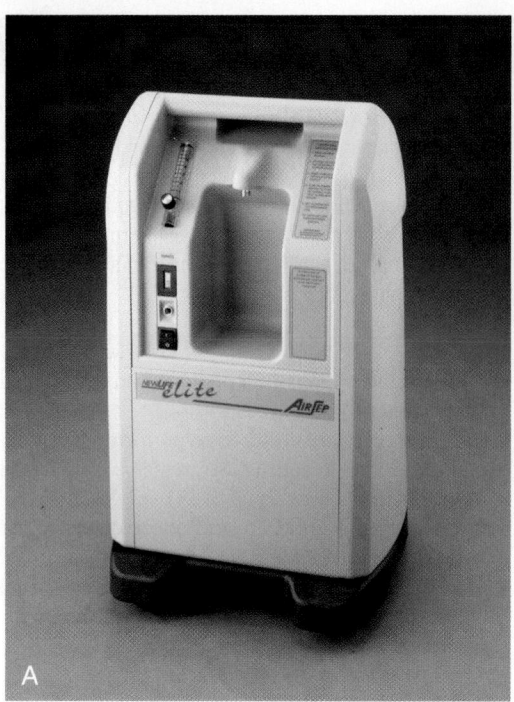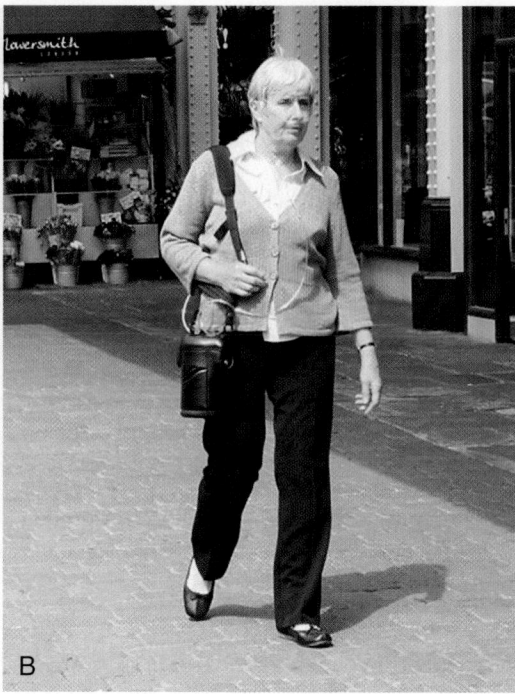

FIG 44.2 A, Portable oxygen concentrator for home use. **B,** Ambulatory tank is small enough to be carried easily. *(Courtesy AirSep Corporation.)*

TABLE 44.2		
Home Oxygen Delivery Systems		
	Advantages	**Disadvantages**
Compressed Oxygen		
Oxygen is stored under pressure in a cylinder equipped with a regulator that controls the flow rate.	An oxygen-conserving device may be attached to the system to avoid waste; device releases gas only on inhalation and cuts it off with exhalation; does not require an electrical source; smaller tanks are available.	Large tanks are heavy and only suitable for stationary use. Client must know how to read regulator and understand when to call medical supplier for replacement cylinder.
Liquid Oxygen System		
Oxygen is stored as a very cold liquid in a vessel very similar to a thermos. When released, the liquid converts to a gas and is breathed in just like compressed gas.	Storage method takes up less space than the compressed gas cylinder; it can transfer the liquid to a small, portable vessel at home.	It is more expensive than compressed gas, and the vessel vents when it is not in use. An oxygen-conserving device may be built into the vessel to conserve the oxygen.
Oxygen Concentrator		
It separates the oxygen out of the air, concentrates it, and stores it.	It does not have to be resupplied, and it is not as costly as liquid oxygen. Extra tubing permits the user to move around with minimal difficulty. Small, portable systems have been developed that afford even greater mobility.	It must have a cylinder of oxygen as a backup in the event of a power failure.

Compressed oxygen requires a regulator and flowmeter. The client receives delivery of several large oxygen tanks to the home. The size of the tank and flow rate determine how long compressed oxygen tanks will last (Table 44.3). Liquid systems take up less space because oxygen is stored in a liquid state. Liquid oxygen is stored at or below −183°C (−297°F) and requires the use of a small ambulatory tank that is filled from a reservoir in the home (Fig. 44.3). Table 44.4 shows how long a liquid oxygen system will last, depending on the prescribed flow rate. The oxygen concentrator method extracts oxygen from room air and supplies oxygen to the client at prescribed flow rates. Oxygen concentrators deliver a lower percentage of oxygen to the flowmeter. Therefore, if a client is switched to a concentrator, the flow rate usually needs to be adjusted. The client who uses a concentrator needs to have a backup system such as a portable oxygen tank in case of power failure.

Home oxygen equipment and supplies are designated as durable medical equipment (DME) by Medicare; a certificate of medical necessity (CMN) is required for clients who receive Medicare (DHSS, 2015). Governmental or private insurance often pays for home oxygen therapy if there is a written order from the health care provider.

Clients and their family caregivers need extensive teaching to use oxygen therapy correctly and safely. Instruct a client to have an all-purpose fire extinguisher nearby and learn how to use it and

TABLE 44.3

Oxygen Cylinder Timetable*

| L/min | Large (H-K) Tank | | Small (E) Tank | |
	2200 lbs Full	1000 lbs ½ Full	625 L Full	284 L ½ Full
1	115 h	52 h	10 h	5 h
2	56 h	26 h	5 h	2 h
3	37 h	17 h	3 h	1 h
4	28 h	13 h	3 h	1 h
5	22 h	10 h	2 h	54 min
6	18 h	8 h	<2 h	47 min

The following formulas can also be used to determine the length of time a tank will last:

For E Cylinders

Pressure on cylinder gauge (psi): 500 psi (safety factor) × 0.3 (E cylinder factor) ÷ L/min = minutes

For H Cylinders

Pressure on cylinder gauge (psi): 500 psi (safety factor) × 3.1 (H cylinder factor) ÷ L/min = minutes

EXAMPLE: If E cylinder reads 1500 psi and liter flow rate is 4 L/min:
Time left: 1500 − 500 × 0.3 ÷ 4 = 1000 × 0.3 ÷ 4 = 300 ÷ 4 = 75 minutes (1 h 15 min)

NOTE: Do not allow oxygen cylinder pressure to fall below 500 psi, or the client may run out of oxygen.
*All times are approximate.

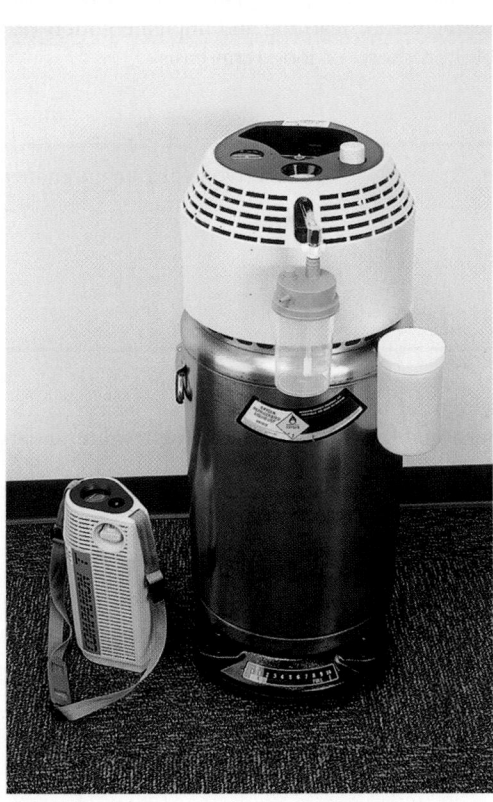

FIG 44.3 Oxygen reservoir and ambulatory tank.

to keep the oxygen supplier's number handy. In addition, provide client education about the safe use of oxygen in the home (Box 44.3). When initiating and managing ongoing oxygen therapy, collaborate with the client, health care provider, family caregivers, DME provider, and payer.

TABLE 44.4

Liquid Oxygen Timetable

| L/min | Stationary Reservoirs | | Portable Units | |
	41 L	31 L	½ L	1 L
0.25	1400 h	1060 h	28 h	44 h
0.50	1125 h	850 h	18 h	27 h
1	560 h	425 h	9 h	15½ h
1.5	375 h	283½ h	6 h	11½ h
2	281 h	213 h	4½ h	8½ h
3	187½ h	142 h	3 h	6 h

BOX 44.3

Safe Home Oxygen Therapy

Fire Safety
Although oxygen is not flammable, if it comes in contact with fire it will burn; therefore:

- Use and store oxygen in a well-ventilated area.
- Keep cylinders and vessels at least 5 feet from heat sources, open flames, or electrical devices.
- Do not use open flames (e.g., matches, fireplaces, stoves, space heaters, candles) when oxygen is in use.
- Do not allow smoking in the house. Post "No Smoking" signs inside and outside the house.
- Install smoke detectors and have a fire extinguisher available in the home. Test smoke detectors twice a month.
- Help client or family caregiver plan a fire evacuation route. Have two routes out of every room and an outside meeting place.

Oxygen Storage and Handling
- Store oxygen tanks upright in carts or stands to prevent tipping or falling or place tanks flat on the floor when not in use.
- Do not store oxygen tanks in the trunk of a car.
- When transporting oxygen in a vehicle, ensure that tanks are secured properly in the passenger area with the windows opened 5 to 7.5 cm (2 to 3 inches) to allow adequate ventilation.

Concentrator Safety
- Plug concentrators into properly grounded outlets.
- Do not use extension cords, power strips, or multi-outlet adapters with concentrators.
- Ensure that power supply or circuit meets or exceeds the amperage requirements of the concentrator.

Liquid Oxygen Safety
- Avoid direct contact with liquid oxygen because it can cause frostbite. The vapors are also extremely cold; can damage delicate tissues such as eyes.
- Do not touch connectors that are frosted or icy.
- Keep ambulatory tanks upright; do not lay them down or place on their side.

Adapted from Lewis S, et al: *Medical-surgical nursing: assessment and management of clinical problems,* ed 10, St Louis, 2017, Elsevier; National Fire Protection Association, 2015, http://www.nfpa.org/safety-information/safety-tip-sheets. Accessed April 13, 2016.

Delegation and Collaboration

- The skill of teaching clients how to use home oxygen equipment cannot be delegated to nursing assistive personnel (NAP).

Equipment

- Nasal cannula, oxygen mask (see Chapter 23), OCD, or other prescribed delivery device

- Oxygen tubing
- Home oxygen-delivery system (compressed oxygen, oxygen concentrator, or liquid oxygen) with all required equipment (varies with supplier and system used)

- "No Smoking/Oxygen in Use" sign for each entrance to the home

STEP	RATIONALE

ASSESSMENT

1. Identify client using at least two identifiers during hospital and first home visit. Facial recognition can be used as one of two identifiers for ongoing subsequent home visits.	Ensures client safety (TJC, 2016).
2. While client is still in hospital, determine client's or family caregiver's ability to apply and regulate oxygen equipment correctly. In home setting reassess for appropriate use of equipment.	Physical or cognitive impairments indicate need to teach caregiver how to operate home oxygen equipment. Determines specific components of skill that client and family caregiver are able to complete easily. Home assessment is critical for client and community safety (Wiles, 2015).
3. Determine appropriate resources in community for equipment and assistance, including maintenance and repair services and medical equipment supplier.	Ensures readily available help for clients with home oxygen systems (Wiles, 2015). Home oxygen risk assessment is priority with home oxygen therapy (TJC, 2015).
4. Determine appropriate backup systems for compressor in event of power failure (e.g., notify local emergency medical services [EMS]). Have spare oxygen tank available for emergency use.	Many municipalities require that clients who have home oxygen equipment notify EMS before putting equipment in home. In case of power outage, EMS will call home, and in some cases home is on priority list for having power restored.
5. Assess client's learning readiness and ability to concentrate; consider presence of pain, nausea, or fatigue and client interest in instruction.	Presence of significant illness, frailty, or confusion affects client's ability to attend to teaching plan. Indicates need to rely on family caregiver for learning and implementation (if available) on short- or long-term basis.

NURSING DIAGNOSES

- Anxiety
- Deficient knowledge regarding oxygen therapy
- Ineffective health maintenance

Related factors are individualized based on client's condition or needs.

PLANNING

1. Expected outcomes following completion of procedure:	
• Client receives oxygen at prescribed rate.	Oxygen system set up correctly.
• Client or family caregiver verbalizes purpose and correct use of home oxygen.	Provides measurable criteria to determine level of understanding.
• Client or family caregiver demonstrates how to apply, regulate, and maintain oxygen system.	Indicates learning has occurred.
• Client or family caregiver states indications for calling DME provider to replenish oxygen supply and reorder oxygen-delivery supplies.	Client needs constant supply of oxygen at home.
• Client or family caregiver verbalizes safety guidelines for oxygen use (e.g., place "No Smoking/Oxygen in Use" signs at entrances to home; educate about safety for client who continues to smoke) (Wiles, 2015).	Provides measure of understanding of oxygen use.
• Client or family caregiver verbalizes emergency plan of care (Wiles, 2015).	Ensures safe, continuous delivery of home oxygen.
2. Select setting in home where client is most likely to use oxygen equipment and is conducive to a teaching session:	Practicing in same environment where skill is routinely performed facilitates comprehension and learning.
a. Select a room that is well lit with comfortable seating.	
b. Be sure that client is close and can see nurse clearly.	
c. Control sources of noise and distractions.	Room environment needs to minimize existing sensory alterations. Comfortable environment free of distractions promotes client's attention.

STEP	**RATIONALE**

IMPLEMENTATION

1. Teach client or family caregiver how to perform hand hygiene before handling oxygen equipment.	Reduces transmission of microorganisms.
2. Place oxygen-delivery system in clutter-free environment that is well ventilated; away from walls, drapes, curtains, bedding, and combustible materials; and at least 8 feet (2.4 meters) from heat sources.	Keeps system balanced and prevents injury.

Clinical Decision Point *Do not place oxygen delivery system in a closet.*

3. Demonstrate steps for preparation and maintenance of oxygen therapy:	Demonstration is reliable technique for teaching psychomotor skill and enables client to ask questions.
a. Compressed oxygen system:	
(1) Turn cylinder valve counterclockwise two to three turns with wrench.	Turns on oxygen.
(2) Check cylinders by reading amount on pressure gauge.	Verifies adequate oxygen supply for client use.
(3) Store wrench with oxygen tank or in other safe place.	Storing wrench in safe place ensures that it is available whenever needed.
b. Oxygen concentrator system:	
(1) Plug concentrator into appropriate outlet.	Provides power safely to concentrator.
(2) Turn on power switch.	Starts concentrator motor.
(3) Alarm will sound for few seconds.	Alarm turns off when desired pressure inside concentrator is reached.
c. Liquid oxygen system:	
(1) Check liquid system by depressing button at lower right corner and reading dial on stationary oxygen reservoir or ambulatory tank.	Verifies adequate oxygen supply for client use.
(2) Collaborate with DME provider to provide instruction in refilling ambulatory tank when it becomes empty.	Ensures that continuous oxygen therapy is not interrupted.

Clinical Decision Point *Ambulatory tanks are only filled when they are empty. Liquid oxygen is stored at or below −297°F (−183°C) inside reservoir, and the temperature inside the ambulatory tank is warmer. If cold oxygen from the reservoir mixes with warmer oxygen left in the ambulatory tank, the ambulatory tank malfunctions. Keep the DME supplier contact number in a visible location for questions about the equipment.*

(3) To refill liquid oxygen tank:	
(a) Wipe both filling connectors with clean, dry, lint-free cloth.	Removes dust and moisture from system.
(b) Turn off flow selector of ambulatory unit.	
(c) Attach ambulatory unit to stationary reservoir by inserting female adapter from ambulatory tank into male adapter of stationary reservoir (see illustration).	Secures connection between oxygen reservoir and ambulatory tank.

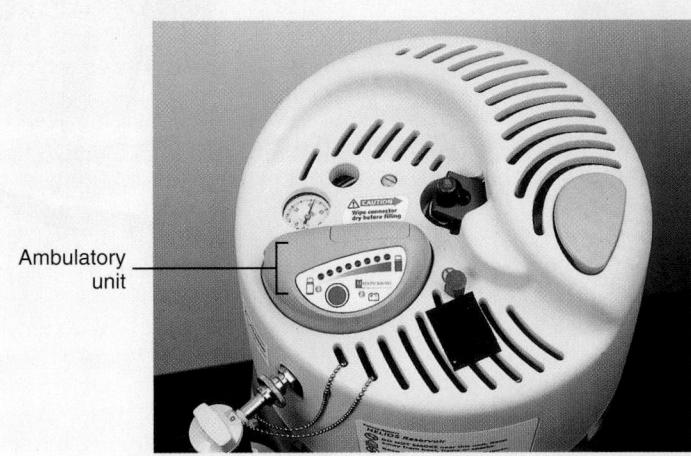

Ambulatory unit

STEP 3c(3)(c) Top view of stationary reservoir.

STEP	RATIONALE
(d) Open fill valve on ambulatory tank (e.g., lever, button, key) and apply firm pressure to top of stationary reservoir (see illustration). Stay with unit while it is filling. You will hear loud hissing noise. Tank should be filled in about 2 minutes.	Prevents leakage of oxygen during filling process. If oxygen leaks during filling process, connection between ambulatory tank and reservoir potentially ices up, and ambulatory and reservoir tanks stick together.
(e) Disconnect ambulatory unit from stationary reservoir when hissing noise changes and vapor cloud begins to form from stationary unit.	Overfilling causes ambulatory unit to malfunction as result of high pressure in tank.

Clinical Decision Point *If ambulatory unit does not separate easily, valves from reservoir and ambulatory unit are frozen together. Wait until valves warm to disengage (about 5 to 10 minutes). Do not touch any frosted areas because contact with skin causes skin damage from frostbite.*

STEP	RATIONALE
(f) Wipe both filling connectors with clean, dry, lint-free cloth.	Ice often forms during filling process. Removes moisture from oxygen system.
4. Connect oxygen-delivery device (e.g., nasal cannula) to oxygen-delivery system (see Chapter 23) (see illustration).	Connects oxygen source to delivery method.
5. Adjust oxygen flow rate (L/min) to ordered rate.	Ensures that ordered oxygen dose is delivered.
6. Have client or family caregiver apply oxygen-delivery device (e.g., nasal cannula) correctly (see Chapter 23). Ensure that client has two sets of oxygen-delivery devices and tubing.	Delivers oxygen to client. Extra set of equipment is used when equipment is cleaned or in case of equipment malfunction.
7. Instruct client and family caregiver not to change oxygen flow rate.	Exceeding prescribed amount of oxygen is sometimes harmful (e.g., client with chronic obstructive pulmonary disease [COPD]).
8. Have client or family caregiver perform each step with guidance. Provide written material for reinforcement and review.	Allows for correction of any errors in technique and discussion of their implications.

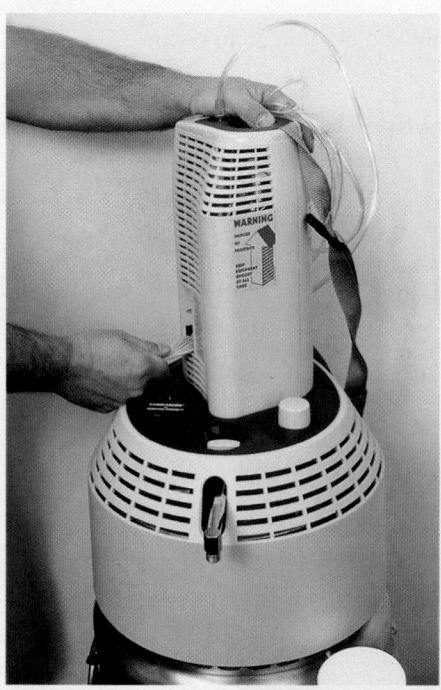

STEP 3c(3)(d) Fill valve on ambulatory tank is opened while applying firm pressure to top of ambulatory tank.

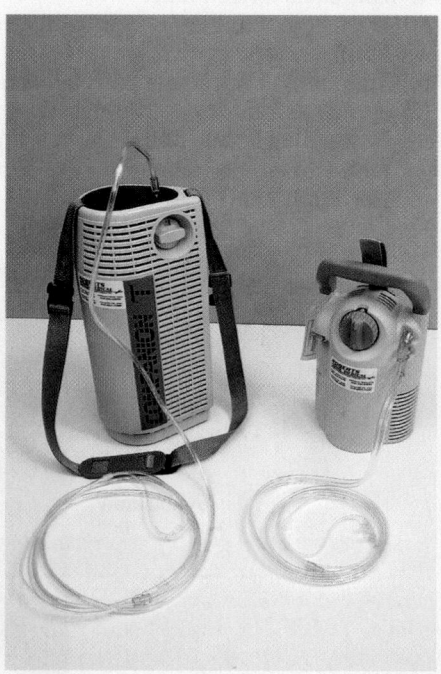

STEP 4 Oxygen-delivery device (nasal cannulas) and tubing attached to ambulatory oxygen tanks.

STEP	RATIONALE
9. Instruct client or family caregiver to notify health care provider if signs or symptoms of hypoxia occur, including apprehension, anxiety, decreased ability to concentrate, decreased levels of consciousness, increased fatigue, dizziness, behavioral changes, increased pulse, increased respiratory rate, pallor, and cyanosis or respiratory tract infection (e.g., fever, increased sputum, change in color of sputum, foul sputum odor).	Hypoxia sometimes occurs at home when client uses oxygen. Possible causes of hypoxia include poor tubing connections; use of long oxygen tubing; or worsening of client's physical problem, with change in respiratory status. Respiratory tract infections increase oxygen demand and often affect oxygen transfer from lungs to blood, creating exacerbation of client's pulmonary disease.
10. Discuss emergency plans for power loss, natural disaster, and acute respiratory distress. Have client or family caregiver call 9-1-1 and notify health care provider and home care agency.	Ensures appropriate response and can prevent worsening of client's condition.
11. Instruct client and family caregiver in safe home oxygen practices, including placing "No Smoking/Oxygen in Use" signs at each entrance to home, not allowing smoking in house, keeping oxygen tanks 8 feet (2.4 meters) away from open flames, and storing oxygen tanks upright.	Ensures safe use of oxygen in home and prevents injury to client and family (Galligan et al., 2015).

EVALUATION

1. Monitor rate at which oxygen is being delivered during each home visit.	Determines if client or family caregiver is regulating oxygen at prescribed rate.
2. Ask client or family caregiver about ease or problems associated with home oxygen.	Determines ability of client or caregiver to deal with stressors associated with home oxygen use. Also indicates client's risk for inappropriate oxygen use.
3. Ask client or family caregiver to state safety guidelines, emergency precautions, and emergency plan.	Determines client's or caregiver's knowledge of what to do if power fails, there is a failure in equipment, or client's status worsens.
4. **Use Teach-Back:** "I want to be sure I explained the importance of oxygen. Tell me in your own words why you need oxygen and the signs and symptoms of hypoxia?" Revise your instruction now or develop a plan for revised client or family caregiver teaching if client or family caregiver is not able to teach back correctly.	Determines client's and family caregiver's level of understanding of instructional topic.

Unexpected Outcomes	Related Interventions
1. Client has signs and symptoms associated with hypoxia.	• Determine if oxygen-delivery device and oxygen source are delivering oxygen properly. • Determine if prescribed oxygen flow rate is set properly. • Assess client for change in respiratory status such as airway plugging, respiratory tract infection, or bronchospasm. • Teach client or family caregiver when to notify health care provider or activate EMS because of signs of hypoxia.
2. Client uses unsafe practices with oxygen therapy, uses oxygen around fire or cigarette smoking, or sets incorrect flow rate.	• Reinforce client education and perform follow-up reassessment (see Box 44.3). • Include caregiver in instruction and set up problem-solving exercises with client.
3. Client is unable to fill ambulatory system.	• Identify and instruct family caregiver who can help client fill tank.

Recording and Reporting

- Record teaching plan, information provided to client, and client's and family caregiver's ability to discuss information in home care record.
- Communicate client's or family caregiver's learning progress to other health care providers involved in client's care.
- Record oxygen-delivery system, related supplies, and prescribed oxygen flow rate in home care record.

- Report respiratory complications/concerns to health care provider.

Special Considerations
Teaching

- Potential for oxygen desaturation and decreased oxygen delivery to brain impairs client's ability to remember previous learning. Provide frequent teaching sessions and written or

pictorial instructions to reinforce previous learning of teaching plan.
- Teach client or caregiver that oxygen is a medication (Hart, 2015).
- Explain to client and family caregiver signs of hypoxia. Hypoxia sometimes occurs at home when client uses oxygen. Possible causes of hypoxia include poor tubing connections, use of long oxygen tubing, or worsening of client's physical problem, with change in respiratory status.
- Teach the client or family caregiver not to smoke within the home for the safety of all occupants. Post "Oxygen in Use" signs on all exterior doors and on bedroom door.
- Instruct client or family caregiver in appropriate cleaning, disinfecting, and maintaining all oxygen-delivery systems and supplies. Verify instructions with manufacturer guidelines and DME provider's instructions.
- Instruct client or family caregiver to check mask and tubing by placing hands or face over mask or cannula to feel airflow and check that mask is not too tight; tight mask often leaves marks on skin.

- Always leave a phone number and instructions about how to reach home care nurse if needed.

Pediatric
- Keep equipment out of reach of any children in home. Do not allow children to handle or operate home oxygen equipment.
- Keep children away from fire and flames at all times; as appropriate, educate about dangers of oxygen coming into contact with fire (Wiles, 2015).

Gerontological
- Older adults have less efficient respiratory systems and less surface area for gas exchange; thus they are at greater risk for cerebral anoxia and confusion when they experience decreased oxygen levels. They may be unable to recognize respiratory problems or problems with their oxygen-delivery system; therefore they need frequent contact with a designated family caregiver.

◆ SKILL 44.5   Teaching Home Tracheostomy Care and Suctioning

Performing tracheostomy care and suctioning in the home is similar to performing them in the hospital except for one key variable: the use of *medical asepsis* or *clean technique*. The home environment has fewer germs than hospitals; therefore clean technique can be used. Aseptic technique is used in the hospital because the client is more susceptible to infection and more virulent or pathogenic microorganisms are usually present. In the home setting the majority of clients use clean technique. Use judgment in choosing the correct technique for each client (e.g., use aseptic technique with clients who are immunocompromised; are infected [not colonized]; or have family caregivers infected with viral, bacterial, or fungal microorganisms). Clients living in unclean conditions also need to be suctioned with aseptic technique whenever possible to try to prevent infection. All family caregivers need to use standard precautions when suctioning with either clean or aseptic technique.

Caring for a tracheostomy at home begins in the hospital (see Chapter 25) with teaching and return demonstration. The client or family caregiver usually learns better when instruction in less invasive techniques such as tracheal stoma care precedes more invasive techniques such as inner cannula care and suctioning. Continually develop, implement, and evaluate the teaching plan based on client performance. It is imperative that clients and their caregivers have the ability to practice suctioning frequently before discharge to develop confidence with skill performance; otherwise arrangements to provide 24-hour care are necessary before discharge.

Delegation and Collaboration

The skill of teaching home tracheostomy care and suctioning cannot be delegated to nursing assistive personnel (NAP). The nurse instructs the NAP to:

- Report changes in client's level of consciousness, irritability, vital signs, or decreased pulse oximetry.
- Report increased airway secretions.

Equipment
- Suction machine with connecting tube
- Clean or sterile gloves
- Three small basins
- Hydrogen peroxide
- Normal saline
- Appropriate-size sterile or clean and disinfected suction catheter (diameter no greater than half the diameter of the tracheostomy tube [e.g., if tracheostomy tube is 8 mm (0.3 inches), use 16-Fr or smaller suction catheter])
- Tracheostomy care kit or clean 4 × 4–inch gauze pads (nonshredding)
- Small nylon bottle brush or pipe cleaners or disposable inner cannula
- Cotton-tipped applicators
- Tracheostomy ties (twill tape [⅛-inch preferably] or Velcro-type tie holders)
- Mirror
- Wet washcloth or paper towel (*optional*)
- Dry cloth, towel, or paper towel (*optional*)
- Protective eyewear (*optional*)
- Trash bag (plastic, leak proof preferred)
- Disposable apron (*optional*)
- Bag-valve-mask (BVM) with oxygen supply (*optional*)

STEP	RATIONALE

ASSESSMENT

| 1. Identify client using at least two identifiers during first home visit. Facial recognition can be used as one of two identifiers for ongoing subsequent home visits. | Ensures client safety (TJC, 2016). |

STEP	RATIONALE
2. Assess client's or family caregiver's vision and fine motor function for ability to perform tracheostomy care and suctioning properly. Also assess client's level of consciousness, ability to attend and problem solve.	Instructing family caregiver is essential if client's physical and cognitive impairment prevents ability to perform tracheostomy care and suctioning. Emergency situations usually require family caregiver or significant other to suction.
3. Assess client's or family caregiver's knowledge of indications for the need to perform:	
a. Tracheostomy care, including presence of excess peristomal secretions, excess intratracheal secretions, soiled or damp tracheostomy dressing/ties, and diminished airway through tracheostomy tube.	Knowledge needed for client or caregiver to accurately assess need to provide tracheostomy care. Signs and symptoms are related to presence of secretions at stoma site or within tracheostomy tube.
b. Suctioning, including client's perceived need for suctioning, presence of gurgling, wheezes on inspiration or expiration, restlessness, ineffective coughing, tachypnea, cyanosis, acutely decreased level of consciousness, tachycardia or bradycardia, acutely shallow respirations, or acute dyspnea.	Knowledge allows client or family caregiver to accurately determine need to perform tracheostomy tube suctioning. Physical signs and symptoms result from lower-airway obstruction and tissue hypoxia.
4. Assess client's or family caregiver's ability to assess pulse rate and respirations.	Necessary for appropriate monitoring in the home.
5. Assess client's learning readiness and ability to concentrate; consider presence of pain, nausea, or fatigue and client interest in instruction.	Presence of significant illness, frailty, or confusion affects client's ability to attend to teaching plan. Indicates need to rely on family caregiver for learning and implementation (if available) on short- or long-term basis.
6. Observe client or family caregiver perform complete tracheostomy tube care and suctioning.	Determines which specific components of skill that client or caregiver can complete easily and which are more difficult and require reinforcement.

NURSING DIAGNOSES

- Deficient knowledge regarding tracheostomy care
- Ineffective breathing pattern
- Ineffective health maintenance
- Risk for family caregiver role strain
- Risk for infection

Related factors/Risk factors are individualized based on client's condition or needs.

PLANNING

1. Expected outcomes following completion of procedure:	
• Client or family caregiver identifies signs and symptoms indicating need for tracheostomy care and suctioning.	Client or caregiver is able to institute preventive means to maintain airway.
• Client or family caregiver states factors that influence tracheostomy airway functioning.	Tracheostomy often impairs normal airway clearance, humidification, and gas exchange.
• Client or family caregiver correctly demonstrates complete tracheostomy tube care and suctioning in controlled setting.	Provides validation of ability to perform procedure.
• Client or family caregiver identifies signs of stoma inflammation or respiratory tract infection and when to notify health care provider.	Measures cognitive learning.
• Lower and upper airways are cleared of secretions, as evidenced by absent or diminished wheezes and gurgles in large airways, normalization of pulse and respiratory rate, increased depth of respirations, absence of cyanosis, improved color, and decreased dyspnea.	Suctioning by client or family caregiver is successful.
• Stoma site is clean and free of an infection and transesophageal fistula. Signs of transesophageal fistula include frequent coughing when eating, aspiration, and/or fever.	Tracheostomy care is successful.
• Inner cannula is free of secretions.	
2. Select setting in home that client or family caregiver is most likely to perform tracheostomy tube care.	Practicing skill in same setting where skill will be routinely performed facilitates comprehension and learning.
a. Select room that is well lit with comfortable seating.	
b. Be sure that client is close and can see nurse clearly.	

STEP	RATIONALE

c. Control sources of noise and distractions.

Room environment needs to minimize existing sensory alterations. Comfortable environment free of distractions promotes client's attention.

3. Discuss and demonstrate with client or family caregiver proper position for procedure (high-Fowler's position in front of mirror).

Promotes understanding of comfort and safety principles and facilitates visibility.

IMPLEMENTATION

1. **Suctioning:**

   a. Verify health care provider's orders for suctioning. Ensure that client and family caregiver understand suctioning order.

   Invasive procedure requires order.
   Order may be written for as-needed suctioning; ensures that client and family caregiver understand what this means.

   b. Teach client or family caregiver techniques for hand hygiene and application of clean gloves.

   Reduces transmission of microorganisms.

   c. Explain and demonstrate step-by-step preparation and completion of tracheostomy tube suctioning using either open or closed suctioning (see Chapter 25) (see illustration).

   Demonstration is reliable technique for teaching psychomotor skill and enables client or family caregiver to ask questions throughout procedure. Steps used to suction clients in hospital are also used in home.

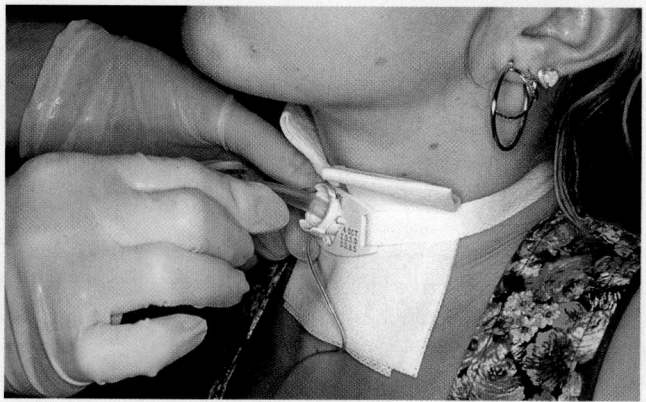

STEP 1c Insertion of suction catheter into tracheostomy tube.

Clinical Decision Point *Instillation of normal saline before suctioning, once a common practice, is no longer recommended. Use of normal saline adversely affects arterial and global tissue oxygenation (Ayhan et al., 2015).*

d. After client or family caregiver suctions tracheostomy, teach how to suction nasal and oral pharynx and perform mouth care. Encourage client or family caregiver to brush teeth with small soft toothbrush 2 times a day and use mouth moisturizer to moisturize lips every 2 to 4 hours.

Suctioning removes secretions from trachea and lower airway that clients are not able to clear by coughing (Lamb, 2014). Dental plaque harbors microorganisms.

e. At conclusion of procedure, have client take two to three deep breaths; reassess status of breathing.

Deep breathing reduces oxygen loss and prevents hypoxia. Expect client's respiratory status to improve following suctioning.

f. Demonstrate how to disconnect suction catheter; coil and discard catheter in appropriate receptacle. If catheter is to be cleaned and disinfected, set aside. Have client or family caregiver remove soiled gloves and dispose in appropriate container; perform hand hygiene.

Prevents transmission of microorganisms.

2. **Tracheostomy care:**

   a. Have client sit at table with mirror. Instruct client or family caregiver how to perform hand hygiene and apply clean gloves with you. Teach skills of tracheostomy care, including cleaning stoma and tracheostomy tube and changing tracheostomy ties and dressing (see illustrations and Chapter 25). *Exception:* Clean inner cannula with hydrogen peroxide and small brush (Cleveland Clinic, 2015).

   Prevents transmission of microorganisms. Steps used to provide tracheostomy care in hospital are also used in home.

STEP	RATIONALE

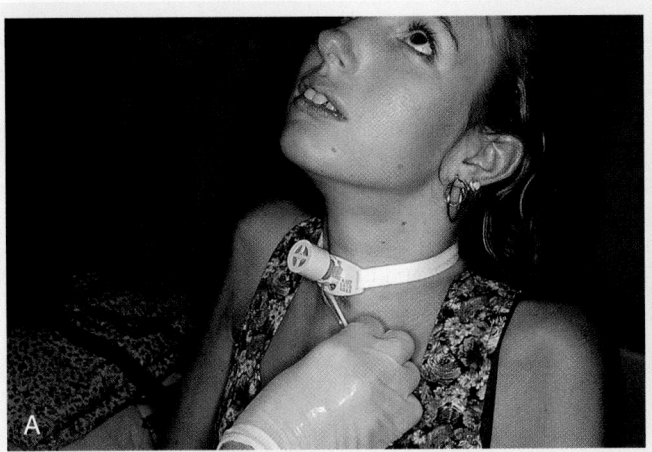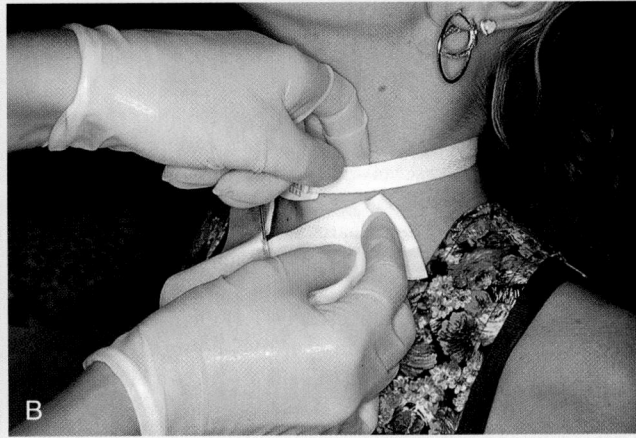

STEP 2a A, Cleaning area around tracheal stoma. **B,** Applying clean tracheostomy dressing.

Clinical Decision Point *During tracheostomy care a client is at risk for the tracheostomy tube coming out. Instruct client or family caregiver to never remove the old tracheostomy tube ties until the new ties are secured properly. Keep two tracheostomy tubes, one the same size as the client's and one a size smaller, accessible to the client so he or she can insert a new tube if the tube comes out.*

b. Have client or family caregiver remove and dispose of gloves. Perform hand hygiene.	Reduces transmission of microorganisms.
c. Instruct client or family caregiver to apply clean gloves. Demonstrate technique for cleaning reusable supplies in warm soapy water. Rinse thoroughly and dry between two layers of clean paper towels. Store supplies in loosely closed clear plastic bag; label bag.	Prevents transmission of microorganisms. Air must circulate, or humidity in bag can promote microorganism growth.
d. Have client or family caregiver remove and discard gloves. Perform hand hygiene.	Reduces transmission of microorganisms.
3. Disinfecting supplies:	
a. Explain procedure for disinfecting reusable supplies. This needs to be done at least weekly. To disinfect supplies use one of following methods:	Removes organisms and reduces risk for infection.
(1) *Method 1:* Boil reusable (boilable) supplies for 15 minutes. Allow to cool and dry.	
(2) *Method 2:* Soak reusable supplies in equal parts of vinegar and water for 30 minutes. Remove, rinse thoroughly, and dry.	
(3) *Method 3:* Soak reusable supplies in prepared solutions of quaternary ammonium chloride compounds according to manufacturer instructions. Rinse and dry.	
4. Have client or family caregiver perform each step with guidance from you.	Adults learn psychomotor skills best by active participation, and you can correct any errors in technique as they occur and discuss their implications.
5. Teach client or family caregiver signs and symptoms of the following:	Client or caregiver must be able to recognize onset of complications associated with long-term tracheostomy use early so medical treatment can begin, reducing risk for more serious negative outcomes. Emphasize importance of notifying health care provider when signs and symptoms of complications occur.
a. Stoma infection (redness, tenderness, drainage)	
b. Respiratory tract infection (fever, increased sputum, change in color of sputum, foul sputum odor, increased cough, chills, night sweats)	
c. Transesophageal fistula (air leaking through stoma, nose, or mouth with cuff properly inflated; more air needed to inflate cuff; aspiration of food or liquid during suctioning; excessive belching; coughing when swallowing)	

STEP	RATIONALE

EVALUATION

1. Observe client or family caregiver demonstrate technique for tracheostomy tube care and suctioning.

2. Ask client or family caregiver to describe signs and symptoms indicating need for tracheostomy care and suctioning and the factors that influence tracheostomy airway functioning.

3. Have client and family caregiver explain the problems that need to be reported to their health care provider.

4. **Use Teach-Back:** "I want to be sure I explained how you will feel and what you may see if you develop problems or complications with your tracheostomy. Tell me the signs and symptoms for needing to suction your tracheostomy." Revise your instruction now or develop a plan for revised client or family caregiver teaching if client or family caregiver is not able to teach back correctly.

Feedback through independent demonstration of psychomotor skill is reliable method to evaluate learning.

Demonstrates learning and client and family caregiver's ability to respond when airway problems develop.

Demonstrates client's ability to take steps for emergent care.

Determines client's and family caregiver's level of understanding of instructional topic.

Unexpected Outcomes	Related Interventions
1. Stoma site is reddened or hard, with or without drainage.	• Evaluate client's or family caregiver's technique. • Increase frequency of tracheostomy care. • Have client use sterile technique for suctioning and tracheostomy care.
2. Copious colored secretions are present around stoma or when client or family caregiver suctions tracheostomy.	• Secretions may be pink, rust colored, or blood tinged, depending on problem; documenting color helps health care provider diagnose problem. • Evaluate for adequate humidity (use room humidifier or tracheostomy collar humidity, if needed) (see Chapter 25). • Notify health care provider.
3. Bloody secretions are suctioned.	• Evaluate suctioning technique, suctioning frequency, and size of catheter used. • Usual length to insert catheter is length of tracheostomy tube plus $\frac{1}{4}$ inch. • Assess for signs of infection. • Assess client for use of anticoagulant medications.
4. No secretions are suctioned.	• Evaluate client's fluid status, need for increased humidity. • Determine if appropriate-size suction catheter is used. • Reassess need to suction.
5. Skin breakdown is present at stoma site.	• Assess site for pressure areas or site infection. • Remove pressure source.

Recording and Reporting

• Record client instruction and client's and family caregiver's ability to demonstrate tracheostomy care, suctioning skills, and disinfecting skills in home health record.

• Develop a system of recording home care for client or family caregiver to document and keep track of tracheostomy care provided.

Special Considerations
Teaching

• The nose and mouth normally provide warmth, filtering, and moisture for the air we breathe. A tracheostomy tube bypasses these mechanisms. Humidification must be provided to keep secretions thin and to avoid mucous plugs.

• Caution clients and family caregivers against using alcohol-based products to clean supplies because it can cause the materials to become hard and brittle. Do not place equipment or supplies in the dishwasher .

• Always leave a phone number and instructions about how to reach home care nurse if needed.

Pediatric

• Encourage parents to give tracheostomy care as soon as child is stable in the hospital. The more time they have to practice these skills, the more comfortable they become in caring for the child at home.

• Children with tracheostomies need to socialize and play with other children who are close to their own age. Encourage family caregivers to take children out of the home. However, an additional adult needs to travel with the child to help if problems arise while in the car (Hockenberry and Wilson, 2015).

• To prevent hypoxia, teach family caregivers that suctioning needs to last no more than 5 seconds. Allow the child to rest for at least 30 to 60 seconds between suctioning passes and do not suction more than 3 times (Hockenberry and Wilson, 2015).

• Teach family caregivers pediatric cardiopulmonary resuscitation, including use of BVM or mouth-to-tracheostomy technique. They also need to notify the local EMS of the child's condition and the presence of a tracheostomy and provide EMS with a list of equipment in the home (Hockenberry and Wilson, 2015).

- Encourage family caregivers to have a cool-mist humidifier in same room as child; humidity helps keep secretions thin and decreases the likelihood of mucus plugging (Hockenberry and Wilson, 2015).
- Caring for a child with a tracheostomy often disrupts family caregivers' ability to socialize and can cause sleep deprivation. Develop a plan that includes respite care to allow caregivers time to meet their own needs (Hockenberry and Wilson, 2015).
- Teach family caregivers to avoid dressing the child in clothes that could cover the tracheostomy opening such as turtlenecks and clothes that have a tight-fitting collar. Avoid clothing, toys, and pets that shed fine hair or lint because they could get into the tracheostomy and cause breathing problems (Hockenberry and Wilson, 2015).

Gerontological

- Older adults lose some properties of elastic recoil and often have greater difficulty clearing airway secretions through cough. As a result they require more suctioning and airway care and have increased risk for infection (Ebersole et al., 2015).
- Assess for cognitive, mobility, or sensory impairments that impair ability to manage artificial airway at home and teach family caregiver if client is unable to manage airway independently.
- Anxiety accompanies decreased ability to breathe and may cause the older adult to become too nervous to perform suctioning independently.

✦ SKILL 44.6 Teaching Medication Self-Administration

Approximately 50% of prescribed medications are used incorrectly, and some clients do not choose to take their prescribed medication (CDC, 2013). The nurse finds resources and addresses issues that can influence clients' adherence to their medication regimen (e.g., ability to purchase medications, transportation to pharmacy, side effects). Teaching clients how to correctly administer medications is very important, but first the nurse identifies and addresses any issues that are of concern.

Compliance was used in the past to describe if clients' behaviors matched that of health care providers' recommendations when it came to taking prescribed medications or adhering to prescribed treatments (CDC, 2013). Recent literature supports the term *adherence* since this emphasizes a client's role in decision making, taking into account freedom of choice (Iihara et al., 2014). One method that has been identified to increase adherence is to understand and then support clients' decisions in how to take their medications. Use teaching methods that incorporate active listening so you can adapt clients' needs and concerns into their medication regimen.

Some barriers to medication adherence include fear of adverse reactions from medications, belief that a medication does not help, inconvenience of taking medication, cost of medication, inadequate knowledge, forgetfulness, and relationship with health care provider (Müller et al., 2015). Considering these potential barriers,

you can provide information and support to ensure that a client or family caregiver is making a well-informed decision when it comes to whether or not to take a medication. Once a client has mastered the skill of administering medications, you must continue to validate that the skill is being performed correctly and assess for new issues and concerns.

Delegation and Collaboration

The skill of teaching clients medication self-administration cannot be delegated to nursing assistive personnel (NAP). The nurse directs the NAP to:

- Communicate to the nurse problems that client reports having with medication self-administration.

Equipment

- Medication
- Liquid to take with medication
- Medication administration record or other up-to-date list of current medications from health care provider
- Medication log
- Container for daily or weekly preparation
- Measuring devices as needed (e.g., medicine cup, teaspoon)
- Teaching tools (e.g., charts, written instructions, color codes for medicine containers)

STEP	RATIONALE

ASSESSMENT

1. Identify client using at least two identifiers during first home visit. Facial recognition can be used as one of two identifiers for ongoing subsequent home visits.

Ensures client safety (TJC, 2016).

2. Assess client's cognitive, sensory, and motor function: level of consciousness, sight, hearing, touch, health literacy level, swallowing ability, mobility, activity tolerance, social support, and willingness to cooperate.

Cognitive, sensory, and motor deficits frequently influence client's ability to take or prepare prescribed medication correctly and participate in instruction.

3. Assess resources client or family caregiver has to obtain medications when needed (e.g., finances, social support, and transportation).

Lack of resources is major factor that negatively affects adherence with medication self-administration regimen (Müller et al., 2015).

4. Assess client's learning readiness and ability to concentrate (consider presence of pain, nausea, or fatigue and client interest in instruction) and learning style preference.

Presence of significant illness, frailty, or confusion affects person's ability to attend to teaching plan. Indicates need to rely on family caregiver for learning and implementation (if available) on short- or long-term basis. Learning style affects choice of teaching resources.

STEP	RATIONALE
5. Assess client's and family caregiver's knowledge regarding medication therapy: names of drugs, how to administer, purpose or action, daily doses and times to be taken, side effects to expect, and what to do if problems occur.	Clients need to be able to understand information about their medications and remember it (Kornburger et al., 2013). Family caregivers' self-confidence in administering medication influences their ability to manage medication for client (Kornburger et al., 2013).
6. Assess client's belief in need for medication therapy. Consider prior experiences, ethnic values, religious beliefs, personal experiences with medications, and significant others' values about medications.	Many factors influence client's willingness to follow drug regimen.
7. Assess client's prescribed and over-the-counter (OTC) medications, including use of herbal supplements: Has more than one health care provider prescribed medications? Are labels clearly marked? Are time schedules confusing? Do different drugs look alike? Does client store medications together or out of original containers? Are expiration dates on bottles still current?	Determines sources of confusion affecting client's adherence. Adherence with medication therapy (especially in older adults) is often complicated by polypharmacy (multiple chronic conditions are often treated with multiple medications, sometimes prescribed by more than one health care provider). Adherence is more complicated when medication regimens are complex.
8. Be sure that family caregiver knows client's drug allergies.	As new drugs are prescribed, the family caregiver often becomes the one to monitor for inappropriate drug prescription.
9. Consult with health care provider to review medications that client is receiving and simplify regimen if possible.	Review of medications helps minimize risk for drug interactions from multiple medications and ensures accuracy of medication regimen. Simplification of regimen improves adherence, particularly related to daily frequency of prescribed doses.

NURSING DIAGNOSES

- Anxiety
- Deficient knowledge regarding medication self-administration
- Ineffective health maintenance
- Readiness for enhanced knowledge

Related factors are individualized based on client's condition or needs.

PLANNING

1. Expected outcomes following completion of procedure:	
• Client or family caregiver is able to state purpose of each medication and why it is beneficial. If medication has been discontinued, client or family caregiver correctly explains why this was done.	Demonstrates cognitive learning.
• Client or family caregiver identifies common adverse effects and relief measures.	Encourages adherence to medication therapy.
• Client or family caregiver is able to state when to notify health care provider about medication problems.	Empowers client to participate in care.
• Client or family caregiver reads each label and explains when each medication should be taken.	Prevents medication administration errors.
• Client or family caregiver demonstrates self-administration of medication by prescribed route.	Demonstrates skill achieved.
2. Prepare environment for teaching session:	Improves likelihood of client and family caregiver being attentive to instruction.
a. Select room that is well lit and offers comfortable seating.	
b. Be sure that client is close and can see nurse clearly.	
c. Control sources of noise and distractions.	Room environment needs to minimize existing sensory alterations. Comfortable environment free of distractions promotes client's attention.
3. Prepare teaching materials:	Client-centered care focuses on working in partnership with clients to provide high-quality, appropriate, and cost-effective health care (Hyrkas and Wiggins, 2014).
a. Plan approach that matches client's learning preference (visual, auditory, read or write, kinesthetic):	Using an instructional approach that matches client's learning style in the context in which learning occurs allows for an individualized approach that incorporates teaching modalities to maximize client learning (Inott and Kennedy, 2011).

STEP	RATIONALE

(1) Written materials printed in large bold letters (set in 14-point or larger type)

Assists clients with visual limitations.

(2) DVD or Internet instructional programs

(3) Illustrations of medication safety guidelines

(4) Handling equipment and supplies

4. Ensure that client is wearing glasses or hearing aids if needed during teaching session.

Use of glasses or hearing aids increases client's sensory perception and likelihood of attending to teaching session and understanding content.

5. Arrange teaching time to allow participation of family caregivers (see illustration).

Caregiver can serve as positive resource to client and often reinforce information provided (Hyrkas and Wiggins, 2014).

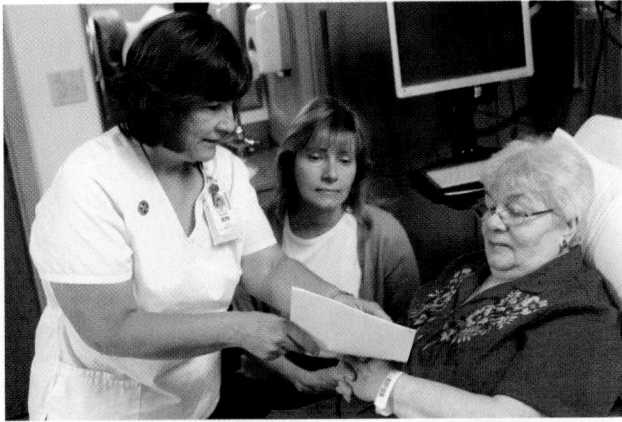

STEP 5 Client and family caregiver participate in medication self-administration teaching program.

IMPLEMENTATION

1. Instruct client or family caregiver about importance of performing hand hygiene before medication self-administration.

Reduces transmission of microorganisms.

2. Present information clearly and concisely:

Improves client's ability to attend and understand (Kornburger et al., 2013).

  a. Face learner in well-lit room.

Allows visualization of client's nonverbal responses to education. Client with hearing loss or visual problem is able to see your expressions, read written information, and hear your voice more clearly.

  b. Use short sentences and speak in slow, low-pitched voice.

Enhances understanding of information.

  c. Provide descriptions in understandable terms.

Prevents confusion of terminology. Clients learn more quickly when you present information at level of learner (Kornburger et al., 2013).

3. Provide frequent pauses so client or family caregiver can ask questions and express understanding of content.

Increases learner participation. Ongoing feedback ensures that client is acquiring information.

4. Instruct client or family caregiver on following content: purpose of regularly scheduled and prn (as needed) medications and their desired effects, how medication works and why it helps, dosage schedules and rationale, common side effects, what to do to relieve side effects, what to do if dose is missed, when to call health care provider with problems, who to call with problems, medication safety guidelines, and implications when medications are not taken.

Provides client or caregiver with sufficient information to understand and take medications safely at home.

5. Instruct client or family caregiver in appropriate route of medication delivery, including oral, subcutaneous, intramuscular, inhalation, and topical.

Client needs to be proficient in all routes of medication administration. Adverse effects often occur if medications are administered incorrectly.

6. Provide frequent, short teaching sessions. Plan to have several teaching sessions, especially if client needs to take multiple medications.

Frequent sessions improve client's attention and retention of information discussed.

STEP	RATIONALE
7. Provide teaching about OTC medications and herbal supplements.	Clients may not understand effects of OTC and herbal supplements (Werner, 2014).
8. Provide client with written schedules or individualized instruction sheets for review. Offer special charts, diagrams, learning aids, written information, weekly pill organizers, and Internet/Intranet resources (see illustration).	Clear written information, charts, and other resources such as Internet/Intranet enhance client learning and allow for reinforcement of information (Kornburger et al., 2013).

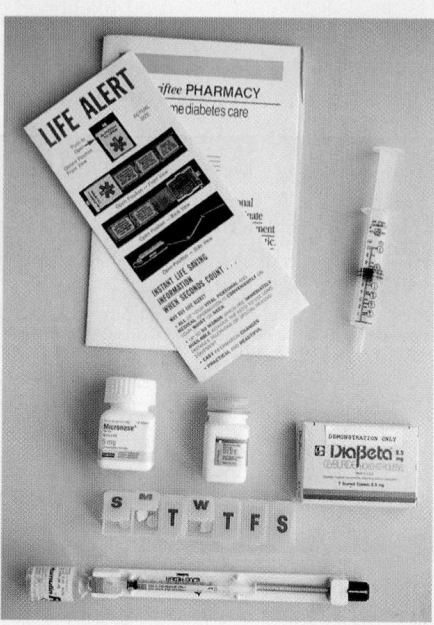

STEP 8 Examples of aids for client self-administration of medication.

STEP	RATIONALE
9. Offer help as client practices preparing medication (e.g., "Let's prepare the medications you will take with your meals or the medicines you take first in the morning").	Allows for observation of client's ability to read labels correctly and prepare all medications for prescribed times.
10. Have pharmacy provide clear, large-print labels for medication bottles and medication teaching handouts if appropriate.	Improves client's ability to read and follow directions.
11. Have pharmacy provide containers that client can open independently if manual dexterity is limited.	Most pharmacies dispense pills in "childproof" containers, which client with limited mobility of fingers/hands often find difficult to manipulate or open.

Clinical Decision Point *If there are pets or small children in the home or children who frequently visit the home, help client establish a "safe place" for medication storage to reduce risk for accidental ingestion by pets or children.*

STEP	RATIONALE
12. Facilitate arrangements for pharmacy to receive written prescriptions in timely fashion if required for dispensing. Arrange for pharmacy to deliver medications to home if client is unable to arrange for transportation to pharmacy.	Availability of drugs influences adherence.
13. Discuss with client or family caregiver how to dispose of discontinued or expired medications.	Ensures safe disposal.

EVALUATION

1. Ask client or family caregiver to explain information about each drug: purpose; actions; routes; timing of medications and maximum frequency of use of either prescribed or OTC medications; side effects and interactions; and foods, herbals, or OTC medications to avoid.	Clients and caregivers need to be able to understand information they are given and remember this information (Tamura-Lis, 2013).
2. Ask client or family caregiver to describe when to call health care provider or refer to printed information for resources.	Developing techniques to gain information and solve problems helps client adherence and reduces potential problems from medication regimen (Kornburger et al., 2013).

STEP	RATIONALE
3. Have client or family caregiver prepare and administer doses for all prescribed medications.	Indicates understanding of medication dosages and schedules.
4. **Use Teach-Back:** "I want to be sure I explained how to safely dispose of medicines you are no longer taking. Tell me in your own words the correct way to dispose of your tablets here in the home." Revise your instruction now or develop a plan for revised client or family caregiver teaching if client or family caregiver is not able to teach back correctly.	Determines client's and family caregiver's level of understanding of instructional topic.

Unexpected Outcomes	Related Interventions
1. Client or family caregiver makes errors in preparing medications or is unable to recall and/or explain information discussed in teaching sessions.	• Provide additional instruction and/or teaching materials for consultation when information is forgotten or unclear.
	• Ensure that written instructions are at client's level of understanding. Some commercially prepared booklets contain instructions that are too complex or contain medical jargon that is difficult to understand.
	• Consider use of different pictures, color coding, diagrams, and tape-recorded instructions for clients with visual impairment or a reading disability.
	• Consider use of weekly pill organizers.
	• Periodically observe client or caregiver prepare and administer medications.
2. Medication self-administration plan is not possible because of client's self-care deficits. This is very common when client develops cognitive changes.	• Develop alternative plan, which often relies on family caregivers to provide safe administration of home medication regimen.
3. Client refuses to take medications as prescribed.	• Explore and identify reasons for nonadherence, which often include the following: cost, side effects, complexity of regimen, problems with swallowing or other side effects, and cultural preferences.
	• See Box 44.4.

Recording and Reporting

- Document instruction provided and learning outcomes achieved by client and family caregiver in home care record.
- Develop a system of recording (client diary) for client or family caregiver to use to document adherence to dosage schedules and self-monitoring of any problems.
- Always leave a phone number and instructions about how to reach home care nurse if needed.

Special Considerations
Teaching

- See Chapter 43 for guidelines for medication safety.
- If it is difficult to plan a separate teaching session, teach client while administering medications.
- Examples of learning aids include homemade calendars for each week that contain plastic bags containing medications to take at specific times, egg cartons divided into color-coded sections with medications for the day, clock faces for clients who cannot read or see clearly, color coding for drug types (e.g., blue for sedative, red for pain pill), and pillboxes that identify days of the week and times of day.

Pediatric

- Instruct adults to keep all medications locked and securely out of reach of children.
- Encourage family caregivers not to tell children that medications are treats because this increases the risk for child overdosing by mistaking medicine for candy.
- Successful medication teaching involves the child's parents or other caregivers and the child and siblings whenever possible.

BOX 44.4

Evidence-Based Nursing Interventions to Enhance Adherence to Medication Therapy

- Involve clients as partners in collaboration. Encourage them to express their views and share in the decision making with you.
- Encourage clients to take medications.
- Use medication reminders and devices such as smartphone alarms and pill boxes.
- Be empathetic regarding clients' feelings.
- Encourage a sense of control for the client by providing information about diagnosis and treatment.
- Recognize family caregiver needs and provide information and support. Understand that caregiver may have competing responsibilities (e.g., employment, other dependents).
- Client's attitude will affect his or her willingness to work with health care providers and be compliant with treatments.

Modified from Kinney RL et al: The association between patient activation and medication adherence, hospitalization, and emergency room utilization in patients with chronic illnesses: a systematic review, *Patient Educ Counsel* 98(5):545, 2015; Mantri P: Patient adherence to medication, *Pract Nurs* 25(12):590, 2014; Shin, Habermann, and Pretzer-Aboff: Challenges and strategies of medication adherence in Parkinson's disease: a qualitative study, *Geriatr Nurs* 36(3):191, 2015.

To provide effective medication teaching to children, take the child's developmental and cognitive abilities into consideration when planning teaching sessions (Hockenberry and Wilson, 2015).

- Family caregivers need to supervise older children as they begin taking responsibility for their own treatment.

Gerontological

- Capacity for learning new information remains as people age (in the absence of dementia); however, older clients often need additional time to accomplish learning. Allow adequate time and number of teaching sessions to support successful learning. Effective teaching strategies for older adults include memory aids, information written in large letters, involvement of family caregiver, follow-up teaching sessions either over the telephone or in person, and computer-assisted teaching guides (Ebersole et al., 2015).
- Cognition problems coupled with complexity of medication regimens have a negative effect on older adults' ability to self-administer medication safely. Try to decrease the complexity of medication regimens in clients with cognitive deficits whenever possible to promote safe medication self-administration practices.
- Older adults often have to take medications in multiple routes (e.g., oral, inhaled, injections). Many times problems with physical dexterity, eyesight, cognitive skills, and memory negatively affect adherence to medication schedules. Establish a therapeutic nurse-client relationship to help clients overcome these barriers to adherence.

♦ SKILL 44.7 Managing Feeding Tubes in the Home

Over 1.3 million clients in the United States receive enteral feedings at home (ASPEN, 2015). Clients benefit when they are able to see tube-feeding equipment and devices when learning how to administer home enteral nutrition. Provide hands-on experience and client involvement with decision making about home enteral nutrition whenever possible. Enteral nutrition therapy in the home setting is usually effective when a client tolerates at least 70% of feeding intake without complications and is medically stable, the client or family caregiver is able to administer feedings, and there is sufficient time in a controlled environment to learn the skill.

This procedure in the home setting follows the guidelines and skills described in Chapter 32. Most clients who receive enteral nutrition in the home have either gastrostomy or jejunostomy tubes. This skill focuses on teaching the client or family caregiver how to administer such feedings in the home. Frequently in the home setting the nurse is responsible for reinsertion of gastrostomy feeding tubes, and the health care provider is responsible for reinsertion of jejunostomy tubes.

Delegation and Collaboration

The skill of teaching clients and family caregivers how to manage feeding tubes in the home cannot be delegated to nursing assistive personnel (NAP). The nurse directs the NAP to:
- Report when client has difficulty with feeding, coughing, gagging, respiratory distress, discomfort, or vomiting.

Equipment

See Skills 32.1 through 32.4 and Procedural Guideline 32.1 for lists of equipment.
- Log to record daily weights, intake and output (I&O), temperature, feeding residuals

STEP	RATIONALE

ASSESSMENT

1. Identify client using at least two identifiers during first home visit. Facial recognition can be used as one of two identifiers for ongoing subsequent home visits.

Ensures client safety (TJC, 2016).

2. Assess client's current health status and tolerance to enteral feedings (if already being administered).

Determines if any changes are needed in feeding schedule.

3. Assess client's and family caregiver's physical (visual, fine motor) function. Also assess emotional, financial, and community resources.

Determines client's and family caregiver's ability to manipulate equipment. Availability of resources increases ability for self-care home management.

4. Assess environmental conditions of home (sanitation, storage of equipment, work area, supplies, and power source).

Determines if home environment is safe for enteral feeding, with minimal risks for infection and complications.

5. Assess client's and family caregiver's understanding of purpose of enteral feedings and positive expected outcomes.

Understanding rationale of treatment is critical to enhancing participation and cooperation in care.

6. Assess client's and family caregiver's understanding of storage and management of equipment and supplies and where and how to obtain supplies.

Ensures safe home management and decreases risk for complications.

Home care delivery companies usually deliver a month's supply at a time. If client stores feeding containers in garage, they must be brought into the house a couple hours before using in colder months to warm to room temperature (Best, 2012). Garage is not a good storage place during hot weather; use basement if possible.

7. Assess client's learning readiness and ability to concentrate (consider presence of pain, nausea, or fatigue and client interest in instruction); and learning style preference.

Presence of significant illness, frailty, or confusion affects client's ability to attend to teaching plan. Indicates need to rely on family caregiver for learning and implementation (if available) on short- or long-term basis. Learning style affects choice of teaching resources.

STEP	RATIONALE
8. Observe client or family caregiver administer an enteral feeding (when already ordered).	Determines which specific components of skill that client or caregiver can complete easily and which are more difficult and require reinforcement.

NURSING DIAGNOSES

- Anxiety
- Deficient knowledge regarding tube feeding self-administration
- Feeding self-care deficit
- Imbalanced nutrition: less than body requirements
- Ineffective health maintenance
- Risk for aspiration

Related factors/Risk factors are individualized based on client's condition or needs.

PLANNING

1. Expected outcomes following completion of procedure: • Client or family caregiver verbalizes purpose of enteral feedings and enhanced nutritional health. • Client or family caregiver demonstrates proper use of equipment and handling of formulas. • Client or family caregiver demonstrates accurate administration of enteral feedings and medications. • Client or family caregiver verbalizes understanding of signs, symptoms, and management of complications of feeding. 2. Prepare environment for teaching session: a. Select room that is well lit with comfortable seating. b. Be sure that client is close and can see nurse clearly. c. Control sources of noise and distractions.	Provides measurable criteria to determine level of cognitive understanding. Provides demonstration of skills needed to manage home enteral nutrition. Provides demonstration of skills needed to administer home enteral nutrition and medications. Confirms that client or caregiver has knowledge needed to respond when problems with feedings develop. Improves likelihood of client and family caregiver being attentive to instruction. Room environment needs to minimize existing sensory alterations. Comfortable environment free of distractions promotes client's attention.

IMPLEMENTATION

1. Have client or family caregiver perform hand hygiene with you and explain the importance of skill. 2. Discuss with client or family caregiver purpose of enteral feeding and enhanced nutritional health. 3. Help client or family caregiver determine feeding schedule that will maintain nutritional requirements, fit within client's or family's schedule, and fit health care provider's order.	Reduces transmission of microorganisms. Reinforces importance of infection control. Reinforces importance of regular feedings. Promotes adherence to enteral nutrition therapy. Client-centered approach increases client confidence in managing his or her own feedings (Best, 2012).

Clinical Decision Point *Explain that family caregiver needs to communicate to home health or health care provider any changes in feeding schedules made to fit daily routine.*

4. Have client or family caregiver apply clean gloves with you. If a client has a nasoenteral tube, demonstrate how to identify placement of feeding tube: aspirating gastric fluid, checking pH of gastric fluid, and acceptable pH range (see Skill 32.2).	Reduces transmission of microorganisms. Some nasally placed tubes are inadvertently placed in respiratory system and migrate to esophagus or into respiratory tract. In these cases, check pH periodically (Best, 2013; Taylor et al., 2015). Aspirated secretions with low pH are strong indicator of gastric placement. However, high pH cannot differentiate between aspirated secretions obtained from respiratory and intestinal tube placements.

Clinical Decision Point *Instruct client or family caregiver to avoid administration of all feedings, flushes, or medications if there is any doubt as to placement of enteral feeding tube.*

5. Observe client or family caregiver demonstrate placement of nasally placed tube.	Return demonstration identifies if there are areas for further teaching.

STEP	RATIONALE
6. When client has a gastrostomy or jejunostomy tube, observe client or family caregiver check for gastric residual volume by aspirating gastric contents (Best, 2013; Stepter, 2012). Have client return aspirated contents to stomach unless volume exceeds 250 mL (see agency policy) (Metheny et al., 2011).	Checking gastric residual in a small-bore nasogastric tube can easily lead to occlusion or displacement. Gastric residual volumes in the range of 200 to 500 mL should raise concern and lead to implementation of measures to reduce the risk of aspiration, such as changing from intermittent to continuous feedings, evaluating possibility of decreasing opioid analgesics, and starting medication that enhances gastric motility (e.g., metoclopramide). Automatic cessation of feeding should not occur for GRV less than 500 mL in the absence of other signs of intolerance (McCarthy et al., 2015).
7. Discuss use of medical asepsis in setting up and changing administration sets, mixing formulas (do not add formula to hanging bag), refrigerating unused formula, limiting amount of formula "hung" at one time to amount that can be infused in 4- to 6-hour period (less time in warmer weather), and maintaining and caring for bag.	Medical aseptic technique minimizes risk for microorganism contamination. Refrigeration and limiting "hang" time reduce microorganisms. Changing administration sets every 24 hours reduces microorganism growth.
8. Instruct client or family caregiver that client needs to sit up in chair or have head of bed elevated at least 30 degrees, preferably 45 degrees, while receiving feedings or medications or when tube is flushed.	Decreases risk for aspiration. Aspiration is indicated by increased coughing, difficulty in breathing, or increased sputum (Metheny and Frantz, 2013).
9. Observe client or family caregiver mixing, administering, and storing formulas. Discuss flushing of tube after administration of feedings or medications.	Identifies competence and need for further teaching. Regular flushing of tube prevents clogging.
10. Observe client or family caregiver change administration sets and clean bags. Have them dispose of supplies, remove gloves, and perform hand hygiene.	Reduces transmission of infection.
11. Observe client or family caregiver administering medications and flushing tube (see Skill 21.2).	Ensures that medications are given correctly.

Clinical Decision Point *Verify that medications do not include any sublingual, enteric-coated, or sustained-release medications. These medications cannot be crushed for administration.*

STEP	RATIONALE
12. Discuss and observe use of infusion pump if client is receiving continuous feeding (see Chapter 32).	Use of tube-feeding infusion pumps is complex and requires reinforcement.
13. Discuss measures to stabilize feeding tube in clients with abdominal tubes and to clean and protect skin insertion site (see Chapter 32).	Prevents tube from dislodging and skin breakdown.
14. Provide contact information for ordering equipment and supplies or who to call in case of equipment failure.	Ensures that family caregiver is able to respond in an emergency.
15. Discuss emergency plan and actions to take for signs and symptoms of aspiration such as elevating head of bed, oral suctioning, and calling health care provider.	Ensures understanding of management of equipment, supplies, emergency plan, and collaboration.
16. Discuss who to contact and when for signs of diarrhea, constipation, or weight loss.	Provides support to client or caregiver.

EVALUATION

1. Ask client or family caregiver to state purpose of home enteral nutrition therapy.	Demonstrates cognitive learning.
2. Observe client or family caregiver performing medical asepsis techniques, checking tube placement, aspirating residuals, administering medications and feedings, and using/cleaning equipment.	Demonstrates psychomotor learning.
3. Ask client or family caregiver to state measures used to prevent complications (e.g., verification of tube position before each feeding, elevation of client's head during feeding, stabilization and flushing of tubing).	Ensures safe home management and identification of areas for teaching.
4. Ask client or family caregiver how to care for open formula cans.	Ensures safe home management for preventing foodborne illness.

STEP	RATIONALE
5. **Use Teach-Back:** "I want to be sure I explained how to manage complications that can occur with your tube feedings. Tell me how to manage nausea, stomach fullness or distention, and diarrhea." Revise your instruction or develop a plan for revised client or family caregiver teaching if client or family caregiver is not able to teach back correctly.	Determines client's and family caregiver's level of understanding of instructional topic.

Unexpected Outcomes	Related Interventions
1. Feeding tube becomes displaced.	• Instruct client or family caregiver to stop feeding and notify home care nurse. • Nurse or health care provider will reposition feeding tube and verify placement before initiating any enteral feeding.
2. Signs and symptoms of aspiration are present.	• Stop feeding. Raise head of bed. • Verify tube position. • Notify health care provider.
3. Client develops diarrhea.	• Notify health care provider. • Collaborate with dietitian and health care provider to consider change in strength, type, or rate of enteral feeding, soluble fiber; review medications; or use antidiarrheal medications (Blumenstein et al., 2014).
4. Skin surrounding stoma breaks down, or drainage around insertion site develops.	• Clean stoma area more frequently. • Apply antibiotic ointment around stoma as ordered. • Contact health care provider.

Recording and Reporting

- Record instructions given to client and family caregiver and their response in home care record.
- Record specifics of enteral feeding plan, including type and size of tube in home, formula, and amounts to be administered in specific time frames.
- Client or family caregivers need to document I&O, daily weights, amount of gastric fluid aspirated before each feeding (or every 4 hours if receiving continuous feeding), date and time of feedings, amount and type of formula, any additives, and date and time that administration sets are changed.

Special Considerations
Teaching

- Performing skill without nurse in attendance provokes anxiety. Always leave a phone number and instructions about how to reach home care nurse if needed.
- Teach client and family caregiver the maximum hang time for any enteral feeding. After a can of formula has been opened, it should remain at room temperature for no longer than 8 to 12 hours,
- If the client has a nasoenteral tube, encourage frequent mouth care to prevent dryness of oral mucous membranes.

Pediatric

- Children are at risk for aspiration and fluid and electrolyte imbalance; thus teach parent to monitor child carefully (Hockenberry and Wilson, 2015).
- Children who receive long-term home enteral feedings often experience developmental and growth delays. Other common problems include sleep disturbance, tube blockages, problems with delivery of equipment, and equipment malfunction. Therefore these children require close follow-up and frequent nutritional monitoring.
- Teach family caregiver to position children who cannot sit up during or after a tube feeding on their right side during the tube feeding and for approximately 1 hour after it (Hockenberry and Wilson, 2015).

Gerontological

- Assess for changes and limitations in sensory function, mobility, or dexterity that indicate a need to teach a family caregiver how to administer feedings.
- Clients with dementia who are receiving enteral tube feeding are at higher risk for restraint use (Bentur et al., 2015).

◆ **SKILL 44.8** **Managing Parenteral Nutrition in the Home**

Parenteral nutrition (PN) in the home is indicated for clients who cannot take adequate nutrition by mouth and when enteral feedings are contraindicated (e.g., cancer, renal failure, motor neuron disorders, cardiac disease, chronic respiratory or gastrointestinal disorders [Wilson and Blackett, 2012]). Nurses who manage PN in the home collaborate frequently with registered dietitians and other health care providers to ensure that clients receive sufficient calories, protein, and fluid. PN is administered through a long-term central venous catheter (CVC) such as a tunneled CVC (e.g., Groshong or Hickman catheter), an implantable port, or a peripherally inserted central catheter (PICC) (see Chapter 29). Potential complications are associated with PN infusion, including intravenous (IV)–related blood clots and bloodstream infection.

PN is individually formulated and includes a mixture of amino acids, dextrose, fat emulsions, vitamins, electrolytes, minerals, and trace elements. Administering PN in the home requires an inter-professional approach and a client and/or family caregiver who demonstrates competency in its preparation and administration (Durfee et al., 2014).

Usually administration of PN in the home takes about 12 hours; thus many clients choose to receive their PN during the night. Because of the risks involved with PN and because manage-ment in the home is very complex, clients receive their first infusion in an acute care setting. After discharge a home care nurse visits frequently. The home care nurse will need to carefully assess the reaction of the client or family caregiver to the use of the technology needed to administer PN at home and provide emotional support. Although administering PN in the home increases clients' autonomy, it often interferes with their ability to maintain their normal routines. Work with the client or family caregiver to stress the benefits and offer support in dealing with related issues.

Delegation and Collaboration

The skill of managing PN in the home cannot be delegated to nursing assistive personnel (NAP). The nurse instructs the NAP to:

- Report findings of fingerstick blood glucose monitoring.
- Report vital signs outside of normal range to nurse.
- Report client complaints of shortness of breath, headache, weakness, or discomfort.
- Report if the catheter dressings are wet or bleeding at the site.

Equipment

- IV solution of PN
- IV tubing with optional filter
- Electronic IV infusion pump with alarms and protection from free flow
- Home blood glucose monitoring equipment
- Alcohol swabs
- Clean gloves
- Log

STEP	RATIONALE

ASSESSMENT

1. Identify client using at least two identifiers during first home visit. Facial recognition can be used as one of two identifiers for ongoing subsequent home visits.

Ensures client safety (TJC, 2016).

2. Assess client's ongoing nutritional status and risk for malnutrition by using nutrition screening tool (see Chapter 31) and performing physical examination. Identify signs and symptoms of malnutrition (e.g., weight loss or weight below ideal level; muscle atrophy, wasting, or weakness; lethargy; unable to eat for more than 6 days). Include measurement of vital signs.

Nutritional assessment helps to identify client's baseline to determine response to parenteral nutrition.

3. Assess client's fluid and electrolyte levels, serum albumin, total protein, transferrin, prealbumin, triglycerides, and glucose levels.

Provides additional baseline assessment data (Durfee et al., 2014).

4. Assess client's venous access device for edema, drainage, tenderness, and signs of inflammation (see Chapter 29). Measure circumference of upper arm if client has PICC; mark place on arm where measurement was taken.

Infection is common complication when client has venous access device. Measurement of arm helps detect infiltration of PICC. Mark on arm ensures consistent measurements over time.

5. Verify health care provider's order for PN, including amino acids, dextrose, fat emulsions, vitamins, minerals, trace elements, electrolytes, and flow rate.

Ensures safe and accurate PN administration.

6. Assess client's learning readiness, anxiety and ability to concentrate (consider presence of pain, nausea, or fatigue and client interest in instruction), and learning style preference.

Presence of significant illness, frailty, or confusion affects client's ability to attend to teaching plan. Indicates need to rely on family caregiver for learning and implementation (if available) on short- or long-term basis. Learning style affects choice of teaching resources.

7. Assess client's or family caregiver's previous knowledge and experience in managing PN in home. Have client or caregiver perform return demonstration if able to perform skill.

Determines level of understanding before beginning teaching session.

NURSING DIAGNOSES

- Adult failure to thrive
- Anxiety
- Caregiver role strain
- Deficient knowledge regarding total parenteral nutrition

- Fatigue
- Imbalanced nutrition: less than body requirements

- Readiness for enhanced nutrition
- Risk for infection
- Social isolation

Related factors/Risk factors are individualized based on client's condition or needs.

STEP	RATIONALE

PLANNING

1. Expected outcomes following completion of procedure:
  - Client or family caregiver is able to administer PN correctly.
  - Client or family caregiver demonstrates proper care of CVC.
  - Client or family caregiver explains how to properly store and maintain formulas for feeding.
  - Client or family caregiver states signs and symptoms of alterations that need to be reported to health care provider.
  - Client or family caregiver demonstrates correct measurement of blood glucose.

2. Select setting in home where client is most likely to administer PN and is conducive to a teaching session.
  a. Select room that is well lit with comfortable seating.
  b. Be sure that client is close and can see nurse clearly.
  c. Control sources of noise and distractions.

Indicates that skills are effectively learned.

Prevents infection and ensures patency of venous access device.

Knowledge of infection control principles prevents foodborne illness.
Ensures safe administration of PN in home.

Necessary for safe monitoring of client's response to parenteral nutrition therapy.
Practicing in same environment where skill is routinely performed facilitates comprehension and learning.

Room environment needs to minimize existing sensory alterations. Comfortable environment free of distractions promotes client's attention.

IMPLEMENTATION

1. Provide name and phone number of people or resources available 24 hours a day, 7 days a week in case problems arise.

2. Explain type/name of infusion, volume and infusion rate, expected outcomes, and components of PN. Explain that PN needs to be stored in refrigerator.

3. Have client or family caregiver perform each of the following steps with guidance from nurse. Do not rush client.

4. Instruct client or family caregiver to inspect the intravenous solution bag label, ensure that client's name is on label, ensure that solution has not expired, and check bag for leaks.

5. Suggest taking PN solution out of refrigerator for 30 to 60 minutes before scheduled infusion time.

6. Explain need to inspect fluid in bag for color and precipitates.

Provides assurance and allows client or family caregiver to troubleshoot problems and answer questions.

Allows client or caregiver to verify that correct PN is infused and that client or caregiver understands expected outcomes of care. Refrigeration maintains integrity of PN.
Allows you to correct errors in technique as they occur and discuss implications.

Ensures that client or family caregiver knows how to check pharmacy-prepared solution to ensure right client receives right PN. Bag needs to be intact to maintain closed system and ensure that client receives all prescribed nutrients.
Chilled solution often causes discomfort; allowing solution to warm enhances comfort during infusion.
Changes in color or precipitates in bag indicate disruption in PN.

Clinical Decision Point *If precipitate appears, components of mixture are separated, or color changes, explain that solution needs to be discarded.*

7. Have client or family caregiver perform hand hygiene and apply clean gloves with you. Demonstrate how to attach IV tubing to bag, how to attach filter to IV tubing (*optional*), how to prime IV tubing, and how to load IV tubing into electronic infusion pump (see Chapter 29).

8. Wipe CVC port with alcohol and show how to flush CVC and connect IV tubing to port (see Chapter 29). Use needleless system whenever possible.

9. Explain how to determine appropriate rate of infusion and program infusion pump (see Skill 29.2). Caution client and family caregiver against changing rate to "catch up."

10. Have client and family caregiver remove and dispose of gloves; perform hand hygiene.

11. When infusion is completed, explain and demonstrate how to disconnect IV tubing and flush CVC (see Chapter 29). Ensure that client or family caregiver performs hand hygiene before and after disconnecting line.

Reduces transmission of infection. Prepares PN solution for IV administration.

CVC needs to be patent, and IV tubing needs to connect to CVC to allow PN to be administered. Needleless systems prevent needlestick injuries.
Ensures that PN is administered at appropriate rate.

Prevents spread of microorganisms.

Flushing CVC following infusion maintains patency of vascular access device. Meticulous hand hygiene prevents infection.

STEP	RATIONALE
12. Describe appropriate use and storage of infusion pump and supplies. Explain appropriate tubing replacement schedules (e.g., every 24 hours for total nutrition admixture (TNA), 72 hours for three-in-one solutions).	Maintains integrity of equipment; appropriate timing of tubing changes prevents infection.
13. Help to develop plan for appropriate disposal of supplies, including needles, syringes, and unused medications or solutions, using principles of standard precautions.	Implementation of standard precautions is necessary to prevent transmission of communicable diseases and needlestick injuries.
14. Demonstrate appropriate care of CVC site; discuss how to change dressings, frequency of dressing changes, and signs of infection (see Skill 29.6).	Prevents infection at CVC insertion site.
15. Teach client and/or family caregiver about signs and symptoms that indicate potential complications from PN therapy (e.g., infection and phlebitis at CVC site, refeeding syndrome, hyperglycemia, hypernatremia, hypophosphatemia, hypokalemia, hypomagnesemia) and when to call for help.	Knowledge of complications of PN therapy allows for early detection and appropriate action.
16. Demonstrate use of self–blood glucose monitor. Explain frequency of testing, normal glucose values, and what to do if values fall outside of expected range (see Chapter 7).	PN increases blood glucose levels, which negatively affects client outcomes. Frequent monitoring of glucose level helps detect problems early. Expect testing frequency to decrease as client's condition and response to PN stabilizes.
17. Provide client with logbook to record administration of PN, weights, intake and output, and blood glucose levels.	Allows health care providers and clients to evaluate outcomes and detect adverse effects of nutritional therapy.
18. Help client develop plan to reorder supplies, PN fluid, and prescribed additives; for emergencies (e.g., what to do if electricity goes out); and for home safety plan (e.g., how to get to bathroom without tripping over IV tubing).	Plans allow for continuous, safe, and effective administration of PN.

EVALUATION

1. Have client or family caregiver independently demonstrate initiation, infusion, and discontinuation of PN infusion and CVC site care.

Feedback through return demonstration of psychomotor skill is best means of evaluating mastery of skill.

2. Watch client or family caregiver clean and store PN, equipment, and supplies.

Proper cleaning and storage prevents bacterial growth.

3. Ask client or family caregiver to identify expected outcomes of nutritional therapy.

Measures client cognitive learning and confirms understanding of information.

4. Have client or family caregiver independently demonstrate blood glucose monitoring and recording.

Ensures mastering of skill needed for effective evaluation of client status.

5. Watch client or family caregiver record information in log. Review client's or caregiver's log periodically to ensure that information is being recorded correctly.

Health care providers make changes in client care based on information provided by client. To ensure that changes are made appropriately, client needs to record accurate information.

6. **Use Teach-Back:** "I want to be sure I explained the common signs and symptoms of infection and other potential complications of PN. Tell me the signs and symptoms of infection." Revise your instruction now or develop a plan for revised client or family caregiver teaching if client or family caregiver is not able to teach back correctly.

Determines client's and family caregiver's level of understanding of instructional topic.

Unexpected Outcomes	Related Interventions
1. Client or family caregiver is unable to manage home PN therapy or verbalize information that was taught.	• Ask client or caregiver to describe difficulties experienced while performing skill. • Use different teaching strategy. • Teach caregiver further and evaluate need to increase frequency of home visits to ensure safe administration of PN at home.
2. Client or family caregiver reports signs and symptoms of complications from PN or CVC.	• Inform health care provider. • Tell client or caregiver to call emergency medical services (EMS) if signs and symptoms are severe.

Recording and Reporting

- Record information taught, client's and family caregiver's response, and outcomes of PN therapy (e.g., weight, electrolyte and glucose levels, physical assessment findings) in home care log.
- Record appearance of CVC site, infusions, glucose monitoring results, client's weight in home care log.

Special Considerations
Teaching

- Assess client's psychosocial status while providing information. Many clients experience a decrease in the quality of life when PN feedings are started in the home, which often increases anxiety and decreases comprehension of information.
- Eating is often a social event. When clients do not eat, they tend to feel socially isolated. Teach clients and family caregivers the importance of maintaining social relationships and enhancing social support during PN therapy. Refer client to support groups and other resources such as the Oley Foundation (http://oley.org/index.html) (Hockenberry and Wilson, 2015).

- Always leave a phone number and instructions about how to reach home care nurse if needed.

Pediatric
- The risk for displacement of the CVC increases as the child grows. Ensure that the placement of the venous access device is confirmed with x-ray film examination as the child grows.
- Teach the family caregiver to socialize child with other children to enhance development (Hockenberry and Wilson, 2015).

Gerontological
- Frail older adults are at high risk for electrolyte disturbances. Frequently assess and monitor their response to PN and their laboratory values.
- Carefully assess client's ability to perform skill. Management of PN at home is complex and requires manual dexterity, visual acuity, and high-level critical thinking and decision-making skills. Include family caregiver in teaching plan to help with management of home PN.

▶ CLINICAL DEBRIEF

You are scheduled to visit an 86-year-old retired engineer who lives in a private home with his 84-year-old wife. The client is currently hospitalized for an acute episode of bronchitis and is newly diagnosed with chronic obstructive pulmonary disease. He will be sent home on oral antibiotics and oxygen therapy. When you contact his wife about an initial home assessment, you find that, in addition to his new diagnosis and oxygen therapy, his adult son who smokes one pack of cigarettes per day lives in the home. This is your first home visit.

1. What information would you like to have about the client's home environment before he is discharged to help him safely manage his new home oxygen therapy?

2. During your initial home visit with the client, wife, and son, you reassess the home environment and discover that oxygen cylinders are being stored in the bedroom closet. What should you do?

3. You schedule a follow up visit to the home and discover that the son smokes near his father. How will you address the son's smoking status and the importance of maintaining a nonsmoking environment?

4. Providing medication information when his daughter and infant grandchild are visiting him
5. Using medication caps that the client can open independently

3. An older adult is receiving home enteral nutrition because of dysphagia (swallowing difficulty). Which action(s) will the nurse instruct the family caregiver to take with enteral feeding? (Select all that apply.)
   1. Have family caregiver perform hand hygiene before initiating the enteral feeding.
   2. Have client's head of bed elevated at least 10 to 20 degrees while receiving feedings.
   3. Verify tube placement.
   4. Schedule feedings to maintain nutritional requirements.
   5. Use teach-back to verify the family caregiver's understanding of signs and symptoms of complications such as aspiration with enteral tube feeding.

ⓔ *Visit the Evolve site for a complete list of Clinical Debrief and Review Questions answers.*

▶ REVIEW QUESTIONS

1. A client is being taught self-administration of medications. Which of the following are assessments to be completed before the teaching session? (Select all that apply.)
   1. Purpose of regularly scheduled medications and their desired effects
   2. Explanation of dosage schedules and rationale
   3. Knowledge regarding medication therapy
   4. Learning readiness and ability to concentrate
   5. Client's belief in need for medication therapy

2. A 94-year-old client is discharged from the hospital to his home after treatment for bronchitis. The client lives independently, and his closest family is 100 miles away. Which nursing intervention will enhance adherence to his medication regimen? (Select all that apply.)
   1. Teaching everything he needs to know in 1 day and returning in 2 weeks
   2. Including him in deciding the system used to help him remember to take his medications
   3. Providing 12-point font instructions that are written in red ink

REFERENCES

American Academy of Pediatricians (AAP): *How to take a child's temperature*, 2015, https://www.healthychildren.org/English/health-issues/conditions/fever/Pages/How-to-Take-a-Childs-Temperature.aspx. Accessed April 13, 2016.

American Heart Associations (AHA): *How to monitor and record your blood pressure*, 2015, http://www.heart.org/HEARTORG/Conditions/HighBloodPressure/SymptomsDiagnosisMonitoringofHighBloodPressure/How-to-Monitor-and-Record-Your-Blood-Pressure_UCM_303323_Article.jsp. Accessed April 13, 2016.

American Nurses Association (ANA): *Home health nursing: scope and standards of practice*, ed 2, Silver Springs, 2014, ANA.

American Society for Parenteral and Enteral Nutrition (ASPEN), *Nutrition support patient data*, 2015, http://www.nutritioncare.org/About_Clinical_Nutrition/Nutrition_Support_Patient_Data_Fact_Sheet/ Accessed September 3, 2016.

American Thoracic Society: *Oxygen sources and delivery devices*, 2015, http://www.thoracic.org/clinical/copd-guidelines/for-health-professionals/management-of-stable-copd/long-term-oxygen-therapy/oxygen-sources-and-delivery-devices.php. Accessed April 13, 2016.

Ashton K, Oermann M: Patient education in home care: strategies for success, *Home Healthc Nurse* 32(5):289, 2014.

Ayhan H, et al: Normal saline instillation before endotracheal suctioning: "What does the evidence say? What do the nurses think?" Multimethod study, *J Crit Care* 30(4):762, 2015.

Bentur N, et al: Feeding tubes for older people with advanced dementia living in the community in Israel, *Am J Alzheimers Dis Other Demen* 30(2):165, 2015.

Best C: Supporting home eternal tube feeding: some considerations, *Br J Community Nurs* S6, November 2012.

Best C: Nasogastric feeding in the community: safe and effective practice, *Br J Community Nurs* S8, October 2013.

Blumenstein I, et al: Gastroenteric tube feeding: techniques, problems and solutions, *World J Gastroenterol* 20(26):8512, 2014.

Bolinger R, Engberg S: Barriers, complications, adherence, and self-reported quality of life for people using clean intermittent catheterization, *J Wound Ostomy Continence Nurs* 40(1):83, 2013.

Buscombe C: Using Gagne's theory to teach procedural skills, *Clin Teach* 10(5):303, 2013.

Camicia M, et al: The essential role of the rehabilitation nurse in facilitating care transitions: a white paper by the Association of Rehabilitation Nurses, *Rehabil Nurs* 39(1):10, 2014.

Centers for Disease Control and Prevention (CDC): *Medication adherence*, 2013, http://www.cdc.gov/primarycare/materials/medication/docs/medication-adherence-01ccd.pdf. Accessed August 29, 2016.

Center for Health Care Strategies (CHCS): *Health literacy fact sheets*, 2015, http://www.chcs.org/resource/health-literacy-fact-sheets. Accessed on April 13, 2016.

Cleveland Clinic: *Tracheostomy*, 2015, http://my.clevelandclinic.org/services/head-neck/treatments-services/tracheostomy-care. Accessed April 13, 2016.

Crabtree M, Stuart-Shor E: Implementing home blood pressure monitoring into usual care, *J Nurse Pract* 10(8):607, 2014.

Dean G: Are single-use catheters worth the expense?, *J Urol* 194(1):12, 2015.

Department of Health & Human Services (DHHS): *Home oxygen therapy*, 2015, https://www.cms.gov/Outreach-and-Education/Medicare-Learning-Network-MLN/MLNProducts/Downloads/Home-Oxygen-Therapy-Text-Only.pdf. Accessed April 13, 2016.

Durfee S, et al: ASPEN standards for nutrition support: home and alternate site care, *Nutr Clin Pract* 29(4):545–552, 2014.

Eadie C: Health literacy: a conceptual review, *Medsurg Nurs* 23(1):10, 2014.

Ebersole P, et al: *Toward healthy aging: human needs and nursing response*, ed 9, St Louis, 2015, Mosby.

Environmental Protection Agency (EPA): *Thermometers*, 2014, http://www.epa.gov/mercury/thermometer-main.html. Accessed August 28, 2016.

Fallon N: The challenge of measuring blood pressure accurately, *Br J Cardiac Nurs* 10(3):136, 2015.

Frese E, et al: Blood pressure measurement guidelines for physical therapists, *Cardiopulm Phys Ther J* 22(2):5, 2011.

Galligan CJ, et al: A growing fire hazard concern in communities: home oxygen therapy and continued smoking habits, *New Solut* 24(4):549, 2015.

Hart M: Safety considerations when transitioning the elderly from hospital to home, *AARC Times* 39(2):10, 2015.

Heiss G: Health teaching. In Maurer F, Smith C, editors: *Community health nursing practice for families and populations*, ed 5, St Louis, 2013, Mosby.

Hockenberry MJ, Wilson D: *Wong's nursing care of infants and children*, ed 10, St Louis, 2015, Mosby.

Home Health Quality Improvement (HHQI): *Welcome to the HHQI national campaign*, 2015, http://www.homehealthquality.org/Home.aspx. Accessed April 13, 2016.

Hyrkas K, Wiggins M: A comparison of usual care, a patient-centered education intervention and motivational interviewing to improve medication adherence and readmissions of adults in an acute-care setting, *J Nurs Manag* 22(3):350, 2014.

Iihara N, et al: Comparing patient dissatisfaction and rational judgment in intentional medication non-adherence versus unintentional non-adherence, *J Clin Pharm Ther* 39(1):45, 2014.

Inott T, Kennedy B: Assessing learning styles: practical tips for patient education, *Nurs Clin North Am* 46(3):313–320, 2011.

Jett KF: Culture and aging. In Touhy TT, Jett KF, editors: *Ebersole and Hess' gerontological nursing and healthy aging*, ed 4, St Louis, 2014, Mosby.

Jung M, et al: Reliability of home blood pressure monitoring: in the context of validation and accuracy, *Blood Press Monit* 20(4):5, 2015.

Kantarci G: Home and ambulatory blood pressure monitoring: When? Who?, *Kidney Int Suppl* 3(4):337, 2013.

Knier S, et al: Patients' perceptions of the quality of discharge teaching and readiness for discharge, *Rehabil Nurs* 40(1):30, 2015.

Kornburger C, et al: Using "teach-back" to promote a safe transition from hospital to home: an evidence-based approach to improving the discharge process, *J Pediatr Nurs* 28(3):284–290, 2013.

Lamb B: The hazards of suctioning, *AARC Times* 38(11):7, 2014.

Lewis S, et al: *Medical-surgical nursing: assessment and management of clinical problems*, ed 10, St Louis, 2017, Elsevier.

Mager D: Hospitalization of home care patients: adverse drug events, *Home Health Care Manag Pract* 26(1):15, 2014.

Marrelli T: Update on home health care: how it's changing, *Am Nurse Today* 9(6):4, 2014.

McBride M, Andrews GJ: The transition from acute care to home: a review of issues in discharge teaching and a framework for better practice, *Can J Cardiovasc Nurs* 23(3):22, 2013.

McCarthy MS, Martindale RG: What's on the menu? Delivering evidence-based nutritional therapy, *Nursing* 45(8):36, 2015.

Metheny NA, et al: Relationship between feeding tube site and respiratory outcomes, *JPEN J Parenter Enteral Nutr* 35:346, 2011.

Metheny NA, Frantz RA: Head-of-bed elevation in critically ill patients: a review, *Crit Care Nurse* 33(3):55, 2013.

Müller S, et al: Validation of the adherence barriers questionnaire: an instrument for identifying potential risk factors associated with medication-related non-adherence, *BMC Health Serv Res* 15(1):2, 2015.

National Institute of Health (NIH): *Health literacy*, 2015, http://www.nlm.nih.gov/medlineplus/healthliteracy.html. Accessed August 28, 2016.

Newman D, Willson M: Review of intermittent catheterization and current best practices, *Urol Nurs* 31(1):12, 2011.

Nies MA, McEwen M: *Community public health nursing*, ed 6, St Louis, 2015, Elsevier.

Parker E, et al: Exploring best practices in home health care: a review of available evidence on select innovations, *Home Health Care Manag Pract* 26(1):17, 2014.

Pereira K, et al: Internet delivered diabetes self-management education: a review, *Diabetes Technol Ther* 17(1):55, 2015.

Peter D, et al: Reducing readmissions using teach-back: enhancing patient and family education, *J Nurs Adm* 45(1):36, 2015.

Rosa MA, et al: The interdisciplinary approach to the implementation of a diabetes home care disease management program, *Home Healthc Nurse* 32(2):109, 2014.

Seth JH, et al: Ensuring patient adherence to clean intermittent self-catheterization, *Patient Prefer Adherence* 8:193, 2014.

Sheldon P: Successful intermittent self-catheterization teaching: one nurse's strategy of how and what to teach, *Urol Nurs* 33(3):113, 2013.

Society of Urologic Nurses and Associates (SUNA): *Adult intermittent self-catheterization: client fact sheet*, 2010, https://www.suna.org/download/members/selfCatheterization.pdf. Accessed April 13, 2016.

Stepter C: Maintaining placement of temporary enteral feeding tubes in adults: a critical appraisal of the evidence, *Medsurg Nurs* 21(2):67, 2012.

Sund-Levander M, Grodzinsky E: Assessment of body temperature measurement options, *Br J Nurs* 22(15):880, 2013.

Tamura-Lis W: Teach-back for quality education and patient safety, *Urol Nurs* 33(6):267, 2013.

Taylor SJ, et al: The efficacy of feeding tubes: confirmation and loss, *Br J Nurs* 24(7):371, 2015.

The Joint Commission (TJC): *National Patient Safety Goals: home accreditation program*, 2016, http://www.jointcommission.org/assets/1/6/2016_NPSG_OME.pdf. Accessed on September 3, 2016.

Tiep B, et al: Long-term supplemental oxygen therapy. In Post TW, editor: *UpToDate*, Waltham, MA, 2015, UpToDate.

United States Department of Health & Human Services (USDHHS): *Quick guide to health literacy*, 2015, http://www.health.gov/communication/literacy/quickguide/factsliteracy.htm. Accessed August 28, 2016.

Werner SM: Patient safety and the widespread use of herbs and supplements, *Front Pharmacol* 5:1, 2014.

Wiles KS: Oxygen safety in the home…a growing concern, *AARC Times* 39(5):5, 2015.

Wilson M: Clean intermittent self-catheterisation: working with patients, *Br J Nurs* 24(2):80, 2015.

Wilson N, Blackett B: Parenteral nutrition: considerations for practice, *Br J Community Nurs* S18, May 2012.

Wyndaele JJ: Self-intermittent catheterization in multiple sclerosis, *Ann Phys Rehabil Med* 5(57):315, 2014.

Appendix A

NANDA DEFINITIONS FROM *NURSING DIAGNOSES: DEFINITIONS AND CLASSIFICATION 2015-2017,* 10TH EDITION.

Activity intolerance: Insufficient physiological or psychological energy to endure or complete required or desired daily activities.

Acute confusion: Abrupt onset of reversible disturbances of consciousness, attention, cognition, and perception that develop over a short period of time.

Acute pain: An unpleasant sensory and emotional experience associated with actual or potential tissue damage, or described in terms of such damage (International Association for the Study of Pain); sudden or slow onset of any intensity from mild to severe with an anticipated or predictable end.

Anxiety: Vague, uneasy feeling of discomfort or dread accompanied by an autonomic response (the source is often nonspecific or unknown to the individual); a feeling of apprehension caused by anticipation of danger. It is an alerting sign that warns of impending danger and enables the individual to take measures to deal with threat.

Autonomic dysreflexia: Life-threatening, uninhibited sympathetic response of the nervous system to a noxious stimulus after a spinal cord injury at T7 or above.

Bathing self-care deficit: Impaired ability to perform or complete bathing activities for self.

Bowel incontinence: Change in normal bowel habits characterized by involuntary passage of stool.

Caregiver role strain: Difficulty in performing family/significant other caregiver role.

Chronic confusion: Irreversible, long-standing, and/or progressive deterioration of intellect and personality characterized by decreased ability to interpret environmental stimuli and decreased capacity for intellectual thought processes, and manifested by disturbances of memory, orientation, and behavior.

Chronic functional constipation: Infrequent or difficult evacuation of feces, which has been present for at least three of the prior 12 months.

Chronic low self-esteem: Longstanding negative self-evaluating/feelings about self or self-capabilities.

Chronic pain syndrome: Recurrent or persistent pain that has lasted at least three months, and that significantly affects daily functioning or well-being.

Chronic pain: Unpleasant sensory and emotional experience associated with actual or potential tissue damage, or described in terms of such damage (International Association for the Study of Pain); sudden or slow onset of any intensity from mild to severe, constant or recurring without an anticipated or predictable end and a duration of greater than three (>3) months.

Chronic sorrow: Cyclical, recurring, and potentially progressive pattern of pervasive sadness experienced (by a parent, caregiver, individual with chronic illness or disability) in response to continual loss throughout the trajectory of an illness or disability.

Complicated grieving: A disorder that occurs after the death of a significant other, in which the experience of distress accompanying bereavement fails to follow normative expectations and manifests in functional impairment.

Compromised family coping: A usually supportive primary person (family member, significant other, or close friend) provides insufficient, ineffective, or compromised support, comfort, assistance, or encouragement that may be needed by the client to manage or master adaptive tasks related to his or her health challenge.

Constipation: Decrease in normal frequency of defecation accompanied by difficult or incomplete passage of stool and/or passage of excessively hard, dry stool.

Contamination: Exposure to environmental contaminants in doses sufficient to cause adverse health effects.

Death anxiety: Vague, uneasy feeling of discomfort or dread generated by perceptions of a real or imagined threat to one's existence.

Decisional conflict: Uncertainty about course of action to be taken when choice among competing actions involves risk, loss, or challenge to values and beliefs.

Decreased cardiac output: Inadequate blood pumped by the heart to meet the metabolic demands of the body.

Decreased intracranial adaptive capacity: Intracranial fluid dynamic mechanisms that normally compensate for increases in intracranial volumes are compromised, resulting in repeated disproportionate increases in intracranial pressure (ICP) in response to a variety of noxious and non-noxious stimuli.

Defensive coping: Repeated projection of falsely positive self-evaluation based on a self-protective pattern that defends against underlying perceived threats to positive self-regard.

Deficient community health: Presence of one or more health problems or factors that deter wellness or increase the risk of health problems experienced by an aggregate.

Deficient diversional activity: Decreased stimulation from (or interest or engagement in) recreational or leisure activities.

Deficient fluid volume: Decreased intravascular, interstitial, and/or intracellular fluid. This refers to dehydration, water loss alone without change in sodium level.

Deficient knowledge: Absence or deficiency of cognitive information related to a specific topic.

Delayed surgical recovery: Extension of the number of postoperative days required to initiate and perform activities that maintain life, health, and well-being.

Diarrhea: Passage of loose, unformed stools.

Disabled family coping: Behavior of primary person (family member, significant other, or close friend) that disables his or her capacities and the client's capacities to effectively address tasks essential to either person's adaptation to the health challenge.

Disorganized infant behavior: Disintegrated physiological and neurobehavioral responses of infant to the environment.

Disturbed body image: Confusion in mental picture of one's physical self.

Disturbed personal identity: Inability to maintain an integrated and complete perception of self.

Disturbed sleep pattern: Time limited interruptions of sleep amount and quality due to external factors.

Dressing self-care deficit: Impaired ability to perform or complete dressing activities for self.

Dysfunctional family processes: Psychosocial, spiritual, and physiological functions of the family unit are chronically disorganized, which leads to conflict, denial of problems, resistance to change, ineffective problem-solving, and a series of self-perpetuating crises.

Dysfunctional gastrointestinal motility: Increased, decreased, ineffective, or lack of peristaltic activity within the gastrointestinal system.

Dysfunctional ventilatory weaning response: Inability to adjust to lowered levels of mechanical ventilator support that interrupts and prolongs the weaning process.

Excess fluid volume: Increased isotonic fluid retention.

Fatigue: An overwhelming, sustained sense of exhaustion and decreased capacity for physical and mental work at the usual level.

Fear: Response to perceived threat that is consciously recognized as a danger.

Feeding self-care deficit: Impaired ability to perform or complete self-feeding activities.

Frail elderly syndrome: Dynamic state of unstable equilibrium that affects the older individual experiencing deterioration in one or more domain of health (physical, functional, psychological, or social) and leads to increased susceptibility to adverse health effects, particularly disability.

Functional urinary incontinence: Inability of a usually continent person to reach the toilet in time to avoid unintentional loss of urine.

Grieving: A normal complex process that includes emotional, physical, spiritual, social, and intellectual responses and behaviors by which individuals, families, and communities incorporate an actual, anticipated, or perceived loss into their daily lives.

Hopelessness: Subjective state in which an individual sees limited or no alternatives or personal choices available and is unable to mobilize energy on own behalf.

Hyperthermia: Core body temperature above the normal diurnal range due to failure of thermoregulation.

Hypothermia: Core body temperature below normal diurnal range due to failure of thermoregulation.

Imbalanced nutrition: less than body requirements: Intake of nutrients insufficient to meet metabolic needs.

Impaired bed mobility: Limitation of independent movement from one bed position to another.

Impaired comfort: Perceived lack of ease, relief, and transcendence in physical, psychospiritual, environmental, cultural and/or social dimensions.

Impaired dentition: Disruption in tooth development/eruption patterns or structural integrity of individual teeth.

Impaired emancipated decision-making: A process of choosing a health care decision that does not include personal knowledge and/or consideration of social norms, or does not occur in a flexible environment, resulting in decisional dissatisfaction.

Impaired gas exchange: Excess or deficit in oxygenation and/or carbon dioxide elimination at the alveolar-capillary membrane.

Impaired home maintenance: Inability to independently maintain a safe growth-promoting immediate environment.

Impaired memory: Inability to remember or recall bits of information or behavioral skills.

Impaired mood regulation: A mental state characterized by shifts in mood or affect and which is comprised of a constellation of affective, cognitive, somatic, and/or physiological manifestations varying from mild to severe.

Impaired oral mucous membrane: Injury to the lips, soft tissue, buccal cavity, and/or oropharynx.

Impaired parenting: Inability of the primary caretaker to create, maintain, or regain an environment that promotes the optimum growth and development of the child.

Impaired physical mobility: Limitation in independent, purposeful physical movement of the body or of one or more extremities.

Impaired religiosity: Impaired ability to exercise reliance on beliefs and/or participate in rituals of a particular faith tradition.

Impaired resilience: Decreased ability to sustain a pattern of positive responses to an adverse situation or crisis.

Impaired sitting: Limitation of ability to independently and purposefully attain and/or maintain a rest position that is supported by the buttocks and thighs, in which the torso is upright.

Impaired skin integrity: Altered epidermis and/or dermis.

Impaired social interaction: Insufficient or excessive quantity or ineffective quality of social exchange.

Impaired spontaneous ventilation: Decreased energy reserves resulting in an inability to maintain independent breathing that is adequate to support life.

Impaired standing: Limitation of ability to independently and purposefully attain and/or maintain the body in an upright position from feet to head.

Impaired swallowing: Abnormal functioning of the swallowing mechanism associated with deficits in oral, pharyngeal, or esophageal structure or function.

Impaired tissue integrity: Damage to the mucous membrane, cornea, integumentary system, muscular fascia, muscle, tendon, bone, cartilage, joint capsule, and/or ligament.

Impaired transfer ability: Limitation of independent movement between two nearby surfaces.

Impaired urinary elimination: Dysfunction in urine elimination.

Impaired verbal communication: Decreased, delayed, or absent ability to receive, process, transmit, and/or use a system of symbols.

Impaired walking: Limitation of independent movement within the environment on foot.

Impaired wheelchair mobility: Limitation of independent operation of wheelchair within environment.

Ineffective activity planning: Inability to prepare for a set of actions fixed in time and under certain conditions.

Ineffective airway clearance: Inability to clear secretions or obstructions from the respiratory tract to maintain a clear airway.

Ineffective breastfeeding: Difficulty providing milk to an infant or young child directly from the breasts, which may compromise nutritional status of the infant/child.

Ineffective breathing pattern: Inspiration and/or expiration that does not provide adequate ventilation.

Ineffective childbearing process: Pregnancy and childbirth process and care of the newborn that does not match the environmental context, norms, and expectation.

Ineffective community coping: A pattern of community activities for adaptation and problem solving that is unsatisfactory for meeting the demands or needs of the community.

Ineffective coping: Inability to form a valid appraisal of the stressors, inadequate choices of practiced responses, and/or inability to use available resources.

Ineffective denial: Conscious or unconscious attempt to disavow the knowledge or meaning of an event to reduce anxiety and/or fear, leading to the detriment of health.

Ineffective family health management: A pattern of regulating and integrating into family processes a program for the treatment of illness and its sequelae that is unsatisfactory for meeting specific health goals.

Ineffective health maintenance: Inability to identify, manage, and/or seek out help to maintain health.

Ineffective health management: Pattern of regulating and integrating into daily living a therapeutic regimen for the treatment of illness and its sequelae that is unsatisfactory for meeting specific health goals.

Ineffective impulse control: A pattern of performing rapid, unplanned reactions to internal or external stimuli without regard for the negative consequences of these reactions to the impulsive individual or to others.

Ineffective infant feeding pattern: Impaired ability of an infant to suck or coordinate the suck/swallow response resulting in inadequate oral nutrition for metabolic needs.

Ineffective peripheral tissue perfusion: Decrease in blood circulation to the periphery that may compromise health.

Ineffective protection: Decrease in the ability to guard self from internal or external threats such as illness or injury.

Ineffective relationship: A pattern of mutual partnership that is insufficient to provide for each other's needs.

Ineffective role performance: A pattern of behavior and self-expression that does not match the environmental context, norms, and expectations.

Ineffective sexuality pattern: Expressions of concern regarding own sexuality.

Ineffective thermoregulation: Temperature fluctuation between hypothermia and hyperthermia.

Insomnia: A disruption in amount and quality of sleep that impairs functioning.

Insufficient breast milk: Low production of maternal breast milk.

Interrupted breastfeeding: Break in the continuity of providing milk to an infant or young child directly from the breasts, which may compromise breastfeeding success and/or nutritional status of the infant/child.

Interrupted family processes: Change in family relationships and/or functioning.

Labile emotional control: Uncontrollable outbursts of exaggerated and involuntary emotional expression.

Labor pain: Sensory and emotional experience that varies from pleasant to unpleasant, associated with labor and childbirth.

Latex allergy response: A hypersensitive reaction to natural latex rubber products.

Moral distress: Response to the inability to carry out one's chosen ethical/moral decision/action.

Nausea: A subjective phenomenon of an unpleasant feeling in the back of the throat and stomach, which may or may not result in vomiting.

Neonatal jaundice: The yellow-orange tint of the neonate's skin and mucous membranes that occurs after 24 hours of life as a result of unconjugated bilirubin in the circulation.

Noncompliance: Behavior of person and/or caregiver that fails to coincide with a health-promoting or therapeutic plan agreed on by the person (and/or family and/or community) and health care professional. In the presence of an agreed-on, health-promoting,

or therapeutic plan, person's or caregiver's behavior is fully or partly non-adherent and may lead to clinically ineffective or partially effective outcomes.

Obesity: A condition in which an individual accumulates abnormal or excessive fat for age and gender that exceeds overweight.

Overflow urinary incontinence: Involuntary loss of urine associated with overdistention of the bladder.

Overweight: A condition in which an individual accumulates abnormal or excessive fat for age and gender.

Parental role conflict: Parental experience of role confusion and conflict in response to crisis.

Perceived constipation: Self-diagnosis of constipation combined with abuse of laxatives, enemas, and/or suppositories to ensure a daily bowel movement.

Post-trauma syndrome: Sustained maladaptive response to a traumatic, overwhelming event.

Powerlessness: The lived experience of lack of control over a situation, including a perception that one's actions do not significantly affect an outcome.

Rape-trauma syndrome: Sustained maladaptive response to a forced, violent, sexual penetration against the victim's will and consent.

Readiness for enhanced breastfeeding: A pattern of providing milk to an infant or young child directly from the breasts, which may be strengthened.

Readiness for enhanced childbearing process: A pattern of preparing for and maintaining a healthy pregnancy, childbirth process, and care of the newborn for ensuring well-being, which can be strengthened.

Readiness for enhanced comfort: A pattern of ease, relief, and transcendence in physical, psychospiritual, environmental, and/or social dimensions, which can be strengthened.

Readiness for enhanced communication: A pattern of exchanging information and ideas with others, which can be strengthened.

Readiness for enhanced community coping: A pattern of community activities for adaptation and problem-solving for meeting the demands or needs of the community, which can be strengthened.

Readiness for enhanced coping: A pattern of cognitive and behavioral efforts to manage demands related to well-being, which can be strengthened.

Readiness for enhanced decision-making: A pattern of choosing a course of action for meeting short- and long-term health-related goals, which can be strengthened.

Readiness for enhanced emancipated decision-making: A process of choosing a healthcare decision that includes personal knowledge and/or consideration of social norms, which can be strengthened.

Readiness for enhanced family coping: A pattern of management of adaptive tasks by primary person (family member, significant other, or close friend) involved with the client's health change, which can be strengthened.

Readiness for enhanced family processes: A pattern of family functioning to support the well-being of family members, which can be strengthened.

Readiness for enhanced fluid balance: A pattern of equilibrium between the fluid volume and chemical composition of body fluids, which can be strengthened.

Readiness for enhanced health management: A pattern of regulating and integrating into daily living a therapeutic regimen for treatment of illness and its sequelae, which can be strengthened.

Readiness for enhanced hope: A pattern of expectations and desires for mobilizing energy on one's own behalf, which can be strengthened.

Readiness for enhanced knowledge: A pattern of cognitive information related to a specific topic, or its acquisition, which can be strengthened.

Readiness for enhanced nutrition: A pattern of nutrient intake, which can be strengthened.

Readiness for enhanced organized infant behavior: A pattern of modulation of the physiological and behavioral systems of functioning (i.e., autonomic, motor, state-organization, self-regulatory, and attentional-interactional systems) in an infant, which can be strengthened.

Readiness for enhanced parenting: A pattern of providing an environment for children or other dependent person(s) to nurture growth and development, which can be strengthened.

Readiness for enhanced power: A pattern of participating knowingly in change for well-being, which can be strengthened.

Readiness for enhanced relationship: A pattern of mutual partnership to provide for each other's needs, which can be strengthened.

Readiness for enhanced religiosity: A pattern of reliance on religious beliefs and/or participation in rituals of a particular faith tradition, which can be strengthened.

Readiness for enhanced resilience: A pattern of positive responses to an adverse situation or crisis, which can be strengthened.

Readiness for enhanced self-care: A pattern of performing activities for oneself to meet health-related goals, which can be strengthened.

Readiness for enhanced self-concept: A pattern of perceptions or ideas about the self, which can be strengthened.

Readiness for enhanced sleep: A pattern of natural, periodic suspension of relative consciousness to provide rest and sustain a desired lifestyle, which can be strengthened.

Readiness for enhanced spiritual well-being: A pattern of experiencing and integrating meaning and purpose in life through connectedness with self, others, art, music, literature, nature, and/or a power greater than oneself, which can be strengthened.

Readiness for enhanced urinary elimination: A pattern of urinary functions for meeting eliminatory needs, which can be strengthened.

Reflex urinary incontinence: Involuntary loss of urine at somewhat predictable intervals when a specific bladder volume is reached.

Relocation stress syndrome: Physiological and/or psychosocial disturbance following transfer from one environment to another.

Risk for activity intolerance: Vulnerable to insufficient physiological or psychological energy to endure or complete required or desired daily activities, which may compromise health.

Risk for acute confusion: Vulnerable to reversible disturbances of consciousness, attention, cognition, and perception that develop over a short period of time, which may compromise health.

Risk for adverse reaction to iodinated contrast media: Vulnerable to noxious or unintended reaction associated with the use of iodinated contrast media that can occur within seven days after contrast agent injection, which may compromise health.

Risk for allergy response: Vulnerable to exaggerated immune response or reaction to substances, which may compromise health.

Risk for aspiration: Vulnerable to entry of gastrointestinal secretions, oropharyngeal secretions, solids, or fluids to the tracheobronchial passages, which may compromise health.

Risk for autonomic dysreflexia: Vulnerable to life-threatening, uninhibited response of the sympathetic nervous system postspinal shock, in an individual with spinal cord injury or lesion at T6 or above (has been demonstrated in patients with injuries at T7 and T8), which may compromise health.

Risk for bleeding: Vulnerable to a decrease in blood volume, which may compromise health.

Risk for caregiver role strain: Vulnerable to difficulty in performing the family/significant other caregiver role, which may compromise health.

Risk for chronic functional constipation: Vulnerable to infrequent or difficult evacuation of feces, which has been present nearly 3 of the prior 12 months, which may compromise health.

Risk for chronic low self-esteem: Vulnerable to longstanding negative self-evaluating/feelings about self or self-capabilities, which may compromise health.

Risk for complicated grieving: Vulnerable to a disorder that occurs after death of a significant other in which the experience of distress accompanying bereavement fails to follow normative expectations and manifests in functional impairment, which may compromise health.

Risk for compromised human dignity: Vulnerable for perceived loss of respect and honor, which may compromise health.

Risk for constipation: Vulnerable to a decrease in normal frequency of defecation accompanied by difficult or incomplete passage of stool, which may compromise health.

Risk for contamination: Vulnerable to exposure to environmental contaminants which may compromise health.

Risk for corneal injury: Vulnerable to infection or inflammatory lesion in the corneal tissue that can affect superficial or deep layers, which may compromise health.

Risk for decreased cardiac output: Vulnerable to inadequate blood pumped by the heart to meet metabolic demands of the body, which may compromise health.

Risk for decreased cardiac tissue perfusion: Vulnerable to a decrease in cardiac (coronary) circulation, which may compromise health.

Risk for deficient fluid volume: Vulnerable to experiencing decreased intravascular, interstitial, and/or intracellular fluid volumes, which may compromise health.

Risk for delayed development: Vulnerable to delay of 25% or more in one or more of the areas of social or self-regulatory behavior, or in cognitive, language, gross, or fine motor skills, which may compromise health.

Risk for delayed surgical recovery: Vulnerable to an extension of the number of postoperative days required to initiate and perform activities that maintain life, health, and well-being, which may compromise health.

Risk for disorganized infant behavior: Vulnerable to alteration in integration and modulation of the physiological and behavioral systems of functioning (i.e., autonomic, motor, state-organization, self-regulatory, and attentional-interactional systems), which may compromise health.

Risk for disproportionate growth: Vulnerable to growth above the 97th percentile or below the 3rd percentile for age, crossing two percentile channels, which may compromise health.

Risk for disturbed maternal–fetal dyad: Vulnerable to disruption of the symbiotic maternal-fetal dyad as a result of comorbid or pregnancy-related conditions, which may compromise health.

Risk for disturbed personal identity: Vulnerable to the inability to maintain an integrated and complete perception of self, which may compromise health.

Risk for disuse syndrome: Vulnerable to deterioration of body systems as the result of prescribed or unavoidable musculoskeletal inactivity, which may compromise health.

Risk for dry eye: Vulnerable to eye discomfort or damage to the cornea and conjunctiva due to reduced quantity or quality of tears to moisten the eye, which may compromise health.

Risk for dysfunctional gastrointestinal motility: Vulnerable to a decrease in normal frequency of defecation accompanied by difficult or incomplete passage of stool, which may compromise health.

Risk for electrolyte imbalance: Vulnerable to changes in serum electrolyte levels, which may compromise health.

Risk for falls: Vulnerable to increased susceptibility to falling, which may cause physical harm and compromise health.

Risk for frail elderly syndrome: Vulnerable to a dynamic state of unstable equilibrium that affects the older individual experiencing deterioration in one or more domains of health (physical, functional, or social) and leads to increased susceptibility to adverse health effects, in particular disability.

Risk for hypothermia: Vulnerable to a failure of thermoregulation that may result in a core body temperature below the normal diurnal range, which may compromise health.

Risk for imbalanced body temperature: Vulnerable to failure to maintain body temperature within normal parameters, which may compromise health.

Risk for imbalanced fluid volume: Vulnerable to a decrease, increase, or rapid shift from one to the other of intravascular, interstitial, and/or intracellular fluid, which may compromise health. This refers to body fluid loss, gain, or both.

Risk for impaired attachment: Vulnerable to disruption of the interactive process between parent/significant other and child that fosters the development of a protective and nurturing reciprocal relationship.

Risk for impaired cardiovascular function: Vulnerable to internal or external causes that can damage one or more vital organs and the circulatory system itself.

Risk for impaired emancipated decision-making: Vulnerable to a process of choosing a healthcare decision that does not include personal knowledge and/or considerations of social norms, or does not occur in a flexible environment resulting in decisional satisfaction.

Risk for impaired liver function: Vulnerable to a decrease in liver function, which may compromise health.

Risk for impaired oral mucous membrane: Vulnerable to injury to the lips, soft tissues, buccal cavity, and/or oropharynx, which may compromise health.

Risk for impaired parenting: Vulnerable to inability of the primary caretaker to create, maintain, or regain an environment that promotes the optimum growth and development of the child, which may compromise the well-being of the child.

Risk for impaired religiosity: Vulnerable to an impaired ability to exercise reliance on religious beliefs and/or participate in rituals of a particular faith tradition, which may compromise health.

Risk for impaired resilience: Vulnerable to decreased ability to sustain a pattern of positive response to an adverse situation or crisis, which may compromise health.

Risk for impaired skin integrity: Vulnerable to alteration in epidermis and/or dermis, which may compromise health.

Risk for impaired tissue integrity: Vulnerable to damage to the mucous membrane, cornea, integumentary system, muscular fascia, muscle, tendon, bone, cartilage, joint capsule, and/or ligament, which may compromise health.

Risk for ineffective activity planning: Vulnerable to an inability to prepare for a set of actions fixed in time and under certain conditions, which may compromise health.

Risk for ineffective cerebral tissue perfusion: Vulnerable to a decrease in cerebral tissue circulation, which may compromise health.

Risk for ineffective childbearing process: Vulnerable to not matching environmental context, norms and expectations of pregnancy, childbirth process, and the care of the newborn.

Risk for ineffective gastrointestinal perfusion: Vulnerable to decrease in gastrointestinal circulation, which may compromise health.

Risk for ineffective peripheral tissue perfusion: Vulnerable to a decrease in blood circulation to the periphery, which may compromise health.

Risk for ineffective relationship: Vulnerable to developing a pattern that is insufficient for providing a mutual partnership to provide for each other's needs.

Risk for ineffective renal perfusion: Vulnerable to a decrease in blood circulation to the kidney, which may compromise health.

Risk for infection: Vulnerable to invasion and multiplication of pathogenic organisms which may compromise health.

Risk for injury: Vulnerable to physical damage due to environmental conditions interacting with the individual's adaptive and defensive resources, which may compromise health.

Risk for latex allergy response: Vulnerable to a hypersensitive reaction to natural latex rubber products, which may compromise health.

Risk for loneliness: Vulnerable to experiencing discomfort associated with a desire or need for more contact with others, which may compromise health.

Risk for neonatal jaundice: Vulnerable to the yellow orange tint of the neonate's skin and mucous membranes that occur after 24 hours of life as a result of unconjugated bilirubin in the circulation, which may compromise health.

Risk for other-directed violence: Vulnerable to behaviors in which an individual demonstrates that he or she can be physically, emotionally, and/or sexually harmful to others.

Risk for overweight: Vulnerable to abnormal or excessive fat accumulation for age and gender, which may compromise health.

Risk for perioperative hypothermia: Vulnerable to an inadvertent drop in core body temperature below 36° C/96.8° F occurring one hour before to 24 hours after surgery, which may compromise health.

Risk for perioperative positioning injury: Vulnerable to inadvertent anatomical and physical changes as a result of posture or equipment used during an invasive/surgical procedure, which may compromise health.

Risk for peripheral neurovascular dysfunction: Vulnerable to disruption in the circulation, sensation, and motion of an extremity, which may compromise health.

Risk for poisoning: Vulnerable to accidental exposure to, or ingestion of, drugs or dangerous products in sufficient doses, which may compromise health.

Risk for post-trauma syndrome: Vulnerable to sustained maladaptive response to a traumatic, overwhelming event, which may compromise health.

Risk for powerlessness: Vulnerable to the lived experience of lack of control over a situation, including a perception that one's actions do not significantly affect the outcome, which may compromise health.

Risk for pressure ulcer: Vulnerable to localized injury to the skin and/or underlying tissue usually over a bony prominence as a result of pressure, or pressure in combination with shear.

Risk for relocation stress syndrome: Vulnerable to physiological and/or psychosocial disturbance following transfer from one environment to another that may compromise health.

Risk for self-directed violence: Vulnerable to behaviors in which an individual demonstrates that he or she can be physically, emotionally and/or sexually harmful to self.

Risk for self-mutilation: Vulnerable to deliberate self-injurious behavior causing tissue damage with the intent of causing non-fatal injury to attain relief of tension.

Risk for shock: Vulnerable to an inadequate blood flow to the body's tissues that may lead to life-threatening cellular dysfunction, which may compromise health.

Risk for situational low self-esteem: Vulnerable to developing a negative perception of self-worth in response to a current situation, which may compromise health.

Risk for spiritual distress: Vulnerable to an impaired ability to experience and integrate meaning and purpose in life through connectedness within self, literature, nature, and/or a power greater than oneself, which may compromise health.

Risk for sudden infant death syndrome: Vulnerable to unpredicted death of an infant.

Risk for suffocation: Vulnerable to inadequate air availability for inhalation, which may compromise health.

Risk for suicide: Vulnerable to self-inflicted, life threatening injury.

Risk for thermal injury: Vulnerable to extreme temperature damage to skin and mucous membranes, which may compromise health.

Risk for trauma: Vulnerable to accidental tissue injury (e.g., wound, burn, fracture), which may compromise health.

Risk for unstable blood glucose level: Vulnerable to variation in blood glucose/sugar levels from the normal range, which may compromise health.

Risk for urge urinary incontinence: Vulnerable to involuntary passage of urine occurring soon after a strong sensation or urgency to void, which may compromise health.

Risk for urinary tract injury: Vulnerable to damage of the urinary tract structures from use of catheters, which may compromise health.

Risk for vascular trauma: Vulnerable to damage to vein and its surrounding tissues related to the presence of a catheter and/or infusion solutions, which may compromise health.

Risk-prone health behavior: Impaired ability to modify lifestyle/behaviors in a manner that improves health status.

Sedentary lifestyle: Reports a habit of life that is characterized by a low physical activity level.

Self-mutilation: Deliberate self-injurious behavior causing tissue damage with the intent of causing nonfatal injury to attain relief of tension.

Self-neglect: A constellation of culturally framed behaviors involving one or more self-care activities in which there is a failure to maintain a socially accepted standard of health and well-being.

Sexual dysfunction: A state in which an individual experiences a change in sexual function during the sexual response phases of desire, excitation, and/or orgasm, which is viewed as unsatisfying, unrewarding, or inadequate.

Situational low self-esteem: Development of a negative perception of self-worth in response to a current situation.

Sleep deprivation: Prolonged periods of time without sleep (sustained natural, periodic suspension of relative consciousness).

Social isolation: Aloneness experienced by the individual and perceived as imposed by others and as a negative or threatening state.

Spiritual distress: A state of suffering related to the impaired ability to experience meaning in life through connections with self, others, world, or a superior being.

Stress overload: Excessive amounts and types of demands that require action.

Stress urinary incontinence: Sudden leakage of urine with activities that increase intra-abdominal pressure.

Toileting self-care deficit: Impaired ability to perform or complete self-toileting activities.

Unilateral neglect: Impairment in sensory and motor response, mental representation, and spatial attention of the body, and the corresponding environment, characterized by inattention to one side and overattention to the opposite side. Left -side neglect is more severe and persistent than right-side neglect.

Urge urinary incontinence: Involuntary passage of urine occurring soon after a strong sense of urgency to void.

Urinary retention: Incomplete emptying of the bladder.

Wandering: Meandering, aimless or repetitive locomotion that exposes the individual to harm; frequently incongruent with boundaries, limits, or obstacles.

Appendix B

TERMINOLOGY/COMBINING FORMS: PREFIXES AND SUFFIXES

Medical terminology is similar to a foreign language. Many medical terms are derived from Latin and Greek sources. They often consist of two or more simple words or word elements. A word root or *combining form* may be put together with a *prefix* and a *suffix*.

Root—the basis of a word
 Example: *nephr/o/tic* (degenerative changes in the kidney)
 Root: nephr- (kidney)

Linking vowel—a vowel that joins the combining form to the suffix or another combining form
 Example: nephr/*o*/sis (disease of the kidneys)
 Linking vowel: o

Prefix—the beginning of a word
 Example: *hyper*/active (excessively active)
 Prefix: hyper- (excessive)

Suffix—the ending of a word
 Example: nephr/*itis* (inflammation of the kidney)
 Suffix: -itis (inflammation)

Combining form—the union of a word root with a linking vowel
 Example: *hepato*/megaly (enlargement of the liver)
 Combining form: hepato- (liver)

The following table provides some of the most commonly used terminology for your reference.

COMMON PREFIXES

Prefix	Definition
a-	without
ab-	away from
abd-	abdominal
acu-	sharp
ad-	toward
adip-	fat
ad lib-	freely, as wanted
aero-	air, gas
al-	toward
ambi-	both
an-	not
ana-	up
ante-	before, in front of
anti-	against
arteri-	artery
arthro-	joint
auto-	self
bi-	two
brady-	slow
cata-	down
chole-	bile
cili-	eyelid
circum-	around
co-	with, together
cogni-	know
colo-	colon

Prefix	Definition
con-	with, together
contra-	against
crani-	skull
cut-	skin
cyt-	cell
de-	from, lack of
demi-	half
dent-	tooth
derm-	skin
dia-	through, across
diplo-	double, twofold
dis-	to free or undo
dors-	back
dur-	hard
dy-	two
dys-	bad, painful, difficult, abnormal
ec-	out, out from
ecto-	outside
em-	in
embol-	to insert
encephalo-	brain
endo-	in, within
entero-	intestine
epi-	above, on
erythro-	red
eso-	within, inward
et-	and
eu-	good, normal
ex-	out, away from
exo-	outside
extra-	outside
faci-	face
fiss-	split, cleft
fore-	before, in front of
gastro-	stomach
glosso-	relating to the tongue
glyco-	sugar
haplo-	simple, single
heme-	iron-based
hemi-	one half
hepat-	liver
hetero-	different
histo-	tissue
homo-	same
hydro-	wet, water
hyper-	excessive, above normal
hypo-	under, below
im-	not
in-	in, not
infra-	under, below
inter-	between
intra-	in, within
isch-	deficiency

Prefix	Definition	Suffix	Definition
iso-	equal, alike	-al	pertaining to
lapis-	stone	-algia	painful condition, pain
lapra-	loin or flank, sometimes abdomen	-apheresis	removal
latero-	side	-ar	pertaining to
macro-	large	-ary	pertaining to
mal-	bad	-ase	enzyme
meato-	opening	-bi	two, double
medi-	middle	-blast	developing cell
melano-	black	-cele	hernia, swelling, sac
mesa-	middle	-centesis	puncture of a cavity
meso-	middle	-clasis	break, fracture
meta-	beyond, change	-clysis	irrigation, washing
micro-	small	-coccus	berry shaped
mono-	one	-crit	to separate
morpho-	form, structure	-cyte	cell
multi-	many, much	-desis	fusion, binding, fixation
neo-	new	-drome	to run
nephro-	kidney	-dynia	pain
oculo-	eye	-ectasis	expansion, dilation
onco-	tumor	-ectomy	excision, removal of a body part
oro-	mouth	-emesis	vomiting
osteo-	bone	-emia	blood
pan-	all	-er	one who
para-	beside, beyond	-gen	forming, producing, origin
per-	through, by	-genesis	forming, producing, origin
peri-	around	-genic	origin, formation
phago-	eating	-grade	to go
poly-	many, much	-gram	the record made, mark
post-	after, behind	-graph	instrument for recording, machine
pre-	before, in front of	-graphy	the process, process of recording
primi-	first	-ia	condition
pro-	before, in front of	-iasis	morbid condition
pseudo-	false	-iatry	treatment, medicine
quadri-	four	-ic/-ical	pertaining to
re-	again, backward	-icle	small, minute
retro-	backward, behind	-ism	condition
rhabdo-	rod-shaped, striated	-ist	one who specializes in, specialist
rhodo-	red	-itis	inflammation
scler-	hardening	-lith	stone, calculus
semi-	one half	-logist	specialist in the study of
stetho-	chest	-logy	process of study
sub-	under, below	-lysis	dissolution, setting free
super-	above, excessive	-malacia	softening, soft
supra-	above, excessive	-megaly	enlargement
sym-	together	-meter	instrument for measuring
syn-	union, together, joined	-metry	act of measuring
tachy-	rapid	-odynia	pain
tetra-	four	-oid	form, shape
therm-	heat	-ole	small, minute
trans-	through, across	-ology	study or science of
tri-	three	-oma	tumor
ultra-	beyond, excess	-opsy	to view
uni-	one	-or	one who
vas-	vessel or duct	-orrhea	flow, discharge
xantho-	yellow	-osis	condition or state
xero-	dry	-ous	pertaining to
		-para	to bear (offspring)
		-paresis	partial paralysis

COMMON SUFFIXES

Suffix	Definition		
-ac	pertaining to	-pathy	disease, suffering
-agra	excessive pain	-penia	deficiency, lack of, decrease
		-pexy	fixation

Suffix	Definition	Suffix	Definition
-phagia	eating, swallowing	-sepsis	infection
-phasia	speech	-sis	state of, condition
-philia	attraction for	-spasm	involuntary spasm
-phobia	fear	-stalsis	constriction
-physis	to grow	-stasis	control, constant level, stop
-plasia	formation, growth	-stenosis	narrowing, stricture
-plasm	growth, formation	-stomy	creation of an opening
-plasty	mold, shape, repair	-therapy	treatment
-plegia	paralysis	-tic	pertaining to
-poiesis	formation, production	-tome	instrument for cutting
-ptosis	downward displacement, falling	-tomy	process of cutting, incision
-ptysis	spitting	-toxic	poison
-rrhage	bursting forth, rupture	-tresia	opening
-rrhaphy	suturing in place	-tripsy	surgical crushing
-rrhea	flow, discharge	-trophy	nourishment
-rrhexis	rupture	-ula	small, minute
-scope	instrument to visually examine	-ule	small, minute
-scopy	process of examining, visual examination	-y	process

Index

Page numbers followed by *b* indicates boxes, *f* indicates illustrations, and *t* indicates tables.

Index of Skills and Procedural Guidelines